VIRAL PATHOGENESIS

VIRAL PATHOGENESIS

Editor-in-Chief
Neal Nathanson, M.D.
Department of Microbiology
University of Pennsylvania Medical Center
Philadelphia, Pennsylvania

Associate Editors
Rafi Ahmed, Ph.D.
Department of Microbiology and Immunology
Emory University
Atlanta, Georgia

Francisco Gonzalez-Scarano, M.D.
Departments of Neurology and Microbiology
University of Pennsylvania School of Medicine
Philadelphia, Pennsylvania

Diane E. Griffin, M.D., Ph.D.
Department of Molecular Microbiology and Immunology
The Johns Hopkins University
School of Public Health
Baltimore, Maryland

Kathryn V. Holmes, Ph.D.
Department of Microbiology
University of Colorado Health Sciences Center
Denver, Colorado

Frederick A. Murphy, D.V.M., Ph.D.
School of Veterinary Medicine
University of California, Davis
Davis, California

Harriet L. Robinson, Ph.D.
Department of Pathology
University of Massachusetts Medical Center
Worcester, Massachusetts

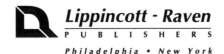

Lippincott - Raven
PUBLISHERS
Philadelphia • New York

Acquisitions Editor: Vickie E. Thaw
Senior Developmental Editor: Judith E. Hummel
Project Editor: Ellen M. Campbell
Production Manager: Caren Erlichman
Senior Production Coordinator: Kevin P. Johnson
Design Coordinator: Kathy Luedtke
Indexer: Sandra King
Compositor: Compset Inc.
Printer: Quebecor/Kingsport

Cover photo: Marburg virus in the liver of an African green monkey (*Cercopithecus aethiops*) infected 7 days previously with 200 guinea pig LD50 by the intraperitoneal route, and sacrificed when moribund. Characteristic filovirus virions are seen accumulating within a bile canaliculus after budding upon the lateral plasma membrane of a hepatocyte (*front cover*). Virions are also seen accumulating within an invagination of the plasma membrane of a neighboring hepatocyte (*back cover*). The liver tissue illustrated here contained $10^{9.2}$ guinea pig LD50 per gm. [Single transmission electron microscopic image spanning the front and back covers, uranyl acetate and lead citrate stain, approximate magnification $\times$ 75,000. After studies in Murphy FA, Simpson DIH, Whitfield SG, Slotnick I, and Carter GB. Marburg virus infection in monkeys: ultrastructural studies. Laboratory Investigation 1971:24:279–291. Photograph provided by C.S. Goldsmith, DVRD, NCID, CDC.]

Library of Congress Cataloging-in-Publication Data
Viral pathogenesis / editor-in-chief, Neal Nathanson ; associate
    editors, Rafi Ahmed . . . [et al.].
        p.   cm.
    Includes bibliographical references and index.
    ISBN 0-7817-0297-6 (alk. paper)
    1. Virus diseases—Pathogenesis.   I. Nathanson, Neal.   II. Ahmed,
Rafi.
    [DNLM: 1. Viruses—pathogenicity.   2. Virus Diseases—etiology.
QZ 65 V813 1996]
QR201.V55V53   1996
616.9'2507—dc20
DNLM/DLC
for Library of Congress   96-23106
                                                                   CIP

9 8 7 6 5 4 3 2 1

Care has been taken to confirm the accuracy of the information presented and to describe generally accepted practices. However, the authors, editors, and publisher are not responsible for errors or omissions or for any consequences from application of the information in this book and make no warranty, express or implied, with respect to the contents of the publication.

The authors, editors, and publisher have exerted every effort to ensure that drug selection and dosage set forth in this text are in accordance with current recommendations and practice at the time of publication. However, in view of ongoing research, changes in government regulations, and the constant flow of information relating to drug therapy and drug reactions, the reader is urged to check the package insert for each drug for any change in indications and dosage and for added warnings and precautions. This is particularly important when the recommended agent is a new or infrequently employed drug.

Some drugs and medical devices presented in this publication have Food and Drug Administration (FDA) clearance for limited use in restricted research settings. It is the responsibility of the health care provider to ascertain the FDA status of each drug or device planned for use in their clinical practice.

Contributors

Gordon L. Ada, D.Sc.
Professor
Division of Immunology and Cell Biology
John Curtin School of Medical Research
Australian National University
Canberra City, ACT 2601
Australia

Rafi Ahmed, Ph.D.
Department of Microbiology
Rollins Research Center
Emory University School of Medicine
Atlanta, GA 30322

Ann M. Arvin, M.D.
Department of Pediatrics
Stanford University School of Medicine
300 Pasteur Drive
Stanford, CA 94305-5119

Stephen W. Barthold, D.V.M., Ph.D.
Professor of Comparative Medicine
Yale University School of Medicine
P.O. Box 208016
New Haven, CT 06520-8016

Persephone Borrow, Ph.D.
Department of Neuropharmacology
The Scripps Research Institute
10550 North Torrey Pines Road
La Jolla, CA 92037

Margo A. Brinton, Ph.D.
Department of Biology
Georgia State University
Box 4010
Atlanta, GA 30302-4010

Thomas R. Broker, Ph.D.
Department of Biochemistry
University of Alabama at Birmingham
1918 University Boulevard
Birmingham, AL 35294-0005

R. Mark L. Buller, Ph.D.
Department of Molecular Microbiology
& Immunology
St. Louis University Health Sciences Center
1042 South Grand Boulevard
St. Louis, MO 63104

Yahia Chebloune, Ph.D.
Department of Microbiology
Ecole Nationale Veterinaire de Lyon
1, Avenue Bourgelat
69280 Marcy l'Etoile
France

Francis V. Chisari, M.D.
Department of Molecular and Experimental
Medicine
The Scripps Research Institute
10550 North Torrey Pines Road
La Jolla, CA 92037

Louise T. Chow, Ph.D.
Department of Biochemistry
University of Alabama at Birmingham
1918 University Boulevard
Birmingham, AL 35294-0005

Janice E. Clements, Ph.D.
Division of Comparative Medicine
School of Medicine
The Johns Hopkins University
720 Rutland Ave
Baltimore, MD 21205–2196

Margaret E. Conner, Ph.D.
Division of Molecular Virology
Baylor College of Medicine
One Baylor Plaza
Houston, TX 77030-3498

Richard T. D'Aquila, M.D.
Infectious Disease Unit
Massachusetts General Hospital
149 Thirteenth Street
Charlestown, MA 02129

Terence S. Dermody, M.D.
Department of Pediatrics
Vanderbilt University Medical Center
Nashville, TN 37232–2581

Peter C. Doherty, Ph.D.
Department of Immunology
St. Jude's Children's Research Hospital
332 North Lauderdale
Memphis, TN 38105

Frank Fenner, M.D.
John Curtin School of Medical Research
Australian National University
Canberra City, ACT 0200
Australia

Carlo Ferrari, M.D.
Department of Infectious Diseases
The University of Parma
Via A. Gramsci 14
43100 Parma
Italy

Donald H. Gilden, M.D.
Department of Neurology
University of Colorado Health Sciences Center
4200 East Ninth Avenue
Denver, CO 80262

Francisco Gonzalez-Scarano, M.D.
Department of Neurology
University of Pennsylvania Medical Center
Clinical Research Building
Philadelphia, PA 19104-6146

Diane E. Griffin, M.D., Ph.D.
Department of Molecular Microbiology
*   and Immunology*
School of Hygiene and Public Health
The Johns Hopkins University
615 N. Wolfe Street
Baltimore, MD 21205-2179

Ashley T. Haase, M.D.
Department of Microbiology
University of Minnesota Medical School
420 Delaware Street, SE
Minneapolis, MN 55455-0312

J. Marie Hardwick, Ph.D.
Department of Molecular Microbiology and
*   Immunology*
School of Hygiene and Public Health
The Johns Hopkins University
615 N. Wolfe Street
Baltimore, MD 21205–2179

Martin S. Hirsch, M.D.
Department of Medicine
Massachusetts General Hospital
Fruit Street
Boston, MA 02114

Kathryn V. Holmes, Ph.D.
Department of Microbiology
University of Colorado Health Sciences Center
4200 East 9th Avenue
Denver, CO 80262

Alan C. Jackson, M.D.
Department of Medicine
Queen's University
78 Barrie Street
Kingston, Ontario, K7L 3J7
Canada

Sanjay V. Joag, M.D., Ph.D.
Department of Microbiology
University of Kansas Medical Center
3901 Rainbow Boulevard
Kansas City, KS 66160-7424

Joan C. Kaplan, Ph.D.
Infectious Disease Unit
Massachusetts General Hospital
149 Thirteenth Street
Charlestown, MA 02129

David M. Knipe, Ph.D.
Professor of Microbiology and Molecular Genetics
Harvard Medical School
200 Longwood Avenue
Boston, MA 02115

Hsing-Jien Kung, Ph.D.
Department of Molecular Biology and
*   Microbiology*
School of Medicine
Case Western Reserve University
10900 Euclid Avenue
Cleveland, OH 44106–4960

Howard L. Lipton, M.D.
Division of Neurology
Evanston Hospital
2650 Ridge Avenue
Evanston, IL 60201-1797

Juinn-Lin Liu, D.V.M., Ph.D.
Department of Molecular Biology and
*   Microbiology*
School of Medicine
Case Western Reserve University
10900 Euclid Avenue
Cleveland, OH 44106–4960

Grant McFadden, Ph.D.
Department of Biochemistry
University of Alberta
Edmonton, Alberta, T6G 2H7
Canada

Philip D. Minor, Ph.D.
Division of Virology
National Institute for Biological Standards and
*   Control*
Blanche Lane, South Mimms, Potters Bar
Hertfordshire, EN6 3QG
United Kingdom

Lynda A. Morrison, Ph.D.
Department of Molecular Microbiology and
*   Immunology*
St. Louis University School of Medicine
1402 S. Grand Boulevard
St. Louis, MO 63104

Frederick A. Murphy, D.V.M., Ph.D.
School of Veterinary Medicine
University of California, Davis
Haring Hall
Davis, CA 95616

Opendra Narayan, D.V.M., Ph.D.
Department of Microbiology
University of Kansas Medical Center
3901 Rainbow Boulevard
Kansas City, KS 66160-7424

Neal Nathanson, M.D.
Department of Microbiology
University of Pennsylvania Medical Center
Clinical Research Building
Philadelphia, PA 19104-6146

William A. O'Brien, M.S., M.D.
Division of Infectious Diseases
West Los Angeles Veterans Affairs Medical Center
11301 Wilshire Boulevard
Los Angeles, CA 90073

Michael B. A. Oldstone, M.D.
Department of Neuropharmacology
The Scripps Research Institute
10550 North Torrey Pines Road
La Jolla, CA 92037

Clarence J. Peters, M.D.
Division of Viral and Rickettsial Diseases
Center for Infectious Diseases
Centers for Disease Control
1600 Clifton Road
Atlanta, GA 30333

Roger J. Pomerantz, M.D.
Department of Medicine
Jefferson Medical College
Thomas Jefferson University
1020 Locust Street
Philadelphia, PA 19107

Stanley B. Prusiner, M.D.
Department of Neurology
School of Medicine
University of California, San Francisco
San Francisco, CA 94143-0518

Glenn F. Rall, Ph.D.
Division of Basic Science
The Fox Chase Cancer Center
7701 Burholme Avenue
Fox Chase, PA 19111

Robert F. Ramig, Ph.D.
Division of Molecular Virology
Baylor College of Medicine
One Baylor Plaza
Houston, TX 77030-3498

Alan R. Rein, Ph.D.
National Cancer Institute
Frederick Cancer Research and Development
*   Center*
P.O. Box 13
Frederick, MD 21703

Harriet L. Robinson, Ph.D.
Department of Pathology
University of Massachusetts Medical Center
55 Lake Avenue North
Worcester, MA 01655

Ganes C. Sen, Ph.D.
Department of Molecular Biology
Cleveland Clinic Foundation
9500 Euclid Avenue
Cleveland, OH 44195–5001

Abigail L. Smith, Ph.D.
Department of Epidemiology and Public Health
Yale University School of Medicine
P.O. Box 208016
New Haven, CT 06520-8016

Nancy A. Speck, Ph.D.
Department of Biochemistry
Dartmouth Medical School
Vail Building
Hanover, NH 21701

Kenneth L. Tyler, M.D.
Department of Neurology
Denver Veterans Affairs Medical Center
1055 Clermont Street
Denver, CO 80262

Herbert W. Virgin IV, M.D., Ph.D.
Department of Pathology
Washington University School of Medicine
660 S. Euclid Avenue
St. Louis, MO 63110-1093

Scott C. Weaver
Department of Pathology
University of Texas Medical Branch
Galveston, TX 77555-0605

Raymond M. Welsh, Ph.D.
Department of Pathology
University of Massachusetts Medical Center
55 Lake Avenue North
Worcester, MA 01655

Peter Wright, M.D.
Department of Pediatrics
Vanderbilt University Medical Center
1121 South 21st Avenue
Nashville, TN 37232-2581

M. Christine Zink, D.V.M., Ph.D.
Division of Comparative Medicine
The Johns Hopkins Medical School
720 Rutland Avenue
Baltimore, MD 21205

Rolf M. Zinkernagel, M.D., Ph.D.
Institute for Experimental Immunology
University of Zürich
Schmelzbergstrasse 12
CH-8901 Zürich
Switzerland

Preface

"In the field of observation, chance favors only the prepared mind."
Louis Pasteur, 1854*

Humans have always been fascinated with the cause of illness, either driven by curiosity or by the hope to treat or prevent disease. Viruses first made themselves known by the diseases they caused, long before they were recognized as unique life forms, existing at the boundary between inert matter and free-living organisms. The development of the methods of modern biology made it possible to study these agents in increasingly intimate detail, and to apply that information to the ways in which these agents cause disease. It is the aim of this book to set down the current state of knowledge in this area of biology, which is often called viral pathogenesis.

Viral pathogenesis has recently evolved at an accelerated tempo, reflecting the explosive growth of cellular and molecular biology. Furthermore, within the community of virologists there has been a concomitant recognition of the importance of a better understanding of disease causation. A thorough comprehension of pathogenesis is critical for the rational development of preventive vaccines or therapeutic drugs, and for epidemiologic control of transmission. For these reasons, we judged that it was timely to attempt to assemble in one place our current knowledge of viral pathogenesis.

Viral Pathogenesis was conceived to provide graduate and professional students, postdoctoral fellows, research investigators, and infectious disease specialists in human and veterinary medicine with a detailed exposition of learning in this field. Furthermore, it was designed to complement existing texts, particularly *Fields Virology* (Third Edition, 1996), which has become the standard research reference for animal virology. For this reason, *Viral Pathogenesis* has been organized in a different manner from most existing virology, microbiology, or infectious disease books that utilize a virus-by-virus or disease-by-disease treatment. Instead, we have adopted a holistic approach and have divided the book into four major components.

Part I is devoted to the *principles of viral pathogenesis,* with attention to topics such as the dissemination of viruses, tropism and localization, virulence, virus–cell interactions, persistence, viral oncology, host determinants of susceptibility, nonspecific hose defenses, immune responses, immune suppression, and immunopathology. Part II focuses on *experimental pathogenesis,* with an atlas that illustrates salient aspects of pathogenesis, followed by three chapters on methods in viral pathogenesis. This section reviews classic procedures for animal studies, plus current techniques for identifying viral genes and gene products in individual cells in vivo, and recently introduced methods involving manipulation of the host genome by inactivating normal host genes or introducing novel genes. Part III, on *classic models of viral pathogenesis,* brings together information on several experimental models. In the aggregate, these models have yielded many of the important concepts in this field. Some of these models, such as lymphocytic choriomeningitis virus and reovirus, do not involve diseases of great importance to humans or animals, and are not thoroughly treated in most standard texts. Although others, such as poliovirus, ectromelia, and rabies, are important pathogens, detailed descriptions of their pathogenesis are not readily available. Part IV, *systems pathogenesis,* provides a view of the common features of pathogenesis that characterize viral infection of specific systems, such as the respiratory tract, the gastrointestinal tract, the liver, the nervous systems, and the fetus.

Also, it should be noted that *Viral Pathogenesis* is devoted mainly to the viruses of humans and animals. Plant and bacterial viruses are mentioned only occasionally, and insect viruses are considered in the context of vectors that transmit arboviruses to animal hosts. Since the book is designed primarily as a reference, the authors have attempted to make each chapter comprehensible when read by itself, even though this involves occasional repetition of information in other chapters. The detailed bibliographies which follow each chapter will direct the interested reader to the original literature.

The Editors

---

*Vallery-Radot R, editor. *Oeuvres de Pasteur.* Paris: Masson et Cie, 1939.

Acknowledgment

The Editors would like to acknowledge the highly professional support which they received from the staff of Lippincott–Raven Publishers. Vickie Thaw played a key role in planning this undertaking, and Judy Hummel has maintained a consistent level of commitment, punctuated with a fine sense of humor, to the multitude of details required to acquire individual chapters and bring them to a high level of editorial quality. To sum up the experience, Judy provided an excerpt from an old *New York Times* article:

> It is one of those hoary musical anecdotes that, no matter how preposterous, survive and even find their way into college classrooms: With an operatic premiere looming, the notoriously laggard composer Giaocchino Rossini was spirited off to a tower by his noble patron to complete the overture, long overdue. His guards were instructed to drop the pages from a window as completed, for copying; if production stalled, they were to pitch out the composer himself.

Their enthusiasm for this project and expertise in overseeing it have played a vital role in the development and completion of this book.

Contents

xiii

VIRAL
PATHOGENESIS

PART I

Principles of Viral Pathogenesis

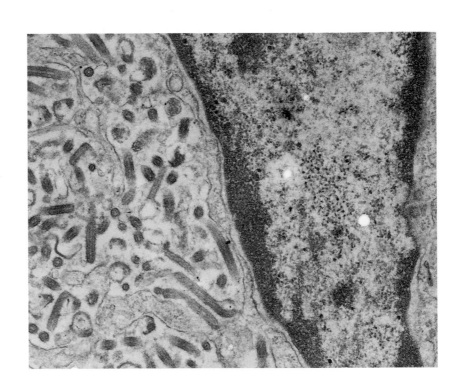

Viral Pathogenesis,
edited by Neal Nathanson, et al.
Lippincott–Raven Publishers, Philadelphia © 1997

CHAPTER 1

Introduction and History

Neal Nathanson

Scientists at work have the look of creatures following genetic instructions; they seem to be under the influence of a deeply placed human instinct. It sometimes looks like a lonely activity, but it is as much the opposite of lonely as human behavior can be. There is nothing so social, so communal, so interdependent. An active field of science is like an immense intellectual anthill; the individual almost vanishes into the mass of minds tumbling over each other, carrying information from place to place, passing it around at the speed of light. There is nothing to touch the spectacle. In the midst of what seems a collective derangement of minds in total disorder, with bits of information being scattered about, torn to shreds, disintegrated, reconstituted, engulfed, in a kind of activity that seems as random and agitated as that of bees in a disturbed part of the hive, there suddenly emerges, with the purity of a slow phrase of music, a single new piece of truth about nature.

Lewis Thomas, 1974[105]

INTRODUCTION

For those with the time and inclination, it may be of interest to understand the roots of viral pathogenesis, its development, and its current status. This chapter attempts to do that, recognizing that any one individual's view of these mattters is colored by his or her personal experiences as an investigator. The reader may also wish to consult other treatments of the history of virology.[30,36,53,54,113]

AN HISTORICAL VIEW OF VIRAL PATHOGENESIS

The Beginnings: Ancient Times to 1900

Historically, knowledge of viral disease has evolved in sequential stages but at an ever increasing pace. The initial stage was the identification of certain diseases as distinct nosologic entities, attendant on the gradual evolution of clinical medicine from ancient times to the 19th century. With the identification of various clinical entities, it was recognized that some diseases were transmissible from person to person or from animals to humans, as suggested by a sequential chain of illnesses or the occurrence of an outbreak of clinically similar cases.

Rabies

Rabies is a particularly notable example, because hydrophobia and associated symptoms, in both the rabid dog or wolf and humans, are unique and unmistakable. In the 4th century BC, Aristotle wrote in the *Natural History of Animals*

N. Nathanson: Department of Microbiology, University of Pennsylvania Medical Center, Philadelphia, PA 19104.

"that dogs suffer from the madness. This causes them to become very irritable and all animals they bite become diseased." Accounts from the middle ages of periodic outbreaks when rabid wolves, foxes, dogs, or bears invaded a village and bit many inhabitants provide dramatic testimony to the mode of transmission.[94]

Smallpox

Smallpox is a distinctive disease with its characteristic skin lesions and its ability to cause epidemics, and it probably existed in ancient civilizations such as Egypt. The mummy of Ramses V, who died in 1157 BC, had skin lesions which were probably those of smallpox, and historians speculate that a number of the notable plagues of the ancient world were smallpox. The plague of Athens that occurred in 430 BC was reported by Thucydides to have originated in Ethiopia and spread to Egypt and Libya before crossing the Mediterranean to the port of Piraeus and thence to Athens. Although it is debatable whether the plague of Athens was actually smallpox,[59] accounts of this kind clearly indicate that some observers recognized the communicable nature of infectious diseases at this time.[28,69]

Measles

Measles provides another example in which epidemiologic observations led to the inference of a transmissible agent of disease. As summarized by Lilienfeld in his classic *Foundations of Epidemiology*:[55]

> An early example of the epidemiologic analysis of a disease is Panum's report of an epidemic of measles that occurred in the Faroe Islands in 1846 [69]. A cabinetmaker from Copenhagen landed in the Faroe Islands on March 28, 1846, and developed symptoms of measles early in April. The population of the Faroes at the time numbered 7,864; 6,100 came down with measles between the end of April and October and 170 deaths occurred. The islanders had experienced measles in the past but there had been no cases between 1781 and 1846. The Danish government sent a twenty-six-year-old physician, P. L. Panum, to deal with the epidemic situation; to his observations, we owe much of our knowledge of measles. Panum personally visited fifty-two villages and made observations on several thousand cases of measles of which he personally treated 1,000. He obtained information on "the circumstances and dates of their exposure to infection, the dates on which the exanthem [rash] appeared on them and the time that elapsed thereafter before other residents broke out with the exanthem." From these observations, he concluded that the period from exposure to development of the rash (the incubation period) is usually thirteen-fourteen days and that the patient is infectious at the time that the rash is breaking out, or had just broken out, and possibly for a few days prior to the eruption, although he was not certain about this. He did not find the disease to be transmissible during the period of desquamation (when the rash disappears with shedding of the skin), which was the prevalent view at the time. From these observations on personal contacts, he concluded that measles can be transmitted only by direct contact between infected and susceptible individ-

ual. It is not conveyed by miasma nor does it arise spontaneously, at least not in the Faroe Islands.

Germ Theory

After establishing the concept of transmissibility, the next important milestone was the development of the germ theory of infectious diseases in the late 19th century. Pasteur, in his studies of fermentation conducted from 1857 to 1865, put forward the concept that each fermentative process could be traced to a specific living microbe, simultaneously dispensing with the theory of spontaneous generation and setting the stage for the concept that each disease was caused by a specific microbial agent.[47] Duvaine, in 1865, demonstrated that anthrax was due to a bacillus present in the blood or serum of an infected animal; this provided important evidence for Pasteur's germ theory. With the development of the first methods for the culture of bacteria in the mid-19th century, it became possible to isolate individual bacteria in pure culture and to demonstrate that some of these bacteria were responsible for specific infectious diseases. With this technology available, Koch and Henle developed the following postulates designed to test the hypothesis that a specific agent caused a particular disease:

The incriminated agent can be cultured from the disease lesions.
The organism can be grown in pure culture.
The organism reproduces the disease when introduced into an appropriate host.
The organism can be recultured from the experimental disease.

Discussion of the Henle-Koch postulates and their modern reworking in relation to viruses and molecular genetics are provided elsewhere.[19,20,78]

As a direct outgrowth of these pioneering studies on bacterial diseases, filterable viruses were discovered, first as plant pathogens and then as animal pathogens. Subsequent to the introduction of Chamberland candles, which are porcelain filters with a pore size of 100 to 500 nm that exclude bacteria, Mayer, Ivanovsky, and Beijerinck, working independently from 1886 to 1898, found that the agent of mosaic disease of tobacco could be transmitted by filtrates prepared from the sap of infected plants and could multiply when serially passaged on tobacco leaves, although the filtrate could not be grown on bacterial media. The first animal viruses, foot and mouth disease virus, a picornavirus,[56] and yellow fever virus, a flavivirus, were discovered shortly thereafter.

Yellow Fever

Yellow fever, in contrast to some other important human pathogens, was not reported in antiquity, perhaps because it was maintained as a zoonosis of jungle monkeys either in South America or Africa.[97] Yellow fever was initially recognized as a disease entity in the 17th century, and the first recorded use of the name was by Hughes in his *Natural History of the Barbadoes*, published in 1750. Urban yellow fever became endemic in major cities of South America, from whence it was imported to North American seaports by mosquitoes carried on sailing vessels beginning in the late 17th century. During the 18th and 19th centuries, major epidemics recurred periodically in the United States; Philadelphia suffered 20 epidemics.[73]

Yellow fever was the first human disease shown to be caused by a virus, a demonstration that occurred under dramatic circumstances. In June 1900, Walter Reed, a surgeon in the United States Army, was sent to Cuba as president of a commission to study yellow fever.[74] The commission was activated at the Columbia Barracks in Quemados, Cuba, during an ongoing epidemic. The investigators initially focused on the possibility that yellow fever was caused by *Bacillus icteroides*, a hypothesis that had been proposed in 1897 by Giuseppe Sanarelli. Based on the study of clinical cases and autopsies, they concluded that *B icteroides* was a secondary invader and not the causal agent.[75] The commission then investigated the proposal that yellow fever was transmitted by mosquitoes, which had been suggested in 1881 by Carlos Finlay, a Cuban physician. Using colonized *Aedes aegypti* provided by Finlay, they were able to transmit the disease by mosquitoes that fed first on patients and then, about 2 weeks later, on human volunteers.[76] Furthermore, they showed that yellow fever could be transmitted to volunteers by blood obtained from patients in the first 2 days of illness but not by exposure to patients' fomites. At this time, William Welch, a famous pathologist at the Johns Hopkins Medical School, called Reed's attention to the work of Loeffler and Frosch, which indicated that foot-and-mouth disease was caused by a filterable virus. Reed and Carroll injected three volunteers with serum obtained from patients in the early phase of yellow fever which had been diluted and passed through a bacteria-retaining Berkefeld filter; two of the volunteers developed the disease.[77]

The word virus, derived from the Latin word for poison, has been used since ancient times for the causal agents of transmissible diseases. With the discovery of filtration as a means to exclude bacteria, the term filterable virus was introduced and subsequently shortened to virus. Only later were viruses defined in modern biochemical and molecular terms.[54]

From Virus Isolation to Cell Culture: 1900 to 1950

With the recognition that viruses are distinct from bacteria and other transmissible pathogens, the first era of modern virology began. From the mid-19th century, bacteria could be grown on solid or liquid media, permitting a wide variety of experimental studies. However, prior to the introduction of cell culture, viruses, because they are obligate intracellular parasites, could be propagated only in complex hosts such as tobacco plants (tobacco mosaic virus) or primates (yellow fever virus). This technical limitation was a constraint in experimental virology for the first half of the 20th century. The necessity of using animal hosts for the propagation and assay of viruses had several consequences. First, it focused research on viruses of great medical importance that justified cumbersome and costly experimentation or on research that could be carried out in relatively inexpensive small animals, particularly rodents or embryonated eggs. Second, there were severe limitations in the ability to follow the course of a viral in-

fection, and observations were often limited to clinically detectable signs of illness, such as paralysis, tumor formation, or death, or to histologic descriptions of pathologic changes in infected tissues. Poliomyelitis, rabies, yellow fever, and Rous sarcoma virus (RSV) are examples of viruses that were the object of extensive study even under these relatively adverse circumstances.

Poliomyelitis

Poliovirus was first isolated in 1908 by Landsteiner and Popper,[49,50] who homogenized the spinal cord from a human with a fatal case of the disease, showed that it was bacteriologically sterile, and then inoculated the homogenate intraperitoneally into one monkey and one baboon, both of which developed paralysis with typical poliomyelitic lesions in their spinal cords. Several laboratories quickly confirmed these results, and Flexner and Lewis[32,33] at the Rockefeller Institute demonstrated that the transmissible agent was a filterable virus. Although these experiments did not meet the strict requirements of the Henle-Koch postulates in full, it was generally accepted that the causal agent of poliomyelitis had been isolated. Among the early findings was the observation that the agent could be serially transmitted to primates by several routes of injection but could not be transmitted to subprimate laboratory animals. This meant that research on poliomyelitis, including its pathogenesis, would require resources that could only be found at a few well-endowed and well-equipped research institutes and academic laboratories. For this reason, Landsteiner, who had only modest resources at his disposal, abandoned this line of research and turned to immunologic investigations that won him an appointment at the Rockefeller Institute in the 1920s and a Nobel Prize in 1930.[71] However, Landsteiner and collaborators[48] did make some additional important observations regarding the distribution of poliovirus by showing that it could be isolated from nasal secretions, the tonsils, and mesenteric lymph nodes, all evidence of the systemic distribution of infection and the pantropic nature of the virus.

Research on the pathogenesis of poliomyelitis was pursued by Flexner, who quickly became one of the leaders in this field. An initial requirement for experimental studies was the preparation of stocks of virus. Monkeys were inoculated intracerebrally, sacrificed at the time of acute paralysis, and the spinal cord homogenized and stored in the frozen state. To prepare new stocks, the virus was passaged serially. At the time, it was not appreciated that Flexner's procedure led to the neuroadaptation of the virus, thereby altering its biologic properties. This was a critical mistake that led Flexner and his associates into an erroneous view of the pathogenesis of the disease. Many of their experiments were performed with the mixed virus (MV) strain, a type 2 poliovirus, which was later shown to be an obligatory neurotrope.[41,62] With the MV strain, the only way in which monkeys could be consistently infected was to drip virus into the nose of an animal held in an inverted posture, a procedure that was thought to simulate the natural portal of infection. Investigators were also misled by their reliance on the rhesus macaque as an experimental animal, because this species is much less susceptible to feeding of poliovirus than is the cynomolgus macaque or the chimpanzee. Following intranasal administration, the virus infected the first-order sensory neurons in the olfactory mucosa and then travelled to the olfactory bulb, the brainstem, and down the spinal cord to destroy motor neurons in the anterior horn, a sequence of dissemination inferred by histologic studies of lesions in the central nervous system. This scheme of pathogenesis had been widely accepted by 1931 when it was summarized by Flexner.[31]

The conviction that poliovirus was exclusively neurotropic was so strong that it led to the development of a method for prevention of the disease in humans. Following the demonstration that an astringent nasal spray could protect monkeys from paralysis,[2] a trial of a zinc sulfate spray was conducted in children in the summer of 1936. Although the spray produced anosmia in some recipients, it failed to prevent disease.[106]

This experience led to a reexamination of the pathogenesis of poliomyelitis. Careful autopsies of humans who had fatal cases of the disease failed to reveal evidence of the olfactory bulb lesions that were characteristic of poliomyelitis following intranasal inoculation of rhesus monkeys with the MV strain of virus.[88] A revised view of the pathogenesis of poliomyelitis became possible only after the introduction by Enders and colleagues[18] of tissue culture methods for cultivating poliovirus. A discussion of the long duration of the nasal portal of entry theory is provided elsewhere.[71]

Rous Sarcoma Virus

Experimental transplantation of tumors was first attempted in the late 19th century but was rarely successful. However, early in this century, Ehrlich[17] established several lines of mouse mammary carcinomas, which were adapted so that they could be transplanted to many strains of mice. From these early trials, it was observed that transplantation was favored with the use of newborn or young animals, the intraperitoneal rather than other routes of inoculation, and cell suspensions rather than solid tumor fragments. Building on these observations, Rous began his studies of sarcomas of the domestic chicken. Rous made several seminal observations in his original series of studies.[79–82] The sarcoma could be readily transplanted serially by subcutaneous injection of tumor cells to Plymouth Rock chickens, a partially inbred strain of animals, and with passage the tumors became more aggressive. Most importantly, extracts of tumor cells could transmit the tumor, and these extracts were still active after passage through a bacteria-retaining filter, implying that the sarcoma was induced by a virus.

Rous' initial observations were extended in several directions. It was shown that tumors were most readily transplanted to young chickens or embryonated eggs and that a larger number of cells was required to transplant tumors to adult chickens. With passage, the tumors could be transplanted to a wider range of chickens and other fowl, and even to mammals under certain circumstances, although tumors more frequently regressed in less susceptible hosts. Additionally, Rous was able to distinguish immunity to the tumor cells from immunity to the viral agent. However, over the next 40 years, further progress was constrained by the technical limitations of experimental virology. Perhaps the most significant observation during this period of limited progress was made by Keogh,[45] who exploited Rous' observations on embryonated eggs to introduce a quantitative assay for the virus, which proved that a single virus particle was sufficient to initiate a single pock. Reviews of the early history of tumor virology are provided elsewhere.[37,108]

Mousepox

In the 1940s, there was little understanding of the sequential events that took place during the course of a typical viral infection, partly as a result of the technical limitations noted previously. Mousepox was originally called infectious ectromelia when it was first described by Marchal in the 1930s, because it often led to amputation of a foot and required differentiation from congenital ectromelia (i.e., the deformity of one or more limbs). In 1931, Marchal identified the causal agent of infectious ectromelia as a virus, and in 1936, Burnet showed that the virus could be titrated on the chorioallantoic membrane of embryonated chicken eggs, providing a quantitative bioassay well before Dulbecco's introduction of plaque assays for animal viruses in 1952.[16] Furthermore, two assays for antibodies against ectromelia were developed: neutralization using the chorioallantoic membrane system or inhibition of hemagglutination. With these tools in hand, in the late 1940s Fenner did a series of studies[21–23,25–27] that systematically described the course of mousepox infection, including the portal of entry, the viremic spread of the virus, the seeding of target organs (i.e., the liver and skin), and the mode of transmission from desquamated skin. Fenner's studies of mousepox represented a pioneering effort that provided a prototype for characterization of the pathogenesis of an acute viral infection.[24] Subsequently, these studies were expanded by Mims using fluorescent tagged antibody to visualize viral antigen.[60] Based on his studies of several experimental viral infections, Mims[60,61] and others[44] published some landmark reviews that encoded the knowledge of viral pathogenesis through the mid-1960s. The pathogenesis of ectromelia is reviewed in Chapter 22.

From Cell Culture to Molecular Genetics: 1950 to 1980

The announcement by Enders and coworkers[18] that it was possible to cultivate poliovirus in primary cultures prepared from a variety of human embryonic tissues catalyzed a new era in tissue culture methods for viruses. The use of transformed cell lines, usually derived from tumors of humans or animals, and the development of nontransformed cell strains provided a wide variety of culture systems.[34,38,90,91,107,108] Over the following 15 years, cell culture added several important methods to the armamentarium of the experimental virologist:

It became easy to make primary isolates of natural wild-type strains of many but not all viruses.

It became much easier to measure infectivity using either a quantal (endpoint) or a particle (plaque) assay.

The plaque assay made it possible to obtain genetically pure populations of virions derived from a single infectious particle.[16]

Sera and other body fluids could be readily assayed for their content of neutralizing antibodies.

The transforming capacity of some tumor viruses could be demonstrated in vitro, permitting the analysis of some essential biologic properties of such agents.

It became possible to obtain large quantities of purified virus, which is a prerequisite for many biochemical, structural, and molecular studies.

Almost simultaneously with the introduction of cell culture, methods were introduced for the identification of viral antigens in infected cultures and animal tissues. Additionally, electron microscopy[87] was refined into a relatively routine technique that could be used to visualize virions and some subvirion structures in cells and tissues, as well as demonstrate the intimate details of virus-induced cellular pathology. Together, these methods made it possible to localize virus infection to individual cells and subcellular compartments. Concurrently, immunologic methods for measurement of antibody were rapidly expanded to increase their specificity, sensitivity, variety, and ease of application. In the 1970s, in vitro methods for assay of cell-mediated immune responses, such as cytolytic T-lymphocyte and lymphocyte proliferation assays, were introduced and rapidly quantified. Furthermore, assays for other host defenses, such as interferon, became available.

The application of methods for animal genetics increased the availability of inbred animals, particularly many strains of mice, leading to the investigation of host genetic determinants of disease susceptibility and of genetic variation in host immune responses to viruses. Certain models of pathogenesis were discovered only through the use of special inbred mouse strains. Additionally, the use of specific pathogen–free or germ-free (gnotobiotic) strains of mice offered additional opportunities for studies of viral pathogenesis.

In aggregate, the introduction of these techniques (see Chaps. 19 and 20) opened the modern era of viral pathogenesis, which may be illustrated with a few examples.

Poliovirus

With the introduction of tissue culture, it became relatively easy to isolate poliovirus from the stool and pharyngeal swabs of infected persons; this led to a revival of the view that poliovirus was an enterovirus, a hypothesis originally proposed by Swedish investigators in 1912.[46,71] Furthermore, the recovery of virus from patients provided fresh field isolates with the properties of wild-type virus. It was then shown that cynomolgus monkeys and chimpanzees could be infected by virus feeding, and that the virus consistently produced a viremia.[6] This led to the modern view of the pathogenesis of poliomyelitis: the virus enters the nasopharynx and small intestine, probably by infecting microvilli or microfold (M) cells overlying lymphatic accumulations (i.e., tonsils in the nasopharynx and Peyer's patches in the small intestine), replicates there in macrophages, and travels through the afferent lymphatic circulation to regional lymph nodes and thence through afferent lymphatics to enter the circulation as a plasma viremia. In some individuals, the virus then invades the central nervous system, either directly across the blood-brain barrier or indirectly through invasion of peripheral nerve ganglia, with subsequent neural spread to the central nervous system (see Chap. 23).[7,89] The revised view of pathogenesis

with its emphasis on viremia led directly to a renewed investigation of the ability of antibody to protect animals when administered prior to virus challenge, which in turn formed the biologic rationale for the development of an inactivated poliovirus vaccine.[8]

The development of simple methods for the measurement of neutralizing antibodies opened the field of serologic epidemiology.[72] Several critical facts were elucidated. It was shown that poliovirus strains could be grouped into three antigenic types; there was cross immunity within each type but little immunity among types. This finding laid the basis for subsequent studies of immune protection and also was essential for interpretation of epidemiologic observations. Serologic surveys for antibody to poliovirus verified an important but previously unproven hypothesis: that most infections with poliovirus were subclinical but conferred protection against subsequent exposure to the virus. The occurrence of inapparent immunizing infections established an important principle in viral pathogenesis and indicated the potential for an attenuated live poliovirus vaccine.

Rous Sarcoma Virus

The period from 1950 to 1980 was one of great progress in tumor virology, and many of the seminal discoveries were made using RSV as a model system.[108,115] With the introduction of cell cultures, it was shown that RSV produced foci on chicken fibroblast monolayers.[104] The number of foci was proportional to the concentration of the inoculum, confirming that transformation could be induced by a single infectious virion.[57,104] Extending this work to other strains of RSV, it was shown that the Bryan high-titer strain produced transformed foci but not progeny virus when cells were infected with limiting dilutions of virus. This was shown to be attributable to the presence of two agents in the virus stocks: a defective sarcoma virus and a replication-competent avian leukosis virus, Rous-associated virus, which acted as a helper for replication of RSV.[98,111] This was an important discovery, because it clarified many confusing observations regarding the biology of replication-defective retroviruses.

Using cell culture, it was possible to apply biochemical tests that distinguished DNA viruses from RNA viruses using inhibitors of DNA synthesis (e.g., cytosine arabinoside, fluorodeoxyuridine) and inhibitors of DNA-dependent RNA polymerase (e.g., actinomycin D). Unexpectedly, these inhibitors blocked replication of RSV,[3,99] leading Temin to propose the existence of a DNA intermediate (DNA provirus) in the replication of RSV.[10,100] Because it violated the central tenet of molecular biology—that information flowed from DNA to RNA to protein—the provirus hypothesis received little support until Temin and Mitzutani[102,103] and Baltimore[4] showed that mature particles of RSV and murine leukemia virus both had reverse transcriptase activity.

The discovery of the provirus led to formulation of the protovirus hypothesis of Temin,[101] which focussed on the origin of RNA tumor viruses from cellular genes, emphasizing a dynamic process of genetic modification leading to neoplastic potential. The protovirus hypothesis followed the oncogene hypothesis of Huebner and Todaro,[42] which suggested that normal cellular DNA contained the complete genomes of

RNA tumor viruses, which were composed of a virogene required for replication and an oncogene with transforming activity. Genetic evidence for the existence of a transforming oncogene was provided by temperature-sensitive mutants, one class of which was transformation defective but replication competent at the restrictive temperature.[58a] Physical evidence for a potential transforming gene arose from the observation that RSV strains that were replication and transformation competent contained a larger genome than did viruses that were replication competent but transformation defective.[15] Based on this information, a probe was prepared that was specific for the putative transforming sequences,[95] and a comparison was made between normal and transformed fibroblasts to demonstrate that the src open reading frame was present in transformed but not in normal cells. Surprisingly, the src probe hybridized to normal as well as to transformed cells.[96] This observation supported the protovirus hypothesis that transforming genes were cellular genes that had been acquired by the viral genome in a process of recombination involving an exchange of viral and cellular genetic information.

These findings stimulated a search for the product of the putative oncogene in RSV-transformed cells and led to the discovery of a protein, pp60[src], which was encoded in the RSV genome and which mediated transformation.[11] The discovery of this protein confirmed that the virus was transforming because it contained an open reading frame encoding an oncogene; only later did it become clear that in those strains of RSV that were replication defective there had been a major deletion of virion structural genes as a result of a recombination event which resulted in the insertion of the open reading frame encoding the oncogene. Subsequently, it was found that pp60[v-src] had some sequence differences from its cellular counterpart, pp60[c-src], and that only the viral protein had transforming activity.[43,70] The discovery of pp60[src] opened the field of retroviral oncogenes and led to an explosion of work that continues to this day.[5,110] Chapter 26 provides a review of avian tumor viruses, and Chapter 11 reviews oncogenic mechanisms of RNA tumor viruses. *The DNA Provirus: Howard Temin's Scientific Legacy[14]* provides a fine summary of the discovery of the provirus.

Application of cell culture to RSV permitted the elucidation of one other enigmatic phenomenon: the patterns of infectivity of different RSV isolates in different strains of chickens or other birds. Rubin[86] reported that some chick embryos carry a virus that can convert RSV-susceptible cells to a state of resistance (i.e., Rous-interfering factor), and further investigation showed that the interfering virus was an avian leukosis virus that blocked cellular receptors.[92,93] Based on patterns of interference, chicken leukemia viruses were classified into five subgroups, with the viruses within each subgroup being related by host range and antigenicity.[108] The basis of the interference phenomenon was further explored using viral pseudotypes, which are phenotypically mixed virions that carry the envelope of RSV encapsidating the genome of vesicular stomatitis virus.[9,114] Pseudotype viruses showed the same host range as the RSV strain that contributed the viral envelope, confirming Rubin's hypothesis that different RSV strains carry envelope proteins that bind to different cellular receptors. This work provided an important model of the interaction between viral attachment proteins and their counterpart cellu-lar receptors which has informed parallel investigations of many other viruses.

Lymphocytic Choriomeningitis Virus

Lymphocytic choriomeningitis virus (LCMV) has played a special role in the evolution of viral pathogenesis because it has provided seminal insights in viral immunology and in immunobiology.[1,51,52,63,64] LCMV was first isolated in the 1930s by Rivers and Scott from patients with aseptic meningitis, by Armstrong and Lillie during the passage of St. Louis encephalitis virus in mice, and by Traub from a colony of laboratory mice. Traub[109] studied enzootic LCMV infection in a mouse colony and showed that the virus produced congenital infections with lifelong persistence of the virus but without apparent disease, subsequently called persistent tolerant infection, whereas intracerebral infection of adult mice caused an acutely fatal lymphocytic choriomeningitis for which the virus was named. The occurrence of persistent tolerant infection and Owen's observations on chimerism in cattle, stimulated Burnet and Fenner[12] in the late 1940s to propose the immunologic concept of self and nonself. In the 1950s, Rowe and colleagues[83–85] studied LCMV in mice and discovered that the acute disease could be prevented by immunosuppression, resulting in the novel proposal that LCMV disease was mediated by the immune response to the virus and not produced by a direct virus effect on cells. In the 1960s, Hotchin[39,40] extended these observations and described the late disease that occurred in virus-carrier mice infected when newborn.

In the 1970s, it was shown that LCMV carriers actually made antiviral antibody and that late disease was caused by deposition of immune complexes in the kidney to produce glomerulonephritis.[66–68] LCMV was one of the systems used to pioneer the development of cytolytic T-cell assays for cell-mediated immunity,[13,58] and it played a central role in the discovery of cytolytic T-cell restriction—namely, the requirement for two unique and separate signals necessary for the lysis of infected target cells.[116,117] These discoveries in turn led to the modern understanding of antigen presentation and antigen recognition by the T-cell receptor. In addition, it was shown that LCMV-immune T cells could mediate acute LCMV disease[35] and also could clear carriers of a persistent infection.[112] These discoveries and their intellectual progeny have done much to elucidate the multiple roles played by the immune response in the pathogenesis of viral infection and the mechanisms of cellular immunity. Chapter 25 provides a detailed description of lymphocytic choriomeningitis.

The Current Era: 1980 to the Present

In the past 15 years there has been a renaissance of interest in viral pathogenesis that may be traced to the explosion of molecular genetics research, comprising techniques that can be applied either to viruses or to their hosts.[65] It is now possible to sequence the genome of even the largest viruses and to construct a complete physical map of open reading frames. For DNA viruses and positive-stranded RNA viruses, specific point mutations, substitutions, insertions, or deletions can be engineered into the viral genome; these techniques are being extended to negative-stranded RNA viruses. In this manner it is possible to explore the influence of specific viral genes, protein domains, and even individual amino acids, as well as noncoding regions of the viral genome, on the virulence of the agent and pathogenesis of the disease. Additionally, molecular genetics has been adapted to the in vivo detection of viral genomes through in situ hybridization and polymerase chain reaction in situ hybridization, which make it possible to localize viral genomes to individual cells, to quantitate genomes and their transcripts, and to identify which sequences are being transcribed (see Chap. 19).

Simultaneously, a new epoch has dawned in animal genetics with the introduction of methods for the insertion of novel transgenes and the deletion (knockout) of existing genes using embryonic stem cell technology (see Chap. 21). These methods provide a powerful approach to determining the role of different host defenses, such as antibodies, cellular immunity, interferon, and a variety of cytokines and interleukins, on the response of animals to different viruses. The role of critical cellular proteins such as viral receptors and of individual viral proteins, when expressed as constitutive host components, can now be teased apart, and the complexities of virus-initiated autoimmune diseases can be dissected. Even more exotic models, such as the severe combined immunodeficiency mouse, the nude mouse, and the hairless mouse, have also been developed.

The burgeoning molecular technology has led to a resurgence of interest in pathogenesis, which is reflected in the recent introduction of sections dealing with viral pathogenesis, viral immunology, and virus-cell interactions into the leading journals in virology. Examples of these developments in viral pathogenesis are reflected in many chapters of this book.

It is also worthy of mention that, despite these advances in biomedical knowledge, there still remain many fundamental, challenging, and important unsolved questions in viral pathogenesis. For instance, it is sobering to reflect that in 1996, when we are on the verge of global eradication of human polioviruses, there are still many aspects of the pathogenesis of poliomyelitis that are incompletely understood, such as the initial site of enteric invasion and replication, the cellular sites of replication in lymphoid tissue, the role of the monocyte-macrophage in pathogenesis, the mechanism of central nervous system invasion, the reason for localization in anterior horn motor neurons, the precise role of the poliovirus receptor and other accessory molecules in cellular tropism, and the mechanism of cell killing (see Chap. 23). The human immunodeficiency virus provides another example in which the understanding of pathogenesis and immunity is still insufficient to deal effectively with problems of immense significance, such as the requirements for an effective preexposure vaccine or the potential for a postexposure vaccine.[29]

ABBREVIATIONS

LCMV: lymphocytic choriomeningitis virus
M cells: microvilli or microfold cells
MV: mixed virus
RSV: Rous sarcoma virus

ACKNOWLEDGEMENTS

I would like to thank David Boettiger, Gary Cohen, Francisco Gonzalez-Scarano, Michael Malim, and Frederick Murphy for their comments and suggestions.

REFERENCES

1. Anonymous. International symposium on arenaviral infections of public health importance. Bull World Health Organ 1975;52:381–765.
2. Armstrong C, Harrison WT. Prevention of intranasally inoculated encephalitis virus (St. Louis type) and of poliomyelitis in monkeys by means of chemicals instilled into the nostrils. Public Health Rep 1936;51:1105–1110.
3. Bader JP. The requirements for DNA synthesis in the growth of Rous sarcoma and Rous-associated virions. Virology 1965;26:253–265.
4. Baltimore D. Viral RNA-dependent DNA synthesis. Nature 1970;226:1209–1211.
5. Bishop JM. Nobel lecture. Retroviruses and oncogenes II. Biosci Rep 1990;10:473–491.
6. Bodian D. A reconsideration of the pathogenesis of poliomyelitis. Am J Hygiene 1952;55:414–438.
7. Bodian D. Emerging concept of poliomyelitis infection. Science 1955;122:105–108.
8. Bodian D. Poliomyelitis and the sources of useful knowledge. Johns Hopkins Medical Journal 1976;138:130–136.
9. Boettiger D. Animal virus pseudotypes. Prog Med Virol 1979;25:37–68.
10. Boettiger D, Temin HM. Light inactivation of focus formation by chicken embryo fibroblasts infection with avian sarcoma virus in the presence of 5-bromodeoxyuridine. Nature 1970;228:622–624.
11. Brugge JS, Erikson RL. Identification of a transformation-specific antigen induced by an avian sarcoma virus. Nature 1977;269:346–348.
12. Burnet FM, Fenner F. The production of antibodies. Melbourne: Macmillan, 1949.
13. Cole GA, Prendergast RA, Henney CS. In vitro correlates of LCM virus-induced immune response. In: Lehmann-Grube F, ed. Lymphocytic choriomeningitis virus and other arenaviruses. New York: Springer-Verlag, 1973:61–72.
14. Cooper GM, Temin RG, Sugden B, eds. The DNA provirus: Howard Temin's scientific legacy. Washington: ASM Press, 1995.
15. Duesberg PH, Vogt PK. Differences between the ribonucleic acids of transforming and nontransforming avian tumor viruses. Proc Natl Acad Sci U S A 1970;67:1673–1680.
16. Dulbecco R. Production of plaques in monolayer tissue cultures caused by single particle of an animal virus. Proc Natl Acad Sci U S A 1952;38:747–752.
17. Ehrlich P. Experimental studies of mouse tumors (German). Z Krebforschung 1907;5:59–69.
18. Enders JF, Weller TH, Robbins FC. Cultivation of the Lansing strain of poliomyelitis virus in cultures of various human embryonic tissues. Science 1949;109:85–87.
19. Evans AS. Causation and disease: the Henle-Koch postulates revisited. Yale J Biol Med 1976;49:175–195.
20. Falkow S. Molecular Koch's postulates applied to microbial pathogenicity. Rev Infect Dis 1988;10:274–276.
21. Fenner F. Studies in infectious ectromelia in mice. I. Immunization of mice against ectromelia with living vaccinia virus. Aust J Exp Biol Med 1947;25:257–274.
22. Fenner F. Studies in infectious ectromelia in mice. II. Natural transmission: the portal of entry of the virus. Aust J Exp Biol Med 1947;25:275–282.
23. Fenner F. Studies in infectious ectromelia in mice. III. Natural transmission: elimination of the virus. Aust J Exp Biol Med 1947;25:327–335.
24. Fenner F. Mousepox (infectious ectromelia of mice): a review. J Immunol 1949;63:341–373.

25. Fenner F. Studies in mousepox (infectious ectromelia in mice). IV. Quantitative investigations on the spread of virus through the host in actively and passively immunized animals. Aust J Exp Biol Med 1949;27:1–17.

26. Fenner F. Studies in mousepox (infectious ectromelia in mice). VI. A comparison of the infectivity and virulence of three strains of ectromelia virus. Aust J Exp Biol Med 1949;27:31–43.

27. Fenner F. Studies in mousepox (infectious ectromelia in mice). VII. The effect of the age of the host upon the response to infection. Aust J Exp Biol Med 1949;27:45–53.

28. Fenner F, Henderson DA, Arita I, Jezek Z, Ladnyi ID. Smallpox and its eradication. Geneva: World Health Organization, 1988.

29. Fields BN. AIDS: time to turn to basic science. Nature 1994;369:95–96.

30. Fields BN, Knipe DM. Introduction. In: Fields BN, Knipe DM, eds. Virology. New York: Raven Press, 1990:3–7.

31. Flexner S. Poliomyelitis (infantile paralysis). Science 1931;74:251–256.

32. Flexner S, Lewis PA. The nature of the virus of poliomyelitis. JAMA 1909;53:2095–2096.

33. Flexner S, Lewis PA. The transmission of poliomyelitis to monkeys. JAMA 1909;53:1639–1641.

34. Gey G, Coffman W, Kubicek M. Tissue culture studies of the proliferative capacity of cervical carcinoma and normal epithelium. Cancer Res 1952;12:264–278.

35. Gilden DH, Cole GA, Nathanson N. Immunopathogenesis of acute central nervous system disease produced by lymphocytic choriomeningitis virus. II. Adoptive immunization of virus carriers. J Exp Med 1972;135:874–889.

36. Grafe A. A history of experimental virology. Berlin: Springer-Verlag, 1991.

37. Gross L. Oncogenic viruses. New York: Pergammon Press, 1970.

38. Hayflick L, Moorhead P. The serial cultivation of human diploid cell strains. Exp Cell Res 1961;25:585–598.

39. Hotchin J. The biology of lymphocytic choriomeningitis virus infection: virus-induced immune disease. Cold Spring Harbor Symp Quant Biol 1962;27:479–500.

40. Hotchin J. Tolerance to lymphocytic choriomeningitis virus. Ann N Y Acad Sci 1971;181:159–181.

41. Howe HA, Bodian D. Neural mechanisms in poliomyelitis. New York: The Commonwealth Fund, 1942.

42. Huebner RJ, Todaro GJ. Oncogenes of RNA tumor viruses as determinants of cancer. Proc Natl Acad Sci U S A 1969;64:1087–1092.

43. Iba H, Takeya T, Cross F, Hanafusa T, Hanafusa H. Rous sarcoma virus variants which carry the cellular src gene instead of the viral src gene cannot transform chicken embryo fibroblasts. Proc Natl Acad Sci U S A 1984;81:4424–4428.

44. Johnson RT, Mims CA. Pathogenesis of viral infections of the nervous system. N Engl J Med 1968;278:23–30.

45. Keogh EV. Ectodermal lesions produced by the virus of Rous sarcoma. Br J Exp Pathol 1938;19:1–14.

46. Kling C, Pettersson A, Wernstedt W. The presence of the microbe of infantile paralysis in human beings. Comunications Institut Medicine Etat 1912;3:5–12.

47. Koprowski H, Plotkin SA, eds. World's debt to Pasteur. New York: Alan R Liss, 1985.

48. Landsteiner K, Levaditi C, Pastia C. Experimental study of acute poliomyelitis (Heine-Medin disease). Annales Institut Pasteur 1911;25:805–820.

49. Landsteiner K, Popper E. Microscopic specimens from one human and two monkey spinal cords. Wien Klin Wochenschr 1908;21:1830–1834.

50. Landsteiner K, Popper E. Transmission of acute poliomyelitis to monkeys (German). Z Immunitatsforsch Exp Ther 1909;2:377–381.

51. Lehmann-Grube F. Lymphocytic choriomeningitis virus. New York: Springer-Verlag, 1971.

52. Lehmann-Grube F, ed. Lymphocytic choriomeningitis virus and other arenaviruses. New York: Springer-Verlag, 1973.

53. Levine AJ. Viruses. New York: Scientific American Library, 1992.

54. Levine AJ. The origins of virology. In: Fields BN, Knipe DM, Howley PM, eds. Fields' virology. Philadelphia: Lippincott-Raven Publishers, 1996:1–14.

55. Lilienfeld AM. Foundations of epidemiology. New York: Oxford University Press, 1976.

56. Loeffler FA, Frosch P. Studies of the commission for research in foot-and-mouth disease of the Institute for Infectious Diseases in Berlin. Centralblatt fur Bakteriologie 1898;23:371–391.

57. Manaker RA, Groupe V. Discrete foci of chicken embryo cells associated with Rous sarcoma virus in tissue culture. Virology 1956;2:838–840.

58. Marker O, Volkert M. In vitro measurement of the time course of cellular immunity to LCM virus in mice. In: Lehmann-Grube F, ed. Lymphocytic choriomeningitis virus and other arenaviruses. New York: Springer-Verlag, 1973:207–216.

58a. Martin GS, Rous sarcoma virus: a function required for maintenance of the transformed state. Nature 1970;227:1021–1023.

59. McNeill WH. Plagues and peoples. New York: Doubleday, 1977.

60. Mims CA. Aspects of the pathogenesis of virus diseases. Bacteriol Rev 1964;28:30–71.

61. Mims CA. Pathogenesis of rashes in virus diseases. Bacteriol Rev 1966;30:739–760.

62. Nathanson N, Bodian D. Experimental poliomyelitis following intramuscular virus injection. I. The effect of neural block on a neurotropic and a pantropic strain. Bulletin of the Johns Hopkins Hospital 1961;108:308–319.

63. Oldstone MBA. Arenaviruses: biology and immunotherapy. Curr Top Microbiol Immunol 1987;134:1–242.

64. Oldstone MBA. Arenaviruses: genes, proteins, and expression. Curr Top Microbiol Immunol 1987;133:1–256.

65. Oldstone MBA. Animal virus pathogenesis: a practical approach. Oxford: IRL Press, 1990.

66. Oldstone MBA, Dixon FJ. Pathogenesis of chronic disease associated with persistent lymphocytic choriomeningitis virus infection. I. Relationship of antibody production to disease in neonatally infection mice. J Exp Med 1969;129:483–505.

67. Oldstone MBA, Dixon FJ. Pathogenesis of chronic disease associated with persistent lymphocytic choriomeningitis virus infection. II. Relationship of the anti-lymphocytic choriomeningitis immune response to tissue injury in chronic lymphocytic choriomeningitis disease. J Exp Med 1970;131:1–19.

68. Oldstone MBA, Dixon FJ. Persistent lymphocytic choriomeningitis virus infection. III. Virus-anti-viral antibody complexes and associated chronic disease following transplacental infection. J Immunol 1970;105:829–837.

69. Panum PL. Observations made during the epidemic of measles on the Faroe Islands in the year 1846. New York: American Public Health Association, 1940.

70. Parker R, Varmus HE, Bishop JM. Expression of v-src and c-src in rat cells demonstrates qualitative differences between pp60v-src and pp60c-src. Cell 1984;37:131–139.

71. Paul J. A history of poliomyelitis. New Haven: Yale University Press, 1971.

72. Paul JR, White C. Serological epidemiology. New York: Academic Press, 1973.

73. Powell JH. Bring out your dead: the great plague of yellow fever in Philadelphia in 1793. Philadelphia: University of Pennsylvania Press, 1993.

74. Reed W. Recent researches concerning etiology, propagation and prevention of yellow fever, by the United States Army Commission. J Hygiene 1902;2:101–119.

75. Reed W, Carroll J, Agramonte A. Etiology of yellow fever; additional note. JAMA 1901;36:431–440.

76. Reed W, Carroll J, Agramonte A, Lazear JW. Etiology of yellow fever: preliminary note. Philadelphia Medical Journal 1900;6:790–796.

77. Reed W, Carroll J. Etiology of yellow fever: supplemental note. Am Med 1902;3:301–305.

78. Rivers TM. Viruses and Koch's postulates. J Bacteriol 1937;33:1–6.

79. Rous P. A transmissible avian neoplasm: sarcoma of the common fowl. J Exp Med 1910;12:696–714.

80. Rous P. A sarcoma of the fowl transmissible by an agent separable from the tumor cells. J Exp Med 1911;13:397–412.

81. Rous P. Resistance to a tumor-producing agent as distinct from the tumor cells. J Exp Med 1913;18:416–428.

82. Rous P. The challenge to man of the neoplastic cell. Science 1967;157:24–28.

83. Rowe WP. Studies on pathogenesis and immunity in lymphocytic choriomeningitis infection of the mouse. Research Reports of the Naval Medical Research Institute 1954;12:167–220.

84. Rowe WP. Protective effect of pre-irradiation on lymphocytic choriomeningitis infection in mice. Proc Soc Exp Biol Med 1956;92:194–198.

85. Rowe WP, Black PH, Levey RH. Protective effect of neonatal thymectomy on mouse LCM infection. Proc Soc Exp Biol Med 1963;114:248–251.

86. Rubin H. A virus in chick embryos which induces resistance in vitro to infection with Rous sarcoma virus. Proc Natl Acad Sci U S A 1960;46:1105–1109.

87. Ruska H. Visualization of lytic bacteriophage in the ultramicroscope. Naturwissenschaften 1940;28:45–46.

88. Sabin AB. Olfactory bulb in human poliomyelitis. Am J Dis Child 1940;60:1313–1317.

89. Sabin AB. Pathogenesis of poliomyelitis: reappraisal in the light of new data. Science 1956;123:1151–1157.

90. Sanford KK, Earle W, Likely GD. The growth in vitro of single isolated tissue cells. J Natl Cancer Inst 1948;9:229–240.

91. Shannon J, Earle W, Walts H. Massive tissue cultures prepared from whole chick embryos planted as a cell suspension on glass substrate. J Natl Cancer Inst 1952;13:349–362.

92. Steck FT, Rubin H. The mechanism of interference between an avian leukosis virus and Rous sarcoma virus. I. Establishment of interference. Virology 1966;29:628–641.

93. Steck FT, Rubin H. The mechanism of interference between avian leukosis virus and Rous sarcoma virus. II. Early steps in infection under conditions of interference. Virology 1966;29:642–656.

94. Steele JH. History of rabies. In: Baer GM, ed. The natural history of rabies. New York: Academic Press, 1975:1–32.

95. Stehelin D, Guntaka RV, Varmus HE, Bishop JM. Purification of DNA complementary to sequences required for neoplastic transformation of fibroblasts by avian sarcoma viruses. J Mol Biol 1976;101:341–365.

96. Stehelin D, Varmus HE, Bishop JM, Vogt PK. DNA related to the transforming gene(s) of avian sarcoma viruses is present in normal avian DNA. Nature 1976;260:170–173.

97. Strode GK, ed. Yellow fever. New York: McGraw-Hill, 1951.

98. Temin HM. Separation of morphological conversion and virus production in Rous sarcoma virus infection. Cold Spring Harbor Symp Quant Biol 1962;27:407–415.

99. Temin HM. The effects of actinomycin D on growth of Rous sarcoma virus in vitro. Virology 1963;20:577–588.

100. Temin HM. Nature of the provirus of Rous sarcoma. Natl Cancer Inst Monogr 1964;17:557–570.

101. Temin HM. The protovirus hypothesis: speculations on the significance of RNA-directed DNA synthesis for normal development and for carcinogenesis. J Natl Cancer Inst 1971;46:3–12.

102. Temin HM. Nobel speech: the DNA provirus hypothesis. Science 1976;192:1075–1080.

103. Temin HM, Mizutani S. RNA-dependent DNA polymerase in the virions of Rous sarcoma virus. Nature 1970;226:1211–1214.

104. Temin HM, Rubin H. Characteristics of an assay for Rous sarcoma virus and Rous sarcoma cells in tissue culture. Virology 1958;6:669–680.

105. Thomas L. Natural science. New York: Viking Press, 1974.

106. Tisdall FF, Brown A, deFries RD. Zinc sulphate nasal spray in prophylaxis of poliomyelitis. Can J Public Health 1937;28:523–530.

107. Todaro G, Green H. Quantitative studies on the growth of mouse embryo cells in culture and their development into established lines. J Cell Biol 1963;17:299–314.

108. Tooze J, ed. The molecular biology of tumour viruses. Cold Spring Harbor: Cold Spring Harbor Laboratory, 1973.

109. Traub E. Persistence of lymphocytic choriomeningitis virus in immune animals and its relation to immunity. J Exp Med 1936;63:847–861.

110. Varmus HE. Nobel speech: retroviruses and oncogenes I. Biosci Rep 1990;10:413–430.

111. Vogt PK. Phenotypic mixing in the avian tumor virus group. Virology 1967;32:708–714.

112. Volkert M. Studies on immunological tolerance to LCM virus. II. Treatment of virus carrier mice by adoptive immunization. Acta Pathol Microbiol Scand 1963;57:465–487.

113. Waterson AP, Wilkinson L. An introduction to the history of virology. Cambridge: Cambridge University Press, 1978.

114. Weiss R. Rhabdovirus pseudotypes. In: Bishop DHL, ed. Rhabdoviruses. Orlando: CRC Press, 1977:52–65.

115. Weiss R, Teich N, Varmus HE, Coffin J, eds. RNA tumor viruses: molecular biology of tumor viruses. Cold Spring Harbor: Cold Spring Harbor Laboratory, 1982.

116. Zinkernagel R, Doherty P. Immunological surveillance against altered self-components by sensitized T lymphocytes in lymphocytic choriomeningitis. Nature 1974;251:547–548.

117. Zinkernagel R, Doherty P. MHC-restricted cytotoxic T cells: studies on the biological role of polymorphic major transplantation antigens determining T-cell restriction specificity, function, and responsiveness. Adv Immunol 1979;27:51–177.

Viral Pathogenesis,
edited by Neal Nathanson, et al.
Lippincott–Raven Publishers, Philadelphia © 1997

CHAPTER 2

Entry, Dissemination, Shedding, and Transmission of Viruses

Neal Nathanson and Kenneth L. Tyler

INTRODUCTION

One of the cardinal differences between viral infection of a simple cell culture and infection of an animal host is the much greater structural complexity of the multicellular organism. The virus must overcome a number of barriers to accomplish stepwise infection of the host, beginning with entry, usually through a single portal, followed by dissemination, localization in a few target tissues, shedding, and transmission to other hosts (Fig. 2-1). This chapter describes this stepwise process, with the exception of localization of infection, which is discussed in Chapter 3. Host defenses, both nonspecific and immune, have an important modulating role in dissemination, and they are discussed in Chapters 6 and 7.

ENTRY

Skin and Mucous Membranes

Selected viruses replicate in cells of the skin or mucous membranes. Prominent examples are papillomaviruses, poxviruses, and herpes simplex viruses (HSV; Table 2-1). It is likely that these viruses cannot initiate infection when placed

N. Nathanson: University of Pennsylvania Medical Center, Philadelphia, Pennsylvania 19104.
K.L. Tyler: University of Colorado Health Sciences Center, Denver, Colorado 80262.

on intact skin, which constitutes a hostile environment for viruses because of its dryness, mild acidity, and surface bacteria. Viruses, therefore, can only obtain access through a break in the epithelium, just as the skin must be scratched to facilitate a "take" by vaccinia virus. Mucous membranes probably present a less obstructive physical barrier but are bathed in a liquid covering that provides protection by virtue of its viscous nature or contained immunoglobulin, particularly secreted IgA. Following infection of skin, viruses may spread by passage of intact virions or virus-infected phagocytic cells (macrophages and dendritic cells) to the regional lymph nodes.

The epidermis consists of several layers. From the deepest to the most superficial, these are the basal germinal layer of dividing cells (stratum Malpighi), the granular layer of dying cells (stratum granulosum), and the superficial layer of keratin (stratum corneum).

Papillomaviruses

Papillomaviruses have a selective tropism for the epidermis and an unusual pattern of gene expression in its successive layers.[142] The papillomavirus initially infects basal cells that express only the early viral genes, whereas cells in the granular and keratinized layers express later viral genes and produce mature virions.[2,147] Papillomaviruses replicate exclusively in the nucleus of the cell, and each localized lesion (i.e., wart) appears to be clonal, representing initial infection of a single germinal cell.

Poxviruses

The skin is the principal portal of entry for some poxviruses, such as ectromelia virus, whereas other poxviruses enter mainly through the respiratory route. Ectromelia is transmitted by infected scabs and depends on the presence of abrasions for introduction. Once they are introduced, poxviruses infect cells in the germinal layer of the epidermis and fibroblasts and macrophages in the dermis, and infection spreads to contiguous cells to produce an enlarging area of infection.[134] Typically, poxviruses spread from skin to regional lymph nodes, probably by movement of infected phagocytic cells through the afferent lymphatics. Chapter 22 contains a discussion of mousepox.

Herpes Simplex Virus

HSV is usually transmitted by intimate contact that exposes skin and mucosal surfaces to infectious oral or genital fluids or secretions. It is postulated that the virus usually enters the skin through abrasions but that it can infect intact mucosal surfaces. HSV is quite promiscuous; it replicates in multiple cell types in the epidermis and dermis, including germinal epithelium, fibroblasts, and macrophages, and spreads to contiguous cells to cause an ulcerating lesion.[22] The unique feature of HSV is its almost inevitable invasion of neural endings in skin and subsequent spread along sensory dendrites to trigeminal and spinal ganglia (see Neural Spread).

Conjunctiva

There are a few viruses that are regularly associated with conjunctivitis, and the conjunctiva may represent a primary portal of entry in such instances. Selected adenovirus serotypes frequently cause outbreaks of conjunctivitis, particularly "swimming pool conjunctivitis" and "shipyard eye," and it appears that the conjunctiva is directly infected from virus-contaminated water or by inadvertent transmission during treatment of workers for eye injuries.[68] Selected enteroviruses, particularly coxsackievirus A24 and enterovirus type 70, also have been associated with massive pandemics of conjunctivitis.[90] In this case, it is postulated that the eyes are inoculated by touching them with virus-contaminated fingers. Many other viruses (e.g., vaccinia, HSV, some enteroviruses) also spread to the conjunctiva on occasion, probably through mechanical inoculation. In these situations, the conjunctiva usually constitutes a secondary site of infection rather than a primary portal of entry.

Urogenital Tract

A considerable number of viruses cause sexually transmitted disease, which is usually acquired by exposure to virus-containing secretions. Infection is initiated either by penetration of the virus through breaks in the skin or by direct infection of the superficial epithelium of the mucous membranes. For papillomaviruses and HSV, which cause lesions of the skin or mucous membranes, the initial sites of replication parallel those discussed previously and usually involve the germinal layer of the epidermis, with or without infection of fibroblasts and phagocytes in the dermis.

An additional group of viruses that are sexually transmitted are those associated with persistent viremia, such as hepatitis B and human immunodeficiency virus (HIV). These agents may invade by different mechanisms than those used by viruses that replicate in the skin and mucous membranes. Virus-contaminated blood, semen, or secretions may introduce virus or virus-infected cells directly into the circulation through breaks in the skin and membranes. Consistent with this mechanism is the well established increase in risk of transmission of HIV conferred by the presence of superficial lesions associated with other sexually transmitted diseases.[81] Alternatively, HIV may establish initial infection in dendritic macrophages (Langerhans cells) in the epidermis or in epithelial cells of the cervix, although the latter cells lack the CD4 receptor.[80,124,149] The uncertainty about the precise mode of HIV entry is highlighted by the debate on prevention of transmission to women.[34]

Transcutaneous and Intravenous Injection

Although the skin is a formidable barrier, mechanical injection that breaches the barrier is a "natural" route of entry for many viruses.

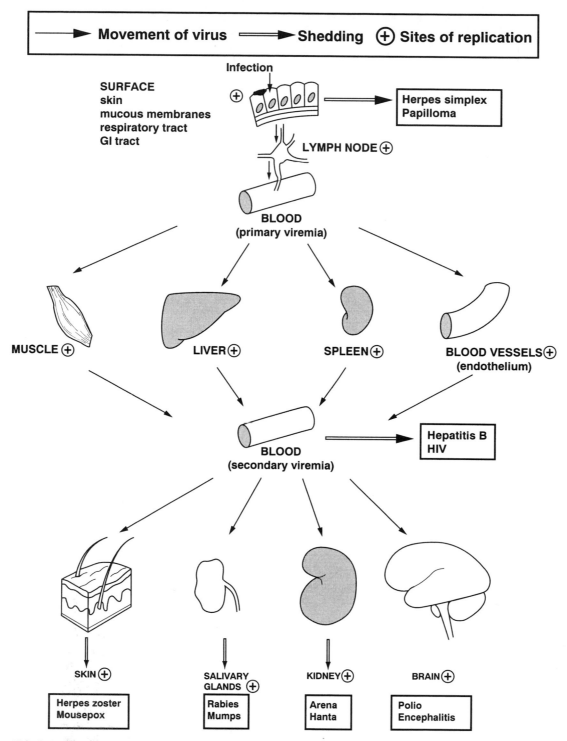

FIG. 2-1. The life cycle of the virus in the infected host includes entry, dissemination, and shedding of blood-borne viruses. This generalized scheme emphasizes the sequential sites of and steps in virus replication: at the point of entry, in regional lymph nodes, production of primary viremia, replication in other tissues (different tissues for different viruses), production of secondary viremia, and invasion of target organs (different ones for different viruses), often leading to pathologic lesions and clinical disease. This scheme applies to many but not all viruses and does not illustrate neural spread. Only a few examples are listed. GI, gastrointestinal; HIV, human immunodeficiency virus. (Adapted from Mims CA. The pathogenesis of infectious disease. London: Academic Press, 1987.)

TABLE 2-1. *Viruses that initiate infection via the skin or mucous membranes*

Site of infection	Route of infection	Virus family	Example*
Skin	Minor breaks	Papovaviridae	Papillomavirus
		Herpesviridae	Herpes simplex 1
		Poxviridae	Mouse ectromelia
		Hepadnaviridae	Hepatitis B
Skin and deeper tissues	Animal bite	Rhabdoviridae	Rabies
		Herpesviridae	Herpes B
	Vector bite, mechanical	Poxviridae	Rabbit myxoma
	Vector bite, biologic	Flaviviridae	Yellow fever
		Togaviridae	Eastern encephalitis
		Bunyaviridae	Rift Valley fever
		Reoviridae	Colorado tick fever
	Injection	Flaviviridae	Hepatitis C
		Retroviridae	Human immunodeficiency virus
		Hepadnaviridae	Hepatitis B
		Herpesviridae	Cytomegalovirus
Conjunctiva	Contact	Picornaviridae	Enterovirus 70
		Adenoviridae	Adenovirus
Genital tract	Contact	Flaviviridae	Hepatitis C
		Retroviridae	Human immunodeficiency virus
		Papovaviridae	Papillomavirus
		Hepadnaviridae	Hepatitis B
		Herpesviridae	Herpes simplex 2

*Examples are viruses of humans except where otherwise indicated.
Adapted from Mims CA, White DO. Viral pathogenesis and immunology. Oxford: Blackwell, 1984.

Arboviruses

A large number of animal viruses are maintained in nature through a cycle that involves a vector and a vertebrate host.[100] These arboviruses include more than 500 individual viruses, mainly in the families Bunyaviridae, Flaviviridae, Reoviridae, Rhabdoviridae, and Togaviridae. When the infected vector takes a blood meal, virus contained in the salivary gland is injected. During the feeding process, which involves probing for a capillary, most of the salivary fluids are deposited in the subcutaneous tissue; feeding primarily involves subcutaneous rather than intravenous injection of virus. The volume of saliva and the amount of virus injected depend on the vector and the virus. Samples from in vitro–induced salivation by experimentally infected mosquitoes typically contain 10^4 plaque-forming units (PFU) of an arbovirus. If a mosquito deposits 10^{-3} mL of saliva and if the fluid contains a titer of 10^7 PFU/mL, the injected saliva would contain 10^4 infectious virions. Transmission of arboviruses is discussed in more detail in Chapter 14.

Mechanical Transmission by the Vector

Although most viruses that are transmitted by an insect vector replicate within the vector, there are a few instances in which the vector acts only as a "flying pin" and apparently does no more than mechanically carry the virus from one vertebrate host to another. The most notable example is myxoma virus of rabbits, which is transmitted by mosquitoes or mites even though it does not cause an active infection of the vec-

tor[52]; rabbit papillomatosis is transmitted by a similar mechanism.[40]

Intramuscular Injection: Rabies

Rabies is the only virus that is maintained in many of its natural cycles by the bite of a sick animal (see Chap. 24).[12] Following transcutaneous and intramuscular injection, the virus may either enter the processes of peripheral nerves directly or replicate in striated muscle. It can then cross the neuromuscular junction and spread along peripheral nerves to the central nervous system. The sequence of events depends on the biologic properties of the virus strain. Laboratory strains that have been neuroadapted by intracerebral passage in animals move very quickly into peripheral nerves, whereas field isolates with minimum laboratory passage remain in the periphery for many days before they undergo neural spread. The sequence of events can be inferred from experiments involving peripheral virus injection followed by interruption of neural spread at various times after infection (Table 2-2).

Injection or Transfusion

Virus may be accidentally transmitted by repeated use of contaminated needles, injection of a virus-contaminated therapeutic agent, or transfusion with virus-contaminated blood or blood products. There are a sufficient number of instances of this kind of "unnatural" infection to justify comment, particularly because many of the implicated viruses are important hu-

TABLE 2-2. *Incubation period following footpad injection of rabies virus and protection by neurectomy**

Virus and dose	Time from infection to amputation	Dead/total	Survival time (d)	
			Median	Range
Neuroadapted	0.25 h	1/27		
(CVS) strain	1 h	0/25		
$10^{6.5}$ LD50[†]	2 h	0/26		
	4 h	8/25		
	8 h	30/30		
	12 h	29/30		
	24 h	28/29		
	Control	27/30	7	(6–9)[‡]
Natural field	0.003 d	0/15		
(bobcat)	1 d	2/18	13.5	13–14
isolate	3 d	1/13	14	
$10^{3.5}$ LD50[†]	5 d	3/18	15	14–16
	9 d	3/18	17	15–22
	18 d	3/18	27	14–29
	Controls	22/43	27	17–120

*This table shows that rabies virus spreads to the central nervous system by the neural route, and contrasts a fixed (neuroadapted) strain (challenge virus standard, CVS) that appears to enter the neural pathway shortly after infection and a natural field (bobcat) isolate with a long incubation period that appears to remain in the periphery for many days.

†Virus titered intracerebrally in mice.

‡Estimated median and range of survival times; actual times not recorded in publication.

Data from references 9 and 42.

man pathogens. The agents most frequently involved are those that produce persistent viremias, such as hepatitis B, C, and D; cytomegalovirus; and HIV. Contaminated needles play a major role in initiating infection under two circumstances: parenteral injection of drugs by abusers in developed countries and re-use of needles in developing countries. The same group of viruses can also be injected inadvertently as contaminants of infected therapeutic agents, such as hepatitis B in yellow fever vaccine[137] or HIV in blood products,[81] or be introduced in virus-contaminated blood transfusions. Following parenteral injection, virus appears to be widely disseminated, reaching cells for which it has a tropism, which may be either cells in the circulation (e.g., HIV, cytomegalovirus) or in the parenchyma of a target organ (e.g., hepatitis B).

Oropharynx and Gastrointestinal Tract

The oropharynx and gastrointestinal tract are important portals of entry for many viruses, and enteric viruses may invade the host in a variety of sites from the oral cavity to the colon. Some viruses produce localized infections that remain confined to the gastrointestinal tract, whereas others disseminate to produce systemic infection (Table 2-3).

Most enteric viruses, such as rotaviruses, produce localized infections of the epithelium of the small or large intestine.[85,136] However, some enteroviruses, such as poliovirus, can also replicate in lymphoid tissue of the nasopharynx. Following oral virus ingestion, the course of infection in susceptible cells

of the oropharynx and gastrointestinal tract can be followed indirectly by determining the titers of excreted virus, as shown in Figure 2-2, for chimpanzees fed a wild strain of poliovirus.[24]

Barriers to Infection

There are numerous barriers to infection through the enteric route. First, much of the ingested inoculum remains trapped in the luminal contents and never reaches the wall of the gut. Second, the lumen constitutes a hostile environment because of the acidity of the stomach, the alkalinity of the small intestine, the array of potent digestive enzymes found in the saliva and pancreatic secretions, and the lipolytic action of bile. Third, the mucus that lines the intestinal epithelium presents a physical barrier that protects the intestinal surface. Finally, phagocytic scavenger cells and secreted antibodies in the lumen can reduce the titer of infectious virus.

Thus, viruses that are acid labile, such as rhinoviruses, cannot infect by the intestinal route. Hepatitis A and B viruses illustrate this point. Both viruses are excreted in the bile into the intestinal tract, but hepatitis A virus survives and is excreted in an infectious form in the feces, whereas hepatitis B virus is inactivated.[39,59,66,67,131] As a consequence, hepatitis A behaves epidemiologically as an enterovirus, whereas hepatitis B does not. Viruses that are successful in using the enteric portal to gain entry tend to be resistant to acid pH, proteolytic attack, and bile, and some may actually exploit the hostile environment to enhance their infectivity.[33,49]

TABLE 2-3. *Viruses that initiate infection via the gastrointestinal tract**

Localization of disease	Virus family	Example†
Gastroenteritis	Astroviridae	Astrovirus
	Caliciviridae	Norwalk
	Toroviridae	Bovine Breda
	Coronaviridae	Transmissible gastroenteritis of swine
	Rotaviridae	Rotavirus
	Parvoviridae	Canine parvovirus
	Adenoviridae	Adenovirus 40, 41
No enteric illness	Picornaviridae	Poliovirus
		Coxsackievirus
		Enterovirus
		Hepatitis A
	Adenoviridae	Adenovirus
	Caliciviridae	Hepatitis E

*See Chapter 30 for a detailed discussion.
†Examples are viruses of humans except when otherwise indicated.
Adapted from Mims CA, White DO. Viral pathogenesis and immunology. Oxford: Blackwell, 1984.

Reovirus

The intimate details of the initial steps in gastrointestinal invasion are probably better studied for reovirus than for any other enteric virus. A detailed description of reovirus pathogenesis is presented in Chapter 28. Reovirus is an example of a virus that undergoes conversion by proteolytic enzymes in the small intestine to an infectious subvirion particle (ISVP).[4,18,25] After inoculation into the upper gastrointestinal tract of mice, reovirus selectively adsorbs to microvilli or microfold (M) cells, which form a specialized epithelium overlying Peyer's patches (i.e., focal areas of lymphoid tissue in the gut wall), and ISVPs are more efficiently taken up than intact virus. Virions are endocytosed into M cells, transported across these cells within cytoplasmic vesicles, and released on the basal surface by exocytosis.[19] Virions may then disseminate further, either locally to intestinal epithelial cells that are infected via their basal surface, or systemically by neural or lymphatic-hematogenous pathways, depending on the biologic properties of the reovirus type. A similar route of infection may be used by poliovirus.[144]

Lower Gastrointestinal Tract

The importance of anal intercourse as a risk factor for hepatitis B and HIV infection has led to the recognition that some viruses can gain entry through the lower gastrointestinal tract. HIV has been detected in bowel epithelium[81] and also replicates in continuous cell lines derived from human colonic carcinomas,[1,50,81,110] but the exact mechanism of HIV infection through the anocolonic portal remains to be determined.

Respiratory Tract

Many viruses are transmitted by the respiratory route. Important groups of viruses transmitted in this manner include the rhinoviruses, the myxoviruses, the adenoviruses, the herpesviruses, and the poxviruses (Table 2-4). It is important to point out that respiratory infection may be initiated either by virus contained in aerosols that are inhaled by the recipient host or by virus that is contained in nasopharyngeal fluids and is transmitted by hand-to-hand contact.

Aerosolized droplets are deposited at different levels in the respiratory tract depending on their size; those larger than $10\ \mu$ are deposited in the nose, those 5 to $10\ \mu$ are deposited in the airways, and those smaller $5\ \mu$ are deposited in the alveoli.[83] Once deposited in the respiratory tract, the virus must bypass several effective barriers before it can initiate infection, including a covering layer of mucus, the action of ciliated epithelial cells which clears the respiratory tree of foreign particles, and the surveillance of phagocytic cells in the respiratory lumen. Additionally, the temperature of the respiratory tract varies from about 33°C in the nasal passages to core body temperature (37°C) in the alveoli. Therefore, those viruses (e.g., rhinoviruses) that can replicate well at 33°C but not at 37°C tend to be limited to the upper respiratory tract and, conversely, viruses that replicate well at 37°C but not at 33°C (e.g., influenza virus) infect mainly the lower respiratory tract.

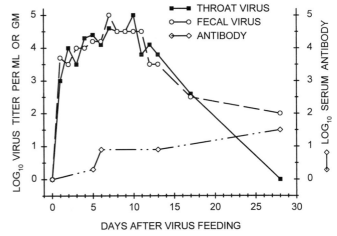

FIG. 2-2. The course of infection at the sites of entry of a typical enterovirus, as reflected in excretion from tissues representing the portals of entry. Chimpanzees were fed poliovirus type 2 Wallingford strain (a low-passage field isolate), $10^{4.6}$ TCD100, and pharyngeal swabs and stools were collected and assayed for infectivity. Virus titers are expressed per milliliter or gram and represent geometric means of data on four animals, whereas antibody titers represent neutralization of 100 TCD100/0.25 mL serum. Note that virus shedding persists for about 1 month, well after the appearance of neutralizing antibody in the circulation at about 1 week after infection. (Data from Bodian D, Nathanson N. Inhibitory effects of passive antibody on virulent poliovirus excretion and on immune response in chimpanzees. Bull Johns Hopkins Hospital 1960;107:143.)

TABLE 2-4. *Viruses that initiate infection via the nasopharynx, respiratory tract, or both**

Localization of disease	Virus family	Example†
Upper respiratory tract	Picornaviridae Adenoviridae	Rhinovirus Adenovirus
Lower respiratory tract	Coronaviridae Orthomyxoviridae Paramyxoviridae Bunyaviridae	Bovine corona Influenza Respiratory syncytial Sin Nombre
No respiratory illness	Togaviridae Paramyxoviridae Bunyaviridae Arenaviridae Reoviridae Papovaviridae Herpesviridae Poxviridae	Rubella Mumps Hantavirus Lassa fever Reovirus Murine polyoma Varicella zoster Variola

*See Chapter 29 for a detailed discussion.
†Examples are viruses of humans except where indicated.
Adapted from Mims CA, White DO. Viral pathogenesis and immunology. Oxford: Blackwell, 1984.

Most respiratory viruses initiate infection by replicating in the epithelial lining of the alveoli or the respiratory tree. In some cases, the virus will also replicate in phagocytic cells free in the respiratory lumen or in subepithelial spaces.

Rhinoviruses

Detailed studies by Couch[38] and Douglas and colleagues[45] have documented the parameters of infection for rhinoviruses, and have shown that a typical rhinovirus exhibits a gradient from high to low infectivity, from nasopharynx, to anterior nares, to tongue, to internal nares. Biopsy specimens indicate that virus initially replicates in the epithelium of the nasal mucosa.

Poxviruses

Respiratory infection with ectromelia (i.e., mousepox) virus has been studied in some detail.[133] On the first day after infection, the virus infects free alveolar macrophages and epithelial cells of small bronchioles. Two days after infection, there is evidence of contiguous spread to adjacent cells. By day three postinfection, there is extension to endothelial cells of afferent lymphatic channels and a few macrophages in regional nodes and in the spleen, followed by systemic viremia and generalized dissemination. Concomitant with infection of the lower respiratory tract, there is infection of olfactory mucosa and submucosal macrophages, with spread to regional lymph nodes.

Reoviruses

Reoviruses can infect by way of the respiratory tract, and it has been shown that in mice, initial infection involves the M cells that overlie bronchus-associated lymphoid tissue,[101] a route that is similar to that used by reovirus when it infects by way of the gastrointestinal tract.

DISSEMINATION

Local Spread

Following establishment at the site of entry, most viruses spread locally by cell-to-cell transmission of infection. Simultaneously, virus is carried through afferent lymphatic drainage from the site of initial infection to the regional lymph nodes, either as free virions or in virus-infected phagocytic cells; this is usually the first step in dissemination of the infection. Some viruses remain localized near their site of entry, whereas others spread widely. One determinant of infection sequence is the intracellular polarization of viral maturation and release, which in epithelial cells can be to the apical surface, the basolateral surface, or both. Viruses that are released only at the apical surface tend to remain localized, whereas those that are released at the basal surface tend to disseminate.[154]

Viremia

The most important mechanism for dissemination is the circulation, which can potentially carry the virus to any organ or tissue. Viruses can circulate either free in the plasma phase of the blood or associated with formed elements; these two types of viremia have different characteristics and implications.

Sources of Viremia

Virus can enter the circulation from a number of different sites, including the efferent lymphatics, vascular endothelium, and peripheral blood monocytic cells such as monocytes and lymphocytes.

Lymphatics

Many viruses are carried by afferent lymphatic channels from their initial site of entry to regional lymph nodes, from which they may move through efferent lymphatics to the thoracic duct to reach the circulation. This is a critical phase in the process of infection, because it may be a necessary precursor to viremia and generalized spread of virus. Some viruses replicate within regional lymph nodes, which amplifies virus titers and increases the potential for significant levels of viremia. However, viruses that appear to be unable to replicate in any lymphoid organ can still produce high-titer viremias.

Thus, La Crosse virus, a bunyavirus whose extraneural replication appears confined to striated and cardiac muscle, produces a substantial viremia.[73] In such instances, it is presumed that virus is conveyed through the lymphatic system into the circulation, although it is possible that it moves directly from muscle across the capillary wall to the circulation.

Endothelium

A number of viruses replicate in endothelial cells lining the vasculature and are shed directly into the circulation. An example is the hemorrhagic encephalopathy of rats (HER) strain of rat virus.[15,35]

Blood Cells

As discussed later, under cell-associated viremia, many viruses such as HIV replicate in mononuclear cells, both cells found in the circulation and cells found in the lymphoreticular tissues. A few viruses, such as Colorado tick fever virus,[114] replicate in erythroblasts in the bone marrow and circulate in association with erythrocytes.

Plasma Viremia

"Plasma" viremia is the term usually used for blood-borne virus that is not associated with any of the formed elements of blood. There are several sources of plasma viremia. "Passive" viremia is viremia that results from entry of a virus inoculum directly into the circulation following injection by intravenous, intraperitoneal, intracerebral, intradermal, intramuscular, or subcutaneous routes without any intervening stage of replication. Figure 2-3 shows an example of passive viremia following subcutaneous injection; characteristically, the viremia appears about 3 to 6 hours after injection and disappears by 12 to 24 hours postinoculation. It is calculated that perhaps 10^{-3} (0.1%) of the inoculum appears in the blood following a subcutaneous infection; however, given a sufficiently large dose of virus, the passive viremia alone may be sufficient to deliver a potentially lethal amount of virus to a critical target organ (see Fig. 2-3).

"Active" viremia is viremia caused by the active replication of virus in the host. In some instances, active viremia may occur in two phases: "primary" viremia, in which virus spreads from a focal site of entry, and "secondary" viremia, which is generated after widespread infection has occurred, with replication of virus in peripheral tissues such as endothelium, tissue macrophages, liver, muscle, or other sites. This distinction is shown in Figure 2-1, and is illustrated for ectromelia in Figure 22-5 in Chapter 22.

An example of active viremia is shown in Figure 2-4, in which the virus appears in the plasma a few days after infection and lasts for about 1 week. The initial lag period is the interval required for tissue replication and shedding into the circulation. Termination of viremia is often quite abrupt and coincides with the appearance of neutralizing antibody in the serum (see Fig. 2-4). The importance of the immune response in terminating viremia is brought out by immunosuppression. When an infected animal is treated with an immunosuppressive regimen, the viremia may persist for long periods rather than being cleared quickly.[108,158]

Plasma viremia reflects a dynamic process in which virus continually enters the circulation and is removed. The rate of turnover of virus within the plasma compartment may be measured either in terms of physical virions using labeled virus or in terms of infectivity using a titration assay; infectivity is probably a more biologically relevant measure. Turnover is

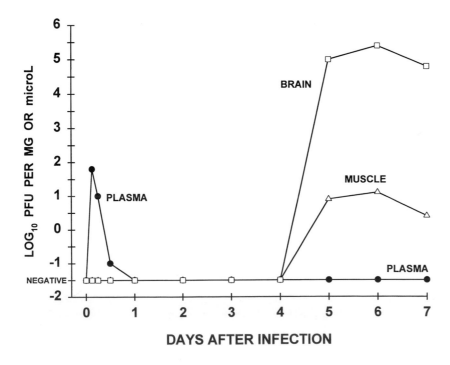

FIG. 2-3. Passive viremia following intraperitoneal injection of La Crosse virus, a California serogroup virus of the family Bunyaviridae, in 4-week-old mice. Because there is no active viremia in mice of this age, the passive viremia stands out in profile as a sharp peak limited mainly to the first 12 hours after injection. Mice were injected with 10^8 plaque-forming units (PFU). If the plasma volume was about 400 µL, it would require no more than 10^5 PFU to produce a peak viremia of 100 PFU/µl, suggesting that no more 10^{-3} of the injected virus entered the circulation. Even this small fraction of the inoculum and this transient viremia were sufficient to deliver enough virus to the target organ (in this instance, the brain) to initiate lethal encephalitis. (Adapted from Pekosz A, Griot C, Stillmock K, Nathanson N, Gonzalez-Scarano F. Protection from La Crosse virus encephalitis with recombinant glycoproteins: role of neutralizing anti-G1 antibodies. J Virol 1995;69:3475.)

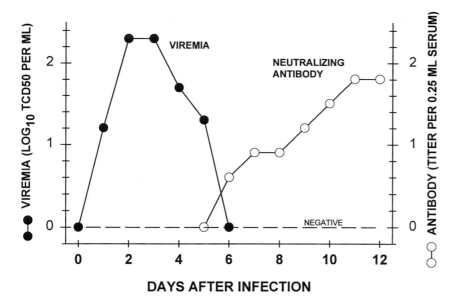

FIG. 2-4. The course of active plasma viremia. A group of 19 cynomolgus monkeys (*Macaca irus*) were infected with poliovirus type 1 Mahoney strain, a pantropic virulent strain, by intramuscular injection of about 10^5 TCD50. Viremia lasts for about 1 week, and the clearance of viremia coincides with the appearance of neutralizing antibody in the serum. Viremia is expressed as TCD50/mL serum, and antibody is expressed as as neutralizing dose 100 (ND100)/0.25 mL serum. (Data from Nathanson N, Bodian D. Experimental poliomyelitis following intramuscular virus injection. II. Viremia and the effect of antibody. Bull Johns Hopkins Hospital 1961;108: 308.)

best expressed as transit time, the average duration of a virion in the blood compartment. Experimentally, turnover can be estimated in two ways: by following the disappearance of virus after intravenous injection of a single bolus of virus or by determining the steady-state level of viremia produced by a continual intravenous infusion of virus. The steady-state method produces more reliable results because many individual titrations can be averaged to determine the steady-state level and because the die-away curve in clearance studies is not linear. Figure 2-5 illustrates an experimental determination of transit time using the steady-state method, and Figure 2-6 illustrates clearance curves following intravenous injection of a single dose of virus. Typically, transit times range from 1 to 60 minutes and tend to decrease in inverse proportion to increasing size of the virion.[27,92,94,95,139] Circulating virus is removed by the reticuloendothelial system, primarily

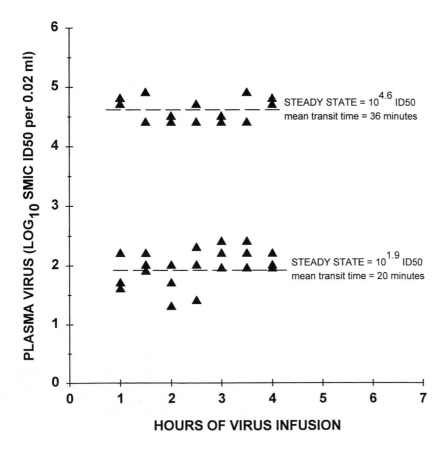

FIG. 2-5. Measurement of transit time of Langat virus, a flavivirus, using the steady-state method. Virus was infused continually through an intravenous cannula into spider monkeys (genus *Ateles*), and blood samples were obtained at 30-minute intervals over a 4-hour period. Two or three monkeys were used for each of two different concentrations of virus, producing two different steady-state levels. In each instance, the transit time, *t* (mean lifetime of circulating virions), was computed as $\log t = \log V_{ss} - \log V_1 + \log 2400$, where V_{ss} is the titer of steady-state viremia (TCD50/ 0.02 mL), V_i is the titer of infused virus (TCD50/0.02 mL), and the rate of infusion is 1/2400 blood volume per minute. Estimated transit times were 36 ± 10 minutes for the higher and 20 ± 9 minutes for the lower level of virus infusion (i.e., about 30 minutes at either virus dose). If *t* is 30 minutes, the half-life ($t_{1/2}$) would be about 27 minutes and the decilife ($t_{1/10}$) would be about 90 minutes. (Data from Nathanson N, Harrington B. Experimental infection of monkeys with Langat virus. II. Turnover of circulating virus. Am J Epidemiol 1967;85:494.)

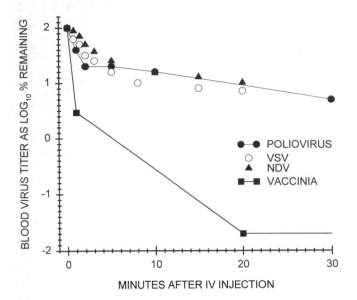

FIG. 2-6. Disappearance of virus from the circulation following an intravenous injection of a single bolus of virus. Virus was injected in the tail vein of mice, and blood was titered periodically. Viruses injected included poliovirus, a picornavirus, measured as infectivity; Newcastle disease virus (NDV) an orthomyxovirus; and vesicular stomatitis virus (VSV), a rhabdovirus, measured as P32-labeled purified virus; and vaccinia virus, a poxvirus, measured as infectivity. All of the curves show an early, rapid phase of clearance followed by at least one slower phase, illustrating the difficulty of determining the transit time, t (mean lifetime of circulating virions), by this technique. Vaccinia is cleared rapidly (decilife about 2.5 minutes, t about 0.8 minutes) and completely. The other three viruses follow clearance curves (decilife about 30 minutes, t about 10 minutes) similar to that determined for Langat virus (see Fig. 2-4). (Data from references 27, 95, and 139.)

by the Kupffer cells of the liver, and to a lesser extent in the lung, spleen, and lymph nodes.[27,95] Following uptake by sessile macrophages that monitor the blood, there are several alternate consequences which are diagramed in Figure 2-7. The virus may be degraded, transit macrophages to underlying parenchyma without replicating, or replicate in macrophages with or without spread of infection to underlying parenchymal cells.

After the host has developed circulating antibody, plasma virus is rapidly neutralized in the circulation, and virus-anti-

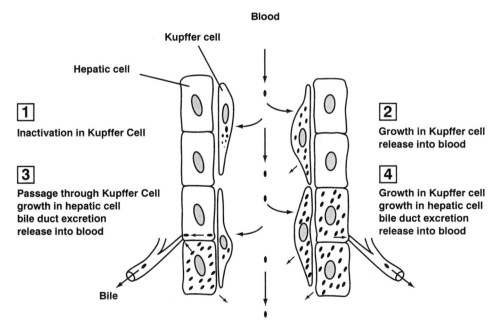

FIG. 2-7. Interaction between viruses and macrophages is exemplified by Kupffer cells in the liver, which are the primary site of clearance of circulating virus. A variety of outcomes can occur with different viruses. (**1**) The virus may be phagocytosed by Kupffer cells and degraded, as in La Crosse virus, a bunyavirus, and reovirus. (**2**) The virus may replicate in Kupffer cells and be shed back into the circulation to enhance the viremia, as in lactic dehydrogenase virus, a flavivirus. (**3**) The virus may be taken up by Kupffer cells but, rather than replicate, be transcytosed to exit their basolateral surface and infect hepatocytes to produce a severe hepatitis, with subsequent shedding into the bile, as in Rift Valley fever virus, a bunyavirus, or hepatitis B, a hepadnavirus. (**4**) The virus may replicate in Kupffer cells and in hepatocytes, producing a high-titer viremia and severe hepatitis with subsequent shedding into the bile, as in yellow fever, a flavivirus. (Adapted from Mims CA. The pathogenesis of infectious disease. London: Academic Press, 1976.)

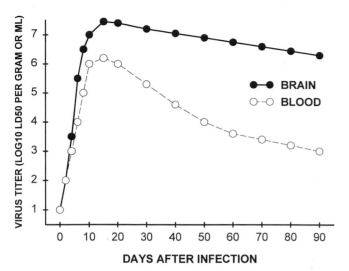

FIG. 2-8. Persistent plasma viremia associated with immunologic hyporesponsiveness to the viral antigens. Adult mice were infected with lymphocytic choriomeningitis virus intracerebrally and were immunosuppressed with aminopterin, 4 mg/kg, on days 4 and 6 after infection. The mice developed a persistent asymptomatic infection of the brain and a prolonged viremia. Mice infected in the same way but not treated with aminopterin died of acute choriomeningitis about 8 days after infection. (Data from Hotchin J. The biology of lymphocytic choriomeningitis infection: virus-induced immune disease. Cold Spring Harb Symp Quant Biol 1962;27:479.)

body complexes bind to Fc receptors, facilitating removal by sessile macrophages lining the vessels. Under these circumstances, it can be assumed that transit time is greatly reduced compared with the ranges described previously.

Although plasma viremias are usually short-lived, there are some notable exceptions. Some viruses are bound by antibody but the immune complex retains infectivity (e.g., Aleutian mink disease virus, a parvovirus, and lactic dehydrogenase virus, a togavirus). In such instances, plasma infectivity resists neutralization with exogenous antibody but may be reduced by the addition of anti-Ig antibodies.[111,112,125–127] Other exceptions are instances where the infected host is "tolerant" of the viral antigens and fails to develop a sufficient level of antibody to clear viremia; examples are hepatitis B virus and lymphocytic choriomeningitis virus, both of which may be associated with long-term plasma viremias in the absence of readily detectable circulating antibody (see Chaps. 25 and 31).[66,113] The persistent viremia of lymphocytic choriomeningitis virus in adult mice immunosuppressed with aminopterin at the time of infection is illustrated in Figure 2-8.

Cell-Associated Viremia

A number of viruses replicate in cells that are found in the circulation, particularly monocytes, B or T lymphocytes, or rarely, erythrocytes. Table 2-5 lists some of the viruses that replicate in circulating blood cells. Under these circumstances, virus is said to be "cell-associated," although it may also be found free in the plasma compartment. Cell-associated viremias associated with acute infections may be of short du-

TABLE 2-5. *Viruses that replicate in circulating blood cells*

Cell type	Virus family	Example*	Duration of viremia
Monocytes	Flaviviridae	Dengue	Acute
	Togaviridae	Rubella	Acute
	Coronaviridae	Mouse hepatitis	Acute
	Orthomyxoviridae	Influenza	Acute
	Paramyxoviridae	Measles	Acute
	Arenaviridae	Lymphocytic choriomeningitis	Persistent
	Retroviridae	Human immunodeficiency virus	Persistent
		Ovine maedivisna	Persistent
	Herpesviridae	Cytomegalovirus	Persistent
	Poxviridae	Mousepox	Acute
		Rabbit myxoma	Acute
B lymphocytes	Retroviridae	Murine leukemia	Persistent
	Herpesviridae	Epstein-Barr	Persistent
T lymphocytes	Retroviridae	Human immunodeficiency virus	Persistent
		Human T-cell leukemia I	Persistent
	Herpesviridae	Human herpes 6, 7	Acute
Erythroblasts†	Reoviridae	Colorado tick fever	Acute

*Examples are viruses of humans except where indicated.
†Colorado tick fever virus replicates in erythroblasts in bone marrow and circulates in mature erythrocytes.

ration, as in the case of ectromelia and other poxviruses (see Figs. 22-4 and 22-9 in Chap. 22). Cell-associated viremias often have features that are quite different from those of plasma viremias. In many instances of cell-associated viremias, blood virus titers are low, virus may be difficult to isolate from the blood, and viremia persists for the life of the host rather than terminating when neutralizing antibody appears.

A typical example of persistent cell-associated viremia involving infection of sheep with maedi/visna virus is shown in Figure 2-9. Infectious virus can be recovered by co-cultivation of circulating monocytes but virus cannot be isolated from the plasma phase, either because the virus is latent in infected circulating monocytes or because any cell-free virus is rapidly neutralized by plasma antibody.[121]

HIV provides an important instance of cell-associated viremia (Table 2-6) that has probably been investigated in more detail than any other example.[81] HIV infects both CD4+ T lymphocytes and monocytes in the blood, but most infected cells are CD4+ T lymphocytes. The frequency of infected peripheral blood CD4+ T lymphocytes varies from 0.2% to 10% in asymptomatic persons to 2% to 60% in symptomatic patients,[13,71,118,138] and 50% to 90% of infected T lymphocytes contain the genome in a latent state.[118] In typical asymptomatic individuals, it is estimated that there are about 5000 infected cells/mL blood (0.1% of 5×10^6 leukocytes/mL).[81]

In addition to infected cells, free infectious HIV is also present in the plasma; the amount varies with the stage of disease (see Table 2-6). Plasma viremia levels are highest in the early, transient, acute stage of infection and then drop markedly, presumably with the appearance of circulating antibody, only to rise again in the terminal stages of infection, when CD4+ cell counts diminish.[116] In typical asymptomatic individuals, it is estimated that there are about 100 tissue culture infectious doses (TCD) per milliliter of plasma,[81] which

is considerably fewer than the number of infected cells. The ability to isolate infectious virus from plasma, which presumably contains antiviral antibody, some of which has neutralizing activity, presents an apparent paradox. However, these low levels of infectivity in the plasma may represent only a small fraction of the virus shed into the circulation, a fraction that survives as infectious immune complexes. Circumstantial evidence for this theory is provided by the finding, using quantitative competitive polymerase chain reaction, that there are 10^4 to more than 10^6 total virions, compared with 10^2 to 10^3 TCD/mL plasma.[81,122]

It should be noted that in some instances a virus that does not replicate in blood cells may be cell associated because it is adsorbed to erythrocytes or other formed elements. This phenomenon has been reported for Rift Valley fever and influenza viruses, both of which are hemadsorbing viruses.[93,95]

Antibody-Dependent Enhancement of Infection

Antibody-dependent enhancement of infection is a special aspect of cell-associated viremia, which has been described mainly for dengue virus and other flaviviruses.[57,62] Dengue virus replicates primarily, perhaps exclusively, in monocytes and macrophages, but it does not enter these cells readily. However, in the presence of low concentrations of antibody, viral infection is markedly enhanced, presumably because the virus-antibody complex is bound to the Fc receptors on monocytes, initiating productive infection rather than virus degradation. There are four dengue virus serotypes, and severe disease (i.e., shock syndrome) is associated with reinfection with a second virus serotype in persons who were previously infected with another serotype. It is postulated that antibody-dependent enhancement may play a role in this phenomenon.

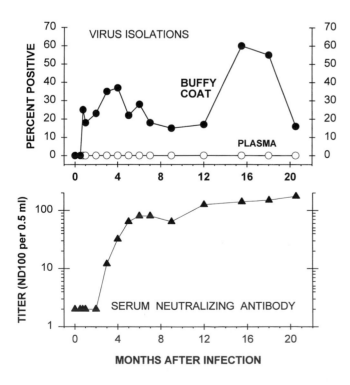

FIG. 2-9. Cell-associated viremia in sheep (the natural host) infected with maedi/visna virus, a lentivirus. A group of 19 sheep were injected intracerebrally with virus strain 1514, and buffy coat, plasma, and serum were tested at regular intervals for virus and antibodies. Virus was isolated by co-cultivation of buffy coat cells with indicator cells (sheep choroid plexus cells); virus was never isolated from the plasma. Virus was isolated from about 30% of more than 200 specimens collected 1 month or more after infection, and viremia was demonstrated in 17 of 19 animals, but patterns of isolation were irregular. Note that the frequency of buffy coat isolations was unrelated to the presence of serum neutralizing antibodies. (Data from Petursson G, Nathanson N, Georgsson G, Panitch H, Palsson PA. Pathogenesis of visna. I. Sequential virologic, serologic, and pathologic studies. Lab Invest 1976; 35:402.)

TABLE 2-6. *Simultaneous plasma and cell-associated viremia**

CD4+ cells per 0.001 mL[†]	Plasma HIV TCD/mL[†]	Stage of infection[‡]	% CD4+ cells infected[‡]
>500	114 (1–500)	II	2.7 (0.2–11)
300–499	205 (1–500)	III	21 (2–35)
200–299	381 (25–500)		
<200	1466 (25–5000)	IV	30 (2–65)

*The titer of HIV-1 in the plasma of infected persons according to CD4+ cell count, and the frequency of infected CD4+ T lymphocytes in blood according to clinical stage of infection.

[†]Mean and range plasma HIV titer is based on cell culture assay. Data from Pan L-Z, Wein A, Levy JA. Detection of plasma viremia in individuals at all clinical stages. J Clin Microbiol 1993;13:283.

[‡]CDC infection stage: II, asymptomatic; III, persistent generalized lymphadenopathy; IV, clinical AIDS. Mean and range percent CD4+ cells infected based on in situ polymerase chain reaction. Data from Bagasra O, Seshamma T, Oakes JW, Pomerantz RJ. High percentages of CD4-positive lymphocytes harbor the HIV-1 provirus in the blood of certain infected individuals. AIDS 1993;7:1419.

Viral Transport Across the Vascular Barrier

The localization of viruses to specific organs, tissues, and cells is the subject of Chapter 3, but it is appropriate to mention in this chapter the mechanisms by which virus leaves the circulation to enter potential target organs. There are several ways in which a virus can cross the vascular wall,[76] but the precise mechanism for penetrating the blood-tissue barrier is unknown in most instances, even though this an almost universal attribute of pathogenic viruses.

In some tissues, the capillary is fenestrated and virus can pass between endothelial cells that line the vessel. One example is the fenestrated capillaries of the choroid plexus of the central nervous system. Penetration at this site provides access to the epithelial cells of the choroid plexus and can be followed by entry into the cerebrospinal fluid and spread to the ependymal lining of the ventricles. Several viruses replicate in either choroid plexus (e.g., lymphocytic choriomeningitis virus,[56] maedi/visna virus[121]) or in the ventricular ependyma (e.g., mumps virus[64,84]) suggesting that they use this route of transcapillary tissue invasion.

Virus can be transported through the endothelial cell by a process of endocytosis followed by translocation of virus-containing vesicles and release by exocytosis at the basal surface of the endothelial cell.[14,76,117]

Some viruses are capable of replicating within endothelial cells and potentially can "grow" across the blood-tissue barrier. Many viruses can infect primary cultures of endothelial cells,[54] and in vivo studies have identified capillary infection for a number of agents, including picornaviruses, retroviruses, alphaviruses, and parvoviruses.[15,35,75,87,123,161]

Viruses that cause a cell-associated viremia may invade by an alternate mechanism, as "passengers" in infected lymphocytes or monocytes. Infected mononuclear cells can cross the blood-tissue barrier as part of their normal trafficking pattern or they may be actively recruited into sites of inflammation. Dubbed the "Trojan horse" route of invasion, this mechanism has been postulated to explain the invasion of the central nervous system by HIV.[61] This hypothesis rests on the observations that HIV infects circulating monocytes, invades the brain early in infection, and in the neuroparenchyma is localized primarily in microglia or macrophages, particularly in perivascular sites where macrophage-derived giant cells are prominent.[78,81,91,143,157]

Neural Spread

Some viruses can disseminate by spreading along peripheral nerves (Table 2-7). Although less important than viremia, neural spread plays an essential role for certain viruses (e.g., rabies viruses, several herpesviruses), whereas other viruses (e.g., poliovirus, reovirus) can spread by both neural and viremia mechanisms. Different strains of the same virus may differ markedly in their ability to spread by the neural route.[106,132] Several viruses that usually produce viremia have been laboratory adapted to replicate in nervous tissue, and these neuroadapted clones may use neural spread. Table 2-8 contrasts two strains of poliovirus that represent an example of this phenomenon. In some instances, natural isolates of the same virus may differ markedly in their relative use of neural or viremia routes of spread, as exemplified by type 1 and type 3 reoviruses (see Fig. 28-4 in Chap. 28).[155]

The mechanisms of neural spread are well understood. The earliest studies showed that neural spread could be blocked by cutting, freezing, or otherwise interrupting a peripheral nerve (see Table 2-2)[8–10,106] and led to calculations of the rate of neural spread, which is estimated at about 5 to 7 cm per 24 hours.[42,70,72,79,153,155] Subsequent studies established that spread occurs within the axons and dendrites of neurons[7,8,10,11,29,65,74,104,129] and does not depend upon the myelin-producing cells, Schwann cells, or other cells of the endoneurium, perineurium, and epineurium, even though virus may eventually spread from neurons to such supporting cells.

More recent reports using pseudorabies virus[29,47] and HSV[160] demonstrated the exquisite specificity of intraneuronal and transneuronal spread, which can be used as a powerful method for tracing multineuronal pathways. Additionally,

TABLE 2-7. *Viruses that spread by the neural route*

Virus family	Example	Notes	Investigators
Picornaviridae	Polio	Neuroadapted clones only Natural isolates viremic Transgenic mice*	Nathanson and Bodian, 1961[106] Bodian, 1955[23] Racaniello, 1988[130] Ren and Racaniello, 1992[132]
Flaviviridae	Yellow fever	Neuroadapted clones only† Natural isolates viremic	Strode, 1951[148]
Alphaviridae	Venezuelan equine encephalitis	Hematogenous invasion of peripheral nerves	Charles et al, 1995[32]
Coronaviridae	Mouse hepatitis	Neural spread after intranasal infection	Perlman et al, 1989[120] Barnett and Cassell, 1993[17]
Rhabdoviridae	Rabies	Exclusively neural	Baer, 1991[12]
Reoviridae	Reovirus	Type 3 uses neural spread Type 1 spreads by blood	Tyler et al, 1986[155] Morrison et al, 1991[102]
Herpesviridae	Herpes simplex 1,2	Exclusively neural in adults Pantropic in newborns	Stevens and Cook, 1973[37] Stevens and Cook, 1974[146]
	Pseudorabies	Used for neural pathways	Enquist, 1994[47]

*In transgenic mice bearing the poliovirus receptor, the Mahoney strain of type 1 virus behaves like an obligatory neurotropic strain, spreading exclusively by the neural route.

†The French neurotropic strain of yellow fever, virus was neuroadapted by multiple intracerebral passages in mice. This virus, which was never cloned, produced encephalitis in monkeys but also retained some viremic and viscerotropic properties.

these studies have shown that different viruses or virus strains exhibit different patterns of neural spread[17,30,160] and have begun to dissect the role of various viral genes and proteins in determining these patterns.[30,48]

It appears that virus enters neurons by mechanisms similar to those involving entry into other cell types. The uncoated nucleocapsid is then carried passively along the neural process, probably by fast axoplasmic flow. Subsequent to the transport process, the virus may replicate in axons or dendrites, but this is a slow process and is not required for neural spread. Evidence for this pattern of neural spread is provided by several lines of evidence:

The rate of neural spread (>5 cm/day) is similar to the rate of axoplasmic transport (>10 cm/day), although neural spread tends to be a little slower, perhaps as a result of technical inaccuracies in the in vivo estimates of the speed of neural spread.[42,70,72,79,153,155]

Drugs that block fast axoplasmic transport (e.g., colchicine) also block transport of viral genomes.[8,20,31,152]

Temperature-sensitive strains of herpesvirus, which cannot replicate at body temperature, are able to move from a peripheral site of inoculation to a sensory ganglion such as the trigeminal ganglion and may be recovered by culturing the

TABLE 2-8. *Comparison of a neuroadapted and a natural pantropic isolate of poliovirus**

	Neuroadapted MV strain		Pantropic Mahoney strain	
	Control	Block	Control	Block
Paralysis	25/26	0/11	19/19	18/20
Site of initial paralysis				
Injected leg	24		3	5
Other	1		16	13
Incubation to paralysis	5 d		7 d	7.5 d

*The neuroadapted virus spreads only by the neural route, causes initial paralysis in the injected limb, and fails to paralyze after a nerve block, whereas the pantropic strain spreads by viremia, does not cause localized initial paralysis, and is not impeded by nerve block. The type 2 MV strain was a laboratory strain that was neuroadapted by many intracerebral passages in monkeys, whereas the type 1 Mahoney strain was a pantropic natural field isolate that was passaged a few times in cell culture. Viruses were injected into the left gastrocnemius muscle (MV strain, $>10^5$ PD50; Mahoney strain, 10^5–10^6 TCD50). Neural block was done just prior to virus injection by freezing the sciatic nerve with dry ice proximal to the site of virus injection.

Data from Nathanson N, Bodian D. Experimental poliomyelitis following intramuscular virus injection. I. The effect of neural block on a neurotropic and a pantropic strain. Bull Johns Hopkins Hospital 1961;108:308.

explanted ganglion at temperatures that are permissive for temperature-sensitive clones.[36,86,141]

Several days after initiation of neural spread, viruses such as rabies virus, HSV, and pseudorabies virus (an alphaherpesvirus) can be seen replicating within axons (Fig. 2-10)[8,29,65,74,104,129]

Centripetal and Centrifugal Movement of Virus

Axoplasmic flow is a bidirectional process, transporting constituents both toward and away from the neuronal cell body. Molecular studies have defined distinct "motors" for anterograde and retrograde transport and have shown that the rates differ between the two directions. Neural spread not only conducts virus from the periphery to the central nervous system but also produces centrifugal spread from the central nervous system to the periphery.[7,8] In this manner, neurotropic viruses can be disseminated widely along peripheral neural pathways (see Chap. 18). It has been shown that for a single virus clone the rate of anterograde and retrograde neuronal

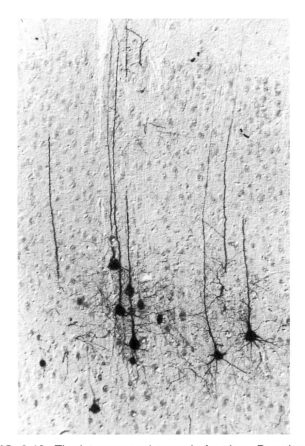

FIG. 2-10. The intraneuronal spread of a virus. Pseudorabies virus, Bartha strain, is seen in neurons in the perirhinal cortex of a rat following virus injection into the prefrontal cortex. Peroxidase staining has been used to visualize viral antigen. (From Card JP, Enquist LW. Use of pseudorabies virus for definition of synaptically linked populations of neurons. Methods Mol Genet 1994;4:363.)

spread may vary, whereas different virus clones may move at distinct rates or in only one direction.[30,48,160]

Neural Versus Viremic Spread

Viremic and neural spread have been contrasted as alternative modes of dissemination; however for some viruses, a scheme of pathogenesis has been proposed that invokes both mechanisms in sequential steps of infection with a single virus. One proposal for the pathogenesis of poliomyelitis postulates that viremia delivers virus to peripheral autonomic or other peripheral ganglia, from whence the virus spreads by neural routes to the central nervous system (see Fig. 23-6 in Chap. 23).[135] An hypothesis regarding the pathogenesis of varicella-zoster postulates that the virus, which produces a viremia, invades the skin and then moves along neural pathways to lodge in first-order sensory ganglia. It has been suggested that several arboviruses produce viremia, invade specific sites in the peripheral nervous system such as the olfactory mucosa or trigeminal ganglion, and then use neural spread to invade the central nervous system.[32,99]

LOCALIZATION

Localization of infection and tropism of viruses are discussed in Chapter 3.

SHEDDING

Acute viral infections are characterized by brief periods of intensive virus shedding. Virus may be shed into respiratory aerosols, feces, urine, or other bodily secretions or fluids; each of these sources is important for the transmission of selected viruses. Although shedding may be well documented, often the exact cellular origin of the shed virus is less clear. Additionally, a given virus may be excreted from several portals, only a few of which are relevant for transmission. Persistent viruses may be shed at relatively low levels, but these low levels may be adequate for transmission over the prolonged duration of infection.

Oropharynx and Gastrointestinal Tract

The course of shedding of enteric viruses can be easily followed. Figure 2-2 illustrates the excretion of wild poliovirus from the pharynx and in the feces following feeding of chimpanzees, which constitute a good model for the natural human host. In contrast to viremia, which terminates about 1 week after infection concomitant with the appearance of circulating antibody (see Fig. 2-4), poliovirus continues to be shed in the pharynx for 2 to 4 weeks and in the feces for 1 to 2 months after infection. Pathogenesis studies suggest that excreted poliovirus is derived from virus that replicates in lymphoid tissue of the pharynx and small intestine (Peyer's patches).[23] Other enteroviruses exhibit similar patterns.[90] Hepatitis A virus is excreted in the feces for 1 to 2 months after infection, presumably from virus that replicates in the liver, enters the bile, and is discharged into the small intestine.[67,150,151] Rotaviruses replicate in the superficial epithelial cells of the small intestine, associated with a relatively acute enteric infection leading to virus shedding into the feces that lasts only 1 to 2 weeks after infection.[77]

Respiratory Tract

Respiratory viruses may be transmitted by aerosols generated by coughing or sneezing or by virus-containing nasopharyngeal fluids that are transmitted by hand-to-hand contact. Most acute respiratory viruses are excreted over a relatively short period, and infected persons are potential transmitters for only about 1 week; transmission may begin a few days before onset of symptoms. Detailed studies of rhinoviruses by Couch[38] and by Douglas and colleagues[45] have documented the course of virus shedding into nasopharyngeal fluids for rhinovirus type 15 (Fig. 2-11).

Skin

Although many viruses cause skin lesions that contain infectious virus, relatively few viruses are actually spread from skin lesions. Exceptions are HSV, which is spread by labial transmission; varicella-zoster, which, rarely, spreads from zoster to cause chickenpox[28]; and papillomaviruses, all of which are transmitted by mechanical contact. Additionally, some poxviruses can be spread by virus aerosolized from infected, desquamated skin, and there are apocryphal 18th century accounts of the deliberate use of smallpox fomites as the first instance of "biological warfare."[53,89]

Mucous Membranes and Oral and Genital Fluids

Viruses that cause sexually transmitted disease, such as HSV type 2 and papillomaviruses, are often shed from lesions of the genital mucous membranes. Viruses that infect the oral mucous membranes, such as HSV type 1, can be shed into the oropharyngeal fluids. Additionally, some viruses, such as mumps and Epstein-Barr viruses, replicate in the salivary glands and are discharged into the saliva to enter the oral cavity. Of these, the most important is rabies virus, which has a propensity to replicate in the salivary gland and is usually transmitted by introduction of contaminated saliva from the bite of a rabid animal (see Chap. 24).[51]

Semen

Several human viruses are shed in the semen under circumstances in which this plays an important role in sexual transmission. Hepatitis B antigen is often found in seminal fluid of carriers of HBsAg,[3,140] consistent with its transmission from men to partners of either sex.[66] HIV can be isolated from seminal fluids in a considerable proportion of infected men (10 to 50 infectious units/mL in one third of those tested).[5,26,81] In addition, 0.01% to 5% of mononuclear cells in semen are HIV genome–positive; an average ejaculate contains about 10^6 mononuclear cells or 10^2 to 10^4 virus-positive cells. Murine retroviruses have also been reported to be transmitted by infected semen.[82,128]

Milk

A number of human viruses are excreted in colostrum and milk, including cytomegalovirus, mumps, and rubella virus;

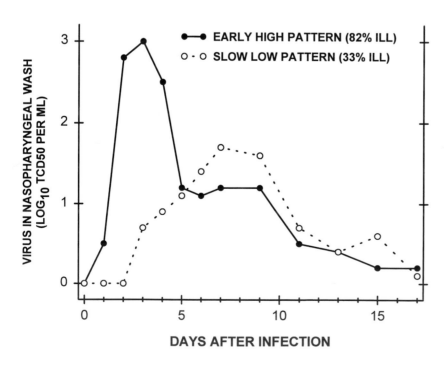

FIG. 2-11. The excretion of a typical respiratory virus, rhinovirus type 15, following inoculation of human volunteers by the transnasal route. The subjects demonstrated two patterns of virus excretion: an early onset, high-concentration pattern associated with a high frequency of respiratory symptoms, and a late onset, low-concentration pattern associated with a low frequency of symptoms. (Data from Douglas RG Jr, Cate TR, Gerone JP, Couch RB. Quantitative rhinovirus shedding patterns in volunteers. Am Rev Respir Dis 1966;94:159.)

this is probably a significant route of perinatal transmission of cytomegalovirus.[46,145] Perinatal transmission of hepatitis B virus is important in countries where there is a high prevalence of antigenemic women of childbearing age, but transmission is thought to occur during delivery rather than be associated with breast feeding.[66] Excretion of virus in milk is also a notable mode of transmission for certain viral infections of animals. Maedi/visna virus is frequently transmitted from infected ewes to newborn lambs, but if lambs born of infected ewes are removed from the mother before they can take colostrum and sequestered from infected sheep, they escape infection entirely.[41] Milk also plays a key role in the transmission of mouse mammary tumor virus.[21,60,103]

Blood

Blood is also an important source of transmitted virus, particularly for those viruses that produce persistent plasma or cell-associated viremias. Hepatitis B, C, and D viruses, HIV, human T-cell leukemia viruses I and II, and cytomegalovirus are among the important human pathogens that are transmitted in this manner. Persistent viremias vary in titer. For instance, HIV is commonly found at levels of 100 TCD/mL plasma and 1000 infected cells/mL blood, but hepatitis B can reach levels of 10^7 infectious units/mL blood (see Chap. 31).[16]

Arboviruses usually cause short-term acute viremias and are transmissible only if an appropriate vector ingests a blood meal during this brief interval. In view of the limited amount of blood taken, the viremia must reach considerable levels if it is to be transmitted. For instance, if a mosquito ingests 1 to 2 μL, a viremia of 10^4 PFU/mL would lead to the uptake of 10 PFU. Vector transmission is discussed in Chapter 14.

Urine

A number of viruses have been isolated in urine, including mumps, HIV, hepatitis B, and polyomaviruses,[6,156] and it may be that any virus that produces sufficient viremia will also cause viruria.[139] However, viruria is probably not important for the transmission of most viruses. A special exception are certain zoonotic viruses, such as arenaviruses and Hantaviruses, which cause lifelong viruria in their natural rodent hosts, putatively leading to human infection through exposure to aerosolized dried urine.[58,88]

Survival in the Environment

The probability that a virus will be transmitted depends on both the intensity and duration of shedding and its ability to survive in the environment. Viruses differ in their ability to survive in aerosols; somewhat surprisingly, under conditions of low humidity, enveloped viruses appear to be better able to retain viability than nonenveloped viruses.[43,44,63] This may account for the fact that most viruses that infect the lower respiratory tract are enveloped. To be excreted in an infectious form, enteric viruses must be able to survive the harsh environment of the gastrointestinal tract (see Entry).

TRANSMISSION

Once shed, there are a several means by which a virus is transmitted from host to host in a propagated chain of infection. Probably the most important mechanism is contamination of the hands of the infected transmitter from feces, oral fluids, or respiratory secretions. The virus is then passed by hand-to-hand contact, leading to oral, gastrointestinal, or respiratory infection. A second common route is inhalation of aerosolized virus. A third significant mechanism involves direct person to person contact by one of four means: oral-oral, genital-genital, oral-genital, or skin-skin. Finally, indirect person-to-person transmission can occur via blood or contaminated needles. Common-source transmissions are less common but can produce dramatic outbreaks through contaminated water, food products, or biological agents such as blood products and vaccines.

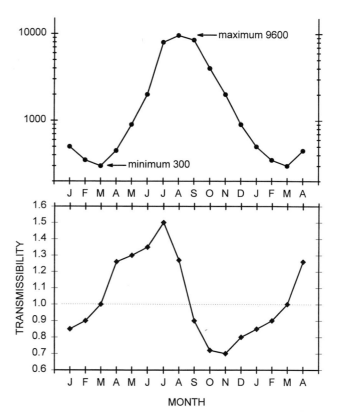

FIG. 2-12. Transmissibility of poliomyelitis by season, based on reported cases in the United States from 1953 to 1955, before the introduction of poliovirus vaccines. (**A**) Average monthly numbers of poliomyelitis cases. (**B**) Estimated transmissibility by month. Transmissibility is defined as the number of new infections produced per existing infection for each successive generation period and is estimated by a computerized bookkeeping method. Transmissibility of poliomyelitis varies around a mean of 1, with a seasonal high of 1.5 and a low of 0.75. (Data from Yorke JA, Nathanson N, Pianigiani G, Martin JR. Seasonality and the requirements for perpetuation and eradication of viruses in populations. Am J Epidemiol 1979;109:103.)

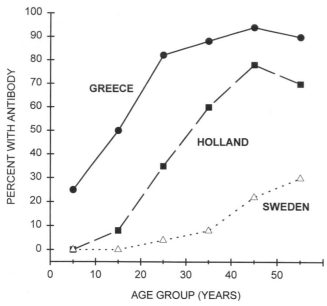

FIG. 2-13. Differences in transmissibility of hepatitis A virus among three European countries, as reflected in the different age-specific profiles of antibody prevalence. (Data from Frosner GG, Papaevangelou G, Butler R, et al. Antibody against hepatitis A in seven European countries. I. Comparison of prevalence data in different age groups. Am J Epidemiol 1979;110:63.)

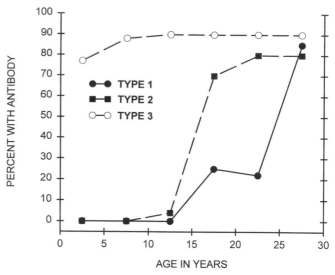

FIG. 2-14. Disappearance of a virus is the expression of reduced transmissibility as a result of exhaustion of the susceptible population. Age-specific prevalence of three types of poliovirus are shown for Narssak, Greenland, an isolated Eskimo village. There is no evidence of infection with type 1 virus in those younger than 25 years of age and no evidence of infection with type 2 virus in those younger than 15 years of age, implying that these two viruses have disappeared from this population. In contrast, type 3 virus has infected all age groups. (Data from Paffenbarger RS, Bodian D. Poliomyelitis immune status in ecologically diverse populations, in relation to virus spread, clinical incidence, and virus disappearance. Am J Hygiene 1961;74:311.)

The success of a virus as a life form can be defined as its ability to be perpetuated over the millennia. In turn, perpetuation of a virus depends in part on its efficient transmission, particularly for viruses that cause only acute infections. For viruses that can persist in individual hosts, perpetuation is determined by transmission over the lifetime of the host and in some instances by the ability to be vertically passed to offspring of the host by transplacental or perinatal routes or as germline genes.

There are various ways to measure the transmissibility of a virus in a host population. Epidemiologically, transmissibility is often defined as the number of new infections initiated by each existing infection[105] without regard to the duration of the infection. If transmissibility is more than 1, the number of infected individuals is increasing; conversely, if transmissibility is less than 1, the number of infected individuals is falling. Within a given population, transmissibility may cycle above and below 1, but it must average close to 1 over a long time period if the virus is to be perpetuated in the specified population. This is illustrated in Figure 2-12, which models seasonal variation in the transmission rate of poliovirus in the United States in the prevaccine era.[159]

For acute virus infections, one simple measure of overall efficiency of transmission in a population is the age distribution of infections. Assuming that the initial infection confers lifelong immunity and lifelong detectable antibody, the age-specific antibody prevalence profile provides a sensitive reflection of transmission efficiency. Figure 2-13 shows age profiles for hepatitis A in several different populations and illustrates the subtle but unmistakable differences in transmissi-

bility of a single virus in different populations. Likewise, in a single population, there are marked differences in the transmissibility of different viruses.

If transmissibility is reduced sufficiently, then a given virus will disappear from a defined population. This can happen in nature when a virus spreads so widely in a specific population that it eliminates most susceptible hosts and "burns out." This phenomenon is illustrated in Figure 2-14 for poliovirus (see Fig. 15-4 in Chap. 15, which represents the same phenomenon for measles in Iceland). Transmissibility can also be reduced by immunization, which, under certain circumstances, can be used to eradicate a virus from its host population. Smallpox is the seminal example of planned eradication,[53] and the elimination of wild poliovirus from the western hemisphere is another important illustration.

ABBREVIATIONS

HER: hemorrhagic encephalopathy of rats
HIV: human immunodeficiency virus
HSV: herpes simplex virus
ISVP: infectious subvirion particle
M cells: microvilli or microfold cells
PFU: plaque-forming unit
TCD: tissue culture infectious doses

REFERENCES

1. Adachi A, Koenig S, Gendelman HE, et al. Productive, persistent infection of human colorectal cell lines with human immunodeficiency virus. J Virol 1987;61:209–213.
2. Almeida JD, Howatson AF, Williams MG. Electron microscopic study of human warts, sites of virus production, and the nature of the inclusion bodies. J Invest Dermatol 1962;38:337–345.
3. Alter HJ, Purcell RH, Gerin JL. Transmission of hepatitis B surface antigen positive saliva and semen. Infect Immun 1977;16:928–933.
4. Amerongen HM, Wilson GAR, Fields BN, Neutra MR. Proteolytic processing of reovirus is required for adherence to intestinal M cells. J Virol 1994;68:8428–8432.
5. Anderson DJ, O'Brien TR, Politch JA, et al. Effects of disease stage and zidovudine therapy on the detection of human immunodeficiency virus type 1 in semen. JAMA 1992;267:2769–2774.
6. Arthur RR, Shah KV. Occurrence and significance of papovavirus BK and JC in the urine. Prog Med Virol 1989;36:42–61.
7. Baer GM. Pathogenesis to the central nervous system. In: Baer GM, ed. The natural history of rabies. New York: Academic Press, 1975:181–198.
8. Baer GM. Rabies pathogenesis to the central nervous system. In: Baer GM, ed. The natural history of rabies. 2nd ed. Boca Raton: CRC Press, 1991:105–120.
9. Baer GM, Cleary WF. A model in mice for the pathogenesis and treatment of rabies. J Infect Dis 1972;125:520–529.
10. Baer GM, Shantha TR, Bourne GH. The pathogenesis of fixed rabies virus in rats. Bull World Health Organ 1968;38:119–125.
11. Baer GM, Shanthaveerappa TR, Bourne GH. Studies on the pathogenesis of fixed rabies virus in rats. Bull World Health Organ 1965;33:783–790.
12. Baer GM, ed. The natural history of rabies. 2nd ed. Boca Raton: CRC Press, 1991.
13. Bagasra O, Seshamma T, Oakes JW, Pomerantz RJ. High percentages of CD4-positive lymphocytes harbor the HIV-1 provirus in the blood of certain infected individuals. AIDS 1993;7:1419–1425.
14. Bang F, Luttrell C. Factors in the pathogenesis of virus diseases. Adv Virus Res 1961;8:199–244.
15. Baringer JR, Nathanson N. Parvovirus hemorrhagic encephalopathy of rats: electron microscopic observations of the vascular lesions. Lab Invest 1972;27:514–522.
16. Barker LF, Murray R. Relationship of virus dose to incubation time of clinical hepatitis and time of appearance of hepatitis-associated antigen. Am J Med Sci 1972;263:27–33.
17. Barnett EM, Cassell MD. Two neurotropic viruses, herpes simplex virus type 1 and mouse hepatitis virus, spread along different neural pathways from the main olfactory bulb. Neuroscience 1993;57:1007–1025.
18. Bass DM, Bodkin D, Danbrauskas R, Trier JS, Fields BN, Wolf JL. Intraluminal proteolytic activation plays an important role in replication of type 1 reovirus in the intestines of neonatal mice. J Virol 1990;64:1830–1833.
19. Bass DM, Trier JS, Danbrauskas R, Wolf JL. Reovirus type 1 infection of small intestinal epithelium in suckling mice and its effect on M cells. Lab Invest 1988;55:226–235.
20. Bijenga G, Heaney T. Post-exposure local treatment of mice infected with rabies virus with two axonal flow inhibitors, colchicine and vinblastine. J Gen Virol 1978;39:381–390.
21. Bittner JJ. Some possible effects of nursing on the mammary gland tumor incidence in mice. Science 1936;162:164.
22. Blank H, Burgoon CF, Baldridge GD, McCarthy PL, Urback F. Cytologic smears in diagnosis of herpes simplex, herpes zoster, and varicella. JAMA 1951;146:1410–1412.
23. Bodian D. Emerging concepts of poliomyelitis infection. Science 1955;122:105–108.
24. Bodian D, Nathanson N. Inhibitory effects of passive antibody on virulent poliovirus excretion and on immune response in chimpanzees. Bull Johns Hopkins Hospital 1960;107:143–162.
25. Bodkin D, Nibert ML, Fields BN. Proteolytic digestion of reovirus in the intestinal lumens of neonatal mice. J Virol 1989;63:4676–4681.
26. Borzy MS, Connell RS, Kiessling AA. Detection of human immu-
nodeficiency virus in cell-free seminal fluid. J Acquir Immune Defic Syndr 1988;1:419–424.
27. Brunner KT, Hurez D, McCluskey RT, Benacerraf B. Blood clearance of P32 labeled vesicular stomatitis and Newcastle disease viruses by the reticuloendothelial system in mice. J Immunol 1960;85:99–105.
28. Bruusgaard E. The mutual relation between zoster and varicella. Br J Dermatol 1932;44:1–24.
29. Card JP, Enquist LW. Use of pseudorabies virus for definition of synaptically linked populations of neurons. Methods Mol Genet 1994;4:363–382.
30. Card JP, Whealy ME, Robbins AK, Enquist LW. Two alphavirus strains are transported differentially in the rodent visual system. Neuron 1992;6:957–969.
31. Ceccaldi PE, Gillet JP, Tsiang H. Inhibition of the transport of rabies virus in the central nervous system. J Neuropathol Exp Neurol 1989;48:620–630.
32. Charles PC, Walters E, Margolis F, Johnston RE. Mechanism of neuroinvasion of Venezuelan equine encephalitis virus in the mouse. Virology 1995;208:662–671.
33. Clark SM, Roth JR, Clark ML. Tryptic enhancement of rotavirus infectivity: mechanism of enhancement. J Virol 1981;39:816–822.
34. Cohen J. Women: absent term in the AIDS research equation. Science 1995;269:777–780.
35. Cole GA, Nathanson N, Rivet H. Viral hemorrhagic encephalopathy of rats. II. Pathogenesis of hemorrhagic lesions. Am J Epidemiol 1970;91:339–350.
36. Cook ML, Bastone VB, Stevens JG. Evidence that neurons harbor latent herpes simplex virus. Infect Immun 1974;9:946–951.
37. Cook ML, Stevens JG. Pathogenesis of herpetic neuritis and ganglionitis in mice: evidence of intra-axonal transport of infection. Infect Immun 1973;7:272–288.
38. Couch RB. Rhinoviruses. In: Fields BN, Knipe DM, eds. Virology. 2nd ed. New York: Raven Press, 1990:607–629.
39. Coulepis AG, Locarnini SA, Lehmann NI, Gust ID. Detection of hepatitis A virus in the feces of patients with naturally acquired infections. J Infect Dis 1980;141:151–156.
40. Dalmat H. Arthropod transmission of rabbit papillomatosis. J Exp Med 1958;108:9–20.
41. de Boer GF, Houwers DJ. Epizootology of maedi/visna in sheep. In: Tyrrell DAJ, ed. Aspects of slow and persistent virus infections. The Hague: Martinus Nijhoff, 1979:198–220.
42. Dean DJ, Evans WM, McClure RC. Pathogenesis of rabies. Bull World Health Organ 1963;29:803–811.
43. DeJong JG. The survival of measles virus in air in relation to the epidemiology of measles. Arch Gesamte Viruschforsch 1965;16:97–102.
44. DeJong JG, Winkler KC. The inactivation of poliovirus in aerosols. J Hygiene 1968;66:557–565.
45. Douglas RG Jr, Cate TR, Gerone JP, Couch RB. Quantitative rhinovirus shedding patterns in volunteers. Am Rev Respir Dis 1966;94:159–167.
46. Dworsky ME, Yow M, Stagno S. Cytomegalovirus infection of breast milk and transmission in infancy. Pediatrics 1983;72:295–299.
47. Enquist LW. Infection of the mammalian nervous system by pseudorabies virus (PRV). Semin Virol 1994;5:221–231.
48. Enquist LW, Dubin J, Whealy ME, Card JP. Complementation analysis of pseudorabies virus gE and gI mutants in retinal ganglion cell neurotropism. J Virol 1994;68:5275–5279.
49. Estes MK, Graham DY, Mason BB. Proteolytic enhancement of rotavirus infectivity: molecular mechanisms. J Virol 1981;39:879–888.
50. Fantini J, Yahi N, Baghdiguian S, Chermann J-C. Human colon epithelial cells productively infected with human immunodeficiency virus show impaired differentiation and altered secretion. J Virol 1992;66:580–585.
51. Fekadu M, Shadduck JH, Baer GM. Excretion of rabies virus in the saliva of dogs. J Infect Dis 1982;145:715–719.
52. Fenner F. Biological control as exemplified by smallpox eradication and myxomatosis. Proc R Soc Lond 1983;218:259–285.
53. Fenner F, Henderson DA, Arita I, Jezek Z, Ladnyi ID. Smallpox and its eradication. Geneva: World Health Organization, 1988.

54. Friedman H, Macarek E, MacGregor RA. Virus infection of endothelial cells. J Infect Dis 1981;143:266–273.

55. Frosner GG, Papaevangelou G, Butler R, et al. Antibody against hepatitis A in seven European countries. I. Comparison of prevalence data in different age groups. Am J Epidemiol 1979;110:63–69.

56. Gilden DH, Cole GA, Monjan AA, Nathanson N. Immunopathogenesis of acute central nervous system disease produced by lymphocytic choriomeningitis virus. I. Cyclophosphamide-mediated induction of the virus-carrier state in adult mice. J Exp Med 1972; 135:860–873.

57. Gollins SW, Porterfield JS. Flavivirus infection enhancement in macrophages: radioactive and biological studies on the effect of antibody on viral fate. J Gen Virol 1984;65:1261–1272.

58. Gonzalez-Scarano F, Nathanson N. Bunyaviruses. In: Fields BN, Knipe DM, eds. Virology. 2nd ed. New York: Raven Press, 1990: 1195–1228.

59. Grabow WOK, Prozesky OW, Applebaum PC, Lecatsas G. Absence of hepatitis B antigens from feces and sewage as a result of enzymatic destruction. J Infect Dis 1975;131:658–664.

60. Gross L. Oncogenic viruses. Oxford: Pergammon Press, 1970.

61. Haase AT. Pathogenesis of lentivirus infections. Nature 1986;322: 130–136.

62. Halstead SB, O'Rourke EJ. Dengue viruses and mononuclear phagocytes. I. Infection enhancement by non-neutralizing antibody. J Exp Med 1977;146:201–217.

63. Hemmes HH, Winklerk KC, Kool SM. Virus survival as a seasonal factor in influenza and poliomyelitis. Nature 1960;188:430–431.

64. Herndon RM, Johnson RT, Davis LE. Ependymitis in mumps virus meningitis: electron microscopic studies of the cerebrospinal fluid. Arch Neurol 1974;30:475–479.

65. Hill T, Field H, Roome A. Intra-axonal location of herpes simplex virus particles. J Gen Virol 1972;15:253–255.

66. Hollinger FB. Hepatitis B virus. In: Fields BN, Knipe DM, eds. Virology. 2nd ed. New York: Raven Press, 1990:2171–2238.

67. Hollinger FB, Ticehurst J. Hepatitis A virus. In: Fields BN, Knipe DM, eds. Virology. 2nd ed. New York: Raven Press, 1990:631–667.

68. Horwitz MS. Adenoviruses. In: Fields BN, Knipe DM, eds. Virology. 2nd ed. New York: Raven Press, 1990:1723–1742.

69. Hotchin J. The biology of lymphocytic choriomeningitis infection: virus-induced immune disease. Cold Spring Harb Symp Quant Biol 1962;27:479–500.

70. Howe HA, Bodian D. Neural mechanisms in poliomyelitis. New York: The Commonwealth Fund, 1942.

71. Hsia K, Spector SA. Human immunodeficiency virus DNA is present in a high percentage of CD4+ lymphocytes of seropositive individuals. J Infect Dis 1991;164:470–475.

72. Iwasaki Y, Liu D, Yamamoto T. On the replication and spread of rabies virus in the human central nervous system. J Neuropathol Exp Neurol 1985;44:185–195.

73. Janssen R, Gonzalez-Scarano F, Nathanson N. Mechanisms of bunyavirus virulence: comparative pathogenesis of a virulent strain of La Crosse virus and an avirulent strain of Tahyna virus. Lab Invest 1984;50:447–455.

74. Jenson A, Raben E, Bentinck D. Rabiesvirus neuronitis. J Virol 1969;3:265–269.

75. Johnson RT. Virus invasion of the central nervous system: a study of Sindbis virus infection in the mouse using fluorescent antibody. Am J Pathol 1965;46:929–943.

76. Johnson RT, Mims CA. Pathogenesis of virus infections of the nervous system. N Engl J Med 1968;278:23–92.

77. Kapikian AZ, Chanock RM. Rotaviruses. In: Fields BN, Knipe DM, eds. Virology. 2nd ed. New York: Raven Press, 1990:1353–1404.

78. Koenig S, Gendelman HE, Orenstein JM, et al. Detection of AIDS virus in macrophages in brain tissue from AIDS patients with encephalopathy. Science 1986;233:1089–1093.

79. Kristensson K, Lycke E, Sjostand J. Spread of herpes simplex virus in peripheral nerves. Acta Neuropathol 1971;17:44–53.

80. Langhoff E, Terwilliger EF, Bos J, et al. Replication of human immunodeficiency virus type 1 in primary dendritic cell cultures. Proc Natl Acad Sci U S A 1991;88:7998–8002.

81. Levy JA. HIV and the pathogenesis of AIDS. Washington: ASM Press, 1994.

82. Levy JA, Joyner J, Borenfreund E. Mouse sperm can horizontally transmit type C viruses. J Gen Virol 1980;51:439–443.

83. Lippmann M, Yeates DB, Albert RE. Deposition, retention, and clearance of inhaled particles. Br J Indust Med 1980;37:337–362.

84. Lipton HL, Johnson RT. The pathogenesis of rat virus infections in the newborn hamster. Lab Invest 1972;27:508–513.

85. Little LM, Shadduck JA. Pathogenesis of rotavirus infection in mice. Infect Immun 1982;38:755–763.

86. Lofgren KW, Stevens JG, Marsden HS, Subak-Sharpe JH. Temperature sensitive mutants of herpes simplex virus differ in their capacity to establish latent infections in mice. Virology 1977;76:440–443.

87. Masuda M, Hoffman PM, Ruscetti SK. Viral determinants that control the neuropathogenicity of PVC-211 murine leukemia virus in vivo determine brain capillary endothelial cell tropism in vitro. J Virol 1993;67:4580–4587.

88. McCormick JB. Arenaviruses. In: Fields BN, Knipe DM, eds. Virology. 2nd ed. New York: Raven Press, 1990:1245–1267.

89. McNeill WH. Plagues and peoples. New York: Doubleday, 1977.

90. Melnick JL. Enteroviruses: polioviruses, coxsackieviruses, echoviruses, and newer enteroviruses. In: Fields BN, Knipe DM, eds. Virology. 2nd ed. New York: Raven Press, 1990:549–606.

91. Meyenhofer MF, Epstein LG, Cho E-S, Sharer LR. Ultrastructural morphology and intracellular production of human immunodeficiency virus (HIV) in brain. J Neuropathol Exp Neurol 1987;46: 474–484.

92. Mims CA. The response of mice to large intravenous injections of ectromelia virus. I. The fate of injected virus. Br J Exp Pathol 1959;40:533–128.

93. Mims CA. Rift Valley fever virus in mice. II. Adsorption and multiplication of virus. Br J Exp Pathol 1956;37:110–119.

94. Mims CA. Rift Valley fever virus in mice. III. Further quantitative features of the infective process. Br J Exp Pathol 1956;37:120–542.

95. Mims CA. Aspects of the pathogenesis of virus diseases. Bacteriological Reviews 1964;28:30–71.

96. Mims CA. The pathogenesis of infectious disease. London: Academic Press, 1976.

97. Mims CA. The pathogenesis of infectious disease. 3rd ed. London: Academic Press, 1987.

98. Mims CA, White DO. Viral pathogenesis and immunology. Oxford: Blackwell, 1984.

99. Monath TR, Cropp CB, Harrison AK. Mode of entry of a neurotropic arbovirus into the central nervous system: reinvestigation of an old controversy. Lab Invest 1983;48:399–410.

100. Monath TR, ed. The arboviruses: epidemiology and ecology. Boca Raton: CRC Press, 1988.

101. Morin MJ, Warner A, Fields BN. A pathway for the entry of reovirus into the host through M cells of the respiratory tract. J Exp Med 1994;180:1523–1527.

102. Morrison LA, Sidman RL, Fields BN. Direct spread of reovirus from intestinal lumen to the central nervous system through the autonomic vagal nerve fibers. Proc Natl Acad Sci U S A 1991;88: 2852–2856.

103. Muhlbock O, Bentvelzen O. The transmission of the mammary tumor viruses. Perspect Virol 1968;6:75–90.

104. Murphy FA, Bauer SP, Harrison AK, Winn WC Jr. Comparative pathogenesis of rabies and rabies-like viruses: viral infection and transit from inoculation site to the central nervous system. Lab Invest 1973;28:361–374.

105. Nathanson N. Epidemiology. In: Fields BN, Knipe DM, eds. Virology. 2nd ed. New York: Raven Press, 1990:267–291.

106. Nathanson N, Bodian D. Experimental poliomyelitis following intramuscular virus injection. I. The effect of neural block on a neurotropic and a pantropic strain. Bull Johns Hopkins Hospital 1961;108:308–319.

107. Nathanson N, Bodian D. Experimental poliomyelitis following intramuscular virus injection. II. Viremia and the effect of antibody. Bull Johns Hopkins Hospital 1961;108:308–319.

108. Nathanson N, Cole GA. Immunosuppression: a means to assess the role of the immune response in acute virus infection. Fed Proc 1971;30:1822–1830.

109. Nathanson N, Harrington B. Experimental infection of monkeys with Langat virus. II. Turnover of circulating virus. Am J Epidemiol 1967;85:494–502.

110. Nelson J, Wiley CA, Reynolds-Kohler C, Reese CE, Margaretten W, Levy JA. Human immunodeficiency virus detected in the bowel ep-

ithelium from patients with gastrointestinal symptoms. Lancet 1988; 1:259–262.

111. Notkins AL, Mage M, Ashe WK, Mahar S. Neutralization of sensitized lactic dehydrogenase virus by anti-gamma-globulin. J Immunol 1968;100:314–320.

112. Notkins AL, Mahar S, Scheele C, Goffman J. Infectious virus-antibody complexes in the blood of chronically infected mice. J Exp Med 1966;124:81–97.

113. Oldstone MBA. Immunotherapy for virus infection. Curr Top Microbiol Immunol 1987;134:211–229.

114. Oshiro LS, Dondero DV, Emmons RW, Lennette EH. The development of Colorado tick fever virus within cells of the haemopoietic system. J Gen Virol 1978;39:73–79.

115. Paffenbarger RS, Bodian D. Poliomyelitis immune status in ecologically diverse populations, in relation to virus spread, clinical incidence, and virus disappearance. Am J Hygiene 1961;74:311–325.

116. Pan L-Z, Werner A, Levy JA. Detection of plasma viremia in individuals at all clinical stages. J Clin Microbiol 1993;13:283–288.

117. Pathak S, Webb HE. Possible mechanisms for the transport of Semliki Forest virus into and within mouse brain: an electron microscopic study. J Neurol Sci 1974;23:175–184.

118. Patterson BK, Till M, Otto P, et al. Detection of HIV-1 DNA and messenger RNA in individual cells by PCR-driven in situ hybridization and flow cytometry. Science 1993;260:976–979.

119. Pekosz A, Griot C, Stillmock K, Nathanson N, Gonzalez-Scarano F. Protection from La Crosse virus encephalitis with recombinant glycoproteins: role of neutralizing anti-G1 antibodies. J Virol 1995; 69:3475–3481.

120. Perlman S, Jacobsen G, Afifi A. Spread of a neurotropic murine coronavirus into the CNS via the trigeminal and olfactory nerves. Virology 1989;170:556–560.

121. Petursson G, Nathanson N, Georgsson G, Panitch H, Palsson PA. Pathogenesis of visna. I. Sequential virologic, serologic, and pathologic studies. Lab Invest 1976;35:402–412.

122. Piatek M Jr, Saag S, Yang IC, et al. High levels of HIV 1 in plasma during all stages of infection determined by competitive PCR. Science 1993;259:1749–1754.

123. Pitts O, Powers M, Billelo JE. Ultrastructural changes associated with retroviral replication in central nervous system capillary endothelial cells. Lab Invest 1987;56:401–409.

124. Pomerantz RJ, de la Monte SM, Donegan SP, et al. Human immunodeficiency virus (HIV) infection of the uterine cervix. Ann Intern Med 1988;108:321–327.

125. Porter DD. Persistence of viral infection in the presence of immunity. In: Notkins AL, ed. Viral immunology and immunopathology. New York: Academic Press, 1975:189–200.

126. Porter DD, Cho HJ. Aleutian disease of mink: a model for persistent infection. In: Fraenkel-Conrat H, Wagner RR, eds. Virus-host interactions. New York: Plenum Press, 1980:233–256.

127. Porter DD, Larsen AE. Aleutian disease of mink: infectious virus-antibody complexes in the serum. Proc Soc Exp Biol Med 1967; 126:680–682.

128. Portis JL, McAtee F, Haynes S. Horizontal transmission of murine retroviruses. J Virol 1987;61:1037–1044.

129. Rabin E, Jenson A, Melnick J. Herpes simplex virus in mice: electron microscopy of neural spread. Science 1968;162:126–129.

130. Racaniello VR. Poliovirus neurovirulence. Adv Virus Res 1988; 34:217–246.

131. Rakela J, Moseley JW. Fecal excretion of hepatitis A virus in humans. J Infect Dis 1977;135:933–938.

132. Ren R, Racaniello VR. Poliovirus spreads from muscle to the central nervous system by neural pathways. J Infect Dis 1992; 166: 747–752.

133. Roberts JA. Histopathogenesis of mousepox. I. Respiratory infection. Br J Exp Pathol 1962;43:451–461.

134. Roberts JA. The histopathogenesis of mousepox. II. Cutaneous infection. Br J Exp Pathol 1962;43:462–470.

135. Sabin AB. Pathogenesis of poliomyelitis: reappraisal in light of new data. Science 1956;123:1151–1157.

136. Saif LJ. Comparative aspects of enteric virus infection. In: Saif LJ, Theil KW, eds. Viral diarrheas of man and animals. Boca Raton: CRC Press, 1990:9–31.

137. Sawyer WA, Meyer KF, Eaton MD, Bauer JH, Putnam P, Schwentker FF. Jaundice in army personnel in the western region of the United States and its relation to vaccination against yellow fever. Am J Hygiene 1944;39:337–387.

138. Schnittman SM, Greenhouse JJ, Psallidopoulos MC, et al. Increasing viral burden in CD4± T cells from patients with human immunodeficiency virus (HIV) infection reflects rapidly progressive immunosuppression and clinical disease. Ann Intern Med 1990; 113:438–443.

139. Schultz I, Neva FA. Relationship between blood clearance and viruria after intravenous injection of mice and rats with bacteriophage and polioviruses. J Immunol 1965;94:833–841.

140. Scott RM, Snitbhan R, Bancroft WH. Experimental transmission of hepatitis B virus by semen and saliva. J Infect Dis 1980;142:67–71.

141. Sederati F, Margolis TP, Stevens JG. Latent infection can be established with drastically restricted transcription and replication of the HSV-1 genome. Virology 1993;192:687–691.

142. Shah KV, Howley PM. Papillomaviruses. In: Fields BN, Knipe DM, eds. Virology. 2nd ed. New York: Raven Press, 1990:1651–1678.

143. Sharer LR. Pathology of HIV-1 infection of the central nervous system: a review. J Neuropathol Exp Neurol 1992;51:3–11.

144. Sicinski P, Rowinski J, Warchol JB, et al. Poliovirus type 1 enters the human host through intestinal M cells. Gastroenterology 1990; 98:56–58.

145. Stagno S, Reynolds DW, Pass RF. Breast milk and the risk of cytomegalovirus infection. N Engl J Med 1980;302:1073–1076.

146. Stevens JG, Cook ML. Latent herpes simplex virus in sensory ganglia. Perspect Virol 1974;8:171–185.

147. Stone RH, Shope RE, Moore DH. Electron microscope study of the development of the papilloma virus in the skin of the rabbit. J Exp Med 1959;10:543–546.

148. Strode GK, ed. Yellow fever. New York: McGraw-Hill, 1951.

149. Tan X, Pearce-Pratt R, Phillips DM. Productive infection of a cervical epithelial cell line with human immunodeficiency virus: implications for sexual transmission. J Virol 1993;67:6447–6452.

150. Tassopoulos NC, Papaevangelou GJ, Ticehurst JR, Purcell RH. Fecal excretion of Greek strains of hepatitis A in patients with hepatitis A and in experimentally infected chimpanzees. J Infect Dis 1986; 154:231–237.

151. Ticehurst J, Feinstone SM, Chestnut T, Tassopoulos NC, Popper H, Purcell RH. Detection of hepatitis A virus by extraction of viral RNA and molecular hybridization. J Clin Microbiol 1987;25: 1822–1829.

152. Tsiang H. Evidence for an intraaxonal transport of fixed and street rabies virus. J Neuropathol Exp Neurol 1979;38:286–295.

153. Tsiang H. Pathophysiology of rabies virus infection of the nervous system. Adv Virus Res 1993;42:375–412.

154. Tucker SP, Compans RW. Virus infection of polarized epithelial cells. Adv Virus Res 1992;42:187–247.

155. Tyler K, McPhee D, Fields BN. Distinct pathways of viral spread in the host determined by reovirus S1 gene segment. Science 1986; 233:770–774.

156. Utz JP. Viruria in man. Prog Med Virol 1964;6:71–81.

157. Watkins BA, Dorn HH, Kelly WB, et al. Specific tropism of HIV-1 for microglial cells in primary human brain cultures. Science 1990;249:549–553.

158. Worthington M, Baron S. Host defenses during primary vaccinia virus infection in mice. Fed Proc 1971;30:241.

159. Yorke JA, Nathanson N, Pianigiani G, Martin JR. Seasonality and the requirements for perpetuation and eradication of viruses in populations. Am J Epidemiol 1979;109:103–123.

160. Zemanick MC, Strick PL, Dix RD. Direction of transneuronal transport of herpes simplex virus 1 in the primate motor system is strain-dependent. Proc Natl Acad Sci U S A 1991;88:8048–8051.

161. Zurbriggen A, Fujinami R. Theiler's virus infection in nude mice: viral RNA in vascular endothelial cells. J Virol 1988;62:3589–3596.

Viral Pathogenesis,
edited by Neal Nathanson, et al.
Lippincott–Raven Publishers, Philadelphia © 1997

CHAPTER 3

Localization of Viral Infections

Kathryn V. Holmes

INTRODUCTION

Fortunately, no virus infects all species or all tissues within its hosts. Largely because of their profound dependence on the biochemical processes and structural characteristics of various potential host cells, most viruses cause disease only in a small number of species. For the same reason, within its infected host a virus generally causes pathology in only one or a small number of the many potential target tissues. Therefore, a virus is often characterized or even named for its usual host and the tissue that it most commonly or most obviously affects (e.g., human hepatitis virus, feline infectious peritonitis virus).

The terms species specificity and tissue tropism are often used to describe these important differences in the epidemiology and pathology of different viruses.[115] It is important to define these commonly used terms more precisely, because careful studies often show that a virus can replicate in many other tissues in addition to the one in which its major pathologic changes are observed, and that it may be able to infect several other species in addition to its commonly identified host,

causing little or no apparent disease. For example, acute systemic virus diseases such as measles are often initiated by inapparent virus replication in the upper respiratory tract before the virus spreads systemically and causes its characteristic febrile disease with rash. For many viruses, some lucky individuals develop only subclinical infections, in which the virus replicates at the site of entry but does not cause the characteristic disease syndrome. Like those with clinically apparent infections, these asymptomatic individuals may also develop virus-specific antibodies and cell-mediated immune responses that may protect them from the same virus in the future. Thus, to aid in understanding the pathophysiology of viral diseases, the definition of virus tissue tropism should be expanded to include all tissues that can be infected by a virus, regardless of whether or not pathologic changes occur in these tissues. Similarly, the concept of virus species specificity should include all of the species that a virus can infect, whether or not infection leads to disease in all of these species.

This chapter addresses the various levels in virus replication that can affect the species specificity and tissue tropism of virus infection. Related concepts are found in Chapters 2 and 13. Because of their genetic variability, viruses can sometimes overcome species-specific and tissue-specific barriers to infection and jump to a new host[85,133,153,179] or develop

K.V. Holmes: Department of Microbiology, University of Colorado Health Sciences Center, Denver, Colorado 80262.

altered tissue tropism within the original host and cause a different disease.[50,151] Analysis of such naturally occurring host-range and tissue-tropism virus variants often reveals how virus replication is restricted in particular host cells. Cell and organ cultures also provide useful model systems for the identification of molecular determinants of virus tissue tropism and species specificity. It is possible to modify the genomes of many viruses by site-directed mutagenesis and to modify host animals by introducing genes from other species or by knocking out genes that may affect virus susceptibility. These genetically engineered viruses and hosts provide powerful experimental models for the study of the mechanisms of virus tissue tropism and species specificity.

For a virus, there are obvious disadvantages to being restricted to replicating in only one or a few tissues in only a few species. To survive in nature, the virus must be very successful in infecting these limited targets. It is probable that many host-range or tissue-tropism virus mutants arise but quickly become extinct because they are not efficiently transmitted to new susceptible hosts. Either cytocidal or noncytocidal viruses could be selected against if they are not shed efficiently. Fenner's classic studies of the events following the intentional introduction of virulent myxoma virus into the highly susceptible population of European rabbits in Australia (see Chap. 15) showed that virus variants with decreased virulence and rabbits with increased resistance to virus were rapidly selected.[51,52,164] Thus, a highly virulent virus that causes overwhelming infection and rapidly kills its host may not survive in nature as well as a virus variant that causes milder, more prolonged infection.

As a virus repeatedly replicates in a particular type of host cell, its life cycle becomes adapted to the characteristic biochemical and structural features of that cell. This adaptation is generally accomplished over time through the selection of a series of subtle mutations in many viral genes that optimize virus replication, assembly, and release from that cell type. This adapted virus consequently becomes less well adapted to growth in any cell that differs from its customary host cell. In this way, species-specific or tissue-specific differences among cells can restrict virus replication.

Virologists take advantage of the process of viral adaptation when they make an attenuated live-virus vaccine by repeatedly passaging a virulent virus through a new cell type such as tissue culture cells or embryonated eggs. As the virus adapts to the new host cell type, it becomes increasingly inefficient in infecting its original host cells in vivo.[26,27] The passaged virus variant selected as a vaccine is one that has become sufficiently attenuated in replication in vivo in its original host, so that it no longer causes disease. However, the viral vaccine candidate must still retain the antigens and T-cell epitopes that stimulate a protective immune response in the natural host. Until recently, the development of attenuated live-virus vaccines against human or veterinary pathogens depended on this process of repeated passage followed by testing of virus stocks for virulence and antigenicity. It is now possible to introduce specific mutations into viral genes and test the effects of the mutations on virus virulence and antigenicity. The genomes of vaccine strains and virulent virus strains are sequenced to identify all mutations in the vaccine strain, then each of these mutations is introduced separately into the genome of the virulent virus. The resultant virus progeny are

then tested for virulence. Using this strategy, it is possible to identify specific mutations in viral genes that are associated with attenuation of virulence.[116] The characterization of some of these mutations can help to identify host-dependent mechanisms that restrict virus replication.

Not only must a successful virus be well adapted to growth in a specific host and target tissues, but to survive in nature, it must be transmitted from an infected individual to new susceptible hosts. Some of the virions shed from the tissues of the infected host must survive long enough in the environment to reach the susceptible target tissues in the new host. Successful viruses have solved the problem of transmission in myriad ways. The structure of the virion, which is determined by viral genes, is an important determinant of the virus' resistance to inactivation by factors in the environment such as proteases, alterations in pH, osmotic shock, drying, or heat. In general, nonenveloped viruses are considerably more resistant to inactivation by these factors than are enveloped viruses. For example, enteroviruses and reoviruses retain infectivity in contaminated water considerably longer than do most enveloped viruses, and papillomaviruses are more resistant to inactivation by drying than are influenzaviruses. Some viruses that cause sexually transmitted diseases, such as human immunodeficiency virus (HIV) or herpes simplex virus (HSV), may require close contact for effective transmission because they are readily inactivated outside the body, partly as a result of their lipid-containing envelopes. The genetic adaptations that optimize virus replication in the host cell must be compatible with those needed for stability of virions during transmission to a new susceptible host. Thus, each successful virus achieves a genetically optimized equilibrium between the features required for efficient transmission and the characteristics needed for infection of particular target cells.

Cells in different tissues vary in many ways that can affect their susceptibility to virus infection and their ability to support virus production. Although expression of genes that control common essential functions is similar for all cells within a species, each type of cell in the body also expresses a different constellation of genes that confer their unique properties. Similarly, within each cell lineage, the program of gene expression changes markedly during development. Species-specific differences among cells can also affect virus replication. Divergence of species occurs over millions of years and involves numerous mutations in genes that determine many cellular structures and functions. Proteins required for functions common to different species tend to conserve elements that are essential for their structure and molecular associations while showing considerable drift in the amino acid sequences of some other domains. Cell-dependent differences in many cellular functions can either be exploited by viruses or hinder virus replication. Virus tissue tropism can be affected by cell-dependent differences in any of the following: plasma membranes, which can affect virus binding, entry, uncoating, or release; transcription factors, enhancers, or polymerases, which can affect virus gene expression; nucleases and proteases, which can destroy or activate virus components; mechanisms for the transport and sorting of macromolecules, which can affect the replication, sorting, assembly, and release of viral macromolecules and virions; and structural and microenvironmental differences among cells, which may affect their availability to virus infection or their ability to release virions. This chapter describes many fascinating examples of the diverse ways in which differences among host cells determine their permissivity for the replication of particular viruses.

ROLE OF RECEPTORS IN VIRUS TROPISM

Receptors as Determinants of Tissue Tropism

There are many examples of naturally occurring or laboratory selected mutations in a virus attachment protein that alter the tissue tropism, virulence, or both of virus infection. Even without identifying the receptor for a virus, studies of mutations in the receptor-binding proteins of the virus illustrate the importance of virus-receptor interactions in determining virus tissue tropism and virulence in vivo. A classic example is the analysis of the tissue tropism in mice of a panel of genetic reassortants between a neuronotropic strain of reovirus, type 3 Dearing, and the type 1 Lang strain of reovirus, which shows marked tropism for ependymal cells in the brain. Taking advantage of the facts that each of the 10 segments of the double-stranded viral RNA genome encodes only one protein (except for S1, which encodes 2 proteins)[9] and that the genome segments in the progeny of cells infected with two strains of reovirus are randomly inherited from each parental virus, Weiner and collaborators[189] showed that the tissue tropisms of the reassortant viruses correlate with the parental origin of the S1 genome segment that encodes the hemagglutinin (HA) protein of the virus. Thus, the reovirus attachment protein determines the tissue tropism of reovirus disease in the central nervous system.

Similar observations have been made for naturally occurring mutations of virus attachment proteins of viruses with monopartite genomes. The porcine coronavirus (PRCV) transmissible gastroenteritis virus (TGEV) causes enteric disease in piglets and replicates in epithelial cells of the small intestine and in the lung. A new PRCV that causes only respiratory infection of swine first appeared in Europe in the early 1980s and then spread rapidly, causing severe economic losses. The PRCV strains are very closely related to TGEV but have either a deletion of 224 amino acids or amino acid substitutions in the N-terminal domain of the viral attachment glycoprotein S.[151] Thus, differences in tropism and pathogenesis between TGEV and PRCV correlate with alterations in the receptor-binding protein.

Several retroviruses develop mutations in their envelope glycoproteins, the virus attachment glycoproteins that show tropism for replication in brain capillary endothelial cells (BCEC). A neuropathogenic variant of murine Friend leukemia virus was selected by passage of the murine virus through rats. It caused a progressive neurologic disease when inoculated into in rats or some inbred mice before 6 days of age. Although histologic changes in the brain involved many cell types, including vacuolation and degeneration of neurons and proliferation of astroglia, the virus replicated only in BCECs.[74] Thus, virus infection of a critical tissue such as capillary endothelial cells in the brain can cause a degenerative disease that indirectly affects other cell types. A feline leukemia virus recombinant in the envelope glycoprotein with an endogenous retrovirus sequence also developed the ability to replicate in BCECs, unlike the parental virus.[30]

Virus variants capable of replicating in the brain also develop during the course of infection with simian immunodeficiency virus (SIV-1) or HIV-1, both of which are in the lentivirus group of retroviruses. These variants also have specific changes in the envelope glycoprotein that adapt them for growth in BCEC in vivo and in vitro.[101,157] The virus variants may enter the central nervous system either by being carried in by infected macrophages or via infection of BCECs.[59,79,126,139] Once in the central nervous system, however, HIV-1 variants with macrophage-tropic envelope glycoproteins replicate primarily in microglial cells.[98,157] Thus, development in vivo of virus envelope glycoprotein variants capable of infecting BCECs, macrophages, or microglial cells appears to be essential to allow SIV-1 and HIV-1 to enter the brain and cause neurologic disease.

Viruses with mutations in their virus attachment proteins can be selected either by incubation with neutralizing monoclonal antibodies (Mabs) or soluble receptors or by site-directed mutagenesis. Analysis of such mutants shows the importance of virus-receptor interactions in determining viral tissue tropism.[39,87] Mutation in a highly exposed loop on the surface of the poliovirus capsid can extend the host range of the type 1 Mahoney strain so that, in addition to replicating in primate cells like the parental virus, the mutant virus can also replicate in murine cells.[34] Similarly, the host range of canine parvovirus (CPV) is determined by several amino acid residues on the surface of the virus capsid.[132] Variants of type 3 reovirus selected by Mabs directed against the viral HA protein can replicate only in a subset of the neurons that are susceptible to the parental virus. These Mab escape variants, unlike the parental virus, are not neurotropic and will not invade the central nervous system after peripheral inoculation.[166]

Virus Receptor Identification

The outer surface of virions is studded with an array of organelles used for attachment to cells. These viral surface elements are composed of one or more virus-encoded proteins, and they take different forms in the various virus groups. However, each of these surface elements is naturally selected for the ability to attach to a specific cell surface receptor molecule to initiate the delivery of the virus genome into a susceptible cell. A single virus attachment protein may suffice for some small viruses, whereas large viruses such as the herpesviruses may have several alternative or cooperative ways to interact with the cell membrane. Some viruses encode several different attachment proteins and display them on the virion surface, whereas other viruses encode a single surface protein that has several different domains that recognize alternative receptors expressed on different cell types. Viruses may initiate infection of susceptible cells by a programmed sequence of several specific virus-binding events. Such sequential binding events could provide multiple determinants of tissue or species specificity if cell types differ in their expression of the essential virus-binding ligands.

Carbohydrate Receptors

Some of the first virus receptors identified were the sialic acid (SA)-containing receptors of myxoviruses.[174] Influenza A virus and parainfluenza viruses bind to receptors on erythrocyte membranes, causing hemagglutination. Myxovirus envelope glycoproteins bind specifically to glycoconjugates that are found on the membranes of many cell types, including erythrocytes, respiratory epithelial cells, cells of the chorioallantoic membranes (CAMs) of embryonated eggs, and tissue culture cells. However, myxoviruses cannot bind to erythrocytes that have been pretreated with the receptor-destroying enzyme neuraminidase. This enzyme was first isolated from *Vibrio cholerae* and was later found to be a function of the NA glycoprotein spike on the influenza virus envelope and the HN glycoproteins of parainfluenzavirus envelopes. The neuraminidase cleaves terminal N-acetylneuraminic acid (Neu5Ac), or SA, residues from glycoconjugates on the cell surface so that the virus attachment proteins cannot bind. The enzyme removes SA residues from N-linked and O-linked sialyloligosaccharides on membrane glycoproteins and from sialyloligosaccharides on gangliosides. After SA has been enzymatically removed from the cell membranes, susceptibility to myxovirus infection can be restored by treating the cells with purified sialyl transferases, which replace terminal SAs on the oligosaccharides, or by incubation of the cells with purified gangliosides containing Neu5Ac residues, which insert into the lipid bilayer of the plasma membrane.[174] X-ray crystallographic studies of the HA glycoprotein of influenza A co-crystallized with sialosides identified the amino acids that bind to the SA residue in the principal receptor-binding pocket, located at the tip of the HA glycoprotein.[189a] The amino acids in the receptor-binding pocket are largely conserved among influenza HA glycoproteins of different antigenic subtypes, despite significant differences in amino acid sequences of other parts of the HA glycoprotein. The HA glycoproteins of avian, equine, and human H3 strains of influenza A have a common structure but differ markedly in their binding affinities for a variety of sialyloligosaccharides of defined structure that were enzymatically introduced onto cell membranes. For example, the HA of human influenza A virus strain H3 binds strongly to cells whose complex N-linked oligosaccharides contain the terminal SAα2,6Gal linkage but poorly to cells expressing SAα2,3Gal as the terminal sugar on oligosaccharides linked to serine or threonine residues. In contrast, the HA glycoproteins of avian and equine viruses bind preferentially to cells containing the SAα2,3Gal linkage.[146] Specific sialyloligosaccharides expressed on cells of different species thus may play an important role in determining the host range of viruses that use them as receptors.[147]

In contrast to influenza A viruses, which infect humans, birds, and other mammals, influenza C virus causes disease only in humans. The HA glycoprotein of influenza C specifically binds N-acetyl-9-O-acetylneuraminic acid (Neu5,9Ac$_2$).[145] Removal of this residue from susceptible cells by treatment with either neuraminidase or neuraminate 9-O-acetylesterase makes the cells resistant to influenza C infection.[71] When these cells or other influenza C–resistant cell lines are incubated with brain gangliosides containing Neu5,9Ac$_2$, their susceptibility to influenza C virus is restored.[70] These experiments show that, at least in vitro, the cell tropism of influenza C is determined by whether or not the cells express the specific Neu5,9Ac$_2$ residue which serves as the receptor for this virus.[70] However, this receptor moiety is also expressed on the membranes of cells from species that are not susceptible to influenza C virus infection. Thus, the species

specificity of influenza C virus is determined, at least in part, by other factors in addition to its Neu5,9Ac$_2$ receptor specificity.

Some coronaviruses, including bovine coronavirus, human coronavirus (HCV-OC43), hemagglutinating encephalomyelitis virus of swine, and some strains of mouse hepatitis virus (MHV), encode a hemagglutinin esterase (HE) glycoprotein with significant homology to that of influenza C virus.[100,155,184,185] Coronavirus HE, like influenza C hemagglutinin, binds specifically to Neu5,9Ac$_2$ and has acetyl esterase activity that destroys the receptor on the cell membrane. In several hemagglutinating coronaviruses, the spike glycoprotein S also has Neu5,9Ac$_2$-binding activity.[155] Enzymatic removal of this moiety from cell membranes makes the cells resistant to virus infection, as shown for influenza C.[184] It is not yet clear whether binding of the virions to this carbohydrate moiety on cell membranes is the only molecular recognition event required for virus infection, or whether binding to Neu5,9Ac$_2$ represents a preliminary step that must be followed by interaction with a different receptor to initiate infection.

Many other viruses also encode virion-associated HA proteins that bind to carbohydrate moieties found on membranes of erythrocyte and other cell types and cause hemagglutination. These include both enveloped viruses like those described previously, and nonenveloped viruses such as encephalomyocarditis virus, polyomavirus, and parvoviruses.[37,118] SA residues are often involved in binding these viruses to cells. Polyomavirus is an icosahedral virus that recognizes SA-containing receptors on erythrocytes and cultured cells by means of its capsid protein. The structure of murine polyomavirus bound to 3'-sialyl lactose was determined by x-ray crystallography, and the binding site for its sialyloligosaccharide receptor was found within a shallow groove in the capsid subunit containing the VP1 protein.[168] The valine residue at position 296 of VP1 binds by van der Waals forces to the SA ring of the receptor. A polyomavirus variant, LID, with increased virulence for newborn C3H/Bi mice had an alanine substituted for valine 296, which resulted in reduced binding affinity for SA.[8] In the newborn mouse model of polyomavirus infection, this variant spread more rapidly, grew to higher titers, and infected some tissues that are not normally infected by the wild type virus.[8] Thus, in this model, the binding affinity of the virus attachment protein for its oligosaccharide receptor is an important variable that affects virus tissue tropism and virulence.

CPV binds to SA-containing moieties and causes hemagglutination of erythrocytes. The three-dimensional structure of the CPV capsid shows a canyon and a dimple, which are candidates for binding sites.[180] Mutations that introduce amino acid substitutions in the canyon have no effect on SA binding to capsids or infectivity of recombinant mutant virions.[178] In contrast, amino acid substitutions in the walls of the dimple-yield capsids bind little or no SA but can still bind to CPV-susceptible feline lymphoblastoid cells at the same level that wild-type capsids bind to neuraminidase-treated cells. These observations suggest that the CPV capsid has two different binding sites: one for SA moieties and another for an as yet unidentified receptor moiety. Perhaps CPV infection requires cooperative or sequential binding of the dimple domain to SA-containing oligosaccharides and to another putative cellular receptor at a different site on the capsid.[178] Viruses that bind to oligosaccharide moieties that are expressed on many cell types and by many species yet cause only disease in one species must limit their tissue tropism and species specificity by other host-dependent factors that follow the initial virus-binding event.

Glycolipid moieties on the cell membrane can be used as portals of entry into the cell for several types of viruses. Paramyxoviruses bind to sialoglycolipids, and resistant cells can be made susceptible by incubation with these glycolipids.[135,174] Rotavirus SA11 binds to GA2, a neutral glycolipid extracted from infant mouse intestine, and to cholesterol 3 sulfate, which is found in the cell membrane.[167] Preincubation of rotavirus with immobilized GA1 glycolipid prevents infection of MA104 cells, and treatment of these cells with anti-GA-1 antibody blocks rotavirus infection.[195] HIV-1 uses as its principal receptor CD4, a glycoprotein in the immunoglobulin superfamily (discussed later), but HIV-1 can also infect some cell types in which expression of CD4 cannot be demonstrated, including neurons, brain endothelium, cell lines from the cervix or colon, and the SK-N-MC line of human peripheral neuroblastoma cells.[68,201,202] Several lines of evidence suggest that the alternative HIV-1 receptor on these cells is a neutral glycolipid, perhaps galactosyl ceramide or its sulfated derivative 3'-sulfo-galactosyl ceramide. Antibodies to galactosyl ceramide prevent infection of CD4-negative, HIV-1–susceptible cell lines, and the HIV-1 spike glycoprotein gp120 binds specifically and with high affinity to these glycolipids in vitro.

Human parvovirus B19 also uses a glycolipid moiety as its receptor. The virus binds to globoside, also known as erythrocyte P antigen, a neutral glycosphingolipid that is expressed in the target cells for B19.[18,37] Bone marrow cultures from individuals who lack this antigen are completely resistant to B19 infection.[118] Thus, the erythrocyte P antigen plays a role in the tissue tropism of B19 infection and even determines the virus susceptibility of individuals within the same species.

Some viruses have attachment proteins that bind specifically to oligosaccharide moieties on the cell membrane but also require one or more subsequent membrane recognition steps for entry of the viral genome into the cell. Several lines of experimental evidence demonstrate the sequential events at the membrane during herpesvirus infections. For HSV-1 and HSV-2, the virions initially bind to target cells by their gC glycoproteins, which interact with a cell surface glycosaminoglycan, heparan sulfate.[69,198] Removal of heparan sulfate from cell membranes by treatment with heparatinase prevents HSV infection, and soluble heparin competitively inhibits HSV infection of susceptible cells in culture. HSV is unable to attach to mutant Chinese hamster ovary cells that fail to synthesize heparan sulfate, and the gC glycoprotein of HSV binds directly to heparan sulfate. Similarly, other alphaherpesviruses, including pseudorabies virus and bovine herpesvirus, bind to heparin-related molecules on the cell surface.[114,128] In addition, human cytomegalovirus (hCMV), a betaherpesvirus, also binds first to cell surface heparan sulfate.[36] A series of subsequent events takes place at the membrane, including binding of an hCMV spike glycoprotein to a high-affinity glycoprotein receptor, followed by fusion of the viral envelope with cell membranes, which is probably mediated by a different viral glycoprotein. Heparan sulfate is widely distributed on the extracellular matrix of tissues and cultured cells of many species. Its presence on the cells is required for initiation of infection with HSV-1, HSV-2, and cytomegalovirus, but heparan sulfate cannot initiate infection without the subsequent series of interactions at the host cell membrane.

The concept of several sequential steps associated with virion binding and penetration probably also applies to many other groups of viruses. Binding of the first virus attachment protein to a widely distributed membrane moiety such as heparan sulfate or SA may concentrate virions on the cell membrane and position the second virus attachment protein (or another domain of the same attachment protein) close enough to its cell surface ligand, such as a receptor glycoprotein, to promote specific binding. Penetration of the viral genome into the cytoplasm by fusion of the viral envelope with the cell membrane are discussed later.

Glycoprotein Receptors

During the past decade, receptors for many viruses have been shown to be cell membrane glycoproteins (Table 3-1; Fig. 3-1). In general, the proof that a cellular glycoprotein is a receptor for a particular virus depends on cloning the cDNA encoding the putative receptor, expressing it in cells that are normally resistant to the virus, and demonstrating that these cells become susceptible to virus infection. Additional support comes from evidence that monoclonal antibodies directed against the binding domain of the putative receptor protein bind to susceptible cells and prevent virus infection.

If resistant cells become susceptible to infection by a virus when they express a recombinant virus receptor glycoprotein, then their natural resistance to virus infection must be the result of a lack of a functional receptor for the virus. Experiments with recombinant receptor glycoproteins for many different viruses have shown that the species specificity of virus infection is often the result, at least in part, of the failure of receptor homologs on the resistant species to serve as virus receptors. The specific domains and amino acids of a receptor glycoprotein that bind to a virus attachment protein can then be identified by comparison of the amino acid sequences of the receptor with homologous glycoproteins from species that are resistant to that virus. Chimeric proteins between the receptor and its inactive receptor homolog are made, or individual mutations corresponding to each amino acid substitution in the homolog are introduced into the cDNA encoding the natural receptor glycoprotein, and naturally resistant cells expressing these chimeric or recombinant proteins are then tested for the ability to bind the virus and for susceptibility to virus infection.[81] The domain that determines the virus-binding specificity of the receptor glycoprotein is sometimes found in a region that is highly polymorphic among species. As shown for the virus-binding domains of CD4[187] and the poliovirus receptor (PVR),[140] these virus-binding sites frequently represent domains of the glycoprotein that are in variable regions on the surface rather than at conserved residues required for the proper conformation of the glycoprotein.

The cell membrane glycoproteins that serve as virus receptors vary markedly in structure and serve many unrelated cellular functions (see Fig. 3-1). Some virus receptors are enzymes, others are permeases or transporters, and still others are cell adhesion molecules. Cell membrane receptors for hormones, growth factors, neurotransmitters, and cytokines or

TABLE 3-1. *Receptors for some animal viruses*

Virus family		Virus	Receptor
DNA VIRUSES			
Nonenveloped	*Parvoviridae*	Human parvovirus B19	Erythrocyte P antigen (globoside)[24]
		Canine parvovirus	Sialic acid–containing oligosaccharides[132]
	Adenoviridae	Adenovirus	Integrin $\alpha_v\beta_5$, $\alpha_v\beta_3$ (for internalization)[148]
	Papovaviridae	Polyomavirus	Sialic acid–containing oligosaccharides
Enveloped	*Herpesviridae*	Herpes simplex type 1	Heparan sulfate[198]
		Human cytomegalovirus	Heparan sulfate[36]
			Human aminopeptidase N (for penetration)[165]
			30-kD glycoprotein[38]
		Epstein-Barr virus	CR2[108]
		Murine cytomegalovirus	MHC class I[199]
	Poxviridae	Vaccinia virus	Epidermal growth factor receptor type 1[103]
RNA VIRUSES			
Nonenveloped			
	Picornaviridae	Echovirus 1, 8	α2 subunit of integrin VLA-2[10,13,14]
		Echovirus 7, 13, 21, 29, 33	Decay-accelerating factor CD55[11,33,188]
		Coxsackievirus B1, B3, B5	Decay-accelerating factor[12,156]
		Coxsackievirus A9	Integrin $\alpha_v\beta_5$[148]
		Foot-and-mouth disease virus	Integrin[14]
		Human rhinoviruses	Major receptor group (ICAM-1)[63]
			Minor receptor group, (LDLR)[65,73]
		Poliovirus	Poliovirus receptor[91,113]
	Reoviridae	Reovirus type 3	Sialic acid–containing oligosaccharides[53]
		Rotavirus SA11	Sialic acid–containing oligosaccharides[149]
Enveloped	*Alphaviridae*	Sindbis virus	High-affinity laminin receptor[170]
			Glycoprotein[182]
	Arenaviridae	Lymphocytic choriomeningitis virus	100-kDa glycoprotein[17]
	Orthomyxoviridae	Influenza A	Sialic acid–containing oligosaccharides[135]
		Influenza C	9-O-acetylated neuraminic acid[71]
	Paramyxoviridae	Parainfluenza viruses	Sialic acid–containing oligosaccharides[135]
			Glycosphingolipids[174]
		Measles	CD46[43]
	Coronaviridae	Mouse hepatitis virus	Biliary glycoproteins[49]
		Bovine coronavirus	9-O-acetylated sialic acid–containing oligosaccharides[185]
		Human coronavirus OC43	9-O-acetylated sialic acid–containing oligosaccharides[185]
		Human coronavirus 229E	Human aminopeptidase N[203]
		Transmissible gastroenteritis virus, porcine coronavirus	Porcine aminopeptidase N[42]
	Retroviridae	Gibbon ape leukemia virus	Sodium-dependent phosphate transporter[84,129,136,183]
		Amphotropic mouse leukemia virus	Sodium-dependent phosphate transporter[84,196]
		Mouse leukemia virus E	Cationic amino acid transporter[4]
		Human immunodeficiency virus type 1	CD4[89]

ICAM-1, intercellular adhesion molecule 1; LDLR, low-density lipoprotein receptor.

cofactors that regulate complement activities on the membrane can also be co-opted for use as receptors by specific viruses. The kind of glycoprotein adopted for use by a particular virus appears to be rather random, but receptor choice may profoundly affect the tissue tropism and species specificity of the virus. Related viruses may utilize homologous receptors; for example, porcine and human coronaviruses use porcine or human aminopeptidase N, respectively,[42,203] and gibbon ape leukemia virus and amphotropic murine retrovirus bind to the phosphate permeases of their respective species.[190] Some-

times, however, related viruses bind to entirely different types of cellular glycoproteins. For example, different members of the *Retroviridae* family use as receptors either immunoglobulin-like molecules such as CD4 for HIV and SIV, the cationic amino acid transporter, or the inorganic phosphate transporter.[190] Members of the *Picornaviridae* family are also specialized to recognize very diverse receptors. The intercellular adhesion molecule 1 (ICAM-1) is the receptor for the major receptor group of rhinoviruses; the low-density lipoprotein receptor is the receptor for the minor group of rhinoviruses;

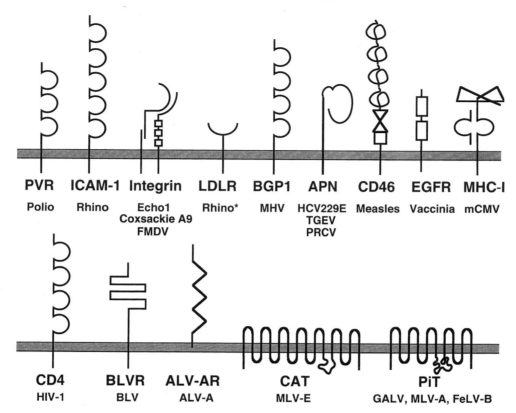

FIG. 3-1. Molecular models of glycoprotein receptors for some animal viruses. Many different types of cell surface glycoproteins serve as specific receptors for viruses. The structures of some of these receptor glycoproteins are schematically illustrated. In some cases, several isoforms of a glycoprotein can have virus receptor activity, or the receptor may be expressed on the membrane as an oligomer (not shown). The receptors are named in large type, and the virus that uses each receptor to infect cells is named in smaller type. Many of these cell surface glycoproteins have known cellular functions, such as the intercellular adhesion molecules (ICAM-1), integrins, biliary glycoprotein (BGP1), MHC class I, and CD4. Aminopeptidase N (APN) degrades peptides in the intestine and at synaptic junctions. Virus receptors can be ligands for growth factors, such as epidermal growth factor receptor (EGFR), or for complement proteins, such as CD46. Some of these glycoproteins also have transmembrane signaling functions (not shown). The cellular functions for some virus receptor glycoproteins are not yet known. Related viruses can be adapted to use quite different receptors; for example, poliovirus (PVR), ICAM-1, integrins, low density lipoprotein receptor (LDLR), and the decay-accelerating factor (DAF; not shown) are recognized by different members of the *Picornavirus* family, and each of the receptors on the bottom row is recognized by a retrovirus. Semicircles, immunoglobulin-like domains; boxes, serine-threonine–rich areas; rectangles, cysteine-rich domains; shaded area, the lipid bilayer of the plasma membrane; *, minor receptor group of rhinoviruses; ALV-AR, receptor for avian leukosis virus A; BLVR, receptor for Bovine leukemia virus; CAT, cationic amino acid transporter; FeLV, feline leukemia virus; FMDV, foot and mouth disease virus; GALV, Gibbon ape leukemia virus; HCV229E, human coronavirus 229E; HIV-1, human immunodeficiency virus type 1; MHV, mouse hepatitis virus; MLV, murine leukemia virus; PiT, inorganic phosphate transporters; PRCV, porcine respiratory coronavirus; TGEV, transmissible gastroenteritis virus. (Adapted from Weiss RA, Tailor CS. Retrovirus receptors. Cell 1995;82:531–533.)

integrins are the receptors for some echoviruses, coxsackieviruses, and possibly foot-and-mouth disease virus (FMDV); decay accelerating factor CD55 is the receptor for other echoviruses; and an immunoglobulin superfamily member, PVR, is the receptor for poliovirus. Perhaps coincidentally, several unrelated viruses can compete for the same receptor glycoprotein on one cell type. For example, incubation of human cells with adenovirus type 2 partially blocks attachment of human rhinovirus type 2 and completely blocks attachment of coxsackie B viruses.[99]

There seems to be no single specific structural element that is common for all virus receptor glycoproteins, just as there are no common features for the attachment proteins of different viruses. A small domain of each virus attachment protein binds to a small region of the receptor glycoprotein, usually but not always near the distal tip of the glycoprotein. The amino acids of the receptor that bind to the virus attachment protein may either be contiguous, as in the sequences recognized by gibbon ape leukemia virus,[84,197] or in a conformationally determined complex of noncontiguous binding residues.[7,107] Important elements of the receptor recognition site may include charged residues, hydrophobic interactions, or both. Although there appears to be little actual molecular mimicry of the receptor's natural cellular ligands by the virus attachment proteins, viruses often bind near the attachment site for the cellular ligand of the receptor, perhaps because this region is exposed to the external milieu.

Closely related viruses that use homologous receptor glycoproteins often have different amino acids at the receptor-binding domain on the virus attachment protein. Virus variants containing mutations in the receptor-binding domain of the virus attachment protein are naturally selected to optimize both receptor binding and penetration into the cell. Mutations experimentally introduced into the receptor-binding region of a virus attachment protein can result in viruses with little or no infectivity or viruses with altered species specificity.[110]

Cell membrane glycoproteins have several different mechanisms of recycling in the membrane. For example, when the transferrin receptor is bound to transferrin, it is taken up into pinocytic vesicles where the bound transferrin is released; then the receptor is recycled onto the plasma membrane by vesicular transport. Some cell surface glycoproteins are inserted into the membrane and then remain there, like many of the glycoproteins on the apical surface of epithelial cells in the small intestine. Other receptor glycoproteins that bind a ligand are taken up into vesicles in the same manner as the transferrin receptor, but they then are digested within the cell without recycling to the cell membrane. These different forms of trafficking of cell membrane proteins may affect their utilization as virus receptors.

Receptor Dynamics and Regulation of Receptor Expression

Binding of a single virus attachment protein on a virion to a glycoprotein receptor on the plasma membrane is generally not a high-affinity interaction.[29] Consequently, the virion may detach or elute from the cell membrane unless additional attachment proteins on the virion also bind to receptors, forming a multivalent, cooperative interaction with increased affinity. The ability to recruit additional receptors to the membrane underlying a bound virus probably depends on several host cell–dependent factors including membrane fluidity, the freedom of movement of the receptor glycoprotein within the plane of the membrane, and the surface density of the receptor glycoprotein. The amount of receptor expressed on the membrane can affect the susceptibility of a cell to virus infection.[83] If too little receptor is expressed, the opportunity to form multivalent virus-receptor complexes is reduced, and virions are more likely to elute. Tissues that express high levels of a receptor glycoprotein are likely to be more susceptible to virus infection than tissues that express low levels. Expression of some virus receptor glycoproteins or glycolipids can be modulated by cell differentiation. In this case, cells are susceptible to viral infection only at the specific stage in their development when the receptor is expressed.

Expression of receptors may be reduced following virus infection, perhaps because of intracellular interactions of virus attachment proteins with nascent receptors. When this happens, the cells become resistant to superinfection with the same virus, although they remain susceptible to infection with viruses that utilize a different receptor. A fascinating example of this is the avian retroviruses, which fall into five different subgroups referred to as A through E.[190] Chickens that inherit endogenous proviruses encoding the A virus glycoprotein are resistant to infection with the A strain of avian leukosis virus (ALV) because the virus glycoprotein blocks the receptors, but they are susceptible to infection with strains B through E. Persistent infection in vitro can also result in the development or selection of cells that express little or no virus receptor. In murine cells persistently infected with the coronavirus MHV, the expression of the virus receptor glycoprotein Bgp1a is markedly reduced, perhaps because of intercellular interactions with virus spike glycoprotein or because cells that express higher levels of receptor are selectively killed by virus infection.[152]

Some cells are resistant to infection by virions but nevertheless can be infected with the same virus if they are co-cultivated with infected cells. This receptor-independent spread of virus infection has been demonstrated for MHV-JHM. Virions infect only murine cells in vitro, and the BHK21 line of hamster cells is susceptible to infection with virions only if the cells are transfected with cDNA encoding a murine Bgp1 glycoprotein that serves as a virus receptor.[49] However, seeding of a BHK21 cell monolayer with a small number of MHV-JHM–infected murine cells results in extensive fusion of the hamster cells and virus replication.[57] The plasma membrane of the infected murine cells used as the inoculum is covered with large amounts of the virus attachment glycoprotein S, as well as numerous adsorbed virions. It is possible that this barrage of virus attachment proteins allows a hamster homolog of the Bgp1a receptor to serve as a functional, low-affinity receptor, even though it has such poor receptor activity that single virions cannot use it to infect the cells. Alternatively, the intimate proximity of the infected cell membrane with that of the hamster cells may bring together the viral S glycoprotein with a hamster cell membrane component that is required for cell fusion, bypassing the need for a specific virus receptor binding interaction. In the infected animal, it is possible that a virus may initially infect cells that express higher levels of receptor; then infection may spread by cell-to-cell contact to other tissues that express either less of the same receptor or a less-efficient alternative receptor. Once a virus genome is introduced by any mechanism into a cell that normally is resistant to the virus because it does not express an appropriate receptor, there is an opportunity for the selection of virus mutants better adapted for growth in that cell type. Perhaps this is one way that virus variants adapted to growth in different tissues can arise during persistent infection in vivo, as shown for the arenavirus lymphocytic choriomeningitis virus (LCMV).[3]

Entry of Antibody-Coated Virions by Way of Fc Receptors or Polymeric Ig Receptors

Virus infection does not always depend on interaction of a virus attachment protein with a specific receptor on the cell membrane. Certain cells (e.g., macrophages) express a membrane glycoprotein that is a specific receptor for the Fc domain of IgG. Some viruses may enter cells that lack specific virus receptors if they are first complexed with antiviral IgG antibody and then the virus-antibody complex adsorbs to cells via the Fc receptor. This unusual process of virus entry, called antibody-dependent enhancement of infection, was first shown for dengue virus, a member of the flaviviruses,[67] and has also been demonstrated with FMDV, a picornavirus in Chinese hamster ovary cells expressing a recombinant Fc receptor.[105] This antibody-dependent mechanism of virus entry can even rescue the infectivity of a genetically engineered FMDV mutant that cannot bind to its normal receptor.[105] In contrast, although poliovirus coated with antiviral antibody can also bind to poliovirus-negative, resistant cells that express the recombinant Fc receptor, virus infection does not result.[104] Therefore, the postbinding steps associated with virus penetration and uncoating may differ between these two picornaviruses.

Although Epstein-Barr virus (EBV) normally infects human B cells by interaction of a viral glycoprotein with the complement receptor CR2 (also called CD21),[108] EBV can also infect some human epithelial cell types that do not express CD21. A unique route of entry for EBV into some mucosal epithelial cells occurs when EBV virions coated with specific antiviral polymeric IgA are bound to the polymeric Ig receptor expressed on the basolateral pole of the cells, and then internalized and uncoated.[162]

Alternative Receptors

Some viruses can utilize several alternative receptors to enter cells, a marked advantage over viruses that require several different hosts for transmission or replicate in many tissues. An excellent example is Sindbis virus, an alphavirus that alternates between mosquito and vertebrate hosts. Sindbis virus has a wide host range and can infect many different vertebrates, including birds and mammals, as well as many tissues within *Aedes albopictus* mosquitoes.[19] The virus has been shown to bind to the high-affinity laminin receptor, a membrane protein that is very highly conserved among different species,[170] and a different, as yet unidentified receptor for Sindbis is found on mouse neural cells.[182] The receptor for this virus in insect cells is not yet known.

Reovirus type 3 can utilize two different domains of the viral HA protein to enter two murine cell types by way of different receptors.[150] Reovirus type 2 can grow in murine erythroleukemia cells, and its attachment to and growth in these cells is prevented by an anti-HA Mab that blocks hemagglutination. This MAb does not prevent reovirus type 3 infection of murine fibroblasts. A variant virus expressing an altered HA protein that lacks hemagglutinating activity still infects fibroblasts but does not infect the erythroleukemia cells. Studies of genetic reassortants of reoviruses have shown that infection of both cell types is determined by the HA protein. These experiments suggest that the HA domain of the HA protein reacts with a receptor on erythroleukemia cells, and a different part of the same protein recognizes another receptor on fibroblasts.

Some of the cellular glycoproteins selected as receptors by viruses are expressed in several isoforms as a result of differential splicing or differences in glycosylation or other processing events. In this case, it is important to know whether all isoforms can serve as receptors for the virus, and, if so, whether all are equally efficient receptors. For MHV-A59 and poliovirus, which bind to receptors in the immunoglobulin superfamily, alternative splicing of cDNAs encoding the receptors yields several glycoprotein isoforms. These were tested and found to function as receptors that differ in their efficacy in leading to virus infection.[48,64,91,206] Mouse strain differences were found in the gene encoding the MHV receptor Bgp1. Adult SJL mice, which are highly resistant to infection with MHV-A59, express a receptor glycoprotein called Bgp1b,[48,125,205] which differs in 29 of 108 amino acids in the N-terminal virus-binding domain. This glycoprotein does not bind virus as well as the receptor glycoprotein from susceptible BALB/c mice,[21] although it can serve as a receptor when the recombinant protein is expressed at high levels in hamster cells.

Viruses of several different groups can compete for receptors on the same cell type.[99] Adenovirus and coxsackievirus may share a common receptor; however, coxsackieviruses have been found to have several different receptor specificities. Coxsackie B binds to one receptor on HeLa cells and to a different membrane glycoprotein on the RD line of human rhabdosarcoma cells.[12,200] Viruses that are able to bind only to one or the other of these two receptors have been selected by serial passage in these cells.

Receptor Distribution in Vivo

The distribution of specific virus receptors on various tissues of susceptible or resistant animals can be studied by several techniques, including immunolabeling with polyclonal or monoclonal antireceptor antibodies, direct virus binding to tissues,[60] measurement of receptor glycoproteins in membrane extracts,[194] and measurement of mRNA that encodes the receptor.[83] In general, receptors are detected on cells at the portal of entry and on the principal target tissues for each virus[40,56,60,77,95,96,142]; however, some tissues that express specific receptors for a virus are never infected with the virus in vivo.[60] It may be that during infection the virus fails to reach the receptor on these tissues, or perhaps there is a different block in virus replication in these cells at a stage after virus attachment.

In some cases, tissues that are infected in vivo do not show detectable levels of virus receptor expression. Perhaps the virus genome is delivered to these tissues by infected cells rather than by free virions, as discussed previously, or else an alternative receptor is used in these tissues. Tissue cultures prepared from some virus-resistant, receptor-negative organs are found to express the receptor and to be susceptible to virus infection. For example, the primate kidney is resistant to poliovirus infection in vivo, but monkey kidney cells in vitro express a functional receptor and are excellent producers of the virus.[55] Expression of different membrane glycoproteins can be either induced or repressed on explantation into tissue culture.

ROLE OF VIRUS UNCOATING ON TISSUE TROPISM

After a virus binds to a specific receptor on a cell membrane, one or more additional steps are needed to release the viral genome into the host cell. The genome must get across the membrane and out of the virion to be replicated. These important steps are handled in a variety of ways by different viruses. Interaction with the virus-specific receptor often triggers a preprogrammed sequence of events that lead, in the case of enveloped virions, to fusion of the virus envelope with cell membranes or, in the case of nonenveloped virions, to penetration of the membrane and disassembly of the virion. Host cell–dependent blocks in these vital processes in virus disassembly and entry can determine whether or not a virus can infect a cell that expresses the appropriate virus receptor. For example, HIV-1 is not able to infect murine cells, even if they are expressing recombinant human CD4. This restriction is at an early stage in virus replication prior to genome replication and is probably associated with the steps immediately following receptor binding.

Fusion of the Viral Envelope With Host Membranes

Once an enveloped virion and host cell membrane are brought into close contact, either through the binding of a virus attachment protein to a specific receptor or by means of a nonspecific agent such as polyethylene glycol, the viral fusion glycoprotein comes close to the cell membrane, where it will initiate fusion. The fusion domain of the glycoprotein can be either a component of the virus attachment glycoprotein, as it is for influenza viruses, alphaviruses, coronaviruses, and retroviruses, or it can be on a separate viral envelope glycoprotein, such as the F glycoprotein of paramyxoviruses. Complementation studies show that some recombinant paramyxovirus F proteins can fuse membranes whether they are delivered to the target membrane by the HA of the same or a different virus.[169] Host cell specificity of canine distemper virus is determined by the viral attachment protein HN rather than the viral fusion protein F.[169]

To initiate membrane fusion, conformational changes take place in the viral envelope glycoprotein, the receptor, or both. Such fusion-activating conformational changes following receptor binding are beautifully illustrated by structural studies of two membrane-fusing viral glycoproteins, the influenza HA glycoprotein[131] and the envelope glycoproteins of alphaviruses.[86]

The envelope glycoproteins of different isolates of HIV-1 show extensive amino acid sequence variation, particularly in several variable domains. The third variable domain, called the V3 loop, plays an indirect role in macrophage tropism of HIV-1 or SIV-1 isolates by influencing the postbinding steps in viral entry.[80,88,98,161] Mabs to V3 neutralize virus infectivity. Although they do not prevent binding of virions to CD4 receptor glycoproteins, they do block fusion of the viral envelope with the plasma membrane.[72] Mutations in the V3 loop can affect the kinetics of virus binding to CD4+ T-cell lines and the dissociation of the HIV-1 envelope glycoprotein gp120 from gp41.[193] The HIV-1 envelope glycoprotein undergoes conformational changes after binding to its CD4 receptor.[112,163] Apparently, the V3 loop affects this conformational change and plays a role in the antigenicity and stability of the virions and in their membrane-fusing activities for different cell types.[31,193]

Protease Activation of Membrane Fusion

To activate their membrane fusing activity, some viral fusion glycoproteins require specific cleavage by proteolytic enzymes before the required conformational change can occur. This cleavage of the fusion glycoprotein is a host-dependent reaction of a host enzyme either in the Golgi or plasma membrane of the cell that produced the virus or at the tissue site of infection (e.g., the lumen of the small intestine). Cells or tissues that lack the required protease activity produce virions with uncleaved fusion glycoproteins, which are consequently noninfectious.

Virus tissue tropism in vivo can also be determined by the availability of a host protease that activates the membrane fusing activity of a viral glycoprotein.[75,127] The fusion proteins of virulent strains of orthomyxoviruses or paramyxoviruses are usually cleaved in the Golgi apparatus by the cellular protease furin, whereas the nascent viral protein moves toward the plasma membrane where virions bud.[78] If a variant fusion protein has an amino acid sequence that makes it resistant to furin cleavage, then it can still be activated if the virions are exposed to a secreted host protease in extracellular fluids.[62] Finally, in some but not all cell types, an uncleaved viral fusion protein can be activated at the stage of virus entry.[20] Virulent and attenuated strains of Newcastle disease virus (NDV) differ in their tissue tropisms in birds and in embryonated chicken eggs. The virulent strains, which cause systemic infection, encode F glycoproteins with several arginine residues at the cleavage.[124] These F proteins are readily cleaved by furin in all avian cells. In contrast, avirulent strains that cause only local infection have a single arginine at the cleavage site of F, and these variant glycoproteins are cleaved by proteases found only in the respiratory or alimentary tracts.

Sendai virus, another parainfluenza virus, also has strains that differ markedly in virulence depending on the susceptibility of their viral F proteins to cleavage by cellular proteases. Only strains whose F proteins are susceptible to cleavage by a protease in mouse lung can cause pneumonia in mice.[119,176] Similarly, influenza A viruses show different tissue tropisms, depending on the amino acid sequences at the cleavage sites of the HA fusion glycoproteins.[90] In chick embryos, attenuated strains of NDV, Sendai virus, and influenza A virus replicate only in the endoderm of the CAM, whereas virulent strains of these viruses with several arginine residues at their cleavage sites can also replicate in the mesoderm and ectoderm, leading to death of the embryo. The chorioallantoic fluid contains a protease related to blood clotting factor X and prothrombin that can activate the infectivity of all three attenuated viruses by cleaving the variant fusion glycoproteins that have a single arginine at the cleavage site.[62] A specific inhibitor of this enzyme blocks replication in the CAM of the three attenuated viruses but not of the virulent strain of NDV.[62] Thus, differences in the cellular expression of several proteases that cleave the viral fusion proteins can determine the tissue tropisms of some strains of orthomyxoviruses and paramyxoviruses.

Cellular Determinants of Membrane Fusion

As described previously, HIV-1 isolates show strong tropism for either human macrophages or CD4+ T cells. This host restriction occurs at an early step, after binding and before provirus DNA synthesis, and can be overcome by transfecting the cells with viral genetic material.[173] In addition to differences in the V3 loop, another important determinant of the tropism of different HIV-1 strains is the cellular specificity of the membrane fusion activity of the envelope glycoproteins. Recombinant envelope proteins derived from either T-cell–tropic or macrophage-tropic HIV-1 strains were expressed in cells containing a plasmid encoding β-galactosidase under under the T7 promoter and then incubated with either macrophages or T-cell lines expressing recombinant T7 RNA polymerase.[22] The blue reporter protein is synthesized only after env-CD4–mediated cell fusion. Macrophages fuse only with cells expressing env glycoproteins from macrophage-tropic viruses, and CD4+ T-cell lines fuse only with cells expressing env from T-cell–tropic viruses. Thus, HIV-1 strains specific for each cell type have mutations that somehow optimize the membrane fusion activities of the envelope glycoprotein for that cell type.

Another observation also suggests that a second host cell–dependent factor in the plasma membrane determines whether or not HIV-1 can enter a CD4+ cell. HIV-1 can bind to murine cells expressing recombinant human CD4, but the virions do not fuse with the plasma membrane of these murine cells. Apparently, the membranes of the murine cells lack a factor found only in primate cells that is required for fusion of the viral envelope with the plasma membrane.

The lipid composition of the host cell membrane can affect cellular permissivity for infection with an enveloped virus. For example, Semliki Forest virus requires cholesterol in the host plasma membrane for fusion to occur.[138]

In addition to protease cleavage of fusion glycoproteins, some enveloped viruses also require an acidic environment to activate their membrane-fusing activity. These viruses, including influenza viruses, vesicular stomatitis virus (VSV), and alphaviruses, bind to receptors on the plasma membrane and are carried into endosomes, which are then acidified by fusion with lysosomes, allowing fusion of the viral envelope with the endosomal membrane.[102] The acidification of the endosomes can be inhibited by lysosomotropic drugs such as chloroquine, and membrane fusion is also blocked by bafilomycin A1, a selective inhibitor of the vacuolar H^+-ATPase pump.[137] Treatment of cells with these agents prevents infection by viruses that require acidic conditions to trigger membrane fusion. In contrast, other enveloped viruses, including paramyxoviruses, lentiviruses (e.g,. HIV-1), coronaviruses, poxviruses, and HSV can cause fusion at neutral or mildly alkaline pH and are able to fuse with the plasma membrane without requiring additional activation steps.[22,58,93,175]

Following binding of the viral glycoprotein to receptors on the membrane and fusion of the viral envelope with host cell membranes, the viral nucleocapsid enters the cytoplasm, and additional, as yet rather poorly defined host cell–dependent steps must occur before virus genomes are replicated. Such a step that occurs after virus binding but before genome replication has been implicated in restriction of MHV-JHM infection in cells from the MHV-resistant SJL/J mouse.[204]

Penetration of Nonenveloped Virions Across Host Membranes

The mechanisms by which nonenveloped virions either pass through the host membranes or permit their genomes to enter the host cytoplasm are not yet clearly understood. Some insight into this question is provided by studying the effects of purified specific virus receptor glycoproteins such as ICAM-1 or PVR on nonenveloped virions such as rhinoviruses or poliovirus, respectively.[28,61,76] After the receptor binds to the canyon in the VP1 protein of the capsid, a concerted conformational change of the entire capsid occurs that liberates VP4 proteins from within the capsid and exposes the viral RNA genome to the medium. Virus mutants that have increased resistance to these in vitro uncoating effects of recombinant soluble receptors or to growth in a drug that inhibits uncoating have been isolated and found to have mutations in the receptor binding site that change receptor binding affinity, mutations that affect binding of sphingosine in the pocket beneath the floor of the canyon, or mutations at the borders between capsomers, which lead to tighter interactions and increased resistance to uncoating.[34,123] Soluble receptor-resistant mutants also show increased resistance to uncoating by susceptible cells that express the anchored virus receptor. These experiments indicate that some receptors function not only to bind virions to the membrane but also to initiate uncoating of the viral genome.

Virions of reoviruses are nonenveloped and are very stable outside the body. However, when they are ingested and enter the small intestine, the virions are changed to infectious subvirion particles (ISVPs) by host proteases in the lumen that act on several capsid proteins. The μ1 protein and its cleavage product μ1C are further cleaved, the σ3 protein is released from the virion, and the attachment protein, σ1, is extended on the tip of a long projection from each vertex of the capsid.[46] The ISVPs are much less stable in the environment than virions, but they have developed the ability to bind to receptors on M cells in the intestine and to penetrate into the M cells, from where they can initiate infection of lymphoid cells in the underlying Peyer's patches.[5] Some differing susceptibilities of host species could be related to differences in the availability of host proteases to convert virions into infectious ISVPs.

Adenoviruses are nonenveloped virions that bind to as yet unidentified host cell receptors by means of long fibers that extend from the vertices of the icosahedral virus[60,111,130]; this binding is necessary but not sufficient to initiate infection of the cells. Penetration of the virus through the endocytic membrane depends on subsequent binding of the penton base protein of the viral capsid to the vitronectin receptors, the $\alpha_V\beta_3$ and $\alpha_V\beta_5$ integrins, on the cell membrane.[2,192] Cells lacking these integrins are not susceptible to infection, but they become susceptible after transfection with cDNA encoding $\alpha_V\beta_5$.[191,192] The mechanism for this second step in adenovirus penetration is not understood. Following membrane penetration, the adenovirus core enters the cell cytoplasm and is carried to the nuclear pores, undergoing programmed disassembly as it delivers its genomic DNA into the nucleus.[111]

EFFECTS OF TRANSCRIPTION FACTORS, ENHANCERS, AND HORMONES ON VIRUS TROPISM

For some DNA viruses and retroviruses, transcription of viral genes can be affected by tissue-specific enhancers or transcription factors. Even if a cell contains appropriate virus receptors and permits virus penetration, virus replication can be blocked at the level of transcription of viral genes if the host cell fails to express the particular enhancers, transcription factors, or activators of inactive transcription factors that are required for transcription of specific virus genes. The role of cellular enhancers in determining the permissivity of cells for polyomavirus replication is clearly defined.[8] Some transcription factors are present in inactive form in many cell types but are activated only to bind to a specific site on the DNA by interaction with a specific ligand such as a steroid hormone. Thus, specific transcription factors active in a particular cell type may determine which viral genes are expressed. In addition, specific binding of hormones or other ligands to certain transcription factors can further modulate expression of virus genes.

Papillomaviruses exhibit marked tissue tropisms. They replicate only in epithelial cells of one host species; each human papillomavirus propagates only in a small region of the epithelium; and within the epithelial tissues, infectious virions can be formed only in differentiated keratinocytes and not in basal cells (see Chap. 12). Generally, in basal and parabasal cells, the papillomavirus genome is present only at low levels, only some early virus proteins are made, and no viral capsid proteins or virions are made. In these cells, the early E2 virus proteins and host transcription factors bind to the upstream regulatory region of the E6 promoter and repress transcription of the E6 and E7 genes. There is some degree of tissue specificity in the regulation of virus gene expression.[41,44,45,109] As papillomavirus-infected basal cells differentiate into the midspinous layer of the epithelium, the cellular differentiation program in each type of epithelium turns on a combination of transcription factors which then promote transcription of the papillomavirus late genes encoding capsid proteins. As described previously, high levels of papillomavirus DNA are also made in the differentiated cells, because virus infection upregulates DNA synthesis in these cells.[32] Consequently, only in specific differentiated keratinocytes are large amounts of papillomavirus structural proteins and viral genomic DNA synthesized and infectious virions assembled.

The tissue tropism of retroviruses is determined by several factors, including the receptor specificities of their virus envelope glycoproteins and their membrane fusion specificities (discussed previously),[190] and also by variations in the long terminal repeat (LTR) sequences of the proviruses.[23,143] Recombinant ALV with different envelope glycoproteins and LTRs show unexpected tissue tropisms in 1-day-old chicks. Some infect bursal lymphocytes like the parental viruses, but others also replicate in skeletal muscle or thymus. Both the envelope glycoprotein and LTR sequences affect this tissue tropism.[23]

ROLE OF POLYMERASES IN VIRUS TROPISM

A classic example of the dependence of a virus on host cell factors involving a nucleic acid polymerase is the host-dependent replication of bacteriophage Qβ. This phage can replicate only in bacteria whose genomes encode a protein that can form an enzymatically active complex with the viral replicase proteins. Among animal viruses, the autonomous parvoviruses replicate only in dividing host cells that provide DNA polymerase activity.[177,186] For this reason, in adult animals, these viruses exhibit an apparent tropism for rapidly dividing cell populations such as the intestinal epithelium or bone marrow progenitors. In fetal or young animals that are rapidly growing, dependoviruses such as canine or feline parvovirus can also cause disease in other tissues, including the myocardium and cerebellum.[134] This dependence of the virus on host cell DNA synthesis explains, at least in part, the tissue tropism and age dependence of parvovirus replication.

Cellular DNA replication requires many enzymes, as well as the synthesis and transport of deoxyribonucleotides into the nucleus. Papillomaviruses require these host enzymes and nucleotide pools for replication of virus DNA.[171] In the nondividing differentiated cells of the suprabasal layers of the epithelium where the papillomaviruses replicate, this machinery is not active. Cellular differentiation stimulates the expression of the viral gene encoding the E7 early protein, which in turn upregulates cellular DNA replication, moving cells from the G_O state into the S phase so that the viral DNA can be replicated.[32]

Many DNA viruses encode their own DNA-dependent DNA polymerases but may nevertheless rely on other cellular factors for the replication of the viral genome. For example, HSV-1 encodes a viral thymidine kinase that is required to facilitate viral DNA replication in nondividing cells in vivo but not in tissue culture cells.[54] If all of the other cellular factors needed to permit the full lytic cycle of virus replication are available in the cell, then infection generally leads to cell death. However, if some other host cell factors required for production of the virus, such as transcription factors, are unavailable, then the virus early genes may stimulate uncontrolled cell division or immortalization. For example, EBV infection of human B lymphocytes establishes a persistent latent infection in which only early proteins are expressed, but the cells are stimulated to enter the cell cycle and undergo unrestrained cell division.[172]

The RNA polymerase of influenza A virus, a negative-strand RNA virus, requires nascent host cell mRNAs to prime the synthesis of viral mRNAs in the nuclei of infected cells.[92] This unusual requirement for host cell mRNA synthesis would probably cause influenza virus to replicate best in cells that are synthesizing high levels of cellular mRNAs. In vivo, influenza A virus replicates in the respiratory epithelium of humans or pigs and the respiratory or enteric epithelium of birds. These epithelial cells turn over rapidly and exhibit active mRNA synthesis.

Mutations in viral polymerase genes can affect the cell tropism of virus infection. For example, in LCMV, a single amino acid change in the RNA-dependent RNA polymerase is a major determinant of virus yield from macrophages.[106]

The RNA-dependent RNA polymerases of many plus-strand RNA viruses such as picornaviruses or alphaviruses require the elaboration of intracytoplasmic membranes.[25] Although the mechanisms for stimulating the proliferation of these membranes and their roles in viral RNA replication are not yet fully understood, this may provide another possible host cell–dependent process that could affect the replication of some RNA viruses.

ROLE OF MACROMOLECULAR TRANSPORT ON VIRUS TISSUE TROPISM

As intracellular parasites, all viruses depend upon the host cell for the timely and accurate intracellular transport of viral macromolecules and macromolecular complexes during a productive virus infection. Although many intracellular transport processes are shared by all cell types, some differ substantially from one cell type to another. For example, some cells are specialized for high levels of endocytosis, whereas other cells have much less of this activity. Cells can be specialized for secretion of proteins, for transcytosis, for maintenance of barriers to the extracellular environment, or for many other activities that require unusual or exaggerated intracellular transport functions. Viruses that replicate in such specialized cell types may be dependent on these intracellular transportation mechanisms.

After adenoviruses bind with high affinity to as yet unidentified receptors on the host cell membrane by the tip of the fiber protein,[60] the 5 Arg-Gly-Asp sequences on the adenovirus penton base protein interacts with vitronectin-binding integrins $\alpha_v\beta_3$ or $\alpha_v\beta_5$ on the cell membrane.[192] This second specific interaction mediates the penetration of the virus across the cell membrane, which occurs in the endosomes.[191] The viral nucleocapsid is then transported by host cell mechanisms through the cytoplasm to the nuclear pore complex, where disassembly of the viral nucleocapsid occurs and the DNA genome enters the nucleus.[6] This directed transport of the viral nucleocapsid is an essential prelude to adenovirus replication.

Mouse leukemia virus in the retrovirus family requires mitosis for integration into the host cell chromosomes of the provirus DNA. A complex consisting of viral DNA and proteins forms and remains in the cytoplasm until the cells undergo mitosis. Apparently, only when the nuclear envelope disassembles during mitosis can the provirus complex come into contact with cellular chromosomes so that integration can occur.[144] Thus, cells in the resting G_0 state are unlikely to allow murine leukemia virus provirus DNA to integrate into their chromosomes. In contrast, lentiviruses in the retrovirus family do not require mitosis of host cells for integration of the provirus into host chromosomes.[97]

Viruses that replicate in the cell nucleus, including most DNA viruses and influenza viruses, can take advantage of many host cell activities that take place there, such as DNA-dependent DNA polymerase and DNA-dependent RNA polymerase activities and mRNA splicing. However, the viral mRNAs must be transported from the nucleus into the cytoplasm to be translated, and some virus-encoded enzymes and capsid proteins must be transported into the nucleus from their sites of synthesis in the cytoplasm. To accomplish this, the viral genomes encode proteins that carry motifs that mimic or duplicate the nuclear transport motifs of cellular proteins destined for localization in the nucleus. Indeed, the first nuclear transport motif was identified on the T antigens of papovaviruses.[82,94] It is possible that the transport of viral macromolecules into and out of the nucleus is more efficiently coordinated in some cell types than others, facilitating virus replication in those cells with efficient transport.

Other important host cell transport mechanisms usurped by viruses are the targeting of viral mRNAs that encode membrane glycoproteins to the rough endoplasmic reticulum (RER) and the transport of viral glycoproteins through the complex machinery for vesicular transport to the Golgi and to the plasma membrane. Again, the study of the intracellular transport of viral glycoproteins provided important insight into these cellular mechanisms for glycoprotein synthesis and targeting.[121,122] Differentiated cells in various tissues show marked differences in the sizes and enzymatic activities of their RER and Golgi complexes. Such differences could affect the yield of viruses from cells of different tissues.

The plasma membranes of epithelial cells in vivo are polarized by the presence of tight junctions between cells. Viral envelope glycoproteins may be transported either to the apical membrane, as for the influenza A HA and NA glycoproteins, or to the basolateral membranes, as for the VSV G glycoprotein.[16] The localization of the viral envelope glycoproteins determines where infectious virions can bud and be released from infected epithelial cells.[35,181] This may have important consequences for virus tropism. If viruses bud only from the apical surface of epithelial cells, and if the epithelium is not destroyed by infection, then the virus is likely to spread to other cells by way of secretions on the luminal side of the epithelium. These viruses, such as influenza A virus or some strains of Sendai virus, would then apparently show tropism for epithelial cells. In contrast, viruses that are released preferentially from the basolateral membranes, such as VSV, measles, and virulent variants of Sendai virus, would potentially be more likely to spread from infected epithelial cells to underlying cells in the lamina propria, possibly resulting in viremia and systemic infection. Because of the way their glycoproteins are designed to be transported and sorted by the cellular glycoprotein transport vesicles, such viruses would have a broader tissue tropism than the viruses that bud only from apical membranes.

Poliovirus infection of human cells in vitro can be blocked by monoclonal antibodies directed against the PVR,[117] and expression of recombinant PVR makes transgenic mice susceptible to poliovirus infection.[142] However, in vivo PVR is expressed on the membranes of many human cells and tissues that are resistant to poliovirus infection. Therefore, an additional host factor, besides PVR expression, may affect the tissue tropism of poliovirus in vivo. A candidate for this second host factor is CD44H, an isoform of the lymphocyte homing receptor.[159,160] Expression of this protein in human tissues closely reflects their susceptibility to poliovirus infection,[158] and monoclonal antibody to CD44H can block poliovirus infection, although recombinant CD44H does not serve as a PVR. A molecular interaction between CD44H and PVR in the plasma membrane is postulated to occur and to enhance the receptor activity of PVR in vivo in the tissues, where CD44H is expressed. Interestingly, a different isoform, CD44S, has also been shown to affect the production of HIV-1 from CD4+ human leukocytes.[47] Thus, host cell membrane components, in addition to specific virus receptors, can affect the susceptibility of differentiated cell types to virus infection.

ROLE OF THE CELL CYCLE ON VIRUS RELEASE AND YIELD

Many cell types exist in vivo in either of two states: as cells that are actively cycling through the cell cycle, or as resting cells held in the G_0 phase of the cell cycle. The expression of various cellular proteins associated with cell cycling is regulated by host cell transcription factors. The productive infection of papillomaviruses in differentiated keratinocytes in the epithelium is an excellent example of the importance of the cell cycle in virus replication. The differentiated cells which are in G_0 and no longer cycling cannot provide host polymerase functions needed for virus replication unless the virus stimulates the cells to enter the cell cycle and initiate DNA.[32] Many other DNA viruses also express proteins that alter the cell cycle of their host cells and facilitate virus replication.

Although some RNA viruses can bind specifically to their target cells and enter them whether or not they are cycling, replication and production of infectious virions may only occur in cells that are cycling. When infected cells in G_0 are stimulated to enter the cell cycle by cytokines, growth factors, or other modulators, virus replication is activated. Several examples of this cell activation–dependent arrest of RNA virus synthesis are known. For example, the rhabdovirus VSV can enter resting T lymphocytes but replicates in them only if they have been activated by exposure to specific antigens or mitogens.[15] Lentiviruses such as HIV-1 or maedi/visna virus can enter resting macrophages that bear appropriate receptors, but infectious virus is produced only after the cells have been activated.[154] Such growth-arrested cells may provide an in vivo reservoir for the persistence of genomes from HIV-1 and various other viruses, and later reactivation of the cells by host factors may result in release of infectious virus.

DIFFERENTIAL CLEARANCE OF VIRUS FROM DIFFERENT TISSUES

As discussed previously, tissue tropism can be determined by many factors that make a cell type permissive for replication of a particular virus. However, tissue tropism can also result from differences in clearance of a virus from several infected tissues. One of the best understood examples of this is LCMV, which can cause persistent infection of some tissues after being cleared from other tissues by the host immune response.[3]

Mosquitoes infected with the alphavirus Sindbis have several patterns of virus replication in different tissues as a result of differential clearance of virus from some tissues.[19] Some organs, such as ovarioles, are not infected; others, including salivary glands, midgut, and thoracic muscle, are transiently infected; and the fat bodies, hemolymph, hindgut, and tracheole-associated cells become persistently infected.[19] Although the mechanism for the differential clearance of virus from different tissues of the mosquito is not yet understood, it is possible that an extracellular antiviral protein induced by virus infection may play a role.[99a]

NATURAL AND EXPERIMENTAL ALTERATIONS OF VIRUS TROPISM

Natural selection of virus variants that have altered tissue tropism or host range happens rarely and may result in the emergence of "new" viral diseases.[50,133] As described previously, analysis of mutations in such virus variants can provide valuable information about the determinants of species specificity and tissue tropism. It is possible to genetically manipulate the hosts of virus infection to identify factors that can affect the localization of virus infection. An exciting example is the study of human poliovirus infection in transgenic mice expressing human PVR.[1,77,141] Neurotropism and neurovirulence in this model reflect those observed in experimentally infected primates and can therefore facilitate analysis of determinants of tissue tropism and virulence. These experiments show that the tropism of poliovirus for the anterior horn cells is not solely the result of expression of the receptor PVR. In addition, experimental inoculation of virus by different routes also allows exploration of how poliovirus spreads to the central nervous system.[142]

Mice with severe combined immunodeficiency (SCID) can be used to explore the tropism of virus strains for different tissues in vivo in the absence of an antigen-specific immune response. Reovirus reassortants were introduced into adult SCID mice to identify the genome segments associated with increased virulence of type 1 reovirus.[66] Four virus proteins associated with the vertex of the viral capsid were found to play an important role in organ tropism. Interestingly, organs such as liver, brain, or intestine differed in regard to which combination of these four virus genome segments was associated with virulence and virus replication. Further analysis may indicate what host cell factors determine the permissivity of these tissues for reovirus infection in vivo.

A powerful tool for the study of the tissue tropism of human viruses that cannot be propagated in any animal models is the SCID-hu mouse. Because these animals are immunosuppressed, they can tolerate implants of human fetal thymus, liver, or skin. Varicella zoster virus (VZV) injected into thymus and liver implants under the kidney capsule was able to replicate in human T cells, and skin lesions similar to those seen in human VZV infections were obtained by inoculation of virus into subcutaneous fetal skin implants.[120]

An extensive discussion of the uses of genetically altered animals in experimental virus pathogenesis is included in Chapter 20. A new understanding of the molecular mechanisms underlying virus tissue tropism and species specificity is beginning to emerge from studies using genetically altered host animals, molecular genetics and structural analysis of viral variants, and structural and biochemical analysis of age-dependent and tissue-dependent differences between host cells.

ABBREVIATIONS

ALV: avian leukosis virus
BCEC: brain capillary endothelial cells
CAM: chorioallantoic membrane
CPV: canine parvovirus
EBV: Epstein-Barr virus
FMDV: foot-and-mouth disease virus
HA: hemagglutinin
hCMV: human cytomegalovirus
HCV: human coronavirus
HE: hemagglutinin esterase
HIV: human immunodeficiency virus
HSV: herpes simplex virus
ICAM-1: intercellular adhesion molecule 1
ISVP: infectious subvirion particle

LCMV: lymphocytic choriomeningitis virus
LTR: long terminal repeat
Mab: monoclonal antibodies
MHV: mouse hepatitis virus
NDV: Newcastle disease virus
Neu5,9Ac$_2$: N-acetyl-9-O-acetylneuraminic acid
Neu5Ac: N-acetylneuraminic acid
PRCV: porcine coronavirus
PVR: poliovirus receptor
RER: rough endoplasmic reticulum
SA: sialic acid
SCID: severe combined immunodeficiency
SIV: simian immunodeficiency virus
TGEV: transmissible gastroenteritis virus
VSV: vesicular stomatitis virus
VZV: varicella zoster virus

ACKNOWLEDGEMENTS

I am grateful to Drs. Bruce Zelus, Dina Tresnan, and Rebecca Holmes for their thoughtful suggestions about this chapter, and to Dr. Zelus for preparing Figure 3-1. I also thank John Schneider, James Ahn, and Thomas Chamberlin for their help in the preparation of this chapter. This work was supported in part by NIH grant #25231.

REFERENCES

1. Abe S, Ota Y, Doi Y, et al. Studies on neurovirulence in poliovirus-sensitive transgenic mice and cynomolgus monkeys for the different temperature-sensitive viruses derived from the Sabin type 3 virus. Virology 1995;210:160–166.
2. Adzhar AB, Shaw K, Britton P, Cavanagh D. Avian infectious bronchitis virus: Differences between 793/B and other strains. Vet Rec 1995;136:548. Letter
3. Ahmed R, Hahn CS, Somasundaram T, Villarete L, Matloubian M, Strauss JH. Molecular basis of organ-specific selection of viral variants during chronic infection. J Virol 1991;65:4242–4247.
4. Albritton LM, Tseng L, Scadden D, Cunningham JM. A putative murine ecotropic receptor gene encodes a multiple membrane-spanning protein and confers susceptibility to virus infection. Cell 1989; 57:659.
5. Amerongen HM, Wilson GAR, Fields BN, Neutra MR. Proteolytic processing of reovirus is required for adherence to intestinal M cells. J Virol 1994;68:8428–8432.
6. Anton IM, Sune C, Meloen RH, Borras-Cuesta F, Enjuanes L. A transmissible gastroenteritis coronavirus nucleoprotein epitope elicits T helper cells that collaborate in the in vitro antibody synthesis to the three major structural viral proteins. Virology 1995;212:746–751.
7. Aoki J, Koike S, Ise I, Sato-Yoshida Y, Nomoto A. Amino acid residues on human poliovirus receptor involved in interaction with poliovirus. J Biol Chem 1994;269:8431–8438.
8. Bauer PH, Bronson RT, Fung SC, et al. Genetic and structural analysis of a virulence determinant in polyomavirus VP1. J Virol 1995;69:7925–7931.
9. Belli BA, Samuel CE. Biosynthesis of reovirus-specified polypeptides: Identification of regions of the bicistronic reovirus S1 mRNA that affect the efficiency of translation in animal cells. Virology 1993;193:16–27.
10. Bergelson JM, Chan BM, Finberg RW, Hemler ME. The integrin VLA-2 binds echovirus 1 and extracellular matrix ligands by different mechanisms. J Clin Invest 1993;92:232–239.
11. Bergelson JM, Chan M, Solomon KR, St. John NF, Lin H, Finberg RW. Decay-accelerating factor (CD55), a glycosylphosphatidyl-inositol-anchored complement regulatory protein, is a receptor for several echoviruses. Proc Natl Acad Sci U S A 1994;91:6245–6249.
12. Bergelson JM, Mohanty JG, Crowell RL, St. John NF, Lublin DM, Finberg RW. Coxsackievirus B3 adapted to growth in RD cells binds to decay-accelerating factor (CD55). J Virol 1995;69:1903–1906.
13. Bergelson JM, St. John N, Kawaguchi S, et al. Infection by echoviruses 1 and 8 depends on the alpha 2 subunit of human VLA-2. J Virol 1993;67:6847–6852.
14. Berinstein A, Roivainen M, Hovi T, Mason PW, Baxt B. Antibodies to the vitronectin receptor (integrin alpha V beta 3) inhibit binding and infection of foot-and-mouth disease virus to cultured cells. J Virol 1995;69:2664–2666.
15. Bloom BR, Jimenez L, Marcus PI. A plaque assay for enumerating antigen-sensitive cells in delayed type hypersensitivity. J Exp Med 1970;132:16.
16. Bok D, O'Day W, Rodriguez-Boulan E. Polarized budding of vesicular stomatitis and influenza virus from cultured human and bovine retinal pigment epithelium. Exp Eye Res 1992;55:853–860.
17. Borrow P, Oldstone MB. Characterization of lymphocytic choriomeningitis virus-binding protein(s): A candidate cellular receptor for the virus. J Virol 1992;66:7270–7281.
18. Bousquet F, Martin C, Girardeau JP, et al. CS31A capsule-like antigen as an exposure vector for heterologous antigenic determinants. Infect Immun 1994;62:2553–2561.
19. Bowers DF, Abell BA, Brown DT. Replication and tissue tropism of the alphavirus Sindbis in the mosquito *Aedes albopictus*. Virology 1995;212:1–12.
20. Boycott R, Klenk HD, Ohuchi M. Cell tropism of influenza virus mediated by hemagglutinin activation at the stage of virus entry. Virology 1994;203:313–319.
21. Boyle JF, Weismiller DG, Holmes KV. Genetic resistance to mouse hepatitis virus correlates with absence of virus-binding activity on target tissues. J Virol 1987;61:185–189.
22. Broder CC, Berger EA. Fusogenic selectivity of the envelope glycoprotein is a major determinant of human immunodeficiency virus type 1 tropism for CD4+ T-cell lines vs. primary macrophages. Proc Natl Acad Sci U S A 1995;92:9004–9008.
23. Brown DW, Robinson HL. Influence of env and long terminal repeat sequences on the tissue tropism of avian leukosis viruses. J Virol 1988;62:4828–4831.
24. Brown KE, Young NS, Liu JM. Molecular, cellular and clinical aspects of parvovirus B19 infection. Crit Rev Oncol Hematol 1994; 16:1–31.
25. Butterworth BE, Shimshick EJ, Yin FH. Association of the polioviral RNA complex with phospholipid membranes. J Virol 1976; 19: 457–466.
26. Cao JX, Ni H, Wills MR, et al. Passage of Japanese encephalitis virus in HeLa cells results in attenuation of virulence in mice. J Gen Virol 1995;76:2757–2764.
27. Carpenter S, Chesebro B. Change in host cell tropism associated with in vitro replication of equine infectious anemia virus. J Virol 1989;63:2492–2496.
28. Casasnovas JM, Springer TA. Pathway of rhinovirus disruption by soluble intercellular adhesion molecule 1 (ICAM-1): An intermediate in which ICAM-1 is bound and RNA is released. J Virol 1994; 68:5882–5889.
29. Casasnovas JM, Springer TA. Kinetics and thermodynamics of virus binding to receptor: Studies with rhinovirus, intercellular adhesion molecule-1 (ICAM-1), and surface plasmon resonance. J Biol Chem 1995;270:13216–13224.
30. Chakrabarti R, Hofman FM, Pandey R, Mathes LE, Roy-Burman P. Recombination between feline exogenous and endogenous retroviral sequences generates tropism for cerebral endothelial cells. Am J Pathol 1994;144:348–358.
31. Chavda SC, Griffin P, Han-Liu Z, Keys B, Vekony MA, Cann AJ. Molecular determinants of the V3 loop of human immunodeficiency virus type 1 glycoprotein gp120 responsible for controlling cell tropism. J Gen Virol 1994;75:3249–3253.
32. Cheng S, Schmidt-Grimminger DC, Murant T, Broker TR, Chow LT. Differentiation-dependent up-regulation of the human papillomavirus E7 gene reactivates cellular DNA replication in suprabasal differentiated keratinocytes. Genes Dev 1995;9:2335–2349.

33. Clarkson NA, Kaufman R, Lublin DM, et al. Characterization of the echovirus 7 receptor: Domains of CD55 critical for virus binding. J Virol 1995;69:5497–5501.

34. Colston E, Racaniello VR. Soluble receptor-resistant poliovirus mutants identify surface and internal capsid residues that control interaction with the cell receptor. EMBO J 1994;13:5855–5862.

35. Compans RW. Virus entry and release in polarized epithelial cells. Curr Top Microbiol Immunol 1995;202:209–219.

36. Compton T, Nowlin DM, Cooper NR. Initiation of human cytomegalovirus infection requires initial interaction with cell surface heparan sulfate. Virology 1993;193:834–841.

37. Cooling LL, Koerner TA, Naides SJ. Multiple glycosphingolipids determine the tissue tropism of parvovirus B19. J Infect Dis 1995; 172:1198–1205.

38. Cooper NR, Nowlin D, Taylor HP, Compton T. Cellular receptor for human cytomegalovirus. Transplant Proc 1994;23:56–59.

39. Cordonnier A, Montagnier L, Emerman M. Single amino-acid changes in HIV envelope affect viral tropism and receptor binding. Nature 1989;340:571–574.

40. Dalgleish AG, Habeshaw J, Manca F. HIV and tropism: Implications for pathogenesis. Mol Aspects Med 1991;12:267–282.

41. de Villiers EM. Human pathogenic papillomavirus types: An update. Curr Top Microbiol Immunol 1994;186:1–12.

42. Delmas B, Gelfi J, L'Haridon R, et al. Aminopeptidase N is a major receptor for the entero-pathogenic coronavirus TGEV. Nature 1992; 357:417–420.

43. Doerig RE, Marcil A, Chopra A, Richardson CD. The human CD46 molecule is a receptor for measles virus (Edmonton strain). Cell 1993; 75:295.

44. Dollard SC, Broker TR, Chow LT. Regulation of the human papillomavirus type 11 E6 promoter by viral and host transcription factors in primary human keratinocytes. J Virol 1993;67:1721– 1726.

45. Dong G, Broker TR, Chow LT. Human papillomavirus type 11 E2 proteins repress the homologous E6 promoter by interfering with the binding of host transcription factors to adjacent elements. J Virol 1994;68:1115–1127.

46. Dryden KA, Wang G, Yeager M, et al. Early steps in reovirus infection are associated with dramatic changes in supramolecular structure and protein conformation: Analysis of virions and subviral particles by cryoelectron microscopy and image reconstruction. J Cell Biol 1993;122:1023–1041.

47. Dukes CS, Yu Y, Rivadeneira ED, et al. Cellular CD44S as a determinant of human immunodeficiency virus type 1 infection and cellular tropism. J Virol 1995;69:4000–4005.

48. Dveksler GS, Dieffenbach CW, Cardellichio CB, et al. Several members of the mouse carcinoembryonic antigen-related glycoprotein family are functional receptors for the coronavirus mouse hepatitis virus-A59. J Virol 1993;67:1–8.

49. Dveksler GS, Pensiero MN, Cardellichio CB, et al. Cloning of the mouse hepatitis virus (MHV) receptor: Expression in human and hamster cell lines confers susceptibility to MHV. J Virol 1991; 65: 6881–6891.

50. Enjuanes L, Sanchez C, Mendez A, Ballesteros ML. Tropism and immunoprotection in transmissible gastroenteritis coronaviruses. Dev Biol Stand 1995;84:145–152.

51. Fenner F, Poole WE, Marshall ID, Dyce AL. Studies on the epidemiology of infectious myxomatosis of rabbits. VI. The experimental introduction of the European strain of virus into Australian wild rabbit populations. J Hyg 1957;55:192.

52. Fenner F, Woodroofe BM. Changes in the virulence and antigenic structure of strains of myxoma virus recovered from Australian wild rabbits between 1950 and 1964. Aust J Exp Biol Med Sci 1965; 43: 359.

53. Fernandes J, Tang D, Leone G, Lee PW. Binding of reovirus to receptor leads to conformational changes in viral capsid proteins that are reversible upon detachment. J Biol Chem 1994;269:17043.

54. Field HJ, Wildy P. The pathogenicity of thymidine kinase-deficient mutants of herpes simplex virus in mice. J Hyg 1978;81:267–277.

55. Freistadt MS, Kaplan G, Racaniello VR. Heterogeneous expression of poliovirus receptor-related proteins in human cells and tissues. Mol Cell Biol 1990;10:5700–5706.

56. Freistadt MS, Stoltz DA, Eberle KE. Role of poliovirus receptors in the spread of the infection. Ann N Y Acad Sci 1995;753:37–47.

57. Gallagher TM, Buchmeier MJ, Perlman S. Cell receptor-independent infection by a neurotropic murine coronavirus. Virology 1992; 191:517–522.

58. Gallagher TM, Escarmis C, Buchmeier MJ. Alteration of the pH dependence of coronavirus-induced cell fusion: Effect of mutations in the spike glycoprotein. J Virol 1991;65:1916–1928.

59. Gilles PN, Lathey JL, Spector SA. Replication of macrophage-tropic and T-cell-tropic strains of human immunodeficiency virus type 1 is augmented by macrophage-endothelial cell contact. J Virol 1995; 69:2133–2139.

60. Godfraind C, Langreth SG, Cardellichio CB, et al. Tissue and cellular distribution of an adhesion molecule in the carcinoembryonic antigen family that serves as a receptor for mouse hepatitis virus. Lab Invest 1995;73:615–627.

61. Gomez Yafal A, Kaplan G, Racaniello VR, Hogle JM. Characterization of poliovirus conformational alteration mediated by soluble cell receptors. Virology 1993;197:501–505.

62. Gotoh B, Ogasawara T, Toyoda T, Inocencio NM, Hamaguchi M, Nagai Y. An endoprotease homologous to the blood clotting factor X as a determinant of viral tropism in chick embryo. EMBO J 1990; 9: 4189–4195.

63. Greve JM, Davis G, Meyer AM, et al. The major human rhinovirus receptor is ICAM-1. Cell 1989;56:839.

64. Gromeier M, Lu HH, Bernhardt G, Harber JJ, Bibb JA, Wimmer E. The human poliovirus receptor: Receptor-virus interaction and parameters of disease specificity. Ann N Y Acad Sci 1995;753:19–36.

65. Gruenberger M, Wandl R, Nimpf J, et al. Avian homologs of the mammalian low-density lipoprotein receptor family bind minor receptor group human rhinovirus. J Virol 1995;69:7244–7247.

66. Haller BL, Barkon ML, Vogler GP, Virgin HW. Genetic mapping of reovirus virulence and organ tropism in severe combined immunodeficient mice: Organ-specific virulence genes. J Virol 1995;69: 357– 364.

67. Halstead SB. Pathogenesis of dengue: Challenges to molecular biology. Science 1988;239:476–481.

68. Harouse JM, Collman RG, Gonzalez-Scarano F. Human immunodeficiency virus type 1 infection of SK-N-MC cells: Domains of gp120 involved in entry into a CD4-negative, galactosyl ceramide/3' sulfo-galactosyl ceramide-positive cell line. J Virol 1995;69: 7383–7390.

69. Herold BC, WuDunn D, Soltys N, Spear PG. Glycoprotein C of herpes simplex virus type 1 plays a principal role in the adsorption of virus to cells and in infectivity. J Virol 1991;65:1090–1098.

70. Herrler G, Klenk HD. The surface receptor is a major determinant of the cell tropism of influenza C virus. Virology 1987;159:102–108.

71. Herrler G, Rott R, Klenk HD, Muller HP, Shukla AK, Schauer R. The receptor-destroying enzyme of influenza C virus is neuraminate-O-acetylesterase. EMBO J 1985;4:1503–1506.

72. Hiscox JA, Mawditt KL, Cavanagh D, Britton P. Investigation of the control of coronavirus subgenomic mRNA transcription by using T7-generated negative-sense RNA transcripts. J Virol 1995;69: 6219–6227.

73. Hofer F, Gruenberger M, Kowalski H, et al. Members of the low density lipoprotein receptor family mediate cell entry of a minor-group common cold virus. Proc Natl Acad Sci U S A 1994;91: 1839–1842.

74. Hoffman PM, Cimino EF, Robbins DS, Broadwell RD, Powers JM, Ruscetti SK. Cellular tropism and localization in the rodent nervous system of a neuropathogenic variant of Friend murine leukemia virus. Lab Invest 1992;67:314–321.

75. Hohdatsu T, Yamada H, Ishizuka Y, Koyama H. Enhancement and neutralization of feline infectious peritonitis virus infection in feline macrophages by neutralizing monoclonal antibodies recognizing different epitopes. Microbiol Immunol 1993;37:499–504.

76. Hoover-Litty H, Greve JM. Formation of rhinovirus-soluble ICAM-1 complexes and conformational changes in the virion. J Virol 1993; 67:390–397.

77. Horie H, Koike S, Kurata T, et al. Transgenic mice carrying the human poliovirus receptor: New animal models for study of poliovirus neurovirulence. J Virol 1994;68:681–688.

78. Huang R, Guo J, Li X, Faustman DL. Elimination of self-peptide major histocompatibility complex class I reactivity in NOD and beta 2-microglobulin-negative mice. Diabetes 1995;44:1114–1120.

79. Hurwitz AA, Berman JW, Lyman WD. The role of the blood-brain barrier in HIV infection of the central nervous system. Adv Neuroimmunol 1994;4:249–256.

80. Hwang SS, Boyle TJ, Lyerly HK, Cullen BR. Identification of the envelope V3 loop as the primary determinant of cell tropism in HIV-1. Science 1991;253:71–74.

81. Johann SV, van Zeijl M, Cekleniak J, O'Hara B. Definition of a domain of GLVR1 which is necessary for infection by gibbon ape leukemia virus and which is highly polymorphic between species. J Virol 1993;67:6733–6736.

82. Kalderon D, Roberts B, Richardson WD, Smith AE. A short amino acid sequence able to specify nuclear localization. Cell 1994;39: 499–509.

83. Kaplan G, Racaniello VR. Down regulation of poliovirus receptor RNA in HeLa cells resistant to poliovirus infection. J Virol 1991; 65: 1829–1835.

84. Kavanaugh MP, Miller DG, Zhang W, et al. Cell-surface receptors for gibbon ape leukemia virus and amphotropic murine retrovirus are inducible sodium-dependent phosphate symporters. Proc Natl Acad Sci U S A 1994;91:7071–7075.

85. Keil W, Geyer R, Dabrowski J, et al. Carbohydrates of influenza virus. Structural elucidation of the individual glycans of the FPV hemagglutinin by two-dimensional 1H n.m.r. and methylation analysis. EMBO J 1985;4:2711–2720.

86. Kenney JM, Sjoberg M, Garoff H, Fuller SD. Visualization of fusion activation in the Semliki Forest virus spike. Structure 1994;2: 823–832.

87. Kim CH, Winton JR, Leong JC. Neutralization-resistant variants of infectious hematopoietic necrosis virus have altered virulence and tissue tropism. J Virol 1994;68:8447–8453.

88. Kirchhoff F, Mori K, Desrosiers RC. The V3 domain is a determinant of simian immunodeficiency virus cell tropism. J Virol 1994; 68:3682–3692.

89. Klatzmann D, Champagne E, Chamaret S, et al. T-lymphocyte T4 molecule behaves as the receptor for human retrovirus LAV. Nature 1984;312:767–768.

90. Klenk HD, Rott R. The molecular biology of influenza virus pathogenicity. Adv Virus Res 1988;34:247–281.

91. Koike S, Horie H, Ise I, et al. The poliovirus receptor protein is produced both as membrane-bound and secreted forms. EMBO J 1990; 9:3217–3224.

92. Krug RM. Priming of influenza virus RNA transcription by capped heterologous RNAs. Curr Top Microbiol Immunol 1981;93:125–149.

93. Lamb RA. Paramyxovirus fusion: A hypothesis for changes. Virology 1993;197:1–11.

94. Lanford RE, Butel JS. Construction and characterization of an SV40 mutant defective in nuclear transport of T antigen. Cell 1984;37: 801–813.

95. Leon-Monzon ME, Illa I, Dalakas MC. Expression of poliovirus receptor in human spinal cord and muscle. Ann N Y Acad Sci 1995; 753:48–57.

96. Levy JA. Viral and cellular factors influencing HIV tropism. Adv Exp Med Biol 1991;300:1–15.

97. Lewis PF, Emerman M. Passage through mitosis is required for oncoretroviruses but not for the human immunodeficiency virus. J Virol 1994;68:510–516.

98. Liu ZQ, Wood C, Levy JA, Cheng-Mayer C. The viral envelope gene is involved in macrophage tropism of a human immunodeficiency virus type 1 strain isolated from brain tissue. J Virol 1990;64: 6148–6153.

99. Lonberg-Holm K, Crowell RL, Philipson L. Unrelated animal viruses share receptors. Nature 1976;259:679.

99a. Luo T, Brown DT. Purification and characterization of a Sinbis virus-induced peptide which stimulates its own production and blocks viral RNA synthesis. Virology 1993;94:44–49.

100. Luytjes W, Bredenbeek PJ, Noten AF, Horzinek MC, Spaan WJ. Sequence of mouse hepatitis virus A59 mRNA2: Indications for RNA recombination between coronaviruses and influenza C virus. Virology 1988;166:415–422.

101. Mankowski JL, Spelman JP, Ressetar HG, et al. Neurovirulent simian immunodeficiency virus replicates productively in endothelial cells of the central nervous system in vivo and in vitro. J Virol 1994;68:8202–8208.

102. Marsh M, Helenius A. Virus entry into animal cells. Adv Virus Res 1989;36:107–151.

103. Marsh YV, Eppstein DA. Vaccinia virus and the EGF receptor: A portal for infectivity? J Cell Biochem 1987;34:239.

104. Mason PW, Baxt B, Brown F, Harber J, Murdin A, Wimmer E. Antibody-complexed foot-and-mouth disease virus, but not poliovirus, can infect normally insusceptible cells via the Fc receptor. Virology 1993;192:568–577.

105. Mason PW, Rieder E, Baxt B. RGD sequence of foot-and-mouth disease virus is essential for infecting cells via the natural receptor but can be bypassed by an antibody-dependent enhancement pathway. Proc Natl Acad Sci U S A 1994;91:1932–1936.

106. Matloubian M, Kolhekar SR, Somasundaram T, Ahmed R. Molecular determinants of macrophage tropism and viral persistence: Importance of single amino acid changes in the polymerase and glycoprotein of lymphocytic choriomeningitis virus. J Virol 1993;67: 7340–7349.

107. McClelland A, deBear J, Yost SC, Meyer AM, Marlor CW, Greve JM. Identification of monoclonal antibody epitopes and critical residues for rhinovirus binding in domain 1 of intercellular adhesion molecule 1. Proc Natl Acad Sci U S A 1991;88:7993–7997.

108. McClure JE. Cellular receptor for Epstein-Barr virus. Prog Med Virol 1992;39:116.

109. McDougall JK. Immortalization and transformation of human cells by human papillomavirus. Curr Top Microbiol Immunol 1994;186: 101–119.

110. McKenna TS, Lubroth J, Rieder E, Baxt B, Mason PW. Receptor binding site-deleted foot-and-mouth disease (FMD) virus protects cattle from FMD. J Virol 1995;69:5787–5790.

111. Mei YF, Wadell G. Molecular determinants of adenovirus tropism. Curr Top Microbiol Immunol 1995;199:213–228.

112. Mello IG, Vassao RC, Pereira CA. Virus specificity of the antiviral state induced by IFN gamma correlates with resistance to MHV 3 infection. Arch Virol 1993;132:281–289.

113. Mendelsohn CL, Wimmer E, Racaniello VR. Cellular receptor for poliovirus: Molecular cloning, nucleotide sequence, and expression of a new member of the immunoglobulin superfamily. Cell 1989; 56:855–865.

114. Mettenleiter TC, Zsak L, Zuckermann F, Sugg N, Kern H, Ben-Porat T. Interaction of glycoprotein gIII with a cellular heparinlike substance mediates adsorption of pseudorabies virus. J Virol 1990;64: 278–286.

115. Mims CA. The pathogenetic basis of viral tropism. Am J Pathol 1989;135:447–455.

116. Minor PD. The molecular biology of poliovaccines. J Gen Virol 1992;74:3065–3077.

117. Minor PD, Pipkin PA, Hockley D, Schild GC, Almond JW. Monoclonal antibodies which block cellular receptors for poliovirus. Virus Res 1984;1:203.

118. Mochizuki M, Nakatani H, Yoshida M. Inhibitory effects of recombinant feline interferon on the replication of feline enteropathogenic viruses in vitro. Vet Microbiol 1994;39:145–152.

119. Mochizuki Y, Tashiro M, Homma M. Pneumopathogenicity in mice of a Sendai virus mutant, TSrev-58, is accompanied by in vitro activation with trypsin. J Virol 1988;62:3040–3042.

120. Moffat JF, Stein MD, Kaneshima H, Arvin AM. Tropism of varicella-zoster virus for human CD4+ and CD8+ T lymphocytes and epidermal cells in SCID-hu mice. J Virol 1995;69:5236–5242.

121. Morrison TG, McQuain C. Assembly of viral membranes. I. Association of vesicular stomatitis virus membrane proteins and membranes in a cell-free system. J Virol 1977;21:451–458.

122. Morrison TG, McQuain CO. Assembly of viral membranes: Nature of the association of vesicular stomatitis virus proteins to membranes. J Virol 1978;26:115–125.

123. Mosser AG, Sgro JY, Rueckert RR. Distribution of drug resistance mutations in type 3 poliovirus identifies three regions involved in uncoating functions. J Virol 1994;68:8193–8201.

124. Nagai Y. Virus activation by host proteinases: A pivotal role in the spread of infection, tissue tropism and pathogenicity. Microbiol Immunol 1995;39:1–9.

125. Nedellec P, Dveksler GS, Daniels E, et al. Bgp2, a new member of the carcinoembryonic antigen-related gene family, encodes an alter-

native receptor for mouse hepatitis viruses. J Virol 1994;68:4525–4537.

126. Nottet HS, Persidsky Y, Sasseville VG, et al. Mechanisms for the transendothelial migration of HIV-1-infected monocytes into brain. J Immunol 1996;156:1284–1295.

127. Ogasawara T, Gotoh B, Suzuki H, et al. Expression of factor X and its significance for the determination of paramyxovirus tropism in the chick embryo. EMBO J 1992;11:467–472.

128. Okazaki K, Matsuzaki T, Sugahara Y, et al. BHV-1 adsorption is mediated by the interaction of glycoprotein gIII with heparinlike moiety on the cell surface. Virology 1991;181:666–670.

129. Olah Z, Lehel C, Anderson WB, Eiden MV, Wilson CA. The cellular receptor for gibbon ape leukemia virus is a novel high affinity sodium-dependent phosphate transporter. J Biol Chem 1994;269:25426–25431.

130. Opstelten DJ, Raamsman MJ, Wolfs K, Horzinek MC, Rottier PJ. Envelope glycoprotein interactions in coronavirus assembly. J Cell Biol 1995;131:339–349.

131. Parr RL, Collissor EW. Epitopes on the spike protein of a nephropathogenic strain of infectious bronchitis virus. Arch Virol 1993;133:369–383.

132. Parrish CR. Mapping specific functions in the capsid structure of canine parvovirus and feline panleukopenia virus using infectious plasmid clones. Virology 1991;183:195–205.

133. Parrish CR. The emergence and evolution of canine parvovirus: An example of recent host range mutation. Semin Virol 1994;5: 121–132.

134. Parrish CR. Pathogenesis of feline panleukopenia virus and canine parvovirus. Baillieres Clin Haematol 1995;8:57–71.

135. Paulson JC, Rogers GN. Resialylated erythrocytes for assessment of the specificity of sialyloligosaccharide binding proteins. Methods Enzymol 1987;138:162–168.

136. Pedersen L, Johann SV, van Zeijl M, Pedersen FS, O'Hara B. Chimeras of receptors for gibbon ape leukemia virus/feline leukemia virus B and amphotropic murine leukemia virus reveal different modes of receptor recognition by retrovirus. J Virol 1995;69:2401–2405.

137. Perez L, Carrasco L. Involvement of the vacuolar H(+)-ATPase in animal virus entry. J Gen Virol 1994;75:2595–2606.

138. Phalen T, Kielian M. Cholesterol is required for infection by Semliki Forest virus. J Cell Biol 1991;112:615–623.

139. Poland SD, Rice GP, Dekaban GA. HIV-1 infection of human brain-derived microvascular endothelial cells in vitro. J Acquir Immune Defic Syndr Hum Retrovirol 1995;8:437–445.

140. Racaniello VR. Cell receptors for picornaviruses. Curr Top Microbiol Immunol 1990;161:1–22.

141. Racaniello VR, Ren R, Bouchard M. Poliovirus attenuation and pathogenesis in a transgenic mouse model for poliomyelitis. Dev Biol Stand 1993;78:109–116.

142. Ren R, Racaniello VR. Human poliovirus receptor gene expression and poliovirus tissue tropism in transgenic mice. J Virol 1992;66:296–304.

143. Robinson HL, Ramamoorthy L, Collart K, Brown DW. Tissue tropism of avian leukosis viruses: Analyses for viral DNA and proteins. Virology 1993;193:443–445.

144. Roe T-Y, Reynolds TC, Yu G, Brown PO. Integration of murine leukemia virus DNA depends on mitosis. EMBO J 1993;12:2099–2108.

145. Rogers GN, Herrler G, Paulson JC, Klenk HD. Influenza C virus uses 9-O-acetyl-N-acetylneuraminic acid as a high affinity receptor determinant for attachment to cells. J Biol Chem 1986;261:5947–5951.

146. Rogers GN, Paulson JC. Receptor determinants of human and animal influenza virus isolates: Differences in receptor specificity of the H3 hemagglutinin based on species of origin. Virology 1983;127:361–373.

147. Rogers GN, Pritchett TJ, Lane JL, Paulson JC. Differential sensitivity of human, avian, and equine influenza A viruses to a glycoprotein inhibitor of infection: selection of receptor specific variants. Virology 1983;131:394–408.

148. Roivainen M, Piirainen L, Hovi T, et al. Entry of coxsackievirus A9 into host cells: Specific interactions with alpha v beta 3 integrin, the vitronectin receptor. Virology 1994;203:357–365.

149. Rolsma MD, Gelberg HB, Kuhlenschmidt MS. Assay for evaluation of rotavirus-cell interactions: Identification of an enterocyte ganglioside fraction that mediates group A rotavirus recognition. J Virol 1994;68:258.

150. Rubin DH, Wetzel JD, Williams WV, Cohen JA, Dworkin C, Dermody TS. Binding of type 3 reovirus by a domain of the sigma 1 protein important for hemagglutination leads to infection of murine erythroleukemia cells. J Clin Invest 1992;90:2536–2542.

151. Sanchez CM, Gebauer F, Sune C, Mendez A, Dopazo J, Enjuanes L. Genetic evolution and tropism of transmissible gastroenteritis coronaviruses. Virology 1992;190:92–105.

152. Sawicki SG, Lu JH, Holmes KV. Persistent infection of cultured cells with mouse hepatitis virus (MHV) results from the epigenetic expression of the MHV receptor. J Virol 1995;69:5535–5543.

153. Scholtissek C, Rohde W, von Hoyningen V, Rott R. On the origin of the human influenza virus subtypes H2N2 and H3N2. Virology 1978; 7:13–20.

154. Schuitemaker H, Koostra NA, Fourchier RAM, Hooibrin B, Miedema F. Productive HIV-1 infection of macrophages restricted to the cell fraction with proliferative capacity. Cell 1994;13:5929–5936.

155. Schultze B, Herrler G. Recognition of N-acetyl-9-O-acetylneuraminic acid by bovine coronavirus and hemagglutinating encephalomyelitis virus. Adv Exp Med Biol 1993;342:299–304.

156. Shafren DR, Bates RC, Agrez MV, Herd RL, Burns GF, Barry RD. Coxsackieviruses B1, B3, and B5 use decay accelerating factor as a receptor for cell attachment. J Virol 1995;69:3873–3877.

157. Sharpless NE, O'Brien WA, Verdin E, Kufta CV, Chen IS, Dubois-Dalcq M. Human immunodeficiency virus type 1 tropism for brain microglial cells is determined by a region of the env glycoprotein that also controls macrophage tropism. J Virol 1992;66:2588–2593.

158. Shepley M, Sherry B, Weiner H. Monoclonal antibody identification of a 100 kD membrane protein in HeLa cells and human spinal cord involved in poliovirus attachment. Proc Natl Acad Sci U S A 1988; 85:7743.

159. Shepley MP. Lymphocyte homing receptor CD44 and poliovirus attachment. In: Wimmer E, ed. Cellular receptors for animal viruses. Cold Spring Harbor, NY: Cold Spring Harbor Laboratory Press, 1944:481–491.

160. Shepley MP, Racaniello VR. A monoclonal antibody that blocks poliovirus attachment recognizes the lymphocyte homing receptor CD44. J Virol 1994;68:1301.

161. Shioda T, Levy JA, Cheng-Mayer C. Small amino acid changes in the V3 hypervariable region of gp120 can affect the T-cell-line and macrophage tropism of human immunodeficiency virus type 1. Proc Natl Acad Sci U S A 1992;89:9434–9438.

162. Sixbey JW, Yao QY. Immunoglobulin A-induced shift of Epstein-Barr virus tissue tropism. Science 1992;255:1578–1580.

163. Sizun J, Soupre D, Legrand MC, et al. Neonatal nosocomial respiratory infection with coronavirus: A prospective study in a neonatal intensive care unit. Acta Paediatr 1995;84:617–620.

164. Sobey WR. Selection for resistance to myxomatosis in domestic rabbits (Oryctolagus cuniculus). J Hyg 1969;67:743.

165. Soderberg C, Giugni TD, Zaia JA, Larsson S, Wahlberg JM, Moller E. CD13 (human aminopeptidase N) mediates human cytomegalovirus infection. J Virol 1993;67:6576–6585.

166. Spriggs DR, Bronson RT, Fields BN. Hemagglutinin variants of reovirus type 3 have altered central nervous system tropism. Science 1983;220:505–507.

167. Srnka CA, Tiemeyer M, Gilbert JH, et al. Cell surface ligands for rotavirus: Mouse intestinal glycolipids and synthetic carbohydrate analogs. Virology 1992;190:794–805.

168. Stehle T, Yan Y, Benjamin TL, Harrison SC. Structure of murine polyomavirus complexed with an oligosaccharide receptor fragment. Nature 1994;369:160–163.

169. Stern LB, Greenberg M, Gershoni JM, Rozenblatt S. The hemagglutinin envelope protein of canine distemper virus (CDV) confers cell tropism as illustrated by CDV and measles virus complementation analysis. J Virol 1995;69:1661–1668.

170. Strauss JH, Wang KS, Schmaljohn AL, Kuhn RJ, Strauss EG. Host-cell receptors for Sindbis virus. Arch Virol Suppl 1994;9:473–484.

171. Sueyoshi M, Tsuda T, Yamazaki K, et al. An immunohistochemical investigation of porcine epidemic diarrhoea. J Comp Pathol 1995; 113:59–67.

172. Sugden B, Mark W. Clonal transformation of adult human leukocytes by Epstein-Barr virus. J Virol 1977;23:503–508.

173. Sun N, Grzybicki D, Castro RF, Murphy S, Perlman S. Activation of astrocytes in the spinal cord of mice chronically infected with a neurotropic coronavirus. Virology 1995;213:482–493.

174. Suzuki Y. Gangliosides as influenza virus receptors: Variation of influenza viruses and their recognition of the receptor sialo-sugar chains. Prog Lipid Res 1994;33:429–457. Review.

175. Taguchi F. The S2 subunit of the murine coronavirus spike protein is not involved in receptor binding. J Virol 1995;69:7260–7263.

176. Tashiro M, Homma M. Pneumotropism of Sendai virus in relation to protease-mediated activation in mouse lungs. Infect Immun 1983; 39:879–888.

177. Tattersall P. Replication of the parvovirus MVM. I. Dependence of virus multiplication and plaque formation on cell growth. J Virol 1972;10:586.

178. Tresnan DB, Southard L, Weichert W, Sgro JY, Parrish CR. Analysis of the cell and erythrocyte binding activities of the dimple and canyon regions of the canine parvovirus capsid. Virology 1995; 211:123–132.

179. Truyen U, Agbandje M, Parrish CR. Characterization of the feline host range and a specific epitope of feline panleukopenia virus. Virology 1994;200:494–503.

180. Tsao J, Chapman MS, Agbandje M, et al. The three-dimensional structure of canine parvovirus and its functional implications. Science 1991;251:1456–1464.

181. Tucker SP, Compans RW. Virus infection of polarized epithelial cells. Adv Virus Res 1993;42:187–247.

182. Ubol S, Griffin DE. Identification of a putative alphavirus receptor on mouse neural cells. J Virol 1991;65:6913–6921.

183. van Zeijl M, Johann SV, Closs E, et al. A human amphotropic retrovirus receptor is a second member of the gibbon ape leukemia virus receptor family. Proc Natl Acad Sci U S A 1994;91:1168– 1172.

184. Vlasak R, Luytjes W, Leider J, Spaan W, Palese P. The E3 protein of bovine coronavirus is a receptor-destroying enzyme with acetylesterase activity. J Virol 1988;62:4686–4690.

185. Vlasak R, Luytjes W, Spaan W, Palese P. Human and bovine coronaviruses recognize sialic acid-containing receptors similar to those of influenza C viruses. Proc Natl Acad Sci U S A 1988; 85: 4526–4529.

186. Walter S, Richards R, Armentrout RW. Cell cycle-dependent replication of the DNA of minute virus of mice, a parvovirus. Biochim Biophys Acta 1996;607:420.

187. Wang JH, Yan YW, Garrett TP, et al. Atomic structure of a fragment of human CD4 containing two immunoglobulin-like domains. Nature 1990;348:411–418. Comments

188. Ward T, Pipkin PA, Clarkson NA, Stone DM, Minor PD, Almond JW. Decay-accelerating factor CD55 is identified as the receptor for echovirus 7 using CELICS, a rapid immuno-focal cloning method. EMBO J 1994;13:5070–5074.

189. Weiner HL, Powers ML, Fields BN. Absolute linkage of virulence and central nervous system cell tropism of reoviruses to viral hemagglutinin. J Infect Dis 1980;141:609–616.

189a. Weis W, Brown JH, Cusack S, Paulson JC, Skehel JJ, Wiley DC. Structure of the influenza virus hemagglutinin complexed with its receptor, siatic acid. Nature 1988;333:426–431.

190. Weiss RA, Tailor CS. Retrovirus receptors. Cell 1995;82:531– 533.

191. Wickham TJ, Filardo EJ, Cheresh DA, Nemerow GR. Integrin alpha v beta 5 selectively promotes adenovirus mediated cell membrane permeabilization. J Cell Biol 1994;127:257–264.

192. Wickham TJ, Mathias P, Cheresh DA, Nemerow GR. Integrins alpha v beta 3 and alpha v beta 5 promote adenovirus internalization but not virus attachment. Cell 1993;73:309–319.

193. Willey RL, Theodore TS, Martin MA. Amino acid substitutions in the human immunodeficiency virus type 1 gp120 V3 loop that change viral tropism also alter physical and functional properties of the virion envelope. J Virol 1994;68:4409–4419.

194. Williams RK, Jiang GS, Holmes KV. Receptor for mouse hepatitis virus is a member of the carcinoembryonic antigen family of glycoproteins. Proc Natl Acad Sci U S A 1991;88:5533–5536.

195. Willoughby RE, Yolken RH, Schnaar RL. Rotaviruses specifically bind to the neutral glycospingolipid asialo GM1. J Virol 1990; 64:4830–4835.

196. Wilson CA, Eiden MV, Anderson WB, Lehel C, Olah Z. The dual-function hamster receptor for amphotropic murine leukemia virus (MuLV), 10A1 MuLV, and gibbon ape leukemia virus is a phosphate symporter. J Virol 1995;69:534–537.

197. Wilson CA, Farrell KB, Eiden MV. Comparison of cDNAs encoding the gibbon ape leukaemia virus receptor from susceptible and nonsusceptible murine cells. J Gen Virol 1994;75:1901–1908.

198. WuDunn D, Spear PG. Initial interaction of herpes simplex virus with cells is binding to heparan sulfate. J Virol 1989;63:52–58.

199. Wykes MN, Shellam GR, McCluskey J, Kast WM, Dallas PB, Price P. Murine cytomegalovirus interacts with major histocompatibility complex class I molecules to establish cellular infection. J Virol 1993;67:4182–4189.

200. Xu R, Mohanty JG, Crowell RL. Receptor proteins on newborn Balb/c mouse brain cells for coxsackievirus B3 are immunologically distinct from those on HeLa cells. Virus Res 1995;35:323– 340.

201. Yahi N, Baghdiguian S, Moreau H, Fantini J. Galactosyl ceramide (or a closely related molecule) is the receptor for human immunodeficiency virus type 1 on human colon epithelial HT29 cells. Journal of Virology 1992;66:4848–4854.

202. Yahi N, Spitalnik SL, Stefano KA, De Micco P, Gonzalez-Scarano F, Fantini J. Interferon-gamma decreases cell surface expression of galactosyl ceramide, the receptor for HIV-1 GP120 on human colonic epithelial cells. Virology 1994;204:550–557. Erratum in Virology 1995;207(1):343.

203. Yeager CL, Ashmun RA, Williams RK, et al. Human aminopeptidase N is a receptor for human coronavirus 229E. Nature 1992; 357:420–422.

204. Yokomori K, Asanaka M, Stohlman SA, Lai MM. A spike protein-dependent cellular factor other than the viral receptor is required for mouse hepatitis virus entry. Virology 1993;196:45–56.

205. Yokomori K, Lai MM. Mouse hepatitis virus S RNA sequence reveals that nonstructural proteins ns4 and ns5a are not essential for murine coronavirus replication. J Virol 1991;65:5605–5608.

206. Yokomori K, Lai MMC. Mouse hepatitis virus utilizes two carcinoembryonic antigens as alternative receptors. J Virol 1992;66: 6194–6199.

Viral Pathogenesis,
edited by Neal Nathanson, et al.
Lippincott–Raven Publishers, Philadelphia © 1997

CHAPTER 4

Viral Effects on Cellular Functions

J. Marie Hardwick and Diane E. Griffin

INTRODUCTION

Being obligate intracellular parasites, viruses are intimately linked in every aspect of their life cycle to the host cell. Viruses weave their way through a myriad of cellular processes, beginning with the first virus–host cell receptor interaction. They

J. M. Hardwick and D. E. Griffin: Department of Molecular Microbiology and Immunology, Johns Hopkins University School of Public Health, Baltimore, Maryland 21205.

employ cellular transcription and replication factors, cellular translational machinery, and intracellular targeting and trafficking tools. Along this pathway, viruses also leave their mark on the cell, ending with the establishment of lifelong persistence, cell death, or clearance of the viral genome. Viruses can encode genes that induce, mimic, or modulate cellular functions for their own benefit (see Chap. 5). The effects of viruses on the host cell vary from essentially undetectable to tolerated manipulation to complete destruction. The viral and cellular factors that determine the outcome of virus infection often are delicately balanced, and a single amino acid change can dramatically alter subsequent events. The disruption of normal cellular functions, the induction of cell death, and activation of inappropriate immune responses by viruses are manifested as disease in the host organism. An increased understanding of the virus–host cell interactions that determine the outcome of virus infection is essential to the understanding of viral pathogenesis.

CELLULAR RESPONSES TO VIRUS–HOST CELL RECEPTOR INTERACTIONS

To gain access to the cell, viruses must first bind to a cellular receptor. A variety of cell surface molecules, including carbohydrates, glycolipids and proteins, can serve as receptors that specifically bind viral surface components (see Chaps. 2 and 3). The viral surface components of many, if not all, viruses mimic natural ligands; thus, viruses gain entry into cells by exploiting a previously existing cellular mechanism. Because many natural ligands mediate their action through receptor-signalling pathways, it is conceivable that the interaction of a virus with its cellular receptor is sufficient to trigger an alteration in host cell function. Thus, many viruses may elicit cellular responses prior to entering the cell.

Epstein-Barr Virus

The cellular receptor for Epstein-Barr virus (EBV) is CD21 (CR2), a 145-kD glycoprotein expressed on the cell surface.* CD21 normally serves as a receptor for components of the complement cascade iC3b, C3dg, and C3d.[468,517] Both C3d and a subset of anti-CD21 antibodies are capable of enhancing activation of B lymphocytes.[138,322,349] This information, together with the observation that B-cell activation occurs early following infection with EBV, suggested that the binding of EBV virions to their cellular receptor may also trigger a response similar to that of the natural ligand C3d. Subsequently, it was demonstrated that ultraviolet (UV)-inactivated EBV, which can bind cells but not express viral genes, was capable of initiating the activation of B cells.[165,204,314] The virion component responsible for directly contacting the receptor is gp350/220.[350,465] The region of gp350/220 involved in binding to CD21 was successfully predicted by virtue of its amino acid sequence similarity to a short segment of C3dg.[260,348] Thus, using a strategy of molecular mimicry, the virus can carry out some of the functions of the cell's natural ligands.

CD21 has a short cytoplasmic tail and probably does not transmit a signal. However, CD21 complexes with CD19, TAPA-1, and Leu-13 to mediate signal transduction.[46,122,459,469] Binding of gp350/220 to CD21 increases tyrosine phosphorylation on CD19.[443] This signal transduction pathway is apparently not required for virus entry but is important for efficient expression of EBV genes in primary B cells.[443] Thus, it appears that EBV can create an environment for successful infection by triggering a cell surface receptor and upregulating a signal

transduction pathway leading to the activation of quiescent B cells capable of expressing EBV genes.

Human Immunodeficiency Virus

The cellular receptor for the retrovirus human immunodeficiency virus (HIV) is the CD4 molecule that is expressed on a subset of T cells. The HIV-encoded glycoprotein responsible for binding to the cellular receptor is gp120. Acquired immunodeficiency syndrome (AIDS), the disease that results from HIV infection of humans, is characterized by the gradual depletion of CD4+ T cells. Although a direct infection of cells with the HIV virus may account for some cell loss, it has become evident that the majority of cells that die are uninfected. Only about 0.1% of peripheral blood T cells are infected with HIV, yet peripheral blood T cells from HIV-positive individuals are much more prone to undergo apoptotic cell death compared with cells from uninfected individuals when activated in vitro by engagement of the T-cell receptor (apoptosis is discussed later).[9,114,325] One of the mechanisms proposed to explain the loss of CD4+ T cells in AIDS is inappropriate signaling through the CD4 molecule. Crosslinking of the CD4 molecule on normal human CD4+ T cells by the HIV glycoprotein gp120 triggers apoptotic cell death.[18,81,266,301,368] This inappropriate cell death can be induced by gp120 expressed on transfected T cells[81,266] and by immune complexes of gp120 and anti-gp120 antibodies.[18,352,368] Injection of mice with crosslinking anti-CD4 antibodies also leads to CD4+ T-cell deletion by apoptosis.[200,510]

Other Viruses

The reovirus s1 protein is responsible for binding this nonenveloped virus to the cell surface. The interaction of strain T3D s1 protein with the cell surface appears to be sufficient to cause the rapid induction of apoptotic cell death in murine L929 cells.[491] This was determined by generating reassortant viruses with strain T1L, which induces cell death much less efficiently than T3D. The rapid-cell-death phenotype mapped to the S1 gene segment that encodes two proteins: s1 and s1s. UV-inactivated T3D virus is also capable of inducing cell death, eliminating a role for the nonstructural protein s1s. Thus, binding of s1 protein to a yet unknown reovirus receptor triggers the cell death pathway.

One of the host cell defense mechanisms against viruses is the production of interferons (IFN). IFN-α can be induced by cell surface contact with a variety of infectious agents. Induction of IFN-α by inactivated virus particles, isolated viral glycoproteins, or virus-infected cells fixed with glutaraldehyde has been demonstrated for several viruses, including herpes simplex virus (HSV), coronavirus, Sendai virus, adenovirus, and dengue virus.[61,161,212,254,481] The transmembrane glycoprotein M of the coronavirus-transmissible gastroenteritis virus is responsible for induction of IFN-α. Sequence analysis of 13 mutant viruses with impaired abilities to induce IFN-α mapped the important region of mature M protein to amino acids 6 through 22.[265]

---

*References 133, 137, 286, 311, 331, 351, 441, 477.

MODULATION OF HOST CELL TRANSCRIPTION

Inhibition of Cellular Transcription

The inhibition of cellular macromolecular synthesis is a common mechanism by which viruses selectively express their own genes at the expense of the cell. Many different classes of viruses, including poxviruses,[22] rhabdoviruses,[516,539] reoviruses,[439] paramyxoviruses,[530] and picornaviruses[318] have been shown to inhibit cellular RNA transcription; however, the molecular mechanisms for this inhibition are not well understood. In some cases, inhibition of transcription may be the indirect consequence of viral effects on protein synthesis, which decrease the availability of transcription factors required for RNA polymerase (pol) activity.

Vesicular Stomatitis Virus

Two mechanisms have been put forth to explain the potent inhibition of cell transcription by the rhabdovirus vesicular stomatitis virus (VSV). Early studies demonstrated that synthesis of viral RNA was required for inhibition of host transcription and attention was focused on the 45-nucleotide plus strand leader RNAs (complementary to the 3' end of the viral genome), which are capable of inhibiting transcription in vitro.[319,506] It was suggested that the leader RNA was capable of sequestering cellular proteins required for transcription.[171] Similar mechanisms were proposed for paramyxoviruses.[405] More recent work has focused on the matrix (M) protein of VSV, which appears to be primarily responsible for inhibition of host cell transcription.[38] This function is consistent with the observation that a fraction of the M protein is localized to the nucleus of infected cells.[304] A temperature-sensitive mutant of VSV ts082 defective in shutting off host cell function has a mutation in the M gene.[88] Furthermore, expression of M protein alone in transfected cells efficiently inhibits RNA transcription.[38,372]

M protein also has other functions, such as binding to cell membranes and facilitating the interaction between the ribonucleoprotein core and the transmembrane G protein. M is also potently cytopathic; this trait may correspond to its membrane-binding activity rather than to its inhibition of cellular transcription.[39,42,540] Deletions near the N-terminus of M abolish interactions with nucleocapsid and cellular membranes[540] but do not impair inhibition of host-directed pol II transcription or translocation of M to the nucleus.[39,372,540] In contrast, deletion of the 56 C-terminal residues abolished the ability of M to inhibit transcription from a nuclear reporter plasmid.[372] The mechanism by which M inhibits transcription is not known but probably does not involve inhibition of translation of factors critical for the transcription machinery, because M does not appear to affect cellular translation.[37]

Poliovirus

Poliovirus-induced inhibition of pol I, pol II, and pol III transcription is correlated with inactivation of specific transcription factors. Within hours after infection, cellular extracts are unable to transcribe pol II templates.[90] Inhibition of pol II is dependent on viral protein synthesis[401] and is associated with a reduction in the active form of pol II, which is bound to chromatin.[400] Binding of upstream stimulatory factor, a 46-kD general host transcription factor that binds 60 base pairs upstream from the pol II transcription start site, is impaired in poliovirus-infected cells.[269] Nuclear extracts from poliovirus-infected cells are deficient in the ability to transcribe from the adenovirus major late promoter probably as a result of inactivation of TFIID, a complex of the TATA-binding protein (TBP), and a collection of associated proteins called TAFs (TBP-associated factors).[96,243] TFIID inactivation and inhibition of pol II transcription are correlated with cleavage of TBP by the viral protease 3C.[75,95]

Transcription of pol I and pol III is also inhibited in poliovirus-infected cells. Decreased pol I transcription of rRNA correlates with a deficiency in initiation factors[418] and with an alteration in the pol I promoter DNA-protein complexes that is apparently the result of cleavage of pol I transcription factors by the 3C protease.[419] Inhibition of pol III transcription appears to be mediated by a decrease in the activities of transcription factors IIIC (TFIIIC) and IIIB (TFIIIB).[73,139] TFIIIC and is cleaved by the 3C protease. Polioviruses with mutations in this protease have a limited ability to inhibit pol III transcription.[74]

The foot-and-mouth disease virus (FMDV) protease 3C cleaves histone H3, resulting in deletion of the N-terminal domain, which is involved in the regulation of transcriptionally active chromatin. The C-terminal portion of H3 (Pi) remains associated with chromatin.[119] This cleavage correlates with decreased RNA transcription.[471]

Lymphocytic Choriomeningitis Virus Auxiliary Function

Infection of newborn mice with lymphocytic choriomeningitis virus (LCMV) causes growth retardation and low serum glucose levels due to growth hormone deficiency.[364,365] The anterior pituitary cells that produce growth hormone are targets of LCMV. Infection of these cells with LCMV does not result in cell death or obvious structural injury but instead results in a persistent infection in which the cells survive but progeny virus continues to be produced.[364,365] Persistent LCMV results in decreased transcription of growth hormone mRNA in mouse pituitary.[242,497] Despite a decrease in growth hormone gene expression, expression of other pituitary genes, thyroid-stimulating hormone and prolactin, and several housekeeping genes was minimally affected.[99,242] Even in cultured PC rat pituitary cells that express both prolactin and growth hormone, growth hormone transcription was selectively downregulated by LCMV infection.[99] A region of the growth hormone promoter containing the binding sites for growth hormone transactivation factor GHF1/Pit1 appears to be responsible for the selective reduction in growth hormone gene expression.[99] This is somewhat surprising, because GHF1/Pit1 also regulates its own promoter and that of prolactin, both of which are only modestly affected by LCMV infection.[99] Although GHF1/Pit1 is sufficient to activate the growth hormone promoter in transient transfection assays in HeLa cells, other factors may also modulate growth hormone gene expression to explain the observed promoter specificity. Furthermore, a splice variant of

GHF1/Pit1, GHF2, which contains a 26–amino acid insertion in the activation domain, can enhance the expression of growth hormone but not prolactin or itself.[474]

LCMV also establishes a persistent infection in neurons of the brain. Although LCMV is a noncytolytic virus and neurons of infected animals do not show structural damage or deletion, these mice exhibit behavioral abnormalities.[163] Infected mice were deficient in their ability to learn a Y-maze discrimination. Although the molecular mechanism of this abnormality is not known, the effect of scopolamine on infected mice suggests a cholinergic defect.[163] Neuroblastoma cells persistently infected with LCMV have suppressed levels of acetyl cholinesterase.[363] Persistence of LCMV in thyroid gland epithelial cells also downregulates thyroglobulin mRNA and reduces circulating thyroid hormones.[240,241] Thus, disease states can result from persistent virus infections in which the cells remain viable but have impaired auxiliary functions.

Inhibition of Processing of Cellular mRNAs

VSV, influenza virus, and HSV are known to interfere with splicing of pre-mRNAs to form mature mRNAs. VSV inhibits the maturation of U1 and U2 snRNPs necessary for splicing of cellular pre-mRNAs, but the mechanism by which it does this has not been determined.[91,140] The influenza RNA-binding protein NS1 inhibits pre-mRNA splicing.[136,347] Spliceosomes are formed, but subsequent catalytic steps are inhibited.[299] Spliceosomes contain NS1 bound to a purine-containing bulge in the stem structure of the key U6 spliceosomal RNA, inhibiting U6-U2 and U6-U4 snRNA interactions.[299,396] The ICP27 protein of HSV suppresses RNA splicing by an unknown mechanism, leading to reduced amounts of cellular mRNAs from intron-containing genes and accumulation of pre-mRNAs.[179]

Direct Activation of Cellular Transcription by Viral Proteins

Many viruses encode transcription factors for the purpose of regulating expression of their own genes. For example, all herpesviruses encode proteins that bind directly to specific viral DNA sequences and regulate the transcription of other viral genes. Some viral transcription factors have been found to modulate the expression of cellular genes as well.

Epstein-Barr Virus

The Epstein-Barr nuclear antigen 2 (EBNA2) protein is a transcription factor that activates the expression of the viral latency membrane protein (LMP) genes[1,512,558] and the latency Cp promoter[215,413,455] as well as several cellular genes, including CD21,[264] CD23,[288,511] and c-fgr.[244] The transactivation activity of EBNA2 correlates with the ability of EBV to induce growth transformation in B lymphocytes.[82,83,177] Studies have provided clues to the mechanism by which EBNA2 regulates gene expression. EBNA2 does not bind to DNA directly but rather is tethered to DNA by a cellular factor CBF1/RBPJk, the mammalian homolog of the *Drosophila* gene.† CBF1/-

RBPJk facilitates downregulation of cellular gene transcription, and this repression is counteracted by the direct interaction of EBNA2 with CBF1/RBPJk.[201] In addition to its CBF1/RBPJk-binding domain, EBNA2 contains an acidic activation domain that directly contacts the cellular transcriptional machinery to facilitate initiation of transcription.[290,486] Thus, EBNA2 induces the expression of cellular genes that would otherwise be turned off by CBF1/RBPJk. In this regard, EBNA2 is a functional homolog of the cellular *Notch* gene product.

Human T-Cell Lymphotropic Virus Type I

Tax is a transcription factor encoded by the retrovirus human T-cell lymphotropic virus type I (HTLV-I), which causes adult T-cell leukemia and tropical spastic paraparesis.[34,158,447,531] Tax is important in regulating viral gene expression and is a key factor in pathogenesis, because Tax alone can transform human T lymphocytes.[93,166,463] Tax induces expression of viral genes via a 21–base pair repeat in the viral long terminal repeat (LTR). Tax does not appear to bind DNA directly[148,160,308] but instead binds to the cellular transcription factor CREB, which recognizes the cAMP response element (CRE) within the LTR.[24,28,456,543] Tax appears to stimulate transcription by two mechanisms: increasing the binding affinity of CREB for the LTR and directly activating transcription through its own activation domain.[160,435,507,552] However, Tax does not activate all promoters containing CREs.[147] Furthermore, Tax activates other viral and cellular promoters through different transcription factors. For example, Tax activates expression of the IL-2 receptor through an NFkB-binding site[277] and activates the c-*fos* gene through SRF and AP-2 sites.[144,145] It is not known how Tax can achieve selective transcription regulation through such a wide variety of cellular factors.

CREB itself belongs to an extended basic-zipper (bZIP) transcription factor family. The conserved basic region of bZIP proteins binds directly to DNA and is immediately adjacent to the zipper dimerization domain. Because the basic region of bZIP proteins makes direct contact with DNA, it was surprising to discover that the basic region also binds to Tax.[19,383] Furthermore, Tax can modulate the binding affinity of a particular bZIP factor for a particular DNA sequence, presumably leading to the selective regulation of transcription. However, the versatility of Tax must extend beyond bZIP proteins to explain its interaction with NFkB components and p67SRF[146,196]

Induction of Cellular Transcription by Indirect Mechanisms

A number of RNA viruses induce the synthesis of alpha and beta IFN-α and IFN-β, including some IFN-responsive proteins and heat shock proteins. Synthesis of these cellular proteins is the result of virus infection but may not be directly the result of viral transactivators.

---

† References 172, 187, 268, 289, 509, 557.

Interferons Alpha and Beta

Synthesis of IFN-α and IFN-β are not detectable in uninfected cells because of active repression but can be induced by virus binding to the cell surface (discussed previously), virus infection, or dsRNA.[94,390,436] The control of IFN induction is primarily at the level of transcription, although the rate of IFN mRNA turnover can also be regulated. Transcriptional activation of IFN by virus infection does not require host cell protein synthesis, suggesting that latent cellular factors become activated.[94,390] Induction of IFN-β requires transport of the transcriptional activators interferon regulatory factor (IRF)-1, NFkB, and 4MG-1 to the nucleus.[436] IFN-α gene expression also requires translocation of IRF-1 to the nucleus, but the IFN-α promotor contains the GAAAGT sequence rather than NFkB-binding sites and requires binding of 68- and 96-kD TG proteins.[436] IFN-α is induced primarily in lymphoid and monocytoid cells. Both IRF-1 and IRF-2 mRNAs are constitutively expressed, but binding to the promotor by the negative regulator IRF-2 predominates because it is the more stable protein.[164,464] After exposure to dsRNA and activation of IFN-β transcription, IRF-2 is proteolytically cleaved, leaving an N-terminal DNA-binding domain with increased affinity for the promotor and postinduction repression of IFN-β expression.[527] Some IFN-inducible genes can be transactivated directly by virus or dsRNA without requiring IFN synthesis through activation of dsRNA-activated factors.[94] Activation is dependent on phosphorylation, because inhibitors of tyrosine kinase and protein kinase C block activation.[94]

Cellular Stress Proteins

Cells induce production of a number of proteins in response to environmental stresses such as heat shock. These proteins play major roles in protein folding, translocation, and formation of macromolecular complexes. Members of the 70-kD family of stress protein genes are particularly likely to be induced.[385] Adenoviruses,[223,385] SV40 and polyoma viruses,[234] HSV-1,[356,385] and cytomegalovirus (CMV)[428] induce expression of hsp70, whereas paramyxoviruses SV5 and Sendai induce expression of grp78 (Bip).[378,514] Induction of these proteins does not appear to be a generalized cellular response to the stress of viral infection but rather a specific response with induction of only selected members of these protein families.[385] For instance, adenovirus and HSV-1 induce hsp70 but not other members of the 70-kD family or hsp90, which is also highly heat inducible, do so.[385] In contrast, paramyxoviruses induce grp78 but not hsp70, and this appears to occur in response to synthesis of large amounts of the viral hemagluttinin-neuraminidase (HN) glycoprotein and subsequent flux of proteins through the endoplasmic reticulum.[378,514] Activation of hsp70 is associated primarily with DNA viruses that replicate in the nucleus and encode promiscuous immediate early transactivators that may activate this gene directly.[223,356,467,529] The responsible adenovirus transactivator appears to be the product of the E1A 13S message.[223,467,532] Polyoma virus large T antigen transactivates the hsp70 promotor indirectly.[237]

MODULATION OF HOST PROTEIN SYNTHESIS

Inhibition of Translation of Cellular Proteins

Shutoff of host protein synthesis while viral protein synthesis continues is a characteristic of many, but not all, virus infections. Most of the viruses that inhibit translation of host mRNA affect global protein synthesis, but some viruses decrease synthesis of only a few cellular proteins. The best studied examples of viruses that inhibit cellular protein synthesis globally are the picornaviruses, alphaviruses, orthomyxoviruses, rhabdoviruses, adenoviruses, and herpesviruses. Viruses in each of these families alter translation of cellular mRNAs in different ways, and each has evolved a mechanism for assuring that mRNAs for viral proteins, usually the late structural proteins needed for virion assembly, continue to be translated. Many of these viruses inhibit the primary mechanism of translational initiation used by cells and then employ alternative mechanisms of initiation for which viral mRNAs are better suited than most cellular mRNAs.

Shutoff mechanisms employed by viruses include inactivation of translation factors, degradation of host cell mRNAs, production of factors that specifically inhibit cellular mRNA translation or facilitate viral mRNA translation, viral mRNAs that outcompete cellular mRNAs for the translation machinery, and changes in the intracellular ionic environment that favor translation of viral mRNAs.[226,432] Many viruses employ multiple mechanisms to control translation of cellular mRNAs, so that often no one mechanism completely explains the effect of the virus on cellular protein synthesis. In turn, cells have mechanisms for inhibiting translation of virus proteins and many viruses encode proteins or RNAs that suppress these cellular defenses.

Overview of Cellular mRNA Translation

Protein synthesis is divided into three phases: initiation, elongation, and termination (Fig. 4-1). The rate-limiting steps occur primarily during initiation. There are four major steps in the initiation of translation: dissociation of 80S ribosomes into 40S and 60S subunits, binding of initiator Met-tRNA to 40S ribosomes, binding of mRNA to the 43S ribosomal initiation complex, and junction of the 60S subunit with the mRNA-containing 48S initiation complex.[190]

Dissociation of 80S ribosomes to free the 40S subunit for initiation involves eukaryotic initiation factor (eIF)-1A and eIF-3 and does not appear to be a tightly regulated or rate-limiting step. Binding of initiator Met-tRNA to 40S ribosomal subunits requires the formation of a complex of Met-tRNA, eIF-2, and GTP, as well as subsequent binding and stabilization of this complex onto the 40S subunit by eIF-3 and eIF-1A (see Fig. 4–1). This step is highly regulated by variable phosphorylation of the participating initiation factors and is rate limiting. It is a frequent site for virus-induced inhibition.[112,191]

The eIF-2 translation factors are essential for GTP-dependent Met-tRNA binding to the 40S ribosomal subunit and for recycling of initiation factors. To function in another round of initiation, eIF-2 must exchange GDP for GTP. This reaction requires catalysis by eIF-2B and is dependent on the phosphory-

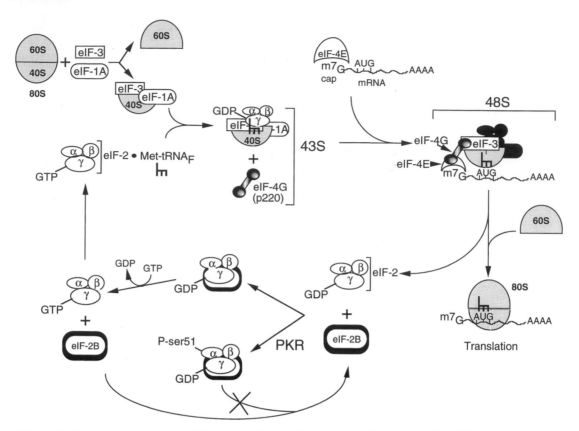

FIG. 4-1. Overview of cellular mRNA translation initiation. In the first phase, the 40S ribosomal subunit is freed by eIF-1A and eIF-3. In the second phase, met-tRNA, eIF-2, and GTP complex and bind to the ribosome to form the 43S initiation complex. In the third phase, mRNA binding to the 43S complex is facilitated by association of the mRNA with the cap-binding complex and results in the formation of the 48S initiation complex. In the fourth phase, the 60S ribosomal subunit joins with the 48S complex to begin formation of peptide bonds and releases most of the initiation factors, including eIF-2-GDP, which is recycled back to eIF-2-GTP by guanine nucleotide exchange factor eIF-2B. PKR, protein kinase RNA-dependent; eIF, eukaryotic initiation factor.

lation state of the α subunit of eIF-2. When eIF-α is phosphorylated a stable complex of GDP, eIF-2 and eIF-2B forms. Phosphorylation of eIF-2α has negative effects on the initiation of protein synthesis, because this prevents recycling of eIF-2-GDP to eIF-2-GTP by recycling factor eIF-2B, because eIF-2B is trapped in an inactive complex with eIF-2-GDP. Because eIF-2B is present in limiting amounts, translation is inhibited. Translation, therefore, can be regulated by controlling the extent to which eIF-2α is phosphorylated (see Fig. 4–1).[426]

The protein kinase responsible for phosphorylation of eIF-2α is protein kinase RNA-dependent (PKR; also known as p68 and DAI), a 68-kD cAMP-independent serine/threonine kinase associated with ribosomes.[33,199] The PKR protein has two well-characterized domains: an N-terminal regulatory domain that contains the dsRNA-binding site and a C-terminal catalytic domain that contains all of the conserved motifs for protein kinase activity.[20,324] PKR is activated in a dose-dependent manner by dsRNA, which leads to ATP-dependent autophosphorylation. The active form of PKR is postulated to be a dimer with two PKR molecules binding a molecule of dsRNA. When large amounts of dsRNA are present, PKR activation is decreased, because saturation of dsRNA-binding

sites shift the equilibrium toward monomers. Although some RNAs are more potent activators than others,[188] there are no sequence requirements for the dsRNA; however there are size requirements, because at least 50 base pairs of duplex appear to be necessary.[315] Phosphorylated PKR, in turn, phosphorylates eIF-2α on Ser-51.[199] PKR control of cellular protein synthesis is regulated by a 97-kD phosphoprotein that can dephosphorylate PKR in response to growth signals[211] and by a 58-kD repressor that prevents PKR and eIF-2α phosphorylation.[273] The 58-kD PKR inhibitor is a highly conserved member of the tetratricopeptide repeat family of proteins[272] and is activated during influenza virus infection.[273]

Binding of the mRNA to the loaded 43S ribosomal initiation complex in mammalian cells occurs primarily through a scanning mechanism.[251] Most cellular mRNAs are capped and polyadenylated. The cap at the 5' end is composed of 7mGppp (m⁷ GTP) covalently linked to the first nucleotide of the mRNA. Translation is initiated when the m7G-cap structure is recognized by the eIF-4 cap-binding protein complex. The eIF-4 group of translation initiation factors includes eIF-4A, a 46-kD ATP-dependent helicase; eIF-4B, a 70-kD RNA-binding phosphoprotein that enhances eIF-4A activity; eIF-4E, a

25-kD cap-binding phosphoprotein, and eIF-4G (p220), a 154-kD phosphoprotein that complexes with eIF-4A, eIF-4B, eIF-4E, and eIF-3. Data suggest that eIF-4G is present in the 43S ribosomal initiation complex and that free eIF-4E binds to capped mRNA with subsequent binding of the eIF-4E-mRNA complex to the 43S complex through eIF-4G (Fig. 4–1).[220] Cellular translational activity can be controlled by altering the phosphorylation state of eIF-4E. eIF-4E is underphosphorylated at times of restricted protein synthesis (e.g., during mitosis, after serum deprivation, after heat shock) and becomes phosphorylated on Ser-53 after mitogen stimulation or serum activation.[191] This step in translation is vulnerable to virus-induced control through cleavage of eIF-4G by viral proteases and alteration of the level of phosphorylation of eIF-4E.

The structure of the 5' nontranslated region (NTR) of the mRNA is an important determinant of translation efficiency in different circumstances.[250,251] Secondary structure may determine initial interactions with the ribosome, binding of cellular proteins that facilitate or inhibit translation, and recognition of the initiator AUG. However, the initiation complex appears to have a limited ability to melt duplex regions of RNA, so that mRNAs with extensive secondary structure in the 5'NTR may be inefficiently translated.[250,251] Reduced 5' secondary structure enhances translation initiation and decreases the requirement for the cap-binding complex, because eIF-4A and 4B can bind to unstructured RNA in a cap-independent fashion.[2,3] This property is used to advantage by a number of viruses that have unstructured 5'NTRs.

Protein synthesis is also dependent on the intracellular concentrations of K^+ and Ca^{2+}, pH, and redox potential.[302] Alterations in membrane integrity that allow K^+ to leak from the cell and intracellular $[K^+]$ to decrease are associated with decreased protein synthesis, which can be restored by increasing the concentration of K^+ in the extracellular fluid.[302] The mechanism by which these ionic changes affect translation is not known.

Picornaviruses

Most picornaviruses shut down host cell protein synthesis within a few hours after infection, whereas synthesis of viral proteins continues. Multiple mechanisms are employed to accomplish this task, and these include cleavage of initiation factor eIF-4G, phosphorylation of eIF-2α, and alteration of the intracellular ionic environment of the cell.

Initiation Factor Cleavage

Early studies of picornavirus-infected cells localized the defect in cellular protein synthesis to the initiation step of translation of host mRNAs.[275,528] Subsequently, it was shown that capped mRNAs were unable to associate with the 40S ribosomal subunits from infected cells. These cellular mRNAs remained intact and translatable in vitro but were not translated in infected cells.[130,247] During poliovirus infection, this defect is due at least in part to the inactivation of the cap-binding protein complex (eIF-4) during poliovirus infection.[116,270] Decline in host protein synthesis is preceded by cleavage of eIF-4G (also known as eIF-4γ and p220) to peptides of 100 to 130 kD,[117] which separates the functional domains of eIF-4G. The N-terminal portion contains the binding site for eIF-4E (cap-binding protein), and the C-terminal portion contains the binding sites for eIF-3 (ribosome-binding protein) and eIF-4A (helicase). Therefore, eIF-4G cleavage during poliovirus infection uncouples cap recognition and ribosome binding (Fig. 4-2).[261]

eIF-4G can be cleaved by calcium-dependent cellular enzymes,[533] and initial studies suggested that viral infection activated a cellular protease[292]; however, more recent data indicate that viral proteases are directly responsible for eIF-4G cleavage.[274] Poliovirus encodes 2 proteases, 3C, and 2A.[391] Several pieces of evidence indicate that the small cysteine protease 2A mediates cleavage of eIF-4G. Synthesis of 2A correlates with eIF-4G cleavage, and 2A cleaves eIF-4G in vitro.[253] Mutation of 2A results in viruses that cannot inhibit host protein synthesis early in infection or induce cleavage of eIF-4G.[32] Cleavage of eIF-4G in cellular extracts requires the presence of eIF-3, but the reason for this is not clear,[534,535] and eIF-3 is not required when purified components are used in vitro.[262]

The 2A proteases of enteroviruses and rhinoviruses contain an active site that recognizes the sequence Ile/Leu-X-Thr-X*Gly and processes the viral polyprotein between VP1 and 2A.[180,181,448] This amino acid sequence corresponds to the mapped site of rhinovirus- and coxsackievirus 2A–induced cleavage of eIF-4G, further suggesting that 2A acts directly on eIF-4G.[262]

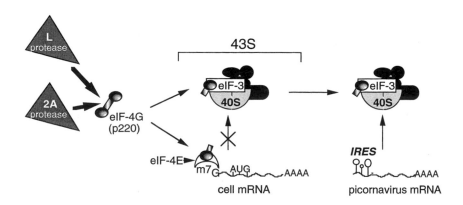

FIG. 4-2. Selective translation of picornavirus RNAs. Cleavage of eIF-4G by the 2A protease of enteroviruses and rhinoviruses or the L protease of foot and mouth disease virus (FMDV) separates the cap-binding and ribosome-binding functions of eIF-4G so that capped cellular mRNAs are no longer bound efficiently to the 43S ribosomal initiation complex. Picornavirus RNAs with an internal ribosomal entry site (IRES) are preferentially translated.

Not all picornaviruses encode a 2A with the conserved 18–amino acid cysteine protease sequence in the C-terminal portion of 2A required for eIF-4G cleavage. FMDV 2A contains only 16 of the 18 necessary conserved active site amino acids.[291] However, a similar protease function is present within protein L, which is encoded within the FMDV leader sequence. L is a protease that induces cleavage of eIF-4G (see Fig. 4–2).[103] The L cleavage site is distinct from the 2A cleavage site, but both are in the same region of the eIF-4G protein, suggesting conservation of function in the evolution of these viruses.[238] FMDV strains with a mutation that prevents expression of the L gene induce shutoff of host protein synthesis more slowly than do viruses with a functional L and grow to a lower titer than wild-type virus.[386] The cardioviruses do not encode either a 2A or an L protease and do not induce cleavage of eIF-4G.[291]

The RNAs of enteroviruses (e.g., poliovirus), cardioviruses (e.g., encephalomyocarditis virus [EMCV]), and apthoviruses (e.g., FMDV) all lack the methylated cap structures that are found on most cellular mRNAs and are required for efficient translation of cellular mRNA.[130] Picornaviruses initiate translation of viral RNA through a cap-independent mechanism that uses an internal ribosomal entry site (IRES) in the 5'NTR of the uncapped viral RNA.[431] The 5'NTR binds the cellular RNA-binding protein La, which appears to be involved in facilitating internal initiation of translation.[321] Capped cellular mRNAs with reduced secondary structure can also initiate translation in poliovirus-infected cells, demonstrating the reduced need of such mRNAs for the cap-binding complex. Translation of uncapped mRNAs with a 5'IRES is more efficient when eIF-4G is cleaved, suggesting decreased competition from capped cellular mRNAs.[274,556]

Activation of PKR and Phosphorylation of eIF-2a

Cleavage of eIF-4G appears to be necessary, but not sufficient, for complete shutoff of host mRNA translation during picornavirus infection.[45,96,380] Viruses with mutations in 2A exhibit delayed inhibition of protein synthesis,[32] and this later inhibition correlates with the phosphorylation of eIF-2α.[361] PKR is activated during poliovirus infection, apparently by dsRNA replicative intermediates, which bind PKR and induce autophosphorylation at four sites (Fig. 4-3).[41,475] PKR is also significantly degraded in poliovirus-infected cells.[41] The protease responsible for PKR degradation, which requires divalent cations and RNA, has not been identified but does not appear to be a viral protease.[40] It has also been reported that poliovirus induces an 80- to 100-kD cellular inhibitor of PKR-mediated phosphorylation of eIF-2α.[402]

Alteration of Intracellular Cation Concentrations

The cardioviruses EMCV and Theiler's murine encephalomyelitis virus do not encode a protease that cleaves eIF-4G but

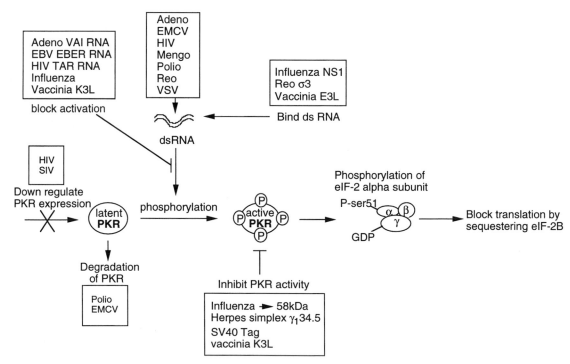

FIG. 4-3. Regulation of protein kinase RNA-dependent (PKR) activity by viral functions. Latent PKR is activated by binding dsRNA and undergoing autophosphorylation. Phosphorylation of the alpha subunit of eIF-2 by activated PKR leads to a stable complex between eIF-2 and the guanine nucleotide exchange factor eIF-2B, thereby blocking initiation of translation. Many viruses encode functions that regulate the production, degradation, activation, and activity of PKR. EBER, Epstein-Barr virus–encoded small RNA; EBV, Epstein–Barr virus.

do shut off host protein synthesis.[213,334] This shutoff is probably linked to altered cation transport. Infection with picornaviruses alters cation flux[120,342] with dramatic decreases in K+ flux beginning 4 to 5 hours after infection.[55,120] Changes in K+ flux parallel decreases in host protein synthesis.[295] Increased intracellular [Na+] decreases cellular mRNA translation but improves the translation of picornaviral RNA.[55] Treatment of poliovirus-infected cells with the ionophores monensin and nigericin prevents the inhibition of host translation.[209]

Alphaviruses

Alphaviruses, such as Sindbis virus and Semliki Forest virus, dramatically decrease host protein synthesis within 3 hours after infection of a susceptible cell.[340] As with the picornaviruses, multiple mechanisms may contribute to this shutoff. Competition of viral mRNA for the translation machinery has been postulated, but competition is unlikely to be the sole mechanism.[451] The capsid protein binds to ribosomes and can inhibit translation of cellular RNA and viral genomic RNA in vitro,[498] but there is little evidence that this is important in infected cells. Expression of the nonstructural proteins alone is sufficient to inhibit host protein synthesis.[142] Changes in intracellular cation concentrations correlate most closely with decreases in host protein synthesis.[86,154,155] Intracellular [K+] decreases and [Na+] increases during infection.[154] These changes in ionic environment are dependent on synthesis of the viral glycoproteins[495] and appear to be due to inhibition of cellular Na+,K+-ATPase activity.[156,496] Treatment of infected cells with tunicamycin prevents inhibition of Na+,K+-ATPase, but partial inhibition of host protein synthesis still occurs, suggesting that altered ionic conditions are only partially responsible for decreased translation of host mRNAs.[167,495]

Late during infection, initiation factors for translation lose the ability to support translation of host and 42S genomic RNA, which encodes nonstructural proteins, but can translate 26S subgenomic RNA, which encodes the structural proteins, and EMCV RNA.[29,499] Translational capacity is restored with addition of eIF-4B and eIF-4E. The cap structure of subgenomic 26S RNA binds more efficiently to eIF-4B and eIF-4E than to 42S RNA[29] and therefore requires lower concentrations of eIF-4B and eIF-4E for optimal translation.[500] In addition, sequences downstream from the initiator AUG have a predicted hairpin-like structure. This structure enhances translation in infected cells but not uninfected cells, possibly by causing the ribosome to pause, thus allowing initiation factors present in low concentrations to bind to the translation complex.[141,143] Sindbis virus infection activates PKR, suggesting that phosphorylation of eIF-2α may also play a role in decreased protein synthesis.[424]

Orthomyxoviruses

Influenza virus induces the shutoff of host protein synthesis, and this is associated with an inhibition of elongation as well as initiation of translation of cellular mRNAs.[152,227] Multiple mechanisms are used to effect this shutoff. Influenza virus infection is associated with dephosphorylation and inactivation of eIF-4E[123] and hyperphosphorylation of eIF-4G. Viral mRNAs appear to require smaller amounts of active eIF-2 and eIF-4E than cellular mRNAs, a surprising observation because the cap and the first 10 to 15 nucleotides of influenza viral mRNAs are "snatched" from cellular mRNAs.[153] However, cellular RNA segments with the least secondary structure, which are therefore the most efficiently translated, are selectively snatched. In addition, the NS1 RNA-binding protein prevents export of spliced mRNAs to the cytoplasm by binding to poly(A) tails of mRNAs in the nucleus[8,394,395] and enhances the translation of viral RNAs.[98]

Infected cells contain a protein that interferes with the activation of PKR.[229] It was originally postulated that the PKR inhibitor was a viral protein,[231] but subsequent studies revealed that influenza virus infection activates a 58-kD cellular inhibitor of PKR.[273] This inhibitor represses phosphorylation of eIF-2α by activated PKR and autophosphorylation of PKR.[273] The RNA-binding protein NS1 can also bind dsRNA and prevent activation of PKR (see Fig. 4–3).[300]

Rhabdoviruses

VSV infection of cells results in rapid inhibition of cellular protein synthesis.[518] This inhibition requires synthesis of viral proteins[313] and is mediated, at least in part, by activation of PKR (see Fig. 4–3).[58] In this environment, viral mRNAs are preferentially translated because of sequences residing in the 5' end of the viral mRNA.[30] The exact mechanism of inhibition of translation is unclear, but it is separable from the effect of VSV on cellular transcription, which is effected by the VSV M protein.[37]

Adenoviruses

Adenoviruses inhibit cellular protein synthesis late in the replication cycle, and viral mRNAs are preferentially translated.[26] Adenovirus infection induces underphosphorylation of eIF-4E, providing further evidence for cap-independent translation of late adenovirus mRNAs.[203] Inhibition of eIF-4E phosphorylation occurs in response to synthesis of the late adenovirus proteins.[550] mRNAs for the late adenovirus proteins are produced from a single long primary transcript that is differentially spliced to produce 3' coterminal mRNAs with a common 5'NTR. This 5' region is coded in three separate segments of the viral DNA which are joined by splicing of the primary late transcript, and the final product is termed the tripartite leader.[31] This 200-nucleotide leader significantly enhances the efficiency of translation of mRNAs late, but not early in infection.[294] The first segment of the tripartite leader is unstructured, a property consistent with its ability to enhance translation and provide independence from the cap-binding complex.[106,549] The second and third portions of the leader have significant secondary structure, which may enhance the binding of cellular elongation factors. The tripartite leader allows translation in poliovirus-infected cells[107] and therefore is not dependent on intact eIF-4G.

Adenoviruses also inhibit the export of cellular mRNAs from the nucleus to the cytoplasm through the action of the E1b 55-kD and E4 34-kD proteins.[16,26] This transport block is selective[330] and does not contribute significantly to the decrease in cellular protein synthesis because mRNAs already in the cytoplasm are abundant but untranslated,[15] and 2-aminopurine prevents suppression of cellular mRNA translation without disrupting the transport block.[202]

Adenoviruses with mutations that prevent production of virus-associated RNA-I (VAI), a small (160-nucleotide) pol III transcript, do not synthesize viral or cellular proteins efficiently late after infection because of activation of PKR, which leads to phosphorylation of eIF-2α.[360,408,442] Activation of PKR occurs late in infection, presumably through production of viral transcripts with extensive secondary structure.[359] VAI-RNA binds PKR efficiently[317] and inhibits PKR activation and subsequent eIF-2a phosphorylation.[239,433] Low levels of VAI-RNA activate PKR, whereas high levels inactivate this kinase.[150] VAI-RNA is produced in abundance late in infection and may prevent activation of PKR by complexing with it in large amounts[150,159,228] or by physically interfering with the kinase domain.[323] VAI-RNA cannot inhibit PKR activity once PKR has been activated.[360] VAI-RNA may also interact with a cellular PKR inhibitor[411] and may even encode a protein that stabilizes ribosome-bound mRNAs.[452] Shutoff of host protein synthesis is prevented by 2-aminopurine without impairing PKR activation or phosphorylation of eIF-2α.[202] This suggests that activation of PKR and phosphorylation of eIF-2α may be required, but are not sufficient, for inhibition of host cell protein synthesis during adenovirus infection.

Herpesviruses

HSV, particularly type 2, infection of permissive cells is characterized by rapid cessation of cellular protein synthesis while viral mRNA continues to be translated.[129,412] Complete shutoff of host protein synthesis is probably a multistep process.[124] Initial shutoff is mediated by a structural component of the HSV virion[129] that leads to degradation of host mRNA and disaggregation of polyribosomes.[127,255,446] Mutations in the virion host shutoff (vhs) gene result in viruses that can still induce shutoff, but it is delayed and incomplete.[118,125,126,256] The vhs protein, a 58-kD polypeptide that can be phosphorylated, induces rapid turnover of viral mRNAs as well as host mRNAs.[255,256] The less phosphorylated form of vhs is incorporated into the virion, where it is complexed with the virion transactivator VP16 in the tegument.[407,445] Vhs is the only viral gene product needed for increased degradation of mRNA[219,373] and probably acts by interacting with a cellular factor.[256] However, in vivo, an intact UL13 gene is also necessary for vhs-induced shutoff.[367] Vhs mutant viruses are viable but have a 5- to 10-fold reduction in virus yield and exhibit altered patterns of viral protein synthesis during infection.[406,446] Although the stability of both host and viral mRNAs are decreased by vhs, there is some evidence that a newly synthesized viral protein may allow accumulation of viral mRNAs after host mRNAs have been degraded.[128]

The secondary stage of host shutoff further reduces host protein synthesis and requires prior viral gene expression.[124,412] Viruses with mutations in ICP27 have a decreased ability to shutoff host protein synthesis,[423] suggesting that a decrease in pre-mRNA splicing contributes to decreases in host protein synthesis (discussed previously). The $\gamma_1$34.5 protein of HSV blocks the premature shutoff of host protein synthesis that oc-

curs with the onset of viral DNA synthesis.[70] PKR associates with a phosphorylated 90-kD protein, leading to phosphorylation of eIF-2α in cells infected with viruses that lack the functional C-terminus of $\gamma_1$34.5.[69]

Other Viruses

Coronaviruses decrease cellular protein synthesis and enhance viral protein synthesis by inducing degradation of some (e.g., actin), but not all, cellular mRNAs[193,257] and by producing viral mRNAs with a leader sequence that competes effectively with cellular mRNAs for translation.[458]

The HIV tat-responsive sequence has a stable stem-bulge-loop structure with an intrinsic ability to bind and activate PKR,[317,320] inducing phosphorylation of eIF-2α. This activation is downregulated by expression of the Tat regulatory protein, which binds this region of RNA.[417] HIV-infected lymphoid cells have decreased amounts of cellular mRNAs, apparently as a result of increased degradation.[4]

Vaccinia virus probably employs multiple virion-associated and virus-encoded mechanisms for inhibiting host protein synthesis.[336] These include a decrease in the stability of cellular mRNAs, production of small nontranslated polyadenylated RNAs that sequester poly(A)-binding proteins, and preferential translation of viral RNAs that have a 5' capped poly(A) leader adjacent to the translation initiation codon.[17,205,434] Vaccinia virus is resistant to the antiviral effects of IFN,[370] and extracts of vaccinia virus–infected cells are able to reverse the translation block mediated by activation of PKR[410,520] and inhibit the activity of the 2-5A system.[371]

Regulation of Activation of Protein Kinase RNA-Dependent

Viruses have a variety of strategies to prevent inhibition of viral protein synthesis by PKR-mediated phosphorylation of eIF-2α (see Fig. 4-3).[225,315] Poliovirus induces degradation of PKR, apparently by activating a cellular protease[41] that cleaves PKR in the dsRNA-binding domain.[225] Adenoviruses and EBV synthesize small RNAs (VAI-RNA and EBERs, respectively) in large amounts that bind to, but do not activate, PKR and thus prevent PKR activation by dsRNA.[315,438] The reovirus s3, influenza NS1, and vaccinia p25 proteins bind dsRNA to prevent activation of PKR.[293,300,515] Binding of dsRNA has been mapped to an 85–amino acid domain in the C-terminal portion of s3.[326] In addition to p25, which is a product of the E3L gene,[60,112] vaccinia virus also encodes an 88–amino acid protein in the K3L gene that is a homolog of eIF-2a but lacks the phosphorylation site of eIF-2α and is postulated to bind PKR and prevent phosphorylation of eIF-2α.[225] Influenza virus activates p58, a cellular inhibitor of PKR,[273] by dissociating it from its own inhibitor.[225]

Altered Processing and Transport of Cellular Proteins

Viral proteins may inhibit transport of cellular proteins from the endoplasmic reticulum, and this inhibition often leads to the degradation of these proteins. The vpu protein of

HIV inhibits transport of CD4.[504] The adenovirus E3/19K binds and retains the heavy chain of the major histocompatibility complex (MHC) class I molecule in the endoplasmic reticulum.[369] The CMV UL18 protein binds the light chain of the MHC class I molecule, β_2 microglobulin, preventing its association with the heavy chain and its subsequent transport to the plasma membrane.[48] Sequestration of these immunologically important proteins may prevent immune recognition of infected cells by the host (see Chap. 10).

Some viruses encode serpins and other protease inhibitors that block proteolytic processing of cellular proteins. For instance, the vaccinia virus protein crmA is a serpin that inhibits the processing of pro IL-1β to IL-1β by the cysteine protease IL-1β converting enzyme (ICE; discussed later).[59,246,404,478]

ALTERATIONS IN CELLULAR MEMBRANES

Cellular membranes participate in many phases of viral replication, from entry to formation of replication complexes to assembly. Viruses may alter plasma membrane permeability, affect ion exchange and membrane potential, induce synthesis of new intracellular membranes, and induce rearrangement of previously existing membranes. Replication complexes are often membrane-bound. Enveloped viruses incorporate cellular membrane lipids into virions, and the insertions of viral proteins into the plasma membrane may lead to cellular membrane fusion and syncytia formation.

Membrane Synthesis and Rearrangement

Many viruses form replication complexes associated with cellular membranes, and membranous vesicles are often formed during infection.[35,173,280,379,381] The effect of virus infection on lipid metabolism has been examined in selected systems. Both picornaviruses and alphaviruses stimulate the synthesis of phospholipids.[5,501] Inhibition of phospholipid synthesis decreases and stimulation of smooth membrane formation increases replication of viral RNA.[173,376,381] Poliovirus also induces extensive proliferation and rearrangement of smooth membranes to generate vesicles on which viral RNA replication occurs. The 2C and 2BC proteins are associated with vesicles, but the mechanism by which they induce these changes is unknown.[5,21,68]

The relative contributions of new membrane synthesis and rearrangement of existing membranes is not clear. In poliovirus-infected or 2BC- or 2C-expressing cells, Golgi stacks are disassembled, suggesting that the components of these membranes are redistributed to new sites.[36,68] Inhibition of vesicle transport by brefeldin A inhibits RNA synthesis, suggesting a necessary maturation of membranous vesicles from a vesicular compartment for formation of replication complexes.[207] There is also evidence for increased phospholipid synthesis in poliovirus-infected cells. Increased cytoplasmic CTP catalyzes phosphocholine cytidyltransferase to increase phosphatidyl choline synthesis for new membranes.[71,501] Poliovirus infection also inhibits transport of cellular plasma membrane and secretory proteins. This appears to be a function of the 2B and 3A viral proteins.[105]

HSV infection of some, but not all, cells is associated with fragmentation and dispersal of the Golgi apparatus.[51] The breakdown and dispersal of the Golgi apparatus coincides with virion assembly, is dependent on the expression of viral late genes, and may reflect a disequilibrium between anterograde and retrograde Golgi transport caused by the large flux of viral proteins through the exocytic pathway.[51]

Membrane Permeability and Control of Ion Flux

A generalized increase in membrane permeability, detected by entry into cells of normally excluded macromolecules or release by intracellular molecules, occurs during entry of picornaviruses, alphaviruses, reoviruses, rhabdoviruses, and adenoviruses.[53,102,131,135] Uptake may be linked in part to co-internalization of macromolecules during receptor-mediated endocytosis of these viruses, but more specific effects have also been documented and linked to specific viral proteins.[54,135] In mammalian cells, poliovirus uncoating is required for permeabilization to some, but not all, normally excluded molecules to occur.[7] The adenovirus 23K protease is necessary for membrane disruption and entry.[87] Interaction of the u1 capsid protein of the infectious form of reovirus (i.e., the intermediate subviral particle) at the cell surface is sufficient to increase membrane permeability.[198,303]

Many viruses probably encode transmembrane proteins that can function as channels. A few have been identified. The influenza M2 protein is inserted into the endosomal membrane at the time of virus entry and serves as a channel for H+.[389] Poliovirus 3A, alphavirus 6K, and HIV gp41 proteins increase membrane permeability when expressed in *Escherichia coli* or form pores in planar lipid bilayers, suggesting that they may act similarly in infected cells.[11,65,259,429]

Changes in the intracellular concentrations of both monovalent and divalent cations also occur as a consequence of viral infection. In uninfected cells, there is a high concentration of K+ and low concentration of Na+ compared with concentrations in the extracellular fluid. These cation gradients and plasma membrane potential are maintained through active ion transport, executed primarily by the Na+,K+-ATPase. Altered intracellular cation concentrations may result from a generalized increase in membrane permeability, virus-encoded ion channels, or interference with the function of the Na+,K+-ATPase or other cellular ion channels involved in active ion transport.[54]

Development of cell enlargement (cytomegaly) in CMV-infected cells is dependent on increases in intracellular Na+. Treatment of infected cells with amiloride blocks cell enlargement, suggesting that CMV activates the Na+/H+ exchanger to increase Na+ entry into the cell.[355]

K+ flux is dramatically reduced in cells infected with picornaviruses and alphaviruses beginning a few hours after infection.[55,342] In picornavirus-infected cells, this appears to be due to a generalized increase in membrane permeability.[295] This increase was originally hypothesized to be the result of changes in the cellular membrane as a consequence of insertion of coat proteins during infection.[52] Studies with a variety of drugs suggest that there is a generalized increase in cell membrane permeability induced by synthesis of virus proteins rather than specific virus-induced changes in ion channel function.[86] This is further suggested by studies indicating that K+ flux is not sensitive to inhibitors of ion channel function.[295] This change may be effected by the nonstructural proteins 2B and 3A[258] and may be linked to a virus-induced increase in phospholipase C (PLC) activity.[174] Changes in intracellular [Ca^{2+}] may also be associated with activation of phospholipases. Poliovirus stimulates the activity of PLC while inhibiting phospholipase A2 (PLA2).[174,208] Cells infected with Semliki Forest virus or VSV have increased activity of both PLA2 and PLC.[382]

Changes in free intracellular Ca^{2+} occur during infections with a number of viruses at different stages in the virus life cycle. Enveloped viruses such as Sendai and influenza induce an increase during virus entry.[175] CMV increases Ca^{2+} entry into intracellular stores, probably by affecting the function of Ca^{2+} channels.[354] Rotavirus morphogenesis is dependent on Ca^{2+},[437] and the nsP4 protein increases cytosolic Ca^{2+} by mobilizing Ca^{2+} from endoplasmic reticulum stores.[479,480] Poliovirus infection increases intracellular Ca^{2+} about 10-fold within 4 hours after infection, primarily by increasing entry of extracellular Ca^{2+}.[206] This change is dependent on synthesis of viral proteins.

Membrane Fusion

Enveloped viruses enter cells by fusing the viral membrane with the cell membrane through the action of a fusogenic viral protein. Viruses such as paramyxoviruses and lentiviruses have virion fusion proteins that fuse the viral membrane to the cell plasma membrane. These fusion proteins are activated by proteases late in the replication cycle. Viruses such as alphaviruses, rhabdoviruses, and orthomyxoviruses require exposure to low pH to activate the fusion protein and fuse with the endosomal membrane.[236,508,526] Cells infected by viruses that can fuse at neutral pH often have fusogenic proteins expressed on the cell surface late in infection. Cell membranes modified in this way can fuse to neighboring infected or uninfected cells to form syncytia.[263,306] The viral proteins responsible for cell-to-cell fusion are transmembrane proteins and include the gp41 protein of HIV[329] and the fusion protein of paramyxoviruses, which induces fusion in concert with the hemagglutinin attachment protein.[333] Strains of HIV vary in the efficiency with which they induce fusion, and these differences often map to the gp120 envelope protein,[100] suggesting that the attachment protein is an important contributor to syncytia formation for lentiviruses as well as paramyxoviruses. Reviews on virus-cell fusion are available elsewhere.[27,235]

CHANGES IN THE CYTOSKELETON

Changes in cell shape are one of the common signs of virus-induced cytopathic effect, and the cytoskeleton is often an important participant in entry, formation of replication complexes and assembly sites, and virus release.[276,339] The cytoskeleton is not a static structure, and polymerization and depolymerization of cytoskeletal proteins are ongoing processes. In the uninfected cell, polyribosomes are associated with the cytoskeleton, and mRNAs and initiation factors are particularly enriched in the cytoskeletal cellular fraction. Cellular mRNAs remain associated with the cytoskeleton in influenza- and adenovirus-infected cells despite their failure to be translated[230] but

are dissociated in poliovirus-infected cells.[230,276] Vaccinia virus can induce the formation of polymerized actin tails that propel the virus particles from the infected cell into an adjacent cell.[92]

The cytoskeleton is composed of the major filament systems: microfilaments (e.g., actin), microtubules (e.g., tubulin), and intermediate filaments (e.g., vimentin, keratin). Actin filaments increase in Newcastle disease virus–infected cells, whereas they decrease in VSV-infected cells.[420]

Adenovirus infections are associated with changes in the intermediate filaments vimentin, lamin, and cytokeratin. Early after infection with subgroup C adenoviruses, the vimentin network of intermediate filaments condenses in the perinuclear region and subsequently degenerates,[102,548] apparently through viral activation of a cellular protease.[25] Collapse of the vimentin and lamin networks are linked to expression of the E1b 19-kD protein.[523] The L3 23-kD late-acting viral protease degrades cytokeratins K18 and K7, resulting in disassembly of the cytokeratin system.[63,551] HIV protease cleaves a number of components of the cytoskeleton in vitro,[197] but the in vivo importance of these observations is not clear.

Poliovirus infection induces extensive cytoskeletal changes.[276] These changes are associated with cleavage of a cytoskeletal protein, microtubule-associated protein 4 (MAP-4).[216] MAP-4 is cleaved by the 3C proteases of poliovirus and rhinovirus, but cleavage does not occur in EMCV-infected cells or in cells infected with VSV or adenoviruses.[217] Cleavage of MAP-4 results in collapse of microtubules.

In HSV-infected cells, fragmentation of microtubules, particularly at the periphery of the cell, is an early event that is independent of the onset of DNA synthesis and is followed by reformation of microtubules into perinuclear bundles.[14]

VIRUS-INDUCED CELL DEATH: APOPTOSIS VERSUS NECROSIS

Classically, virologists have assumed that viruses kill cells by usurping their transcriptional and translational machinery and disrupting membrane integrity. That is, the infected cell is accosted to such a degree that it cannot go on living, and the cell dies by necrosis, or "murder." Whereas some viruses are clearly capable of such lethal parasitism, other viruses kill cells by triggering cellular "suicide," or programmed cell death. Most cells that have activated their programmed cell death pathway undergo characteristic morphologic changes referred to as apoptosis. The striking morphologic changes and biochemical events that occur during apoptosis are distinguishable from necrosis. Cells dying by apoptosis exhibit severe chromatin condensation around the periphery of the nucleus that is detectable using DNA stains and electron microscopy. A cellular endonuclease activated during apoptosis cleaves cellular DNA into nucleosome-length fragments detectable as 180– to 200–base pair ladders on agarose gels. The membrane of an apoptotic cell actively blebs but remains intact. Ultimately, the cell blebs apart into membrane-bound apoptotic bodies that contain cytoplasmic material, nuclear material, or both. In tissues, these apoptotic bodies are engulfed by adjacent, normally nonphagocytic cells. In contrast, necrotic cell death is typified by early loss of membrane integrity, allowing cytosolic spillage, and DNA is degraded randomly. Representatives of many virus groups, including herpesviruses,[210,232,245,544] adenoviruses,[521] poxviruses,[47] parvoviruses,[332] retroviruses,[114,267,325,362,409] rhabdoviruses,[249] paramyxoviruses,[113,488] myxoviruses,[132,195,462] alphaviruses,[281,494] and picornaviruses,[484] are capable of inducing apoptosis in one cultured cell type or another. The relevance of apoptosis and programmed cell death in viral pathogenesis is an active area of research.

Inhibition of Virus-Induced Apoptosis

Apoptosis is recognized as an essential mechanism in multicellular organisms for the elimination of unwanted, no longer needed, or potentially harmful cells. Cells between digits must die during fetal development for the formation of fingers,[176] approximately 50% of the neuron population dies during maturation of the mammalian nervous system,[89,399] autoreactive lymphocytes must be eliminated to protect the host,[449,450] and cytotoxic T lymphocytes kill their target cells by inducing apoptosis.[84] A number of cellular genes have been identified that regulate and modulate the cell death pathway, including the *bcl-2* gene family, but little is known about their molecular mechanisms of action.

It has also been suggested that apoptosis is a protective host response to eliminate virus-infected cells.[502] This hypothesis is supported by the finding that many viruses encode genes that inhibit the apoptotic pathway (Table 4-1). The ability to inhibit programmed cell death allows the virus to complete its replication cycle before the cell expires. Adenoviruses and baculoviruses with defective anti-apoptotic genes are severely impaired for progeny virus production, apparently because the cell dies prematurely from apoptosis. In contrast, small viruses with rapid life cycles may not need to inhibit apoptotic cell death to achieve efficient progeny production. The alphavirus Sindbis appears to prefer apoptotic cells, because inhibitors of apoptosis appear to impair Sindbis virus replication.[494] Virus-induced apoptosis may also be harmful to the host in cases in which the virus itself does not kill the cell or in which the virus infects a cell population that cannot be replenished. In these situations, virus-induced programmed cell death may contribute to the pathogenesis of disease.

TABLE 4-1. *Viral proteins that modulate the apoptotic pathway*

Induce cell death	Inhibit cell death
Adenovirus E1A	Adenovirus E1b 19K
Adenovirus E3/ADP	Adenovirus E1b 55K
Chicken anemia virus VP3/apoptin	Baculovirus p35
Human immunodeficiency virus gp120	Baculovirus iap
Human immunodeficiency virus tat	Cytomegalovirus IE1
Human T-cell lymphotropic virus type I	Cytomegalovirus IE2
Reovirus σ1	Epstein-Barr virus BHRF1
Sindbis virus E2	Herpesvirus saimiri ORF16
	Poxvirus crmA (SPI-2)
	Poxvirus SPI-1

The bcl-2 Oncogene

The *bcl-2* oncogene was first identified at t(14;18) translocations that occur in the majority of follicular B-cell lymphomas.[489] This translocation event results in overexpression of *bcl-2*, which allows B cells to survive when they would normally die by apoptosis. Bcl-2 protects a wide variety of cell types, both in vivo and in vitro, from many death-inducing stimuli, including serum and growth factor withdrawal, treatment with calcium ionophores, glucose withdrawal, membrane peroxidation, glucocorticoid treatment, chemotherapeutic agents, and virus infection.[††] Transgenic mice overexpressing *bcl-2* in the B-cell lineage exhibit prolonged survival of responsive B cells[358] and develop an autoimmune disease resembling systemic lupus erythematosus.[450] In *bcl-2*–deficient mice, the immune system initially appears to develop normally, but with time, massive apoptosis takes place in the spleen and thymus.[222,343,344,503] Defects are also detectable in the small intestine and in epithelial cells, which normally express substantial levels of *bcl-2*.[222] In addition, these animals have delayed growth and early mortality. Although *bcl-2* is also abundantly expressed in the nervous system during development, no neurologic abnormalities have been detected in bcl-2–deficient mice. However, because *bcl-2* is a member of a growing family of related genes, including *bcl-x* and *mcl-1*,[44,252] these genes may substitute or compensate for the lack of *bcl-2*. However, mice that are *bcl-x*–deficient die during embryogenesis, with severe apoptosis of neurons and hematopoietic cells.[337] No molecular function has been assigned to any of the bcl-2–related proteins, and the mechanism by which they block apoptosis is unknown.

Herpesvirus, BHRF1

Several viruses encode homologs of the cellular *bcl-2* gene. When *bcl-2* was initially cloned, it was found to have sequence similarity with a previously identified gene, BHRF1, encoded by EBV.[76] BHRF1 shares 23% amino acid sequence identity with bcl-2 and has a similar topographical organization. Like bcl-2, BHRF1 appears to be anchored to cytoplasmic membranes via a C-terminal hydrophobic transmembrane domain.[178,192,377] In gene transfer experiments, BHRF1 protects B-lymphoma cell lines and Chinese hamster ovary cells from apoptosis induced by a variety of stimuli.[183,466] However, a role for BHRF1 in the life cycle of EBV is not yet clear. BHRF1 protein is expressed abundantly in the early phase of the lytic cycle by way of a lytic cycle promoter.[121,178] In infected individuals, lytic virus replication occurs predominantly in epithelial cells of the oropharynx.[444] SCC12F nontumorigenic human squamous cell carcinoma cultures mimic stratified epithelium in that the upper layers express differentiation markers and undergo apoptosis.[97] Expression of BHRF1 in SCC12F cells significantly delays terminal differentiation, as evidenced by the accumulation of underdifferentiated cells into a multilayered epithelium.[97] The ability of BHRF1 to inhibit apoptosis is presumably responsible for the prolonged survival and delayed differentiation of SCC12F cells. BHRF1 is abundantly expressed in oral hairy leukoplakia, an EBV in-

---

†† References 6, 110, 151, 195, 281, 305, 328, 553.

fection of the tongue in AIDS patients characterized by epithelial thickening and hyperkeratosis similar to that observed with SCC12F cells overexpressing BHRF1.[168,427,545] These observations draw a potential link between BHRF1 and the epithelial tumors associated with EBV infection, such as nasopharyngeal carcinoma.[285,397] The conservation of BHRF1 in natural isolates of EBV further indicates an important role for BHRF1 in the virus life cycle.[182]

EBV establishes a latent infection in B lymphocytes and induces growth transformation through the action of five latent-cycle EBV genes: EBNA-1, 2, 3A, and 3C and LMP-1.[83,177,233,485] Although latent-cycle transcripts that contain the BHRF1 open reading frame have been identified by several laboratories,[12,43] no BHRF1 protein expression has been detected during latency. Furthermore, EBV mutants with engineered defects in BHRF1 are competent to infect and immortalize B lymphocytes in culture.[271,307,384] The multimembrane-spanning EBV protein LMP-1 activates expression of the cellular bcl-2 gene during the latent cycle, resulting in protection of B cells from apoptosis.[134,169,184,416] Although LMP-1 expression correlates with bcl-2 expression in posttransplant lymphoproliferative disorders,[338] there is no correlation in nasopharyngeal carcinoma.[297]

The apparent independent acquisition of a bcl-2 homolog by the more distantly related gamma herpesvirus, herpesvirus saimiri, further supports an important role for anti-apoptotic genes. BHRF1 and ORF16 of herpesvirus saimiri are distantly related to members of the bcl-2 family, and ORF16 was recently demonstrated to have anti-apoptotic function.[345] Viral homologs of bcl-2 are not limited to herpesviruses. A pox-like virus, African swine fever virus, also encodes a bcl-2 homolog LMW5-HL,[346] but the role of LMW5-HL in the virus life cycle in unknown.

Adenovirus, E1b

The adenovirus function required to prevent premature cell death of adenovirus-infected cells was mapped to E1b 19K, one of two E1b gene products.[388,460,525] Subsequently, it was demonstrated that E1b 19K protects infected cells by inhibiting apoptosis.[403,524] Viruses with a mutation in 19K produce 10-fold fewer progeny compared with wild-type viruses because of premature cell death.[388] The other E1b gene product, E1b 55K, was also shown to inhibit apoptosis, although less potently. It was presumed that 19K and 55K functioned by blocking cell death induced by another viral protein. Subsequently, the adenovirus-transforming gene E1A was shown to be responsible for the apoptotic phenotype.[403,524] Expression of E1A increases the intracellular levels of tumor suppressor p53 through stabilization of p53, contributing to the induction of apoptosis.[194,296] Whereas E1A was shown to induce apoptosis in a p53-dependent manner in rat kidney cells,[101,422] others have observed p53-independent induction of apoptosis by E1A.[470] E1A modulates cellular transcription and drives the cell into S phase. In this manner, adenoviruses convert a quiescent cell into a suitable environment for adenovirus replication. E1A accomplishes this goal in part because it binds directly to the retinoblastoma protein (Rb), freeing the E2F transcription factor normally bound to Rb. E2F activates the expression of several cellular genes involved in DNA synthesis, but the attempt by quiescent fibroblasts to enter S phase triggers apoptosis.[248] Thus, expression of E1A alone is insufficient to transform cells, and the developing cell foci wither and die. The transforming phenotype of E1A requires the anti-apoptotic function of E1b. Although E1b 19K and 55K have no sequence similarity, either is sufficient to mediate cell transformation by E1A.[101]

E1b 55K appears to inhibit p53-dependent cell death by binding directly to p53 and inhibiting p53-mediated transcription activation.[425,541,542] E1b 19K can inhibit both p53-dependent and p53-independent apoptosis, but the mechanism of action is not known.[62,101,453,522] Although 19K has only limited amino acid sequence similarity to the bcl-2 family, bcl-2 can substitute for 19K to facilitate transformation by E1A and can protect cells during adenovirus infection.[67,403] Because 19K can block p53-mediated cell death, it seems reasonable that 19K may alter the action of p53, which is presumed to function as a transcription regulator. Although E1b 19K fails to alter p53-mediated transcriptional activation, it can abolish p53-mediated transcriptional repression, causing p53 to activate genes that it normally represses.[421,440] These data suggest the possibility that transcriptional repression by p53 may lead to apoptosis. In contrast to 55K, there is no evidence that 19K binds to p53 or affects intracellular levels of p53.

Viral Transcription Regulatory Proteins

Viral transcription regulatory proteins have been shown to block apoptotic cell death. Human papillomavirus E6 protein and the SV40 T antigen inhibit cell death by inactivating p53.[316,375,457] CMV immediate early transcription regulators IE1 and IE2, encoded by alternately spliced mRNAs, inhibit apoptotic cell death induced by tumor necrosis factor alpha (TNF-α) and by infection with E1b 19K-deficient adenovirus.[554] The ability of CMV IE1 and IE2 to inhibit cell death is consistent with the lengthy replication cycle and the lifelong persistent infections caused by this virus.

Poxvirus, crmA

Poxviruses are unique among viruses in that they encode members of the serpin superfamily. Serpins are highly conserved serine protease inhibitors that serve as multipurpose regulators of cellular responses.[56,309,392,393] CrmA (SPI-2) is one of several serpins encoded by poxviruses and is the first serpin identified that functions as a cysteine protease inhibitor.[404] CrmA is a specific inhibitor of the cellular protease ICE, which cleaves proIL-1β to produce the active proinflammatory cytokine IL-1β.[59,404,478] Like other serpins, crmA serves as a pseudosubstrate that stably complexes with ICE but ultimately is cleaved and released from the ICE protease. In contrast to the red, hemorrhagic pocks chorioallantoic membranes of embryonated eggs infected with wild-type cowpox virus, mutant viruses with a defective crmA gene form white viral lesions.[374,387,476] The white pocks phenotype is due to infiltration of neutrophils, indicating that crmA inhibits the inflammatory response of the host.[72,374]

ICE shares significant amino acid sequence homology to CED-3, encoded by the nematode *Caenorhabditis elegans*.[547] In *C elegans*, CED-3 has pro-apoptotic activity that is inhibited by CED-9, a homolog of mammalian bcl-2.[185,186,546] Mutations in CED-3 yield adult worms with 131 extra somatic cells that failed to die by programmed cell death during development.[109] These studies suggest a role for ICE in apoptosis; this is supported by the ability of the cowpox virus ICE inhibitor crmA to block apoptosis induced by a wide variety of death stimuli in cultured cells.[149,327,472,473] However, the role of ICE in cell death is controversial, and crmA has not been shown to inhibit cell death in poxvirus-infected cells.[47,476] ICE is a member of a growing family of mammalian ICE-like proteases, and crmA's ability to block apoptosis may be due to inhibition of one or more of these related enzymes. Thus, the study of cowpox virus crmA has been revealing and has significantly contributed to the concept that ICE-like proteases are part of a common cell death pathway. In contrast to crmA, another poxvirus serpin, SPI-1, inhibits poxvirus-induced apoptosis.[47] SPI-1 mutant virus initiates the virus replication cycle but does not complete it, apparently because of premature cell death.[47] The cellular protease targeted by SPI-1 is not known.

Baculovirus, p35 and iap

Genetic analysis of baculoviruses led to the identification of two anti-apoptotic genes, p35 and iap, that are distinct from the genes described previously. *Autographa californica* nuclear polyhedrosis virus (AcMNPV), the widely used expression vector, completes its replication cycle in lepidopteran insect cells over a period of several days, ending in necrotic cell death and release of progeny virus.[78] A spontaneous mutant of AcMNPV called the annihilator was identified because of its rapid cytolytic phenotype.[77] The genetic determinant for the annihilator phenotype was mapped to the *p35* gene,[77] which is expressed both early and late after infection and is required for efficient production of late viral genes and progeny virus.[79,189,353] P35 protein inhibits apoptosis induced by a wide variety of stimuli when expressed in mammalian as well as invertebrate cells, suggesting an evolutionarily conserved molecular pathway.[23,312,398,454,454] Interestingly, p35 represents a new class of protease inhibitors that binds to and is cleaved by members of the ICE protease family, blocking their ability to induce apoptosis.[50,536]

In a search for p35 homologs, a new class of anti-apoptotic genes was identified. The baculovirus inhibitor of apoptosis (*iap*) gene protects baculovirus-infected cells from apoptosis. The predicted amino acid sequence of iap reveals two N-terminal repeats (BIR repeats) containing putative zinc fingers and a ring finger motif near the C-terminus. Baculovirus iap can also function to protect mammalian cells from apoptosis induced by Sindbis virus infection,[111] implying that, like p35, the iap pathway is evolutionarily conserved. This was verified by the identification of several human homologs.[78,415] Human iap proteins bind to cellular TNF receptor–associated factor (TRAF) proteins, which have been implicated in receptor-mediated transduction and apoptosis.[66,366,415,538] Thus, it is possible that iap proteins modulate the TRAF pathway leading to cell death. It is interesting to note that the EBV LMP-1 protein also binds directly to TRAF proteins.[335]

How Viruses Induce Programmed Cell Death, or Apoptosis

There are several potential mechanisms by which viruses activate the apoptotic pathway (see Table 4-1). Some viruses may do so through the direct action of a specific viral protein. As discussed previously, adenovirus E1A alone is sufficient to induce apoptotic cell death. Chicken anemia virus has a 2.3-kb single-strand circular DNA genome with three overlapping open reading frames encoding VP1, VP2, and VP3. The 121–amino acid VP3/apoptin protein localizes to the nucleus and can induce apoptosis independent of other viral proteins.[357,555] Other virus-encoded proteins, including Tat and gp120 of HIV,[284,298] HTLV-I Tax protein,[537] and the E2 glycoprotein of Sindbis virus,[218] have been shown to induce apoptotic cell death. The mechanisms by which these proteins induce apoptosis is under investigation.

The adenovirus death protein, ADP (E3 11.6K), is made in low abundance early after infection but is produced abundantly late in the infection.[483] Viruses with mutant ADP are not defective for viral replication but are impaired for virus production. ADP, a glycosylated nuclear envelope transmembrane protein, is required for cell lysis and release of progeny virus.[430,482] The onset of cell lysis normally occurs at 2 to 3 days postinfection with wild-type virus but does not begin until 5 to 6 days after infection with the ADP mutant. Without ADP, the nucleus becomes swollen and laden with virus.[482] The programmed cell death induced by ADP is morphologically like necrosis and does not exhibit the characteristics of apoptosis.[482]

Another possibility is that viruses induce apoptosis indirectly through their effects on other cellular processes. Baculovirus-mediated cessation of cellular RNA transcription has been suggested to be the stimulus for apoptosis in baculovirus-infected SF-21 insect cells.[80] The shutoff of host protein synthesis has been postulated as the mechanism by which nonpermissive polioviruses activate the death pathway in HeLa cells.[484] The observation that uninfected SF-21 and HeLa cells, used for studying these viruses, undergo apoptosis following treatment with metabolic inhibitors supports the hypothesis that viruses could trigger apoptosis in this manner.[80,484] The implication from these studies is that SF-21 and HeLa cells require ongoing synthesis of a protective protein to avoid activating the death pathway. In contrast to these cell types, neurons, baby hamster kidney (BHK) cells, and a number of other cells are protected from apoptosis by metabolic inhibitors,[282,310] implying that these cells require the expression of new genes to facilitate the death pathway. Genes that are activated during neuronal cell death are beginning to be identified.[115]

The alphavirus Sindbis targets neurons in vivo and is propagated in cultured BHK cells. Although Sindbis virus has the capacity to potently inhibit host protein synthesis, it seems unlikely that Sindbis virus would induce apoptosis in neurons and BHK cells via inhibition of host protein synthesis and may induce expression of a cellular death gene. Like many other viruses, infection with Sindbis virus activates the cellular transcription factor NFkB within 1 to 2 hours after infection.[287] Upon activation, NFkB is released from its cytoplasmic retainer IkB and translocates to the nucleus, where it binds to specific DNA sequence motifs to activate gene transcription. Treatment of cells with oligonucleotide decoys that bind NFkB and prevent activation of downstream genes protects AT-3 cells from Sindbis virus–induced apoptosis, indicating that NFkB plays a role in the death pathway activated by Sindbis virus, at least in some cell types.[287] The requirement for new gene expression, through the action of NFkB, to activate the death pathway seems contrary to the observation that Sindbis virus efficiently shuts off host protein synthesis. Yet it is conceivable that some cellular transcripts escape the inhibitory effects of the virus just as viral transcripts escape these effects (discussed previously).

Fas/APO-1 (CD95) is abundantly expressed on activated mature lymphocytes and on lymphocytes infected with HTLV-I, HIV, or EBV.[341] Fas is a member of the TNF receptor family and activates apoptotic cell death following interaction with its ligand FasL or anti-Fas antibodies.[487] Like TNF, Fas appears to transmit a signal involving TRADD/FADD family proteins.[66] Fas plays an important role in apoptosis of activated T cells, and mutations in either Fas or FasL lead to autoimmune disease.[49,85,104,221,513] Influenza virus infection induces the expression of Fas, and Fas-mediated cell death has been suggested to be an important mechanism of influenza virus killing.[461,505] HIV-1 Tat protein upregulates FasL expression in T cells and sensitizes T cells to apoptosis triggered by T-cell receptor engagement or binding of HIV-1 gp120 to CD4.[224,519]

Role of Apoptosis in Viral Pathogenesis

Apoptotic cell death may be an important host defense mechanism for eliminating virus-infected cells from the body, thereby slowing the spread of virus.[502] The observation that some viruses have acquired one or more anti-apoptotic genes (described previously) to prolong cell survival during infection supports the hypothesis. In contrast, other viruses appear to thrive in apoptotic cells, perhaps in part because their replication cycle is completed prior to cell death.[283,494] Apoptosis induced by these viruses may be an important mechanism of pathogenesis.

Induction of Apoptosis Versus Viral Persistence

The alphavirus Sindbis causes encephalitis and hind limb paralysis in mice. The ability of Sindbis virus to induce apoptotic cell death of infected neurons in mouse brains and spinal cords was confirmed by in situ terminal deoxynucleotidy/transferase-mediated dUTP nick end-labeling (TUNEL) assays on mouse tissues and the detection of DNA fragmentation in extracts of infected mouse brains.[283] Induction of apoptosis by Sindbis virus in neurons of mouse brains and spinal cords correlates with mortality. That is, neurovirulent strains induce abundant apoptosis in vivo compared with less virulent strains.[283] However, neurovirulent Sindbis viruses also replicate more efficiently in mouse brains and spinal cords. Thus, it appears that a viral determinant allows neurovirulent strains to replicate more efficiently, leading to the induction of apoptosis. In fact, a single amino acid change in the E2 glycoprotein of Sindbis virus converts an avirulent virus to a neurovirulent virus.[490,494] However, both virulent and avirulent strains

replicate equally efficiently in BHK cell lines,[490] implying that a host cell determinant in mouse brains is also important in distinguishing between the neurovirulent and avirulent viruses. Thus, a factor in mouse brains may be responsible for suppressing replication of avirulent viruses. For example, the neurovirulent strain may bind to a neuronal receptor more efficiently than the avirulent strain.[493] Alternatively, anti-apoptotic genes could modulate the outcome of virus infection.[170] The anti-apoptotic bcl-2 and bcl-x_L proteins (discussed previously) are normally expressed in neurons of the brain and spinal cord. AT-3 and LNcap cells overexpressing bcl-2 are protected from apoptosis induced by the less virulent Sindbis virus strains, but these cells are readily killed by the neurovirulent strains.[281,494]

A potential role for cellular anti-apoptotic genes in suppression of virus-induced apoptosis was further tested by inserting a copy of the *bcl-2* gene into the Sindbis virus genome. Bcl-2 protein expressed from the recombinant Sindbis virus protects cultured cells from Sindbis virus–induced apoptosis.[64] Furthermore, bcl-2 protects recombinant virus–infected mice from fatal encephalitis.[278] Importantly, bcl-2 appears to suppress Sindbis virus replication.[278,494] Taken together, these data support the attractive hypothesis that failure to activate the death pathway following virus infection could lead to a persistent infection.[281] Such a mechanism could explain persistence of avirulent Sindbis virus strains in neurons of mouse brains for extended periods of time.[279,280,492] In support of this possibility, cell lines expressing bcl-2 were able to sustain a low-grade Sindbis virus infection during months of passaging.[281] Similar mechanisms may exist for other viruses.

The induction of bcl-2 expression by latent cycle genes in EBV-infected B cells appears to support persistence of EBV in the latent state.[169,184,416] Influenza virus–infected cells are also protected from apoptosis by overexpression of bcl-2, although these cells eventually died.[195] Furthermore, bcl-2 impairs influenza virus replication, perhaps by altering glycosylation of the viral hemagglutinin protein.[366]

E1b 19K expressed in CD4+ Jurkat T cells blocks apoptosis induced following infection with HIV facilitating a persistent infection. In contrast to Sindbis and influenza viruses, inhibition of apoptosis in HIV-infected cells led to increased virus production presumably due to increased cell survival.[10] Thus, cells that fail to activate their cell death pathway following virus infection may provide prime sites of viral persistence even if the mechanism of viral persistence differs for different viruses.

Direct and Indirect Induction of Apoptosis

In some disease states, apoptosis occurs only in those cells that are infected with the virus; for example, Sindbis virus infection of neurons in vivo.[283] Chicken anemia virus causes complete depletion of the thymic cortex in hatchlings.[214] Although thymic epithelial cells are spared, direct infection of cortical thymocytes by this lymphotropic virus results in massive apoptosis.[214]

It is also conceivable that a virus-infected cell could cause apoptosis in an adjacent uninfected cell by a number of possible mechanisms, including the shutoff of growth factor production or secretion of factors that activate the death program.

Measles virus infection of human thymus tissue implanted into SCID mice also induces apoptosis in thymocytes.[13] In contrast to chicken anemia virus, measles virus replicates primarily in the thymic epithelial stroma, with no evidence of measles antigens in thymocytes. Thus, apoptosis induced by measles virus appears to result from an indirect mechanism.[13] Likewise, apoptosis of CD4+ T cells and neurons in AIDS pathogenesis, and thymocyte depletion following infection with murine CMV or mouse hepatitis virus, appear to be an indirect result of virus infection, because the dying cells are largely uninfected.[9,115,157,162,245] Although indirect mechanisms appear to be the rule for several viruses in vivo, most of these viruses are capable of directly inducing apoptotic cell death in cultured cells.[113,267,362,409]

Apoptosis and Autoimmune Disease

Apoptotic cell death induced by virus infections as well as other stimuli results in the formation of two distinct types of apoptotic bodies: those that arise from the nucleus and contain condensed chromatin, and small blebs that contain components of the endoplasmic reticulum.[57] Autoantigens targeted in systemic lupus erythematosus are specifically packaged into one or the other of these apoptotic compartments.[57] A subset of autoantigens co-clusters with Sindbis virus proteins into the small blebs that form during virus-induced apoptosis.[414] The formation of complexes of viral and self antigens in apoptotic bodies has been suggested as a potential mechanism for breaking tolerance to these specific self-molecules leading to autoimmune disease.[108,414] The association of Sindbis virus with inflammatory illnesses and arthritis in humans is consistent with such a mechanism. Viral persistence with occasional reactivation and induction of apoptotic cell death that elicits an inappropriate immune response could result in a disease state whose origin would be difficult to trace.

ABBREVIATIONS

AcMNPV: *Autographa californica* nuclear polyhedrosis virus
AIDS: acquired immunodeficiency syndrome
BHK: baby hamster kidney
BIR: baculovirus IAP repeat
bZIP: basic zipper
CMV: cytomegalovirus
CRE: cAMP response element
EBNA: Epstein-Barr nuclear antigen
EBV: Epstein-Barr virus
eIF: eukaryotic initiation factor
EMCV: encephalomyocarditis virus
FMDV: foot-and-mouth disease virus
HIV: human immunodeficiency virus
HSV: herpes simplex virus
HTLV: human T-cell lymphotropic virus
ICE: IL-1β converting enzyme
IFN: interferon
IRF: interferon regulatory factor
IRES: internal ribosomal entry site
LCMV: lymphocytic choriomeningitis virus
LMP: latency membrane protein

LTR: long terminal repeat
MAP: microtubule-associated protein
MHC: major histocompatibility complex
NTR: nontranslated region
PKR: protein kinase RNA-dependent
PL: phospholipase
pol: polymerase
TBP: TATA-binding protein
TF: transcription factor
TNF: tumor necrosis factor
TRAF: TNF–associated factor
TUNEL: terminal deoxynucleotidy/transferase-mediated dUTP nick end–labeling
VAI: virus-associated RNA-I
VSV: vesicular stomatitis virus

REFERENCES

1. Abbot SD, Rowe M, Cadwallader K, et al. Epstein-Barr virus nuclear antigen 2 induces expression of the virus-encoded latent membrane protein. J Virol 1990;64:2126–2134.
2. Abramson RD, Dever TE, Lawson TG, Ray BK, Thach RE, Merrick WC. The ATP-dependent interaction of eukaryotic initiation factors with mRNA. J Biol Chem 1987;262:3826–3832.
3. Abramson RD, Dever TE, Merrick WC. Biochemical evidence supporting a mechanism for cap-independent and internal initiation of eukaryotic mRNA. J Biol Chem 1988;263:6016–6019.
4. Agy MB, Wambach M, Foy K, Katze MG. Expression of cellular genes in CD4 positive lymphoid cells infected by the human immunodeficiency virus, HIV-1: Evidence for a host protein synthesis shut-off induced by cellular mRNA degradation. Virology 1990; 177: 251–258.
5. Aldabe R, Carrasco L. Induction of membrane proliferation by poliovirus proteins 2C and 2BC. Biochem Biophys Res Commun 1995; 206:64–76.
6. Allsopp TE, Wyatt S, Paterson HF, Davies AM. The proto-oncogene bcl-2 can selectively rescue neurotrophic factor-dependent neurons from apoptosis. Cell 199373:295–307.
7. Almela MJ, Gonzalez ME, Carrasco L. Inhibitors of poliovirus uncoating efficiently block the early membrane permeabilization induced by virus particles. J Virol 1991;65:2572–2577.
8. Alonso-Caplen FV, Nemeroff ME, Qiu Y, Krug RM. Nucleocytoplasmic transport: The influenza virus NS1 protein regulates the transport of spliced NS2 mRNA and its precursor NS1 mRNA. Genes Dev 1992;6:255–267.
9. Ameisen JC, Estaquier J, Idziorek T, De Bels F. The relevance of apoptosis to AIDS pathogenesis. Trends Cell Biol 1995;5:27–32.
10. Antoni BA, Sabbatini P, Rabson AB, White E. Inhibition of Apoptosis in human immunodeficiency virus-infected cells enhances virus production and facilitates persistent infection. J Virol 1995;69: 2384– 2392.
11. Arroyo J, Boceta M, Gonzalez ME, Michel M, Carrasco L. Membrane permeabilization by different regions of the human immunodeficiency virus type 1 transmembrane glycoprotein gp41. J Virol 1995;69:4095–4102.
12. Austin PJ, Flemington E, Yandava CN, Strominger JL, Speck SH. Complex transcription of the Epstein-Barr virus *Bam*HI fragment H rightward open reading frame 1 (BHRF1) in latently and lytically infected B lymphocytes. Proc Natl Acad Sci U S A 1988;85:3678– 3682.
13. Auwaerter PG, Kaneshima H, McCune JM, Wiegand G, Griffin DE. Measles virus infection in the SCID-hu mouse: Disruption of the human thymic microenvironment. J Cell Biochem 1995;S19(A):288. Abstract.
14. Avitabile E, Di Gaeta S, Torrisi MR, Ward PL, Roizman B, Campadelli-Fiume G. Redistribution of microtubules and golgi apparatus in herpes simplex virus-infected cells and their role in viral exocytosis. J Virol 1995;69:7472–7482.
15. Babich A, Feldman LT, Nevins JR, Darnell JE Jr, Weinberger C. Effect of adenovirus on metabolism of specific host mRNAs: Trans-

port control and specific translational discrimination. Mol Cell Biol 1983;3:1212–1221.

16. Babiss LE, Ginsberg HS. Adenovirus type 5 early region 1b gene product is required for efficient shutoff of host protein synthesis. J Virol 1984;50:202–212.

17. Bablanian R, Goswami SK, Esteban M, Banerjee AK, Merrick WC. Mechanism of selective translation of vaccinia virus mRNAs: Differential role of poly(A) and initiation factor in the translation of viral and cellular mRNAs. J Virol 1991;65:4449–4460.

18. Banda NK, Bernier J, Kurahara DK, et al. Crosslinking CD4 by human immunodeficiency virus gp120 primes T cells for activation-induced apoptosis. J Exp Med 1992;176:1099–1106.

19. Baranger AM, Palmer CR, Hamm MK, et al. Mechanism of DNA binding enhancement by the human T-cell leukaemia virus transactivator Tax. Nature (London) 1995;376:606–608.

20. Barber GN, Tomita J, Garfinkel MS, Meurs E, Hovanessian A, Katze MG. Detection of protein kinase homologues and viral RNA-binding domains utilizing polyclonal antiserum prepared against a baculovirus-expressed ds RNA-activated 68,000-Da protein kinase. Virology 1992;191:670–679.

21. Barco A, Carrasco L. A human virus protein, poliovirus protein 2BC, induces membrane proliferation and blocks the exocytic pathway in the yeast Saccharomyces cerevisiae. EMBO J 1995;14:3349–3364.

22. Becker Y, Joklik WK. Messenger RNA in cells infected with vaccinia virus. Biochemistry 1964;51:577–585.

23. Beidler DR, Tewari M, Friesen PD, Poirier G, Dixit VM. The baculovirus p35 protein inhibits Fas and tumor necrosis factor-induced apoptosis. J Biol Chem 1995;270:16526–16528.

24. Beimling P, Moelling K. Direct interaction of CREB protein with 21 bp Tax-response elements of HTLV-I LTR. Oncogene 1992;7:257–262.

25. Belin MT, Boulanger P. Processing of vimentin occurs during the early stages of adenovirus infection. J Virol 1987;61:2559–2566.

26. Beltz GA, Flint SJ. Inhibition of HeLa cell protein synthesis during adenovirus infection: Restriction of cellular messenger RNA sequences to the nucleus. J Mol Biol 1979;131:353–373.

27. Bentz J, ed. Viral fusion mechanisms. Boca Raton: CRC Press, 1993.

28. Beraud C, Lonbard-Platet G, Michal Y, Jalinot P. Binding of the HTLV-I Tax1 transactivator to the inducible 21 bp enhancer is mediated by the cellular factor HEB1. EMBO J 1991;10:3795–3803.

29. Berben-Bloemheuvel G, Kasperaitis MA, van Heugten H, Thomas AA, Van Steeg H, Voorma HA. Interaction of initiation factors with the cap structure of chimaeric mRNA containing the 5'-untranslated regions of Semliki Forest virus RNA is related to translational efficiency. Eur J Biochem 1992;208:581–587.

30. Berg DT, Grinnell BW. 5' sequence of vesicular stomatitis virus N-gene confers selective translation of mRNA. Biochem Biophys Res Commun 1992;189:1585–1590.

31. Berget SM, Moore C, Sharp PA. Spliced segments at the 5' terminus of adenovirus 2 late mRNA. Proc Natl Acad Sci U S A 1977;74:3171–3175.

32. Bernstein HD, Sonenberg N, Baltimore D. Poliovirus mutant that does not selectively inhibit host cell protein synthesis. Mol Cell Biol 1985;5:2913–2923.

33. Berry MJ, Knutson GS, Lasky SR, Munemitsu SM, Samuel CE. Mechanism of interferon action. Purification and substrate specificities of the double-stranded RNA-dependent protein kinase from untreated and interferon-treated mouse fibroblasts. J Biol Chem 1985;260:11240–11247.

34. Bhagavati S, Ehrlich G, Kula RW, et al. Detection of human T-cell lymphoma/leukemia virus type I DNA and antigen in spinal fluid and blood of patients with chronic progressive myelopathy. N Engl J Med 1988;318:1141–1147.

35. Bienz K, Egger D, Pasamontes L. Association of polioviral proteins of the P2 genomic region with the viral replication complex and virus-induced membrane synthesis as visualized by electron microscopic immunocytochemistry and autoradiography. Virology 1987;160:220–26.

36. Bienz K, Egger D, Troxler M, Pasamontes L. Structural organization of poliovirus RNA replication is mediated by viral proteins of the P2 genomic region. J Virol 1990;64:1156–1163.

37. Black BL, Brewer G, Lyles DS. Effect of vesicular stomatitis virus matrix protein on host-directed translation in vivo. J Virol 1994;68:555–560.

38. Black BL, Lyles DS. Vesicular stomatitis virus matrix protein inhibits host cell-directed transcription of target genes in vivo. J Virol 1992;66:4058–4064.

39. Black BL, Rhodes RB, McKenzie M, Lyles DS. The role of vesicular stomatitis virus matrix protein in inhibition of host-directed gene expression is genetically separable from its function in virus assembly. J Virol 1993;67:4814–4821.

40. Black TL, Barber GN, Katze MG. Degradation of the interferon-induced 68,000-Mr protein kinase by poliovirus requires RNA. J Virol 1993;67:791–800.

41. Black TL, Safer B, Hovanessian A, Katze MG. The cellular 68,000-Mr protein kinase is highly autophosphorylated and activated yet significantly degraded during poliovirus infection: Implications for translational regulation. J Virol 1989;63:2244–2251.

42. Blondel D, Harmison GG, Schubert M. Role of matrix protein in cytopathogenesis of vesicular stomatitis virus. J Virol 1990;64:1716–1725.

43. Bodescot M, Perricaudet M. Epstein-Barr virus mRNAs produced by alternative splicing. Nucl Acids Res 1986;14:7103–7114.

44. Boise LH, Gonz˘A0lez-Garcia M, Postema CE, et al. Bcl-x, a bcl-2-related gene that functions as a dominant regulator of apoptotic cell death. Cell 1993;74:597–608.

45. Bonneau A-M, Sonenberg N. Proteolysis of the p220 component of the cap-binding protein complex is not sufficient for complete inhibition of host cell protein synthesis after poliovirus infection. J Virol 1987;61:986–991.

46. Bradbury LE, Kansas GS, Levy S, Evans RL, Tedder TF. The CD19/21 signal transducing complex of human B lymphocytes includes the target of antiproliferative antibody-1 and Leu-13 molecules. J Immunol 1992;149:2841–2850.

47. Brooks MA, Ali AN, Turner PC, Moyer RW. A rabbitpox virus serpin gene controls host range by inhibiting apoptosis in restrictive cells [SPI-1, not SPI-2]. J Virol 1995;69:7688–7698.

48. Browne H, Smith G, Beck S, Minson T. A complex between the MHC class I homologue encoded by human cytomegalovirus and beta 2 microglobulin. Nature (London) 1990;347:770–772.

49. Brunner T, Mogil RJ, LaFace D, et al. Cell-autonomous Fas (CD95)/Fas-ligand interactions mediates activation-induced apoptosis in T-cell hybridomas. Nature (London) 1995;373:441–444.

50. Bump NJ, Hackett M, Hugunin M, et al. Inhibition of ICE family proteases by baculovirus antiapoptotic protein p35. Science 1995;269:1885–1888.

51. Campadelli G, Brandimarti R, Di Lazzaro C, Ward PL, Roizman B, Torrisi MR. Fragmentation and dispersal of Golgi proteins and redistribution of glycoproteins and glycolipids processed through the Golgi apparatus after infection with herpes simplex virus 1. Proc Natl Acad Sci U S A 1993;90:2798–2802.

52. Carrasco L. The inhibition of cell functions after viral infection. FEBS Lett 1977;76:11–15.

53. Carrasco L. Modification of membrane permeability by animal viruses. Adv Vir Res 1995;45:61–113.

54. Carrasco L, Otero MJ, Castrillo JL. Modification of membrane permeability by animal viruses. Pharm Ther 1989;40:171–212.

55. Carrasco L, Smith AE. Sodium ions and the shut-off of host cell protein synthesis by picornaviruses. Nature (London) 1976;264:807–809.

56. Carrell RW, Pemberton PA, Boswell DR. The serpins: Evolution and adaptation in a family of protease inhibitors. Cold Spring Harb Symp Quant Biol 1987;3:527–535.

57. Casciola-Rosen LA, Anhalt G, Rosen A. Autoantigens targeted in systemic lupus erythematosus are clustered in two populations of surface structures on apoptotic keratinocytes. J Exp Med 1994;179:1317–1330.

58. Centrella M, Lucas-Lenard J. Regulation of protein synthesis in vesicular stomatitis virus-infected mouse L-929 cells by decreased protein synthesis initiation factor 2 activity. J Virol 1982;41:781–791.

59. Cerretti DP, Kozlosky CJ, Mosely B, et al. Molecular cloning of the interleukin-1-beta converting enzyme. Science 1992;256:97–100.

60. Chang HW, Watson JC, Jacobs BL. The E3L gene of vaccinia virus encodes an inhibitor of the interferon-induced, double-stranded RNA-dependent protein kinase. Proc Natl Acad Sci U S A 1992;89:4825–4829.

61. Charley B, Laude H. Induction of alpha interferon by transmissible gastroenteritis coronavirus: Role of transmembrane glycoprotein E1. J Virol 1988;62:8–11.

62. Chen G, Branton PE, Shore GC. Induction of p53-independent apoptosis by hygromycin B: Suppression by Bcl-2 and adenovirus E1B 19-KDa protein. Exp Cell Res 1995;221:55–59.

63. Chen PH, Ornelles DA, Shenk T. The adenovirus L3 23-kilodalton proteinase cleaves the amino-terminal head domain from cytokeratin 18 and disrupts the cytokeratin network of HeLa cells. J Virol 1993;67:3507–3514.

64. Cheng EH-Y, Levine B, Boise LH, Thompson CB, Hardwick JM. Bax-independent inhibition of apoptosis by Bcl-x_L. Nature (London) 1996;379:554–556.

65. Chernomordik L, Chanturiya N, Suss-Toby E, Nora E, Zimmerberg J. An amphipathic peptide from the C-terminal region of the human immunodeficiency virus envelope glycoprotein causes pore formation in membranes. J Virol 1994;68:7115–7123.

66. Chinnaiyan AM, Tepper CG, Seldin MF, et al. FADD/MORT1 is a common mediator of CD95 (Fas/APO-1)-and TNF-receptor-induced apoptosis. J Biol Chem 1996;271:4573–4576.

67. Chiou S-K, Tseng C-C, Rao L, White E. Functional complementation of the adenovirus E1B 19-kilodalton protein with Bcl-2 in the inhibition of apoptosis in infected cells. J Virol 1994;68:6553–6566.

68. Cho MW, Teterina N, Egger D, Bienz K, Ehrenfeld E. Membrane rearrangement and vesicle induction by recombinant poliovirus 2C and 2BC in human cells. Virology 1994;202:129–145.

69. Chou J, Chen J-J, Gross M, Roizman B. Association of a M_r90,000 phosphoprotein with protein kinase PKR in cells exhibiting enhanced phosphorylation of translation initiation factor eIF-2a and premature shutoff of protein synthesis after infection with $g_1$34.5$^-$ mutants of herpes simplex virus I. Proc Natl Acad Sci U S A 1995; 92:10516–10520.

70. Chou J, Roizman B. The gamma-1-34.5 gene of herpes simplex virus 1 precludes neuroblastoma cells from triggering total shutoff of protein synthesis characteristic of programed cell death in neuronal cells. Proc. Natl. Acad. Sci. 1992;89:3266–3270.

71. Choy PC, Paddon HB, Vance DE. An increase in cytoplasmic CTP accelerates the reaction catalyzed by CTP: Phosphocholine cytidylyltransferase in poliovirus-infected HeLa cells. J Biol Chem 1980; 255:1070–1073.

72. Chua TP, Smith CE, Reith RW, Williamson JD. nflammatory responses and the generation of chemoattractant activity in cowpox virus-infected tissues. Immunology 1990;69:202–208.

73. Clark ME, Dasgupta A. A transcriptionally active form of TFIIIC is modified in poliovirus-infected HeLa cells. Mol Cell Biol 1990; 10:5106–5113.

74. Clark ME, Hammerle T, Wimmer E, Dasgupta A. Poliovirus proteinase 3C converts an active form of transcription factor IIIC to an inactive form: A mechanism for inhibition of host cell polymerase III transcription by poliovirus. EMBO J 1991;10:2941–2947.

75. Clark ME, Lieberman PM, Berk AJ, Dasgupta A. Direct cleavage of human TATA-binding protein by poliovirus protease 3C in vivo and in vitro. Mol Cell Biol 1993;13:1232–1237.

76. Cleary ML, Smith SD, Sklar J. Cloning and structural analysis of cDNAs for bcl-2 and a hybrid bcl-2/immunoglobulin transcript resulting from the t(14;18) translocation. Cell 1986;47:19–28.

77. Clem RJ, Fechheimer M, Miller LK. Prevention of apoptosis by a baculovirus gene during infecton of insect cells. Science 1991;254: 1388–1390.

78. Clem RJ, Hardwick JM, Miller LK. Anti-apoptotic genes of baculoviruses. Cell Death Differ 1996;3:9–16.

79. Clem RJ, Miller LK. Apoptosis reduces both the in vitro replication and the in vivo infection of a baculovirus. J Virol 1993;67:3730–3738.

80. Clem RJ, Miller LK. Control of programmed cell death by the baculovirus gene. Mol Cell Biol 1994;14:5212–5222.

81. Cohen DI, Tani Y, Tian H, Boone E, Samelson LE, Lane HC. Participation of tyrosine phosphorylation in the cytopathic effect of human immunodeficiency virus-1. Science 1992;256:542–545.

82. Cohen JI, Kieff E. An Epstein-Barr virus nuclear protein 2 domain essential for transformation is a direct transcriptional activator. J Virol 1991;65:5880–5885.

83. Cohen JI, Wang F, Mannick J, Kieff E. Epstein-Barr virus nuclear protein 2 is a key determinant of lymphocyte transformation. Proc Natl Acad Sci U S A 1989;86:9558–9562.

84. Cohen JJ, Duke RC, Fadok VA, Sellins KS. Apoptosis and programmed cell death in immunity. Annu Rev Immunol 1992;10: 267–293.

85. Cohen PL, Eisenberg RA. The *lpr* and *gld* genes in systemic autoimmunity: Life and death in the *Fas* lane. Immunol Today 1992;13: 427–428.

86. Contreras A, Carrasco L. Selective inhibition of protein synthesis in virus-infected mammalian cells. J Virol 1979;29:114–1221.

87. Cotten M, Weber JM. The adenovirus protease is required for virus entry into host cells. Virology 1995;213:494–502.

88. Coulon P, Deutsch V, Lafay F, et al. Genetic evidence for multiple functions of the matrix protein of vesicular stomatitis virus. J Gen Virol 1990;71:991–996.

89. Cowan WM, Fawcett JW, O'Leary DDM, Stanfield BB. Regressive events in neurogenesis. Science 1984;225:1258–1265.

90. Crawford N, Fire A, Samuels M, Sharp PA, Baltimore D. Inhibition of transcription factor activity by poliovirus. Cell 1981;27:555–561.

91. Crone DE, Keene JD. Viral transcription is necessary and sufficient for vesicular stomatitis virus to inhibit maturation of small nuclear ribonucleoproteins. J Virol 1989;63:4172–4180.

92. Cudmore S, Cossart P, Griffiths G, Way M. Actin-based motility of vaccinia virus. Nature (London) 1995;378:636–638.

93. Cullen BR. Mechanism of action of regulatory proteins encoded by complex retroviruses. Microbiol Rev 1992;56:375–394.

94. Daly C, Reich NC. Double-stranded RNA activates novel factors that bind to the interferon-stimulated response element. Mol Cell Biol 1993;13:3756–3764.

95. Das S, Dasgupta A. Identification of the cleavage site and determinants required for poliovirus 3CPro-catalyzed cleavage of human TATA-binding transcription factor TBP. J Virol 1993;67:3326–3331.

96. Davies MV, Pelletier J, Meerovitch K, Sonenberg N, Kaufman RJ. The effect of poliovirus proteinase 2A(pro) expression on cellular metabolism. J Biol Chem 1991;266:14714–14720.

97. Dawson CW, Eliopoulos AG, Dawson J, Young LS. BHRF1, a viral homologue of the Bcl-2 oncogene, disturbs epithelial cell differentiation. Oncogene 1995;9:69–77.

98. de la Luna S, Fortes P, Beloso A, Ortin J. Influenza virus NS1 protein enhances the rate of translation initiation of viral mRNAs. J Virol 1995;69:2427–2433.

99. de la Torre JC, Oldstone MBA. Selective disruption of growth hormone transcription machinery by viral infection. Proc Natl Acad Sci U S A 1992;89:9939–9943.

100. De Mareuil J, Salaun D, Chermann JC, Hirsch I. Fusogenic determinants of highly cytopathic subtype D Zairian isolate HIV-1 NDK. Virology 1995;209:649–653.

101. Debbas M, White E. Wild-type p53 mediates apoptosis by E1A, which is inhibited by E1B. Genes Dev 1993;7:546–554.

102. Defer C, Belin MT, Caillet-Boudin ML, Boulanger P. Human adenovirus-host cell interactions: Comparative study with members of subgroups B and C. J Virol 1990;64:3661–3673.

103. Devaney MA, Vakharia VN, Lloyd RE, Ehrenfeld E, Grubman MJ. Leader protein of foot-and-mouth disease virus is required for cleavage of the p220 component of the cap-binding protein complex. J Virol 1988;62:4407–4409.

104. Dhein J, Walczak H, Baumler C, Debatin K-M, Krammer PH. Autocrine T-cell suicide mediated by APO-1/(Fas/CD95). Nature (London) 1995;373:438–441.

105. Doedens JR, Kirkegaard K. Inhibition of cellular protein secretion by poliovirus protein 2B and 3A. EMBO J 1995;14:894–907.

106. Dolph PJ, Huang J, Schneider RJ. Translation by the adenovirus tripartite leader: Elements which determine independence from cap-binding protein complex. J Virol 1990;64:2669–2677.

107. Dolph PJ, Racaniello V, Villamarin A, Palladino F, Schneider RJ. The adenovirus tripartite leader may eliminate the requirement for cap-binding protein complex during translation initiation. J Virol 1988;62:2059–2066.

108. Dong X, Hamilton KJ, Satoh M, Wang J, Reeves WH. Initiation of autoimmunity to the p53 tumor suppressor protein by complexes of p53 and SV40 large T antigen. J Exp Med 1994;179:1317–1330.

109. Driscoll M. Molecular genetics of cell death in the nematode *Caenorhabditis elegans*. J Neurobiol 1992;23:1327–1351.

110. Duboisdauphin M, Frankowski H, Tsujimoto Y, Huarte J, Martinou JC. Neonatal motoneurons overexpressing the bcl-2 protooncogene in transgenic mice are protected from axotomy-induced cell death. Proc Natl Acad Sci U S A 1994;91:3309–3313.

111. Duckett CS, Nava VE, Gedrich RW, et al A conserved family of apoptosis inhibitors related to the baculovirus *iap* gene. EMBO J 1996;15:2685–2694.

112. Duncan RF. Protein synthesis initiation factor modifications during viral infections: Implications for translational control. Electrophoresis 1990;11:219–227.
113. Esolen LM, Park SW, Hardwick JM, Griffin DE. Apoptosis as a cause of death in measles virus-infected cells. J Virol 1995;69: 3955–3958.
114. Estaquier J, Idziorek T, De Bels F, et al. Programmed cell death and AIDS: Significance of T-cell apoptosis in pathogenic and nonpathogenic primate lentiviral infections. Proc Natl Acad Sci U S A 1994; 91:9431–9435.
115. Estus S, Zaks WJ, Freeman RS, Gruda M, Bravo R, Johnson EM Jr. Altered gene expression in neurons during programmed cell death: Identification of c-Jun as necessary for neuronal apoptosis. J Cell Biol 1994;127:1717–1727.
116. Etchison D, Hansen J, Ehrenfeld E, et al. Demonstration in vitro that eucaryotic initiation factor 3 is active but that a cap-binding protein complex is inactive in poliovirus-infected HeLa cells. J Virol 1984; 51:832–837.
117. Etchison D, Milburn SC, Edery I, Sonenberg N, Hershey JW. Inhibition of HeLa cell protein synthesis following poliovirus infection correlates with the proteolysis of a 220,000-dalton polypeptide associated with eucaryotic initiation factor 3 and a cap binding protein complex. J Biol Chem 1982;257:14806–14810.
118. Everett RD, Fenwick ML. Comparative DNA sequence analysis of the host shutoff genes of different strains of herpes simplex virus: Type 2 strain HG52 incodes. J Gen Virol 1990;71:1387–1390.
119. Falk MM, Grigera PR, Bergmann IE, Zibert A, Multhaup G, Beck E. Foot-and-mouth disease virus protease 3C induces specific proteolytic cleavage of host cell histone H3. J Virol 1990;64:748–756.
120. Farnham AE, Epstein W. The influence of encephalomyocarditis (EMC) virus infection on potassium transport in L cells. Virology 1963; 21:436–447.
121. Farrell PJ. Epstein-Barr virus genome. In Klein G, ed. Advances in viral oncology: Tumorigenic DNA viruses, vol 8. New York: Raven Press, 1989:103–132.
122. Fearon DT. The CD19-CR2-TAPA-1 complex, CD45 and signaling by the antigen receptor of B lymphocytes. Curr Biol 1993;5:341–348.
123. Feigenblum D, Schneider RJ. Modification of eukaryotic initiation factor 4F during infection by influenza virus. J Virol 1993;67: 3027–3035.
124. Fenwick ML, Clark J. Early and delayed shut-off of host protein synthesis in cells infected with herpes simplex virus. J Gen Virol 1982; 61:121–125.
125. Fenwick ML, Everett RD. Transfer of UL41, the gene controlling virion-associated host cell shutoff, between different strains of herpes simplex virus. J Gen Virol 1990;71:411–418.
126. Fenwick ML, Everett RD. Inactivation of the shutoff gene (UL41) of herpes simplex virus types 1 and 2. J Gen Virol 1990;71:2961–2967.
127. Fenwick ML, McMenamin MM. Early virion-associated suppression of cellular protein synthesis by herpes simplex virus is accompanied by inactivation of mRNA. J Gen Virol 1984;65:1225–1228.
128. Fenwick ML, Owen SA. On the control of immediate early (alpha) mRNA survival in cells infected with herpes simplex virus. J Gen Virol 1988;69:2869–2877.
129. Fenwick ML, Walker MJ. Suppression of the synthesis of cellular macromolecules by herpes simplex virus. J Gen Virol 1978;41: 37–51.
130. Fernandez-Munoz R, Darnell JE. Structural difference between the 5' termini of viral and cellular mRNA in poliovirus-infected cells: Possible basis for the inhibition of host protein synthesis. J Virol 1976;126:719–726.
131. Fernandez-Puentes C, Carrasco L. Viral infection permeabilizes mammalian cells to protein toxins. Cell 1980;20:769–775.
132. Fesq H, Bacher M, Nain M, Gemsa D. Programmed cell death (apoptosis) in human monocytes infected by influenza A virus. Immunobiology 1994;190:175–182.
133. Fingeroth JD, Weis JJ, Tedder TF, Strominger JL, Biro PA, Fearon DT. Epstein-Barr virus receptor of human B lymphocytes is the C3d receptor CR2. Proc Natl Acad Sci U S A 1984;81:4510–4514.
134. Finke J, Fritzen R, Ternes P, et al. Expression of bcl-2 in Burkitt's lymphoma cell lines: Induction by latent Epstein-Barr virus genes. Blood 1992;80:459–469.
135. FitzGerald DJP, Padmanabhan R, Pastan I, Willingham MC. Adenovirus-induced release of epidermal growth factor and pseudomonas toxin in the cytosol of KB cells during receptor-mediated endocytosis. Cell 1983;32:607–617.
136. Fortes P, Beloso A, Ortin J. Influenza virus NS1 protein inhibits pre-mRNA splicing and blocks mRNA nucleocytoplasmic transport. EMBO J 1994;13:704–712.
137. Frade R, Barel M, Ehlin-Henriksson B, Klein G. gp140, the C3d receptor of human B lymphocytes, is also the Epstein-Barr virus receptor. Proc Natl Acad Sci U S A 1985;82:1490–1493.
138. Frade R, Crevon MC, Barel M, et al. Enhancement of human B cell proliferation by an antibody to the C3d receptor, the gp140 molecule. Eur J Immunol 1985;15:73–76.
139. Fradkin LG, Woshinaga SK, Berk AJ, Dasgupta A. Inhibition of host cell RNA polymerase III-mediated transcription by poliovirus: Inactivation of specific transcription factors. Mol Cell Biol 1987;7: 3880–3887.
140. Fresco LD, Kurilla MG, Keene JD. Rapid inhibition of processing and assembly of small nuclear ribonucleoproteins after infection with vesicular stomatitis virus. Mol Cell Biol 1987;7:1148–1155.
141. Frolov I, Schlesinger S. Translation of Sindbis virus mRNA: Effects of sequences downstream of the initiating codon. J Virol 1994;68: 8111–8117.
142. Frolov I, Schlesinger S. A comparison of the effects of Sindbis virus and Sindbis virus replicons on host cell protein synthesis and cytopathogenicity in BHK cells. J Virol 1994;68:1721–1727.
143. Frolov I, Schlesinger S. Translation of Sindbis virus mRNA: Analysis of sequences downstream of the initiating AUG codon that enhance translation. J Virol 1996;70:1182–1190.
144. Fujii M, Niki T, Mori T, et al. HTLV-I Tax induces expression of various immediate early serum responsive genes. Oncogene 1991;6: 2349–2352.
145. Fujii M, Sassone-Corsi P, Verma IM. c-fos promoter transactivation by the tax1 protein of human T-cell leukemia virus type I. Proc Natl Acad Sci U S A 1988;85:8526–8530.
146. Fujii M, Tsuchiya H, Chujoh T, Akizawa T, Seiki M. Interaction of HTLV-I Tax1 with p67SRF causes the aberrant induction of cellular immediate early genes through CArG boxes. Genes Dev 1992;6: 2066–2076.
147. Fujisawa J, Toita M, Yoshida M. A unique enhancer element for the *trans* activator (p40tax) of human T-cell leukemia virus type I that is distinct from cyclic AMP and 12-O-tetradecanoylphorbol-13-acetate-responsive elements. J Virol 1989;63:3234–3239.
148. Fujisawa J, Toita M, Yoshimura T, Yoshida M. The indirect association of human T-cell leukemia virus Tax proteins with DNA results in transcriptional activation. J Virol 1991;65:4525–4528.
149. Gagliardini V, Fernandez P-A, Lee RKK, et al. Prevention of vertebrate neuronal death by the crmA gene. Science 1994;263:826–828.
150. Galabru J, Katze MG, Robert N, Hovanessian AG. The binding of double-stranded RNA and adenovirus VAI RNA to the interferon-induced protein kinase. Eur J Biochem 1989;178:581–589.
151. Garcia I, Martinou I, Tsujimoto Y, Martinou J-C. Prevention of programmed cell death of sympathetic neurons by the bcl-2 proto-oncogene. Science 1992;258:302–304.
152. Garfinkel MS, Katze MG. Translational control by influenza virus. Selective and cap-dependent translation of viral mRNAs in infected cells. J Biol Chem 1992;267:9383–9390.
153. Garfinkel MS, Katze MG. Translational control by influenza virus. Selective translation is mediated by sequences within the viral mRNA 5'-untranslated region. J Biol Chem 1993;268:22223–22226.
154. Garry RF, Bishop JM, Parker S, Westbrook K, Lewis G, Waite MRF. Na+ and K+ concentrations and the regulation of protein synthesis in Sindbis virus-infected chick cells. Virology 1979;96:108–120.
155. Garry RF, Waite MRF. Na+ and K+ concentrations and the regulation of the interferon system in chick cells. Virology 1979;96: 121–128.
156. Garry RF, Westbrook K, Waite MRF. Differential effects of ouabain on host- and Sindbis virus-specific protein synthesis. Virology 1979; 99:179–182.
157. Gelbard HA, James HJ, Sharer LR, et al. Apoptotic neurons in brains from paediatric patients with HIV-1 encephalitis and progressive encephalopathy. Neuropathol Appl Neurobiol 1995;21:208–217.
158. Gessain A, Vernant JC, Maurs L, et al. Antibodies to human T-lymphotropic virus type I in patients with tropical spastic paraparesis. Lancet 1985;2:407–410.

159. Ghadge GD, Swaminathan S, Katze MG, Thimmapaya B. Binding of the adenovirus VAI RNA to the interferon-induced 68-kDa protein kinase correlates with function. Proc Natl Acad Sci U S A 1991;88:7140–7144.

160. Giam CZ, Xu YL. HTLV-I tax gene product activates transcription via pre-existing cellular factors and cAMP responsive element. J Biol Chem 1995;264:15236–15241.

161. Gobl AE, Funa K, Alm GV. Different induction patterns of mRNA for IFN-a and -b in human mononuclear leukocytes after in vitro stimulation with herpes simplex virus-infected fibroblasts and Sendai virus. J Immunol 1988;140:3605–3609.

162. Godfraind C, Holmes K, Coutelier J-P. Thymus involution induced by mouse hepatitis virus A59 in BALB/c mice. J Virol 1995;69:6541–6547.

163. Gold LH, Brot MD, Polis I, et al. Behavioral effects of persistent lymphocytic choriomeningitis virus infection in mice. Behav Neural Biol 1994;62:100–109.

164. Goodbourn S, Maniatis T. Overlapping positive and negative regulatory domains of the human beta-interferon gene. Proc Natl Acad Sci U S A 1988;85:1447–1451.

165. Gordon J, Walker L, Guy G, Brown G, Rowe M, Rickinson A. Control of human B-lymphocyte replication. II. Transforming Epstein-Barr virus exploits three distinct viral signals to undermine three separate control points in B-cell growth. Immunology 1986;58:591–595.

166. Grassmann R, Dengler C, Muller-Fleckenstein I, et al. Transformation to continuous growth of primary human T lymphocytes by human T-cell leukemia virus type I X-region transduced by a herpesvirus saimiri vector. Proc Natl Acad Sci U S A 1989;86:3351–3355.

167. Gray MA, Micklem KJ, Paternak CA. Protein synthesis in cells infected with Semliki Forest virus is not controlled by intracellular cation changes. Eur J Biochem 1983;135:299–302.

168. Greenspan JS, Greenspan D, Lennette ET, et al. Replication of Epstein-Barr virus within the epithelial cells of oral "hairy" leukoplakia, an AIDS-associated lesion. N Engl J Med 1985;313:1564–1571.

169. Gregory CD, Dive C, Henderson S, et al. Activation of Epstein-Barr latent genes protects human B cells from death by apoptosis. Nature (London) 1991;349:612–614.

170. Griffin DE, Levine B, Ubol S, Hardwick JM. The effects of alphavirus infection on neurons. Ann Neurol 1994;35:S23–S27.

171. Grinnell BW, Wagner RR. Inhibition of DNA-dependent transcription by the leader RNA of vesicular stomatitis virus: Role of specific nucleotide sequences and cell protein binding. Mol Cell Biol 1985;5:2502–2513.

172. Grossman SR, Johannsen E, Tong X, Yalamanchili R, Kieff E. The Epstein-Barr virus nuclear antigen 2 transactivator is directed to response elements by the J kappa recombination signal binding protein. Proc Natl Acad Sci U S A 1994;91:7568–7572.

173. Guinea R, Carrasco L. Phospholipid biosynthesis and poliovirus genome replication, two coupled phenomena. EMBO J 1990;9:2011–2016.

174. Guinea R, Lopez-Rivas A, Carrasco L. Modification of phospholipase C and phospholipase A2 activities during poliovirus infection. J Biol Chem 1989;264:21923–21927.

175. Hallett MB, Fuchs P, Campbell AK. Sendai virus causes a rise in intracellular free Ca2+ before cell fusion. Biochem J 1982;206:671–674.

176. Hammar SP, Mottet NK. Tetrazolium salt and electronmicroscopic studies of cellular degeneration and necrosis in the interdigital areas of the developing chick limb. J Cell Sci 1971;8:229.

177. Hammerschmidt W, Sugden B. Genetic analysis of immortalizing functions of Epstein-Barr virus in human B lymphocytes. Nature (London) 1989;340:393–397.

178. Hardwick JM, Lieberman PM, Hayward SD. A new Epstein-Barr virus transactivator, R, induces expression of a cytoplasmic early antigen. J Virol 1988;62:2274–2284.

179. Hardwicke MA, Sandri-Goldin RM. The herpes simplex virus regulatory protein ICP27 contributes to the decrease in cellular mRNA levels during infection. J Virol 1994;68:4797–4810.

180. Hellen CU, Facke M, Krausslich HG, Lee CK, Wimmer E. Characterization of poliovirus 2A proteinase by mutational analysis: Residues required for autocatalytic activity are essential for induction of cleavage of eukaryotic initation factor 4F polypeptide. J Virol 1991;65:4226–4231.

181. Hellen CU, Lee CK, Wimmer E. Determinants fo substrate recognition by poliovirus 2A prteinase. J Virol 1992;66:3330–3338.

182. Heller M, Dambaugh T, Kieff E. Epstein-Barr virus DNA. IX. Variation among viral DNAs from producer and nonproducer infected cells. J Virol 1982;38:632–648.

183. Henderson S, Hue D, Rowe M, Dawson C, Johnson G, Rickinson A. Epstein-Barr virus-coded BHRF1 protein, a viral homologue of bcl-2, protects human B cells from programmed cell death. Proc Natl Acad Sci U S A 1993;90:8479–8483.

184. Henderson S, Rowe M, Gregory C, et al. Induction of bcl-2 expression by Epstein-Barr virus latent membrane protein 1 protects infected B cells from programmed cell death. Cell 1991;65:1107–1115.

185. Hengartner MO, Ellis RE, Horvitz HR. Caenorhabditis elegans gene ced-9 protects cells from programmed cell death. Nature (London) 1992;356:494–499.

186. Hengartner MO, Horvitz HR. C. elegans cell survival gene ced-9 encodes a functional homolog of the mammalian proto-oncogene bcl-2. Cell 1994;76:665–676.

187. Henkel T, Ling PD, Hayward SD, Peterson MG. Mediation of Epstein-Barr virus EBNA2 transactivation by recombination signal-binding protein J kappa. Science 1994;265:92–95.

188. Henry GL, McCormack SJ, Thomis DC, Samuel CE. Mechanism of interferon action. Translational control and the RNA-dependent protein kinase (PKR): Antagonists of PKR enhance the translational activity of mRNAs that include a 161 nucleotide region from reovirus S1 mRNA. J Biol Regul Homeost Agents 1994;8:15–24.

189. Hershberger PA, LaCount DJ, Friesen PD. The apoptotic suppressor P35 is required early during baculovirus replication adn is targeted to the cytosol of infected cells. J Virol 1994;68:3467–3477.

190. Hershey JWB. Translational control in mammalian cells. Annu Rev Biochem 1991;60:717–755.

191. Hershey JWB. Introduction to translational initiation factors and their regulation by phosphorylation. Virology 1993;4:201–207.

192. Hickish T, Robertson D, Clarke P, et al. Ultrastructural localization of BHRF1: An Epstein-Barr virus gene product which has homology with bcl-2. Cancer Res 1994;54:2808–2811.

193. Hilton A, Mizzen L, MacIntyre G, Sheley S, Anderson R. Translational control in murine hepatitis virus infection. J Gen Virol 1986;67:923–932.

194. Hinds PW, Weinberg RA. Tumor suppressor genes. Curr Opin Genet Dev 1994;4:135–141.

195. Hinshaw VS, Olsen CW, Dybdahl-Sissoko N, Evans D. Apoptosis: A mechanism of cell killing by influenza A and B viruses. J Virol 1994;68:3667–3673.

196. Hirai H, Suzuki T, Fujisawa J-I, Inoue J-I, Yoshida M. Tax protein of human T-cell leukemia virus type I binds to the ankyrin motifs of inhibitory factor kB and induces nuclear translocation of transcription factor NF-kB proteins for transcriptional activation. Proc Natl Acad Sci U S A 1994;91:3584–3588.

197. Honer B, Shoeman RL, Traub P. Degradation of cytoskeletal proteins by the human immunodeficiency virus type 1 protease. Cell Biol Int Rep 1992;16:603–612.

198. Hooper JW, Fields BN. Role of the mu1 protein in reovirus stability and capacity to cause chromium release from host cells. J Virol 1996;70:459–467.

199. Hovanessian AG. Interferon-induced dsRNA-activated protein kinase (PKR): Antiproliferative, antiviral and antitumoral functions. Virology 1993;4:237–245.

200. Howie SEM, Sommerfield AJ, Gray E, Harrison DJ. Peripheral T lymphocyte depletion by apoptosis after CD4 ligation in vivo: Selective loss of CD44− and "activating" memory T cells. Clin Exp Immunol 1994;95:195–200.

201. Hsieh JJ, Hayward SD. Masking of the CBF1/RBPJ kappa transcriptional repression domain by Epstein-Barr virus EBNA2. Science 1995;268:560–563.

202. Huang J, Schneider RJ. Adenovirus inhibition of cellular protein synthesis is prevented by the drug 2-aminopurine. Proc Natl Acad Sci U S A 1990;87:7115–7119.

203. Huang J, Schneider RJ. Adenovirus inhibition of cellular protein synthesis involves inactivation of cap-binding protein. Cell 1991;65:271–280.

204. Hutt-Fletcher LM. Synergistic activation of cells by Epstein-Barr virus and B-cell growth factor. J Virol 1987;61:774–781.

205. Ink BS, Pickup DJ. Vaccinia virus directs the synthesis of early mRNAs containing 5' poly(A) sequences. Proc Natl Acad Sci U S A 1990;87:1536–1540.

206. Irurzun A, Arroyo J, Alvarez A, Carrasco L. Enhanced intracellular calcium concentration during poliovirus infection. J Virol 1995;69: 5142–5146.
207. Irurzun A, Perez L, Carrasco L. Involvement of membrane traffic in the replication of poliovirus genomes: Effects of brefeldin A. Virology 1992;191:166–175.
208. Irurzun A, Perez L, Carrasco L. Enhancement of phospholipase activity during poliovirus infection. J Gen Virol 1993;74:1063–1071.
209. Irurzun A, Sanchez-Palomino S, Novoa I, Carrasco L. Monensin and Nigericin prevent the inhibition of host translation by poliovirus, without affecting p220 cleavage. J Virol 1995;69:7453– 7460.
210. Ishii HH, Gobe GC. Epstein-Barr virus infection is associated with increased apoptosis in untreated and phorbol ester-treated human Burkitt's lymphoma (AW-Ramos) cells. Biochem Biophys Res Commun 1993;192:1415–1423.
211. Ito T, Jagus R, May WS. Interleukin 3 stimulates protein synthesis by regulating double-stranded RNA-dependent protein kinase. Proc Natl Acad Sci U S A 1994;91:7455–7459.
212. Ito Y, Nishiyama Y, Shimokata K, Nagata J, Takcyama II, Kunu A. The mechanism of interferon induction in mouse spleen cells stimulated with HVJ. Virology 1978;88:128–137.
213. Jen G, Detjen BM, Thach RE. Shutoff of HeLa cell protein synthesis by encephalomyocarditis virus and poliovirus: A comparative study. J Virol 1980;35:150–156.
214. Jeurissen SHM, Wagenaar F, Pol MA, van der Eb AJ, Noteborn MHM. Chicken anemia virus causes apoptosis of thymocytes after in vivo infection and of cell lines after in vitro infection. J Virol 1992; 66:7383–7388.
215. Jin XW, Speck SH. Identification of critical *cis* elements involved in mediating Epstein-Barr virus nuclear antigen 2-dependent activity of an enhancer located upstream of the viral BamHI C promoter. J Virol 1992;66:2846–2852.
216. Joachims M, Etchison D. Poliovirus infection results in structural alteration of a microtubule-associated protein. J Virol 1992;66: 5797–5804.
217. Joachims M, Harris KS, Etchison D. Poliovirus protease 3C mediates cleavage of microtuble-associated protein 4. Virology 1995; 211: 451–461.
218. Joe AK, Griffin DE, Chiu H, Hardwick JM, Levine B. Induction of apoptosis by the Sindbis virus E2 envelope glycoprotein. American Society for Virology 14th Annual Meeting, Austin, TX July 8–12, 1995. Abstract.
219. Jones FE, Smibert CA, Smiley JR. Mutational analysis of the herpes simplex virus virion host shutoff protein: Evidence that vhs functions in the absence of other viral proteins. J Virol 1995;69:4863–4871.
220. Joshi B, Yan R, Rhoads RE. In vitro synthesis of human protein synthesis initiation factor 4G and its localization on 43 and 48 S initiation complexes. J Biol Chem 1994;269:2048–2055.
221. Ju S-T, Panka DJ, Cui H, et al. Fas(CD95)/FasL interactions required for programmed cell death after T-cell activation. Nature (London) 1995;373:444–448.
222. Kamada S, Shimono A, Shinto Y, et al. bcl-2 deficiency in mice leads to pleiotropic abnormalities: Accelerated lymphoid cell death in thymus and spleen, polycystic kidney, hair hypopigmentation, and distorted small intestine. Cancer Res 1995;55:354–359.
223. Kao HT, Nevins JR. Transcriptional activation and subsequent control of the human heat shock gene during adenovirus infection. Mol Cell Biol 1983;3:2058–2065.
224. Katsikis PD, Wunderlich ES, Smith CA, Herzenberg LA, Herzenberg LA. Fas antigen stimulation induces marked apoptosis of T lymphocytes in human immunodeficiency virus-infected individuals. J Exp Med 1995;181:2029–2036.
225. Katze MG. Games virues play: A strategic initiative against the interferon-induced dsRNA activated 68,000 Mr protein kinase. Virology 1993;4:259–268.
226. Katze MG, Agy MB. Regulation of viral and cellular RNA turnover in cells infected by eukryotic viruses including HIV-1. Enzyme 1990;44:332–346.
227. Katze MG, DeCorato D, Krug RM. Cellular mRNA translation is blocked at both initiation and elongation after infection by influenza virus or adenovirus. J Virol 1986;60:1027–1039.
228. Katze MG, DeCorato D, Safer B, Galabru J, Hovanessian AG. Adenovirus VAI RNA complexes with the 68,000 Mr protein kinase to regulate its autophosphorylation and activity. EMBO J 1987;6:689–697.
229. Katze MG, Detjen BM, Safer B, Krug RM. Translational control by influenza virus: Suppression of the kinase that phosphorylates the alpha subunit of initiation factor eIF-2 and selective translation of influenza viral mRNAs. Mol Cell Biol 1986;6:1741–1750.
230. Katze MG, Lara J, Wambach M. Nontranslated cellular mRNAs are associated with the cytoskeletal framework in influenza virus or adenovirus infected cells. Virology 1989;169:312–322.
231. Katze MG, Tomita J, Black T, Krug RM, Safer B, Hovanessian A. Influenza virus regulates protein synthesis during infection by repressing autophosphorylation and activity of the cellular 68, 000-Mr protein kinase. J Virol 1988;62:3710–3717.
232. Kawanishi M. Epstein-Barr virus induces fragmentation of chromosomal DNA during lytic infection. J Virol 1993;67:7654–7658.
233. Kaye KM, Izumi KM, Kieff E. Epstein-Barr virus latent membrane protein 1 is essential for B-lymphocyte growth transformation. Proc Natl Acad Sci U S A 1993;90:9150–9154:
234. Khandjian EW, Turler H. Simian virus 40 and polyoma virus induce synthesis of heat shock protein in permissive cells. Mol Cell Biol 1983;3:1–8.
235. Kielian M. Membrane fusion and the alphavirus life cycle. Adv Virus Res 1995;45:113–151.
236. Kielian M, Helenius A. pH-induced alterations in the fusogenic spike protein of Semliki forest virus. J Cell Biol 1985;101:2284–2291.
237. Kingston RE, Cowie A, Morimoto RI, Gwinn KA. Binding of polyomavirus large T antigen to the human hsp70 promoter is not required for trans activation. Mol Cell Biol 1986;6:3180–3190.
238. Kirchweger R, Zielger E, Lamphear BJ, et al. Foot-and-mouth disease virus leader proteinase: Purification of the Lb form and determination of its cleavage site on eIF-4gamma. J Virol 1994;68:5677–5684.
239. Kitajewski J, Schneider RJ, Safer B, Munemitus SM, Samuel CE. Adenovirus VAI RNA antagonizes the antiviral action of interferon by preventing activation of the interferon-induced eIF-2 alpha kinase. Cell 1986;15:195–200.
240. Klavinskis LS, Notkins AL, Oldstone MBA. Persistent viral infection of the thyroid gland: Alteration of thyroid function in the absence of tissue injury. Endocrinology 1988;122:567–575.
241. Klavinskis LS, Oldstone MBA. Lymphocytic choriomeningitis virus can persistently infect thyroid epithelial cells and perturb thyroid hormone production. J Gen Virol 1987;68:1867–1873.
242. Klavinskis LS, Oldstone MBA. Lymphocytic choriomeningitis virus selectively alters differentiated but not housekeeping functions: Block in expression of growth hormone gene is at the level of transcriptional initiation. Virology 1989;168:232–235.
243. Kliewer S, Dasgupta A. An RNA polymerase II transcription factor inactivated in poliovirus-infected cells copurifies with transcription factor TFIID. Mol Cell Biol 1988;8:3175–3182.
244. Knutson JC. The level of c-fgr RNA is increased by EBNA-2, an Epstein-Barr virus gene required for B-cell immortalization. J Virol 1990;64:2530–2536.
245. Koga Y, Tanaka K, Lu Y, et al. Priming of immature thymocytes to CD3-mediated apoptosis by infection with murine cytomegalovirus. J Virol 1994;68:4322–4328.
246. Komiyama T, Ray CA, Pickup DJ, Howard AD, Thornberry NA, Peterson EP, Salvesen G. Inhibition of the interleukin-1 beta converting enzyme by the cowpox virus sepin CrmA: An example of cross-class inhibition. J Biol Chem 1994;269:19331–19337.
247. Koschel K. Poliovirus infection and poly(A) sequences of cytoplasmic cellular RNA. J Virol 1974;13:1061–1066.
248. Kowalik TF, DeGregori J, Schwarz JK, Nevins JR. E2F1 overexpression in quiescent fibroblasts leads to induction of cellular DNA synthesis and apoptosis. J Virol 1995;69:2491–2500.
249. Koyama AH. Induction of apoptotic DNA fragmentation by the infection of vesicular stomatitis virus. Virus Res 1995;37:285– 290.
250. Kozak M. Influences of mRNA secondary structure on initiation by eukaryotic ribosomes. Proc Natl Acad Sci U S A 1986;83:2850–2854.
251. Kozak M. An analysis of vertebrate mRNA sequences: Intimations of translational control. J Cell Biol 1991;115:887–903.
252. Kozopas KM, Yang T, Buchan HL, Zhou P, Craig RW. MCL1, a gene expressed in programmed myeloid cell differentiation, has se-

quence similarity to BCL2. Proc Natl Acad Sci U S A 1993;90: 3516–3520.

253. Krausslich HG, Nicklin MJH, Toyoda H, Etchison D, Wimmer E. Poliovirus proteinase 2A induces cleavage of eucaryotic initiation factor 4F polypeptide p220. J Virol 1987;61:2711–2718.

254. Kurane I, Meager A, Ennis FA. Induction of interferon alpha and gamma from human lymphocytes by dengue virus-infected cells. J Gen Virol 1986;67:1653–1661.

255. Kwong AD, Frenkel N. Herpes simplex virus-infected cells contain a function(s) that destabilizes both host and viral mRNAs. Proc Natl Acad Sci U S A 1987;84:1926–1930.

256. Kwong AD, Frenkel N. The herpes simplex virus virion host shutoff function. J Virol 1989;63:4834–4839.

257. Kyuwa S, Cohen M, Nelson G, Tahara SM, Stohlman SA. Modulation of cellular macromolecular synthesis by coronavirus: Implication for pathogenesis. J Virol 1994;68:6815–6819.

258. Lama J, Carrasco L. Expression of poliovirus nonstructural proteins in *Escherichia coli* cells. J Biol Chem 1992;267:15932–15937.

259. Lama J, Carrasco L. Mutations in the hydrophobic domain of poliovirus protein 3AB abrogate its permeabilizing activity. FEBS Lett 1995;367:5–11.

260. Lambris JD, Ganu VS, Hirani S, Muller-Eberhard HJ. Mapping of the C3d receptor (CR2)-binding site and a neoantigenic site in the C3d domain of the third component of complement. Proc Natl Acad Sci U S A 1985;82:4235–4239.

261. Lamphear BJ, Kirchweger R, Skern T, Rhoads RE. Mapping functional domains in eukaryotic protein synthesis initiation factor 4G (eIF4G) with picornaviral proteases. J Biol Chem 1995;270:21975–21983.

262. Lamphear BJ, Yan R, Yang F, et al. Mapping the cleavage site in protein synthesis initiation factor eIF-4gamma o the 2A proteases from human coxsackievirus and rhinovirus. J Biol Chem 1993;268:19200–19203.

263. Lanzrein M, Kasermann N, Weingart R, Kempf C. Early events of Semliki forest virus-induced cell-cell fusion. Virology 1993;196:541–547.

264. Larcher C, Kempkes B, Kremmer E, et al. Expression of Epstein-Barr virus nuclear antigen-2 (EBNA2) induced CD21/CR2 on B and T cell lines and shedding of soluble CD21. Eur J Immunol 1995;25:1713–1719.

265. Laude H, Gelfi J, Lavenant L, Charley B. Single amino acid changes in the viral glycoprotein M affect induction of alpha interferon by the coronavirus transmissible gastroenteritis virus. J Virol 1992;66:743–749.

266. Laurent-Crawford AG, Bernard K, Riviere Y, et al. Membrane expression of HIV envelope glycoproteins triggers apoptosis in CD4 cells. AIDS Res Hum Retroviruses 1993;9:761–773.

267. Laurent-Crawford AG, Krust B, Muller S, et al. The cytopathic effect of HIV is associated with apoptosis. Virology 1991;185:829–839.

268. Laux G, Adam B, Strobl LJ, Moreau-Gachelin F. The Spi-1/PU.1 and Spi-B ets family transcription factors and the recombination signal binding protein RBP-J kappa interact with an Epstein-Barr virus nuclear antigen 2 responsive cis-element. EMBO J 1994;13:5624–5632.

269. Lazard D, Fernandez-Tomas C, Gariglio P, Weinmann R. Modification of an adenovirus major late promoter-binding factor during poliovirus infection. J Virol 1989;63:3858–3864.

270. Lee KA, Sonenberg N. Inactivation of cap-binding proteins accompanies the shut-off of host protein synthesis by poliovirus. Proc Natl Acad Sci U S A 1982;79:3447–3451.

271. Lee M-A, Yates JL. BHRF1 of Epstein-Barr virus, which is homologous to human proto-oncogene *bcl-2*, is not essential for transformation of B cells or for virus replication in vitro. J Virol 1992;66:1899–1906.

272. Lee TG, Tang N, Thompson S, Miller J, Katze MG. The 58,000-dalton cellular inhibitor of the interferon-induced double-stranded RNA-activated protein kinase (PKR) is a member of the tetratricopeptide repeat family of proteins. Mol Cell Biol 1994;14:2331–2342.

273. Lee TG, Tomita J, Hovanessian AG, Katze MG. Purification and partial characterization of a cellular inhibitor of the interferon-induced protein kinase of Mr 68,000 from influenza virus-infected cells. Proc Natl Acad Sci U S A 1990;87:6208–6212.

274. Leibig HD, Ziegler E, Yan R, et al. Purification of two picornaviral 2A proteinases: Interaction with eIF-4 gamma influence on in vitro translation. Biochemistry 1993;32:7581–7588.

275. Leibowitz R, Penman S. Regulation of protein synthesis in HeLa cells. J Virol 1971;8:661–668.

276. Lenk R, Penman S. The cytoskeletal framework and poliovirus metabolism. Cell 1979;16:289–301.

277. Leung K, Nabel GJ. HTLV-I transactivator induces interleukin-2 receptor expression through an NF-kappa B-like factor. Nature (London) 1988;333:776–778.

278. Levine B, Goldman JE, Jiang HH, Griffin DE, Hardwick JM. Bcl-2 protects mice against fatal alphavirus encephalitis. Proc Natl Acad Sci U S A 1996;93:4810–4815.

279. Levine B, Griffin DE. Persistence of viral RNA in mouse brains after recovery from acute alphavirus encephalitis. J Virol 1992;66:6429–6435.

280. Levine B, Hardwick JM, Trapp BD, Crawford TO, Bollinger RC, and Griffin DE. Antibody-mediated clearance of alphavirus infection from neurons. Science 1991;254:856–860.

281. Levine B, Huang Q, Isaacs JT, Reed JC, Griffin DE, Hardwick JM. Conversion of lytic to persistent alphavirus infection by the bcl-2 cellular oncogene. Nature (London) 1993;361:739–742.

282. Lewis J, Hardwick JM. Sindbis virus-induced cell death does not require inhibition of host protein synthesis. American Society for Virology 14th Annual Meeting, Austin, TX, July 8–12, 1995. Abstract.

283. Lewis J, Wesselingh SL, Griffin DE, Hardwick JM. Sindbis virus-induced apoptosis in mouse brains correlates with neurovirulence. J Virol 1996;70:1828–1835.

284. Li CJ, Friedman DJ, Wang C, Metelev V, Pardee AB. Induction of apoptosis in uninfected lymphocytes by HIV-1 tat protein. Science 1995;268:429–431.

285. Liebowitz D. Nasopharyngeal carcinoma: The Epstein-Barr virus association. Semin Oncol 1994;21:376–381.

286. Liebowitz D, Kieff E. Epstein-Barr virus. In Roizman B, Whitley RJ, Lopez C, eds. The human herpesviruses. New York: Raven Press, 1993:107–172.

287. Lin K-I, Lee S-H, Narayanan R, Baraban JM, Hardwick JM, Ratan RR. Thiol agents and Bcl-2 identify an alphavirus-induced apoptotic pathway that requires activation of the transcription factor NF-kappa B. J Cell Biol 1995;131:1149–1161.

288. Ling PD, Hsieh JJ, Ruf IK, Rawlins DR, Hayward SD. EBNA-2 up-regulation of Epstein-Barr virus latency promoters and the cellular CD23 promoter utilizes a common targeting intermediate CBF1. J Virol 1994;68:5375–5383.

289. Ling PD, Rawlins DR, Hayward SD. The Epstein-Barr virus immortalizing protein EBNA-2 is targeted to DNA by a cellular enhancer-binding protein. Proc Natl Acad Sci U S A 1993;90:9237–9241.

290. Ling PD, Ryon JJ, Hayward SD. EBNA-2 of herpesvirus papio diverges significantly from the type A and type B EBNA-2 proteins of Epstein-Barr virus but retains an efficient transactivation domain with a conserved hydrophobic motif. J Virol 1993;67:2990–3003.

291. Lloyd RE, Grubman MJ, Ehrenfeld E. Relationship of p220 cleavage during picornavirus infection to 2A proteinase sequencing. J Virol 1988;62:4216–4223.

292. Lloyd RE, Toyoda H, Etchison D, Wimmer E, Ehrenfeld E. Cleavage of the cap binding protein complex polypeptide p220 is not effected by the second poliovirus protease 2A. Virology 1986;150:299–303.

293. Lloyd RM, Shatkin AJ. Translational stimulation by reovirus polypeptide sigma 3: Substitution for VAI RNA and inhibition of phosphorylation of the alpha subunit of eukaryotic initiation factor 2. J Virol 1992;66:6878–6884.

294. Logan J, Shenk T. Adenovirus tripartite leader sequence enhances translation of mRNAs late after infection. Proc Natl Acad Sci U S A 1984;81:3655–3659.

295. Lopez-Rivas A, Castrillo JL, Carrasco L. Cation content in poliovirus-infected HeLa cells. J Gen Virol 1987;68:335–342.

296. Lowe SW, Ruley HE. Stabilization of the p53 tumor suppressor is induced by adenovirus E1A and accompanies apoptosis. Genes Dev 1993;7:535–545.

297. Lu QL, Elia G, Lucas S, Thomas JA. Bcl-2 proto-oncogene expression in Epstein-Barr virus-associated nasopharyngeal carcinoma. Int J Can 1996;87:706–711.

298. Lu Y-Y, Koga Y, Tanaka K, Sasaki M, Kimura G, Nomoto K. Apoptosis induced in CD4+ cells expressing gp160 of human immunodeficiency virus type 1. J Virol 1994;68:390–399.

299. Lu Y, Qian X-Y, Krug RM. The influenza virus NS1 protein: A novel inhibitor of pre-mRNA splicing. Genes Dev 1994;8:1817–1828.

300. Lu Y, Wambach M, Katze MG, Krug RM. Binding of the influenza virus NS1 protein to double-stranded RNA inhibits the activation of the protein kinase that phosphorylates the eIF-2 translation initiation factor. Virology 1995;214:222–228.

301. Lu Y-Y, Koga Y, Tanaka K, Sasaki M, Kimura G, Nomoto K. Apoptosis induced in CD4+ cells expressing gp160 of human immunodeficiency virus type 1. J Virol 1994;68:390–399.

302. Lubin M. Intracellular potassium and macromolecular synthesis in mammalian cells. Nature (London) 1967;213:451–453.

303. Lucia-Jandris P, Hooper JW, Fields BN. Reovirus M2 gene is associated with chromium release from mouse L cells. J Virol 1993;67:5339–5345.

304. Lyles DS, Puddington L, McCreedy BJ. Vesicular stomatitis virus M protein in nuclei of infected cells. J Virol 1988;62:4387–4392.

305. Mah SP, Zhong LT, Liu Y, Roghani A, Edwards RH, Bredesen DE. The protooncogene bcl-2 inhibits apoptosis in PC12 cells. J Neurochem 1993;60:1183–1186.

306. Mann E, Edwards J, Brown DT. Polycaryocyte formation mediated by Sindbis virus glycoproteins. J Virol 1983;45:1083–1089.

307. Marchini A, Tomkinson B, Cohen JI, Kieff E. BHRF1, the Epstein-Barr virus gene with homology to Bcl-2, is dispensable for B-lymphocyte transformation and virus replication. J Virol 1991;65:5991–6000.

308. Marriott SJ, Boros I, Duvall JF, Brady JN. Indirect binding of human T-cell leukemia virus type 1 tax, to a responsive element in the viral long terminal repeat. Mol Cell Biol 1989;9:4152–4160.

309. Marshall CJ. Evolutionary relationships among the serpins. Phil Trans R Soc Lond B 1993;342:101–119.

310. Martin DP, Schmidt RE, DiStefano PS, Lowry OH, Carter JG, Johnson EM Jr. Inhibitors of protein synthesis and RNA synthesis prevent neuronal death caused by nerve growth factor deprivation. J Cell Biol 1988;106:829–844.

311. Martin DR, Yuryev A, Kalli RK, Fearon T, Ahearn JM. Determination of the structural basis for selective binding of Epstein-Barr virus to human complement receptor type 2. J Exp Med 1991;174:1299–1311.

312. Martinou I, Fernandez P-A, Missotten M, et al. Viral proteins E1B19K and p35 protect sympathetic neurons from cell death induced by NGF deprivation. J Cell Biol 1995;128:201–208.

313. Marvaldi JL, Lucas-Lenard J, Sekellick MJ, Marcus PI. Cell killing by viruses. Virology 1977;79:267–280.

314. Masucci MG, Szigeti R, Ernberg I, et al. Activation of B lymphocytes by Epstein-Barr virus/CR2 receptor interaction. Eur J Immunol 1987;17:815–820.

315. Mathews MB. Viral evasion of cellular defense mechanisms: Regulation of the protein kinase DAI by RNA effectors. Virology 1993;4:247–257.

316. McCarthy SA, Symonds HS, Van Dyke T. Regulation of apoptosis in transgenic mice by simian virus 40 T antigen-mediated inactivation of p53. Proc Natl Acad Sci U S A 1994;91:3979–3983.

317. McCormack SJ, Samuel CE. Mechanism of interferon action: RNA-binding activity of full-length and R-domain forms of the RNA-dependent protein kinase PKR—determination of KD values for VAI and TAR RNAs. Virology 1995;206:511–519.

318. McCormick W, Penman S. Inhibition of RNA synthesis in HeLa and L cells by mengovirus. Virology 1967;31:135–141.

319. McGowan JJ, Emerson SU, Wagner RR. The plus-strand leader RNA of VSV inhibits DNA-dependent transcription of adenovirus and SV40 genes in a soluble whole-cell extract. Cell 1982;28:325–333.

320. McMillan NAJ, Chun RF, Siderovski DP, et al. HIV-1 tat directly interacts with the interferon-induced, double-stranded RNA-dependent kinase, PKR. Virology 1995;213:413–424.

321. Meerovitch K, Svitkin YV, Lee HS, et al. La autoantigen enhances and corrects aberrant translation of Poliovirus RNA in reticulocyte lysate. J Virol 1993;67:3798–3807.

322. Melchers F, Erdei A, Schulz T, Dierich MP. Growth control of activated, synchronized murine B cells by the C3d fragment of human complement. Nature (London) 1985;317:264–267.

323. Mellits KH, Kostura M, Mathews MB. Interaction of adenovirus VA RNA(I) with the protein kinase DAI: Nonequivalence of binding and function. Cell 1990;61:843–852.

324. Meurs E, Chong K, Galabru J, Thomas MS, Kerr IM, Williams BR. Molecular cloning and characterization of the human double-stranded RNA-activated protein kinase induced by interferon. Cell 1990;62:379–390.

325. Meyaard L, Otto SA, Jonker RR, Miinster MJ, Keet RPM, Miedema F. Programmed death of T cells in HIV-1 infection. Science 1992;257:217–219.

326. Miller JE, Samuel CE. Proteolytic cleavage of the reovirus sigma 3 protein results in enhanced double-stranded RNA-binding activity: Identification of a repeated basic amino acid motif within the C-terminal binding region. J Virol 1992;66:5347–5356.

327. Miura M, Friedlander RM, Yuan J. Tumor necrosis factor-induced apoptosis is mediated by a CrmA-sensitive cell death pathway. Proc Natl Acad Sci U S A 1995;92:8318–8322.

328. Miyashita T, Reed JC. bcl-2 gene transfer increases relative resistance of S49.1 and WEH17.2 lymphoid cells to cell death and DNA fragmentation induced by glucocorticoids and multiple chemotherapeutic drugs. Cancer Res 1992;52:5407–5411.

329. Mobley PW, Lee HF, Curtain CC, Kirkpatrick A, Waring AJ, Gordon LM. The amino-terminal peptide of HIV-1 glycoprotein 41 fuses human erythrocytes. Biochim Biophys Acta 1995;1271:304–314.

330. Moore M, Schaack J, Baim SB, Morimoto RI, Shenk T. Induced heat shock mRNAs escape the nucleocytoplasmic transport block in adenovirus-infected HeLa cells. Mol Cell Biol 1987;7:4505–4512.

331. Moore MD, Cooper NR, Tack BF, Nemerow GR. Molecular cloning of the cDNA encoding the Epstein-Barr virus/C3d receptor (complement receptor type 2) of human B lymphocytes. Proc Natl Acad Sci U S A 1987;84:9194–9198.

332. Morey AL, Ferguson DJP, Fleming KA. Ultrastructural features of fetal erythroid precursors infected with parvovirus B19 in vitro: Evidence of cell death by apoptosis. J Pathol 1993;169:213–220.

333. Morrison T, McQuain C, McGinnes L. Complementation between avirulent Newcastle disease virus and a fusion protein gene expressed from a retrovirus vector: Requirements for membrane fusion. J Virol 1991;65:813–822.

334. Mosenkis J, Daniels-McQueen S, Janovec S, et al. Shutoff of host translation by encephalomyocarditis virus infection does not involve cleavage of the eucaryotic initiation factor 4F polypeptide that accompanies poliovirus infection. J Virol 1985;54:643–645.

335. Mosialos G, Birkenbach M, Yalamanchili R, VanArsdale T, Ware C, Kieff E. The Epstein-Barr virus transforming protein LMP1 engages signaling proteins for the tumor necrosis factor receptor family. Cell 1995;80:389–399.

336. Moss B. Inhibition of HeLa cell protein synthesis by the vaccinia virion. J Virol 1968;2:1028–1037.

337. Motoyama N, Wang F, Roth KA, et al. Massive cell death of immature hematopoietic cells and neurons in Bcl-x-deficient mice. Science 1995;267:1506–1510.

338. Murray PG, Swinnen LJ, Constandinou CM, Pyle JM, Hardwick JM, Ambinder RF. Bcl-2 but not its Epstein-Barr virus-encoded homologue, BHRF1, is commonly expressed in posttransplantation lymphoproliferative disorders. Blood 1996;87:706–711.

339. Murti KG, Goorha R. Interaction of frog virus-3 with the cytoskeleton. I. Altered organization of microtubules, intermediate filaments, and microfilaments. J Cell Biol 1983;96:1248–1257.

340. Mussgay M, Enzmann P-J, Horst J. Influence of an arbovirus infection (Sindbis Virus) on the protein and ribonucleic acid synthesis of cultivated chick embryo cells. Arch Gesamte Virusforsch 1970;31:81–92.

341. Nagata S, Golstein P. The Fas death factor. Science 1995;267:1449–1456.

342. Nair CN. Monovalent cation metabolism and cytopathic effects of poliovirus-infected HeLa cells. J Virol 1981;37:268–273.

343. Nakayama K-I, Nakayama K, Negishi I, et al. Disappearance of the lymphoid system in bcl-2 homozygous mutant chimeric mice. Science 1993;261:1584–1588.

344. Nakayama K, Nakayama K-I, Negishi I, Kuida K, Sawa H, Loh DY. Targeted disruption of Bcl-2ab in mice: Occurrence of gray hair, polycystic kidney disease, and lymphocytopenia. Proc Natl Acad Sci U S A 1994;91:3700–3704.

345. Nava VE, Cheng EH-Y, Clem RJ, Hardwick JM. ORF16 of herpesvirus Saimiri encodes a homolog of Bcl-2 with anti-apoptotic activity. 1996. (Submitted for publication)

346. Neilan JG, Lu Z, Afonso CL, Kutish GF, Sussman MD, Rock DL. An African swine fever virus gene with similarity to the proto-oncogene bcl-2 and the Epstein-Barr virus gene BHRF1. J Virol 1993; 67:4391–4394.

347. Nemeroff ME, Utans U, Kramer A, Krug RM. Identification of cis-acting intron and exon regions in influenza virus NS1 mRNA that inhibit splicing and cause the formation of aberrantly sedimenting presplicing complexes. Mol Cell Biol 1992;12:962–970.

348. Nemerow GR, Houghten RA, Moore MD, Cooper NR. Identification of an epitope in the major envelope protein of Epstein-Barr virus that mediates viral binding to the B lymphocyte EBV receptor (CR2). Cell 1989;56:369–377.

349. Nemerow GR, McNaughton ME, Cooper NR. Binding of monoclonal antibody to the Epstein Barr virus (EBV)/CR2 receptor induces antivation and differentiation of human B lymphocytes. J Immunol 1985;135:3068–3073.

350. Nemerow GR, Mold C, Keivens-Schwend V, Tollefson V, Cooper NR. Identification of gp350 as the viral glycoprotein mediating attachment of Epstein-Barr virus (EBV) to the EBV/C3d receptor of B cells: Sequence homology of gp350 and C3 complement fragment C3d. J Virol 1987;61:1416–1420.

351. Nemerow GR, Wolfert R, McNaughton ME, Cooper NR. Identification and characterization of the Epstein-Barr virus receptor on human B lymphocytes and its relationship to the C3d complement receptor (CR2). J Virol 1985;55:347–351.

352. Newell MK, Haughn LJ, Maroun CR, Julius MH. Death of mature T cells by separate ligation of CD4 and the T-cell receptor for antigen. Nature (London) 1990;347:286–289.

353. Nissen MS, Friesen PD. Molecular analysis of the transcriptional regulatory region of an early baculovirus gene. J Virol 1989;63: 493–503.

354. Nokta M, Eaton D, Steinsland OS, Albrecht T. Ca2+ responses in cytomegalovirus-infected fibroblasts of human origin. Virology 1987; 157:259–267.

355. Nokta M, Fons MP, Eaton DC, Albrecht T. Cytomegalovirus: Sodium entry and development of cytomegaly in human fibroblasts. Virology 1988;164:411–419.

356. Notarianni EL, Preston CM. Activation of cellular stress protein genes by herpes simplex virus temperature-sensitive mutants which overproduced immediate early polypeptides. Virology 1982;123: 113–122.

357. Noteborn MHM, Todd D, Verschueren CAJ, et al. A single chicken anemia virus protein induces apoptosis. J Virol 1994;68: 346–351.

358. Nῠῆez G, Hocknebery D, McDonnell TJ, Sorensen CM, Korsmeyer SJ. Bcl-2 maintains B cell memory. Nature (London) 1991;353:71–73.

359. O'Malley R, Duncan RF, Hershey JWB, Mathews MB. Modification of protein synthesis initiation factors and the shut-off of host protein synthesis in adenovirus-infected cells. Virology 1989;168: 112–118.

360. O'Malley RP, Mariano TM, Siekierka J, Mathews MB. A mechanism for the control of protein synthesis by adenovirus VA RNAI. Cell 1986;44:391–400.

361. O'Neill RE, Racaniello VR. Inhibition of translation in cells infected with a poliovirus 2A-pro mutant correlates with phosphorylation of the alpha subunit of eucaryotic initiation factor 2. J Virol 1989;63:5069–5075.

362. Ohno K, Okamoto Y, Miyazawa T, et al. Induction of apoptosis in a T lymphoblastoid cell line infected with feline immunodeficiency virus. Arch Virol 1994;135:153–158.

363. Oldstone MBA, Holmstoen J, Welsh RM Jr. Alterations of acetylcholine enzymes in neuroblastoma cells persistently infected with lymphocytic choriomeningitis virus. J Cell Physiol 1977;91:459–472.

364. Oldstone MBA, Rodriguez M, Daughaday WH, Lampert PW. Viral perturbation of endocrine function: Disorder of cell function leading to disturbed homeostasis and disease. Nature (London) 1984;307: 278–280.

365. Oldstone MBA, Sinha YN, Blount P, et al. Virus-induced alterations in homeostasis: Alterations in differentiated functions of infected cells in vivo. Science 1982;218:1125–1127.

366. Olsen CW, Kehren JC, Dybdahl-Sissoko NR, Hinshaw VS. bcl-2 alters influenza virus yield, spread, and hemagglutinin glycosylation. J Virol 1996;70:663–666.

367. Overton H, McMillan D, Hope L, Wong-Kai-In P. Production of host shutoff-defective mutants of herpes simplex virus type 1 by inactivation of the UL13 gene. Virology 1994;202:97–106.

368. Oyaizu N, McCloskey TW, Coronesi M, Chirmule N, Kalyanaraman VS, Pahwa S. Accelerated apoptosis in peripheral blood mononuclear cells (PBMCs) from human immunodeficiency virus type-1 infected patients and in CD4 cross-linked PBMCs from normal individuals. Blood 1993;82:3392–3400.

369. Paabo S, Severinsson L, Andersson M, Martens I, Nilsson T, Peterson PA. Adenovirus proteins and MHC expression. Adv Cancer Res 1989;52:151–163.

370. Paez E, Esteban M. Resistance of vaccinia virus to interferon is related to an interference phenomenon between the virus and the interferon system. Virology 1984;134:12–28.

371. Paez E, Esteban M. Resistance of vaccinia virus to interferons: Modulation of the 2-5A system in interferon-treated, vaccinia virus infected cells. Microbiologia 1987;3:163–178.

372. Paik S-Y, Banerjea AC, Harmison GG, Chen C-J, Schubert M. Inducible and conditional inhibition of human immunodeficiency virus proviral expression by vesicular stomatitis virus matrix protein. J Virol 1995;69:3529–3537.

373. Pak AS, Everly DN, Knight K, Read GS. The virion host shutoff protein of herpes simplex virus inhibits reporter gene expression in the absence of other viral gene products. Virology 1995;211:491–506.

374. Palumbo GJ, Pickup DJ, Fredrickson TN, McIntyre LJ, Buller RML. Inhibition of an inflammatory response is mediated by a 38-kDa protein of cowpox virus. Virology 1989;172:262–273.

375. Pan H, Griep AE. Altered cell cycle regulation in the lens of HPV-16 E6 or E7 transgenic mice: Implication for tumor suppressor gene function in development. Genes Dev 1994;8:1285–1299.

376. Pathak S, Webb HE. Effect of myocrisin (sodium auro-thio-malate) on the morphogenesis of avirulent Semliki forest virus in mouse brain: An electron microscopical study. Neuropathol Appl Neurobiol 1983;9:313–327.

377. Pearson GR, Luka J, Petti L, et al. Identification of an Epstein-Barr virus early gene encoding a second component of the restricted early antigen complex. Virology 1987;160:151–161.

378. Peluso RW, Lamb RA, Choppin PW. Infection with paramyxoviruses stimulates synthesis of cellular polypeptides that are also sitmulated in cells transformed by Rous sarcoma virus or deprived of glucose. Proc Natl Acad Sci U S A 1978;75:6120–6124.

379. Peranen J, Kaariainen L. Biogenesis of type I cytopathic vacuoles in Semliki Forest virus-infected BHK cells. J Virol 1991;65:1623–1627.

380. Perez L, Carrasco L. Lack of direct correlation between p220 cleavage and the shut-off of host translation after poliovirus infection. Virology 1992;189:178–186.

381. Perez L, Guinea R, Carrasco L. Synthesis of Semliki forest virus RNA requires continuous lipid synthesis. Virology 1991;183:74–82.

382. Perez L, Irurzun A, Carrasco L. Activation of phospholipase activity during Semliki Forest virus infection. Virology 1993;194:28–36.

383. Perini G, Wagner S, Green MR. Recognition of bZIP proteins by the human T-cell leukaemia virus transactivator Tax. Nature (London) 1995;376:602–605.

384. Pfitzner AJ, Tsai E, Strominger JL, Speck SH. Isolation and characterization of cDNA clones corresponding to transcripts from the BamHI H and F regions of the Epstein-Barr virus genome. J Virol 1987; 61:2902–2909.

385. Phillips B, Abravaya K, Morimoto RI. Analysis of the specificity and mechanism of transcriptional activation of the human hsp70 gene during infection by DNA viruses. J Virol 1991;65:5680–5692.

386. Piccone ME, Rieder E, Mason PW, Grubman MJ. The foot-and-mouth disease virus leader proteinase gene is not required for viral replication. J Virol 1995;69:5376–5382.

387. Pickup DJ, Ink BS, Hu W, Ray CA, Joklik WK. Hemorrhage in lesions caused by cowpox virus in induced by a viral protein that is related to plasma protein inhibitors of serine proteases. Proc Natl Acad Sci U S A 1986;83:7698–7702.

388. Pilder S, Logan J, Shenk T. Deletion of the gene encoding the adenovirus 5 early region 1B 21,000-molecular-weight polypeptide leads to degradation of viral and host cell DNA. J Virol 1984;52:664–671.

389. Pinto LH, Holsinger LJ, Lamb RA. Influenza virus M2 protein has ion channel activity. Cell 1992;69:517–528.

390. Pitha PM, Au WC. Induction of interferon alpha genes expression. Semin Virol 1995;6:151–159.

391. Porter AG. Picornavirus nonstructural proteins: Emerging roles in virus replication and inhibition of host cell function. J Virol 1993; 67:6917–6921.

392. Potempa J, Korzus E, Travis J. The serpin superfamily of proteinase inhibitors: Structure, function, and regulation. J Biol Chem 1994;2 69: 15957–15960.

393. Pratt CW, Church FC. General features of the heparin-binding serpins antithrombin, heparin cofactor II and protein C inhibitor. Blood Coagul Fibrinolysis 1993;4:479–490.

394. Qian XY, Alonso-Caplen F, Krug RM. Two functional domains of the influenza virus NS1 protein are required for regulation of nuclear export of mRNA. J Virol 1994;68:2433–2441.

395. Qiu Y, Krug RM. The influenza virus NS1 protein is a poly(A)-binding protein that inhibits nuclear export of mRNAs containing poly(A). J Virol 1994;68:2425–2432.

396. Qiu Y, Nemeroff M, Krug RM. The influenza virus NS1 protein binds to a specific region in human U6 snRNA and inhibits U6-U2 and U6-U4 snRNA interactions during splicing. RNA 1995;1:304–316.

397. Raab-Traub N. Epstein-Barr virus and nasopharyngeal carcinoma. Semin Cancer Biol 1992;3:297–307.

398. Rabizadeh S, LaCount DJ, Friesen PD, Bredesen DE. Expression of the baculovirus p35 gene inhibits mammalian neural cell death. J Neurochem 1993;61:2318–2321.

399. Raff MC. Social controls on cell survival and cell death. Nature (London) 1992;356:397–400.

400. Rangel LM, Gernandez-Tomas C, Dahmus ME, Gariglio P. Modification of RNA polymerase IIO subspecies after poliovirus infection. J Virol 1987;61:1002–1006.

401. Rangel LM, Gernandez-Tomas C, Dahmus ME, Gariglio P. Poliovirus-induced modification of host cell RNA polymerase IIO is prevented by cycloheximide and zinc. J Biol Chem 1988;263: 19267–19269.

402. Ransone LJ, Dasgupta A. A heat-sensitive inhibitor in poliovirus-infected cells which selectively blocks phosphorylation of the alpha subunit of eucaryotic initiation factor 2 by the double-stranded RNA-activated protein kinase. J Virol 1988;62:3551–3557.

403. Rao L, Debbas M, Sabbatini P, Hockenbery D, Korsmeyer S, White E. The adenovirus E1A proteins induce apoptosis, which is inhibited by the E1B 19-kDa and Bcl-2 proteins. Proc Natl Acad Sci U S A 1992;89:7742–7746.

404. Ray CA, Black RA, Kronheim SR, et al. Viral inhibition of inflammation:cowpox virus encodes an inhibitor of the interleukin-1-beta converting enzyme. Cell 1992;69:597–604.

405. Ray J, Whitton JL, Fujinami RS. Rapid accumulation of measles virus leader RNA in the nucleus in infected HeLa cells and human lymphoid cells. J Virol 1991;65:7041–7045.

406. Read GS, Frenkel N. Herpes simplex virus mutants defective in the virion-associated shutoff of host polypeptide synthesis and exhibiting abnormal synthesis of alpha (immediate early) viral polypeptides. J Virol 1983;46:498–512.

407. Read GS, Karr BM, Knight K. Isolation of a herpes simplex virus type 1 mutant with a deletion in the virion host shutoff gene and identification of multiple forms of the vhs (UL41) polypeptide. J Virol 1993;67:7149–7160.

408. Reichel PA, Merrick WC, Siekierka J, Mathews MB. Regulation of a protein synthesis initiation factor by adenovirus-associated RNA. Nature (London) 1985;313:196–200.

409. Rey-Cuille M-A. HIV-2 EHO isolate has a divergent envelope gene and induces single cell killing by apoptosis. Virology 1994;202: 471–476.

410. Rice AP, Kerr IM. Interferon-mediated, double-stranded RNA-dependent protein kinase is inhibited in extracts from vaccinia virus-infected cells. J Virol 1984;50:229–236.

411. Rice AP, Kostura M, Mathews MB. Identification of a 90-kDa polypeptide which associates with adenovirus VA RNA(I) and is phosphorylated by the double-stranded RNA-dependent protein kinase. J Biol Chem 1989;264:20632–20637.

412. Roizman B, Borman GS, Rousta M-K. Macromolecular synthesis in cells infeced with herpes simplex virus. Nature (London) 1965; 206:1374–1375.

413. Rooney CM, Brimmell M, Buschle M, Allan G, Farrell PJ, Kolman JL. Host cell and EBNA-2 regulation of Epstein-Barr virus latent-cycle promoter activity in B lymphocytes. J Virol 1992;66:496–504.

414. Rosen A, Casciola-Rosen L, Ahearn J. Novel packages of viral and self-antigens are generated during apoptosis. J Exp Med 1995;181: 1557–1561.

415. Rothe M, Pan M-G, Henzel WJ, Ayres TM, Goeddel DV. The TNFR2-TRAF signaling complex contains two novel proteins related to baculoviral inhibitor of apoptosis proteins. Cell 1995;83: 1243–1252.

416. Rowe M, Peng-Pilon M, Huen DS, et al. Upregulation of bcl-2 by the Epstein-Barr virus latent membrane protein LMP1: A B-cell-specific response that is delayed relative to NF-kB activation and to induction of cell surface markers. J Virol 1994;68:5602–5612.

417. Roy S, Katze MG, Parkin NT, Edery I, Hovanessian AG, Sonenberg N. Control of the inteferon-induced 68-kilodalton protein kinase by the HIV-1 tat gene product. Science 1990;247:1216–1219.

418. Rubinstein SJ, Dasgupta A. Inhibition of rRNA synthesis by poliovirus: Specific inactivation of transcription factors. J Virol 1989; 63:4689–4696.

419. Rubinstein SJ, Hammerle T, Wimmer E, Dasgupta A. Infection of HeLa cells with polivirus results in modification of a complex that binds to the rRNA promoter. J Virol 1992;66:3062–3068.

420. Rutter G, Mannweiler K. Alterations of actin-containing structures in BHK21 cells infected with Newcastle disease virus and vesicular stomatitis virus. J Gen Virol 1977;37:233–242.

421. Sabbatini P, Chiou S-K, Rao L, White E. Modulation of p53-mediated transcriptional repression and apoptosis by the adenovirus E1B 19K protein. Mol Cell Biol 1995;15:1060–1070.

422. Sabbatini P, Lin J, Levine AJ, White E. Essential role for p53-mediated transcription in E1A-induced apoptosis. Genes Dev 1995;9: 2184–2192.

423. Sacks WR, Greene CC, Aschman DP, Schaffer PA. Herpes simplex virus type 1 ICP27 is an essential regulatory protein. J Virol 1985; 55:796–805.

424. Saito S. Enchancement of the interferon-induced double-stranded RNA-dependent protein kinase activity by Sindbis virus infection and heat-shock stress. Microbiol Immunol 1990;34:859–870.

425. Samow P, Ho YS, Williams J, Levine AJ. Adenovirus E1B-58kd tumor antigen and SV40 large tumor antigen are physically associated with the same 54kd cellular protein. Cell 1982;28:387–395.

426. Samuel CE. The eIF-2 alpha protein kinases, regulators of translation in eukaryotes from yeasts to humans. J Biol Chem 1993;268: 7603–7606.

427. Sandvej K, Krenacs L, Hamilton-Dutoit SJ, Rindum JL, Pindborg JJ, Pallesen G. Epstein-Barr virus latent and replicative gene expression in oral hairy leukoplakia. Histopathology 1992;20:387–395.

428. Santomenna LD, Colberg-Poley AM. Induction of cellular hsp70 expression by human cytomegalovirus. J Virol 1990;64:2033–2040.

429. Sanz MA, Perez L, Carrasco L. Semliki forest virus 6K protein modifies membrane permeability after inducible expression in Escherichia coli cells. J Biol Chem 1994;269:12106–12110.

430. Scaria A, Tollefson AE, Saha SK, Wold WSM. The E3-11.6K protein of adenovirus is an asn-glycosylated integral membrane protein that localizes to the nuclear membrane. Virology 1992;191:743–753.

431. Schmid M, Wimmer E. IRES-controlled protein synthesis and genome replication of poliovirus. Arch Virol 1994;9:279–289.

432. Schneider RJ. Impact of virus infection on host cell protein synthesis. Ann Rev Biochem 1987;56:317–332.

433. Schneider RJ, Safer B, Munemitsu SM, Samuel CE, Shenk T. Adenovirus VAI RNA prevents phosphorylation of the eukaryotic initiation factor 2-alpha subunit subsequent to infection. Proc Natl Acad Sci U S A 1985;82:4321–4325.

434. Schnierle BS, Moss B. Vaccinia virus-mediated inhibition of host protein synthesis involves neither degradation nor underphosphorylation of components of the cap-binding eukaryotic translation initiation factor complex eIF-4F. Virology 1992;188:931–933.

435. Semmes OJ, Jeang K-T. Definition of a minimal activation domain in human T-cell leukemia virus type I Tax. J Virol 1995;69:1827–1833.

436. Sen GC, Ransohoff RM. Interferon-induced antiviral actions and their regulation. Adv Vir Res 1993;42:57–103.

437. Shahrabadi MS, Babiuk LA, Lee PW. Further analysis of the role of calcium in rotavirus morphogenesis. Virology 1987;158:103–111.

438. Sharp TV, Schwemmle M, Jeffrey I, et al. Comparative analysis of the regulation of the interferon-inducible protein kinase PKR by Epstein-Barr virus RNAs EBER-1 and EBER-2 and adenovirus VAI RNA. Nucleic Acids Res 1993;21:4483–4490.

439. Sharpe AH, Fields BN. Reovirus inhibition of cellular RNA and protein synthesis: Role of the S4 gene. Virology 1982;122:381–391.

440. Shen Y, Shenk T. Relief of p53-mediated transcriptional repression by the adenovirus E1B 19kDa protein or the cellular Bcl-2 protein. Proc Natl Acad Sci U S A 1994;91:8940–8944.

441. Siaw MFE, Nemerow GR, Cooper NR. Biochemical and antigenic analysis of the Epstein Barr virus/C3d receptor (CR2). J Immunol 1986;136:4146–4151.

442. Siekierka J, Mariano TM, Reichel PA, Mathews MB. Translational control by adenovirus: Lack of virus-associated RNAI during adenovirus infection results in phosphorylation of initiation factor eIF-2 and inhibition of protein synthesis. Proc Natl Acad Sci U S A 1985;82:1959–1963.

443. Sinclair AJ, Farrell PJ. Host cell requirements for efficient infection of quiescent primary B lymphocytes of Epstein-Barr virus. J Virol 1995;69:5461–5468.

444. Sixbey JW, Nedrud JG, Raab-Traub N, Hanes RA, Pagano JS. Epstein-Barr virus replication in oropharyngeal epithelial cells. N Engl J Med 1984;310:1225–1230.

445. Smibert CA, Popova B, Xiao P, Capone JP, Smiley JR. Herpes simplex virus VP16 forms a complex with the virion host shutoff protein vhs. J Virol 1994;68:2339–2346.

446. Smibert CA, Smiley JR. Differential regulation of endogenous and transduced beta-Globin genes during infection of erythroid cells with a herpes simplex virus type 1 recombinant. J Virol 1990;64: 3882–3894.

447. Sodroski JG. The human T-cell leukemia virus (HTLV) transactivator (Tax) protein. Biochim Biophys Acta 1992;1114:19–29.

448. Sommergruber W, Ahorn H, Klump H, et al. 2A proteinases of coxsackie- and rhinovirus cleave peptides derived from eIF-4gamma via a common recognition motif. Virology 1994;198:741–745.

449. Strasser A, Harris AW, Cory S. Bcl-2 transgene inhibits T cell death and perturbs thymic self-censorship. Cell 1991;67:889–899.

450. Strasser A, Whittingham S, Vaux DL, et al. Enforced BCL2 expression in B-lymphoid cells prolongs antibody responses and elicits autoimmune disease. Proc Natl Acad Sci U S A 1991;83:8661–8665.

451. Strauss JH, Strauss EG. The alphaviruses: Gene expression, replication, evolution. Microbiol Rev 1994;58:491–562.

452. Strijker R, Fritz DT, Levinson AD. Adenovirus VAI-RNA regulates gnee expression by controlling stability of ribosome-bound RNAs. EMBO J 1989;8:2669–2675.

453. Subramanian T, Tarodi B, Chinnadurai G. p53-independent apoptotic and necrotic cell deaths induced by adenovirus infection: Suppression by E1B 19K and Bcl-2 proteins. Cell Growth Differ 1995; 6:131–137.

454. Sugimoto A, Friesen PD, Rothman JH. Baculovirus p35 prevents developmentally programmed cell death and rescues a ced-9 mutant in the nematode Caenorhabditis elegans. EMBO J 1994;13:2023–2028.

455. Sung NS, Kenney S, Gutsch D, Pagano JS. EBNA-2 transactivates a lymphoid-specific enhancer in the BamHI C promoter of Epstein-Barr virus. J Virol 1991;65:2164–2169.

456. Suzuki T, Fujisawa JI, Toita M, Yoshida M. The transactivator tax of human T-cell leukemia virus type 1 (HTLV-I) interacts with cAMP-responsive element (CRE) binding and CRE modulator proteins that bind to the 21-base-pair enhancer of HTLV-I. Proc Natl Acad Sci U S A 1993;90:610–614.

457. Symonds H, Krall L, RemingtonL, et al. p53-dependent apoptosis suppresses tumor growth and progression in vivo. Cell 1994;78: 703–711.

458. Tahara SM, Dietlin TA, Bergmann CC, et al. Coronavirus translational regulation: Leader affects mRNA efficiency. Virology 1994; 202: 621–630.

459. Takahashi S, Doss C, Levy S, Levy R. TAPA-1, the target of an antiproliferative antibody, is associated on the cell surface with the Leu-13 antigen. J Immunol 1990;145:2207–2213.

460. Takemori N, Cladaras C, Bhat B, Conley A, Wold WSM. *Cyt* gene of adenovirus 2 and 5 is an oncogene for transforming function in early region E1B and encodes the E1B 19,000-molecular-weight polypeptide. J Virol 1984;52:793–805.

461. Takizawa T, Fukuda R, Miyawaki T, Ohashi K, Nakanishi Y. Activation of the apoptotic Fas antigen-encoding gene upon influenza virus infection involving spontaneously produced beta-interferon. Virology 1995;209:288–296.

462. Takizawa T, Matsukawa S, Higuchi Y, Nakamura S, Nakanishi Y, Fukuda R. Induction of programmed cell death (apoptosis) by influenza virus infection in tissue culture cells. J Gen Virol 1993;74: 2347–2355.

463. Tanaka A, Takahashi C, Yamaoka S, Nosaka T, Maki M, Hatanaka M. Oncogenic transformation by the tax gene of human T-cell leukemia virus type I in vitro. Proc Natl Acad Sci U S A 1990;87: 1071–1075.

464. Tanaka N, Kawakami T, Taniguchi T. Recognition DNA sequences of interferon regulatory factor 1 (IRF-1) and IRF-2, regulators of cell growth and the interferon system. Mol Cell Biol 1993;13:4531–4538.

465. Tanner J, Weis J, Fearon D, Whang Y, Kieff E. Epstein-Barr virus gp350/220 binding to the B lymphocyte C3d receptor mediates adsorption, capping, and endocytosis. Cell 1987;50:203–213.

466. Tarodi B, Subramanian T, Chinnadurai G. Epstein-Barr virus BHRF1 protein protects against cell death induced by DNA-damaging agents and heterologous viral infection. Virology 1994;201: 404– 407.

467. Taylor IC, Kingston RE. E1a transactivation of human HSP70 gene promoter substitution mutants is independent of the composition of upstream and TATA elements. Mol Cell Biol 1990;10:176–183.

468. Tedder TF, Clement LT, Cooper MD. Expression of C3d receptors during human B cell differentiation: Immunofluorescence analysis with the HB-5 monoclonal antibody. J Immunol 1984;133:678.

469. Tedder TF, Zhou L-J, Engel P. The CD19/CD21 signal transduction complex of B lymphocytes. Immunol Today 1994;15:437–442.

470. Teodoro JG, Shore GC, Branton PE. Adenovirus E1A proteins induce apoptosis by both p53-dependent and p53-independent mechanisms. Oncogene 1995;11:467–474.

471. Tesar M, Marquardt O. Foot-and-mouth disease virus protease 3C inhibits cellular transcription and mediates cleavage of histone H3. Virology 1990;174:364–374.

472. Tewari M, Beidler DR, Dixit VM. CrmA-inhibitable cleavage of the 70-kDa protein component of the U1 small nuclear ribonucleoprotein during fas- and tumor necrosis factor-induced apoptosis. J Biol Chem 1995;270:18738–18741.

473. Tewari M, Telford WG, Miller RA, Dixit VM. CrmA, a poxvirus-encoded serpin, inhibits cytotoxic T-lymphocyte-mediated apoptosis. J Biol Chem 1995;270:22705–22708.

474. Theill LE, Hattori K, Lazzaro D, Castrillo JL, Karin M. Differential splicing of the GHF1 primary transcript gives rise to two functionally distinct homeodomain proteins. EMBO J 1992;11:2261– 2269.

475. Thomis DC, Samuel CE. Mechanism of interferon action: Characterization of the intermolecular autophosphorylation of PKR, the interferon-inducible, RNA-dependent protein kinase. J Virol 1995;69: 5195–5198.

476. Thompson JP, Turner PC, Ali AN, Crenshaw BC, Moyer RW. The effects of serpin gene mutations on the distinctive pathobiology of cowpow and rabbitpox virus following intranasal inoculation of Balb/c mice. Virology 1993;197:328–338.

477. Thorley-Lawson DA. Basic virological aspects of Epstein-Barr virus infection. Semin Hematol 1988;25:247–260.

478. Thornberry NA, Bull HG, Calaycay JR, et al. A novel heterodimeric cysteine protease is required for interleukin-1-beta processing in monocytes. Nature (London) 1992;356:768–774.

479. Tian P, Estes MK, Hu Y, Ball JM, Zeng CQ, Schilling WP. The rotavirus nonstructural glycoprotein NSP4 mobilizes Ca2+ from the endoplasmic reticulum. J Virol 1995;69:5763–5772.

480. Tian P, Hu Y, Schiling WP, Lindsay DA, Eiden J, Estes MK. The nonstructural glycoprotein of the rotavirus affects intracellular calcium levels. J Virol 1994;68:251–257.

481. Tiensiwakul P, Khoobyarian N. Adenovirus fiber protein produces synthesis of interferon in mouse spleen and macrophage cultures. Intervirology 1983;20:52–55.

482. Tollefson AE, Scaria A, Hermiston TA, Ryerse JS, Wold LJ, Wold WSM. The adenovirus death protein (E3-11.6K) is required at very late stages of infection for efficient cell lysis and release of adenovirus from infected cells. J Virol 1996;70:2296–2306.

483. Tollefson AE, Scaria A, Saha SK, Wold WSM. The 11,600-M_w protein encoded by region E3 of adenovirus is expressed early but is greatly amplified at late stages of infection. J Virol 1992;66:3633– 3642.

484. Tolskaya EA, Romanova LI, Kolesnikova MS, et al. Apoptosis-inducing and apoptosis-preventing functions of poliovirus. J Virol 1995; 69:1181–1189.

485. Tomkinson B, Robertson E, Kieff E. Epstein-Barr virus nuclear proteins EBNA-3A and EBNA-3C are essential for B-lymphocyte growth transformation. J Virol 1993;67:2014–2025.

486. Tong X, Wang F, Thut CJ, Kieff E. The Epstein-Barr virus nuclear protein 2 acidic domain can interact with TFIIB, TAF40, and RPA70 but not with TATA-binding protein. J Virol 1995;69:585–588.

487. Trauth BC, Klas C, Peters AMJ, et al. Monoclonal antibody-mediated tumor regression by induction of apoptosis. Science 1989;245: 301–305.

488. Tropea F, Troiano L, Monti D, et al. Sendai virus and herpes virus type 1 induce apoptosis in human peripheral blood mononuclear cells. Exp Cell Res 1995;218:63–70.

489. Tsujimoto Y, Bashir MM, Givol I, Cossman J, Jaffe E, Croce CM. DNA rearrangements in human follicular lymphoma can involve the 5' or the 3' region of the bcl-2 gene. Proc. Natl. Acad. Sci. 1987; 84: 1329–1331.

490. Tucker PC, Strauss EG, Kuhn RJ, Strauss JH, Griffin DE. Viral determinants of age-dependent virulence of Sindbis virus for mice. J Virol 1993;67:4605–4610.

491. Tyler KL, Squier MKT, Rodgers SE, et al. Differences in the capacity of reovirus strains to induce apoptosis are determined by the viral attachment protein s1. J Virol 1995;69:6972–6979.

492. Tyor WR, Wesselingh SL, Levine B, Griffin DE. Longterm intraparenchymal immunoglobulin secretion after acute viral encephalitis in mice. J Immunol 1992;149:4016–4020.

493. Ubol S, Griffin DE. Identification of a putative alphavirus receptor on mouse neural cells. J Virol 1991;65:6913–6921.

494. Ubol S, Tucker PC, Griffin DE, Hardwick JM. Neurovirulent strains of alphavirus induce apoptosis in bcl-2-expressing cells; Role of a single amino acid change in the E2 glycoprotein. Proc Natl Acad Sci U S A 1994;1:5202–5206.

495. Ulug ET, Bose HR. Effect of tunicamycin on the development of the cytopathic effect in Sindbis virus-infected cells. Virology 1985;143: 546–557.

496. Ulug ET, Garry RF, Bose HR. The role of monovalent cation transport in Sindbis virus maturation and release. Virology 1989;172:42– 50.

497. Valsamakis A, Riviere Y, Oldstone MBA. Perturbation of differentiated functions in vivo during persistent viral infection. III. Decreased growth hormone mRNA. Virology 1987;156:214–220.

498. Van Steeg H, Kasperaitis M, Voorma HO, Benne R. Infection of neuroblastoma cells by Semliki Forest virus. The interference of viral capsid protein with the binding of host messenger RNAs into initation complexes is the cause of the shut-off of host protein synthesis. Eur J Biochem 1984;138:473–478.

499. Van Steeg H, Thomas A, Verbeek S, Kasperaitis M, Voorma HO. Shutoff of neuroblastoma cell protein synthesis by Semliki Forest virus: Loss of ability of crude initation factors to recognized early Semliki Forest virus and host mRNA's. J Virol 1981;38:728–736.

500. Van Steeg H, Van Grinsven M, Van Mansfeld F, Voorma HO, Benne R. Initiation of protein synthesis in neuroblastoma cells infected by Semliki Forest virus. FEBS Lett 1981;129:62–66.

501. Vance DE, Trip EM, Paddon HB. Poliovirus increases phosphatidylcholine biosynthesis in HeLa cells by stimulation of the rate-limiting reaction catalyzed by CTP: Phosphocholine cytidyltransferase. J Biol Chem 1980;255:1064–1069.

502. Vaux DL. Toward an understanding of the molecular mechanisms of physiological cell death. Proc Natl Acad Sci U S A 1993;90:786– 789.

503. Veis DJ, Sorenson CM, Shutter SR, Korsmeyer SJ. Bcl-2-deficient mice demonstrate fulminant lymphoid apoptosis, polycystic kidneys, and hypopigmented hair. Cell 1993;75:229–240.

504. Vincent MJ, Jabbar MA. The human immunodeficiency virus type 1 Vpu protein: A potential regulator of proteolysis and protein transport in the mammalian secretory pathway. Virology 1995;213:639– 649.

505. Wada N, Matsumura M, Ohba Y, Kobayashi N, Takizawa T, Nakanishi Y. Transcription stimulation of the Fas-encoded gene by nuclear factor for interleukin-6 expression upon influenza virus infection. J Biol Chem 1995;270:18007–18012.

506. Wagner RR, Thomas JR, McGowan JJ. Rhabdovirus cytopathology: Effects on cellular macromolecular synthesis. In Frankel-Conrat H, Wagner RR, eds. Comprehensive virology, vol 19. New York: Plenum, 1984:223–295.

507. Wagner S, Green MR. HTLV-I tax protein stimulation of DNA binding of bZIP proteins by enhancing dimerization. Science 1993;262: 395–399.

508. Wahlberg JM, Garoff H. Membrane fusion process of Semliki forest virus. I. Low pH-induced rearrangement in spike protein quaternary structure precedes virus penetration into cells. J Cell Biol 1992;116: 339–348.

509. Waltzer L, Logeat F, Brou C, Israel A, Sergeant A, Manet E. The human J kappa recombination signal sequence binding protein (RBP-Jk) targets the Epstein-Barr virus EBNA2 protein to its DNA responsive elements. EMBO J 1994;13:5633–5638.

510. Wang A-Q, Dudhane A, Orlikowsky T, et al. CD4 engagement induced Fas antigen-dependent apoptosis of T cells in vivo. Eur J Immunol 1994;24:1549–1552.

511. Wang F, Kikutani H, Tsang S, Kishimoto T, Kieff E. Epstein-Barr virus nuclear protein 2 transactivates a cis-acting CD23 DNA element. J Virol 1991;65:4101–4106.

512. Wang F, Tsang SF, Kurilla MG, Cohen JI, Kieff E. Epstein-Barr virus nuclear antigen 2 transactivates the latent membrane protein (LMP1). J Virol 1990;64:3407–3416.

513. Watanabe-Fukunaga R, Brannan CI, Copeland NG, Jenkins NA, Nagata S. Lymphoroliferation disorder in mice explained by defects in Fas antigen that mediates apoptosis. Nature (London) 1992;356: 314–317.

514. Watowich SS, Morimoto RI, Lamb RA. Flux of the paramyxovirus hemagglutinin-neuraminidase glycoprotein through the endoplasmic reticulum activates transcription of the GRP78-BiP gene. J Virol 1991;65:3590–3597.

515. Watson JC, Chang HW, Jacobs BL. Characterization of a vaccinia virus-encoded double-stranded RNA-binding protein that may be involved in inhibition of the double-stranded RNA-dependent protein kinase. Virology 1991;185:206–216.

516. Weck PK, Wagner RR. Inhibition of RNA synthesis in mouse myeloma cells infected with vesicular stomatitis virus. J Virol 1978; 25: 770–780.

517. Weis JJ, Tedder TF, Fearon DT. Identification of a 145,000 Mr membrane protein as the C3d receptor (CR2) of human B lymphocytes. Proc Natl Acad Sci U S A 1984;81:881.

518. Wertz GW, Youngner JS. Interferon production and inhibition of host synthesis in cells infected with vesicular stomatitis virus. J Virol 1970;6:476–484.

519. Westendorp MO, Frank R, Ochsenbauer C, et al. Sensitization of T cells to CD95-mediated apoptosis by HIV-1 Tat and gp120. Nature (London) 1995;375:497–500.

520. Whitaker-Dowling P, Youngner JS. Vaccinia rescue of VSV from interferon-induced resistance: Reversal of translation block and inhibition of protein kinase activity. Virology 1983;131:128–136.

521. White E. Regulation of apoptosis by the transforming genes of the DNA tumor virus adenovirus. Proc Soc Exp Biol Med 1993;204:30– 39.

522. White E. Function of the adenovirus E1B oncogene in infected an transformed cells. Virology 1994;5:341–348.

523. White E, Cipriani R. Specific disruption of intermediate filaments and the nuclear lamina by the 19-kDa product of the adenovirus E1B oncogene. Proc Natl Acad Sci U S A 1989;86:9886–9890.

524. White E, Cipriani R, Sabbatini S, Denton A. Adenovirus E1B 19-kilodalton protein overcomes the cytotoxicity of E1A proteins. J Virol 1991;65:2968–2978.

525. White E, Grodzicker T, Stillman BW. Mutations in the gene encoding the adenovirus early region 1B 19,000-molecular weight tumor antigen cause the degradation of chromosomal DNA. J Virol 1984; 52:410–419.

526. White J, Matlin K, Helenius A. Cell fusion by Semliki forest, influenza, and vesicular stomatitis viruses. J Cell Biol 1981;89:674– 679.

527. Whiteside ST, King P, Goodbourne S. A truncated form of the IRF-2 transcription factor has the properties of a postinduction repressor of interferon-beta gene expression. J Biol Chem 1994;269:27059– 27065.

528. Willems M, Penman S. The mechanism of host cell protein synthesis inhibition by poliovirus. Virology 1966;30:355–367.

529. Williams GT, McClanahan TK, Morimoto RI. E1a transactivation of the human HSP70 promoter is mediated through the basal transcriptional complex. Mol Cell Biol 1989;9:2574–2587.

530. Wilson DE. Inhibition of host-cell protein and ribonucleic acid synthesis by Newcastle disease virus. J Virol 1968;2:1–6.

531. Wong-Staal F, Gallo RC. The family of human T-lymphotropic leukemia viruses: HTLV-I as a cause of adult T cell leukemia and HTLV-III as the cause of acquired immunodeficiency syndrome. Blood 1991;65:253–263.

532. Wu BJ, Hurst HC, Hones NC, Morimoto RI. The E1A 13S product of adenovirus 5 activates transcription of the cellular human HSP70 gene. Mol Cell Biol 1986;6:2994–2999.

533. Wyckoff EE, Croall DE, Ehrenfeld E. The p220 component of eukaryotic initiation factor 4F is a substrate for multiple calcium-dependent enzymes. Biochemistry 1990;29:10055–10061.

534. Wyckoff EE, Hershey JW, Ehrenfeld E. Eukaryotic initiation factor 3 is required for poliovirus 2A protease-induced cleavage of the p220 component of eukaryotic initiation factor 4F. Proc Natl Acad Sci U S A 1990;87:9529.

535. Wyckoff EE, Lloyd RE, Ehrenfeld E. Relationship of eukaryotic initiation factor 3 to poliovirus-induced p220 cleavage activity. J Virol 1992;66:2943–2951.

536. Xue D, Horvitz R. Inhibition of the *Caenorhabditis elegans* cell-death protease CED-3 by a CED-3 cleavage site in baculovirus p35 protein. Nature (London) 1995;377:248–251.

537. Yamada T, Yamaoka S, Goto T, Nakai M, Tsujimoto Y, Hatanaka M. The human T-cell leukemia virus type I Tax protein induces apoptosis which is blocked by the Bcl-2 protein. J Virol 1994;68:3374–3379.

538. Yang E, Zha J, Jockel J, Boise LH, Thompson CB, Korsmeyer SJ. Bad, a heterodimeric partner for Bcl-xL and Bcl-2, displaces Bax and promotes cell death. Cell 1995;80:285–291.

539. Yaoi Y, Mitsui H, Amano M. Effect of U.V.-irradiated vesicular stomatitis virus on nucleic acid synthesis in chick embryo cells. J Gen Virol 1970;8:165–172.

540. Ye Z, Sun W, Suryanarayana K, Justice P, Robinson D, Wagner RR. Membrane-binding domains and cytopathogenesis of the matrix protein of vesicular stomatitis virus. J Virol 1994;68:7386–7396.

541. Yew P, Liu X, Berk AJ. Adenovirus E1B oncoprotein tethers a transcriptional repression domain to p53. Genes Dev 1994;8:190–202.

542. Yew PR, Berk AJ. Inhibition of p53 transactivation required for transformation by adenovirus early 1B protein. Nature (London) 1992;357:82–85.

543. Yin M-J, Paulssen EJ, Seeler S-J, Gaynor RB. Protein domains involved in both in vivo and in vitro interactions between human T-cell leukemia virus type I Tax and CREB. J Virol 1995;69:3420–3432.

544. Yoshida H, Sumichika H, Hamano S, et al. Induction of apoptosis of T cells by infecting mice with murine cytomegalovirus. J Virol 1995;69:4769–4775.

545. Young LS, Lau R, Rowe M, et al. Differentiation-associated expression of the Epstein-Barr virus BZLF1 transactivator protein in oral hairy leukoplakia. J Virol 1991;65:2868–2874.

546. Yuan J, Horvitz HR. The Caenorhabditis elegans genes ced-3 and ced-4 act cell autonomously to cause programmed cell death. Dev Biol 1990;138:33–41.

547. Yuan J, Shaham S, Ledoux S, Ellis HM, Horvitz HR. The *C. elegans* cell death gene *ced-3* encodes a protein similar to mammalian interleukin-1-beta-converting enzyme. Cell 1993;75:641–652.

548. Zhai ZH, Wang X, Qian XY. Nuclear matrix-intermediate filament system and its alteration in adenovirus infected HeLa cell. Cell Biol Int Rep 1988;12:99–108.

549. Zhang Y, Dolph PJ, Schneider RJ. Secondary structure analysis of adenovirus tripartite leader. J Biol Chem 1989;264:10679–10684.

550. Zhang Y, Feigenblum D, Schneider RJ. A late adenovirus factor induces eIF-4E dephosphorylation and inhibition of cell protein synthesis. J Virol 1994;68:7040–7050.

551. Zhang Y, Schneider RJ. Adenovirus inhibition of cell translation facilitates release of virus particles and enhances degradation of the cytokeratin network. J Virol 1994;68:2544–2555.

552. Zhao L, Giam C. Human T-cell lymphotropic virus type I (HTLV-I) transcriptional activator, Tax, enhances CREB binding to HTLV-I 21-base-pair repeats by protein-protein interaction. Proc Natl Acad Sci U S A 1992;89:7070–7074.

553. Zhong L-T, Sarafian T, Kane DJ, et al. Bcl-2 inhibits death of central neural cells induced by multiple agents. Proc Natl Acad Sci U S A 1993;90:4533–4537.

554. Zhu H, Shen Y, Shenk T. Human cytomegalovirus IE1 and IE2 proteins block apoptosis. J Virol 1995;69:7960–7970.

555. Zhuang S-M, Shvarts A, van Ormondt H, et al. Apoptin, a protein derived from chicken anemia virus, induces p53-independent apoptosis in human osteosarcoma cells. Cancer Res 1995;55:486–489.

556. Ziegler E, Borman AM, Deliat FG, et al. Picornavirus 2A proteinase-mediated stimulation of internal initiation of translation is dependent on enzymatic activity and the cleavage products of cellular proteins. Virology 1995;213:549–557.

557. Zimber-Strobl U, Strobl LJ, Meitinger C, et al. Epstein-Barr virus nuclear antigen 2 exerts its transactivating function through interaction with recombination signal binding protein RBP-J kappa, the homologue of Drosophila Suppressor of Hairless. EMBO J 1994;13:4973–4982.

558. Zimber-Strobl U, Suentzenich K-O, Laux G, et al. Epstein-Barr virus nuclear antigen 2 activates transcription of the terminal protein gene. J Virol 1991;65:415–423.

Viral Pathogenesis,
edited by Neal Nathanson, et al.
Lippincott–Raven Publishers, Philadelphia © 1997

CHAPTER 5

Viral Virulence

Neal Nathanson and Grant McFadden

INTRODUCTION

Virulence refers to the ability of a virus to cause illness or death in an infected host relative to other isolates or variants of the same agent. Interest in virulence arises from the empiri-

cal observation that this feature, like other biological characteristics, is subject to natural variation. It has been recognized since the beginnings of experimental virology that different strains of a given virus may differ in their ability to cause disease, although the significance of this variation in studies of viral pathogenesis has sometimes been overlooked. Interest in virulence has been enhanced by the application of molecular genetics, which has made it possible to deliberately alter the virulence determinants of the viral genome, either to analyze mechanisms or to construct attenuated-virus variants for use as vaccines.

N. Nathanson: Department of Microbiology, University of Pennsylvania Medical Center, Philadelphia, PA 19104.
G. McFadden: Department of Biochemistry, University of Alberta, Edmonton, Alberta, Canada T6G 2H7.

There are two distinct yet complementary approaches to the study of virulence. If virulence is regarded as a property of the virus, it is of interest to map the genetic determinants of this property, a field that has blossomed in the last decade with the development of increasingly sophisticated methods in molecular genetics. Mapping of genetic determinants defines proteins, or noncoding sequences, of importance and raises questions regarding the biochemical or structural mechanisms that underlie the phenotype.

The other approach to virulence is through study of pathogenesis to describe the differences in infections with viral variants of different virulence. Virulence differences may be quantitative, involving the rate of viral replication or number of cells infected, or they may be qualitative. It is important to recognize the qualitative aspect of viral variation at the outset, because it confers a multidimensional character on virus virulence that cannot always be measured along a simple linear axis. Variants of a single virus may differ markedly in their cellular tropism, their impact on the cells that they infect, their mode of dissemination in the infected host, and the disease phenotype that they produce.

Virulence is intimately intertwined with pathogenesis. Not only can the study of virulence variants provide important insights into pathogenesis, but variation in viral phenotype must be given consideration in design and interpretation of in vivo studies of the dissemination, localization, and pathologic consequences of viral infection. Historically, the failure to understand this point has led to important misunderstanding about the pathogenesis of viruses such as poliovirus (see Chaps. 1 and 23).[129] Study of virulence also has practical implications, because it carries the potential for the development of attenuated live virus variants that could be used as vaccines. The potential for this approach was initially demonstrated in 1798 by Jenner and colleagues[50] when he introduced vaccinia virus for the prevention of smallpox, although vaccinia is not an attenuated strain of variola but a distinct virus of bovines.

MEASURES OF VIRAL VIRULENCE

Relative Nature of Viral Virulence

Virulence is not an absolute property of a virus strain; it depends on the dose of virus, the route of infection, and the age, gender, and genetic susceptibility of the host. Two viruses that differ in virulence in one experimental paradigm may exhibit similar virulence in another paradigm. This point is illustrated in Table 5-1, which compares a virulent wild-type clone of La Crosse virus, a bunyavirus, with a laboratory-derived attenuated bunyavirus clone. When the two viruses are injected intracerebrally in adult mice, the differences in their virulence are striking; one plaque-forming unit (PFU) of the wild-type virus initiates a fatal encephalitis, whereas 10^6 PFU of attenuated clone B.5 fails to cause illness. Conversely, both viruses are highly virulent when injected intracerebrally in suckling mice (about 1 PFU of either virus is lethal) and can scarcely be distinguished from each other in this regard. Likewise, when injected subcutaneously (the natural route of entry for an arbovirus) in suckling mice, wild-type La Crosse virus is highly virulent, whereas clone B.5 is very attenuated, although both viruses are equally innocuous when injected by the subcutaneous route in adult mice.

Clinical, Pathologic, and Functional Indicators of Disease

The conventional measure of viral virulence is the production of disease in the host, defined either by death or by some specific constellation of signs and symptoms caused by the infection. For poliovirus, this measure is paralysis; for hepatitis virus, the intensity of jaundice or period of hospitalization; for variola virus, the extent and severity of pox. Measurement of viral virulence is illustrated for poliovirus in Table 5-2, which

TABLE 5-1. *The relative virulence of viruses depends on the context within which they are assessed**

Virus clone	IC Infection; suckling mice	SC Infection; suckling mice	IC Infection; adult mice	SC Infection; adult mice
Wild-type La Crosse original	~1	~1	~1	>10^7
Attenuated B.5 clone	~1	>10^5	>10^6	>10^7

*Illustrated by two variants of La Crosse virus (a bunyavirus) when injected by different routes in suckling and adult mice. One clone, La Crosse/original, is a wild-type isolate; the other, B.5, is a laboratory-derived attenuated strain. The two viruses exhibit striking differences in virulence upon intracerebral (IC) injection of adult mice or subcutaneous (SC) injection of suckling mice, but both appear similar in their high virulence for suckling mice inoculated intracerebrally and in their low virulence for adult mice inoculated subcutaneously. Virulence is expressed as the ratio of PFU per LD50; the lower the number, the more virulent the virus.

Data from Endres MJ, Valsamakis A, Gonzalez-Scarano F, Nathanson N. Neuroattenuated bunyavirus variant: derivation, characterization, and revertant clones. J Virol 1990;64: 1927–1933.

TABLE 5-2. *Virulence expressed as the comparative ability of different strains of a virus to produce clinical illness**

Virus	Study period	Rate per 1,000,000 primary infections (range)	Relative rates
Wild-type[†] (mainly type 1)	1931–1954	7000 (2000–20,000)	~10,000
OPV[††] (mainly type 3)	1961–1978	0.62	1

*Table shows the comparative paralytic rate for wild-type polioviruses circulating in nature compared with the attenuated oral polioviruses (OPV) that are included in the vaccine formulated by Sabin.

†Natural poliomyelitis: the ranges are derived either from studies of outbreaks where infection was determined by serological surveys or from lifetime risk studies; the overall average was about 7000 per 1,000,000 infections, or 1 case per 150 infections. These estimates mainly represent the risk for infection with type 1 virus; which accounted for about 75% of paralytic cases, whereas type 2 caused about 15% and type 3 about 10% of cases.[120]

††Vaccine-associated poliomyelitis: the population represents first infections with the vaccine virus, and the numerator is limited to recipient cases (contact cases are omitted). Among 135,000,000 vaccine recipients, there were 84 paralytic cases. These estimates mainly represent the risk for infection with type 3 virus, which accounted for about 70% of paralytic cases, whereas type 2 caused about 5% and type 1 about 25% of cases.[116,120,122,145]

contrasts the paralytic rate following primary infection with wild-type virus with that following administration of oral poliovirus vaccine (OPV). In this instance, the paralytogenic potential of the vaccine viruses is estimated to be about 10,000-fold lower than that of wild-type polioviruses. The incubation period to onset of illness or survival time to death are subsidiary measures that usually vary directly with virulence, as shown in a comparison of strains of myxoma virus (a leporipoxvirus) (Table 5-3).

The data in Table 5-3 illustrate another fundamental concept in viral pathogenesis: virulence is not a static parameter. The virus-host interaction is a dynamic process subject to continuous, powerful pressures exerted by natural selection. In

the case of myxoma virus, within 10 years after the field release of grade I virulence virus, there was an overall reduction in virulence levels of individual isolated viruses, coupled with the emergence of rabbit populations that were inherently more resistant to the development of myxomatosis, even when exposed to the parental grade I virus. These issues are discussed in Chapter 15.

An alternative measure of virulence is an assessment of pathologic lesions, as exemplified by the comparison of the severity of encephalitis produced by a range of neurotropic flaviviruses (Fig. 5-1). Figure 5-1 also demonstrates that virulence is not necessarily a unidimensional property; in this case, Japanese encephalitis and the 17D strain of yellow fever virus are most pathogenic for the forebrain, West Nile virus for the midbrain, and Langat virus for the spinal cord. Another set of virulence measures may be provided by laboratory tests that reflect virus-induced pathophysiologic changes. For instance, the severity of hepatitis can be assessed by the serum titer of alanine or aspartate aminotransferase that signals release of hepatocellular proteins, and the severity of acquired immunodeficiency syndrome (AIDS) can be assessed by the reduction in the the blood concentration of CD4+ T lymphocytes caused by human immunodeficiency virus (HIV) infection.

For precise estimation of virulence, it is important to adjust for virus dose, because dose can influence outcome. This is illustrated in Table 5-4, which shows the influence of dose on survival time. To correct for variation in virus dose, it is convenient to titrate different virus strains in a permissive cell culture system as well as in animals. From these titrations, the ratio of PFU per 50% lethal dose can be computed, and the PFU per LD50 can then be recorded for the different virus variants under comparison. An example of such quantitation is shown in Figure 5-2 for reassortants of virulent and attenuated

TABLE 5-3. *Virulence measured by differences in survival time**

Virulence grade	Case fatality rate (%)	Mean survival time (d)	Percent of isolates
I	>99	<13	4.1
II	95–99	14–16	17.6
IIIA	90–95	17–22	38.8
IIIB	70–90	23–28	24.8
IV	50–70	29–50	14.0
V	<50	NC	0.9

NC, not calculable.

*Survival time tends to correlate with lethality, as exemplified by different natural isolates of myxoma virus (a leporipoxvirus). Rabbits were injected subcutaneously with a large number of field isolates, collected 10 years after release of grade I virulence virus, and an overall fatality rate and mean survival time was recorded for groups of animals infected with each isolate.

Data from references 39, 48, 49, and 104.

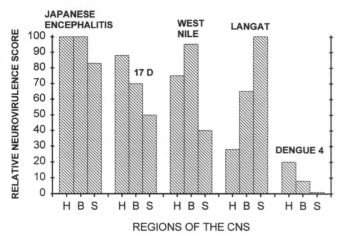

FIG. 5-1. Histologic lesions can be used to compare viruses of different virulence. In this instance, monkeys were injected intracerebrally with five different neurotropic flaviviruses, and the severity of lesions were evaluated for different regions of the central nervous system to produce a neurovirulence profile for each virus. Each virus produced a distinct profile depending on its relative affinity for different parts of the nervous system, illustrating that virulence can be a multidimensional parameter. B, brain stem, including midbrain and hindbrain; CNS, central nervous system; H, hemispheres, including forebrain; S, spinal cord. (Data from Nathanson N, Gittelsohn AM, Thind IS, Price WH. Histological studies of the monkey neurovirulence of group B arboviruses. III. Relative virulence of selected viruses. Am J Epidemiol 1967;85:503–517.)

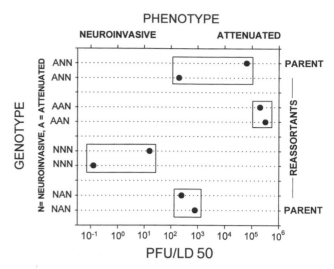

FIG. 5-2. An example of a quantitative comparison of virulence. Each virus clone has been titrated in tissue culture and in suckling mice by subcutaneous injection to determine the ratio of plaque-forming units (PFU) per 50% lethal dose (LD50), which is plotted on a log scale. This quantitative approach permits a more precise expression of the relative virulence of different variants, which can vary over a range of about 1 million–fold. In this example, reassortants were constructed between two partially attenuated clones which contained one attenuated RNA segment (A) and two neuroinvasive RNA segments (N). With this range of virulence, it is possible to demonstrate that some reassortant variants (genotype NNN) are more virulent than either parental clone and some (genotype AAN) are less virulent than either parental clone, consistent with their number of attenuated gene segments. (Data from Griot C, Pekosz A, Davidson R, et al. Replication in cultured C2C12 muscle cells correlates with the neuroinvasiveness of California serogroup bunyaviruses. Virology 1994;201:399–403.)

strains of California serogroup viruses (bunyaviruses). Figure 5-2 illustrates that quantitative measurement can differentiate various degrees of virulence and can be used to detect the additive effect of several genetic determinants. Chapter 20 provides further discussion of experimental variables in the assay of virulence.

EXPERIMENTAL MANIPULATION OF VIRULENCE

A prerequisite to the study of virulence is the availability of viral variants that differ in virulence phenotype. In some instances, natural isolates may differ sufficiently in virulence to provide a basis for the study of the genetics or pathogenesis of virulence. An example is the human reoviruses, in which serotype 1 and serotype 3 viruses differ remarkably in their biological properties, even though they are so closely related genetically that reassortants between the two types are readily constructed. In many instances, laboratory manipulation must be used to obtain virulence variants. Almost invariably, the procedures commonly used in the laboratory, such as passage in cell culture or viral mutagenesis, select for attenuated variants of reduced virulence.

Passage in Animal Hosts

In the early period of experimental virology, before the advent of routine cell culture, viruses were often maintained by

TABLE 5-4. *Survival time varies inversely with dose*

Virus dose ($\log_{10}$ LD50)	Mortality rate (%)	Median survival time (d)
7.6	100	2.4
6.6	100	2.4
5.6	100	3.3
4.6	100	2.7
3.6	100	4.6
2.6	100	5.2
1.6	100	5.6
0.6	100	5.8
−0.4	10	7.0

Data from ElDadah AH, Nathanson N, Sarsitis R. Pathogenesis of West Nile virus encephalitis in mice and rats. I. Influence of age and species on mortality and infection. Am J Epidemiol 1967;86:765–775.

serial animal passage. On occasion, it was noted that passage altered viral virulence, and this adventitious finding was sometimes used to identify or isolate variants with different properties. In general, passage by a defined route in a particular species enhanced the virulence of the virus when assessed under the conditions of passage but often reduced the virulence in other animals or by alternate routes of infection. Human polioviruses usually do not infect rodents but on occasion have been adapted to mice; repeated mouse passage of monkey neurovirulent isolates produces variants that often have high intracerebral and intraspinal virulence for mice but may exhibit relatively low intracerebral virulence for monkeys.[97,132,140]

Yellow fever virus provides another example of attenuation by laboratory passage.[156] Theiler[158] found that yellow fever virus would infect adult mice by intracerebral inoculation and that the virus could be passed serially in this manner. On prolonged passage (>20 serial transmissions), several changes consistently occurred in the properties of the virus. It was reduced in its parenteral virulence for rhesus monkeys; the wild-type virus routinely caused fatal yellow fever, but the passaged virus produced an immunizing infection with transient fever but without other symptoms.[144] Meanwhile, the virus became neuroadapted for mice. The Asibi wild-type virus killed mice after an interval of 8 to 30 days, depending on dose, whereas the mouse-adapted French neurotropic strain killed mice after an interval of 4 to 8 days, depending on dose. Furthermore, the French neurotropic strain appeared to spread exclusively by the neural route in mice, and little if any viremia could be demonstrated.[51]

Passage in Cell Culture

Even before the introduction of modern methods of cell culture, it had been established that virus could be passaged in embryonated eggs or cultures composed of tissue explants and that such passage might, on occasion, lead to the selection of attenuated virus strains. A prominent example was the successful search by Theiler and Smith[159] for an attenuated variant of yellow fever virus, which culminated in the selection of the 17D strain.

With the advent and widespread use of cell culture, serial passage became frequently used for the selection of attenuated virus variants. An example is given in Table 5-5, which gives the history of the identification of an attenuated clone of a reassortant California serogroup virus.[41] A number of different virus stocks were passaged in cell culture, and the uncloned virus pools were then tested for virulence. Several passage lines showed some evidence of reduced virulence, and the line exhibiting the greatest attenuation was used to derive 10 plaque-purified variants which were then retested. One of these 10 variants showed a marked attenuation that was confirmed on more extensive study. In the course of study it was found that this clone was a temperature-sensitive variant with an attenuating mutation in the large gene segment encoding the viral polymerase. This example illustrates several common observations:

Apparently identical passage protocols can yield stocks with different degrees of attenuation; there is an element of unpredictability in this approach to attenuation.

TABLE 5-5. *Derivation of an attenuated virus clone through tissue culture passage of several cloned parental virus strains*

	Mortality (dead/tested)
EACH VIRUS PASSED 25 TIMES THEN TESTED FOR VIRULENCE	
La Crosse/original, pass A	5/5
La Crosse/original, pass B	3/5
La Crosse/p10, pass A	3/5
La Crosse/p10, pass B	4/5
La Crosse/pp31, pass A	5/5
La Crosse/pp31, pass B	4/5
Tahyna/181-57, pass A	5/5
Tahyna/181-57, pass B	5/5
La Crosse/RFC, pass A	1/5
La Crosse/RFC, pass B	**0/5**
LA CROSSE/RFC B PASSAGE SERIES CLONES TESTED FOR VIRULENCE	
1	5/5
2	4/5
3	5/5
4	3/5
5	**0/5**
6	4/5
7	2/5
8	1/5
9	5/5
10	1/5

Upper panel: Each of five virus stocks was passed in BHK-21 cells 25 times; the uncloned stocks were then tested for neurovirulence by intracerebral injection of 100 plaque-forming units into adult mice. Each virus was passed in two identical series, designated A or B.

Lower panel: Stock RFC, passage line B, was used to derive 10 plaque-purified variants that were retested for neurovirulence by intracerebral injection of 10,000 plaque-forming units into adult mice. One clone, number 5, exhibited marked avirulence. Note the unpredictability of the effect of prolonged cell culture passage and the variable degree of attenuation of variants derived from the uncloned virus stock.

Data from Endres MJ, Valsamakis A, Gonzalez-Scarano F, Nathanson N. Neuroattenuated bunyavirus variaent: derivation, characterization, and revertant clones. J Virol 1990;64:1927–1933.

Viral stocks often represent a "swarm" of genetically diverse variants that differ in their degree of attenuation.

Attenuated variants may be temperature sensitive, even when they were not selected for this phenotype.

Although passage in cell culture often results in attenuation of virulence in vivo, this is not always the case. For instance, when several different attenuated strains of rabies virus were passaged in murine or human neuroblastoma cell lines, there was a consistent selection for virus of increased virulence.[27] Passage in other cell types cells did not enhance virulence, suggesting that neuroblastoma cell passage exerted the same selective pressures seen with intracerebral passage in animals.

TABLE 5-6. *Selection of attenuated virus variants of La Crosse virus using neutralizing monoclonal antibodies**

Epitope group	Epitope number	Frequency of variants ($\log_{10}$)	Fusion efficiency	Virulence (intraperitoneal; weanling mice)
1	09	−3.7	+	+
	13	−5.9	+	+
	15	−6.2	+	+
	18	−5.3	+	+
	31	−6.0	+	+
	35	−5.3	+	+
2	260	−5.4	+	+
3	12	−5.0	R	R
	33	−4.1	R	R
4	25	NR	+	+
5	22	−6.1	RR	RR

*A panel of antibodies was used to select a corresponding panel of monoclonal antibody resistant (MAR) variant viruses from an uncloned mouse brain pool of La Crosse virus, original strain. Each of the antibodies and variants was antigenically unique based on cross-neutralization tests. Variants were tested for fusion efficiency and for neuroinvasiveness after intraperitoneal injection of weanling mice. Clone 22 is shown (Figure 2-3) to have reduced neuroinvasiveness in suckling mice but normal neurovirulence in adult mice.

+, wild-type level; NR, not recorded; R, slightly reduced; RR: markedly reduced. Data from references 58 and 61.

Monoclonal Antibody–Resistant Mutants

With the development of panels of monoclonal antibodies for most viruses, it became possible to select variants that escape neutralization. Such variants often represent point mutations and occur naturally at a frequency of about 10^{-5}, depending on the virus.[69,155] When a panel of such variants, selected with different monoclonal antibodies, are tested in vivo, it is often observed that a few of the escape mutants are attenuated. Table 5-6 shows an example of a panel of 11 monoclonal antibody–resistant (MAR) mutants of La Crosse virus, in which one of these (variant 22) is attenuated. Figure 5-3 shows that variant 22 has reduced neuroinvasiveness but wild-type neurovirulence.[58,61] It is also possible to select viral mutants that escape recognition by epitope-specific cytolytic T cells,[96] and it is plausible that some such escape variants might exhibit altered virulence.

Mutagenesis and Temperature-Sensitive Mutants

A standard strategy for the definition of viral genes is the deliberate exposure of a virus stock to a mutagenizing treatment, following which variants are selected. One convenient way to select mutants is to look for viral variants that are temperature sensitive and that will replicate well at the lower permissive temperature of 33°C to 37°C but not at an elevated nonpermissive temperature such as 40°C, where the wild-type parent virus will still replicate well.

Many temperature-sensitive mutants exhibit reduced virulence in animals. It should be emphasized that reduced virulence is not necessarily a direct consequence of temperature

sensitivity, because the body temperature of the host is frequently within the range of permissive temperatures. More likely, such temperature-sensitive mutants are also host-range restricted in certain cell types even at the permissive temperature, thus explaining their in vivo attenuation. An example of these phenomena is shown in Figure 5-4 for the California serogroup attenuated mutant clone B.5, described previously. Clone B.5 replicates well at 37°C in BHK-21 cells, the culture system in which it was selected, but it is markedly restricted at 40°C. In addition, clone B.5 exhibits host-range restriction at 37°C in most mouse cell lines such as mouse neuroblastoma cells, which are usually permissive for California serogroup viruses. Finally, clone B.5 barely replicates when injected intracerebrally into adult mice, whereas the wild-type virus replicates rapidly and consistently kills mice.

Temperature-sensitive variants do not necessarily show reduced virulence. A temperature-sensitive variant, *ts*1, of Moloney murine leukemia virus (MuLV), has been studied in detail by Wong and colleagues.[60] The variant *ts*1 does not cause lymphoma, but it does cause a neurodegenerative disease associated with increased viral titers in the central nervous system and infection and death of astrocytes. The altered phenotype of *ts*1 has been mapped to a codon of the *env* gene involving amino acid 25 of the major glycoprotein (wild-type gp70env is converted to mutant gp80env). It appears that, under nonpermissive conditions (i.e., elevated temperature in culture cells or 37°C in astrocytes), the mutant protein is misfolded and accumulates in the endoplasmic reticulum; how accumulation leads to neurodegeneration remains to be elucidated.

Although random mutagenesis is a convenient way to produce attenuated viruses, there may be mutations in several viral genes that are "silent" in cell culture but influence the in

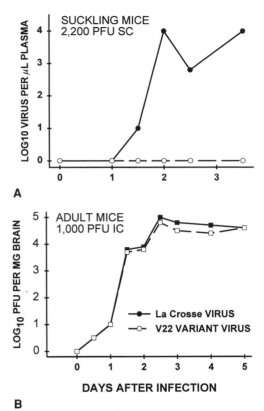

A

B

FIG. 5-3. Reduced virulence of a monoclonal antibody–resistant mutant clone. Clone V22 is a variant of La Crosse virus, selected as described in Table 5-6. (A) This variant has reduced neuroinvasiveness, as evidenced by the difference in viremia following subcutaneous (SC) infection of suckling mice. (B) Variant V22 resembles wild-type La Crosse virus in its neurovirulence, as shown by its replication in adult mouse brain after intracerebral (IC) infection. PFU, plaque-forming unit. (Data from Gonzalez-Scarano F, Janssen R, Najjar JA, Pobjecky N, Nathanson N. An avirulent G1 glycoprotein variant of La Crosse bunyavirus with defective fusion function. J Virol 1985;54:757–763.)

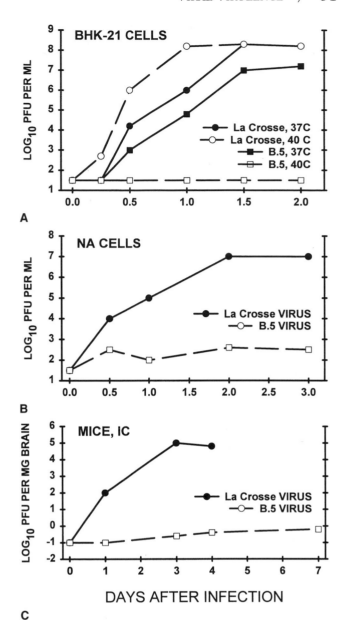

A

B

C

FIG. 5-4. Phenotype of an attenuated, temperature-sensitive La Crosse virus clone. Clone B.5 is a California serogroup virus that was derived from passage in cell culture and then selected for reduced virulence as described in Table 5-5. (A) Replication of clone B.5 in a standard cell culture (BHK-21 cells) at permissive (37°C) and restrictive temperatures (40°C). (B) Replication of clone B.5 in mouse NA neuroblastoma cells shows its host range restriction at 37°C. (C) Replication in brains of adult mice after intracerebral injection shows in vivo neuroattenuation. In each instance, clone B.5 is compared with a prototype virulent clone, wild-type La Crosse–original virus, at a multiplicity of infection of 0.01 plaque-forming units (PFU) in cell culture or 700 PFU with intracerebral injection. (Data from reference 41.)

vivo phenotype, which may complicate conclusions about the mechanism of attenuation.

Cold-Adapted Mutants

Many viruses can be cold adapted by passage at a reduced temperature (traditionally 25°C), and such variants are often attenuated in animals.[100] Maassab and DeBorde[100] conducted extensive studies of cold adaptation of influenza viruses in the hope of developing candidate strains to use as live attenuated vaccines. These studies have shown that passage at 25°C consistently yields cold-adapted influenza viral variants. Cold-adapted influenza variants replicate as well at 37°C and much better at 25°C than wild-type virus (Table 5-7), but are usually temperature sensitive at 40°C. When tested intranasally in ferrets, cold-adapted influenza viruses have markedly reduced pneumopathogenicity. Genetic analysis of cold-adapted influenza viruses indicates that they have mutations in many or all of their eight gene segments, but reassortant viruses bear-

TABLE 5-7. *Selection of attenuated virus variants by cold adaptation**

Character	Not adapted (1 passage at 25°C)	Cold adapted (6 passages at 25°C)
Replication at	Log_{10} (PFU/mL)	Log_{10} (PFU/mL)
37°C	$10^{7.3}$	$10^{7.3}$
30°C	$10^{4.6}$	$10^{6.4}$
25°C	$10^{2.0}$	$10^{6.5}$
Temperature sensitive (at 40°C)	No	Yes
Virulence for ferrets (intranasally)	High	Reduced

*Influenza A virus AA/2/65 (previously grown at 37°C) was passed repeatedly at 25°C in primary chicken kidney cells, and different passage levels were characterized for the ability to grow at several temperatures. Note that once the virus was adapted to 25°C, it still replicated well at 37°C but had become temperature-sensitive at 40°C. The adapted virus was attenuated when inoculated intranasally in ferrets.

Data from Maassab HF, DeBorde DC. Development and characterization of cold-adapted viruses for use as live virus vaccines. Vaccine 1985;3:355–369.

ing only a few segments from cold-adapted variants exhibit the cold-adapted attenuated phenotype.[32,82,124]

Specifically Designed Mutations

With the development of methods for introducing mutations into DNA, it became possible to design mutants of DNA viruses and some positive- and negative-strand RNA viruses. Several different kinds of mutations can be introduced, including point mutations involving substitution of a single or several individual amino acids; construction of genetic chimeras between two viral variants by exchange of a larger genetic sequence; and inactivation of an open reading frame by introduction of a stop codon, insertion of a selectable marker cassette, or deletion of part of the open reading frame. In some instances, noncoding domains of the viral genome carry major determinants of virulence, which can be mapped by similar methods.

An example of the use of these methods is provided by HIV and simian immunodeficiency virus (SIV), in which genetic modifications have been used to address various aspects of virulence.[95] For example, chimeric viruses have been used to map macrophage tropism to the *env* gene,[24,25,99,123] and point mutations have been used to map tropism within the fine structure of the V3 loop of the SU (gp120) glycoprotein.[25,72,149,165] Introduced stop codons and deletions have been

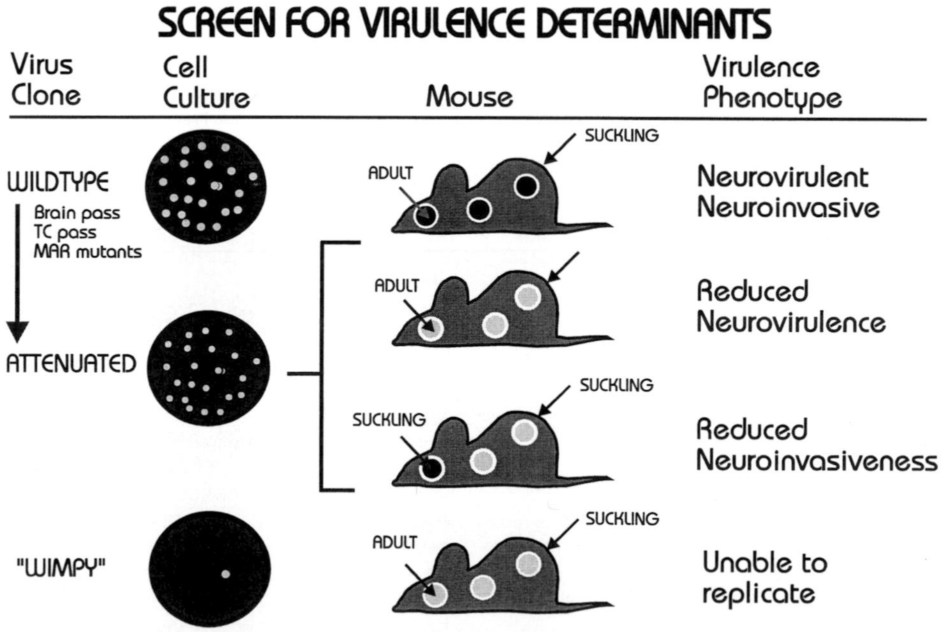

FIG. 5-5. Protocol for the selection of attenuated La Crosse virus variants, as developed for California serogroup viruses. A parental, virulent, wild-type virus is passed a number of times (typically 10 to 50 times) in cell culture or in animals, and plaque-purified clones are prepared. Alternatively, a neutralizing monoclonal antibody is used to select resistant variants that are plaque purified. Candidate viral clones are then tested for virulence in vivo and replication in cell culture. Two in vivo tests are used: intracerebral injection of adult mice tests for neurovirulence, and subcutaneous injection of suckling mice tests for neuroinvasiveness. Dark circles signify virulence, and light circles signify attenuation. Variants that replicate well in cell culture and show the greatest reduction in virulence based on the plaque-forming units (PFU) per LD50 ratio are selected for further study. Viruses that replicate poorly in cell culture (i.e., "wimpy" variants) are discarded because they do not identify viral genetic determinants that are specific for in vivo virulence. MAR, monoclonal antibody–resistant; TC pass, passage in tissue culture.

used in SIV to explore the role of the *nef* gene, resulting in the finding that *nef* deletions do not affect the ability of the virus to replicate in cell culture but markedly reduce the ability of a virulent clone, 239, to induce AIDS in rhesus monkeys.[34,83]

Selection of Attenuated Variants

In selecting variants of reduced virulence, several points should be kept in mind. First, as noted previously, most virus pools consist of a mixture of variants that may differ markedly in their biological phenotype. It is therefore necessary to plaque purify and characterize a number of variants before selecting virus stocks for study. Second, the mutations of greatest interest are those that specifically impair virulence in vivo without affecting the ability of a virus to replicate in a defined reference cell culture system. Such mutants can be considered to be "host-range" variants, in contrast to "global" mutants that impair replication in all cell hosts. An example of the strategy employed to select virulence mutants is diagrammed in Figure 5-5 as adapted for California serogroup viruses. Similar but more elaborate strategies have been developed for the identification of bacterial virulence genes.[66,103]

PATHOGENIC MECHANISMS OF VIRULENCE OR ATTENUATION

There are many sequential steps in viral infection, as described in Chapter 2. In theory, a difference in the comparative replication or spread of two virus variants at any one of these steps could explain their relative degrees of virulence. In practice, attenuated variants usually replicate or spread less briskly in one or several tissues associated with the pathogenic process. Additionally, variant viruses may differ qualitatively in their cell and tissue tropism or in their mode of dissemination. Regrettably, there is a relative paucity of studies that localize the precise differences in pathogenesis of attenuated virus variants.

Viremia

Viremia, either free extracellular virions or virus associated with circulating cells, is an obligatory step in the dissemination of most viruses that cause systemic infection. Therefore, a reduction in viremia can be an important mechanism for the reduction in virulence. Figure 5-6 compares a virulent and an avirulent California serogroup virus, La Crosse virus original clone and Tahyna virus 181-57 clone, respectively.[79] In suckling mice injected subcutaneously, wild-type La Crosse original virus is virulent (PFU/LD50~1), whereas avirulent Tahyna 181-57 virus has a PFU/LD50 ratio of more than 10^4. The viremia produced by these two viruses is illustrated in Figure 5-6A, which shows that at a low inoculum, the attenuated Tahyna 181-57 clone produces no viremia, fails to reach the brain (the target organ) and does not cause illness. In this model, the major site of peripheral virus replication is striated muscle, and the attenuated virus replicates very poorly in that tissue compared with the virulent La Crosse virus.[62] Because

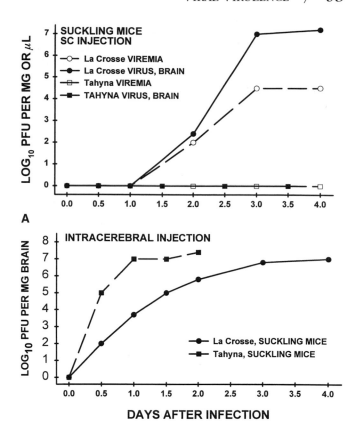

FIG. 5-6. Viremia as a determinant of viral virulence. Two California serogroup viruses are compared: virulent, wild-type La Crosse–original virus and attenuated Tahyna/181-57 virus. (**A**) Infection following subcutaneous (SC) injection of 700 plaque-forming units (PFU) of either virus shows that the virulent virus causes a viremia, invades the brain, and replicates to a high titer, producing a lethal encephalitis, whereas the attenuated Tahyna clone produces no viremia, fails to reach the brain, and does not cause illness. (**B**) The reduced peripheral virulence of the attenuated Tahyna clone is the result of its inability to produce viremia and not of any reduced tropism for the target organ (in this case, the central nervous system). This is demonstrated by its augmented replication after intracerebral injection of 700 PFU, reflecting its history of neural adaptation by repeated brain-to-brain passage. (Data from Janssen R, Gonzalez-Scarano F, Nathanson N. Mechanisms of bunyavirus virulence: comparative pathogenesis of a virulent strain of La Crosse and an attenuated strain of Tahyna virus. Lab Invest 1984;50:447–455.)

the attenuated Tahyna 181-57 virus was derived by serial brain-to-brain passage in mice, it has maintained high tropism for the central nervous system, as shown in Figure 5-6*B*. In this instance, avirulence can be attributed to reduced ability replicate in peripheral tissues with consequent reduction in viremogenicity because there is no reduction in virulence for the target organ.

Poliomyelitis is another example in which viremia can play a role in virulence. This is most clearly demonstrated under somewhat artificial conditions, in which monkeys are infected by intravascular injection with virus strains that produce different levels of viremia.[15,16] It was found that one strain, type

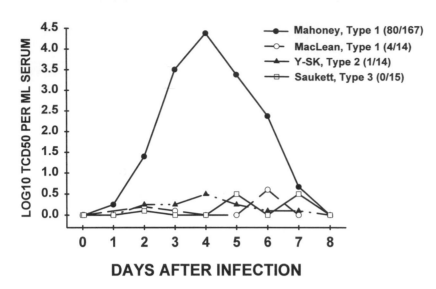

FIG. 5-7. Viremia as a determinant of viral virulence. A similar dose (10^5 TCD50) of four different poliovirus isolates were injected by the intracardiac route in cynomolgus monkeys; the animals were bled periodically to determine the level of serum virus and the frequency of paralysis was observed. Of these strains, type 1 Mahoney virus produced the highest level of viremia and the highest frequency of paralysis (48%), whereas the other three low-viremia strains produced an aggregate paralytic rate of 12%. The four virus strains and the paralytic rates that they produced (in parentheses) are identified. (Data from Bodian D. Viremia in experimental poliomyelitis. I. General aspects of infection after intravascular inoculation with strains of high and low invasiveness. Am J Hygiene 1954;60:339–357.)

1 Mahoney virus, caused a much higher viremia and paralytic rate than did several other strains that were less viremogenic (Fig. 5-7).

Neural Spread

Some viruses, such as rabies virus, disseminate only by neural spread, because they do not produce a viremia (see Chap. 2). Attenuated variants can also be derived for such viruses. Many attenuated strains of rabies virus have been developed by cell culture passage to be used as live-virus vaccines.[10] In general, these attenuated strains exhibit reduced neurovirulence, so that the intracerebral PFU/LD50 ratio (~ 1 for virulent rabies viruses) is increased to 10^4 to 10^6.[27] Interestingly, these attenuated strains undergo a sublethal round of replication in the brain, because their PFU/ID50 ratio is usually close to 1.

The attenuation of rabies virus has been further investigated using MAR mutants of virulent parent viruses. It was found that some of the MAR variants in one epitope group (but not those in other epitope groups) were markedly attenuated, and the attenuating mutation was mapped to amino acid residue 333 of the rabies glycoprotein, where the virulent phenotype was associated with an arginine or lysine and the avirulent phenotype with a glycine, glutamine, methionine, or lysine.[37,147,161] Some MAR variants at the same epitope had point mutations at amino acids other than 333; interestingly, none of these viruses were attenuated.

After intramuscular injection, variant RV194-2, an attenuated mutant with a mutation at site 333, spread centripetally to the brain and then throughout the neuraxis at a rate similar to virulent parent challenge virus standard (CVS) virus.[76] However, following initial dissemination within the central nervous system, CVS virus spread rapidly to many contiguous neurons, whereas clone RV194-2 spread only to relatively few neurons and the infection was aborted, presumably by the intervention of the immune response (see Fig. 24-6 in Chap. 24). Thus, attenuation of the RV194-2 clone appears to be associated with reduced neuron-to-neuron spread within the nervous system, and similar observations were made with an-

other MAR variant, Av01.[31,94] When compared in mouse neuroblastoma cell culture, the avirulent clone RV194-2 was inhibited in its internalization into cells and in its ability to spread from cell to cell compared with virulent CVS virus, although the two viruses infected and replicated in BHK-21 cells with identical kinetics (Fig. 5-8). These observations strengthened the impression that the difference between virulent and attenuated MAR viruses lay in their differential efficiency in entry into neuronal cells, probably associated with differences in the binding of their glycoproteins to cellular receptors. Chapter 24 provides a detailed discussion of rabies pathogenesis.

MAR variants have also been used to study neural spread to the central nervous system.[31,90] After intraocular injection, virulent CVS rabies virus followed three different pathways to the central nervous system: along the trigeminal (sensory) nerve, through the autonomic (parasympathetic) pathway, and through the optic (visual) pathway. By contrast, the MAR variant Av01 used only the trigeminal pathway (see Fig. 24-9 in Chap. 24). Thus, there may be anatomic restrictions on the neural spread of an avirulent compared with a virulent rabies virus.

An attenuated variant of pseudorabies virus, a neurotropic herpesvirus, also exhibits specific restrictions in neural spread.[42] After intraocular injection, wild-type pseudorabies virus spreads along several optic pathways in the brain, but a variant that does not express the viral glycoproteins E (gE) and I (gI) will use some but not all of these pathways.

Tropism and Host Range

Different variants of a single virus can exhibit differences in their tropism for organs, tissues, and cell types, which confers a multidimensional character on virulence. A variant virus may be reduced in its ability to cause one type of pathology but enhanced in its ability to cause another. For instance, some wild-type strains of mouse hepatitis virus, a coronavirus, replicate in both neurons and oligodendroglia (the cells that produce myelin) and produce an acutely fatal encephalomyelitis as a result of neuronal destruction. Variant clones, selected by monoclonal

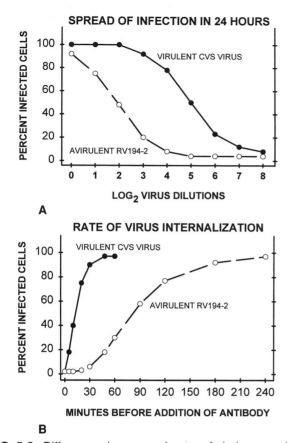

SPREAD OF INFECTION IN 24 HOURS

VIRULENT CVS VIRUS

AVIRULENT RV194-2

LOG$_2$ VIRUS DILUTIONS

A

RATE OF VIRUS INTERNALIZATION

VIRULENT CVS VIRUS

AVIRULENT RV194-2

MINUTES BEFORE ADDITION OF ANTIBODY

B

FIG. 5-8. Differences in neuronal entry of virulence variants of a neurotropic virus. An avirulent monoclonal antibody–resistant (MAR) mutant of rabies virus is less efficient in its ability to infect and spread among neuronal cells than is its neurovirulent counterpart. The avirulent variant, RV194-2, was selected from parent virulent CVS virus by its ability to escape neutralization with monoclonal antibody 194-2 and was shown to differ from the parent virus by a single amino acid at position 333 on the viral glycoprotein. **(A)** C1300 NA neuroblastoma cells were exposed to serial dilutions of either virus and were examined 24 hours later for the proportion of infected cells; both viruses had a titer of 10$^{7.6}$ plaque-forming units (PFU) per mL on BHK-21 cells. On NA cells, the avirulent virus spread much less efficiently than did the virulent virus. Both viruses spread equally well when BHK-21 cells were infected. **(B)** To determine the kinetics of internalization, NA cells were exposed to virus for different intervals at 10 PFU/cell. The cells were washed and antibody was added; 18 hours later, the proportion of infected cells was determined. The avirulent virus was internalized more slowly than the virulent virus. (Data from Dietzschold B, Wunner WH, Wiktor TJ, et al. Characterization of an antigenic determinant of the glycoprotein that correlates with pathogenicity of rabies virus. Proc Natl Acad Sci U S A 1983;80:70–74.)

antibodies against glycoprotein E2 or as temperature-sensitive mutants, may show marked reduction in their neuronotropism. Such attenuated viruses do not kill mice acutely but produce persistent infections of oligodendroglia leading to demyelination and chronic paralysis.[33,52,88]

HIV presents another example of tropism differences. Most strains of HIV can be classified into one of two categories, according to their ability to replicate in T-cell lines (T-tropic) or in primary macrophages (M-tropic). Essentially all HIV isolates can replicate well in primary blood leukocyte (PBL) cultures, but only the M-tropic viruses will grow well in primary cultures of blood monocytes/macrophages (Table 5-8). Tropism has been mapped to the envelope (gp120 or SU) protein, and studies of the initial steps in infection suggest a difference in the efficiency of virus entry.[25,72,95,148,165] However, the CD4 molecule acts as the viral receptor for both T cells and macrophages,[28] and the mechanism of differential tropism remains enigmatic. The role of the two tropism biotypes of HIV in disease pathogenesis is only partly understood, but it is known that M-tropic strains dominate during the prolonged period of clinical latency, and the T-tropic strains are more frequently isolated from the blood of patients with clinical AIDS. T-tropic strains are considered more virulent based on their greater syncytium-inducing ability, their "high rapid" pattern of replication in PBLs, and their dominance during the period of progressive clinical deterioration. It is not clear whether both biotypes are involved in patient-to-patient transmission, although it has been suggested that M-tropic strains are preferentially transmitted, because strains isolated within the first 2 months after infection are usually M-tropic.[146,169]

Reoviruses are classified into three serotypes, which are sufficiently closely related that genetic reassortants can be constructed among them. Despite this genetic compatibility, reovirus serotype 1 (Lang strain) and serotype 3 (Dearing strain) viruses exhibit striking differences in their in vivo tropism when characterized in mice (see Chap. 28). When injected intracerebrally in mice, the type 1 Lang strain infects the ependymal lining of the brain and causes ependymitis and hydrocephalus, whereas the type 3 Dearing strain replicates in neurons in the brain, causing a lethal encephalitis. These differences are mainly conferred by the σ1 protein, which is the viral attachment protein that binds to cellular receptors. A number of other in vivo properties of reoviruses have been mapped to other viral genes (discussed later).

Virulence for Target Organs

Different variants of a specific virus may show different degrees of virulence for a key target organ. Figure 5-9 compares four California serogroup variants and shows their different rates of replication after intracerebral injection of identical virus inocula. These variable replication rates produce differences in intracerebral virulence as reflected in the PFU/LD50 ratio.

Virulence after peripheral infection reflects both virulence for the target organ and the ability of each virus clone to move through the sequential steps in infection that deliver it to the target organ, and these two properties are not necessarily associated. This point is illustrated in Table 5-1, which compares two California serogroup viruses. Attenuated clone B.5 and virulent wild-type La Crosse virus are almost equally virulent on intracerebral injection into suckling mice, but on subcutaneous injection into suckling mice, clone B.5 is much less virulent because it fails to cause a viremia after peripheral injection.

TABLE 5-8. *Virus isolates may vary in their host range**

Viral biotype	HIV-1 isolate	Growth in each cell type†			
		Peripheral blood leukocytes	Monocyte-derived macrophages	Monocytoid cell line U937	T-cell line Sup-T1
T-tropic	IIIB	++++	+	++++	++++
	DV	++++	++	++++	++++
M-tropic	SF162	++++	+++	—	—
	89.6	++++	+++	—	—

*HIV strains can be classified into two major biotypes, M-tropic (replicating in macrophages) and T-tropic (replicating in T lymphocytoid cell lines) as shown for several different virus strains.

†Replication is indicated by peak level of p24 antigen production.

++++, >100 ng/mL; +++, 10–100 ng/mL; ++, 1–10 ng/mL; +, <1 ng/mL; —, <10 pg/mL. Data from references 29 and 30.

Sabin,[140,141] when developing attenuated vaccine candidate strains, noted that there was a dissociation between peripheral infectivity and central nervous system virulence. Field isolates were often virulent when introduced by feeding or by intracerebral injection; however, some natural isolates were highly infectious after feeding but had low intracerebral virulence, whereas strains that had low infectivity after feeding but were virulent after intracerebral injection could be obtained by passage in the laboratory.

The three attenuated strains of poliovirus used in OPV provide an example in which virulence for the target organ appears to be the determinant of peripheral virulence. The relative virulence of the type 1, type 2, and type 3 strains when administered orally can be measured by the relative numbers of vaccine-recipient cases; the relative ability of the three strains to produce viremia was documented in early studies of OPV, and the relative neurovirulence of the three virus strains has been determined in monkey neurovirulence tests. Table 5-9 provides selected data on all these parameters. The type 3 strain has the greatest virulence after virus feeding under field conditions, but the type 2 strain is clearly the most viremogenic in children. Furthermore, the type 3 strain appears to have a lower average neurovirulence than does the type 1 strain; however, severe cord lesions, which are rarely seen with any OPV strain, are produced at a higher frequency by the type 3 than by the type 1 strain. This paradoxical neurovirulence test profile may reflect the tendency for the type 3 strain to undergo a higher frequency of mutations that produce a reversion to a virulent phenotype. In this instance, it appears that virulence is an expression of the relative frequency of revertants that are virulent for the target organ; it has not been determined whether these revertant clones might also have an increase in their viremogenicity.

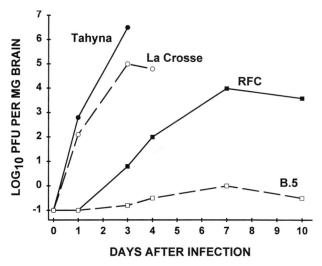

FIG. 5-9. Viral variants can show different degrees of virulence for a target organ. Four California serogroup viruses (La Crosse virus, Tahyna virus, and two reassortants between them) were injected intracerebrally in adult mice at a dose of 700 plaque-forming units (PFU) and observed for their rates of replication in the brain. The differences in replication rates were also reflected in the quantitative virulence differences in mice when expressed as $\log_{10}$ PFU/LD50. These ratios were: Tahyna/181-57, 0; La Crosse–original, 0.1; clone RFC, 1.5; and clone B.5, >6.1). (Data from Endres MJ, Valsamakis A, Gonzalez-Scarano F, Nathanson N. Neuroattenuated bunyavirus variant: derivation, characterization, and revertant clones. J Virol 1990;64:1927–1933.)

Immune-Mediated Mechanisms

The expression of virulence may involve the host response to infection. If a virus can dampen a component of the host response that acts as a natural defense mechanism, this may alter the course of the infection and the nature and severity of associated disease. It has long been known that certain viruses have the ability to suppress the immune response and that immunosuppression may be associated with persistent infection (see Chap. 10). Furthermore, different variants of a single virus may differ in their immunosuppressive activity, and this may influence their ability to persist and alter their virulence phenotype.

Lymphocytic choriomeningitis virus (LCMV), an arenavirus, illustrates this mechanism.[1–5,17,18,35,44,85,106,107,125,142,143,163] If newborn mice are infected with the neurovirulent Armstrong strain of LCMV, a persistent infection is established in multiple organs. When virus clones are isolated from the brain, they have the neurovirulent phenotype of parental Armstrong virus;

TABLE 5-9. *Virulence in vivo, viremogenicity, and intraspinal neurovirulence for oral poliovirus vaccine strains*

	Type 1	Type 2	Type 3
IN VIVO VIRULENCE: CASES OF PARALYTIC POLIOMYELITIS IN RECIPIENTS OF ORAL POLIOVIRUS VACCINE			
Number of cases	22	13	62
VIREMOGENICITY: VIREMIA IN INFANTS FED MONOVALENT ORAL POLIOVIRUS VACCINE			
Frequency of viremia	0/16	17/19	0/16
NEUROVIRULENCE: MONKEY NEUROVIRULENCE SCORES FOLLOWING INTRASPINAL INJECTION OF ORAL POLIOVIRUS VACCINE			
Mean lesion score	1.05		0.79
Percent severe lesions	0.05		1.15

Top panel: paralytic poliomyelitis cases in vaccine recipients associated with types 1, 2, or 3 oral poliovirus vaccine. Family and community contact cases are excluded. Based on data for cases reported from 1961–1984 for the United States.[122,145]

Middle panel: The frequency of viremia in triple-negative infants fed monovalent oral poliovirus vaccines and shown to have an immune response.[71]

Bottom panel: Monkey neurovirulence tests following intraspinal injection of type 3 or type 1 oral poliovirus vaccine (type 2 was not included in this study), summarized as the mean lesion score or the percent of animals with severe lesions (grades 3/3 or 4).[119]

however, when variants are isolated from other organs such as the spleen, they have a markedly altered phenotype, being M-tropic, immunosuppressive, and nonneurovirulent (i.e., not lethal for adult mice after intracerebral injection). Following infection with neurotropic Armstrong virus, M-tropic variants replace the injected virus in the spleen in about 30 days; this occurs more slowly in the kidney and not at all in the brain.

When neurovirulent and M-tropic variants are compared, the M-tropic variants infect a higher proportion of macrophages, replicate to a higher titer, and in vivo, suppress the cytolytic T-cell response, whereas the neurovirulent Armstrong virus replicates more briskly in neuronal cell lines. Sequence comparison of neurotropic and M-tropic variants has identified two critical point mutations, involving single amino acids in the polymerase and glycoprotein genes, as the only consistent differences between the two phenotypes. At position 260 of the glycoprotein, a phenylalanine in neurotropic variants is replaced by a leucine in M-tropic variants, and at position 1079 of the polymerase gene, a lysine in neurotropic variants is replaced by a glutamine or asparagine in M-tropic variants.

It appears that conversion from an acutely neurovirulent phenotype to a nonneurovirulent phenotype is produced by a change in cellular host range from neurotropic to M-tropic, and that the M-tropic virus suppresses the cellular immune response, which helps to initiate a persistent "tolerant" infection. The pathogenesis of LCMV is reviewed in Chapter 28.

Tumorigenesis

When applied to tumor viruses, virulence can be expressed in several different ways. The most common differences among the oncogenic viruses involve either the latent period from infection to development of a neoplasm or the cell type that is transformed. These points are illustrated with examples from the transforming retroviruses. Chapters 11 and 26 provide detailed discussions of oncogenesis and retroviruses, respectively.

Acute Versus Long-Latency Retroviruses

In general, the transforming retroviruses can be divided into two major classes according to whether they cause tumors with a long latency or are acutely transforming. The long-latency viruses are often replication competent and do not carry a transduced oncogene. They act as insertional mutagens when their proviruses are integrated into the host DNA. On rare occasions, insertion occurs at a site where the promoter, enhancer, or terminator sequences in the viral genome can influence the transcription of a host protooncogene. Upregulation or deregulation of such a protooncogene leads to transformation of the infected cell, which can result in neoplasia, usually after a long latency period.

Acute transforming retroviruses carry in their genomes a transduced cellular protooncogene that has replaced viral sequences so that the virus is replication incompetent and requires a helper virus to supply the missing viral gene products. Often the transduced cellular protooncogene undergoes mutations that enhance its transforming potential. Retroviruses carrying a transduced oncogene are acutely oncogenic, causing a high frequency of neoplasms with an incubation period of 2 to 8 weeks. The nature of the neoplasm is often determined by the identity of the oncogene; Rous sarcoma virus carrying the *src* gene causes sarcomas in chickens, and avian leukosis viruses carrying the *erbB* gene cause erythroleukemias in chickens.

Role of the Long Terminal Repeat in Cellular Tropism

MuLVs are replication-competent, long-latency oncogenic retroviruses. Different MuLV isolates induce different kinds of neoplasms involving T lymphocytes, B lymphocytes, erythroid precursor cells, or myeloid precursor cells. Genetic studies, including the production of viral chimeras, have allowed the genetic determinants to be mapped to the viral U3 region, a noncoding part of the viral genome just upstream from the transcriptional start site.[47,70] The U3 region has a domain that contains a number of transcriptional enhancer sites, and tissue specificity has been mapped to this domain.[153] Thus, exchange of a 200–base pair region within the U3 enhancer domain will reciprocally convert a Moloney MuLV, which causes T-cell lymphomas, and a Friend MuLV, which causes erythroleukemias, to the opposite phenotype.[23,57,75,98] Tropism is thought to correlate with relative ability to replicate in different potential target cells; this has been borne out, at least in part, by in vivo studies of the relative replication rates of different MuLVs in different tissues.[46,77,139] Thus, T-lymphoma–inducing viruses replicate preferentially in the thymus. Transient or stable transcriptional assays have shown that long terminal repeats bearing different enhancer domains and a reporter gene are preferentially transcribed in different cell types,[19,22,68,150,168] although the detailed mechanisms, such as differences in transacting nuclear proteins, have not been elucidated.

Role of Viral Attachment Proteins in Host Range

The avian sarcoma and leukosis viruses (ASLV) can be classified into groups depending on their viral attachment proteins, which bind only to cells from chicken strains that bear the corresponding receptor molecules.[46,164] For domestic chickens, there are six ASLV subgroups (A, B, C, D, E, and J) and at least three groups of receptors (transforming virus or tv-a, tv-b, and tv-c). Thus, subgroup A viruses infect only cells and chickens bearing the tv-a receptor. Similar receptor and viral attachment protein specificities occur for all retroviruses. A virus must encode an attachment protein that will bind to the receptors expressed by the host if the virus is to initiate a potentially oncogenic infection.

GENETIC DETERMINANTS OF VIRULENCE AND ATTENUATION

Viral virulence, or more broadly, the biologic phenotype of the virus, is encoded in the viral genome and expressed through structural proteins, nonstructural proteins, or noncoding sequences. Over the past 20 years, a large body of information has been assembled regarding the viral genetic determinants of virulence. These studies have established several important points:

The use of mutants has made it possible to identify the role of individual genes and proteins as determinants of the biologic behavior of many viral variants.
There is no "master" gene or protein that determines virulence, and attenuation may be associated with changes in any of the structural or nonstructural proteins or in the noncoding regions of the genome.
The virulence phenotype can be altered by very small changes in the genome if they occur at "critical sites." At such sites, a single point mutation leading to the substitution of a specific amino acid or base is often sufficient to alter virulence. For most viruses with small genomes (<20 kb), only a few discrete critical sites have been discovered, usually fewer than 10 per genome.
It is possible to create variants with attenuating mutations at several critical sites, and these may be more attenuated than single point mutants. Additionally, reversion to virulence is less frequent in variants with several discrete attenuating mutations.
Attenuating mutations are often host-range mutations that affect replication in some cells but not in others. This is partly a reflection of the fact that most well-characterized mutants have been deliberately selected because they replicate well in a convenient cell culture system.
Although many attenuating mutations have been identified, relatively few have been characterized at a biochemical or structural level regarding their mechanism of action.
Reversion to virulence may be the result of mutations at a site of attenuation, at another site in the same protein, or even at a site in a different protein.

Polioviruses

Information on the virulence of polioviruses has been primarily derived from detailed studies of the three attenuated strains of type 1, type 2, and type 3 polioviruses that constitute the OPV originally developed by Sabin.[141] The three vaccine strains are much less virulent than most wild-type polioviruses (by about 10,000-fold; see Table 5-2). The genomes of the vaccine viruses can be compared with the the wild-type viruses from which they were derived, but they differ at a considerable number of sites, reflecting their complex passage history, and many of these differences are not relevant to the attenuated phenotype. Virulent revertants of the vaccine strains occur with passage in animals, humans, or cell culture. Because there are relatively few sequence differences between attenuated and revertant virulent variants, it is easier to identify sites relevant to attenuation. Using reverse genetics,[134] infectious DNA clones of poliovirus genomes can be used to construct chimeric viruses, and these clones can then be transfected into permissive cells to reconstitute mutated infectious virus. The same approach can be used to engineer point mutatinos for fine mapping of virulence determinants.

Viral phenotypes can be characterized by intracerebral or intraspinal injection in monkeys, by intracerebral injection in transgenic mice bearing the poliovirus receptor,[135,137] and in various cell cultures at standard and restrictive temperatures. One limitation of the methods used to characterize virulence[133] is that they focus on neurovirulence and do not necessarily detect changes in neuroinvasiveness (i.e., the ability to spread from sites of initial replication in the gut to the nervous system), which involves spread to regional lymph nodes, initiation of viremia, or spread along peripheral neuronal pathways. Chapter 23 provides a detailed account of the pathogenesis and genetics of poliovirus.

From an extensive series of investigations, several generalizations can be made about the attenuation of the vaccine strains of poliovirus.[7,112,113,132,133,135]

The 5′ Nontranslated Region

Each of the three strains of trivalent oral poliovirus vaccine (T-OPV) carry critical point mutations in the nontranslated region (NTR), at positions 480, 481, or 472 in types 1, 2, and 3, respectively.[20,45,101,102,111,138,166] Attenuating mutations at these sites are associated with reduced neurovirulence and reduced ability to replicate in the central nervous system of transgenic mice bearing the poliovirus receptor. Attenuated variants are temperature-sensitive host-range mutants that replicate well in primate fibroblast cell lines such as HeLa cells but have reduced ability to replicate in neuroblastoma cells.[93] The bases at attenuating sites in the 5′ NTR are thought to be involved in an RNA stem loop, based on computer models of their predicted secondary structure. When mutations are introduced in the region of the critical site, there is a rough correlation between the degree of predicted disruption of the secondary structure and the temperature sensitivity and degree of attenuation. It is believed that the stem structure at positions 470 to 540 is involved in the initiation of translation involving binding of ribosomal complexes. Presumably, initiation factors must differ, either quantitatively or qualitatively, in different cell types to explain the cellular host-range restriction of the vaccine strains.

Structural and Nonstructural Proteins

It appears that each of the OPV strains carries at least one mutation that is associated with an alteration in a viral structural or nonstructural protein and that confers temperature sensitivity and reduced neurovirulence. However, in contrast to the mutations in the 5' NTR, these mutations involve different proteins for the three OPV strains. For type 1 OPV, mutations associated with increased virulence are found in the virus capsid proteins and in the nonstructural 3D polymerase.[20,26,56,126] For type 2 OPV, it appears that neurovirulence in the mouse is associated with VP1, but other proteins may also be involved in neurovirulence, particularly in primates.[91,92,102,115,131,138] For type 3 OPV, sites in VP3 (amino acid 91) and in VP1 (amino acid 6) confer temperature sensitivity and neuroattenuation.[157] It is not clear how mutations in the structural proteins result in attenuation, but it has been suggested that these are involved in structural transitions that occur either during virion assembly or virion uncoating.

Bunyaviruses

Bunyaviruses are negative-stranded, or ambisense, RNA viruses with a trisegmented genome. The large (L) RNA segment contains a single open reading frame that encodes the viral polymerase; the middle (M) RNA segment contains a single open reading frame that encodes two glycoproteins (G1 and G2) and a nonstructural protein, Ns_m; the small (S) segment encodes the nucleoprotein and a nonstructural protein, Ns_s.[59,78]

The following discussion is limited to the California serogroup of the *Bunyavirus* genus of the family Bunyaviridae, because most studies of virulence have used this group of viruses. Members of the California serogroup reassort readily with each other. Beginning with two parent viruses, panels of reassortants containing all possible combinations of gene segments can be constructed. Given two parental virus variants with a difference in phenotype, it is possible to map the phenotype to a specific gene segment. In addition, MAR mutants have been used to identify variants in the major G1 glycoprotein that are associated with differences in virulence. Although all three RNA segments have been cloned and sequenced, it has not yet been possible to use "reverse genetics" to introduce mutations into the genome of this negative-stranded virus.

The Middle RNA Segment and the Large Glycoprotein

A detailed comparison has been made of the wild-type La Crosse virus original clone with an attenuated laboratory-passaged strain of Tahyna virus 181-57 clone.[62,78,79] The attenuated virus was obtained by multiple intracerebral passages in mice and therefore is highly neurovirulent, but it has markedly reduced neuroinvasiveness after subcutaneous injection in suckling mice. The reduction in neuroinvasiveness is associated with a reduced ability to cause viremia (see Fig. 5-6), which in turn is associated with a reduced ability to replicate in striated muscle, the major extraneural site of replication of this group of viruses. Attenuation maps to the M RNA segment (see Fig. 5-2) encoding the viral glycoproteins, suggesting that there is an alteration in the entry phase of infection of myocytes but not of neurons. When reassortants were made between these two viruses, parent and reassortant viruses plaqued equally well on BHK-21 cells; however, on a murine myocyte cell line (C2C12), viral variants bearing the M RNA segment of the attenuated parent failed to plaque, whereas variants bearing the M RNA segment of the virulent parent plaqued well.[62] Studies using other sets of reassortant California serogroup viruses have shown that differences in infectivity for mosquitoes can also map to the M RNA segment.[13]

MAR mutants of the La Crosse virus are readily obtained, at a frequency suggesting that they are point mutations (see Table 5-6). Mutants at one epitope site but not at other sites, exemplified by clone V22, exhibited reduced neuroinvasiveness and wild-type neurovirulence (see Fig. 5-3).[58,61] Furthermore, clone V22 showed strikingly reduced fusion efficiency at acid pH compared with parental wild-type La Crosse virus. These observations suggest that attenuation may be associated with an alteration in the major glycoprotein that reduces efficiency in the infection of myocytes.

The Large RNA Segment and the Viral Polymerase

The attenuated clone B.5, derived from a reassortant California serogroup virus by passage in BHK-21 cells (see Table 5-5), has been shown to bear an attenuated L RNA segment, which presumably reflects an alteration of the viral polymerase.[41,63] This clone is a temperature-sensitive host-range mutant that replicates poorly in C1300 NA neuroblastoma and other murine cell lines, although it grows well in BHK-21 cells (see Fig. 5-4). Clone B.5 shows a striking reduction in its ability to replicate in the central nervous system of adult mice (see Fig. 5-9), although it retains virulence after intracerebral injection of suckling mice (see Table 5-1). Revertants of clone B.5 can be obtained at the restrictive temperature at a frequency of about 10^{-5}, implying that the revertants are point mutations,[41] and the responsible mutation has been mapped to the L RNA segment. Revertants lose their temperature-sensitive phenotype and also exhibit wild-type neurovirulence, indicating that the reverting mutation has a pleiotropic effect.

Arenaviruses

Arenaviruses are negative-stranded, or ambisense, bisegmented RNA viruses. The L RNA segment encodes an L protein, the viral polymerase, in the viral complementary sense, whereas the S RNA segment is ambisense and encodes a nucleoprotein in the viral complementary sense and a glycoprotein in the viral sense. Most studies of arenavirus virulence have used LCMV, which has served as an important model for virus immunobiology and viral persistence for the past 50 years; LCMV is reviewed in detail in Chapter 25. Information on the role of viral genes and proteins in virulence has arisen from studies of viral variants that differ qualitatively in their tropism and ability to induce or suppress the immune response. As described previously, M-tropic variants have the ability to replicate in macrophages and dendritic cells, leading to immunosuppression and persistent infection, whereas neurotropic variants replicate well in neurons but poorly in macrophages, inducing a brisk immune response and acute neurologic disease rather than persistent infection.

Two viral genes and proteins have been shown to carry determinants of this specific type of LCMV tropism: the L RNA segment and the L protein, and the S RNA segment and the glycoprotein. The L protein or polymerase carries a determinant at amino acid 1079 that influences tropism; at this position, a lysine in neurotropic variants is replaced by a glutamine or asparagine in M-tropic variants. At position 260 of the glycoprotein, a phenyl alanine in neurotropic variants is replaced by a leucine in M-tropic variants.

Reoviruses

Reoviruses are double-stranded, 10-segmented RNA viruses. Both the genetic segments and the proteins that they encode have been characterized in detail. Although cDNA copies of the segments have been made, it is not yet possible to introduce mutagenized DNA clones into the viral genome. Nevertheless, the large number of segments have made reoviruses an attractive model system for study of the genetic determinants of viral phenotypes. These studies have been facilitated by major differences in the biologic phenotypes of naturally occurring reovirus serotypes, particularly serotypes 1 and 3. The reovirus pathogenesis model, which was developed and exploited by Fields and colleagues, is discussed in detail in Chapter 28.

Biologic functions have been ascribed to many of the reovirus genes and proteins (see Table 28-4 and Fig. 28-8 in Chap. 28). Most data have been drawn from comparisons of reovirus type 1 Lang strain (T1L) and type 3 Dearing strain (T3D), which differ markedly in the diseases that they cause in suckling mice and adult severe combined immunodeficiency (SCID) mice. Virulence differences represent both qualitative differences in tissue and organ tropism and quantitative differences in disease severity. Proteins that carry important viru-

lence determinants include the S1 segment encoding the σ1 and σ1s proteins, the M1 segment encoding the μ2 protein, the M2 segment encoding the m1 protein, the L1 segment encoding the λ3 protein, and the L2 segment encoding the λ2 protein.

The S1 Segment Encoding the σ1 and σ1s Proteins

The σ1 protein is the viral attachment protein that binds to receptors on permissive cells, binds erythrocytes acting as the viral hemagglutinin, and is a major target for neutralizing and hemagglutination inhibiting (HI) antibodies. T1L disseminates through the blood and causes an ependymitis in the brain, whereas T3D disseminates via the neural route, replicates in neurons in the brain, and causes encephalitis. The S1 segment is the major determinant of dissemination and brain cell tropism. In addition, the S1 segment is a determinant of virulence in adult SCID mice, myocarditis in neonatal mice, replication levels in the intestine, efficiency of inhibition of DNA replication, and apoptosis in infected cells.

The M1 Segment Encoding the μ2 Protein

The M1 segment influences replication in cardiac myocytes and myocarditis, as well as the virulence and severity of hepatitis in adult SCID mice.

The M2 Segment Encoding the μ1 Protein

The M2 segment affects the protease sensitivity of the virion, apoptosis induction in cell culture, and quantitative neurovirulence.

The L1 Segment Encoding the λ3 Protein

The L1 segment influences replication in cardiac myocytes and myocarditis, as well as virulence in adult SCID mice.

The L2 Segment Encoding the λ2 Protein

The L2 segment acts as a guanylyl transferase in cell culture and influences replication levels in the intestine, titers of shed virus, horizontal transmission between mice, and virulence in adult SCID mice.

VIRAL VIRULENCE GENES OF CELLULAR ORIGIN

Over the past 10 years, a new class of virus-encoded proteins has been recognized. These virus-encoded proteins contribute to the virulence of viruses by mimicking normal cellular proteins. This group of cell-derived genes has been identified primarily within the genomes of large DNA viruses that probably have a greater capacity to maintain accessory genes than do viruses with small genomes. Because these genes are homologs of cellular genes, it is hypothesized that they were acquired by recombination and modification. Thus, from an evolutionary viewpoint, they resemble viral oncogenes, but instead of endowing the virus with the ability to transform cells, these viral genes generally function by subverting or modulating various antiviral mechanisms of the infected host.

Cell-derived viral genes encode proteins that enhance virulence by many different mechanisms. Virokines are secreted from virus-infected cells and mimic cytokines, thereby perturbing normal host responses, whereas viroceptors resemble cellular receptors for cytokines that are thereby diverted from their normal cellular targets. Some virus-encoded proteins bind antibodies or complement components, preventing or deferring the lysis of virus-infected cells, whereas others interfere with antigen presentation and immune induction, prevent apoptosis, or interrupt intracellular signaling initiated by cytokines or interferons. Selected cell-derived genes that have been described for poxviruses and herpesviruses serve as examples of this group of viral genes and illustrates how they contribute to viral virulence.[110]

Poxviruses

Tumor Induction

Several poxviruses cause either benign or malignant tumors; however, it appears that the mechanism of oncogenesis is different from that associated with classic DNA or RNA tumor viruses, because there is no evidence that viral sequences are incorporated into the genome of transformed cells. Virus strains may gain or lose tumorigenicity independent of their ability to replicate, and continued productive replication of the virus appears to be required for tumor growth. It was postulated in the 1960s that these viruses may produce a growth factor that accounts for their induction of tumors.[81] Since then, a large body of research has documented that several poxviruses encode a protein that can be classified as a member of the epidermal growth factor–like (EGF-like) family of growth factors.[109] Shope fibroma virus and malignant rabbit fibroma virus both encode a very similar protein, Shope fibroma growth factor (SFGF), whereas myxoma virus encodes a related myxoma growth factor (MGF). These proteins contain the functional domains (six characteristically spaced cysteines) shared by members of the EGF family. Furthermore, when these genes are deleted from the virus genomes, the MGF and SFGF viruses replicate normally in cell culture but show a much reduced ability to induce tumors in rabbits.[127] Even highly cytolytic poxviruses such as vaccinia express related growth factor homologs, indicating that their role in poxvirus pathogenesis undoubtedly extends beyond the capacity to stimulate tumor-like proliferations in infected tissues.

Receptors for Antiviral Cytokines: Tumor Necrosis Factor, Interferon, and Interleukin 1

Tumor necrosis factor (TNF) is a potent proinflammatory cytokine that is produced by activated macrophages and T cells. There are three homologous molecular forms of TNF: TNFα, lymphotoxin a (TNFβ), and lymphotoxin b. These TNFs act by binding to two related but distinct cellular receptors that are both type 1 integral membrane proteins characterized by multiple cysteine-rich exodomains. Through their receptors on myeloid and lymphoid cells, the TNFs exert complex pleiotropic effects on immune networks and host responses to infection. A number of poxviruses encode a protein, designated T2 in the case of Shope fibroma virus, that is a soluble form of the cellular p75 TNF receptor.[151,162] It is presumed that this protein binds and inactivates TNF, thereby modulating TNF-mediated cellular responses to infection, although it may also bind to cell-associated TNF, thereby reducing the release of free TNF or the cytolytic activity of cells bearing TNF on their surface.[152] It is postulated that T2 may enhance replication of poxviruses in vivo by downmodulating antiviral defenses of the infected host, although T2 may simultaneously favor the host by reducing the severity of virus-induced inflammatory lesions.

Since the discovery of the poxvirus TNF viroceptors in 1990, similar receptor-like proteins that are secreted from poxvirus-infected cells have been described that are specific for three other host cytokines: interferon-γ, interleukin-1β, and interferon-α/β.[6,108,154] Because dozens of secreted poxvirus proteins are known but have not yet been biochemically characterized, it is likely that more examples of viroceptors targeted for other specific immune ligands remain to be discovered.

Vaccinia Virus Complement Control Protein

The complement system is a complex group of proteins that act in a cascade that forms one of the initial host defenses against microbial pathogens. The complement system is potent, and when uncontrolled, has the potential to cause severe damage. It is therefore tightly regulated by several different mechanisms, including C4-BP, a plasma protein that binds C4b2a, one of the complexes formed in the course of complement activation. Vaccinia virus encodes a protein, vaccinia virus complement control protein (VCP), that is homologous to C4-BP.[74] VCP binds human C4b, and a VCP-mutant of vaccinia virus fails to inhibit complement-mediated lysis of sensitized sheep erythrocytes, whereas wild-type vaccinia virus has an inhibitory effect.[89] When wild-type and VCP- vaccinia viruses were compared in vivo, the wild-type virus was more virulent on intracerebral injection of mice and, as shown in Figure 5-10, produced larger skin lesions after intradermal inoculation in rabbits.[73]

Herpes Simplex Viruses

Herpes Simplex Virus Complement Receptors

The importance of the complement cascade and its regulation were mentioned previously. Because C3b plays a key role in initiating the formation of the membrane attack complex, the last part of the complement cascade, its regulation is important. A number of cell types, including monocytes/macrophages, neutrophils, and some T cells, express receptors for C3b that downmodulate the complement cascade by reducing the levels of C3b and enhancing its inactivation by cleavage to iC3b. Glycoprotein C (gC) of HSV-1, but not of HSV-2, binds

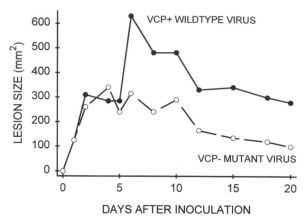

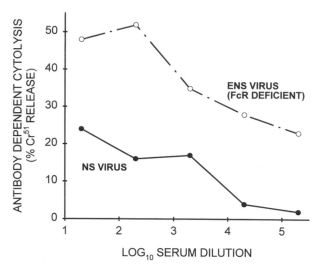

FIG. 5-10. Cell-derived viral genes as virulence factors. The effect of deleting the vaccinia complement control (VCP) gene from vaccinia virus. Rabbits received intradermal injections of 10^6 plaque-forming units (PFU) of VCP− or VCP+ wild-type vaccinia virus at different sites on the back, and the sizes of the lesions were recorded. The lesions caused by VCP+ wild-type virus were consistently larger, indicating that the VCP gene enhances the virulence of vaccinia virus. (Data [the median for three animals] from Isaacs SN, Kotwal GJ, Moss B. Vaccinia virus complement-control protein prevents antibody-dependent complement-enhanced neutralization of infectivity and contributes to virulence. Proc Natl Acad Sci U S A 1992;89:628–632.)

FIG. 5-11. Cell-derived viral genes as virulence factors. Glycoprotein E (gE) of herpes simplex virus (HSV), which functions as an Fc receptor (FcR), influences the susceptibility of HSV-infected cells to antibody-dependent cell-mediated cytotoxicity (ADCC). This plot compares the degree of ADCC in target cells infected with the NS (FcR+) strain of HSV, or with an FcR-deficient mutant of NS virus (strain ENS) expressing an altered gE, at different dilutions of anti-HSV antibody. Cells infected with parent NS (FcR+) virus show lower percent lysis, indicating that the viral-encoded FcR can reduce the susceptibility of HSV-infected cells to ADCC. (Data from Dubin G, Socolof E, Frank I. Herpes simplex virus type 1 Fc receptor protects infected cells from antibody-dependent cellular cytotoxicity. J Virol 1991;65:7046–7050.)

C3b and iC3b and provides protection against complement-mediated neutralization of HSV and complement-mediated lysis of HSV-infected cells.[54,65,167] Although it has not yet been demonstrated that gC mutants are less virulent in vivo, the conservation of gC in natural isolates of HSV suggests that this protein and its complement-binding activity play a role in HSV survival in nature.

Herpes Simplex Virus Fc Receptors

HSV-infected cells express receptors (FcR) for the Fc domain of the immunoglobulin (IgG) molecule.[12] A considerable body of work[167] has identified glycoproteins gE and gI of HSV as the molecules that bind IgG. It has been suggested that the presence of FcR on the herpes simplex virion or on the surface of HSV-infected cells leads to bipolar bridging of the IgG molecule that may reduce secondary effects of antibody binding such as the ability to initiate the complement cascade. Comparison of an FcR-deficient mutant expressing an altered gE protein with wild-type HSV has shown that FcR-deficient virus is less resistant to complement-mediated neutralization and lysis of virus-infected cells (Fig. 5-11).[38,53] Furthermore, gE- HSV exhibits reduced virulence in mice.[121,136]

ATTENUATED VIRUSES AS VACCINES

The most important practical application of the study of viral virulence is the development of attenuated viral variants as vaccines. Many of the established and effective viral vaccines are live attenuated variants, including vaccines for variola,

poliomyelitis, yellow fever, measles, rubella, mumps, and varicella. Viral vaccines are discussed in detail in Chapter 16; this section is limited to the principles of viral virulence as applied to an attenuated-virus vaccine.

There are several requirements for an attenuated virus suitable for use as a vaccine.

The virus must be sufficiently attenuated so that it does not cause clinically significant disease in humans. In practice, a very low level of significant vaccine-associated disease is caused by many established live-virus vaccines, on the order of one case per 1 million primary immunizations.

The vaccine virus must be sufficiently infectious so that it can stimulate humoral and cellular immune responses.

The vaccine strain should be genetically uniform to the maximal extent practical and should not produce virulent revertants.

If the vaccine virus is administered by a natural route, such as the enteric or respiratory portal, it should be able to replicate even when vaccine recipients are undergoing intercurrent infections with other enteric or respiratory viruses.

The vaccine virus should be reasonably stable under field conditions.

The vaccine should be sold at a price that makes it available to developing countries.

In practice, it is the first three requirements that pose the most difficult challenge to vaccine development. In selecting attenuated virus strains for use in immunization, virus variants have often been obtained that are excessively attenuated, so that they fail to cause an immunizing infection even though they replicate well in cell culture. Conversely, there have been repeated problems with disease caused by attenuated virus variants that are immunogenic but retain residual virulence. It appears that the most effective approach to these problems is to exploit the observation that different strains of the same virus vary in their relative tropism for different tissues and organs. This suggests that a search should be made for a virus variant that replicates poorly in the target organ associated with disease production but replicates more briskly in cells, tissues, or organs that are involved in inducing an immunizing response.

The problem of genetic reversion to increased virulence has plagued some attenuated vaccines, such as 17D yellow fever and OPV; however, modern molecular genetic methods offer a rational approach to this problem. Often, there are relatively few critical point mutations that are major determinants of virulence. The identification of these critical sites can enable the construction of attenuated variants that are unlikely to revert in phenotype because they bear several independent attenuating mutations. The challenges involved in developing attenuated viral vaccines is briefly illustrated using poliovirus and HIV as examples.

Polioviruses

Of all live vaccine viruses, OPV has been the subject of the most sophisticated and elegant analysis of the genetic determinants of its virulence and attenuation.[21] However, only recently have the virus isolates from the central nervous system of vaccine-associated poliomyelitis patients been adequately characterized. In a study of eight vaccine-associated poliomyelitis cases, all isolates (four type 2 and four type 3) from the spinal fluid or central nervous system exhibited increased (moderate or severe) neurovirulence.[55] The neural isolates were no more virulent than fecal isolates from the same patients, suggesting that reversion had occurred in the gut prior to systemic dissemination. Revertant mutations were consistently found in the 5′ NTR critical site (discussed previously), and many isolates also had one or more revertant mutations in structural or nonstructural proteins. In addition, the majority of isolates were recombinants containing sequences of two OPV virus types. Similar data have been reported for stool isolates from vaccine-associated cases.[43,114,128]

It seems clear that vaccine-associated poliomyelitis cases are caused by reversion of the attenuated phenotype to a more neurovirulent one as a result of reversion mutations. Although revertants frequently can be isolated from the feces of children fed OPV, vaccine-associated disease is a relatively rare event (see Table 5-2) occurring at a rate of less than 1 per 10^6 vaccine recipients (i.e., 10,000-fold less frequently than disease caused by naturally occurring wild polioviruses). Furthermore, the frequency of vaccine-associated poliomyelitis is considerably lower for type 1 and type 2 OPV virus than for the type 3 OPV virus (see Table 5-9). This observation correlates with the smaller number of attenuating mutations in the type 3 strain and with its higher frequency of reversion after oral virus administration. Based on this information, some candidate viruses have been developed that represent anti-

genic chimeras (type 3 antigenic sequences introduced into the type 1 OPV virus) or have genetically stable attenuating mutations in the 5′ NTR and at sites that determine the temperature-sensitive phenotype.[8,87] These efforts have set a new standard for the rational design of attenuated viruses that can achieve high levels of safety without sacrificing immunogenicity. Unfortunately, the complexity of the regulatory process for the approval of new attenuated viral vaccines has made it unlikely that these potentially improved vaccine strains will be adopted for widespread use in humans.

Human Immunodeficiency Virus

HIV has proved to be a major challenge to vaccinology.[118] There is no promising vaccine candidate on the immediate horizon, despite an intense and well-funded effort to develop such a vaccine. In view of the disappointing results with noninfectious vaccines, some investigators have turned to the development of attenuated infectious HIV variants as vaccine candidates. The following comments are designed to illustrate the challenges of developing suitable attenuated viruses as vaccines and are not meant to be a complete or balanced discussion of the multiple potential approaches to an HIV vaccine.[86] There are several reasons to consider an attenuated strain of HIV as a vaccine candidate.

Efficacy

There is considerable evidence that humans infected with one strain of HIV are relatively resistant to superinfection with other strains, because infected persons who have had multiple exposures to HIV usually carry a single virus that may be inferred from the microheterogeneity of sequences obtained by polymerase chain reaction.[14,64] Also, humans infected with HIV-2 appear to be at reduced risk of infection with HIV-1 compared with those not infected with either virus.[160]

Safety

There is some evidence that HIV strains differ in their virulence for humans,[95] and HIV infections do not necessarily lead to disease, as evidenced by long-term survivors who are asymptomatic for up to 15 years after infection. Of particular interest is a recent report of a blood donor infected with a nef− strain of HIV-1 and a cohort of six individuals infected from this donor, all of whom have remained free from disease for 10 to 14 years after infection.[36] Furthermore, HIV-2 may be less virulent than HIV-1.[80,130] Also, strains of SIV exhibit marked variation in virulence for monkeys, producing infections that range from acutely lethal to asymptomatic.[67,105] These observations suggest that HIV strains of relatively lower virulence may occur in nature, and that attenuated strains may be identified or created.

HIV has a number of accessory genes that are common to lentiviruses but are not found in other groups of retroviruses. Some of these genes are not necessary for replication of the virus in certain cell lines,[11,84] but it may be assumed that they are conserved because they are required for successful perpetuation of the virus in humans or other primate hosts. Particular attention has focussed on the *nef* gene, based on the work of Desrosiers and colleagues.[34] SIV clones that are *nef*− replicate well in certain cell cultures, but the *nef* gene appears to be of greater importance in vivo because SIV bearing a point mutation in *nef* always reverts to a *nef*+ genotype after infection of monkeys. When rhesus monkeys were infected with a pathogenic SIV that was altered by a major nonrevertable deletion in the *nef* gene, the animals underwent an immunizing infection that did not progress to AIDS over a 3-year observation period, whereas controls infected with the virulent parent virus uniformly developed clinical disease within about 3 months. When animals previously infected with the *nef*− virus were challenged with a potentially pathogenic SIV, they did not develop AIDS. However, it has been reported that the *nef*− SIV caused AIDS in newborn rhesus monkeys exposed by the oral route.[9] Thus, as with other viruses, the virulence of attenuated strains of primate lentiviruses are dependent on the age of the host, the route of infection, and the size of the inoculum. Much additional work is required to determine whether a strain of HIV can be developed that is sufficiently attenuated to meet safety criteria while maintaining sufficient infectivity to be immunogenic and that does not revert or recombine to increase its virulence during persistent infection.

ABBREVIATIONS

AIDS: acquired immunodeficiency syndrome
ASLV: avian sarcoma and leukosis viruses
EGF: epidermal growth factor
FcR: Fc receptor
gC: glycoprotein C
gE: glycoprotein E
gI: glycoprotein I
HIV: human immunodeficiency virus
IgG: immunoglobulin
L RNA segment: large RNA segment
LCMV lymphocytic choriomeningitis virus
M RNA segment: middle RNA segment
MAR: monoclonal antibody–resistant
MGF: myxoma growth factor
MuLV: murine leukemia virus
NTR: nontranslating region
OPV: oral poliovirus vaccine
PBL: primary blood leukocyte
PFU: plaque-forming units
S RNA segment: small RNA segment
SCID: severe combined immunodeficiency
SFGF: Shope fibroma growth factor
SIV: simian immunodeficiency virus
TNF: tumor necrosis factor
VCP: vaccinia virus complement control protein

ACKNOWLEDGEMENTS

We would like to thank Rafi Ahmed, Francisco Gonzalez-Scarano, Alan Jackson, Vincent Racaniello, Harriet Robinson, and Herbert Virgin III for their numerous constructive suggestions.

REFERENCES

1. Ahmed R, Hahn CS, Somasundaram T, Villarete L, Matloubian N, Strauss JM. Molecular basis of organ-specific selection of viral variants during chronic infection. J Virol 1991;65:4242–4247.
2. Ahmed R, King CC, Oldstone MBA. Virus-lymphocyte interaction: T cells of the helper subset are infected with lymphocytic choriomeningitis virus during persistent infection in vivo. J Virol 1987; 61:1571–1576.
3. Ahmed R, Oldstone MBA. Organ specific selection of viral variants during chronic infection. J Exp Med 1988;167:1719–1724.
4. Ahmed R, Salmi A, Butler LD, Chiller J, Oldstone MBA. Selection of genetic variants of lymphocytic choriomeningitis virus in spleens of persistently infected mice: role in suppression of cytotoxic T lymphocytic response and viral persistence. J Exp Med 1984; 60: 521–540.
5. Ahmed R, Simon RD, Matloubian N, Kolhekar SR, Southern PJ, Freedman DM. Genetic analysis of in vivo selected viral variants causing chronic infection: importance of mutation in the L RNA segment of lymphocytic choriomeningitis virus. J Virol 1988; 62:3301–3308.
6. Alcami A, Smith GL. Cytokine receptors encoded by poxviruses: a lesson in cytokine biology. Immunol Today 1995;16:474–478.
7. Almond JW. Poliovirus neurovirulence. Semin Neurosci 1991; 3:101–108.
8. Almond JW, Stone D, Burke K, et al. Approaches to the construction of new candidate poliovirus type 3 vaccine strains. Dev Biol Standard 1993;78:161–170.
9. Baba RW, Jeong YS, Pennicnck D, Bronson R, Greene MF, Ruprecht RM. Pathogenicity of live, attenuated SIV after mucosal infection of neonatal macaques. Science 1995;267:1820–1824.
10. Baer GM, ed. The natural history of rabies. Boca Raton: CRC Press, 1991.
11. Balliet JW, Kolson DL, Eiger G, et al. Distinct effects in primary macrophages and lymphocytes of the simian immunodeficiency virus type 1 accessory genes vpr, vpu, and nef: mutational analysis of a primary HIV-1 isolate. Virology 1994;200:623–631.
12. Baucke RB, Spear PG. Membrane proteins specified by herpes simplex virus. V. Identification of an Fc-binding glycoprotein. J Virol 1979;32:779–789.
13. Beaty BJ, Miller BR, Shope RE, Rohzon EJ, Bishop DH. Molecular basis of bunyavirus per os infection of mosquitoes: role of the middle-sized RNA segment. Proc Natl Acad Sci U S A 1982; 79:1295–1297.
14. Benn S, Rutledge R, Folks T, et al. Genomic heterogeneity of AIDS retroviral isolates from North American and Zaire. Science 1985; 230:949–951.
15. Bodian D. Viremia in experimental poliomyelitis. I. General aspects of infection after intravascular inoculation with strains of high and low invasiveness. Am J Hygiene 1954;60:339–357.
16. Bodian D. The enhancement of susceptibility of monkeys to polioviruses of high and of low virulence. Am J Hygiene 1956; 64: 92–103.
17. Borrow P, Evans CF, Oldstone MBA. Virus-induced immunosuppression: immune system-mediated destruction of virus-infected dendritic cells results in generalized immune suppression. J Virol 1995;69:1059–1070.
18. Borrow P, Tishon A, Oldstone MBA. Infection of lymphocytes by a virus that aborts cytotoxic T lymphocyte activity and establishes persistent infection. J Exp Med 1991;174:203–212.
19. Bosze Z, Thiesen HJ, Charnay P. A transcriptional enhancer with specificity for erythroid cells is located in the long terminal repeat of the Friend murine leukemia virus. EMBO J 1986;5:1615–1623.
20. Bouchard MJ, Lam D-H, Racaniello VR. Determinants of attenuation and temperature sensitivity in the type 1 poliovirus Sabin vaccine. J Virol 1995;69:4972–4978.
21. Brown F, Lewis BP, eds. Poliovirus attenuation: molecular mechanisms and practical aspects. Basel: Karger, 1993.

22. Celander D, Haseltilne WA. Tissue-specific transcription preference as a determinant of cell tropism and leukemogenic potential of murine retroviruses. Nature 1984;312:159–162.

23. Chatis PA, Holland CA, Silver JE, Fredericksen TN, Hopkins N, Hartley JW. A 3´ end fragment encompassing the transcriptional enhancer of nondefective Friend virus confers erythroleukemogenicity on Moloney leukemia virus. J Virol 1984;52:248–254.

24. Cheng-Mayer C, Quiroga M, Tung JW, Dina D, Levy JA. Viral determinants of HIV-1 T-cell/macrophage tropism, cytopathicity, and CD4 antigen modulation. J Virol 1990;64:4390–4398.

25. Chesebro B, Nishio J, Perryman S, et al. Identification of human immunodeficiency virus envelope gene sequences influencing viral entry into CD4-positive HeLa cell, T-leukemia cells, and macrophages. J Virol 1991;65:5782–5789.

26. Christodoulou C, Cobaree-Garapin F, Macadam AJ, et al. Mapping of mutations associated with neurovirulence in monkeys infected with Sabin 1 poliovirus revertants selected at high temperature. J Virol 1990;64:4922–4929.

27. Clark HF. Rabies viruses increase in virulence when propagated in neuroblastoma cell culture. Science 1978;199:1072–1075.

28. Collman R, Godfrey B, Cutilli J, et al. Macrophage tropic strains of human immunodeficiency virus type 1 utilize the CD4 receptor. J Virol 1990;64:4468–4476.

29. Collman R, Hassan NF, Walker R, et al. Infection of monocyte-derived macrophages with human immunodeficiency virus type 1 (HIV-1): monocyte- and lymphocyte-tropic strains of HIV-1 show distinctive patterns of replication in a panel of cell types. J Exp Med 1989;170:1149–1163.

30. Collman R, Nathanson N. Human immunodeficiency virus type-1 infection of macrophages. Semin Virol 1992;3:185–202.

31. Coulon P, Derbin C, Kucera P, Lafay F, Prehaud C, Flamand A. Invasion of the peripheral nervous system of adult mice by the CVS strain of rabies virus and its avirulent derivative Av01. J Virol 1989; 63:3550–3554.

32. Cox NJ, Kendal AP, Maassab HF, Scholtissek C, Spring SB. Genetic synergism between matrix protein and polymerase protein required for temperature sensitivity of the cold-adapted influenza A/Ann Arbor/6/60 mutant virus. In: Bishop DHL, Compans RW, eds. The replication of negative strand viruses. New York: Elsevier, 1981: 405–413.

33. Dalziel RG, Lampert PW, Talbot PJ, Buchmeier MJ. Site specific alteration of murine hepatitis virus type 4 peplomer glycoprotein E2 results in reduced neurovirulence. J Virol 1986;59:463–471.

34. Daniel MD, Kirchhoff F, Czajak PK, Sehgal PK, Desrosiers R. Protective effects of a live attenuated SIV vaccine with a deletion in the nef gene. Science 1992;258:1938–1941.

35. de la Torre C, Rall G, Oldstone C, Sanna PP, Borrow P, Oldstone MBA. Replication of lymphocytic choriomeningitis virus is restricted in terminally differentiated neurons. J Virol 1993;67: 7350–7359.

36. Deacon NJ, Tsykin A, Solomon A, et al. Genomic structure of an attenuated quasi species of HIV-1 from a blood transfusion donor and recipients. Science 1995;270:988–991.

37. Dietzschold B, Wunner WH, Wiktor TJ, et al. Characterization of an antigenic determinant of the glycoprotein that correlates with pathogenicity of rabies virus. Proc Natl Acad Sci U S A 1983;80:70–74.

38. Dubin G, Socolof E, Frank I. Herpes simplex virus type 1 Fc receptor protects infected cells from antibody-dependent cellular cytotoxicity. J Virol 1991;65:7046–7050.

39. Edmonds JW, Nolan IF, Shephard RC, Gocs A. Myxomatosis: the virulence of field strains of myxoma virus in a population of wild rabbits (Oryctolagus cuniculus L.) with high resistance to myxomatosis. J Hygiene (Cambridge) 1975;74:417–418.

40. ElDadah AH, Nathanson N, Sarsitis R. Pathogenesis of West Nile virus encephalitis in mice and rats. I. Influence of age and species on mortality and infection. Am J Epidemiol 1967;86:765–775.

41. Endres MJ, Valsamakis A, Gonzalez-Scarano F, Nathanson N. Neuroattenuated bunyavirus variant: derivation, characterization, and revertant clones. J Virol 1990;64:1927–1933.

42. Enquist LW. Circuit-specific infection of the mammalian nervous system. ASM News 1995;61:633–638.

43. Equestre M, Genovese D, Cavalieri F, Fiore L, Santoro R, Perez Bercoff R. Identification of a consistent pattern of mutations in neurovirulent variants derived from the Sabin vaccine strain of poliovirus 2. J Virol 1991;65:2707–2710.

44. Evans CF, Borrow P, de la Torre C, Oldstone MBA. Virus-induced immunosuppression: kinetic analysis of the selection of a mutation associated with viral persistence. J Virol 1994;68:7367–7373.

45. Evans DMA, Dunn G, Minor PD, et al. Increased neurovirulence associated with a single nucleotide change in a noncoding region of the Sabin type 3 poliovaccine genome. Nature 1985;314:548–550.

46. Evans L, Morrey J. Tissue-specific replication of Friend and Moloney mouse leukemia viruses in infected mice. J Virol 1987;61: 1350–1357.

47. Fan H. Influences of the long terminal repeats on retrovirus pathogenicity. Semin Virol 1990;1:165–174.

48. Fenner F. Biological control as exemplified by smallpox eradication and myxomatosis. Proceedings of the Royal Society, Series B (London) 1983;218:259–285.

49. Fenner F, Chapple PJ. Evolutionary changes in myxoma viruses in Britain. An examination of 222 naturally occurring strains obtained from 80 counties during the period October-November 1962.J Hygiene (Cambridge) 1965;63:175–185.

50. Fenner F, Henderson DA, Arita I, Jezek Z, Ladnyi ID. Smallpox and its eradication. Geneva: World Health Organization, 1988.

51. Findlay GM, Mahaffy AF. Paths of infection of central nervous system in yellow fever. Trans R Soc Trop Med Hygiene 1936;30: 355–362.

52. Fleming JO, Trousdale MD, El-Zaatari FAK, Stohlman SA, Weiner LP. Pathogenicity of antigenic variants of murine coronavirus JHM selected with monoclonal antibodies. J Virol 1986;58:869–875.

53. Frank I, Friedman H. A novel function of the herpes simplex virus type 1 Fc receptor: participation of bipolar bridging of antiviral immunoglobulin. J Virol 1989;63:4479–4488.

54. Friedman HM, Cohen GH, Eisenberg RJ. Glycoprotein C of herpes simplex virus 1 acts as a receptor for the C3b complement on infected cells. Nature 1984;309:633–635.

55. Georgescu M-M, Delpeyroux F, Tardy-Panit M, et al. High diversity of poliovirus strains isolated from the central nervous system from patients with vaccine-associated paralytic poliomyelitis. J Virol 1995;68:8089–8101.

56. Georgescu M-M, Tardy-Panit M, Guillot S, Crainic R, Delpeyroux F. Mapping of mutations contributing to the temperature sensitivity of the Sabin 1 vaccine strain of poliovirus. J Virol 1995;69: 5278–5286.

57. Golemis E, Fredericksen TN, Hartley JW, Hopkins N. Distinct segments within the enhancer region collaborate to identify the type of leukemia induced by non defective Friend and Moloney viruses. J Virol 1989;63:328–337.

58. Gonzalez-Scarano F, Janssen R, Najjar JA, Pobjecky N, Nathanson N. An avirulent G1 glycoprotein variant of La Crosse bunyavirus with defective fusion function. J Virol 1985;54:757–763.

59. Gonzalez-Scarano F, Nathanson N. Bunyaviruses. In: Fields BN, Knipe DM, eds. Virology. 3rd ed. Philadelphia: Lippincott-Raven Publishers, 1995:1473–1504.

60. Gonzalez-Scarano F, Nathanson N, Wong PKY. Retroviruses and the nervous system. In: Levy JA, ed. The retroviridae. New York: Plenum Press, 1995:409–490.

61. Gonzalez-Scarano F, Shope RE, Calisher CH, Nathanson N. Monoclonal antibodies against the G1 and nucleocapsid proteins of La Cross and Tahyna viruses. In: Calisher CH, ed. California serogroup viruses. New York: Alan R Liss, 1983:145–156.

62. Griot C, Pekosz A, Davidson R, et al. Replication in cultured C2C12 muscle cells correlates with the neuroinvasiveness of California serogroup bunyaviruses. Virology 1994;201:399–403.

63. Griot C, Pekosz A, Lukac D, et al. Polygenic control of neuroinvasiveness in California serogroup viruses. J Virol 1993;67: 3861–3867.

64. Hahn BH, Shaw GM, Taylor ME, et al. Genetic variation in HTLV-III-LAV over time in patients with AIDS or at risk for AIDS. Science 1986;232:1548–1553.

65. Harris SL, Frank I, Yee A. Glycoprotein C of herpes simplex virus type 1 prevents complement-mediated cell lysis and virus neutralization. J Infect Dis 1990;162:331–337.

66. Hensel M, Shea JE, Gleeson C, Jones MD, Dalton E, Holden DW. Simultaneous identification of bacterial virulence genes by negative selection. Science 1995;269:400–403.

67. Hirsch VM, Johnson PR. Pathogenic diversity of simian immunodeficiency viruses. Virus Res 1994;32:183–203.

68. Holland CA, Anklesaria P, Sakakeeny MA, Greenberger JS. Enhancer sequences of a retroviral vector determine expression of gene in multipotent hematopoietic progenitors and committed erythroid cells. Proc Natl Acad Sci U S A 1987;84:8662–8666.

69. Holland JJ, Spindler K, Horodyski F, Grabau E, Nichol S, Vandepol S. Rapid evolution of RNA genomes. Science 1982;215:1577–1585.

70. Hopkins N, Golemis E, Speck N. Role of enhancer regions in leukemia induction by nondefective murine C type retroviruses. In: Notkins AL, Oldstone MBA, eds. Concepts in viral pathogenesis. New York: Springer-Verlag, 1989:41–49.

71. Horstmann DM, Opton EM, Klemperer R, Llado B, Vignec AJ. Viremia in infants vaccinated with oral poliovirus vaccine (Sabin). Am J Hygiene 1964;79:47–63.

72. Hwang SS, Boyle TJ, Lyerly HK, Cullen BR. Identification of the envelope V3 loop as the primary determinant of cell tropism in HIV-1. Science 1991;253:71–74.

73. Isaacs SN, Kotwal GJ, Moss B. Vaccinia virus complement-control protein prevents antibody-dependent complement-enhanced neutralization of infectivity and contributes to virulence. Proc Natl Acad Sci U S A 1992;89:628–632.

74. Isaacs SN, Moss B. Inhibition of complement activation by vaccinia virus. In: McFadden G, ed. Viroceptors, virokines, and related immune modulators encoded by DNA viruses. Austin: RG Landes, 1995:55–66.

75. Ishimoto A, Takimoto M, Adachi A, et al. Sequences responsible for erythroid and lymphoid leukemia in the long terminal repeats of Friend mink cell focus-forming and Moloney murine leukemia viruses. J Virol 1987;61:1861–1866.

76. Jackson A. Biological basis of rabies virus neurovirulence in mice: comparative pathogenesis study using the immunoperoxidase technique. J Virol 1991;65:537–540.

77. Jaenisch R. Retroviruses and embryogenesis: microinjection of Moloney leukemia virus into midgestation mouse embryos. Cell 1980;19:181–188.

78. Janssen R, Endres MJ, Gonzalez-Scarano F, Nathanson N. Virulence of La Crosse virus is under polygenic control. J Virol 1986;59:1–7.

79. Janssen R, Gonzalez-Scarano F, Nathanson N. Mechanisms of bunyavirus virulence: comparative pathogenesis of a virulent strain of La Crosse and an attenuated strain of Tahyna virus. Lab Invest 1984;50:447–455.

80. Kanki P, M'Boup S, Marlink R. Prevalence and risk determinants of human immunodeficiency virus type 2 (HIV-2) in West African female prostitutes. Am J Epidemiol 1992;136:895–907.

81. Kato S, Miyamoto H, Takahashi M. Shope fibroma and rabbit myxoma viruses. II. Pathogenesis of fibromas in domestic rabbits. Biken J 1963;6:135–143.

82. Kendal AP, Maassab HF, Alexandrova I, Ghendon Y. Development of cold adapted recombinant live-attenuated influenza A vaccines in the US and USSR. Antiviral Res 1981;1:339–350.

83. Kestler H, Kodoma T, Ringler D, et al. Induction of AIDS in rhesus monkeys by molecularly cloned simian immunodeficiency virus. Science 1990;248:1109–1112.

84. Kestler H, Ringler DJ, Mori K, et al. Importance of the nef gene for maintenance of high virus loads and for development of AIDS. Cell 1991;65:651–662.

85. King CC, de Fries R, Kolhekar SR, Ahmed R. In vivo selection of lymphocyte-tropic and macrophage-tropic variants of lymphocytic choriomeningitis virus during persistent infection. J Virol 1990;64:5611–5616.

86. Koff WC. The next steps toward a global AIDS vaccine. Science 1994;266:1335–1337.

87. Kohara M, Abe S, Yoshioka I, Nomoto A. Development of candidates for new type 2 and type 3 oral poliovirus vaccines. Dev Biol Stand 1993;78:141–148.

88. Koolen MJM, Osterhaus ADME, van Steenis G, Horzinek MC, van den Zeijst BAM. Temperature sensitive mutants of mouse hepatitis virus strain A59: isolation, characterization, and neuropathogenic properties. Virology 1983;125:393–402.

89. Kotwal GJ, Isaacs SN, McKenzie R, Frank MM, Moss B. Inhibition of the complement cascade by the major secretory protein of vaccinia virus. Science 1990;250:827–830.

90. Kucera P, Dolivo M, Coulon P, Flamand A. Pathways of the early propagation of virulent and avirulent rabies strains from the eye to the brain. J Virol 1985;55:158–162.

91. La Monica N, Almond JW, Racaniello VR. A mouse model for poliovirus neurovirulence identifies mutations that attenuate the virus for humans. J Virol 1987;61:2917–2920.

92. La Monica N, Meriam C, Racaniello VR. Mapping of the sequences required for mouse neurovirulence of poliovirus type 2 Lansing. J Virol 1986;57:515–525.

93. La Monica N, Racaniello VR. Differences in replication of attenuated and neurovirulent polioviruses in human neuroblastoma cell line SH-SY5Y. J Virol 1989;63:2357–2360.

94. Lafay F, Coulon P, Astic L, Flamand A. Spread of the CVS strain of rabies virus and of the avirulent mutant Av01 along the olfactory pathways of the mouse after intranasal inoculation. Virology 1991;183:320–330.

95. Levy JA. HIV and the pathogenesis of AIDS. Washington: ASM Press, 1994.

96. Lewick H, Tishon A, Borrow P, et al. CTL escape viral variants. I. Generation and molecular characterization. Virology 1995;210: 29–40.

97. Li CP, Schaeffer M, Nelson DB. Experimentally produced variants of poliomyelitis virus combining in vivo and in vitro techniques. Ann N Y Acad Sci 1955;61:902–910.

98. Li Y, Golemis E, Hartley JW, Hopkins N. Disease specificity of nondefective Friend and Moloney murine leukemia viruses is controlled by a small number of nucleotides. J Virol 1987;61:696–700.

99. Liu Z-Q, Wood C, Levy JA, Cheng-Mayer C. The viral envelope gene is involved in the macrophage tropism of an HIV-1 strain isolated from the brain. J Virol 1990;64:6143–6153.

100. Maassab HF, DeBorde DC. Development and characterization of cold-adapted viruses for use as live virus vaccines. Vaccine 1985;3:355–369.

101. Macadam AJ, Pollard SR, Ferguson G, et al. The 5′ noncoding region of the type 2 poliovirus vaccine strain contains determinants of attenuation and temperature sensitivity. Virology 1991;181:451–458.

102. Macadam AJ, Pollard SR, Ferguson G, et al. Genetic basis of the attenuation of the Sabin type 2 vaccine strain of poliovirus in primates. Virology 1993;192:18–26.

103. Mahan MJ, Slauch JM, Mekalanos JJ. Selection of bacterial virulence genes that are specifically induced in host tissue. Science 1993;259:686–688.

104. Marshall ID, Fenner F. Studies in the epidemiology of infectious myxomatosis of rabbits. VII. The virulence of strains of myxoma virus recovered from Australian wild rabbits between 1951 and 959. J Hygiene (Cambridge) 1960;58:485–488.

105. Marthas ML, Van Rompay KKA, Otsyula M, et al. Viral factors determine progression to AIDS in simian immunodeficiency virus-infected newborn rhesus macaques. J Virol 1995;69:4198–4205.

106. Matloubian N, Kolhekar SR, Somasundaram T, Ahmed R. Molecular determinants of macrophage-tropism and viral persistence: importance of single amino acid changes in the polymerase and glycoprotein of lymphocytic choriomeningitis virus. J Virol 1993;67:7340–7349.

107. Matloubian N, Somasundaram T, Kolhekar SR, Selvukamar R, Ahmed R. Genetic basis of viral persistence: single amino acid change in the viral glycoprotein affects ability of lymphocytic choriomeningitis virus to persistent in adult mice. J Exp Med 1990;172:1043–1048.

108. McFadden G, Graham K. Modulation of cytokine networks by poxvirus: the myxoma virus model. Semin Virol 1995;5:421–429.

109. McFadden G, Graham K, Opgenorth A. Poxvirus growth factors. In: McFadden G, ed. Viroceptors, virokines, and related immune modulators encoded by DNA viruses. Austin: RG Landes, 1995:1–16.

110. McFadden G, ed. Viroceptors, virokines, and related immune modulators encoded by DNA viruses. Austin: RG Landes, 1995.

111. McGoldrick A, Macadam AJ, Dunn G, et al. Role of mutations G-480 and C-6203 in the attenuation phenotype of Sabin type 1 poliovirus. J Virol 1995;69:7601–7605.

112. Minor PD. The molecular biology of poliovaccines. J Gen Virol 1992;73:3065–3077.

113. Minor PD. Attenuation and reversion of the Sabin strains of poliovirus. Dev Biol Stand 1993;78:17–26.

114. Minor PD, John A, Ferguson M, Icenogle JP. Antigenic and molecular evolution of the vaccine strain type 3 poliovirus during the period of excretion by a primary vaccinee. J Gen Virol 1986;67:693–706.

115. Moss EG, O'Neill RE, Racaniello VR. Mapping of attenuating sequences of an avirulent poliovirus type 2 strain. J Virol 1989;63:1884–1890.

116. Nathanson N. Eradication of poliomyelitis in the United States. Rev Infect Dis 1984;4:940–945.

117. Nathanson N, Gittelsohn AM, Thind IS, Price WH. Histological studies of the monkey neurovirulence of group B arboviruses. III. Relative virulence of selected viruses. Am J Epidemiol 1967;85:503–517.

118. Nathanson N, Gonzalez-Scarano F. Human immunodeficiency virus, an agent which defies vaccination. Adv Vet Science Comp Med 1989;33:397–412.

119. Nathanson N, Horn SD. Neurovirulence tests of type 3 oral poliovirus vaccine manufactured by Lederle Laboratories, 1964–1988. Vaccine 1992;10:469–475.

120. Nathanson N, Martin JR. The epidemiology of poliomyelitis: enigmas surrounding its appearance, epidemicity, and disappearance. Am J Epidemiol 1979;110:672–692.

121. Neidhardt H, Schroder CH, Kaerner HC. Herpes simplex virus type 1 glycoprotein E is not indispensable for viral infectivity. J Virol 1987;61:600–603.

122. Nkowane BM, Wassilak SGF, Orenstein WA, et al. Vaccine-associated paralytic poliomyelitis, United States: 1973 through 1984. JAMA 1987;257:1335–1340.

123. O'Brien WA, Koyanagi Y, Namazie A, et al. HIV-1 tropism for mononuclear phagocytes can be determined by regions of gp120 outside the CD4-binding domain. Nature 1990;348:69–73.

124. Odagiri T, DeBorde DC, Maassab HF. Cold-adapted recombinants of influenza A virus in MDCK cells. Virology 1982;119:82–90.

125. Oldstone MBA, Salvato M, Tishon A, Lewicki H. Virus-lymphocyte interactions. III. Biological parameters of a viral variant that fails to generate CTL and establishes persistent infection in immunocompetent hosts. Virology 1988;164:507–516.

126. Omata T, Kohara M, Kuge S, et al. Genetic analysis of the attenuation phenotype of poliovirus type 1. J Virol 1986;58:348–358.

127. Opgenorth A, Strayer D, Upton C. Deletion of the growth factor gene related to EGF and TGFa reduces virulence of malignant rabbit fibroma virus. Virology 1992;186:175–191.

128. Otolea D, Guillot S, Furione M, et al. Genomic modifications in naturally occurring neurovirulent revertants of Sabin 1 polioviruses. Dev Biol Stand 1993;78:33–38.

129. Paul J. A history of poliomyelitis. New Haven: Yale University Press, 1971.

130. Pepin J, Morgan G, Dunn D, et al. HIV-2 induced immunosuppression among asymptomatic West African prostitutes: evidence that HIV-2 is pathogenic, but less so than HIV-1. AIDS 1991;5: 1165–1172.

131. Pollard SR, Dunn G, Cammack N, Minor PD, Almond JW. Nucleotide sequence of a neurovirulent variant of the type 2 oral poliovirus vaccine. J Virol 1989;63:4949–4951.

132. Racaniello VR. Poliovirus neurovirulence. Adv Virus Res 1988;34:217–246.

133. Racaniello VR. The molecular and functional basis of poliovirus attenuation and host range. In: Notkins AL, Oldstone MBA, eds. Concepts in viral pathogenesis. New York: Springer-Verlag, 1989: 30–37.

134. Racaniello VR, Baltimore D. Cloned poliovirus complementary DNA is infectious in mammalian cells. Science 1981;214:914–919.

135. Racaniello VR, Ren R, Bouchard MJ. Poliovirus attenuation and pathogenesis in a transgenic mouse model for poliomyelitis. Dev Biol Stand 1993;78:109–116.

136. Rajcani J, Herget U, Kaerner HC. Spread of herpes simplex virus (HSV) strains SC16, ANG, ANGpath and its glyC minus and GlyE minus mutants in DBA-2 mice. Acta Virol 1990;34:305–320.

137. Ren R, Constantini FJ, Gorgacz EJ, Lee JJ, Racaniello VR. Transgenic mice expressing a human poliovirus receptor: a new model for poliomyelitis. Cell 1990;63:353–362.

138. Ren R, Moss EG, Racaniello VR. Identification of two determinants that attenuate vaccine-related type 2 poliovirus. J Virol 1991;65:1377–1382.

139. Rosen C, Haseltine WA, Lenz J, Ruprecht R, Cloyd MW. Tissue selectivity of murine leukemia virus infection is determined by long terminal repeat sequences. J Virol 1985;55:862–866.

140. Sabin AB. Characteristics and genetic potentialities of experimentally produced and naturally occurring variants of poliomyelitis virus. Ann N Y Acad Sci 1955;61:924–938.

141. Sabin AB. Oral poliovirus vaccine: history of its development and use and current challenge to eliminate poliomyelitis from the world. J Infect Dis 1985;151:420–436.

142. Salvato M, Borrow P, Shimomaye E, Oldstone MBA. Molecular basis of viral persistence: a single amino acid change in the glycoprotein of lymphocytic choriomeningitis virus is associated with suppression of the antiviral cytotoxic T-lymphocyte response and establishment of persistence. J Virol 1991;65:1863–1869.

143. Salvato M, Shimomaye E, Southern P, Oldstone MBA. Virus-lymphocyte interactions. IV. Molecular characterization of LCMV Armstrong (CTL+) small genomic segment and that of its variant clone 13 (CTL−). Virology 1988;164:517–522.

144. Sawyer WA, Kitchen SF, Lloyd W. Vaccination against yellow fever with immune serum and virus fixed for mice. J Exp Med 1932;55:945–969.

145. Schonberger LB, McGowan JE Jr, Gregg MB. Vaccine-associated poliomyelitis in the United States, 1961–1972. Am J Epidemiol 1976;104:202–211.

146. Schuitemaker H, Koot M, Kootsra NA, et al. Biological phenotype of HIV-1 clones at different stages of infection: progression of disease is associated with a shift from monocytotropic to T-cell-tropic populations. J Virol 1992;66:1354–1360.

147. Seif I, Coulon P, Rollin PE, Flamand A. Rabies virulence: effect on pathogenicity and sequence characterization of rabies virus mutations affecting antigenic site III of the glycoprotein. J Virol 1985;53:926–934.

148. Shioda T, Levy JA, Cheng-Mayer C. Macrophage and T-cell line tropisms of HIV-1 are determined by specific regions of the envelope gp120 gene. Nature 1991;349:167–169.

149. Shioda T, Levy JA, Cheng-Mayer C. Small amino acid changes in the V3 hypervariable region of gp120 can affect the T cell line and macrophage tropisms of human immunodeficiency virus type 1. Proc Natl Acad Sci U S A 1992;89:9434–9438.

150. Short MK, Okenquist SA, Lenz J. Correlation of leukemogenic potential of murine retroviruses with transcriptional tissue preference of the viral long terminal repeats. J Virol 1987;61:1067–1072.

151. Smith CA, Davis T, Anderson D. A receptor for tumor necrosis factor defines an unusual family of cellular and viral proteins. Science 1990;248:1019–1023.

152. Smith CA, Goodwin RG. Tumor necrosis factor receptors in the poxvirus family: biological and genetic implications. In: McFadden G, ed. Viroceptors, virokines and related immune modulators encoded by DNA viruses. Austin: RG Landes, 1995:29–40.

153. Speck N, Renjifo O, Golemis E, Fredericksen TN, Hartley JW, Hopkins N. Mutation of the core or adjacent LVb elements of the Moloney murine leukemia virus enhancer alters disease specificity. Genes Dev 1990;4:233–242.

154. Spriggs M. Poxvirus-encoded soluble cytokine receptors. Virus Res 1994;33:1–10.

155. Steinhauer DA, Holland JJ. Rapid evolution of RNA viruses. Ann Rev Microbiol 1987;41:409–433.

156. Strode GK, Bugher JC, Kerr JA, et al. Yellow fever. New York: McGraw-Hill, 1951.

157. Tatem JM, Weeks-Levy C, Georgiu A, et al. A mutation present in the amino terminus of Sabin 3 poliovirus VP1 protein is attenuating. J Virol 1992;66:3194–3197.

158. Theiler M. Studies on the action of yellow fever virus in mice. Ann Trop Med 1930;24:249–272.

159. Theiler M, Smith HH. Effect of prolonged cultivation in vitro upon pathogenicity of yellow fever virus. J Exp Med 1937;65:767–786.

160. Travers K, Mboup S, Marlink R, et al. Natural protection against HIV-1 infection provided by HIV-2. Science 1995;268:1612–1615.

161. Tuffereau C, Leblois H, Benejean J, Coulon P, Lafay F, Flamand A. Arginine or lysine in position 333 of ERA and CVS glycoprotein is necessary for rabies virulence in adult mice. Virology 1989;172: 206–212.

162. Upton C, Delange A, McFadden G. Tumorigenic poxviruses: genomic organization and DNA sequence of the telomeric region of the Shope fibroma virus genome. Virology 1987;180:20–30.

163. Villarete L, Somasundaram T, Ahmed R. Tissue-mediated selection of viral variants: correlation between glycoprotein mutation and growth in neuronal cells. J Virol 1994;68:7490–7496.

164. Weiss RA. Cellular receptor and viral glycoproteins involved in retrovirus entry. In: Levy JA, ed. The retroviridae. New York: Plenum Press, 1992:1–108.

165. Westervelt P, Trowbridge DB, Epstein LG, et al. Macrophage tropism determinants of human immunodeficiency virus type 1 in vivo. J Virol 1992;66:2577–2582.

166. Westroop GD, Wareham KA, Evans DMA, et al. Genetic basis of attenuation of the Sabin type 3 oral poliovirus vaccine. J Virol 1989;63:1338–1344.

167. York IA, Johnson DC. Inhibition of humoral and cellular immune recognition by herpes simplex viruses. In: McFadden G, ed. Viroceptors, virokines, and related immune modulators encoded by DNA viruses. Austin: RG Landes, 1995:89–110.

168. Yoshimura F, Davison B, Chaffin K. Murine leukemia virus long terminal repeat sequences can enhance gene activity in a cell-type-specific manner. Mol Cell Biol 1985;5:2832–2835.

169. Zhu T, Mo H, Wang N, et al. Genotypic and phenotypic characterization of HIV-1 in patients with primary infection. Science 1993;261:1179–1181.

Viral Pathogenesis,
edited by Neal Nathanson, et al.
Lippincott–Raven Publishers, Philadelphia © 1997

CHAPTER 6

Nonspecific Host Responses to Viral Infections

Raymond M. Welsh and Ganes C. Sen

INTRODUCTION

Natural immunity refers to the ability of preexisting or rapidly inducible host effector systems to combat infectious agents against which the host has not been previously immu-

R. M. Welsh: Department of Pathology, University of Massachusetts Medical Center, Worcester, Massachusetts 01655.
G. C. Sen: Department of Molecular Biology, Cleveland Clinic Foundation, Cleveland, Ohio 44195-5285.

nized. A successful retardation of the replication of the invading pathogen by the natural immune system may provide time for the development of specific antibody and T-cell responses to successfully control the infection. Conversely, an impaired natural immune system occurring as a consequence of genetic deficiency, physiologic state, or infection with another pathogen can result in life-threatening infections by otherwise mild infectious agents. On entry into its host, a virus must first avoid inactivation by humoral factors such as antibody and complement and then replicate in macrophages or other cells that may be under the influence of preexisting levels of antiviral cytokines such as the interferons (IFNs). As a consequence of viral infection, additional cytokines are made, including more antiviral cytokines and activation and chemotactic factors for leukocytes such as macrophages, natural killer (NK) cells, and granulocytes (Table 6-1). These inflammatory cytokines contribute to many of the symptoms of disease but also play roles in maximizing the effectiveness of the natural immune system and initiating the development of specific immunity. This chapter addresses these various aspects of natural immunity, critically evaluates their importance in host resistance to viral infections, and describes how these components interact with each other to produce an effective nonspecific host response.

ROLE OF HUMORAL IMMUNITY FACTORS IN NATURAL RESISTANCE

Natural Antibody

Serum contains many antibodies that are reactive with infectious agents to which the host has not been previously immunized. Some of these are natural antibodies, whose definition in recent years has been narrowed to that of antibodies of IgM, IgG, or IgA isotypes, often having polyspecific low-affinity autoreactivity and produced by B cells lacking germline rearrangements or somatic mutations in the immunoglobulin

TABLE 6-1. *Cytokines associated with nonspecific host responses*

Name	Abbreviation	Amino acids	Cell source	Major functions
Interferon type I	IFNα, IFNβ	165, 166	Many types	Antiviral NK cell activation MHC upregulation
Interferon type II	IFNγ	146 (dimer)	T cells NK cells	Antiviral Macrophage activation MHC upregulation
Interleukin 1	IL-1α, IL-1β	153–159	Many types Macrophages Stromal cells	Inflammation Fever
Interleukin 2	IL-2	133	T cells	T and NK activation Induction of IFNγ
Interleukin 6	IL-6	184	Macrophages Stromal cells Endothelia Hepatocytes	Inflammation Fever
Interleukin 8	IL-8	69–79 (dimer)	Endothelia Macrophages Neutrophils Stromal cells	Chemotaxis
Interleukin 10	IL-10	160	Keratinocytes Macrophages T and B cells	Immune suppression
Interleukin 12	IL-12	197, 306 (heterodimer)	Macrophages B cells	NK cell activation IFNγ secretion
Monocyte chemoattractant protein	MCP	76	B cells Endothelia Macrophages Stromal cells	Chemotaxis
Macrophage inflammatory proteins	MIPα, MIPβ	66–69	B and T cells Basophils Macrophages Mast cells	Chemotaxis
Transforming growth factor β	TGFβ	112 (isoforms)	Many types	Immune suppression
Tumor necrosis factor α	TNFα	157	Endothelia Macrophages Neutrophils NK cells Stromal cells T cells	Inflammation Chemotaxis Apoptosis Macrophage activation Neutrophil activation

This is an incomplete list of cytokines involved in nonspecific responses to infection. Many of these cytokines have pleotropic functions and have diverse biologic activities in addition to those listed. Emphasis is placed on the activities the cytokines have on the nonspecific host responses to viral infections. IL-2 is normally associated with specific T-cell responses to infection, but it is included because of its effects in stimulating IFNγ production.

MHC, major histocompatibility complex; NK, natural killer.

coding regions.[10,11,230] These natural antibodies may be produced in the absence of infectious agents or other environmental antigens and may be a product of the normal immunoregulatory network of the immune system. These antibodies can react with proteins, but many can react with lipids or carbohydrate structures. Examples of these include natural antibodies to blood group antigens (i.e., A, B), as originally described by Landsteiner.[165] Serum is also replete with more conventional natural antibodies bearing somatic mutations as a consequence of specific selection against environmental antigens or infectious agents. Either of these types of antibodies can be cross-reactive with infectious agents, and there is substantial evidence to indicate that natural antibodies may play a role, along with complement, in the opsonization of bacteria, such that the bacteria are phagocytosed by macrophages or granulocytes, which have receptors for antibody (FcR) and complement (CR) molecules.[10,269]

The significance of natural antibody in resistance to viral infections is not well understood, but some evidence suggests that it could be a factor. Obvious roles for such putatively cross-reactive antibodies include the direct neutralization of the virion, the sensitization of the virion to attack by complement proteins, and the opsonization of the virion, perhaps with complement, such that it is cleared from the system by macrophages and other FcR- or C3R-bearing cells. Human IgM natural antibody of otherwise unknown specificity mediates the human complement-dependent inactivation and lysis of vesicular stomatitis virus (VSV) virions; this activity has been found in all tested human sera and occurs in a completely homologous system in that serum from an individual inactivates virus grown in cells isolated from that same individual.[20]

Natural antibodies generated as a consequence of a related virus infection may influence infection by another member of a virus group but are usually not strongly neutralizing. There is considerable antigenic cross-reactivity among different serotypes of influenza virus and among different species of viruses within the enterovirus, paramyxovirus, and togavirus groups, and the specificity of the antibody response that is induced is skewed as a consequence of previous infection status. This phenomenon, sometimes referred to as original antigenic sin, leads to a preferential stimulation of antibodies that are cross-reactive between the two viruses.[291,306] This is simply an example of cross-reactive memory responses and not a function of narrowly defined natural antibody, but the effect is the same in that it may influence the outcome of an infection by binding to viruses on their entry into the host.

Natural antibodies frequently react with lipid and carbohydrate structures.[10,165,225a,260a] Some of these antibodies are autoreactive, but strong cross-species reactivities can occur. For example, humans have strong natural antibody responses to mouse cells, whereas guinea pigs do not. Enveloped viruses acquire cellular lipid and carbohydrate determinants as they bud through the plasma membrane,[154,245] and antibodies generated against a cell type or against purified carbohydrates isolated from that cell type can inactivate budding viruses propagated in those cells.[164] Inactivation of budding viruses by anti–host cell antibody can be greatly augmented in the presence of complement, and anti–host cell antibody that is otherwise nonneutralizing may mediate substantial reductions in viral titers when complement is present.[293] Inactivation of

virions by antibodies to host cell membrane determinants has also been observed in studies with vaccines against immunodeficiency viruses.[9] The host modification of viruses by the cells in which it is passed may influence its inactivation by natural antibody. Humans have high levels of natural antibody directed against the mouse L-929 cell line but low levels of natural antibody against the human HeLa cell line or against the hamster BHK21 cell line. Passage of lymphocytic choriomeningitis virus (LCMV) in L-929 cells resulted in a virus that was inactivated by human serum natural antibody and complement, but LCMV passaged in HeLa or BHK cells was resistant to inactivation.[293] This leads to speculation that a level of natural immunity could result against enveloped viruses grown in one species but not another, and it is of interest that outbreaks of LCMV in humans are often associated with infections of hamsters.[101]

A natural antibody specificity that may be of profound interspecies importance is that directed against the disaccharide Gal (α1-3) Gal. This anti–α-galactosyl antibody is present at high levels in the serum of humans and other old world primates. The old world primates lack the enzyme (α1-3) galactosyl transferase, which is present in many other mammalian species, and this antibody facilitates the human complement-mediated lysis of xenogeneic cells and of murine retroviruses grown in such cells.[227a,262a]

In addition to direct effects on viruses, naturally occurring autoimmune antibodies have in some cases been found to influence infection by binding to virus-infected cells. In one study with fish antibodies, which have a limited specificity repertoire, antibodies reacted with cell surface determinants exposed by viral infection and inhibited viral replication by unknown mechanisms.[92] In another study, a hybridoma-produced mouse monoclonal natural autoantibody enhanced VSV infection by inhibiting the interaction of IFN-α and IFN-β with the cell surface.[181] Experimental data are lacking to demonstrate the significance of natural antibodies in resistance to viral infections in vivo, but some role for them is suggested by the in vitro data.

Complement

Complement, acting alone or in concert with natural antibody, may contribute to natural resistance to infections. Complement can neutralize viral infectivity by a variety of mechanisms, including coating of the virion with protein, agglutination of virions resulting in a net loss in infectivity, opsonization of virions for degradation by C3-receptor–bearing phagocytes, and lysis of enveloped virions.[52] Such lysis of an antibody- and complement-treated virion (LCMV) is captured in the electron micrographs shown in Figure 6-1, which illustrates the binding of complement protein, the swelling of the virion membrane, and membrane rupture and release of virion core material.[300]

Some viruses have innate sensitivity to inactivation by complement in the absence of antibody and can directly trigger either the classic or the alternative complement pathway (Fig. 6-2). Mammalian cells are protected to a degree from complement-mediated destruction by regulatory membrane proteins such as complement receptor type 1 (CR1), membrane cofactor protein, and decay accelerating factor (DAF), which inactivate or dissociate complement proteins on the cell surface.[49] Virions, with some

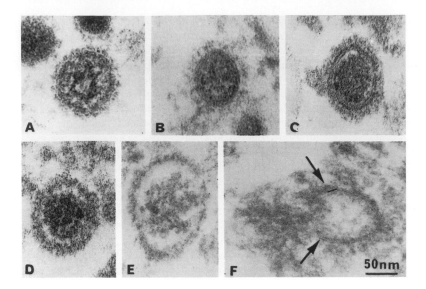

FIG. 6-1. Antibody and complement-mediated disruption of lymphocytic choriomeningitis virus (LCMV). Electron micrographs of LCMV treated with (**A**) normal control serum, (**B**) heated guinea pig serum containing antibody to LCMV, or (**C–F**) guinea pig serum containing antibody and complement. Note the swelling and rupture of the antibody and complement-treated virion. Arrows point to the disrupted viral envelope releasing virion core material. (From Welsh RM, Lampert PW, Burner PA, Oldstone MBA. Antibody-complement interactions with purified lymphocytic choriomeningitis virus. Virology 1976;73:59–71.

exceptions (e.g., human immunodeficiency virus [HIV]), are thought to lack these regulatory molecules and often are quite sensitive to complement-mediated inactivation and lysis. The significance of complement in resistance to viral infections is unclear, and the mouse, which is the most important model for examining the control of viral infections by the immune response, may be unsuitable to examine the role of complement because of the low levels of complement in laboratory strains of mice. Humans with genetic deficiencies in complement tend to be more sensitive to bacterial infection than to viral infection, but species-dependent

inactivations of retroviruses (discussed later) suggest that complement may be important in resistance to infection.

Retroviruses from mice, rats, birds, and cats are lysed by complement in human serum[240,297,299]; lysis of the virion can be detected by the release of radiolabeled virion RNA in density gradients or release of reverse transcriptase activity from serum-treated virions. In the case of murine leukemia viruses, the virion is able to directly activate the human classic complement pathway in the absence of antibody.[50,297] Purified components of C1 were added to the virion; C1q bound to

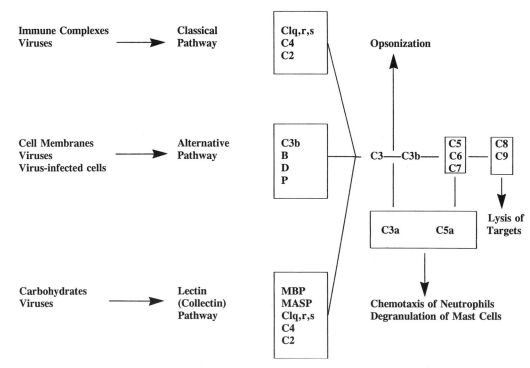

FIG. 6-2. Complement activation pathways and effector mechanisms.

the virus, probably to the p15e virion membrane protein, and catalyzed the cleavage of C1s by the proteolytic C1r enzyme.[17,50,52] Sera from many other species, including guinea pigs, mice, rats, and birds, did not lyse murine retroviruses.[299] Studies with hybrid C1 molecules containing different combinations of human and guinea pig C1q, r, and s, showed that human C1s was needed for complement activation, and guinea pig C1q and C1r were interchangeable with human C1q and r.[16] Interestingly, human and guinea pig C1s molecules were interchangeable in immune-complex–mediated complement activation, suggesting that human C1s may interact directly with virion components.

The human complement inactivation and lysis of retroviruses grown in nonhuman cells may be substantially enhanced by the anti–α-galactosyl natural antibody that is present in high quantities in human serum (see Natural Antibody). Murine retroviruses grown on nonhuman cells incorporate onto the virion the Gal (α1-3) Gal disaccharide. These virions bind the natural antibody, which renders them markedly more susceptible to complement-mediated lysis.[227a,262a]

Prior to the discovery of human retroviruses in 1979, it was hypothesized that human complement provided a natural resistance factor against retroviral infections,[297] and the human retroviruses subsequently discovered are resistant to inactivation and lysis by human complement.[12,66,127] In contrast to the failure of murine retroviruses to activate guinea pig complement, human T-cell leukemia virus IIIB (HTLV-IIIB), HIV-1, and HIV-2 bind to and activate C1, but inactivation or lysis of the virions does not ensue. This resistance to complement may be due to the fact that these virions assimilate host cell membrane complement-inhibitory factors, such as DAF[176a,194a,228a] and membrane cofactor protein.[194a] Studies with recombinant HIV gp160 and synthetic peptides revealed that, analogous to the murine retrovirus p15e, HIV gp41 sequences bound to C1q and activated the complement cascade.[73] Opsonization of retroviruses with human complement in the absence of virion lysis could possibly enhance the uptake of virus into degradative pathways of phagocytic cells and play an important role in natural immunity, but in fact it may have the opposite effect and enhance the infectivity of the virus. The addition of human complement to HTLV-IIIB, HIV-1, or HIV-2 enhanced the productive infection of cells bearing CR1 or CR3.[265] Thus, instead of human complement being a profound barrier to infection with retroviruses, it serves to enhance infection by those retroviruses that have evolved to resist inactivation by it.

In addition to retroviruses, many other viruses (e.g., Newcastle disease virus [NDV], Sindbis virus, VSV, Epstein-Barr virus [EBV]) can directly activate either the classic or alternative human complement pathway.[51] The susceptibility of viruses such as NDV and Sindbis to complement inactivation can vary with the cells in which they are propagated.[123,293] This host modification effect may reflect the assimilation of complement-inhibitory factors onto the virion, but in the case of Sindbis virus, this was shown to be a function of sialic acid content. Differences in virion sialation occur as a function of the host cell used for propagation. Treatment of complement-resistant high–sialic acid–containing Sindbis virions with neuraminidase cleaved off the sialic acid and rendered the virions sensitive to complement-mediated inactivation.[123] This may be important for natural resistance to this virus in vivo, because the levels of Sindbis virus in the blood of in-

fected outbred mice 18 hours postinfection correlated with erythrocyte and muscle sialic acid levels in the individual mice tested.[124]

Human cells infected with a variety of viruses, such as measles virus, EBV, herpes simplex virus (HSV), and respiratory syncytial virus, activate the alternative complement pathway in the absence of antibody.[51] In vitro, however, this activation is insufficient to lead to lysis of the target cell unless the kinetics of complement deposition to decay are shifted by the addition of antiviral antibody. Nevertheless, it is possible that this antibody-independent alternative complement pathway deposition on virus-infected target cells may be sufficient to lyse target cells in vivo or to release chemotactic factors such as C3a and C5a, which would attract phagocytes to the virus-infected cells.

Alternative complement pathway interactions with EBV and EBV-infected cells have been examined in detail. EBV encodes a major virion surface attachment glycoprotein, gp350, which mediates the binding of EBV to CR2 on cells.[204] Purified virions, purified gp350, and EBV-infected cells expressing gp350 all activate the alternative complement pathway in the absence of antiviral antibody if the alternative pathway component properdin is present.[192] This does not necessarily imply virion or virus-infected cell lysis, however, because purified EBV can act as a cofactor for factor I–mediated breakdown of C3b and C4b intermediates,[193] thereby inhibiting later stages of complement activation. Similarly, the gC glycoprotein of HSV-1 binds to C3b and possesses decay-accelerating activity for the alternative complement pathway C3 convertase[84]; the HSV-1 gC inhibits both antibody-dependent and antibody-independent complement-mediated inactivation of HSV.

Collectins

Other plasma proteins may also affect the ability of viruses to successfully infect cells. Of note is a group of proteins known as collectins, which are collagenous C-type lectins bearing some structural and functional homology with C1q.[125] These carbohydrate-binding proteins include conglutinin, mannose-binding protein (MBP), CL-43, and the pulmonary surfactant proteins SP-A and SP-D. Collectins bind to carbohydrate structures on the surfaces of mammalian cells, bacteria, and presumably viruses, and can sometimes substitute for C1q in the initiation of the complement cascade (see Fig. 6-2). MBP, for example, can stimulate the complement-mediated lysis of bacteria.[149] Studies suggest that collectins may either inhibit or enhance infectivity of different viruses. A bovine conglutinin can bind to and inhibit the infectivity of influenza A virus subtypes H1 and H3,[112] and human MBP, in the absence of complement, inhibits the infectivity of HIV-1.[77] MBP added to HIV gp120 stimulates classic complement pathway activation,[118] and this may lead to enhanced infectivity, as discussed previously.

THE MACROPHAGE BARRIER TO INFECTION

Different cell types serve as initial sites for viral replication, depending on the portal of entry for the virus and its spe-

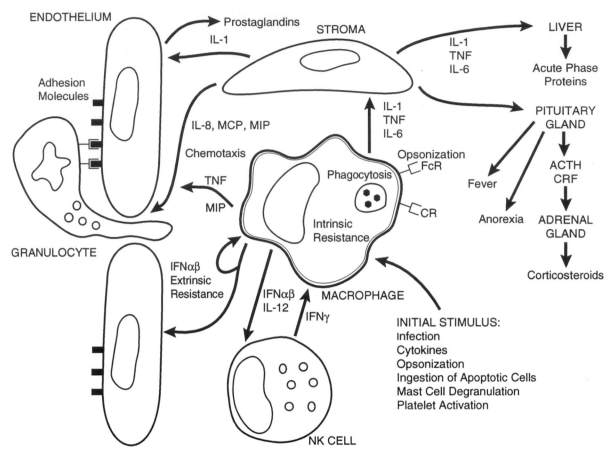

FIG. 6-3. The central role of the macrophage in the early response to viral infection. ACTH, adreno-corticotropic hormone; CR, complement receptor; CRF, corticotropin release factor; FcR, Fc receptor; IFN, interferon; IL, interleukin; MCP, membrane cofactor protein; MIP, macrophage inflammatory proteins; NK cell, natural killer cell; TNF, tumor necrosis factor.

cific cellular tropism (Fig. 6-3). Macrophages, however, are thought to be of particular importance in natural resistance because of their ability to accumulate invading pathogens by phagocytosis and to restrict the pathogens' replication or degrade them. Macrophages, such as the alveolar macrophages in the lung, are strategically located at various portals of entry and are in close contact with circulating blood entering the different organs. Poxviruses injected intravenously into nonimmune mice are cleared rapidly from the blood by macrophages and concentrate in Kupffer cells, which are differentiated macrophages lining the liver sinusoids.[189] Macrophages are also rapidly recruited into sites of viral infection and become the major cell type present by 24 hours postinfection (Figs. 6-4 and 6-5.)[184] The uptake of virions by macrophages is a function of particle size (larger virions are assimilated faster), but virion uptake also involves factors such as availability of viral attachment sites on the macrophage and whether or not a virus has been opsonized by antibody, complement, or both. The fate of an opsonized virus in a macrophage can be different from that of a nonopsonized one. Addition of a nonneutralizing antibody to vaccinia virus causes it to degrade rather than productively replicate in macrophages bearing FcR.[244] Antibody or complement may also enhance the infectivity of HIV and other viruses such as dengue by a process known as immune enhancement;

FcR or CR promote the infection of cells by antibody, complement-coated virions, or both.[190]

Intrinsic Resistance

The antiviral activity of macrophages is usually considered in terms of two mechanisms: the restriction of viral replication within macrophages (intrinsic resistance) and the capacity of macrophages to secrete antiviral substances (e.g., IFN-α and IFN-β) that control viral infections in other cells (extrinsic resistance).[197,315] Many viruses replicate poorly in primary macrophage or monocyte cultures, and interest in the intrinsic resistance of macrophages to viral infections comes from studies in a variety of animal models that correlate macrophage resistance to infection with that of the whole host.[191] Macrophages are actually a diverse population of cells, and they differ in their intrinsic and extrinsic antiviral activity as a function of age, organ of origin, activation state, and differentiation state. The distinction between activation and differentiation may be blurred, because many of the same cytokines can induce both states. By definition, an activation state refers to a cell's transient change in morphology, biochemical state, and function that can revert to the resting preactivation state, whereas differ-

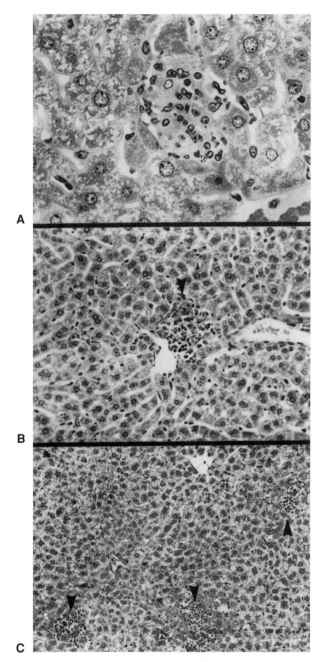

FIG. 6-4. Leukocyte infiltrate within virus-infected tissue. Liver sections from murine cytomegalovirus (MCMV)-infected mice show inflammatory foci at magnifications of (**A**) ×100, (**B**) ×160, and (**C**) ×400. The leukocyte infiltrates, which at day 3 postinfection are predominantly composed of macrophages and lymphocytes, are arranged around degenerating hepatocytes, which are infected with MCMV. (From Bukowski JF, Woda BA, Habu S, Okumura K, Welsh RM. Natural killer cell depletion enhances virus synthesis and virus-induced hepatitis in vivo. J Immunol 1983;131:1531–1538.)

entiation refers to a relatively irreversible stage of development.[316] IFN-γ and tumor necrosis factor alpha (TNF-α) are among a variety of cytokines important for macrophage activation during viral infections.[119] A primary monocyte-macrophage population usually contains a heterogenous population of cells at different stages of activation and differentiation. This is re-

flected in HSV-1 studies, which show that about 15% of peritoneal mouse macrophages are nonproductively infected yet express the HSV-1 immediate early antigen ICP4, whereas the remaining cells are completely nonpermissive and expressed no HSV gene products.[196] Exposure of macrophages to various activating agents (e.g., *Corynebacterium parvum*, thioglycolate, lipopolysaccharide) or cytokines (e.g., TNF-α, granulocyte-macrophage colony-stimulating factor, macrophage colony-stimulating factor) may either enhance or inhibit HSV replication.[316] The situation is complicated and probably involves changes in cellular transcription factors needed for productive viral infection.

A major mechanism for the intrinsic macrophage resistance against many viruses, including VSV, encephalomyocarditis virus (EMCV), and influenza virus, is the antiviral state established in these cells by endogenous levels of IFN-α and IFN-β. Freshly isolated macrophages are usually more resistant to viral infection than are macrophages cultivated for several days in vitro. Cultivated macrophages are probably under the influence of endogenous levels of IFN, because expression of the IFN-induced enzyme 2′,5′-oligoadenylate synthetase [2-5(A)] is high in freshly isolated cells and wanes thereafter.[67] Treatment of mice with antibody to IFN-α and IFN-β 1 day prior to removal of peritoneal macrophages results in increased VSV replication in vitro.[21] Expression of the *Mx* gene, whose IFN-induced gene product confers selective resistance to orthomyxovirus infections, is also found in freshly isolated macrophages, which are resistant to influenza virus; incubation of the cells in vitro leads to decreased Mx protein levels and susceptibility to influenza virus infection.[106,250–252] IFN is therefore of fundamental importance, although it is not the only mechanism of the refractory state of macrophages to viral infection.

Interest in intrinsic resistance to viral infections by macrophages has stemmed from a series of studies correlating this intrinsic resistance in vitro with resistance to viral infections in vivo.[4,191] Studies with a number of viruses showed that virus strains that grew well in macrophages were more pathogenic in vivo; macrophages from genetically resistant strains of mice restricted viral replication better than those from genetically susceptible strains; and macrophages from baby mice, which are highly susceptible to viral infections, displayed less intrinsic resistance to infection. The caveat in the interpretation of these studies is that other cells in the body may have the same intrinsic resistance that the macrophages do. In general, peritoneal macrophages can be easily isolated and used in primary cultures before IFN-mediated–resistance has waned. Isolation of other cells into primary culture is more difficult and usually requires proteolytic enzyme treatment and time-consuming procedures to obtain a pure culture. Older studies, for the most part, did not compare macrophages with another primary cell isolate. For example, classic studies correlating mouse strain–related resistance of macrophages to mouse hepatitis virus (MHV) infection with the resistance of the host[14] required reinterpretation when it was found that all the cells in the resistant host lacked receptors for MHV.[310] Similarly, a genetic resistance of macrophages to influenza virus was found to be the result of differences in Mx gene expression, which also occurred in hepatocytes and other cells.[106,250–252] Age-related differences in macrophage intrinsic resistance may relate to age-dependent differences in endogenous IFN production, because suckling mice produce very

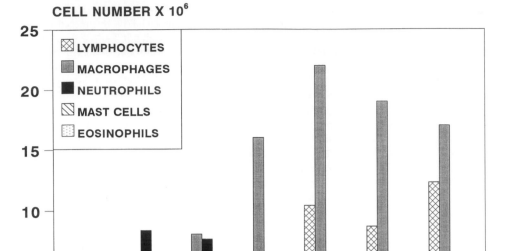

FIG. 6-5. Leukocyte infiltration into a virus-infected peritoneal cavity. Numbers represent the total number of leukocytes infiltrating the peritoneal cavity of C57BL/6 mice after intraperitoneal infection with mouse hepatitis virus. (Data from Natuk RJ, Welsh RM. Accumulation and chemotaxis of natural killer/large granular lymphocytes to sites of virus replication. J Immunol 1987;138:877–883.)

low levels of IFN. An ability to replicate in macrophages is nevertheless a virulence factor for a virus, because virtually all viruses that establish a persistent infection replicate in macrophages, and mutations that cause an enhanced tropism for macrophages can lead to substantially greater viral synthesis in vivo.[4,180]

Extrinsic Resistance

Macrophages also may contribute to the natural resistance to infections by the phenomenon of extrinsic resistance, which refers to their ability to protect other cells in the environment. Macrophages are major producers of IFN-α and IFN-β, which can inhibit viral replication in surrounding tissue (see Fig. 6-3). Macrophages also can produce substantial levels of TNF-α, which can be preferentially toxic to cells infected with any of several viruses, including HSV-1[156] and HIV-1.[182] Antibodies to TNF-α administered to mice in vivo can elevate the titers of viruses such as murine cytomegalovirus (MCMV).[119] Macrophages can also enhance infections in some cell types by the secretion of TNF-α and other cytokines that promote viral replication; a notable example is HIV-1, in which the same cytokine (TNF-α) that lyses some HIV-infected cell types promotes HIV replication in other cells types.[182]

Interaction of Macrophages With Other Leukocytes

Macrophages undoubtedly also contribute to viral infections by their influence on other leukocytes (see Figs. 6-3 and 6-4;

see Table 6-1). Macrophages release chemotactic factors such as macrophage inflammatory proteins (MIPs)[307] which attract lymphocytes into areas of infection, and they, along with dendritic cells, present antigen to T and B cells. Notable in the natural immune response is the interaction between macrophages and NK cells. It is believed that IFN-α/β production by macrophages is a major contributor to NK cell activation.[68,271] Macrophages also secrete TNF-α and interleukin 12 (IL-12; NK stimulatory factor), which can also contribute to NK cell activation by stimulating the synthesis of IFN-γ,[23,209a,b] which in turn further activates macrophages and causes them to produce nitric oxide (NO). Inhibitors of NO synthase counteract the antiviral effect of IFN-γ in macrophages against vaccinia and other viruses.[23] Macrophages and the IFN system may interact in several ways to establish antiviral states. Intrinsic resistance of macrophages to viruses at the beginning of infection is, at least in part, mediated by preexisting endogenous levels of IFN-α/β. Extrinsic resistance is partly mediated by the secretion of IFN-α/β by virus-infected macrophages, and this IFN then acts back on the macrophages themselves. Exposure of macrophages to IFN-γ then induces additional antiviral mechanisms.

Experiments Examining the Antiviral Functions of Macrophages in Vivo

Experimental manipulations of mice produced evidence that macrophages provide natural resistance to viral infections in vivo, although much of this work is either subject to other interpretation or else does not distinguish between intrinsic and extrinsic antiviral activity. The adoptive transfer of adult macrophages into suckling mice provided protection against HSV-1 infection.[139] This protection was probably mediated by IFN, as shown in subsequent experiments.[37,122] Suckling mice produce much lower levels of early IFN in response to HSV infection than do adult mice, and antibody to IFN makes mice much more susceptible to HSV.[322] Although it is clear that macrophages mediated the protective effect, the protection may have primarily been a function of the capacity of adult cells of any type to make higher levels of IFN than did suckling mouse cells, because protection of suckling mice from HSV-1 could even be mediated by adoptive transfer of cell lines, such as L-929 cells.[37]

Agents that deplete macrophages break resistance to many viral infections. A commonly used compound is silica, which is selectively toxic to macrophages after they ingest it. In mice, silica treatment has been shown to enhance the synthesis or pathology of HSV, yellow fever virus, coxsackievirus B-3, MCMV, Friend leukemia virus, rabies virus, influenza virus, and several other viruses.[5,190] A problem with the interpretation of these experiments is that whereas silica specifically targets macrophages, the macrophages secrete immunosuppressive factors after ingesting the silica particles, thereby depressing other immune functions involving NK cells and T cells. Treatment with antimacrophage antisera led to elevated titers of VSV,[121] but in general it has been difficult to selectively eliminate macrophages in vivo with antisera or monoclonal antibodies. Biologic response modifiers (e.g., pyran copolymer, bacterial adjuvants) that target and activate macrophages provide resistance to viral infection by mechanisms likely to involve extrinsic effects of cytokines on many of the cells of the host.[191,197]

THE VERY EARLY GRANULOCYTE RESPONSE

Neutrophils are a major component of the leukocyte infiltrate into tissue at early stages (<24 hours) of viral infection (Fig. 6-5),[199] and virus-infected cells, reacting with antibody, complement, or both, release factors that are chemotactic to neutrophils.[248] Neutrophils express FcR and CR and can phagocytose virions opsonized with antibody, complement, or both[283]; this phagocytic activity is enhanced by TNF. In the presence of antiviral antibody, complement, or both, neutrophils can also lyse cells infected with viruses such as HSV-1 and varicella zoster virus (VZV).[209]

Neutrophils produce and release peptide defensins, which are antimicrobial and cytotoxic cationic peptides of 29 to 35 amino acids. They are generated from 93– to 95–amino acid precursor peptides and, by virtue of disulfide bond formation between six invariant cysteines, fold into a complex triple-stranded β-pleated sheet conformation.[169] Purified defensins fuse and lyse negatively charged liposomes while maintaining their β-pleated sheet conformation, but they have little activity on neutral liposomes.[86] Defensins can permeabilize membranes of mammalian cells and induce single-strand breaks in the DNA of these cells.[88,89] Defensins have been extensively studied regarding their antibacterial and antifungal properties, but their ability to permeabilize membranes enables them to be antiviral agents as well. Defensins can inhibit HIV replication in vitro,[201] and purified defensins can neutralize a variety of enveloped viruses, including HSV-1, HSV-2, cytomegalo-

virus (CMV), VSV, and influenza A virus, but not unenveloped viruses, including echovirus type 11 and reovirus type 3.[54,168] Serum or serum albumin interferes with the defensin-dependent neutralization of HSV-1, and the importance of these two components in the control of infection is unclear. Neutrophils from mice have very low levels of defensin activity, making them poor models for examining the role of defensins in vivo.[76]

Despite these potential antiviral activities, neutrophils have usually been ignored as mediators of natural resistance to viral infections. This is because they seem better designed for controlling bacterial infections, and other effector cells (e.g., NK cells) seem better equipped to attack virus-infected targets. Neutrophils are often absent from areas of virus-infected tissue after the initial time points of infection, and neutropenia is a common consequence of severe viral infection as a result of a deterioration of bone marrow function.[29,266]

In the case of influenza virus infection, however, neutrophils may be important in both natural resistance to infection and in the ultimate severe pathology caused by bacterial invasion at later stages of disease. Studies have shown that influenza A virions or cells infected with influenza A virus can cause an intense activation and then ultimate dysfunction of neutrophils.[43,114] The influenza virus hemagglutinin protein binds to sialic acid–containing structures on the neutrophil and induces a respiratory burst associated with oxygen consumption and the generation of peroxide. Influenza A virus activates neutrophil phospholipase C, resulting in intermediates that cause a rise in intracellular Ca^{++}, Ca^{++} efflux without a Ca^{++} influx, and activation of protein kinase C. This then results in a deactivation of neutrophils, because subsequent challenge of the neutrophil with other neutrophil-activating agents such as F-met-leu-phe peptide or bacteria resulted in reduced superoxide production and Ca^{++} efflux response.[113] The partial activation of neutrophils by influenza virus may thus lead to deactivation on exposure to another stimulus as a result of the impaired availability of Ca^{++} stores. Purified influenza HA protein causes first an activation and then a depression in neutrophil function, similar to that of whole virus. In many respects, this binding of influenza A virus to neutrophils and their subsequent activation is similar, although with some differences, to the activation of neutrophils mediated by lectins such as wheat germ agglutinin or concanavalin A. The binding of influenza A virus to neutrophils is lessened in the presence of antiviral antibodies, indicating that FcR-dependent binding is less efficient than the direct binding of influenza A virus to its neutrophil receptor.[219] The collectin MBP binds to the influenza virus HA and inhibits hemagglutination, but in the presence of neutrophils, MBP acts as an opsonin, facilitating the uptake of influenza A virus by the neutrophils via a mechanism that does not lead to neutrophil dysfunction.[115] Thus, the dynamics between virus and neutrophil in vivo may be quite complex due to serum factors modulating the interaction.

It is well established that depressed neutrophil function during influenza virus infection may lead to bacterial invasion of the lung, because neutrophils are of major importance in natural resistance to bacteria.[114] It is not clear how much of this dysfunction is due to direct viral effects on neutrophils and how much is due to modulation of neutrophils by virus-induced cytokines and mediators. Whether neutrophils are important in natural resistance to influenza virus infection is less clear. A potential role for granulocytes has been demonstrated by experiments showing that adoptive transfer of syngeneic neutrophils into gamma-irradiated mice prevented an increase in viral titers in the liver and lung at early stages after intravenous infection.[278] Additionally, a biologic response modifier, Y-19995, caused a rapid reconstitution of neutrophils in immunosuppressed mice and restored resistance to influenza virus in parallel with the reconstitution of neutrophils.[279]

THE ACUTE PHASE RESPONSE

The response of the host to infection and to tissue damage involves a complex cascade of inflammatory cytokine, hormone, and cellular responses directed toward the repair of tissue damage and control of the infectious agent (Table 6-2; Fig. 6-6; see Table 6-1; see Fig. 6-3). The rapid early response that occurs before substantial T- and B-cell responses are mobilized is referred to as the acute phase response.[18] In the context of a

viral infection, the acute phase response could be initiated by the activation of complement by virions or virus-infected cell surfaces, by the induction of cytokines in virus-infected cells, or by the virus-induced lysis of cells, which are ingested by phagocytes and whose degraded products can activate the complement system. Damage to cells and tissue can also stimulate mast cell degranulation and platelet activation, causing the release of various chemotactic factors and inflammatory mediators. Central to the initiation of the acute phase response are monocytes and macrophages, which, when activated, release early alarm cytokines such as IL-1 and TNF-α that mediate pleotropic local and systemic effects (see Figs. 6-3 and 6-6; see Table 6-2).[254] In the areas of infection, these cytokines act locally on stromal cells (fibroblasts), endothelial cells, and leukocytes, causing them to produce a second wave of cytokines and other mediators that amplify the acute phase response. These include chemotactic factors, such as IL-8 and monocyte chemoattractant protein, which attract more phagocytes into the area of infection, further amplifying the system. The inflammatory response to influenza virus and coxsackievirus is greatly inhibited in mice whose MIP-1α gene has been genetically disrupted.[47a] Neutrophils are present in the early stages (i.e., the first 24 hours) of viral lesions but frequently give way to macrophages, which can become the dominant cell type as early as 1 day postinfection (see Fig. 6-5).[202] Endothelial cells responding to the cytokines upregulate the expression of integrins and intercellular adhesion molecules such as ICAM-1, and various metabolites act to permeabilize blood vessel walls, resulting in edema and changes in leukocyte circulation and migration. This acute phase response results in the release of various mediators, including histamine, serotonin, platelet-activating factor, prostaglandins, and leukotrienes.

An important feature during many viral infections is fever, which is modulated by a variety of cytokines, including IL-1, IL-6, and TNF. These cytokines target the hypothalamus; IL-6 is an upregulator of fever, and TNF serves to downregulate body temperature that is already elevated.[155] The cytokine-mediated induction of prostaglandin E_2 regulates fever and also reduces the pain-perception threshold in neurons, leading to the characteristic aches and pains associated with viral infections. IL-1 and IL-6 also act on the pituitary gland, causing the release of corticotropin release factor and adrenocorticotropic hormone, which acts on the adrenal glands, leading to the secretion of corticosteroids, which have the effect of downregulating the acute phase response (see Fig. 6-3). Early in the viral infection, there can be marked thymic atrophy associated with a major reduction of thymocytes that probably have undergone corticosteroid-induced apoptosis.[103,107] Additionally, during the early stages of a severe acute viral infection there is a less-understood deterioration of bone marrow function, reflected in a reduction in granulocytes in the peripheral blood (i.e., neutropenia) and a failure of bone marrow cells to give rise to clones in colony-forming unit (CFU) assays.[29] This diminished bone marrow function is likely a consequence of direct cytokine effects, corticosteroid exposure, and lysis of CFU progenitors by activated NK cells.[266] Corticosteroids also target the sexual organs, leading to decreased sexual interest, and local exposure of the hypothalamus to low concentrations of TNF can cause anorexia (i.e., loss of appetite).

TABLE 6-2. *Acute phase proteins produced by the liver*

Major acute phase reactants	Serum amyloid A
	C-reactive protein
	Serum amyloid P component
Complement proteins	B, C2, C3, C4, C5, C9
	C1 inhibitor; C4 binding protein
Coagulation proteins	Fibrinogen
	von Willebrand factor
Proteinase inhibitors	α_1-antichymotrypsin
	α_1-antitrypsin
	α_1-antiplasmin
	Heparin cofactor II
	Plasminogen activator inhibitor
Metal–binding proteins	Ceruloplasmin
	Haptoglobin
	Hemopexin
	Manganese superoxide dismutase
Miscellaneous other proteins	α_1-acid glycoprotein
	Heme oxygenase
	Leukocyte protein I
	Lipopolysaccharide-binding protein
	Lipoprotein
	Mannose-binding protein
Negative acute phase reactants	α_2-HS glycoprotein
	Albumin
	apoA1
	apoA2
	Histidine-rich glycoprotein
	Inter-α-trypsin inhibitor
	Prealbumin
	Transferrin

Adapted from Steel DM, Whitehead AS. The major acute phase reactants: C-reactive protein, serum amyloid P component and serum amyloid A protein. Immunol Today 1994;15:81–88.

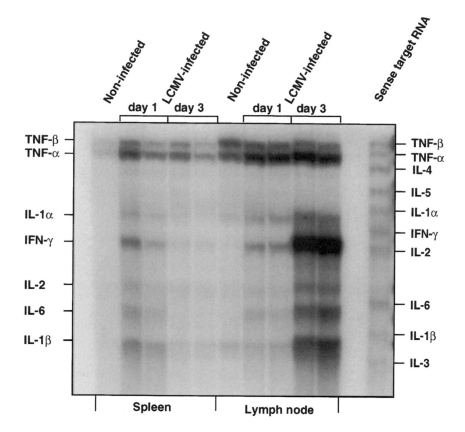

FIG. 6-6. Cytokine gene expression in virus-infected mice. Levels of cytokine-specific mRNA in the spleen and lymph nodes following lymphocytic choriomeningitis virus (LCMV) infection of mice. Male Balb/c mice were injected intraperitoneally with either vehicle or vehicle containing 5×10^5 plaque-forming units of LCMV, Armstrong 53b strain. At day 1 and day 3 postinfection, the spleens and mesenteric lymph nodes were removed, and poly A + RNA was prepared. Determination of cytokine RNA levels was performed on 2.5 μg of RNA using an RNase protection assay.[40] This assay permits the detection of multiple cytokine mRNA targets in a single sample. The composition of the probe set and its reaction with a synthetic sense target RNA set are shown on the right. The specific cytokine mRNAs detected in the experimental samples are shown on the left. IFN, interferon; IL, interleukin; TNF, tumor necrosis factor. (Courtesy of Iain Campbell, MD, and Ana Samimi, Scripps Clinic and Research Fdn., La Jolla, CA.)

IL-1, TNF, IL-6, a variety of growth factors, and cortisol also target liver hepatocytes, which produce a variety of acute phase proteins, including fibrinogen, antiproteases, complement proteins, and other proteins that serve to enhance the body's repair process (see Table 6-2). Pathology and physiology textbooks provide more details on the inflammatory processes that are common to many types of infections. Additional acute phase cytokines that are induced by viruses to reach high levels and are of great importance in the control of viral infections are IFN-α and IFN-β. Inoculation of human subjects with IFN can lead to fatigue, anorexia, vomiting, fever; central nervous system, renal, and cardiac toxicity; and muscle aches and pains.[215] Thus, in addition to being a potent antiviral cytokine (discussed later), IFN may be responsible for some of the clinical symptoms of infection.

A consequence of this acute phase response is that the host becomes ill. The symptoms of illness, including fever, aching muscles, decreased sexual interest, and anorexia may have evolutionary significance by causing the host to rest and not be distracted by other activities that would use the energy required to fight infection and repair damaged tissue.

THE INTERFERON SYSTEM

Properties of Interferons

The IFNs are a family of cytokines that share the property of inhibiting virus replication.[135] These cytokines have, in ad-

dition, many other biologic effects, including those on the immune system. IFNs are not constitutively synthesized by cells, but external stimuli, such as virus infections, trigger their transient synthesis and secretion. The secreted IFN is distributed locally or is carried by the circulation to other cells in the body and interacts with them. This interaction is mediated by specific cell surface receptors that are ubiquitous but IFN type–specific. Binding of IFN to its receptor elicits signals that induce the transcription of a set of genes in the nucleus. These IFN-inducible genes encode proteins, which carry out the diverse functions of the IFN system.

Interferon Genes and Proteins

IFNs were originally classified by their sources as leukocyte, fibroblast, and immune IFNs. The first two were grouped as type I IFN and the third as type II.[63] The current nomenclature is based on the primary structures of the proteins (Table 6-3). The type I superfamily is subdivided into IFN-α, IFN-β, IFN-ω and IFN-τ. The genes and proteins of this family are structurally related. These genes are believed to have evolved from a single ancestral gene, because they are clustered in a single locus which, in humans, is on the short arm of chromosome 9.[292] Additionally all type I IFNs lack introns. In humans, there are at least 18 IFN-α nonallelic genes, 4 of which are pseudogenes, and at least 6 IFN-ω nonallelic genes, 5 of which are pseudogenes. The single IFN-β gene shows about 45% homology at the DNA level and 25% to

TABLE 6-3. *Human interferons and their characteristics*

Type	Class	Subtype	Chromosome	Protein amino acid	Receptor
I	α	14	9	165	All have
	β	1	9	166	at least 2
	ϖ	1	9	172	subunits
	τ	1	9	172	
II	γ	1	12	146	2 subunits

30% homology at the protein level with the IFN-α genes. It has been estimated that the IFN-α and IFN-β genes diverged before the emergence of vertebrates, whereas the members of the IFN-α and IFN-ω subfamilies have separated more recently. The 5'-flanking regulatory regions of the IFN-α and IFN-β genes also have significant homology, reflecting the fact that they are often coordinately regulated.[60]

All IFN proteins have signal peptides, which are cleaved off prior to their secretion. The mature type I IFNs are 165 to 172 amino acids long. Human IFN-αs are not glycosylated, and they contain four conserved cysteine residues, which are thought to form two intramolecular disulfide bonds.[302] Human IFN-β is glycosylated, and its crystal structure shows the presence of five alpha-helices.[281] Both IFN-α and IFN-β function as monomers.

There is no structural homology between type I and type II IFNs. A single gene containing three introns encodes IFN-γ, the sole known member of type II IFN family. Mature human IFN-γ has 146 amino acids and is N-glycosylated. IFN-γ is active as a homodimer, and the sites binding the receptor are likely to contain segments from the amino and carboxyl termini of the two subunits.[276]

Biologic Properties of Interferons

As indicated previously, IFNs are multifunctional biologic response modifiers[63,237]; these biologic activities include the following:

- Inhibition of virus replication
- Inhibition of cell growth
- Activation of monocyte-macrophages, NK cells, and cytotoxic T lymphocytes (CTLs)
- Induction of major histocompatibility complex (MHC) class I and class II antigens and Fc receptors
- Inhibitors of nonviral intracellular pathogens
- Pyrogenic action
- Antitumor action

The major function of IFNs is in the host defense against viral and parasitic infections and in the growth of certain tumors. IFNs were discovered by their antiviral actions in vitro,[135] and their importance in the resistance of viral infections in vivo was initially shown by injecting mice with antibodies to IFNs. All viruses are, however, not equally susceptible to the action of IFNs, because many of them have evolved means to counteract them.

The second major common property of IFNs is the inhibition of cell growth. The particular cell lineage, its growth characteristics, and the type of IFN all determine the magnitude of this effect.

The third prominent effect of IFNs is on the immune system. This effect is brought about by activating monocytes-macrophages, NK cells, and CTLs. Induction of both MHC class I and class II antigens and FcR contribute to the activation of the cells of the immune system. Many immune-enhancing properties, such as the upregulation of MHC class I antigens and the activation of NK cells, are mediated by all IFN types, but some functions, such as the stimulation of MHC class II antigens and the complete activation of macrophages to cytotoxic and to antiviral states by virtue of NO synthase induction, are properties exclusively of type II IFN (i.e., IFN-γ). IFN-γ is also important for the antiparasitic action of macrophages against nonviral intracellular pathogens. One distinct member of the type I superfamily, IFN-τ, or trophoblast IFN, may be responsible for the preservation of the corpus luteum, which is needed for successful completion of pregnancy in cattle and sheep. However, IFN-τ uses a receptor in common with that of IFN-α, and gestation is normal in IFN-α receptor knockout mice.[200]

Interferon Biosynthesis

IFN-α and IFN-β synthesis can be induced in almost all cells, and viral infection is the most effective cause of IFN induction. Double-stranded RNA (dsRNA), which is often a side product of virus replication, is a potent inducer of IFN and is thought to be the intracellular mediator of the induction process in virus-infected cells.[63] In addition to viruses, bacteria, mycoplasma, and protozoa also can induce IFN synthesis by diverse mechanisms. Cytokines and growth factors, such as colony-stimulating factor 1 (CSF-1), IL-1, IL-2, and TNF, can also induce IFNs. IFN-τ is produced by the epithelial cells of the preimplantation embryo in large quantities; the inducing agent in this case is yet to be identified. Only T lymphocytes and NK cells have been shown to synthesize IFN-γ. There are multiple inducers of IFN-γ, including crosslinking of the TcR of T cells by a foreign antigen–self MHC complex or by the cytokine IL-2, which induces IFN-γ in both T and NK cells. Infection or stimulation of monocytes with bacteria and protozoa can induce IL-12, which acts on NK cells and stimulates the production of IFN-γ. A variety of mediators, such as IL-1, IL-2, IL-12, estrogen, and IFN-γ itself increase

IFN-γ induction, whereas others, such as glucocorticoids, transforming growth factor beta (TGF-β), and IL-10 downregulate the process.[321]

The regulation of IFN synthesis is primarily at the level of transcription, although posttranscriptional processes such as mRNA stabilization also contribute to the process.[177] The induction is transient, even in the continuous presence of inducers. Inhibitors of protein synthesis cause superinduction of IFN mRNA synthesis, presumably by blocking the synthesis of putative repressor proteins. The induction process is also enhanced by the pretreatment of cells with a low dose of IFN, a phenomenon called priming. The molecular basis of priming remains unknown.

IFN-β Gene Induction

The transcriptional regulation of IFN-α and IFN-β genes is complex, and it involves multiple positive and negative regulatory factors.[166,235] These factors bind to various cis-elements present in the 5'-flanking regions of the genes. Different factors can bind to the same element and have opposite effects on transcription. The human IFN-β gene regulatory region consists of about 200 base pairs located upstream of the transcription initiation site. The region contains four positive regulatory domains (PRD), PRDI through PRDIV, and one negative regulatory domain.[93,206] Some of these elements structurally overlap. The PRDI element resembles the interferon-stimulated response element (ISRE), and multimerized PRDI can respond not only to virus infection but also to IFNs. Interferon regulatory factors 1 and 2 (IRF-1 and IRF-2) can bind to PRDI. They are structurally related but have different effects on transcription; IRF-1 is an inducer, whereas IRF-2 is a repressor.[108,263] A third member of the family is interferon consensus sequence-binding protein (ICSBP), an IFN-γ-induced protein expressed in T cells.[70] Another PRDI-binding protein that does not belong to the IRF-1 family is PRDIBF1, which has five zinc finger motifs and is a potent repressor of the IFN-β gene.[150]

The role of IRF-1 in IFN-β induction is unclear. The lack of IFN-induction in undifferentiated embryonal carcinoma cells can be attributed to the absence of IRF-1,[110] but IFN-β induction in differentiated cells does not require IRF-1.[183] IRF-1 synthesis is induced by many cytokines, such as IFN-α, IFN-γ, TNF, IL-1, IL-6, and prolactin,[87] and the functional activity of the IRF-1 protein appears to be regulated by a posttranslational process induced by virus infection.[289] IRF-1 is involved in many other regulatory processes, including the induction of NO synthase and guanylate-binding protein (GBP).[141] Overexpression of IRF-1 causes death of B cells,[317] but overexpression of IRF-2 in NIH 3T3 cells causes cellular transformation, which is prevented by concomitant overexpression of IRF-1.[109] In certain types of human leukemia, the genetic locus encompassing the IRF-1 gene is frequently deleted, suggesting a possible role of IRF-1 as a tumor suppressor.[311]

The PRDII site of the IFN-β gene binds the transcription factor nuclear factor kappa B (NFkB).[264] This factor is activated by dsRNA, among many other agents.[288] The activation of NFkB by dsRNA is caused by the dissociation of its inhibitor, inhibitor kappa B (IkB), as a result of its phosphoryla-

tion by protein kinase RNA-dependent (PKR).[159,178] Induction of the IFN-β gene requires binding of another protein, HMGI (Y), which in turn stimulates the binding of a virus-inducible complex containing activating transcription factor (ATF-2) to the PRDIV element.[71] Thus, optimum transcription of the IFN-β promoter requires the assembly of a multiprotein complex, many of whose components are activated by dsRNA or by virus infection.

IFN-α and IFN-γ Gene Induction

The IFN-α genes, which are also induced by virus infection, contain PRDI-like elements but no NFkB binding sites. In addition to the activation of PRDI-binding proteins, activation of DNA-binding TG proteins, which bind to the GAAATG sequence, is required for the induction of IFN-α mRNAs.[174] Differences have been noted in the virus-inducibility of different IFN-α genes. Such a difference between mouse α4 and α6 genes is the result of a two-nucleotide sequence difference in their regulatory regions. The regulation of induction of the IFN-γ gene is poorly understood. Its enhanced transcription is regulated by cis-elements present in both the 5'-flanking region and the introns of the gene.[321]

IFN Receptors and Signal Transduction

Type I and type II IFNs bind to two different cell surface receptors that are present in almost all cell types.[79] Each receptor is composed of at least two different protein components. These proteins have single transmembrane domains, extracellular ligand-binding domains, and intracellular cytoplasmic signaling domains. They belong to the type II cytokine receptor family, which includes tissue factor receptor and the IL-10 receptor.[19] In general, IFNs bind specifically, or at least preferentially, to receptors of the same species. This property of species specificity has been profitably exploited to identify receptor components by transfection of human genes into mouse cells and vice versa.

IFN-α/β Receptor

Two components of the human type I IFN receptors have been cloned so far,[207,282] and current evidence indicates that there could be additional, as yet unidentified, components of this receptor. The genes of all these proteins are clustered on chromosome 21. The first component, designated HuIFN-αR, when expressed in mouse cells, conferred partial response to one human IFN-α species but not to other IFN-α species or to IFN-β.[282] The importance of this protein in the IFN response was, however, firmly established in the murine system. Mice lacking the gene for MuIFN-αR cannot respond to any type I IFN.[200] A second component of the human type I receptor complex has been cloned. When this protein, designated HuIFN-α/βR, was expressed in murine cells, it conferred binding ability to all human type I IFNs.[207] This binding, however, did not induce a biologic response, suggesting that additional human proteins may be required for the reconstitution of a fully active type I receptor.

HuIFN-αR is a monomeric protein of 554 residues, whereas HuIFN-α/βR is a disulfide-linked homodimer of two 51-kD subunits. The IFN-α/βR has been shown to be associated with the tyrosine kinase Janus kinase (JAK1; discussed later), which is required for IFN-elicited transcriptional signaling.[207] Several alternative or ancillary candidate proteins are thought to serve as receptors for IFN-α. Among them is the complement receptor CR2 and a related protein that is expressed in B lymphoma cells.[61]

IFN-γ Receptor

The IFN-γR is composed of two proteins. The binding component (i.e., IFN-γRα) has a single transmembrane domain, and its extracellular domain dictates the species-specific binding of the ligand.[3,98] Experiments using human-mouse chimeric IFN-γRα revealed that there is an additional species-specific component. This component of the receptor (IFN-γRβ) has been identified in both human and mouse systems.[120,249] It also is a transmembrane protein associated with IFN-γRα. Human cells expressing mouse IFN-γRα and mouse IFN-γRβ can fully respond to mouse IFN-γ, but mouse cells expressing human IFN-γRα and human IFN-γRβ can only partially respond to human IFN-γ; MHC class I genes are induced, but EMCV replication is not blocked. The latter observation suggests either that in humans there are alternative IFN-γRβ proteins that elicit different signals or that additional components (perhaps IFN-γR-γ) of the receptor complex exist. Binding of IFN-γ, which is a dimeric protein, to its receptor leads to enhanced tyrosine phosphorylation of IFN-γRα and to its dimerization.[99,100] Within the intracellular domain of this protein, specific residues whose mutations cause a loss of the IFN-γ signaling activity have been identified. These residues probably interact with the cytoplasmic components of the signaling machinery.[48,78]

Signal Transduction

The pathways used for transmitting the transcriptional signals from the IFN receptor complex on the cell surface to the cognate IFN-inducible genes in the nucleus have been thoroughly investigated (Fig. 6-7). These studies have led to the discovery of the JAK-STAT pathways, which are used for signaling not only by IFNs but also by many other cytokines and growth factors.[57] The receptors for these cytokines, like the IFN receptors, lack any intrinsic protein kinase activities. They are, however, closely associated with specific members of the JAK family of protein tyrosine kinases. Ligand binding to the receptors results in the activation and tyrosine phosphorylation of the associated JAKs, which in turn tyrosine-phosphorylate members of the signal transducers and activators of transcription (STAT) family of proteins. The phosphorylated STATs translocate to the nucleus, where they themselves, or in combination with other proteins, bind to specific DNA sequences and boost transcription of the corresponding genes.

Transcription of IFN-α/β–activated genes starts within minutes of cells coming in contact with the cytokine and does not require new protein synthesis.[224,236,309] The induction is

transient and usually declines after a few hours. Although receptor downregulation contributes to the observed decline of transcription, additional mechanisms of desensitization must exist. Inhibitors of protein synthesis prolong the period of transcription, suggesting that IFN-induced proteins may participate in repressing the induced transcription.

All IFN-α/β–inducible genes contain a specific sequence, ISRE, in their 5'-flanking regions.[57] This element is both necessary and sufficient to confer IFN-α/β responsiveness to any attached gene. It was identified by comparing the sequence of the 5' upstream regions of many IFN-inducible genes and by testing the IFN-responsiveness of transfected reporter genes driven by this element. Mutation of individual nucleotides of ISRE has revealed their importance in driving IFN-induced gene transcription. These studies have led to the definition of a consensus ISRE: AGTTTCNNTTTCNC/T. However, there are several IFN-inducible genes whose ISRE sequences resemble but do not strictly conform to the consensus ISRE sequence. It remains possible that these genes use a partially overlapping pathway of transcriptional activation.[237]

Three ISRE-binding protein complexes formed in the nuclear extract of most IFN-α–treated cells and separated by electrophoretic mobility shift assays are called interferon-stimulated gene factors (ISGFs) 1, 2, and 3.[253] The ISGF-1 complex is also found in the extracts of untreated cells and thus is thought not to be involved in the IFN-mediated signal transduction. The ISGF-2 complex is heterogeneous, and it contains IRF-1,[108] but its role in the IFN-α–mediated signal transduction, if any, remains to be delineated. ISGF-3 is the crucial complex whose formation is required for IFN-α–induced gene transcription. This complex is composed of three proteins: p48 is the ISRE-binding component, which has structural homology with IRF-1; p113 is the STAT2 protein, which is tyrosine-phosphorylated in IFN-α–treated cells; and either p91 (STAT1α) or p84 (STAT1β), which are alternative splicing products of the same gene and are tyrosine-phosphorylated like STAT2 in response to IFN-α.[57,243] The crucial event triggering ISGF3 formation is IFN-α–induced tyrosine phosphorylation of STAT1 and STAT2, which are related in structure and contain the src-homology 2 (SH2) domain.[85,233] Two tyrosine kinases, JAK1 and Tyk2, are also tyrosine phosphorylated in response to IFN-α–treatment of cells.[199,286] Both of these kinases are required for IFN-α–induced STAT1 and STAT2 tyrosine phosphorylation, ISGF3 formation, and gene activation. As expected, mutant cells lacking functional Tyk2, JAK1, STAT1, STAT2, or p48 protein fail to transmit IFN-α's signal to ISRE.[57]

IFN-β is thought to activate essentially the same signal transduction pathway as IFN-α, although some bifurcation in the two pathways may be expected from the observation that cells lacking functional Tyk2 can respond partially to IFN-β but not at all to IFN-α.[286]

The IFN-γ–responsive genes do not fall into one homogeneous category. Their kinetics of induction and requirements of ongoing protein synthesis are different. It is conceivable that different cis-elements mediate the different types of responses. Indeed, a variety of such sequences have been identified in various IFN-γ–inducible genes. For the gene encoding GBP, the IFN-γ–responsive element has been identified.[171] This element, called gamma-activated sequence (GAS), is present in several other IFN-γ–inducible genes, and its con-

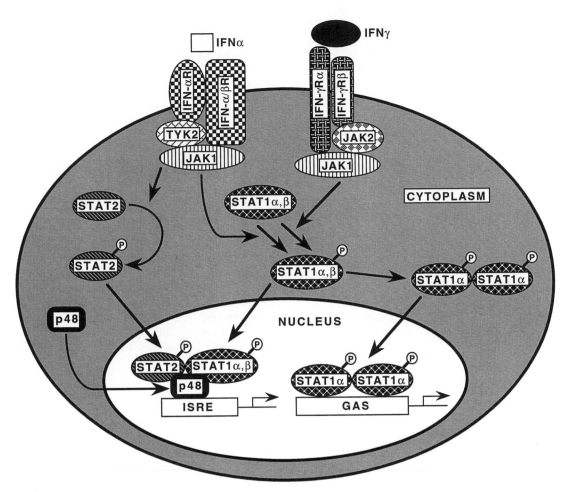

FIG. 6-7. Transcriptional signaling by interferons (IFNs). Both type I and type II IFNs use Janus kinase–signal transducer and activators of transcription (JAK-STAT) pathways to activate transcription of specific cellular genes. The IFNα-inducible genes are activated through the cis-element gamma-activated sequence (GAS). Binding of the two types of IFNs to their respective receptors causes tyrosine phosphorylation of specific members of the JAK and the STAT protein families. Activated STAT proteins translocate to the nucleus and form the transcription complexes that bind to the genes and stimulate their transcription. ISRE, IFN-stimulated response element; TYK, tyrosine kinase.

sensus sequence is TTNNNNNAA. Conversely, the IFN-γ induction of the 9-27 gene (Table 6-4), one of several sequenced IFN-induced genes of unknown function that are designated with numbers, is mediated by an ISRE.[223] In another set of IFN-γ–inducible genes, such as MHC class II and the invariant chain genes, there are no ISRE or GAS sequences. Instead, the well-defined Z, Y, and X boxes of class II regulatory regions are required for the IFN-γ response.[277]

Among the IFN-γ–activated trans-acting factors, only the GAS-binding factor GAF has been identified. GAF consists of a homodimer of tyrosine-phosphorylated STAT1α.[242] IFN-γ binding to its receptor leads to tyrosine phosphorylation of STAT1 but not STAT2. Tyrosine-phosphorylated STAT1α can form homodimers, translocate into the nucleus, bind to GAS, and boost transcription. Two JAK kinases, JAK1 and JAK2, are required for this process.[290] Thus, two components of the IFN-α and the IFN-γ signal transduction pathways are common, JAK1 and STAT1. Moreover, the same tyrosine residue

of STAT1 gets phosphorylated in response to either IFN-α or IFN-γ.

Cross-Talk Among the Interferons

The partial overlap of the signal transduction pathways used by IFN-α and IFN-γ suggests a means of cross-talk between the two cytokines. Such a cross-talk may lead to either synergistic induction of genes or antagonistic repression. Examples of both situations are known. This type of cross-talk is not restricted only to the IFNs; many other cytokines and growth factors activate different members of the STAT family, and members of the JAK kinase family are known to be associated with the receptors of some of these biologic response modifiers.[57] Although this opens an avenue of mutual interaction, it also makes the maintenance of specificity of a biologic response a demanding task. An added layer of complexity arises from the fact that genes encoding the STATs and the ISRE-binding proteins are themselves induced by IFNs and other cytokines. Thus, a specific cytokine may activate one of these proteins to its DNA-binding state, but others may elevate the cellular level of the protein, thus helping or hindering the functioning of the activated protein. In the context of a viral infection, where high levels of IFNs are produced in conjunction with many other acute phase cytokines and growth factors, predicting the molecular response of cells to these stimuli is a challenging task. Fortunately, cells under these conditions can usually mount an effective antiviral response.

Interferon-Induced Proteins and Their Antiviral Activities

The variety of biologic effects of IFNs are mediated by the individual IFN-induced proteins (see Table 6-4).[235] Some of these proteins participate in the antiviral mechanisms of IFNs, but others are important in the metabolism of uninfected cells. An example is the family of IFN-induced enzymes, the 2-5(A) synthetases, which are not only required for IFN-induced inhibition of picornavirus replication but also are involved in

cellular processes as diverse as growth regulation and pre-mRNA splicing. Although the exact number of IFN-induced proteins is not known, it is estimated to be between 50 and 100. The specific set of genes whose transcription is enhanced by IFN treatment depends on the cell type and the type of IFN. The lists of type I and type II IFN-inducible genes are partially overlapping. They include several enzymes, a family of GBPs, major histocompatibility antigens, several transcription factors, and a multitude of proteins of unknown biologic functions. IFNs can also downregulate the expression of specific cellular proteins, including several mitochondrial gene products.

Antiviral Actions

Studies of the antiviral effects of IFNs have revealed that several steps in the replicative cycle of a virus may be independently inhibited by IFN; that viral gene products, such as dsRNA, may be required for triggering some of the IFN-induced antiviral pathways; that different pathways may be primarily responsible for inhibiting different families of viruses; and that the different antiviral pathways are mediated by different IFN-induced proteins.[229,235] The steps of viral

TABLE 6-4. *Interferon-induced proteins*

Protein	Function	Inducer
2-5(A) synthetase	Antiviral and anticellular	α, β, γ, dsRNA
Protein kinase PNA–dependent	Antiviral, antigrowth	$\alpha, \beta > \gamma$
Indoleamine-2, 3-dioxygenase	Tryptophan degradation protozoan inhibition	$\gamma > \alpha, \beta$
Inducible nitric oxide synthetase	Macrophage effector	γ
Tryptophanyl-tRNA synthetase, g56	Trp-tRNA synthetase	$\gamma > \alpha, \beta$
Leucine amino peptidase	Exopeptidase	γ
Mn-leucine amino peptidase	Mitochondrial superoxide scavenger	γ
RNase L	Degradation of cellular and viral RNAs	α, β
IRF-1	Trans-acting factor	$\gamma > \alpha, \beta$, dsRNA
IRF-2	Negative regulator of transcription	γ, α, β, dsRNA
ICSBP	Negative regulator	γ
β_2-Microglobulin	MHC class I light chain	α, β, γ
Invariant chain	MHC class II assembly	γ
MHC class I	Antigen presentation	α, β, γ
MHC class II	Antigen presentation	γ
RING 12	Proteasome complex	γ
RING 14	Putative peptide transporter	γ
MxA	Inhibition of influenza and vesicular stomatitis viruses	$\alpha, \beta > \gamma$, dsRNA
MxB	Unknown	$\alpha, \beta > \gamma$, dsRNA
IP-10	Platelet factor 4–related	$\gamma > \alpha, \beta$
IP-30	Unknown	$\gamma > \alpha, \beta$
CRG-2	Monokine-like	α, β, γ
FcgRI	Binds IgG-Fc	γ
GBP, g67	GTP binding	$\gamma > \alpha, \beta$
ISG-15	Ubiquitin–like	$\alpha, \beta > \gamma$, dsRNA
IFP-35	Leucine zipper protein	α, β, γ
ISG 54, PIF-2	Unknown	α, β, γ, dsRNA
C56, 561, PIF-2	Unknown	α, β, dsRNA
Phagocyte gp91-phox	NADPH oxidase cytochrome β subunit	γ
g.1	Unknown	γ
202	Unknown	α, β
204	Unknown	α, β
1-8/9-27/Rbp-27	Unknown	α, β, γ
6-16	Unknown	$\alpha, \beta > \gamma$

MHC, major histocompatibility complex.

replication that are affected by IFNs have been identified for several viruses. For VSV and influenza virus, both primary transcription and translation are inhibited. For reoviruses, translation is affected, whereas for EMCV and Mengo virus, the steady-state level of viral mRNA is reduced. Retroviruses are inhibited at the early stage of DNA synthesis and at the late stage of viral morphogenesis. For the DNA viruses, multiple steps of the viral cycle are affected by IFN.

Two IFN-induced enzymatic pathways require dsRNA, a common viral byproduct, and both lead to protein synthesis inhibition (Fig. 6-8). The IFN-induced enzyme 2-5(A) synthetase oligomerizes ATP into 2'-5' linked oligoadenylates 2-5(A), which in turn activates a latent RNase, RNase L, leading to mRNA degradation. Another dsRNA-activated IFN-induced enzyme, PKR, phosphorylates the translation initiation factor eIF-2, thus inhibiting its ability to be reused in continuing cycles of initiation of translation. The full functioning of both of these pathways requires the IFN-induced synthesis of the key enzymes 2-5(A) synthetase and PKR and the presence of the obligatory cofactor dsRNA, whose pro-

duction is dependent on virus infection. These enzyme systems may be selectively activated at sites of virus replication in infected cells and thereby eliminate the viral infection while preserving cellular integrity. However, in the case of high-multiplicity infection, there may be such widespread activation of these enzymes that the infected cell will, in effect, commit suicide, thus preventing further spreading of new virus infection in the body.

2-5(A) Synthetases

The 2-5(A)synthetases are a family of proteins of small (40- to 46-kD), medium (69-kD), and large (100-kD) molecular weights.[235,308] All are induced by IFNs, and all require dsRNA as a cofactor, although the concentration of dsRNA required for the optimum activation of the different coenzymes varies. The family of small synthetases are encoded by more than one gene, and each gene, due to alternative splicing, gives rise to more than one mRNA and a corresponding protein.[130] Differ-

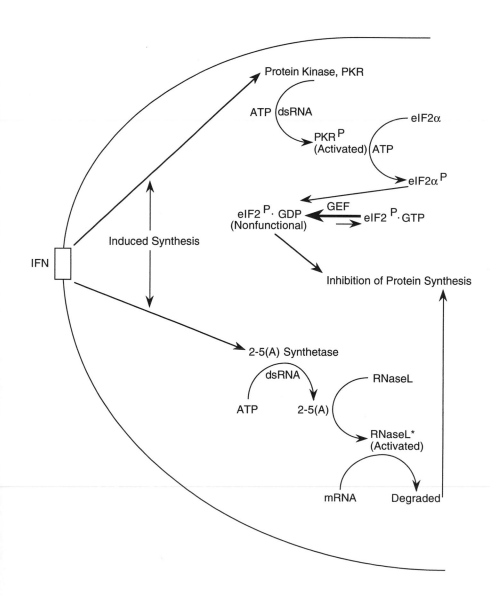

FIG. 6-8. Interferon (IFN)-induced dsRNA-activated pathways leading to inhibition of protein synthesis. IFNs induce the synthesis of both RNA-dependent protein kinase (PKR) and 2-5(A) synthetase. PKR is activated by autophosphorylation in the presence of dsRNA. Activated PKR phosphorylates eIF2α and blocks its recycling from the inactive (eIF2-GDP) to the active (eIF2-GTP) form by guanosine exchange factor (GEF), thus causing protein synthesis inhibition. 2-5(A) synthetase polymerizes adenosine triphosphate (ATP) into 2-5(A) in the presence of dsRNA. 2-5(A) activates a latent ribonuclease, RNase L, that in turn degrades mRNA.

ent isozymes have been shown to be present in different sub-cellular compartments. The affinity of the small synthetase for dsRNA is low, and its dsRNA-binding domain has no apparent structural homology to that of PKR.[90] This enzyme can be activated by perfect dsRNA as well as by viral RNAs of partial double-stranded structures such as adenoviral VAI RNA[64] and HIV-1 TAR RNA.[175] The 69-kD isozyme is myristoylated and has strong structural homology with the smaller isozymes.

The second enzyme of this pathway, RNase L, has nine ankyrin-like repeats and a cysteine-rich domain.[323] Ankyrin repeats have been found in the regions of adhesion molecules that mediated protein-protein interactions. 2-5(A) binds to and activates this enzyme.[69] RNase L is present constitutively in most cells, but its level is enhanced by IFN treatment.

The 2-5(A) synthetase–RNase L pathway is responsible for inhibiting the replication of picornaviruses. Cells transfected with 2-5(A) synthetase expression vectors do not support the replication of these viruses, even without IFN-treatment.[46] Conversely, in cells expressing a trans-dominant inhibitory mutant of RNase L, IFN fails to inhibit the replication of EMCV.[117] Viral dsRNA complexes with 2-5(A) synthetase in EMCV-infected cells and thereby activates the enzyme. The possible role of this pathway in inhibiting the replication of many other viruses remains to be evaluated; however, it is neither necessary nor sufficient for inhibiting the replication of the rhabdovirus VSV.

Protein Kinase RNA-Dependent

The IFN-inducible protein kinase PKR also requires dsRNA as an activator.[131] Activation of PKR by dsRNA results in its autophosphorylation, which probably occurs intermolecularly between two PKR molecules.[211] High concentrations of dsRNA inhibit this process, as do many viral RNAs such as VAI RNA and TAR RNA.[235] Other known activators of PKR include polyanions such as heparin. The dsRNA-binding domain of PKR lies at its N-terminus, and PKR has structural homology with many other dsRNA-binding proteins.[81,187,210,255] Specific mutations within this domain eliminate the dsRNA-binding ability.[212]

Activated PKR can phosphorylate eukaryotic initiation factor 2α (eIF-2α) and thereby inhibit protein synthesis. This mode of translation inhibition involving activation of PKR is used not only by the IFN system but also by many viruses to preferentially inhibit cellular protein synthesis. PKR is also involved in the transduction of transcriptional signaling by dsRNA.[267,324] One of these signaling pathways involves the activation of the transcription factor NFkB by dsRNA. DsRNA-activated PKR phosphorylates IkB, causing its release from and the resultant activation of NFkB.[159] In cells lacking PKR, dsRNA cannot activate NFkB.[178] PKR has also been implicated in growth suppression of insect, yeast, and mammalian cells, as well as in adipocytic differentiation and cellular apoptosis.[15,158,188]

Other Interferon-Induced Proteins

Another family of IFN-induced proteins, the Mx proteins, is responsible for inhibiting the replication of influenza virus.[250–252] Some members of this family can also inhibit VSV. Some of these proteins are nuclear, whereas others are cytoplasmic. They bind GTP and have an intrinsic GTPase activity that is required for their antiviral effects.[126] The human MxA protein can bind to cytoskeletal proteins such as actin and tubulin and has homology with the yeast protein, Vps1, which is implicated in vacuolar protein sorting.[228] Other IFN-induced proteins, such as MHC class I and class II proteins, the proteasomes, and the permeases,[151] although not antiviral at the cellular level, are extremely important in the recognition of virus-infected cells by the cells of the immune system. Another IFN-γ–induced protein, NO synthase, may be involved in inhibiting poxvirus and HSV-1 replication.[145]

The Interferon System's Interactions With dsRNA

Double-stranded RNA is not a common cellular component. Cells contain many nuclear and cytoplasmic RNA molecules which can, in principle, form intramolecular double-stranded stem structures. They are, however, present in the cell as ribonucleoproteins. The proteins bound to these RNAs presumably prevent their self-annealing and keep them in a single-stranded conformation. When isolated from cells and deproteinized, however, total cellular RNA has enough double-stranded structure to activate the dsRNA-dependent enzymes. Whether such activation takes place in cells under specific physiologic conditions remains to be determined. In contrast, the presence of dsRNA in virus-infected cells has been convincingly demonstrated. RNA viruses either contain dsRNA as their genetic material or they produce it in the course of the replication cycle if their genomes are single-stranded. Partially double-stranded viral RNAs have been isolated from poliovirus-infected cells, and similar RNAs have been shown to be present in EMCV-infected cells. Many DNA viruses, such as adenoviruses and vaccinia virus, produce complementary RNA molecules in the infected cells, presumably due to symmetrical transcription of the complementary strands of parts of their genome. Thus, dsRNA can operationally be considered as a chemical signature of virus infection.[236]

dsRNA and the IFN system interact with each other at many levels (see Fig. 6-8). First, exogenously added dsRNA or dsRNA produced during viral infection is the most potent inducer of transcription of the IFN genes. Second, transcription of many IFN-inducible genes is directly induced by dsRNA.[268] As a result, the encoded proteins are induced in virus-infected cells without an involvement of IFNs. Third, two IFN-induced enzymes, PKR and 2-5(A) synthetase, require dsRNA as an obligatory cofactor. Because these enzymes are known to mediate some of the antiviral actions of IFN, their activation must take place in IFN-treated virus-infected cells. Indeed, such activation has been well demonstrated in EMCV-infected cells. Cross-linking and immunoprecipitation experiments have demonstrated the existence of complimentary RNA strands of EMCV bound to 2-5(A) synthetase. Similarly, it has been shown convincingly that 2-5(A) is produced in IFN-treated EMCV-infected cells and activates RNase L.[235]

Transcriptional induction by dsRNA is mediated by multiple cis-elements. Two such elements have been clearly defined: kB and ISRE.[13,178] The dsRNA-inducible IFN-β gene contains the kB-like PRDII element and the ISRE-like PRDI element, both of which are required for efficient gene activation. In contrast, other dsRNA-inducible genes, such as TNF, contain only kB elements, and genes such as 561, an IFN-inducible gene with unknown function, contain only ISRE but no kB. Thus, it is clear that dsRNA can elicit at least two distinct transcriptional signaling pathways. The major trans-acting protein mediating the response through the kB element of the IFN-β gene is a heterodimer of the P65 and P50 NFkB proteins.[264] The mechanism of activation of these proteins involves phosphorylation and dissociation of the inhibitory protein IkB from the NFkB-IkB complex. DsRNA apparently brings this about by activating PKR, which can phosphorylate IkB.[178] The ISRE-mediated transcriptional induction also appears to involve PKR, although the relevant target of PKR phosphorylation is unknown. It is clear that although the same cis-element, ISRE, is used by IFNs and dsRNA to activate the 561 gene, different signal transduction pathways are used. This gene can be induced well by dsRNA in mutant cell lines that cannot respond to IFN-α due to defects in various components of the IFN signal transduction pathway. IRF-1, conversely, seems to be important in 561 mRNA induction by dsRNA. Another interesting observation is that all IFN-inducible genes are not equally induced by dsRNA. For example, the 6-16 gene (function unknown) is induced better than the 561 gene by IFN-α, but, unlike the latter, is poorly induced by dsRNA. The molecular basis of this discrimination is unknown.[13]

Viral Strategies to Neutralize the Actions of Interferons

Because activation of the IFN system is one of the most common and potent cellular antiviral responses, many viruses have developed means to evade it or to partially neutralize it (Table 6-5).[170,235] The viral defense mechanisms use two general strategies. Virus-encoded proteins globally shut down IFN signaling and the resultant expression of the IFN-inducible proteins, or viral and cellular inhibitors blocking the action of specific IFN-induced antiviral proteins are produced.

Shutoff of Signaling

Many DNA viruses are relatively resistant to the actions of IFNs. Adenovirus and hepatitis B virus (HBV) accomplish this by blocking IFN-induced signaling. As a result, in adenovirus-infected cells, IFN is unable to inhibit not only adenovirus replication but also VSV replication. Experiments with adenovirus mutants established that the viral E1A proteins are responsible for blocking IFN action.[1,104,140] Both E1A 289R and E1A 243 isoforms are functional in this respect. Mutational analysis of the E1A proteins revealed that the conserved region 1, but not regions 2 and 3, is required for this action. The p300 protein, which binds to E1A proteins, is a homolog of the transcriptional adapter protein CBP, which links the cAMP response element–binding protein to the basal transcription factor TFIIB.[163] Mutations in E1A that abolish the binding of the p300 protein also abolish its effect on IFN signaling.

Two E1A-expressing transfected cell lines, HeLa and HT1080, have been used to identify the specific step in IFN signaling which is blocked by E1A. IFN-α signaling through ISRE requires the formation of the active trans-acting factor ISGF3. In both cell lines expressing exogenous E1A, IFN-α fails to activate ISGF3, and as a result, transcription of the IFN-inducible genes is not enhanced. Further analyses revealed that the gamma component of ISGF3, which is now known to be composed of the p48 protein, is nonfunctional in both E1A-expressing cell lines, although the IFN receptors are functional. In the HeLa E1A cell line, IFN-α also fails to activate ISGF3α, which is composed of STAT1 and STAT2, and GAS-element–mediated signaling by IFN-γ is also blocked. As a result, IFN-γ cannot induce the IRF-1 gene in these cells. Similarly, induction of the 9-27 and HLA-DRα genes by IFN-γ is blocked in E1A-expressing HT1080 cells. It remains to be seen if the E1A-elicited blocks in the pathways of IFN-α and IFN-γ signaling are caused by a common mechanism.

In transient transfection assays, HBV polymerase protein was shown to inhibit the responses of cells to both IFN-α and IFN-γ.[83] Cells stably expressing the terminal protein domain of the HBV polymerase did not respond to IFN-α or IFN-γ but did respond normally to TNF-α. IFNs bound to these cells but did not activate ISGF3α or ISGF3-γ. The HBV-elicited block in IFN-action may have clinical implications in chronic HBV infections.

Inhibition of Interferon-Induced Enzymes

In addition to a shutoff of IFN signaling, many viruses cope with IFN's effects by producing inhibitors of the antiviral proteins induced by IFNs. These inhibitors are either virally coded or are cellular products induced in virus-infected cells. The activity of RNase L is inhibited in EMCV-infected or HSV-infected cells.[147,235]

TABLE 6-5. *Viral resistance to IFN action*

Mechanism	Virus	Responsible agent
Blocks transcriptional signaling	HBV	Terminal protein
	Adenovirus	E1A
Blocks RNase L activation	HSV-1	2-5(A) analogs
Blocks anticellular action	EBV	EBNA2
Neutralizes IFNγ	Myxoma	MT2
Blocks PKR activation	Adenovirus	VA1 RNA
	EBV	EBER
	HIV-1	TAR
	Influenza virus	Cellular P58
Degrades PKR	Poliovirus	Unknown
Sequesters dsRNA	Reovirus	σ3
	Vaccinia virus	E3L
Decoy for eIF-2	Vaccinia virus	K3L

EBV, Epstein-Barr virus; HIV-1, human immunodeficiency virus type 1; HSV-1, herpes simplex virus type 1; PKR, protein kinase DNA-dependent.

The most common target of viral inhibition of IFN-induced proteins is PKR. Several independent strategies are used by different viruses to accomplish this goal. Picornaviruses, such as poliovirus, cause its degradation,[28] whereas influenza virus activates a 58-kD cellular protein that inhibits PKR activation.[167] Another strategy is used by the vaccinia virus E3L protein[45] and the reovirus Â3 protein[134]; these bind and sequester dsRNA, which is the physiologic activator of PKR. Vaccinia virus also encodes a K3L protein, which has homology with eIF-2α and can serve as a decoy substrate for PKR.[58]

Several viruses encode RNA inhibitors, which probably compete with dsRNA for binding to the PKR enzyme. Some of these RNA inhibitors can also activate the enzyme, depending on their concentrations; thus, the nature of their effect on PKR activity can be subtly controlled during the progression of viral infection. The most well-studied RNA in this group is the adenoviral VAI RNA, which is a potent inhibitor of PKR.[179] Genetic analysis with adenovirus mutants lacking the VA gene has established the requirement of this RNA for efficient viral protein synthesis. VAI RNA has several double-stranded stem structures, which are required for its binding to PKR and blocking its activation by dsRNA. Correction of occasional base mismatches present in these stems makes VAI RNA even more efficient at inhibiting PKR. Surprisingly, VAI RNA does not inhibit the other IFN-inducible dsRNA-dependent enzyme, 2-5(A) synthetase, but instead activates it.[64] HIV-1 TAR RNA also activates 2-5(A) synthetase; it also activates PKR at a low concentration but inhibits it at higher concentrations.[175]

Myxoma virus uses a different strategy to block the action of IFN-γ. It encodes a protein, M-T7, that is homologous to the extracellular ligand binding domain of the IFN-γ receptor. As a result, this protein can bind to IFN-γ and neutralize its cellular activity.[280] This strategy is used by many members of the poxvirus family to neutralize several important cytokines.

Interferon-Mediated Antiviral Activity in Vivo

The importance of the IFN system in the host resistance to viral infections in vivo has been established by three different types of investigation: analysis of mouse strains that differ in their susceptibility to specific viruses, determination of the effects of administering antibodies of IFN on the course of virus infection, and studying the effects of targeted disruption of mouse genes encoding IFN, IFN receptors, or IFN-induced proteins. Such studies have shown the importance of the Mx proteins in blocking influenza virus replication.[250,251] Antibody administration studies revealed an involvement of IFN in the host response to infection by EMCV, HSV-1, HSV-2, Semliki Forest virus, murine leukemia virus, polyomavirus, influenza virus, Sindbis virus, MCMV, and MHV-3.[102] In fact, in nearly every tested system, the depletion of type I IFN with antibodies led to viral titers that were orders of magnitude higher than controls.

Several studies have examined viral replication in mice carrying experimentally disrupted genes for IFN-αR, IFN-γ, IFN-γR, and the interferon response transcription factor IRF-1. Mice disrupted in IFN-αR, which is used by all type I IFNs, were highly susceptible to infection by several viruses, including VSV, Semliki Forest virus, vaccinia virus, and LCMV.[200] Mice disrupted in the IFN-γ gene failed to induce NO production in macrophages and were very susceptible to the intracellular parasite *Mycobacterium bovis*,[55] but influenza virus infection was controlled normally in these mice,[97] even though the specific immune response to influenza became more heavily biased in the Th[2] direction. Mice disrupted in IFN-γR had increased sensitivity to the intracellular bacterium *Listeria monocytogenes*[132] and to vaccinia virus,[132] but the course of the VSV infection was unaltered.[132] Mice disrupted in the IRF-1 gene, whose product is involved not only in the transcription of IFN-α and IFN-β genes but also in the transcription of a number of IFN-induced genes, were more susceptible to infection with EMCV and with coxsackievirus B3.[153]

In certain cases, IFN production due to virus infection can be deleterious to the host. Suckling mice infected with a strain of LCMV developed renal and hepatic toxicity, which could be prevented by antiserum to type I IFN.[226] This is consistent with some human studies showing renal toxicity in patients treated with IFN.[215] An extreme and unusual example of potential harmful effects of IFN occurs in mice infected intracranially with a strain of LCMV that normally induces a lethal T-cell–dependent meningoencephalitis by that route. Administration of antibody to IFN to these mice decreases disease symptoms and mortality,[213] and mice bearing a disruption in the IFN-αR gene did not die on intracranial infection.[200] In contrast, in mice infected with a strain of LCMV that normally does not induce encephalitis, treatment with IFN inducers resulted in encephalitic symptoms.[137] The explanation for this is that an overwhelming viral load occurring in the absence of IFN causes a rapid clonal exhaustion or apoptotic deletion of the virus-specific T cells, thereby precluding the lethal T-cell–dependent encephalitis.[200,221] These mice then become persistently infected for a protracted period thereafter.

TUMOR NECROSIS FACTORS

TNF-α and TNF-β are cytokines that can have direct antiviral and immunomodulatory activities (see Table 6-1). TNF-β is produced mainly by T cells, whereas TNF-α is produced by macrophages, NK cells, and other cell types.[285] Macrophages respond to activation stimuli by synthesizing and secreting TNF-α, but viral infections can directly induce TNF-α synthesis in macrophages and other cells.[2,285] The TNF promotor includes a region which, like the IFN-β promotor, responds to dsRNA; this is due to an NFkB-binding site. The dsRNA activates the PKR enzyme, which in turn phosphorylates the inhibitory protein IkB, which normally binds and sequesters NFkB. Phosphorylation of IkB results in the release of the bound NFkB, which is then free to interact with the TNF promoter. TNF itself induces the synthesis of NFkB, thereby amplifying this system.

TNF binds to one of two receptors on the cell membrane, p55-60 or p75-80. These receptors have different intracellular domains. Signaling through the p55-60 receptor can induce apoptosis in target cells.[287,312] TNFR has homology with Fas, which is a cell surface receptor for the apoptosis-inducing Fas ligand, which itself has homology with TNF.[262,272] TNF has many functions; it can act as a growth factor, differentiation agent, or inducer of cell death, depending on the target cell. TNF can induce a variety of genes under control of transcription factors such as NFkB, Fos, and Jun, and in certain cell types it can actually enhance the synthesis of some viruses, such as HIV-1 and rat CMV.[72,105,270] In some virus-cell combinations, TNF can inhibit virus production either by interfering with virus synthesis or by inducing apoptosis in the infected cell. Some of the antiviral properties of TNF have been linked to its ability to induce IFN-β, and TNF can synergize with the antiviral effect of IFN-γ against HSV-1 infection by inducing IFN-β.[80] Transcription is not required for the initiation of apoptosis by TNF, and, in fact, TNF-induced gene products such as manganous superoxide dismutase (MnSOD) may serve to inhibit apoptosis in TNF-treated cells.[313]

Virus-infected cells may have either enhanced sensitivity or enhanced resistance to TNF-induced apoptosis. HSV-1– and feline immunodeficiency virus–infected cells are, by undefined mechanisms, much more sensitive to TNF.[156,182,208] Adenovirus E1A gene products can function as oncogenes and stimulate cell-cycle progression, but in the presence of the tumor-suppressor protein p53, which drives abnormally cycling cells into apoptosis, adenovirus E1A gene products render cells sensitive to spontaneous apoptosis. The adenovirus E1B 55K gene product, however, binds and inactivates p53, prevents E1A/p53-induced apoptosis, and thereby promotes cell transformation.[221,303–305] Cells expressing adenovirus E1A gene products by themselves are extremely sensitive to TNF-induced apoptosis, but the whole virus-infected target cell is relatively resistant to TNF-induced apoptosis, because E1B 55K and no fewer than four other adenovirus gene products (E3-14.7K, E3-10.4/14.5K, E1B-19K) inhibit the process.[59,94–96] The function of the E3 gene products is unclear, but E1B-19K may inhibit TNF-induced apoptosis by enhancing expression of MnSOD, which degrades toxic oxygen free radicals.[116] It is interesting to note that productive HIV infection inhibits MnSOD production, and the reduction of this apoptosis inhibitor may render these cells more sensitive to virus-induced apoptotic mechanisms.[314]

Apoptosis induced by T cells and NK cells involves the targeting of proteolytic enzymes to p34^{cdc2}, a serine-threonine kinase that complexes with cyclins A and B and is important for entry of the cells into mitosis. This entry of cells into mitosis involves characteristics in common with apoptosis, such as chromatin condensation and dissolution of the nuclear membrane.[241] Cells in cycle are more susceptible to the apoptotic mechanisms of T cells, and infection of cells with a variety of DNA viruses that do not transform cells, such as HSV-1, also render target cells more susceptible to CTL-induced apoptosis.[205] Induction of cell-cycle–related proteins to make a more suitable environment for DNA viral replication may be involved in this enhanced sensitivity. It is noteworthy that HSV-1 infection renders cells more sensitive to apoptosis induced by either TNF or by CTLs, suggesting that a common mechanism may be involved.

Through induction of transcription factors, TNF may augment the replication of some viruses, such as HIV-1.[72] In man, NK cells can be subdivided into CD8+ and CD8−, and these subtypes respond differently to HIV infection. Exposure of HIV to IL-2–treated CD8− NK cells leads to IFN-γ and IFN-α production and to an inhibition in virus synthesis. Exposure of IL-2–treated CD8+ NK cells to HIV-1 leads to IFN-

γ and TNF-α production, enhanced HIV synthesis, and lysis of the NK cells. During persistent HIV-1 infection in humans, there is a selective loss in NK cells that express CD8.[270]

The importance of TNF in natural resistance to viral infections is being addressed in gene knockout mice and in mice depleted of TNF with antibodies. Mice deleted in the p55 receptor are markedly more susceptible to infection by *L monocytogenes*, but they can control infections with LCMV and vaccinia virus (VV). However, changes in viral synthesis early in infection were not evaluated in this study, and these mice still expressed the p75 TNFR.[227] Mice depleted of TNF-α with antibody synthesize higher titers of some viruses, such as MCMV.[119]

THE NATURAL KILLER CELL SYSTEM

Whereas macrophages are central to most immune responses and granulocytes are well designed to combat bacterial infections, NK cells represent an early host response mechanism particularly suited to control viral infections.[295,301] Because much of what has been learned about NK cell activation, proliferation, and functions was from work done in viral systems, NK cells are discussed in detail in this chapter.

NK cells are large lymphocytes harboring cytoplasmic granules that contain a group of serine proteases, or granzymes, and the membrane pore-forming molecule perforin.[257,273,274] These granules are cytotoxic when released onto the surface of target cells; perforin can mediate osmotic lysis of targets by the insertion of pores into the plasma membrane, whereas the granzymes, notably granzyme B (fragmentin), initiate apoptosis and nuclear DNA fragmentation of the target.[241] NK cells also secrete a limited number of cytokines, including IFN-γ, TNF-α, colony-stimulating factors, IL-1, and possibly IL-8.[274] NK cells lack T-cell receptor and immunoglobulin expression and gene rearrangement and contain on their surface a number of activation or adhesion molecules, including CD2, CD11a (LFA-1), CD11b (Mac-1), CD45, CD56, and the Fc gamma receptor CD16, which enables them to mediate antibody-dependent cell-mediated cytotoxicity (ADCC).[246,257]

Importantly, NK cells have been shown to express a cluster of natural killer cell receptor proteins (NKR-P), which are type 2 integral membrane proteins with considerable structural homology with C-type animal lectins.[91,129,273,319] These proteins are encoded by several genes, thereby providing a potential for considerable heterogeneity in their cell surface expression. Studies have indicated that the genes may be expressed in alternatively spliced forms, leading to further complexity and heterogeneity.[247] Some antibodies to these proteins (e.g., NK1.1 in the mouse, 3.2.3 in the rat) can stimulate NK cell–mediated lysis of FcR-bearing target cells by adhering to the FcR on the target cell and to the natural killer cell receptor (NKR) on the effector cell (reverse ADCC), thereby indicating that these are NK cell triggering molecules.

Natural Killer Cell Specificity

NK cell specificity studies with macrophages, lymphocytes, and hematopoietic precursor cells have revealed some selectivities in target cells lysed, and clear preference for certain targets has been shown with cloned human NK cell lines.[47,143,152,238] In general, NK cells, in contrast to CTLs, lyse targets expressing low levels of MHC class I antigens better than those expressing higher levels.[172] Additionally, similar to CTLs, NK cells lyse allogeneic targets better than syngeneic targets.[152] Expression of certain NKR-P–related gene products render an NK cell incapable of killing targets expressing a specific, defined MHC class I allotype.[47,143] For example, a subset of C57BL/6 mouse (H-2b) NK cells expressing Ly-49 do not lyse target cells expressing H-2Dd due to a negative signal delivered to the NK cell. The Ly49 NK receptor molecule has been shown to directly bind to MHC class I antigens.[142] Exon-shuffling and point mutation experiments with target cells transfected with class I molecules have indicated that the α1 and α2 domains and possibly the peptide-binding regions are important for delivery of the negative signal to NK cells.[256] Although some experiments have suggested that this interaction may be modified by antigenic peptides displayed by the MHC class I antigens,[44,174a,258] others have suggested that the specificity of the peptide does not matter as long as the class I molecules stay displayed in mature conformation on the cell surface.[32,53]

Studies have indicated that at least some NKR proteins bind to oligosaccharide structures on the cell surface,[22] that such structures might be displayed by MHC molecules,[56] and that there is a glycosylation site in the class I molecule α1 domain near residues required for NK cell recognition.[56] Coating of NK-resistant target cells with liposomes containing certain oligosaccharides enhanced lysis by NK cells, whereas in other cases, oligosaccharides inhibited the lysis of sensitive targets.[22] By virtue of the expression of a variety of NKR molecules, a complex series of positive and negative signals can be stimulated on target cell engagement, and the relative balance between these positive and negative signals may determine whether the NK cell will be triggered to lyse the target. This interaction with carbohydrates is consistent with the observation that some NKR proteins have homology with lectin molecules.

Cytokines Regulating the Virus-Induced Natural Killer Cell Response

Superimposed on these subtle specificities is the phenomenon that NK cell cytotoxic activity can be greatly augmented by a variety of cytokines, including IFN-α, IFN-β, IFN-γ, IL-2, and IL-12 (NK cell stimulatory factor).[23,275,301] The IFNs and IL-2 also have the ability to stimulate NK cell proliferation, particularly when administered in vivo.[25–27] During an acute viral infection, there is a profound augmentation of NK cell cytotoxic activity and proliferation at early stages of infection when there are high levels of IFN-α and IFN-β, produced as a consequence of direct induction of IFN by the virus (Fig. 6-9).[26,294] IFNs are not normally considered mitogenic, but they cause marked alterations in the pattern of leukocyte distribution in organs such as the spleen and may attract NK cells into areas rich in mitogenic factors.[136] NK cells respond chemotactically to IFNs, IL-2, TNF-α, MIP, and other cytokines,[203,214] and they accumulate at high levels in virus-infected tissue, where they may mediate antiviral effects.[186] IFN-α/β is probably produced by many types of cells, but macrophages and possibly dendritic cells contribute signifi-

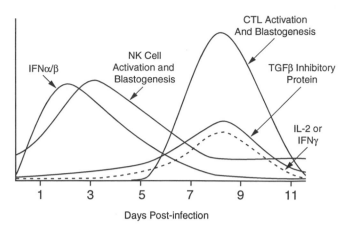

FIG. 6-9. Kinetics of cytokine production and cytolytic lymphocyte activation during lymphocytic choriomeningitis virus (LCMV) infection of mice. This figure depicts the peaks in cytokine production and natural killer (NK) cell and cytotoxic T-lymphocyte (CTL) activity in mice infected with LCMV. IFN, interferon; IL, interleukin; TGF, tumor growth factor. (Data from references 23, 259, 293, and 301.)

cantly to the IFN production.[68,271] Macrophages also release IL-12, which can contribute to NK cell activation and stimulate IFN-γ production.[23] Not all viruses induce significant levels of IL-12 early in infection. Both LCMV and MCMV stimulate high levels of NK cell activation during infection of mice, and their NK cells express transcripts for IFN-γ. However, only the MCMV-induced NK cells synthesize IFN-γ protein; this is because MCMV induces high levels of IL-12, which stimulates the translation of the IFN-γ message.[209a,209b]

The NK cell response, at least in the mouse, usually wanes as the specific immune response develops. This may seem surprising, given that activated T cells produce the NK cell–activating agents IFN-γ and IL-2, but it can be explained by the precipitous decline in the profound IFN-α and IFN-β response, which initially stimulated the NK cells (see Fig. 6-9).[301] In addition, high levels of TGF-β are produced late in infection, and NK cell proliferation is exquisitely sensitive to inhibition by that cytokine.[259,260] IL-10 can also inhibit the NK cell response.[198] It is noteworthy that EBV, a virus considered sensitive to NK cells, encodes a molecule, BCRF1,[195] which has strikingly high homology to IL-10, and a recombinant VV expressing the gene for mouse IL-10 induced a significantly lower NK cell response than a control VV lacking the IL-10 insertion.[162]

TGF-β is produced by macrophages and many other cell types, but during an acute viral infection, much of the TGF-β production may be a CD8 T-cell–dependent event.[259–261] Mice that lack CD8 cells as a consequence of disruption of the gene for β2-microglobulin, which results in diminished surface expression of normally conformed MHC class I antigens and the lack of positive selection for CD8 cells in the thymus,[157] continue to have high levels of NK cell activity associated with NK cells expressing high-affinity IL-2 receptors and presumably responding to IL-2 made by CD4 cells.[261] Thus, in experimental viral infections that ultimately stimulate a strong CD8 cell response, NK cell activation and proliferation are primarily driven by IFN-α/β and not by IL-2; under conditions of a weak CD8 response, NK cell activation and proliferation can be driven by IL-2 produced by CD4 cells.[146] In this regard, CD8 cells can act as suppressor cells for NK cells.

Evidence for the Antiviral Activity of Natural Killer Cells in Vivo

Considerable evidence derived from human clinical studies and experimental animal studies has established a role for NK cells in natural resistance to viral infections. Correlations have been made between decreased human NK cell activity as a consequence of disease or drug therapy and susceptibility to infections with CMV and with HSV-1.[173,216] Examples of individuals with complete NK cell defects are very rare, perhaps attesting to the importance of NK cells, but one adolescent with a complete and selective deficiency in NK cell number and activity presented with unusually severe infections with VZV, CMV, and HSV-1[24]; although the VZV and human CMV infections were life-threatening, each infection resolved completely, probably due to the fact that T-cell and B-cell immunity was normal in this individual.

Definitive studies on the role of NK cells in viral infections have been performed in the mouse model. Depletion of NK cells in vivo by administration of anti–NK cell antibodies leads to enhanced synthesis of some viruses, such as MCMV and VV, but not of other viruses, such as LCMV.[301] Mice bearing the beige mutation have decreased NK cell cytotoxic capacity and are very sensitive to MCMV.[239] Biologic response modifiers that augment NK cell activity in vivo, such as OK432 or MVE-2, enhance resistance to MCMV.[74,160] An age-dependent resistance to MCMV occurs in mice at about the third week of age and correlates with the maturation of the NK cell response; adoptive transfers of NK cells into suckling mice protect them from severe MCMV infection.[34] Lymphokine activated killer (LAK) cells, which are NK cells that are highly activated by growth in culture in the presence of IL-2, provide marked resistance to MCMV in suckling mice.[39] An innate genetic resistance of mice to MCMV is conferred by a single gene locus, Cmv-1, which genetically maps near the NKR complex, very close to the NK1.1 NKR protein gene.[231,232] The effect of the Cmv-1 gene seems to be mediated by NK cells, perhaps expressing an undefined NKR protein with some specificity for MCMV-infected cells.

NK cell–sensitive and –resistant strains of Pichinde virus (PV) have been defined[284]; the establishment of an infection in severe combined immunodeficient (SCID) mice with the NK-sensitive strain led to the production of NK-resistant virus after 2 months of persistent infection.[296] The related arenavirus LCMV normally causes a persistent infection in mice in nature and is also NK cell resistant. Thus, it appears that the continued pressure of an elevated NK cell response during persistent infection may force a selection for NK escape variants.

Mechanisms of the Antiviral Activity of Natural Killer Cells

It is not understood how NK cells control viral infections in vivo. Possible mechanisms include the direct lysis of virus-infected cells; the secretion of antiviral cytokines such as IFN-γ and TNF-α, which inhibit viral replication or lyse virus-infected cells; or the influencing of the function of other leukocytes through the release of these and similar cytokines. In the case of VV and ectromelia virus infections in mice, it has been suggested that the production of IFN-γ by NK cells causes macrophages to resist infection through a NO-dependent mechanism.[144,218] Infection of mice with a vaccinia–IL-2 recombinant virus was shown to be controlled in nude mice, which lack T cells, but treatment of the mice with antibodies to either NK cells or to IFN-γ abrogated the resistance.[144] Mice with disrupted IFN-γR genes are very sensitive to VV infection, consistent with that hypothesis.[132]

The replication of MCMV in normal mice and in SCID mice, whose primary source of IFN-γ is the NK cells, is elevated by administration of antibody to IFN-γ,[119,209b,300a] and E26 mice, which lack NK or T cells and cannot produce IFN-γ, are very sensitive to MCMV infection.[209b] Genetic studies on the susceptibility of mice to MCMV have noted that the NK cell–associated resistance to MCMV mediated by the Cmv-1 locus relates to MCMV replication in the spleen, but not in the liver.[231,232] Because NK cells can control MCMV replication in both organs, this suggests that there may be different mechanisms of resistance in each organ. Administration of antibodies to IFN-γ led to a greater enhancement in MCMV titers in the liver than in the spleen, and mice with a disrupted perforin gene synthesized proportionally more MCMV in the spleen than in the liver.[300a] A hypothesis to explain these data would be that NK cell recognition events mediated by a putative though as yet undefined NKR-like protein encoded by Cmv-1 might be important to control infection in the spleen, but cytokine-dependent mechanisms (e.g., IFN-γ) not dependent on receptor recognition may have greater significance in the liver.

Many in vitro studies have demonstrated the lysis of virus-infected cells by NK cells. Often this lysis was due to a virus-induced IFN-mediated activation of NK cells that lysed target cells without any selectivity. In other cases, virus-infected target cells were clearly shown to be more sensitive to lysis at discrete time points postinfection.[31,301] Several mechanisms could account for enhanced lysis of virus-infected cells by NK cells. Some viral glycoproteins, such as those of Sendai virus, bind to NK cells and augment the binding of NK cells to the virus-infected target cell.[298] However, several studies have shown that the triggering rather than the binding function of NK cells may be more important for target cell lysis, and the enhanced lysis of VSV- or VV-infected targets by NK cells is likely to be due to a postbinding triggering step.[32,194] Purified virion surface glycoproteins isolated from mumps virus, measles virus, influenza virus, and LCMV were shown to enhance the levels of human NK cell–mediated lysis directed against K562 cells, and in some cases, antisera to surface glycoproteins inhibited the lysis of virus-infected cells.[8,42,111] Evidence that NKR proteins bind to oligosaccharides suggests that the carbohydrate moieties of these glycoproteins may be involved in this NK cell activation.

Virus-infected target cells can be rendered more resistant to NK cell–mediated lysis late in infection when the plasma membrane has been sufficiently altered to remove NK cell–binding determinants.[31,298] Virus-infected cells may be vulnerable to NK cell attack only during a discrete time period postinfection, but it is not well understood what renders these cells sensitive. One explanation may be that virus infections often downregulate the expression of MHC class I proteins, which protect targets from NK cell–mediated lysis.[172] Viruses can interfere with MHC class I mRNA transcription, translation, or protein processing.[225] For example, the adenovirus 12 E1A gene product inhibits the transcription of MHC class I, and its E3 19-kD gene product complexes with the MHC class I α-chain in the cytoplasm and prevents its transport to the cell surface.[7] The HSV type 1 ICP47 gene product causes immature MHC class I molecules to accumulate in the endoplasmic reticulum.[320] A second means by which viruses may alter MHC class I is by the insertion of viral peptides into the antigen-binding groove.[44,176a,258] Cells infected with VV lose their alloreactivity; at a time when they are sensitive to VV-specific CTLs, they have lost their sensitivity to allospecific CTLs, an observation consistent with replacement of endogenous alloreactive peptides with viral peptides.[31] At the same time, these targets have enhanced sensitivity to NK cells. Target cells expressing class I human leukocyte antigen (HLA) are rendered more sensitive to NK cells when infected with HSV-1 under conditions in which there is no reduction in overall MHC class I expression, whereas targets lacking MHC class I do not become more sensitive to NK cells after infection with HSV-1.[148] These findings also may be consistent with a peptide-insertion hypothesis,[44,176a] but work challenging the significance of peptide specificity in NK cell recognition

suggests that other mechanisms may also be responsible for these observations.[32,53]

An additional factor of great significance during the course of viral infections in vivo is the ability of virus-induced IFN to upregulate MHC class I antigens (Fig. 6-10). With the exception of mature leukocytes and antigen-presenting cells, most of the cells in the uninfected host express rather low levels of class I antigens, but this expression is greatly elevated during infection.[36] IFN protects target cells from NK cell–mediated lysis as it upregulates MHC class I expression[275]; the consequence of this upregulation is that target cells in the body become increasingly sensitive to CD8 CTLs as they become increasingly resistant to NK cells.[36] Many cytopathic viral infections interfere with the ability of IFN to function in virus-infected cells, and the inability of IFN to protect virus-infected cells from NK cells may be a mechanism by which NK cells can selectively lyse virus-infected cells during infections in vivo. IFN, for example, fails to protect MCMV-infected cells from NK cell–mediated lysis.[35] An alternative role for IFN in protecting targets from lysis by NK cells could be its ability to alter cell surface expression of oligosaccharides, which are a factor in delivering signals to NK cells.[22,56,318]

More work is necessary to clearly define the roles of MHC class I antigens in the NK cell–mediated control of viral infections, but a host response can be envisioned in which, at early stages of infection, the NK cells attack the virus-infected

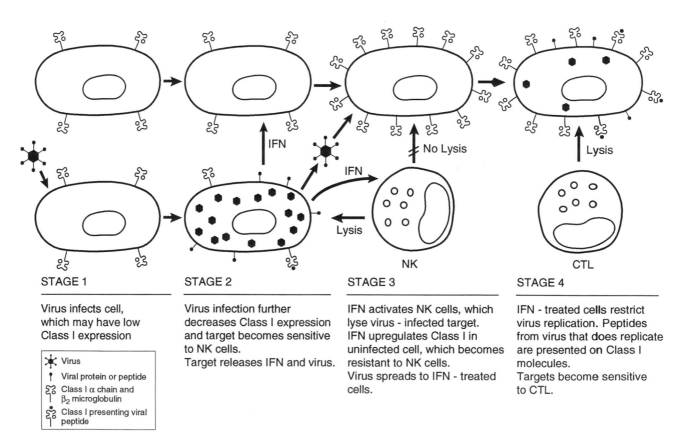

STAGE 1

Virus infects cell, which may have low Class I expression

- ✳ Virus
- ⌁ Viral protein or peptide
- ⧉ Class I α chain and β₂ microglobulin
- ⧉ Class I presenting viral peptide

STAGE 2

Virus infection further decreases Class I expression and target becomes sensitive to NK cells.
Target releases IFN and virus.

STAGE 3

IFN activates NK cells, which lyse virus-infected target. IFN upregulates Class I in uninfected cell, which becomes resistant to NK cells. Virus spreads to IFN-treated cells.

STAGE 4

IFN-treated cells restrict virus replication. Peptides from virus that does replicate are presented on Class I molecules.
Targets become sensitive to CTL.

FIG. 6-10. Susceptibility of target cells to cytotoxic lymphocytes. CTL, cytotoxic T lymphocyte; IFN, interferon; NK cells, natural killer cells.

cells, which express low levels of MHC class I antigen. The continued IFN response elevates MHC class I antigens on other cells in the body, which the virus then infects. These may partially resist viral replication and lysis by NK cells, but they will be highly sensitive targets to the CTLs that are generated later in infection (see Figs. 6-9 and 6-10).

NATURAL IMMUNITY MEDIATED BY T CELLS

Non–MHC-restricted Cytotoxic T Lymphocytes

Some evidence suggests that different classes of T cells may also provide natural resistance to viral infections. A subpopulation of T cells in human peripheral blood mediate NK cell–like nonspecific cytotoxicity and selectively lyse target cells infected with certain viruses, such as Sendai and dengue.[6,161] These effector cells, termed non–MHC-restricted CTLs, express TcR, CD3, usually CD8, and the human NK cell marker antigen CD56.[82] The origin of these cells is unclear, but they may be derived from memory cells, which are at higher states of activation and may be under the influence of endogenous IL-2 production.

Exposure of human peripheral blood lymphocytes (PBL) PBL or mouse splenocytes to high levels of IL-2 in the absence of added antigen leads to the expansion in culture of LAK cells, which are mixtures of both highly cytotoxic TcR−, CD3− NK cells and TcR+, CD3+, CD8+ non–MHC-restricted T cells.[82] CD8 memory cells have been shown to express CD11b (Mac-1) as well as IL-2R,[185] and the T-cell progenitors of these non–MHC-restricted CTLs express CD11b.[65] Adoptive transfer of nonimmune CD8+ T LAK cells into suckling mice protects the mice against the NK-sensitive virus MCMV but not against the NK-resistant virus LCMV,[39] thereby demonstrating the capacity of these effector cells to control viral infections.

Cross-Reactive Memory T Cells

It is difficult to discern the nonspecific activity from the specific activity of T cells in vivo, and cells of the memory CTL phenotype may be able to contribute to the natural resistance against viruses by more specific mechanisms. Studies have shown that relatively unrelated viruses stimulate memory T cells specific for viruses from previous infections and selectively mobilize and expand cross-reactive subsets of the memory pool as a part of the repertoire of T cells responding to that infection.[234] The ability to stimulate these memory cells may reflect the fact that memory cells express high levels of adhesion molecules and IL-2R and may be easy to stimulate with low-affinity peptides.[185,222] Three days after influenza virus infection, as many as 30% of the T cells in the mediastinal lymph nodes express IFN-γ mRNA transcripts, a number too great to be produced by the expanding clones of influenza virus–specific T cells.[41] Cytokine production by CD4 T cells early during a viral infection can be substantially greater in mice that have a history of other viral infections.[300a] Mice having a history of one virus infection, such as LCMV, are more resistant than naive mice to other virus infections such as PV or VV, and the resistance to PV can be transferred

with T cells from the LCMV-immune mice. This can cause substantial 10-fold reductions in viral titers as early as 3 days postinfection.[300a] Thus, this rapidly mobilized memory T-cell response, which is a phenomenon somewhat similar to the original antigenic sin in antibody responses,[291,306] can be considered as a contributor to natural immunity.

γδ T Cells

T cells expressing γδ TcR are a more primitive form of T cell expressing a less diverse group of receptors. Targets for γδ expressing T cells have not been well defined, but several studies have shown γδ expressing T-cell clones selectivity lyse virus-infected targets.[138,176] These clones may not be highly specific—some recognize induced cellular antigens in cells transformed by viruses such as EBV[62]—but one clone was reported to specifically recognize HSV glycoprotein I.[138] γδ expressing T cells are generally not MHC-restricted in their cytotoxicity.[220] The number of γδ T cells expands during infection of mice with influenza virus,[75] Sendai virus,[128] and VV,* and in the case of VV infection, γδ T cells are lytic to a wide range of targets. It has been suggested that part of the coxsackievirus B3–induced autoimmune T-cell response directed against myocytes is mediated by γδ T cells.[133] The role of γδ T cells in natural immunity is not well studied, but given their ability to lyse virus-infected cells in vitro as well as their ability to secrete the antiviral cytokine IFN-γ, it is likely that they play a part.

REDUNDANCIES AND INTERRELATIONS OF THE COMPONENTS OF NATURAL IMMUNITY

A virus can encounter a variety of effector systems contributing to the natural resistance of the host against infection. Different effector systems may have greater or lesser significance against a given virus, but there undoubtedly are a number of backup systems or redundancies available to provide defenses for the host. Examples of these backup systems include the complement inactivation of viruses initiated by the classic complement pathway, alternative complement pathway, or collectin-dependent mechanisms; the secretion of IFN-γ by NK cells, γδ expressing T cells, or memory α/β T cells; phagocytosis by macrophages or granulocytes; and the production by many cells of antiviral cytokines such as IFN-α, IFN-β, TNF-α, TNF-β, and IL-6. A role for a given component of the natural immune system in resistance to viral infection may be inapparent in the presence of these many redundant systems but may take on greater significance in their absence. Substantial work has shown that NK cells can lyse HSV-1–infected targets in vitro, but selective depletion of NK cell activity in mice does not lead to enhanced HSV synthesis, probably because the antiviral properties of IFN and other effector mechanisms more than suffice to control the spread of virus.[37] However, in mice whose immune system was suppressed with cyclophosphamide, adoptive transfer of NK cells provided protection.[217] Treatment of mice with high

---

*Selin LK, Welsh RM, unpublished data March 1996.

doses of IFN-α or with biologic response modifiers such as poly I:C or OK-432 provided protection against MCMV in the absence of NK cells. However, under conditions of lower-level IFN treatment or induction, a role for NK cells became apparent.[33,160]

It has also become clear that that the various effector mechanisms of the natural immune system can not only reinforce each other in combating infection but also can antagonize each other. Collectins, for example, can interfere with the ability of granulocyte defensins to inactivate viruses. Macrophages may contribute to NK cell activation by secreting IFN-α and IL-12, but they influence NK cell downregulation by secreting TGF-β or prostaglandins. Activated NK cells, in turn, can stimulate macrophages by secreting IFN-γ, but they also are capable of attacking and lysing macrophages as well as other cytotoxic lymphocytes.[30] Activated NK cells can inhibit the generation of neutrophils by attacking hemopoietic bone marrow cell precursors[266]; granulocytes, in turn, can inhibit NK cell function through the production of oxidative intermediates such as hydrogen peroxide. Interactions between the cytokines are enormously complex, because they modulate effector function in both positive and negative manners to maintain homeostasis. The pathogen, of course, must have evolved at least in part to resist these diverse mechanisms so that it would be perpetuated in nature.

ABBREVIATIONS

2-5(A): 2'-5'-oligoadenylate
ADCC: antibody-dependent cell-mediated cytotoxicity
CFU: colony-forming unit
CMV: cytomegalovirus
CR: complement receptor
CSF: colony-stimulating factor
CTL: cytotoxic T lymphocyte
DAF: delay accelerating factor
EBV: Epstein-Barr virus
eIF: eucaryotic initiation factor
EMCV: encephalomyocarditis virus
FcR: receptor for Fc region of antibody molecule
GAS: gamma-activated sequence
GBP: guanylate-binding protein
HBV: hepatitis B virus
HIV: human immunodeficiency virus
HSV: herpes simplex virus
HTLV: human T-cell leukemia virus
IFN: interferon
IkB: inhibitor kappa B
IL: interleukin
IRF: interferon regulatory factor
ISGF: interferon-stimulated gene factor
ISRE: interferon-stimulated response element
JAK: Janus kinase
LAK: lymphokine activated killer (cell)
LCMV: lymphocytic choriomeningitis virus
MBP: mannose-binding protein
MCMV: murine cytomegalovirus
MHC: major histocompatibility complex
MHV: mouse hepatitis virus
MIP: macrophage inflammatory protein
MnSOD: manganous superoxide dismutase

NDV: Newcastle disease virus
NFkB: nuclear factor kappa B
NK: natural killer (cell)
NKR: natural killer (cell) receptor
NKR-P: natural killer (cell) receptor protein
NO: nitric oxide
PKR: protein kinase RNA-dependent
PRD: positive regulatory domain
PV: Pichinde virus
SCID: severe combined immunodeficient (mouse)
STAT: signal transducers and activators of transcription
TGF: transforming growth factor
TNF: tumor necrosis factor
VSV: vesicular stomatitis virus
VV: vaccinia virus
VZV: varicella zoster virus

REFERENCES

1. Ackrill AM, Foster GR, Laxton CD, Flavell DM, Stark GR, Kerr IM. Inhibition of the cellular response to interferons by products of the adenovirus type 5 E1A oncogene. Nucl Acids Res 1991;19:4387–4393.
2. Aderka D, Holtmann H, Toker L, Hahn T, Wallach D. Tumor necrosis factor induction by Sendai virus. J Immunol 1986;136:2938–2942.
3. Aguet M, Dembic Z, Merlin G. Molecular cloning and expression of the human interferon-γ receptor. Cell 1988;55:273–-280.
4. Allison AC. Interactions of antibodies, complement components and various cell types in immunity against viruses and pyogenic bacteria. Transplant Rev 1974;19:3–55.
5. Allison AC, Harington JS, Birbeck M. An examination of the cytotoxic effects of silica on macrophages. J Exp Med 1966;124:141–153.
6. Alsheikhly A-R, Andersson T, Perlmann P. Virus-dependent cellular cytotoxicity (VDCC) in vitro: Mechanisms of induction and effector cell characterization. Scand J Immunol 1985;21:329–335.
7. Andersson M, Paabo S, Nilsson T, Peterson PA. Impaired intracellular transport of class I MHC antigens as a possible means for adenovirus to evade immune surveillance. Cell 1985;43:215–222.
8. Arora DJS, House M, Justewicz DM, Mandeville R. In vitro enhancement of human natural killer cell-mediated cytotoxicity by purified influenza virus glycoproteins. J Virol 1984;52:839–845.
9. Arthur LO, Bess JW, Sowder RC, et al. Cellular proteins bound to immunodeficiency viruses: Implications for pathogenesis and vaccines. Science 1992;258:1935–1938.
10. Avrameas S. Natural autoantibodies: from 'horror autotoxicus' to 'gnothi seauton.' Immunol Today 1991;12:154–159.
11. Baccala R, Quang TV, Gilbert M, Ternynck T, Avrameas S. Two murine natural polyreactive antibodies are encoded by nonmutated germ-like genes. Proc Natl Acad Sci U S A 1989;86:4624–4628.
12. Banapour B, Sernatinger J, Levy JA. The AIDS-associated retrovirus is not sensitive to lysis or inactivation by human serum. Virology 1986;152:268–271.
13. Bandyopadhyay S, Leonard G, Bandyopadhyay T, Stark GR, Sen GC. Transcriptional induction by double-stranded RNA mediated by interferon-stimulated response elements without activation of interferon-stimulated gene factor 3. J Biol Chem 1995;270:19624–19629.
14. Bang FB, Warwick A. Mouse macrophages as host cells for the mouse hepatitis virus and the genetic basis of their susceptibility. Proc Natl Acad Sci U S A 1960;46:1065–1075.
15. Barber GN, Thompson S, Lee TG, et al. The 58 kDa inhibitor of the interferon induced dsRNA activated protein kinase is a TPR protein with oncogenic properties. Proc Natl Acad Sci U S A 1994;91:4278–4282.
16. Bartholomew RM, Esser AF. Differences in activation of human and guinea pig complement by retroviruses. J Immunol 1978;121:1748–1751.

17. Bartholomew RM, Esser AF, Muller-Eberhard HJ. Lysis of oncornaviruses by human serum: Isolation of the viral component (C1) receptor and identification as p15E. J Exp Med 1978;147:844–853.

18. Baumann, H, Gauldie, J. The acute phase response. Immunol Today 1994;15:74–80.

19. Bazan JR. Structural design and molecular evolution of a cytokine receptor superfamily. Proc Natl Acad Sci U S A 1990;87:6934–6938.

20. Beebe DP, Cooper NR. Neutralization of vesicular stomatitis virus (VSV) by human complement requires a natural IgM antibody present in human serum. J Immunol 1981;126:1562–1568.

21. Belardelli F, Vignaux F, Proietti E, Gresser I. Injection of mice with antibody to interferon renders peritoneal macrophages permissive for vesicular stomatitis virus and encephalomyocarditis virus. Proc Natl Acad Sci U S A 1984;81:602–606.

22. Bezouska K, Yuen C-T, O'Brien JO, et al. Oligosaccharide ligands for NKR-P1 protein activate NK cells and cytotoxicity. Nature 1994;372:150–157.

23. Biron CA. Cytokines in the generation of immune responses to, and resolution of, virus infection. Curr Opin Immunol 1994;6:530–538.

24. Biron CA, Byron KS, Sullivan JS. Severe herpes virus infections in an adolescent without natural killer cells. N Engl J Med 1989;320:1731–1735.

25. Biron CA, Sonnenfeld G, Welsh RM. Interferon induces natural killer cell blastogenesis in vivo. J Leukocyte Biol 1984;35:31–37.

26. Biron CA, Welsh RM. Blastogenesis of natural killer cells during viral infection in vivo. J Immunol 1982;129:2788–2795.

27. Biron CA, Young HA, Kasaian MT. Interleukin 2-induced proliferation of murine natural killer cells in vivo. J Exp Med 1990;171:173–188.

28. Black TL, Safer B, Hovanessian A, Katze MG. The cellular 68,000-Mr protein kinase is highly autophosphorylated and activated yet significantly degraded during poliovirus infection: Implications for translational regulation. J Virol 1989;63:2244–2251.

29. Bro-Jorgensen K. The interplay between lymphocytic choriomeningitis virus, immune function, and hemopoiesis in mice. Adv Virus Res 1978;22:327–369.

30. Brubaker JO, KT Chong, Welsh RM. Lymphokine-activated killer (LAK) cells are rejected in vivo by activated natural killer cells. J Immunol 1991;147:1439–1444.

31. Brutkiewicz RR, Klaus SJ, Welsh RM. Window of vulnerability of vaccinia virus-infected cells to natural killer cell-mediated cytolysis correlates with enhanced NK cell triggering and is concomitant with a decrease in H-2 Class I antigen expression. Natural Immun 1992;11:203–214.

32. Brutkiewicz RR, Welsh RM. Class I MHC antigens and the control of viral infections by natural killer cells. J Virol 1995;69:3967–3971.

33. Bukowski JF, McIntyre KW, Yang H, Welsh RM. Natural killer cells are not required for interferon-mediated prophylaxis against vaccinia or murine cytomegalovirus infections. J Gen Virol 1987;68:2219–2222.

34. Bukowski JF, Warner JR, Dennert G, Welsh RM. Adoptive transfer studies demonstrating the antiviral effect of natural killer cells in vivo. J Exp Med 1985;161:40–52.

35. Bukowski JF, Welsh RM. Susceptibility of virus-infected targets to natural killer cell-mediated lysis in vitro correlated with natural killer cell-mediated antiviral effects in vivo. J Immunol 1985;135:3537–3541.

36. Bukowski JF, Welsh RM. Enhanced susceptibility to cytotoxic T lymphocytes of target cells isolated from virus-infected or interferon-treated mice. J Virol 1986;59:735–739.

37. Bukowski JF, Welsh RM. The role of natural killer cells and interferon in resistance to acute infection of mice with herpes simplex virus type 1. J Immunol 1986;136:3481–3485.

38. Bukowski JF, Woda BA, Habu S, Okumura K, Welsh RM. Natural killer cell depletion enhances virus synthesis and virus-induced hepatitis in vivo. J Immunol 1983;131:1531–1538.

39. Bukowski JF, Yang H, Welsh RM. The antiviral effect of lymphokine-activated killer (LAK) cells. 1. Characterization of the effector cells mediating prophylaxis. J Virol 1988;62:3642–3648.

40. Campbell IL, Hobbs MV, Kemper P, Oldstone MBA. Cerebral expression of multiple cytokine genes in mice with lymphocytic choriomeningitis virus. J Immunol 1994;152:716–723.

41. Carding SR, Allan W, McMickle A, Doherty PC. Activation of cytokine genes in T cells during primary and secondary murine influenza pneumonia. J Exp Med 1993;177:475–482.

42. Casali P, Sissons JGP, Buchmeier MJ, Oldstone MBA. In vitro generation of human cytotoxic lymphocytes by virus. Viral glycoproteins induce nonspecific cell-mediated cytotoxicity without release of interferon. J Exp Med 1981;154:840–855.

43. Cassidy LT, Lyles DS, Abramson JA. Depression of polymorphonuclear leukocyte functions by purified influenza virus hemagglutinin and sialic acid binding lectins. J Immunol 1989;142:4401–4406.

44. Chadwick BS, Sambhara SR, Sasakura Y, Miller RG. Effect of class I MHC binding peptides on recognition by natural killer cells. J Immunol 1992;149:3150–3156.

45. Chang H-W, Watson JC, Jacobs BL. The E3L gene of vaccinia virus encodes an inhibitor of the interferon-induced, double-stranded RNA-dependent protein kinase. Proc Natl Acad Sci U S A 1992;89:4825–4829.

46. Chebath J, Benech P, Revel M, Vigneron M. Constitutive expression of (2'-5') oligo A synthetase confers resistance to picornavirus infection. Nature 1987;330:587–588.

47. Ciccone E, Pende D, Viale O, et al. Involvement of HLA class I alleles in natural killer (NK) cell-specific functions: Expression of HLA-Cw3 confers selective protection from lysis by alloreactive NK clones displaying a defined specificity. J Exp Med 1992;176:963–972.

47a. Cook DN, Beck MA, Coffman TM, et al. Requirement of MIP-1α for an inflammatory response to viral infection. Science 1995;269:1583–1585.

48. Cook JR, Jung V, Schwartz B, Wang P, Pestka S. Structural analysis of the human IFN-γ receptor: A small segment of the intracellular domain is specifically required for class I major histocompatibility complex antigen induction and antiviral activity. Proc Natl Acad Sci U S A 1992;89:11317–11321.

49. Cooper NR. Complement evasion strategies of microorganisms. Immunol Today 1991;12:327–331.

50. Cooper NR, Jensen FC, Welsh RM Jr, Oldstone MBA. Lysis of RNA tumor viruses by human serum: Direct antibody independent triggering of the classical complement pathway. J Exp Med 1976;144:970–984.

51. Cooper NR, Nemerow GR. Complement and infectious agents: A tale of disguise and deception. Complement Inflamm 1989;6:249–258.

52. Cooper NR, Welsh RM. Antibody and complement dependent viral neutralization. Semin Immunopathol 1979;2:285–310.

53. Correa I, Raulet DH. Binding of diverse peptides to MHC class I molecules inhibits target cell lysis by activated natural killer cells. Immunity 1995;2:61–71.

54. Daher KA, Selsted ME, Lehrer RI. Direct inactivation of viruses by human granulocyte defensins. J Virol 1986;60:1068–1074.

55. Dalton DK, Pitts-Meek S, Keshav S, Figari IS, Bradley A, Stewart TA. Multiple defects of immune cell function in mice with disrupted interferon-γ genes. Science 193;259:1739–1742.

56. Daniels BF, Nakamura MC, Rosen SD, Yokoyama WM, Seaman WE. Ly49A, a receptor for H-2Dᵈ, has a functional carbohydrate recognition domain. Immunity 1994;1:785–792.

57. Darnell Jr JE, Kerr IM, Stark GR. JAK-STAT pathways and transcriptional activation in response to interferons and other extracellular signaling proteins. Science 1994;264:1415–1421.

58. Davies MV, Chang HW, Jacobs BL, Kaufman RJ. The E3L and K3L vaccinia virus gene products stimulate translation through inhibition of the double-stranded RNA-dependent protein kinase by different mechanisms. J Virol 1993;67:1688–1692.

59. Debbas M, White E. Wild-type p53 mediates apoptosis by E1A which is inhibited by E1B. Genes Dev 1993;7:546–554.

60. Degrave W, Derynck R, Tavernier J, Haegeman G, Fiers W. Nucleotide sequence of the chromosomal gene for human fibroblast (β1) interferon and of the flanking regions. Gene 1981;14:137–143.

61. Delcayre A, Salas F, Mathur S, Kovats K, Lotz M, Lernhardt W. Epstein Barr virus/complement C3d receptor is an interferon receptor. EMBO J 1991;10:919–926.

62. Del Porto P, Mami-Chouaib F, Bruneau JM, et al. TCT.1, a target molecule for gamma/delta T cells, is encoded by an immunoglobulin superfamily gene (Blast-1) located in the CD1 region of human chromosome 1. J Exp Med 1991;173:1339–1344.

63. DeMaeyer E, DeMaeyer-Guignard J. Interferon and other regulatory cytokines. New York: John Wiley & Sons, 1988.

64. Desai SY, Patel RC, Sen GC, Malhotra P, Ghadge GD, Thimmapaya B. Activation of interferon-inducible 2'-5' oligoadenylate synthetase by adenoviral VAI RNA. J Biol Chem 1995; 270:3454–3461.

65. Dianzani U, Zarcone D, Pistoia V, et al. CD8+CD11b+ peripheral blood T lymphocytes contain lymphokine-activated killer cell precursors. Eur J Immunol 1989;19:1037–1044.

66. Dierich MP, Ebenbichler CF, Marschang P, Fust G, Thielens NM, Arlaud. HIV and human complement: Mechanisms of interaction and biological implication. Immunol Today 1993;14:435–440.

67. Difrancesco P, Coccia EM, Gessani S, et al. Studies on the mechanism of the interferon-mediated antiviral state to vesicular stomatitis virus in resting mouse peritoneal macrophages. J Gen Virol 1989; 70:1899–1905.

68. Djeu JY, Heinbaugh JA, Holden HT, Herberman RB. Role of macrophages in the augmentation of mouse natural killer cell activity by poly I:C and interferon. J Immunol 1979;122:182–188.

69. Dong B, Silverman RH. 2-5(A) dependent RNase molecules dimerize during activation by 2-5(A). J Biol Chem 1995;270:4133–4137.

70. Driggers P, Ennist D, Gleason S, et al. An interferon-γ-regulated protein that binds the interferon-inducible enhancer element of major histocompatibility complex class 1 genes. Proc Natl Acad Sci U S A 1991;87:3743–3747.

71. Du W, Thanos D, Maniatis T. Mechanisms of transcriptional synergism between distinct virus-inducible enhancer elements. Cell 1993;74:887–898.

72. Duh EJ, Maury WJ, Folks TM, Fauci AS, Rabson AB. Tumor necrosis factor α activates human immunodeficiency virus type (look up) through induction of nuclear factor binding to the NK-kB sites in the long terminal repeat. Proc Natl Acad Sci U S A 1989;86:5974–5978.

73. Ebenbichler CF, Thielens NM, Vornhagen R, Marschang P, Arlaud GJ, Dierich MP. Human immunodeficiency virus type 1 activates the classical pathway of complement by direct C1 binding through specific sites in the transmembrane glycoprotein gp41. J Exp Med 1991;174:1417–1424.

74. Ebihara K, Minimashima Y. Protective effect of biological response modifiers on human cytomegalovirus infection. J Virol 1984;51: 117–122.

75. Eichelberger M, Allan W, Carding SR, Bottomly K, Doherty PC. Activation status of the CD4-8-gamma delta-T cells recovered from mice with influenza pneumonia. J Immunol 1991;147:2069–2074.

76. Eisenhauer PB, Lehrer RI. Mouse neutrophils lack defensins. Infect Immun 1992;60(8):3446–3447.

77. Ezekowitz RAB, Kuhlman M, Groopman JE, Byrn RA. A human serum mannose-binding protein inhibits in vitro infection by human immunodeficiency virus. J Exp Med 1989;185–196.

78. Farrar MA, Campbell JD, Schreiber RD. Identification of a functionally important sequence in the C terminus of the interferon-γ receptor. Proc Natl Acad Sci U S A 1992;89:11706–11710.

79. Farrar MA, Schreiber RD. The molecular cell biology of interferon-γ and its receptor. Ann Rev Immunol 1993;11:571–611.

80. Feduchi E, Carrasco L. Mechanism of inhibition of HSV-1 replication by tumor necrosis factor and IFN-γ. Virology 1991;180:822–825.

81. Feng GS, Chong K, Kumar A, Williams BR. Identification of double-stranded RNA-binding domains in the interferon-induced double-stranded RNA-activated p68 kinase. Proc Natl Acad Sci U S A 1992;89:5447–5451.

82. Fitzgerald-Bocarsly P, Herberman R, Hercend T, et al. A definition of natural killer cells. Immunol Today 1988;9:292.

83. Foster GR, Ackrill AM, Goldin RD, Kerr IM, Thomas HC, Stark GR. Expression of the terminal protein region of hepatitis B virus inhibits cellular responses to interferons α and γ and double-stranded RNA. Proc Natl Acad Sci U S A 1991;88:2888–2892.

84. Fries LF, Friedman HM, Cohen GH, Eisenberg RJ, Hammer CH, Frank MM. Glycoprotein C of herpes simplex virus is an inhibitor of the complement cascade. J Immunol 1986;137:1636–1641.

85. Fu XY. A transcription factor with SH2 and SH3 domains is directly activated by an interferon a-induced cytoplasmic protein tyrosine kinase(s). Cell 1992;70:323—335.

86. Fujii G, Selsted ME, Eisenberg D. Defensins promote fusion and lysis of negatively charged membranes. Protein Sci 1993:2(8):1301–1312.

87. Fujita T, Reis LFL, Watanabe N, Kimura Y, Taniguchi T, Vilcek J. Induction of the transcription factor IRF-1 and interferon-b mRNAs by cytokines and activators of second messenger pathways. Proc Natl Acad Sci U S A 1989;86:9936–9940.

88. Ganz T, Liu L, Valore EV, Oren A. Posttranslational processing and targeting of transgenic human defensin in murine granulocyte, macrophage, fibroblast, and pituitary adenoma cell lines. Blood 1993; 82(2):641–650.

89. Gera JF, Lichenstein A. Human neutrophil peptide defensins induce single strand DNA breaks in target cells. Cell Immunol 1991; 138(1): 108–120.

90. Ghosh SK, Kusari J, Bandyopadhyay S, Kumar R, Sen GC. Cloning, sequencing and expression of two murine 2'-5' oligoadenylate synthetases: Structure-function relationships. J Biol Chem 1991;266: 15293–15299.

91. Giorda R, Weisberg EP, Tagge EP, Trucco M. Molecular characterization of a novel NK cell signal transduction molecule:NKR-P1. In: Lotzova E, Herberman RB, eds. NK cell mediated cytotoxicity: Receptors, signaling, and mechanisms. Boca Raton: CRC Press, 1992.

92. Gonzales R, Matsioto P, Torchy C, de Kinkelin P, Avrameas S. Natural anti-TNP antibodies from rainbow trout interfere with viral infection in vitro. Res Immunol 1989;140:675–684.

93. Goodbourn S, Maniatis T. Overlapping positive and negative regulatory domains of the human β-interferon gene. Proc Natl Acad Sci U S A 1988;85:1447–1451.

94. Gooding LR, Aquino L, Duersken-Hughes PJ, et al. The E1B 19,000-molecular-weight protein of group C adenoviruses prevents tumor necrosis factor cytolysis of human cells but not of mouse cells. J Virol 1991;65:3083–3094.

95. Gooding LR, Elmore LW, Tollefson AE, Brady HA, Wold WSM. A 14,700 MW protein from the E3 region of adenovirus inhibits cytolysis by tumor necrosis factor. Cell 1988;53:341–346.

96. Gooding LR, Ranheim TS, Tollefson AE, et al. The 10,400- and 14,500-dalton proteins encoded by region E3 of adenovirus function together to protect many but not all mouse cell lines against lysis by tumor necrosis factor. J Virol 1991;65:4114–4123.

97. Graham MB, Dalton, DK, Giltinan D, Braciale VL, Stewart TA, Braciale TJ. Response to influenza infection in mice with a targeted disruption in the interferon-γ gene. J Exp Med 1993;178:1725–1732.

98. Gray PW, Leong S, Fennie E, et al. Cloning and expression of the cDNA for the murine interferon γ receptor. Proc Natl Acad Sci U S A 1989;86:8479–8501.

99. Greenlund AC, Farrar MA, Viviano BL, Schreiber RD. Ligand-induced IFN-γ receptor tyrosine phosphorylation couples the receptor to its signal transduction system (p91). EMBO J 1994;13:1591–1600.

100. Greenlund AC, Schreiber RD, Goeddel DV, Pennica D. Interferon-γ induces receptor dimerization in solution and on cells. J Biol Chem 1993;268:18103–18110.

101. Gregg MB. Recent outbreaks of lymphocytic choriomeningitis virus in the United States of America. Bull World Health Organ 1975;52: 549–554.

102. Gresser I. Role of interferon in resistance to viral infection in vivo. In: Vilcek J, DeMaeyer E, eds. Interferon: Interferons and the immune system, vol, 2. Amsterdam: Elsevier, 1984:221–247.

103. Gruber J, Sgonc R, Hu YH, Beug H, Wick G. Thymocyte apoptosis induced by elevated endogenous corticosterone levels. Eur J Immunol 1994;24:1115–1121.

104. Gutch MJ, Reich NC. Repression of the interferon signal transduction pathway by the adenovirus E1A oncogene. Proc Natl Acad Sci U S A 1991;88:7913–7917.

105. Haagsmans BL, Stals FS, van der Meide PH, Bruggeman CA, Horzinek MC, Schijns VECJ. Tumor necrosis factor alpha promotes replication and pathogenicity of rat cytomegalovirus. J Virol 1994;68:2297–2304.

106. Haller O. Inborn resistance of mice to orthomyxoviruses. Curr Top Microbiol Immunol 1981;92:25–52.

107. Hamaoka M, Suzuki S, Hotchin J. Thymus-dependent lymphocytes: Destruction by lymphocytic choriomeningitis virus. Science 1969; 163:1216–1219.

108. Harada H, Fujita T, Miyamoto M, et al. Structurally similar, but functionally distinct factors, IRF-1 and IRF-2, bind to the same reg-

ulatory elements of IFN and IFN-inducible genes. Cell 1989; 58:729–739.

109. Harada H, Kitagawa M, Tanaka N, et al. Anti-oncogenic and oncogenic potentials of interferon regulatory factors -1 and -2. Science 1993;259:971–974.

110. Harada H, Willison K, Sakakibara J, Miyamoto M, Fujita T, Taniguchi T. Absence of the type 1 IFN system in EC cells: Transcriptional activator (IRF-1) and repressor (IRF-2) genes are developmentally regulated. Cell 1990;63:303–312.

111. Harfast B, Orvell C, Alsheikhly A, Andersson T, Perlmann P, Norrby E. The role of viral glycoproteins in mumps virus-dependent lymphocyte-mediated cytotoxicity in vitro. Scand J Immunol 1980;11: 391–400.

112. Hartley CA, Jackson DC, Anders EM. Two distinct serum mannose-binding lectins function as β inhibitors of influenza virus: Identification of bovine serum β inhibitor as conglutinin. J Virol 1992;66: 4358–4363.

113. Hartshorn KL, Collamer M, Auerbach M, Myers JB, Pavlotsky N, Tauber AI. Effects of influenza A virus on human neutrophil calcium metabolism. J Immunol 1988;141:1295–1301.

114. Hartshorn KL, Karnad AB, Tauber AI. Influenza A virus and the neutrophil: a model of natural immunity. J Leuk Biol 1990;47:176–186.

115. Hartshorn KL, Sastry K, White MR, et al. Human mannose-binding protein functions as an opsonin for influenza A viruses. J Clin Invest 1993;91:1414–1420.

116. Hashimoto S, Ishii A, Yonehara S. The E1b oncogene of adenovirus confers cellular resistance to cytotoxicity of tumor necrosis factor and monoclonal anti-Fas antibody. Int Immunol 1991;3:343–351.

117. Hassel BA, Zhou A, Sotomayar C, Maran A, Silverman RH. A dominant negative mutant of 2-5(A)-dependent RNase suppresses antiproliferative and antiviral effects to interferon. EMBO J 1993;12: 3297–3304.

118. Haurum JS, Thiel S, Jones IM, Fischer PB, Laursen SB, Jensenius JC. Complement activation upon binding of mannan-binding protein to HIV envelope glycoproteins. AIDS 1993;7:1307–1313.

119. Heise MT, Virgin HW. The T-cell-independent role of gamma interferon and tumor necrosis factor alpha in macrophage activation during murine cytomegalovirus and herpes simplex virus infections. J Virol 1995;69:904–909.

120. Hemmi S, Bohni R, Stark G, DiMarco F, Aguet M. A novel member of the interferon receptor family complements functionality of the murine interferon-γ receptor in human cells. Cell 1994;76:803–810.

121. Hirsch MS, Gary GW, Murphy FA. In vitro and in vivo properties of anti-macrophage sera. J Immunol 1969;102:656–661.

122. Hirsch MS, Zisman B, Allison AC. Macrophages and age-dependent resistance to herpes simplex virus in mice. J Immunol 1970;104: 1160–1165.

123. Hirsch RL, Griffin DE, Winkelstein JA. Host modification of Sindbis virus sialic acid content influences alternative complement pathway activation and virus clearance. J Immunol 1981;127:1740–1743.

124. Hirsch RL, Griffin DE, Winkelstein JA. Natural immunity to Sindbis virus is influenced by host tissue sialic acid content. Proc Natl Acad Sci U S A 1983;80:548–550.

125. Holmskov U, Malhotra R, Sim RB, Jensenius JC. Collectins: Collagenous C-type lectins of the innate immune defense system. Immunol Today 1994;15:67–74.

126. Horisberger MA. Interferon-induced human protein MxA is a GTPase which binds transiently to cellular protein. J Virol 1992;66: 4705–4709.

127. Hoshino H, Tanaka H, Miwa M, Okada H. Human T-cell leukemia virus is not lysed by human serum. Nature 1984;310:324–325.

128. Hou S, Katz JM, Doherty PC, Carding SR. Extent of gamma delta T cell involvement in the pneumonia caused by Sendai virus. Cell Immunol 1992;143:183–193.

129. Houchins JP, Yabe T, McSherry C, Bach FH. DNA sequence analysis of NKG2, a family of related cDNA clones encoding type II integral membrane proteins on human natural killer cells. J Exp Med 1991;173:1017–1020.

130. Hovanessian A. RNA-activated enzymes: A specific protein kinase and 2'-5'-oligoadenylate synthetases. J Interferon Res 1991;11: 199–205.

131. Hovanessian A. The double-stranded RNA activated protein kinase induced by interferon. J Interferon Res 1989;9:641–647.

132. Huang S, Hendriks W, Althage A, et al. Immune response in mice that lack the interferon-γ receptor. Science 1993;259:1742–1745.

133. Huber SA, Moraska A, Choate M. T cells expressing the gamma delta T-cell receptor potentiate coxsackievirus B-induced myocarditis. J Virol 1992;66:6541–6546.

134. Imani F, Jacobs BL. Inhibitory activity for the interferon-induced protein kinase is associated with the reovirus serotype 1-sigma 3 protein. Proc Natl Acad Sci U S A 1988;85:7887–7891.

135. Isaacs A, Lindenmann J. Virus interference. I. The interferon. Proc R Soc London 1957;147(Ser B):258–267.

136. Ishikawa R, Biron CA. IFN induction and associated changes in splenic leukocyte distribution. J Immunol 1993;150:3713–3727.

137. Jacobson S, Friedman RM, Pfau CJ. Interferon induction by lymphocytic choriomeningitis virus correlates with maximum virulence. J Gen Virol 1981;57:275–283.

138. Johnson RM, Lancki DW, Sperling AI, et al. A murine CD4−, CD8− T cell receptor-gamma delta T lymphocyte clone specific for herpes simplex glycoprotein I. J Immunol 1992;148:983–988.

139. Johnson RT. The pathogenesis of herpes virus encephalitis. II. A cellular basis for the development of resistance with age. J Exp Med 1964;120:359–374.

140. Kalvakolanu DVR, Bandyopadhyay S, Harter ML, Sen GC. Inhibition of interferon-inducible gene expression by adenoviral E1A proteins: Block in transcriptional complex formation. Proc Natl Acad Sci U S A 1991;88:7459–7463.

141. Kamijo R, Harada H, Matsuyama T, et al. Requirement for transcription factor IRF-1 in NO synthase induction in macrophages. Science 1994;263:1612–1615.

142. Kane KP. Ly-49 mediates EL4 lymphoma adhesion to isolated class I major histocompatibility complex molecules. J Exp Med 1994: 179:1011–1015.

143. Karlhofer FM, Ribaudo RK, Yokoyama WM. MHC class I alloantigen specificity of Ly-49+ IL-2-activated natural killer cells. Nature 1992;358:66–70.

144. Karupiah G, Blanden RV, Ramshaw IA. Interferon gamma is involved in the recovery of athymic nude mice from recombinant vaccinia virus/interleukin 2 infection. J Exp Med 1990;172:1495–1503.

145. Karupiah G, Xie Q-W, Buller RM, Nathan C, Duarte C, MacMicking JD. Inhibition of viral replication by interferon-γ-induced nitric oxide synthase. Science 1993;261:1445–1448.

146. Kasaian MT, Biron CA. Cyclosporine A inhibition of interleukin 2 gene expression, but not natural killer cell proliferation, after interferon induction in vivo. J Exp Med 1990;171:745–762.

147. Katze MG. The war against the interferon-induced dsRNA-activated protein kinase: Can viruses win? J Interferon Res 1992;12: 241–248.

148. Kaufman DS, Schoon RA, Leibson PJ. Role for major histocompatibility complex class I in regulating natural killer cell-mediated killing of virus-infected cells. Proc Natl Acad Sci U S A 1992;89: 8337–8341.

149. Kawasaki N, Kawasaki T, Yamasina I. A serum lectin (mannan-binding protein) has complement-dependent bactericidal activity. J Biochem 1989;106:483–489.

150. Keller A, Maniatis T. Identification and characterization of a novel repressor of β-interferon gene expression. Genes Dev 1991;5:868–879.

151. Kelly A, Powis S, Glynne R, Radley E, Beck S, Trowsdale J. Second proteasome-related gene in the human MHC class II region. Nature 1991;353:667–668.

152. Kiessling R, Welsh RM. Killing of normal cells by activated mouse natural killer cells: Evidence for two patterns of genetic regulation of lysis. Int J Cancer 1980;25:611–615.

153. Kimura T, Nakayama K, Penninger J, et al. Involvement of the IRF-1 transcription factor in antiviral responses to interferons. Science 1994;264:1921–1924.

154. Klenk H-D, Rott R, Becht H. On the structure of the influenza virus envelope. Virology 1972;47:579–591.

155. Klir JJ, Roth J, Szelenyi Z, McClellan JL, Kluger MJ. Role of hypothalamic interleukin-6 and tumor necrosis factor-α in LPS fever in rat. Am J Physiol 1993;265:R512–R517.

156. Koff WC, Fann AV. Human tumor necrosis factor-alpha kills herpesvirus-infected but not normal cells. Lymphokine Res 1986;5: 215–221.

157. Koller BH, Marrack P, Kappler JW, Smithies O. Normal development of mice deficient in β_2M, MHC class I proteins, and CD8+ T cells. Science 1990;248:1227–1230.

158. Koromilas AE, Roy S, Barber GN, Katze MG, Sonenberg N. Malignant transfection by a mutant of the IFN-inducible dsRNA-dependent protein. Science 1992;257:1685–1689.

159. Kumar A, Haque J, Lacoste J, Hiscott J, Williams BRG. Double-stranded RNA-dependent protein kinase activates transcription factor by phosphorylating IkB. Proc Natl Acad Sci U S A 1994;91: 6288–6292.

160. Kunder SC, Morahan PS. Role of NK cells in immunomodulator-mediated resistance to herpesvirus infection. Antiviral Res 1993;21: 103–118.

161. Kurane I, Hebblewaite D, Brandt WE, Ennis FE. Lysis of dengue virus-infected cells by natural cell-mediated cytotoxicity and antibody-dependent cell-mediated cytotoxicity. J Virol 1984;52:223–230.

162. Kurilla MG, Swaminathan S, Welsh RM, Kieff E, Brutkiewicz RR. Effects of virally expressed interleukin-10 on vaccinia virus infection in mice. J Virol 1993;67:7623–7628.

163. Kwok RPS, Lundbland JR, Chrivia JC, et al. Nuclear protein CBP is a coactivator for the transcription factor CREB. Nature 1994;370: 223–226.

164. Laver WG, Webster RG. The structure of influenza viruses. IV. Chemical studies on the host antigen. Virology 1966;30:104–115.

165. Landsteiner K. Zur Kenntnis der antifermentativen, lytischen und agglutinierenden Wirkungen des Blutserums und der Lymphe. Centralbl F Bacterol Parasitenk, Jena 1900;28:357–362.

166. Leblanc J-F, Cohen L, Rodrigues M, Hiscott J. Synergism between distinct enhasion domains in viral induction of the human beta interferon gene. Mol Cell Biol 1990;10:3987–3993.

167. Lee TG, Tomita J, Hovanessian AG, Katze MG. Purification and partial characterization of a cellular inhibitor of the interferon-induced protein kinase of Mr 68,000 from influenza virus-infected cells. Proc Natl Acad Sci U S A 1990;87:6208–6212.

168. Lehrer RI, Daher K, Ganz T, Selsted ME. Direct inactivation of viruses by MCP-1 and MCP-2, natural peptide antibiotics from rabbit leukocytes. J Virol 1985;54:467–472.

169. Lehrer RI, Lichenstein AK, Ganz T. Defensins: Antimicrobial and cytotoxic peptides of mammalian cells. Ann Rev Immunol 1993;11: 105–128.

170. Lengyel P. Tumor-suppressor genes: News about the interferon connection. Proc Natl Acad Sci U S A 1993;90:5893–5895.

171. Lew DJ, Decker T, Strehlow I, Darnell JE. Overlapping elements in the guanylate-binding protein gene promoter mediate transcriptional induction by α and γ interferons. Mol Cell Biol 1991;11:182–191.

172. Ljunggren H-G, Karre K. In search of the 'missing self': MHC molecules and NK cell recognition. Immunol Today 1990;11:237–244.

173. Lopez C, Kirkpatrick D, Reid SE, et al. Correlation between low natural killing of fibroblasts infected with herpes simplex virus type 1 and susceptibility to herpesvirus infections. J Infect Dis 1983;147: 1030–1035.

174. MacDonald N, Kuhl D, Maguire D, et al. Different pathways mediate virus inducibility of the human IFN-α1 and IFN-β genes. Cell 1990;60:767–779.

175. Maitra RK, McMillan N, Desai S, et al. HIV-1 TAR RNA has an intrinsic ability to activate interferon-inducible enzymes. Virology 1994;204:823–827.

176. Malkovsky M, Bartz SR, MacKenzie D, et al. Are $\gamma\delta$ expressing T cells important for the elimination of virus-infected cells? J Med Primatol 1992;21:113–118.

176a. Malnati MS, Paruzzi M, Parkere KC, et al. Peptide specificity in the recognition of MHC class I by natural killer cell clones. Science 1995;267:1016–1018.

177. Maniatis T, Whittemore LA, Du W, et al. In: McKnight SL, Yamamoto K, eds. Transcriptional regulation, part 2. New York: Cold Spring Harbor, 1992:1193–1220.

178. Maran A, Maitra RK, Kumar A, et al. Blockage of signaling by selective ablation of an mRNA target by 2-5(A) antisense chimeras. Science 1994;215:789–792.

178a. Marschang P, Sodroski J, Wurzner R, Dierich MP. Decay-accelerating factor (CD55) protects human immunodeficiency virus type 1 from inactivation by human complement. Eur J Immunol 1995;25: 285–290.

179. Mathews MB, Shenk T. Adenovirus-associated RNA and translation control. J Virol 1991;65:5657–5662.

180. Matloubian M, Kolhekar SR, Somasundaram T, Ahmed R. Molecular determinants of macrophage tropism and viral persistence: Importance of single amino acid changes in the polymerase and glycoprotein of lymphocytic choriomeningitis virus. J Virol 1993;67: 7340–7349.

181. Matsiota P, Saron M-S, Guillon J-C, Avrameas S. Mouse natural autoantibodies can interfere with murine alpha and beta interferons. J Virol 1989;63:955–956.

182. Matsuyama T, Hamamoto Y, Soma G, Mizuno D, Yamamoto N, Kobayashi N. Cytocidal effect of tumor necrosis factor on cells chronically infected with human immunodeficiency virus (HIV): Enhancement of HIV replication. J Virol 1989;63:2504–2509.

183. Matsuyama T, Kimura T, Kitagawa M, et al. Targeted disruption of IRF-1 or IRF-2 results in abnormal type 1 IFN gene induction and aberrant lymphocyte development. Cell 1992;75:83–97.

184. McFarland HF, Griffin DE, Johnson RT. Specificity of the inflammatory response in viral encephalitis. I. Adoptive immunization of immunosuppressed mice infected with Sindbis virus. J Exp Med 1972;136:216–220.

185. McFarland HI, Nahill SR, Maciaszek JW, Welsh RM. CD11b (Mac-1): A marker for CD8+ cytotoxic T cell activation and memory in virus infection. J Immunol 1992;149:1326–1333.

186. McIntyre KW, Natuk RJ, Biron CA, Kase K, Greenberger J, Welsh RM. Blastogenesis and proliferation of large granular lymphocytes in non-lymphoid organs. J Leukocyte Biol 1988;43:492–501.

187. Meurs EF, Chong K, Galabru J, et al. Molecular cloning and characterization of the human double-stranded RNA-activated protein kinase induced. Cell 1990;62:379–390.

188. Meurs EF, Galabru J, Barber GN, Katze MG, Hovanessian AG. Tumor suppressor function of the interferon-induced double-stranded RNA-activated protein kinase. Proc Natl Acad Sci U S A 1993;90: 232–236.

189. Mims CA. Aspects of the pathogenesis of virus diseases. Bacteriol Rev 1964;28:30–71.

190. Mogensen SC. Role of macrophages in natural resistance to virus infections. Microbiol Rev 1979;43:1–26.

191. Mogensen SC, Virelizier J-L. The interferon-macrophage alliance. Interferon 1987;8:55–84.

192. Mold C, Bradt BM, Nemerow GR, Cooper NR. Activation of the alternative complement pathway by EBV and the viral envelope glycoprotein, gp350. J Immunol 1988;140:3867–3874.

193. Mold C, Bradt BM, Nemerow GR, Cooper NR. Epstein-Barr virus regulates activation and processing of the third component of complement. J Exp Med 1988;168:949–969.

194. Moller JR, Rager-Zisman B, Quan P, et al. Natural killer cell recognition of target cells expressing different antigens of vesicular stomatitis virus. Proc Natl Acad Sci U S A 1985;82:2456–2459.

194a. Montefiori DC, Cornell RJ, Zhou JY, Zhou JT, Hirsch VM, Johnson PR. Complement control proteins, CD46, CD55, and CD59, as common surface constituents of human and simian immunodeficiency viruses and possible targets for vaccine protection. Virology 1994; 205:85–92.

195. Moore KW, Vieira P, Fiorentino DF, Trounstine ML, Khan TA, Mosmann TR. Homology of cytokine synthesis inhibitory factor (IL-10) to the Epstein-Barr virus gene BCRF1. Science 1990;248: 1230–1234.

196. Morahan PS, Mama S, Anaraki F, Leary K. Molecular localization of abortive infection of resident peritoneal macrophages by herpes simplex virus type 1. J Virol 1989;63:2300–2307.

197. Morahan PS, Morse SS. Macrophage-virus interactions. In: Proffitt M, ed. Virus-lymphocyte interactions: Implications for disease. New York: Elsevier, 1979:17–35.

198. Mosmann TR, Moore KW. The role of IL-10 in crossregulation of Th1 and Th2 responses. Immunol Today 1991;12:A49.

199. Muller M, Briscoe J, Laxton C, et al. The protein tyrosine kinase Jak1 complements defects in interferon-α/β and -γ signal transduction. Nature 1993;366:129–135.

200. Muller U, Steinhoff U, Reis LFL, et al. Functional role of type I and type II interferons in antiviral defense. Science 1994;264:1918–1921.

201. Nakashima HY, Hamamoto N, Masuda M, Fujii N. Defensins inhibit HIV replication in vitro. AIDS 1993;7(8):1129.

202. Natuk RJ, Welsh RM. Accumulation and chemotaxis of natural killer/large granular lymphocytes to sites of virus replication. J Immunol 1987;138:877–883.

203. Natuk RJ, Welsh RM. Chemotactic effect of human recombinant interleukin-2 on mouse activated large granular lymphocytes. J Immunol 1987;139:2737–2743.

204. Nemerow GR, Mold C, Keivens Schwend V, Tollefson V, Cooper NR. Identification of gp350 as the viral glycoprotein mediating attachment of Epstein-Barr virus (EBV) to the EBV/C3d receptor of B cells: Sequencing homology of gp350 and the C3 complement fragment C3d. J Virol 1987;61:1416–1420.

205. Nishioka WK, Welsh RM. Susceptibility to CTL-induced apoptosis is a function of the proliferative status of the target. J Exp Med 1994;179:769–774.

206. Nourbakhsh M, Hoffmann K, Hauser H. Interferon-β promoters contain a DNA element that acts as a position-independent silencer on the site. EMBO J 1993;12:451–459.

207. Novick D, Cohen B, Rubinstein M. The human interferon-α/β receptor: Characterization and molecular cloning. Cell 1994;77:391–400.

208. Ohno K, Nakano T, Matsumoto Y, et al. Apoptosis induced by tumor necrosis factor in cells chronically infected with feline immunodeficiency virus. J Virol 1993;67:2429–2433.

209. Oleske JM, Ashman RB, Kohl S, et al. Human polymorphonuclear leukocytes as mediators of antibody-dependent cellular cytotoxicity to herpes simplex virus-infected cells. Clin Exp Immunol 1977;27:446–453.

209a. Orange JS, Biron CA. An absolute and restricted requirement for IL-12 in natural killer cell IFN-γ production and antiviral defense: Studies of natural killer and T cell responses in contrasting viral infections. J Immunol 1996;156:1138–1142.

209b. Orange JS, Wang B, Terhorst C, Biron CA. Requirement for natural killer cell-produced interferon gamma in defense against murine cytomegalovirus infection and enhancement of this defense pathway by interleukin 12 administration. J Exp Med 1995;182:1045–1056.

210. Patel R, Sen G. Identification of the double-stranded RNA binding domain of the human interferon-inducible protein kinase. J Biol Chem 1992;267:7671–7676.

211. Patel RC, Stanton P, McMillan NMJ, Williams BRG, Sen GC. The interferon-inducible double-stranded RNA-activated protein kinase, PKR, self associates in vitro and in vivo. Proc Natl Acad Sci U S A 1995;92:8283–8287.

212. Patel RC, Stanton P, Sen GC. Role of the amino-terminal residues of the interferon-induced protein kinase in its activation by double-stranded RNA and heparin. J Biol Chem 1994;269:18593–18598.

213. Pfau CJ, Gresser I, Hunt KD. Lethal role of interferon in lymphocytic choriomeningitis virus-induced encephalitis. J Gen Virol 1983;64:1827–1830.

214. Pilaro AM, Taub DD, McCormick KL, et al. TNF-α is a principle cytokine involved in the recruitment of NK cells to liver parenchyma. J Immunol 1994;153:333–342.

215. Quesada JR, Talpaz M, Rios A, Kurzrock R, Gutterman JU. Clinical toxicity of interferons in cancer patients: a review. J Clin Oncol 1986;4:234–243.

216. Quinnan GV, Kirmani N, Rook AH, et al. Cytotoxic T cells in cytomegalovirus infection. HLA-restricted T lymphocyte and non-T-lymphocyte cytotoxic responses correlate with recovery from cytomegalovirus infection in bone marrow transplant recipients. N Engl J Med 1983;307:7–13.

217. Rager-Zisman B, Quan P-C, Rosner M, Moller JR, Bloom BR. Role of NK cells in protection of mice against herpes simplex virus-1 infection. J Immunol 1987;138:884–888.

218. Ramsay AJ, Ruby J, Ramshaw IA. A case for cytokines as effector molecules in the resolution of virus infection. Immunol Today 1993;14:155–157.

219. Ratcliffe DR, Michl J, Cramer EB. Neutrophils do not bind to or phagocytize human immune complexes formed with influenza virus. Blood 1993;82:1639–1646.

220. Raulet DH. How γδ expressing T cells make a living. Curr Biol 1994;4:246–248.

221. Razvi ES, Welsh RM. Apoptosis in viral infections. Adv Virus Res 1995;49:1–60.

222. Razvi ES, Welsh RM, McFarland HI. In vivo state of antiviral CTL precursors. Characterization of a cycling cell population containing CTL precursors in immune mice. J Immunol 1995;154:620–632.

223. Reid LE, Brasnett AH, Gilbert CS, et al. A single DNA response element can confer inducibility by both α- and γ-interferons. Proc Natl Acad Sci U S A 1989;86:840–844.

224. Revel M, Chebath J. Interferon-activated genes. Trends Biochem Sci 1986;11:166–170.

225. Rinaldo CR. Modulation of major histocompatibility complex antigen expression by viral infection. Am J Pathol 1994;144:637–650.

226. Riviere Y, Gresser I, Guillon J-C, Tovey MG. Inhibition by anti-interferon serum of lymphocytic choriomeningitis virus disease in suckling mice. Proc Natl Acad Sci U S A 1977;74:2135–2139.

227. Rothe J, Lesslauer W, Lotscher H, et al. Mice lacking the tumor necrosis factor receptor 1 are resistant to TNF-mediated toxicity but highly susceptible to infection by *Listeria monocytogenes*. Nature 1993;364:798–802.

227a. Rother RP, Fodor WL, Springhorn JP, et al. A novel mechanism of retrovirus inactivation in human serum mediated by anti-alpha-galactosyl natural antibody. J Exp Med 1995;182:1345–1355.

228. Rothman J, Raymond C, Gilbert T, O'Hara P, Stevens T. A putative GTP binding protein homologous to interferon-inducible Mx proteins performs an essential function in yeast protein sorting. Cell 1990;61:1063–1074.

228a. Saifuddin M, Parker CJ, Peeples ME, et al. Role of virion-associated glycosylphosphatidylinositol-linked proteins CD55 and CD59 in complement resistance of cell line-derived and primary isolates of HIV-1. J Exp Med 1995;182:501–509.

229. Samuel C. Antiviral actions of interferon: Interferon-regulated cellular proteins and their surprisingly selective antiviral activities. Virology 1991;183:1–11.

230. Sanz I, Casali P, Thomas JW, Notkins AI, Capra JD. Nucleotide sequences of eight human natural autoantibody VH regions reveals apparent restricted use of VH families. J Immunol 1989;142:4054–4061.

231. Scalzo AA, Fitzgerald NA, Simmons A, La Vista AB, Shellam GR. Cmv-1, a genetic locus that controls murine cytomegalovirus replication in the spleen. J Exp Med 1990;171:1469–1483.

232. Scalzo AA, Fitzgerald NA, Wallace CR, et al. The effect of the Cmv-1 resistance gene, which is linked to the natural killer cell gene complex, is mediated by natural killer cells. J Immunol 1992; 149:581–589.

233. Schindler C, Shuai K, Prezioso VR, Darnell JE. Interferon-dependent tyrosine phosphorylation of a latent cytoplasmic transcription factor. Science 1992;257:809–813.

234. Selin LK, Nahill SR, Welsh RM. Cytotoxic T cell cross-reactivity between heterologous viruses during acute viral infections. J Exp Med 1994;179:1933–1943.

235. Sen GC, Ransohoff RM. Interferon-induced antiviral actions and their regulation. Adv Virus Res 1993;42:57–102.

236. Sen GC. Transcriptional regulation of interferon-inducible genes. In Cohen PP, Foulke J, eds. Hormonal regulation of gene transcription. Amsterdam: Elsevier, 1991:349–374.

237. Sen GC, Lengyel P. The interferon system: A bird's eye view of its biochemistry. J Biol Chem 1992;267:5017–5020.

238. Sentman CL, Hackett J, Kumar V, Bennett M. Identification of a subset of murine natural killer cells that mediates rejection of Hh-1^d but not Hh-1^b bone marrow grafts. J Exp Med 1989;170:191–202.

239. Shellam GR, Allan JE, Papadimitriou JM, Bancroft GJ. Increased susceptibility to cytomegalovirus infection in beige mutant mice. Proc Natl Acad Sci U S A 1981;78:5104–5108.

240. Sherwin SA, Benveniste RE, Todaro GJ. Complement-mediated lysis of type-C virus: Effect of primate and human sera on various retroviruses. Int J Cancer 1978;21:6–11.

241. Shi L, Nishioka WK, Th'ng J, Bradbury EM, Litchfield DW, Greenberg AH. Premature p34^{cdc2} activation required for apoptosis. Science 1994;263:1143–1145.

242. Shuai K, Horvath CM, Huang T, Gureshi SA, Cowburn D, Darnell JE Jr. Interferon activation of the transcription factor Stat91 in-

volves dimerization through SH2-Phosphotyrosyl peptide interactions. Cell 1994;76:821–828.

243. Shuai K, Ziemiecki A, Wilks AF, et al. Polypeptide signalling to the nucleus through tyrosine phosphorylation of Jak and Stat protein. Nature 1993;366:580–583.

244. Silverstein S. Macrophages and viral immunity. Semin Haematol 1970;7:185–214.

245. Simpson RW, Hauser RE. Influence of lipids on the viral envelope. I. Interactions of myxoviruses and their lipid constituents with phospholipases. Virology 1966;30:684–697.

246. Sissons JGP, Oldstone MBA. Antibody-mediated destruction of virus-infected cells. Adv Immunol 1980;29:209–260.

247. Smith HRC, Karlhofer FM, Yokoyama WM. Ly-49 multigene family expressed by IL-2-activated NK cells. J Immunol 1994;153:1068–1079.

248. Snyderman R, Wohlenberg C, Notkins AL. Inflammation and viral infection: Chemotactic activity resulting from the interaction of antiviral antibody and complement with cells infected with herpes simplex virus. J Infect Dis 1972;126:207–109.

249. Soh J, Donnelly RJ, Kotenko S, et al. Identification and sequence of an accessory factor required for activation of the human interferon-γ receptor. Cell 1994;76:793–802.

250. Staeheli P, Haller O, Boll W, Lindenmann J, Weissman C. Mx protein: Constitutive expression in 3T3 cells transformed with cloned Mx cDNA confers selective resistance to influenza virus. Cell 1986;44:147–158.

251. Staeheli P, Pravtcheva D, Lundin LG, et al. Interferon-regulated influenza virus resistance gene Mx is localized on mouse chromosome 16. J Virol 1986;58:967–969.

252. Staeheli P. Interferon-induced proteins and the antiviral state. Adv Virus Res 1990;38:147–200.

253. Stark GR, Kerr IM. Regulation of interferon-β gene: Structure and function of cis-elements and transfactors. J Interferon Res 1992;12:147–151.

254. Steel DM, Whitehead AS. The major acute phase reactants: C-reactive protein, serum amyloid P component and serum amyloid A protein. Immunol Today 1994;15:81–88.

255. St. Johnston D, Brown NH, Gall JG, Jantsch M. A conserved double-stranded RNA-binding domain. Proc Natl Acad Sci U S A 1992;89:10979–10983.

256. Storkus WJ, Salter RD, Alexander J, et al. Class I-induced resistance to natural killing: Identification of nonpermissive residues in HLA-A2. Proc Natl Acad Sci U S A 1991;88:5989–5992.

257. Storkus WJ, Dawson JR. Target structures involved in natural killing (NK): Characteristics, distribution, and candidate molecules. Crit Rev Immunol 1991;10:393–416.

258. Storkus WJ, Salter RD, Cresswgll P, Dawson JR. Peptide-induced modulation of target cell sensitivity to natural killing. J Immunol 1992;149:1185–1190.

259. Su HC, Ishikawa R, Biron CA. Transforming growth factor β expression and natural killer cell responses during virus infection of normal, nude, and SCID mice. J Immunol 1993;151:4874–4890.

260. Su HC, Leite-Morris A, Braun L, Biron CA. A role for transforming growth factor-beta 1 in regulating natural killer cell and T lymphocyte proliferative responses during acute infection with lymphocytic choriomeningitis virus. J Immunol 1991;147:2717–2727.

261. Su HC, Orange JS, Fast LD, et al. IL-2-dependent NK cell responses discovered in virus-infected β₂-microglobulin-deficient mice. J Immunol 1994;153:5674–5681.

262. Suda T, Takahashi T, Golstein P, Nagata S. Molecular cloning and expression of the Fas ligand, a novel member of the tumor necrosis family. Cell 1993;75:1169–1178.

262a. Takeuchi Y, Porter CD, Strahan KM, et al. Sensitization of cells and retroviruses to human serum by (α1-3) galactosyltransferase. Nature 1996;379:85–88.

263. Taniguchi T. Regulation of interferon-β gene: Structure and function of cis-elements and trans-factors. J Interferon Res 1989;9:633–640.

264. Thanos D, Maniatis T. Identification of the rel family members required for virus induction of the human beta interferon gene. Mol Cell Biol 1995;15:152–164.

265. Thieblemont N, Haeffner-Cavaillon N, Ledur A, L'Age-Stehr J, Ziegler-Heitbrock HW, Kazatchkine MD. CR1 (CD35) and CR3 (CD11b/CD18) mediate infection of human monocytes and mono-cytic cell lines with complement–opsonized HIV independently of CD4. Clin Exp Immunol 1993; 92:106–113.

266. Thomsen AR, Pisa P, Bro-Jorgensen K, Kiessling R. Mechanisms of lymphocytic choriomeningitis virus-induced hematopoietic dysfunction. J Virol 1986;59:428–433.

267. Tiwari R, Kusari J, Kumar R, Sen G. Gene induction by interferons and double-stranded RNA: Selective inhibition by 2-aminopurine. Mol Cell Biol 1988;8:4289–4294.

268. Tiwari R, Kusari J, Sen G. Functional equivalents of interferon-mediated signals needed for induction of an mRNA can be generated by double-stranded RNA and growth factors. EMBO J 1987;6:3373–3378.

269. Tomer Y, Shoenfeld Y. The significance of natural autoantibodies. Immunol Invest 1988;17:389–424.

270. Toth FD, Mosborg-Petersen P, Kiss J, et al. Differential replication of human immunodeficiency virus type 1 in CD8− and CD8+ subsets of natural killer cells: Relationship to cytokine production pattern. J Virol 1993;67:5879–5888.

271. Tracey DE. The requirement for macrophages in the augmentation of natural killer cell activity by BCG. J Immunol 1979;123:840–845.

272. Trauth BC, Klas C, Peters AMJ, et al. Monoclonal antibody-mediated tumor progression by induction of apoptosis. Science 1989;245:301–305.

273. Trinchieri G. Recognition of major histocompatibility class I antigens by natural killer cells. J Exp Med 1994;180:417–421.

274. Trinchieri G. Natural killer cells in hematopoiesis. In Lewis CE, McGee JO'D. eds. The natural killer cell: The natural immune system. Oxford: IRL Press 1992:41–65.

275. Trinchieri G, Santoli D. Antiviral activity induced by culturing lymphocytes with tumor derived or virus-transformed cells: Enhancement of natural killer activity by interferon and antagonistic inhibition of susceptibility of target cells to lysis. J Exp Med 1978;147:1314–1333.

276. Trotta PP, Nagabhushan TL. Gamma interferon, protein structure and function. In Baron S, Coppenhaver DH, Dianzani F, et al, eds. Interferon: Principles and medical applications. Galveston, TX: The University of Texas Medical Branch at Galveston Department of Microbiology, 1992:117–127.

277. Tsang SY, Nakanishi M, Peterlin BM. Mutational analysis of the DRA promoter: Cis-acting sequences and trans-acting factors. Mol Cell Biol 1990;10:711–719.

278. Tsuru S, Fujisawa H, Taniguchi M, Zinnaka Y, Nomoto K. Mechanism of protection during the early phases of a generalized viral infection. II. Contribution of polymorphonuclear leukocytes to protection against intravenous infection with influenza virus. J Gen Virol 1987;68:419–424.

279. Tsuru S, Shinomiya N, Nomoto K. Depression of early protection against influenza virus infection by cyclophosphamide and its restoration by Y-19995 (2,4'-bis(1-methyl-2-dimethyl-amino-ethoxyl)-3-benzoylpyridine dimaleate). Nat Immun Cell Growth Regul 1991;10:1–11.

280. Upton C, Mossman K, McFadden G. Encoding of a homolog of the IFN-γ receptor by myxoma virus. Science 1992;258:1369–1372.

281. Utsumi J, Shimizu H. Human interferon β, protein structure and function. In Baron S, Coppenhaver DH, Dianzani F, et al, eds. Interferon: Principles and medical applications. Galveston, TX: The University of Texas Medical Branch at Galveston, Department of Microbiology, 1992:107–116.

282. Uze G, Lutfalla G, Gresser I. Genetic transfer of a functional human interferon-a receptor into mouse cells: Cloning and expression of its cDNA. Cell 1990;60:225–234.

283. van Strijp JA, van der Tol ME, Miltenborg LA, van Kessel KP, Verhoef J. Tumour necrosis factor triggers granulocytes to internalize complement-coated viral particles. Immunology 1991;73:77–82.

284. Vargas-Cortes M, O'Donnell CL, Maciaszek JW, Welsh RM. Generation of "natural killer cell-escape" variants of Pichinde virus during acute and persistent infections. J Virol 1992;66:2532–2535.

285. Vassalli P. The pathophysiology of tumor necrosis factors. Annu Rev Immunol 1992;10:411–452.

286. Velazquez L, Fellows M, Stark GR, Pellegrini S. A protein tyrosine kinase in the interferon α/β signaling pathway. Cell 1992;70:313–322.

287. Vilcek J, Lee TH. Tumor necrosis factor. New insights into the molecular mechanisms of its multiple actions. J Biol Chem 1991;226:7313–7316.
288. Visvanathan KV, Goodbourn S. Double-stranded RNA activates binding of to an inducible element in the human β-interferon promoter. EMBO J 1989;8:1129–1138.
289. Watanabe N, Sakakibara J, Hovanessian A, Taniguchi T, Fujita T. Activation of IFN-β element by IRF-1 requires a post translational event in addition to IRF-1 synthesis. Nucl Acids Res 1991;19:4421–4428.
290. Watling D, Guschin D, Muller M, et al. Complementation by the protein tyrosine kinase Jak2 of a mutant cell line defective in the interferon-γ signal transduction pathway. Nature 1993;366:166–170.
291. Webster RG. Original antigenic sin in ferrets. The response to sequential infections with influenza viruses. J Immunol 1966;97:177–183.
292. Weissmann C, Weber H. The interferon genes. Progr Nucl Acids Res Mol Biol 1986;33:251–300.
293. Welsh RM. Host cell modification of lymphocytic choriomeningitis virus and Newcastle disease virus altering viral inactivation by human complement. J Immunol 1977;118:348–354.
294. Welsh RM. Cytotoxic cells induced during lymphocytic choriomeningitis virus infection of mice. 1. Characterization of natural killer cell induction. J Exp Med 1978;148:163–181.
295. Welsh RM. Regulation of virus infections by natural killer cells. Nat Immun Cell Growth Regul 1986;5:169–199.
296. Welsh RM, Brubaker JO, Vargas-Cortes M, O'Donnell CL. Natural killer (NK) cell response to virus infections in mice with severe combined immunodeficiency: The stimulation of NK cells and the NK cell-dependent control of virus infections occur independently of T and B cell function. J Exp Med 1991;173:1053–1063.
297. Welsh RM, Cooper NR, Jensen FC, Oldstone MBA. Human serum lyses RNA tumor viruses. Nature 1975;257:612–614.
298. Welsh RM, Hallenbeck LA. Effect of virus infections on target cell susceptibility to natural killer cell-mediated lysis. J Immunol 1980;124:2491–2497.
299. Welsh RM, Jensen FC, Cooper NR, Oldstone MBA. Inactivation and lysis of oncornaviruses by human serum. Virology 1976;74:432–440.
300. Welsh RM, Lampert PW, Burner PA, Oldstone MBA. Antibody-complement interactions with purified lymphocytic choriomeningitis virus. Virology 1976;73:59–71.
300a. Welsh RM, Tay CH, Varga SM, O'Donnell CL, Vergilis KL, Selin LK. Lymphocyte-dependent 'natural' immunity to virus infections mediated by both natural killer and memory T cells. Semin Virol 1996;7:95–102.
301. Welsh RM, Vargas-Cortes M. Natural killer cells in viral infection. In Lewis CE, McGee JO'D, eds. The natural killer cell: The natural immune system. Oxford: IRL Press, 1992:107–150.
302. Wetzel R. Assignment of the disulphide bonds of leukocyte interferon. Nature 1981;289:606–607.
303. White E, Cipriani R. Specific disruption of intermediate filaments and nuclear lamina by the 19-kDa product of the adenovirus E1B oncogene. Proc Natl Acad Sci U S A 1989;86:9886–9890.
304. White E, Cipriani R. Role of adenovirus E1B proteins in transformation: Altered organization of intermediate filaments in transformed cells that express the 19-kilodalton protein. Mol Cell Biol 1990;10:120–130.
305. White E, Cipriani R, Sabbatini P, Denton A. Adenovirus E1B 19-kilodalton protein overcomes the cytotoxicity of E1A proteins. J Virol 1991;65:2968–2978.
306. White DO, Fenner FJ. Medical virology. Orlando, FL: Academic Press, 1986.
307. Widmer U, Manogue KR, Cerami A, Sherry B. Genomic cloning and promoter analysis of macrophage inflammatory protein (MIP)-2, MIP-1α, and MIP-1β, members of the chemokine superfamily of proinflammatory cytokines. J Immunol 1993;150:4996–5012.
308. Williams BR, Silverman R. The 2-5A system: Clinical and molecular aspects of the interferon regulated pathway. New York: Liss, 1985.
309. Williams BR. Transcriptional regulation of interferon-stimulated genes. Eur J Biochem 1991;200:1–11.
310. Williams RK, Jiang GS, Snyder SW, Frana MF, Holmes KV. Purification of the 110-kilodalton glycoprotein receptor for mouse hepatitis virus (MHV)-A59 from mouse liver and identification of a nonfunctional, homologous protein in MHV-resistant SJL/J mice. J Virol 1990;64:3817–3823.
311. Willman CL, Sever CE, Pallavicini MG, et al. Deletion of IRF-1, mapping to chromosome 5q31.1, in human leukemia and preleukemic myelodysplasia. Science 1993;259:968–971.
312. Wold WSM. Adenovirus genes that modulate the sensitivity of virus-infected cells to lysis by TNF. J Cell Biochem 1993;53:329–335.
313. Wong GH, Elwell JH, Oberley LW, Goeddel DV. Manganous superoxide dismutase is essential for cellular resistance to cytotoxicity of tumor necrosis factor. Cell 1989;58:923–931.
314. Wong GHW, McHugh T, Weber R, Goeddel DV. Tumor necrosis factor α selectively sensitizes human immunodeficiency virus-infected cells to heat and radiation. Proc Natl Acad Sci U S A 1991;88:4372–4376.
315. Wu L, Morahan PS. Macrophages and other nonspecific defenses: Role in modulating resistance against herpes simplex virus. Curr Top Microbiol Immunol 1992;179:89–110.
316. Wu L, Morahan PS, Leary K. Mechanisms of intrinsic macrophage-virus interactions in vitro. Microbiol Pathol 1990;9:293–301.
317. Yamada G, Ogawa M, Akagi K, et al. Specific depletion of the B-cell population induced by aberrant expression of human interferon regulatory factor 1 gene in transgenic mice. Proc Natl Acad Sci U S A 1991;88:532–536.
318. Yogeeswaran G, Fujinami R, Kiessling R, Welsh RM. Interferon induced alterations in cellular sialic acid and glycoconjugates: Correlation with susceptibility to activated natural killer cells. Virology 1982;121:363–371.
319. Yokoyama WM, Ryan JC, Hunter JJ, Smith HRC, Stark M, Seaman WE. cDNA cloning of mouse NKR-P1 and genetic linkage with Ly-49: Identification of a natural killer cell gene complex on mouse chromosome 6. J Immunol 1991;147:3229–3236.
320. York IA, Roop C, Andrews DW, Riddell SR, Graham FL, Johnson DC. A cytosolic herpes simplex virus protein inhibits antigen presentation to CD8+ T lymphocytes. Cell 1994;77:525–535.
321. Young HA, Hardy KJ. Interferon-gamma: Producer cells, activation stimuli, and molecular genetic regulation. Pharmacol Ther 1990;45:137-151.
322. Zawatzky R, Engler H, Kirchner H. Experimental infection of inbred mice with herpes simplex virus. III. Comparison between newborn and adult C57BL/6 mice. J Gen Virol 1982;60:25–29.
323. Zhou A, Hassel BA, Silverman RH. Expression cloning of 2-5A-dependent RNase: A uniquely regulated mediator of interferon action. Cell 1993;72:753–765.
324. Zinn K, Keller Z, Wittemore L-A, Maniatis T. 2-aminopurine selectively inhibits the induction of β-interferon, c-fos, and c-myc gene expression. Science 1988;240:210–213.

Viral Pathogenesis,
edited by Neal Nathanson, et al.
Lippincott–Raven Publishers, Philadelphia © 1997

CHAPTER 7

Immune Responses to Viral Infection

Peter C. Doherty and Rafi Ahmed

INTRODUCTION

Virus infections are dealt with largely by the specific immune response, although early, nonspecific effects (see Chap. 6) mediated by the production of various cytokines (particularly interferon [IFN]-αβ) may be important[149] before the stage that effector T lymphocytes and secreted immunoglobulin (Ig) molecules are available to eliminate infected cells and neutralize free virions, respectively.[56,238] Various other host resistance mechanisms, such as the defensins that may be central to limiting the rapid growth of (for instance) invading bacteria, probably are less involved in viral immunity.[117] This

chapter examines the interaction between viruses and the immune system that leads, if the individual is to survive, to clearance of the invading pathogen or to some biologic compromise between virus and host that permits coexistence.[65]

VIRUSES AND THE EVOLUTION OF THE IMMUNE SYSTEM

Viruses are obligate intracellular parasites, with no capacity to replicate in the extracellular environment. Except under laboratory conditions, most viruses do not survive for long outside living cells. Many of the models studied by viral immunologists subvert the normal means of viral spread and are not subject to the constraints discussed in the remainder of this section. The influenza A viruses, for example, never infect mice in nature, but have proven to be of great value for analyzing viral pathogenesis and T-cell specificity.[14,210,234]

P. C. Doherty: Department of Immunology, St. Jude's Children's Research Hospital, Memphis, Tennessee 38105.
R. Ahmed: Department of Microbiology and Immunology and Emory Vaccine Center, Emory University, Atlanta, Georgia 30322.

Thoughtful dissection of the host response to lymphocytic choriomeningitis virus (LCMV) probably has revealed more about the way the immune system works than any other antigen system[29,92,238] (see Chap. 25). In addition to findings from such experimental models, the natural histories of single-host pathogens also must be considered when discussing the fundamentals of the virus-host interaction in the broadest sense.

The biologic imperative for any virus is transmission, which is reflected in the evolution of the viral genome that in turn dictates the spectra of interactions between the virus and its host or hosts. Some viruses, particularly members of the flavivirus and alphavirus groups, may have part of their life cycle in biting insects, such as mosquitoes (e.g., eastern equine encephalitis) or ticks (e.g., Russian spring/summer encephalitis), but they also depend on replication and viremia in a mammalian or avian species to supply the blood meal for the vector. Infection of humans with these viruses may be incidental to their basic ecology and, as a consequence, can lead to a rapidly lethal conclusion. The classic example is yellow fever virus, which has a sylvatic cycle in nonhuman primates. However, most mammalian viruses, particularly those that infect only a single species, have evolved an accommodation with their hosts so that, even if they are to cause a fatal conclusion, the end will be sufficiently protracted so there will be adequate opportunities for transmission.

The nature of the interaction between virus and mammal, particularly for a single-host virus, should be thought of as an evolving ecosystem. On the one hand are the variety of host resistance mechanisms, particularly the specific immune response, and on the other is the viral genome. The virus, with its short life cycle, has the capacity to vary infinitely more rapidly than the mammal. However, unless such a change promotes the long-term survival and transmission of the virus, it will not have selective advantage and will not persist in nature. Complex biologic systems like mammals, however, are successful only if they live long enough to mature sexually, reproduce, and (at least for humans) nurture their young.

The immune system is the evolutionary result of the need to maintain the milieu interieur of the higher vertebrates in the face of constant challenge by a great variety of potentially parasitic, simpler life forms. An individual may be regarded as an interdependent complex of functioning organ systems, any or all of which may be the target of particular pathogens. Our most intimate parasites (the single-host viruses) and the immune surveillance system that targets effector T lymphocytes to the surface of virally modified cells may be considered to have evolved together. The phylogeny of the thymus and the CD8+ and CD4+ T cells that see aberrant peptide in the context of self class I or class II major histocompatibility complex (MHC) glycoproteins is clearly a consequence of consistent selective pressures exerted, in particular, by viruses and other intracellular pathogens.[66,236]

ORGANIZATION OF THE IMMUNE SYSTEM

It probably is appropriate to introduce the subject of the specific host response by making a few general points about the way the mammalian immune system works. Several excellent immunology texts cover the following basic points in much greater detail, although they do not necessarily deal well with viral immunity.[55] In this chapter, the primary topic is what happens in the secondary lymphoid tissue (lymph nodes and spleen), rather than the events that occur in the thymus or bone marrow during lymphocyte ontogeny.[127,221]

The Lymphocytes

The cellular mediators of specific immunity are the lymphocytes, which, together with the monocytes, make up the great preponderance of the leukocytes in normal individuals. These cells discriminate self from nonself with a high degree of precision mediated by the specific recognition units on the lymphocytes, the T-cell receptors (TCRs) and Ig molecules.[45,50,112] The T-cell population overall is selected in the thymus to allow the survival of precursors expressing TCRs with low avidity for cells expressing self class I (CD8+ subset) or class II (CD4+ subset) MHC glycoproteins, and high avidity for somatic cells (encountered later in the extrathymic environment) signaling abnormality or "danger" through surface MHC molecules that have been modified by the binding of peptides processed from nonself (i.e., viral proteins). The viral proteins are degraded from newly synthesized product in cytoplasm (class I, endogenous pathway).[26,234] or in endosomes/lysosomes subsequent to phagocytosis (class II, exogenous pathway). The MHC molecules are among the most polymorphic known,[35,66,238] reflecting the need of the species to avoid nonresponsiveness to a novel pathogen after failure to develop an appropriate (i.e., antigenic) peptide-MHC glycoprotein complex. The TCR-MHC interaction is true immune surveillance,[34,63] although the term was used initially in the context of preventing oncogenesis.

The spectrum of "self tolerance" is inclusive of self peptide presented in the binding site of the MHC molecules in the thymus, probably leading to the deletion of potential responding clonal precursors. Viruses that are substantially nonlytic and infect the developing thymus (the particular case being LCMV contracted in utero) are essentially treated as self. The mechanisms for maintaining "peripheral" tolerance to self peptides that first are encountered outside the thymus are less well understood, and the interplay between "clonal abortion," "anergy," "exhaustion," and "immune deviation" is the focus of much basic investigation* and of attempts at preventing or inhibiting autoimmunity.[211]

The antigen-specific TCR on both sets of lymphocytes consists of an αβ heterodimer that cannot be assigned *a priori* to a CD8+ or CD4+ T cell simply by looking at sequence variation.[50] Both CD4 and CD8 have ancillary binding function for nonvarying regions of the particular MHC molecule,[135] and there are six other TCR-associated chains (the CD3 complex), all of which are thought to have the capacity to transduce signals to the cytoplasm.[79,180] The alternative TCR, the γδ heterodimer, is expressed on substantial populations of essentially sessile lymphocytes in the skin and various mucosae, and on a fairly low percentage of circulating T cells in mice and humans.[209] The γδ T cells are much more prevalent in

---

*References 4, 5, 23, 53, 140, 175, 205, 211, 237.

chickens, pigs, cattle, and sheep.[30,88,209] However, although they are found in sites of virus-induced inflammatory pathology,[69,98] no functional role in virus infections has been ascribed to them. It is speculated that the γδ TCRs may be much more Ig-like in their binding characteristics with, perhaps, a tendency to recognize heat-shock proteins, which may have bound peptides derived from other proteins.[24]

The B-cell receptor, the Ig molecule, is not interested in self MHC glycoprotein, but binds directly to tertiary structures on proteins. Although surface-bound Ig on precursor B cells is part of a signaling complex that also involves ancillary signaling molecules,[38] the Igs act functionally as secreted product. In general, it is much easier to demonstrate breakage of self tolerance for B cells than for T cells. If B-cell hybridomas are made from mice acutely infected with a virus, for example, hybridoma cell lines are readily generated that secrete Ig that can bind to a variety of self proteins.[166]

CD8+ T Cells

The essential function of the CD8+ T cells in viral immunity is to kill virus-infected cells, preventing the indolent spread of the infection and beginning the end of the initial, antigen-driven phase of the host response.[108,224] These cytotoxic T lymphocytes (CTLs) operate through the polar secretion of perforin, which assembles complement-like channels in the membrane of the virus-infected target subsequent to recognition by the specific (clonotypic) TCR.[165] Other molecules (serine esterases, granzymes) may pass through this channel[52,147] and cause homogenization of the nuclear DNA (apoptosis). The effector CTLs kill many times but, when all the targets are eliminated, may themselves undergo apoptosis and die. The normal consequence of the primary response is to leave a greatly expanded pool of CTL precursors (CTLp) that have the potential to respond more rapidly after secondary challenge.†

The CD8+ CTLs are the major mediators of immune surveillance, detecting changes on the surface of cells expressing specifically modified class I MHC glycoproteins. The class I MHC molecules can be expressed on most cells throughout the body (neurons are an exception) and are upregulated by (in particular) IFN-γ produced by natural killer cells or responder CD4+ (Th1) or CD8+ T cells.[144,231] The capacity of CD8+ T cells to produce IFN-γ and other cytokines has been somewhat underemphasized.[125] In addition, immune responses can be manipulated so that CD8+ T cells assume a Th2 lymphokine production profile secreting, for example, interleukin-4 (IL-4).[124]

Experiments with LCMV have shown that the process of acute virus elimination depends on perforin-dependent cytotoxicity, and cannot be mediated solely by cytokines.[108,224] However, the relative importance of cytotoxicity versus cytokine production in controlling viral infections is likely to vary depending on the nature (cytolytic or noncytolytic) of the virus.[94,108,170,224,236] Cells infected by a noncytolytic virus, such as LCMV, continue to produce virus and the most efficient way of "shutting down" this virus factory is to kill the

infected cell. It is not surprising that CTL-mediated killing of virus-infected cells is necessary for terminating LCMV infection. In contrast, this mechanism (i.e., killing per se) is not essential for controlling cytolytic viruses such as vaccinia, because the virus itself is going to kill the cell. In such instances, the production of antiviral cytokines by T cells to protect uninfected cells may be more important than T-cell–mediated cytotoxicity.

CD4+ T Cells

The CD4+ T cells also can be induced to develop CTL function, particularly in virus-infected mice that lack the CD8+ subset,[17,95,148] although the nature of the lytic mechanism is not understood.[96] In addition, it is far from established that CD4+ CTLs actually do eliminate virus-infected cells in vivo, although both influenza virus and Sendai virus infections (but not LCMV) can be terminated by a CD4-dependent mechanism.[17,61,70,77,95,116,121,126,188] Experiments with the influenza model suggest that such clearance is mediated by help for antibody production rather than by a direct effect of the CD4+ T cells themselves.[188] Mice persistently infected with LCMV that have only CD4+ T cells develop a chronic wasting disease, which presumably is cytokine mediated.[61,77,116]

An important role of the CD4+ subset in virus infections is to provide the help (Th) necessary to promote the clonal expansion and differentiation of virus-specific B lymphocytes.[3] Essentially all the antibody-secreting cells that develop in mice lacking CD4+ T cells are IgM producers.[22,72,222] The CD4+ T-cell response in most virus infections seems to be dominated by a Th1 profile, characterized by IFN-γ and IL-2 production, which leads to a prominent IgG2a response.[84,143,158] However, some viral proteins, specifically the surface glycoprotein[10] of respiratory syncytial virus, apparently induce a Th2 profile (at least in BALB/c mice). Secretion of the Th2 cytokines IL-4 and IL-5, which favor IgE secretion and the allergic reactions that are designed to deal with metazoan parasites, could be the reason for the asthmatic symptoms commonly seen after respiratory syncytial virus infection of infants.[54,155] Influenza virus can be eliminated acutely by adoptively transferred CD4+ Th1, but not Th2, cell lines.[84]

An essential point concerning Th for antibody production is that, at least for the response to a whole virus particle, the CD4+ T cells can be specific for any viral peptide that is appropriately presented by the class II MHC molecules on the B lymphocyte.[187] A B cell expressing surface Ig specific for the hemagglutinin coat protein of an influenza A virus will interiorize the captured virion as a result of crosslinking of the Ig molecules, degrade the virus in the endosomal/lysosomal compartment, and express, for example, nucleoprotein peptide bound to class II MHC molecules. As a result, a nucleoprotein-specific CD4+ Th can promote a hemagglutinin-specific B-cell response.

The need for CD4+ Th to promote the development of virus-specific CD8+ CTLs has been found to vary between experimental systems.‡ Many virus-specific CD8+ CTL re-

---

†References 1, 2, 4, 13, 59, 62, 80, 97, 115, 139, 157.

‡References 3, 20, 33, 56, 99, 102, 110, 168.

sponses proceed perfectly well in the absence of CD4+ T cells or class II MHC glycoproteins. The overall impression is that any positive effect of concurrent CD4+ Th stimulation reflects the fact that the increased availability of cytokines such as IL-2 and IFN-γ contributes to generalized cellular activation in the responding lymphoid tissue. Priming with a viral peptide recognized by CTLs is facilitated by using Freund's adjuvant, which presumably stimulates cytokine production by cells that have no specificity for any viral determinant.[111]

B Cells

The B cells (precursors of the antibody-secreting plasma cells) are generated in the bone marrow in postnatal life, and localize to germinal centers in secondary lymphoid tissue.[85] Their receptor, the Ig molecule, has the capacity to bind directly to tertiary structures on viral protein.[45] During the course of an immune response, viral protein is captured by a cell expressing the appropriate Ig molecule, the highest-affinity ligand present. Concurrent stimulation of the CD4+ set leads to the provision of lymphokines, such as IL-2 and IFN-γ, which promote B-cell proliferation, class-switching to produce (usually) IgG and IgA class antibodies, and maturation of the plasma cell response.[75] A central difference between B-cell and T-cell responses is affinity maturation as a consequence of somatic mutation[43]: the T-cell repertoire (spectrum of available TCRs) is essentially determined at the time the cells leave the thymus.

Analysis with monoclonal antibodies suggests that binding about six Ig molecules results in rhinovirus neutralization in vitro.[196] How this formula translates to the in vivo situation, where other antibody-related mechanisms (e.g., complement fixation) also may be operating, is not known. Virus-specific Ig molecules also may attach to activated macrophages through their Fc regions, and act to promote antibody-dependent cellular cytotoxicity. The antibody-dependent cellular cytotoxicity effect has been known for many years, particularly from experiments with herpesvirus,[167,172,181] but its biologic significance has never been clarified.

Secondary Lymphoid Tissue and the Lymphatics

The secondary lymphoid tissue of mammals consists of the lymph nodes, the spleen, and the mucosa-associated lymphoid tissue. The last of these has received the least amount of attention from viral immunologists,[131] although it probably is enormously important. Aggregates of lymphoid tissue in the nose and around the bronchi must be involved in respiratory infections,[90] although, in the mouse, it is not clear that these aggregates exist before some antigenic challenge to the lung. Bacterial immunologists have focused on the gut-associated lymphoid tissue, which is characterized by well-organized foci (Peyer's patches) in the wall of the gut.[200]

All tissues have two forms of drainage, the venous system and the lymph. The former is monitored by the spleen, the latter by the lymph nodes. Extracellular fluid may be collected into the afferent lymphatics and pumped, as a result of normal movement and muscular contraction, to the regional lymph nodes (e.g., cervical, popliteal, axillary). Intradermal injec-tion, for example, can be regarded as essentially intralymphatic. A virus that invades by this route (i.e., ectromelia; see Chap. 22) may be taken up by dendritic cells (Langerhans cells, veiled cells) or by monocyte/macrophages and transported by the lymph to the regional node, where the primary immune response then develops. For example, the respiratory tract is lined with large numbers of dendritic cells.[134] In contrast, virus that gains direct entry to the blood is removed from the circulation in the spleen, which does essentially the same job as the lymph nodes.

Immunologically naive T and B cells enter the lymph nodes through the specialized high endothelial venules, which express specific ligands for the L-selectin (CD62L) molecule on the lymphocyte membrane.[136,163] Memory T cells, on the other hand, may express little L-selectin,[4,28,93] and transit to the lymph node in afferent lymph after leaving the blood in the postcapillary venules of solid tissues. Access to the spleen is thought not to be controlled by this gating process involving L-selectin, emphasizing the probable importance of the spleen in secondary responses. Constitutive expression of the class II MHC molecules that target the CD4+ helper T lymphocytes tends to be mainly a property of cells that are located in the lymph nodes and spleen, emphasizing that these anatomic niches function to promote interaction between antigen-specific CD4+ T and B cells, optimizing the development of the immune response.

T and B cells exit the lymph nodes through the efferent lymphatics, which cumulate to larger ducts that drain to the vena cava, and (after passage through the lung) are pumped around the body in the arterial circulation. Antigen-stimulated T and B cells can extravasate into tissue sites supporting virus growth,[56,58,141] with B-cell localization being particularly apparent for the viral encephalitides. Locally produced Ig is readily detected[64,174,216] in the "great drain" of the central nervous system, the cerebrospinal fluid, and (because neurons do not express MHC glycoproteins) is clearly important[105,118] for limiting infectious processes in the brain (see Chap. 8). In general, however, the continuing recirculation from blood to tissue to lymph of the primed (see section on Immune Memory) lymphocytes that mediate immune surveillance is essentially a function of the T-cell subsets.[197]

THE PRIMARY RESPONSE

The character of the primary virus-specific response probably is described best (in contemporary terms) for continuing mouse experiments with respiratory viruses,[55,56] particularly the influenza A viruses and the murine parainfluenza type 1 virus (Sendai virus). Productive infection by both viruses is limited almost exclusively to the superficial epithelial cells of the respiratory tract, reflecting the distribution of a trypsin-like enzyme[223] required to cleave the viral hemagglutinin (influenza) or fusion (Sendai) proteins before infectious progeny can be assembled. Defective growth cycles occur in other cell types, such as macrophages and dendritic cells, but this does not lead to the spread of infection, although it probably is important for the dissemination of viral antigen to secondary lymphoid tissue.

The probable pathogenesis is that, after intranasal administration to anesthetized mice, the virus infects epithelial cells, dendritic cells, and macrophages located at the mucosal surface. At least a proportion of these dendritic cells and, perhaps, free virus particles then transit in the afferent lymph to the regional cervical (upper respiratory tract) or mediastinal (lower respiratory tract) lymph nodes. Other nonproductively infected cells may enter the blood and be removed in the spleen, where they also may function to stimulate virus-specific CTLp. At the same time, the process of virus infection itself has induced the production of cytokines such as IFN-αβ. Some of this lymphokine probably drains through the lymph to the regional node.

The mediastinal lymph nodes then begin a process of massive (greater than fivefold) selective enlargement as a consequence of lymphocyte recruitment from the blood, which may cause transient lymphopenia. The increase in cellularity probably is mediated by the local involvement of a cytokine, which has been shown, at least in a vaccinia model, to be IFN-αβ. Another possible candidate is IL-6. The relative prevalence of the various lymphocyte subsets (50% B cells, more CD4+ than CD8+ αβ TCR+ cells, a few γδ T cells) remains much the same as in "resting" lymphoid tissue. Such recruitment usually is less apparent for the cervical lymph nodes, which (even in specific pathogen–free mice) already are large, probably as a consequence of continued exposure to food proteins and low-grade encounters with gastrointestinal tract commensals.[100,123]

CD8+ T Cells

The kinetics of the primary response have been analyzed most thoroughly for the CD8+ CTLp, which can be grown in microcultures and measured by limiting dilution analysis. Virus-specific CTLp are thought to be at low prevalence ($1 : 5 \times 10^5$ to $1 : 10^6$ lymph node cells) in the L-selectin–high naive set.[4,93] Evidence of priming to the point that CTL activity can be detected subsequent to bulk culture with infected stimulator cells is first found from day 3 or day 4 after intranasal exposure to virus. Virus-specific CTLp are readily demonstrated by limiting dilution analysis from day 5, with most or all of these cells being L-selectin–low. The CTLp frequency in the mediastinal lymph node CD8+ L-selectin–low set may be as high as $1 : 1,000$–$1 : 100$ by day 7 or day 8 after priming, reflecting a doubling time of about 10 hours.

With Sendai virus and the less virulent variants of the influenza A viruses, there usually is little evidence of CTL activity in mediastinal lymph nodes, cervical lymph nodes, or spleen analyzed directly after recovery from the mouse.[9,95] This probably reflects the absence of significant productive infection, and resultant relative lack of antigen, in these sites.[72] However, effector CTLs are readily detected in the cervical lymph nodes of mice that have been injected intracerebrally with "neurotropic" LCMV, because the virus also grows in the lymph nodes.[123] Infection with the "viscerotropic" strains of LCMV leads to much more extensive replication in lymphoid and other tissues, with effector CTLs being detected in many sites,[67,235] including the thymus (see Chaps. 8 and 25).

Potent effector CTL activity is readily demonstrated in the respiratory tract of mice infected with Sendai virus and the influenza A viruses from about day 7 to day 9 after infection.[9,95]

The kinetic evidence indicates that these CTLs are the further differentiated state, or the progeny, of the CTLp found earlier in the regional lymphoid tissue.[62] The CTLs themselves may undergo apoptosis and die after the virus-infected epithelium has been eliminated, although this has not been established. What is clear is that a relatively small percentage (perhaps 10% to 20%) of the virus-specific CTLp that can be detected in the lymph nodes or spleen actually enter the site of inflammatory pathology in the lung. Many of the other 80% to 90% of the CTLp probably continue as memory T cells, or serve as the precursors of these memory cells (see Immune Memory). Evidence indicates that the phase of rapid CTLp proliferation in lymphoid tissue is substantially over by day 20 after the initial infection, and is never prominent in the pneumonic lung.

In summary, primary CTL responses to an acute viral infection (e.g., LCMV, influenza, vaccinia) can be broken down into three distinct phases: activation and expansion, death, and stability or memory[4] (Fig. 7-1). During the initial phase, which typically lasts about a week, there is antigen-driven expansion of the specific T cells and their differentiation into effector CTLs (i.e., direct ex vivo killers). In several viral systems examined, there is between 100-fold and 5000-fold expansion of virus-specific CD8+ T cells.[§] A period of death then ensues (between days 7 and 30), during which most of the activated T cells undergo apoptosis and effector activity subsides as the level of antigen declines.[‖] This contraction of the T-cell response is as dramatic as the expansion, and in most instances, 95% or more of the antigen-specific T cells disappear. This phenomenon, termed *activation-induced cell death,* serves as a mechanism for regulating cell numbers and maintaining homeostasis. Apoptosis resulting from fas (CD95)/fas L interactions has been implicated in activation-induced cell death, and a role for tumor necrosis factor in the apoptosis of activated CD8+ T cells has been documented.[235] The third phase of the T-cell response is the phase of memory that is characterized by a stable pool of memory cells that can persist for many years.[4,115] The eventual magnitude and duration of immunity is the sum effect of changes occurring in all three phases of the CTL response.

CD4+ T Cells

Quantitative analysis of the development of virus-specific CD4+ Th precursors through the primary response has not been done for any virus, although the theme probably is fairly similar to that described earlier for the CD8+ set. The problem is that the limiting dilution analysis for these lymphocytes[137] depends on lymphokine production, which may not be a reliable indicator of specific stimulation, particularly for cells from a responding ("activated") lymph node. However, the frequencies of Th precursors that can be detected 10 to 20 days after infection usually are comparable to those found for the CTLp, and the responding lymphocytes all are L-selectin–low.[74]

The CD4+ T cells are the majority lymphokine producers in the lymph nodes, with most viruses inducing a Th1 (IL-2, IFN-γ) profile, even though at least some of the CD4+ T cells

---

[§]References 4, 39, 56, 80, 97, 115, 119, 132, 139, 153, 159, 160, 212, 214, 237.
[‖]References 4, 41, 78, 113, 122, 151, 171, 173, 177, 190, 207, 225.

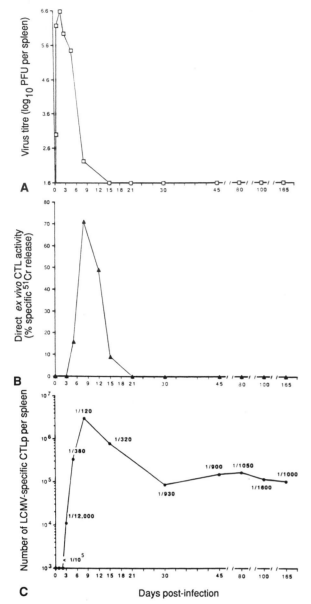

FIG. 7-1. Kinetics of cytotoxic T-lymphocyte (CTL) response after acute viral infection. Adult mice were infected with lymphocytic choriomeningitis virus (LCMV) and, at the indicated time, monitored for virus levels in the spleen (**A**), direct ex vivo CTL activity (**B**; effector response), and number of LCMV-specific CTLs in the spleen (**C**). The numbers on the graph indicate the frequency of LCMV specific CTLP per spleen at various times postinfection. PFU, plaque-forming units. (Adapted from Lau LL, Jamieson BD, Somasundaram T, Ahmed R. Cytotoxic T-cell memory without antigen. Nature 1994;369:648–652.)

may be expressing messenger RNA for Th2 products (IL-4, IL-10), particularly IL-4.[22,40,185] In the virus-infected lung, however, substantial numbers of IL-4 producing inflammatory cells are found concurrently with the predicted Th1 lymphocytes.[138,184] It appears that functional expression of some lymphokine genes is much more controlled in the tightly

packed "headquarters" of the regional lymph node than in the less-controlled "battlefield" of the site of pathology.

B Cells

Clonal expansion of the B-cell precursors has been analyzed, using the ELISPOT assay to detect virus-specific plasma cells producing particular Ig isotypes. The prevalence of these plasma cells in secondary lymphoid tissue peaks during the first 8 to 14 days after infection, and then decreases over the next 2 to 3 weeks.[16,101,106,107,182,192,193] In the long term, virus-specific plasma cells are found at highest frequency in the bone marrow[101,192,193] (Fig. 7-2). The spectrum of Ig isotype switching can be modified in fairly predictable ways by inhibiting the function of various lymphokines.[182,201] In addition, mice that lack CD8+ T cells have been found to make more Sendai virus–specific IgA, at least in the cervical lymph nodes.[100]

IMMUNE MEMORY

Acute viral infections induce both T- and B-cell memory.[1,2,4,56] However, the nature of T- and B-cell memory is different (Fig. 7-3). Antiviral B-cell memory often is manifested by continuous antibody production even after resolution of the disease. Prolonged antibody production (lasting for decades) after infection or vaccination has been observed with many human (Table 7-1) and animal viruses. In contrast, the effector phase of the T-cell response is short-lived (a few weeks) and "memory" in the T-cell compartment results from the presence of memory T cells, which are found at higher frequencies and can respond faster and develop into effector cells (i.e., CTL or cytokine producers) more efficiently than can naive T cells.

Footprints of Memory: Humoral and Cell-Mediated Immunity

Immune memory for CD4+ and CD8+ T cells is characterized by the presence of increased numbers of precursors, usually measured in lymphoid tissue for mice and peripheral blood for humans, and enhanced expression of various "activation" markers on these lymphocytes.[4,86] Detection of CD4+ T-cell memory classically has relied on a skin test, the delayed-type hypersensitivity reaction. In humans, delayed-type hypersensitivity usually is measured 24 or 48 hours after intradermal challenge with antigen, reflecting the localization of memory T cells to the site of antigen presentation, the triggering of these cells to produce cytokines, and the recruitment of monocyte/macrophages from the blood. This response is familiar to older individuals who received multiple doses of smallpox vaccine (vaccinia virus) over the years, but now is normally encountered only by those who are given bacille

---

#Dr. Cedric A. Mims, a prominent scientist in the field of viral pathogenesis and immunity, described this as the "Oedipus assay": the direct translation of Oedipus is swollen foot!

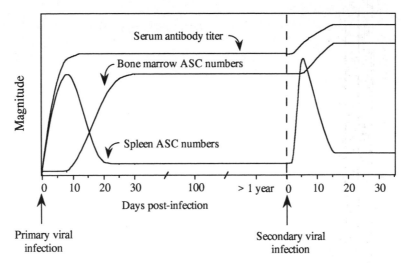

FIG. 7-2. Kinetics and anatomic site of antibody production after acute viral infection. Antibody-secreting cells (ASCs) were measured in the spleen and bone marrow after acute lymphocytic choriomeningitis virus infection of adult mice. The ELISPOT assay was used to identify individual ASCs that spontaneously secrete antiviral antibody directly ex vivo, without any in vitro restimulation. Initial antibody production occurs in the spleen, but after resolving the viral infection, the bone marrow becomes the site of long-term antibody production. After secondary viral infection, the spleen mounts a rapid but transient ASC response, and after returning to homeostasis, the bone marrow is again the predominant source of antiviral ASCs. (Adapted from Slifka MK, Matloubian M, Ahmed R. Bone marrow is a major site of long-term antibody production after acute viral infection. J Virol 1995;69: 1895–1902; and Slifka MK, Ahmed R. Long-term humoral immunity against viruses: revisiting the issue of plasma cell longevity. Trends Microbiol 1996 (in press).

Calmette-Guérin as a diagnostic indicator of exposure to tuberculosis. The protocol has been used extensively in experiments with rodents, in which investigators (at least in the mouse) give the antigen into the footpad and measure the extent of swelling 24 or 48 hours later.[#] T-cell memory is measured best by restimulating cells in culture, then determining proliferation, lymphokine release, or cytotoxicity after several days. Such techniques normally are part of research protocols rather than diagnostic applications.

Virus-specific B-cell memory usually is assayed by measuring Ig, the product of the terminally differentiated end cell of the B-lymphoid series, the plasma cell. These large secretory cells produce the Ig that is readily detected in serum, or by more tedious lavage or enrichment procedures in the respiratory tract or stools. Specific antibody is titrated easily by a range of well-established serologic techniques.

Traditionally, evidence of B-cell memory is considered to reflect established humoral immunity, whereas T-cell memory is thought of as a manifestation of cell-mediated immunity. The basis of both types of immunity is cellular, reflecting clonal expansion and differentiation from naive precursors. However, the distinction between humoral and cell-mediated immunity reflects the fact that the effectors of the B-cell response, the Ig molecules, often function at sites that are remote from where they are produced. The T cells, in contrast, make direct cellular contact, and their secreted products tend to operate at short range, requiring (at least for the CD8+ set) direct cell-to-cell contact.[56,142] Massive secretion of T-cell products induced by exposure of virally activated lymphocytes to bacterial superantigens can lead to lethal systemic shock.[183]

The Essential Difference Between T- and B-Cell Memory

The fact that T-cell products can cause shock when produced in excessive amounts[183] highlights the reason why T- and B-cell memory does not present in the same way (see Fig. 7-3). The Ig molecules themselves are not inherently damaging, although they can be the basic cause of autoimmune disease if directed at essential molecules such as the acetylcholine receptor (myasthenia gravis), at self DNA (systemic lupus erythematosus), or at viral protein[154] that is being produced constantly (some strains of mice persistently infected with LCMV). Activated T cells, in contrast, produce molecules such as lymphotoxin and tumor necrosis factor, which trigger (for example) nitric oxide production in macrophages.[208] These are toxic molecules that are optimally used sparingly to destroy invading pathogens.

The ideal situation for the recall of cell-mediated immunity is the rapid induction of memory T cells to localize to a site of virus growth and destroy virus-infected cells, but otherwise remain in an available but not effector mode. It is important to ensure that CTLp remain at high frequency, perhaps with an enhanced activation state, but do not constitutively express the molecules that are required to mediate cytotoxicity. The net consequence is that CTL effectors usually cannot be found for more than a few days after a virus is cleared. The exception is human immunodeficiency virus, which is not eliminated. Effector CTLs can be detected in blood throughout the initial phases of this infection, but eventually may be lost with the development of the acquired immunodeficiency syndrome. The complex nexus between protection, immunopathology,

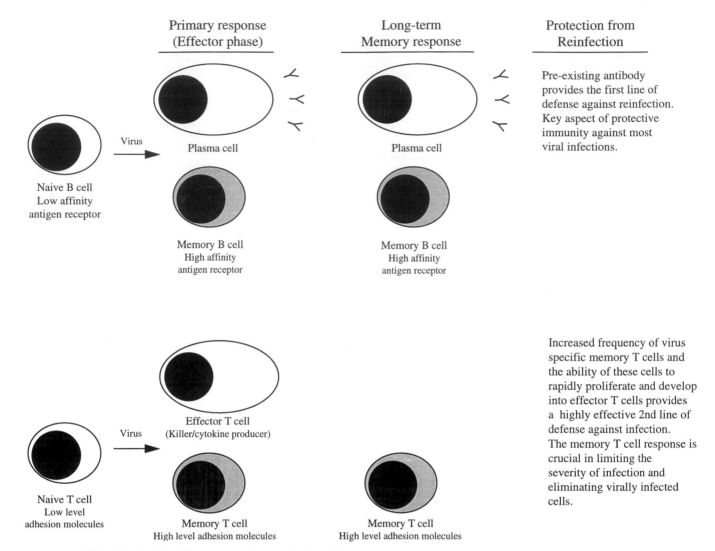

FIG. 7-3. Antiviral immunity after resolution of acute viral infection. The nature of T-cell and B-cell memory is different. B-cell memory is manifested by the presence of memory B cells and by continuous antibody production. In contrast, the effector phase of the T-cell response is short-lived, and long-term T-cell memory is due to the presence of "quiescent" antigen-specific memory T cells that are present at higher frequencies and are able to respond faster on reexposure to virus as a result of increased levels of adhesion molecules. (Adapted from Ahmed R. Virus persistence and immune memory. Semin Virol 1994;5:319–324.)

and eventual immunodeficiency is discussed elsewhere in this volume (see Chaps. 8, 10, 27, and 34).

With the antibody response, it is desirable that the Ig molecules should remain indefinitely in blood. There probably would be a good chance of preventing infections such as papillomavirus in the reproductive tract and the kissing disease (mononucleosis) caused by Epstein-Barr virus (EBV; see Modulating the Immune Response: Immune Evasion) if these mucosae could be bathed constantly in locally produced (or blood-derived) antibody. What is needed optimally from B-cell memory is the continued presence of the Ig molecule. With the CD8+ T cells, however, the requirement is for rapid recall, but no constitutive secretion of product. The situation for the CD4+ T cells is somewhat less clear at our present level of un-

derstanding. Perhaps it is desirable that they should be producing helper lymphokines for B cells, although not effector molecules such as tumor necrosis factor. However, experiments are suggesting alternative mechanisms for ensuring continued Ig production (see discussion on B Cells), and it is possible that the constraints governing CD4+ and CD8+ T-cell memory may be essentially the same.

Characteristics of the Memory Cells

The study of virus-immune memory at the cellular level historically has received remarkably little attention. Part of

TABLE 7-1. *Humoral response to acute viral infection in humans*

Example	Virus family	Serum antibody (y)	Mucosal antibody* (mo)	Reference
SYSTEMIC INFECTIONS				
ACUTE VIRAL INFECTIONS THAT ARE INTRODUCED DIRECTLY INTO THE BLOODSTREAM BY INSECT BITES, NEEDLES, ANIMAL BITES, OR INJURY				
Chikungunya	*Alphaviridae*	30		109
Rift Valley fever virus	*Bunyaviridae*	12		178
Dengue	*Flaviviridae*	32		76
Yellow fever	*Flaviviridae*	75		186
ACUTE VIRAL INFECTIONS OF MUCOSAL SURFACES THAT SPREAD SYSTEMICALLY				
Measles	*Paramyxoviridae*	65		161
Mumps	*Paramyxoviridae*	12		228
Polio	*Picornaviridae*	40		162
Hepatitis A	*Picornaviridae*	25		103
Smallpox	*Poxviridae*	40		36
Vaccinia	*Poxviridae*	15		46
Rubella	*Togaviridae*	14		164
MUCOSAL INFECTIONS				
ACUTE VIRAL INFECTIONS OF MUCOSAL SURFACES LINING THE RESPIRATORY OR GASTROINTESTINAL TRACT				
Coronavirus	*Coronaviridae*		12	37
Influenza virus	*Orthomyxoviridae*		30	104
Respiratory syncytial virus	*Paramyxoviridae*		3	91
Rotavirus	*Reoviridae*		12	47,49

*The secretory antibody response of the respiratory or gastrointestinal tract is shown. The duration of the serum antibody response after a single infection often is difficult to determine because of the high frequency of reinfection by this group of viruses. Serum antibody responses to viral respiratory and gastrointestinal infections are acquired at an early age and identified throughout adulthood.

the reason for this is that the necessary assay systems have been tedious and cumbersome to pursue or simply not available. It is easiest to summarize the situation for the different lymphocyte subsets separately.

B Cells

The analysis of B-cell memory has been greatly advanced by the application of the ELISPOT assay for determining the specificity, numbers, and spectrum of Ig isotype production for virus-specific plasma cells. Studies have established that these plasma cells tend to have a considerably higher frequency in bone marrow than in lymph nodes or spleen, being found for life in mice that have had a single virus infection as young adults.[2,101,193] The situation for lymphoid tissue in mucosal sites has received little attention from viral immunologists. The essential point about the bone marrow is that this is

the one site in the body where there is constitutive production of secreted growth and differentiation factors, necessitated by the requirement for continued hematopoiesis. Perhaps this cytokine-rich milieu favors the long-term survival of plasma cells that seeded to bone marrow at the time of, or soon after, the acute response. The broad alternative is that B-cell clones are maintaining in secondary lymphoid tissue, entering the blood, and lodging (stochastically) in bone marrow, where they differentiate to become antibody-producing cells in the presence of hematopoietic growth factors. Possible mechanisms of maintaining long-term antibody production are shown in Table 7-2.

CD4+ αβ T Cells

The nature of virus-specific CD4+ T-cell memory has received more attention for humans than for experimental ani-

TABLE 7-2. *Mechanisms of long-term antibody production*

Stimulus	Source of antibody	Comment
Reexposure to virus	Continuous differentiation	Conventional view
Persistent viral infection	of memory B cells into short-lived	
Persistent viral antigen on follicular dendritic cells	plasma cells	
Cross-reacting self or environmental antigens		
Idiotypic networks		
None	Long-lived plasma cells in the bone marrow	Possible additional mechanism

mal models, because almost all studies of specificity for human T lymphocytes start with memory cells from peripheral blood. Long-term CD4+ T-cell memory in particular has been analyzed for viruses such as measles and EBV.[194,219] Virus-specific CD4+ T cells in both cases can be induced to become CTL effectors after in vitro stimulation.

Memory CD4+ T cells in mice usually have been shown to maintain an activated L-selectin–low, CD44-high phenotype,[27,31] although this is only now receiving attention for the virus models. Relatively little has been done to measure virus-specific CD4+ T-cell memory using limiting dilution analysis techniques, and the interpretation of such assays (using lymphokine secretion) is not particularly straightforward. Most probably follow the Th1 lymphokine production phenotype characteristic of most acute virus infections, although this may change in some persistent infections (e.g., human immunodeficiency virus) under conditions of continued antigen stimulation.[44] However, where large amounts of the inducing virus continue to be present, it probably is not appropriate to describe particular antigen-specific responders as memory cells.

Hybridoma cell lines and clones that have been used to analyze specificity profiles often have been derived from the memory population.[112] In general, however, there is surprisingly little information available concerning the immunobiology of long-term, virus-specific CD4+ T-cell memory. For example, the extent to which memory CD4+ T cells are required for the maintenance of virus-specific B-cell memory (see discussion on B Cells) is not clear, although it is obvious that they are essential to promote primary and secondary B-cell responses after viral challenge.

CD8+ αβ T Cells

The dissection of CD8+ T-cell memory has benefited from the fact that the limiting dilution analysis technique for measuring virus-specific CTLp has been relatively straightforward.[115,157] This frequency analysis may not give absolute numbers, because the estimates can vary twofold to threefold from assay to assay depending on culture conditions, but it does allow the question of relative prevalence to be explored. In an otherwise specific pathogen–free C57BL mouse, for example, the frequency of naive CTLp specific for a particular class I MHC glycoprotein, (H-2D^b) the 365- to 380-nucleoprotein peptide of an influenza A virus, is less than 1 : 10^6 for the regional lymph node, increases to 1 : 2000 to 1 : 5000 within 7 to 8 days of intranasal priming, and is between 1 : 3000 and 1 : 20,000 in the spleen 2 years later, when the mouse is geriatric.[56,146] Similar prolonged survival of memory CTLp is seen in several other experimental systems, such as LCMV, vaccinia virus, and varicella zoster virus.[2,56] In the LCMV model, the presence of memory CTLp correlates with protection against secondary challenge; mice remain fully protected even 2 years after initial priming.[2,4,56,115] However, in the influenza virus system, protective immunity may wane from 4 or 5 months after initial priming.[120] What may be changing is the activation state, rather than the numbers, of the memory T cells. In culture, memory T cells are considered to require less lymphokine- and TCR-mediated signal,[32,206] and to be minimally dependent on the B7/CD28 interaction[15] that is required to drive naive precursors to become effector CTLs. Whereas

acutely stimulated influenza-specific CTLp express (for example) high levels of the α4 integrin, which is associated with the transit of lymphocytes through various epithelia, many of the T cells revert to the naive α4 integrin–low form within 5 or 6 months of priming. The memory CTLp also tend with time to express higher levels of L-selectin,[93] the molecule that promotes the passage of naive T cells into lymph nodes through the high endothelial venules. Even so, shift from the L-selectin–low phenotype associated with acute stimulation may take more than 12 months and is never absolute.

Epidemiologic evidence from human populations indicates that the heterologous protection associated with recurrent influenza A virus infection tends to wane after about 2 to 4 years.[133] Analysis of individuals who received vaccinia virus as children or young adults has provided indications that memory CTLp clones may persist as long as 50 years, although at low frequency.[51] It is probable that periodic boosting with antigen is important for maintaining effective virus-specific T-cell memory in the long term. Smallpox vaccine was given every 5 to 7 years when this virus was a threat. However, the question of the need for, and frequency of, boosting to maintain cell-mediated immunity merits repeated study with contemporary immunologic approaches.

CD4⁻8⁻α γδ and αβ T Cells, CD4+α⁻β+ T Cells, Suppressor T Cells, and Th1 and Th2 Subsets

Although both CD4⁻8⁻γδ and αβ T cells can be detected as minority subsets in the viral pneumonias, nothing is known about the characteristics of memory for either lymphocyte population.[7,8] Evidence of viral specificity has been shown convincingly for one murine γδ T-cell clone that recognizes a herpesvirus protein.[189] Hybridoma cell lines have been generated that recognize cells infected with an influenza A or B virus and also are stimulated by a heat-shock protein (HSP60). An attempt to show secondary responses for primed γδ T cells was inconclusive,[8,57] principally because measuring population sizes in the absence of a biologic effect (e.g., virus clearance) or the capacity to determine specificity is a futile exercise. The CD4+α⁻β+ T cells have been found at high prevalence in the respiratory tract of influenza virus–infected mice that have been genetically manipulated to "knock out" (−/−) the TCRα gene.[71,215] They showed no evidence of viral specificity, and can be thought of as some sort of immunologic Frankenstein monster.

There are some preliminary indications (M. Eichelberger, The Johns Hopkins University, Baltimore, MD, unpublished) that γδ T cells may be delaying the development of the primary CD8+ T-cell response to an influenza A virus. This could reflect the secretion of an inhibitory lymphokine, such as transforming growth factor-β.[203] In general, it seems that much of the early speculation about the existence of defined suppressor T-cell populations that were distinct from the more classic CD4+ and CD8+ subsets now can be explained by lymphocytes that show conventional class I or class II MHC-restricted specificity patterns, but secrete transforming growth factor-β, IL-4, IL-5 (Th2), or IL-10, rather than IL-2 or IFN-γ (Th1). How virus-specific memory is balanced between the Th1 and Th2 themes, which may be found for both CD4+ and CD8+ subsets, is unclear.

PROTECTION: SYSTEMIC VERSUS MUCOSAL IMMUNITY

Although some viruses are transmitted by biting insects (e.g., Rift Valley fever) or mammals (rabies), most enter through the mucosae. There is a fundamental difference between viruses that grow predominantly in mucosal epithelium and those that have a pathogenesis depending on systemic spread to other tissues. Examples of the former are the influenza A viruses and the parainfluenza type 1 viruses, which, at least in mammals, tend to replicate only in the superficial epithelial cells of the respiratory tract (see The Primary Response). Many other viruses classically invade through the mucosae, but cause disease as a consequence of systemic spread. Poliovirus only constitutes a problem if it enters, and destroys, motor neurons. Measles virus causes a disseminated disease.

Preexisting Antibody

Serum-neutralizing antibody is effective at limiting serum viremia, providing a virus does not continually vary its coat glycoproteins or enter the body in lymphocytes transmitted, for example, during sexual intercourse (both characteristic of human immunodeficiency virus). Such antibody may not necessarily prevent reinfection, and perhaps shedding, from the mucosal epithelium, but it does limit distal spread to key target organs and resultant disease. The consequence is that good vaccines are available for many viruses with a systemic pathogenesis, such as poliovirus and measles virus. Measles virus can transmit from cell to cell without being in the extracellular phase, which probably is the basis of the indolent spread of defective virus that occurs despite the presence of massive amounts of locally secreted Ig in the brains of children in whom subacute sclerosing panencephalitis develops[21,68] (see Chap. 36). However, measles vaccine in general has been effective, indicating that there normally is insufficient dissemination by cell-associated virus to cause a problem.

Antibody-mediated protection against a virus that grows only in superficial epithelium (and causes disease as a consequence) is clearly dependent on maintaining a sufficiently high level of virus-specific Ig at the mucosal surface. This potentially can be supplied by localized plasma cells secreting Ig within the mucosae, or from serum Ig that is at sufficiently high titer to spill across to the mucosal surface or (like IgA) is actively transported across the mucosae. There is some evidence that IgA traveling through respiratory epithelium as a consequence of attaching to the secretory piece on the vascular aspect of the cells can mediate a measure of intracytoplasmic virus neutralization.[128] Although there is a set of assumptions concerning local antibody secretion in sites such as the lung, the amount of solid information concerning the duration of plasma cell localization after (for example) a single episode of respiratory infection is limited.[106,218] As shown in Table 7-1, in contrast to long-lived serum antibody responses, mucosal antibody levels wane rapidly. It probably would be of enormous benefit for preventive medicine if better mechanisms could be developed for maintaining high levels of antibody at mucosal surfaces.

Mice that have been infected with a particular influenza A virus, or with the parainfluenza type 1 virus, Sendai virus,

seem to be substantially protected for life. The same is true for mice immunized with recombinant vaccinia viruses expressing the key viral surface proteins (hemagglutinin and hemagglutinin/neuraminidase) that are the target for neutralizing antibody.[11,73,179] Giving a substantial dose of the same virus again to primed animals causes a transient increase in the number of antibody-secreting cells in the regional lymph nodes, which usually are at minimal to undetectable levels within 3 weeks of priming, but no increase in the number of plasma cells in the bone marrow.

The situation for humans is less clear. The process of antigenic drift for the influenza A viruses leads to changes in the surface hemagglutinin such that new pandemic strains are neutralized much less readily.[226,227] However, all the potential Ig binding sites on, for example, a new variant of the H3 hemagglutinin will not have been modified. On the other hand, the parainfluenza type 1 viruses (the cause of croup in young children) do not show evidence of great antigenic variation, but infect the same children in successive years.[229] The repeated episodes are progressively less severe, but the infection also is seen in contact adults (parents) who all have well-established immunity. Increasingly, it is being realized that these viruses return again as a cause of severe disease problems in the elderly. We know that the influenza A viruses rely on antibody-mediated selection (antigenic drift) or reassortment after random, simultaneous infection of a single cell with two distinct variants (antigenic shift) to promote their survival and cause pandemics, but the strategy used by the much more conserved parainfluenza viruses remains to be deciphered.

The fact that both influenza A viruses and paramyxoviruses that grow in mucosal sites (parainfluenza virus type 1, respiratory syncytial virus) cause illness in the elderly[18,129] probably is a reflection of the general "running down" of the immune system with age. Perhaps this can be circumvented by developing better protocols for boosting immunity. Annual administration of killed or subunit influenza vaccine clearly has some benefit. A possibility worth investigating is that it will be possible to enhance protection by simultaneously administering cytokines that have an "adjuvant" effect.[130,169]

Secondary T-Cell Responses

Most of the available information on secondary virus-specific CD8+ T-cell responses has been generated for the CD8+ subset. Restimulating virus-specific CD8+ T cells usually requires that at least some cells be infected and present viral peptide through the endogenous (class I) MHC pathway. This is not necessarily the case for CD4+ T cells, which recognize peptide-class II MHC glycoprotein: the viral peptide may be derived from endosomal/lysosomal processing of complexes of viral protein with virus-specific Ig molecules. Even so, the difference between CD4+ and CD8+ T cells in this regard may be more conceptual than real. Unless there is some replication, the amount of input viral protein probably will be small. The latter situation can be modified for vaccine-boosting strategies by giving large amounts of viral protein or, for both CD4+ and CD8+ T cells, by injecting the particular viral peptides that bind the individual's class II or class I MHC molecules.

The characteristics of CD8+ T-cell memory are, as discussed earlier (see Immune Memory), that the numbers of CTLp are increased more than 30-fold, and that (at least for some months) these CTLp are much more readily recalled to effector CTL function. The net consequence is that, after secondary intranasal infection with a heterologous (no cross-neutralization) influenza A virus, the recall response to the viral nucleoprotein epitope-H-2D^b is massive.[7,9,56] The inflammatory process in the lung develops more rapidly and to a much greater level, effector CTLs are detected in the respiratory tract from day 5 rather than day 7, and the virus is eliminated 2 to 3 days earlier. The presence of primed T cells ensures a measure of protection, which also seems to operate in human populations. However, the virus still is established in the respiratory tract, and there also is the risk of enhanced immunopathology with the greater secondary response.

The idea has been entertained that the disastrous[48] 1918 to 1919 influenza pandemic (more than 6 million individuals died) could have been a consequence of immunopathology resulting from a greater T-cell response after prior exposure to a different pandemic strain of influenza virus.[60] However, reading the epidemiologic accounts that are available from that time suggests instead that any previous influenza infection was protective. Current speculation (given the unusual pattern of rapid death in otherwise fit adults) is that the acuteness of the clinical phase could reflect the interaction between virally activated CD4+ T cells and a superantigen derived from a secondary bacterial infection.[183]

The essential point about memory CD8+ T-cell responses is that the presence of an expanded pool of CTLp can only cause more rapid elimination of the pathogen. Primed CD8+ T cells, in the absence of neutralizing Ig, cannot prevent the establishment of infection. In addition, although rigorous contemporary comparisons have not been made, the general impression is that CD8+ T-cell memory is more effective at dealing with systemic infections characterized by virus growth in solid tissues[4,42,56,114,115] than in ameliorating high-dose challenge with viruses that replicate essentially in superficial mucosae.

MODULATING THE IMMUNE RESPONSE: IMMUNE EVASION

Viral genomes, particularly those of the large DNA viruses, increasingly are being found to incorporate elements that mimic genes encoding proteins involved in the normal host response.[6,82,198] EBV, for example, carries an IL-10 homolog[202,220]; high levels of IL-10 are a feature of many acute virus infections.[138,185] Vaccinia virus encodes a protein that binds IL-1.[195,199] The adenovirus E3-14.7K protein protects cells from the lethal effects of tumor necrosis factor.[83] Investigators are taking open reading frames of unknown function in EBV and probing the mammalian genome in the search for novel regulatory elements.[198] If it has been to the evolutionary advantage of this virus to assume, or copy, these host genes, it seems probable that they are biologically important. Many further examples of cytokine, or cytokine receptor, homologs are likely to be found in viruses and in more complex microorganisms. However, at this early stage, there is little insight into how such molecules function to promote the evolutionary

advantage of the virus. This area is likely to be a focus of intense study over the next 5 to 10 years.

Other viruses have evolved mechanisms that clearly have the potential to subvert immunity. The adenoviruses have several different strategies for interfering with the cell-surface expression of the peptide-class I MHC glycoprotein complexes that target effector CD8+ T cells.[230] This can lead to tumorigenesis in some animal model systems.[230]

Continued Presence of Virus Within the Host

Different viruses have evolved a variety of mechanisms for persisting within the host and transmitting vertically from mother to fetus or offspring, or horizontally to other members of the same (or different) species (see Chap. 9). Vertical transmission as a sole route of spread is largely confined to a few retroviruses, and is dealt with elsewhere in this volume (see Chaps. 11 and 26). Integrated sequences of mammary tumor viruses are the most "evolved" of such systems, having essentially become self and (as a result of expression in thymus) causing clonal deletion of cells expressing various TCRβ genes as a consequence of "superantigen" effects.[19,23] This phenomenon is of considerable interest to immunologists who are interested in the basis of immune tolerance and anergy. The effort to understand the strategies that viruses use to persist in immunocompetent hosts has revealed, and is still revealing, much about the way the immune system functions. Some of these are dealt with briefly here, the particular virus models being discussed in much greater detail elsewhere in this volume.

Lymphocytic Choriomeningitis Virus: A Virus That Has Evolved to Cause Tolerance

The key feature of LCMV (see Chap. 25) is that the virus is essentially nonlytic, and grows and is released from cells without causing any significant functional defect. This infection provides a clear example of a virus that has evolved to cause central unresponsiveness, or tolerance. Mice carry the virus through life and progeny are infected in utero. At birth, viral protein can be found in almost every tissue throughout the body, including the thymus. This is thought to cause complete T-cell unresponsiveness as a result of clonal deletion in the thymus. However, there is evidence that B-cell tolerance is incomplete, with production of antiviral Ig of a variety of subclasses being detectable in the brain,[141] and late immune-complex disease developing as a consequence of deposition of viral protein bound to Ig in the kidney glomeruli.[154]

Herpesviruses That Hide in Nonreplicating Cells

The herpesviruses are never eliminated from the body after the initial infection.[25] Herpes simplex virus is a highly lytic virus that infects and is shed from epithelia, then lies latent in nonreplicating sensory neurons. The familiar "cold sore" occurs when some form of external stress, such as sunburn or wind burn, damages the lip epithelium and causes virus that is in some sense latent in the innervating trigeminal ganglion to reactivate and transit through normal axonal flow to the lip. The virus then enters replicative cycle in the lip epithelium, leading to the transport of viral antigen (perhaps in dendritic cells or macrophages) to the regional lymph nodes in the neck. Memory herpes simplex virus–specific CD4+ and CD8+ T cells and B cells then are activated to become (at least for the CD8+ set) CTL effectors, which travel through the lymph to the blood and to the lip. This leads to the elimination of the infected epithelial cells and, with time, resolution of the lesion.

A somewhat similar situation is seen for another herpesvirus, varicella zoster virus, which causes chickenpox (usually in children) at the time of initial infection and systemic spread. The general decline in T-cell immunity that occurs with age is thought to lead to the reemergence of varicella zoster virus from sites of latency in the sympathetic ganglia, causing the painful disease known as *shingles* at the nerve endings. The pattern of the lesions tends to follow the distribution of the dermatomes. Most people recover with time, and then are protected against a further recurrence for life. Even in the elderly, boosting T-cell memory can have a powerful protective effect.

Herpesviruses That Are Maintained in Replicating Cells

The gammaherpesviruses tend to persist in T and B lymphocytes, cell populations that are commonly in replicative phase. The best-studied virus is EBV, which usually downregulates the expression of viral genes that encode proteins providing epitopes recognized by the CD8+ "surveillance" T cells.[145,150] Other gammaherpesviruses, such as the murine gammaherpesvirus 68 (GHV68), are maintained in T and B cells.[152,204] Both EBV and GHV68 can cause lymphoproliferative disease in the immunosuppressed, with EBV being a major problem in transplant recipients. This is being treated experimentally by T-cell immunotherapy, which involves growing out EBV-specific T-cell lines from the donor and giving them to the transplant recipient after immunosuppression at the time of organ or bone marrow transplantation.[89] The protocol appears to be effective, but the therapy is cumbersome.

The other major feature of the pathogenesis of the gammaherpesviruses is that they replicate in, and are shed from, mucosal epithelium.[191] In the case of EBV, this is principally the epithelium of the oropharynx. Initial infection with EBV classically results in the development of acute infectious mononucleosis, or "kissing disease" in western teenagers. The protracted confrontation between the immune system and EBV that leads to the prolonged symptoms of acute infectious mononucleosis also is apparent for GHV68 in mouse models, and is being dissected experimentally in this system.

EBV normally is associated with persistent, but low-level, shedding from epithelium in the oropharynx. That this is under immune control is shown clearly by the fact that immunosuppression, which may lead to lymphoproliferative disease, also results in enhanced viral shedding.[87] It is debated whether EBV persists in its downregulated state in the proliferating basal epithelium, entering replicative cycle in the desquamating (and nonreplicating) superficial epithelium. However,

EBV genomes have not been identified in the basal cells, and it also is possible that the virus is delivered back to the epithelial site in infected B lymphocytes.

The lifelong relationship between humans and EBV also illuminates two important characteristics of T-cell memory. The first is that, although immunosuppression may lead to escape from immune surveillance and EBV-induced lymphoproliferative disease (and solid tumors), this normally is not a problem in the elderly. It seems that the CD8+ T cells are able to control the more deleterious consequences of EBV infection well into advanced age. The second, and novel, insight is that the persistent confrontation between this virus and the immune system leads to clonal dominance in the memory T-cell population, matching a single TCR αβ pair with a particular peptide-class I MHC glycoprotein complex.[12] This clonotype, at least, is not "exhausted," in spite of decades of stimulation by the same viral epitope.

Papillomaviruses: An Epithelial Replication Strategy and Tumorigenesis

The human papillomaviruses (HPVs) that infect the reproductive tract normally are even more restricted than EBV, to a productive replication cycle in nonproliferating, desquamating epithelium.[81,156] This means that the virus is relatively, although not absolutely, protected from immune attack. There would be minimal antiviral control associated with an attack of effector CD8+ CTLs on desquamating epithelial cells, which already are dying. The virus is not synthesizing structural proteins in the basal epithelium, and is somewhat sheltered from the immune system.

It is necessary to understand why the CD8+ T cells do not operate to limit the emergence of HPV-associated oncogenesis. The obvious difference from EBV is that there is no persistence in lymphocytes, which, as a consequence of periodic reactivation in secondary lymphoid tissue, may help to maintain a high state of readiness in the T-cell surveillance system. For HPV, immediate practical questions are twofold. The first is whether appropriate T-cell peptide vaccines can be developed to limit the emergence of tumors; this is being tried with EBV, but comparatively little is known about the CD8+ T-cell response to HPV. The other possibility is that a vaccine might be developed that stimulates the production of virus-neutralizing antibody in the reproductive tract of pubescent girls; such a vaccine might prevent the initial infection of the epithelium.

Enhancing Virus Persistence: Applications in Gene Therapy

Historically, research investigators have not sought to promote the long-term presence of viruses. A change in emphasis has resulted from the desire to use viruses as vectors for gene therapy applications.[176,232] Most of the effort that has taken account of contemporary immunologic analysis has been with engineered adenoviruses to correct the defect in cystic fibrosis. This requires the delivery of large doses of nonreplicating, recombinant adenovirus to the respiratory tract, a situation that is different from the normal pathogenesis of a respiratory infection, in which comparatively small numbers of input virions replicate to cause an increasing antigenic load, and then are eliminated.

The adenovirus gene therapists face a range of potential problems, not the least of which are the high mucus content in the cystic fibrosis lung and the fact that the superficial respiratory epithelial cells do not live indefinitely. However, the main constraint is the effectiveness of the primary immune response in eliminating virus-infected cells[233] and the protective effect of antibody, which prevents entry into the epithelium after repeated challenge with the vector. Still, the experiments that are emerging from these studies are of considerable general interest. The investigators are removing components of the virus other than those essential for replication in culture, to produce adequate amounts of the vector and to permit entry of the engineered virus into the respiratory epithelium. Although the need to give large doses of virus and the requirement for viral coat proteins to package the transfected gene tend to subvert the intent of therapy, it will be intriguing to see what the analysis eventually brings forth. So far, there is no evidence that giving large amounts of killed virus intranasally or orally promotes immune tolerance, the claim that is being made for such approaches with putative autoantigens. However, the possibility has not been addressed in much detail for any virus model.

SUMMARY AND CONCLUSIONS

The vertebrate immune system in large measure has evolved to deal with pathogens, the most intimate of which are the viruses. The viruses have evolved to maximize transmission, a process that is essential for their survival.

Immunity is a function of specifically committed sets of lymphocytes, which are stimulated in specialized anatomic niches (secondary lymphoid tissue), move through different body compartments, and can lodge in a variety of tissue sites. The acute elimination of virus-infected cells normally is mediated by CD8+ killer T cells. The promotion of an effective antibody response by lymphocytes of the B-cell lineage is a function of the CD4+ T-helper cells. Common principles of clonal expansion and differentiation govern the primary responses of these three lymphocyte subsets, with the exception that the receptors expressed on the initial clonal precursors of the responding T cells do not change, whereas there is a process of affinity maturation and somatic generation of diversity in the B cells.

Immune memory reflects the continued, long-term presence of increased numbers of T- and B-cell precursors. The additional phenotype of memory for the plasma cells (the end cells of the B-lymphocyte lineage) is persistent antibody production, a prominent feature of the bone marrow that may be regarded as a constitutively activated microenvironment. The memory T cells, in contrast, do not continue to produce secreted product in the absence of further challenge. Ideally, memory T-cell populations remain at high frequency and in a partially activated state that facilitates rapid recall to effector function.

ABBREVIATIONS

CTL: cytotoxic T lymphocyte
CTLp: cytotoxic T-lymphocyte precursors
EBV: Epstein-Barr virus
HPV: human papillomavirus
IFN: interferon
Ig: immunoglobulin
IL: interleukin
LCMV: lymphocytic choriomeningitis virus
MHC: major histocompatibility complex
TCR: T-cell receptor
Th1: CD4+ T cell producing IFN-γ and IL-2
Th2: CD4+ T cell producing IL-4

REFERENCES

1. Ahmed R. Immunological memory against viruses. Semin Immunol 1992;4:105–109.
2. Ahmed R. Virus persistence and immune memory. Seminars in Virology 1994;5:319–324.
3. Ahmed R, Butler LD, Bhatti L. T4+ T helper cell function in vivo: differential requirement for induction of anti-viral cytotoxic T cell and antibody responses. J Virol 1988;62:2102–2106.
4. Ahmed R, Gray D. Immunological memory and protective immunity: understanding their relation. Science 1996;272:54.
5. Ahmed R, Salmi A, Butler LD, Chiller J, Oldstone MBA. Selection of genetic variants of lymphocytic choriomeningitis virus in spleens of persistently infected mice: role in suppression of cytotoxic T lymphocyte response and viral persistence. J Exp Med 1984;160:521–540.
6. Alcamí A, Smith GL. A soluble receptor for interleukin-1β encoded by vaccinia virus: a novel mechanism of virus modulation of the host response to infection. Cell 1992;71:153–167.
7. Allan W, Carding SR, Eichelberger M, Doherty PC. Analyzing the distribution of cells expressing mRNA for T cell receptor gamma and delta chains in a virus-induced inflammatory process. Cell Immunol 1992;143:55–65.
8. Allan W, Carding SR, Eichelberger M, Doherty PC. hsp65 mRNA+ macrophages and gammaδ T cells in influenza virus-infected mice depleted of the CD4+ and CD8+ lymphocyte subsets. Microb Pathog 1993;14:75–84.
9. Allan W, Tabi Z, Cleary A, Doherty PC. Cellular events in the lymph node and lung of mice with influenza: consequences of depleting CD4+ T cells. J Immunol 1990;144:3980–3986.
10. Alwan WH, Record FM, Openshaw PJ. Phenotypic and functional characterization of T cell lines specific for individual respiratory syncytial virus proteins. J Immunol 1993;150:5211–5218.
11. Andrew ME, Coupar BE, Boyle DB, Ada GL. The roles of influenza virus haemagglutinin and nucleoprotein in protection: analysis using vaccinia virus recombinants. Scand J Immunol 1987;25:21–28.
12. Argaet VP, Schmidt CW, Burrows SR, et al. Dominant selection of an invariant T cell antigen receptor in response to persistent infection by Epstein-Barr virus. J Exp Med 1994;180:2335–2340.
13. Askonas BA, Mullbacher A, Ashman RB. Cytotoxic T-memory cells in virus infection and the specificity of helper T cells. Immunology 1982;45:79–84.
14. Askonas BA, Taylor PM, Esquivel F. Cytotoxic T cells in influenza infection. Ann NY Acad Sci 1988;532:230–237.
15. Azuma M, Phillips JH, Lanier LL. CD28-T lymphocytes: antigenic and functional properties. J Immunol 1993;150:1147–1159.
16. Bachmann MF, Kündig TM, Kalberer CP, Hengartner H, Zinkernagel RM. How many specific B cells are needed to protect against a virus. J Immunol 1994;152:4235–4241.
17. Bender BS, Croghan T, Zhang L, Small PA Jr. Transgenic mice lacking class I major histocompatibility complex-restricted T cells have delayed viral clearance and increased mortality after influenza virus challenge. J Exp Med 1992;175:1143–1145.

18. Bender BS, Johnson MP, Small PA. Influenza in senescent mice: impaired cytotoxic T-lymphocyte activity is correlated with prolonged infection. Immunology 1991;72:514–519.

19. Beutner U, Frankel WN, Cote MS, Coffin JM, Huber BT. Mls-1 is encoded by the long terminal repeat open reading frame of the mouse mammary tumor provirus Mtv-7. Proc Natl Acad Sci USA 1992;89:5432–5436.

20. Biasi G, Facchinetti A, Panozzo M, Zanovello P, Chieco-Bianchi L, Collavo D. Moloney murine leukemia virus tolerance in anti-CD4 monoclonal antibody-treated adult mice. J Immunol 1991;147: 2284– 2289.

21. Billeter MA, Cattaneo R, Spielhofer P, et al. Generation and properties of measles virus mutations typically associated with subacute sclerosing panencephalitis. Ann NY Acad Sci 1994;724:367–377.

22. Biron CA. Cytokines in the generation of immune responses to, and resolution of, virus infection. Curr Opin Immunol 1994;6:530–538.

23. Blackman MA, Gerhard-Burgert H, Woodland DL, Palmer E, Kappler JW, Marrack P. A role for clonal inactivation in T cell tolerance to Mls-1a. Nature 1990;345:540–542.

24. Born W, Happ MP, Dallas A, et al. Recognition of heat shock proteins and gamma delta cell function. Immunol Today 1990;11:40–43.

25. Borysiewicz LK, Sissons JGP. Cytotoxic T cells and human herpes virus infections. Curr Top Microbiol Immunol 1994;189:123–150.

26. Braciale TJ. Antigen processing for presentation by MHC class I molecules. Curr Opin Immunol 1992;4:59–62.

27. Bradley LM, Duncan DD, Tonkonogy S, Swain SL. Characterization of antigen-specific CD4+ effector T cells in vivo: immunization results in a transient population of MEL-14−, CD45RB− helper cells that secretes interleukin 2 (IL-2), IL-3, IL-4, and interferon gamma. J Exp Med 1991;174:547–559.

28. Bradley LM, Watson SR, Swain SL. Entry of naive CD4 T cells into peripheral lymph nodes requires L-selectin. J Exp Med 1994;180: 2401–2406.

29. Buchmeier MJ, Welsh RM, Dutko FJ, Oldstone MB. The virology and immunobiology of lymphocytic choriomeningitis virus infection. Adv Immunol 1980;30:275–331.

30. Bucy RP, Chen CH, Cooper MD. Ontogeny of T cell receptors in the chicken thymus. J Immunol 1990;144:1161–1168.

31. Budd RC, Cerottini JC, Horvath C, et al. Distinction of virgin and memory T lymphocytes: stable acquisition of the Pgp-1 glycoprotein concomitant with antigenic stimulation. J Immunol 1987;138: 3120–3129.

32. Budd RC, Cerottini JC, MacDonald HR. Selectively increased production of interferon-gamma by subsets of Lyt-2+ and L3T4+ T cells identified by expression of Pgp-1. J Immunol 1987;138:3583– 3586.

33. Buller RML, Holmes KL, Hugin A, Fredrickson N, Morse HC III. Induction of cytotoxic T cell responses in vivo in the absence of CD4 helper cells. Nature 1987;328:77–79.

34. Burnet FM. Immunological surveillance in neoplasia. Transplant Rev 1971;7:3–25.

35. Burnet FM. Multiple polymorphism in relation to histocompatibility antigens. Nature 1973;245:359–361.

36. Burnet FM, Fenner F. The production of antibodies. Melbourne: Macmillan, 1949.

37. Callow KA, Parry HF, Sergeant M, Tyrrell DAJ. The time course of the immune response to experimental coronavirus infection of man. Epidemiol Infect 1990;105:435–446.

38. Cambier JC, Bedzyk W, Campbell K, et al. The B-cell antigen receptor: structure and function of primary, secondary, tertiary and quaternary components. Immunol Rev 1993;132:85–106.

39. Cao Y, Qin L, Zhang L, et al. Virologic and immunologic characterization of long-term survivors of human immunodeficiency virus type 1 infection. N Engl J Med 1995;332:201–208.

40. Carding SR, Allan W, McMickle A, Doherty PC. Activation of cytokine genes in T cells during primary and secondary murine influenza pneumonia. J Exp Med 1993;177:475–482.

41. Carter LL, Dutton RW. Relative perforin- and Fas-mediated lysis in T1 and T2 CD8 effector populations. J Immunol 1995;155:1028.

42. Castrucci MR, Hou S, Doherty PC, Kawaoka Y. Protection against lethal lymphocytic choriomeningitis virus (LCMV) infection by immunization of mice with an influenza virus containing an LCMV epitope recognized by cytotoxic T lymphocytes. J Virol 1994;68: 3486–3490.

43. Clarke SH, Huppi K, Ruezinsky D, Staudt L, Gerhard W, Weigert M. Inter- and intraclonal diversity in the antibody response to influenza hemagglutinin. J Exp Med 1985;161:687–704.

44. Clerici M, Shearer GM. The Th1-Th2 hypothesis of HIV infection: new sights. Immunol Today 1994;15:575–581.

45. Colman PM, Laver WG, Varghese JN, et al. Three-dimensional structure of a complex of antibody with influenza virus neuraminidase. Nature 1987;326:358–363.

46. Cooney EL, Collier AC, Greenberg PD, et al. Safety of and immunological response to a recombinant vaccinia virus vaccine expressing HIV envelope glycoprotein. Lancet 1991;337:567–572.

47. Coulson BS, Grimwood K, Masendycz PJ, et al. Comparison of rotavirus immunoglobin A coproconversion with other indices of rotavirus infection in a longitudinal study in childhood. J Clin Microbiol 1990;28:1367–1374.

48. Crosby AW. America's forgotten pandemic: the influenza of 1918. New York: Cambridge University Press, 1989.

49. Davidson GP, Hogg RJ, Kirubakaran CP. Serum and intestinal immune response to rotavirus enteritis in children. Infect Immun 1983;40:447–452.

50. Davis MM, Chien Y. Topology and affinity of T-cell receptor mediated recognition of peptide-MHC complexes. Curr Opin Immunol 1993;5:45–49.

51. Demkowicz WE Jr, Ennis FA. Vaccinia virus-specific CD8+ cytotoxic T lymphocytes in humans. J Virol 1993;67:1538–1544.

52. Doherty PC. Cell-mediated cytotoxicity. Cell 1993;75:607–612.

53. Doherty PC. Immune exhaustion: driving virus-specific CD8+ T cells to death. Trends Microbiol 1993;1:207–209.

54. Doherty PC. Vaccines and cytokine-mediated pathology in RSV infection. Trends Microbiol 1994;2:148–149.

55. Doherty PC. Immune response to viruses. In: Rich R, ed. Clinical immunology. St Louis, Mosby-Year Book, 1995:535–549.

56. Doherty PC, Allan W, Eichelberger M, Carding SR. Roles of alpha beta and gamma delta T cell subsets in viral immunity. Annu Rev Immunol 1992;10:123–151.

57. Doherty PC, Allan W, Eichelberger M, Hou S, Bottomly K, Carding S. Involvement of gamma T cells in respiratory virus infections. Curr Top Microbiol Immunol 1991;173:291–296.

58. Doherty PC, Allan JE, Lynch F, Ceredig R. Dissection of an inflammatory process induced by CD8+ T cells. Immunol Today 1990;11: 55–59.

59. Doherty PC, Effros RB, Bennink J. Heterogeneity of the cytotoxic response of thymus-derived lymphocytes after immunization with influenza viruses. Proc Natl Acad Sci USA 1977;74:1209–1213.

60. Doherty PC, Effros RB, Bennink J. Cell-mediated immunity in virus infections: influenza virus and the problem of self-non-self discrimination. In: Pollard M, ed. Perspectives in virology. 1978; 19:73–91.

61. Doherty PC, Hou S, Southern PJ. Lymphocytic choriomeningitis virus induces a chronic wasting disease in mice lacking class I major histocompatibility complex glycoproteins. J Neuroimmunol 1993; 46:11–18.

62. Doherty PC, Hou S, Tripp RA. CD8+ T-cell memory to viruses. Curr Opin Immunol 1994;6:545–552.

63. Doherty PC, Knowles BB, Wettstein PJ. Immunological surveillance of tumors in the context of major histocompatibility complex restriction of T cell function. Adv Cancer Res 1984;42:1–65.

64. Doherty PC, Reid HW, Smith W. Louping-ill encephalomyelitis in the sheep. IV. Nature of the perivascular inflammatory reaction. J Comp Pathol 1971;81:545–549.

65. Doherty PC, Tripp RA, Sixbey JW. Evasion of host immune responses by tumours and viruses. In: Chadwick, DJ, Marsh J, eds. Vaccines against virally induced cancers (Ciba Foundation Symposium 187) Chichester, NY, John Wiley. 1995:245–260.

66. Doherty PC, Zinkernagel RM. A biological role for the major histocompatibility antigens. Lancet 1975;1:1406–1409.

67. Doherty PC, Zinkernagel RM, Ramshaw IA. Specificity and development of cytotoxic thymus-derived lymphocytes in lymphocytic choriomeningitis. J Immunol 1974;112:1548–1552.

68. Dorries R, Liebert UG, Ter Meulen V. Comparative analysis of virus-specific antibodies and immunoglobulins in serum and cerebrospinal fluid of subacute measles virus-induced encephalomyelitis (SAME) in rats and subacute sclerosing panencephalitis (SSPE). J Neuroimmunol 1988;19:339–352.

69. Eichelberger M, Allan W, Carding SR, Bottomly K, Doherty PC. Activation status of the CD4⁻8⁻ gammaδ-T cells recovered from mice with influenza pneumonia. J Immunol 1991;147:2069–2074.

70. Eichelberger M, Allan W, Zijlstra M, Jaenisch R, Doherty PC. Clearance of influenza virus respiratory infection in mice lacking class I major histocompatibility complex-restricted CD8+ T cells. J Exp Med 1991;174:875–880.

71. Eichelberger M, McMickle A, Blackman M, Mombaerts P, Tonegawa S, Doherty PC. Functional analysis of the TCR αβ+ cells that accumulate in the pneumonic lung of influenza virus infected TCRα(−/−) mice. J Immunol 1995;154:1569–1576.

72. Eichelberger MC, Wang M, Allan W, Webster RG, Doherty PC. Influenza virus RNA in the lung and lymphoid tissue of immunologically intact and CD4-depleted mice. J Gen Virol 1991;72:1695–1698.

73. Epstein SL, Misplon JA, Lawson CM, Subbarao EK, Connors M, Murphy BR. β2-Microglobulin-deficient mice can be protected against influenza A infection by vaccination with vaccinia-influenza recombinants expressing hemagglutinin and neuraminidase. J Immunol 1993;150:5484–5493.

74. Ewing C, Topham D, Doherty PC. Prevalence and activation phenotype of Sendai virus-specific CD4+ T cells. Virology 1995;210:179–185.

75. Finkelman FD, Holmes J, Katona IM, et al. Lymphokine control of in vivo immunoglobulin isotype selection. Annu Rev Immunol 1990;8:303–333.

76. Fujita N, Yoshida K. Follow-up studies on dengue endemic in Nagasaki, Japan: detection of specific antibodies in serum taken more than 30 years after a single attack of dengue. Kobe J Med Sci 1979;25:217–224.

77. Fung-Leung WP, Kundig TM, Zinkernagel RM, Mak TW. Immune response against lymphocytic choriomeningitis virus infection in mice without CD8 expression. J Exp Med 1991;174:1425–1429.

78. Galvan M, Ahmed R. Lymphocytic choriomeningitis virus infection of *fas* deficient mice. J Virol (submitted 1996).

79. Gauen LKT, Kong A-NT, Samelson LE, Shaw AS. p59ᶠʸⁿ Tyrosine kinase associates with multiple T-cell receptor subunits through its unique amino-terminal domain. Mol Cell Biol 1992;12:5438–5446.

80. Gessner A, Moskophidis D, Lehman-Grube F. Enumeration of single IFN-gamma-producing cells in mice during viral and bacterial infection. J Immunol 1989;142:1292.

81. Gissmann L. Papillomavirus and human oncogenesis. Curr Opin Genet Dev 1992;2:97–102.

82. Gooding LR. Virus proteins that counteract host immune defenses. Cell 1992;71:5–7.

83. Gooding LR, Sofola IO, Tollefson AE, Duerksen-Hughes P, Wold WS. The adenovirus E3-14.7K protein is a general inhibitor of tumor necrosis factor-mediated cytolysis. J Immunol 1990;145:3080–3086.

84. Graham MB, Braciale VL, Braciale TJ. Influenza virus-specific CD4+ T helper type 2 T lymphocytes do not promote recovery from experimental virus infection. J Exp Med 1994;180:1273–1282.

85. Gray D. Understanding germinal centres. Res Immunol 1991;142:237–242.

86. Gray D. Immunological memory. Annu Rev Immunol 1993;11:49–77.

87. Hanto DW, Frizzera G, Purtilo DT, et al. Clinical spectrum of lymphoproliferative disorders in renal transplant recipients and evidence for the role of Epstein-Barr virus. Cancer Res 1981;41:4253–4261.

88. Hein WR, Mackay CR. Prominence of gamma delta T cells in the ruminant immune system. Immunol Today 1991;12:30–34.

89. Heslop HE, Brenner MK, Rooney C. Administration of neomycin resistance gene marked EBV specific cytotoxic T lymphocytes to recipients of mismatched-related or phenotypically similar unrelated donor marrow grafts. Hum Gene Ther 1994;5:381–397.

90. Holt PG. Development of bronchus associated lymphoid tissue (BALT) in human lung disease: a normal host defence mechanism awaiting therapeutic exploitation. Thorax 1993;48:1097–1098.

91. Hornsleth A, Friis B, Grauballe C, Krasilnikof A. Detection by ELISA of IgA and IgM antibodies in secretion and IgM antibodies in serum in primary lower respiratory syncytial virus infection. J Med Virol 1984;13:149–161.

92. Hotchin J. The role of transient infection in arenavirus persistence. Prog Med Virol 1974;18:81–93.

93. Hou S, Doherty PC. Partitioning of responder CD8+ T cells in lymph node and lung of mice with Sendai virus pneumonia by LECAM-1 and CD45RB phenotype. J Immunol 1993;150:5494–5500.

94. Hou S, Doherty PC. Clearance of Sendai virus by CD8+ T cells requires direct targeting to virus-infected epithelium. Eur J Immunol 1995;25:111–116.

95. Hou S, Doherty PC, Zijlstra M, Jaenisch R, Katz JM. Delayed clearance of Sendai virus in mice lacking class I MHC-restricted CD8+ T cells. J Immunol 1992;149:1319–1325.

96. Hou S, Fishman M, Gopal Murti K, Doherty PC. Divergence between cytotoxic effector function and tumor necrosis factor alpha production for inflammatory CD4+ T cells from mice with Sendai virus pneumonia. J Virol 1993;67:6299–6302.

97. Hou S, Hyland L, Ryan KW, Portner A, Doherty PC. Virus-specific CD8+ T-cell memory determined by clonal burst size. Nature 1994;369:652–654.

98. Hou S, Katz JM, Doherty PC, Carding SR. Extent of gamma delta T cell involvement in the pneumonia caused by Sendai virus. Cell Immunol 1992;143:183–193.

99. Hou S, Mo X-Y, Hyland L, Doherty PC. Host response to Sendai virus in mice lacking class II major histocompatibility complex glycoproteins. J Virol 1995;69:1429–1434.

100. Hyland L, Hou S, Coleclough C, Takimoto T, Doherty PC. Mice lacking CD8+ T cells develop greater numbers of IgA-producing cells in response to a respiratory virus infection. Virology 1994;204:234–241.

101. Hyland L, Sangster M, Sealy R, Coleclough C. Respiratory virus infection of mice provokes a permanent humoral immune response. J Virol 1994;68:6083–6086.

102. Jennings SR, Bonneau RH, Smith PM, Wolcott RM, Cervenak R. CD4+ T lymphocytes are required for the generation of the primary but not the secondary CD8+ cytolytic T lymphocyte response to herpes simplex virus in C57BL/6 mice. Cell Immunol 1991;133:234–252.

103. Jia XY, Summers DF, Ehrenfeld E. Host antibody response to viral structural and nonstructural proteins after hepatitis A virus infection. J Infect Dis 1992;165:273–280.

104. Johnson PRJ, Feldman S, Thompson M, Mahoney JD, Wright PF. Comparison of long-term systemic and secretory antibody responses in children given live, attenuated, or inactivated influenza A vaccine. J Med Virol 1985;17:325–335.

105. Joly E, Mucke L, Oldstone MB. Viral persistence in neuron explained by lack of major histocompatibility class I expression. Science 1991;253:1283–1285.

106. Jones PD, Ada GL. Influenza virus-specific antibody-secreting cells in the murine lung during primary influenza virus infection. J Virol 1986;60:614–619.

107. Jones PD, Ada GL. Persistence of influenza virus-specific antibody-secreting cells and B-cell memory after primary murine influenza virus infection. Cell Immunol 1987;109:53–64.

108. Kagi D, Ledermann B, Burki K, et al. Cytotoxicity mediated by T cells and natural killer cells is greatly impaired in perforin-deficient mice. Nature 1994;369:31–37.

109. Kanamitsu M, Taniguchi K, Urasawa S, Ogata T, Wada Y, Saroso JS. Geographic distribution of arbovirus antibodies in indigenous human populations in the indo-australian archipelago. Am J Trop Med Hyg 1979;28:351–363.

110. Kasaian MT, Leite-Morris KA, Biron CA. The role of CD4+ cells in sustaining lymphocyte proliferation during lymphocytic choriomeningitis virus infection. J Immunol 1991;146:1955–1963.

111. Kast WM, Roux L, Curren J, et al. Protection against lethal Sendai virus infection by in vivo priming of virus-specific cytotoxic T lymphocytes with a free synthetic peptide. Proc Natl Acad Sci USA 1991;88:2283–2287.

112. Kavaler J, Caton AJ, Staudt LM, Schwartz D, Gerhard W. A set of closely related antibodies dominates the primary antibody response to the antigenic site CB of the A/PR/8/34 influenza virus hemagglutinin. J Immunol 1990;145:2312–2321.

113. Kawabe Y, Ochi A. Programmed cell death and extrathymic reduction of Vbeta8+ CD4+ T cells in mice tolerant to Staphylococcus areus enterotoxin B. Nature 1991;349:245.

114. Klavinskis LS, Whitton JL, Oldstone MB. Molecularly engineered vaccine which expresses an immunodominant T-cell epitope in-

duces cytotoxic T lymphocytes that confer protection from lethal virus infection. J Virol 1989;63:4311–4316.

115. Lau LL, Jamieson BD, Somasundaram T, Ahmed R. Cytotoxic T-cell memory without antigen. Nature 1994;369:648–652.

116. Lehmann-Grube F, Lohler J, Utermohlen O, Gegin C. Antiviral immune responses of lymphocytic choriomeningitis virus-infected mice lacking CD8+ T lymphocytes because of disruption of the beta 2-microglobulin gene. J Virol 1993;67:332–339.

117. Lehrer RI, Lichtenstein AK, Ganz T. Defensins: antimicrobial and cytotoxic peptides of mammalian cells. Annu Rev Immunol 1993; 11:105–128.

118. Levine B, Hadwick JM, Trapp BD, Crawford TO, Bollinger RC, Griffin DE. Antibody-mediated clearance of alphavirus infection from neurons. Science 1991;254:856–860.

119. Levy JA. HIV pathogenesis and long-term survival. AIDS 1993;7: 1401.

120. Liang S, Mozdzanowska K, Palladino G, Gerhard W. Heterosubtypic immunity to influenza type A virus in mice: effector mechanisms and their longevity. J Immunol 1994;152:1653–1661.

121. Lightman S, Cobbold S, Waldmann H, Askonas BA. Do L3T4+ T cells act as effector cells in protection against influenza virus infection. Immunology 1987;62:139–144.

122. Liu Y, Janeway CA. Interferon gamma plays a critical role in induced cell death of effector cell: a possible third mechanism of self-tolerance. J Exp Med 1990;172:1735–1749.

123. Lynch F, Doherty PC, Ceredig R. Phenotypic and functional analysis of the cellular response in regional lymphoid tissue during an acute virus infection. J Immunol 1989;142:3592–3598.

124. Manetti R, Annunziato F, Biagiotti R, et al. CD30 expression by CD8+ CD30+ T cell clones in human immunodeficiency virus infection. J Exp Med 1994;180:2407–2411.

125. Maraskovsky E, Pech MH, Kelso A. High-frequency activation of single CD4+ and CD8+ T cells to proliferate and secrete cytokines using anti-receptor antibodies and IL-2(1). Int Immunol 1991;3: 255–264.

126. Matloubian M, Concepcion RJ, Ahmed R. CD4+ T cells are required to sustain CD8+ cytotoxic T cell responses during chronic viral infection. J Virol 1994;68:8056–8063.

127. Matzinger P. Tolerance, danger, and the extended family. Annu Rev Immunol 1994;12:991–1045.

128. Mazanec MB, Kaetzel CS, Lamm ME, Fletcher D, Nedrud JG. Intracellular neutralization of virus by immunoglobulin A antibodies. Proc Natl Acad Sci USA 1992;89:6901–6905.

129. Mbawuike IN, Lange AR, Couch RB. Diminished influenza A virus-specific MHC class I-restricted cytotoxic T lymphocyte activity among elderly persons. Viral Immunol 1993;6:55–64.

130. Mbawuike IN, Wyde PR, Anderson PM. Enhancement of the protective efficacy of inactivated influenza A virus vaccine in aged mice by IL-2 liposomes. Vaccine 1990;8:347–352.

131. McGhee JR, Mestecky J, Dertzbaugh MT, Eldridge JH, Hirasawa M, Kiyono H. The mucosal immune system: from fundamental concepts to vaccine development. Vaccine 1992;10:75–88.

132. McHeyzer-Williams MG, Davis MM. Antigen-specific development of primary and memory T cells in vivo. Science 1995;268:106.

133. McMichael A. Cytotoxic T lymphocytes specific for influenza virus. In: Oldstone MBA, ed. Cytotoxic T lymphocytes in human viral and malaria infections. Curr Top Microbiol Immunol 1994:189:75–91.

134. McWilliam AS, Nelson D, Thomas JA, Holt PG. Rapid dendritic cell recruitment is a hallmark of the acute inflammatory response at mucosal surfaces. J Exp Med 1994;179:1331–1336.

135. Miceli MC, Parnes JR. Role of CD4 and CD8 in T cell activation and differentiation. Adv Immunol 1993;53:59.

136. Michie SA, Streeter PR, Bolt PA, Butcher EC, Picker LJ. The human peripheral lymph node vascular addressin: an inducible endothelial antigen involved in lymphocyte homing. Am J Pathol 1993;143:1688–1698.

137. Miller RA, Reiss CS. Limiting dilution cultures reveal latent influenza virus-specific helper T cells in virus-primed mice. Journal of Molecular and Cellular Immunology 1984;1:357–368.

138. Mo XY, Sarawar SR, Doherty PC. Induction of cytokines in mice with parainfluenza pneumonia. J Virol 1995;69:1288–1291.

139. Moskophidis D, Assman-Wischer U, Simon MM, Lehmann-Grube F. The immune response of the mouse to lymphocytic choriomeningitis virus. V. High numbers of cytolytic T lymphoctes are generated

in the spleen during acute infection. Eur J Immunol 1987;17:937–942.

140. Moskophidis D, Lechner F, Pircher H, Zinkernagel RM. Virus persistence in acutely infected immunocompetent mice by exhaustion of antiviral cytotoxic effector T cells. Nature 1993;362:758–761.

141. Moskophidis D, Lohler J, Lehmann-Grube F. Antiviral antibody-producing cells in parenchymatous organs during persistent virus infection. J Exp Med 1987;165:705–719.

142. Mosmann TR. Directional release of lymphokines from T cells. Immunol Today 1988;9:306–307.

143. Mosmann TR, Coffman RL. Heterogeneity of cytokine secretion patterns and functions of helper T cells. Adv Immunol 1989;46:111–147.

144. Mosmann TR, Coffman RL. TH1 and TH2 cells: different patterns of lymphokine secretion lead to different functional properties. Annu Rev Immunol 1989;7:145–173.

145. Moss DJ, Burrows SR, Khanna R, Misko IS, Sculley TB. Immune surveillance against Epstein-Barr virus. Semin Immunol 1992;4:97–104.

146. Mullbacher A. The long-term maintenance of cytotoxic T cell memory does not require persistence of antigen. J Exp Med 1994;179: 317–321.

147. Muller C, Kagi D, Aebischer T, et al. Detection of perforin and granzyme A mRNA in infiltrating cells during infection of mice with lymphocytic choriomeningitis virus. Eur J Immunol 1989;19:1253–1259.

148. Muller D, Koller BH, Whitton JL, LaPan KE, Brigman KK, Frelinger JA. LCMV-specific, class II-restricted cytotoxic T cells in beta 2-microglobulin-deficient mice. Science 1992;255: 1576–1578.

149. Müller U, Steinhoff U, Reis LFL, et al. Functional role of type I and type II interferons in antiviral defense. Science 1994;264:1918–1921.

150. Murray RJ, Kurilla MG, Brooks JM, et al. Identification of target antigens for the human cytotoxic T cell response to Epstein-Barr virus (EBV): implications for the immune control of EBV-positive malignancies. J Exp Med 1992;176:157–168.

151. Nagata S, Goldstein P. The Fas death factor. Science 1995;267: 1449–1456.

152. Nash AA, Sunil-Chandra NP. Interactions of the murine gammaherpesvirus with the immune system. Curr Opin Immunol 1994;6:560–563.

153. Oehen S, Waldner H, Kundig TM, Hengartner H, Zinkernagel RM. Antivirally protective cytotoxic T cell memory to lymphocytic choriomeningitis virus is governed by persisting antigen. J Exp Med 1992;176:1273–1281.

154. Oldstone MB, Dixon FJ. Persistent lymphocytic choriomeningitis viral infection. 3. Virus-anti-viral antibody complexes and associated chronic disease following transplacental infection. J Immunol 1970;105:829–837.

155. Openshaw PJ, Clarke SL, Record FM. Pulmonary eosinophilic response to respiratory syncytial virus infection in mice sensitized to the major surface glycoprotein G. Int Immunol 1992;4:493–500.

156. Orth G, Breiburd F, Favre M, Croissant O. Papillomaviruses: possible role in human cancer. In: Hiatt HH, Watson JD, Winsten JA, eds. Cold Spring Harbor conferences on cell proliferation. Vol 4. Cold Spring Harbor Laboratory, Cold Spring Harbor, NY: 1977:1043–1068.

157. Owen JA, Allouche M, Doherty PC. Limiting dilution analysis of the specificity of influenza-immune cytotoxic T cells. Cell Immunol 1982;67:49–59.

158. Palladino G, Scherle PA, Gerhard W. Activity of CD4+ T-cell clones of type 1 and type 2 in generation of influenza virus-specific cytotoxic responses in vitro. J Virol 1991;65:6071–6076.

159. Pantaleo G, Graziosi C, Fauci AS. New concepts in the immunopathogenesis of human immunodeficiency virus infection. N Engl J Med 1993;328:327.

160. Pantaleo G, Menzo S, Vaccarezza M, et al. N Engl J Med 1995;332: 209–213.

161. Panum PL. Beobachtungen uber das Maserncontagium. Virchows Arch 1847;1:492–503.

162. Paul JR, Riiordan JT, Melnick JL. Antibodies to three different antigenic types of poliomyelitis virus in sera from North Alaskan Eskimos. Am J Hyg 1951;54:275–285.

163. Picker LJ. Control of lymphocyte homing. Curr Opin Immunol 1994;6:394–406.

164. Plotkin SA, Buser F. History of RA27/3 rubella vaccine. Rev Infect Dis 1985;7:S77–78.

165. Podack ER. Perforin: structure, function, and regulation. Curr Top Microbiol Immunol 1992;178:175–184.

166. Prabhakar BS, Saegusa J, Onodera T, Notkins AL. Lymphocytes capable of making monoclonal autoantibodies that react with multiple organs are a common feature of the normal B cell repertoire. J Immunol 1984;133:2815–2817.

167. Rager-Zisman B, Bloom BR. Immunological destruction of herpes simplex virus I infected cells. Nature 1974;251:542–543.

168. Rahemtulla A, Rung-Leung WP, Schilham MW, et al. Normal development and function of CD8+ cells but markedly decreased helper cell activity in mice lacking CD4. Nature 1991;353:180–184.

169. Ramsay AJ, Husband AJ, Ramshaw IA, et al. The role of interleukin-6 in mucosal IgA antibody responses in vivo. Science 1994;264:561–563.

170. Ramsay AJ, Ruby J, Ramshaw IA. A case for cytokines as effector molecules in the resolution of virus infection. Immunol Today 1993;14:155–157.

171. Ramsdell F, Seaman MS, Miller RE, Picha KS, Kennedy MK, Lynch DH. Differential ability of Th1 and Th2 T cells to express Fas ligand and to undergo activation-induced cell death. Int Immunol 1994;6:1545–1553.

172. Ramshaw IA. Lysis of herpesvirus-infected cells by immune spleen cells. Infect Immunol 1975;11:767–769.

173. Razvi ES, Welsh RM. Apoptosis in viral infections. Adv Virus Res 1995;45:1–60.

174. Reid HW, Doherty PC, Dawson AM. Louping-ill encephalomyelitis in the sheep. 3. Immunoglobulins in cerebrospinal fluid. J Comp Pathol 1971;81:537–543.

175. Rocha B, Von Boehmer H. Peripheral selection of the T cell repertoire. Science 1991;251:1225–1228.

176. Rosenfeld MA, Chu C-S, Seth P, et al. Gene transfer to freshly isolated human respiratory epithelial cells in vitro using a replication-deficient adenovirus containing the human cystic fibrosis transmembrane conductance regulator cDNA. Hum Gene Ther 1994;5:331–342.

177. Russell JH, White CL, Loy DY, Meleedy-Rey P. Receptor-stimulated death pathway is opened by antigen in mature T cells. Proc Natl Acad Sci USA 1991;88:2151.

178. Sabin AB, Blumber RW. Human infection with Rift Valley fever: immunity twelve years after single attack. Proc Soc Exp Biol Med 1947;64:385–389.

179. Sakaguchi T, Takao S, Kiyotani K, Fujii Y, Nakayama T, Yoshida T. Expression of the HN, F, NP and M proteins of Sendai virus by recombinant vaccinia viruses and their contribution to protective immunity against Sendai virus infections in mice. J Gen Virol 1993;74:479–484.

180. Samelson LE, Klausner RD. Tyrosine kinases and tyrosine-based activation motifs: current research on activation via the T cell antigen receptor. J Biol Chem 1992;267:24913–24916.

181. Sanchez-Pescador L, Paz P, Navarro D, Pereira L, Kohl S. Epitopes of herpes simplex virus type 1 glycoprotein B that bind type-common neutralizing antibodies elicit type-specific antibody-dependent cellular cytotoxicity. J Infect Dis 1992;166:623–627.

182. Sangster MY, Hyland L, Sealy R, Coleclough C. Distinctive kinetics of the antibody-forming cell response to Sendai virus infection of mice in different anatomical compartments. Virology 1995;207:287–291.

183. Sarawar SR, Blackman MA, Doherty PC. Superantigen shock in mice with an inapparent viral infection. J Infect Dis 1994;170:1189–1194.

184. Sarawar SR, Carding SR, Allan W, et al. Cytokine profiles of bronchoalveolar lavage cells from mice with influenza pneumonia: consequences of CD4+ and CD8+ T cell depletion. Reg Immunol 1993;5:142–150.

185. Sarawar SR, Doherty PC. Concurrent production of interleukin-2, interleukin-10, and gamma interferon in the regional lymph nodes of mice with influenza pneumonia. J Virol 1994;68:3112–3119.

186. Sawyer WA. Persistence of yellow fever immunity. Journal of Preventive Medicine 1931;5:413–428.

187. Scherle PA, Gerhard W. Functional analysis of influenza-specific helper T cell clones in vivo: T cells specific for internal viral proteins provide cognate help for B cell responses to hemagglutinin. J Exp Med 1986;164:1114–1128.

188. Scherle PA, Palladino G, Gerhard W. Mice can recover from pulmonary influenza virus infection in the absence of class I-restricted cytotoxic T cells. J Immunol 1992;148:212–217.

189. Sciammas R, Johnson RM, Sperling AI, et al. Unique antigen recognition by a herpesvirus-specific TCR-gammaδ cell. J Immunol 1994;152:5392–5397.

190. Singer GG, Abbas AK. The Fas antigen is involved in peripheral but not thymic deletion of T lymphocytes in T cell transgenic mice. Immunity 1994;1:365.

191. Sixbey JW, Nedrud JG, Raab-Traub N, Hanes RA, Pagano JS. Epstein-Barr virus replication in oropharyngeal epithelial cells. N Engl J Med 1984;310:1225–1230.

192. Slifka MK, Ahmed R. Long-term humoral immunity against viruses: revisiting the issue of plasma cell longevity. Trends Microbiol 1996 (in press).

193. Slifka MK, Matloubian M, Ahmed R. Bone marrow is a major site of long-term antibody production after acute viral infection. J Virol 1995;69:1895–1902.

194. Slobod KS, Freiberg AS, Allan JE, Rencher SD, Hurwitz JL. T-cell receptor heterogeneity among Epstein-Barr virus-stimulated T-cell populations. Virology 1993;196:179–189.

195. Smith GL, Chan YS. Two vaccinia virus proteins structurally related to the interleukin-1 receptor and the immunoglobulin superfamily. J Gen Virol 1991;72:511–518.

196. Smith TJ, Olson NH, Cheng RH, et al. Structure of human rhinovirus complexed with Fab fragments from a neutralizing antibody. J Virol 1993;67:1148–1158.

197. Sprent J, Webb SR. Function and specificity of T cell subsets in the mouse. Adv Immunol 1987;41:39–133.

198. Spriggs MK. Cytokine and cytokine receptor genes "captured" by viruses. Curr Biol 1994;6:526–538.

199. Spriggs MK, Hruby DE, Maliszewski CR, et al. Vaccinia and cowpox viruses encode a novel secreted interleukin-1-binding protein. Cell 1992;71:153–167.

200. Staats HF, Jackson RJ, Marinaro M, Takahashi I, Kiyono H, McGhee JR. Mucosal immunity to infection with implications for vaccine development. Curr Opin Immunol 1994;6:572–583.

201. Stevens TL, Bossie A, Sanders VM, et al. Regulation of antibody isotype secretion by subsets of antigen-specific helper T cells. Nature 1988;334:255–258.

202. Stewart JP, Behm FG, Arrand JR, Rooney CM. Differential expression of viral and human interleukin-10 (IL-10) by primary B cell tumors and B cell lines. Virology 1994;200:724–732.

203. Su HC, Leite-Morris KA, Braun L, Biron CA. A role for transforming growth factor-beta 1 in regulating natural killer cell and T lymphocyte proliferative responses during acute infection with lymphocytic choriomeningitis virus. J Immunol 1991;147:2717–2727.

204. Sunil-Chandra NP, Efstathiou S, Nash AA. Interactions of murine gammaherpesvirus 68 with B and T cell lines. Virology 1993;193:825–833.

205. Suzuki S, Hotchin J. Initiation of persistent lymphocytic choriomeningitis infection in adult mice. J Infect Dis 1971;123:603–610.

206. Tabi Z, Lynch F, Ceredig R, Allan JE, Doherty PC. Virus-specific memory T cells are Pgp-1+ and can be selectively activated with phorbol ester and calcium ionophore. Cell Immunol 1988;113:268–277.

207. Takahashi T, Tanaka M, Brannan C, et al. Generalized lymphoproliferative disease in mice, caused by a point mutation in Fas ligand. Cell 1994;76:969.

208. Titus RG, Sherry B, Cerami A. The involvement of TNF, IL-1 and IL-6 in the immune response to protozoan parasites. Immunol Today 1991;12:A13–A16.

209. Haas W, Pereira P, Tonegawa S. Gamma/delta cells. Annu Rev Immunol 1993;11:637–685.

210. Townsend AR, Gotch FM, Davey J. Cytotoxic T cells recognize fragments of the influenza nucleoprotein. Cell 1985;42:457–467.

211. Trentham DE, Dynesius-Trentham RA, Orav EJ, et al. Effects of oral administration of type II collagen on rheumatoid arthritis. Science 1993;261:1727–1730.

212. Tripp RA, Hou S, McMickle A, Houston J, Doherty PC. Recruitment and proliferation of CD8+ T cells in respiratory virus infections. J Immunol 1995;154:6013.

213. Tripp RA, Hou S, McMickle A, Houston J, Doherty PC. Recruitment and proliferation of virus-specific CD8+ T cells in respiratory virus infections. J Immunol 1995;154:6013–6021.

214. Tripp RA, Lahti JM, Doherty PC. Laser light suicide of proliferating virus-specific CD8+ T cells in an in vivo response. J Immunol 1995;155:3719.

215. Tsuji M, Mombaerts P, Lefrancois L, Nussenzweig RS, Zavala F, Tonegawa S. Gammaδ T cells contribute to immunity against the liver stages of malaria in αβ T-cell-deficient mice. Proc Natl Acad Sci USA 1994;91:345–349.

216. Tyor WR, Wesselingh S, Levine B, Griffin DE. Long term intraparenchymal Ig secretion after acute viral encephalitis in mice. J Immunol 1992;149:4016–4020.

217. Uehara T, Miyawaki T, Ohta K, et al. Apoptotic cell death of primed CD45RO+ T lymphocytes in Epstein-Barr virus-induced infectious mononucleosis. Blood 1992;80:452–458.

218. Ukkon P, Hovi T, von Bonsdorff C-H, Saikku P, Penttinen K. Age-specific prevalence of complement-fixing antibodies to sixteen viral antigens: a computer analysis of 58,500 patients covering a period of eight years. J Med Virol 1984;13:131–148.

219. Uytdehaag FGCM, van Binnendijk RS, Kenter JH, Osterhaus ADME. Cytotoxic T lymphocyte responses against measles virus. In: Oldstone MBA, ed. Cytotoxic T-lymphocytes in human viral and malaria infections. Curr Top Microbiol Immunol 1994;189:151–167.

220. Vieira P, de Waal-Malefyt R, Dang MN, et al. Isolation and expression of human cytokine synthesis inhibitory factor cDNA clones: homology to Epstein-Barr virus open reading frame BCRFI. Proc Natl Acad Sci USA 1991;88:1172–1176.

221. Von Boehmer H. Developmental biology of T cells in T cell-receptor transgenic mice. Annu Rev Immunol 1990;8:531–556.

222. Waldmann H. Manipulation of T-cell responses with monoclonal antibodies. Annu Rev Immunol 1989;7:407–444.

223. Walker JA, Sakaguchi T, Matsuda Y, Yoshida T, Kawaoka Y. Location and character of the cellular enzyme that cleaves the hemagglutinin of a virulent avian influenza virus. Virology 1992;190:278–287.

224. Walsh CM, Matloubian M, Liu C-C, et al. Immune function in mice lacking the perforin gene. Proc Natl Acad Sci USA 1994;91:10854–10858.

225. Webb S, Morris C, Sprent J. Extrathymic tolerance of mature T cells: clonal elimination as a consequence of immunity. Cell 1990;63:1249.

226. Webster RG, Bean WJ, Gorman OT, Chambers TM, Kawaoka Y. Evolution and ecology of influenza A viruses. Microbiol Rev 1992;56:152–179.

227. Webster RG, Laver WG, Air GM, Ward C, Gerhard W, van Wyke KL. The mechanism of antigenic drift in influenza viruses: analysis of Hong Kong (H3N2) variants with monoclonal antibodies to the hemagglutinin molecule. Ann NY Acad Sci 1980;354:142–161.

228. Weibel RE, Buynak EB, Mclean AA, Hilleman MR. Follow-up surveillance for antibody in human subjects following live attenuated measles, mumps, and rubella virus vaccines (40675). Proc Soc Exp Biol Med 1979;162:328–332.

229. Welliver RC, Ogra PL. Immunology of respiratory viral infections. Annu Rev Med 1988;39:147–162.

230. Wold WS, Gooding LR. Region E3 of adenovirus: a cassette of genes involved in host immunosurveillance and virus-cell interactions. Virology 1991;184:1–8.

231. Wong GH, Bartlett PF, Clark-Lewis I, McKimm-Breschkin JL, Schrader JW. Interferon-gamma induces the expression of H-2 and Ia antigens on brain cells. J Neuroimmunol 1985;7:255–278.

232. Yang Y, Ertl HCJ, Wilson JM. MHC class I-restricted cytotoxic T lymphocytes to viral antigens destroy hepatocytes in mice infected with E1–deleted recombinant adenoviruses. Immunity 1994;1:433–442.

233. Yang Y, Nunes FA, Berencsi K, Furth EE, Gönczöl E, Wilson JM. Cellular immunity to viral antigens limits E1-deleted adenoviruses for gene therapy. Proc Natl Acad Sci USA 1994;91:4407–4411.

234. Yewdell JW, Bennink JR. Cell biology of antigen processing and presentation to major histocompatibility complex class I molecule-restricted T lymphocytes. Adv Immunol 1992;52:1–123.

235. Zheng L, Fisher G, Miller RE, Peschon J, Lynch DH, Lenardo MJ. Induction of apoptosis in mature T cells by tumor necrosis factor. Nature 1995;377:348–351.

236. Zinkernagel R, Doherty PC. The discovery of MHC restriction. Immunol Today 1996 (in press).

237. Zinkernagel RM. Immunology taught by viruses. Science 1996;271:173–178.

238. Zinkernagel RM, Doherty PC. MHC-restricted cytotoxic T cells: studies on the biological role of polymorphic major transplantation antigens determining T-cell restriction-specificity, function, and responsiveness. Adv Immunol 1979;27:51–177.

Viral Pathogenesis,
edited by Neal Nathanson, et al.
Lippincott–Raven Publishers, Philadelphia © 1997

CHAPTER 8

Virus-Induced Immunopathology

Rolf M. Zinkernagel

INTRODUCTION

Protection by immune mechanisms is often accompanied by immunopathology. In cases in which neutralizing antibodies can efficiently mediate protection, immune complex disease can be induced and eventually cause illness. Alternatively, antivirally active CD8+ cytotoxic T lymphocytes (CTLs) protect by destroying virus-producing host cells, optimally during the eclipse phase of virus infection.[102] The balance between the extent and kinetics of virus spread and the kinetics of the immune response directly determine the outcome of infections with cytolytic viruses (Table 8-1). Unimpaired virus growth destroys too many host cells by viral cytolysis and results in disease and death. Infected hosts survive such cytolytic viruses only if immunosurveillance is efficient. For noncytopathic viruses, the situation is quite different; the virus alone does not cause pathology or disease, and the survival of both the virus and the host do not depend on efficient immunosurveillance.

It seems that there are viruses that can shift from a noncytolytic to a cytolytic phenotype within a herd of cattle (e.g., bovine viral diarrhea virus [BVDV])[15]; this illustrates that the varied interplay between viruses and the immune system. Although vaccines can reduce disease incidence by 100- to 10,000-fold, rare vaccinees who are not protected may reveal forms of diseases favored by vaccination.[1,81,83] When discussing the variable nature of virus-host and host-immunity interactions, it must be emphasized that nature uses major pathways and that generalizations are therefore possible.

Several specific viruses that cause immunopathology are discussed in detail in this book; this chapter attempts to outline the general aspects of the immune system, the immune response, and antiviral immunity resulting in pathology, bearing in mind that immunopathology is usually only a minor aspect of immunoprotection, and that information in this field is evolving rapidly.

R. M. Zinkernagel: University Hospital, Department of Pathology, Institute for Experimental Immunology, University of Zurich, CH-8901 Zurich, Switzerland.

TABLE 8-1. *Effects of antiviral cytotoxic T cells*

	Protection	Immunopathology
Cytopathic viruses	+++	Not noticeable
Noncytopathic viruses		
Limited spread	++	±
Widely spread or in essential organs or cells	+	+++
Putative unknown noncytopathic viruses	Not noticeable	+++

± to +++, relative frequencies of the observed phenotype (±, relatively rare, +++, relatively frequent.)

GENERAL IMMUNOLOGIC CONSIDERATIONS

Cellular Versus Humoral Immunity to Viruses

Cellular immunity is mediated mainly by T cells that act locally by way of contact in solid tissue. The specific humoral immune response is expressed by B cells, whose induction generally depends on T helper cells. Antibodies, the biologically active products of B cells, multiply the effector units of one B cell more than 100,000 times. In both T cells and antibodies, uniform and stereotyped mechanisms are focused on the site where the foreign antigen is present. Whereas T cells recognize antigen only when associated with specialized cell surface molecules, B cells may recognize cell surface antigens but are most efficient against soluble antigens. The induction and triggering of effector mechanisms of T cells is guided by way of their specificity for self major histocompatibility complex (MHC) products and by way of accessory molecules. Antibody effector function is mediated through the constant portion, which either binds to Fc receptors (e.g., IgE on mast cells or basophils) or binds C1q, initiating the complement cascade. Therefore, effector functions triggered by way of T-cell or antibody recognition are similar; both link specificity for foreign antigenic determinants with stereotyped receptors and signal cascades for mediating effector functions.

A major problem in the purely analytical approach to immunology, and to the study of viruses, is that immunologic specificity is relative. Specificity of antibodies can be adequately defined by association constants. Although an anti-A antibody may bind to A only 100 to 1000 times better than to B, there is usually no dispute that this antibody, particularly in concert with the rest of the complex anti-A immune response, is specific against A. Because T-cell receptor binding cannot yet be measured quantitatively to any comparable extent,[91] it is important not to overinterpret experimental results in which T-cell responses measured in vitro are often interpreted on a simple plus-minus scale. Differing specificities of T and B cells also reflect topographic characteristics of antigens on cell surfaces, where virally induced antigens usually trigger immune responses. T cells recognize processed epitopes bound by self MHC,[13,95,105] whereas B cells recognize unprocessed three-dimensional antigenic determinants. Calculations evaluating the access of antibody to determinants on influenza virus hemagglutinins suggest that antibody may interact with distal (more variable) determinants but not with the proximal (constant) ones, mainly because of simple space restrictions.[26] Therefore, the relative topography of viral determinants on both infected cells and on virus particles may directly determine B-cell immune responses and specificity. The antigenic structure and topography of relevant viral antigens may co-evolve and be molded by the immune system to permit survival of both viruses and vertebrate hosts.

Role of Antigen and Its Localization in Inducing and Driving an Immune Response

For most antigens, viral determinants must be appropriately expressed by antigen-presenting cells to induce T-cell responses[61,92]; if this is not the case, no immune response is induced (Table 8-2). Viruses that induce an early and efficient CD8+ T-cell response tend to infect antigen-presenting cells, including macrophages, whereas viruses that first replicate in epithelial, mesenchymal, or neuronal cells (e.g., rabies virus[8,82,96]) and are generally poorly cytopathic (e.g., some papillomaviruses)[94] do not induce a measurable or protective immune response.

The more widely spread the antigen is, the more serious may be the consequences of immune reactivities by way of immunologic destruction or indirectly, through inflammation triggered by immune effector mechanisms. For cytopathic viruses, any limitation of virus spread is beneficial to the host; spread cannot really be stopped early enough to limit pathology. For noncytopathic viruses, the more the virus spreads, the more serious will be the pathologic consequences of immune reactions. The longer the immunogenic antigen persists, the more extensive is the immunopathologically caused damage.

Cell-Mediated Effector Mechanism

T cells are instrumental in early antiviral immunity and often determine recovery from viral infections. Their role in protection against reinfection in the primed host is less clear. Infants with severe combined T- and B-cell immunodeficiency (SCID) or thymus or T-cell deficiency alone are dramatically more susceptible to viral infections. Studies in mice

TABLE 8-2. *Viral antigens and antigen-presenting cells*

Antigen distribution	Immune response	Examples
Antigen not on APC, not in lymphoid organ	Indifference (none or minimal)	Rabies virus in neurons Papillomavirus in keratinocytes LCMV in kidney tubular cells
Antigen on few APC in lymphoid organ	Induction (optimal)	Smallpox virus Vaccinia virus LCMV
Antigen on all APC everywhere	Exhaustion (tolerance)	Hepatitis B virus LCMV

APC, antigen-presenting cells; LCMV; lymphocytic choriomeningitis virus.

that are thymus deficient, T-cell deficient, or both (e.g., nude mice[17]; SCID mice; mice depleted of T cells by thymectomy, irradiation, and reconstituted with bone marrow[14]; by treatment with antisera or specific monoclonal antibodies against cell determinants on immunologically important cells[51,58]; or by homologous recombination [gene knockout mice][30,38,60,77]) have confirmed these observations and defined the defects and their consequences more precisely.

Experiments in the early 1970s have shown that T cells are essential for recovery from several viruses. When in vitro cytotoxicity assays that were developed for transplantation immunology[19] were applied to viral immunology, it became obvious that antiviral protection in vivo often correlated with the capacity of T cells to lyse infected but not uninfected or third-party virus–infected target cells in vitro.[53,71] Antiviral CTL responses usually follow virus replication by a few days[14] (Fig. 8-1) and become measurable by 5 to 8 days after spread of the virus to the lymph nodes or spleen.[14] At about the time when T cells can be detected in a direct cytotoxicity test, viral titers usually start to decrease. By the time virus titers are no longer measurable (about 2 to 4 days later), CTL activity declines rapidly, below levels necessary for detection in short-term cytolysis assays.[14,104] Spleen or lymph node cells from virus-immunized animals do, however, regularly respond to restimulation in vivo and in vitro by mounting an accelerated CTL response; this is a direct reflection of increased CTL precursor (CTLp) frequencies.

Not all viruses induce CTL responses to the same extent. For example, CTL responses against herpesvirus and cytomegalovirus are poor, whereas mousepox or lymphocytic choriomeningitis virus (LCMV) induce excellent, strong CTL responses that are detectable early, on day 6 to 10 postinfection in spleen cells directly ex vivo. These latter activities are far greater (>100-fold) than any of the class I MHC-specific CTL alloresponses that have been observed. Because of these great activities of CTLs, analysis of their reactivity and specificity was relatively easy. These studies revealed that antiviral CTLs exhibit a dual specificity for both viral and self MHC class I (MHC restriction)[105] and helped define rules of positive selection for self-recognition of CTLs in the thymus.[104]

Virus replication and spread in antigen-presenting cells and in lymphoid organs is essential for the induction of potent T-cell responses. It is likely that only under these circumstances are enough interleukins, some forms of T help, and organized intercellular contacts properly provided.

The extent to which specific CD4+ T help is needed for the induction of antiviral CTLs is subject to the same variables that determine CD8+ T-cell induction. CD4+ T-cell–depleted mice or CD4−/− knockout mice respond nearly as well as CD4+ T-cell–competent mice by generating a powerful CTL response if the virus replicates optimally in lymphohemopoietic cells.[51,77] For other usually less replicating and less virulent viruses, T help seems more important

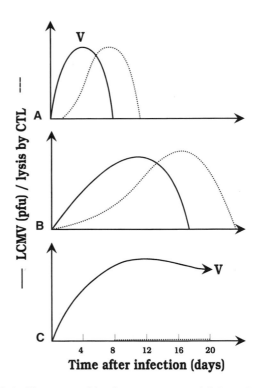

FIG. 8-1. Noncytopathic viruses may establish various balanced states with a host. (**A**) Virus that replicates poorly and induces a rapid CD8+ T-cell response is eliminated rapidly, and immunopathologic damage is limited. (**B**) If virus spreads widely and the T-cell response occurs too late, immunopathologic damage is extensive. (**C**) If T-cell responses are absent, no CD8+ T-cell mediated immunopathology results.

(e.g., vesicular stomatitis virus [VSV], influenza virus, vaccinia, Sendai virus).

Destruction of Infected Host Cells by T Cells

Antiviral CTLs exert their effector function by direct T-cell–mediated lysis[42,48,106] or by way of interleukins.[46,80] The straightforward view is that CTLs recognize relevant class I presented antigen during the eclipse phase of virus infection before virus is assembled; therefore, destruction of the virus-replicating cell also destroys the virus. Experiments in vitro support this view by showing that co-incubation of CTLs with freshly infected target cells results in drastic reduction of virus titer yields[102]; however, if CTLs are added to infected target cells at a time when infectious progeny have already been assembled, antiviral effects are minimal during this particular round of infection. The implication is that during the next round of replication, the effector CTLs will efficiently catch up with the virus. In the case of noncytolytic viruses, CTL-mediated lysis of persistently infected target cells stop the virus from replicating further.

Cytolysis has been thought to reflect activation of lytic enzymes, including perforin and phosphatases released from CTLs, intracellular activation of target cell endonucleases, causing internal disintegration of the nucleus, or some combination of these mechanisms. Studies with mice lacking the perforin gene (deleted by homologous recombination) demonstrated unequivocally that perforin is a key limiting factor in MHC-restricted CD8+ T-cell–mediated target cell lysis in vitro and in vivo against virus-infected target cells, class I

MHC-allogenic target cells, and NK-susceptible targets (Fig. 8-2).[42] There is some lysis against selected target cells that is mediated via the Fas ligand.[12,43,55] Additional mechanisms of CD8+ T-cell–mediated antiviral action, particularly against cytopathic viruses, include release of interferons or other antiviral interleukins such as tumor necrosis factor, to which the infected target cells may be sensitive.

IMMUNE PROTECTION VERSUS IMMUNOPATHOLOGY

Immune T cells function to eliminate cytopathic viruses or intracellular bacteria; in general, they fulfill this task well. After the infectious agents and their antigens are eliminated, the immune responses quickly fade. Rapid increase in the concentration of foreign antigen on specialized cells (i.e., macrophages, antigen-presenting cells, follicular dendritic cells) is sufficient stimulus to provoke a T-cell– or B-cell–mediated immune response; elimination of antigens suffices to stop the immune response. Thus, for acute infectious agents, it is not necessary to invoke sophisticated suppressor cells or cellular circuits to regulate an immune response.

However, some viruses—maybe most—are not acute cytopathic agents; such viruses or bacteria are not highly virulent, and infected hosts may survive independent of the immune response. Such agents may be able to infect immunodeficient hosts or may survive in any host for a long time without causing disease or death. Hepatitis B virus (HBV) infections in humans or LCMV infection in mice (Fig. 8-3 through 8-5) serve as examples of such agents.[23,27,74,106] The majority (>90%) of in-

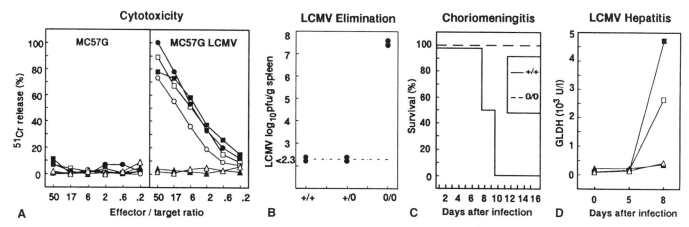

FIG. 8-2. Antiviral protection and immunopathology in mice lacking a functional perforin gene (o/o,). Their effector CD8+ T cells (**A**) cannot lyse infected target cells in vitro, (**B**) cannot eliminate lymphocytic choriomeningitis virus (LCMV) from the spleen, and do not cause (**C**) lethal choriomeningitis or (**D**) hepatitis. (**A**) Cytotoxicity: 8d immune spleen cells were assayed in a 5-hour ^{51}Cr-release assay on H-2 compatible normal or infected target cells. Spleen cells were from perforin +/+ (o,●), +/o (□,■), or o/o (△,▲) mice. (**B**) LCMV elimination: mice were intravenously infected with 2 × 10² plaque-forming units (PFU), and titers were determined on day 12. (**C**) Choriomeningitis: perforin +,+ or o/o mice were infected intracerebrally with 10² PFU of a neurotropic LCMV. (**D**) LCMV hepatitis: perforin +/+ (□,■) or o/o (△,▲) mice were intravenously infected with 10⁵ PFU of a hepatotropic LCMV. Glutamate dehydrogenase (GLDH) values (a measure of liver destruction and dysfunction) were determined in the serum at the times indicated. (From Kägi D, Ledermann B, Bürki K, et al. Cytotoxicity mediated by T cells and natural killer cells is greatly impaired in perforin-deficient mice. Nature 1994;369:31–37.)

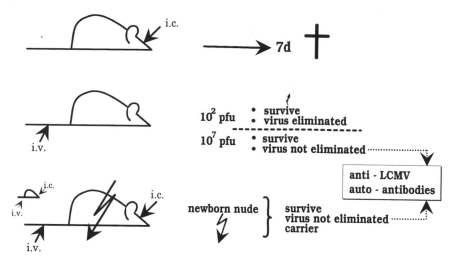

FIG. 8-3. The various virus-host relations between lymphocytic choriomeningitis virus (LCMV) and mice. Mice die 6 to 10 days after intracerebral (i.c.) infection of adult immunocompetent hosts. After intravenous (i.v.) infection with low doses, LCMV is usually eliminated, and mice survive. After infection with high doses of LCMV or certain lymphotropic LCMV isolates, mice survive but fail to clear virus and eventually become virus carriers. If T-cell incompetent mice (e.g., thymus-deficient nude mice, fetuses or newborn mice, irradiated or immunosuppressed mice; *jagged arrows*) are infected, LCMV is not eliminated, and mice become virus carriers. Carrier mice may develop immune complex disease if the antibody response to LCMV is not completely impaired. Such split tolerance (i.e., B-cell responses without obvious T-cell responses) is seen under certain experimental conditions in laboratory mice, but rarely is seen after transplacental infection of wild mice (Data from references 16, 37, 49, and 104.)

fected hosts generate a potent immune response, eliminate the infectious agent efficiently and rapidly, and therefore show no or few symptoms. The few hosts lacking an effective immune response become virus carriers (e.g., HBV carriers, LCMV carriers, polar lepromatous leprosy patients). In a few infected hosts, immune effector mechanisms cannot quite eliminate the infectious agent, and the persistent conflict between immunity and infection results in immunopathologic damage (e.g., aggressive hepatitis, virus-induced wasting disease, tuberculoid leprosy.)

CD8+ T-Cell–Mediated ("Aggressive") Hepatitis

Classic examples of infections with noncytopathic viruses are lymphocytic choriomeningitis (see Fig. 8-3) in mice and hepatitis B in humans. Lymphocytic choriomeningitis in mice develops only in immunocompetent animals; after intracerebral injection of LCMV, mice develop lethal choriomeningitis, after intravenous infection, hepatitis may develop. Mice lacking T cells or those immunosuppressed by irradiation or cytostatic drugs do not develop inflammatory reactions or lymphocytic choriomeningitis, but they fail to eliminate the virus and as a result become LCMV carriers. Lymphocytic choriomeningitis has been carefully analyzed and has been shown to be T-cell mediated.[21] Lethal lymphocytic choriomeningitis apparently depends on effector T cells being preferentially recruited to the acutely infected leptomeninges or liver. The resulting LCMV-induced hepatitis (see Figs. 8-4 and 8-5) in mice has been monitored histologically and by the determination of changes in serum levels of aminotransferases and alkaline phosphatase (see Fig. 8-4). The kinetics of histologic disease

manifestations, increases of liver enzyme levels in the serum, and CTL activities in liver and spleen correlate and are dependent on several parameters, such as the LCMV isolate, the virus dose and route of infection, and the general genetic background of the murine host. The degree of immunocompetence is also important in that T-cell–deficient nu/nu mice never develop hepatitis, whereas nu/+ or +/+ mice always do.[106]

Because the major transplantation antigens generally bind foreign antigen fragments specifically and thus determine whether a T-cell response is efficiently induced, the MHC haplotype may drastically influence the balance between virus and immune-mediated tissue damage (see Fig. 8-5). Among many other variables characteristic for either the virus or the host, severity of disease has been shown to be determined by major transplantation antigens in both HBV infections in humans[74] and in LCMV infections in mice.[50]

These examples suggest that if the causative infectious agent is not known, it may often be difficult to distinguish between autoimmunity and virus-induced immunopathology, because phenotypically, both are similar if not identical. This factor has led to the proposal that unbalanced T-cell responses to known infectious agents may be called immunopathologic, whereas those against unknown or unrecognized agents may be falsely called autoimmune.[108] In addition, viral and host self-antigens exclusively expressed by nonlymphohemopoietic cells and outside of lymphoid organs are usually ignored by T cells.[68] If such antigens themselves, or cross-reactive (i.e., "mimicking") determinants, reach proper antigen-presenting cells in lymphoid organs in sufficient quantities, an immune response may be triggered that causes immunopathology or autoimmunity (discussed later).

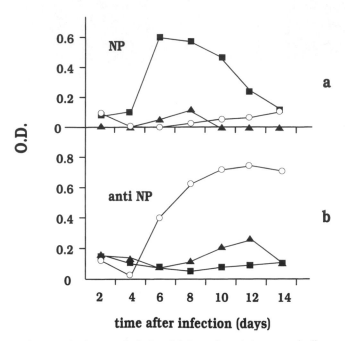

time after infection (days)

FIG. 8-4. Release of viral cell internal protein as an indicator of destruction of infected host cells by antiviral CD8+ T cells. Serum samples of mice infected with lymphocytic choriomeningitis virus (LCMV) WE strain and either injected with CD4-depleting antibodies (■) or anti-CD4 and -CD8– depleting antibodies (▲) or left untreated (○) were tested by enzyme-linked immunosorbent assay (ELISA) to detect LCMV nucleoprotein (NP; a) and by a second ELISA to detect antibodies against NP (b). Optical Density (O.D.) values at a serum dilution of 1 : 2 in a and 1 : 30 in b are shown, with the O.D. of normal serum (0.174) subtracted as background. Because antibodies against LCMV NP prevent detection by ELISA of released NP in serum samples, anti-CD4 treatment was necessary to render possible the demonstration of NP released into blood.

Virus-Triggered Immunosuppression by T-Cell–Mediated Immunopathology

Another example of T-cell–mediated immunopathologic disease is acquired immunosuppression triggered by LCMV.[5,39,52,57,64,100] It has been known for some time that LCMV causes immunosuppression in mice. When this fact was reevaluated, it was found that LCMV suppressed the capacity to mount an IgM or IgG response to VSV (Fig. 8-6). LCMV also rendered mice considerably more susceptible to VSV, which does not replicate extraneuronally in adults and is usually nonpathogenic if injected subcutaneously or intravenously. The extent of immunosuppression by LCMV depends on the virus isolate, the mouse strain, and the MHC haplotype.

The following experimental results suggest that the antiviral T-cell response was responsible for immunosuppression. LCMV carrier mice were found to mount anti-VSV IgM and IgG or antivaccinia virus CTL responses comparable to those of normal control mice. T-cell–deprived nude mice infected with LCMV also had normal IgM responses. This indicated that LCMV alone is not immunosuppressive and that the ob-

served immunosuppression is not caused by the action of interferons on VSV. In contrast, LCMV-infected nude mice inoculated with LCMV immune CTLs exhibited suppressed antibody responses. Additionally, whereas LCMV-infected mice failed to exhibit an anti-VSV IgG antibody response, similarly infected mice treated with anti-CD8 antisera at the time of LCMV infection mounted normal IgM and IgG responses. These results are compatible with the view that antiviral CTLs are responsible for immune suppression in this model of infection. LCMV infects many macrophages or antigen-presenting cells (Fig. 8-7)[5,64] involved in anti-VSV antibody responses; these infected cells are in turn destroyed by anti-LCMV–specific CTLs (see Fig. 8-7).

Impairment of antigen presentation may dampen the antibody response against the triggering virus itself if the antiviral CD8+ T-cell response is generated quickly enough to reduce or stop antigen presentation to T-helper cells or B cells. The neutralizing antibody response against LCMV seems to be at least partially prevented or delayed by this mechanism (Fig. 8-8).[11]

It is possible that a mechanism similar to that described previously may contribute to the development of acquired immunodeficiency syndrome after human immunodeficiency virus (HIV) infection (Fig. 8-9).[107] There is no evidence as yet that HIV is cytolytic in vivo; therefore, CD8+ effector T cells may be responsible for eventually reducing the great number of HIV-infected CD4+ T cells, as well as HIV-infected macrophages and antigen-presenting cells. Because of the progressive destruction of antigen-presenting cells, CD4 T cells may

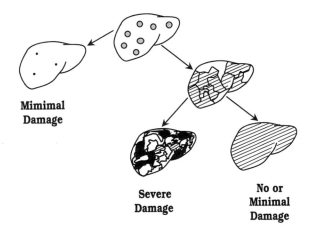

FIG. 8-5. Role of MHC in causing virus-induced T-cell–mediated immunopathology, as exemplified by lymphocytic choriomeningitis virus (LCMV) or hepatitis B virus. Damage of hepatitis B virus–infected or LCMV-infected liver cells is caused by virus-specific cytotoxic T cells. If the immune response is excellent (high responder), replication and spread of virus is halted quickly; only limited tissue damage occurs, with recovery within 3 weeks (*left*). If there is no T-cell response (nonresponder), the virus spreads throughout the liver but does not cause damage because it is noncytopathic; the host will become a virus carrier (*bottom, right*). If there is a low and slow T-cell response (low responder), the immune response will kill the many liver cells infected by virus and cause substantial destruction of liver tissue, possibly resulting in aggressive hepatitis (*lower center*). *Hatched areas,* virus infection; *black areas,* cellular damage.

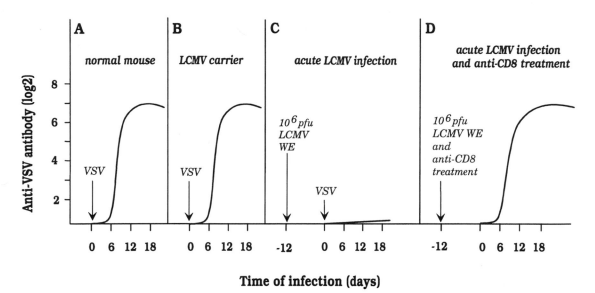

Time of infection (days)

FIG. 8-6. Immune suppression by lymphocytic choriomeningitis virus (LCMV) is not caused by the virus itself but rather by the cytotoxic T-cell response against the virus. **(A)** Normal mice or **(B)** neonatally induced LCMV carrier mice that are immunologically tolerant to LCMV show a normal immune response to vesicular stomatitis virus (VSV). **(C)** LCMV may cause severe immunosuppression in infected mice if the antibody response against VSV is assessed 8 to 10 days after LCMV infection was initiated. **(D)** If acutely LCMV-infected mice are depleted of antiviral cytotoxic T cells by treatment with nonclonal antibody against CD8+ T cells in vivo, the antibody response to VSV is within the normal range. These findings indicate that LCMV–specific cytotoxic T cells destroy LCMV-infected antigen-presenting cells and thus prevent an immune response from being generated. (Data from references 52 and 64.)

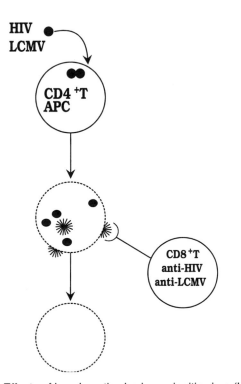

FIG. 8-7. Effects of lymphocytic choriomeningitis virus (LCMV) or human immunodeficiency virus (HIV) infection on CD4+ T cells or antigen-presenting cells (APC). LCMV and HIV are noncytopathic; therefore, they destroy the CD4+ T cells and macrophages or APCs indirectly by infecting APCs, which are then destroyed by antiviral CD8+ T cells (i.e., by immunopathology). (Adapted from references 101 and 107.)

be hampered indirectly by deprivation of growth factors and proper stimulation (see Fig. 8-7). In addition, reduction of monocytes/macrophages has severe consequences for host resistance against many intracellular parasites.

Autoantibody Responses Induced by Immunopathologic T-Cell Help

A T-cell–mediated immunopathologic mechanism comparable to the virus-triggered immunopathology may explain induction of autoantibodies. Tolerance and responsiveness of B cells was studied in transgenic mice expressing VSV-Indiana glycoprotein (Fig. 8-10). When immunized with purified VSV-Indiana glycoprotein mixed with a strong adjuvant, these mice failed to produce IgG antibodies with VSV-Indiana–neutralizing activity[7,89,103]; they also failed to respond to infection with a vaccinia recombinant virus encoding the VSV-Indiana glycoprotein. However, after infection with VSV-Indiana wild-type virus, the VSV transgenic mice promptly mounted an IgG autoantibody response, evidenced by neutralizing antibody against the VSV glycoprotein. The response to the membrane-associated viral antigen demonstrates that reactive B cells have not been eliminated in these VSV-Indiana glycoprotein transgenic mice. Some of the B cells can be induced to produce IgG if direct contact–mediated T-cell help to a linked new helper determinant is provided by other VSV proteins. In this model, unresponsiveness of B cells is maintained by the absence of T help, a concept that has been previously documented as "split tolerance" in LCMV,[37,49,86] lactate dehydrogenase virus (LDV) and retrovirus-infected carrier mice.[70,93] These circumstances

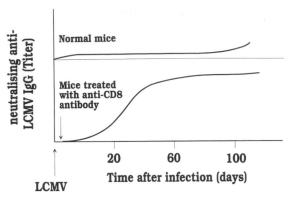

FIG. 8-8. Inhibition of lymphocytic choriomeningitis virus (LCMV)-specific neutralizing antibody responses by CD8+ T cells causes immunopathologic damage of lymphohemopoietic tissues. Whereas normal mice generate neutralizing antibodies to LCMV very slowly, if at all, treatment of mice with anti-CD8 antibodies, which impair the antiviral cytotoxic T-cell response, enhances generation of neutralizing antibodies, despite the fact that virus elimination is also impaired. (Data from references 11 and 101.)

	Anti-VSV-G$_{IND}$ Antibodies		
Immunogen	IgM	IgG	T help (specificity)
G purified + adjuvant	—	—	—
G-carrier protein x	—	++	+ (anti-X)
VSV IND$_{wt}$	++	++	+ (anti NP or M)
vacc-G$_{IND}$	±	—	—

FIG. 8-10. Induction of autoantibodies against a new self-antigen (VSV-G$_{IND}$) introduced as a transgene. Mice expressing VSV-G$_{IND}$ under various promoters as self-antigen were immunized with the indicated immunogens. Neutralizing antibody titers against VSV-IND were monitored on day 4 for IgM and on day 12 for IgG. The specificity of the necessary T help is indicated. G, glycoprotein of vesicular stomatitis virus, Indiana strain; M, matrix protein; NP, nucleoprotein; vacc-G$_{IND}$, recombinant vaccinia virus expressing G$_{IND}$; VSV, vesicular stomatitis virus; VSV$_{IND}$, vesicular stomatitis virus, Indiana strain; wt, wild-type virus. (Data from references 7, 89, 101, and 103.)

may also be associated with chronic immunocomplex disease (Table 8-3).

ANTIBODY-MEDIATED IMMUNOPATHOLOGY TRIGGERED BY VIRUSES

Autoantibodies and Viral Infections

The detection of autoantibodies in certain virus infections has encouraged speculation about the possible role of

viruses and other infectious agents in antibody-dependent autoimmunity.[34,93] The following mechanisms have been proposed:

Viruses mimic structures of self antigen and induce anti-self–reactive antibodies of potential pathogenicity.[63,69]

Because T helper cells usually are tolerant for autoantibody induction, the necessary reactive T help must be brought in by way of a linked foreign "carrier" determinant.[98] Cells infected by cytolytic viruses form cell membrane fragments juxtaposing self antigens with viral antigens; these frag-

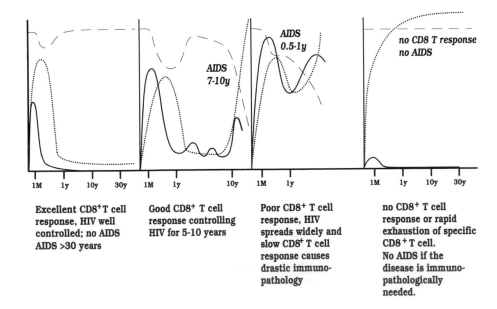

Excellent CD8+ T cell response, HIV well controlled; no AIDS AIDS >30 years

Good CD8+ T cell response controlling HIV for 5-10 years

Poor CD8+ T cell response, HIV spreads widely and slow CD8+ T cell response causes drastic immunopathology

no CD8+ T cell response or rapid exhaustion of specific CD8+ T cell. No AIDS if the disease is immunopathologically needed.

FIG. 8-9. Explanation for the various disease phenotypes caused by human immunodeficiency virus (HIV), with the assumption that HIV is noncytopathic. From left to right, HIV replication is controlled well (*left*) by potent CD8+ T-cell responses or not (*right*) because CD8+ T cell responses are absent or exhausted. *Dotted line*, HIV; *solid line*, CD8+ T cells anti-HIV; *dashed line*, antigen-presenting cells (APC) and CD4+ T cells; AIDS, acquired immunodeficiency syndrome. (Adapted from Zinkernagel RM, Hengartner H. T cell mediated immunopathology versus direct cytolysis by virus: implications for HIV and AIDS. Immunol Today 1994;15:262–268.)

TABLE 8-3. *Immune complex diseases in which viruses are or may be involved*

Host	Disease	References
Mice	LCMV, LDV, leukemia viruses, retroviruses(?), endogenous viruses(?)	37,49,62,70,86,93
Mink	Aleutian mink disease virus	76
Man	Hepatitis B virus, HIV, endogenous viruses(?)	36,56,87,93

HIV, human immunodeficiency virus; LCMV, lymphocytic choriomeningitis virus; LDV, lactate dehydrogenase virus.

ments then may be taken up by antigen-presenting cells and B cells and thereby enable linked recognition of self-specific B cells by T-helper cells specific for the foreign determinant.

Persistent infections by poorly cytopathic viruses may cause chronic inflammation, resulting in lymphoid organ–like organization.[108] Under these conditions, local antigens that have thus far been ignored by T cells are now presented under conditions optimal for the induction of a T-helper immune response. Autoantibody autoimmune responses are facilitated; in fact, they often go hand-in-hand with lymphoid organ formation in situ (e.g., autoimmune thyroiditis [Hashimoto's disease], Sjögren's disease). Induction of an immune response is difficult to achieve and demands proper antigen-presenting lymphoid organs and persistence of antigen. Chronic viral or other infections may provide these conditions and thereby induce autoimmunity in the periphery against autoantigens that are antigenically unrelated to the infectious agents involved.

Immune Complex Diseases

Immune complex–dependent inflammatory disease is induced only if immune complexes are generated in excess. This happens when antigen is not eliminated efficiently or when replicating antigen is not controlled by the immune response and therefore is constantly produced. As discussed in a later section, CD8+ T-cell immune responses against some noncytopathic viruses can be exhausted by overwhelming induction by widely spreading virus infection.[35,59,97] Apparently, this does not readily occur for CD4+ T helper cells and T-help–dependent antibody responses.[37,71] It can be speculated that this process is used by such viruses to limit or avoid lethal immunopathology by way of host cell destruction. Because CD4+ T cells are apparently not lytic in vivo (at least, there is no convincing evidence available thus far, but Fas-dependent mechanisms remain to be analyzed[88]), such limitations are less necessary. Additionally, there is some evidence that induced B cells producing IgG may be less dependent on T help for continuing responses. Thus, virus persistence and production, for whatever reason, may result in prolonged or continuous production of viral antigens, inducing corresponding antibodies and resulting in the production of immune complexes.[93] Such complexes are usually eliminated by phagocytic cells and Fc receptor–positive cells belonging to the functionally defined reticuloendothelial system. Again, it is the balance of immune complex production versus elimination that determines the extent of disease.

Of the various classic immune complex diseases in humans, some are associated with chronic infections of poorly cytopathic or noncytopathic viruses and others with chronic bacterial or parasitic infections, but for many the etiology is not known (Table 8-3). For some chronic virus infections in mice, immune complex disease manifestations have been described and analyzed in kidneys and other organs; they are usually as-

TABLE 8-4. *Viral or self antigen in privileged sites is ignored by cytotoxic T cells*

Mouse strain H-2^b	CTL precursors specific for LCMV-GP	Reactivity to LCMV-GP	Diabetes (at time)		
			Spontaneous	After LCMV iv	After vaccination with LCMV-GP iv
C57BL/6	<10^{-5}	+++	— >300 d	— >300 d	— >300 d
TCRtg 327	>10^{-1}	+++	— >300 d	— >300 d	— >300 d
GP-tg	<10^{-5}	+++	— >300 d	++ 10 d	— >300 d
F$_1$(GP-tg × 327)	>10^{-1}	+++	— >300 d	++ 4 d	++ 10 d

iv, intravenous; LCMV, lymphocytic choriomeningitis virus; PFU, plaque-forming unit.

Control mice or mice expressing a transgenic T-cell receptor specific for LCMV-GP aa33-41 on D^b(TCR tg327) or mice expressing LCMV-GP on β islet cells of the pancreas (GP tg) or mice expressing both transgenes [F$_1$(GP-tg × 327)] express different precursor frequencies of LCMV-GP–specific T cells. The severity (—, ++, +++) and the time of onset of diabetes in untreated LCMV infected (2 × 10^2 PFU iv) or vaccinia virus–expressing LCMV GP infected (2 × 10^6 PFU iv) mice was monitored.[67,68]

sociated with basal membranes of secretory or filtering epithelia and of blood vessels. Typically, many virus and host parameters contribute to disease susceptibility, duration, and phenotype. Only in a few cases have viral antigens been defined in complexes themselves (e.g., chronic HBV infections, LCMV carrier mice).[93] Whether viral antigens other than those derived from chronic exogenous viral infections (e.g., endogenous viral antigens) may be involved has been debated.[93] In this respect, it is interesting to note that inbred strains of mice may be special if not abnormal, because they develop immune complex disease more readily than wild mice. This phenotype is particularly pronounced in NZB, NZW, MRL, BXSB, and some other inbred strains of mice during induced chronic viral infections with LCMV, LDV, and leukemia viruses, among others.[93] How this phenotype results from B-cell hyperexcitability and breaking of B-cell unresponsiveness, limitation of complex elimination, or both remains to be shown. The example of mouse mammary tumor virus transmission[28,35,54] documents how complex the interactions between some of the most successful viruses and the immune system are, and how they may be exaggerated under conditions in which laboratory mice are kept and bred.

ORGAN SPECIFICITY OF VIRUS-INDUCED IMMUNOPATHOLOGY AND THE ROLE OF ANTIGEN-PRESENTING CELLS

The localization of immunologically mediated damage is dependent on the dominant localization of virus infection. This is comparable to direct cytolytic effects of a virus; the only difference is that immunologically mediated mechanisms cause cell damage. However, the requirements of immune induction may dissociate the presence of a virus from the immunologic consequences (see Table 8-2). Noncytopathic viruses may infect cells in immunologically privileged sites such as neurons, which are isolated from lymphocytes by various barriers, including glial cells and the blood-brain barrier. Epithelial and mesenchymal cells are also distant from lymphoid organs. Under these conditions, an antigen, whether self or foreign, cannot induce an immune response and is usually ignored by T cells, so that no antiviral response is induced and there is no resultant immunopathology. This may occur early in a primary infection when noncytopathic viruses exclusively infect those epithelial cells not in contact with lymphohemopoietic cells (e.g., macrophages, dendritic cells). Papillomaviruses infecting basal epidermal cells but replicating only in differentiating keratinocytes at a distance from Langerhans' cells are an excellent example,[94] as is rabies virus, which first infects neuronal cells exclusively.[8,82] These virus infections are initially ignored by the immune system because the obligate conditions for the effective induction of an immune response have not been met.

As previously stated, immune responses are only induced against viruses when they infect antigen-presenting cells or when their antigens reach antigen-presenting cells and lymphoid organs (see Table 8-2). This probably explains why several viruses such as papillomaviruses or rabies viruses can survive in nonlymphoid cells for a long time without inducing immune responses and why postexposure vaccination is pos-

sible, as is classically shown for rabies and may be proposed for control of papillomaviruses. In these infections, the vaccine is considerably better at fulfilling induction conditions by bringing antigen in an optimal form into lymphoid organs and antigen-presenting cells.

Viruses may also persist in privileged sites (e.g. epithelial cells, neuronal cells) after they have been cleared from lymphoid organs and peripheral lymphohemopoietic cells. Efficient persistent sequestration of viruses in such cells has been documented for herpesviruses and for LCMV, most readily in kidney tubular cells and epithelial cells, but also in the parotid gland, testis, and neurons.[16,25,37,41,49]

The following experiments illustrate the concept that viral antigens exposed on non–antigen-presenting cells in the periphery, (i.e., not in lymphoid organs) are ignored by T cells (see Tables 8-2 and 8-4). CTL reactivities and tolerance were studied in transgenic mice.[68,72] The transgenic mouse line expressed the viral glycoprotein LCMV-GP, including the target peptide of the transgenic T-cell receptor, under the rat insulin promoter (RIP) only in pancreatic islet cells. The RIP-GP-islet transgenic mice did not delete antigen-specific thymocytes and T cells in the thymus and did not develop diabetes up to the age of 1 year. However, infection with LCMV induced an antiviral protective CTL response causing the RIP-GP mice to develop diabetes exactly in parallel with the induced LCMV-specific CTL response. These results document an example of absence of specific peripheral tolerance to an exclusively, extrathymically presented self antigen. This model raises the general question of whether such pathogenic T-cell responses against self are frequently a cause of autoimmune diseases. As widely documented, clonal abortion in the thymus is expected to render this possibility unlikely, particularly because tolerance is more sensitive than antigen-stimulated induction of effector T cells.[75] The previous example, and possibly other rare examples of T-cell epitope mimicry, cannot be distinguished operationally or mechanistically from T-cell–mediated immunopathology against foreign antigenic epitopes (see Table 8-1).

Rabies viruses initially localized in the axon of neurons and papillomaviruses in keratinocytes are examples illustrating the concept that any antigen, whether self antigen, viral antigen, or tumor-associated antigen, if expressed exclusively in non–antigen-presenting cells and not in lymphoid tissue, is ignored by the immune system. T cells are neither rendered tolerant nor are they induced to respond unless the antigen reaches antigen-presenting cells in lymphoid organs in sufficient quantities.

MIMICRY AND IMMUNOPATHOLOGY OR AUTOIMMUNITY TRIGGERED BY VIRUSES

The term mimicry was originally coined to describe the possibility that induction of autoimmunity or immunopathology mediated by antibodies could be initiated by way of antigenic epitopes of infectious agents whose structures are identical or related to self antigens.[69] A considerable volume of literature presents evidence in support of this notion. Although the idea is attractive, in no case has convincing evidence yet been produced; there is no example in which an infectious agent can be linked to autoantibody responses of defined and proven pathogenetic activity. Additionally, in no experimental system has virus infection resulted in autoantibody-mediated pathology. In many examples, usually detecting autoantibodies by immunohistology on frozen sections, antibodies (including monoclonal antibodies) have been found that react with both viral and self antigens but do not necessarily exhibit autoimmune pathogenetic activity.[63] The discrepancy between concept and pathogenetic evidence largely lies in misconceptions about antibody specificities and binding qualities, target antigens, and duration of the response. The latter two points are particularly important: a self antigen functions as a target for autoimmunity only if it is accessible to antibodies. Additionally, induction of an effective immune response is difficult to achieve and depends on nontolerant T-cell help and a minimal duration before pathologic consequences are seen. Therefore, most responses initiated by mimicking or cross-reactive antigens are probably not efficient in causing severe pathology.

With the evidence of peptides presented by MHC being recognized by T cells, the concept of mimicry had to be adapted and extended. Accordingly, peptides coded for by infectious agents could be identical or similar (i.e., sharing the crucial anchor residues[31,78]) to peptides of the host. If these self peptides are not presented in sufficient quantities, they do not induce thymic or peripheral tolerance but are simply ignored by T cells. Introduction of such self peptides by way of agents that infect antigen-presenting cells or other cells in lymphoid organs or are produced in great amounts and then taken up by antigen-presenting cells may therefore induce self-reactive effector T cells of the CD8 type or, more often, of the CD4 type. Although well documented in a transgenic model situation, this possibility has not been documented under less artificial situations. Nevertheless, mimicry could explain the pathogenesis of some autoimmunities and may be operational in some of the elusive examples in which infectious agents may have triggered autoimmune-like disease states.

CYTOLYSIS BY VIRUS VERSUS CYTOLYSIS BY IMMUNE MECHANISMS

As previously pointed out, cytopathic viruses destroy cells in which they replicate and thereby cause pathology. Nonlytic viruses have arranged "gentlemen's agreements" with cells and hosts to the advantage of both. In this case, immune effector mechanisms may cause destruction of infected host cells. However, there may be in-between states in which both situations occur to some limited extent. It has been proposed that cells infected with noncytolytic viruses may function quite normally in vitro and in vivo except that they no longer perform certain "luxury" functions. For example, infected neuronal cells may survive but produce less acetylcholine, and it is this diminished function that may cause disease.[73]

Another example may be increased susceptibility of HBV-infected hepatocytes to interferon or other interleukin actions when compared with uninfected hepatocytes.[6,20] In a mouse expressing hepatitis B antigen as transgene in the liver, interferon injection causes liver cell damage, whereas control animals show no disease. Such a mechanism may explain fulminant hepatitis during natural infections with HBV; similar mechanisms in other disease entities have been described.[4,84]

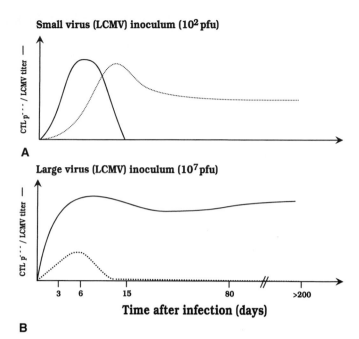

FIG. 8-11. Induction, exhaustion, or both of antiviral CD8+ T-cell responses by overwhelming infections with noncytopathic viruses. (**A**) A small virus inoculum induces a slowly developing but robust cytotoxic T cell (CTL) response that clears the infection. (**B**) A large virus inoculum induces a very rapid but weak CTL response that fails to clear the virus, leading to a state of virus persistence. LCMV, lymphocytic choriomeningitis virus; pfu, plaque-forming unit. (Data from Moskophidis D, Lechner F, Pircher HP, Zinkernagel RM. Virus persistence in acutely infected immunocompetent mice by exhaustion of antiviral cytotoxic effector T cells. Nature 1993;362:758–761.)

COMPLETE INDUCTION AND EXHAUSTION OF THE ANTIGEN-SPECIFIC REPERTOIRE BY EXCESSIVE ANTIGEN

The presence of antigen on too many antigen-presenting cells in the periphery, throughout the lymphoid organs, and probably also on other host cells apparently causes rapid induction of all available precursor T cells. Because induced effector cells normally die within 2 to 3 days, as has been shown in the acute CTL response against viruses, this results in the depletion or clonal abortion of the particular specificity concerned (Fig. 8-11; Table 8-5). Cytopathic viruses cannot overpower the immune system in this way because the result would be death of the host, but some noncytopathic viruses apparently achieve a state of immunologic unresponsiveness by way of exhaustive induction of CTL precursors (CTLp).[59] Peripheral deletion of CTLs helps to establish viral persistence. This is facilitated by relatively low CTLp levels, either because of MHC-linked low-responder status or as a result of immunosuppression or other factors; rapidly replicating virus variants that are more resistant to interferon; or early systemic hematogenous spread of the virus. Only poorly lytic viruses may exhaustively induce specific protective CTLps.

TABLE 8-5. *Induction of LCMV-carrier status in adult mice after infection with 10² PFU of LCMV IV*

Mouse strain	Armstrong WE		Cl-13 DOCILE	
	Persistence of LCMV >200 d	Presence of anti-LCMV CTLs	Persistence of LCMV >200 d	Presence of anti-LCMV CTLs
BALB/$_c$ H-2^{d}L^d	—	++	—	++
BALB/$_c$ H-2^{dm2}	—	++	+	—
DBA/$_2$ H-2^{d}L^d	—	++	+	—

CTL, cytotoxic T-lymphocyte; LCMV, lymphocytic choriomeningitis virus; PFU, plaque-forming unit.

H-2^d and H-2^{dm2} mutant mice lacking the major LCMV-NP$_{aa118-126}$ epitope-presenting L^d were infected with 10² PFU of the indicated viruses. Persistence of virus and presence or absence of LCMV-specific CTLs were monitored on day 250. Mice having fewer (DBA/2) or virtually no LCMV-specific precursor CTLs when compared with BALB/c (L^d is presenting the dominant LCMV-NP peptide 118-126) become carriers after infection with a low dose of rapidly replicating LCMV isolates Cl-13 or DOCILE but not with Armstrong or WE. There is a strict correlation between virus persistence and absence of CTLs. These experiments show that both viral and immune parameters influence the virus-host balance.

Data from Moskophidis D, Lechner F, Hengartner H, Zinkernagel RM. MHC class I and non MHC-linked capacity for generating an antiviral CTL response determines susceptibility to CTL exhaustion and establishment of virus persistence in mice. J Immunol 1994;152:4976–4983.

The response remains deleted if virus infects the thymus and also deletes differentiating specific thymocytes. From an evolutionary viewpoint, it could even be argued that the early induction and turning off of induced CTL minimizes immunopathologic damage and is one way for noncytopathic viruses to prevent the death of too many hosts by immunopathologic disease. If virus spread exhibits intermediate kinetics and extent instead of rapid and wide distribution, mice often die of overwhelming graft-versus-host–like disease 10 to 25 days after infection.[37,49] Thus, induction of a potent CTL response by a more localized virus infection may cause restricted immunopathology in lymphoid tissue.

Earlier studies had shown that specific T-cell epitope peptides given subcutaneously or intraperitoneally with a mild adjuvant such as an oil-in-water emulsion (i.e., incomplete Freund's adjuvant) induced protective CTL responses.[44,85] Several protocols were used to imitate rapid and overwhelming virus infections by applying peptide in incomplete Freud's adjuvant (IFA) three times intraperitoneally.[3,47] When the CTL activity after infection with LCMV was tested against target cells coated with the relevant peptide, the specific activity was absent, although activity against other LCMV T-cell epitopes and vaccinia virus or any third-party virus was present.

The same protocol was evaluated in the diabetes model described previously. Treatment of RIP-LCMV-GP transgenic mice with 100 g of peptide GP$_{33-41}$ in IFA three times intraperitoneally rendered the mice resistant to LCMV-induced CTL-mediated diabetes (Fig. 8-12). These results suggest that peripheral deletion of part of the specific antiviral repertoire by appropriate peptides might be used to prevent induction of immunopathologic disease. Again, the role of the relative balances between antigen distribution, relative precursor frequencies, and immunopathologic consequences of CTL responses cannot be overemphasized. If LCMV-primed mice with increased CTLp are infected with very high doses of virus, they may succumb to a graft-versus-host–like disease in a dose-dependent fashion.

These data suggest that, in addition to conventional vaccination, it might be possible to protect against immunopathologic consequences of noncytopathic viruses by exhaustive induction and deletion of immunopathologically active T cells. Exact knowledge of the relative balances between localization and spread of noncytopathic virus and host immunity is sometimes essential to prevent immunoprotection from causing aggravation of immunopathologically mediated disease.

IMMUNOPATHOLOGIC CONSEQUENCES OF VACCINATION

Immune responses are in general protective, but depending on the various parameters discussed thus far, immunopathology may be more or less prominent. For cytopathic viruses, only immunoprotection by vaccination is observed, but for noncytopathic viruses in which immunopathology may determine disease, vaccination may in rare cases have negative consequences. Under some conditions, vaccination may shift the balance between virus and host immune response such that immunopathology may be enhanced. Such occurrences are relatively rare but may become more frequent if poorly cytopathic and noncytopathic virus infections become targets of prophylaxis by vaccination.[18,22,29,33,90] It must be emphasized that such potentially negative effects of vaccination on disease are exceptions and should not discourage promotion of vaccination in general; nevertheless, physicians should be aware of the potential problems.

Two major pathogenetic pathways leading to disease enhancement by vaccination have become apparent: induction of antiviral CD8+ T cells but not of neutralizing antibodies against a noncytopathic virus, and induction of neutralizing antibodies in the absence of induced CD8+ T-cell memory.

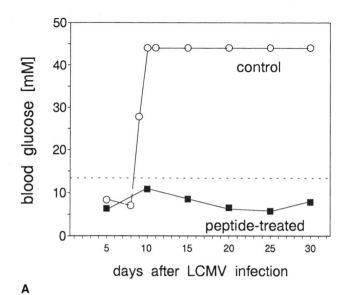

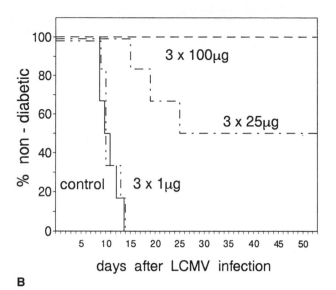

FIG. 8-12. Induction of autoimmune disease and its prevention by immunoprophylaxis through exhaustive induction and deletion of antiviral cytotoxic T cells. Transgenic mice expressing the lymphocytic choriomeningitis virus (LCMV) glycoprotein (GP) under control of the rat insulin promoter (RIP) become diabetic after infection with LCMV, which induces immune-mediated destruction of islet cells expressing the LCMV-GP (control). **(A)** Groups of three RIP-GP mice (H-2bxd) were treated intraperitoneally three times at 3-day intervals with 100 µg of GP33 peptide in IFA (■). Control RIP-GP mice were similarly treated with IFA alone (○). Three days after the last peptide injection, mice were infected with 1000 plaque-forming units (PFU) of LCMV Armstrong, and blood glucose levels were monitored on the days indicated. **(B)** Groups of six RIP-GP mice (H-2bxd) were injected intraperitoneally three times at 3-day intervals with the indicated dose of GP33 peptide. Three days after the last injection, mice were infected with 100 PFU of LCMV Arm, and diabetes incidence was monitored. (Data from Aichele P, Kyburz D, Ohashi PS, Zinkernagel RM, Hengartner H, Pircher H. Peptide induced T cell tolerance to prevent autoimmune diabetes in a transgenic mouse model. Proc Natl Acad Sci U S A 1994;91:444–448.)

Vaccine-Enhanced Disease by Induction of CD8+ T Cells but Not of Protective Antibodies

Optimal vaccines should express neutralizing epitopes and protective T-cell epitopes and persist for a long time.[2] When a vaccine induces T cells, particularly CD8+ T cells, in the absence of neutralizing antibodies, virus spread may not be controlled quickly after reexposure of the host to a noncytopathic virus. Therefore, such a noncytopathic virus (e.g., LCMV, HBV, possibly HIV) may spread widely before being checked by the memory CTL response. Although this memory CTL response eliminates the noncytopathic virus efficiently, it also may cause immunopathology. As shown in Table 8-6, DBA/2 mice that have low CD8+ T-cell concentrations do not succumb to T-cell–mediated lethal choriomeningitis because of exhaustion of the CTL response. However, DBA/2 mice previously vaccinated with either a major or minor T-cell epitope–containing vaccine prevent this exhaustion of CTLs, and subsequent infection with an otherwise innocuous virus dose may aggravate disease and cause lethal immunopathology.[65]

It must be reemphasized that such complications are not seen in infections with cytopathic viruses or when the vaccine induces a potent neutralizing antibody response in addition to CTLs. Overall, enhancement of immunopathologic disease by vaccination is rare. It depends on host genetic determinants

(including the MHC), the virus isolate, the infectious dose, the time after vaccination (i.e., the kinetics of immunologic memory),[32,40,66] the immunocompetence of the host, and many other factors. In such infections, vaccination may shift the balance from low- (i.e., late) to high- (i.e., early) responder status and therefore may prevent immunopathologically mediated disease (see Table 8-6), or it may shift the balance only slightly from a nonresponsive asymptomatic carrier to a low- or intermediate-responder status, thus causing immunopathology. This usually happens not with whole-virus vaccines exhibiting multiple protective T-cell epitopes[2] but when only one or few of the viral epitopes are used for vaccination, as is the case in some peptide or recombinant vaccines. Such strategies should be examined carefully, because in some rare cases vaccination may cause rather than prevent T-cell–mediated immunopathologic disease.

Harmful Effects of Preexisting Neutralizing Antibodies in the Absence of Protective T-Cell Memory

Antibody-dependent enhancement of viral infection and disease has been shown for dengue fever,[33] feline infectious peritonitis,[90] and in vitro HIV.[79] Responsible pathogenic mechanisms include enhancement of infectivity by Fc recep-

TABLE 8-6. *Protective or disease-enhancing effects of active or passive immunization on susceptibility to LCM*

			Percent survival of mice after IC infection				
			Active immunization [BALB/c (H-2^d)]			Passive immunization [C57BL/6 (H-2^b)]	
LCMV isolate	Dose PFU	Replication kinetics	None	Major T-cell epitope vacc-LCMV-NP	Minor T-cell epitope vacc-LCMV-GP	Neutralizing serum	Nonneutralizing serum
Armstrong	10^1–10^2	Slow	Not tested			100	0
	10^5–10^6					0	0
WE	10^1–10^2	Intermediate	0	100	0	0	0
	10^5–10^6		100	100	0	50	100
DOCILE	10^1–10^2	Fast	20	100	0	20	100
	10^5–10^6		100	20	0	20	100

IC, intracerebral; LCMV, lymphocyte choriomeningitis virus; PFU, plaque-forming unit.

Vaccination that induced either extensive (vaccination with the major T-cell epitope-expressing vacc-LCMV-NP) or only partial T-cell responses (vaccination with the minor T-cell epitope-expressing vacc-LCMV-GP) either protected against choriomeningitis after IC infection or caused more extensive disease in some combinations. Transfer of immune sera that did not neutralize LCMV had no influence on the course of choriomeningitis after IC infection. Adoptive transfer of neutralizing sera prevented disease in some combinations but enhanced it in others.

Data from references 10 and 65.

tors or complement activation. Similarly, inactivated respiratory syncytial virus (RSV) or measles vaccines may enhance the pathogenicity of a subsequent infection, apparently by causing more severe cell-mediated immunopathology.[18,22,29]

It is possible that antibodies that influence virus spread and replication could thereby modulate both T-cell–mediated immunity and T-cell–dependent immunopathology. LCMV, a noncytopathic virus, is a powerful model to address this question, because the balance between virus spread and T-cell response is crucial in determining the disease outcome[16,37,49] and because neutralizing antibodies occur only late (20 to 100 days) after infection. Protection against an acute LCMV infection is primarily mediated by CTLs,[37,49] which also can mediate immunopathology. The degree of immunopathology depends on the degree of induction of CTLs and the number of virally infected and consequently lysed cells. For example, after intracerebral infection, the T-cell immune response is protective only when large numbers of T cells are rapidly recruited at a time when relatively few choriomeningeal cells are infected. If the virus can spread efficiently and infect many choriomeningeal cells before effector T cells or neutralizing antibodies reach the brain, then even LCMV-primed mice are not protected.

The protective function of humoral immunity against reinfection with LCMV has not been much appreciated because of the dominance of an early protective CTL response.[9,99] Nevertheless, studies have demonstrated that monoclonal neutralizing antiviral antibody, under certain experimental conditions, attenuated T-cell–mediated immunopathology following LCMV infection. Furthermore, passive transfer of antibodies from immune mothers protected offspring against lymphocytic choriomeningitis.[10] Surprisingly, passive transfer of polyclonal immune serum influenced susceptibility to CTL-mediated choriomeningitis positively or negatively, dependent on both viral (see Table 8-6) properties and host parameters. The intravenous administration of antibodies before infection effi-

ciently reduced hematogenous virus spread to the spleen and therefore drastically lowered the primary CTL response with a neurotropic LCMV strain (Armstrong) but failed to prevent replication of virus in the choriomeninges. Thus, as a result of neutralizing antibodies, cytotoxicity was reduced, T-cell–mediated immunopathology prevented, and mice protected, because a massive influx of activated CTLs is required to mediate lethal choriomeningitis. When the mice were challenged intravenously with LCMV-Armstrong, the strong effect of preexisting antibodies on the CTL response was even more evident; no primary CTL response could be measured. The influence of neutralizing antiviral antibodies on the severity of choriomeningitis caused by faster-replicating LCMV strains (WE and DOCILE) was drastically different (see Table 8-6). Polyclonal sera, with or without neutralizing capacity, were not effective against a low dose intracerebral infection with LCMV-WE; all mice died. However, mice pretreated with the neutralizing but not the nonneutralizing antibodies and challenged with a high dose of LCMV-WE or low dose of LCMV-DOCILE exhibited a drastically enhanced mortality. In contrast, untreated control mice survived intracerebral infection with a high dose of LCMV-WE as well as a challenge with different doses of LCMV-DOCILE as a result of exhaustion of CTLs.

Thus in this specific model, neutralizing but not nonneutralizing anti-LCMV antibodies in the absence of primed CTLs regulate the balance between virus spread relative to the kinetics of the disease-causing CD8+ T-cell responses and thereby change the outcome of immunopathologic disease (see Table 8-6). Neutralizing antibodies protect against low but not high intracerebral doses of the slowly replicating LCMV-Armstrong. In general, neutralizing antibodies are more efficient against LCMV when injected intravenously than when introduced by subcutaneous or intracerebral injection, in which case they may even enhance infection and immunopathology. Antibodies can prevent high virus dose immune paralysis (exhaustion of CTLs) by reducing LCMV replication. Thus, neutralizing antibodies may modulate the CTL response in a beneficial or harmful way dependent on preexisting antibody titers, site of infection, virus strain, and host MHC and non-MHC genes and may decrease, or paradoxically increase, susceptibility to disease.

These results are compatible with the theory that a state of heightened T-cell activity in the absence of locally protective neutralizing antibodies may play an important role in disease potentiation mediated apparently by CD4+ T cells in RSV and possibly also in some cases of measles vaccines.[90] The results presented may help us understand why antibodies specific for HIV mediated neutralization in vitro but conversely often fail to provide efficient protection and prevention of infection despite neutralizing activity. These results also may explain why vaccines failed to induce protective immunity against reinfection with hepatitis C virus.[24] Additionally, the results with LCMV may elucidate why guinea pigs infected intracerebrally with Junin virus, which is also an arenavirus causing Argentine hemorrhagic fever, were partly protected by immune sera although they still had detectable virus in the brain.[45] Similarly, if T-cell memory is short-lived, enhancement of dengue fever by preexisting antibodies may reflect enhancement both of infection and of T-cell–mediated immunopathology.

SUMMARY AND CONCLUSIONS

The studies summarized in this chapter illustrate how analysis of antiviral immunity provides significant insight into the biologic parameters of immunologic tolerance and specificity. Immune protection against viruses and other infectious agents is beneficial to the host, particularly if the infectious agent is cytopathic. However, immunoprotection often causes cell destruction, under some circumstances resulting in immunopathologically mediated disease. If the replicating infectious agent is not eliminated, the continual confrontation with immune defence mechanisms, including antibodies forming antigen-antibody complexes, may cause chronic disease. The balances between infectious agent and host, including the host's immune system, determine the relative impact of protection versus pathology. This balance may be shifted by mutations in the virus or by factors influencing host resistance. Conventional vaccination (i.e., induction and relative increase of protective effector T cells and of protective antibodies) improves protection. Decrease of T cells by nonspecific immunosuppression or by specific peripheral deletion increases the susceptibility of the host to cytopathic viruses. However, this dangerous and unwanted consequence may be beneficial in noncytopathic virus infections, in which T-cell–mediated immunopathology may be reduced. Overall, the balance between viruses and hosts can be intentionally altered to benefit most but not all hosts; in every case, protective benefits and immunopathologic costs must be appreciated, weighed, and optimized for the benefit of the host.

ABBREVIATIONS

BVDV: bovine viral diarrhea virus
CTL: cytotoxic T lymphocyte
CTLp: cytotoxic T lymphocyte promoter
HBV: hepatitis B virus
HIV: human immunodeficiency virus
IFA: incomplete Freud's adjuvant
LCMV: lymphocytic choriomeningitis virus
LDV: lactate dehydrogenase virus
MHC: major histocompatibility complex
RIP: rat insulin promoter
RSV: respiratory syncytial virus
SCID: severe combined immunodeficiency
VSV: vesicular stomatits virus

REFERENCES

1. Ada G. The immunological principles of vaccination. Lancet 1990; 335:523–526.
2. Ada G. Vaccine development: real and imagined dangers. Nature 1991;349:369.
3. Aichele P, Kyburz D, Ohashi PS, Zinkernagel RM, Hengartner H, Pircher H. Peptide induced T cell tolerance to prevent autoimmune diabetes in a transgenic mouse model. Proc Natl Acad Sci U S A 1994;91:444–448.
4. Allison J, Campbell IL, Morahan G, Mandel TE, Harrison LC, Miller JFAP. Diabetes in transgenic mice resulting from overexpression of class I histocompatibility molecules in pancreatic b cells. Nature 1988;333:529–533.
5. Althage A, Odermatt B, Moskophidis D, Kündig Th, Hengartner H, Zinkernagel RM. Immunosuppression by lymphocytic choriomeningitis virus infection: competent effector T and B cells but impaired antigen presentation. Eur J Immunol 1992;22:1803–1812.
6. Ando K, Moriyama T, Guidotti LG, et al. Mechanisms of class I restricted immunopathology: a transgenic mouse model of fulminant hepatitis. J Exp Med 1993;178:1541–1554.
7. Bachmann MF, Hoffmann Rohrer U, Kündig TM, Bürki K, Hengartner H, Zinkernagel RM. The influence of antigen organisation on B cell responsiveness. Science 1993;262:1448–1451.
8. Baer GM, Cleary WF. A model in mice for the pathogenesis and treatment of rabies. J Infect Dis 1972;125:520–527.
9. Baldridge JR, Buchmeier MJ. Mechanisms of antibody-mediated protection against lymphocytic choriomeningitis virus infection: mother-to-baby transfer of humoral protection. J Virol 1992;66: 4252–4257.
10. Battegay M, Kyburz D, Hengartner H, Zinkernagel RM. Enhancement of disease by neutralizing antiviral antibodies in the absence of primed antiviral cytotoxic T cells. Eur J Immunol 1993;23: 3236–3241.
11. Battegay M, Moskophidis D, Waldner H, et al. Impairment and delay of neutralizing antiviral antibody responses by virus specific cytotoxic T cells. J Immunol 1993;151:5408–5415.
12. Berke G. T cell mediated cytotoxicity. Curr Opin Immunol 1991;3: 320–325.
13. Bjorkman PJ, Saper MA, Samraoui B, Bennett WS, Strominger JL, Wiley DC. Structure of the human class I histocompatibility antigen, HLA-A2.Nature 1987;329:506–511.
14. Blanden RV. T cell response to viral and bacterial infection. Transplant Rev 1974;19:56–84.
15. Brownlie J. The pathways for the bovine virus diarrhoea virus biotypes in the pathogenesis of disease. Arch Virol 1991;(Suppl 3): 79–96.
16. Buchmeier MJ, Welsh RM, Dutko FJ, Oldstone MBA. The virology and immunobiology of lymphocytic choriomeningitis virus infection. Adv Immunol 1980;30:275–331.
17. Burns WH, Billups LC, Notkins AL. Thymus dependence of viral antigens. Nature 1975;256:654–656.
18. Cannon MJ, Openshaw PJ, Askonas BA. Cytotoxic T cells clear virus but augment lung pathology in mice infected with respiratory syncytial virus. J Exp Med 1988;168:1163–1168.
19. Cerottini JC, Brunner KT. Cell-mediated cytotoxicity, allograft rejection and tumor immunity. Adv Immunol 1974;18:67–132.
20. Chisari FV, Filippi P, Buras J, et al. Structural and pathological effects of synthesis of hepatitis B virus large envelope polypeptide in transgenic mice. Proc Natl Acad Sci U S A 1987;84:6909–6913.

21. Cole GA, Nathanson N, Prendergast RA. Requirement for theta bearing cells in lymphocytic choriomeningitis virus-induced central nervous system disease. Nature 1972;238:335–337.

22. Connors M, Kulkarni AB, Firestone C-Y, et al. Pulmonary histopathology induced by respiratory syncytial virus (RSV) challenge of formalin-inactivated RSV-immunized BALB/c mice is abrogated by depletion of CD4+ T cells. J Virol 1992;66:7444–7451.

23. Eddleston ALWF, Williams R. HLA and liver disease. Br Med Bull 1978;34:295–300.

24. Farci P, Alter HJ, Govindarajan S, et al. Lack of protective immunity against reinfection with hepatitis C virus. Science 1992;258:135–140.

25. Fazakerley JK, Southern P, Bloom F, Buchmeier MJ. High resolution in situ hybridization to determine the cellular distribution of lymphocytic choriomeningitis virus RNA in the tissues of persistently infected mice: relevance to arenavirus disease and mechanisms of viral persistence. J Gen Virol 1991;72:1611–1625.

26. Fazekas de St. Groth S. Cross recognition and cross-reactivity. Cold Spring Harbor Symp Quant Biol 1967;32:525–536.

27. Ferrari C, Penna A, Giuberti T, et al. Intrahepatic, nucleocapsid antigen-specific T cells in chronic active hepatitis B. J Immunol 1987;139:2050–2058.

28. Frankel WN, Rudy C, Coffin JM, Huber BT. Linkage of Mls genes to endogenous mammary tumour viruses of inbred mice. Nature 1991;349:526–528.

29. Fujinami RS, Oldstone MBA. Antiviral antibody reacting on the plasma membrane alters measles virus expression inside the cell. Nature 1979;279:529–530.

30. Fung-Leung WP, Kündig ThM, Zinkernagel RM, Mak TW. Immune response against lymphocytic choriomeningitis virus infection in mice without CD8 expression. J Exp Med 1991;174:1425–1429.

31. Gautam AM, Lock CB, Smilek DE, Pearson CI, Steinman L, McDevitt HO. Minimum structural requirements for peptide presentation by major histocompatibility complex class II molecules: implications in induction of autoimmunity. Proc Natl Acad Sci U S A 1994;91:767–771.

32. Gray D, Sprent J. Immunological memory. Curr Top Microbiol Immunol 1990;159:1–138.

33. Halstead SB. Pathogenesis of dengue: challenges to molecular biology. Science 1988;239:476–481.

34. Haspel MV, Onodera T, Prabhakar BS, Horita M, Suzuki H, Notkins AL. Virus-induced autoimmunity: monoclonal antibodies that react with endocrine tissues. Science 1983;220:304–306.

35. Held W, Shakhov AN, Waanders G, et al. An exogenous mouse mammary tumor virus with properties of Mls-1a (Mtv-7). J Exp Med 1992;175:1623–1633.

36. Hirsch MS, Allison AC, Harvey JJ. Immune complexes in mice infected neonatally with moloney leukaemogenic and murine sarcoma viruses. Nature 1969;223:739–740.

37. Hotchin J. Persistent and slow virus infections. Monogr Virol 1971;3:1–211.

38. Huang S, Hendriks W, Althage A, et al. Immune response in mice that lack the interferon-gamma receptor. Science 1993;259:1742–1745.

39. Jacobs RP, Cole GA. Lymphocytic choriomeningitis virus-induced immunosuppression: a virus-induced macrophage defect. J Immunol 1976;117:1004–1009.

40. Jamieson BD, Ahmed R. T cell memory: long-term persistence of virus-specific cytotoxic T cells. J Exp Med 1989;169:1993–2005.

41. Jamieson BD, Somasundaram T, Ahmed R. Abrogation of tolerance to a chronic viral infection. J Immunol 1991;147:3521–3529.

42. Kägi D, Ledermann B, Bürki K, et al. Cytotoxicity mediated by T cells and natural killer cells is greatly impaired in perforin-deficient mice. Nature 1994;369:31–37.

43. Kägi D, Vignaux F, Ledermann B, et al. Fas and perforin pathways as major mechanisms of T cell-mediated cytotoxicity. Science 1994;265:528–530.

44. Kast WM, Roux L, Curren J, et al. Protection against lethal Sendai virus infection by in vivo priming of virus-specific cytotoxic T lymphocytes with a free synthetic peptide. Proc Natl Acad Sci U S A 1991;88:2283–2287.

45. Kenyon RH, Green DE, Eddy GA, Peters CJ. Treatment of junin virus-infected guinea pigs with immune serum: development of late neurological disease. J Med Virol 1986;20:207–218.

46. Kündig TM, Hengartner H, Zinkernagel RM. T cell dependent interferon gamma exerts an antiviral effect in the central nervous system but not in peripheral solid organs. J Immunol 1993;150:2316–2321.

47. Kyburz D, Aichele P, Speiser DE, Hengartner H, Zinkernagel R, Pircher H. T cell immunity after a viral infection versus T cell tolerance induced by soluble viral peptides. Eur J Immunol 1993;23:1956–1962.

48. Kyburz D, Speiser DE, Battegay M, Hengartner H, Zinkernagel RM. Lysis of infected cells in vivo by anti-viral cytolytic T-cells demonstrated by release of cell internal viral proteins. Eur J Immunol 1993;23:1540–1545.

49. Lehmann-Grube F. Lymphocytic choriomeningitis virus. Virol Monogr 1971;10:1–173.

50. Leist TP, Althage A, Haenseler E, Hengartner H, Zinkernagel RM. MHC-linked susceptibility or resistance to disease caused by a noncytopathic virus varies with the disease parameter evaluated. J Exp Med 1989;170:269–277.

51. Leist TP, Cobbold SP, Waldmann H, Aguet M, Zinkernagel RM. Functional analysis of T lymphocyte subsets in antiviral host defense. J Immunol 1987;138:2278–2281.

52. Leist TP, Rüedi E, Zinkernagel RM. Virus-triggered immune suppression in mice caused by virus-specific cytotoxic T cells. J Exp Med 1988;167:1749–1754.

53. Marker O, Volkert M. Studies on cell-mediated immunity to lymphocytic choriomeningitis virus in mice. J Exp Med 1973;137:1511–1525.

54. Marrack P, Kushnir E, Kappler J. A maternally inherited superantigen encoded by a mammary tumour virus. Nature 1991;349:524–526.

55. Martz E, Howell DM. CTL: are they virus control cells first, and cytolytic cells second? DNA fragmentation, apoptosis, and the prelytic halt hypothesis. Immunol Today 1989;10:70–80.

56. Miller I, London WT, Sutnick AI, Blumberg BS. Australia antigen-antibody complexes. Nature 1970;226:83–84.

57. Mims CA, Wainwright S. The immunodepressive action of lymphocytic choriomeningitis virus in mice. J Immunol 1968;101:717–724.

58. Moskophidis D, Cobbold SP, Waldmann H, Lehmann-Grube F. Mechanism of recovery from acute virus infection: treatment of lymphocytic choriomeningitis virus-infected mice with monoclonal antibodies reveals that Lyt-2+ T lymphocytes mediate clearance of virus and regulate the antiviral antibody response. J Virol 1987;61:1867–1874.

59. Moskophidis D, Lechner F, Pircher HP, Zinkernagel RM. Virus persistence in acutely infected immunocompetent mice by exhaustion of antiviral cytotoxic effector T cells. Nature 1993;362:758–761.

60. Muller D, Koller BH, Whitton JL, LaPan KE, Brigman KK, Frelinger JA. LCMV-specific, class II-restricted cytotoxic T cells in beta 2-microglobulin-deficient mice. Science 1992;255:1576–1578.

61. Nossal GJV, Ada GL. Antigens, lymphoid cells and the immune response. New York: Academic Press, 1971.

62. Notkins AL, Mahar S, Scheele C, Goffman J. Infectious virus-antibody complex in the blood of chronically infected mice. J Exp Med 1966;124:81–97.

63. Notkins AL, Onodera T, Prabhakar B. Virus-induced autoimmunity. In: Notkins AL, Oldstone MBA, eds. Concepts in viral pathogenesis. New York: Springer-Verlag, 1984:210–215.

64. Odermatt B, Eppler M, Leist TP, Hengartner H, Zinkernagel RM. Virus-triggered acquired immunodeficiency by cytotoxic T-cell dependent destruction of antigen-presenting cells and lymph follicle structure. Proc Natl Acad Sci U S A 1991;88:8252–8256.

65. Oehen S, Hengartner H, Zinkernagel RM. Vaccination for disease. Science 1991;251:195–198.

66. Oehen S, Waldner HP, Kündig Th, Hengartner H, Zinkernagel RM. Antivirally protective cytotoxic T cell memory to lymphocytic choriomeningitis virus is governed by persisting antigen. J Exp Med 1992;176:1273–1281.

67. Ohashi PS, Oehen S, Aichele P, et al. Induction of diabetes is influenced by the infectious virus and local expression of MHC class I and TNF-α. J Immunol 1993;150:5185–5194.

68. Ohashi PS, Oehen S, Bürki K, et al. Ablation of "tolerance" and induction of diabetes by virus infection in viral antigen transgenic mice. Cell 1991;65:305–317.

69. Oldstone MBA. Molecular mimicry and autoimmune disease. Cell 1987;50:819–820.

70. Oldstone MBA, Dixon FJ. Lactic dehydrogenase virus-induced immune complex type of glomerulonephritis. J Immunol 1971;106: 1260–1263.

71. Oldstone MBA, Dixon FJ. Tissue injury in lymphocytic choriomeningitis viral infection: virus-induced immunologically specific release of a cytotoxic factor from immune lymphoid cells. Virology 1970;42:805–813.

72. Oldstone MBA, Nerenberg M, Southern P, Price J, Lewicki H. Virus infection triggers insulin-dependent diabetes mellitus in a transgenic model: role of anti-self (virus) immune response. Cell 1991; 65:319–331.

73. Oldstone MBA, Sinha YN, Blount P, et al. Virus-induced alterations in homeostasis leading to disease alterations in differentiated but not vital function of infected cells in vivo. Science 1982;218: 1125–1127.

74. Peters M, Vierling J, Gershwin ME, Milich D, Chisari FV, Hoofnagle JH. Immunology and the liver. Hepatology 1991;13:977–994.

75. Pircher HP, Hoffmann Rohrer U, Moskophidis D, Zinkernagel RM, Hengartner H. Lower receptor avidity required for thymic clonal deletion than for effector T cell function. Nature 1991;351:482–485.

76. Porter DD, Larsen AE, Porter HG. The pathogenesis of aleutian disease of mink. J Exp Med 1969;130:575–593.

77. Rahemtulla A, Fung-Leung WP, Schilham MW, et al. Normal development and function of CD8+ cells but markedly decreased helper cell activity in mice lacking CD4. Nature 1991;353:180–184.

78. Rammensee H-G, Falk K, Rötzschke O. MHC molecules as peptide receptors. Curr Biol 1993;5:35–44.

79. Robinson W, Montefiori D, Mitchell W. Antibody-dependent enhancement of human immunodeficiency virus type 1 infection. Lancet 1988;1:790–794.

80. Ruby J, Ramshaw I. The antiviral activity of immune CD8+ T cells is dependent on interferon-gamma. Lymphokine Cytokine Res 1992; 10:353–358.

81. Sabin AB. Improbability of effective vaccination against human immunodeficiency virus because of its intracellular transmission and rectal portal of entry. Proc Natl Acad Sci U S A 1992;89:8852–8855.

82. Sabin A, Olitsky P. Pathological evidence of axonal and transsynaptic progression of vesicular stomatitis and eastern equine encephalomyelitis viruses. Am J Pathol 1937;13:615.

83. Salk J. Prospects for the controls of AIDS by immunizing seropositive individuals. Nature 1987;327:473–476.

84. Sarvetnick N, Shizuru J, Liggitt D, et al. Loss of pancreatic islet tolerance induced by beta-cell expression of interferon-gamma. Nature 1990;346:844–847.

85. Schulz M, Zinkernagel RM, Hengartner H. Peptide induced antiviral protection by cytotoxic T cells. Proc Natl Acad Sci U S A 1991; 88:991–993.

86. Schwartz RH. Fugue in T-lymphocyte recognition. Nature 1987; 326:738–739.

87. Shulman NR, Barker LF. Virus-like antigen, antibody, and antigen-antibody complexes in hepatitis measured by complement fixation. Science 1969;165:304–306.

88. Stalder T, Hahn S, Erb P. Fas antigen is the major target molecule for CD4+ T cell-mediated cytotoxicity. J Immunol 1994;152:1127.

89. Steinhoff U, Burkhart C, Arnheiter H, Hengartner H, Zinkernagel RM. Virus or a hapten-carrier complex can activate autoreactive B cells by providing linked T help. Eur J Immunol 1994;24: 773–776.

90. Stott EJ, Taylor G, Ball LA, et al. Immune and histopathological responses in animals vaccinated with recombinant vaccinia viruses that express individual genes of human respiratory syncytial virus. J Virol 1987;61:3855–3861.

91. Sykulev Y, Brunmark A, Jackson M, Cohen RJ, Peterson PA, Eisen HN. Kinetics and affinity of reactions between an antigen-specific T cell receptor and peptide-MHC complexes. Immunity 1994;1: 15–22.

92. Tew JG, Kosco MH, Burton GF, Szakal AK. Follicular dendritic cells as accessory cells. Immunol Rev 1990;117:185–212.

93. Theofilopoulos AN, Dixon FJ. The biology and detection of immune complexes. Adv Immunol 1979;28:89–220.

94. Tindle RW, Frazer IH. Immune response to human papillomaviruses and the prospects for human papillomavirus-specific immunisation. Curr Top Microbiol Immunol 1994;186:217–252.

95. Townsend ARM, Gotch FM, Davey J. Cytotoxic T cells recognize fragments of the influenza nucleoprotein. Cell 1985;42:457–467.

96. Wagner RR. Rhabdoviridae and their replication. In: Fields BN, ed. Virology. New York: Raven Press, 1990:867–879.

97. Webb S, Morris C, Sprent J. Extrathymic tolerance of mature T cells: clonal elimination as a consequence of immunity. Cell 1990; 63:1249–1256.

98. Weigle WO. Analysis of autoimmunity through experimental models of thyroiditis and allergic encephalomyelitis. Adv Immunol 1980;30:159–273.

99. Wright KE, Buchmeier MJ. Antiviral antibodies attenuate T-cell-mediated immunopathology following acute lymphocytic choriomeningitis virus infection. J Virol 1991;65:3001–3006.

100. Wu-Hsieh B, Howard DH, Ahmed R. Virus-induced immunosuppression: a murine model of susceptibility to opportunistic infection. J Infect Dis 1988;158:232–235.

101. Zinkernagel RM. Protection and damage by anti-viral immunity. Harvey Lectures 1993–94:29–51.

102. Zinkernagel RM, Althage A. Antiviral protection by virus-immune cytotoxic T cells: infected target cells are lysed before infectious virus progeny is assembled. J Exp Med 1977;145:644–651.

103. Zinkernagel RM, Cooper S, Chambers J, Lazzarini RA, Hengartner H, Arnheiter H. Virus induced autoantibody response to a transgenic viral antigen. Nature 1990;344:68–71.

104. Zinkernagel RM, Doherty PC. MHC-restricted cytotoxic T cells: studies on the biological role of polymorphic major transplantation antigens determining T cell restriction-specificity, function and responsiveness. Adv Immunol 1979;27:52–142.

105. Zinkernagel RM, Doherty PC. Restriction of in vitro T cell mediated cytotoxicity in lymphocytic choriomeningitis within a syngeneic or semiallogeneic system. Nature 1974;248:701–702.

106. Zinkernagel RM, Haenseler E, Leist TP, Cerny A, Hengartner H, Althage A. T cell mediated hepatitis in mice infected with lymphocytic choriomeningitis virus. J Exp Med 1986;164:1075–1092.

107. Zinkernagel RM, Hengartner H. T cell mediated immunopathology versus direct cytolysis by virus: implications for HIV and AIDS. Immunol Today 1994;15:262–268.

108. Zinkernagel RM, Pircher HP, Ohashi PS, Hengartner H. T cells causing immunological disease. Semin Immunol 1992;14:105–113.

Viral Pathogenesis,
edited by Neal Nathanson, et al.
Lippincott–Raven Publishers, Philadelphia © 1997

CHAPTER 9

Viral Persistence

Rafi Ahmed, Lynda A. Morrison, and David M. Knipe

INTRODUCTION

Virus survival in nature requires continuous infection of susceptible individuals. Within an infected host, viruses can cause short-term, acute infections or they can establish long-term persistence. During acute infections, virus is cleared by the host immune response, necessitating rapid transmission or the capacity for extra-organismal survival. Some acute viruses, such as measles or mumps, survive by continual infection of new human hosts, whereas others, such as influenza, yellow fever, or rabies viruses, circulate in more than one species. Still other viruses possess structural features that permit them to survive the rigors of an extra-organismal environment until contact with a susceptible host occurs. For example, poxviruses are stable in a dried form, whereas enteric viruses, such as poliovirus or rotaviruses, can survive in water supplies until ingested by susceptible individuals. Alternatively, viruses may persist within an individual host organism

R. Ahmed: Department of Microbiology and Immunology and Emory Vaccine Center, Emory University School of Medicine, Atlanta, Georgia 30322.

L .A. Morrison and D. M. Knipe: Department of Microbiology and Molecular Genetics, Harvard Medical School, Boston, Massachusetts 02115.

for extended periods. Such virus infections begin as acute infections but progress to latent or chronic infections during which the virus is transmitted periodically to new host organisms. Viruses that can persist in humans and animals are listed in Tables 9-1 and 9-2. As can be seen from these tables, the ability to persist in vivo is not confined to a particular virus group, and a variety of DNA- and RNA-containing viruses can establish long-term infections.

Persistent viruses cause an increasing proportion of the viral disease burden borne by humans (e.g., the acquired immunodeficiency syndrome [AIDS] caused by human immunodeficiency virus [HIV], chronic hepatitis and hepatocellular carcinoma caused by infection with hepatitis B virus [HBV], anogenital cancer associated with human papillomaviruses [HPVs], disseminated herpes simplex virus [HSV] type 2 infection in the newborn; see Table 9-1). It also is probable that more sensitive techniques, such as polymerase chain reaction, will uncover even more evidence of low-level viral persistence. Additional diseases may be found to be caused by viruses persisting at low levels. As our knowledge of chronic disease associated with viral infections has increased, there has been a greater urgency to understand the mechanisms of viral persistence.

During acute infection of the host, many viruses inhibit the metabolism of the host cells they productively infect so that

TABLE 9-1. *Viruses that persist in humans*

Virus group	Site of persistence	Consequence
DNA VIRUSES		
Adenovirus	Adenoids, tonsils, lymphocytes	None known
Cytomegalovirus	Kidney, salivary glands, lymphocytes? macrophages? stromal cells?	Pneumonia, retinitis
Epstein-Barr virus	Pharyngeal epithelial cells, B cells	Infectious mononucleosis, Burkitt's lymphoma, nasopharyngeal carcinoma, non-Hodgkin's lymphoma, oral hairy leukoplakia
Herpes simplex virus 1 and 2	Sensory ganglia neurons	Cold sores, genital herpes, encephalitis, keratitis
Human herpesvirus 6	Lymphocytes	Exanthem subitum
Varicella zoster virus	Sensory ganglia neurons and/or satellite cells	Varicella, zoster
Hepatitis B virus	Hepatocytes, lymphocytes? macrophages?	Hepatitis, hepatocellular carcinoma
Hepatitis D virus	Hepatocytes	Exacerbation of chronic HBV infection
Papillomavirus	Epithelial skin cells	Papilloma, carcinomas
Parvovirus B19	Erythroid progenitor cell in bone marrow	Aplastic crisis in hemolytic anemia, chronic bone marrow deficiency
Polyomavirus BK	Kidney	Hemorrhagic cystitis
Polyomavirus JC	Kidney, oligodendrocytes in CNS	Progressive multifocal leukoencephalopathy
RNA VIRUSES		
Hepatitis C virus	Hepatocytes, lymphocytes? macrophages?	Hepatitis, hepatocellular carcinoma
Measles virus*	Neurons and supporting cells in CNS	Subacute sclerosing panencephalitis, measles inclusion body encephalitis
Rubella virus*	CNS	Progressive rubella panencephalitis, insulin-dependent diabetes? juvenile arthritis?
Human immunodeficiency virus	CD4+ T cells, monocytes/ macrophages, microglia	AIDS
Human T-cell leukemia virus I	T cells	T-cell leukemia, tropical spastic paraparesis, polymyositis
Human T-cell leukemia virus II	T cells	None known

*Measles and rubella viruses typically cause acute infections. However, in rare instances, these viruses have been shown to persist in the CNS.

AIDS, acquired immunodeficiency syndrome; CNS, central nervous system; HBV, hepatitis B virus.

TABLE 9-2. *Persistent viral infections of animals, selected examples**

Virus family	Virus	Natural host	Associated disease
DNA VIRUSES			
Parvoviridae	Feline parvovirus	Cat	Feline panleukopenia; cerebellar ataxia†
Herpesviridae	B virus	Monkey	Encephalitis
	Cytomegalovirus	Mouse	Cytomegalovirus inclusion disease of multiple organs
Polyomavirinae	Polyomavirus	Mouse	Tumors of multiple tissues
	Simian virus 40	Monkey	Generally none / Progressive multifocal leukoencephalopathy‡
Hepadnaviridae	Duck hepatitis virus	Peking duck	Hepatitis; hepatocellular carcinoma
	Woodchuck hepatitis virus	Woodchuck	Hepatitis; hepatocellular carcinoma
RNA VIRUSES			
Picornaviridae	Theiler's murine encephalitis virus	Mouse	CNS demyelination
Coronaviridae	Mouse hepatitis virus	Mouse	CNS demyelination
Paramyxoviridae	Canine distemper virus	Dog	CNS demyelination
Arenaviridae	Lymphocytic choriomeningitis virus	Mouse	Chronic glomerulonephritis
Lentiviridae	Visna/maedi virus	Sheep	Interstitial pneumonitis; CNS demyelination
	Caprine arthritis encephalitis virus	Goat	Chronic arthritis; encephalomyelitis
	Equine infectious anemia virus	Horse	Recurrent hemolytic anemia
Retroviridae	Avian leukosis virus	Chicken	Leukemia
	Avian sarcoma virus	Chicken	Sarcoma
	Murine leukemia virus	Mouse	Leukemia

*Examples are persistent infections that have been the subject of extensive study.
†In newborn animals.
‡In immunosuppressed primates.
CNS, central nervous system.

cytopathic effects or cell death ultimately result. If a cytolytic virus is going to establish a persistent infection, alternative virus-host cell interactions must occur so that the cytopathic effects of the virus are limited. Much of the story of persistent infections told in this chapter describes the mechanisms by which the effects of a virus on the host cell are attenuated so that the cell can survive and the virus can persist within it. In many ways, this is the classic story of a parasite, needing to survive and persist within a host without harming it, while nonetheless resisting its defenses.

To present the subject of viral persistence, this chapter has been divided into three sections. The first section defines the different patterns of viral infection seen in a host. The second part considers, in general terms, the possible mechanisms and strategies that viruses use to successfully establish and maintain a persistent infection. This section draws on examples from human viral infections and animal model infections to illustrate specific concepts and principles. The third section examines in greater detail the mechanisms by which individual viruses persist within a human host. In this section, rather than discussing all viruses known to persist in humans, representative examples have been selected to illustrate the various types of virus-host interactions that occur during persistent infections. Other chapters within this book examine the implications of viral persistence within the context of specific viral infections, such as arenaviruses, retroviruses, lentiviruses, hepatitis viruses, HIV, neurotropic viruses, and prion diseases.

PATTERNS OF VIRAL INFECTION

Viral infections of a host organism can be divided into several general categories, based on the patterns and levels of infectious virus detectable in the organism at various times after infection (Fig. 9-1). The four types of infection illustrated in Figure 9-1 are as follows:

1. Acute infection followed by viral clearance by the host immune response.
2. Acute infection followed by latent infection in which the virus persists in a noninfectious form with intermittent periods of viral reactivation and shedding. These viruses must be capable of undergoing a productive infection in certain cells or under certain conditions while undergoing a nonpermissive infection in other cells (Table 9-3). The important issues here are the mechanisms by which the cytopathic potential of these viruses is limited so they can establish latency, how they are maintained in a latent form, and how they reactivate.
3. Acute infection followed by persistent infection in which infectious virus is continuously shed from or is present in infected tissues. Persistent infections can be established if the host immune response cannot eliminate virus generated during an acute infection. Productive infection of host cells may be followed by spread to cells that are less permissive, or by evolution of an immune response that dampens viral replication but cannot completely clear the virus from the host.
4. Slow, progressive infection. This pattern is observed only with unconventional agents, such as those causing spongi-

Patterns of Viral Infection in the Host

I. Acute viral infection followed by viral clearance

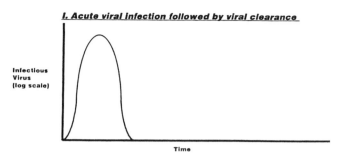

II. Acute viral infection followed by latent infection and periodic reactivation

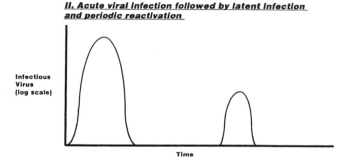

III. Acute viral infection followed by persistent infection

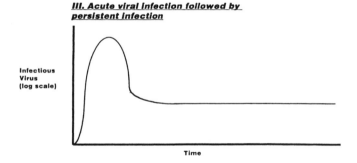

IV. Slow chronic infections

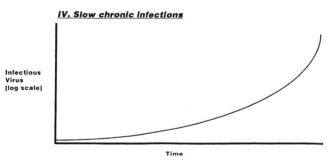

FIG. 9-1. General patterns of viral infection in the host organism.

TABLE 9-3. *Examples of latent infection followed by periodic reactivation*

Example	Mechanism of establishment	Maintenance	Stimulatory mechanism for reactivation
Herpes simplex virus in sensory ganglion neurons	Limited transcription and possibly replication of genome	Nonreplicating episome	Neuronal activation or damage
Epstein-Barr virus in B lymphocytes	Limited transcription of viral genome	Replication of viral DNA as episome	Antigen activation or other stimuli of B cells
Papillomavirus in basal cells of epidermis	Limited transcription of viral genome	Replication of viral DNA as episome	Differentiation of basal cells

form encephalopathies. Because such infections are not caused by any of the known viruses, this pattern is not discussed further here, but additional information on these unconventional agents can be found in Chapter 37.

Idealized patterns of viral infections of the host have been defined, but many viruses show different patterns of infection in different tissues or cell types, or combine these general patterns such that their infection of the host does not fit cleanly within these definitions. Therefore, these patterns should be viewed as themes with variations, and not as rigid definitions.

MECHANISMS OF VIRAL PERSISTENCE

Three general conditions must be fulfilled for a virus to persist long-term in a host. First, the virus must be able to infect host cells without being overtly cytolytic. Second, there must be mechanisms for maintaining the viral genome in host cells. Third, the virus has to avoid detection and elimination by the host's immune system. Viruses have devised various strategies to accomplish these goals, and these general mechanisms are explored in this section. Selected examples are used to illustrate the various concepts involved.

Restriction of Viral Cytolytic Effect

Survival of critical numbers of infected cells is a basic requirement for viral persistence. Therefore, a virus can persist in a host cell only if it does not kill the cell or the animal host. Viruses that cause nonlytic productive infections are well suited for persistence, and these viruses are the ones most likely to establish a chronic infection. For example, most arenaviruses can replicate in a cell without killing it or affecting its growth rate.[30,150] This nonlytic phenotype permits the various arenaviruses to survive in nature as lifelong chronic infections of their respective rodent hosts.[114,148,216] Another example of a nonlytic virus-host cell interaction is chronic infection of liver cells with HBV, which productively infects hepatocytes with minimal to no cell injury. However, for viruses that usually inhibit host cell metabolism and lyse the cell, the lytic phenotype is a potential barrier to the successful establishment of a persistent infection. Conditions under which the cytopathic effect of lytic viruses is limited include infection of nonpermissive cell types or of cells in a nonpermissive environment and evolution of viral variants that are less cytolytic

or interfere with replication of wild-type virus. Another possible mechanism for limitation of viral cytopathic effect would be for the virus to evolve complex regulatory controls that actively shut down viral gene expression in certain cell types, but there are no known examples of this scenario. Instead, certain cell types are nonpermissive, imposing a downregulatory effect on viral gene expression, and it appears that viruses may have merely evolved to persist in this restrictive environment.

In addition, a virus may be lytic for certain cell types but not for others. This is particularly relevant for persistence in vivo, because many different cell types are present in the whole animal. For instance, there is evidence suggesting that HIV is more lytic for T cells than for monocytes/macrophages. Productive infection of T cells can result in cell death, whereas HIV-infected mononuclear phagocytes produce virus for long periods without cell lysis.[83,108,133,146,235] Similarly, Sindbis virus, the prototype alphavirus, causes a lytic infection in neuroblastoma cells or freshly explanted dorsal root ganglion neurons, but establishes a persistent infection in neurons that have differentiated in the presence of nerve growth factor.[156] Although persistence of alphaviruses in humans has not been documented, studies have shown that Sindbis virus can persist in neurons of adult mice without causing overt damage.[155,157]

Infection of Nonpermissive Cells

The best examples of restricted viral gene expression involve the infection of nonpermissive or semi-permissive cells. For example, sensory neurons are nonpermissive for the normally cytolytic HSV, allowing little or no viral gene expression. In these cells, a latent infection is established. Similarly, B lymphocytes are nonpermissive for Epstein-Barr virus (EBV). In this case, selective expression of EBV genes not involved in lytic infection permits viral DNA replication to occur when the host cell divides, while nonetheless maintaining the noncytolytic state. In addition, basal layer skin cells are nonpermissive for papillomaviruses, and latent infections are established in these cells. These viruses remain in the latent state until they are induced to reactivate by perturbations of the host cell environment, such as cell injury or cellular differentiation, which are thought to convert, at least temporarily, a nonpermissive cell type to one that is permissive for viral replication (see Table 9-3). Latent herpesvirus and papillomavirus infections are discussed in more detail in a later section of this chapter.

Another example of restricted gene expression by a normally cytolytic virus comes from in vitro studies on the infection of teratocarcinoma cells by cytomegalovirus (CMV).[69,88] CMV causes a productive infection of differentiated teratocarcinoma cells, but the infection of undifferentiated cells results in incomplete viral transcription. If these nonproductively infected cells are then driven to differentiate by treatment with retinoic acid (or by any other signals leading to differentiation), multiple transcripts associated with lytic infection are produced, viral proteins are synthesized, and infectious progeny are released. In vivo, CMV causes a nonproductive infection of human peripheral blood mononuclear cells.[72,127,181,219] Infection is confined predominantly to monocytes, and viral gene expression appears to be limited to the immediate-early (IE) gene products. There is now some evidence that differentiation of monocytes into macrophages can convert this nonproductive infection into a productive one.[269]

"Smoldering" Infection of Low Numbers of Permissive Cells

Studies on persistent virus infections of cultured cells have shown that lytic viruses also can persist in vitro under conditions in which only a small fraction of the total cells are infected at any one time. In such carrier cultures, the few infected cells release virus and are killed, but the progeny virus again infects only a small number of the total cells, while most of the cells remain uninfected. This restriction could result from a limited number of susceptible cells at a given time or from the presence of soluble inhibitors such as interferon in the culture medium.[285,286,301] This type of "smoldering" or "cycling" infection has been implicated in the persistence of lactic dehydrogenase virus in mice and adenoviruses in humans.[3,165,211] It is possible that such smoldering infections are more common in vivo than has been appreciated.

Evolution of Viral Variants

There is considerable evidence from in vitro studies that viral mutants generated from normally cytocidal wild-type viruses possess modified lytic potential.[112,165,290,301] Several types of viral variants, such as temperature-sensitive and small plaque mutants and defective-interfering particles, have been implicated in the establishment of persistent infections in vitro. In some systems, the genetic basis of attenuation is known, and the viral gene or genes that play a role in persistence have been identified. For example, studies on reovirus persistence have shown that mutations in specific viral genes are crucial for the establishment and maintenance of persistent infection in L-929 cells.[6,7,63,131] In addition, mutational alterations of the glycoproteins of Sindbis virus have been shown to modify the lytic potential of Sindbis virus for neurons.[155] These studies illustrate the concept that a few amino acid changes in selected viral genes can convert a lytic infection into a persistent one.

In addition to selection of viral variants, there also is the possibility of obtaining variants of the host cell. Several reports have described the selection of mutant cells during persistent infection of cell lines in culture. For example, HeLa cells with increased resistance to poliovirus or coxsackievirus A9 were selected in carrier cultures.[1,267,280] The increased resistance of HeLa cell variants resulted from blocks at different steps of the poliovirus life cycle: some cell lines were nonpermissive for poliovirus infections because of decreased levels of expression of the poliovirus receptor, whereas others were nonpermissive for poliovirus replication at intracellular steps.[48,128] Similarly, African green monkey kidney cells partially resistant to simian virus 40 were isolated from persistently infected cell lines.[218,295] A persistently infected cell culture provides a dynamic environment, and co-evolution of both host cells and virus has been described during persistence of reovirus in L cells.[5,63] It was shown that both the original L cells and the parental reovirus had changed, followed by a co-selection of variant cells and virus. During the course of the persistent infection, mutant L cells that were highly resistant to lysis by reovirus were selected, and this was followed by selection of an altered reovirus that grew much better in these mutant cells. These observations on host-virus co-evolution described for reovirus also have been shown to occur during persistent infection of baby hamster kidney cells with foot-and-mouth disease virus and in L cells infected with minute virus of mice.[59–61,228] Although these studies have shown that host cells in culture can evolve to a state allowing persistent infection, it is probable that cells are constrained in their potential for this type of evolution during in vivo infections.

Mechanisms of Viral Genome Maintenance

The second requirement for viral persistence is a mechanism for maintenance of the viral genome in the persistently infected cell. If the host cell is dividing, there must be replication of the viral genome so that it is not diluted out among daughter cells. For retroviruses, the mechanism to achieve this result is a part of the viral replicative process. The DNA copy of the viral RNA genome is integrated into the host chromosome so that the viral genome is propagated with the host chromosomes (for details of this process, see Chap. 26). Integration into the host chromosome is by far the most efficient mechanism for maintaining the viral genome, because replication of the viral DNA is now inherently tied in with replication of host DNA. In addition to retroviruses, some DNA viruses also can persist by integrating their genome into the host chromosome. A well-characterized example of this is adeno-associated virus (AAV). AAV is a member of the dependovirus genus of the *Parvoviridae* family and can persist in a latent form in the human host and in cultured cells. Although there is limited information about the mechanisms by which parvoviruses persist in the human host, the mechanism by which AAV integrates its DNA into host chromosomes is well defined and novel among the DNA viruses. AAV particles contain a single-stranded DNA genome encapsidated in a protein coat. AAV replication requires co-infection with a helper virus such as adenovirus or HSV. Because AAV commonly is found in a latent form within human embryonic kidney cells,[110] latent infection in vivo is believed to be common. All the knowledge about the mechanisms of AAV DNA integration has come from studies of AAV infection of cells in culture. On infection of a host cell in the absence of helper virus, limited AAV gene expression occurs. Viral DNA replication has not been detected after viral entry into the host cell, but the viral DNA sequences become integrated as double-stranded DNA in the host cell DNA in the form of tandem repeats.[47,100] Therefore, at least limited DNA replication must occur. The viral DNA is integrated specifically within one region of chromosome 19, although the precise site of integration may range over several hundred base pairs.[140–142,234] The AAV Rep protein appears to promote integration through downregulation of viral gene expression and DNA replication or by binding to the preintegration site, but is not absolutely essential for integration. AAV can persist within cultured cells, and probably its human host, by integration of its genomic DNA into the host chromosome. On superinfection of latently infected cells with a helper virus,[110] or possibly on other environmental changes, rescue of the latent genome occurs with production of infectious AAV leading to possible transmission to a new host.

Alternatively, viral DNA also can be maintained as episomal circular molecules. This is seen with several persistent DNA viruses, such as papillomaviruses, EBV, and HSV. The maintenance of HSV and EBV genomes is described in more detail later in this chapter. The persistence and replication of papillomavirus DNA is discussed here because it represents a unique example showing how replication of viral DNA can be intimately linked with differentiation of the host cell. HPVs, the causative agents of human warts, undergo a nonproductive infection of basal layer cells in the skin, but replicate productively when basal layer cells or their daughter cells differentiate into keratinized cells of the stratum spinosum and granular layers of the epidermis. Papillomaviruses do not replicate in cultured cells except in specialized systems, so much of the information available on their replication cycle has been pieced together from studies of nonpermissive infections of cultured cells by bovine papillomavirus and, more recently, HPVs, and from histologic analyses of viral gene expression in clinical samples of wart tissue. Infection of basal layer skin cells by HPV is initiated when the virus is introduced into the lower layers of the epidermis as a consequence of trauma to the epithelium. Early viral transcription can occur in these cells,[264] and the viral DNA is retained in them,[238] probably replicated to low copy numbers as an extrachromosomal plasmid. However, the undifferentiated basal layer cells are not permissive for the replication of viral DNA for packaging into progeny particles (a process called *vegetative viral DNA replication*), or for late gene transcription. The early viral gene products stimulate cell growth in the basal layer, leading to the formation of a wart. As the basal layer cells divide and differentiate into keratinocytes, they become permissive for vegetative viral DNA replication, allowing late viral gene expression and the formation of infectious viral particles. Amplified levels of viral DNA and late transcripts and proteins can be found only in the most superficial layers of wart tissue. HPV infection of basal cells could be considered to constitute a form of latent infection during primary infection itself in that the cells contain the viral genome but no viral proteins or infectious virus are produced. These cells are nonpermissive because vegetative viral DNA replication cannot take place. Differentiation of the basal cells leads to the induction of vegetative viral DNA replication, probably because a missing host factor becomes available or an inhibitor is lost. At a low frequency, after a period of 20 to 25 years, a wart or latently infected cell can undergo an oncogenic and, in some cases, malignant conversion. In carcinomas associated with HPV-6 and HPV-11 infections, which usually are at low risk for malignant progression, the viral genome is extrachromosomal and transcriptionally active. In contrast, in neoplasia associated with the more frequently malignant HPV-16 and HPV-18 infections, the viral genome is integrated into host cell chromosomes,[70] often in a way that disrupts the HPV E2 open reading frame.[16,243] This inactivates the repressor function of E2, allowing expression of the E6 and E7 oncogene products.[282]

DNA viruses can maintain their genome in the host cell in an integrated form or as an extrachromosomal plasmid. In some instances, the viral genome also can be maintained in the absence of any viral proteins because the host cell is able to carry out the processes necessary for propagating the viral DNA. In contrast, the host cell is unable to provide on its own the functions necessary for replicating viral RNA. Because of this dichotomy, true latent infections are more common with DNA viruses (or retroviruses), whereas persistence of RNA viruses is characterized by the continuous expression of viral proteins necessary for the replication and maintenance of viral RNA.

Evasion of Host Immunity

The primary function of the host's immune system is recognition and elimination of foreign antigens. A major requirement for viral persistence is evasion of immunologic surveillance. Viruses have developed various strategies to shift the balance so as to avoid elimination by the host's immune system, as summarized in Table 9-4.[3,89,90,167,180,256]

Antiviral Immunity

Antibodies and T cells are the two main antigen-specific effector systems for resolving viral infections.[68] (For a detailed description of the immune response to viruses, see Chap. 7). However, before discussing the various escape mechanisms that viruses have evolved, it is useful to review how T and B cells control viral infections and to define the critical molecules involved in the recognition of viral materials by T cells and antibodies (Table 9-5). Antibodies can recognize free virus or virus-infected cells. They control virus infections by neutralizing virus particles and by killing infected cells through complement-mediated cytotoxicity or antibody-dependent cell-mediated cytotoxicity. The critical viral proteins recognized in these processes are surface glycoproteins or outer capsid proteins, and although antibodies against internal and nonstructural viral proteins also are made, these do not participate in viral neutralization or antibody-mediated killing of infected cells. Antibody binding to viral glycoproteins at the cell surface also can downregulate the expression of viral genes inside the infected cell,[82] but the mechanism by which this effect occurs is not understood. This interesting phenomenon, first described for measles virus (MV)–infected cells in culture,[80,81] also may operate in vivo in controlling Sindbis virus infection in neurons.[157] Similar observations have been

TABLE 9-4. *Viral strategies for evading the immune system*

Escape mechanism	Example*
1. Restricted gene expression; virus remains latent in the cell with minimal to no expression of viral proteins	HSV and VZV in latently infected neurons, EBV in B cells, HIV in resting T cells
2. Infection of sites not readily accessible to the immune system	HSV, VZV, measles, and rubella persistence in neurons/CNS CMV, polyomaviruses BK and JC in the kidney EBV and CMV in the salivary gland Papillomaviruses in the epidermis
3. Antigenic variation; virus rapidly evolves and mutates antigenic sites that are critical for recognition by antibody and T cells	Antibody escape variants in lentiviruses CTL escape variants in HIV, EBV, and HBV T-cell receptor antagonism by HIV and HBV variants
4. Suppression of cell-surface molecules required for T-cell recognition	Suppression of MHC class I molecules by adenoviruses, CMV, HSV, and HIV Decreased expression of cell adhesion molecules LFA-3 and ICAM-1 by EBV Suppression of MHC class II molecules by CMV, HIV, and measles
5. Interference with antigen processing and presentation	HSV ICP47 protein interferes with TAP to inhibit MHC class I antigen presentation
6. Viral "defense" molecules that interfere with the function of antiviral cytokines	Adenovirus proteins (E3-14.7K, E3-10.4K/14.5K, and E1B-19K) protect infected cells from lysis by TNF Adenovirus VA RNA, EBV EBER RNA, and HIV TAR RNA inhibit function of interferon-α/β EBV protein BCRFI (a homolog of IL-10) blocks synthesis of cytokines such as IL-2 and interferon-γ
7. Immunologic tolerance	Clonal deletion/anergy of virus-specific CTLs in HBV carriers, HIV (?)
8. Cell-to-cell spread by syncytia	SSPE caused by measles

*Only examples of viruses known to persist in humans are cited.

HSV, herpes simplex virus; VZV, varicella zoster virus; EBV, Epstein-Barr virus; HIV, human immunodeficiency virus; CNS, central nervous system; CMV, cytomegalovirus; CTL, cytotoxic T lymphocyte; HBV, hepatitis B virus; MHC, major histocompatibility complex; TNF, tumor necrosis factor; IL, interleukin; SSPE, subacute sclerosing panencephalitis.

TABLE 9-5. *Antiviral T-cell and B-cell immunity*

Effector system	Recognition molecule	Mechanism of viral control
Antibody	Surface glycoproteins or outer capsid proteins of virus particles. Viral glycoproteins expressed on membrane of infected cells.	(i) Neutralization of virus (ii) Opsonization of virus particles (i) Antibody-complement–mediated and antibody-dependent cell-mediated cytotoxicity of virus-infected cells (ii) Downregulation of intracellular viral gene expression
CD4+ T cells	Viral peptides (10–20 mers) presented by MHC class II molecules. Peptides presented by MHC class II molecules usually are derived from exogenous proteins. This could be any viral protein (surface, internal, or nonstructural). The limiting factors are the processing and binding to MHC molecules.	(i) Release of antiviral cytokines (interferon-γ, TNF) (ii) Activation/recruitment of macrophages (iii) Help for antiviral antibody production (iv) Help for CD8+ CTL responses (v) Killing of virus-infected cells?
CD8+ T cells	Viral peptides (8–10 mers) presented by MHC class I molecules of infected cells. Peptides presented by MHC class I usually are derived from endogenous proteins. This could be any viral protein, the main limiting factors being the processing and binding affinity of the peptide for MHC molecules.	(i) Killing of virus-infected cells (ii) Release of antiviral cytokines (interferon-γ, TNF) (iii) Activation/recruitment of macrophages

MHC, major histocompatibility complex; TNF, tumor necrosis factor; CTL, cytotoxic T lymphocyte.

made using antibodies to the surface glycoproteins of rabies virus and Sendai virus.[66,174] These studies also have suggested that antibodies can neutralize virus inside the cell.[66,157,174] Thus, antibodies can control viral infections by several different mechanisms, and the critical recognition molecules appear to be viral surface glycoproteins or outer capsid proteins. Changes in the structure or expression of these viral outer capsid or surface glycoproteins could be important mechanisms by which viruses can avoid elimination by antibodies. Alterations in other viral proteins (internal and nonstructural) probably are not critical in escape from humoral immunity. However, there are some reports of antibodies to internal or core proteins also playing a role in protection.[161]

In contrast to antibodies, which recognize viral proteins by themselves, T cells only see viral antigen in association with host major histocompatibility complex (MHC) molecules.[85,303] The antigen-specific T-cell receptor (TCR) recognizes short viral peptides bound to cellular MHC molecules.[57,178] An important consequence of this mode of recognition is that T cells cannot recognize free virus, and their antiviral activities are confined to infected cells. The T-cell arm of the immune system has evolved for the surveillance of infected cells, whereas antibody serves as the primary defense against free virus. T cells are subdivided further into two subsets, CD4+ and CD8+ T cells.[85,160] CD4+ T cells recognize viral peptides in association with MHC class II antigens, whereas CD8+ T cells recognize viral peptides bound to MHC class I antigens.[26,29,163] These peptide fragments can be derived from any viral protein, structural (surface or internal) or nonstructural. All viral proteins can be potential targets for T-cell recognition. The limiting factors are the intracellular processing of the protein and the capability of the peptides to bind to MHC molecules (i.e., their affinity for various MHC molecules). The interaction of virus-specific T cells with virus-infected cells depends on binding of the antigen-specific TCR with the MHC-peptide complex and on several other accessory molecules that increase adherence between T cells and their infected target cells.[257] Molecules involved in adhesion include LFA-1, CD2, CD4, and CD8 on T cells and their corresponding ligands on target cells, ICAM-1, LFA-3, and the MHC class II and I molecules, respectively. Alterations in the structure or expression of any of these proteins can interfere with the effector functions of T cells and provide a possible mechanism of escape from T-cell–mediated immunity.

How do T cells control virus infections? The primary mechanism used by CD8+ T cells is killing of virus-infected cells. These CD8+ cytotoxic T lymphocytes (CTLs) are highly efficient in this process and can kill infected cells by two distinct mechanisms: a secretory and membranolytic pathway involving perforin and granzymes, and a nonsecretory receptor-mediated pathway involving Fas, a protein of the tumor necrosis factor (TNF) receptor family.[20,126,287] Two studies using perforin gene knock-out mice have shown that the perforin pathway is essential for clearing lymphocytic choriomeningitis virus (LCMV) infection in vivo.[125,287] In addition to their killing function, CD8+ T cells also control virus growth by producing antiviral cytokines such as interferon-γ and TNF, which interfere intracellularly with virus replication.[24,68] CD4+ T cells contribute to antiviral immunity in many different ways: they produce antiviral cytokines, are involved in the activation and recruitment of macrophages, and provide cy-

tokine-mediated help for both antibody production and CD8+ CTL responses.[24,68,169,187,205] CD4+ T cells play a central role in antiviral immunity. Virus-specific CD4+ CTLs also have been described in several systems, but their contribution to the control of virus infections in vivo is not clear.[68,149,188]

Viral Evasion Strategies

Viruses use various strategies to evade the immune system.

Restricted Expression of Viral Genes

Restricted viral gene expression reduces the lytic potential of viruses and also provides a simple and highly effective mechanism by which infected cells escape detection by the host's immune response. This strategy is used to varying degrees by nearly all the viruses that cause persistent infections. However, it is exemplified best by the herpesviruses and retroviruses. The most extensively analyzed system is latent infection of neurons by HSV, in which viral gene expression is turned off completely except for transcription from one region of the genome, and there appear to be no viral proteins expressed in the infected neurons.[260,261] Under such conditions, the virus essentially becomes invisible to the immune system because immunity is directed against foreign proteins and is not programmed to distinguish between "self" and "foreign" nucleic acid. Absolute latency is an ideal way of evading the immune system. However, this is not always feasible because, often, certain viral proteins are essential for replicating viral DNA during latency. For example, during latent infection of B cells by EBV, expression of one of the EBV proteins, called *EBNA-1,* is necessary for propagating the episomal EBV genome through cycles of cell division. Further, a permanent state of latency also is not in the best interest of the virus in terms of transmission. Without the production of infectious virus, there can be no horizontal spread—an important mode of viral transmission. As a result, even viruses that are highly efficient in establishing latent infections go through intermittent phases of productive infection.

Infection of Immunologically Privileged Sites

Another strategy used by viruses is infection of tissues and cell types that are not readily accessible to the immune system.[17] A site of persistence favored by many viruses is the central nervous system (CNS). At least two factors favor viral persistence in the CNS: the presence of the blood-brain barrier, which limits lymphocyte trafficking through the CNS, and the presence of specialized cells such as neurons, which express neither MHC class I nor class II molecules and cannot be recognized directly by T cells.[8,118,121,200] The kidney is another organ in which viruses tend to persist.[8,36,119] The human polyomaviruses BK and JC replicate in the kidney, with almost lifelong shedding into the urine. CMV also is found in the kidney and shed for long periods. It is not fully understood why the immune system is less effective in eliminating microbes from the kidney because no blood-kidney barrier exists and extensive trafficking of lymphocytes through the kidney occurs. However, a study has shown that, although T cells infiltrate the kidney, they have limited access to infected epithelial cells. These cells are protected by an intact basement membrane and microvascular endothelium, and this barrier has to be broken before T cells can have direct contact with their target cells.[11] Limited T-cell access also would apply to the epithelial surfaces of other secretory or excretory glands, and it is notable that the salivary gland, a secretory tissue, is a favored site of persistence for viruses such as CMV and EBV. Replication of papillomaviruses in the epidermis provides another example of persistence at an immunologically privileged site. The productive cycle only occurs in differentiating keratinocytes, and as a result, the infected cell and the viral particles are physically separated from the host's immune response by a basement membrane.

Antigenic Variation

The emergence of viral variants during persistence is a well-documented phenomenon.[113,259,301] Viruses, especially those with RNA genomes, can undergo mutation at high frequencies, and under the appropriate selective pressure, variants can arise rapidly.[111] This ability to mutate quickly can provide a means of evading both T-cell and B-cell immunity.

Viral Escape From Antibody Recognition. There are many examples of antibody-resistant variants, and mutation of viral proteins at sites critical for antibody recognition is a highly effective means of escape from neutralizing antibody. The classic example of this is the antigenic "shift" and "drift" seen among influenza viruses.[202,289] These antigenic changes are the result of alterations in the two surface glycoproteins of influenza virus, the hemagglutinin and the neuraminidase. Influenza virus does not establish a persistent infection in individuals, but the emergence of antigenic variants does contribute to the persistence of influenza virus at the population level. The best example of antigenic variation in a given individual during a persistent infection comes from the lentiviruses. Kono and colleagues[136,137] were the first to report antigenic drift of equine infectious anemia virus in chronically infected horses. They showed that sera taken at various times from an infected animal were able to neutralize virus isolates from previous clinical episodes, but failed to effectively neutralize subsequent equine infectious anemia virus isolates. Additional studies have shown that these serologic changes correlate with alterations in the glycoproteins of equine infectious anemia virus.[183,233] Narayan and colleagues[189-192] have demonstrated the presence of antigenic variants in sheep chronically infected with visna virus. The altered neutralization properties of these variants have been correlated with genetic changes in the visna virus glycoproteins. Antigenic variants also have been shown to emerge during persistence of caprine arthritis encephalitis virus in goats, simian immunodeficiency virus in monkeys, and HIV in humans.[34,35,76,192,217,223,294] The appearance of serologically different variants during chronic infection is a common feature of all lentiviruses. However, the biologic importance of antigenic variation in these viruses is not fully understood. With the possible exception of equine infectious anemia

virus, in which the recurrent episodes of disease (clinical symptoms associated with bursts of viremia) correlate with the emergence of antibody escape variants, the phenomenon of antigenic variation among lentiviruses does not seem to be essential for the persistence or induction of disease.[76,162,183,189,233,275] In many cases, the "parental" virus continues to persist along with the variants in the infected host, in spite of the presence of neutralizing antibodies. Although neutralizing antibodies select antigenic variants, they are unable to eliminate completely the parental wild-type virus, and variant and wild-type virus often coexist in the persistently infected host.

Viral Escape From T-Cell Recognition. Antigenic variation in viral peptides at residues involved in the processing and binding of the peptides to MHC molecules or alterations in viral peptides at sequences that directly contact the TCR can result in loss of recognition by the appropriate T cell. Theoretically, such alterations can occur in viral peptides presented by MHC class I or class II molecules, resulting in escape from CD8+ and CD4+ T cells, respectively. Few studies have systematically analyzed antigenic variation within viral epitopes recognized by CD4+ T cells. In large part, this is because of the paucity of information on viral peptides seen by CD4+ T cells. In contrast, there is more information on CD8+ T-cell epitopes, and there are several well-documented examples of antigenic variation resulting in viral escape from CTL recognition.[143] CTL escape variants were first demonstrated using the LCMV system.[210] In this study, it was shown that a single amino acid change can abrogate CTL recognition, leading to persistence of the mutant virus in vivo. However, this profound biologic effect of the CTL escape variant was seen in transgenic mice that expressed a single LCMV-specific TCR and could only make a monoclonal CTL response.[210] It remains to be seen whether CTL escape variants will have a similar advantage under more physiologic conditions when antiviral CTL responses are likely to be polyclonal and multispecific.

CTL escape variants have been shown to occur in several viruses infecting humans, including HIV, EBV, and HBV.[52,56,58,73,143,159,208] There is substantial evidence that CTLs play a role in controlling, at least to some degree, infections by all three of these viruses. It is tempting to propose that, in these cases, generation of CTL escape variants is critical for maintenance of the persistent infection. However, in most of the studies in which CTL escape variants were identified, these variants did not go on to become the predominant viral species.[143] In addition, in a longitudinal study of HIV-infected individuals, no escape variants were detected over a 14-month period, demonstrating that the presence of such variants is not essential for HIV persistence.[179] Similar observations have been made with simian immunodeficiency virus.[46] Although these studies question the role of CTL escape variants in viral persistence, escape from CTLs also can occur by several other mechanisms (see later). CTL lysis also may be avoided if the density of viral peptides present on the cell surface is too low to trigger efficient lysis of the target cells. Tsomides and associates[277] have provided evidence for this by showing that the low density of certain HIV peptides on naturally infected cells limits the effectiveness of HIV-specific CTLs.

Two studies on HIV and HBV have provided evidence for a novel strategy for foiling the CTL response.[22,134] These studies have identified mutants of HIV and HBV that can interfere with CTL function in vitro. These variants have alterations in epitopes recognized by CTLs. However, unlike CTL escape variants that are not recognized by CTLs (i.e., are invisible to the TCR), these mutant epitopes still can interact with the TCR, but instead of giving a stimulatory signal, they act as antagonists and render the CTLs nonfunctional. This phenomenon has been termed *TCR antagonism,* and although the mechanism is not understood, it provides a highly effective means of evading the CTL response.[117,252] An important aspect of this strategy is that the "antagonistic" variants can block CTL-mediated lysis of cells that are co-infected with viruses containing wild-type sequences. This would provide a possible explanation for the survival of wild-type virus in the face of an ongoing CTL response. The one caveat to these exciting observations is that it it not known whether TCR antagonism is effective in vivo.

Suppression of Cell-Surface Molecules Required for T-Cell Recognition

Viruses can escape T-cell recognition by mutation of the sequences encoding the epitope (peptide) seen by the TCR and by downregulation of the expression of any one of the several host molecules that are necessary for efficient T-cell recognition of virus-infected cells. These include host MHC class I (for CD8$^+$ cells) or class II (for CD4$^+$ cells) molecules and several adhesion molecules, such as ICAM-1 and LFA-3. Viruses have developed strategies for disrupting this multimeric interaction by selectively inhibiting the expression of these critical host cell molecules.

The reduction of MHC class I antigen expression on host cells as a consequence of viral infection has been reported for several viruses.[120,168,214,220,242,299] This is an effective means of avoiding recognition by CD8$^+$ T cells. The best-documented example of virus-mediated suppression of MHC class I antigens is by the adenoviruses.[10,32,33,71,101,201,242,249,296] Human adenoviruses can downregulate MHC expression by two distinct mechanisms. One of the early proteins of adenovirus type 2, the E3 19-kilodalton protein, termed *E3/19K,* can bind to and form a complex with MHC antigens. The formation of this E3-MHC class I complex prevents the MHC antigens from being processed correctly by inhibiting their terminal glycosylation. This results in reduced cell-surface expression of the class I antigen. Adenovirus type 12 (an oncogenic serotype) prevents MHC class I expression by a different mechanism that involves a transcriptional block or lack of export of messenger RNA (mRNA) from the nucleus. Another early protein, the E1a protein of adenovirus type 12, has been implicated in this inhibition. The biologic significance of this phenomenon was demonstrated by showing that the adenovirus 12–induced tumors that failed to express their endogenous MHC antigens escaped immunologic surveillance and continued to grow on transfer into an immunocompetent host.[21] When these MHC-negative, adenovirus 12–induced tumors were transfected with an exogenous MHC class I gene (whose expression was not suppressed) and then transferred into immunocompetent animals, the tumors were rejected.[268]

It is possible that adenovirus downregulation of MHC class I antigens also may operate in vivo to promote persistent infection. However, despite the many elegant studies on the suppression of MHC class I by adenoviruses, there is still no evidence that persistence of human adenoviruses during the natural infection is related to the downregulation of MHC class I molecules.

Numerous reports have documented virus-mediated suppression of MHC class II antigens.* Among the viruses infecting humans, CMV, HIV, and MV have been shown to interfere with MHC class II expression. The mechanism of viral interference is not understood, but in all the cases examined, viral infection did not affect the basal level expression of MHC class II molecules. Instead, the viral effect was directed toward inhibiting the interferon-γ–mediated upregulation of MHC class II mRNA transcription. Increased expression of MHC class II by interferon-γ is likely to play a key role in antigen presentation, and interference with this step may prevent the generation of an effective immune response against the virus.

Studies by Gregory and colleagues[93] have shown that downregulation of the cell-surface adhesion molecules LFA-3 and ICAM-1 is involved in the escape of EBV-positive Burkitt's lymphoma cell lines from EBV-specific CTLs. Certain EBV-positive Burkitt's lymphoma cell lines were not killed by MHC-matched, virus-specific CTLs in assays in which EBV-transformed B lymphoblastic cells derived from the normal B cells of the same patients were readily lysed. The resistance of these Burkitt's lymphoma cells to CTL killing did not result from altered expression of MHC class I genes or lack of viral gene expression, but instead correlated with a reduced level of the adhesion molecules, LFA-3 and ICAM-1, on the tumor cell surface. The mechanism involved in selective suppression of the molecules is not known, but these studies nicely illustrate yet another viral strategy of circumventing the immune response.

Interference With Antigen Presentation

Studies have described a novel mechanism by which HSV inhibits antigen presentation by MHC class I molecules.[102,299] ICP47, one of the IE proteins of HSV, binds to TAP, the transporter associated with antigen processing, and prevents peptide translocation into the endoplasmic reticulum. As a result, peptide loading onto MHC class I molecules does not take place and the empty class I molecules remain stuck in the endoplasmic reticulum and are not displayed on the cell surface. It will be of interest to determine the role of ICP47 in HSV persistence and pathogenesis in vivo. Studies with ICP47 mutants in appropriate animal models should shed light on this issue. In this context, it is notable that the site of HSV latency is the neuron—a cell that does not express MHC class I molecules. Residence of HSV in neurons during latency or during primary infection when there is productive infection should not be influenced by the ability of ICP47 to inhibit antigen presentation by MHC class I molecules. It is more probable that this novel function of ICP47 is of importance when HSV

---

*References 31, 124, 154, 171, 172, 207, 220, 241, 248.

replicates in cells (epithelial cells, fibroblasts) that do express MHC class I molecules and otherwise would be recognized and killed by HSV-specific CD8+ CTLs. The ability of ICP47 to interfere with TAP function and inhibit antigen presentation in these cells could result in increased HSV shedding and more efficient transmission to new hosts.

Interference With Cytokine Function

Cytokines are an important part of antiviral immunity.[24,187] Studies have described several viral proteins that act as "defense molecules" by interfering with cytokine function.[90,167,256] Three adenovirus early proteins, E3-14.7K, E3-10.4K/14.5K, and E1B-19K, can protect virus-infected cells from lysis by TNF. The mechanism by which these adenovirus proteins counteract TNF is not known. The poxviruses also encode a protein, T2, that inhibits the action of TNF. The poxvirus T2 protein is a homolog of the cellular receptor for TNF and is released from infected cells, serving as a decoy. T2 binds TNF and prevents TNF from binding its true cellular receptor and destroying virus-infected cells. Other examples of viral defense molecules include the EBV protein BCRF1, which is a homolog of interleukin-10 and can block the synthesis of interleukin-2 and interferon-γ, and a secretory protein encoded by myxoma virus that binds interferon-γ.[184,278] In some instances, viral RNA itself can function as a defense molecule. The adenovirus VA RNA, the HIV TAR RNA, and the EBV EBER RNA can inhibit the antiviral effects of interferon-αβ. Interferons induce the synthesis of a phosphoprotein called DAI that, in the presence of double-stranded RNA, phosphorylates initiation factor eIF-2 and prevents the initiation of translation. The extensive secondary structure of these viral RNAs allows them to bind to DAI, inhibiting double-stranded RNA binding and interfering with the action of interferon.[90]

Several viral "defense" molecules have been identified in many different viruses.[90,256] This rapidly expanding area of research is exciting and provocative, but most of the findings are based on in vitro studies, and it is essential that these observations be put to the test in vivo. In one instance, it already is known that the presence of viral defense molecules is not sufficient to completely evade the host's immune response. Several molecules that interfere with various cytokines have been found in vaccinia virus, yet vaccinia virus does not cause a persistent infection and is efficiently eliminated by the immune system. Although these proteins are likely to play a critical role in the pathogenesis of vaccinia virus, it appears that at least in this instance, they are not sufficient to provide long-term persistence within an individual host.

Immunologic Tolerance

Finally, perhaps the most efficient means of establishing and maintaining a persistent infection is to selectively silence the effector system responsible for clearing the virus. The classic example of this is the suppression of LCMV-specific CTL responses in congenitally infected carrier mice.[30,150] Adult mice infected with LCMV mount a vigorous cellular and humoral response against the virus and clear the infection within 2 weeks. This clearance is mediated primarily by LCMV-specific CD8+ CTLs.[4,37,169,185,304] In contrast to the acute infection seen in adults, mice infected with LCMV at birth or in utero become chronically infected, showing life-long viremia with high levels of infectious virus and viral antigen in most of their major organs. The persistence of LCMV in these carrier mice is accompanied by the lack of a T-cell response to the virus. This is a highly specific defect. Such persistently infected mice exhibit no generalized immune suppression and respond normally to other antigens, but they show no detectable T-cell responses against LCMV because the virus-specific T cells have been clonally deleted within the thymus on seeing viral antigen.[9,30,119,185,209] The inability of the carrier mice to eliminate virus results primarily from this T-cell defect. The best evidence for this comes from experiments showing that adoptive transfer of LCMV-specific T cells results in the clearance of virus from carrier mice.[8,86,118,200,281] Although other viral systems have not been studied as extensively, it is probable that a decreased virus-specific T-cell response is an important factor in the establishment and maintenance of many persistent viral infections.

Immunologic tolerance also plays a role in the establishment of chronic HBV infections. Most children (more than 90%) born to HBV-infected mothers go on to become HBV carriers. It is probable that, in these neonatally infected carriers, at least some of the HBV-specific T cells undergo clonal deletion within the thymus or in the periphery. Even during adult onset of HBV infection, it is possible that some of the virus-specific T cells may be deleted in the periphery as a result of overstimulation by high doses of viral antigen, as has been documented during infection of adult mice with macrophage-tropic and invasive strains of LCMV that rapidly produce a high antigen load in many tissues.[9,170,186] Under these conditions, virus-specific CD8+ CTLs are overstimulated and driven to clonal exhaustion (deletion) in the periphery. Studies have shown that CD4+ T cells play a critical role in sustaining CD8+ CTL responses during chronic infection; under conditions of CD4+ T-cell deficiency, there is rapid exhaustion of LCMV-specific CTLs in the periphery.[19,169] These findings have implications for chronic viral infections in general and may provide a possible explanation for the loss of HIV-specific CTL activity that is seen during the late stages of AIDS, when CD4+ T cells become limiting and their numbers fall below a critical threshold necessary for maintaining CTL function.

The various viral evasion mechanisms that have been discussed are summarized in Table 9-4. Although specific examples have been cited to illustrate the different strategies, it is unlikely that a single mechanism can account for the persistence of a given virus. It is more probable that a combination of these strategies, plus other, unknown, mechanisms, contribute to the persistence of virus in an otherwise immunocompetent host.

SELECTED EXAMPLES OF VIRUSES THAT PERSIST IN HUMANS

This section examines the mechanisms by which several viruses establish persistent infections, using some of the better-studied examples. Please consult the appropriate chapters for discussion of some of the remaining viruses listed in Tables 9-1 and 9-2.

Herpes Simplex Virus

Herpes simplex virus, the most extensively studied of the herpesviruses, persists in its human host by establishing a latent infection in sensory neurons. The two types of HSV, type 1 (HSV-1) and type 2 (HSV-2), usually infect at different sites. HSV-1 undergoes a primary productive infection in the oral mucosa or oral cavity (gingivostomatitis). The virus enters sensory nerve endings and establishes a latent infection in sensory neurons of the trigeminal ganglion. At later times, the virus reactivates from latent infection to cause recurrent lesions commonly known as *cold sores* or *fever blisters*. HSV-1 also can infect the cornea (herpes keratitis) as a result of primary infection or reactivation from latent infection. The host immune response to recurrent infections of the cornea can lead to progressive scarring of the cornea, clouding, and eventual blindness. Some lines of evidence suggest that HSV-1 also may establish a latent infection in corneal keratinocytes.[147] Finally, HSV-1 can travel along neuronal pathways into the CNS during primary infection or reactivation, resulting in a serious encephalitis.

HSV-2 usually is acquired as a sexually transmitted disease. HSV-2 infects the genital mucosa, spreads into nerves, and is transported to sacral ganglia, where it establishes a latent infection. Reactivation of this virus causes the recurrent lesions associated with genital herpes. In addition to genital infection, HSV-2 can spread systemically to cause meningitis in a few cases. More serious, however, is the intrauterine or peripartum transmission of HSV-2 from a productively infected mother to her child, which can result in encephalitis, disseminated herpes infection, or both in the newborn. The mortality of infected newborns is high despite the availability of antiviral agents to limit infection, and survivors frequently experience lifelong sequelae.

Despite the varied manifestations of HSV-induced disease, the stages of pathogenesis of HSV infection are relatively constant (Fig. 9-2). The process begins with productive infection of epithelial cells at the site of inoculation. Infection of these cells involves transcription and expression of IE or "alpha" genes, followed by expression of early (E) or "beta" gene products, viral DNA replication, expression of late (L) or "gamma" genes, and assembly of progeny viral particles. After release from these cells, the virus spreads to surrounding cells and eventually binds to and enters axon termini of sensory neurons. The virus or its nucleocapsid is translocated by retrograde axonal transport to the neuronal cell body, where it can follow one of two infection pathways. It can undergo a productive infection leading to the release of progeny virus and, possibly, further spread through the nervous system. Alternatively, it can establish a latent infection during which limited viral gene expression occurs and no infectious virus can be detected in the tissue. In experimental systems, latent infection is defined as the absence of infectious virus when homogenized ganglion tissue is assayed directly on sensitive cell cultures, but the presence of infectious virus when intact ganglion tissue or neurons are co-cultivated with permissive cells. In contrast to productive infection, during which HSV expresses more than 70 viral gene products, latent infection involves expression of only the latency-associated transcripts (LATs), as detected by in situ hybridization (Fig. 9-3). At later times, on appropriate stimulation of the latently infected neuron, the virus can reactivate, undergo a limited productive infection, and spread down the axon to the site innervated by the sensory neuron. There, the virus is released to undergo a productive infection in the epithelial tissue, resulting in a recurrent lesion at a site approximating that of the primary infection.

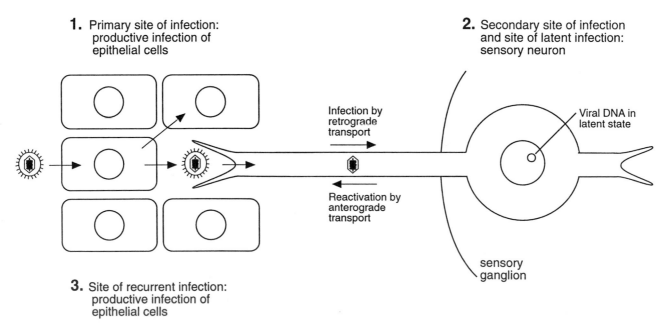

1. Primary site of infection: productive infection of epithelial cells

2. Secondary site of infection and site of latent infection: sensory neuron

Infection by retrograde transport

Reactivation by anterograde transport

Viral DNA in latent state

sensory ganglion

3. Site of recurrent infection: productive infection of epithelial cells

FIG. 9-2. Stages of infection of the host by herpes simplex virus (HSV).

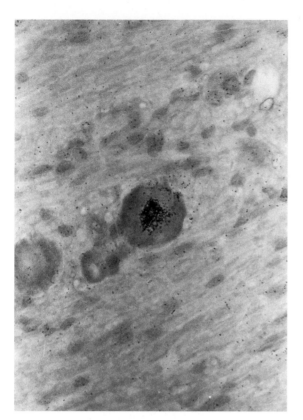

FIG. 9-3. Detection of herpes simplex virus (HSV) LAT RNA in latently infected murine trigeminal ganglion neurons by in situ hybridization. Mice were infected with HSV-1 after corneal scarification. At 30 days after infection, the mice were sacrificed and their trigeminal ganglia were frozen and sectioned. The sections were hybridized with a ³H-labeled DNA probe detecting the LAT RNA as described.[50] (Courtesy of Magdalena Kosz-Vnenchak, Harvard Medical School, Boston, MA.)

Establishment of Latent Infection

In the infected sensory neuron, at least in experimental animal systems, HSV can undergo a productive infection leading to the formation of progeny virus. Alternatively, the virus can establish a latent infection in which viral gene expression is limited and the neuron survives with the viral genome maintained stably in the neuron in a quiescent form. Although the events in an infected neuron that lead to the establishment of latent infection have not been defined, the limited viral gene expression during latent infection led to the idea that restriction of viral IE gene transcription in sensory neurons contributes to or is the sole determinant of the nonpermissive state of these cells.[62,263] Various hypotheses to explain the basis for the limited transcription of IE genes have been proposed. The first is that cellular transcription factors needed for the expression of these viral genes are absent or present at levels too low to support productive infection in these neurons.[227] It also has been proposed that cellular inhibitors of IE gene transcription are present in these neurons.[132] The HSV VP16 virion protein, which normally upregulates the transcription of IE genes, cannot function in these neurons to promote IE gene transcription.[227] However, a study indicates that the lack of VP16 in the neuronal nucleus cannot be the sole factor leading to the nonpermissive state of the neuron and the resultant latent infection.[244] It also has been hypothesized that limited IE gene expression may occur in neurons, but that transactivation of later gene expression cannot take place,[91] or that viral gene products such as ICP4, ICP27, or ICP8 may negatively regulate IE transcription in neurons.[135,199,266] One or more of these mechanisms could contribute to the nonpermissive infection of sensory neurons.

A modified regulatory pathway for HSV gene expression in neurons as compared with epithelial cells also has been proposed.[139] In this model, IE gene transcription is limited on infection of neuronal cells, but if enough IE and E viral gene products are expressed to permit viral DNA replication, IE and other viral gene expression is amplified to levels sufficient for productive infection to occur. If IE and E gene expression and DNA replication cannot occur, the virus would establish a latent infection. This proposed regulatory pathway provides a mechanism for the virus to sense the permissiveness of the host cell and establish a latent infection if the host cell is not permissive for IE and E gene transcription and viral DNA replication.

Viral genetic studies have attempted to address two issues regarding the establishment of latent infection: the stage in infection at which the latent versus productive infection pathways diverge, and the role of viral gene products in affecting this choice of infection pathways. With regard to the stage of infection at which the two infection pathways diverge, it is known that mutant viruses[50,129,138,279] or wild-type viruses, at least in some neuronal cells,[166,247,254] can establish latent infections without complete replication or even substantial viral gene expression in neurons. This has been interpreted to mean that the latent infection pathway deviates early from the productive infection pathway.[50,129,166,279] However, the in situ hybridization techniques used in many of these studies were not sensitive enough to distinguish between the total absence and low levels of viral gene expression during the establishment of latent infection. If low levels of viral gene expression do occur, the productive infection would be aborted at a later stage after limited viral gene expression. With regard to the second issue, the role of viral gene products in the establishment of latency, all viral mutants tested are capable of establishing latent infection, and there is no evidence that the expression of any viral gene product is required for latency.[50,129,151–153,176,245,271] Some viral mutants, including LAT-negative mutant viruses, show reduced efficiency of establishment of latent infection.[236] Although most investigators have interpreted this as being caused by decreased spread of the mutant virus to the neurons, one group has postulated a specific role for LAT in promoting the establishment of latent infection.[236] Because no viral gene product appears to be absolutely essential for the establishment of latent infection, the possibility that the neuron controls the establishment of latency has been raised.[129,166] Nevertheless, it is conceivable that viral gene products may participate in or influence a choice of infection pathways in the neuronal host cell. The other implication of these results is that productive infection is not a prerequisite for the establishment of latent infection.

Maintenance of Latent Infection

During the latent infection, no infectious virus can be detected within sensory ganglia, but viral DNA can be demonstrated, as detected by Southern blot hybridization[224] and by polymerase chain reaction amplification of viral DNA sequences within ganglion tissue.[129] Southern blot hybridization studies have determined that the viral DNA is present in an "endless" form in which the viral DNA termini are not detected.[177,224,225] Detailed studies have permitted the conclusion that the viral DNA probably is in a circular episomal form[177] associated with nucleosomes.[64] Because neurons are nondividing postmitotic cells, the viral DNA would not need to be replicated during the maintenance phase of the latent infection, and viral gene products required for replication would not need to be expressed. The only viral gene products that have been detected within latently infected tissue are the LAT transcripts,[53,62,212,226,262,263] and no protein product in latently infected tissue has been associated with these viral transcripts. The lack of viral protein expression would make the latent infection invisible to the host immune system. Further, sensory neurons express few or no MHC molecules, so T cells could not readily target infected neurons even if viral proteins were expressed.

The major form of the LAT transcript is a 2-kilobase RNA originally detected by in situ hybridization with viral probes. It accumulates within the nuclei of latently infected neurons (see Fig. 9-3). The minor LAT transcript is a large (about 8.5-kilobase) RNA whose coding sequences extend upstream and downstream from those encoding the 2-kilobase major LAT RNA species.[67] The minor LAT is believed to be the primary transcript of this transcriptional unit, which is spliced to give the stable 2-kilobase species.[75]

Genetic studies examining the role of the LAT transcripts in the maintenance of latent infection have demonstrated that the LAT transcripts are not essential for the maintenance of latency in that LAT-negative viruses can still persist in a latent state.[103,152,258,276] The maintenance of latent infection may involve only host cell factors that downregulate viral replication, and HSV gene products may not play an active role.

Reactivation From Latent Infection

The mechanism of HSV reactivation in response to neuronal stimuli has not been defined, but this process must lead in some way to the expression of viral gene products needed for productive infection. One model proposes that an appropriate stimulus leading to the expression of ICP0, an IE-nonspecific transactivator of viral gene expression, may activate the expression of other IE gene products, such as ICP4 and ICP27.[151] These gene products then in turn would activate E and L viral gene expression. However, ICP0 is not absolutely required for reactivation because ICP0-negative mutants can reactivate, albeit less efficiently.[151] Two other models suggest that amplification of HSV DNA in the latently infected neuron may trigger the expression of viral lytic-phase genes.[139,227] One of these postulates that amplification of the viral DNA is accomplished with cellular enzymes[227,246] and the other that viral DNA synthesis uses viral gene products.[139]

With regard to the viral gene products needed for reactivation, ICP0 may play a role in promoting reactivation because ICP0-negative mutants reactivate less frequently than wild-type virus, even though the amount of viral DNA present in the ganglia is about the same for mutant and wild-type virus.[151] Similarly, LAT-negative mutant viruses show reduced efficiency or delayed kinetics of reactivation,[103,152,258,276] leading to the hypothesis that LAT promotes reactivation, even though it is not essential. Ultimately, reactivation involves replication of the virus, so all the gene products essential for productive infection also must be required for the reactivation event.

The stimuli for reactivation in the human host include immunosuppression, hormonal changes, stress, neurectomy, nerve damage, and ultraviolet light exposure. These stimuli are likely to cause changes in the physiologic status of the neuron, and it would be predicted that this could lead to the activation of neuronal signaling pathways, causing the activation of transcription factors or protein kinases. These factors in turn could activate the expression of viral or cellular gene products, leading to an upregulation of expression of viral IE gene products. In experimental animals, reactivation has been achieved by explant of the latently infected tissue into culture and co-cultivation with permissive cells. In addition, in vivo reactivation has been induced by physical trauma to the animal, high temperature, ultraviolet irradiation, iontophoresis of adrenaline into the eye, or neurectomy. These treatments may cause damage to, or physiologic changes in, the neuron that similarly would be predicted to lead to changes in levels of protein kinases or transcription factors within the neuron. HSV seems to have evolved reactivation mechanisms that become operative when the neuronal host cell is perturbed so that the virus can get out of an injured or dying neuron and spread to a new cell or to a new host.

Varicella Zoster Virus

Varicella zoster virus (VZV), a second member of the *Herpesviridae* family, is the causative agent of the acute disease called *chickenpox* (varicella) and the recrudescent disease called *shingles* (herpes zoster). Because VZV remains highly cell-associated during its replication in cultured cells, it has been difficult until recently to obtain high-titer stocks of cell-free virus. This has hampered studies of the replicative mechanisms of VZV. In addition, there is no good animal model system for pathogenesis studies. Nearly all our understanding about the pathogenesis of VZV has been limited to the information derived from clinical samples and studies.

VZV enters an individual by infection of mucosal epithelial cells in the upper respiratory tract, oropharynx, or conjunctiva. After primary replication in the epithelium, the virus is disseminated by the bloodstream to the reticuloendothelial system, where viral replication leads to secondary viremia. Infection of capillary endothelial cells allows spread of the virus to epithelial cells of the epidermis, where focal cutaneous lesions are formed, causing the pocks characteristic of varicella. Host immunity limits the acute disease, but during spread through the epidermal epithelium, the virus also infects sensory nerve endings and is transported to sensory ganglia. Latent infection is established in the ganglia, neurons,[87,115,164] and satellite cells.[54,265] At a later time, reactivation may occur as a consequence of immunosuppression, nerve damage, or other stimuli. If the existing immune response cannot control the reactivating virus, extensive viral replication can occur in the ganglia. Virus also spreads to the periphery by axonal transport through neurons innervating a specific dermatome or dermatomes. There, the virus productively infects the epithelium to cause the lesion characteristic of shingles.

Little is known about the mechanisms of establishment and maintenance of latent infection by VZV. It is believed that latent infection is established in a host cell that is nonpermissive for viral gene transcription. There have been reports of the expression of viral transcripts and proteins from a variety of genes involved in VZV productive infection during what was presumed to be latent infection,[54,115,272] but it is difficult to rule out that these viral gene products were not expressed in cells undergoing limited reactivation. A detailed study has found VZV transcripts only from genes 29 and 62 in latently infected human trigeminal ganglia, suggesting that selected transcription of VZV IE and E genes occurs during latent infection.[175] Similarly, little is known about the mechanisms of reactivation.

Like HSV, which also undergoes a latent infection in sensory ganglia, VZV evades the immune response to establish latency in an immunologically privileged site and downregulates gene expression there. However, the clinical picture of VZV latency and reactivation shows many differences from that of HSV-1. First, most individuals undergo one episode of zoster, whereas HSV recurrences are numerous. Second, the probability of zoster increases with age, whereas the frequency of HSV recurrences decreases with time. Last, neuropathy and cutaneous spread of VZV during zoster can be more extensive than during HSV recurrence. Some have postulated that the capacity of VZV to establish latent infection in satellite cells instead of, or in addition to, neurons could contribute to these differences,[54] but the explanations for these differences will come only with a full understanding of VZV and HSV latent infection.

Epstein-Barr Virus

Epstein-Barr virus, a third member of the *Herpesviridae* family, is the causative agent of infectious mononucleosis and is a cofactor in the induction of the neoplastic diseases of Burkitt's lymphoma, nasopharyngeal carcinoma, posttransplant lymphoproliferative disease, non-Hodgkin's lymphoma, and oral hairy leukoplakia. Limited information exists about the replicative mechanisms of EBV because the virus does not efficiently undergo a productive infection in any cell type in vitro. However, EBV does efficiently establish a latent infection in B lymphocytes in vitro. No animal system faithfully reproduces the many other EBV disease manifestations seen in humans, so much of the knowledge about EBV pathogenesis has been derived from clinical studies and studies on latently infected B cells.

Individuals become infected with EBV by the oral route, possibly by contact with saliva containing infectious virus. EBV can undergo a limited productive infection in oropharyngeal epithelial cells,[252,253] which can continue as a chronic infection in some individuals.[84] By an unknown mechanism,

virus is transmitted to B lymphocytes, where a nonproductive, latent infection usually is established. For entry into B cells, the virus uses the CD21 cell-surface protein as a receptor.[77,79,193] On entry into the cell, the viral DNA is uncoated and circularizes to form the covalently closed circular genome that persists as an episome in the latently infected cell.[2,194]

Unlike the infection of neurons by HSV, EBV establishes latency in dividing cells and, therefore, must retain the potential for replication of its genome during latency. As many as 11 latency gene products are expressed, the number of viral gene products differing somewhat in different latently infected cells. The detection of EBNAs by immunofluorescence is illustrated in Figure 9-4. The EBV nuclear antigen 1, or EBNA-1 protein, is always expressed in latently infected cells because it plays an essential role in viral DNA maintenance in the latently infected B cell. EBNA-1 binds specifically to EBV DNA sequences[215] that serve as the origin for plasmid replication, oriP,[300] and promotes the replication of the viral episome by host cell DNA polymerase during the S phase of the host cell cycle.[2,99] Other EBV latent gene products, such as EBNA-2, stimulate growth of the host B cells, in part by inducing the expression of B-cell activation molecules.[288] This state of continuously stimulated growth often is described as *immortalization*.

A small proportion of latently infected B cells may become permissive for viral replication, in which case viral IE proteins are induced, followed by the expression of E proteins, viral DNA replication, L gene expression, and progeny virus assembly, much as described earlier for HSV. Reactivation of latent virus from B lymphocytes in the human host is thought to allow virus to reinfect epithelial surfaces, including the oropharynx, which would allow viral shedding and transmission. Induction of the lytic cycle in latently infected cells in culture can be achieved by the addition of phorbol esters or halogenated nucleosides.

The mechanisms used by EBV to evade the immune response may differ in latent versus chronic infection, and the virus has been shown to have a broad array of evasion strategies. Viral gene expression is restricted during latent infection of B cells, but some viral proteins are expressed, so the virus must use additional strategies to escape immune detection. The T-cell adhesion molecules LFA-3 and ICAM-1 are downregulated in EBV-transformed lymphoblasts,[93] representing a possible evasion strategy of nontransformed cells latently or chronically infected with EBV. In chronic infection of the nasopharyngeal epithelium by EBV, the virus infects a site that is immunologically privileged because of its relative inaccessibility to T cells. In addition, CTL escape variants also have been demonstrated.[58] Although the involvement of many of these mechanisms in EBV persistence in vivo has yet to be demonstrated, EBV is a fine example of a virus that apparently has evolved multiple strategies to effect persistent infection.

EBV infection of B cells is a classic latent infection with persistence of the viral genome as an episomal plasmid whose replication is tied to the host cell cycle and promoted by the EBNA-1 protein. In addition, it is now clear that the virus can productively infect oropharyngeal epithelial cells, although little is known about the mechanisms underlying this chronic infection. Within the same individual, EBV may persist by two mechanisms: latent and chronic infection.

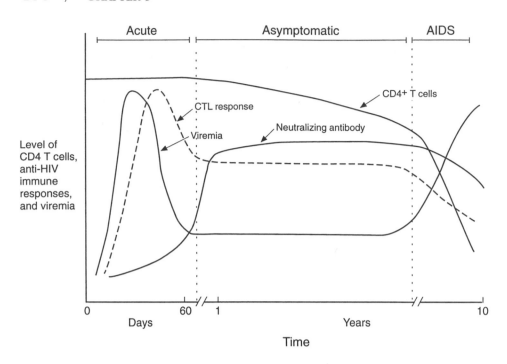

FIG. 9-4. Temporal changes in virus level, anti-human immunodeficiency virus (HIV) immune response, and total CD4+ T-cell count during various stages of HIV infection. AIDS, acquired immunodeficiency syndrome; CTL, cytotoxic T lymphocyte. (Adapted from Koup RA, Ho DD. Shutting down HIV. Nature 1994;370:416.)

Human Immunodeficiency Virus

Human immunodeficiency virus, the causative agent of AIDS, is a human lentivirus in the *Retroviridae* family. Infection can occur by sexual transmission through breaks in the mucosal surface, by direct injection as in puncture of the skin with contaminated needles, or by transfusion of contaminated blood products. Although the principal feature marking the development of AIDS in HIV-infected individuals is a decline in the number of CD4+ T cells and the ensuing impairment of immune responses, current models of HIV pathogenesis describe a complex series of stages of infection that precede the state of immunodeficiency[106,293] (see Fig. 9-4).

Acute Infection

After entry of the HIV into the host, the virus may replicate initially at the site of entry in Langerhans cells or other cells of phagocytic lineage and spread to local lymph nodes. Although the sites and mechanisms of earliest replication and spread are difficult to determine with certainty, the fact that initial isolates during acute infection are predominantly macrophage-tropic supports this conjecture.[229,302] The blood and lymph then disseminate HIV widely through the body, where it becomes sequestered in macrophages or trapped by follicular dendritic cells in the spleen and other lymphoid organs.[13,18,23,78,213,255,270] In these microenvironments, HIV may be concentrated on the surface of follicular dendritic cells from which it could be transmitted to CD4+ lymphocytes as the lymphocytes migrate through the germinal center to the perifollicular mantle and paracortical areas of the lymph nodes and spleen, where most of the HIV-infected lymphocytes have been found.[95]

Dissemination of the virus corresponds to a burst of viremia during the acute infection that may be accompanied by acute clinical illness.[49,55] This phase lasts up to 2 to 4 weeks after infection. The primary viremia then shows a rapid decline, usually between 3 and 6 weeks after infection. This decline correlates with the appearance of a vigorous, HIV-specific CTL response that may play a crucial role in controlling virus replication.[27,145,203,231] In contrast to the CTL response, neutralizing antibody appears much later (at or after 8 weeks). These observations strongly suggest that HIV-specific CTLs are involved in eliminating productively infected cells.

Persistent Infection/Asymptomatic Phase

Despite an impressive control of the acute infection, the host immune response does not completely clear the virus. One crucial consequence of acute infection is the establishment of latency in monocytes and CD4+ T cells in the lymph nodes and other lymphoid organs. Virus often persists for years before any obvious symptoms of immune deficiency are apparent, and infected individuals enter a period that has been called *clinical latency*. Although there is a low level of productively infected lymphocytes circulating in the blood during clinical latency,[76,107] in situ polymerase chain reaction to detect HIV DNA has shown that large numbers of cells within the lymph nodes contain viral DNA in asymptomatic individuals[74,204] (see Chaps. 19 and 34). Studies analyzing HIV infection in vivo have shown that viral load is maintained by a dynamic process involving continuous rounds of de novo virus infection and replication accompanied by rapid turnover of CD4+ T cells.[106,293] These findings imply that there is a constant ongoing battle between HIV and the immune system. Large numbers of infected cells and virus particles are destroyed daily, but a few survive and keep perpetuating the infection.

The infection of CD4+ T cells by HIV involves reverse transcription and integration of the viral DNA in a provirus form. Apparently, if the T cell is incapable of transcribing the provirus, HIV may establish a latent infection. On the other hand, if the cell is able to transcribe viral mRNA from the provirus, a productive infection results, with spread of the infection among CD4+ T cells. Antigen-specific activation of CD4+ T cells may be a key control switch that permits transcription of the viral RNA from the provirus[92] and conversion from latent to productive infection. At early to late stages of infection, Embretson and colleagues[74] observed many provirus-containing cells in lymphoid tissue, but few cells containing viral RNA. In contrast, Pantaleo and associates[204] observed many cells containing viral DNA and RNA, a situation more closely resembling a chronic infection. At this point, it is clear that there are many HIV-infected cells in lymphoid tissues during the asymptomatic phase, but the relative frequency of latently versus chronically infected cells remains to be determined.

During the clinical latency period, infected individuals continue to exhibit vigorous T- and B-cell responses against HIV. They possess antiviral antibody, including neutralizing antibody, and virus-specific CTLs directed against several HIV proteins.[†] Fresh peripheral blood lymphocytes obtained from "healthy" HIV carriers can directly mediate virus-specific CTL activity without any in vitro stimulation. This observation suggests an ongoing effector T-cell response against the virus, which in turn implies chronic, low-level HIV replication during clinical latency.[95]

Why, then, is HIV not eliminated? The various mechanisms that viruses use to evade host immune responses already have been discussed (see Table 9-4), and many of these strategies apply to HIV. Perhaps the most relevant is that HIV can "hide" itself (i.e., become latent), making it difficult for the immune system to completely deplete the reservoir of HIV-infected cells. Periodic activation of these latently infected cells can maintain the HIV reservoir by virus production and spread of the virus to uninfected and perhaps newly generated CD4+ T cells.

Progression to Acquired Immunodeficiency Syndrome

Although the asymptomatic phase can last, in some instances, for many years, eventually CD4+ T-cell numbers decline, possibly through attrition resulting from productive infection of mature CD4+ T cells or their progenitors.[240] Loss of CD4+ T cells also may occur by immunopathologic mechanisms.[76] Disease progression results. A report indicates that the level of HIV mRNA expression in peripheral blood cells predicts disease progression in infected individuals in that those who show high levels of mRNA within circulating T cells appear likely to become symptomatic.[232] Individuals infected with HIV may undergo simultaneously a latent infection and a chronic infection, with the relative proportion of cells exhibiting each type of persistent infection determining

the stage of disease progression. The mechanism or mechanisms by which the latent infection is reactivated or by which the chronic infection of lymph node cells is converted to an infection of circulating lymphocytes, as seen in symptomatic individuals, remain unknown.

Profound immunosuppression and susceptibility to opportunistic infections are "late" events in the pathogenesis of AIDS.[14,76,107] During the later stages of AIDS, the number of productively infected cells increases concomitant with an increase in virus load, while the number of CD4+ T cells declines dramatically and HIV-specific CTL responses are lost. HIV no longer evades the immune response, but overwhelms the defenses it has weakened. Two events may contribute to overt disease progression. First, with impaired immune effectiveness, the opportunistic infections that arise may increase the frequency of T-cell activation that promotes HIV transcription and productive infection. Second, viral variants emerge from the growing virus pool. These variants possess augmented replicative, and in some cases cytopathic, potential in CD4+ T cells as determined from sequential isolates from patients over time.[51] These events set up vicious cycles that contribute to an accelerated decline in most patients with AIDS, and eventually to their demise.

Measles Virus

Measles virus is a member of the *Paramyxoviridae* family of negative-strand RNA viruses that replicate in the cytoplasm of infected cells. Infection of humans results in the acute disease called *measles* and, less commonly, measles pneumonia. Although measles typically is an acute disease, a high incidence of CNS involvement occurs that can lead to the development of acute postinfectious encephalitis or, rarely, subacute sclerosing panencephalitis (SSPE). SSPE is a progressive, dementing disease that develops years after the apparent resolution of acute MV infection and appears to be a consequence of persistent MV infection of the CNS.[274,290]

Humans constitute the only natural host for MV, so much of the information regarding its pathogenesis derives from studies of patient isolates. Many laboratory animals, including monkeys and rodents, also can be infected subclinically with MV and have been used to study acute and persistent infection. From studies in these various systems, it has been determined that MV initiates acute infection in the epithelium of the respiratory tract, oropharynx or nasopharynx, or conjunctiva.[130,222] After replication in the mucosa, virus is transported to draining lymph nodes, possibly within macrophages. Virus undergoes secondary replication in the lymph nodes and then enters the bloodstream in leukocytes.[94,116,122,206] This primary viremia disseminates virus to the reticuloendothelial system, especially the lymphoid tissue, where another round of virus replication causes lymphoid hyperplasia. Multinucleate giant cells pathognomonic of MV infection also form through fusion of infected cells with neighboring uninfected cells.[12,41, 130,250] Secondary viremia disseminates virus to multiple tissue sites, where a generalized infection of the vascular endothelium precedes epithelial infection of the gastrointestinal tract, respiratory tract, and conjunctiva, and the appearance of the characteristic measles rash. Virus probably gains access to the

---

†References 107, 110, 144, 221, 223, 283, 284, 294.

CNS during the secondary viremic phase by infection of capillaries in the meninges, pia, and choroid plexus.[182] In a normal individual, an immune response is induced that effectively controls the acute infection.

Some MV-infected cells may escape immune clearance, however, to become persistently infected. Studies in cell culture indicate that the addition of anti-MV monoclonal antibody to infected lymphocytes induces capping and subsequent shedding of the specific MV antigen,[123] accompanied by selected decreases in other MV antigens.[80,81] Modulation of viral antigens on the surface of infected cells has been postulated to subvert normal viral clearance, allowing MV to establish persistence in the host. MV also has been shown to suppress the expression of MHC class I molecules,[214] and interferon-γ–mediated upregulation of MHC class II molecules.[154] Although these phenomena have been demonstrated only in vitro, generalized decreases in T-cell responsiveness have been observed in MV-infected individuals, suggesting that these or other immune evasion strategies may be operative in vivo. Nonetheless, the establishment and maintenance of chronic infection has a virologic component because cells in culture can be persistently infected in the absence of immune effectors.[195,290,300] These infections with MV represent a special type of persistent infection, however, because virus replicates slowly in the cultures, with little or no production of extracellular virus.[230] Restricted expression of the viral genome may occur through reduced synthesis of one or more structural components[96,251] or selection of defective viruses.[123] These persistently infected cultures resemble infections in the brains of patients with SSPE, in which viral nucleocapsids are retained within the cell but the amount of various membrane antigens is reduced.[15,158] This restricted viral gene expression, and infection of the privileged neuronal site, presumably plays a role in the development of persistent infection in some MV-infected individuals.

The association of measles with SSPE was made first by observations of paramyxovirus nucleocapsids in neurons and glial cells, and high titers of anti-MV antibody in the cerebrospinal fluid of patients with SSPE. Infectious virus has been detected occasionally in SSPE tissue by co-cultivation of infected brain tissue with cells permissive for MV, but more often no infectious virus is found. The mutation of genes encoding MV proteins as a mechanism of persistence was suggested by the observation that many of the viruses isolated from the brain tissue of patients with SSPE show alterations in matrix (M) protein synthesis or expression.[15,28,40,42,291] The M proteins of some SSPE strains are functionally distinct in that they remain cytosolic and cannot bind viral nucleocapsids at the plasma membrane or promote budding.[104,105] M protein coding sequences from SSPE strains show evidence of clustered U-to-C substitutions in the positive-strand sequences (postulated to result from a cellular RNA-modifying activity that alters regions of double-stranded RNA) compared with sequences of acute MV isolates. These biased hypermutation events, originally identified in a case of measles inclusion body encephalitis,[44] are thought to play a role in the evolution of SSPE viruses from acute measles strains.[297,298] Conserved hypermutation events in the coding sequences of cryptic M proteins from several SSPE virus isolates have been associated with the loss of conformation-specific epitopes present in acute measles isolates.[298] Consistent with these observations,

M protein often cannot be detected immunohistochemically in the brain tissue of patients with SSPE,[96,97] and many of these patients mount strong antibody responses to all MV proteins except the M protein,[98,292] Presumably, these SSPE viruses fail to bud from infected cells because of defects in M protein, but the viral genome is amplified and defective virus is disseminated by direct cell-to-cell spread in the face of intact immunity.

M protein expression[15,196] and antibody to M protein[15,65,196–198] have been detected in other cases of SSPE, however, and in these cases, defects in one or more genes encoding envelope proteins suggest a second class of genetic alterations in SSPE viruses. Some SSPE strains encode truncated or elongated fusion proteins with nonconservative amino acid substitutions in the cytoplasmic domain.[45,237] Genetic variability in the gene encoding the hemagglutinin and antigenic variants also has been observed.[25,39,250,273] Finally, multiple strains resistant to the effects of interferon have been identified in acute MV infections and in patients with SSPE.[38]

The role of various viral mutations in the establishment or maintenance of persistent MV infection and the development of the rare cases of SSPE remains to be determined. Restriction of MV gene expression is observed in neurons and glia, and may precede the accumulation of mutations. Evidence indicates that high levels of the antiviral protein, MxA, are induced rapidly on infection of human brain cells, accompanied by marked restriction of MV RNA synthesis.[239] This transcriptional attenuation is cell-type–specific and may contribute to the establishment of MV persistence in the CNS.

One hypothesis to explain the genesis of persistent infection and ultimately of SSPE[43] proposes that host defense mechanisms promote the establishment of persistence through modulation of MV transcription and protein expression. During subsequent rounds of replication, the MV genome may accumulate mutations in multiple viral genes that would impair the assembly of virions, in this case maintaining chronic infection without continual shedding of progeny virus. The selection of genetically altered viruses that are defective for progeny formation eventually may lead to the evolution of a strain possessing a more pathogenic phenotype, shifting the infection from one that is undetectable to one that causes a progressive, degenerative, and eventually fatal disease of the CNS.

ABBREVIATIONS

AAV: adeno-associated virus
AIDS: acquired immunodeficiency syndrome
CMV: cytomegalovirus
CNS: central nervous system
CTL: cytotoxic T lymphocyte
E: early gene products
EBV: Epstein-Barr virus
HBV: hepatitis B virus
HIV: human immunodeficiency virus
HPV: human papillomavirus
HSV: herpes simplex virus
IE: immediate-early genes
L: late genes
LATs: latency-associated transcripts

LCMV: lymphocytic choriomeningitis virus
M: matrix
MHC: major histocompatibility complex
mRNA: messenger RNA
MV: measles virus
SSPE: subacute sclerosing panencephalitis
TCR: T-cell receptor
TNF: tumor necrosis factor
VZV: varicella zoster virus

REFERENCES

1. Ackermann WW, Kurtz H. Observations concerning a persisting infection of HeLa cells with poliomyelitis virus. J Exp Med 1955;102: 555–565.
2. Adams A, Lindahl T. Epstein-Barr virus genomes with properties of circular DNA molecules in carrier cells. Proc Natl Acad Sci USA 1975;72:1477–1481.
3. Ahmed R. Persistent viral infection. Encycl Virol. London: Academic Press, 1994.
4. Ahmed R, Butler LD, Bhatti L. T4+ T helper cell function in vivo: differential requirement for induction of anti-viral cytotoxic T cell and antibody responses. J Virol 1988;62:2102–2106.
5. Ahmed R, Canning WM, Kauffman RS, Sharpe AH, Hallum JV, Fields BN. Role of the host cell in persistent viral infection: coevolution of L cells and reovirus during persistent infection. Cell 1981; 25:325–332.
6. Ahmed R, Chakrabarty PR, Fields BN. Genetic variation during lytic virus infection: high passage stocks of wild type reovirus contain temperature-sensitive mutants. J Virol 1980;34:285–287.
7. Ahmed R, Fields BN. Role of the S4 gene in the establishment of persistent reovirus infection in L cells. Cell 1982;28:605–612.
8. Ahmed R, Jamieson BD, Porter DD. Immune therapy of a persistent and disseminated viral infection. J Virol 1987;61:3920.
9. Ahmed R, Salmi A, Butler LD, Chiller JM, Oldstone MBA. Selection of genetic variants of lymphocytic choriomeningitis virus in spleens of persistently infected mice: role in suppression of cytotoxic T lymphocyte response and viral persistence. J Exp Med 1984;60:521–540.
10. Andersson M, Paabo S, Nilsson T, Peterson PA. Impaired intracellular transport of class I MHC antigens as a possible means for adenoviruses to evade immune surveillance. Cell 1985;43:215–222.
11. Ando K, Guidotti LG, Cerny A, et al. CTL access to tissue antigen is restricted in vivo. J Immunol 1994;153:482–488.
12. Archibald RWR, Weller RO, Meadow SR. Measles pneumonia and the nature of the inclusion bearing giant cells: a light- and electron-microscope study. J Pathol 1971;103:27–34.
13. Armstrong JA, Horne R. Follicular dendritic cells and virus-like particles in AIDS-related lymphadenopathy. Lancet 1984;2:370–372.
14. Auger I, Thomas P, De Gruttola V, et al. Incubation periods for paediatric AIDS patients. Nature 1988;336:575–577.
15. Baczko K, Liebert UG, Billeter M, Cattaneo R, Budka H, ter Meulen V. Expression of defective measles virus genes in brain tissues of patients with subacute sclerosing panencephalitis. J Virol 1986;59:472–478.
16. Baker CC, Phelps WC, Lindgren V, Braun MJ, Gonda MA, Howley PM. Structural and transcriptional analysis of human papillomavirus type 16 sequences in cervical carcinoma cell lines. J Virol 1987;61:962–971.
17. Barker CF, Billingham RE. Immunologically privileged sites. Adv Immunol 1977;25:1–54.
18. Baroni CD, Pezzella F, Mirolo M, Ruco LP, Rossi GB. Immunohistochemical demonstration of p24 HTLV III major core protein in different cell types within lymph nodes from patients with lymphadenopathy syndrome (LAS). Histopathology 1986;10:5–13.
19. Battegay M, Moskophidis D, Rahemtulla A, Hengartner H, Mak TW, Zinkernagel RM. Enhanced establishment of a virus carrier state in adult CD4+ T-cell-deficient mice. J Virol 1994;68;4700–4704.
20. Berke G. The binding and lysis of target cells by cytotoxic lymphocytes: molecular and cellular targets. Annu Rev Immunol 1994;12: 735–773.
21. Bernards R, Schrier PI, Houweling A, et al. Tumorigenicity of cells transformed by adenovirus type 12 by evasion of T-cell immunity. Nature 1983;305:776–779.
22. Bertoletti A, Sette A, Chisari FV, et al. Natural variants of cytotoxic epitopes are T cell receptor antagonists for antiviral cytotoxic T cells. Nature 1994;369:407–410.
23. Biberfeld P, Chayt KJ, Marselle LM, Biberfeld G, Gallo RC, Harper ME. HTLV-III expression in infected lymph nodes and relevance to pathogenesis of lymphadenopathy. Am J Pathol 1986;125: 436–442.
24. Biron CA. Cytokines in the generation of immune responses to and resolution of virus infection. Curr Opin Immunol 1994;6:530–538.
25. Birrer MJ, Bloom BR, Udem S. Characterization of measles polypeptides by monoclonal antibodies. Virology 1981;198:381–390.
26. Bjorkman PJ, Saper MA, Samraoui B, Bennett WS, Strominger JL, Wiley DC. Structure of the human class I histocompatibility antigen, HLA-A2. Nature 1987;329:506–512.
27. Borrow P, Lewicki H, Hahn BH, Shaw GM, Oldstone MBA. Virus-specific CD8+ cytotoxic T-lymphocyte activity associated with control of viremia in primary human immunodeficiency virus type 1 infection. J Virol 1994;68:6103–6110.
28. Brown HR, Goller NL, Thormar H, et al. Measles virus matrix protein gene expression in a subacute sclerosing panencephalitis patient brain and virus isolate demonstrated by cDNA hybridization and immunocytochemistry. Acta Neuropathol (Berl) 1987;75:123–130.
29. Brown JH, Jardetzky TS, Gorga JC, et al. The three-dimensional structure of the human class II histocompatibility antigen HLA-DR1. Nature 1993;364:33–39.
30. Buchmeier MJ, Welsh RM, Dutko FJ, Oldstone MBA. The virology and immunobiology of lymphocytic choriomeningitis virus infection. Adv Immunol 1980;30:275–331.
31. Buchmeier NA, Cooper NR. Suppression of monocyte functions by human cytomegalovirus. Immunology 1989;66:278–283.
32. Burgert H-G, Kvist S. An adenovirus type 2 glycoprotein blocks cell surface expression of human histocompatibility class I antigens. Cell 1985;41:987–997.
33. Burgert H-G, Maryanski JL, Kvist S. E3/19K protein of adenovirus type 2 inhibits lysis of cytolytic T lymphocytes by blocking cell-surface expression of histocompatibility class I antigens. Proc Natl Acad Sci USA 1987;84:1356–1360.
34. Burns DP, Collignon C, Desrosiers RC. Simian immunodeficiency virus mutants resistant to serum neutralization arise during persistent infection of rhesus monkeys. J Virol 1993;67:4104–4113.
35. Burns DP, Desrosiers RC. Selection of genetic variants of simian immunodeficiency virus in persistently infected rhesus monkeys. J Virol 1991;65:1843–1856.
36. Butler JC, Peters CJ. Hantaviruses and hantavirus pulmonary syndrome. Clin Infect Dis 1994;19:387–394.
37. Byrne JA, Oldstone MBA. Biology of cloned cytotoxic T lymphocytes specific for lymphocytic choriomeningitis virus: clearance of virus in vivo. J Virol 1984;51:682–686.
38. Carrigan DR, Knox KK. Identification of interferon-resistant subpopulations in several strains of measles virus: positive selection by growth of the virus in brain tissue. J Virol 64:1606–1615.
39. Carter MJ, Willcocks MM, Loffler S, ter Meulen V. Relationships between monoclonal antibody-binding sites on the measles hemagglutinin. J Gen Virol 1982;63:113–120.
40. Carter MJ, Willcocks MM, ter Meulen V. Defective translation of measles virus matrix protein in a subacute sclerosing panencephalitis cell line. Nature 1983;305:153–155.
41. Cascardo MR, Karzon DT. Measles virus giant cell inducing factor (fusion factor). Virology 1965;26:311–325.
42. Cattaneo R, Rebmann G, Schmid A, Baczko K, ter Meulen V Billeter MA. Altered transcription of a defective measles virus genome derived from a diseased human brain. EMBO J 1987;6: 681–688.
43. Cattaneo R, Schmid A, Billeter MA, Sheppard RD, Udem SA. Multiple viral mutations rather than host factors cause defective measles virus gene expression in a subacute sclerosing panencephalitis cell line. J Virol 1988;62:1388–1397.

44. Cattaneo R, Schmid A, Eschle D, Baczko K, ter Meulen V, Billeter MA. Biased hypermutation and other genetic changes in defective measles viruses in human brain infections. Cell 1988;55:255–265.

45. Cattaneo R, Schmid A, Spielhofer P, et al. Mutated and hypermutated genes of persistent measles viruses which caused lethal human brain diseases. Virology 1989;173:415–425.

46. Chen AX, Shen L, Miller MD, Ghim SH, Hughes AL, Letvin NL. Cytotoxic T lymphocytes do not appear to select for mutations in an immunodominant epitope of simian immunodeficiency virus gag. J Immunol 1992;149:4060–4066.

47. Cheung AK-M, Hoggan MD, Hauswirth WW, Berns KI. Integration of the adeno-associated virus genome into cellular DNA in latently infected human Detroit 6 cells. J Virol 1980;33:739–748.

48. Chinami M, Nakamura E, Kakisako S, Xu B, Shingu M. Poliovirus resistant cells derived from HeLa cells. Kurume Med J 1986;33: 125–129.

49. Clark SJ, Saag MS, Decker WD, et al. High titres of cytopathic virus in plasma of patients with symptomatic primary HIV-1 infection. N Engl J Med 1991;324:954–960.

50. Coen DM, Kosz-Vnenchak M, Jacobson JG, et al. Thymidine kinase-negative herpes simplex virus mutants establish latency in mouse trigeminal ganglia but do not reactivate. Proc Natl Acad Sci USA 1989;86:4736–4740.

51. Conner RI, Ho DD. Transmission and pathogenesis of human immunodeficiency virus type 1. AIDS Res Hum Retroviruses 1994;10: 321–323.

52. Couillin IB, Culmann-Penciolelli B, Gomard E, Levy J-P, Guillet JG, Saragosti S. Impaired CTL recognition due to genetic variations in the main immunogenic region of the HIV-1 nef protein. J Exp Med 1994;180:779–782.

53. Croen KD, Ostrove JM, Dragovic LJ, Smialek JE, Straus SE. Latent herpes simplex virus in human trigeminal ganglia: detection of an immediate-early gene "antisense" transcript by in situ hybridization. N Engl J Med 1987;317:1427–1432.

54. Croen KD, Ostrove JM, Dragovic LJ, Straus SE. Patterns of gene expression and sites of latency in human nerve ganglia are different for varicella-zoster and herpes simplex viruses. Proc Natl Acad Sci USA 1988;85:9773–9777.

55. Daar ES, Moudgil T, Meyer RD, Ho DD. Transient high levels of viremia in patients with primary immunodeficiency virus type 1 infection. N Engl J Med 1991;324:961–964.

56. Dai LC, West K, Littaua R, Takahashi K, Ennis FA. Mutation of the human immunodeficiency virus type 1 at amino acid 585 on gp41 results in loss of killing by CD8+ A24-restricted cytotoxic T lymphocytes. J Virol 1992;66:3151–315.

57. Davis MM, Bjorkman PJ. T-cell antigen receptor genes and T-cell recognition. Nature 1988;334:395–402.

58. de Campos-Lima P-O, Levitsky V, Brooks J, et al. T cell responses and virus evolution: loss of HLA A11-restricted CTL epitopes in Epstein-Barr virus isolates from highly A11-positive populations by selective mutation at anchor residues. J Exp Med 1994;179:1297–1305.

59. de la Torre JC, Davila M, Sabrino F, Ortin J, Domingo E. Establishment of cell lines persistently infected with foot-and-mouth disease virus. Virology 1985;145:24–35.

60. de la Torre JC, Martinez-Salas E, Diez J, et al. Coevolution of cells and viruses in a persistent infection of foot-and-mouth disease virus in cell culture. J Virol 1988;62:2050–2058.

61. de la Torre JC, Martinez-Salas E, Diez J, Domingo E. Extensive cell heterogeneity during persistent infection with foot-and-mouth disease virus. J Virol 1989;63:59–63.

62. Deatly A, Spivack JG, Lavi E, Fraser NW. RNA from an immediate early region of the HSV-1 genome is present in the trigeminal ganglia of latently infected mice. Proc Natl Acad Sci USA 1987;84: 3204–3208.

63. Dermody TS, Nibert ML, Wetzel JD, Tong X, Fields BN. Cells and viruses with mutations affecting viral entry are selected during persistent infections of L cells with mammalian reoviruses. J Virol 1993;67:2055–2063.

64. Deshmane SL, Fraser JW. During latency, herpes simplex virus type 1 DNA is associated with nucleosomes in a chromatin structure. J Virol 1989;63:943–947.

65. Dhib-Jalbut S, McFarland HF, Mingiolo ES, Sever JL, McFarlin DE. Humoral and cellular immune responses to matrix protein of measles virus in subacute sclerosing panencephalitis. J Virol 1988; 62:2483–2489.

66. Dietzschold B, Kao M, Zheng YM, et al. Delineation of putative mechanisms involved in antibody-mediated clearance of rabies virus from the central nervous system. Proc Natl Acad Sci USA 1992;89:7252–7256.

67. Dobson AT, Sedarati F, Devi-Rao G, et al. Identification of the latency-associated transcript promoter by expression of rabbit beta-globin mRNA in mouse sensory nerve ganglia latently infected with a recombinant herpes simplex virus. J Virol 1989;63:3844–3851.

68. Doherty PC, Allan W, Eichelberger M, Carding SR. Roles of ab and gd T cell subsets in viral immunity. Annu Rev Immunol 1992;10: 123–151.

69. Dukto FJ, Oldstone MBA. Cytomegalovirus causes a latent infection in undifferentiated cells and is activated by induction of cell differentiation. J Exp Med 1981;154:1636–1651.

70. Durst M, Kleinheinz A, Hotz M, Gissmann L. The physical state of human papillomavirus type 16 DNA in benign and malignant genital tumors. J Gen Virol 1985;66:1515–1522.

71. Eager KB, Pfizenmaier K, Ricciardi RP. Modulation of major histocompatibility complex (MHC) class I genes in adenovirus 12 transformed cells: interferon-g increases class I expression by a mechanism that circumvents E1A induced-repression and tumor necrosis factor enhances the effect of interferon-g. Oncogene 1989;4:39–44.

72. Einhorn L, Ost A. CMV infection of human blood cells. J Infect Dis 1984;149:207–214.

73. Eisenlohr LC, Yewdell JW, Bennink JR. Flanking sequences influence the presentation of an endogenously synthesized peptide to cytotoxic T lymphocytes. J Exp Med 1992;175:481–487.

74. Embretson J, Supancic M, Ribas JL, et al. Massive covert infection of helper T lymphocytes and macrophages by HIV during the incubation period of AIDS. Nature 1993;362:359–362.

75. Farrell MJ, Dobson AT, Feldman LT. Herpes simplex virus latency associated transcript is a stable intron. Proc Natl Acad Sci USA 1991;88:790–794.

76. Fauci A. Immunopathogenesis of HIV infection. AIDS 1993;6:655–662.

77. Fingeroth JD, Weis JJ, Tedder TF, Strominger JL, Biro PA, Fearon DT. Epstein-Barr virus receptor of human B lymphocytes is the C3d receptor CR2. Proc Natl Acad Sci USA 1984;81:4510–4516.

78. Fox CH, Tenner-Racz K, Racz P, Firpo A, Pizzo PA, Fauci AS. Lymphoid germinal centers are reservoirs of human immunodeficiency virus type 1 RNA. J Infect Dis 1991;164:1051–1057.

79. Frade R, Barel M, Ehlin-Henriksson B, Klein G. gp140, The C3d receptor of human B lymphocytes, is also the Epstein-Barr virus receptor. Proc Natl Acad Sci USA 1985;82:1490–1493.

80. Fujinami RS, Oldstone MBA. Antiviral antibody reacting on the plasma membrane alters measles virus expression inside the cell. Nature 1979;279:935–940.

81. Fujinami RS, Oldstone MAB. Alterations in expression of measles virus polypeptides by antibody: molecular events in antibody-induced antigenic modulation. J Immunol 1980;125:78–85.

82. Fujinami RS, Oldstone MBA. Antibody initiates virus persistence: immune modulation and measles virus infections. In: Nokins AL, Oldstone MBA, eds. Concepts in viral pathogenesis. New York: Springer-Verlag, 1984:187–193.

83. Gartner S, Markovits P, Markovitz DM, Kaplan MH, Gallo RC, Popovic M. The role of mononuclear phagocytes in HTLV-III/LAV infection. Science 1986;233:215–219.

84. Gerber P, Lucas S, Nonoyama M, Perlin E, Goldstein LI. Oral excretion of Epstein-Barr viruses by healthy subjects and patients with infectious mononucleosis. Lancet 1972;2:988–989.

85. Germain RN. MHC-dependent antigen processing and peptide presentation: providing ligands for T lymphocyte activation. Cell 1994; 76:287–299.

86. Gilden DH, Cole GA, Nathanson N. Immunopathogenesis of acute central nervous system disease produced by lymphocytic choriomeningitis virus. II. Adoptive immunization of virus carriers. J Exp Med 1972;135:874–889.

87. Gilden DH, Vafai A, Shtram Y, Becker Y, Devlin M, Wellish M. Varicella-zoster virus DNA in human sensory ganglia. Nature 1983; 306:478–480.

88. Gonczol E, Andres PW, Plotkin SA. Cytomegalovirus replicates in differentiated but not in undifferentiated human embryonal carcinoma cells. Science 1984;224:159–161.

89. Goodglick L, Braun J. Revenge of the microbes: superantigens of the T and B cell lineage. Am J Pathol 1994;144:623–636.

90. Gooding LR. Virus proteins that counteract host immune defenses. Cell 1992;71:5–7.

91. Green MT, Courtney RJ, Dunkel EC. Detection of an immediate early herpes simplex virus type 1 polypeptide in trigeminal ganglia from latently infected animals. Infect Immun 1981;34:987–992.

92. Greene WC. The molecular biology of human immunodeficiency virus type 1 infection. N Engl J Med 1991;324:308–317.

93. Gregory CD, Murray RJ, Edwards CF, Rickinson AB. Down regulation of cell adhesion molecules LFA-3 and ICAM-1 in Epstein-Barr virus-positive Burkitt's lymphoma underlies tumor cell escape from virus-specific T cell surveillance. J Exp Med 1988;167:1811–1824.

94. Gresser J, Chany C. Isolation of measles virus from the washed leucocytic fraction of blood. Proc Soc Exp Biol Med 1963;113:695–698.

95. Haase AT. The role of active and covert infections in lentivirus pathogenesis. Ann NY Acad Sci 1994;724:75–86.

96. Haase AT, Gantz D, Eble B, et al. Natural history of restricted synthesis and expression of measles virus genes in subacute sclerosing panencephalitis. Proc Natl Acad Sci USA 1985;82:3020–3024.

97. Hall WW, Choppin WP. Measles virus proteins in the brain tissue of patients with subacute sclerosing panencephalitis: absence of the M protein. N Engl J Med 1981;394:1152–1155.

98. Hall WW, Lamb RA, Choppin PW. Measles and subacute sclerosing panencephalitis virus protein: lack of antibodies to the M protein in patients with subacute sclerosing panencephalitis. Proc Natl Acad Sci USA 1979;76:2047–2051.

99. Hampar B, Tanaka A, Nonoyama M, Derge JG. Replication of the resident repressed Epstein-Barr virus genome during the early S phase (S-1 period) of nonproducer Raji cells. Proc Natl Acad Sci USA 1974;71:631–635.

100. Handa H, Shiroki K, Shimojo H. Establishment and characterization of KB cell lines latently infected with adeno-associated virus type 1. Virology 1977;82:84–92.

101. Hermiston TW, Tripp RA, Sparer T, Gooding LR, Wold WSM. Deletion mutation analysis of the adenovirus type 2 E3-gp 19K protein: identification of sequences within the endoplasmic reticulum luminal domain that are required for class I antigen binding and protection from adenovirus-specific cytotoxic T lymphocytes. J Virol 1993;67:5289–5298.

102. Hill A, Yugovic P, York I, et al. Herpes simplex virus turns off the TAP to evade host immunity. Nature 1995;375:411–415.

103. Hill JM, Sedarati F, Javier RT, Wagner EK, Stevens JG. Herpes simplex virus latent phase transcription facilitates in vivo reactivation. Virology 1990;174:117–125.

104. Hirano A, Ayata M, Wang AH, Wong TC. Functional analysis of matrix proteins expressed from cloned genes of measles virus variants that cause subacute sclerosing panencephalitis reveals a common defect in nucleocapsid binding. J Virol 1993;67:1848–1853.

105. Hirano A, Wang AH, Gombart AF, Wong TC. The matrix proteins of neurovirulent subacute sclerosing panencephalitis virus and its acute measles virus progenitor are functionally different. Proc Natl Acad Sci USA 1992;89:8745–8749.

106. Ho DD, Neumann AU, Perelson AS, Chen W, Leonard JM, Markowitz M. Rapid turnover of plasma virions and CD4 lymphocytes in HIV-1 infection. Nature 1995;373:123–126.

107. Ho DD, Pomerantz RJ, Kaplan JC. Pathogenesis of infection with human immunodeficiency virus. N Engl J Med 1987;317:278–286.

108. Ho DD, Rota TR, Hirsch MS. Infection of monocyte/macrophages by human T lymphotropic virus type III. J Clin Invest 1986;77:1712–1725.

109. Hoffenback A, Langlade-Demoyen P, Dadaglio G, et al. Unusually high frequencies of HIV-specific cytotoxic T lymphocytes in humans. J Immunol 1989;142:452–462.

110. Hoggan MD, Thomas GF, Thomas FB, Johnson FB. Continuous "carriage" of adenovirus associated virus genome in cell cultures in the absence of helper adenoviruses. In: Silvestri SL, ed. Proceedings of the Fourth Lepetit Colloquium, Cocoyac, Mexico Mexico. Amsterdam: North-Holland, 1972:243.

111. Holland JJ, de la Torre JC, Steinhauer DA. RNA virus populations as quasispecies. Curr Top Microbiol Immunol 1992;176:1–20.

112. Holland JJ, Kennedy SIT, Semmler BL, Jones CL, Roux L, Grabau EA. Defective interfering RNA viruses and the host-cell response. In: Fraenkel-Conrat H, Wagner R, eds. Comprehensive virology. Vol 16. New York: Plenum Press, 1980:137–192.

113. Holland JJ, Spindler K, Horodyski F, Graham E, Nichol S, Vendepol S. Rapid evolution of RNA genomes. Science 1982;215:1577–1585.

114. Howard CR. Arenaviruses. In: Zuckerman AJ, ed. Perspectives in medical virology. Vol 2. Amsterdam: Elsevier, 1986.

115. Hyman RW, Ecker JR, Tenser RB. Varicella-zoster virus RNA in human trigeminal ganglia. Lancet 1983;2:814–816.

116. Hyypia T, Korkiamaki P, Vainionbaa R. Replication of measles virus in human lymphocytes. J Exp Med 1986;161:1261–1271.

117. Jameson SC, Carbone FR, Bevan MJ. Clone-specific T cell receptor antagonists of major histocompatibility complex class-I-restricted cytotoxic T cells. J Exp Med 1993;177:1541–1550.

118. Jamieson BD, Butler LD, Ahmed R. Effective clearance of a persistent viral infection requires cooperation between virus-specific Lyt2+ T cells and nonspecific bone marrow-derived cells. J Virol 1987;61:3930–3937.

119. Jamieson BD, Somasundaram T, Ahmed R. Abrogation of tolerance to a chronic viral infection. J Immunol 1991;147:3521–3529.

120. Jennings SR, Rice PL, Kloszewski ED, Anderson RW, Thompson KL, Tevethia SS. Effect of herpes simplex virus types 1 and 2 on surface expression of class I major histocompatibility antigens on infected cells. J Virol 1985;56:757–766.

121. Joly E, Mucke L, Oldstone MBA. Viral persistence in neurons explained by lack of major histocompatibility class I expression. Science 1991;253:1283–1285.

122. Joseph BS, Lampert PW, Oldstone MBA. Replication and persistence of measles virus in defined subpopulations of human leukocytes. J Virol 1975;16:1638–1649.

123. Joseph BS, Oldstone MBA. Antibody-induced redistribution of measles virus antigens on the cell surface. J Immunol 1974;113:1205–1209.

124. Joseph J, Knobler RL, Lublin FD, Hart MN. Mouse hepatitis virus (MHV-4, JHM) blocks g-interferon-induced major histocompatibility complex class II antigen expression on murine cerebral endothelial cells. J Neuroimmunol 1991;33:181–190.

125. Kägi D, Ledermann B, Bürki K, et al. Cytotoxicity mediated by T cells and natural killer cells is greatly impaired in perforin-deficient mice. Nature 1994;369:31–37.

126. Kägi D, Vignaux F, Ledermann B, et al. Fas and perforin pathways as major mechanisms of T cell-mediated cytotoxicity. Science 1994;265:528–530.

127. Kapasi K, Rice GPA. Cytomegalovirus infection of peripheral blood mononuclear cells: effects of IL-1 and IL-2 production and responsiveness. J Virol 1988;62:3606–3607.

128. Kaplan G, Levy A, Racaniello VR. Isolation and characterization of HeLa cell lines blocked at different steps in the poliovirus life cycle. J Virol 1989;63:43–51.

129. Katz JP, Bodin ET, Coen DM. Quantitative polymerase chain reaction analysis of herpes simplex virus DNA in ganglia of mice infected with replication-incompetent mutants. J Virol 1990;64:4288–4295.

130. Katz SL, Enders JF. Measles virus. In: Horsfall FL Jr, Tamm I, eds. Viral and rickettsial infections of man. 4th ed. Philadelphia: JB Lippincott.

131. Kauffman RS, Ahmed R, Fields BN. Selection of a mutant S1 gene during reovirus persistent infection of L cells: role in maintenance of the persistent state. Virology 1983;131:79–87.

132. Kemp LM, Dent CL, Latchman DS. Octamer motif mediates transcriptional repression of HSV immediate-early genes and octamer-containing cellular promoters in neuronal cells. Neuron 1990;4:215–227.

133. Klatzmann D, Barre-Sinoussi F, Nugeyre MT, et al. Selective tropism of lymphadenopathy associated virus (LAV) for helper-inducer T lymphocytes. Science 1984;225:59–62.

134. Klenerman P, Rowland-Jones S, McAdams S, et al. Cytotoxic T cell activity antagonized by naturally occurring HIV-1 gag variants. Nature 1994;369:403–407.

135. Knipe DM. The role of viral and cellular nuclear proteins in herpes simplex virus replication. Adv Virus Res 1989;37:85–123.

136. Kono Y, Kobayashi K, Fukunaga Y. Serological comparison among various strains of equine infectious anemia virus. Archiv fur die Gesamte Virusforschung 1971;34:202–208.

137. Kono Y, Kobayashi K, Fukunaga Y. Antigenic drift of equine infectious anemia virus in chronically infected horses. Archiv fur die Gesamte Virusforschung 1973;41:1–10.

138. Kosz-Vnenchak M, Coen DM, Knipe DM. Restricted expression of herpes simplex virus lytic genes during establishment of latent infection by thymidine kinase-negative mutant viruses. J Virol 1990; 64:5396–5402.

139. Kosz-Vnenchak M, Jacobson J, Coen DM, Knipe DM. Evidence for a novel regulatory pathway for herpes simplex virus gene expression in trigeminal ganglion neurons. J Virol 1993;67:5383– 5393.

140. Kotin RM, Berns KI. Organization of adeno-associated virus DNA in latently infected Detroit 6 cells. Virology 1989;170:460– 467.

141. Kotin RM, Menninger JC, Ward DC, Berns KI. Mapping and direct visualization of a region-specific viral DNA integration site on chromosome 19q 13-qter. Genomics 1991;10:831–834.

142. Kotin RM, Siniscalco M, Samulski RJ, et al. Site-specific integration by adeno-associated virus. Proc Natl Acad Sci USA 1990;87: 2211–2215.

143. Koup RA. Virus escape from CTL recognition. J Exp Med 1994; 180:779–782.

144. Koup RA, Ho DD. Shutting down HIV. Nature 1994;370:416.

145. Koup RA, Safrit JT, Cao Y, et al. Temporal association of cellular immune responses with the initial control of viremia in primary human immunodeficiency virus type 1 syndrome. J Virol 1994;68: 4650–4655.

146. Koyanagi Y, O'Brien WA, Zhao JQ, Golde DW, Gasson JC, Chen ISY. Cytokines alter production of HIV-1 from primary mononuclear phagocytes. Science 1988;241:1673–1675.

147. Laycock KA, Lee SE, Stulting RD, et al. HSV-1 transcription is not detectable in quiescent human stromal keratitis by in situ hybridization. Invest Ophthalmol Vis Sci 1993;34:285–292.

148. Lehmann-Grube F. Portraits of viruses: arenaviruses. Intervirology 1984;22:121–145.

149. Lehmann-Grube F, Lohler J, Utermohlen O, Gegin C. Antiviral immune responses of lymphocytic choriomeningitis virus-infected mice lacking CD8+ T lymphocytes because of disruption of the b2-microglobulin gene. J Virol 1993;67:332–339.

150. Lehmann-Grube F, Peralta LM, Bruns M, Lohler J. Persistent infection of mice with the lymphocytic choriomeningitis virus. In: Fraenkel-Conrat H, Wagner R, eds. Comprehensive virology. New York: Plenum Press, 1983:43–103.

151. Leib DA, Coen DM, Bogard CL, et al. Immediate-early regulatory gene mutants define different stages in the establishment and reactivation of herpes simplex virus latency. J Virol 1989;63:759– 768.

152. Leib DA, Kosz-Vnenchak M, Jacobson JG, et al. A deletion mutant of the latency-associated transcript of herpes simplex virus type 1 reactivates from the latent state with reduced frequency. J Virol 1989;63:2893–2900.

153. Leist TP, Sandri-Goldin RM, Stevens JA. Latent infections in spinal ganglia with thymidine kinase-deficient herpes simplex virus. J Virol 1989;63:4976–4978.

154. Leopardi R, Ilonen J, Mattila L, Salmi AA. Effect of measles virus infection on MHC class II expression and antigen presentation in human monocytes. Cell Immunol 1993;147:388–396.

155. Levine B, Griffin DE. Molecular analysis of neurovirulent strains of Sindbis virus that evolve during persistent infection of scid mice. J Virol 1993;67:6872–6875.

156. Levine B, Hardwick M, Griffin DE. Persistence of alphaviruses in vertebrate hosts. Trends Microbiol 1994;2:25–28.

157. Levine B, Hardwick JM, Trapp BD, Crawford TO, Bollinger RC, Griffin DE. Antibody-mediated clearance of alphavirus infection from neurons. Science 1991;254:856–860.

158. Liebert UG, Baczko K, Budka H, ter Meulen V. Restricted expression of measles virus proteins in brains from cases of subacute sclerosing panencephalitis. J Gen Virol 1986;67:2435–2444.

159. Lill NL, Tevethia MJ, Hendrickson WG, Tevethia SS. Cytotoxic T lymphocytes (CTL) against a transforming gene product select for transformed cells with point mutations within sequences encoding CTL recognition epitopes. J Exp Med 1992;176:449–457.

160. Littman DR. The structure of the CD4 and CD8 genes. Annu Rev Immunol 1987;5:561–584.

161. Lodmell DL, Esposito JJ, Ewalt LC. Rabies virus antinucleoprotein antibody protects against rabies virus challenge in vivo and inhibits rabies virus replication in vitro. J Virol 1993;67:6080–6086.

162. Lutley R, Petursson G, Palsson PA, Georgsson G, Klein J, Nathanson N. Antigenic drift in visna: virus variation during long-term infection of Icelandic sheep. J Gen Virol 1983;64:1433–1440.

163. Madden DR, Gorga JC, Strominger JL, Wiley DC. The three-dimensional structure of HLA-B27 at 2.1 A resolution suggests a general mechanism for tight peptide binding to MHC. Cell 1992;70:1035– 1048.

164. Mahalingam R, Wellish M, Wolf W, et al. Latent varicella-zoster viral DNA in human trigeminal and thoracic ganglia. N Engl J Med 1990;323:627–631.

165. Mahy BWJ. Strategies of virus persistence. Br Med Bull 1985;41: 50–55.

166. Margolis TP, Sedarati F, Dobson AT, Feldman LT, Stevens JG. Pathways of viral gene expression during acute neuronal infection with HSV-1. Virology 1992;189:150–160.

167. Marrack P, Kappler J. Subversion of the immune system by pathogens. Cell 1994;76:323–332.

168. Masucci MG, Torsteinsdottir S, Colombani J, Brautbar C, Klein E, Klein G. Down-regulation of class I HLA antigens and the Epstein-Barr virus encoded latent membrane protein in Burkitt lymphoma lines. Proc Natl Acad Sci USA 1987;84:4567–4571.

169. Matloubian M, Concepcion RJ, Ahmed R. CD4+ T cells are required to sustain CD8+ cytotoxic T-cell responses during chronic viral infection. J Virol 1994;68:8056–8063.

170. Matloubian M, Kolhekar SR, Somasundaram T, Ahmed R. Molecular determinants of macrophage-tropism and viral persistence: importance of single amino acid changes in the polymerase and glycoprotein of lymphocytic choriomeningitis virus. J Virol 1993;67: 7340–7349.

171. Maudsley DJ, Bateman WJ, Morris AG. Reduced stimulation of helper T cells by Ki-ras transformed cells. Immunology 1991;72: 277–281.

172. Maudsley DJ, Morris AG. Kirsten murine sarcoma virus abolishes interferon g-induced class II but not class I major histocompatibility antigen expression in a murine fibroblast line. J Exp Med 1988;167: 706–711.

173. Maudsley DJ, Morris AG. Regulation of IFN-gamma-induced host cell MHC antigen expression by Kirsten MSV and MLV. II. Effects on class II antigen expression. Immunology 1989;67:26–31.

174. Mazanec MB, Kaetzel CS, Lamm ME, Fletcher D, Nedrud JG. Intracellular neutralization of virus by immunoglobulin A antibodies. Proc Natl Acad Sci USA 1992;89:6901–6905.

175. Meier JL, Holman RP, Croen KD, Smialek JE, Straus SE. Varicella-zoster virus transcription in human trigeminal ganglia. Virology 1993;193:193–200.

176. Meignier B, Longnecker R, Roizman B. In vivo behavior of genetically engineered herpes simplex viruses R7017 and R7020: construction and evaluation in rodents. J Infect Dis 1988;158:602–614.

177. Mellerick DM, Fraser NW. Physical state of the latent herpes simplex virus genome in a mouse model system: evidence suggesting an episomal state. Virology 1987;158:265–275.

178. Meuer SC, Acuto O, Hergend T, Schlossman SF, Reinherz EL. The human T-cell receptor. Annu Rev Immunol 1984;2:23–50.

179. Meyerhans A, Dadaglio G, Vartanian J-P, et al. In vivo persistence of a HIV-1-encoded HLA-B27-restricted cytotoxic T lymphocyte epitope despite specific in vitro reactivity. Eur J Immunol 1991;21: 2637–2640.

180. Mims CA. Parasite survival strategies and persistent infections. In: Mims CA, ed. Medical microbiology. England: Mosby Europe, 1993:15.1–15.2.

181. Minton EJ, Tysee C, Sinclair JH, Sissons JCP. Human cytomegalovirus infection of the monocyte/macrophage lineage in bone marrow. J Virol 1994;68:4017–4021.

182. Moench TR, Griffin DE, Obriecht CR, Vaisberg AJ, Johnson RT. Acute measles in patients with and without neurological involvement: distribution of measles virus antigen and RNA. J Infect Dis 1988;158:433–442.

183. Montelaro CR, Parekh B, Orrego A, Issel CJ. Antigenic variation during persistent infection by equine infectious anemia virus, a retrovirus. J Biol Chem 1984;259:10539–10544.

184. Moore KW, O'Garra A, de Waal Malefyt R, Vieira P, Mosmann TR. Interleukin-10. Annu Rev Immunol 1993;11:165–190.

185. Moskophidis D, Cobbold SP, Waldmann H, Lehmann-Grube F. Mechanism of recovery from acute virus infection: treatment of lymphocytic choriomeningitis virus-infected mice with monoclonal antibodies reveals that Lyt2+T lymphocytes mediate clearance of virus and regulate the antiviral antibody response. J Virol 1987;61: 1867–1874.

186. Moskophidis D, Lechner F, Pircher H, Zinkernagel RM. Viral persistence in acutely infected immunocompetent mice by exhaustion of antiviral cytotoxic effector cells. Nature 1993;362:758–761.

187. Mosmann TR, Coffman RL. TH1 and TH2 cells: different patterns of lymphokine secretion lead to different functional properties. Annu Rev Immunol 1989;7:145–173.

188. Muller D, Koller BH, Whitton JL, LaPan KE, Brigman KK, Frelinger JA. LCMV-specific, class II restricted cytotoxic T cells in b2-microglobulin-deficient mice. Science 1992;255:1576– 1578.

189. Narayan O, Clements JE. Biology and pathogenesis of lentiviruses of ruminant animals. In: Wong-Staal F, Gallo RC, eds. Retrovirus biology: an emerging role in human disease. New York: Marcel Dekker, 1988:1617–1639.

190. Narayan O, Clements J, Griffin DE, Wolinsky JS. Neutralizing antibody spectrum determines the antigenic profiles of emerging mutants of visna virus. Infect Immun 1981;32:1045–1050.

191. Narayan O, Griffin DE, Chase J. Antigenic drift of visna virus in persistently infected sheep. Science 1977;197:376–378.

192. Narayan O, Zink MC, Huso D, et al. Lentiviruses of animals are biological models of the human immunodeficiency viruses. Microbial Pathogenesis 1988;5:149–157.

193. Nemerow G, Wolfert R, McNaughton M, Cooper N. Identification and characterization of the Epstein-Barr virus receptor on human B lymphocytes and its relationship to the C3d complement receptor CR2. J Virol 1985;55:347–351.

194. Nonoyama M, Pagano JS. Separation of Epstein-Barr virus DNA from large chromosomal DNA in non-virus-producing cells. Nature 1972;333:41–45.

195. Norrby E, Chen S-N, Tagoshi T, Sheshberadaran H, Johnson CP. Five measles virus antigens demonstrated by use of mouse hybridoma antibodies in productively infected tissue culture cells. Arch Virol 1982;71:1–11.

196. Norrby E, Kristensson K, Brzosko WJ, Kapsenberg JG. Measles virus matrix proteins detected by immune fluorescence with monoclonal antibodies in the brain of patients with subacute sclerosing panencephalitis. J Virol 1985;56:337–340.

197. Norrby E, Orvell C, Vandvik B, Cherry DJ. Antibodies against measles virus polypeptides in different disease conditions. Infect Immun 1981;34:718–724.

198. Ohara Y, Tashiro M, Takase S, Homma M. Detection of antibody to M protein of measles virus in patients with subacute sclerosing panencephalitis: a comparative study on immunoprecipitation. Microbiol Immunol 1985;29:709–723.

199. O'Hare P, Hayward GS. Three trans-acting regulatory proteins of herpes simplex virus modulate immediate-early gene expression in a pathway involving positive and negative feedback regulation. J Virol 1985;56:723–733.

200. Oldstone MBA, Blount P, Southern P. Cytoimmunotherapy for persistent virus infection reveals a unique clearance pattern from the central nervous system. Nature 1986;321:239–243.

201. Pääbo S, Nilsson T, Peterson PA. Adenoviruses of subgenera B, C, D, and E modulate cell-surface expression of major histocompatibility complex class antigens. Proc Natl Acad Sci USA 1986;83:9665– 9669.

202. Palese P, Young JF. Variation of influenza A, B, and C viruses. Science 1982;215:1468–1474.

203. Pantaleo G, Demarest JF, Soudeyns H, et al. Major expansion of CD8+ T cells with a predominant Vb usage during the primary immune response to HIV. Nature 1994;370:463–467.

204. Pantaleo G, Graziosi C, Demarest JF, et al. HIV infection is active and progressive in lymphoid tissue during the clinically latent stage of disease. Nature 1993;362:355–358.

205. Parker DC. T cell-dependent B-cell activation. Annu Rev Immunol 1993;11:331–360.

206. Peebles TC. Distribution of virus in blood components during the viremia of measles. Archiv fur die Gesamte Virusforschung 1967; 22:43–47.

207. Petit AJC, Terpstra FG, Miedema F. Human immunodeficiency virus infection down-regulates HLA class II expression and induces differentiation in promonocytic U937 cells. J Clin Invest 1987;79: 1883–1889.

208. Phillips RE, Rowland-Jones S, Nixon DF, et al. Human immunodeficiency virus genetic variation that can escape cytotoxic T cell recognition. Nature 1991;354:453–459.

209. Pircher H, Burki K, Lang R, Hengartner H, Zinkernagel RM. Tolerance induction in double specific T-cell receptor transgenic mice varies with antigen. Nature 1989;342:559–561.

210. Pircher H, Moskophidis D, Rohrer U, Burki K, Hengartner H, Zinkernagel RM. Viral escape by selection of cytotoxic T cell-resistant virus variants in vivo. Nature 1990;346:629–633.

211. Porter DD. Persistent infections. In: Baron S, ed. Medical microbiology. 2nd ed. Menlo Park, CA: Addison-Wesley, 1985:784–790.

212. Puga A, Notkins AL. Continued expression of a poly(A)+ transcript of herpes simplex virus type 1 in trigeminal ganglia of latently infected mice. J Virol 1987;61:1700–1703.

213. Racz P, Tenner-Racz K, Kahl C, Feller AC, Kern P, Dietrich M. Spectrum of morphologic changes of lymph nodes from patients with AIDS or AIDS-related complexes. Prog Allergy 1986;37:81– 181.

214. Rager-Zisman B, Ju G, Rajan RV, Bloom BR. Decreased expression of H-2 antigens following acute measles virus infection. Cell Immunol 1981;59:319–329.

215. Rawlins DR, Milman G, Hayward SD, Hayward GS. Sequence specific DNA binding of the Epstein-Barr virus nuclear antigen (EBNA-1) to clustered sites in the plasmid maintenance region. Cell 1985;42:859–868.

216. Rawls WE, Chan MA, Gee SR. Mechanisms of persistence in arenavirus infections: a brief review. Can J Microbiol 1981;27:568– 574.

217. Redfield RR, Markham PD, Salahuddin SZ, et al. Genetic variation in HTLV-III/LAV over time in patients with AIDS or at risk for AIDS. Science 1986;232:1548–1553.

218. Reznikoff C, Tegtmeyer P, Dohan C, Ender JF. Isolation of AGMK cells partially resistant to SV40: identification of the resistant step. Proc Soc Exp Biol Med 1972;141:740–746.

219. Rice GPA, Schrier RD, Oldstone MBA. CMV infects human lymphocytes and monocytes: virus expression is restricted to immediate-early gene products. Proc Natl Acad Sci USA 1984;81:6134– 6138.

220. Rinaldo CR Jr. Modulation of major histocompatibility complex antigen expression by viral infection. Am J Pathol 1994;144:637–650.

221. Riviere Y, Tanneau-Salvadori F, Regnault A, et al. HIV-specific cytotoxic responses of seropositive individuals: distinct types of effector cells mediate killing of targets expressing gag and env proteins. J Virol 1989;63:2270–2277.

222. Robbins FC. Measles: clinical features. Pathogenesis, pathology, and complications. Am J Dis Child 1962;103:266–273.

223. Robert-Guroff M, Brown M, Gallo RC. HTLV-III neutralizing antibodies in patients with AIDS and AIDS-related complex. Nature 1985;316:72–74.

224. Rock DL, Fraser NW. Detection of HSV-1 genome in central nervous system of latently infected mice. Nature 1983;302:523–525.

225. Rock DL, Fraser NW. Latent herpes simplex virus type 1 DNA contains two copies of the virion DNA joint region. J Virol 1985;55: 849–852.

226. Rock DL, Nesburn AB, Ghiasi H, et al. Detection of latency-related viral RNAs in trigeminal ganglia of rabbits latently infected with herpes simplex virus type 1. J Virol 1987;61:3820–3826.

227. Roizman B, Sears AE. An inquiry into the mechanism of herpes simplex virus latency. Annu Rev Microbiol 1987;41:543–571.

228. Ron D, Tal J. Coevolution of cells and virus as a mechanism for the persistence of lymphotropic minute virus of mice in L cells. J Virol 1985;55:424–430.

229. Roos MTL, Lange JMA, DeGoede REY, et al. Viral phenotype and immune response in primary human immunodeficiency virus type 1 infection. J Infect Dis 1992;165:427–432.

230. Rustigian R. Persistent infection of cells in culture by measles virus. II. Effect of measles antibody on persistently infected HeLa sublines and recovery of a HeLa clonal line persistently infected with incomplete virus. J Bacteriol 1966;92:1805–1811.

231. Safrit JT, Andrews CA, Zhu T, Ho DD, Koup RA. Characterization of human immunodeficiency virus type 1-specific cytotoxic T lymphocyte clones isolated during acute seroconversion: recognition of

autologous virus sequences within a conserved immunodominant epitope. J Exp Med 1994;179:463–472.

232. Saksola K, Stevens C, Rubinstein P, Baltimore D. Human immunodeficiency virus type 1 messenger RNA in peripheral blood cells predicts disease progression independently of the numbers of CD4+ lymphocytes. Proc Natl Acad Sci USA 1994;91:1104–1108.

233. Salinovich O, Payne LS, Montelaro RC, Hussain KA, Issel CJ, Schnorr KL. Rapid emergence of novel antigenic and genetic variants of equine infectious anemia virus during persistent infection. J Virol 1986;57:71–80.

234. Samulski RJ, Zhu X, Xiao X, et al. Targeted integration of adeno-associated virus (AAV) into human chromosome 19. EMBO J 1991; 10:3941–3950.

235. Sattentau QJ, Weiss RA. The CD4 antigen: physiologic ligand and HIV receptor. Cell 1988;52:631–633.

236. Sawtell NM, Thompson RL. Herpes simplex virus type 1 latency-associated transcription unit promotes anatomical site-dependent establishment and reactivation from latency. J Virol 1992;66:2157–2169.

237. Schmid A, Spielhofer P, Cattaneo R, Baczko K, ter Meulen V, Billeter MA. Subacute sclerosing panencephalitis is typically characterized by alterations in the fusion protein cytoplasmic domain of the persisting measles virus. Virology 1992;188:910–915.

238. Schneider A, Oltersdorf T, Schneider V, Gissmann L. Distribution of human papillomavirus 16 genomes in cervical neoplasia by molecular in situ hybridization of tissue sections. Int J Cancer 1987;39: 717–721.

239. Schneider-Schaulies S, Schneider-Schaulies J, Schuster A, Bayer M, Pavlovic J, ter Meulen V. Cell type-specific MxA-mediated inhibition of measles virus transcription in human brain cells. J Virol 1994;68:6910–6917.

240. Schnittman SM, Denning SM, Greenhouse JJ, et al. Evidence for susceptibility of intrathymice T-cell precursors and their progeny carrying T-cell antigen receptor phenotypes TCRab+ and TCRgd+ to human immunodeficiency virus infection: a mechanism for CD4+ (T4) lymphocyte depletion. Proc Natl Acad Sci USA 1990; 87:7727–7731.

241. Scholz M, Hamann A, Blaheta RA, Auth MKH, Encke A, Markus BH. Cytomegalovirus- and interferon-related effects on human endothelial cells: cytomegalovirus infection reduces upregulation of HLA class II antigen expression after treatment with interferon g. Hum Immunol 1992;35:230–238.

242. Schrier PI, Bernards R, Vaessen RTMJ, Houweling A, van der Eb AJ. Expression of class I major histocompatibility antigens switched off by highly oncogenic adenovirus 12 in transformed rat cells. Nature 1983;305:771–775.

243. Schwarz E, Freese UK, Gissman L, et al. Structure and transcription of human papillomavirus sequences in cervical carcinoma cells. Nature 1985;314:111–114.

244. Sears AE, Hukkanen V, Labow MA, Levine AJ, Roizman B. Expression of the herpes simplex virus 1 a transinducing factor (VP16) does not induce reactivation of latent virus or prevent the establishment of latency in mice. J Virol 1991;65:2929–2935.

245. Sears AE, Meignier B, Roizman B. Establishment of latency in mice by herpes simplex virus 1 recombinants that carry insertions affecting regulation of the thymidine kinase gene. J Virol 1985;55:410–416.

246. Sears AE, Roizman B. Amplification by host factors of a sequence contained within the herpes simplex virus 1 genome. Proc Natl Acad Sci USA 1990;87:9441–9445.

247. Sedarati F, Margolis TP, Stevens JG. Latent infection can be established with drastically restricted transcription and replication of the HSV-1 genome. Virology 1993;192:687–691.

248. Sedmak DD, Guglielmo AM, Knight DA, Birmingham DJ, Huang EH, Waldman WJ. Cytomegalovirus inhibits major histocompatibility class II expression on infected endothelial cells. Am J Pathol 1994;144:683–692.

249. Shemesh J, Rotem-Yehudar R, Ehrlich R. Transcription and post-transcriptional regulation of class I major histocompatibility complex genes following transformation with human adenoviruses. J Virol 1991;65:5544–5548.

250. Sherman FE, Ruckle G. In vivo and in vitro cellular changes specific for measles. Arch Pathol 1958;65:587–599.

251. Sheshberadaran H, Norrby E, Rammohan KW. Monoclonal antibodies against five structural components of measles virus. II. Characterization of five cell lines persistently infected with measles virus. Arch Virol 1985;83:251–268.

252. Sloan-Lancaster J, Evavold BD, Allen PM. Induction of T-cell anergy by altered T-cell-receptor ligands on live antigen presenting cells. Nature 1993;363:156–159.

253. Sonea S. Bacterial viruses, prophages, and plasmids, reconsidered. Ann NY Acad Sci 1987;503:251–260.

254. Speck PG, Simmons A. Divergent molecular pathways of productive and latent infection with a virulent strain of herpes simplex virus type 1. J Virol 1991;65:4001–4005.

255. Spiegel H, Herbst H, Niedobitek G, Foss HD, Stein H. Follicular dendritic cells are a major reservoir for human immunodeficiency virus type 1 in lymphoid tissues facilitating infection of CD4+ T-helper cells. Am J Pathol 1992;140:15–22.

256. Spriggs MK. Cytokine and cytokine receptor genes captured by viruses. Curr Opin Immunol 1994;6:526–529.

257. Springer TA. Adhesion receptors of the immune system. Nature 1990;346:425–433.

258. Steiner I, Spivack JG, Deshmane SL, Ace CI, Preston CM, Fraser NW. A herpes simplex virus type 1 mutant containing a nontransinducing Vmw65 protein establishes latent infection in vivo in the absence of viral replication and reactivates efficiently from trigeminal ganglia. J Virol 1990;64:1630–1638.

259. Steinhauer D, Holland JJ. Rapid evolution of RNA viruses. Annu Rev Microbiol 1987;41:409–433.

260. Stevens JG. Human herpesviruses: a consideration of the latent state. Microbiol Rev 1989;53:318–332.

261. Stevens JG. Overview of herpesvirus latency. Sem Virol 1994;5: 191–196.

262. Stevens JG, Haarr L, Porter DP, Cook ML, Wagner EK. Prominence of the herpes simplex virus latency-associated transcript in trigeminal ganglia from seropositive humans. J Infect Dis 1988;158:117–123.

263. Stevens JG, Wagner EK, Devi-Rao GB, Cook ML, Feldman LT. RNA complementary to a herpesvirus alpha gene mRNA is prominent in latently infected neurons. Science 1987;253:1056–1059.

264. Stoler MH, Broker TR. In situ hybridization detection of human papilloma virus DNA and messenger RNA in genital condylomas and a cervical carcinoma. Hum Pathol 1986;17:1250–1258.

265. Straus SE. Clinical and biological differences between recurrent herpes simplex virus and varicella-zoster virus infections. JAMA 1989;262:3455–3458.

266. Su L, Knipe DM. Herpes simplex virus a protein ICP27 can inhibit or augment viral gene transactivation. Virology 1989;170:496–504.

267. Takemoto KK, Habel K. Virus-cell relationship in a carrier culture of HeLa cells and coxsackie A9 virus. Virology 1959;7:28–44.

268. Tanaka K, Isselbacher KJ, Khoury G, Jay G. Reversal of oncogenesis by the expression of a major histocompatibility complex class I gene. Science 1985;228:26–30.

269. Taylor-Wiedman J, Sissons P, Sinclair J. Induction of endogenous human cytomegalovirus gene expression after differentiation of monocytes from healthy carriers. J Virol 1994;68:1597–1604.

270. Tenner-Racz K, Racz P, Bofill M, et al. HTLV-III/LAV viral antigens in lymph nodes of homosexual men with persistent generalized lymphadenopathy and AIDS. Am J Pathol 1986;123:9–15.

271. Tenser RB, Hay KA, Edris WA. Latency-associated transcript but not reactivatable virus is present in sensory ganglion neurons after inoculation of thymidine kinase-negative mutants of herpes simplex virus type 1. J Virol 1989;63:2861–2865.

272. Tenser RB, Hyman RW. Latent herpesvirus infections of neurons in guinea pigs and humans. Yale J Biol Med 1987;60:159–167.

273. ter Meulen V, Loffer S, Carter MJ, Stephenson JR. Antigenic characterization of measles and SSPE virus hemagglutinin by monoclonal antibodies. J Gen Virol 1981;57:357–364.

274. ter Meulen V, Stephenson JR, Kreth HW. Subacute sclerosing panencephalitis. Comprehensive Virology 1983;18:105–185.

275. Thormar H, Barshatsky MR, Kozlowski PB. The emergence of antigenic variants is a rare event in long term visna virus infection in vivo. J Gen Virol 1983;64:1427–1432.

276. Trousdale M, Steiner I, Spivack JG, et al. In vivo and in vitro reactivation impairment of a herpes simplex virus type 1 latency-associ-

ated transcript variant in a rabbit eye model. J Virol 1991;65:6989–6993.

277. Tsomides TH, Aldovini A, Johnson RP, Walker BD, Young RA, Eisen HN. Naturally processed viral peptides recognized by cytotoxic T lymphocytes on cells chronically infected by human immunodeficiency virus type 1. J Exp Med 1994;180:1283–1293.

278. Upton C, Mossman K, McFadden G. Encoding of a homolog of the IFN-g receptor by myxoma virus. Science 1992;258:1369–1372.

279. Valyi-Nagi T, Deshmane SL, Spivack JG, et al. Investigation of herpes simplex virus type 1 (HSV-1) gene expression and DNA synthesis during the establishment of latent infection by an HSV-1 mutant, in1814, that does not replicate in mouse trigeminal ganglia. J Gen Virol 1991;72:641–649.

280. Vogt M, Dulbecco R. Properties of HeLa cell culture with increased resistance to poliomyelitis virus. Virology 1958;5:425–434.

281. Volkert M. Studies on immunologic tolerance to LCM virus. 2. Treatment of virus carrier mice by adoptive immunization. Acta Pathol Microbiol Scand 1968;57:465–487.

282. von Knebel-Doeberitz M, Oltersdorf T, Schwarz E, Gissmann L. Correlation of modified human papillomavirus early gene expression with altered growth properties in C4-1 cervical carcinoma cells. Cancer Res 1988;48:3780–3785.

283. Walker BD, Flexner C, Paradis TJ, et al. HIV-1 reverse transcriptase is a target for cytotoxic T lymphocytes in infected individuals. Science 1988;240:64–66.

284. Walker CM, Moody DJ, Stites DP, Levy JA. CD8+ lymphocytes can control HIV infection in vitro by suppressing virus replication. Science 1986;124:1563–1566.

285. Walker DL. The viral carrier state in animal cell cultures. Prog Med Virol 1964;6:111–148.

286. Walker DL. Persistent viral infection in cell cultures. In: Sanders M, Lennette EH, eds. Medical and applied virology. 1968:99–110.

287. Walsh CM, Matloubian M, Liu C-C, et al. Immune function in mice lacking the perforin gene. Proc Natl Acad Sci USA 1996 (in press).

288. Wang F, Gregory CD, Rowe M, et al. Epstein-Barr virus nuclear antigen 2 specifically induces expression of the B-cell activation antigen CD23. Proc Natl Acad Sci USA 1987;83:3452–3457.

289. Webster RG, Laver WG, Air GM, Schild GC. Molecular mechanisms of variation in influenza viruses. Nature 1982;296:115–121.

290. Wechsler S, Meissner HC. Measles and SSPE viruses: similarities and differences. Prog Med Virol 1982;28:65–95.

291. Wechsler SL, Fields BN. Differences between the intracellular polypeptides of measles and subacute sclerosing panencephalitis virus. Nature 1978;272:458–460.

292. Wechsler SL, Weiner HL, Fields BN. Immune responses in subacute sclerosing panencephalitis: reduced antibody response to the matrix protein of measles virus. J Immunol 1979;123:884–889.

293. Wei X, Ghosh SK, Taylor ME, et al. Viral dynamics in human immunodeficiency virus type 1 infections. Nature 1995;373:117–122.

294. Weiss RA, Clapman PR, Cheingsong-Popou R, et al. Neutralization of human T lymphotropic virus type III by sera of AIDS and AIDS-risk patients. Nature 1985;316:69–72.

295. Wilson JH, DePamphilis M, Berg P. Simian virus 40-permissive cell interactions: selection and characterization of spontaneously arising monkey cells that are resistant to simian virus 40 infection. J Virol 1976;20:391–399.

296. Wold WSM, Gooding LR. Region E3 of adenovirus: a cassette of genes involved in host immunosurveillance and virus-cell interactions. Virology 1991;184:1–8.

297. Wong TC, Ayata M, Hirano A, Yoshikawa Y, Tsuruoka H, Yamanouchi K. Generalized and localized biased hypermutation affecting the matrix gene of a measles virus strain that causes subacute sclerosing panencephalitis. J Virol 1989;63:5464–5468.

298. Wong TC, Ayata M, Ueda S, Hirano A. Role of biased hypermutation in evolution of subacute sclerosing panencephalitis virus from progenitor acute measles virus. J Virol 1991;65:2191–2199.

299. York IA, Roop C, Andrews DW, Riddell SR, Graham FL, Johnson DC. A cytosolic herpes simplex virus protein inhibits antigen presentation to CD8+ T lymphocytes. Cell 1994;77:525–535.

300. Young KKY, Heineki BE, Wechsler SL. M protein instability and lack of H protein processing associated with nonproductive persistent infection of HeLa cells by measles virus. Virology 1985;143:536–545.

301. Youngner JS, Preble OT. Viral persistence: evolution of viral populations. In: Fraenkel-Conrat H, Wagner R, eds. Comprehensive virology. Vol 16. New York: Plenum Press, 1980:73–135.

302. Zhu T, Mo H, Wang N, et al. Genotypic and phenotypic characterization of HIV-1 in patients with primary infection. Science 1993;261:1179–1181.

303. Zinkernagel RM, Doherty PC. MHC-restricted cytotoxic T cells: studies on the biological role of polymorphic major transplantation antigens determining T-cell restriction-specificity, function, and responsiveness. Adv Immunol 1979;27:51–177.

304. Zinkernagel RM, Welsh RM. H-2 compatibility requirement for virus-specific T cell-mediated effector functions in vivo. I. Specificity of T cells conferring antiviral protection against lymphocytic choriomeningitis virus is associated with H-2K and H-2D J Immunol 1976;117:1495–1502.

Viral Pathogenesis,
edited by Neal Nathanson, et al.
Lippincott–Raven Publishers, Philadelphia © 1997

CHAPTER 10

Virus-Induced Immune Suppression

Diane E. Griffin

INTRODUCTION

Generalized changes in immune function are common after
many, if not most, viral infections. These changes have been
documented by in vivo observations of increased susceptibility to infections, loss of skin test responses to recall antigens,
altered responses to new immunogens, and remission or prevention of immunologically mediated diseases. Changes in
immune function have also been documented by in vitro studies showing suppression of lymphoproliferative responses
to mitogens and recall antigens, decreased induction of cytotoxic responses, and altered cytokine production. These abnormalities are often present at the same time that vigorous

D. E. Griffin: Department of Molecular Microbiology and Immunology, Johns Hopkins University School of Public Health,
Baltimore, Maryland 21205.

and effective antiviral immune responses are developing.
Some immunosuppressive viruses have confounded studies of
tumor-induced immunity and immunosuppression when they
were unrecognized passengers in tumor cell lines or stocks of
oncogenic viruses.[46,66,372] Some viruses also suppress effective responses to their own antigens and thereby appear to
promote the development of persistent infection. The subject
of virus-induced immune suppression has been reviewed periodically, and these reviews reflect a progressive understanding of the immune system and the viruses that affect its function.[120,324,340,448,527]

HISTORY

The earliest documented recognition of virus-induced immune suppression was in the late 19th century, when text-

books of medicine stated that measles increased the severity of tuberculosis. The first experimental study of virus-induced immunosuppression was carried out by von Pirquet, who reported in 1908 that cutaneous tuberculin reactions became negative during measles.[522] As the study of immune responses moved into the laboratory, it was discovered that leukocytes isolated from the blood of individuals with or recovering from a variety of viral infections failed to proliferate normally in response to T-cell mitogens such as phytohemagglutinin (PHA) and concanavalin A (ConA). Further study on the effects of virus proteins and leukocyte cytokines on immune function has begun to shed light on the mechanisms of this immune suppression.

CHANGES IN IMMUNE FUNCTION DURING VIRAL INFECTIONS

Increased Susceptibility to Other Infections

The change in immune function first recognized by clinicians was an increased susceptibility to other infectious diseases during recovery from a number of common acute viral infections.[339] Pneumonia as a result of bacteria and other viruses is a major complication of measles[20,34,119,384] and influenza,[40,468] and sepsis often complicates varicella.[58] Some of the increase in susceptibility to bacterial infections may be the result of virus-induced damage of respiratory and cutaneous epithelium, but the mechanism is likely to be more complex.[25] Otitis media is a complication of measles, respiratory syncytial virus (RSV), adenovirus, and influenza.[215] Reactivation of previously controlled bacterial, viral, and parasitic infections appears during the acute and convalescent phases of cytomegalovirus (CMV) and measles virus infections.[86,114,117,181,389,453,497]

An increased susceptibility to secondary infections has also been documented as a consequence of a variety of natural and experimental infections of animals, including those caused by lymphocytic choriomeningitis virus (LCMV),[341,442,553] mouse hepatitis virus,[118] lactate dehydrogenase virus (LDV),[214,249] bovine virus diarrhea,[228] reovirus,[271] bovine RSV,[546] a variety of morbilliviruses,[128,135,391] parainfluenza viruses 1 and 3,[115,116,229] bovine herpesvirus 1,[150] CMV,[176] and malignant rabbit fibroma virus.[494]

More recently, chronic viral infections, particularly by retroviruses such as feline leukemia virus (FeLV),[378,428] avian retrovirus,[107] simian retrovirus,[151,268,440] feline immunodeficiency virus,[113,227,402] simian immunodeficiency virus,[32,481] murine leukemia virus (MuLV),[112,163] human T-cell lymphotropic virus type I (HTLV-I),[278,364] and human immunodeficiency virus (HIV)[5] have been recognized to increase host susceptibility to a wide range of opportunistic infections with bacteria, fungi, parasites, and other viruses.

Depressed Skin Test Responses and Graft Rejection

Loss of delayed-type hypersensitivity (DTH) reactions to recall antigens, as reported by von Pirquet in 1908,[522] has been confirmed for measles by multiple investigators[213,489,501,541,543] and also has been reported in association with a number of other acute viral infections, including influenza,[45] varicella,[490,541] Epstein-Barr virus (EBV)- and CMV-induced infectious mononucleosis,[194,315,379] and rubella.[371] Suppression of DTH responses after acute viral infections can persist for months despite apparent recovery from infection. Infection with HIV causes suppression of DTH responses as CD4 counts decrease and the problems of acquired immunodeficiency syndrome (AIDS) appear.[127,179,470] Asymptomatic infection with HTLV-I is often accompanied by loss of DTH skin test reactivity.[364,499] Immunizations with live attenuated measles, yellow fever, and rubella virus vaccines also suppress DTH responses, although more transiently than after infection with wild-type viruses.[52,53,155,217,330,489,563]

In addition, other in vivo parameters of cellular immune responses, such as rejection of allogeneic skin grafts[158,227,231,233,406,548] and induction of contact sensitivity,[203,333,539] may also be suppressed during experimental acute virus infections. Remission of immunologically mediated diseases such as nephrotic syndrome, idiopathic thrombocytopenic purpura, and rheumatoid arthritis have been reported after measles.[298,299,557] Experimental autoimmune encephalomyelitis, glomerulonephritis, and diabetes are more difficult to induce in virus-infected mice.[204,216,246,476]

Depressed Lymphoproliferative and Cytotoxic Responses in Vitro

Depressed in vitro lymphoproliferative responses of peripheral blood mononuclear cells (PBMCs) to ConA, PHA, and specific antigens have been reported during a number of acute human viral infections, including hepatitis A,[367] rubella,[371] measles,[18,97,266,531,532,539] influenza,[74] HIV,[91] hepatitis B,[367] varicella-zoster,[18] herpes simplex virus (HSV),[529] and infectious mononucleosis caused by EBV[307,315,403,457,505] and CMV.[69,71,296,430,431] Live-virus vaccines may also suppress mitogen- and antigen-induced lymphocyte proliferation.[19,100,223,328,363,483,530,563]

Experimental acute virus infections also suppress lymphoproliferative responses. This has been documented for infections with Mengo virus,[479] mouse hepatitis virus,[96] feline immunodeficiency virus,[300] FeLV,[227] Friend leukemia virus,[514] simian retrovirus,[295] avian retrovirus,[108] equine infectious anemia virus,[368] bovine RSV,[546] canine distemper virus,[16] rabies virus,[366] LCMV,[253,461] bovine virus diarrhea,[259] murine CMV,[47,83,231,265] bovine herpesvirus,[150] and malignant rabbit fibroma virus.[493,494]

Abnormalities often persist well beyond the period of clinical disease. For example, suppression of mitogen responses frequently continues for weeks to months in individuals that recover from infection.[231,307,367,532] During persistent infections with rubella,[349,383] Aleutian mink disease virus,[405] feline immunodeficiency virus,[300] HTLV-I,[366] and CMV[398] mitogen responses may remain suppressed for the duration of infection.

Other in vitro parameters of cellular immunity, such as allogeneic and autologous mixed lymphocyte responses[46,231,350,516] and induction of cytotoxic T lymphocytes (CTLs),[65,70,220] may also be suppressed during viral infection. Persistent infections with HTLV-I and HIV are associated with failure to generate normal recall CTL responses in vitro.[252,264,441]

Polyclonal B-cell Activation

An additional immunologic abnormality that frequently accompanies generalized loss of DTH and lymphoproliferative responses is polyclonal activation of B cells leading to increased plasma levels of IgG and autoantibodies. Polyclonal B-cell activation has been described in humans during measles virus,[185,531,539] HIV,[286,317,554] rubella virus,[371] EBV,[226] and CMV[92,379] infections. This polyclonal activation can complicate serologic diagnosis of viral infections based on acute- and convalescent-phase titers.[103,379]

Generalized increases in plasma immunoglobulin levels or in the numbers of antibody-secreting cells have also been described during experimental infections of mink with Aleutian mink disease virus,[302,405] chickens with adenovirus[29] and avian leukosis virus,[121] and mice with LDV,[147,332,334,373] MuLV, and Friend leukemia virus.[222,272] Paradoxically, this polyclonal B-cell activation may be accompanied by decreased[29,47,83,232,302,390,543] or increased[102,230,234,332,373] antibody responses to new antigens. The effect of infection on induction of new antibody responses is dependent on the specific infecting virus, the timing of the virus infection relative to antigen stimulation, and the nature of the antigenic stimulus.[75,76,221,230,234,260,272,302,334,380,381,454,493]

POTENTIAL MECHANISMS OF IMMUNE SUPPRESSION

Descriptions of quantifiable immunologic abnormalities such as loss of DTH responses, decreased mitogen-induced lymphoproliferative responses, and polyclonal activation of B cells have been relatively straightforward. As detailed previously, these abnormalities have been documented during many natural and experimental viral infections. However, determining the mechanisms by which viral infections induce these abnormalities of immune function has been more difficult. This process is not fully understood for any virus infection of any host.

In general, the potential mechanisms for virus-induced immune suppression include changes in immune function as a direct consequence of virus replication in cells that participate in the immune response, changes in immune function as an indirect consequence of the normal host immune response to the infecting virus,[432] and indirect effects of virus replication. For any specific infection, one or more of these mechanisms may contribute to the immune suppression that occurs (Table 10-1).

Virus Replication in Cells Important for Immune Function

Transient abnormalities in immune function may be caused by direct virus infection and depletion of cells of the immune system (e.g., T lymphocytes, B lymphocytes, macrophages, natural killer [NK] cells). As the virus is cleared, these cells are rapidly replenished, and immune function is restored. Longer-term abnormalities in cell numbers may be linked to persistent virus infection of leukocytes or to infection of cells that are important for activation or development of functional lymphocytes and monocytes such as primary antigen-presenting cells (e.g. dendritic cells), stem cells, and stromal cells of the bone marrow and thymus.

Many viruses have been documented to infect cells of the immune system in vivo (Table 10-2). Infection may be productive or nonproductive and may result in virus-induced cell death, cell activation and proliferation, or alterations in the functions of cells that remain viable. The effects of virus infection on cells of the immune system have been studied by identifying the infected cells in vivo and then by isolating these cells from infected individuals and assessing their functional capacities in vitro. In most viral infections, the proportion of cells that can be demonstrated to be infected is 1% or less of the relevant cell population. This small number of infected cells makes it difficult to ascribe all of the immunologic abnormalities observed in vivo or in vitro directly to the loss of function of infected cells.

TABLE 10-1. *Summary of identified immunologic abnormalities and their mechanisms of induction for various virus groups*

Virus group	Immune abnormalities				Mechanisms				
	Increased infections	Decreased DTH	Decreased lymphoproliferation	Increased immunoglobulin	Replication in immune cells	Activation of immune system	Th2 cytokines	Monocyte products	Viral proteins
Picornavirus			+						
Rubivirus		+	+						
Flavivirus		+						+	
Arterivirus	+		+	+	+				
Coronavirus	+		+		+				
Orthomyxovirus	+	+		+				+	+
Paramyxovirus	+	+	+		+	+	+		
Rhabdovirus			+						
Arenavirus	+		+		+	+	+	+	
Reovirus	+							+	
Retrovirus	+	+	+	+	+	+	+	+	+
Hepadnavirus			+						
Parvovirus			+	+	+				
Adenovirus	+		+						+
Herpesvirus	+	+	+	+	+	+	+	+	+
Poxvirus	+		+						+

DTH, delayed-type hypersensitivity.

TABLE 10-2. *Viruses that infect cells of the immune system in vivo*

Cell	Virus
T lymphocyte	Human T lymphotropic virus type 1
	Simian retrovirus
	Feline leukemia virus
	Human immunodeficiency virus
	Simian immunodeficiency virus
	Feline immunodeficiency virus
	Mouse thymic virus
	Human herpesvirus 6
	Human herpesvirus 7
B lymphocyte	Simian retrovirus
	Pancreatic necrosis virus
	Infectious bursal disease virus
	Epstein-Barr virus
	Murine leukemia virus
Monocyte	Venezuelan equine encephalitis virus
	Rubella virus
	Dengue virus
	Lactic dehydrogenase elevating virus
	Murine hepatitis virus
	Lymphocytic choriomeningitis virus
	Influenza virus
	Sendai virus
	Parainfluenza virus
	Measles virus
	Human immunodeficiency virus
	Visna-maedi virus
	Caprine arthritis encephalitis virus
	Cytomegalovirus
	Varicella-zoster virus
Dendritic cell	Human immunodeficiency virus
	Lymphocytic choriomeningitis virus
Stromal cell	Measles virus
	Borna disease virus
	Cytomegalovirus

Interactions between viruses and leukocytes are commonly studied using in vitro infection of PBMCs of humans or spleen cells of experimental animals. These studies often use high multiplicities of infection and laboratory-adapted strains of viruses. The interpretation of these experiments may be further complicated by contamination of virus stocks with other infectious agents or products of infection (e.g., mycoplasma, "passenger" viruses, lipopolysaccharide [LPS]), which have their own effects on immune function.[56,138,382,469] Therefore, relevance of these types of in vitro studies to in vivo virus-cell interactions resulting in altered immune function is uncertain and generally is not emphasized or extensively covered in this chapter.

T Lymphocytes

Human T-Cell Lymphotropic Virus Type I

HTLV-I infects T lymphocytes and induces proliferation of infected cells. The tax regulatory protein of HTLV-I in-creases expression of genes encoding the interleukin-2 (IL-2) receptor, IL-2, and granulocyte-macrophage colony–stimulating factor, leading to spontaneous proliferation of T cells.[31,122, 183,452] Infection also leads to decreased expression of CD3, which is necessary for expression of the T-cell receptor (TCR) on the cell surface.[124] Therefore, HTLV-I–infected cells can proliferate without antigen stimulation and do not respond to antigenic stimulation. In a small percentage of individuals, this virus-induced alteration in control of cell proliferation may be the first step leading to T-cell leukemia. How T-cell infection is linked to immunologic abnormalities (e.g., increased susceptibility to infection, decreased DTH skin test responses) of HTLV-I–infected individuals without leukemia in whom less than 1% of the T cells are infected is not known.

Human Immunodeficiency Virus

A major cellular receptor for HIV is CD4, and CD4-positive T cells in both blood and lymphoid tissue are important target cells for HIV infection.[140,270,325,399] In quiescent T cells, HIV is harbored predominantly as full-length, unintegrated complementary DNA.[57,414] Virus replication requires T-cell activation and integration of viral DNA. Approximately 0.01% to 1% of CD4 T cells in infected blood contain HIV DNA, but only 10% of these infected cells produce virus, as indicated by expression of viral RNA detectable by in situ hybridization.[197,414,464] Therefore, insufficient numbers of CD4 cells are infected to account for the immunologic dysfunction observed, particularly when CD4 T-cell numbers are normal. Some strains of HIV induce syncytia or apoptosis in infected T cells in vitro,[558] thus leading to death of T cells. The protein gp120 on the surface of infected macrophages or T cells can induce fusion of uninfected CD4-positive cells.[106] These processes have been postulated to occur in vivo and to account for the progressive loss of CD4 T cells in HIV-infected individuals (see Chap. 34).[140]

If precursor T cells (i.e., thymocytes) were infected, the effect of infection would be exaggerated by failure to replenish depleted cells. In vitro studies suggest that thymocytes are susceptible to HIV infection,[463] but autopsy studies do not suggest that thymocytes are an important target of infection.[401] Therefore, mechanisms other than elimination of CD4 T cells by direct virus infection have been proposed to account for the abnormalities in CD4 T-cell function observed. These mechanisms include activation-induced apoptosis, production of immunosuppressive cytokines, and superantigen-induced T-cell depletion (discussed later).

Mouse Thymic Virus

Mouse thymic virus is a herpesvirus that infects the thymus of newborn mice (<5 days of age) and causes thymic necrosis and acute immunosuppression 7 to 14 days after infection.[105] CD4+ 8+ thymocytes are decreased by 80%, and CD4+ 8− cells are decreased by more than 98%, suggesting that CD4+ T cells are the main target of infection.[193,355] Two to three weeks after infection, thymic repair begins with infiltration of macrophages and proliferation of stromal cells, followed by repopulation with thymocytes.[105,449] No immune response to the virus is detected, and persistent infection is established. Mice infected as adults develop persistent infection of the salivary glands without thymic abnormalities,[354] indicating that susceptibility of cells to infection is age-dependent.

Human Herpesviruses 6 and 7

Human herpesviruses (HHV) 6 and 7 have been isolated from T cells.[157,500] HHV-7 uses CD4 as a receptor[67] and downregulates its expression in infected cells.[160] The receptor for HHV-6 is not known, but it can replicate lytically in T cells and NK cells in vitro[308,309,439] and decreases expression of the CD3-TCR complex.[308] HHV-6 has been postulated to induce immunodeficiency in infants by progressively destroying peripheral T cells and thymocytes.[275]

B Lymphocytes

Herpesviruses

A primary target of EBV infection in humans and the related herpesvirus papio in baboons is the B lymphocyte. These infections do not usually result in B-cell death or production of infectious virus.[226] In vitro EBV infection immortalizes resting B cells, which often secrete immunoglobulin spontaneously,[269,443] and triggers a complex series of events leading to B-cell proliferation.[343] Production of autoantibodies occurs in vivo during EBV-induced infectious mononucleosis.[55,72] In vitro and in vivo EBV-induced B-cell proliferation is controlled by T cells.[513] If cellular immune responses to EBV are suppressed through genetic defects, drugs, or acquired disease, proliferation of EBV-infected B cells can go unchecked[226] and may be the first step in the induction of B-cell lymphoma.[513]

Birnaviruses

Infectious bursal disease virus of chickens and infectious pancreatic necrosis virus of trout cause lytic infection of dividing B lymphocytes and impaired antibody responses in infected individuals.[61,145,360,458,502] Infection with bursal disease virus results in a rapid and progressive loss of B lymphocytes from the bursa, blood, and thymus.[420,436]

Monocytes/Macrophages

Many viruses that cause immune suppression infect macrophages (see Table 10-2), but the relation between infection and immune suppression is not clear.[521] Macrophages provide important phagocytic control of a number of infectious agents, and any virus-induced decrease in number or in phagocytic or cytocidal function would increase host susceptibility to infection. Monocytes/macrophages are important accessory cells for T-cell function, and infection may induce changes in production of cytokines, antigen presentation, or expression of co-stimulatory cell surface molecules. However, because macrophages can act as antigen-presenting cells for viral antigens, infection of these cells may also be a powerful mechanism for stimulating host antiviral immune responses. Therefore, infected macrophages could have a number of indirect effects on T cells that may lead to immune suppression in vivo. Virus-infected macrophages may also be important for polyclonal B-cell activation.

Arteriviruses

LDV infects macrophages in vivo[245] and in vitro.[495,496] Only a small proportion of macrophages are susceptible to infection.[496] Combined in vitro and in vivo observations suggest that the macrophages that are susceptible to LDV infection are predominantly major histocompatibility complex (MHC) class II–positive and are killed by the infection.[245,495,496] During chronic infection in vivo, an equilibrium appears to be reached between infected and uninfected cells through continuous infection of new susceptible macrophages which evolve from nonsusceptible precursors.[245] Elevation of lactic dehydrogenase and other enzymes in the plasma of infected mice is the result of impairment of the enzyme clearance function of macrophages.[314,372] Decreased enzyme clearance appears to be a direct effect of macrophage infection, because it also occurs in LDV-infected severe combined immunodeficient (SCID) mice.[50,206] Although enzyme clearance is permanently affected by infection, carbon particle clearance is abnormal only during the acute phase,[314] suggesting that two different aspects of macrophage function are differentially affected by infection.

Persistent LDV infection is associated with a number of additional immunologic abnormalities. Macrophages from infected mice have impaired antigen-presenting capacity,[248] perhaps as a result of the preferential lytic infection of MHC class II–positive macrophages.[245] Macrophages from persistently infected mice also release increased amounts of superoxide anion,[205] produce less IL-1 and more prostaglandin E_2 (PGE_2),[202] and are primed to produce more nitric oxide[450] than macrophages from normal mice. Production of IL-6 is normal.[251]

Orthomyxoviruses and Paramyxoviruses

Influenza virus infects human monocytes, but infection is abortive unless lymphocytes are present in the culture, suggesting the need for a T-cell cytokine. Infection of avian macrophage cell lines inhibits production of nitric oxide,[310] a gaseous molecule important for control of bacterial and parasitic pathogens. Influenza virus infection of mice impairs the clearance of bacteria from the lungs. The maximum abnormality in clearance occurs 4 to 10 days after infection, although maximum virus titers are reached within 3 days,[184] raising a question about the importance of direct effects of viral infection for abnormal clearance.

The first thoroughly studied paramyxovirus was parainfluenza 1 (Sendai) virus infection of its normal host, the mouse.

Sendai virus–infected mice show increased susceptibility to bacterial pulmonary infections.[115] Sendai virus replicates in alveolar macrophages, and infected mice have decreased pulmonary phagocytic and bactericidal capacity.[115,116,254,271] Mechanical clearance of bacteria is normal despite extensive destruction of ciliated epithelium,[254] suggesting that increased susceptibility is caused by failure of phagocytes to kill those organisms that are not mechanically cleared. In bovine parainfluenza 3 infection, there is impaired clearance[305] as well as decreased phagocyte function.[482]

In vitro studies have shown that macrophages from parainfluenza virus–infected animals have decreases in Fc receptor function, bactericidal activity, nonimmune and immune-mediated phagocytosis, and phagosome-lysosome fusion.[255,533,534] Infection alters macrophage arachidonic acid metabolism by both the cyclooxygenase and lipoxygenase pathways and inhibits superoxide anion generation in response to zymosan.[136] Studies of macrophages infected in vitro have shown that avian influenza inhibits LPS-induced production of nitric oxide.[310]

RSV infects alveolar macrophages and monocytes in vivo.[129,400] The subpopulation of alveolar macrophages that permit infection are relatively immature cells[90] that express immunocytochemically identifiable MHC class II, IL-1, and tumor necrosis factor (TNF) proteins.[90,336] In vitro infection of macrophages is associated with decreased release of reactive oxygen intermediates, phagocytosis, and killing of protozoa,[180] and with increased production of an IL-1 inhibitor that suppresses mitogen-induced lymphoproliferation.[433,323]

Measles virus infects monocytes in vitro[459] and in vivo,[144,344] and adherent cells often contribute to suppressed mitogen-induced lymphocyte proliferation.[186] Production of IL-1β during measles is normal, whereas production of TNF-α is depressed.[532] Likewise, in vitro infection of monocytes with measles virus enhances IL-1 production and decreases TNF production.[294] Monocytes infected in vitro have impaired presentation of other antigens to T cells despite increased expression of MHC class II molecules.[293]

Arenaviruses

Junin virus and LCMV infect macrophages.[68] In LCMV infection, macrophage dysfunction has been causally linked to depressed mitogen responses.[253] Production of IL-1 is normal.[461] Antigen presentation is impaired.[12] Induction of immune suppression is dependent on the strain of virus and the genetic background and age of the infected mouse.[7,12,377,442,508] Immunosuppressive strains of virus infect macrophages efficiently.[320] It has been postulated that the immune suppression is actually caused by the elimination of infected macrophages and dendritic cells by virus-specific CTLs and consequent destruction of the organization of lymphoid follicles[48,292,377,561] rather than by virus-induced changes in macrophage function.

Lentiviruses

Monocytes/macrophages are major target cells for certain strains of HIV,[82,93] as well as maedi/visna, caprine arthritis-

encephalitis, and equine anemia viruses.[79,168] Tissue macrophages are a reservoir of infection during all stages of disease,[94,168,407] and circulating monocytes are often latently infected.[27] For most lentiviruses, it can be shown that monocytes begin to replicate virus as they differentiate into macrophages.[167,337] In general, replication appears to be without cytopathic effect. Monocyte counts decrease during HIV infection,[306] but phagocytic and microbicidal activity is preserved.[535] Infection of primary monocytes with HIV in vitro has generally shown little effect on production of TNF-α or IL-1 as long as LPS is eliminated as a factor.[345–347,362] However, virus replication is increased by and may be dependent on TNF-α stimulation.[408,523,544]

Herpesviruses

Human and murine CMV, varicella-zoster virus, and HHV-6 infect macrophages.[69,169,201,280,504] Monocytes may also serve as the primary site of latent infection for these viruses.[280,503] Maximal suppression of mitogen responses after infection with murine CMV coincides with maximal infection of adherent cells,[303] and in vitro infection of macrophages results in decreased phagocytic capacity for inert particles[504] and bacteria.[472] Monocytes from patients with CMV can suppress mitogen-induced proliferation of normal lymphocytes.[431] In vitro infection with human CMV leads to production of TNF-α, IL-1-β, and an inhibitor of IL-1.[134,438,485] The CMV immediate early proteins transactivate the TNF-α gene.[166]

Polymorphonuclear Leukocytes

A major contribution to the increased susceptibility to other infections in those who already have a viral infection may come from inefficient function of polymorphonuclear leukocytes (PMNs) as well as mononuclear phagocytes.[3] Viruses rarely have been shown to infect PMNs directly, but decreased bactericidal, chemotactic, oxidative, phagocytic, and secretory functions have been described during a variety of human viral infections.[3] A decreased respiratory burst in response to phorbol esters has been documented for neutrophils from FeLV- and feline immunodeficiency virus–infected cats[125,196] and for PMNs exposed to influenza virus.[2,73] PMN migration into the peritoneal cavity in response to LPS is decreased in LDV-infected mice.[202] The deactivation of PMNs by influenza virus is mediated by binding of the hemagglutinin to sialic-bearing cellular proteins.[200]

Dendritic Cells

Dendritic cells are a population of bone-marrow–derived cells specialized for acquiring and processing antigen for activation of naive and resting T cells. They also promote expansion of already activated memory T cells. Many dendritic-like cells are stationed in tissues where they acquire antigen and migrate to local lymph nodes to interact with T cells. Infection of dendritic cells in vivo has been identified only recently. Determining infection as opposed to sequestration of viral antigen can be difficult, because follicular dendritic cells function in the presence of antibody to concentrate antigens, including intact virus, for subsequent processing and stimulation of T cells.

In humans, HHV-6 has been associated with abnormal proliferation of Langerhans cells.[290] HIV infects follicular dendritic cells in lymphoid tissue,[326] dendritic cells in blood,[312] and Langerhans cells of the skin.[515,423,559] Dendritic cells can also be infected by HIV in vitro.[274] Dendritic cells isolated from HIV-infected individuals are functionally impaired, because they do not stimulate lymphocyte proliferation in a mixed leukocyte reaction.[43,311] It is postulated that loss of ability to stimulate resting T cells may result in a progressive loss of memory T cells.[311] In HIV infection, there are decreased numbers of dendritic cells in blood[104] and of Langerhans cells in skin,[38] suggesting that infection may also lead to cell death of these cells.

In animals, Aleutian mink disease virus, Rauscher leukemia virus, and LCMV infect dendritic cells.[48,161,353] Abnormalities in Rauscher leukemia virus–infected mice include decreased expression of adhesion molecules and failure of migration of Langerhans cells from the skin to lymph nodes after antigenic stimulation of skin.[161] In mice infected with the immunosuppressive clone 13 strain of LCMV, interdigitating dendritic cells in lymphoid tissues are destroyed by cytotoxic lymphocytes, resulting in a decrease in antigen-presenting capacity.[48]

Stromal Cells of the Thymus and Bone Marrow

The thymus is the site of T-cell differentiation; therefore, abnormalities of thymic function could have long-term consequences for peripheral T-cell function. Decreased size and function of the thymus are induced during many virus infections.[195,385,406] In some instances there is demonstrable virus replication in the thymus, and in others there is not. LDV[460] and rabies virus[404] induce thymic involution through the pituitary-adrenocortical axis rather than by direct virus infection, because adrenalectomy prevents thymic involution. Thymocytes are sensitive to corticosteroids, and it is presumed that these cells undergo apoptosis in response to the high levels of corticosteroids induced by the stress of infection with these viruses.

HIV, measles virus, and CMV infect stromal epithelial cells of the thymus in vivo and in vitro.[375,376] The results of thymic infection with these human viruses have been studied using human thymic implants in mice with SCID. HIV infection results in a slow, strain-dependent disruption of the thymic microenvironment, with depletion of thymocytes and degeneration of thymic epithelium over a period of weeks.[279,488] Autopsy studies of fatal cases of measles in humans and experimentally infected monkeys have shown a loss of the thymic cortex.[59,84,542] Thymic destruction in monkeys and the level of measles virus replication in stromal cells of SCID/hu thymic implants correlate with the virulence of the virus. After infection of stromal cells with wild-type strains of measles virus, uninfected thymocytes undergo apoptosis. Polyoma virus and mouse hepatitis virus infections of mice cause thymocyte death as a consequence of functional alteration of infected stromal cells.[243] In vitro infection of thymic stromal cells with CMV, RSV, or cox-sackievirus leads to decreased production of IL-1 activity in the absence of cytopathic effect.[528]

CMV infects stromal cells of the bone marrow and thymus.[277,480] Infection of thymic stromal cells increases the sensitivity of thymocytes to induction of apoptosis by antibody to CD3.[277] Infection of bone marrow stromal cells is associated with myelosuppression and deficiency of production of granulocyte macrophage colony–stimulating factor.[480] Similarly, infectious bursal disease virus may alter function of bursal stromal epithelial cells, disrupting function of that organ in chickens.[420]

Effects of the Host Antiviral Immune Response on Generalized Immune Function

Many of the global abnormalities of immune function occur in the context of a developing virus-specific immune response[265] and may therefore be an unavoidable consequence of the production of an immune response effective for virus clearance and the establishment of long-term protective immunity from reinfection. Evidence of immune activation is common in both acute and chronic viral infections.[99,359] Examples of infections in which a link between immune activation and suppression has been made include measles virus, influenza virus, LCMV, HIV, EBV, and CMV.[99,226,442] Immunologic deficits may be the result of generalized activation of T cells in the absence of appropriate secondary signals, altered cytokine environments, or depletion of virus-specific T cells during attempted control of a persistent infection. These ongoing immune responses may lead to imbalances in the T-cell and macrophage responses to subsequent antigenic challenges. A role for immune activation in the immune suppression associated with viral infections is suggested by the fact that maximum suppression often occurs at the time of the appearance of the immune response and virus clearance rather than at the time of maximum virus replication.[442,492]

Activation-Induced Cell Death

Immune suppression in association with immune activation has been most carefully studied in EBV, HIV, and measles virus infections of humans[21,99,137,365,511] and in LCMV infection of mice.[357,425,442] Antigen-stimulated T cells become activated by signaling through the TCR. As a part of the immune response to a virus, this leads to T-cell proliferation and cytokine production; however, it has become increasingly recognized that these activated cells may also undergo apoptotic cell death.[182] The exact determinants of the outcome of activation are not completely defined, but expression of Fas on the T-cell surface is necessary but not sufficient for induction of apoptosis.[171] Immature T cells and mature T cells activated in the absence of proper co-stimulatory signals are particularly likely to become apoptotic.[182] The latter phenomenon has been described in association with activation by superantigens and during the immune response to viral infection.

CD4 and CD8 T cells from asymptomatic HIV-infected individuals undergo apoptosis in lymph nodes in vivo[365] and following activation in vitro.[177,192,331] The Tat protein of HIV sensitizes T cells to gp120-induced apoptosis by upregulating cell surface expression of the Fas (CD95) molecule.[540] T cells from EBV-infected humans and CMV-infected mice show a high level of apoptosis in vitro.[517,556] T cells from LCMV-infected mice are highly susceptible to activation-induced apoptosis 1 to 3 weeks after infection.[425] Whether activation-induced apoptosis affects only virus-specific T cells or may also involve T cells activated "nonspecifically" during the immune response is not clear. In LCMV and HIV infections, it has been suggested that continuation of this process during persistent infection leads to depletion of virus-specific T cells.[562]

Cytokine-Induced Immune Suppression

Viral infections result in induction of a host immune response to the infecting virus that is designed to eliminate the virus from all sites of replication. Success in elimination depends on the virus, the host, and the site of infection. Many viruses induce production of type I interferons (IFN-α and IFN-β). The virus-specific immune response often results in activation of monocytes and CD4 and CD8 T cells. Spontaneous proliferation of circulating lymphocytes and monocytes,[18,430,531] changes in expression of cell surface molecules,[19,187] and spontaneous production of soluble IL-2 receptor and IL-1β[532] have been documented. Activation of the immune system may also be manifested by increased plasma levels of soluble cell surface molecules such as IL-2 receptor, CD4, and CD8, and products of activated monocytes and lymphocytes such as neopterin, IL-2, IL-4, and IFN-γ.[26,189,190,427,426,509–511] A number of soluble factors that inhibit immune function can be produced by activated lymphocytes and macrophages, and inhibitors of immune function are known to be present in plasma and supernatant fluids of cultured PBMCs.[109,287,289,367,493]

Type I Interferon

Early experiments with LCMV and Newcastle disease virus showed suppression of CTL responses to a second virus and a correlation of suppression with levels of IFN.[51] Subsequent studies with LDV showed that acquisition of contact sensitivity was impaired early after infection and that no impairment was present if mice were treated with anti–IFN-α/β antibody. Contact sensitivity was also inhibited in normal mice treated with IFN-α/β.[203] Type I IFNs have multiple effects on cells, and their interactions with the immune system are complex. IFN alters leukocyte distribution within lymphoid organs, increasing white pulp and decreasing red pulp areas of the spleen, induces leukopenia,[250] and is probably the mechanism by which Newcastle disease virus alters lymphocyte recirculation.[547] In culture, IFN-α contributes to depressed T-cell proliferation[284] and to altered macrophage function.[207]

T-Cell–Induced Suppression

T cells function primarily through the production of soluble factors known as cytokines. Many of the symptoms of viral infections (e.g., fever, myalgias, malaise, somnolence) are caused by the antiviral immune response and the cytokines that are produced and circulating as a consequence of this response. For example, the rash of measles is dependent on a cellular immune response to the virus and may not appear in severely immunocompromised individuals.[141,263,477]

Unstimulated or newly stimulated CD4 and CD8 T cells can produce a wide array of cytokines, but with restimulation, the panel is narrowed, and functional T-cell subtypes emerge. These are referred to as type 1 and type 2 T cells (Fig. 10-1). Type 1 T cells generally produce IFN-γ, IL-2 and TNF-β (lymphotoxin), whereas type 2 T cells produce primarily IL-4, IL-5, IL-6, IL-10, and IL-13. Type 1 cytokines are important for macrophage activation leading to DTH responses (IFN-γ), lymphocyte proliferation (IL-2), and MHC class II–restricted cytotoxicity (TNF-β). Type 2 cytokines are important for macrophage deactivation (IL-4 and IL-10) and B-cell help (IL-4, IL-5, IL-6, IL-10, and IL-13).[358]

The type of T-cell response induced by a particular infectious agent is dependent in part on co-stimulatory signals received from antigen-presenting cells. Production of IL-12 activates type 1 responses and suppresses type 2 responses,[64] whereas production of IL-1 and IL-4 favors development of type 2 responses.[1,536] Production of IFN-γ suppresses activation of type 2 cells,[162] and production of IL-4 suppresses activation of type 1 cells.[1] Thus, the two T-cell types are cross-regulatory, leading to cytokine profiles in response to infection that are often either primarily type 1 (e.g., DTH) or type 2 (e.g., antibody, eosinophilia) in character. Therefore, viruses that induce a type 2 T-cell response are predicted to be associated with suppression of DTH and lymphoproliferative responses but induction of good antibody responses. Viruses that induce a type 1 response are predicted to suppress B-cell responses but induce good DTH and in vitro proliferative responses.[44]

Failure of mitogen-induced proliferation during virus infection has been linked to failure of T cells to produce or bind IL-2. This has been demonstrated after Newcastle disease virus, LCMV, and CMV infection of mice[95,369,461] and measles virus, HIV, and EBV infection of humans.[224,313,403,412,413,467] The decrease in production of IL-2 after in vitro stimulation with mitogens[42,461,512] suggests a suppression of type 1 responses.

CD8 T cells have long been implicated in immune suppression (e.g., suppressor T cells). In measles, spontaneous CD8 T-cell proliferation correlates with low mitogen responses.[531] Some studies have shown increases in the proportion of CD8 lymphocytes,[11,266] whereas others have shown little change.[18,531] In varicella-zoster virus, RSV, CMV, and EBV infections, increases in activated CD8 T cells in peripheral blood are often accompanied by depressed CD4 : CD8 ratios, which are linked to immune suppression.[18,70,71,129,260,283,429,465,537] Activation and increased numbers of CD8 T cells are also observed after measles immunization of infants.[240] CD8 T cells with suppressor activity are induced during rabies virus infection and LCMV infection of mice.[220,292] These cells can suppress lymphocyte proliferation and differentiation of CTLs.[220]

Two T-cell cytokines have been recognized as clearly immunosuppressive and are candidates for inducing global immune suppression: IL-10 and IL-4. IL-10 is an important product of suppressor T cells and is a particularly potent mediator of type 2 responses. IL-10 inhibits the production of

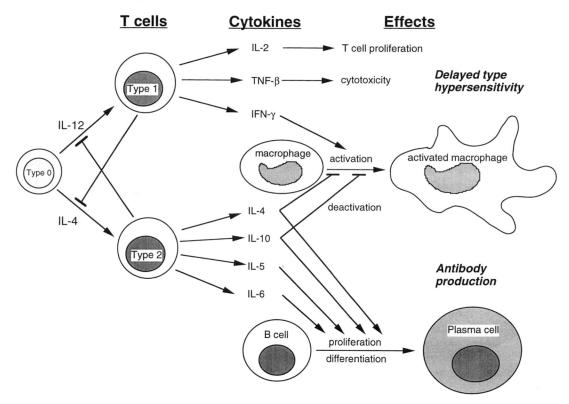

FIG. 10-1. The two types of cross-regulatory cytokine responses produced by type 1 and type 2 T cells.

cytokines by type 1 T cells,[152,154] T-cell proliferation,[123,126] and the production of inflammatory mediators by macrophages.[153,165,392] EBV and equine herpesvirus type 2 encode and produce a viral version of IL-10 that is biologically active.[235,351,435]

IL-4 inhibits the proliferation of and promotes the differentiation of B cells.[322] IL-4 may promote[342] or inhibit[318] the proliferation of T cells in response to mitogens and decreases monocyte production of TNF-α, IL-2, IL-4, PGE$_2$, and IL-1.[36,131,132,143,199] IL-4 also inhibits the effects of IFN-γ and transforming growth factor β (TGF-β) on macrophages[131,291,506,550] and the induction of superoxide.[4,225,291,549] IL-4 production is increased in those with measles[188] and after measles immunization.[530] Increases in IL-4 correlate with the onset of immunosuppression in murine acquired immunodeficiency syndrome (MAIDS),[164] and IL-4–deficient mice have increased survival and delayed development of T-cell abnormalities.[262] Therefore, IL-4 appears to be an important soluble factor associated with immune suppression and immune activation.

In vivo administration of IL-4 and IL-10 inhibit DTH responses,[297,416] suggesting that circulation of increased levels of these cytokines will alter skin test responses independent of the reason for increased cytokine levels. This suggests that if such cytokines are produced as a part of the immune response to a viral infection, generalized immune suppression may result.

Levels of circulating cytokines and spontaneous and antigen-induced production of cytokines by PBMCs have been measured in a limited number of viral infections. Measurement of plasma levels of cytokines during measles has shown

an increase in IL-4 as the rash subsides. These levels remain elevated for weeks after recovery.[188] In HIV and MuLV infections, there is an increase in production of IL-4 and IL-10 by lymphoid cells that coincides with the appearance of immunosuppression.[164,474]

Monocyte/Macrophage Cytokines

"Suppressor" T cells that act by inhibiting the function of antigen-presenting cells have been reported in mice infected with Newcastle disease virus.[301] Therefore, as detailed previously, one mechanism for virus-induced suppression is activation of T cells to produce soluble products that affect macrophage function, such as IL-4 and IL-10. However, macrophages may also produce soluble products that affect T-cell function.

Macrophages and their soluble products have frequently been associated with virus-induced immunosuppression. Suppressor macrophages have been reported in influenza infection of mice,[241] in CMV infection of humans and mice,[41] and in infectious bursal disease virus and reovirus infections of chickens.[473] Macrophages from influenza- and CMV-infected mice suppress in vitro antibody responses.[41,241] Monocytes infected in vitro as well as monocytes taken from patients with CMV mononucleosis suppress mitogen-induced proliferation of normal PBMCs.[69,323]

Immunosuppression has been associated particularly with monocyte and macrophage production of prostaglandins, primarily PGE$_2$, nitric oxide, and TGF-β. PGE$_2$ increases cyclic AMP in cells with PGE$_2$ receptors, resulting in a variety of antiinflammatory effects, including suppression of IL-2 and IFN-γ synthesis by type 1 T lymphocytes.[39,276,374,422,486] Monocyte/macrophage production of PGE$_2$ is increased in HIV infection[149,304,419] and results in inhibition of transendothelial migration of lymphocytes.[388] Treatment with cyclooxygenase inhibitors such as indomethacin often improves in vitro lymphoproliferative responses, suggesting a role for prostaglandins in this indicator of immune suppression.[175]

TGF-β is a multifunctional cytokine produced by a number of cells, including platelets, glial cells, and monocytes.[22] TGF-β was first recognized as an important immunosuppressive factor in patients with glioblastoma, who have suppressed DTH responses.[552] Evaluation of the role and regulation of TGF-β has been complicated by the fact that the gene is constitutively expressed.[22] Control is largely posttranscriptional, and the translated molecule must be activated and secreted to have biologic activity.[526] TGF-β inhibits IL-1–dependent T-cell proliferation,[139,525] NK cell proliferation,[498] T-cell progression into S phase stimulated by IL-2 or IL-4,[455] and generation of CTL activity.[156,421,471] TGF-β promotes class switching of B cells to secrete IgA[520] and production of the integrin cell adhesion molecules[209] and extracellular matrix proteins. Absence of TGF-β1 leads to a fatal multifocal inflammatory disease in mice,[475] providing further evidence of its role in controlling inflammation.

Partly because of the problems in measuring this biologically active molecule, there are limited data on the production of TGF-β in viral disease. The immediate early proteins of CMV can activate transcription of TGF-β1.[335] In LCMV infection of mice, biologically active TGF-β appears 3 days after infection, with peak production at 5 to 9 days postinfection, and correlates with suppression of NK cell proliferation and activity.[498] Macrophages from chickens infected with reovirus produce increased levels of active TGF-β1 and nitric oxide, both of which are potent inhibitors of T-cell proliferation.[348,465] The HIV Tat protein induces synthesis of TGF-β,[560] suggesting possible contributions of TGF-β to HIV-induced immune suppression.

In measles virus and LCMV infections, production of IL-1 is normal.[461,532] In vitro infection of monocytes or macrophages with influenza or RSV induces production of IL-1, TNF-α, and IL-6.[180,433] In vitro infection of macrophages with CMV or RSV, which is not productive of infectious virus or cytotoxic to the infected cells, induces production of an inhibitor of IL-1.[138,323,433,437] Dengue virus–infected monocytes secrete IL-1, TNF, and an IL-1 inhibitor.[77] Mononuclear cells from mice responding to influenza virus reinfection produce a low-molecular-weight factor that suppresses the activity of leukocyte migration inhibition factor.[33]

Effects of Viral Proteins on Immune Function

Viruses encode and direct the synthesis of a wide variety of proteins that can affect host immune responses.[174] Some of these are structural proteins that can bind to cell surface molecules and interfere with function; others are structural and nonstructural proteins that can affect intracellular metabolic processes. Some of these proteins may be released from infected cells and affect the function of cells that are not infected. For example, in vitro studies have suggested that the Newcastle disease viral neuraminidase and the influenza virus hemagglutinin directly affect neutrophil function.[73,146] In ad-

dition, viral proteins may be able to act as superantigens by binding directly to TCR and MHC class II molecules, resulting in activation and subsequent depletion of subsets of T cells.

Viral Proteins That Affect the Function of Immune Cells

In 1979, Mathes and colleagues[319] reported that a 15-kDa virion envelope protein from FeLV (p15E) directly inhibited lymphocyte proliferation of human and feline mononuclear cells in vitro without cellular toxicity and inhibited immune responses to FeLV in vivo.[98,208] This hydrophobic transmembrane envelope protein also inhibits macrophage accumulation in mice[89] and NK and B-cell activation. Similar proteins are encoded by murine retroviruses and human HTLV.[88] Six to seventeen amino acid peptides derived from the conserved region of these proteins contain the suppressive activity and are able to inhibit proliferation of T cells[87,456] and macrophage chemotaxis in vitro.[386] These immunosuppressive proteins or peptides may act by inhibiting signal transduction via protein kinase C.[261]

The gp120 protein of HIV has also been reported to directly affect immune function of uninfected cells.[538] This protein is shed from the surface of HIV-infected cells and virus particles and can bind CD4 on uninfected CD4-positive T cells. Binding CD4 can suppress T-cell activation in a manner similar to the suppressive effect of antibody to CD4[538] and induces monocyte differentiation.[524] Endocytic processing of bound gp120 may also make uninfected cells targets for MHC class II–restricted T-cell cytolysis.[478] Expression of the HIV nef gene as a transgene in T cells causes severe immunodeficiency. These processes are potentially important for immune suppression but have not yet been demonstrated to be important in vivo.

Viral Proteins That Affect Clearance of Infected Cells by Antibody and Complement

Antibody may target virus-infected cells for destruction by cellular or complement-mediated mechanisms. The HSV type 1 (HSV-1) glycoprotein E (gE) and glycoprotein I (gI) proteins together bind the Fc complement-binding domain of IgG.[37,258] Binding of Fc by gE and gI prevents complement-mediated lysis of infected cells or virions and may protect against phagocytosis as well.[133] Disruption of the gI or gE genes decreases virulence in vivo.[30] In addition, the glycoprotein C (gC) protein of HSV-1 binds the C3b fragment of C3, preventing complement activation by both the classic and alternative pathways and complement-mediated neutralization of virion infectivity and lysis of infected cells.[198,329,484]

A major product of vaccinia virus–infected cells is a complement-control protein that binds both C4b and C3b and inhibits both the antibody-dependent classic and antibody-independent alternative complement pathways.[247,282,327] Herpesvirus saimiri, a gammaherpesvirus that causes lymphomas in New World monkeys, encodes two complement regulatory proteins. One, the complement-control protein homolog, is a member of a family of human complement regulatory proteins that interact with C3b or C4b. This gene, like decay-accelerating factor, is differentially spliced, resulting in both a membrane-bound and secreted form associated with infected cells.[9] A second gene (HVS-A15) encodes a protein with significant homology to CD59, a phosphoinositol-linked 18-kDa complement-control glycoprotein. CD59 regulates complement-mediated membrane damage by preventing activation of C9 and assembly of the pore. The product of the HVS-A15 gene has been shown to protect cells from complement-mediated lysis.[444]

Viral Proteins That Affect Recognition of Infected Cells by T Cells

Expression of MHC class I proteins is necessary for CD8 T-cell recognition of virus-infected cells. The first virus that was recognized to decrease expression of MHC class I proteins on infected cells was the oncogenic type 12 adenovirus.[466] Further study has shown that the adenovirus E3/19K protein associates with the MHC class I heavy chain and retains it in the endoplasmic reticulum.[15,60,394,397] Failure to transport class I molecules to the cell surface prevents recognition of these cells by CD8-positive CTLs.[60,395] An additional mechanism, used by subgenus A adenoviruses, suppresses class I expression by decreasing transcription of MHC class I mRNA.[396]

The poxviruses (myxoma virus and malignant rabbit fibroma virus), CMV, and HSV also modulate immune function by decreasing MHC class I protein on the surface of infected cells.[35,49,218,257,555] HSV protein ICP47 binds TAP molecules in the cell, inhibiting peptide transport into the endoplasmic reticulum.[159,219] Empty class I molecules are then retained in the endoplasmic reticulum. Human CMV produces a class 1 heavy chain homolog, UL18, that binds the light chain of the class I molecule, β_2-microglobulin. CMV-infected cells do not express MHC class I molecules on the cell surface, and it is postulated that UL18 sequesters β_2-microglobulin, preventing the maturation of MHC class I molecules and recognition of infected cells by CTLs.[54] CMV may also have a direct effect on the stability of MHC class I heavy chains.[35]

Viral Proteins That Block Cytokine Function

A fascinating array of proteins that modulate immune function are produced by members of the poxvirus family (Table 10-3; see Chap. 22). These gene products are encoded in the termini of the viral genome and are "nonessential" for growth in tissue culture but play important roles in determining viral virulence. A number of these proteins are viroceptors, which are viral-encoded homologs of cellular lymphokine receptors. Shope fibroma, myxoma, and malignant rabbit fibroma viruses encode a TNF-binding protein that competitively inhibits TNF binding to cell surface receptors.[518] Soluble receptors for IFN-γ are secreted from cells infected by at least 17 different orthopoxviruses.[10] Myxoma virus encodes a IFN-γ–receptor homolog and a cell surface protein (M11L) that decreases leukocyte infiltration into areas of virus replication and tumor formation.[178,387,519] Infection with malignant rabbit fibroma virus produces profound immunosuppression that is associated with production of soluble factors by infected cells, suggesting that these viral proteins may have systemic as well as local effects.[491]

Vaccinia virus and cowpox virus encode proteins that bind IL-1, IFN-γ, and TNF,[487] and cowpox virus also encodes a protease inhibitor (crmA) that prevents cleavage of the IL-1β precursor to its active form.[424] Deletion of these genes from vaccinia virus decreases virus virulence but does not inhibit replication in vitro. Tanapox virus produces a 38-kDa protein that binds IFN-γ, IL-2, and IL-5.[142] Homologs of many of these proteins have been identified in smallpox (variola major) virus.[487] The effects of production of these proteins on global immune function in vivo have not been assessed.

TABLE 10-3. *Virus-encoded proteins that interfere with the host immune response*

Host immune response	Virus	Viral protein	Host protein affected
Antibody-dependent complement-mediated lysis	Herpes simplex type 1	gE + gl	Fc portion of IgG
		gC	C3b
	Vaccinia	VCP	C4b + C3b
	Herpes saimiri	HVS-15	C4b Complement activation
		HVS-CD59	
MHC class 1–restricted presentation of viral antigens to cytotoxic T cells	Adenovirus	E3/19K	Class I heavy chain
	Herpes simplex	ICP47	TAP
	Human cytomegalovirus	UL18	β_2-microglobulin
Production of cytokines by macrophages	Shope fibroma	?	TNF
	Myxoma	?	TNF
	Malignant rabbit fibroma	?	TNF
	Vaccinia	?	TNF
			IL-1β
	Cowpox	?	TNF
		crmA	IL-1β
Production of cytokines by T lymphocyte	Orthopox	orf B8R	IFN-γ
	Tanapox	38 kDa	IFN-γ, IL-2 and IL-5
	Myxoma	37 kDa	IFN-γ

Viral Proteins That Act as Superantigens for T Cells

Mouse Mammary Tumor Virus and the Minor Lymphoid-Stimulating Antigens

Several microbial proteins have been demonstrated to be superantigens. These proteins, in conjunction with MHC class II proteins, bind directly to the β chain of the TCR and activate T cells bearing a particular V_β protein (Fig. 10-2). Acute infection with milk-borne mouse mammary tumor virus (MMTV) has long been known to alter immune responses.[191] MMTV infection leads to activation followed by deletion of T cells expressing specific TCR V_β chains in mouse strains with the appropriate MHC class II antigens.[81,316] The murine I-E genes, which are analogous to human DR, appear to be more important for superantigen stimulation than the I-A genes.[256] Deletion is in part the result of elimination of specific V_β T cells in the thymus. In addition, CD4 cells bearing the relevant V_β proteins that escape elimination in the thymus are anergic through exposure to the superantigen and cannot expand in the periphery.[242] MMTV-infected mice have abnormalities in antibody responses and graft rejection,[191,205] but these have not yet been clearly linked to V_β deletion.

The MMTV superantigen is encoded by an open reading frame (ORF) in the 3' long terminal repeat (LTR) of the virus.[85] For MMTV-induced disease to occur, cellular activation is necessary for virus replication.[212] MMTV infects MHC class II–positive B cells, which then activate T cells through expression of the superantigen. The superantigen-activated T cells further stimulate B cells and virus replication,[210,211] increasing the probability of virus infection of mammary epithelial cells and insertional activation of selected protooncogenes (see Chap. 11). Susceptibility to infection is determined by availability of the proper MHC class II antigen and responsive

T cells.[81,173,212] Mice lacking T cells with the relevant TCR V_β protein are immune to MMTV-induced disease.

A consequence of the activation and deletion of a particular V_β subset of T cells is the generation of a "hole" in the T-cell repertoire. The host will then be unable to respond to antigens that are normally recognized by T cells with the deleted V_β.

Endogenous retrovirus sequences that include the 3' LTR and ORF coding region (minor lymphoid-stimulating [mls] antigens) of MMTV are carried by a number of strains of mice.[85] In these mice, there is deletion in the thymus during development of T cells with the V_β subset that reacts with the mls antigen carried by the mouse strain.[85,551] Developing thymocytes bearing TCRs with the particular V_β encounter these endogenous viral superantigens as self molecules in the thymus and are consequently clonally eliminated. Thus far, all superantigens carried in the murine germ line have been mapped to endogenous MMTV proviral integrants. The level of mls expression in the thymus determines the completeness and the stage of development of reactive thymocyte deletion.[352] The function of the 36-kDa glycosylated ORF protein is not clear, but it appears to be a type II transmembrane protein[273,281] that is expressed on the surface of B cells.[545] Sequence comparisons between these proteins suggest that the V_β specificity is determined by the 25 C-terminal amino acids[85,415]; however, divergent C-terminal sequences can mediate deletion of the same V_β T-cell subsets,[172] therefore the exact basis for specificity is not yet clear.

One of the earliest known effects of mls antigens was the suppression of immune responses such as antibody formation and graft rejection on injection of mls-disparate cells into recipient mice. This acute effect appears to be the result of T-cell activation rather than depletion of specific T-cell subsets.[256]

Other Viral Superantigens

There has been an active search for a role for viral superantigens in the pathogenesis of other retrovirus infections associated with immune suppression. The replication-defective MuLV that causes an AIDS-like syndrome in mice is associated with activation of $V_{\beta5}$ T cells responding to gag p30,[239] but immune deficiency can be induced independent of this interaction.[170]

Analysis of the distribution of the percentages of T cells with different TCR V_βs in HIV-infected and uninfected people has led to the hypothesis that HIV acts as a superantigen and may deplete CD4 T cells by this mechanism.[244] $V_{\beta14}$ T-cell lines produce more HIV than $V_{\beta6.7}$ T-cell lines, and $V_{\beta12}$ T cells proliferate in response to HIV-infected antigen-presenting cells, suggesting a superantigen response.[288] However, there is no evidence of $V_{\beta12}$ deletion in HIV-infected individuals. A selective anergy of $V_{\beta8}$ cells to stimulation with bacterial superantigens suggests that these cells were anergized by an HIV superantigen.[110] Studies of twins and neonates have not supported a role for superantigens in HIV-induced immune deficiency.[28,370]

Immunosuppressive strains of FeLV cause depletion of CD4 cells. This is determined by the amino acid composition of the C-terminal portion of gp70,[417] but it is not clear that this is a superantigen effect. A virus-encoded superantigen does not appear to account for depletion of CD4 cells in simian immunodeficiency virus–induced immunodeficiency in rhesus

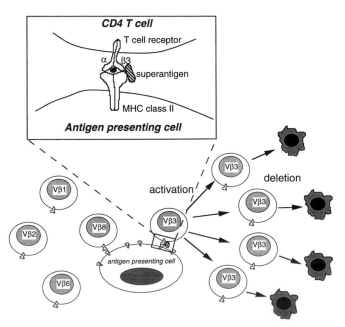

FIG.10-2. Superantigen-mediated deletion of T cells expressing a subset of T-cell receptor variable β (Vβ) chain.

macaques.[81] However, stimulation of $V_{\beta7}$ and $V_{\beta14}$ T cells may play a role in the rapidly lethal disease caused by a simian immunodeficiency virus variant isolated from pigtailed macaques,[80] perhaps by increasing the number of T cells supporting active virus replication.

Because superantigens stimulate T cells with specific $V_\beta s$ in a non–antigen-specific way, they are often mitogenic in culture (i.e., they cause T cells from unimmunized individuals to proliferate). In culture, T cells from unimmunized individuals proliferate in response to the rabies virus nucleocapsid protein in the presence of MHC class II–positive B cells. There is a specific expansion of T cells bearing $V_{\beta8}$.[285] However, there is no indication that rabies or immunization with rabies vaccine leads to deletion of this T-cell subset or to immune deficiency.

Viral Proteins That Stimulate B Cells

EBV infection of B cells stimulates polyclonal activation and immunoglobulin secretion. EBV uses lymphocyte activation pathways to initiate proliferation and encodes and expresses a copy of the IL-10 gene, a B-cell growth factor.[235,351] Equine herpesvirus type 2 also encodes an IL-10 gene.[435]

The mechanism of polyclonal activation of B cells and increased immunoglobulin levels found during infections with other viruses that do not infect B cells is unclear. LDV causes increased levels of IgG and improved antibody responses to various immunogens.[334] The increase in IgG is primarily in the IgG2a subclass and represents a polyclonal activation of B cells producing this isotype.[101,238,332,451] Germinal centers are increased in lymphoid tissue,[373] and increased IgG2a synthesis coincides with the accumulation of LDV RNA in these germinal centers, perhaps trapped by follicular dendritic cells.[14] Immunoglobulin synthesis is not stimulated by LDV infection of athymic nude mice but is stimulated in xid mice.[101]

Some viruses induce cellular proteins that stimulate B cells. For instance, African swine fever virus–infected porcine monocytes release a 36-kDa protein that increases immunoglobulin secretion and antibody responses to new antigens by an unknown mechanism.[17] The hemagglutinin of influenza virus is mitogenic for normal murine spleen cells,[63] and the cells stimulated to proliferate are B cells.[13,411] H2 and H6 subtypes stimulate B cells directly by binding the murine I-Ek MHC class II molecule on the B-cell surface[462]; other hemagglutinin subtypes vary in their ability to activate B cells.[445] This stimulation induces polyclonal immunoglobulin synthesis by a protein kinase C–dependent mechanism.[445,447] The hemagglutinin can stimulate CD5+ B cells as well as conventional B cells, suggesting a mechanism for viruses to expand the pool of autoreactive CD5+ B cells and increase autoantibody production.[446] It is not known whether proteins from other viruses are capable of similar stimulation.

ROLE OF VIRUS STRAINS IN INDUCTION OF IMMUNE DEFICIENCY

For many viruses, it has become clear that induction of immunodeficiency is strain-dependent. Comparative studies of immunosuppressive and nonimmunosuppressive strains of the same virus can be a powerful tool for determining some of the mechanisms of virus-induced immune suppression.

Lymphocytic Choriomeningitis Virus

Immune suppression in LCMV is multifaceted and depends on the strain of virus and genetic background of the host.[442] Immune deficiency is not caused by LCMV directly, as evidenced by normal immune responses in neonatally infected carrier mice.[253,292,341]

Strain-dependent immune suppression in 4- to 8-week-old mice infected with LCMV was first reported in conjunction with the induction of LCMV-specific CTL responses and establishment of virus persistence after infection with the Armstrong strain of LCMV.[7] Strains of LCMV that induce a CTL response leading to clearance of infection (e.g., Armstrong) differ from strains that do not induce a CTL response and cause a persistent infection (e.g., clone 13)[8] by a single amino acid substitution (phenylalanine to leucine) at residue 260 in the envelope glycoprotein.[6,321,381] Ability to persist is also correlated with efficient infection of macrophages[267]; this property is dependent on a single amino acid change at residue 1079 in the polymerase (lysine to glutamine or asparagine).[320] Generalized immune deficiency is induced more effectively by the WE, Docile, and clone 13 strains than by the Armstrong strain in 4- to 8-week-old mice.[442,508]

Feline Leukemia Virus

In FeLV infection, an acute immunodeficiency syndrome (feline acquired immunodeficiency syndrome [FAIDS]) correlates with the replication of a variant (FeLV-FAIDS) that is detected primarily as unintegrated viral DNA in the bone marrow.[227,361] Infection with this variant leads to deficits in colony-forming T cells and depletion of circulating T cells.[418] This variant is replication-defective[393] and differs from the parent virus in its envelope glycoprotein (gp70).[409] Construction of chimeric viruses has identified major determinants of immunodeficiency within a 7–amino acid C-terminal region and a 109–amino acid N-terminal region of gp70.[130,417] These variants fail to block superinfection of T cells in vitro, which results in increased cell death.[130] Changes in gp70 lead to altered processing of the envelope glycoprotein[409,410] and to increased killing of T cells in vitro.[130] T-cell killing can be enhanced further by changes in the U3 region of the LTR.[130]

Chronic immunodeficiency is associated with a predominance of variant genomes with substantial internal deletions.[361] The determinants of delayed cytopathogenicity for T cells and chronic immunodeficiency are different and lie within the extracellular domain of the envelope transmembrane protein.[507] Amino acid changes in this region result in a more severe defect in envelope processing and transport from the endoplasmic reticulum than the determinants of acute immunodeficiency.[62]

Murine Leukemia Virus

Members of the Friend-Moloney-Rauscher subgroup of MuLVs cause leukemia and also immune suppression. The virus stocks used to produce disease contain both defective viruses and replication-competent viruses. Biologically cloned strains have been used to determine the molecular basis of the various biologic phenotypes. Clones of 334C MuLV induce immunosuppression coincident with the in vivo appearance of an immunosuppressive variant[434] in susceptible strains of mice.[237] An immunosuppressive variant of Friend virus, FIS-2, has been isolated from CD4-positive T cells of infected mice.[148] FIS-2 is replication-competent and differs from a nonimmunosuppressive variant (F-MuLV, clone 57) by having a deletion in the LTR region and several point mutations in the gag and env genes.[111] The changes important for immunosuppression have not yet been identified.

The best characterized immunosuppressive strain of MuLV is the LP-BM5 complex, which is derived from Duplan-Laterjet isolate of MuLV[356] and induces MAIDS. This virus mixture contains replication-competent ecotropic and mink cell focus-forming components and a defective virus with a deletion of the pol and env genes.[24] The replication-competent viruses do not induce immunosuppression, whereas preparations containing the 4.8-kb defective virus do.[24,78] The primary gene product of this virus is a 60-kDa gag fusion protein that is not cleaved and is attached to the cell membrane.[236] In B cells, this protein may act as a superantigen inducing activation and proliferation of $V_{\beta 5}$, $V_{\beta 11}$, and $V_{\beta 12}$ CD4 T cells,[239] but it is not clear that this property is crucial to induction of immunosuppression.[170] Production of a type 2 pattern of cytokines is essential for immunosuppression,[164,262] but the role of the defective virus in this process has not been clarified.

Measles

Wild-type and vaccine strains of measles virus both induce immune suppression, but to different degrees.[188,190,530] Reduced DTH skin test responses and lymphoproliferation are more prolonged after natural infection than after immunization. Increased susceptibility to other infections occurs only after natural (wild-type) infection.[34,338] The degree of immune suppression induced is likely to be linked to virus virulence and to the level and perhaps site of virus replication. Immune suppression is associated with activation of CD8 T cells[189,240] and production of type 2 cytokines. Immune activation is most intense during the immune response induced by wild-type infection.[188,190,531] Infected monocytes may contribute directly to immunosuppression through production of suppressive monokines, (e.g., PGE_2, IL-10) or failure to produce proinflammatory cytokines (e.g., TNF),[144,532] or indirectly by influencing the maturation of cytokine-producing T cells toward a type 2 pathway (e.g., low IL-12). Measles virus also replicates in thymic epithelial cells, inducing thymocyte apoptosis. The level of virus replication and the degree of thymocyte death, as studied in monkeys and SCID/hu mice, is greater for wild-type than for vaccine strains of virus.[23] The relative contributions of these different processes to immune suppression is likely to be influenced not only by virus strain, but also by the age and nutritional status of the host.

SUMMARY AND CONCLUSIONS

Viruses that induce immune suppression often replicate in cells of the immune system, but direct lysis of the infected cell has not been shown to be the mechanism of induction of immunosuppression for any virus. It is likely that for most viruses, immune suppression is the result of multiple factors that include host-synthesized cytokines, death of activated cells, and the effects of viral proteins on the immune system.

ABBREVIATIONS

AIDS: acquired immunodeficiency syndrome
CMV: cytomegalovirus
ConA: concanavalin A
CTL: cytotoxic T lymphocyte
DTH: delayed-type hypersensitivity
EBV: Epstein-Barr virus
FAIDS: feline acquired immunodeficiency syndrome
FeLV: feline leukemia virus
HHV: human herpesvirus
HIV: human immunodeficiency virus
HSV: herpes simplex virus
HTLV: human T-cell lymphotropic virus
IFN: interferon
IL: interleukin
LCMV: lymphocytic choriomeningitis virus
LDV: lactate dehydrogenase virus
LPS: lipopolysaccharide
LTR: long terminal repeat
MAIDS: murine acquired immunodeficiency syndrome
MHC: major histocompatibility complex
mls: minor lymphoid-stimulating antigen
MMTV: mouse mammary tumor virus
MuLV: murine leukemia virus
NK: natural killer [cells]
ORF: open reading frame
PBMC: peripheral blood mononuclear cells
PGE_2: prostaglandin E_2
PHA: phytohemagglutinin
PMN: polymorphonuclear leukocyte
RSV: respiratory syncytial virus
SCID: severe combined immunodeficiency
TCR: T-cell receptor
TGF-β: transforming growth factor β
TNF: tumor necrosis factor

ACKNOWLEDGEMENTS

Work from the author's laboratory was supported by a grant from the World Health Organization and by research grants AI23047 and AI35149 from the National Institutes of Health.

REFERENCES

1. Abeshsira-Amar O, Gibert M, Joliy M, Theze J, Jankovic DL. IL-4 plays a dominant role in the differential development of Th0 into Th1 and Th2 cells. J Immunol 1992;148:3820–3829.
2. Abramson JS, Lyles DS, Heller KA. Influenza A virus-induced polymorphonuclear leukocyte dysfunction. Infect Immun 1982;37:794–799.
3. Abramson JS, Mills EL. Depression of neutrophil function induced by viruses and its role in secondary microbial infections. Rev Infect Dis 1988;10:326–341.
4. Abramson SL, Gallin JI. IL-4 inhibits superoxide production by human mononuclear phagocytes. J Immunol 1990;144:625–630.

5. Agostini C, Trentin L, Zambello R, Semenzato G. HIV-1 and the lung: infectivity, pathogenic mechanisms, and cellular immune responses taking place in the lower respiratory tract. Am Rev Respir Dis 1993;147:1038–1049.

6. Ahmed R, Hahn CS, Somasundaram T, Villarete L, Matloubian M, Strauss JH. Molecular basis of organ-specific selection of viral variants during chronic infection. J Virol 1991;65:4242–4247.

7. Ahmed R, Salmi A, Butler LD, Chiller JM, Oldstone MBA. Selection of genetic variants of lymphocytic choriomeningitis virus in spleens of persistently infected mice: role in suppression of cytotoxic T lymphocyte response and viral persistence. J Exp Med 1984;160:521–540.

8. Ahmed R, Simon RS, Matloubian M, Kolhekar SR, Southern PJ, Freedman DM. Genetic analysis of in vivo-selected viral variants causing chronic infection: importance of mutation in the L RNA segment of lymphocytic choriomeningitis virus. J Virol 1988;62:3301–3308.

9. Albrecht JC, Fleckenstein B. New member of the multigene family of complement control proteins in herpesvirus saimiri. J Virol 1992;66:3937–3940.

10. Alcami A, Smith GL. Vaccinia, cowpox, and camelpox viruses encode soluble gamma interferon receptors with novel broad species specificity. J Virol 1995;69:4633–4639.

11. Alpert G, Leibovitz L, Danon YL. Analysis of T lymphocyte subsets in measles. J Infect Dis 1984;149:1018.

12. Althage A, Odermatt B, Moskophidis D, et al. Immunosuppression by lymphocytic choriomeningitis virus infection: competent effector T and B cells but impaired antigen presentation. Eur J Immunol 1992;22:1803–1812.

13. Anders EM, Scalzo AA, White DO. Influenza viruses are T cell-independent B cell mitogens. J Virol 1984;50:960–963.

14. Anderson GW, Rowland RRR, Palmer GA, Even C, Plagemann PGW. Lactate dehydrogenase-elevating virus replication persist in liver, spleen, lymph node, and testis tissues and results in accumulation of viral RNA in germinal centers, concomitant with polyclonal activation of B cells. J Virol 1995;69:5177–5185.

15. Andersson MA, Paabo S, Nilsson T, Peterson PA. Impaired intracellular transport of class I MHC antigens as a possible means for adenoviruses to evade immune surveillance. Cell 1985;43:215–222.

16. Appel MJG, Shek WR, Summers BA. Lymphocyte-mediated immune cytotoxicity in dogs infected with virulent canine distemper virus. Infect Immun 1982;37:592–600.

17. Arala-Chaves MP, Ribeiro, AS, Vilanova M, Porto MT, Santarem MG, Lima M. Correlation between B-cell mitogenicity and immunosuppressor effects of a protein released by porcine monocytes infected with African swine fever virus. Am J Vet Res 1988;49:1955–1961.

18. Arneborn P, Biberfeld G. T lymphocyte subpopulations in relation to immunosuppression in measles and varicella. Infect Immun 1983;39:29–37.

19. Arneborn P, Biberfeld G, Wasserman J. Immunosuppression and alterations of T-lymphocyte subpopulations after rubella vaccination. Infect Immun 1980;29:36–41.

20. Arya LS, Tanna I, Tahiri C, Saidali A, Singh M. Spectrum of complications of measles in Afghanistan: a study of 784 cases. J Trop Med Hygiene 1987;90:117–122.

21. Ascher MS, Sheppard HW. AIDS as immune system activation: a model for pathogenesis. Clin Exp Immunol 1988;73:165–167.

22. Assoian RK, Fluerdelys BE, Stevenson HC, et al. Expression and secretion of type beta transforming growth factor by activated human macrophages. Proc Natl Acad Sci U S A 1987;84:6020–6024.

23. Auwaerter PG, Kaneshima H, McCune JM, Wiegand G, Griffin DE. Measles virus infection in the SCID-hu mouse: disruption of the human thymic microenvironment. J Virol 1996;70:3734–3740.

24. Aziz DC, Hanna Z, Jolicoeur P. Severe immunodeficiency disease induced by a defective murine leukaemia virus. Nature 1989;338:505–508.

25. Babiuk LA, Lawman MJ, Ohmann HB. Viral-bacterial synergistic interaction in respiratory disease. Adv Virus Res 1988;35:219–249.

26. Backman L, Ringden O, Bjorkhem I. Monitoring of serum neopterin levels in renal transplant recipients: increased values during impaired renal function and cytomegalovirus infection. Nephron 1987;46:319–322.

27. Bagasra O, Pomerantz RJ. Human immunodeficiency virus type I provirus is demonstrated in peripheral blood monocytes in vivo: a study utilizing an in situ polymerase chain reaction. AIDS Res Hum Retrovir 1993;9:69–76.

28. Bahadoran P, Rieux-Laucat F, LeDeist F, Blanche S, Fischer A, deVillartay J-P. Lack of selective V-beta deletion in peripheral CD4+ T cells of human immunodeficiency virus-infected infants. Eur J Immunol 1993;23:2041–2044.

29. Bakay M, Beladi I, Berencsi K, et al. Immunoenhancement and suppression induced by adenovirus in chicken. Acta Virol 1992;36:269–276.

30. Balan P, Davis-Poynter N, Bell S, Atkinson H, Browne H, Minson T. An analysis of the in vitro and in vivo phenotypes of mutants of herpes simplex virus type 1 lacking glycoproteins gG, gE, gI or the putative gJ. J Gen Virol 1994;75:1245–1258.

31. Ballard DW, Bohnlein E, Lowenthal JW, Wano Y, Franza R, Greene WC. HTLV-I tax induces cellular proteins that activate the kappa-B element in the IL-2 receptor alpha gene. Science 1988;241:1652–1655.

32. Baskin GB, Murphey-Corb M, Watson EA, Martin LN. Necropsy findings in rhesus monkeys experimentally infected with cultured simian immunodeficiency virus (SIV)/delta. Vet Pathol 1988;25:456–467.

33. Beck MA, Sheridan JF. Regulation of lymphokine response during reinfection by influenza virus: production of a factor that inhibits lymphokine activity. J Immunol 1989;142:3560–3567.

34. Beckford AP, Kaschula ROC, Stephen C. Factors associated with fatal cases of measles: A retrospective autopsy study. S Afr Med J 1985;68:858–863.

35. Beersma MFC, Bijlmakers MJE, Ploegh HL. Human cytomegalovirus down-regulates HLA class I expression by reducing the stability of class I H chains. J Immunol 1993;151:4455–4464.

36. Bello-Fernandez C, Oblakowski P, Meager A, et al. IL-4 acts as a homeostatic regulator of IL-2-induced TNF and IFN-gamma. Immunology 1991;72:161–166.

37. Bell S, Cranage M, Borysiewicz L, Minson T. Induction of immunoglobulin G Fc receptors by recombinant vaccinia viruses expressing glycoproteins E and I of herpes simplex virus type 1. J Virol 1990;64:2181–2186.

38. Belsito DV, Sanchez MR, Baer RL, Valentine F, Thorbecke GJ. Reduced Langerhans' cell Ia antigen and ATPase activity in patients with the acquired immunodeficiency syndrome. N Engl J Med 1984;310:1279–1282.

39. Betz M, Fox BS. Prostaglandin E2 inhibits production of Th1 lymphokines but not of Th2 lymphokines. J Immunol 1991;146:108–113.

40. Bisno AL, Griffin JP, Van Epps KA, Niell HB, Rytel MW. Pneumonia and Hong Kong influenza: a prospective study of the 1968-1969 epidemic. Am J Med Sci 1971;261:251–263.

41. Bixler GS Jr, Booss J. Adherent spleen cells from mice acutely infected with cytomegalovirus suppress the primary antibody response in vitro. J Immunol 1981;127:1294–1299.

42. Blackett S, Mims CA. Studies of depressed interleukin-2 production by spleen cells from mice following infection with cytomegalovirus. Arch Virol 1988;99:1–8.

43. Blauvelt A, Clerici M, Lucey DR, et al. Functional studies of epidermal Langerhans cells and blood monocytes in HIV-infected persons. J Immunol 1995;154:3506–3515.

44. Bloom BR, Salgame P, Diamond B. Revisiting and revising suppressor T cells. Immunol Today 1992;13:131–135.

45. Bloomfield AL, Mateer JG. Changes in skin sensitiveness to tuberculin during epidemic influenza. Am Rev Respir Dis 1919;3:166–168.

46. Bonnard GD, Manders EK, Campbell DA Jr, Herberman RB, Collins MJ Jr. Immunosuppressive activity of a subline of the mouse EL-4 lymphoma: evidence for minute virus of mice causing the inhibition. J Exp Med 1976;143:187–205.

47. Booss J, Wheelock EF. Correlation of survival from murine cytomegalovirus infection with spleen cell responsiveness to concanavalin A. Proc Soc Exp Biol Med 1975;149:443–446.

48. Borrow P, Evans CF, Oldstone MBA. Virus-induced immunosuppression: immune system-mediated destruction of virus-infected dendritic cells results in generalized immune suppression. J Virol 1995;69:1059–1070.

49. Boshkov LK, Macen JL, McFadden G. Virus-induced loss of class I MHC antigens from the surface of cells infected with myxoma virus and malignant rabbit fibroma virus. J Immunol 1992;148:881–887.

50. Bradley DS, Broen JJ, Cafruny WA. Infection of SCID mice with lactate dehydrogenase-elevating virus stimulates B-cell activation. Viral Immunol 1991;4:59–70.

51. Brenan M, Zinkernagel RM. Influence of one virus infection on a second concurrent primary in vivo antiviral cytotoxic T-cell response. Infect Immun 1983;41:470–475.

52. Brody JA, McAlister R. Depression of tuberculin sensitivity following measles vaccination. Am Rev Respir Dis 1964;90:607–611.

53. Brody JA, Overfield T, Hammes LM. Depression of the tuberculin reaction by viral vaccines. N Engl J Med 1964;25:1294–1296.

54. Browne H, Smith G, Beck S, Minson T. A complex between the MHC class I homologue encoded by human cytomegalovirus and beta 2 microglobulin. Nature 1990;347:770–772.

55. Brown N, Smith D, Miller G, Niederman J, Liu C, Robinson J. Infectious mononucleosis: a polyclonal B cell transformation in vivo. J Infect Dis 1984;150:517–522.

56. Buchmeier NA, Cooper NR. Suppression of monocyte functions by human cytomegalovirus. Immunology 1989;66:278–283.

57. Bukrinsky MI, Stanwick TL, Dempsey MP, Stevenson M. Quiescent T lymphocytes as an inducible virus reservoir in HIV-1 infection. Science 1991;254:423–427.

58. Bullowa JGM, Wishik SM. Complications of varicella. Am J Dis Child 1935;49:923–926.

59. Bunting CH. The giant-cells of measles. Yale J Biol Med 1950;22: 513–519.

60. Burgert H-G, Maryanski JL, Kvist S. "E3/19K" protein of adenovirus type 2 inhibits lysis of cytolytic T lymphocytes by blocking cell-surface expression of histocompatibility class I antigens. Proc Natl Acad Sci U S A 1987;84:1356–1360.

61. Burkhardt E, Muller H. Susceptibility of chicken blood lymphoblasts and monocytes to infectious bursal disease virus (IBDV). Arch Virol 1987;94:297–303.

62. Burns CC, Poss ML, Thomas E, Overbaugh J. Mutations within a putative cysteine loop of the transmembrane protein of an attenuated immunodeficiency-inducing feline leukemia virus variant inhibit envelope protein processing. J Virol 1995;2126:2132.

63. Butchko GM, Armstrong RB, Martin WJ, Ennis FA. Influenza A viruses of the H2N2 subtype are lymphocyte mitogens. Nature 1978; 271:66–67.

64. Byun D-G, Demeure CE, Yang LP, et al. In vitro maturation of neonatal human CD8 T lymphocytes into IL-4- and IL-5-producing cells. J Immunol 1994;153:4862–4871.

65. Campbell AE, Slater JS, Futch WS. Murine cytomegalovirus-induced suppression of antigen-specific cytotoxic T lymphocyte maturation. Virology 1989;173:268–275.

66. Campbell DA Jr, Staal SP, Manders EK, et al. Inhibition of in vitro lymphoproliferative responses by in vivo passaged rat 13762 mammary adenocarcinoma cells. II. Evidence that Kilham rat virus is responsible for the inhibitory effect. Cell Immunol 1977;33:378–391.

67. Campetella OE, Galassi NV, Barrios HA. Contrasuppressor cells induced by Junin virus. Immunology 1990;69:629–631.

68. Campetella OE, Sanchez A, Giovanniello OA. In vivo Junin virus-mouse macrophages interaction. Acta Virol 1988;32:198–206.

69. Carney WP, Hirsch MS. Mechanisms of immunosuppression in cytomegalovirus mononucleosis. II. Virus monocyte interactions. J Infect Dis 1981;144:47–54.

70. Carney WP, Iacoviello V, Hirsch MS. Functional properties of T lymphocytes and their subsets in cytomegalovirus mononucleosis. J Immunol 1983;130:390–393.

71. Carney WP, Rubin RH, Hoffman RA, Hansen WP, Healey K, Hirsch MS. Analysis of T lymphocyte subsets in cytomegalovirus mononucleosis. J Immunol 1981;126:2114–2116.

72. Carter RL. Antibody formation in infectious mononucleosis. Br J Haematol 1966;12:268–275.

73. Cassidy LF, Lyles DS, Abramson JS. Depression of polymorphonuclear leukocyte functions by purified influenza virus hemagglutinin and sialic acid-binding lectins. J Immunol 1989;142:4401–4406.

74. Cate TR, Kelly JR. Hong Kong influenza antigen sensitivity and decreased interferon response of peripheral lymphocytes. Antimicrob Agents Chemother 1970;156–160.

75. Ceglowski WS, Friedman H. Immunosuppression by leukemia viruses. I. Effect of Friend disease virus on cellular and humoral hemolysin responses of mice to a primary immunization with sheep erythrocytes. J Immunol 1968;101:594–604.

76. Ceglowski WS, Friedman H. Immunosuppressive effects of Friend and Rauscher leukemia disease viruses on cellular and humoral antibody formation. J Natl Cancer Inst 1968;40:983–995.

77. Chang DM, Shaio MF. Production of interleukin-1 (IL-1) and IL-1 inhibitor by human monocytes exposed to dengue virus. J Infect Dis 1994;170:811–817.

78. Chattopadhyay SK, Morse HC III, Makino M, Ruscetti SK, Hartley JW. Defective virus is associated with induction of murine retrovirus-induced immunodeficiency syndrome. Proc Natl Acad Sci U S A 1989;86:3862–3866.

79. Cheevers WP, McGuire TC. Equine infectious anemia: immunopathogenesis and persistence. Rev Infect Dis 1985;7:83–88.

80. Chen ZW, Kou ZC, Shen L, et al. An acutely lethal simian immunodeficiency virus stimulates expansion of V beta 7- and V beta 14-expressing T lymphocytes. Proc Natl Acad Sci U S A 1994;91:7501–7505.

81. Chen ZW, Kou ZC, Shen L, Reimann KA, Letvin NL. Conserved T-cell receptor repertoire in simian immunodeficiency virus-infected rhesus monkeys. J Immunol 1993;151:2177–2187.

82. Chesebro B, Wehrly K, Nishio J, Perryman S. Macrophage-tropic human immunodeficiency virus isolates from different patients exhibit unusual V3 envelope sequence homogeneity in comparison with T-cell-tropic isolates: definition of critical amino acids involved in cell tropism. J Virol 1992;66:6547–6554.

83. Cheung K-S, Li JKK, Falletta JM, Wagner JL, Lang DL. Murine cytomegalovirus infection: hematological, morphological, and functional study of lymphoid cells. Infect Immun 1981;33:239–249.

84. Chino F, Kodama H, Ohkawa T. Alterations of the thymus and peripheral lymphoid tissues in fatal measles. Acta Pathol Jpn 1979; 29:493–507.

85. Choi Y, Kappler JW, Marrack P. A superantigen encoded in the open reading frame of the 3' long terminal repeat of mouse mammary tumour virus. Nature 1991;350:203–207.

86. Christensen PE, Schmidt H, Bang HO, Andersen V, Jordal B, Jensen O. An epidemic of measles in southern Greenland, 1951: measles in virgin soil. II. The epidemic proper. Acta Med Scand 1953;144: 430–449.

87. Cianciolo GJ, Copeland TD, Oroszlan S, Snyderman R. Inhibition of lymphocyte proliferation by a synthetic peptide homologous to retroviral envelope proteins. Science 1985;230:453–455.

88. Cianciolo GJ, Kipnis RJ, Snyderman R. Similarity between p15E of murine and feline leukaemia viruses and p21 of HTLV. Nature 1984;311:515.

89. Cianciolo GJ, Matthews TJ, Bolognesi DP, Snyderman R. Macrophage accumulation in mice is inhibited by low molecular weight products from murine leukemia viruses. J Immunol 1980;124: 2900–2905.

90. Cirino NM, Panuska JR, Villani A, et al. Restricted replication of respiratory syncytial virus in human alveolar macrophages. J Gen Virol 1993;74:1527–1537.

91. Clerici M, Stocks NI, Zajac RA, et al. Detection of three distinct patterns of T helper cell dysfunction in asymptomatic, human immunodeficiency virus-seropositive patients. J Clin Invest 1989;84: 1892–1899.

92. Cohen JI, Corey GR. Cytomegalovirus infection in the normal host. Medicine 1985;64:100–114.

93. Collman R, Hassan NF, Walker R, et al. Infection of monocyte-derived macrophages with human immunodeficiency virus type 1 (HIV-1). Monocyte-tropic and lymphocyte-tropic strains of HIV-1 show distinctive patterns of replication in a panel of cell types. J Exp Med 1989;1709:1149–1163.

94. Collman R, Nathanson N. Human immunodeficiency virus type-1 infection of macrophages. Virology 1992;3:185–202.

95. Colonna Romano G, Dieli F, Abrignani S, Salerno A, Colizzi V. Inhibition of lymphocyte mitogenesis in mice infected with Newcastle disease virus: viral interference with the interleukin system. Immunology 1986;57:373–378.

96. Cook-Mills JM, Munshi HG, Perlman RL, Chambers DA. Mouse hepatitis virus infection suppresses modulation of mouse spleen T-cell activation. Immunology 1992;75:542–545.

97. Coovadia HM, Wesley A, Brain P, Henderson LG, Hallett AF, Vos GH. Immunoparesis and outcome in measles. Lancet 1977;1:619–621.

98. Copelan EA, Rinehart JJ, Lewis M, Mathes L, Olsen R, Sagone A. The mechanism of retrovirus suppression of human T cell proliferation in vitro. J Immunol 1983;131:2017–2020.

99. Cossarizza A, Ortolani C, Mussini C, et al. Massive activation of immune cells with an intact T cell repertoire in acute human immunodeficiency virus syndrome. J Infect Dis 1995;172:105–112.

100. Coutelier JP, van der Logt JTM, Heessen FWA, Warnier G, Van Snick J. IgG2a restriction of murine antibodies elicited by viral infections. J Exp Med 1987;165:64–69.

101. Coutelier JP, Van Snick J. Isotypically restricted activation of B lymphocytes by lactic dehydrogenase virus. Eur J Immunol 1985; 15:250–255.

102. Craig CP, Reynolds SL, Airhart JW, Staab EV. Alterations in immune responses by attenuated Venezuelan equine encephalitis vaccine. I. Adjuvant effect of VEE virus infection in guinea pigs. J Immunol 1969;102:1220–1227.

103. Cremer NE, Devlin VL, Riggs JL, Hagens SJ. Anomalous antibody responses in viral infection: specific stimulation or polyclonal activation? J Clin Microbiol 1984;20:468–472.

104. Cremer NE, Johnson KP, Fein G, Likosky WH. Comprehensive viral immunology of multiple sclerosis. II. Analysis of serum and CSF antibodies by standard serologic methods. Arch Neurol 1980;37: 610–615.

105. Cross SS, Morse HC, Asofsky R. Neonatal infection with mouse thymic virus: differential effects on T cells mediating the graft-versus-host reaction. J Immunol 1976;117:635–638.

106. Crowe SM, Mills J, Elbeik T, et al. Human immunodeficiency virus-infected monocyte-derived macrophages express surface gp120 and fuse with CD4 lymphoid cells in vitro: a possible mechanism of T lymphocyte depletion in vivo. Clin Immunol Immunopathol 1992; 65:143–151.

107. Cummins TJ, Orme IM, Smith RE. Reduced in vivo nonspecific resistance to Listeria monocytogenes infection during avian retrovirus-induced immunosuppression. Avian Dis 1988;32:663–667.

108. Cummins TJ, Smith RE. Association of persistent synthesis of viral DNA with macrophage accessory cell dysfunction induced by avian retrovirus myeloblastosis-associated virus of subgroup b inducing osteopetrosis in chickens. Cancer Res 1987;47:6033–6039.

109. Cunningham-Rundles S, Michelis MA, Masur H. Serum suppression of lymphocyte activation in vitro in acquired immunodeficiency disease. J Clin Immunol 1983;3:156–165.

110. Dadaglio G, Garcia S, Montagnier L, Gougeon ML. Selective anergy of V beta 8+ T cells in human immunodeficiency virus-infected individuals. J Exp Med 1994;179:413–424.

111. Dai HY, Faxvaag A, Troseth GI, Aarset H, Dalen A. Molecular cloning and characterization of an immunosuppressive and weakly oncogenic variant of Friend murine leukemia virus, FIS-2. J Virol 1994;68:6976–6984.

112. Darban H, Enriquez J, Sterling CR, et al. Cryptosporidiosis facilitated by murine retroviral infection with LP-BM5. J Infect Dis 1991;164:741–745.

113. Davidson MG, Rottman JB, English RV, Lappin MR, Tompkins MB. Feline immunodeficiency virus predisposes cats to acute generalized toxoplasmosis. Am J Pathol 1993;143:1486–1497.

114. Degen JA Jr. Visceral pathology in measles: clinico-pathologic study of 100 fatal cases. Am J Med Sci 1937;194:104.

115. Degre M. Synergistic effect in viral-bacterial infection. Acta Pathol Microbiol Scand 1970;78:41–50.

116. Degre M, Glasgow LA. Synergistic effect in viral-bacterial infection. I. Combined infection of the respiratory tract in mice with parainfluenza virus and Hemophilus influenza. J Infect Dis 1968; 118:449–462.

117. DeMol P, Mukashema S, Bogaerts J, Hemelhof W, Butzler J-P. Cryptosporidium related to measles diarrhoea in Rwanda. Lancet 1984;2:42–43.

118. Dempsey WL, Smith AL, Morahan PS. Effect of inapparent murine hepatitis virus infection on macrophages and host resistance. J Leukoc Biol 1986;39:559–565.

119. Denton J. The pathology of fatal measles. Am J Med Sci 1925; 169:531–543.

120. Dent PB. Immunodepression by oncogenic viruses. Prog Med Virol 1972;14:1–35.

121. Dent PB, Cooper MD, Payne LN, Solomon JJ, Burmester BR, Good RA. Pathogenesis of avian lymphoid leukosis. II. Immunologic reactivity during lymphomagenesis. J Natl Cancer Inst 1968;41:391–401.

122. Depper JM, Leonard WJ, Kronke M, Waldmann TA, Greene WC. Augmented T cell growth factor receptor expression in HTLV-1-infected human leukemic T cells. J Immunol 1984;133:1691–1695.

123. de Waal Malefyt R, Yssel H, deVries JE. Direct effects of IL-10 on subsets of human CD4+ T cell clones and resting T cells. J Immunol 1993;150:4754–4765.

124. de Waal Malefyt R, Yssel H, Spits H, et al. Human T cell leukemia virus type I prevents cell surface expression of the T cell receptor through down-regulation of the CD3-gamma-delta-epsilon, and-zeta genes. J Immunol 1990;145:2297–2303.

125. Dezzutti CS, Wright KA, Lewis MG, Lafrado LJ, Olsen RG. FeLV-induced immunosuppression through alterations in signal transduction: downregulation of protein kinase C. Vet Immunol Immunopathol 1989;21:55–67.

126. Ding L, Shevach EM. IL-10 inhibits mitogen-induced T cell proliferation by selectively inhibiting macrophage costimulatory function. J Immunol 1992;148:3133–3139.

127. Dobozin BS, Judson FN, Cohn DL, et al. The relationship of abnormalities of cellular immunity to antibodies to HTLV-III in homosexual men. Cell Immunol 1986;98:156–171.

128. Domingo M, Visa J, Pumarola M, et al. Pathologic and immunocytochemical studies of morbillivirus infection in striped dolphins (Stenella coeruleoalba). Vet Pathol 1992;29:1–10.

129. Domurat F, Roberts NJ Jr, Walsh EE, Dagan R. Respiratory syncytial virus infection of human mononuclear leukocytes in vitro and in vivo. J Infect Dis 1985;152:895–902.

130. Donahue PR, Quackenbush SL, Gallo MV, et al. Viral genetic determinants of T-cell killing and immunodeficiency disease induction by the feline leukemia virus FeLV-FAIDS. J Virol 1991;65:4461–4469.

131. Donnelly RP, Fenton MJ, Finbloom DS, Gerrard TL. Differential regulation of IL-1 production in human monocytes by IFN-gamma and IL-4. J Immunol 1990;145:569–575.

132. Donnelly RP, Fenton MJ, Kaufman JD, Gerrard TL. IL-1 expression in human monocytes is transcriptionally and posttranscriptionally regulated by IL-4. J Immunol 1991;146:3431–3436.

133. Dubin G, Socolof E, Frank I, Friedman HM. Herpes simplex virus type 1 Fc receptor protects infected cells from antibody-dependent cellular cytotoxicity. J Virol 1991;65:7046–7050.

134. Dudding L, Haskill S, Clark BD, Auron PE, Sporn S, Huang E-S. Cytomegalovirus infection stimulates expression of monocyte-associated mediator genes. J Immunol 1989;143:3343–3352.

135. Dunkin GW, Laidlaw PP. Studies in dog-distemper. II. Experimental distemper in the dog. J Comp Pathol 1926;39:213–221.

136. Dyer RM, Majumdar S, Douglas SD, Korchak HM. Bovine parainfluenza-3 virus selectively depletes a calcium-independent, phospholipid-dependent protein kinase C and inhibits superoxide anion generation in bovine alveolar macrophages. J Immunol 1994;153: 1171–1179.

137. Edelman AS, Zolla-Pazner S. AIDS: a syndrome of immune dysregulation, dysfunction and deficiency. FASEB J 1989;3:22–30.

138. Einhorn L, Ost A. Cytomegalovirus infection of human blood cells. J Infect Dis 1984;149:207–214.

139. Ellingsworth LR, Nakayama D, Segarini P, Dasch J, Carrillo P, Waegell W. Transforming growth factor-betas are equipotent growth inhibitors of interleukin-1-induced thymocyte proliferation. Cell Immunol 1988;114:41–54.

140. Embretson J, Zupancic M, Ribas JL, et al. Massive covert infection of helper T lymphocytes and macrophages by HIV during the incubation period of AIDS. Nature 1993;362:359–362.

141. Enders JF, McCarthy K, Mitus A, Cheatham WJ. Isolation of measles virus at autopsy in cases of giant cell pneumonia without rash. N Engl J Med 1959;261:875–881.

142. Essani K, Chalasani S, Eversole R, Beuving L, Birmingham L. Multiple anti-cytokine activities secreted from tanapox virus-infected cells. Microb Pathog 1994;17:347–353.

143. Essner R, Rhoades K, McBride WH, Morton DL, Economou JS. IL-4 down-regulates IL-1 and TNF gene expression in human monocytes. J Immunol 1989;142:3857–3861.

144. Esolen LM, Ward BJ, Moench TR, Griffin DE. Infection of monocytes during measles. J Infect Dis 1993;168:47–52.

145. Ezeokoli CD, Ityondo EA, Nwannenna AI, Umoh JU. Immunosuppression and histopathological changes in the bursa of Fabricius associated with infectious bursal disease vaccination in chicken. Comp Immunol Microbiol Infect Dis 1990;13:181–188.

146. Faden H, Humbert J, Lee J, Sutyla P, Ogra PL. The in vitro effects of Newcastle disease virus on the metabolic and antibacterial functions of human neutrophils. Blood 1981;58:221–227.

147. Falgout B, Bray M, Schlesinger JJ, Lai C-J. Immunization of mice with recombinant vaccinia virus expressing authentic dengue virus nonstructural protein NS1 protects against lethal dengue virus encephalitis. J Virol 1990;64:4356–4363.

148. Faxvaag A, Dai HY, Aarseth H, Dalen AB. A low oncogenic variant of Friend murine leukemia virus with strong immunosuppressive properties. Arch Virol 1993;131:265–275.

149. Fernandez-Cruz E, Gelpi E, Longo N, et al. Increased synthesis and production of prostaglandin E2 by monocytes from drug addicts with AIDS. AIDS 1989;3:91–96.

150. Filion LG, McGuire RL, Babiuk LA. Nonspecific suppressive effect of bovine herpesvirus type 1 on bovine leukocyte functions. Infect Immun 1983;42:106–112.

151. Fine DL, Landon JC, Pienta RJ, et al. Responses of infant rhesus monkeys to inoculation with Mason-Pfizer monkey virus materials. J Natl Cancer Inst 1975;54:651–658.

152. Fiorentino DF, Bond MW, Mosmann TR. Two types of mouse T helper cell IV. Th2 clones secrete a factor that inhibits cytokine production by Th1 clones. J Exp Med 1989;170:2081–2095.

153. Fiorentino DF, Zlotnik A, Mosmann TR, Howard M, O'Garra A. IL-10 inhibits cytokine production by activated macrophages. J Immunol 1991;147:3815–3822.

154. Fiorentino DF, Zlotnik A, Vieira P, et al. IL-10 acts on the antigen-presenting cell to inhibit cytokine production by Th1 cells. J Immunol 1991;146:3444–3451.

155. Fireman P, Friday G, Kumate J. Effect of measles virus vaccine on immunologic responsiveness. Pediatrics 1969;43:264–272.

156. Fontana A, Frei K, Bodmer S, et al. Transforming growth factor-beta inhibits the generation of cytotoxic T cells in virus-infected mice. J Immunol 1989;143:3230–3234.

157. Frenkel N, Schirmer EC, Wyatt LS, et al. Isolation of a new herpesvirus from human CD4+ T cells. Proc Natl Acad Sci U S A 1990;87:748–752.

158. Friedman H, Melnick H, Mills L, Ceglowski WS. Depressed allograft immunity in leukemia virus infected mice. Transplant Proc 1973;5:981–986.

159. Fruh K, Ahn K, Djaballah H, et al. A viral inhibitor of peptide transporters for antigen presentation. Nature 1995;375:415–418.

160. Furukawa M, Yasukawa M, Yakushijin Y, Fujita S. Distinct effects of human herpesvirus 6 and human herpesvirus 7 on surface molecule expression and function of CD4+ T cells. J Immunol 1994; 152:5768–5775.

161. Gabrilovich DI, Woods GM, Patterson S, Harvey JJ, Knight SC. Retrovirus-induced immunosuppression via blocking of dendritic cell migration and down-regulation of adhesion molecules. Immunology 1994;82:82–87.

162. Gajewski TF, Fitch FW. Anti-proliferative effect of IFN-gamma in immune regulation. I. IFN-gamma inhibits the proliferation of Th2 but not Th1 murine helper T lymphocyte clones. J Immunol 1988;140:4245–4252.

163. Gazzinelli RT, Hartley JW, Fredrickson TN, Chattopadhyay SK, Sher A, Morse HC III. Opportunistic infections and retrovirus-induced immunodeficiency: studies of acute and chronic infections with Toxoplasma gondii in mice infected with LP-BM5 murine leukemia viruses. Infect Immun 1992;60:4394–4401.

164. Gazzinelli RT, Makino M, Chattopadhyay SK, et al. CD4+ subset regulation in viral infection: preferential activation of Th2 cells during progression of retrovirus-induced immunodeficiency in mice. J Immunol 1992;148:182–188.

165. Gazzinelli RT, Oswald IP, James SL, Sher A. IL-10 inhibits parasite killing and nitrogen oxide production by IFN-gamma-activated macrophages. J Immunol 1992;148:1792–1796.

166. Geist LJ, Hunninghake GW. Cytomegalovirus as a trans-activator of cellular genes. Virology 1994;5:415–420.

167. Gendelman HE, Narayan O, Kennedy-Stoskopf S, et al. Tropism of sheep lentiviruses for monocytes: susceptibility to infection and virus gene expression increase during maturation of monocytes to macrophages. J Virol 1986;58:67–74.

168. Gendelman HE, Narayan O, Molineaux S, Clements JE, Ghotbi Z. Slow, persistent replication of lentiviruses: role of tissue macrophages and macrophage precursors in bone marrow. Proc Natl Acad Sci U S A 1985;82:7086–7090.

169. Gilden DH, Devlin M, Wellish M, et al. Persistence of varicella-zoster virus DNA in blood mononuclear cells of patients with varicella or zoster. Virus Genes 1988;2:291–297.

170. Gilmore GL, Cowing C, Mosier DE. LP-BM5 murine retrovirus-induced immunodeficiency disease in allogenic SCID chimeric mice: inability to recognize a putative viral superantigen does not prevent induction of disease. J Immunol 1993;150:185–189.

171. Glickstein LJ, Huber BT. Karoushi: death by overwork in the immune system. J Immunol 1995;155:522–524.

172. Gollob KJ, Palmer E. Divergent viral superantigens delete V-beta-5+ T lymphocytes. Proc Natl Acad Sci U S A 1992;89:5138–5141.

173. Golovkina TV, Chervonsky A, Dudley JP, Ross SR. Transgenic mouse mammary tumor virus superantigen expression prevents viral infection. Cell 1992;69:637–645.

174. Gooding LR. Virus proteins that counteract host immune defenses. Cell 1992;71:5–7.

175. Gordon D, Henderson DC, Westwick J. Effects of prostaglandins E2 and I2 on human lymphocyte transformation in the presence and absence of inhibitors of prostaglandin biosynthesis. Br J Pharmacol 1979;67:17–22.

176. Gosselin J, Flamand L, D'Addario M, et al. Modulatory effects of Epstein-Barr, herpes simplex, and human herpes-6 viral infections and coinfections on cytokine synthesis: a comparative study. J Immunol 1992;149:181–187.

177. Gougeon ML, Garcia S, Heeney J, et al. Programmed cell death in AIDS-related HIV and SIV infections. AIDS Res Hum Retroviruses 1993;9:553–563.

178. Graham KA, Opgenorth A, Upton C, McFadden G. Myxoma virus M11L ORF encodes a protein for which cell surface localization is critical in manifestation of viral virulence. Virology 1992;191:112–124.

179. Graham NM, Nelson KE, Solomon L, et al. Prevalence of tuberculin positivity and skin test anergy in HIV-1-seropositive and -seronegative intravenous drug users. JAMA 1992;267:369–373.

180. Granke-Ullmann G, Pfortner C, Walter P, et al. Alteration of pulmonary macrophage function by respiratory syncytial virus infection in vitro. J Immunol 1995;154:268–280.

181. Greenberg BL, Sack RB, Salazar-Lindo LE, et al. Measles-associated diarrhea in hospitalized children in Lima, Peru: pathogenic agents and impact on growth. J Infect Dis 1991;163:495–502.

182. Green DR, Scott DW. Activation-induced apoptosis in lymphocytes. Curr Opin Immunol 1994;6:476–487.

183. Greene WC, Leonard WJ, Wano Y, et al. Trans-activator gene of HTLV-II induces IL-2 receptor and IL-2 cellular gene expression. Science 1986;232:877–880.

184. Green GM. Patterns of bacterial clearance in murine influenza. Antimicrob Agents Chemother 1966;26–29.

185. Griffin DE, Cooper SJ, Hirsch RL, et al. Changes in plasma IgE levels during complicated and uncomplicated measles virus infections. J Allergy Clin Immunol 1985;76:206–213.

186. Griffin DE, Johnson RT, Tamashiro VG, et al. In vitro studies of the role of monocytes in the immunosuppression associated with natural measles virus infections. Clin Immunol Immunopathol 1987; 45:375–383.

187. Griffin DE, Moench TR, Johnson RT, Lindo de Soriano I, Vaisberg A. Peripheral blood mononuclear cells during natural measles virus infection: cell surface phenotypes and evidence for activation. Clin Immunol Immunopathol 1986;40:305–312.

188. Griffin DE, Ward BJ. Differential CD4 T cell activation in measles. J Infect Dis 1993;168:275–281.

189. Griffin DE, Ward BJ, Jauregui E, Johnson RT, Vaisberg A. Immune activation during measles. N Engl J Med 1989;320:1667–1672.

190. Griffin DE, Ward BJ, Jauregui E, Johnson RT, Vaisberg A. Immune activation during measles: interferon-gamma and neopterin in plasma and cerebrospinal fluid in complicated and uncomplicated disease. J Infect Dis 1990;161:449–453.

191. Griswold DE, Heppner GH, Calabresi P. Alteration of immunocompetence by mammary tumor virus. J Natl Cancer Inst 1973;50:1035–1038.

192. Groux H, Torpier G, Monte D, Mouton Y, Capron A, Ameisen JC. Activation-induced death by apoptosis in CD4+ T cells from human immunodeficiency virus-infected asymptomatic individuals. J Exp Med 1992;175:331–340.

193. Guignard R, Potworowski EF, Lussier G. Mouse thymic virus-mediated immunosuppression: association with decreased helper T cells and increased suppressor T cells. Viral Immunol 1989;2:215–220.

194. Haider S, Coutinho MdeL, Emond RTD, Sutton RNP. Tuberculin anergy and infectious mononucleosis. Lancet 1973;2:74.

195. Hanaoka M, Suzuki S, Hotchin J. Thymus-dependent lymphocytes: destruction by lymphocytic choriomeningitis virus. Science 1969; 163:1216–1219.

196. Hanlon MA, Marr JM, Hayes KA, et al. Loss of neutrophil and natural killer cell function following feline immunodeficiency virus infection. Viral Immunol 1993;6:119–124.

197. Harper ME, Marselle LM, Gallo RC, Wong-Staal F. Detection of lymphocytes expressing human T-lymphotropic virus type III in lymph nodes and peripheral blood from infected individuals by in situ hybridization. Proc Natl Acad Sci U S A 1986;83:772–776.

198. Harris SL, Frank I, Yee A, Cohen GH, Eisenberg RJ, Friedman HM. Glycoprotein C of herpes simplex virus type 1 prevents complement-mediated cell lysis and virus neutralization. J Infect Dis 1990;162:331–337.

199. Hart PH, Vitti GF, Burgess DR, Whitty GA, Piccoli DS. Potential antiinflammatory effects of interleukin 4: suppression of human monocyte tumor necrosis factor alpha, interleukin 1, and prostaglandin E2. Proc Natl Acad Sci U S A 1989;86:3803–3807.

200. Hartshorn KL, Liou LS, White MR, Kazhdan MM, Tauber JL, Tauber AI. Neutrophil deactivation by influenza A virus. J Immunol 1995;154:3952–3960.

201. Hayashi K, Saze K, Uchida Y. Studies of latent cytomegalovirus infection: the macrophage as a virus-harboring cell. Microbiol Immunol 1985;29:625–634.

202. Hayashi T, Iwata H, Hasegawa T, Ozaki M, Yamamoto H, Onodera T. Decrease in neutrophil migration induced by endotoxin and suppression of interleukin-1 production by macrophages in lactic dehydrogenase virus-infected mice. J Comp Pathol 1991;104:161–170.

203. Hayashi T, Koike Y, Hasegawa T, et al. Inhibition of contact sensitivity by interferon in mice infected with lactic dehydrogenase virus. J Comp Pathol 1991;104:357–366.

204. Hayashi T, Noguchi Y, Kameyama Y. Suppression of development of anti-nuclear antibody and glomerulonephritis in NZB × NZWF1 mice by persistent infection with superoxide anion as a progressive effector. Int J Exp Pathol 1993;74:553–560.

205. Hayashi T, Ozaki M, Ami Y, Onodera T, Yamamoto H. Increased superoxide anion release by peritoneal macrophages in mice with a chronic infection of lactic dehydrogenase virus. J Comp Pathol 1992;106:93–98.

206. Hayashi T, Ozaki M, Mori I, Saito M, Itoh T, Yamamoto H. Enhanced clearance of lactic dehydrogenase-5 in severe combined immunodeficiency (SCID) mice: effect of lactic dehydrogenase virus on enzyme clearance. Int J Exp Pathol 1982;73:173–181.

207. Hayashi T, Ozaki M, Onodera T, Ami Y, Yamamoto H. Macrophage function in the acute phase of lactic dehydrogenase virus-infection of mice: suppression of superoxide anion production in normal mouse peritoneal macrophages by interferon-alpha in vitro. J Comp Pathol 1992;106:183–193.

208. Hebebrand LC, Olsen RG, Mathes LE, Nichols WS. Inhibition of human lymphocyte mitogen and antigen response by a 15,000-dalton protein from feline leukemia virus. Cancer Res 1979;39:443–447.

209. Heino J, Ignotz RA, Hemler ME, Crouse C, Massague J. Regulation of cell adhesion receptors by transforming growth factor-beta. J Biol Chem 1989;264:380–388.

210. Held W, Acha-Orbea H, MacDonald HR, Wanders GA. Superantigens and retroviral infection: insights from mouse mammary tumor virus. Immunol Today 1994;15:184–190.

211. Held W, Shakhov AN, Izui S, et al. Superantigen-reactive CD4+ T cells are required to stimulate B cells after infection with mouse mammary tumor virus. J Exp Med 1993;177:359–366.

212. Held W, Waanders GA, Shakhov AN, Scarpellino L, Acha-Orbea H, MacDonald HR. Superantigen-induced immune stimulation amplifies mouse mammary tumor virus infection and allows virus transmission. Cell 1993;74:529–540.

213. Helms S, Helms P. Tuberculin sensitivity during measles. Acta Tubercubea Scand 1958;35:166–171.

214. Henderson DC, Tosta CE, Wedderburn N. Exacerbation of murine malaria by concurrent infection with lactic dehydrogenase-elevating virus. Clin Exp Immunol 1979;33:357–359.

215. Henderson FW, Collier AM, Sanyal MA, et al. A longitudinal study of respiratory viruses and bacteria in the etiology of acute otitis media with effusion. N Engl J Med 1982;306:1377–1383.

216. Hermitte L, Vialettes B, Naquet P, Atlan C, Payan MJ, Vague P. Paradoxical lessening of autoimmune processes in non-obese diabetic mice after infection with the diabetogenic variant of encephalomyocarditis virus. Eur J Immunol 1990;2097:1297–1303.

217. Hildreth EA, Frederic MW, Randall P. Alterations in delayed hypersensitivity produced by live attenuated measles virus in man. Trans Am Clin Climatol Assoc 1963;75:37–51.

218. Hill AB, Barnett BC, McMichael AJ, McGeoch DJ. HLA class I molecules are not transported to the cell surface in cells infected with herpes simplex virus types 1 and 2. J Immunol 1994;152:2736–2741.

219. Hill A, Jugovic P, York I, et al. Herpes simplex virus turns off the TAP to evade host immunity. Nature 1995;375:411–415.

220. Hirai K, Kawano H, Mifune K, et al. Suppression of cell-mediated immunity by street rabies virus infection. Microbiol Immunol 1992;36:1277–1290.

221. Hirano S, Ceglowski WS, Allen JL, Friedman H. Effect of friend leukemogenic virus on antibody-forming cells to a bacterial somatic antigen. J Natl Cancer Inst 1969;43:1337–1345.

222. Hirano S, Friedman H, Ceglowski WS. Immunosuppression by leukemia viruses. VII. Stimulatory effects of Friend leukemia virus on pre-existing antibody forming cells to sheep erythrocytes and Escherichia coli in non-immunized mice. J Immunol 1971;107:1400–1409.

223. Hirsch RL, Mokhtarian F, Griffin DE, Brooks BR, Hess J, Johnson RT. Measles virus vaccination of measles seropositive individuals suppresses lymphocyte proliferation and chemotactic factor production. Clin Immunol Immunopathol 1981;21:341–350.

224. Hofmann B, Odum N, Jakobsen BK, et al. Immunological studies in the acquired immunodeficiency syndrome. II. Active suppression or intrinsic defect investigated by mixing AIDS cells with HLA-DR identical normal cells. Scand J Immunol 1986;23:669–678.

225. Ho JL, He SH, Rios MJC, Wick EA. Interleukin-4 inhibits human macrophage activation by tumor necrosis factor, granulocyte-monocyte colony-stimulating factor, and interleukin-3 for antileishmanial activity and oxidative burst capacity. J Infect Dis 1992;165:344–351.

226. Ho M. The lymphocyte in infections with Epstein-Barr virus and cytomegalovirus. J Infect Dis 1981;143:857–862.

227. Hoover EA, Mullins JI, Quackenbush SL, Gasper PW. Experimental transmission and pathogenesis of immunodeficiency syndrome in cats. Blood 1987;70:1880–1892.

228. Howard CJ. Immunological responses to bovine virus diarrhoea virus infections. Rev Sci Tech 1990;9:95–103.

229. Howard CJ, Stott EJ, Taylor G. The effect of pneumonia induced in mice with Mycoplasma pulmonis on resistance to subsequent bacterial infection and the effect of a respiratory infection with Sendai virus on the resistance of mice to Mycoplasma pulmonis. J Gen Microbiol 1978;109:79–87.

230. Howard RJ, Craig CP, Trevino GS, Dougherty SF, Mergenhagen SE. Enhanced humoral immunity in mice infected with attenuated Venezuelan equine encephalitis virus. J Immunol 1969;103:699–707.

231. Howard RJ, Miller J, Najarian JS. Cytomegalovirus-induced immune suppression. II. Cell-mediated immunity. Clin Exp Immunol 1974;18:119–126.

232. Howard RJ, Najarian JS. Cytomegalovirus-induced immune suppression. I. Humoral immunity. Clin Exp Immunol 1974;18:109–118.

233. Howard RJ, Notkins AL, Mergenhagen SE. Inhibition of cellular immune reactions in mice infected with lactic dehydrogenase virus. Nature 1969;221:873–874.

234. Hruskova J, Rychterova V, Kliment V. The influence of infection with Venezuelan equine encephalomyelitis virus on antibody response against sheep erythrocytes. I. Experiments on mice. Acta Virol 1972;16:115–124.

235. Hsu DH, de Waal Malefyt R, Fiorentino DF, et al. Expression of interleukin-10 activity by Epstein-Barr virus protein BCRF1. Science 1990;250:830–832.

236. Huang M, Jolicoeur P. Characterization of the gag/fusion protein encoded by the defective duplan retrovirus inducing murine acquired immunodeficiency syndrome. J Virol 1990;64:5764–5772.

237. Huang M, Simard C, Jolicoeur P. Susceptibility of inbred strains of mice to murine AIDS (MAIDS) correlates with target cell expansion and high expression of defective MAIDS virus. J Virol 1992;66:2398–2406.

238. Hu B, Even C, Plagemann PG. Immune complexes that bind to ELISA plates not coated with antigen in mice infected with lactate

dehydrogenase-elevating virus: relationship to IgG2a- and IgG2b-specific polyclonal activation of B cells. Viral Immunol 1992;5:27–38.

239. Hugin AW, Vacchio MS, Morse HC III. A virus-encoded "superantigen" in a retrovirus-induced immunodeficiency syndrome of mice. Science 1991;252:424–427.

240. Hussey GD, Goddard EA, Hughes J, et al. The effect of Edmonston-Zagreb and Schwarz measles vaccines on immune responses in infants. J Infect Dis 1995;

241. Ichikawa K, Miura R. The role of suppressive macrophages in influenza virus-induced immunosuppression. Acta Virol 1989;33:262–269.

242. Ignatowicz L, Kappler J, Marrack P. The effects of chronic infection with a superantigen-producing virus. J Exp Med 1992;175:917–923.

243. Imamura M, Matsuyama T, Toh K, Okuyama T. Electron microscopic study on acute thymic involution induced by polyoma virus infection. J Natl Cancer Inst 1971;47:289–299.

244. Imberti L, Sottini A, Bettinardi A, Puoti M, Primi D. Selective depletion in HIV infection of T cells that bear specific T cell receptor V-beta sequences. Science 1991;254:860–862.

245. Inada T, Mims CA. Pattern of infection and selective loss of Ia positive cells in suckling and adult mice inoculated with lactic dehydrogenase virus. Arch Virol 1985;86:151–165.

246. Inada T, Mims CA. Infection of mice with lactic dehydrogenase virus prevents development of experimental allergic encephalomyelitis. J Neuroimmunol 1986;11:53–56.

247. Isaacs SN, Kotwal GJ, Moss B. Vaccinia virus complement-control protein prevents antibody-dependent complement-enhanced neutralization of infectivity and contributes to virulence. Proc Natl Acad Sci U S A 1992;89:628–632.

248. Isakov N, Feldman M, Segal S. Acute infection of mice with lactic dehydrogenase virus (LDV) impairs the antigen-presenting capacity of their macrophages. Cell Immunol 1982;66:317–332.

249. Isakov N, Segal S. A tumor-associated lactic dehydrogenase virus suppresses the host resistance to infection with Listeria monocytogenes. Immunobiology 1983;164:402–416.

250. Ishikawa R, Biron CA. IFN induction and associated changes in splenic leukocyte distribution. J Immunol 1993;150:3713–3727.

251. Iwata H, Hayashi T. Interleukin-6 production by macrophages from BALB/c mice with a chronic infection of lactic dehydrogenase virus. Exp Animals 1994;43:559–562.

252. Jacobson S, Gupta A, Mattson D, Mingioli E, McFarlin DE. Immunological studies in tropical spastic paraparesis. Ann Neurol 1990;27:149–156.

253. Jacobs RP, Cole GA. Lymphocytic choriomeningitis virus-induced immunosuppression: a virus-induced macrophage defect. J Immunol 1976;117:1004–1009.

254. Jakab GJ, Green GM. The effect of Sendai virus infection on bactericidal and transport mechanisms of the murine lung. J Clin Invest 1972;51:1989–1998.

255. Jakab GJ, Warr GA, Sannes PL. Alveolar macrophage ingestion and phagosome-lysosome fusion defect associated with virus pneumonia. Infect Immun 1980;27:960–968.

256. Janeway CA Jr. Selective elements of the Vβ regions of the T cell receptor: mls and the bacterial toxic mitogens. Adv Immunol 1991;50: 1–53.

257. Jennings SR, Rice PL, Kloszewski ED, Anderson RW, Thompson DL, Tevethia SS. Effect of herpes simplex virus types 1 and 2 on surface expression of class I major histocompatibility complex antigens on infected cells. J Virol 1985;56:757–766.

258. Johnson DC, Frame MC, Ligas MW, Cross AM, Stow ND. Herpes simplex virus immunoglobulin G Fc receptor activity depends on a complex of two viral glycoproteins, gE and gI. J Virol 1988;62:1347–1354.

259. Johnson DW, Muscoplat CC. Immunologic abnormalities in calves with chronic bovine viral diarrhea. Am J Vet Res 1973;34:1139–1141.

260. Junker AK, Ochs HD, Clark EA, Puterman ML, Wedgwood RJ. Transient immune deficiency in patients with acute Epstein-Barr virus infection. Clin Immunol Immunopathol 1986;40:436–446.

261. Kadota J, Cianciolo GJ, Synderman R. A synthetic peptide homologous to retroviral transmembrane envelope proteins depresses pr tein kinase C mediated lymphocyte proliferation and directly inactivates protein kinase C: a potential mechanism for immunosuppression. Microbiol Immunol 1991;35:443–459.

262. Kanagawa O, Vaupel BA, Gayama S, Koehler G, Kopf M. Resistance of mice deficient in IL-4 to retrovirus-induced immunodeficiency syndrome (MAIDS). Science 1993;262:240–244.

263. Kaplan LJ, Daum RS, Smaron M, McCarthy CA. Severe measles in immunocompromised patients. JAMA 1992;267:1237–1241.

264. Katsuki T, Katsuki K, Imai J, Hinuma Y. Immune suppression in healthy carriers of adult T-cell leukemia retrovirus (HTLV-I): impairment of T-cell control of Epstein-Barr virus-infected B-cells. Jpn J Cancer Res 1987;78:639–642.

265. Kelsey DK, Overall JC Jr, Glasgow LA. Correlation of the suppression of mitogen responsiveness and the mixed lymphocyte reaction with the proliferative response to viral antigen of splenic lymphocytes from cytomegalovirus-infected mice. J Immunol 1978;121: 464–470.

266. Kiepeila P, Coovadia HM, Coward P. T helper cell defect related to severity in measles. Scand J Infect Dis 1987;19:185–192.

267. King CC, de Fries R, Kolhekar SR, Ahmed R. In vivo selection of lymphocyte-tropic and macrophage-tropic variants of lymphocytic choriomeningitis virus during persistent infection. J Virol 1990;64:5611–5616.

268. King NW, Hunt RD, Letvin NL. Histopathologic changes in macaques with an acquired immunodeficiency syndrome (AIDS). Am J Pathol 1983;113:382–388.

269. Kirchner H, Tosato G, Blaese RM, Broder S, Magrath IT. Polyclonal immunoglobulin secretion by human B lymphocytes exposed to Epstein-Barr virus in vitro. J Immunol 1979;122:1310–1313.

270. Klatzmann D, Barre-Sinoussi F, Nugeyre MT, et al. Selective tropism of lymphadenopathy associated virus (LAV) for helper-inducer T lymphocytes. Science 1984;225:59–62.

271. Klein JO, Green GM, Tilles JG, Kass EH, Finland, M. Effect of intranasal reovirus infection on antibacterial activity of mouse lung. J Infect Dis 1969;199:43–50.

272. Klinman DM, Morse HC. Characteristic of B cell proliferation and activation in murine AIDS. J Immunol 1989;142:1144–1149.

273. Knight AM, Harrison GB, Pease RJ, Robinson PJ, Dyson PJ. Biochemical analysis of the mouse mammary tumor virus long terminal repeat product: evidence for the molecular structure of an endogenous superantigen. Eur J Immunol 1992;22:879–882.

274. Knight SC, Patterson S, Macatonia SE. Stimulatory and suppressive effects of infection of dendritic cells with HIV-1. Immunol Lett 1991;30:213–218.

275. Knox KK, Pietryga D, Harrington DJ, Franciosi R, Carrigan DR. Progressive immunodeficiency and fatal pneumonitis associated with human herpesvirus 6 infection in an infant. Clin Infect Dis 1994;20:406–413.

276. Knudsen PJ, Dinarello CA, Strom TB. Prostaglandins posttranscriptionally inhibit monocyte expression of interleukin 1 activity by increasing intracellular cyclic adenosine monophosphate. J Immunol 1986;137:3189–3194.

277. Koga Y, Tanka K, Lu Y-Y, et al. Priming of immature thymocytes to CD3-mediated apoptosis by infection with murine cytomegalovirus. J Virol 1994;68:4322–4328.

278. Kohno S, Koga H, Kaku M, et al. Prevalence of HTLV-I antibody in pulmonary cryptococcosis. Tohoku J Exp Med 1992;167:13-18.

279. Kollmann TR, Kim A, Pettoello-Mantovani M, et al. Divergent effects of chronic HIV-1 infection on human thymocyte maturation in SCID-hu mice. J Immunol 1995;154:907–921.

280. Kondo K, Kondo T, Okuno T, Takahashi M, Yamanishi K. Latent human herpesvirus 6 infection of human monocytes/macrophages. J Gen Virol 1991;72:1401–1408.

281. Korman AJ, Bourgarel P, Meo T, Rieckhof GE. The mouse mammary tumour virus long terminal repeat encodes a type II transmembrane glycoprotein. EMBO J 1992;11:1901–1905.

282. Kotwal GJ, Isaacs SN, McKenzie R, Frank MM, Moss B. Inhibition of the complement cascade by the major secretory protein of vaccinia virus. Science 1990;250:827–830.

283. Labalette M, Salez F, Pruvot FR, Noel C, Dessaint JP. CD8 lymphocytosis in primary cytomegalovirus (CMV) infection of allograft recipients: expansion of an uncommon CD8(+) CD57(−) subset and its progressive replacement by CD8(+) CD57(+) T cells. Clin Exp Immunol 1994;95:465–471.

284. Lachgar A, Bizzini B. Contribution of alpha interferon (alpha-IFN) to HIV-induced immunosuppression. Cell Mol Biol 1995;41:431–437.

285. Lafon M, Lafage M, Martinez-Arends A, et al. Evidence for a viral superantigen in humans. Nature 1992;358:507–510.

286. Lane HC, Masur H, Edgar LC, Whalen G, Rook AH, Fauci AS. Ab-

normalities of B-cell activation and immunoregulation in patients with the acquired immunodeficiency syndrome. N Engl J Med 1983;309:453–458.

287. Laurence J, Gottlieb AB, Kunkel HG. Soluble suppressor factors in patients with acquired immune deficiency syndrome and its prodrome: elaboration in vitro by T lymphocyte adherent cell interactions. J Clin Invest 1983;72:2072–2081.

288. Laurence J, Hodtsev AS, Posnett DN. Superantigen implicated in dependence of HIV-1 replication in T cells on TCR V-beta expression. Nature 1992;358:255–259.

289. Laurence J, Mayer L. Immunoregulatory lymphokines of Tybridomas from AIDS patients: constitutive and inducible suppressor factors. Science 1984;225:66–69.

290. Leahy MA, Krejci SM, Friednash M, et al. Human herpesvirus 6 is present in lesions of Langerhans cell histiocytosis. J Invest Dermatol 1993;101:642–645.

291. Lehn M, Weiser WY, Engelhorn S, Gillis S, Remold HG. IL-4 inhibits H2O2 production and antileishmanial capacity of human cultured monocytes mediated by IFN-gamma. J Immunol 1989;143: 3020–3024.

292. Leist TP, Ruedi E, Zinkernagel RM. Virus-triggered immune suppression in mice caused by virus-specific cytotoxic T cells. J Exp Med 1988;167:1749–1754.

293. Leopardi R, Ilonen J, Mattila L, Salmi AA. Effect of measles virus infection on MHC class II expression and antigen presentation in human monocytes. Cell Immunol 1993;147:388–396.

294. Leopardi R, Vainionpaa R, Hurme M, Siljander P, Salmi AA. Measles virus infection enhances IL-1beta but reduces tumor necrosis factor-alpha expression in human monocytes. J Immunol 1992; 149:2397–2401.

295. Letvin NL, Eaton KA, Aldrich WR, et al. Acquired immunodeficiency syndrome in a colony of macaque monkeys. Proc Natl Acad Sci U S A 1983;80:2718–2722.

296. Levin MJ, Rinaldo CR Jr, Leary PL, Zaia JA, Hirsch MS. Immune response to herpesvirus antigens in adults with acute cytomegaloviral mononucleosis. J Infect Dis 1979;140:851–857.

297. Li L, Elliott JF, Mosmann TR. IL-10 inhibits cytokine production, vascular leakage, and swelling during T helper 1 cell-induced delayed-type hypersensitivity. J Immunol 1994;153:3967–3978.

298. Lin CY, Hsu HC. Histopathological and immunological studies in spontaneous remission of nephrotic syndrome after intercurrent measles infection. Nephron 1986;42:110–115.

299. Lin CY, Lin MT, Hsieh YL, Tsao LY. Transient disappearance of immunologic disorders and remission after intercurrent measles infections in children with chronic idiopathic thrombocytopenic purpura. J Clin Immunol 1988;8:207–213.

300. Lin DS, Bowman DD, Jacobson RH, et al. Suppression of lymphocyte blastogenesis to mitogens in cats experimentally infected with feline immunodeficiency virus. Vet Immunol Immunopathol 1990; 26:183–189.

301. Lio D, Dieli F, Cillari E, Salerno A. Suppression of contact sensitivity by a plastic adherent T-cell, induced in mice infected with Newcastle disease virus (NDV). Br J Exp Pathol 1987;68:663–674.

302. Lodmell DL, Hadlow WJ, Munoz JJ, Whitford HW. Hemagglutinin antibody response of normal and Aleutian disease-affected mink to keyhole limpet hemocyanin. J Immunol 1970;104:878–887.

303. Loh L, Hudson JB. Murine cytomegalovirus infection in the spleen and its relationship to immunosuppression. Infect Immun 1981;32: 1067–1072.

304. Longo N, Zabay JM, Sempere MJ, Navarro J, Fernandez-Cruz E. Altered production of PGE2, IL-1B, and TNF-a by peripheral blood monocytes from HIV-positive individuals at early stages of HIV infection. J Acquir Immune Defic Syndr 1993;6:1017–1023.

305. Lopez A, Thomson RG, Savan M. The pulmonary clearance of *Pasteurella hemolytica* in calves infected with bovine parainfluenza-3 virus. Can J Comp Med 1976;40:385–391.

306. Lucey DR, Hensley RE, Ward WW, Butzin CA, Boswell RN. CD4+ monocyte counts in persons with HIV-1 infection: an early increase is followed by a progressive decline. J Acquir Immune Defic Syndr 1991;4:24–30.

307. Lumio J, Welin M-G, Hirvonen P, Weber T. Lymphocyte subpopulations and reactivity during and after infectious mononucleosis. Med Biol 1983;61:208–213.

308. Lusso P, Malnati M, DeMaria A, et al. Productive infection of CD4+ and CD8+ mature human T cell populations and clones by

human herpesvirus 6. Transcriptional down-regulation of CD3. J Immunol 1991;147:685–691.

309. Lusso P, Malnati MS, Garzino-Demo A, Crowley RW, Long EO, Gallo RC. Infection of natural killer cells by human herpesvirus 6. Nature 1993;362:458–462.

310. Lyon JA, Hinshaw VS. Inhibition of nitric oxide induction from avian macrophage cell lines by influenza virus. Avian Dis 1993; 37:868–873.

311. Macatonia SE, Gompels M, Pinching AJ, Patterson S, Knight SC. Antigen presentation by macrophages but not by dendritic cells in human immunodeficiency virus (HIV) infection. Immunology 1992; 75:576–581.

312. Macatonia SE, Lau R, Patterson S, Pinching AJ, Knight SC. Dendritic cell infection, depletion and dysfunction in HIV-infected individuals. Immunology 1990;71:38–45.

313. Maggi E, Macchia D, Parronchi P, et al. Reduced production of interleukin-2 and interferon-gamma and enhanced helper activity for IgG synthesis by cloned CD4+ T cells from patients with AIDS. Eur J Immunol 1987;17:1685–1690.

314. Mahy BWJ. Action of Riley's plasma enzyme-elevating virus in mice (discussion and preliminary reports). Virology 1964;24:481–483.

315. Mangi RJ, Niederman JC, Kelleher JE Jr, Dwyer JM, Evans AS, Kantor FS. Depression of cell-mediated immunity during acute infectious mononucleosis. N Engl J Med 1974;291:1149–1153.

316. Marrack P, Kushnir E, Kappler J. A maternally inherited superantigen encoded by a mammary tumour virus. Nature 1991;349:524–526.

317. Martinez-Maza O, Crabb E, Mitsuyasu RT, Fahey JL. Infection with the human immunodeficiency virus (HIV) is associated with an in vivo increase in B lymphocyte activation and immaturity. J Immunol 1987;138:3720–3724.

318. Martinez OM, Gibbons RS, Garovoy MR, Aronson FR. IL-4 inhibits IL-2 receptor expression and IL-2 dependent proliferation of human T cells. J Immunol 1990;144:2211–2215.

319. Mathes LE, Olsen RG, Hebebrand LC, et al. Immunosuppressive properties of a virion polypeptide, a 15,000-dalton protein, from feline leukemia virus. Cancer Res 1979;39:950–955.

320. Matloubian M, Kolhekar SR, Somasundaram T, Ahmed R. Molecular determinants of macrophage tropism and viral persistence: importance of single amino acid changes in the polymerase and glycoprotein of lymphocytic choriomeningitis virus. J Virol 1993;67: 7340–7349.

321. Matloubian M, Somasundaram T, Kolhekar SR, Selvakumar R, Ahmed R. Genetic basis of viral persistence: single amino acid change in the viral glycoprotein affects ability of lymphocytic choriomeningitis virus to persist in adult mice. J Exp Med 1990;172: 1043–1048.

322. Matsui M, Mori KJ, Saida T. Cellular immunoregulatory mechanisms in the central nervous system: characterization of non-inflammatory and cerebrospinal fluid lymphocytes. Ann Neurol 1990;27: 647–651.

323. McCarthy DO, Domurat F, Nichols JE, Roberts NJ Jr. Interleukin-1 inhibitor production by human mononuclear leukocytes and leukocyte subpopulations exposed to respiratory syncytial virus: analysis and comparison with the response to influenza virus. J Leukoc Biol 1989;46:189–198.

324. McChesney MB, Oldstone MB. Viruses perturb lymphocyte functions: selected principles characterizing virus-induced immunosuppression. Ann Rev Immunol 1987;5:279–304.

325. McElrath MJ, Pruett JE, Cohn ZA. Mononuclear phagocytes of blood and bone marrow: comparative roles as viral reservoirs in human immunodeficiency virus type 1 infections. Proc Natl Acad Sci U S A 1989;86:675–679.

326. McIlroy D, Autran B, Cheynier R, et al. Infection frequency of dendritic cells and CD4+ T lymphocytes in spleens of human immunodeficiency virus-positive patients. J Virol 1995;69:4737–4745.

327. McKenzie R, Kotwal GJ, Moss B, Hammer CH, Frank MM. Regulation of complement activity by vaccinia virus complement-control protein. J Infect Dis 1992;166:1245–1250.

328. McMorrow LE, Vesikari T, Wolman SR, Giles JP, Cooper LZ. Suppression of the response of lymphocytes to phytohemagglutinin in rubella. J Infect Dis 1974;130:464–469.

329. McNearney TA, Odell C, Holers VM, Spear PG, Atkinson JP. Herpes simplex virus glycoproteins gC-1 and gC-2 bind to the third

component of complement and provide protection against complement-mediated neutralization of viral infectivity. J Exp Med 1987; 166:1525–1535.

330. Mellman WJ, Wetton R. Depression of the tuberculin reaction by attenuated measles virus vaccine. J Lab Clin Med 1963;61:453–458.

331. Meyaard L, Otto SA, Jonker RR, Mijnster MJ, Keet RP, Miedema F. Programmed death of T cells in HIV-1 infection. Science 1992;257: 217–219.

332. Michaelides MC, Simms ES. Immune responses in mice infected with lactic dehydrogenase virus. I. Antibody response to DNP-BGG and hyperglobulinaemia in BALB/c mice. Immunology 1977;32: 981–988.

333. Michaelides MC, Simms ES. Immune responses in mice infected with lactic dehydrogenase virus. II. Contact sensitization to DNFB and characterization of lymphoid cells during acute LDV infection. Cell Immunol 1977;29:285–294.

334. Michaelides MC, Simms ES. Immune responses in mice infected with lactic dehydrogenase virus. III. Antibody response to a T-dependent and a T-independent antigen during acute and chronic LDV infection. Cell Immunol 1980;50:253–260.

335. Michelson S, Alcami J, Kim SJ, et al. Human cytomegalovirus infection induces transcription and secretion of transforming growth factor beta-1. J Virol 1994;68:5730–5737.

336. Midulla F, Villani A, Panuska JR, et al. Respiratory syncytial virus lung infection in infants: immunoregulatory role of infected alveolar macrophages. J Infect Dis 1993;168:1515–1519.

337. Mikovits JA, Lohrey NC, Schulof R, Courtless J, Ruscetti FW. Activation of infectious virus from latent human immunodeficiency virus infection of monocytes in vivo. J Clin Invest 1992;90:1486–1491.

338. Miller DL. Frequency of complications of measles, 1963. Br Med J 1964;2:75–78.

339. Mills EL. Viral infections predisposing to bacterial infections. Ann Rev Med 1984;35:469–479.

340. Mims CA. Interactions of viruses with the immune system. Clin Exp Immunol 1986;66:1–16.

341. Mims CA, Wainwright S. The immunodepressive action of lymphocytic choriomeningitis virus in mice. J Immunol 1968;101:717–724.

342. Mitchell LC, Davis LS, Lipsky PE. Promotion of human T lymphocyte proliferation by IL-4. J Immunol 1989;142:1548–1557.

343. Miyazaki I, Cheung RK, Dosch H-M. The role of vIL-10 and other EBV latency genes early during B cell growth transformation. Virology 1994;5:405–414.

344. Moench TR, Griffin DE, Obriecht CR, Vaisberg AJ, Johnson RT. Acute measles in patients with and without neurological involvement: distribution of measles virus antigen and RNA. J Infect Dis 1988;158:433–442.

345. Molina J-M, Scadden DT, Amiraulty C, et al. Human immunodeficiency virus does not induce interleukin-1, interleukin-6, or tumor necrosis factor in mononuclear cells. J Virol 1990;64:2901–2906.

346. Molina J-M, Scadden DT, Byrn R, Dinarello CA, Groopman JE. Production of tumor necrosis factor alpha and interleukin 1-beta by monocytic cells infected with human immunodeficiency virus. J Clin Invest 1989;84:733–737.

347. Molina J-M, Schinler R, Ferriani R, et al. Production of cytokines by peripheral blood monocytes/macrophages infected with human immunodeficiency virus type (HIV-1). J Infect Dis 1990;161:888–893.

348. Moncada S, Palmer RM, Higgs EA. Nitric oxide: physiology, pathophysiology, and pharmacology. Pharmacol Rev 1991;43:109–142.

349. Montgomery JR, South MA, Rawls WE, Melnick JL. Viral inhibition of lymphocyte response to phytohemagglutinin. Science 1967; 157:1068–1070.

350. Moody CE, Casazza BA, Christenson WN, Weksler ME. Lymphocyte transformation induced by autologous cells. VIII. Impaired autologous mixed lymphocyte reactivity in patients with acute infectious mononucleosis. J Exp Med 1979;150:1448–1455.

351. Moore KW, Vieira P, Fiorentino DF, Trounstine ML, Khan TA, Mosmann TR. Homology of cytokine synthesis inhibitory factor (IL-10) to the Epstein-Barr virus gene BCRFI. Science 1990;248:1230–1234.

352. Morishima C, Norby-Slycord C, McConnell KR, et al. Expression of two structurally identical viral superantigens results in thymic elimination at distinct developmental stages. J Immunol 1994;153: 5091–5103.

353. Mori S, Wolfinbarger JB, Miyazawa M, Bloom ME. Replication of Aleutian mink disease parvovirus in lymphoid tissues of adult mink: involvement of follicular dendritic cells and macrophages. J Virol 1991;65:952–956.

354. Morse SS. Mouse thymic necrosis virus: a novel murine lymphotropic agent. Lab Animal Sci 1987;37:717–725.

355. Morse SS, Valinsky JE. Mouse thymic virus (MTLV): a mammalian herpesvirus cytolytic for CD4+ (L3T4+) T lymphocytes. J Exp Med 1989;169:591–596.

356. Mosier DE, Yetter RA, Morse HC III. Retroviral induction of acute lymphoproliferative disease and profound immunosuppression in adult C57BL/6 mice. J Exp Med 1985;161:766–784.

357. Moskophidis D, Pircher H, Ciernik I, Odermatt B, Hengartner, H, Zinkernagel RM. Suppression of virus-specific antibody production by CD8+ class I-restricted antiviral cytotoxic T cells in vivo. J Virol 1992;66:3661–3668.

358. Mosmann TR, Coffman RL. Two types of mouse helper T cell clone: implications for immune regulation. Immunol Today 1987;8:223–227.

359. Mukae H, Kohno S, Morikawa N, Kadota J, Matsukura S, Hara K. Increase in T-cells bearing CD25 in bronchoalveolar lavage fluid from HAM/TSP patients in HTLV-I carriers. Microbiol Immunol 1994;38:55–62.

360. Muller H. Replication of infectious bursal disease virus in lymphoid cells. Arch Virol 1986;87:191–203.

361. Mullins JI, Hoover EA, Quackenbush SL, Donahue PR. Disease progression and viral genome variants in experimental feline leukemia virus-induced immunodeficiency syndrome. J Acquir Immune Defic Syndr 1991;4:547–557.

362. Munis JR, Richman DD, Kornbluth RS. Human immunodeficiency virus-1 infection of macrophages in vitro neither induces tumor necrosis factor (TNF)/cachectin gene expression nor alters TNF/cachectin induction by lipopolysaccharide. J Clin Invest 1990;85: 591–596.

363. Munyer TP, Mangi RJ, Dolan T, Kantor FS. Depressed lymphocyte function after measles-mumps-rubella vaccination. J Infect Dis 1975;132:75–78.

364. Murai K, Tachibana N, Shioiri S, et al. Suppression of delayed-type hypersensitivity to PPD and PHA in elderly HTLV-I carriers. J Acquir Immune Defic Syndr 1990;3:1006–1009.

365. Muro-Cacho CA, Pantaleo G, Fauci AS. Intensity of apoptosis correlates with the general state of activation of the lymphoid tissue and not with stage of disease or viral burden. J Immunol 1995;154: 5555–5566.

366. Nakasone T, Araki K, Masuda M, et al. Immune responses and serum levels of cytokines in adult T-cell leukemia patients and human T-cell leukemia virus type-I carriers. Eur J Haematol 1992;48: 99–104.

367. Newble DI, Holmes KT, Wangel AG, Forbes IJ. Immune reactions in acute viral hepatitis. Clin Exp Immunol 1975;20:17–28.

368. Newman MJ, Issel CJ, Truax RE, Powell MD, Horohov DW. Transient suppression of equine immune responses by equine infectious anemia virus (EIAV). Virology 1991;184:55–66.

369. Nicholas JA, Levely ME, Brideau RJ, Berger AE. During recovery from cytomegalovirus infection T-lymphocyte subsets become selectively responsive to activation and have depressed interleukin 2 (IL2) secretion and IL2 receptor expression. Microb Pathog 1987; 2:37–47.

370. Nisini R, Aiuti A, Matricardi PM, et al. Lack of evidence for a superantigen in lymphocytes from HIV-discordant monozygotic twins. AIDS 1994;8:443–449.

371. Niwa Y, Kanoh T. Immunological behaviour following rubella infection. Clin Exp Immunol 1979;37:470–476.

372. Notkins AL. Lactic dehydrogenase virus. Bacteriol Rev 1965;29: 143–160.

373. Notkins AL, Mergenhagen SE, Rizzo AA, Scheele C, Waldmann MD. Elevated gamma-globulin and increased antibody production in mice infected with lactic-dehydrogenase virus. J Exp Med 1966;123:347–364.

374. Novak TJ, Rothenberg EV. cAMP inhibits induction of interleukin 2 but not of interleukin 4 in T cells. Proc Natl Acad Sci U S A 1990;87:9353–9357.

375. Numazaki K, Goldman H, Bai X-Q, Wong I, Wainberg MA. Effects of infection by HIV-1, cytomegalovirus, and human measles virus on cultured human thymic epithelial cells. Microbiol Immunol 1989;33:733–745.

376. Numazaki K, Goldman H, Wong I, Wainberg MA. Replication of measles virus in cultured human thymic epithelial cells. J Med Virol 1989;27:52–58.

377. Odermatt B, Eppler M, Leist TP, Hengartner H, Zinkernagel RM. Virus-triggered acquired immunodeficiency by cytotoxic T-cell-dependent destruction of antigen-presenting cells and lymph follicle structure. Proc Natl Acad Sci U S A 1991;88:8252–8256.

378. Ogilvie GK, Tompkins MB, Tompkins WA. Clinical and immunologic aspects of FeLV-induced immunosuppression. Vet Microbiol 1988;17:287–296.

379. Oill PA, Fiala M, Schofferman J, Byfield PE, Guze LB. Cytomegalovirus mononucleosis in a healthy adult: association with hepatitis, secondary Epstein-Barr virus antibody response and immunosuppression. Am J Med 1977;62:413–417.

380. Oldstone MBA, Tishon A, Chiller JM. Chronic virus infection and immune responsiveness. II. Lactic dehydrogenase virus infection and immune response to non-viral antigens. J Immunol 1974;112:370–375.

381. Oldstone MBA, Tishon A, Chiller JM, Weigle WO, Dixon FJ. Effect of chronic viral infection on the immune system. I. Comparison on the immune responsiveness of mice chronically infected with LCM virus with that of noninfected mice. J Immunol 1973;110:1268–1278.

382. Olson GB, Dent PB, Rawls WE, et al. Abnormalities of in vitro lymphocyte response during rubella virus infections. J Exp Med 1968;128:47.

383. Olson GB, South MA, Good RA. Phytohaemagglutinin unresponsiveness of lymphocytes from babies with congenital rubella. Nature 1967;214:696.

384. Olson RW, Hodges GR. Measles pneumonia: bacterial suprainfection as a complicating factor. JAMA 1975;232:363–365.

385. Onodera T, Taniguchi T, Tsuda T, et al. Thymic atrophy in type 2 reovirus infected mice: immunosuppression and effects of thymic hormone; thymic atrophy caused by reo-2. Thymus 1991;18:95–109.

386. Oostendorp RA, Schaaper WM, Post J, Meloen RH, Scheper RJ. Synthetic hexapeptides derived from the transmembrane envelope proteins of retroviruses suppress N-formylpeptide-induced monocyte polarization. J Leukoc Biol 1992;51:282–288.

387. Opgenorth A, Graham K, Nation N, Strayer D, McFadden G. Deletion analysis of two tandemly arranged virulence genes in myxoma virus, M11L and myxoma growth factor. J Virol 1992;66:4720–4731.

388. Oppenheimer-Marks N, Kavanaugh AF, Lipsky PE. Inhibition of the transendothelial migration of human T lymphocytes by prostaglandin E2. J Immunol 1994;152:5703–5713.

389. Orren A, Kipps A, Moodie JW, Beatty DW, Dowdle EB, McIntyre JP. Increased susceptibility to herpes simplex virus infections in children with acute measles. Infect Immun 1981;31:1–6.

390. Osborn JE, Blazkovec AA, Walker DL. Immunosuppression during acute murine cytomegalovirus infection. J Immunol 1968;100:835–844.

391. Osterhaus A. A morbillivirus causing mass mortality in seals. Vaccine 1989;7:483–484.

392. Oswald IP, Wynn TA, Sher A, James SL. Interleukin 10 inhibits macrophage microbicidal activity by blocking the endogenous production of tumor necrosis factor-alpha required as a costimulatory factor for interferon-gamma-induced activation. Proc Natl Acad Sci U S A 1992;89:8676–8680.

393. Overbaugh J, Donahue PR, Quackenbush SL, Hoover EA, Mullins JI. Molecular cloning of a feline leukemia virus that induces fatal immunodeficiency disease in cats. Science 1988;239:906–910.

394. Paabo S, Bhat BM, Wold WS, Peterson PA. A short sequence in the COOH-terminus makes an adenovirus membrane glycoprotein a resident of the endoplasmic reticulum. Cell 1987;50:311–317.

395. Paabo S, Nilsson T, Peterson PA. Adenoviruses of subgenera B, C, D, and E modulate cell-surface expression of major histocompatibility complex class I antigens. Proc Natl Acad Sci U S A 1986;83:9665–9669.

396. Paabo S, Severinsson L, Andersson M, Martens I, Nilsson T, Peterson, PA. Adenovirus proteins and MHC expression. Adv Cancer Res 1989;52:151–163.

397. Paabo S, Weber F, Nilsson T, Schaffner W, Peterson PA. Structural and functional dissection of an MHC class I antigen-binding adenovirus glycoprotein. EMBO J 1986;5:1921–127.

398. Pahwa S, Kirkpatrick D, Ching C, et al. Persistent cytomegalovirus infection: association with profound immunodeficiency and treatment with interferon. Clin Immunol Immunopathol 1983;28:77–89.

399. Pantaleo G, Graziosi C, Demarest JF, et al. HIV infection is active and progressive in lymphoid tissue during the clinically latent stage of disease. Nature 1993;362:355–358.

400. Panuska JR, Hertz MI, Taraf H, Villani A, Cirino NM. Respiratory syncytial virus infection of alveolar macrophages in adult transplant patients. Am Rev Respir Dis 1992;145:934–939.

401. Papiernik M, Brossard Y, Mulliez N, et al. Thymic abnormalities in fetuses aborted from human immunodeficiency virus type 1 seropositive women. Pediatrics 1992;89:297–301.

402. Pedersen NC, Ho EW, Brown ML, Yamamoto JK. Isolation of a T-lymphotropic virus from domestic cats with an immunodeficiency-like syndrome. Science 1987;235:790–793.

403. Perez-Blas M, Regueiro JR, Ruiz-Contreras J, Arnaiz-Villena A. T lymphocyte anergy during acute infectious mononucleosis is restricted to the clonotypic receptor activation pathway. Clin Exp Immunol 1992;89:83–88.

404. Perry LL, Hotchkiss JD, Lodmell DL. Murine susceptibility to street rabies virus is unrelated to induction of host lymphoid depletion. J Immunol 1990;144:3552–3557.

405. Perryman LE, Banks KL, McGuire TC. Lymphocyte abnormalities in Aleutian disease virus infection of mink: decreased T lymphocyte responses and increased B lymphocyte levels in persistent viral infection. J Immunol 1975;115:22–27.

406. Perryman LE, Hoover EA, Yohn DS. Immunologic reactivity of the cat: immunosuppression in experimental feline leukemia. J Natl Cancer Inst 1972;49:1357–1365.

407. Poli G, Fauci AS. The role of monocyte/macrophages and cytokines in the pathogenesis of HIV infection. Pathobiology 1992;60:246–251.

408. Poli G, Kinter A, Justement JS, et al. Tumor necrosis factor alpha functions in an autocrine manner in the induction of human immunodeficiency virus expression. Proc Natl Acad Sci U S A 1990;87:782–785.

409. Poss ML, Mullins JI, Hoover EA. Posttranslational modifications distinguish the envelope glycoprotein of the immunodeficiency disease-inducing feline leukemia virus retrovirus. J Virol 1989;63:189–195.

410. Poss ML, Quackenbush SL, Mullins JI, Hoover EA. Characterization and significance of delayed processing of the feline leukemia virus FeLV-FAIDS envelope glycoprotein. J Virol 1990;64:4338–4345.

411. Poumbourios P, Anders EM, Scalzo AA, White DO, Hampson AW, Jackson DC. Direct role of viral hemagglutinin in B-cell mitogenesis by influenza viruses. J Virol 1987;61:214–217.

412. Prince HE, Czaplicki CD. In vitro activation of T lymphocytes from HIV-seropositive blood donors. II. Decreased mitogen-induced expression of interleukin 2 receptor by both CD4 and CD8 cell subsets. Clin Immunol Immunopathol 1988;48:132–139.

413. Prince HE, Kermani-Arab V, Fahey JL. Depressed interleukin 2 receptor expression in acquired immune deficiency and lymphadenopathy syndromes. J Immunol 1984;133:1313–1317.

414. Psallidopoulos MC, Schnittman SM, Thompson LM, et al. Integrated proviral human immunodeficiency virus type 1 is present in CD4+ peripheral blood lymphocytes in healthy seropositive individuals. J Virol 1989;63:4626–4631.

415. Pullen AM, Choi Y, Kushnir E, Kappler J, Marrack P. The open reading frames in the 3' long terminal repeats of several mouse mammary tumor virus integrants encode V beta 3-specific superantigens. J Exp Med 1992;175:41–47.

416. Pwrie F, Menon S, Coffman RL. Interleukin-4 and interleukin-10 synergize to inhibit cell-mediated immunity in vivo. Eur J Immunol 1993;23:3043–3049.

417. Quackenbush SL, Donahue PR, Dean GA, et al. Lymphocyte subset alterations and viral determinants of immunodeficiency disease induction by the feline leukemia virus FeLV-FAIDS. J Virol 1990;64:5465–5474.

418. Quackenbush SL, Mullins JI, Hoover EA. Colony forming T lymphocyte deficit in the development of feline retrovirus induced immunodeficiency syndrome. Blood 1989;73:509–516.

419. Ramis I, Rosello-Catafau J, Gomez G, Zabay JM, Fernandez-Cruz E, Gelpi E. Cyclooxygenase and lipoxygenases arachidonic acid metabolism by monocytes from human immune deficiency virus-infected drug users. J Chromatogr 1991;557:507–513.

420. Ramm HC, Wilson TJ, Boyd RL, Ward HA, Mitrangas K, Fahey KJ. The effect of infectious bursal disease virus on B lymphocytes and bursal stromal components in specific pathogen-free (SPF) white Leghorn chickens. Dev Comp Immunol 1991;15:369–381.

421. Ranges GE, Figari IS, Espevik T, Palladino MA Jr. Inhibition of cytotoxic T cell development by transforming growth factor beta and reversal by recombinant tumor necrosis factor alpha. J Exp Med 1987;166:991–998.

422. Rappaport RS, Dodge GR. Prostaglandin E inhibits the production of human interleukin 2. J Exp Med 1982;155:943–948.

423. Rappersberger K, Gartner S, Schenk P, et al. Langerhans' cells are an actual site of HIV-1 replication. Intervirology 1988;29:185–194.

424. Ray CA, Black RA, Kronheim SR, et al. Viral inhibition of inflammation: cowpox virus encodes an inhibitor of the interleukin-1-beta converting enzyme. Cell 1992;69:597–604.

425. Razvi ES, Welsh RM. Programmed cell death of T lymphocytes during acute viral infection: a mechanism for virus-induced immune deficiency. J Virol 1993;67:5754–5765.

426. Reddy MM, Lange M, Grieco MH. Elevated soluble CD8 levels in sera of human immunodeficiency virus-infected populations. J Clin Microbiol 1989;27:257–260.

427. Reddy MM, Vodian M, Grieco MH. Elevated levels of CD4 antigen in sera of human immunodeficiency virus-infected populations. J Clin Microbiol 1990;28:1744–1746.

428. Reinacher M. Diseases associated with spontaneous feline leukemia virus (FeLV) infection in cats. Vet Immunol Immunopathol 1989; 21:85–95.

429. Reinherz EL, O'Brien C, Rosenthal P, Schlossman SF. The cellular basis for viral-induced immunodeficiency: analysis by monoclonal antibodies. J Immunol 1980;125:1269–1274.

430. Rinaldo CR, Black PH, Hirsch MS. Interaction of cytomegalovirus with leukocytes from patients with mononucleosis due to cytomegalovirus. J Infect Dis 1977;136:667–678.

431. Rinaldo CR, Carney WP, Richter BS, Black PH, Hirsch MS. Mechanisms of immunosuppression in cytomegaloviral mononucleosis. J Infect Dis 1980;141:488–495.

432. Roberts NJ Jr. The concept of immunofocusing illustrated by influenza virus infection. Rev Infect Dis 1988;10:1071–1074.

433. Roberts NJ Jr, Prill AH, Mann TN. Interleukin-1 and interleukin-1 inhibitor production by human macrophages exposed to influenza virus or respiratory syncytial virus: respiratory syncytial virus is a potent inducer of inhibitor activity. J Exp Med 1986;163:511–519.

434. Robinson MK, Manly KF, Evans MJ. Immunosuppression by 334C murine leukemia virus: viral specificity and the activation of immunosuppressive effects during cloned viral leukemogenesis. J Immunol 1980;124:1022–1027.

435. Rode HJ, Janssen W, Rosen-Wolff A, et al. The genome of equine herpesvirus type 2 harbors an interleukin 10 (IL10) -like gene. Virus Genes 1993;7:111–116.

436. Rodenberg J, Sharma JM, Belzer SW, Nordgren RM, Naqi S. Flow cytometric analysis of B cell and T cell subpopulations in specific-pathogen-free chickens infected with infectious bursal disease virus. Avian Dis 1994;38:16–21.

437. Rodgers BC, Scott DM, Mundin J, Sissons JG. Monocyte-derived inhibitor of interleukin 1 induced by human cytomegalovirus. J Virol 1985;55:527–532.

438. Rodgers BC, Scott DM, Sissons JGP. A monocyte-derived inhibitor of interleukin 1 induced by human cytomegalovirus. Trans Assoc Am 1985;98:334–343.

439. Roffman E, Frenkel N. Replication of human herpesvirus-6 in thymocytes activated by anti-CD3 antibody. J Infect Dis 1991;164:617–618.

440. Rohwer RG. A new type D retrovirus isolated from macaques with an immunodeficiency syndrome. Science 1984;223:602–603.

441. Rook AH, Manischewitz JE, Frederick WR, et al. Deficient, HLA-restricted, cytomegalovirus-specific cytotoxic T cells and natural killer cells in patients with the acquired immunodeficiency syndrome. J Infect Dis 1985;152:627–630.

442. Roost H, Gobet R, Hengartner H, Zinkernagel RM. An acquired immune suppression in mice caused by infection with lymphocytic choriomeningitis virus. Eur J Immunol 1988;18:511–518.

443. Rosen A, Gergely P, Jondal M, Klein G, Britton S. Polyclonal Ig production after Epstein-Barr virus infection of human lymphocytes in vitro. Nature 1977;267:52–54.

444. Rother RP, Rollins SA, Fodor WL, et al. Inhibition of complement-mediated cytolysis by the terminal complement inhibitor of herpesvirus saimiri. J Virol 1994;68:730–737.

445. Rott O, Cash E. Influenza virus hemagglutinin induces differentiation of mature resting B cells and growth arrest of immature WEHI-231 lymphoma cells. J Immunol 1994;152:5381–5391.

446. Rott O, Charreire J, Mignon-Godefroy K, Cash E. B cell superstimulatory influenza virus activates peritoneal B cells. J Immunol 1995;155:134–142.

447. Rott O, Charreire J, Semichon M, Bismuth G, Cash E. B cell superstimulatory influenza virus (H2-subtype) induces B cell proliferation by a PKR-activating, Ca(2+)-independent mechanism. J Immunol 1995;154:2092–2103.

448. Rouse BT, Horohov DW. Immunosuppression in viral infections. Rev Infect Dis 1986;8:850–873.

449. Rowe WP, Capps WI. A new mouse virus causing necrosis of the thymus in newborn mice. J Exp Med 1960;113:831–844.

450. Rowland RR, Butz EA, Plagemann PGW. Nitric oxide production by splenic macrophages is not responsible for T cell suppression during acute infection with lactate dehydrogenase-elevating virus. J Immunol 1994;152:5785–5795.

451. Rowland RR, Even C, Anderson GW, Chen Z, Hu B, Plagemann PG. Neonatal infection of mice with lactate dehydrogenase-elevating virus results in suppression of humoral antiviral immune response but does not alter the course of viraemia or the polyclonal activation of B cells and immune complex formation. J Gen Virol 1994;75:1071–1081.

452. Ruben S, Poteat H, Tan TH, et al. Cellular transcription factors and regulation of IL-2 receptor gene expression by HTLV-I tax gene product. Science 1988;241:89–92.

453. Rubin RH, Cosimi AB, Tolkoff-Rubin NE, Russell PS, Hirsch MS. Infectious disease syndromes attributable to cytomegalovirus and their significance among renal transplant recipients. Transplantation 1977;24:458–464.

454. Ruedi E, Hengartner H, Zinkernagel RM. Immunosuppression in mice by lymphocytic choriomeningitis virus infection: time dependence during primary and absence of effects on secondary antibody responses. Cell Immunol 1990;130:501–512.

455. Ruegemer JJ, Ho SN, Augustine JA, et al. Regulatory effects of transforming growth factor-beta on IL-2 and IL-4-dependent T cell-cycle progression. J Immunol 1990;144:1767–1776.

456. Ruegg CL, Monell CR, Strand M. Identification, using synthetic peptides, of the minimum amino acid sequence from the retroviral transmembrane protein p15E required for inhibition of lymphoproliferation and its similarity to gp21 of human T-lymphotropic virus types I and II. J Virol 1989;63:3250–3256.

457. Russell AS, Percy JS, Grace M. The relationship of autoantibodies to depression of cell mediated immunity in infectious mononucleosis. Clin Exp Immunol 1975;20:65–71.

458. Saif YM. Immunosuppression induced by infectious bursal disease virus. Vet Immunol Immunopathol 1991;30:45–50.

459. Salonen R, Ilonen J, Salmi A. Measles virus infection of unstimulated blood mononuclear cells in vitro: antigen expression and virus production preferentially in monocytes. Clin Exp Immunol 1988;71:224–228.

460. Santisteban GA, Riley V, Fitzmaurice MA. Thymolytic and adrenal cortical responses to the LDH-elevating virus. Proc Soc Exp Biol Med 1972;139:202–206.

461. Saron M-F, Shidani B, Nahori MA, Guillon J-C, Truffa-Bachi P. Lymphocytic choriomeningitis virus-induced immunodepression: inherent defect of B and T lymphocytes. J Virol 1990;64:4076–4083.

462. Scalzo AA, Anders EM. Influenza viruses as lymphocyte mitogens. II. Role of I-E molecules in B cell mitogenesis by influenza A viruses of the H2 and H6 subtypes. J Immunol 1985;135:3524–3529.

463. Schnittman SM, Denning SM, Greenhouse JJ, et al. Evidence for susceptibility of intrathymic T-cell precursors and their progeny carrying T-cell antigen receptor phenotypes TCR alpha beta + and TCR gamma delta + to human immunodeficiency virus infection: a mechanism for CD4+ (T4) lymphocyte depletion. Proc Natl Acad Sci U S A 1990;87:7727–7731.

464. Schnittman SM, Psallidopoulos MC, Lane HC, et al. The reservoir for HIV-1 in human peripheral blood is a T cell that maintains expression of CD4. Science 1989;245:305–308.

465. Schooley RT, Hirsch MS, Colvin RB, et al. Association of herpesvirus infections with T-lymphocyte-subset alterations, glomerulopathy, and opportunistic infections after renal transplantation. N Engl J Med 1983;308:307–313.

466. Schrier PI, Bernards R, Vaessen RTMJ, Houweling A, van der Eb AJ. Expression of class I major histocompatibility antigens switched off by highly oncogenic adenovirus 12 in transformed rat cells. Nature 1983;305:771–775.

467. Schulick RD, Clerici M, Dolan MJ, Shearer GM. Limiting dilution analysis of interleukin-2-producing T cells responsive to recall and alloantigens in human immunodeficiency virus-infected and uninfected individuals. Eur J Immunol 1993;23:412–417.

468. Schwarzmann SW, Adler JL, Sullivan RJ Jr, Marine WM. Bacterial pneumonia during the Hong Kong influenza epidemic. Arch Intern Med 1971;127:1037–1041.

469. Scott DM, Rodgers BC, Freeke C, Buiter J, Sissons JG. Human cytomegalovirus and monocytes: limited infection and negligible immunosuppression in normal mononuclear cells infected in vitro with mycoplasma-free virus strains. J Gen Virol 1989;70:685–694.

470. Sears SD, Fox R, Brookmeyer R, Leavitt R, Polk BF. Delayed hypersensitivity skin testing and anergy in a population of gay men. Clin Immunol Immunopathol 1987;45:177–183.

471. Shalaby MR, Ammann AJ. Suppression of immune cell function in vitro by recombinant human transforming growth factor-beta. Cell Immunol 1988;112:343–350.

472. Shanley JD, Persanti EL. Replication of murine cytomegalovirus in lung macrophages: effect on phagocytosis of bacteria. Infect Immun 1980;29:1152–1159.

473. Sharma JM, Karaca K, Pertile T. Virus-induced immunosuppression in chickens. Poultry Sci 1994;73:1082–1086.

474. Shearer GM, Clerici M. T helper cell immune dysfunction in asymptomatic, HIV-1-seropositive individuals: the role of Th1-Th2 cross-regulation. Chem Immunol 1992;54:21–43.

475. Shull MM, Ormsby I, Kier AB, et al. Targeted disruption of the mouse transforming growth factor-beta-1 gene results in multifocal inflammatory disease. Nature 1992;359:693–699.

476. Shyp S, Tishon A, Oldstone MB. Inhibition of diabetes in BB rats by virus infection. II. Effect of virus infection on the immune response to non-viral and viral antigens. Immunology 1990;69:501–507.

477. Siegel C, Johnston S, Adair S. Isolation of measles virus in primary rhesus monkey cells from a child with acute interstitial pneumonia who cytologically had giant-cell pneumonia without a rash. Am J Clin Pathol 1990;94:464–469.

478. Siliciano RF, Lawton T, Knall C, et al. Analysis of host-virus interactions in AIDS with anti-gp120 T cell clones: effect of HIV sequence variation and a mechanism for CD4+ cell depletion. Cell 1988;54:561–575.

479. Silver SA, Olson GB. Responsiveness of lymphocytes from Mengo virus treated mice to phytohaemagglutinin stimulation in vitro. Microbios 1974;9:233–238.

480. Simmons P, Kaushansky K, Torok-Storb B. Mechanisms of cytomegalovirus-mediated myelosuppression: perturbation of stromal cell function versus direct infection of myeloid cells. Proc Natl Acad Sci U S A 1990;87:1386–1390.

481. Simon MA, Chalifoux LV, Ringler DJ. Pathologic features of SIV-induced disease and the association of macrophage infection with disease evolution. AIDS Res Hum Retroviruses 1992;8:327–337.

482. Slauson DO, Lay JC, Castleman WL, Neilsen NR. Alveolar macrophage phagocytic kinetics following pulmonary parainfluenza-3 virus infection. J Leukoc Biol 1987;41:412–420.

483. Smedman L, Joki A, daSilva AP, Troye-Blomberg M, Aronsson B, Perlmann P. Immunosuppression after measles vaccination. Acta Paediatr 1994;83:164–168.

484. Smiley ML, Friedman HM. Binding of complement component C3b to glycoprotein C is modulated by sialic acid on herpes simplex virus type 1-infected cells. J Virol 1985;557:857–861.

485. Smith PD, Saini SS, Raffeld M, Manischewitz JF, Wahl SM. Cytomegalovirus induction of tumor necrosis factor-alpha by human monocytes and mucosal macrophages. J Clin Invest 1992;90:1642–1648.

486. Snijdewint FGM, Kalinski P, Wierenga EA, Bos JD, Kapsenberg ML. Prostaglandin E2 differentially modulates cytokine secretion profiles of human T helper lymphocytes. J Immunol 1993;150:5321–5329.

487. Spriggs MK, Hruby DE, Maliszewski CR, et al. Vaccinia and cowpox viruses encode a novel secreted interleukin-1-binding protein. Cell 1992;71:145–152.

488. Stanley SK, McCune JM, Kaneshima H, et al. Human immunodeficiency virus infection of the human thymus and disruption of the thymic microenvironment in the SCID-hu mouse. J Exp Med 1993;178:1151–1163.

489. Starr S, Berkovich S. Effects of measles, gamma-globulin-modified measles and vaccine measles on the tuberculin test. N Engl J Med 1964;270:386–391.

490. Starr S, Berkovich S. The depression of tuberculin reactivity during chickenpox. Pediatrics 1964;33:769–772.

491. Strayer DS, Korber K, Dombrowski J. Immunosuppression during viral oncogenesis. IV. Generation of soluble virus-induced immunologic suppressor molecules. J Immunol 1988;140:2051–2059.

492. Strayer DS, Leibowitz JL. Virus-lymphocyte interactions during the course of immunosuppressive virus infection. J Gen Virol 1987;68:463–472.

493. Strayer DS, Sell S, Skaletsky E, Leibowitz JL. Immunologic dysfunction during viral oncogenesis. I. Nonspecific immunosuppression caused by malignant rabbit fibroma virus. J Immunol 1983;131:2595–2600.

494. Strayer DS, Skaletsky E, Cabirac GF, et al. Malignant rabbit fibroma virus causes secondary immunosuppression in rabbits. J Immunol 1983;130:399–404.

495. Stueckemann JA, Holth M, Swart WJ, et al. Replication of lactate dehydrogenase-elevating virus in macrophages. 2. Mechanism of persistent infection in mice and cell culture. J Gen Virol 1982;59:263–272.

496. Stueckemann JA, Ritzi DM, Holth M, et al. Replication of lactate dehydrogenase-elevating virus in macrophages. 1. Evidence for cytocidal replication. J Gen Virol 1982;59:245–262.

497. Suga S, Yoshikawa T, Asano Y, Nakashima T, Kobayashi I, Yazaki T. Activation of human herpesvirus-6 in children with acute measles. J Med Virol 1992;38:278–282.

498. Su HC, Leite-Morris KA, Braun L, Biron CA. A role for transforming growth factor-beta-1 in regulating natural killer cell and T lymphocyte proliferative responses during acute infection with lymphocytic choriomeningitis virus. J Immunol 1991;147:2717–2727.

499. Tachibana N, Okayama A, Ishizaki J, et al. Suppression of tuberculin skin reaction in healthy HTLV-I carriers from Japan. Int J Cancer 1988;42:829–831.

500. Takahashi K, Sonoda S, Higashi K, et al. Predominant CD4 T-lymphocyte tropism of human herpes virus 6-related virus. J Virol 1989;63:3161–3163.

501. Tamashiro VG, Perez HH, Griffin DE. Prospective study of the magnitude and duration of changes in tuberculin reactivity during complicated and uncomplicated measles. Pediatr Infect Dis J 1987;6:451–454.

502. Tate H, Kodama H, Izawa H. Immunosuppressive effect of infectious pancreatic necrosis virus on rainbow trout (Oncorhynchus mykiss). Nippon Juigaku Zasshi 1990;52:931–937.

503. Taylor-Wiedeman J, Sissons JGP, Borysiewicz LK, Sinclair JH. Monocytes are a major site of persistence of human cytomegalovirus in peripheral blood mononuclear cells. J Gen Virol 1991;72:2059–2064.

504. Tegtmeyer PJ, Craighead JE. Infection of adult mouse macrophages in vitro with cytomegalovirus. Proc Soc Exp Biol Med 1968;129:690–694.

505. ten Napel CHH, The TH. Lymphocyte reactivity in infectious mononucleosis. J Infect Dis 1980;141:716–723.

506. te Velde AA, Huijbens RJF, de Vries JE, Figdor CG. IL-4 decreases Fc-gamma-R membrane expression and Fc-gamma-R-mediated cytotoxic activity of human monocytes. J Immunol 1990;144:3046–3051.

507. Thomas E, Overbaugh J. Delayed cytopathicity of a feline leukemia virus variant is due to four mutations in the transmembrane protein gene. J Virol 1993;67:5724–5732.

508. Tishon A, Borrow P, Evans C, Oldstone MBA. Virus-induced immunosuppression. 1. Age at infection relates to a selective or generalized defect. Virology 1993;195:397–405.

509. Tomar RH, Hennig AK, Oates RP, Yuille MAR, John PA. Serum factors in the progression of human immunodeficiency virus type 1 infection to AIDS. J Clin Lab Anal 1990;4:218–223.

510. Tomkinson BE, Brown MC, Ip SH, Carrabis S, Sullivan JL. Soluble CD8 during T cell activation. J Immunol 1989;142:2230–2236.

511. Tomkinson BE, Wagner DK, Nelson DL, Sullivan JL. Activated lymphocytes during acute Epstein-Barr virus infection. J Immunol 1987;139:3802–3807.

512. Tompkins MB, Ogilvie GK, Gast AM, Franklin R, Weigel R, Tompkins WA. Interleukin-2 suppression in cats naturally infected with feline leukemia virus. J Biol Res Mod 1989;8:86–96.

513. Tosato G. The Epstein-Barr virus and the immune system. Adv Cancer Res 1987;49:75–125.

514. Toy ST, Wheelock EF. In vitro depression of cellular immunity by friend virus leukemic spleen cells. Cell Immunol 1975;17:57–73.

515. Tschachler E, Groh V, Popovic M, et al. Epidermal Langerhans cells: a target for HTLV-III/LAV infection. J Invest Dermatol 1987;88:233–237.

516. Twomey JJ. Abnormalities in the mixed leukocyte reaction during infectious mononucleosis. J Immunol 1974;112:2278–2281.

517. Uehara T, Miyawaki T, Ohta K, Tamaru Y, Yokoi T. Apoptotic cell death of primed CD45RO+ T lymphocytes in Epstein-Barr virus-induced infectious mononucleosis. Blood 1992;80:452–458.

518. Upton C, Macen JL, Schreiber M, McFadden G. Myxoma virus expresses a secreted protein with homology to the tumor necrosis factor receptor gene family that contributes to viral virulence. Virology 1991;184:370–382.

519. Upton C, Mossman K, McFadden G. Encoding of a homolog of the IFN-gamma receptor by myxoma virus. Science 1992;258:1369–1372.

520. vanVlasselaer P, Punnonen J. Transforming growth factor-beta directs IgA switching in human B cells. J Immunol 1992;148:2062–2067.

521. Virelizier JL. Mechanisms of immunodepression induced by viruses: possible role of infected macrophages. Biomedicine 1975;22:255–261.

522. von Pirquet C. Verhalten der kutanen tuberkulin-reaktion wahrend der Masern. Deutsch Med Wochenschr 1908;34:1297–1300.

523. Vyakarnam A, McKeating J, Meager A, Beverley PC. Tumor necrosis factor (alpha,beta) induced by HIV-1 in peripheral blood mononuclear cells potentiate virus replication. AIDS 1990;4:21–27.

524. Wahl SM, Allen JB, Gartner S, et al. HIV-1 and its envelope glycoprotein down-regulate chemotactic ligand receptors and chemotactic function of peripheral blood monocytes. J Immunol 1989;142:3553–3559.

525. Wahl SM, Hunt DA, Wong HL, et al. Transforming growth factor-beta is a potent immunosuppressive agent that inhibits IL-1-dependent lymphocyte proliferation. J Immunol 1988;140:3026–3032.

526. Wahl SM, McCartney-Francis N, Mergenhagen SE. Inflammatory and immunomodulatory roles of TGF-beta. Immunol Today 1989;10:258–262.

527. Wainberg MA, Mills EL. Mechanisms of virus-induced immune suppression. Can Med Assoc J 1985;132:1261–1267.

528. Wainberg MA, Numazaki K, Destephano L, Wong I, Goldman H. Infection of human thymic epithelial cells by human cytomegalovirus and other viruses: effect on secretion of interleukin 1-like activity. Clin Exp Immunol 1988;72:415–421.

529. Wainberg MA, Portnoy JD, Clecner B, et al. Viral inhibition of lymphocyte proliferative responsiveness in patients suffering from recurrent lesions caused by herpes simplex virus. J Infect Dis 1985;152:441–448.

530. Ward BJ, Griffin DE. Changes in cytokine production after measles virus vaccination: predominant production of IL-4 suggests induction of a Th2 response. Clin Immunol Immunopathol 1993;67:171–177.

531. Ward BJ, Johnson RT, Vaisberg A, Jauregui E, Griffin DE. Spontaneous proliferation of peripheral mononuclear cells in natural measles virus infection: identification of dividing cells and correlation with mitogen responsiveness. Clin Immunol Immunopathol 1990;55:315–326.

532. Ward BJ, Johnson RT, Vaisberg A, Jauregui E, Griffin DE. Cytokine production in vitro and the lymphoproliferative defect of natural measles virus infection. Clin Immunol Immunopathol 1991;61:236–248.

533. Warr GA, Jakab GJ. Alterations in lung macrophage antimicrobial activity associated with viral pneumonia. Infect Immun 1979; 26:492–497.

534. Warr GA, Jakab GJ, Chan TW, Tsan MF. Effects of viral pneumonia on lung macrophage lysosomal enzymes. Infect Immun 1979;24:577–579.

535. Washburn RG, Tuazon CU, Bennett JE. Phagocytic and fungicidal activity of monocytes from patients with acquired immunodeficiency syndrome. J Infect Dis 1985;151:565–566.

536. Weaver CT, Hawrylowicz CM, Unanue ER. T helper cell subsets require the expression of distinct costimulatory signals by antigen-presenting cells. Proc Natl Acad Sci U S A 1988;85:8181–8185.

537. Weigle KA, Sumaya CV, Montiel MM. Changes in T lymphocyte subsets during childhood Epstein-Barr virus infectious mononucleosis. J Clin Immunol 990;3:151–155.

538. Weinhold KJ, Lyerly HK, Stanley SD, Austin AA, Matthews TJ, Bolognesi DP. HIV-1 GP120-mediated immune suppression and lymphocyte destruction in the absence of viral infection. J Immunol 1989;142:3091–3097.

539. Wesley A, Coovadia HM, Henderson L. Immunological recovery after measles. Clin Exp Immunol 1978;32:540–544.

540. Westendorp MO, Frank R, Ochsenbauer C, et al. Sensitization of T cells to CD95-mediated apoptosis by HIV-1 Tat and gp120. Nature 1995;375:497–500.

541. Westwater JS. Tuberculin allergy in acute infectious diseases: a study of the intracutaneous test. Quart J Med 1935;4:203–225.

542. White RG, Boyd JF. The effect of measles on the thymus and other lymphoid tissue. Clin Exp Immunol 1973;13:343–357.

543. Whitley RJ, Soong S-J, Linneman C Jr, et al. Herpes simplex: clinical assessment. J Am Med Assoc 1982;247:317–320.

544. Wilt SG, Milward E, Shou JM, et al. In vitro evidence for a dual role of TNF alpha in HIV-1 encephalopathy. Ann Neurol 1995;37:381–394.

545. Winslow GM, Scherer MT, Kappler JW, Marrack P. Detection and biochemical characterization of the mouse mammary tumor virus 7 superantigen (Mls-la). Cell 1992;171:719–130.

546. Woldehiewt Z, Sharma R. Evidence of immunosuppression by bovine respiratory syncytial virus. Scand J Immunol 1992;11:75–80.

547. Woodruff JF, Woodruff JJ. Virus-induced alterations of lymphoid tissues. I. Modification of the recirculating pool of small lymphocytes by Newcastle disease virus. Cell Immunol 1970;1:333–354.

548. Woodruff JF, Woodruff JJ. Prolonged allograft survival in Newcastle disease virus-treated mice. Infect Immun 1974;9:969–970.

549. Wong HL, Lotze MT, Wahl LM, Wahl SM. Administration of recombinant IL-4 to humans regulates gene expression, phenotype, and function in circulating monocytes. J Immunol 1992;148:2118–2125.

550. Wong HL, Welch GR, Brandes ME, Wahl SM. IL-4 antagonizes induction of Fc-gamma-RIII (CD16) expression by transforming growth factor-beta on human monocytes. J Immunol 1991;147:1843–1848.

551. Woodland DL, Lund FE, Happ MP, Blackman MA, Palmer E, Corley RB. Endogenous superantigen expression is controlled by mouse mammary tumor proviral loci. J Exp Med 1991;174:1255–1258.

552. Wrann M, Bodmer S, deMartin R, et al. T cell suppressor factor from human glioblastoma cells is a 12.5-kd protein closely related to transforming growth factor-beta. EMBO J 1987;6:1633–1636.

553. Wu-Hsieh B, Howard DH, Ahmed R. Virus-induced immunosuppression: a murine model of susceptibility to opportunistic infection. J Infect Dis 1988;158:232–235.

554. Yarchoan R, Redfield RR, Broder S. Mechanisms of B cell activation in patients with acquired immunodeficiency syndrome and related disorders. J Clin Invest 1986;78:439–447.

555. York IA, Roop C, Andrews DW, Riddell SR, Graham FL, Johnson DC. A cytosolic herpes simplex virus protein inhibits antigen presentation to CD8+ T lymphocytes. Cell 1994;77:525–535.

556. Yoshida H, Sumichika H, Hamano S, et al. Induction of apoptosis of T cells by infecting mice with murine cytomegalovirus. J Virol 1995;69:4769–4775.

557. Yoshioka K, Miyata H, Maki S. Transient remission of juvenile rheumatoid arthritis after measles. Acta Paediatr Scand 1981;70:419–420.

558. Zagury D, Bernard J, Leonard R, et al. Long-term cultures of HTLV-III-infected T cells: a model of cytopathology of T-cell depletion in AIDS. Science 1986;231:850–853.

559. Zambruno G, Mori L, Marconi A, et al. Detection of HIV-1 in epidermal Langerhans cells of HIV-infected patients using the polymerase chain reaction. J Invest Dermatol 1991;96:979–982.

560. Zauli G, Davis BR, Re MC, Visani G, Furlini G, LaPlaca M. tat protein stimulates production of transforming growth factor-beta-1 by marrow macrophageΔs: a potential mechanism for human immunodeficiency virus-1-induced hematopoietic suppression. Blood 1992; 80:3036–3043.

561. Zinkernagel RM, Hengartner H. Virally induced immunosuppression. Curr Opin Immunol 1992;4:408–412.

562. Zinkernagel RM, Hengartner H. T-cell-mediated immunopathology versus direct cytolysis by virus-implication for HIV and AIDS. Immunol Today 1994;15:262–268.

563. Zweiman B, Pappagianis D, Maibach H, Hildreth EA. Effect of measles immunization on tuberculin hypersensitivity and in vitro lymphocyte reactivity. Int Arch Allergy Appl Immunol 1971;40: 834–841.

Viral Pathogenesis,
edited by Neal Nathanson, et al.
Lippincott–Raven Publishers, Philadelphia © 1997

CHAPTER 11

Retroviral Oncogenesis

Hsing-Jien Kung and Juinn-Lin Liu

INTRODUCTION

Retroviruses induce a variety of diseases, including acquired immunodeficiency syndrome (AIDS) and cancers. The cancer-inducing retroviruses, or oncornaviruses, are prevalent in nature and have been isolated from virtually every species in which viral isolation has been attempted. The oncornaviruses differ substantially in their oncogenic potency, tumor tropisms, latency of tumor induction, and mechanisms of oncogenesis. Based on the latency of tumor induction, oncornaviruses can be broadly divided into nonacute transforming retroviruses, acute transforming retroviruses, and trans-acting transforming viruses. Nonacute retroviruses induce neoplasia after a long incubation period of months to decades, and the tumors induced are of monoclonal or oligoclonal origin. This is also the case with trans-acting retroviruses, the two prominent examples of which are human T-cell leukemia virus

H. J. Kung: Department of Molecular Biology and Microbiology, Case Western Reserve University, Cleveland, Ohio 44106-4960.

J. L. Liu: Department of Molecular Biology and Microbiology, Case Western Reserve University, Cleveland, Ohio 44106-4960.

(HTLV) and bovine leukemia virus (BLV). In contrast, it takes acute retroviruses only weeks to induce polyclonal tumors in experimental animals. Although classification based on latency is not always reliable, because it depends on viral titer, host genetic background, and other external factors, increasing evidence suggests that these groups differ fundamentally in their mechanisms of oncogenesis (discussed later) and can be differentiated by their genome structure. As described later, most of the retroviruses that are widespread in nature are either nonacute or trans-acting retroviruses; both types are replication competent and have lifelong association with the hosts. The acute retroviruses are mostly products of laboratory manipulation and are derived from nonacute retroviruses through recombination with host protooncogenes. All these acute viruses induce neoplastic transformation by perturbing the growth machinery and deregulating the growth signals of the host. Historically, these are the viruses that have helped researchers uncover oncogenes and protooncogenes. In the past decade, research in the areas of oncornaviruses have greatly affected the understanding of signal transduction and oncogenic processes. In this chapter, we first focus on the mechanisms of oncogenesis by oncornaviruses and then present representative examples to illustrate the oncogenic processes.

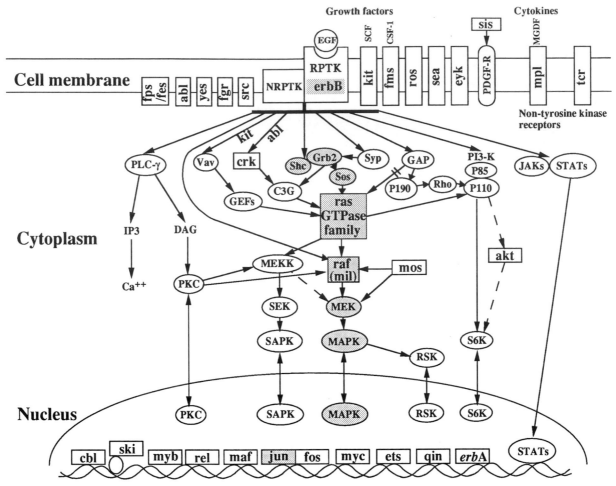

FIG. 11-1. Signal transduction pathways involved in retroviral oncogenesis. On ligand stimulation, receptor protein tyrosine kinases (RPTKs) such as erbB, kit, and fms (*open rectangles on the cell membrane*), become dimerized, phosphorylated, and activated. The activated RPTKs, along with associated non–receptor protein tyrosine kinases (NRPTKs) such as src, fgr, and yes (*small rectangles on the left side of the cell membrane*), then trigger a network of signal transduction pathways through different SH2-containing downstream substrates and effectors. Only the pathways involved in retroviral oncogenes are illustrated. The major pathway mediated through the Shc/Grb2-Sos-ras-raf-MEK-MAPK cascade is shaded and is discussed in detail in the text. Other pathways include ras–GTPase accelerating protein (ras-GAP). This pathway's main function is to downregulate ras activity, but it can also turn on the phosphatidylinositol 3-kinase (PI3-K) through p190 and Rho.[336,357] P85, a subunit of PI3-K, binds to RPTK, and the p110 catalytic subunit is then activated to engage in the turnover of phospholipid; the final product, phosphatidylinositol-1,4,5-triphosphate (PIP3) is involved in actin rearrangement and vesicular trafficking.[192a,425a] In addition, p110 can also activate S6K.[71,77] Phospholipase C-γ (PLC-γ) breaks down phosphatidylinositol-4,5-diphosphate (PIP2) to 1,2-diacylglycerol (DAG) and 1,4,5-triphosphate (IP3). DAG stimulates protein kinase C (PKC) kinase activity, whereas IP3 increases the release of intracellular calcium. The Janus kinase (JAK) family of PTKs utilizes a novel pathway in which their downstream targets, signal transducers and activators of transcription (STATs), are phosphorylated and translocated into nucleus to bind to the interferon-gamma (IFN-γ) response elements. Protein tyrosine phosphatase (PTPase) or SH2-containing tyrosine phosphatase (SYP) can behave like Shc to serve as a bridge factor to interact with Grb2.[240] Vav is an adapter protein specifically expressed in hematopoietic cells and is associated with guanine nucleotide exchange factors (GEFs) to activate the ras pathway.[145] Crk is preferentially activated by abl,[330] and it can enhance ras activity through C3G, a GEF.[398] Akt has been implicated in the PI3-K and S6K signaling pathway,[118] whereas mos has been shown to be the activator of raf and MEK.

The final destination of signal transduction pathways is the nucleus, where transcription factors are phosphorylated by upstream kinases to regulate the expression of genes involved in growth and differentiation. Therefore, it is not surprising that many of the retroviral oncogenes have turned out to be transcription factors, such as jun, fos, and myc. Rectangular boxes indicate signal molecules originally identified as retroviral oncogenes.

RETROVIRUSES AS CARCINOGENS AND MUTAGENS

It is necessary to consider briefly why retroviruses represent a major class of oncogenic viruses and what properties make retroviruses such effective carcinogens. In Chapter 26, the properties and replication of avian and murine retroviruses is discussed in more detail. There are two features that distinguish retroviruses from other viruses and make them potent carcinogens. First, many retroviruses have evolved ways to coexist with the host cells, and unlike most other RNA viruses, they are not cytotoxic or cytolytic to the infected cells. Second, all retroviruses are equipped with integration machinery as part of their replication cycle, and they can efficiently and stably associate with host chromosomes. The survival of the infected cells and the genetic stability of oncogenic information are fundamental requirements for neoplastic transformation. In addition, the retroviruses replicate through both RNA and DNA intermediates. Retroviruses have the high mutation and recombination rates of RNA viruses and the strong promoters of DNA viruses. All these contribute to the oncogenic properties of retroviruses. Furthermore, in comparison with chemical mutagens or carcinogens, retroviruses are much more effective and versatile, because a retroviral mutagen is self-propagating and contains regulatory elements that affect gene expression. The presence of viral sequences that are integrated into the host genome not only disrupts host genes but also profoundly affects the transcription and translation of host genes, some of which are several kilobases distant. Together, these properties make retroviruses potent carcinogens.

CELL GROWTH AND SIGNAL TRANSDUCTION

Before the detailed mechanisms of oncogenesis by oncornaviruses is described, it may be helpful to review the concept of growth signals in normal cells. It is generally postulated that subversion of the normal growth pathways by mutations and activations of key signal molecules or protooncogenes can lead to abnormal growth, which is an important step in neoplastic transformation.

The control of cell growth and differentiation is governed by highly intricate and exquisitely controlled signal transduction pathways.[61] Figure 11-1 presents an updated summary of the current understanding of these pathways. Figure 11-1 serves to emphasize the connection between retroviral oncogenesis and perturbation of signal transduction pathways. Only a selected few of these pathways are discussed in detail in this chapter.

The growth signals are a phosphorylation cascade transmitted from cytoplasm to nucleus, from tyrosine kinases to protein serine/threonine kinases (PS/TKs), and from receptors to transcription factors. A growth signal begins with the binding of growth factors such as epidermal growth factor (EGF) to cell surface receptors such as the erbB/EGF receptor. The receptor then dimerizes and is activated and autophosphorylated.[64,112,350,420] The activated kinase domain of the receptor can bind immediate substrates, such as nonreceptor protein tyrosine kinases,[91,214] protein tyrosine phosphatase,[225,239] phospholipase C gamma (PLC-γ),[255,261] phosphatidylinositol

3-kinase (PI-3K),[36,110,306] GAP,[193,195,243] Janus kinase–signal transducers and activators of transcription (JAK/STATs),[95,177,445] Shc,[316,344] and Grb2,[56,246,343,373] and often phosphorylates them. Although they are diverse in structure and function, a common feature of these substrates is the presence of an src-homology 2 domain, which is recognized by phosphorylated tyrosine residues.[86,201,311a,349] The binding of these molecules to activated receptor or nonreceptor kinases translocates them to plasma membrane and initiates the signal transduction process. For the sake of brevity, we illustrate this process using Grb2/ras/raf/MEK/MAPK as an example. Grb2 is an adapter molecule that connects activated receptor kinases to Sos or guanine nucleotide exchange factor,[44,56,68,108,128,239] which in turn activates ras by converting it from the GTP-bound inactive form to the GTP-bound state. Ras-GTP then activates a group of PS/TKs, such as raf-1 and MEKK (MAPK/ERK kinase kinase).* Subsequently, these PS/TKs activate a family of dual kinases, collectively called MAPK/ERK kinase (MEK) and SAPK/ERK kinase (SEK).[100,174,215,256,347,451,459] MEK/SEKs can phosphorylate both tyrosine and threonine residues and in so doing activate yet another group of PS/TKs, including mitogen-activated protein kinase (MAPK), also called extracellular signal-regulated kinase (ERK),[40,220,331,332] stress-activated protein kinase (SAPK), and jun N-terminal kinase.[97,99,160,216,265,444] MAPK, and presumably SAPK, can translocate into nucleus and phosphorylate key transcription factors involved in growth and differentiation. Thus, MAPK phosphorylates transcription factor elk, which activates the transcription of fos,[183,211] and SAPK activates transcription factor jun.[216] Jun and fos form a heterodimer that binds to AP-1 motif, an enhancer present in the promoters of a number of genes.[8,93] Presumably, some of these genes are crucial components that trigger DNA synthesis and cell division. This completes one of the circuits of signal transduction. Other parallel circuits are provided by signals initiated from PLC-γ, PI-3 kinase, and JAK/STATs, which also end up in the nucleus and function to activate genes.

MECHANISMS OF ONCOGENESIS

Nonacute Retroviruses

As described previously, the nonacute retroviruses are naturally abundant and have been isolated from many species, including humans. Nonacute retroviruses cause a variety of cancers; leukemias and lymphomas are the most prevalent (Table 11-1). All these viruses are replication competent and contain a full complement of viral replicative and structural genes. Some of these viruses have additional open reading frames and accessory proteins, but none of them have incorporated sequences of completely cellular origin, in stark contrast to acute retroviruses. The nonacute retroviruses induce cancers by integrating their viral DNA at or near host protooncogenes or genes involved in growth control, a process referred to as insertional mutagenesis. As a result, host protooncogenes are transcriptionally activated or deregulated. In some cases, the protooncogene product is structurally altered as a result of

---

* References 102, 203, 272, 419, 432, 436, 446, 448, 457.

TABLE 11-1. *Common insertion sites in nonacute retrovirus-mediated oncogenesis*

Action	Class	Locus	Retrovirus	Neoplasia/tumor cell line (species)	Predominant mode of activation	References
Activation	GF/cytokine	CSF-1	MuLV (Ecotropic)	Monocyte-macrophage tumor (m)	E	20, 21
		GM-CSF	R-MuLV	Myeloid precursor line DIND4 (m)	E	387
			SFFV	Myeloid precursor lines DIND5,9(m)	E	387
			IAP	Myeloid precursor line DIND1 (m)/ WEHI-274 cell line (m)	E	107, 156, 229, 387
		IL-2	GaLV	T-leukemic cell line MLA144 (a)	E	73, 168
		IL-3	IAP	Myelomonocytic leukemia cell lines(m)/ mast cell tumor (m)	E	107, 156, 167, 229, 386, 453
		IL-5	IAP	Hematopoietic progenitor cell line K-5 (m)		402
		IL-6	IAP	Plasmacytoma (m)		38
		k-FGF/hst-1	MMTV	Mammary carcinoma (m)	E	320, 358
		wnt-1/int-1	MMTV	Mammary carcinoma (m)	E	79, 299–301
		FGF-3/int-2	MMTV	Mammary carcinoma (m)	E	79, 299–301
		FGF-8	MMTV	Mammary carcinoma (wnt-1 transgenic m)		79, 80, 103, 104, 319, 320, 358
		int-3	MMTV	Mammary carcinoma (m)	E	250
		wnt-3/int-4	MMTV	Mammary carcinoma (m)		129
		wnt-4/int-5	MMTV	Mammary carcinoma (m)		298, 337
			MMTV	Mammary carcinoma (m)		277
	Receptor	CD8-α/lyt-2	SL3-3	T-lymphoma cell line (m)	E	10
		EPO R	SFFV	Erythroleukemia (m)	3'P or 5'P	163, 217
		IL-2 R	IAP	EL-4 T-lymphoma cell line (m)		208
		IL-6 R	IAP	Plasmacytoma (m)		390
		IL-9 R/Gfi-2	MCF/xenotropic	T-lymphoma cell line (r)		116
		Prolactin R	M-MuLV	T lymphoma (r)		17
	RPTK	c-erbB	RAV-1 (ALV)	Erythroblastosis (ch)	5'P	127, 264, 296
		evi-2	BXH2-MuLV	Myeloid tumor (m)	5'P, 3'P, E	55
		C-FMS/FIM-2	F-MuLV	Myeloblastic leukemia (m)	E	138
	PTK	c-fes	HIV	T lymphoma (h)		367
		c-lck/fps	M-MuLV	LSTRAT-cell line (m)	5'P	4, 257, 453
			M-MuLV	T lymphoma (r)	3'P or 5'P	366
	PS/TK	tpl-2	M-MuLV	T lymphoma (m)		252
		cyclin D1/fis-1	F-MuLV	Lymphoma (m)		219, 370
		cyclin D2/vin-1	BL/VL3 RadLV	T leukemia (m,r)		150, 405
		c-mos	IAP	Plasmacytoma (m)		86, 133, 435
		pim-1	M-MuLV/MCF-MuLV	B lymphoma (Eμ-myc transgenic m)	E	94, 280, 354
			M-MuLV (SV40-E)	Erythroleukemia (m)	E	149, 153, 424
			F-MuLV	T lymphoma (c)		106
			FeLV			408
	GTPase	c-Ha-ras	MAV (ALV)	Nephroblastoma (ch)	3'P or 5'P	176, 315, 378, 442
			M-MuLV	Myelomonocytic leukemia line DA-2(m)	3'P	176
		c-Ki-ras	F-MuLV	Myeloid line 416B (m)	3'P	135, 407
	TF	bmi-1/flvi-2	M-MuLV	B lymphoma (Eμ-myc m)		153, 424
			FeLV/LC-FeLV	T lymphoma (c)		231, 233
		c-ets-1/tpl-1	M-MuLV	T lymphoma (r)		22
		fim-3/CB-1/evi-1	F-MuLV	Myeloblastic leukemia (m)		18, 19, 47

Gene	Virus	Tumor	Insertion site	References
	M-MuLV	Myeloid cell lines DA1,3,34(m)	E	276
	AKXD-23 (ecotropic)	Myeloid tumor (m)		281
	Car-Br-E-MuLV	Non-T, non-B lymphoma (m)		31
fli-1	SFFV/F-MuLV	Erythroleukemia (m)	3'P or 5'P	24, 25, 172, 153
	Cas-Br-E-MuLV	Non-T, non-B lymphoma (m)		31, 32
c-fos	RAV-1 (ALV)	Erythroblastosis (ch)		88
Hox-2,4	IAP	Myeloid leukemia (m)	3'P or 5'P	39, 207
meis-1	MuLV (Ecotropic)	Myeloid leukemia (m)		278
c-myb	RAV-1/EU8 (ALV)	B lymphoma (ch)	5'P	192, 322
	A-MuLV	Plasmacytoid lymphosarcoma (m)	E	288
	Cas-Br-M-MuLV	Myeloid cell line NFS60 (m)	3'P or 5'P	362
	M-MuLV	Myeloid leukemia (m)	5'P	140, 339, 363, 364, 438, 439
	Ampho-4070A/F-MuLV-FB29	Promonocytic leukemia (m)	5'P	283, 447
c-myc	RAV-1,-2 (ALV)/REV/RPV	B lymphoma (ch)	3'	125, 126, 155, 241a, 290, 312, 334, 442
	REV	T lymphoma (ch)	3'P or E	181, 297, 371
	M-MuLV/MCF-MuLV	T lymphoma (m)	E	90, 236, 259, 302, 355, 329
	M-MuLV	T lymphoma (r)	E	223, 224, 383, 411
	F-MuLV	Erythroleukemia (m)		106
	A-MuLV/MSV-3611	Plasmacytoma (m)		360
	IAP	Plasmacytoma (m)	E	144
	FeLV	T lymphoma (c)	E	117, 232, 267, 284, 292
	Kpn-1 repet. element (LINE)	Canine venereal tumor (d)	E	194
	SMRV-H	Burkitt lymphoma line—Namalwa (h)		263
N-myc	M-MuLV	T lymphoma (m)	E	442, 423, 452
	MLRV	Macrophage hybridoma (m)	E	356
	MCF247	T lymphoma (m)		43, 105
	FeLV	T lymphoma (c)		234, 235
PU.1/spi-1/spfi-1	SFFV/F-MuLV/R-MuLV	Erythroleukemia (m)	E	273–275, 311, 381
gfi-1	M-MuLV	T lymphoma (r)		137
c-rel	ALV-F42	Pre-B lymphoma (ch)		190
SCL	IAP	Myeloid cell line-WEHI-3BD (m)	3'P	399
ahi-1	A-MuLV	Pre-B lymphoma (m)		324
asi	A-MuLV	T lymphoma (Eμ-myc-transgenic m)		186
c-bic	RAV-1/UR2AV	Chronic myeloproliferative disease (m)		147
bla-1	M-MuLV	B lymphoma (ch)		83
dsi-1	M-MuLV	B lymphoma (Eμ-myc transgenic m)		424
emi-1	M-MuLV	T lymphoma (r)		427
evi-3	AKXD-MuLV	B lymphoma (Eμ-myc transgenic m)		153
fim-1	Cas-Br-M-MuLV	B lymphoma (m)		189
fit-1	F-MuLV	Pre-B lymphoma cell line (m)		189
flvi-1	FeLV-myc	Myeloid leukemia (m)		377
	FeLV	T lymphoma (c)		416
	FeLV	Spleen lymphoma (c)		230

Others

continued

TABLE 11-1. *Continued*

Action	Class	Locus	Retrovirus	Neoplasia/tumor cell line (species)	Predominant mode of activation	References
		fre-1,2 & 3	F-MuLV	Erythroleukemia (m)		426
		gin-1	G-MuLV	T lymphoma (m)		428
		his-1, his-2	Cas-Br-M/M-MuLV	Myeloid leukemia (m)		12
		int-41	MMTV	Mammary carcinoma (m)/kidney carcinoma (m)		132
	Others	int-6	MMTV	Mammary carcinoma (m)	E	254
		int-H	MMTV	Hyperplastic alveolar nodule (m)		143
		mdr-3	MMTV/IAP	P388 lymphoid tumor (m)		228a
		mis-2	M-MuLV	T leukemia (m)		429
		mis-6	M-MuLV	T lymphoma (Eμ-myc-transgenic m)		186
		mit-1	M-MuLV	T lymphoma (CD2-myc-transgenic m)		384
		mlvi-1/mis-1/pvt-1	M-MuLV	B and T lymphoma (m)	E	202, 412, 413, 430
		mlvi-2	M-MuLV	T lymphoma (r)		414
		mlvi-3	M-MuLV	T lymphoma (r)		414
		mlvi-4	M-MuLV	T lymphoma (m and r)	E or 5'P	223, 411
		mml-1	Ampho-MuLV (4070)	Myeloid leukemia (m)		205
		nov	MAV-1 (ALV)	Nephroblastoma (ch)		187
		pal-1	M-MuLV	B lymphoma (Eμ-myc transgenic m)		424
		pim-2	M-MuLV	T lymphoma (Eμ-myc transgenic m)		51, 153, 424
		tblvi-1	TBLV	T lymphoma (m)		282
Inactivation	TF	NF-E2/fli-2	F-MuLV/SFFV	Erythroleukemia (m)		248
	Tumor suppressor gene	p53	F-MuLV/SFFV	Erythroleukemia (m)		26, 27, 75, 106, 172, 222, 279, 286, 342
			A-MuLV	Pre–B lymphoma (m)		340
			E Tn	Osteosarcoma (m)		266

3'P, 3' long terminal repeat promotion; 5'P, 5' long terminal repeat promotion; a, ape; A-MuLV, Abelson-MuLV; ALV, avian leukosis virus; c, cat; ch, chicken; d, dog; E, enhancer insertion; E Tn, endogenous retrovirus-like element; F-MuLV, Friend murine leukemia virus; FeLV, feline leukemia virus; G-MuLV, Gross-MuLV; GaLV, Gibbon ape leukemia virus; GF, growth factor; GM-CSF, granulocyte-macrophage colony-stimulating factor; h, human; HIV, human immunodeficiency virus; IAP, intracisternal A particles; IL, interleukin; m, mouse; M-MuLV, Moloney murine leukemia virus; MCF, mink cell focus-inducing virus; MLRV, Moloney MuLV-like retrovirus; MMTV, mouse mammary tumor virus; MuLV, murine leukemia virus; PS/TK, protein protein serine/threonine kinase; PTK, protein tyrosine kinase; r, rat; R-MuLV, REV, reticuloendotheliosis virus; RPTK, receptor protein tyrosine kinase, RPV, Ring-neck pheasant virus; SFFV, spleen focus-forming virus; SMRV-H, Squirrel-mouse retrovirus-H; TBLV, Type B leukemogenic virus; TF, transcription factor.

viral DNA insertion. There is also at least one instance in which a tumor suppressor gene is inactivated. All these features contribute to genetic alterations that unleash growth controls and lead to neoplastic transformation. Insertional mutagenesis is reviewed elsewhere.[13,213,311a,410,421]

Table 11-1 lists the protooncogenes identified as common insertion sites in individual neoplasms caused by nonacute retroviruses. At least 79 such sites have been identified; many of these encode homologs of viral oncogenes previously identified in acute transforming viruses (Table 11-2; discussed later). Other activated loci represent genes that were unknown before their discovery as nonacute retroviral common insertion sites but subsequently have been shown to have oncogenic properties. Indeed, retrovirus tagging is used as a general method to identify novel oncogenes. Several other features of Table 11-1 are noteworthy. First, all four types of retroviruses—type A (e.g., intracisternal A particles), B (e.g., mouse mammary tumor virus [MMTV]), C (e.g., avian leukosis virus [ALV]) and D (e.g., simian type D retrovirus)—can serve as insertional mutagens and are involved in protooncogene activation.[85] Second, different viruses can induce similar tumors by interacting with the same oncogene (e.g., ALV+, reticuloendotheliosis virus (REV), and ring-neck pheasant virus (RPV) induce B-cell lymphomas by activating c-*myc*). Third, a single virus can induce different kinds of neoplasia by interacting with different oncogenes (e.g., ALV can induce B-cell lymphoma and erythroblastosis by activating c-*myc* and c-*erb*B protooncogenes, respectively). Thus, tissue-specific transformation is mediated by activation of specific oncogenes, and the oncogenic spectrum of a nonacute retrovirus is determined not only by the viral tissue tropism, which is usually controlled by the viral env gene or long terminal repeat (LTR), but also by the particular oncogenes that the virus is capable of activating. Finally, multiple protooncogenes may be identified in a given type of tumor. For example, in murine T-cell lymphoma, c-*myc*, N-*myc*, *pim*-1, and *pim*-2 are potential oncogenes. These represent either oncogenes functioning in different stages of T-cell lineage or cooperating oncogenes acting in the same T cell to effect transformation.

Insertional Activation of Protooncogenes

Retroviral DNA carries two LTRs at the termini. The LTR contains a promoter, an enhancer, and a poly(A) signal (see Chap. 26) used for the efficient expression of viral RNA; when properly juxtaposed with cellular genes, the LTR can significantly enhance the expression of cellular genes. In addition, the virus carries efficient splice sites and translational start sites, as well as signal sequences that could facilitate the processing of the messages and the proteins. These features make retroviral DNAs powerful insertional mutagens. There are three major pathways by which a retrovirus can insertionally activate host protooncogenes.

5′ Long Terminal Repeat Promotion (Readthrough Activation). During retrovirus replication, the viral RNA is first reverse transcribed into a DNA molecule with its terminal sequences duplicated (i.e., the 5′ and 3′LTR). The linear DNA molecule is then integrated into the host genome and serves as the template for transcription (see Chap. 26).[249] The 5′LTR is used in this process as a promoter, and the transcription begins at the U3/R boundary and proceeds along and beyond the viral

genome. The poly(A) signal present at the 3′LTR then directs the cleavage and polyadenylation of the RNA at the R/U5 boundary, giving rise to the genomic RNA. Occasionally, however, the cleavage at the 3′LTR is bypassed, and a downstream poly(A) site belonging to the adjacent cellular sequences is used instead. In this case, a cellular gene adjoining the integration site is transcribed and expressed. It is estimated that of all the 5′LTR-directed transcripts, about 10% to 15% escape polyadenylation with the potential to activate a downstream host gene.[158] Considering the extraordinary strength of retroviral 5′LTR, which can produce as many as 10,000 copies of viral RNA per cell, the 10% level is not trivial. Several protooncogenes are activated in this fashion (see Table 11-1; 5′P). We use the activation of EGF receptor locus by ALV in erythroleukemia as an example of readthrough activation.

The EGF receptor, or *erb*B, is a transmembrane protein involved in growth of many cell types, including erythroblasts in chickens.[307] The entire locus has 28 exons and can be separated into extracellular and intracellular halves by the transmembrane domain.[59] The intracellular domain contains a tyrosine kinase domain and, when activated, phosphorylates signal molecules and turns on a growth pathway. This activation requires ligand stimulation and dimerization. In avian erythroleukemia, ALV DNA integrates in intron 16 and disrupts the continuity of the receptor.[127,326,335] By the 5′LTR promotion mechanism, a transcript that carries the entire viral genome and exons 17 to 28 of *erb*B is generated.[296] This transcript is then processed via the viral gag 5′ splice site and the 3′ splice site of erbB exon 17. As a consequence, the AUG translational start site of the viral gag gene is inframe spliced into the erbB gene, which facilitates its translation and processing.[54] This decapitated receptor kinase no longer binds ligand and is constitutively active and leukemogenic when placed in a retroviral vector.[226,289,317,368,369] This example shows that retroviral DNA can truncate a gene by insertion, transcriptionally activate a gene by the provision of its 5′LTR, and translationally activate a gene by the provision of a viral translational initiation site via inframe splicing.

In addition to erbB activation, there are numerous examples of 5′LTR promotion (see Table 11-1). In every case in which complete information is available, the protooncogene product is truncated, and the initiation codon of the truncated protein is provided by viral sequences through inframe splicing. Those protooncogenes that require N-terminal truncation to enhance their activity are frequently the target of 5′LTR promotion. To achieve 5′LTR promotion and to effectively transcribe the gene, the proviral DNA must be inserted upstream from and in the same orientation as the protooncogene sequence (Fig. 11-2).

3′ Long Terminal Repeat Promotion (Promoter Insertion). Given the sequence identity of the 5′LTR and the 3′LTR, it is not surprising to find that the 3′LTR is also capable of activating host protooncogenes; however, examples of this kind are infrequent (see Table 11-1; 3′P). One of the first and perhaps the best example is c-*myc* activation by ALV and REV DNA in B-cell lymphomas (see Fig. 11-2).[127,155,290, 297,312,334] In these cases, the proviruses are situated upstream from the coding exons (second and third exons) of c-*myc*, and the majority are oriented in the same direction as c-*myc*. Many of the proviruses suffer deletions of the viral sequences close to or at the 5′LTR.[126,139,291,313,334,395] The 3′LTR remains intact and is used to transcribe the c-*myc* gene to a level 20- to 50-fold higher than normal.[155] It is thought that this high level is due to the strong

5' LTR promotion (readthrough activation)

ALV erythroleukemia

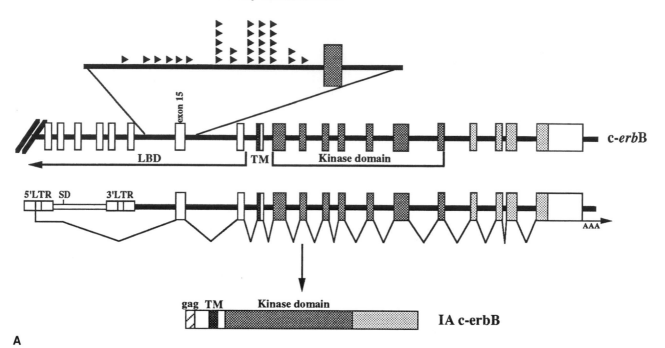

3'LTR promotion (promoter insertion)

ALV B-lymphoma

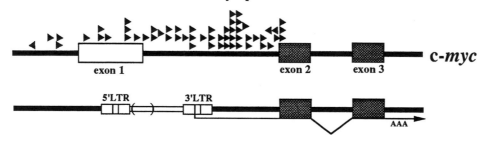

Enhancer insertion

MMTV Mammary tumor

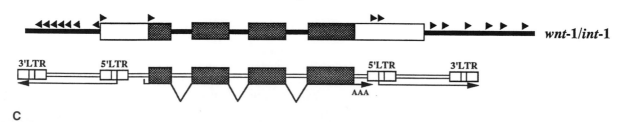

FIG. 11-2.

3'LTR promoter as well as the removal of negative regulatory elements residing in the first exon/intron, which is a polymerase pausing site.[380] The c-*myc* gene is nevertheless translated with the authentic initiation codon, and as such, the gene product is identical to the normal myc protein. Thus, deregulation of its expression, rather than structural alteration of the gene product, underlies the mechanism for c-*myc* activation.

Because the position and the orientation of the provirus relative to the protooncogene are the same for both the 5'LTR and 3'LTR promotion, the immediate questions are how does the provirus differentiate these two promoters, and why does the provirus use 5'LTR promoter to activate some genes such as c-*erb*B and 3'LTR promoter for others such as c-*myc*? To answer the first question, it is necessary to consider how the provirus is transcribed into viral genomic and message RNAs. As described previously, the 5'LTR and 3'LTR serve different roles in viral transcription; the former is the sole promoter, and the latter provides the poly(A) signal. It is estimated that, during viral transcription, the 5'LTR is used about 50 times more often than the 3'LTR, despite their complete sequence identity.[158] As a result, viral transcription is greatly favored over transcription of the downstream cellular sequence. It has long been recognized that when two promoters are situated in tandem, the transcription from the upstream promoter interferes with that of the downstream promoter, presumably by blocking the accessibility of transcription factors and polymerase II to the downstream promoter.[3,92] This is called promoter occlusion, and it makes the upstream promoter stronger than the downstream promoter by about 10-fold. Another factor that contributes to the different strengths of the 5'LTR and 3'LTR is the presence of viral internal sequences, usually in the gag leader, that unidirectionally enhance the strength of the 5'LTR promoter but not the 3'LTR. This was first reported in the avian REV genome[41] and has since been extended to MuLV.[130] The nature of this type of activator sequence is unclear, but its function in a position- and orientation-dependent manner bears resemblance to the TAR sequence of human immunodeficiency virus (HIV), which suggests that it may be an RNA enhancer.[359] The combination of promoter interference and the presence of a putative RNA enhancer close to the 5'LTR contribute to the 50-fold increase in power of the 5'LTR over the 3'LTR promoters in the intact provirus. This is perhaps why proviruses involved in 3'LTR promotion of the c-*myc* gene suffer deletions close to or at the 5'LTR with little transcription from the 5'LTR.[139,155,395] In one detailed study, the defective provirus with the adjoining c-*myc* gene was cloned and the missing viral sequence restored.[41] The restored provirus contained an 87-nucleotide putative RNA enhancer, had high 5'LTR activity, and could no longer activate c-*myc* expression by the 3'LTR. These experiments suggest that a requirement for 3'LTR promotion is the removal of 5'LTR activity by proviral deletion. This added step may explain why 3' LTR promotion mode of protooncogene activation is less frequently observed than 5'LTR promotion.

FIG. 11-2. The mechanisms of insertional activation of protooncogenes by retroviruses. There are three major mechanisms that retroviruses utilize to insertionally activate protooncogenes. (**A**) 5' long terminal repeat (5´LTR) promotion, or readthrough activation, is often associated with cases in which truncation of the protooncogene is necessary for its activation. The example illustrated here is avian leukosis virus (ALV) provirus activation of the c-erbB locus. The 30 leukemic samples analyzed (*triangles*) are all integrated in exon 15 and are in the same orientation as the c-erbB gene. these insertions disrupt the continuity of exons encoding the ligand binding domain (LBD). The transmembrane (TM) and the kinase domain are all downstream from the insertion sites. The inserted provirus is intact, with 5'LTR, 3'LTR, and splice donor (SD) site present. Transcription is initiated in the 5'LTR and proceeds through the entire viral genome, TM, and kinase domain exons, all the way to the end of the c-erbB locus. Splicing joins the viral SD site to the acceptor of c-erbB exon 16. This joins six amino acids of gag and the remaining erbB sequence containing transmembrane and the entire intracellular domain. This "decapitated" receptor molecule no longer binds ligand and is constitutively active. (**B**) The 3'LTR promotion mode of activation is associated with cases in which a high level of expression of the protooncogene is necessary for oncogenesis. The use of the 3'LTR promoter usually gives a 50-fold or higher augmented expression of the protooncogene. The example illustrated is ALV insertional activation of the c-myc gene. Among the 56 B-lymphoma samples analyzed, all the proviruses (*solid triangles*) are integrated upstream from exon 2 of c-myc. Because exon 1 is a noncoding exon, none of the integrations disrupt the coding sequences. The great majority of proviruses are oriented in the same transcriptional direction as the c-myc locus. The transcription of the c-myc gene starts in the 3'LTR promoter. The resulting transcripts contain RU5 of ALV LTR and exons 2 and 3 of c-myc. No other viral sequences are transcribed. Interestingly, the majority of the proviruses involved in 3'LTR promotion suffer internal deletions (*brackets*) close to or at the 5'LTR, which often result in the shut-off of 5'LTR promoter activity, eliminating the interference of the 3'LTR promotion by the 5'LTR directed transcription. (**C**) Enhancer insertion. The LTRs contain enhancer elements that can bind transcription factors or factors engaged in transcription machinery to facilitate transcription. This mode of activation does not possess stringent requirements for position, orientation, or distance. Thus, enhancer insertion represents by far the most prevalent mode of insertional activation of protooncogenes. As shown for the insertional activation of wnt-1/int-1 locus by mouse mammary tumor virus (MMTV), the proviruses are integrated either upstream or downstream of the gene. In most cases, the activated wnt-1/int-1 transcripts are initiated from the natural cellular promoter, and the transcript size is the same as the normal counterpart, except that the transcription level is significantly higher. Triangles indicate the insertion sites and the orientations of the proviruses within individual tumors. Arrowheads represent the direction of transcription. ( ), deletion; $\vee$, splicing; AAA, poly(A) signal.

The question of why the virus must go through the additional deletion step to use 3'LTR promotion when 5'LTR promotion is also capable of activating a protooncogene such as c-*erb*B remains. The answer may lie in the level of expression that can be achieved by these two activation schemes. The overexpression of c-*myc* by 3'LTR promotion in B-cell lymphoma is much higher than that of *erb*B by 5'LTR promotion in erythroleukemia. Only 10% to 15% of the 5'LTR transcripts escape the viral poly(A) signal and have the potential to activate the downstream protooncogene, whereas all 3'LTR-directed transcripts, in the absence of 5'LTR interference, are potential protooncogene transcripts. Thus, in cases in which a high level of protooncogene expression is needed, 3'LTR promotion is selected. Conversely, 3'LTR-directed transcripts do not contain any viral translational and splicing signals. In cases in which the protooncogene coding sequence is interrupted, requiring an exogenous initiation codon, 5'LTR promotion is the only mechanism that can provide a translatable oncogene product.

Enhancer Insertion. Enhancers are DNA sequences that bind transcription factors or activators, engaging RNA polymerase in and facilitating transcription.[196] They exert the enhancing effect in a position- and orientation-independent manner and over a long distance, sometimes more than hundreds of kilobases. Retrovirus LTRs contain many enhancer motifs,[111,249] and their insertions have the potential to activate the adjacent cellular promoters. The proviruses involved do not have as stringent position, orientation, and distance requirements as in LTR promotion. Perhaps as a consequence, enhancer insertion represents the most prevalent mode of insertional activation of protooncogenes (see Table 11-1; E). As shown for the insertional activation of *wnt*-1/*int*-1 locus by MMTV, the proviruses are integrated upstream or downstream from the gene (see Fig. 11-2). In most cases, the activated *wnt*-1/*int*-1 transcripts are initiated from the natural cellular promoter, and the transcript size is the same as that of the normal counterpart. The wnt-1/int-1 protein in tumor cells is identical to that in normal cells, except the level is significantly higher. In some cases, the insertions are located within the 3' untranslated region of the protooncogene and in the same transcriptional direction, the transcript being cleaved at the poly(A) site of the 5'LTR. Such a truncation of the 3' untranslated sequences of the protooncogene may enhance expression at the posttranscriptional level by providing a more efficient viral poly(A) signal or by removing the instability element of cellular messages.[361] Although isolated enhancers function in an orientation-independent manner, the proviruses apparently have preferences. For example, the majority of proviruses flanking the wnt-1/int-1 locus are directed away from the locus. It is postulated that enhancer sequences work best for a promoter that is encountered first in cis. The other orientations would interpose the promoter of MMTV LTR in between the *wnt*-1/*int*-1 promoter and the viral enhancer. This may explain the nonrandom orientation of proviruses involved in enhancer insertion of protooncogenes.

Insertional Inactivation of the Tumor Suppressor Gene

Oncogenesis is usually induced by a combination of activation of protooncogenes and inactivation of tumor suppressor genes. As Table 11-1 shows, there are numerous examples

of protooncogene activation by proviruses, and there are far fewer cases of tumor suppressor gene inactivation by proviruses. Thus far, only p53 gene inactivation by A-MuLV,[340] F-MuLV[†] and endogenous retrovirus-like element (E Tn)[266] have been reported. The paucity of reports is probably because of the recessive nature of the tumor suppressor gene action, which requires two hits for inactivation of both alleles of the tumor suppressor gene—an unlikely scenario for proviral insertions. However, in at least in one cell line this has happened; both p53 alleles were knocked out by independent proviral insertions.[161] In other cases, the second p53 allele was rearranged or deleted by other mechanisms.[26,27] In the remaining cases, the p53 mutations induced by proviral insertions act in a dominant negative fashion, which abolishes the function of wild-type p53 by forming inactive oligomers.[114] In the past several years, the list of tumor suppressor genes has grown rapidly to reach about 10. It is possible that some of the uncharacterized common insertion sites listed in Table 11-1 may prove to involve tumor suppressor genes.

Acute Retroviruses

Under experimental conditions, acute retroviruses often cause polyclonal tumor growth within days. The rapidity and the potency of tumor induction exceed those of any other tumor viruses or carcinogens. Many of these viruses can transform normal embryo fibroblasts or hemopoietic cells in vitro with one-hit mechanisms. These viruses induce foci or colonies in cultures of the recipient cells, providing a convenient assay for acute retroviruses.

The extraordinary ability of acute retroviruses to transform normal cells in vitro and to induce rapid tumors in vivo is conferred by the viral oncogenes present in their genomes (see Table 11-2). Thus far, about 32 viral oncogenes have been identified. All these viral oncogenes are derived from host protooncogenes through recombinations, and their presence serves to structurally distinguish acute retroviruses from nonacute retroviruses. During the recombination process or subsequent selection for tumor phenotypes, many of the viral oncogenes acquire mutations and deletions that enhance the oncogenicity of the protooncogenes. These activating mutations provide important clues regarding how protooncogenes are regulated and how their activities unleashed. As shown in Table 11-2, some viruses (e.g., AEV, Mill Hill no. 2 [MH2]) have captured two oncogenes, and some oncogenes (e.g., *mil/raf*, *fps/fes*) have been captured by more than one type of virus. There are also occasions, as exemplified by *fgr*, when the viral oncogene is a fusion of multiple host genes.

The viral oncogenes assume a variety of functions, ranging from tyrosine kinases, serine kinases, and G-proteins to transcriptional factors.[35,425] Despite these diverse forms, with few exceptions, they all fit into the signal transduction scheme outlined previously (see Fig. 11-1). Indeed, the concept of signal transduction owes a great deal to the intensive pursuit of the function of the viral oncogenes. However, there is an important distinction between viral oncogenes and their host counterparts; the viral oncogenes, in nearly every case examined, are hyperactive and no longer subject to the upstream

---

† References 26, 27, 75, 106, 161, 172, 222, 279, 286.

TABLE 11-2. *Acute retroviruses and their transduced oncogenes*

Species	Retrovirus	Oncogene	Function	Neoplasm
Avian	RSV, B77, S1 and S2	*src*	PTK	Sarcoma
	FuSV, PRCII, PRCIV, UR1	*fps*	PTK	Sarcoma
	Y73ASV, EshASV	*yes*	PTK	Sarcoma
	RPL-30	*eyk*	RPTK	Sarcoma
	UR2ASV	*ros*	RPTK	Sarcoma
	S13 AEV	*sea*	RPTK	Sarcoma
	AEV-H	*erb*-B	RPTK (EGF)	{ Sarcoma { Erythroblastosis
	AEV-ES4 (AEV-R)	{ *erb*-B { *erb*-A	RPTK (EGF) THR	{ Sarcoma { Erythroblastosis
	CT10	*crk*	AP	Sarcoma
	MH2	{ *mil* { *myc*	PS/TK (raf) TF	Endothelioma
	MC29	*myc*	TF	{ Myelocytoma, carcinoma { Endothelioma
	CMII AMV	*myc*	TF	Myelocytoma
	OK10 ALV	*myc*	TF	Endothelioma
	AMV	*myb*	TF	Myeloblastosis
	E26 AMV	{ *myb* { *ets*	TF TF	{ Myeloblastosis { Erythroblastosis
	REV-T	*rel*	TF	Pre–B/T-cell lymphoma
	SKV ASV	*ski*	TF	Carcinoma*
	ASV17	*jun*	TF	Sarcoma
	AS42	*maf*	TF	Sarcoma
	ASV31	*qin*	TF	Sarcoma
Rodent	Ableson MuLV	*abl*	PTK	Pre–B/T-cell lymphoma
	Myeloproliferative LV	*mpl*	MGDF-R	Myeloproliferative disease
	AKT-8 MuLV	*akt*	PS/TK	T-cell lymphoma
	MSV-3611	*raf*	PS/TK	{ Sarcoma { Erythroleukemia
	Gazdar MSV	*mos*	PS/TK	Sarcoma
	Moloney MSV	*mos*	PS/TK	Sarcoma
	Myeloproliferative SV	*mos*	PS/TK	{ Sarcoma { Myeloproliferative disease
	BALB MSV	Ha-*ras*	GTPase	Hemangiosarcoma
	Histiocytosis virus	Ha-*ras*	GTPase	Histiocytosis
	Harvey MSV, Rat SV	Ha-*ras*	GTPase GTPase	{ Sarcoma { Erythroleukemia
	C58 MSV-1	*ras*	GTPase	Erythroleukemia
	Kirstern MSV	Ki-*ras*	GTPase	Erythroleukemia
	FBJ MSV, FBR MSV	*fos*	TF	Osteosarcoma
	Cas-NS-1	*cbl*	TF	Pre–B-cell lymphoma
	Cas-SFFV	*env*†	Mimic EPO	Erythroleukemia
	Friend SFFV	*env*	Mimic EPO	Erythroleukemia
	Rauscher SFFV	*env*	Mimic EPO	Erythroleukemia
Feline	ST-FeSV, GA-FeSV, HZ1-FeSV	*fes*	PTK	Fibrosarcoma
	GR-FeSV, TP1-FeSV	*fgr*	PTK	Fibrosarcoma
	HZ2-FeSV	*abl*	PTK	Fibrosarcoma
	SM-FeSV, HZ5-FeSV	*fms*	RPTK (CSF-1)	Fibrosarcoma
	HZ4-FeSV	*kit*	RPTK (SCF)	Fibrosarcoma
	PI-FeSV	*sis*	PDGF-β	Fibrosarcoma
	NY-FeSV	Ki-*ras*	GTPase	Fibrosarcoma
	FeLV	*myc*	TF	T lymphosarcoma
	FeLV-T17	*tcr*	TCR-β chain	T lymphosarcoma
Simian	Simian sarcoma virus	*sis*	PDGF-β	Sarcoma

*When SKV producing CEFs instead of cell-free virus filtrate were injected into chicken wing webs, carcinoma was observed at the site of innoculation.

†*env* Gene is transduced as a result of recombination between MLV and endogenous virus.

AEV, avian erythroleukemia virus; ALV, avian leukosis virus; AMV, avian meyloblastosis virus; AP, adaptor protein; ASV, avian sarcoma virus; CSF, colony-stimulating factor; EGF, epidermal growth factor; EPO, erythropoietin; FeLV, feline leukemia virus; FeSV, feline sarcoma virus; FuSV, Fujinami sarcoma virus; LV, leukemia virus; MGDF, megakaryocyte growth and development factor; MSV, murine sarcoma virus; MuLV, murine leukemia virus; PDGF, platelet-derived growth factor; PS/TK, protein serine/threonine kinase; PTK, protein tyrosine kinase; R, receptor; RPL, regional poultry laboratory; RPTK, receptor protein tyrosine kinase; RSV, Rous sarcoma virus; SCF, stem cell factor; SFFV, spleen focus-forming virus; TCR, T-cell receptor; TF, transcription factor; THR, thyroid hormone receptor.

controls. For example, v-erbB receptor is constitutively active without its ligand, v-ras is in the GTP-bound state without the action of Sos, and v-raf maintains its high kinase activity toward MEK, independent of ras association. As such, the viral oncogenes overpower the cellular machinery and override growth signals, leading to the uncontrolled proliferation of the infected cells.

As can be seen in Table 11-2, most of the acute retroviruses induce sarcomas or leukemias/lymphomas rather than carcinomas. This is curious and remains to be explained. It is possible that the isolation procedures, sometime involving co-cultivation with fibroblasts, favor the isolation of sarcoma viruses. It has also been postulated, at least for leukemia/lymphomas, that their development may require fewer genetic mutations than carcinomas, because leukemias and lymphomas tend to arise earlier in life.[2] Many of the transduced viral oncogenes are also found as common insertion targets for nonacute retroviruses, and the neoplasias induced in both cases are similar, except for the difference in latency. However, there are a few cases in which the transduced oncogenes have an expanded tumor tropism as a result of the acquisition of additional mutations (described later).

Genesis of Acute Retroviruses: Oncogene Transduction

Acute retroviruses arise through recombination of host protooncogenes and the genome of nonacute retroviruses. In all except two cases (Rous sarcoma virus[341,351] and eyk virus[185]), the acquisition of the host gene is at the expense of viral genes; as a consequence, the recombinant virus becomes replication defective and requires a similar replication-competent retrovirus as helper. The host range of the acute retroviruses is determined primarily by the helper viruses. Once the protooncogene (more appropriately, the mutated copy thereof) is captured by the virus, it is transmitted to another cell; upon subsequent infection, the process is referred to as oncogene transduction.

The oncogene-capturing process is complex and requires both DNA and RNA intermediates.[159] It begins in tumor cells, when nonacute retroviral DNA inserts near a host protooncogene and transcriptionally activates the protooncogene (Fig. 11-3). The initial readthrough transcript carries both the viral genome and the protooncogene sequences. This readthrough transcript is co-packaged with viral genomic RNA, also generated from the same transcription process, to form a heterodimer. During the

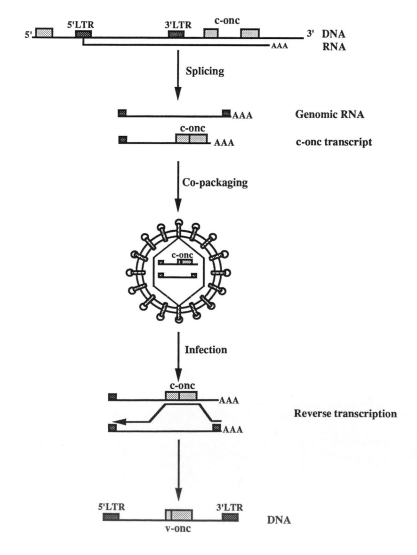

FIG. 11-3. Oncogene transduction by retroviruses. The process of oncogene transduction requires both DNA and RNA intermediates. When nonacute retroviral DNA inserts near a host protooncogene (c-onc) and transcriptionally activates the protooncogene by its 5' long terminal repeat (5'LTR), a readthrough transcript that carries both the viral and the protooncogene sequences is synthesized. Cleavage at the 3'LTR poly(A) signal (AAA) yields wild-type genomic RNA. Cleavage at the poly(A) site of the protooncogene generates the c-onc transcript. The c-onc transcript is processed by joining the viral splice donor site and acceptor site of the c-onc exon. In both cases, the packaging signals (ᴜ) are preserved, and both transcripts are co-packaged into the virion to form a heterodimer. During the second round of infection, the heterodimer RNA is reverse transcribed by a copy-choice mechanism to generate a DNA that incorporates the protooncogene in the middle of the viral genome. The reverse transcriptase must switch strands twice, resulting in two recombination junctions. The location of the junctions is dependent on where the enzyme switches strands, and the extent of viral gene deletion also varies. The consequence of this process is the incorporation of a processed c-onc in the middle of the retroviral genome. The translation of c-onc is often, but not always, initiated by viral gag or env initiation codons, and the polypeptides terminates in the viral sequence (v-onc).

second round of infection, the heterodimer RNA is reverse transcribed by a copy-choice mechanism to generate a DNA that incorporates the protooncogene in the middle of viral sequences. The reverse transcriptase must switch strands at least twice, resulting in two recombination junctures.[333] The locations of these junctures depend on where the enzyme switches strands and varies significantly from virus to virus. As a consequence, the extent of viral gene deletion also varies. Sequences encoding trans-functions (e.g., gag, pol, env products) that can be provided by the co-infecting helper virus may be deleted, whereas those acting in cis in viral replication (e.g., the LTR, the primer binding sites, the package signal, sometimes the splice site) are always retained. A variation of this model is the occurrence of deletion at the provirus level, which removes portion of the genome and the 3'LTR, thereby fusing together the 5'LTR, the cis-signals, and the protooncogene. In this manner, the transcript initiates at the 5'LTR would carry both viral packaging signal and protooncogene sequence, bypassing the need for readthrough transcription.[84,159]

Not every instance of insertional activation of a protooncogene leads to the genesis of an acutely transforming retrovirus; proviruses involved in enhancer insertion are usually in the wrong orientation to promote readthrough transcription, and the transcript generated by 3'LTR promotion will not have the signal for co-packaging. However, in cases in which the proviruses are arranged in the optimum orientation, such as the c-erbB activation by ALV, the frequency of generating acute retroviruses can be as high as 50%.[264] Analysis of a collection of v-erbB oncogenes captured by these viruses reveal that the strand switch sometimes, but not always, involves homologous sequences, and in one particular case, the switch takes place between the poly(A) sequence of the c-erbB transcript and the two consecutive lysine codons (AAA AAA) of the env gene.[327] The presence of a poly(A) sequence within this viral genome, and in that of another acute virus that carries the v-fps oncogene,[173] provides conclusive evidence that the transduction process involves an RNA intermediate, as the previously described model suggests.

Viral Oncogenes and Protooncogene Activation

As discussed previously, reverse transcription is a key process involved in oncogene recombination and transduction. Reverse transcriptase is an enzyme that has a relatively high error rate, and the resulting transduced genes often suffer mutations or deletions. In addition, depending on where the strand switches, it is not uncommon for the protooncogene to lose either its N-terminus or C-terminus during the recombination process and fuse to viral gag or env coding sequences. It is presumed that these mutations and deletions occur somewhat randomly throughout the genome; however, if transformation phenotypes are to be selected, as was the case during the isolation of the sarcoma or leukemia viruses, mutations contributing to oncogenicity would also be selected. Thus, by examining the mutations and deletions accumulated in the viral oncogenes, invaluable information regarding the activation of protooncogenes can be obtained. In the ensuing sections, we select several extensively studied oncogenes of different classes to illustrate the principles of oncogene activation (Fig. 11-4).

c-erbB to v-erbB

c-erbB encodes a growth factor receptor with tyrosine kinase activity. About 30 acute retroviruses carrying v-erbB oncogenes have been identified. Some of these (v-erbB 9134[328] and v-erbB 5005[131]) are identical to the cDNA identified from the leukemic cells with provirus insertion in this locus (i.e., insertionally activated c-erbB). Compared to the intact c-erbB gene, v-erbB 9134 lacks the majority of the ligand-binding domain and consequently cannot bind ligand. This truncation alone is sufficient to activate the constitutive tyrosine kinase activity and erythroleukemogenic potential. The v-erbB 9134 virus is strictly leukemogenic. In contrast, v-erbB AAV5005,[131] v-erbB S3[327] and v-erbB of AEV H[450] have accumulated additional mutations and deletions to cause either sarcoma (v-erbB AAV5005 and S3) or both erythroleukemia and sarcoma (AEV-H). Systematic analyses reveal that the inframe deletion after the kinase domain found in AAV 5005 and S3 apparently removes a negative regulatory region and enhances the kinase's interaction with crucial substrates in fibroblasts. The point mutations within the kinase domain found in v-erbB-H is within a glycine motif involved in ATP binding and phosphate-transfer reaction.[369] This point mutation upregulates the intrinsic kinase activity and induces a higher level of MAP kinase activity in fibroblasts.[368] These additional mutations in the intracellular domain are responsible for the sarcomagenic potential. The fact that leukemogenic and sarcomagenic potentials are activated by different mutations suggest the existence of cell-type–specific oncogenic pathways.

c-ras to v-ras

C-ras encodes a 21-kD GDP/GTP-binding protein with an intrinsic GTPase activity.[247,258,260] There are two related genes in this family that have been transduced by retroviruses: v-ras-H by Harvey sarcoma virus[152] and v-ras-K by Kirsten sarcoma virus.[199] The ras gene family is characterized by several homologous domains and also regions unique to each molecule. For instance, c-ras-H has one effector-binding domain (amino acid 26 to amino acid 45), four GTP-binding domains, one farnesylation site on Cys186, and one heterogeneous region (amino acids 164 through 185). The effector domain is the binding site for downstream signal molecules such as raf-1.[76,457] The GTP-binding domain with the GXXGXGKS (amino acids 10 through 17), DXXG (amino acids 57 through 60), and NKXD (amino acids 57 through 60) motifs forms a GTP-binding pocket and catalyzes the hydrolysis of GTP. The farnesylation takes place by way of a cysteine residue at the C-terminus, through which ras is associated with the plasma membrane (an association that is crucial to ras activity).[58,66,148] C-ras is regulated by GTP binding and is active in the GTP-bound state. The GTP binding is catalyzed by Sos[44,56,68, 108,128,239] and is down-modulated by its intrinsic GTPase activity, in conjunction with GTPase-activating protein (GAP).[456] To counteract the intrinsic GTPase activity in normal cells, c-ras is significantly GTP-bound only if Sos is translocated (via binding to Grb2) to the plasma membrane to be close to ras. In the oncogenic v-ras-H and v-ras-K, mutations invariably affect the GTP-binding pocket such that the GTPase activity is diminished. Thus, Ala59 and Gly12 are found to be hot spots of mutations in v-ras onco-

248

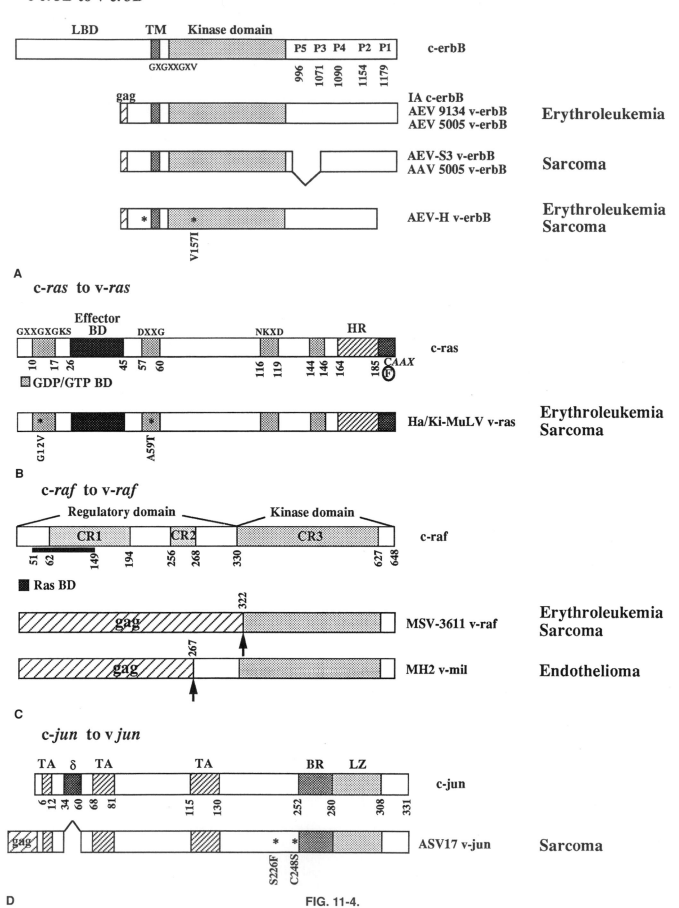

FIG. 11-4.

genes.[247] Such mutations make ras hyperactive and independent of growth factor stimulation.

c-raf to v-raf

C-raf is activated by binding to ras-GTP and translocated to the plasma membrane, where it phosphorylates MEK. The v-*raf* of MSV-3611 and v-*mil* (the chicken homolog of *raf*) of MH2 were both derived from the c-*raf*-1 locus through truncations and point mutations.[45] C-raf-1 is composed of two functional domains, regulatory domain and the C-terminal kinase domain.[96,446] The N-terminal regulatory domain binds ras-GTP, and presumably this binding opens up the kinase domain and translocates raf to the plasma membrane.[76,436] In both v-ras and v-mil, the N-terminal domain is truncated and therefore becomes constitutively active. However, more recent findings suggest that association with the plasma membrane is a key step for activation of c-raf[227,388] by PS/TK phosphoryla-tion (protein kinase C [PKC] or c-mos), PTK (c-src, lck, or lyn) phosphorylation, or both.[65,81,157,204] In addition, several raf-binding proteins have been identified; these include hsp70, p50,[382] and protein 14-3-3.[119,121,180] Whether and how these proteins contribute to c-raf activation and why v-raf is constitutively activated remain to be elucidated.

c-jun to v-jun

C-*jun* belongs to a multigene family of short-lived transcription factors whose transcription rises transiently before S-phase. C-*jun* is the prototype of molecules carrying the basic and leucine zipper (bZIP) domain.[8,93] C-*jun* forms a heterodimer with c-fos, another oncogene with bZIP domain, and is part of the AP-1 complex.[7,42] AP-1 binds a TGAc/gTCA (TPA-response element [TRE]) motif enhancer to regulate transcription. In addition to the bZIP domain, which is involved in DNA binding, nuclear translocation, and dimeri-

FIG. 11-4. Examples of oncogenic conversion by retroviruses. (**A**) c-erbB to v-erbB. c-erbB encodes a tyrosine kinase receptor for epidermal growth factor (EGF). In its native form, it has an extracellular ligand binding domain (LBD), a transmembrane domain (TM), a kinase domain, and a C-terminal domain with five autophosphorylation sites (P1 to P5). The leukemogenic potential of erbB is activated by proviral insertion and the removal of the LBD (IA c-erbB, see Fig. 11-3). All v-erbBs found in acute retroviruses lack the LBD. Thirty acute retroviruses carrying various v-erbBs have been isolated. Some of them (v-erbB 9134 and 5005) are identical to insertionally activated c-erbB (IA c-erbB) and are strictly leukemogenic. By contrast, v-erbB of AEV H is both leukemogenic and sarcomagenic. There are in-frame deletions after the kinase domain found in AAV 5005 and S3 that presumably remove a negative regulatory region and enhance the interaction of kinase with crucial substrates in fibroblasts. v-erbB of AEV H carries two point mutations (*) and a 72–amino acid deletion at the C-terminus. The point mutation (valine 157 to isoleucine) within the kinase domain found in v-erbB H is within a glycine motif involved in the adenosine triphosphate– binding (ATP-binding) pocket. This mutation increases the intrinsic activity of erbB and is responsible for the sarcomagenic potential of the v-erbB of AEV H. (**B**) c-ras to v-ras. The protooncogene c-ras encodes a 21-kD GDP/GTP–binding protein with an intrinsic GTPase activity. P21 ras possesses an effector-binding domain (*heavily shaded area*), four GTP-binding domains (*lightly shaded area*), a farnesylation site (FCAAX), and a heterogeneous region (HR). The effector domain is the binding site for raf-1. The CTP-binding domains form a GTP-binding pocket and catalyze the hydrolysis of CTP. The farnesylation is mediated by Cys 186, through which ras is associated with the plasma membrane. The activity of c-ras is regulated by GTP binding and is active in the CTP-bound state. This GTP binding is catalyzed by Sos and downregulated by its intrinsic GTPase activity in conjunction with GTPase accelerating protein (GAP). In the oncogenic v-ras-H (Harvey) or v-ras-K (Kirsten), mutations such as Ala 59 Thr and Gly 12 Val, located at the GTP-binding pocket, result in diminution of the GTPase activity, and ras becomes hyperactive and independent of growth factor stimulation. (**C**) c-raf to v-raf. The protooncogene c-raf is composed of two functional domains: the N-terminal regulatory domain and the C-terminal kinase domain. There are three regions, CR1 to CR3, that are conserved among the raf family. The regulatory domain contains a binding site (amino acids 51 to 149) for ras-GTP, through which c-raf is translocated to the plasma membrane and activated by protein serine/threonine kinases (PS/TKs) or protein tyrosine kinases (PTKs) phosphorylations. The v-raf of MSV-3611 and v-mil (the chicken homolog of raf) of MH2, which were both derived from c-raf-1 locus, have truncations at the N-terminal domain and become constitutively active. Both molecules are fused to viral gag genes, although the gag portion is not important for its oncogenic properties. (**D**) c-jun or v-jun. The protooncogene c-jun belongs to a multigene family of short-lived transcription factors that is characterized by a basic region (BR), a leucine zipper (LZ), and three activation domains (TA). In the course of c-jun transduction to become v-jun in ASV17, the 27–amino acid delta region (δ) is deleted, and three point mutations have accumulated. Ser 226 to Phe mutation allows v-jun to override the negative regulation of DNA-binding activity by glycogen synthase 3 (GSK3), and Cys 248 to Ser mutation renders the DNA-binding activity of v-jun independent of redox regulation. The delta region has been found to coincide with the stress-activated protein kinase (SAPK) binding site and S63 and S73 are the phosphorylation sites for SAPK in c-jun. Conversely, v-jun does not bind SAPK, and S63 and S73 residues are not phosphorylated by SAPK. The delta region may be involved in ubiquitin-dependent degradation, thereby significantly prolonging the half-life of v-jun.

zation, c-jun contains three activation domains, which are mapped at the N-terminal amino acids 6 through 12, 68 through 81, and 115 through 130.[9] There is also a delta region located at the N-terminus, which is deleted in the oncogenic v-jun and supposedly involved in negative regulation of c-jun.[15] The activity of c-jun is clearly regulated by phosphorylation; it can be phosphorylated by a number of PS/TKs, including casein kinase II (CKII), glycogen synthase 3 (GSK3) and SAPK.[16,99,241,444] The phosphorylation of c-jun at S63 and S73 (in the activation domain) by SAPK is particularly important in the transactivation potential of c-jun, and it is through SAPK that c-jun positively responds to growth factors and other stimuli such as ultraviolet light, heat shock, and TPA.[99,265] C-jun is also negatively regulated by phosphorylation at S243 (in the basic domain), which abolishes its DNA-binding activity. PKC or TPA treatment inactivates GSK3 and upregulates c-jun.[49]

In addition to phosphorylation, c-jun is also regulated by redox reaction on cysteine 248.[1] Under oxidative conditions, c-jun fails to bind TRE; however, in the presence of reducing agents or redox protein Ref-1, c-jun's binding activity is restored.[449] The short half-life of c-jun is in part attributed to an destabilizing element present in the 3' untranslated region of the message; thus, c-jun is subject to multiple regulation. In the course of c-jun transduction to become v-jun, the 3' destabilizing element is truncated, the 27–amino acid delta region is lost, and there are other point mutations, the most significant of which are C248S (cysteine 248 to serine) and S226F (serine 226 to phenylalanine).[251] The former point mutation renders v-jun's binding to DNA independent of redox regulation[303] and the newly acquired serine apparently is the target of PS/TKs, such that v-jun's nuclear translocation becomes cell-cycle dependent.[74] The latter mutation allows v-jun to override a negative regulation by GSK3. It has been determined that SAPK binds to the delta region (amino acids 34 through 60).[404] The c-jun delta peptide can competitively inhibit the phosphorylation of c-jun at S63 and S73 by SAPK,[5]

and v-jun has little ability to bind SAPK nor is it phosphorylated by SAPK.[37,160] It has also been suggested that this region may be involved in ubiquitin-dependent degradation, and v-jun's half-life is significantly prolonged by deletion of this region.[404] The available evidence suggests that v-jun is oncogenic, not because it has higher transactivating ability than c-jun but because of its prolonged half-life and resistance to regulation.[154,404] It has also been suggested that v-jun's binding specificity is altered by the accumulated mutations and may thus affect genes not normally regulated by c-jun.[146]

Trans-Acting Retroviruses

HTLV[374,385] and BLV[57] induce long-latency monoclonal T- or B-cell leukemias; however, their modes of leukemia induction differ from those of acute and nonacute retroviruses. They do not insert their proviruses near protooncogenes in tumor cells nor do they capture host protooncogenes. A comparison of the genome structure of HTLV/BLV with those of acute and nonacute retroviruses reveals additional genes, including tax and rex. Figure 11-5 shows the genomic structure and transcriptional pattern of HTLV (BLV has a similar genetic organization and is not discussed here). In addition to gag, pol, and env found in nonacute retroviruses, there is a unique region designated pX. The transcriptional pattern of HTLV is more complex than nonacute retroviruses involving both single and double splicing. The genomic and singly spliced messages are used for translating gag, pol, and env genes. The doubly spliced messages encode pX-related regulatory proteins. Through different modes of splicing, 10 open reading frames can be assigned, of which at least six have been shown to encode polypeptides; these are Tax, pp27-Rex, pp21-Rex, p12[I], p13[II] and p30[II].[33,62,78,209,210,346] Among these open reading frames, Tax and Rex are the best understood and are discussed in more detail later. In HTLV-trans-

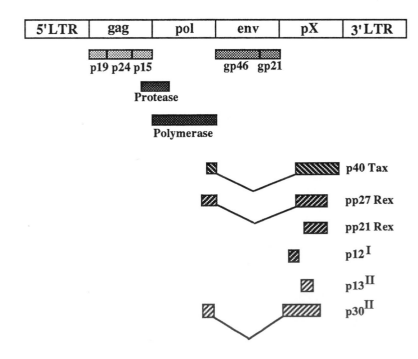

FIG. 11-5. The genomic structure and viral protein of human T-cell leukemia virus type 1 (HTLV-1). In addition to gag, pol, and env found in nonacute retroviruses, there is a unique region designated pX. The mature polypeptides encoded by gag, pol, and env are indicated. The transcription of the HTLV genome is initiated within the 5' long terminal repeat (5'LTR), and the transcripts are processed by both single and double splicing. The genomic and singly spliced messages are used for translating gag, pol, and env genes. The doubly spliced messages encode pX-related regulatory proteins. Through different modes of splicing, 10 open reading frames can be assigned, of which at least six have been shown to encode polypeptides. These are Tax, pp27 Rex, pp21 Rex, p12[I], p13[II], and p30[II].

formed T cells, the provirus is usually in the latent state, and it is thought that only the regulatory proteins from pX region, especially Tax, are important in the immortalization or transformation of T cells.

Structure and Function of Tax and Rex

Rex is a nucleolar, RNA-binding phosphoprotein[200] that is required for the efficient expression of *gag, pol,* and *env* genes because it facilitates the transport of the nonspliced and single-spliced transcripts.[162,178,179] Early after infection and before Rex is made in sufficient quantities, only the complete or double-spliced transcripts are transported to the cytoplasm, from which Tax, Rex, and other pX-related gene products are made. Once Rex accumulates to a high concentration, the ge-

nomic and singly spliced transcript are translocated into cytoplasm.[191,197] Viral gag and env proteins are then made, and the virions are assembled. Thus, although Rex is critical in the lytic cycle of HTLV replication, its direct role in oncogenesis remains to be determined.

In contrast, Tax provides essential functions for both HTLV replication and oncogenesis. Tax is a nuclear protein that is generally hydrophobic, with a hydrophilic and acidic domain at the C-terminus.[376] An unorthodox nuclear localization signal is located within the first 48 amino-terminal residues.[375] In addition, the two cysteines and two histidines at the amino-terminus form a functional zinc-binding motif, and additional four cysteines (amino acids 153, 174, 212, and 261) are involved in multimer formation.[415] Tax is a promiscuous trans-activator that enhances the transcription of the viral LTR as well as other cellular genes (Table 11-3).[113,376] It does not bind

TABLE 11-3. *Genes and their promoters that are transregulated by Tax*

Mechanism of regulation	Gene category	Examples
Trans-activation	Viruses	LTR (21-bp repeat) of HTLV-I and -II LTR of HIV CMV major immediate-early enhancer SV40 enhancer Adenovirus early region promoter
	Cytokines	IL-2 IL-3 IL-4 IL-5 IL-6 IFN-γ
	Growth factors	GM-CSF/G-CSF TNF-α and -β1 c-sis (PDGF-β) NGF
	Cytokine receptors	IL-2Rα
	Immediate-early genes	c-jun jun-B jun-D c-fos fra-1 c-myc egr-1 egr-2
	Other genes	c-rel NF-κB-2 lyn Vimentin gp34 LFA-3 CD30 Proenkephalin Calpain II Integrins Zinc finger 225 Human globin–β and –π PHRP Human IG kappa light chain
Trans-repression		Human polymerase-β

CMV, cytomegalovirus; G-CSF, granulocyte colony-stimulating factor; GM-CSF, granulocyte-macrophage colony-stimulating factor; HIV, human immunodeficiency virus; HTLV, human T-cell leukemia virus; IFN, interferon; IG, immunoglobulin; IL, interleukin; LTR, long terminal repeat; NGF, nerve growth factor; PDGF, platelet-derived growth factor; PHRP, parathyroid hormone-related protein; TNF, tumor necrosis factor.

DNA directly, but complexes with CREB family proteins (e.g., CREB,[392,458] ATF3,[245] CREM[392]), and targets these factors to bind a subset of their cognitive CRE motifs, thus providing additional specificities. This high-affinity CRE motif is present in the HTLV LTR (i.e., the 21–base pair repeat) and accounts for the ability of Tax to autoregulate its own expression.[‡] Tax also interacts directly with components of the basic transcriptional machinery (e.g., TBP,[63] and TFIIA[82]) and thus provides a bridge between CREB-like transcription factors and RNA polymerase II. In addition to being a transactivation partner of CREB family members, Tax also facilitates transactivation by the nuclear factor kappa B (NFkB) family of transcriptional factors through direct interaction with NFkB p50 and p65.[218,393,394] Alternatively, Tax can bind NFkB precursors p100 and p105,[30,165,285,318] as well as inhibitor kappa B (IkB),[166,391] the cytoplasmic inhibitor of NFkB; in so doing, it releases active NFkB p65 and p50 for translocation into the nucleus for transactivation by way of the kB enhancers. This is important because the kB enhancer has been found in the promoters of c-myc, c-rel, interleukin 2 (IL-2), IL-2 receptor, granulocyte-macrophage colony-stimulating factor (GM-CSF) and others. Almost certainly, this property connects Tax to the growth signal pathway. Tax is also reported to be able to interact directly with serum response factor[122,393] and to catalyze the dimer formation of bZIP proteins.[11,434] It appears that Tax is a multifunctional transactivator, and it is no surprise that Tax augments the expression of a variety of genes, including protooncogenes (c-jun, c-fos, c-myc, c-sis, c-rel), cytokines (IL-2, IL-3, IL-4 and IL-6; GM-CSF; tumor growth factor beta [TGF-β]) and cytokine receptors (IL-2 receptor). Thus, although HTLV (and likewise, BLV) does not activate protooncogenes by proviral insertion in cis, it produces a viral product that can activate protooncogenes in trans. The simultaneous transcriptional activation of IL-2 and the IL-2 receptor by Tax is of particular relevance to the initial step of T-cell immortalization, because this sets up an autocrine growth loop that no longer requires external growth signals. Furthermore, Tax has been shown to repress the expression of the β-polymerase gene,[184] possibly through the basic helix loop helix (bHLH) family of transcription factors,[418] and thus may contribute to the genomic instability of HTLV-transformed cells, allowing other genetic changes to occur.

ONCOGENESIS BY NONACUTE RETROVIRUSES

Avian Leukosis Virus and Reticuloendotheliosis Virus

ALV induces a variety of neoplasias in chickens, including erythroleukemia, nephroblastoma, and bursal lymphoma, depending on the insertion sites of the proviruses and the protooncogenes they activate.[213,314] Thus, for erythroleukemia it is c-erbB, for nephroblastoma it is nov, and for B-cell lymphoma it is myc, bic, and myb (see Table 11-1). Among these, B-cell lymphomas of the bursa of Fabricius species are the

most prevalent and have been extensively characterized. At least two stages of lymphomagenesis can be defined for this disease. The enlargement of bursal follicles, usually numbering 50 to 100, is first observed and is considered to represent preneoplastic hyperplasia.[89,175,293] This step is thought to be caused by proviral insertional activation of c-myc[125,155,312] and can be experimentally mimicked by infection with v-myc-containing viruses.[14,294] Subsequently, one or a few of these enlarged follicles develop into frank lymphomas. The oncogenes involved in the latter process have not been fully defined, although c-bic is likely to be one of them.[83] Double infection by ALV of different subgroups was shown to shorten the latency of bursal lymphoma development, and a significant fraction of tumors contain two proviruses, integrating in the c-myc and c-bic loci. In tumors that do not have proviruses inserted in the bic locus, the bic expression is also elevated. This represents a classic example of how insertional activation of two oncogenes contribute to two stages of tumorigenesis. B-cell lymphoma without bursal involvement has also been detected on ALV infection of chicken embryos, and in this case, insertional activation of c-myb is involved, suggesting that different oncogenes (or more appropriately, protooncogenes) are operating at different stages of B-cell development.[192,322] Because ALV induced lymphomas depend on insertional activation of protooncogenes, it follows that the ability of ALV to induce lymphomas critically depends on the strength of the LTR enhancers. This is indeed the case; all ALVs with strong LTR promoters (e.g., Rous-associated virus [RAV]-1.2) are strongly oncogenic, whereas an endogenous virus (RAV-0) with a weak LTR is relatively ineffective in tumor induction. REV is an avian retrovirus that is distinct from ALV, but in a manner similar to ALV, it can effectively induce bursal lymphoma by insertional activation of c-myc.[297] On rare occasions, REV also induces T-cell lymphomas, which also involve c-myc activation by proviruses.[181]

Murine Leukemia Virus

There are two major classes of MuLVs; classification is based on their etiology. Moloney murine leukemia virus (M-MuLV)[271] effectively induces T-cell lymphoma, and Friend (F) MuLV[120] induces erythroleukemia. A major determinant of the disease specificity of MuLV resides in the LTRs of these subclasses.[101,228,410] The enhancer motifs have divergent sequences that presumably bind different transcriptional factors in a cell-type–specific manner.[46,244,379,401] By switching these enhancers, M-MuLV can be converted to induce erythroleukemia and vice versa.[69,70] Likewise, the highly leukemogenic SL3-MuLV can be attenuated by modifying the enhancer sequence, mimicking that of a closely related but nonleukemogenic AKV-MuLV.

Despite the different disease spectrums of M-MuLV and F-MuLV, there are certain similarities in the mechanisms of multistage disease processes. The disease development involves at least two stages.[23,212,410,421] First, on MuLV infection of hemopoietic cells, recombinant viruses with altered env genes are generated. This recombination occurs between the infecting viral genome and an endogenous provirus resident in the host.[52,53,151,389] The resulting recombinant viruses have expanded tropisms and can infect appropriate target cells. More

---

‡ References 50, 123, 124, 304, 308, 309, 365.

importantly, in both cases, the recombinant *env* gene products apparently are mitogens for target cells, leading to polyclonal hyperplasia or the preleukemic phase.[233,238,409,440] The second stage involves insertional activation of protooncogenes by either the parental infecting virus or the recombinant virus. For M-MuLV, the recombinant virus generated is mink cell focus (MCF) inducing, and the target cells are thymic lymphocytes.[151] The protooncogenes found to be associated with this disease include c-*myc*, N-*myc*, *pim*-1, *Mlvi*-1, *Mlvi*-2, and others (see Table 11-1). The multiplicity of protooncogenes activated implies a diversity of transformed T cells but may also represent cooperating protooncogenes involved in multistep transformation processes. The latter was best illustrated by experiments using transgenic mice bearing one activated protooncogene (e.g., *pim*-1 driven by strong promoter) that was subsequently challenged by M-MuLV.[2] The resulting thymic lymphomas invariably carry proviruses inserting in the other protooncogene loci (e.g., c-*myc*, N-*myc*).[422] These tumors developed with exceptionally short latency (about 8 weeks), indicating the rate-determining step of M-MuLV leukemogenesis is not necessarily insertional mutagenesis per se but rather the induction of the preleukemic phase. For F-MuLV, the recombinant virus produced is spleen focus-forming virus (SFFV),[406] whose *env* gene product gp55 can constitutively activate the erythropoietin receptor and expand the erythroblast population.[238] This is followed by F-MuLV/SFFV proviral integration within the p53 locus, a tumor suppressor gene.[75,279,342]

The insertional mutagenesis of p53 is especially interesting and remains the only reported case in which a tumor suppressor gene is inactivated by retroviral provirus during oncogenesis. This was initially surprising because of the recessive nature of p53, which requires that both alleles be simultaneously inactivated—an unlikely scenario for retrovirus insertions. Investigations of five F-MuLV—induced erythroleukemic cell lines revealed that in one line, both alleles had been inactivated by two independent insertions.[279] In the other four cell lines, one allele was inactivated by provirus, and the other was rearranged by mechanisms yet to be defined. Regardless, the consequences are the same—no normal p53 is expressed. In addition to proviral insertions in p53, activations by F-MuLV and SFFV DNA are also found. In more than 95% of tumors harboring proviruses, DNA is found to integrate near the *Spi-1/Spfi1/Pu.1*.[273–275,311,381] In contrast, in more than 75% of tumors with F-MuLV proviral integrations, F-MuLV DNA tends to cluster around *fli-1* locus.[23,24,172,353] A much less frequent common insertion site for both F-MuLV and SFFV proviral DNA is *fli-2/NF E2*.[248 Spi] *Spi*-1, *Fli*-1, and *Fli*-2 are all transcriptional factors implicated in erythroid differentiation. Spi-1 and Fli-1 belong to the Ets family of transcription factors.[25,310] *Ets* was originally uncovered as a viral oncogene in avian erythroleukemia virus E26. The insertional activation of *spi-1* and *fli-1* are mutually exclusive, indicating that they exert an overlapping function. The inactivation of p53 accompanies both *spi-1* and *fli-1* activation. These data permit a tentative assignment of the several steps involved in F-MuLV infections: generation of an SFFV recombinant; gp55 induced erythroblast expansion; proviral activation of *fli-1* or *spi-1*/proviral inactivation of p53; and inactivation of the second p53 allele by mutation or recombination. The order of the latter three steps has not been worked out in detail.

Mouse Mammary Tumor Virus

MMTV has several unique characteristics not shared by other retroviruses. MMTV is a type B virus, and its LTR is regulated by a hormone (glucocorticoid). Perhaps related to its hormone-dependent LTR, the virus has a propensity to induce tumors of mammary epithelial origin. The oncogenesis induced by MMTV apparently does not involve the generation of recombinant viruses but instead depends on insertional activation of protooncogenes.[290] There are at least seven *int* or *wnt* loci that are frequent insertion targets for MMTV. *Wnt-1/int*-1 and *FGF-4/int*-2 are common insertion sites of MMTV initially identified in different strains of mice (C3H versus BR6) that developed mammary carcinomas. Subsequently, it was found that in 50% of BR6 tumors, both *wnt-1/int*-1 and *FGF-4/int*-2 loci are rearranged as a result of MMTV proviral insertions. Concerted activation of two potential protooncogenes in carcinomas induced by MMTV[321] indicates cooperation of these two oncogenes. In addition, int-2 and hst, oncogenes originally identified by transfection of NIH 3T3 cells with DNA from Kaposi's sarcoma (KS)[98] or stomach carcinoma,[396,454] are adjacent to one another. Proviruses that activate *int*-2 often activate *hst* concomitantly. All these loci are growth factor–like polypeptides, which can exert their action in both autocrine and paracrine fashion. It is therefore interesting to note that Gray and colleagues[142,143] and Mester and colleagues[262] reported that mammary tumor clones with individual *int* loci activated apparently enhance the growth of one another in a paracrine fashion.

Feline Leukemia Virus

Feline leukemia virus (FeLV) is associated with proliferative, degenerative, and malignant diseases in domestic cats. The neoplasias induced by FeLV include leukemia-lymphosarcoma, erythroid leukemia, and myeloid leukemia; T lymphosarcoma is the most prevalent. Based on the *env* serotypes, FeLV has been classified into A, B, and C subgroups. FeLV-A is the most prevalent and is the parental type. FeLV-B and FeLV-C are thought to be the MCF counterparts and result from recombination between ecotropic FeLV-A and endogenous retroviruses. Indeed, the *env* gene of FeLV-B and MCF-MuLV show a remarkable resemblance in nucleotide sequence within the xenotropic portion of the MCF-MuLV *env*. The other process thought to occur during tumorigenesis process is the amplification of the LTR enhancer; most of the LTRs that integrate near a protooncogene appear to have undergone duplication or triplication. The protooncogene that is the frequent insertion target for FeLV proviruses in T lymphosarcomas is c-*myc*.[117,232,267,284,292] The insertion event often leads to the generation of *myc*-containing acute FeLV, or FeLV-myc. FeLV-myc then infects and integrates near other protooncogenes to advance the tumorigenic processes. The next most common insertion site is *flvi-2/bim-1*,[231,233] whose gene product is a zinc-finger transcriptional factor.[234,235] This site is followed by *fit-1*[416] and *pim-1*.[408] Another common insertion site, *flvi-1*,[230] is found in a non-B, non-T lymphoma of the spleen; the LTRs that interrupt this locus always contain triplication of the enhancer (Levy LS, personal communication, February 1995), suggesting cell-type specificity of the amplified enhancers.

ONCOGENESIS BY ACUTE RETROVIRUSES

Acute retroviruses are undisputedly the most potent carcinogens. They induce polyclonal tumors in vivo, with rapid kinetics and transformation of normal embryo fibroblasts in vitro with single-hit kinetics. This exceptional potency is partly the result of the high level of oncoprotein expression directed by the viral LTR and partly the result of the continual selection of mutations that enhance oncoprotein activity during serial propagation. Because both of these properties are carried by the viral genome, there is no requirement for specific cellular site of integrations (unlike the nonacute retroviruses), which may explain the rapid kinetics and polyclonal nature of the tumors. A long-standing puzzle is how the acute retroviruses induce neoplasia in a single step when there is overwhelming evidence that oncogenesis is usually a multistage process requiring multiple genetic changes. There are no ready answers to this question; however, it should be recognized that many of the experiments with acute retroviruses were carried out with a high titer in young animals, which do not have fully developed immune systems. Viral replication could be so extensive that it is possible to select for cells that are at a stage that is prone to transformation (e.g., high myc level). In vitro, it has been shown that if individual viral oncogenes are introduced into embryo fibroblasts by transfection protocol rather than by infection, they are incapable of inducing transformation unless a second complementing viral oncogene or selectable marker such as neomycin-resistant gene is co-transfected. These results are interpreted to mean that for the transformation of normal cells, at least two genetic mutations or oncogene activations are required: one to turn on the growth-stimulating signal and the other to shut off the growth-inhibitory signal. The inhibitory signals are generated by the neighboring normal cells, and if G-418 selection is imposed to remove all the neighboring untransfected normal cells, cells successfully transfected with the oncogene and the neomycin-resistant gene will then form colonies. In the case of viral infections, almost all cells could be infected and become transformed, a situation similar to that of transfection with drug selection imposed, in which there are few normal cells left and the transformed cells will form colonies. This may explain the single-hit kinetics of transformation by acute retroviruses and why no other carcinogens can accomplish such a feat.

ONCOGENESIS BY HUMAN T-CELL LEUKEMIA VIRUS

HTLV-I was the first human retrovirus discovered.[323] HTLV-I infection has been etiologically associated with adult T-cell leukemia/lymphoma (ATL),[417] which is endemic in southern Japan, Africa, South America, the Carribean basin, and southeastern parts of United States .[60,169] ATL is a monoclonal or oligoclonal malignancy involving CD4+ T helper cells, most of which are IL-2 receptor-positive and require IL-2 for growth.[352,417,454] The characteristics of the disease include hypercalcemia, skin lesions caused by invasion of leukemic cells,

lymphadenopathy, lymphomatous meningitis, osteolysis, and immunodeficiency.[206,287] The majority of HTLV-I–infected individuals are asymptomatic, and only 0.5% to 2% of them eventually develop ATL several decades following infection. Other human diseases have also been linked to HTLV-I infections; these include HTLV-I–associated myelopathy, also known as tropical spastic paraparesis.[34,136,182,305] Several other members of HTLV have been identified, namely HTLV-II, HTLV-V, and simian T-cell leukemia virus type I (STLV-I). HTLV-II has not been directly implicated in any human disease but was originally isolated from patients with hairy cell leukemia and myelopathies.[338,348] HTLV-V was isolated from patients with cutaneous T-cell leukemia (CTL),[253] but the causal relation needs to be confirmed. STLV-I is a close relative of HTLV-I, and its association with leukemia/lymphoma in Old World nonhuman primates has been established.[170,269,437] Some of the strongest evidence that HTLV is a causative agent for ATL comes from in vitro studies. HTLV-I and HTLV-II infections of peripheral blood leukocytes (PBLs) leads to immortalization of CD4+ T-helper cells.[72,268,325] This process is not limited to human cells; T cells of monkeys,[269] rabbits,[270] cats,[171] and rats[400] can be immortalized as well. Furthermore, a nononcogenic variant of herpesvirus saimiri, when manipulated to incorporate the HTLV-I *Tax* gene,[141] become capable of immortalizing human PBL, providing evidence for the role of Tax in leukemogenesis. These studies, however, also showed that Tax alone is not sufficient to induce full malignancy, because the immortalized T cells are not oncogenic in athymic mice. It has been suggested that the HTLV-I *env* gene product also plays a role in the initial phase of leukemia induction. In a manner similar to that of gp55 of SFFV and *env* of MCF, HTLV-I gp46 exhibits mitogenic activity in resting T cells.[134,455] This activity can be blocked by anti-gp46 but not by ultraviolet irradiation of the virions. The LFA/CD2 pathway, in conjunction with CD3, has been implicated in this mitogenic signaling.[6,198] The decade-long latency and the monoclonal origin of ATL suggest that other genetic changes are required in the development of frank leukemia. Thus far, no consistent chromosomal aberration has been detected; the protooncogenes and tumor suppressor genes involved remain to be identified.

ONCOGENESIS BY HUMAN IMMUNODEFICIENCY VIRUS

HIV is not considered an oncogenic retrovirus but rather a cytopathic virus for CD4+ T lymphocytes and other cells. HIV-infected individuals are predisposed to develop polyclonal B-cell lymphoproliferative disorders, aggressive B-cell non-Hodgkin's lymphoma (NHL), KS, and anogenital neoplasia.[441] In most cases, the incidences of HIV-associated neoplasia are not caused by HIV infections directly but rather are a result of the immunosuppression caused by HIV, which undoubtedly facilitates the growth of other oncogenic viruses and tumor progression. However, in some circumstances, HIV may contribute to oncogenesis in ways that cannot be explained by immunosuppression alone.

KS is the most striking neoplasm to occur in HIV-infected patients, especially among homosexual males, and most of the patients develop KS far in advance of other AIDS symptoms.[28]

Although the exact nature and cause of KS has not been clarified, it has been suggested that HIV infection stimulates CD4+ T cells and macrophages to release ATL-derived factor (ADF) and other cytokines, which activate the KS precursor cells (most likely endothelial cells) to produce growth factors (i.e., IL-1, bFGF, GM-CSF, TGF-β, platelet-derived growth factor) and angiogenesis factor,[372] setting up autocrine growth loops. Consistent with this notion is the lack of HIV genomes found in KS cells. The HIV genome encodes a transactivator Tat (analogous to the Tax of HTLV),[115] which, when expressed as a transgene under the regulation of the HIV LTR, induces KS-like lesions in mice.[295,431] In this instance, the expression of the *tat* gene was not detected in KS cells but in the surrounding skin cells, suggesting again that Tat, in conjunction with cytokines released from other cell types, induces the proliferation of KS cells. Indeed, *tat* and bFGF, when added in vivo, induce transformation of cells into KS-like morphology.[109] These results implicate *tat* as a factor in the higher incidence of KS in HIV-infected individuals. Tat is also known to be a promiscuous transactivator and can activate the expression of a number of herpesvirus genes.[221] A novel herpesvirus has been implicated as a cofactor in KS[67]; how and whether HIV interacts with this herpesvirus remains to be determined.

Regarding HIV-associated lymphomas, the B-cell NHLs are the most common.[29] These tumors often harbor an Epstein-Barr virus (EBV) genome and exhibit *c-myc* translocation and deregulation. Because EBV latent proteins have been shown to be able to transactivate the HIV LTR promoter, and HIV occasionally infects B cells, it has been postulated that HIV provirus insertion may provide one step in the development of HIV-associated NHLs. Laurence and Astrin[221] demonstrated that HIV itself can infect NHL cell lines in vitro and potentiates their oncogenicity. This interesting result notwithstanding, HIV genomes have not yet been identified within NHL tumor samples. Perhaps the most striking result that links HIV insertion to tumorigenesis comes from the study of HIV-associated T-cell lymphomas. A common insertion site, *fur*, which is located upstream from protooncogene *fps/fes*, was identified in four tumors.[367] A detailed molecular characterization of the activated gene is required to determine the potential of *fur* or *fes* to cause T-cell lymphoma and of HIV to serve as an insertional mutagen.

Anogenital neoplasia (i.e., cervical cancer and anal neoplasia) associated with human papillomavirus (HPV) infection arises with increased frequency in patients with HIV infection and exhibits an aggressive clinical course, with frequent occurrence of high-grade anal and cervical neoplastic changes.[242] These precancerous changes are likely to take place before AIDS develops. It has been suggested that HIV *tat* can transactivate the HPV gene expression[403] and therefore potentiate the transformation of anogenital neoplasia by HPV.

DISEASE SPECIFICITIES AND TUMOR TROPISMS

Although most oncogenic retroviruses cause multiple diseases, usually, one type of neoplasia predominates (e.g., T-cell leukemia for HTLV-I, B-lymphoma for ALV, T-cell lymphoma for M-MuLV). This tissue specificity can be attributed to several factors:

Viral *env* Gene Product

Specific env/receptor interaction is required for virus entry and infection. The cell- and species-specific distribution of the receptor undoubtedly contributes to the observed tissue tropism. In addition, several of the viral env products are mitogenic and require specific cell surface receptors to respond to their signal.

Viral Long Terminal Repeat Enhancer

LTR contains sites where cell-type–specific transcription factors can bind. The switch of F-MuLV from erythroleukemogenic to lymphomagenic by base substitutions in the LTR enhancer region dramatically illustrates this point.

Type of Protooncogenes Activated

ALV inserts its provirus near c-*erb*B and *myc* to induce erythroleukemia and B lymphoma, respectively. Clearly, the protooncogenes that are activated determine the type of tumors formed. This is probably not due to the insertion specificities of the provirus in different cell types but rather the result of different tumors selecting for successful insertional activation of different protooncogenes. The question then is why, in the same tumor type, different proviruses select different protooncogenes to activate. For example, SFFV inserts near *Spi*-1, whereas F-MuLV provirus inserts near *Fli*-2 in erythroleukemia. Is this due to heretofore unrecognized insertion specificities of individual viral LTRs? Are there subtle differences in the transcriptional activity and LTR strength of individual proviruses that ultimately determine which loci are successfully activated? In the case of c-*erb*B activation, it is known that the ALV provirus is uniquely suited; ALV has a gag AUG preceding the splice donor site, allowing inframe splicing and provision of the initiation codon to efficiently translate the truncated receptor.

Types of Mutations on Protooncogenes

Mutations on protooncogenes are best illustrated by leukemogenic and sarcomagenic *erb*B mutants, which are likely to assume different configurations and interact with cell-type–specific substrates. The other interesting example is v-*myc*, which carries a *gag* gene at its N-terminus; the *gag* sequence influences the oncogene's ability to induce sarcomas but not myeloid tumors.

There are a number of factors that may contribute to disease specificities and tumor tropisms; the lists given previously are by no means inclusive. Host genetic backgrounds, including the MHC haplotypes, are known to influence the susceptibility as well as the tissue types of retrovirus-induced neoplasia. All these point to the complexity of neoplasia and retroviral oncogenesis.

SUMMARY AND CONCLUSIONS

This chapter reviewed retroviral oncogenesis, focusing on oncogene activation and the mechanisms of oncogenesis.

Based on mechanisms, these viruses can be classified into three groups: nonacute retroviruses, acute retroviruses, and trans-acting retroviruses. The nonacute retroviruses activate host protooncogenes in cis by proviral insertion, whereas trans-acting retroviruses accomplish the same feat by providing promiscuous transactivators in trans. The acute retroviruses have captured the activated protooncogenes and subjected them to further mutations to increase their oncogenic potency and broaden the tumor tropisms. These viral oncogenes are invariably hyperactive forms of the protooncogenes, and when returned to the cell, they override, if not overwhelm, cellular controls. Thus, although the strategies used by these three types of retroviruses are different, they all involve protooncogene activation, perturbation of growth signals, and overriding of cellular controls.

The common insertion sites of nonacute retroviruses and the pirated cellular genes of acute retroviruses are rich sources for the identification of protooncogenes. Thus far, 79 common insertion sites and 32 viral oncogenes have been identified. About one third of these overlap each other. Most of these genes, alone or in combination, have been shown to be oncogenic in vivo and transforming in vitro. Furthermore, many of these loci have been found to be mutated by nonviral mutagens in human cancers. The use of retrovirus DNA as a tag continues to be a fruitful approach to identify novel oncogenes.

Retroviruses are quite versatile and can act as mutagens that can inactivate or activate genes and provide transcriptional promoters, translational start sites, splice sites, and signal peptides. In addition, because of their dual lifestyles as both RNA and DNA viruses, retroviruses can recombine with DNA and RNA. Thus, they can package transcribed cellular messages, eventually leading to transduction of cellular genes. They can also integrate themselves in host genomes as well as in genomes of DNA viruses.[188] Retroviruses are remarkable agents for the exchange of genetic information.

In the past two decades, studies of retroviral oncogenesis have significantly advanced the understanding of oncogene activation and the mechanisms of neoplastic transformation. Retroviruses are recognized as mutagens, carcinogens, gene transducers, and gene deliverers. A full understanding of retroviral oncogenesis will support the possible design of intervention strategies as well as the use of retroviruses as vehicles for gene therapy.

ABBREVIATIONS

AIDS: acquired immunodeficiency syndrome
ALV: avian leukosis virus
ATL: adult T-cell leukemia/lymphoma
BLV: bovine leukemia virus
bZIP: basic and leucine zipper
EBV: Epstein-Barr virus
EGF: epidermal growth factor
ERK: extracellular signal–regulated kinase
E Tn: endogenous retrovirus-like element
F-MuLV: Friend murine leukemia virus
FeLV: feline leukemia virus
GAP: GTPase-activating protein
GM-CSF: granulocyte-macrophage colony-stimulating factor
GSK3: glycogen synthase 3

HIV: human immunodeficiency virus
HPV: human papillomavirus
HTLV: human T-cell leukemia virus
IkB: inhibitor kappa B
IL: interleukin
JAK: Janus kinase
KS: Kaposi's sarcoma
LTR: long terminal repeat
M-MuLV: Moloney murine leukemia virus
MAPK: mitogen-activated protein kinase
MCF: mink cell focus
MEK: mitogen-activated protein kinase kinase
MEKK: mitogen-activated protein kinase kinase kinase
MMTV: mouse mammary tumor virus
NFkB: nuclear factor kappa B
NHL: non-Hodgin's lymphoma
PBL: peripheral blood leukocytes
PKC: protein kinase C
PLC-γ: phospholipase C gamma
PS/TK: protein serine/threonine kinase
REV: reticuloendotheliosis virus
SAPK: stress-activated protein kinase
SEK: stress-activated protein kinase kinase
SFFV: spleen focus-forming virus
STAT: signal transducers and activators of transcription
STLV: simian T-cell leukemia virus
TGF-β: tumor growth factor beta

REFERENCES

1. Abate C, Patel L, Rauscher III FJ, Curran T. Redox regulation of fos and jun DNA-binding activity in vitro. Science 1990;249:1157–1161.
2. Adams J, Cory S. Oncogene cooperation in leukemogenesis. Cancer Surv 1992;15:119–141.
3. Adhya HT, Grottesman M. Promoter occlusion: transcription through a promoter may inhibit activity. Cell 1982;29:939–944.
4. Adler HT, Reynolds PJ, Kelley CM, Sefton BM. Transcriptional activation of lck by retrovirus promoter insertion between two lymphoid-specific promoters. J Virol 1988;62:4113–4122.
5. Adler V, Unlap T, Kraft AS. A peptide encoding the c-jun δ domain inhibits the activity of a c-jun amino-terminal protein kinase. J Biol Chem 1994;269:11186–11191.
6. Akagi T, Shimotohno K. Proliferative response of Tax1-transduced primary human T cells to anti-CD3 antibody stimulation by an interleukin-2-independent pathway. J Virol 1993;67:1211–1217.
7. Angel P, Allegretto EA, Okino ST, et al. Oncogene jun encodes a sequence-specific trans-activator similar to AP-1. Nature (Lond) 1988;332:166–171.
8. Angel P, Karin M. The role of Jun, Fos and the AP-1 complex in cell-proliferation and transformation. Biochim Biophys Acta 1991; 1072:129–157.
9. Angel P, Smeal T, Meek J, Karin M. Jun and v-jun contain multiple regions that participate in transcriptional activation in an independent manner. New Biol 1989;1:35–43.
10. Anson DS, Clarkin K, Hyman R. Activation of lyt-2 associated with distant upstream insertion of an SL3-3 provirus. Immunogenetics 1992;36:3–14.
11. Armstrong AP, Franklin AA, Uittenbogaard MN, Giebler HA, Nyborg JK. Pleiotropic effect of the human T-cell leukemia virus Tax protien on the DNA binding activity of eukaryotic transcription factors. Proc Natl Acad Sci U S A 1993;90:7303–7307.
12. Askew DS, Bartholomew C, Buchberg AM, Valentine MB, Jenkins NA. His-1 and His-2: identification and chromosomal mapping of two commonly rearranged sites of viral integration in a myeloid leukemia. Oncogene 1991;6:2041–2047.

13. Askew DS, Bartholomew C, Ihle JN. Insertional mutagenesis and the transformation of hematopoietic stem cells. Hematol Pathol 1993;7:1–22.

14. Baba TW, Humphries EH. Formation of a transformed folicle is necessary but not sufficient for development of an avian leukosis virus-induced lymphoma. Proc Natl Acad Sci U S A 1985;82:213–216.

15. Baichwal VR, Tjian R. Control of c-jun activity by interaction of a cell-specific inhibitor with regulatory domain δ: differences between v- and c-jun. Cell 1990;63:815–825.

16. Baker SJ, Kerppola TK, Luk D, et al. Jun is phosphorylated by several protein kinases at the same sites that are modified in serum-stimulated fibroblasts. Mol Cell Biol 1992;12:4694–4705.

17. Barker CS, Bear SE, Keler T, et al. Activation of the prolactin receptor gene by promoter insertion in a Moloney murine leukemia virus-induced rat thymoma. J Virol 1992;66:6763–6768.

18. Bartholomew C, Ihle JN. Retroviral insertions 90 kilobases proximal to the Evl-1 myeloid transforming gene activate transcription from the normal promoter. Mol Cell Biol 1991;11:1820–1828.

19. Bartholomew C, Morishita K, Askew D, et al. Retroviral insertions in the CB-1/Fim-3 common site of integration active expression of the Evl-1 gene. Oncogene 1989;4:529–534.

20. Baumbach WR, Colston EM, Cole MD. Intergration of the BALB/c ecotropic provirus into the colony-stimulating factor-1-growth factor locus in a myc retrovirus-induced murine monocyte tumor. J Virol 1988;62:3151–3155.

21. Baumbach WR, Stanley ER, Cole MD. Induction of clonal monocyte-macrophage tumors in vivo by a mouse c-myc retrovirus: rearrangement of the CSF-1 gene as a secondary transforming event. Mol Cell Biol 1987;7:664–671.

22. Bear SE, Bellacosa A, Lazo PA, et al. Provirus insertion in Tpl-1, an Ets-1- related onogene, is associated with tumor progression in Moloney murine leukemia virus-induced rat thymic lymphomas. Proc Natl Acad Sci U S A 1989;86:7495–7499.

23. Ben-David Y, Bernstein A. Friend virus-induced erythroleukemia and the multistage nature of cancer. Cell 1991;66:831–834.

24. Ben-David Y, Giddens EB, Bernstein A. Identification and mapping of a common proviral integration site Fli-1 in erythroleukemia cells induced by Friend murine leukemia virus. Proc Natl Acad Sci U S A 1990;87:1332–1336.

25. Ben-David Y, Giddens EB, Letwin K, Bernstrin A. Erythroleukemia induction by Friend murine leukemia virus: insertional activation of a new member of the ets gene family, Fli-1, closely linked to c-ets-1. Genes Dev 1991;5:908–918.

26. Ben-David Y, Lavigueur A, Cheong GY, Bernstein A. Insertional inactivation of the p53 gene during friend leukemia: a new strategy for identifying tumor suppressor genes. New Biol 1990;2:1015–1023.

27. Ben-David Y, Prideaux VR, Chow V, Benchimol S, Bernstein A. Inactivation of the p53 oncogene by insertional deletion or retroviral integration in erythroleukemic cell lines induced by Friend leukemia virus. Oncogene 1988;3:179–185.

28. Beral V. Epidemiology of Kaposi's sarcoma: cancer HIV and AIDS (Imperial Cancer Research Fund). Cancer Surv 1991;10:5–22.

29. Beral V, Peterman T, Berkelman R, Jaffe H. AIDS-associated non-Hodgkin's lymphoma. Lancet 1991;337:805–809.

30. Beraud C, Sun SC, Ganchi P, Ballard DW, Greene WC. Human T-cell leukemia virus type I Tax associates with and is negatively modulated by the NF-kappa B2 100 gene product: implications for viral latency. Mol Cell Biol 1994;14:1374–1382.

31. Bergeron D, Poliquin L, Houde J, Barbeau B, Rassart E. Analysis of proviruses integrated in Fli-1 and Evi-1 regions in Cas-Br-E MuLV induced non-T, non-B-cell leukemias. Virology 1992;191:661–669.

32. Bergeron D, Poliquin L, Kozak CA, Rassart E. Identification of a common viral integration region in Cas-Br-E murine leukemia virus-induced non-T, non-B-cell lymphomas. J Virol 1991;65:7–15.

33. Berneman ZN, Gartenhaus RB, Reitz JMS, et al. Expression of alternatively spliced human T-lymphotropic virus type I pX mRNA in infected cell lines and in primary uncultured cells from patients with adult T-cell leukemia/lymphoma and healthy carriers. Proc Natl Acad Sci U S A 1992;89:3005–3009.

34. Bhagavati S, Ehrlich G, Kula RW, et al. Detectio of human T-cell lymphoma/leukemia virus type I DNA and antigen in spinal fluid and blood of patients with chronic progressive myelopathy. New Engl J Med 1988;318:1141–1147.

35. Bishop JM. Molecular themes in oncogenesis. Cell 1991;64:235–248.

36. Bjorge JD, Chan TO, Antczak M, Kung H-J, Fujita DJ. Activated type 1 phosphatidylinositol kinase is associated with the epidermal growth factor (EGF) receptor following EGF stimulation. Proc Natl Acad Sci U S A 1990;87:3816–3820.

37. Black EJ, Catling AD, Woodgett JR, Kilbey A, Gillespie DAF. Transcriptionsl activation by the v-jun oncoprotein is independent of positive regulatory phosphorylation. Oncogene 1994;9:2363–2368.

38. Blankenstein T, Qin Z, Li W, Diamantstein T. DNA rearrangement and constitutive expression of the interleukin 6 gene in a mouse plasmacytoma. J Exp Med 1990;171:965–970.

39. Blatt C, Aberdam D, Schwartz R, Sachs L. DNA rearrangement of a homeobox gene in myeloid leukemia cells. EMBO J 1988;7:4283–4290.

40. Blenis J. Siganl transduction via the MAP kinases: proceed at your own RSK. Proc Natl Acad Sci U S A 1993;90:5889–5892.

41. Boerkoel CF, Kung H-J. Transcriptional interaction between retroviral long terminal repeats (LTRs): mechanism of 5' LTR suppression and 3' LTR promoter activation of c-myc in avian B-cell lymphomas. J Virol 1992;66:4814–4823.

42. Bohmann D, Bos TJ, Admon A, Nishimura T, Vogt PK, Tjian R. Human proto-oncogene c-jun encodes a DNA binding protein with structural and functional properties of transcription factor AP-1. Science 1987;238:1386–1392.

43. Boiocchi M, Doketti R, Maestro R, Feriotto G, Rizzo S, Soriego F. A coordinated proto-oncogene expression characterizes MCF 247 murine leukemia virus-induced T-cell lymphomas irrespectively of proviral insertion affecting myc loci. Leuk Res 1990;14:549–558.

44. Bonfini L, Karlovich CA, Dasgupta C, Banerjee U. The son of sevenless gene product: a putative activator of ras. Science 1992;255:603–606.

45. Bonner TI, Kerby SB, Sutrave P, Gunnell MA, Mark G, Rapp UR. Structure and biological activity of human homologs of the raf/mil oncogene. Mol Cell Biol 1985;5:1400–1407.

46. Boral AL, Okenquist SA, Lenz J. Identification of the SL3-3 virus enhancer core as a T-lymphoma cell-specific element. J Virol 1989;63:76–84.

47. Bordeaux D, Fichelson S, Sola B, Tambourin PE, Gisselbrecht S. Frequnt involvement of the fim-3 region in Friend murine leukemia virus-induced mouse myeloblastic leukemias. J Virol 1987;61:4043–4045.

48. Bos TJ, Monteclaro FS, Mitsunobu F, et al. v-jun encodes a nuclear protein with enhancer binding properties of AP-1. Cell 1988;52:705–712.

49. Boyle WJ, Smeal T, Defiez LHK, et al. Activation of protein kinase C decreases phosphorylation of c-jun at sites that negatively regulate its DNA-binding activity. Cell 1991;64:573–584.

50. Brady J, Jeang KT, Durall J, Khoury G. Identification of the p40x-responsive regulatory sequences within the human T-cell leukemia virus type I long terminal repeat. J Virol 1987;61:2175–2181.

51. Breuer ML, Cuypers HT, Berns A. Evidence for the involvement of pim-2, a new common insertion site, in progression of lymphomas. EMBO J 1989;8:743–747.

52. Brightman BK, Farmer C, Fan H. Escape from in vivo restriction of Moloney mink cell focus-inducing viruses driven by the Mo+PyF101 long terminal repeat (LTR) by LTR alterations. J Virol 1993;67:7140–7148.

53. Brightman BK, Rein A, Trepp, Fan H. An enhancer mutant of Moloney murine leukemia virus defective in leukomogenesis does not generate mink cell focus-forming virus in vivo. Proc Natl Acad Sci U S A 1991;88:2264–2268.

54. Bruskin A, Jackson J, Bishop JM, Mc Carley DJ, Schatzman RC. Six amino acids from retroviral gene gag greatly enhance the transforming potential of the oncogene v-erbB. Oncogene 1990;5:15–24.

55. Buchberg AM, Bedigian HG, Jenkins NA, Copeland NG. Evi-2, a common integration site involved in murine myeloid leukemogenesis. Mol Cell Biol 1990;10:4658–4666.

56. Buday L, Downward J. Epidermal growth factor regulates p21 ras through the formation of a complex of receptor, Grb2 adaptor protein, and Sos nucleotide exchange factor. Cell 1993;13:7248–7256.

57. Burny A, Willems L, Callebaut I, et al. Bovine leukemia virus: biology and mode of transformation. In: Minson A, Neil J, McCrae M, eds. Viruses and cancer. Cambridge: Cambridge University Press, 1994:213–234.

58. Cadwallader KA, Paterson H, MacDonald SG, Hancock JF. N-terminally myristoylated ras proteins require palmitoylation or polyba-

sic domain for plasma membrane localization. Mol Cell Biol 1994;14:4722–4730.

59. Callaghan T, Antczak M, Flickinger T, Raines MB, Meyers M, Kung H-J. A complete description of the EGF-receptor exon structure: implications in oncogenic activation and domain evolution. Oncogene 1993;8:2939–2948.

60. Cann AJ, Chen ISY. Human T-cell leukemia virus types I and II. In: Fields BN, Knipe DM, eds. Virology. 2nd ed. New York: Raven Press, 1990:1501–1527.

61. Cantley LC, Auger KR, Carpenter C, et al. Oncogenes and signal transduction. Cell 1991;64:281–302.

62. Caputo A, Haseltine WA. Reexamination of the coding potential of the HTLV-1 pX region. Virology 1992;188:618–627.

63. Caron C, Rousset R, Beraud C, Moncollin V, Egly JM, Jalinot P. Functional and biochemical interaction of the HTLV-I Tax 1 transactivator with TBP. EMBO J 1993;12:4269–4278.

64. Carpenter G. Receptor tyrosine kinase substrates: src homology domains and signal transduction. FASEB J 1992;6:3283–3289.

65. Carroll MP, May WS. Protein kinase C-mediated serine phosphorylation directly activates raf-1 in murine hematopoietic cells. J Biol Chem 1994;269:1249–1256.

66. Casey PJ, Solski PA, Der CJ, Buss JE. p21ras is modified by a farnesl isoprenoid. Proc Natl Acad Sci U S A 1989;86:8323–8327.

67. Chang Y, Cesarman E, Pessin MS, et al. Identification of Herpesvirus-like DNA sequences in AIDS-associated Kaposi's sarcoma. Science 1994;266:1865–1869.

68. Chardin P, Camonis JH, Gale NW, et al. Human Sos1: a guanine nucleotide exchange factor for Ras that binds to GRB2. Science 1993;260:1338–1343.

69. Chatis PA, Holland CA, Hartley JW, Rowe WP. Role for the 3' end of the genome in determining disease specificity of Friend and Moloney murine leukemia viruses. Proc Natl Acad Sci U S A 1983;80:4408–4411.

70. Chatis PA, Holland CA, Silver JE, Frederickson TN, Hopkins N, Harley JW. A 3' end fragment encompassing the transcriptional enhancers of nondefective Friend virus confers erythroleukemogenicity on Moloney leukemia virus. J Virol 1984;52:248–254.

71. Cheatham B, Vlahos CJ, Cheatham L, Wang L, Blenis J, Kahn CR. Phosphatidylinositol 3-kinase activation is required for insulin stimulation of pp70 S6 kinase, DNA synthesis, and glucose transporter translocation. Mol Cell Biol 1994;14:4902–4911.

72. Chen ISY, Quan SG, Golde DW. Human T-cell leukemia virus type II transforms normal lymphocytes. Proc Natl Acad Sci U S A 1983;80:7006–7009.

73. Chen SJ, Holbrook NJ, Mitchell KF, et al. A viral long terminal repeat in the interleukin-2 gene of a cell line that constitutively produces interleukin-2. Proc Natl Acad Sci U S A 1985;82:7284–7288.

74. Chida K, Vogt PK. Nuclear translocation of viral jun but not of cellular jun is cell cycle dependent. Proc Natl Acad Sci U S A 1992;89:4290–4294.

75. Chow V, Ben-David Y, Bernstein A, Benchimol S, Mowat M. Multiatage Friend erythroleukemia: independent origin of tumor clones with normal or rearranged p53 cellular oncogenes. J Virol 1987;61:2777–2781.

76. Chuang E, Barnard D, Hettich L, Zhang X-F, Avruch J, Marshall MS. Critical binding and regulatory interactions between ras and raf through a small, stable N-terminal domain of raf and specific ras effector residues. Mol Cell Biol 1994;14:5318–5325.

77. Chung J, Grammer TC, Lemon KP, Kazlauskas A, Blenis J. PDGF- and insulin-dependent pp70S6K activation by phosphatidylinositol-3-OH kinase. Nature (Lond) 1994;370:71–75.

78. Ciminale V, Pavlakis GN, Derse D, Cunningham CP, Felber BK. Complex splicing in the human T-cell leukemia virus (HTLV) family of retroviruses: novel mRNAs and proteins produced by HTLV type I. J Virol 1992;66:1737–1745.

79. Clausse N, Baines D, Moore R, Brookes S, Dickson C, Peters G. Activation of both Wnt-1 and Fgf-3 by insertion of mouse mammary tumor virus downstream in the reverse orientation: a reappraisal of the enhancer insertion model. Virology 1993;194:157–165.

80. Clausse N, Smith R, Calberg-Bacq CM, Peters G, Dickson C. Mouse-mammary tumor virus activates Fgf-3/Int-2 less frequently in tumors from virgin than from parous mice. Int J Cancer 1993;55:157–163.

81. Cleghon V, Morrison DK. Raf-1 interacts with fyn and src in a non-phosphotyrosine-dependent manner. J Biol Chem 1994;269:17749–17755.

82. Clemens K, Radonovich M, Piras G, et al. Interaction of the HTLV-I Tax₁ protein with the basal transcription factor TFIIA. In: Lenz J, MorseIII HC, Ruscentti S, Tsichlis PN, eds. Pathogenesis of animal retroviruses. Philadelphia: Fox Chase Cancer Center, 1994:32.

83. Clurman BE, Hayward WS. Multiple proto-oncogene activations in avian leukosis virus-induced lymphomas: reidence for stage-specific events. Mol Cell Biol 1989;9:2657–2664.

84. Coffin JM. Retroviridae and their replication. In: Fields BN, Knipe DM, eds. Virology. 2nd ed. New York: Raven Press, 1990:1437–1500.

85. Coffin JM. Structure and classification of retroviruses. In: Levy JA, ed. Retroviridae. vol 1. New York: Plenum Press, 1992:19–49.

86. Cohen JB, Unger T, Rechavi G, Camaani E, Givol D. Rearrangement of the oncogene c-mos in mouse myeloma NSI and hybridomas. Nature (Lond) 1983;306:797–799.

87. Cohen GB, Ren R, Baltimore D. Molecular binding domains in signal transduction proteins. Cell 1995;80:237–248.

88. Collart KL, Aurigemma R, Smith RE, Kawai S, Robinson HL. Infrequent invovement of c-fos in avian leukosis virus-induced nephroblastoma. J Virol 1990;64:3541–3544.

89. Cooper MD, Payne LN, Dent PB, Burmester BR, Good RA. Pathogenesis of avian lymphoid leukosis. J Natl Cancer Inst 1968;41:373–378.

90. Corcoran LM, Adams JM, Dunn AR, Cory S. Murine T lymphomas in which the cellular myc oncogene has been activated by retroviral insertion. Cell 1984;37:113–122.

91. Coutneidge S, Dhand R, Pilat D, Twamley GM, Waterfield MD, Roussel MF. Activation of Src family kinases by colony stimulating factor-1, and their association with its receptor. EMBO J 1993;12:943–950.

92. Cullen BR, Lomedico PT, Ju G. Transcriptional interference in avian retroviruses-implications for the promoter insertion model of leukaemogenesis. Nature (Lond) 1984;307:241–245.

93. Curran T, Vogt PK. Dangerous liasons: Fos and Jun, oncogenic transcription factors. In: McKnight SL, Yamamota K, eds. Transcriptional regulation. Cold Spring Harbor, NY: Cold Spring Harbor Laboratory, 1992:797–831.

94. Cuypers HTM, Selter G, Quint W. Murine leukemia virus-induced T-cell lymphomagenesis: integration of proviruses in a distinct chromosomal region. Cell 1984;37:141–150.

95. Darnell JE, Kerr IM, Stark GR. Jak-STAT pathways and transcriptional activation in response to IFNs and other extracellular signaling proteins. Science 1994;264:1415–1421.

96. Daum G, Eisenmann-Tappe I, Fries H-W, Troppmair J, Rapp UR. The ins and outs of Raf kinases. TIBS 1994;19:474–480.

97. Davis R. MAPKs: new JNK expands the group. TIBS 1994;19:470–473.

98. Deli-Bovi P, Curatola AM, Newman KM, et al. Processing, secretion, and biological properties of a novel growth factor family with oncogenic potential. Mol Cell Biol 1988;8:2933–2941.

99. Derijard B, Hibi M, Wu I-H, et al. JNK1: a protein kinases stimulated by UV light and Ha-ras that binds and phosphorylates the c-jun activation domain. Cell 1994;76:1025–1037.

100. Derijard B, Raingcaud J, Barrett T, et al. Independent human MAP kinase signal transduction pathways defiend by MEK and MKK isoforms. Science 1995;267:682–685.

101. Des Groseillers L, Jolicoeur P. The tandem direct repeats within the long terminal repeat of murine leukemia viruses are the primary determinant of their leukemogenic potential. J Virol 1984;52.

102. Dickson B, Sprenger F, Morrison D, Hafen E. Raf functions downstream of ras 1 in the sevenless signal transduction pathway. Nature (Lond) 1992;360:600–603.

103. Dickson C, Smith R, Brookes S, Peters G. Proviral insertions within the int-2 gene can generate multiple anomalous transcripts but leave the protein-coding domain intact. J Virol 1990;64:784–793.

104. Dickson C, Smith R, Brookes S, Peters G. Tumorigenesis by mouse mammary tumor virus: proviral activation of a cellular gene in the common integration region int-2. Cell 1988;37:529–536.

105. Dolcetti R, Rizzo S, Viel A, et al. N-myc activation by proviral insertion in MCF247-induced murine T-cell lymphomas. Oncogene 1989;4:1009–1014.

106. Dreyfus F, Sola S, Fichelson S, et al. Rearrangements of the Pim-1, c-myc, and p53 genes in Friend helper virus-induced mouse erythroleukemias. Leukemia 1990;4:590–594.

107. Duhrsen U, Stahl J, Gough NM. In vivo transformation of factor-dependent hematopoietic cells: role of intracisternal A-particle transposition for growth factor gene activation. EMBO J 1990;9:1087–1096.

108. Egan SE, Giddings BW, Brooks MW, Buday L, Sizeland AM, Weinberg RA. Association of Sos Ras exchange protein with Grb2 is implicated in tyrosine kinase signal transduction and transformation. Nature (Lond) 1993;363:45–51.

109. Ensoli B, Gendelman R, Markham P, et al. Synergy between basic fibroblast growth factor and HIV-1 Tat protein in induction of Kaposi's sarcoma. Nature (Lond) 1994;371:674–680.

110. Escobedo JA, Navankasattusas S, Kavanaugh WM, Milfay D, Fried VA, Williams LT. cDNA cloning of a novel 85 kd protein that has SH2 domains and regulates binding of PI3-Kinase to the PDGF beta-receptor. Cell 1991;65:75–82.

111. Fan H. Influences of the long terminal repeats within on retroviral pathogenecity. Semin Virol 1990;1:165–174.

112. Fantl WJ, Johnson DE, Williams LT. Signalling by receptor tyrosine kinases. Annu Rev Biochem 1993;62:453–481.

113. Feuer G, Chen ISY. Mechanisms of human T-cell leukemia virus-induced leukemogennesis. Biochim Biophys Acta 1992;1114:223–233.

114. Finlay CA, Hinds PW, Levine AJ. The p53 proto-oncogene can act as a suppressor of transformation. Cell 1989;57:1083–1093.

115. Fisher AG, Feinberg MB, Josephs SF, et al. The trans-activator gene of HTLV-III is essential for virus replication. Nature (Lond) 1986;320:367–371.

116. Flubacher MM, Bear SE, Tsichlis PN. Replacement of IL-2 generated mitogenic signals by an MCF or xenotropic virus-indued IL-9 dependent autocrine loop. Implications for MCF virus-induced leukemogenesis. In: Lenz J, Morse HC III, Ruscetti S, Tsichlis PN, eds. Pathogenesis of animal retroviruses. Philadelphia: Fox Chase Cancer Center, 1994:24.

117. Forrest D, Onions D, Lees G, Neil JC. Altered structure and expression of c-myc in feline T-cell tumours. Virology 1987;158:194–205.

118. Franke TF, Chan TO, Yang SI, et al. The Akt protein kinase is a downstream mediator of Phosphatidylinositol-3(OH) kinase activated by PDGF. Role of the Akt homology/Pleckstrin homology domain. In: Lenz J, Morse HC III, Ruscetti S, Tsichlis PN, eds. Pathogenesis of animal retroviruses. Philadelphia: Fox Chase Cancer Center, 1994:73.

119. Freed E, Symons M, Macdonald SG, McMormick F, Ruggieri R. Binding of 14-3-3 proteins to the protein kinase raf and effects on its activation. Science 1994;265:1713–1716.

120. Friend C. Cell-free transmission in adult Swiss mice of a disease having the character of a leukemia. J Exp Med 1957;105:307.

121. Fu H, Xia K, Pallas DC, et al. Interaction of the protein kinase raf-1 with 14-3-3 proteins. Science 1994;266:126–129.

122. Fujii M, Tsuchiya H, Chuhjo T, Akizawa T, Seiki M. Interaction of HTLV-1 Tax1 with p67SRF causes the aberrant induction of cellular immediate early genes through CArG boxes. Genes Dev 1992;6:2066–2076.

123. Fujisawa JI, Seiki M, Sato M, Yoshida M. A transcriptional enhancer sequence of HTLV-I is responsible for trans-activation mediated by p40x of HTLV-I. EMBO J 1986;5:713–718.

124. Fujisawa J, Toita M, Yoshida M. A unique enhancer element for the transactivator (p40tax) of human T-cell leukemia virus type I that is distinct from cyclic AMP- and 12-o-tetradecanoylphorbol-13-acetate-responsive elements. J Virol 1989;63:3234–3239.

125. Fung Y-KT, Crittenden LB, Kung H-J. Orientation and position of avian leukosis virus DNA relative to the cellular oncogene c-myc in B-lymphoma tumors of highly susceptible 151_5X7_2 chickens. J Virol 1982;44:742–746.

126. Fung Y-KT, Fadly AM, Crittenden LM, Kung H-J. On the mechanism of retrovirus-induced avian lymphoid leukosis: deletion and integration of the proviruses. Proc Natl Acad Sci U S A 1981;78:3418–3422.

127. Fung Y-KT, Lewis WG, Crittenden LB, Kung H-J. Activation of the cellular oncogene c-erbB by LTR insertion: molecular basis for induction of erythroblastosis by avian leukosis virus. Cell 1983;33:357–368.

128. Gale NW, Kaplan S, Lowenstein EJ, Schlessinger J, Bar-Sagi D. Grb2 mediates the EGF-dependent activation of guanine nucleotide exchange on Ras. Nature (Lond) 1993;363:88–92.

129. Gallahan D, Callahan R. Mammary tumorigenesis in fetal mice: identification of a new int locus in mouse mammary tumor virus (Czech II)-induced mammary tumors. J Virol 1987;61:66–74.

130. Gama Sosa MA, Rosas DH, DeGasperi E, Morita E, Hutchinson MR, Ruprecht RM. Negative regulation of the 5' long terminal repeat (LTR) by the 3'LTR in the murine proviral genome. J Virol 1994;68:2662–2670.

131. Gamett DC, Tracy SE, Robinson HL. Differences in sequences encoding the carboxyl-terminal domain of the epidermal growth factor receptor correlate with differences in the disease potential of viral erbB genes. Proc Natl Acad Sci U S A 1986;76:6053–6057.

132. Garcia M, Wellinger R, Vessaz A, Digglemann H. A new site of integration for mouse mammary tumor virus proviral DNA common to Balb/c (C3H) mammary and kidney adenocarcinomas. EMBO J 1986;5:127–134.

133. Gattoni-Celli S, Hsiao W-LW, Weinstein IB. Rearranged c-mos locus in a MOPC21 murine myeloma cell line and its persistence in hybridomas. Nature (Lond) 1983;306:795–796.

134. Gazzolo L, Duc Dondon M. Direct activation of resting T lymphocytes by human T-lymphotropic virus type I. Nature (Lond) 1987;326:714–717.

135. George DL, Glick B, Trusko S, Freeman N. Enhanced c-Ki-ras expression associated with Friend virus integration in a bone marrow-derived mouse cell line. Proc Natl Acad Sci U S A 1986;83:1651–1655.

136. Gessain A, Barin F, Vernant JC, Maurs L, Giordano C, Malone G, Tournie-Lasserve E, De The G. Antibodies to human T-lymphotropic virus type I in patients with tropical spastic pararesis. Lancet 1985;2:407–409.

137. Gilks CB, Bear SE, Grimes HL, Tsichlis PN. Progression of interleukin-2 (IL-2)-dependent rat T cell lymphoma lines to IL-2-independent growth following activation of a gene (Gfi-1) encoding a novel zinc finger protein. Mol Cell Biol 1993;13:1759–1768.

138. Gisselbrecht S, Fichelson S, Sola B. Frequent c-fms activation by proviral insertion in mouse myeloblastic leukaemias. Nature (Lond) 1987;329:259–261.

139. Goddenow MM, Hayward WS. 5' Long terminal repeats of myc-associated proviruses appear structurally intact but are functionally impaired in tumors induced by avian leukosis virus. J Virol 1987;61:2489–2498.

140. Gonda TJ, Cory S, Sobieszczuk P, Holtzman D, Adams JM. Generation of altered transcripts by retroviral insertion in the c-myb gene in two murine monocytic leukemias. J Virol 1987;61:2754–2763.

141. Grassmann R, Berchtold S, Radant I, et al. Role of human T-cell leukemia virus type 1 X region proteins in immortilazation of primary human lymphocytes in culture. J Virol 1992;66:4570–4575.

142. Gray DA, Jackson DP, Percy DH, Morris VL. Activation of int-1 and int-2 loci in GRF mammary tumors. Virology 1986;154:271–278.

143. Gray DA, McGrath CM, Jones RF, Morris VL. A common mouse tumor virus integration site in chemically induced precancerous mammary hyperplasias. Virology 1986;148:360–368.

144. Greenberg R, Hawley R, Marcu KB. Acquisition of an insertional A-particle element by a translocated c-myc gene in a murine plasma cell tumor. Mol Cell Biol 1985;5:3625–3628.

145. Gulbins E, Coggeshall KM, Baler G, et al. Direct stimulation of vav guanine nucleotide exchange activity for ras by phorbol esters and diglycerides. Mol Cell Biol 1994;14:4749–4758.

146. Hadman M, Loo M, Bos TJ. In vivo viral and cellular jun complexes exhibit differential interaction with a number of in vitro generated "AP-1- and CREB-like" target sequences. Oncogene 1993;8:1895–1905.

147. Han XD, Wong PM, Chung SW. Chronic myeloproliferative disease induced by site-specific integration of Aberison murine leukemia virus-infected hemopoietic cells. Proc Natl Acad Sci U S A 1991;88:10129–10133.

148. Hancock JF, Magee AI, Childs JE, Marshall CJ. All ras proteins are polyisoprenylated but only some are palmitoylated. Cell 1989;57:1167–1177.

149. Hanecak R, Pattengale PH, Fan H. Addition or substitution of simian virus 40 enhancer sequences into the Moloney murine leukemia. J Virol 1988;62:2427–2436.

150. Hanna Z, Jankoski M, Tremblay P, et al. The Vin-1 gene, identied by provirus insertional mutagenesis, is the cyclin D2. Oncogene 1993;8:1661–1666.

151. Hartley J, Wolford NK, Old LJ, Rowe WP. A new class of murine leukemia virus associated with the development of spontaneous lymphomas. Proc Natl Acad Sci U S A 1977;74:789–792.

152. Harvey JJ. An unidentified virus which cause the rapid production of tumors in mice. Nature (Lond) 1964;204:1104–1105.

153. Haupt Y, Alexander WS, Barri G, Kilnken SP, Adams JM. Novel zinc finger gene implicated as myc collaborator by retrovirally accelerated lymphomagenesis in Eμ-myc transgenic mice. Cell 1991; 65:753–763.

154. Havarstein LS, Morgan IM, Wong W-Y, Vogt PK. Mutations in the jun delta region suggest as inverse correlation between transformation and transcriptional activation. Proc Natl Acad Sci U S A 1992; 89:618–622.

155. Hayward WS, Neel BG, Astrin SM. Activation of a cellular onc gene by promoter insertion in ALV-induced lymphoid leukosis. Nature (Lond) 1981;290:475–480.

156. Heberlein C, Kawai M, Franz M-J, et al. Retrotransposons as mutagens in the induction of growth autonomy in hematopoietic cells. Oncogene 1990;5:1799–1807.

157. Heidecker G, Kolch W, Morrison DK, Rapp UR. The role of raf-1 phosphorylation in siganl transduction. Adv Cancer Res 1992;53–73.

158. Herman SA, Coffin JM. Differential transcription from the long terminal repeats of integrated avian leukosis virus DNA. J Virol 1986;60:497–505.

159. Herman SA, Coffin JM. Efficient packaging of readthrough RNA in ALV: implication for oncogene transduction. Science 1987;236: 845–848.

160. Hibi M, Lin A, Smeal T, Minden A, Karin M. Identification of an oncoprotein- and UV-responsive protein kinase that binds and potentiates the c-jun activation domain. Genes Dev 1993;7:2135–2148.

161. Hicks GG, Mowat M. Integration of Freind murine leukemia virus into both allels of the p53 oncogene in an erythroleukemic cell line. J Virol 1988;62:4752–4755.

162. Hidaka M, Inoue J, Yoshida M, Seiki M. Post-transcriptional regulator (rex) of HTLV-I initiates expression of viral structural proteins but suppresses expression of regulatory proteins. EMBO J 1988; 7:519–523.

163. Hino M, Tojo A, Misawa Y, Moril H, Takaku F, Shibuya M. Unregulated expression of the erythropoietin receptor gene caused by insertion of spleen focus-forming virus long terminal repeat in a murine erythroleukemia cell line. Mol Cell Biol 1991;11:5527–5533.

164. Hinrichs SH, Nerenberg M, Renolds RK, Khoury G, Jay G. A transgenic mouse model for human neurofibromatosis. Science 1987; 237:1340–1343.

165. Hiral H, Fujisawa J, Suzuki T, et al. Transcriptional activator Tax of HTLV-1 binds to the NF-kappa B precursor p 105. 1992;7:1737–1742.

166. Hirai H, Suzuki T, Fugisawa J-I, Inooue J-I, Yoshida M. Tax protein of human T-cell leukemia virus type I binds to the ankyrin motifs of inhibitory factor κB and induces nuclear translocation of transcription factor NF-κB proteins for transcriptional activation. Proc Natl Acad Sci U S A 1994;91:3584–3588.

167. Hirsch HH, Nair AP, Moroni C. Suppressible and nonsuppressible autocrine mast cell tumors are distinguished by insertion of an endogenous retroviral element (IAP) into the interleukin 3 gene. J Exp Med 1993;178:403–411.

168. Holbrook NJ, Gulino A, Durand D, Lin Y, Crabtree GR. Transcriptional activity of the gibbon ape leukemia virus in the interleukin 2 gene of MLA 144 cells. Virology 1987;159:178–182.

169. Hollsberg P, Whafler DA. Seminars in medicine of the Beth Israel Hospital, Boston. Pathogenesis of disease induced by human lymphotropic virus type I infection. N Engl J Med 1993;328:1173–1182.

170. Homma T, Kanki P, King N, et al. Lymphoma in macaques: association with virus of human T lymphotropic family. Science 1984; 225:716–718.

171. Hoshino H, Tanaka H, Shimotohno K, Miwa M, Nagal T, Yoshiki T, Koike T. Immortalization of peripheral blood lymphocytes of cats by human T-cell leukemia virus. Int J Cancer 1984;34:513–517.

172. Howard JC, Yousefi S, Cheong G, Bernstein A, Ben-David Y. Temporal order and functional analysis of mutations within the Fli-1 and p53 genes during the erythroleukemias induced by F-MuLV. Oncogene 1993;8:2721–2129.

173. Huang CC, Hay N, Bishop JM. The role of RNA molecules in transduction of the proto-oncogene c-fps. Cell 1986;44:935–940.

174. Huang W, Alessandrini A, Crews CM, Erikson RL. Raf-1 forms a stable complex with Mek1 and activates Mek1 by serine phosphorylation. Proc Natl Acad Sci U S A 1993;90:10947–10951.

175. Humphries EH, Baba TW. Folicular hyperplasia in the prelymphomatous avian bursa: relationship to the incidence of B-cell lymphoma. Curr Top Microbiol Immunol 1986;113:47–55.

176. Ihle JN, Smith-White B, Sisson B. Activation of the C-H-ras protooncogene by retrovirus insertion and chromosomal rearrangement in Molonney leukemia virus-induced T-cell leukemia. J Virol 1989; 63:2959–2966.

177. Ihle JN, Witthun BA, Quelle FW, et al. Signaling by the cytokine receptor superfamily: JAKs and STATs. TIBS 1994;19:222–227.

178. Inoue J, Seiki M, Yoshida M. The second pX product p27xIII of HTLV01 is required for gag gene expression. FEBS Lett 1986;209: 187–190.

179. Inoue J, Yoshida M, Seiki M. Transcriptional (p40x) and post-transcriptionasl (p27xIII) regulators are required for the expression and replication of human T-cell leukemia virus type I genes. Proc Natl Acad Sci U S A 1987;84:3653–3657.

180. Irie K, Gotoh Y, Yashar BM, Errede B, Nishida E, Mataumoto K. Stimulatory effects of yeast and mammalian 14-3-3 proteins on the raf protein kinase. Science 1994;265:1716–1719.

181. Isfort R, Witter RL, Kung H-J. c-myc activation in an unusual retrovirus-induced avain T-lymphoma resembling Marek's disease: proviral insertion of 5' exon one enhances the expression of an intron promoter. Oncogene Res 1987;2:81–94.

182. Jacobson S, Raine CS, Mingioli ES, McFarlin DE. Isolation of an HTLV-1-like retrovirus from patients with tropical spastic pararesis. Nature (Lond) 1988;331:540–543.

183. Jankenecht R, Ernst WH, Pingoud V, Nordheim A. Activation of TCF Elk-1 by MAP kinases. EMBO J 1993;12:5097–5104.

184. Jeang KT, Widen SG, Semmes IV OJ, Wilson SH. HTLV-1 transactivator protein, tax, is a trans-repressor of the human beta-polymerase gene. Science 1990;247:1082–1084.

185. Jia R, Mayer BJ, Hanafusa T, Hanafusa H. A novel oncogene,v-ryk, encoding a trucated receptor tyrosine kinase is transduced into the RPL30 virus without loss of viral sequences. J Virol 1992;66:5975–5987.

186. Jolicoeur P, Girard L, Jiang X, Hanna Z, Takac M, Huang M. Insertional mutagenesis in MULV-induced tumors. In: Lenz J, Morse HC III, Ruscetti S, Tsichlis PN, eds. Pathogenesis of animal retroviruses. Philadelphia: Fox Chase Cancer Center, 1994:61.

187. Joliot V, Martinerie C, Dambrine G, Plassiart G, Brisac M, Crochet J. Proviral rearrangements and overexpression of a new cellular gene (nov) in myeloblastosis-associated virus type 1-induced nephroblastosis. Mol Cell Biol 1992;12:10–21.

188. Jones D, Brunovskis P, Kung H-J. Characterization of novel viruses derived from retroviral insertion into herpesvirus. In: Kung H-J, Wood C, eds. Interaction between retroviruses and herpesviruses. NJ: World Scientific, 1994:10–22.

189. Justice MJ, Morse HC III, Jenkins NA, Copeland NG. A novel common site of retroviral integration in mouse AKXD B-cell lymphomas. J Virol 1994;68:1293–1300.

190. Kabrun N, Bumstead N, Hayman MJ. Characterization of a novel promoter insertion in the c-rel locus. Mol Cell Biol 1990;10:4788–4794.

191. Kalland KH, Langhoff E, Bos JH, Gottlinger H, Haseltine WA. Rex-dependent nucleolar accumulation of HTLV-I mRNAs. New Biol 1991;3:389–397.

192. Kanter MR, Smith RE, Hayward WS. Rapid induction of B-cell lymphomas: insertional activation of c-myb by avian leukosis virus. J Virol 1988;62:1423–1432.

192a. Kapeller R, Cautley LC. Phosphatidylinositol 3-kinase. Bioessays 1994;16:565–576.

193. Kaplan DR, Morrison DK, Wong G, McCormick F, Williams LT. PDGF beta-receptor stimulates tyrosine phosphorylation of GAP

and association of GAP with a signaling complex. Cell 1990;61: 125–133.

194. Katzi N, Rechavi G, Cohen JB, et al. "Retroposon" insertion into the cellular oncogene c-myc in canine transmissible venereal tumor. Proc Natl Acad Sci U S A 1985;82:1054–1058.

195. Kazlauskas A, Ellis C, Pawson T, Cooper JA. Binding of GAP to activated PDGF receptors. Science 1990;247:1578–1581.

196. Khoury G, Gruss P. Enhancer elements. Cell 1983;33:313–314.

197. Kim JH, Kaufman PA, Hanley SM, Rimsky LT, Green WC. Rex transregulation of human T-cell leukemia virus type II gene expression. J Virol 1991;65:405–414.

198. Kimata JT, Palker TJ, Ratner L. The mitogenic activity of human T-cell leukemia virus type I is T-cell associated and requires the CD2/LFA-3 activation pathway. J Virol 1993;67:3134–3141.

199. Kirsten WH, Mayer LA. Morphological responses to a murine erythroblastosis. J Natl Cancer Inst 1967;39:311–319.

200. Kiyokawa T, Seiki M, Iwashita S, Imagawa K, Shimizu F, Yoshida M. P27ˣIII and p21ˣIII, proteins encoded by the pX sequence of human T-cell leukemia virus type I. Proc Natl Acad Sci U S A 1985; 82:8359–8363.

201. Koch CA, Anderson D, Moran MF, Ellis C, Pawson T. SH2 and SH3 domains: elements that control interactions of cytoplasmic signaling proteins. Science 1991;252:668–674.

202. Koehne CF, Lazo PA, Alves K, Lee JS, Tsichlis PN, O'Donnell PV. The Mivi-1 locus involved in the induction of rat T-cell lymphoma and pvt-1/mis-1 locus are identical. J Virol 1989;63:2366-2369.

203. Koide H, Satoh T, Nakafuku M, Kaziro Y. GTP-dependent association of Raf-1 with Ha-Ras: identificiation of Raf as a target downstream of Ras in mammalian cells. Proc Natl Acad Sci U S A 1993; 90:8683–8686.

204. Kolch W, Heldecker G, Kochs G, et al. Protein kinase Cα activates raf-1 by direct phosphorylation. Nature (Lond) 1993;364:249–252.

205. Koller R, Krall M, Mock B, Wolff L. Identification of a common integration site in MML-induced by amphotropic MuLV in DBA/2 mice. In: Lenz J, Morse HC III, Ruscetti S, Tsichlis PN, eds. Pathogenesis of animal retroviruses. Philadelpha: Fox Chase Cancer Center, 1994:71.

206. Kondo T, Kono H, Nonaka H, et al. Risk of adult leukemia/lymphoma in HTLV-I carriers. Lancet 1987;2:159.

207. Kongsuwan K, Allen J, Adams JM. Expression of Hox-2,4 homeobox gene directed by proviral insertion in a myeloid leukemia. Nucl Acids Res 1989;17:1881–1892.

208. Kono T, Doi T, Yamada G, et al. Murine interleukin 2 receptor β chain: dysregulated gene expression in lymphoma line EL-4 caused by a promoter insertion. Proc Natl Acad Sci U S A 1990;87:1806–1810.

209. Koralnik IJ, Fullen J, Franchini G. The p12I, p13II, p30III proteins encoded by human T-cell leukemia/lymphotropic virus type I open reading frames I and II are localized in three different cellular components. J Virol 1993;67:2360–2366.

210. Koralnik IJ, Gessain A, Klotman ME, Lo-Monico A, Berneman ZN, Franchini G. Protein isoforms encoded by the pX egion of human T-cell leukemia/lymphotropic virus type I. Proc Natl Acad Sci U S A 1992;89:8813–8817.

211. Kortenjann M, Thomae O, Shaw PE. Inhibition of v-raf-dependent c-fos expression and transformation by a kinase-defective mutant of the mitogen-activated protein kinase Erk2. Mol Cell Biol 1994;14: 4815–4824.

212. Kozak C, Ruscetti S. Retroviruses in Rodents. In: Levy JA, ed. Retroviridae. vol 1. New York: Plenum Press, 1992:405–481.

213. Kung H-J, Boerkoel C, Carter T. Retroviral mutagenesis of cellular oncogenes: a review with insights into the mechanisms of insertional activation. Curr Top Microbiol Immunol 1991;171: 1–25.

214. Kypta RM, Goldberg Y, Ulug ET, Courtneidge SA. Association between the PDGF receptor and members of the src family of tyrosine kinases. Cell 1990;62:481–492.

215. Kyriakis JM, App H, Zhang XF, et al. Raf-1 activates MAP kinasekinase. Nature (Lond) 1992;358:417–421.

216. Kyriakis JM, Banerjee P, Nikolakaki E, et al. The stress-activated protein kinase subfamily of c-jun kinases. Nature (Lond) 1994;369: 156–160.

217. Lacombe C, Chretien S, Lemarchandel V, Mayeux P, Romeo P-H, Gisselbrecht S. Spleen focus-forming virus long terminal repeat insertional activation of the murine erythropoietin receptor gene in the T3C1-2 friend leukemia cell line. J Biol Chem 1991;266:6952–6956.

218. Lacoste J, Lanoix J, Pepin N, Hiscott J. Interactions between HTLV-1 Tax and NF-κB/Rel proteins in T cells. Leukemia 1994;8:S71–S75.

219. Lammi GA, Smith R, Silver J, Brookes S, Dickson C, Peters G. Proviral insertions near cyclin D1 in mouse lymphomas: a parallel for BCL1 translocations in human B-cell neoplasms. Oncogene 1992;7(12):2381–2387.

220. Lange-Carter CA, Pleiman CM, Gardner AM, Blumer KJ, Johnson GL. A divergence in the MAP kinase regulatory network dcfined by MEK kinase and raf. Science 1993;260:315–319.

221. Laurence J, Astrin SM. Human immunodeficiency virus induction of malignant transformation in human B lymphocytes. Proc Natl Acad Sci U S A 1991;88:7635–7639.

222. Lavigueur A, Bernstein A. p53 mutations increase resistance to ionizing radiation. Oncogene 1991;6:831–834.

223. Lazo PA, Lee JS, Tsichlis PN. Long distance activation of the c-myc protein oncogene by provirus insertion in Mlvi-1 or Mlvi-4 in rat T-cell lymphomas. Proc Natl Acad Sci U S A 1990;87:170–173.

224. Lazo PA, Tsichlis PN. Recombination between two integrated proviruses, one of which was inserted near c-myc in a retrovirus-induced rat thymoma: implications for tumor progression. J Virol 1988;62:788–794.

225. Lechleider RJ, Sugimoto S, Bennet AM, et al. Activation of the SH2-containing phosphotyrosine phosphatase SH-PTP2 by its binding site phosphotyrosine 1009 on the PDGF receptor. J Biol Chem 1993;268:21478–21481.

226. Lee EB, Beug H, Hayman MJ. Mutational analysis of the role of the carboxy-terminal egion of the v-erbB protein in erythroid cell transformation. Oncogene 1993;8:1317–1327.

227. Leevers SJ, Paterson HF, Marshall CJ. Requirement for ras in raf activation is overcome by targeting raf to the plasma membrane. Nature (Lond) 1994;369:411–420.

228. Lenz J, Celander D, Crowther RL, Patarca D, Perkins W, Haseltine WA. Determination of the leukemogenicity of a murine retrovirus by sequences with the long terminal repeat. Nature (Lond) 1984; 308:467–470.

228a. Lepage P, Devaute A, Gros P. Activation of the mouse mdro3 gene by insertion of retroviruses in multidry-resistant tumor cells. Mol Cell Biol 1993;13:7380–7392.

229. Leslie KB, Lee F, Schrader JW. Intracisternal A-type particle-mediated activations of cytokine genes in a murine myelomonocytic leukemia: generation of functional cytokine mRNAs by retroviral splicing events. Mol Cell Biol 1991;11:5562–5570.

230. Levesque KS, Bonham L, Levy LS. fivi-1 A common integration domain of feline leukemia virus in naturally occurring lymphomas of a particular tupe. J Virol 1990;64:3455–3462.

231. Levy LS, Fish RE, Baskin GB. Tumorigenic potential of a myc-containing strin of feline leukemia virus in domestic cats. J Virol 1988; 62:4770–4773.

232. Levy LS, Gardner MB, Casey JW. Isolation of a feline leukemia provirus containing the oncogene myc from a feline lymphosarcoma. Nature (Lond) 1984;308:853–856.

233. Levy LS, Lobelle-Rich PA. Insertional mutagenisis of fivi-2 in tumors induced by infection with LC-FeLV, a myc- containing strain of feline leukemia virus. J Virol 1992;66:2885–2892.

234. Levy LS, Lobelle-Rich PA, Overbaugh J, Abkowitz JL, Fulton R, Roy-Burman P. Coincident involvement of fivi-2, c-myc, and novel env genes on natural and experimental lymphosarcomas induced by feline leukemia virus. Virology 1993;196:892–895.

235. Levy LS, Lobelle-Rich PA, Overbaugh J. fivi-2, a target of retroviral insertional mutagenesis in feline thymic lymphosarcomas, encodes bmi-1. Oncogene 1993;8:1833–1838.

236. Li Y, Holland CA, Hartley JW, Hopkins N. Viral integration near c-myc in 10–20% of MCF 247-induced AKR lymphomas. Proc Natl Acad Sci U S A 1984;81:6808–6811.

237. Li J, Baltimore D. Mechanism of leukemogenesis induced by mink cell focus-forming murine leukemia viruses. J Virol 1991;65:2408–2414.

238. Li J, D'Andrea D, Lodish HF, Baltimore D. Activation of cell growth

by binding of Friend spleen focus-forming virus gp55 glycoprotein to the erythropoietin receptor. Nature (Lond) 1990;343:762– 764.

239. Li N, Batzer A, Daly R, et al. Guanine-nucleotide-releasing factor hSos1 binds to Grb2 and links receptor tyrosine kinases to Ras signalling. Nature (Lond) 1993;363:85–88.

240. Li W, Nishimura R, Kashishian A, et al. A new function for a phosphotyrosine phosphatase: linking GRB2-Sos to a receptor tyrosine kinase. Mol Cell Biol 1994;14:509–517.

241. Lin A, Frost J, Deng T, et al. Casein kinase II is a negative regulator of c-jun DNA binding and AP-1 activity. Cell 1992;70:777–789.

242. Lipsey LR, Northfelt DW. Anogenital neoplasia in patients with HIV infection. Curr Opin Oncol 1993;5:861–866.

241a. Linial M, Groudine M. Transcription of three c-myc exons is enhanced in chicken bursal lymphoma cell lines. Proc Natl Acad Sci USA 1985;82:53–57.

243. Liu XQ, Pawson T. The epidermal growth factor receptor phosphorylates GTPase-activating protein (GAP) at Tyr-460,adjacent to GAP SH2 domains. Mol Cell Biol 1991;11:2511–2516.

244. LoSardo JE, Boral AL, Lenz J. Relative importance of elements within the SL3-3 virus enhancer for T-cell specificity. J Virol 1990; 64:1756–1763.

245. Low KG, Chu H-M, Tan Y, et al. Novel interactions between human T-cell leukemia virus type I Tax and activating transcription factor 3 at a cyclic AMP-responsive element. Mol Cell Biol 1994;14:4958– 4974.

246. Lowenstein EJ, Daly RJ, Batzer G, et al. The SH2 and SH3 domain-containg protein GRB2 links receptor tyrosine kinases to ras signaling. Cell 1992;70:431–442.

247. Lowy DR, Willumsen BM. Function and regulation of ras. Annu Rev Biochem 1993;62:851–891.

248. Lu S-J, Rowan S, Bani MR, Ben-David Y. Retroviral integration within the Fli-2 locus results in inactivation of the erythroid transcription factor NF-E2 in Friend eryhtroleukemias: evidence that NF-E2 is essential for globin expression. Proc Natl Acad Sci U S A 1994;91:8398–8402.

249. Luciw PA, Leung AJ. Mechanisms of retrovirus replication. In: Levy JA, ed. Retroviridae. vol 1. New York: Plenum Press, 1992: 259–298.

250. MacArthur CA, Shankar DB, Shackleford GM. Fgf-8, activated by proviral insertion, cooperates with the wnt-1 transgene in murine mammary tumorigenesis. J Virol 1995;69:2501–2507.

251. Maki Y, Bos TJ, Davis C, Starbuck M, Vogt PK. Avian sarcoma virus 17 carries the jun oncogene. Proc Natl Acad Sci U S A 1987; 84:2848–2852.

252. Makris A, Patriotis C, Bear SE, Tsichlis PN. Genomic organization and expression of Tpl-2 in normal cells and Moloney murine leukemia virus-induced rat T-cell lymphomas: activation by provirus insertion. J Virol 1993;67:4283–4289.

253. Manzari V, Gismaoni A, Barillari G, et al. HTLV-V: a new human retrovirus isolated in a TAC-negative T cell lymphoma/leukemia. Science 1987;238:1581–1585.

254. Marchetti A, Buttitta F, Miyazaki S, Gallahan D, Smith GH, Callahan R. Int-6, a highly conserved, widely expressed gene, is mutated by mouse mammary tumor virus in mammary preneoplasia. J Virol 1995;69:1932–1938.

255. Margolis B, Rhee SG, Felder S, et al. EGF induces tyrosine phosphorylation of phospholopase C-II: a potential mechanism for EGF signalling. Cell 1989;57:1101–1107.

256. Marshall CJ. Specificity of receptor tyrosine kinase signaling: transient versus sustained extracellular signal-regulated kinase activation. Cell 1995;80:179–185.

257. Marth JD, Peet R, Krebs EG, Perlmutter RM. A lymphocyte-specific protein-tyrosine kinase gene is rearranged and overexpressed in the murine T cell lymphoma LSTRA. Cell 1985;43:393–404.

258. Maruta H, Burgess W. Regulating of the ras signaling network. BioEssays 1994;16:489–496.

259. Matthews EA, Vasmel WL, Schoenmakers HJ, Melief CJ. Retrovirally induced murine B-cell tumors rarely show proviral integration in sites common in T-cell tumors. Int J Cancer 1989;43:1120–1125.

260. Medema RH, Bos JL. The role of p21ras in receptor tyrosine kinase signaling. Crit Rev Oncol 1993;4:615–661.

261. Meisenhelder J, Suh PG, Rhee SG, Hunter T. Phospholipase C-γ is a substrate for the PDGF and EGF receptor protein-tyrosine kinase in vivo and in vitro. Cell 1989;57:1109–1122.

262. Mester J, Wagenaar E, Sluyser M, Nusse R. Activation of the int-1 and int-2 mammary oncogenes in hormone-dependent and independent mammary tumors of GR mice. J Virol 1987;61:1073–1078.

263. Middleton PG, Miller S, Ross JA, Stell CM, Guy K. Insertion of SMRV-H viral DNA at the c-myc gene locus of a BL cell line and presence in established cell lines. Int J Cancer 1992;52:451–454.

264. Miles BD, Robinson HL. High-frequency transduction of c-erbB in avian leukosis virus-induced erythroblastosis. J Virol 1985;54:295–303.

265. Minden A, Lin A, Smeal T, et al. c-jun N-terminal phosphorylation correlates with activation of the JNK subgroup but not the ERK subgroup of mitogen-activated protein kinases. Mol Cell Biol 1994;14: 6683–6688.

266. Mitreiter K, Schmidt J, Luz A, et al. Disruption of the murine p53 gene by insertion of an endogenous retrovirus-like element (ETn) in a cell line from radiation-induced osteosarcoma. Virolgy 1994;200: 837–841.

267. Miura T, Shibuya M, Tsujimoto H, Fukasawa M, Hayami M. Molecular cloning of a feline leukemia provirus integrated adjacent to the c-myc in a feline T-cell leukemia cell line and the unique structure of its long terminal repeat. Virology 1989;169:458–461.

268. Miyoshi I, Kubonishi I, Yoshimoto S, et al. Type C virus particles in a cord T-cell line deried by co-cultivating normal human cord leukocytes and human leukaemic T cells. Nature (Lond) 1983;294:770– 771.

269. Miyoshi I, Taguchi H, Fujishita M, et al. Transformation of monkey lymphocytes with adult T-cell leukemia virus. Lancet 1982;1:1016.

270. Miyoshi I, Yoshimoto S, Taguchi H, et al. Transformation of rabbit lymphocytes with T-cell leukemia virus. Gann 1983;74:1–4.

271. Moloney JB. Biological studies on a lymphoid-leukemia virus extracted from sarcoma 37. J Natl Cancer Inst Monogr 1960;24:933.

272. Moodie SA, Willumsen BM, Webber MJ, Wolfman A. Complexs of Ras.GTP with Raf-1 and mitogen-activated protein kinase kniase. Science 1993;260:1658–1661.

273. Moreau-Gachelin F, Ray D, deBoth NJ, van der Feltz MJ, Tambourin P, Tavitian A. Spi-1 oncogene activation in Rauscher and Friend murine virus-induced acute erythroleukemias. Leukemia 1990;4:20–23.

274. Moreau-Gachelin F, Ray D, Mattel MG, Tambourin P, Tavitian A. The putative oncogene Spi-1; murine chromosomal location and transcriptional activation in murine acute erythroleukemias. Oncogene 1989;4:1449–1456.

275. Moreau-Gachelin F, Tavitian A, Tambourin P. Spi-1 is a putative oncogene in virally induced murine erythroleakaemias. Nature (Lond) 1988;331:277–280.

276. Morishida K, Parker DS, Mucenski ML, et al. Retroviral activation of a novel gene encoding a zinc finger protein in IL-3-dependent myeloid leukemia cell line. Cell 1988;54:831–840.

277. Morris VL, Rao TR, Kozak CA, et al. Characterization of Int-5, a locus associated with early events in mammary carcinogenesis. Oncogene Res 1991;6:53–63.

278. Moskow JJ, Bullrich F, Huebner K, Buchberg AM. Meis 1, a novel homeobox gene involved in myeloid leukemogenesis. In: Lenz J, Morse HC III, Ruscetti S, Tsichlis PN, eds. Pathogenesis of animal retroviruses. Philadelphia: Fox Chase Cancer Center, 1994:60.

279. Mowat M, Cheng A, Kimura N, Bernstein A, Benchimol S. Rearrangements of the cellular p53 gene in erythroleukemic cells transformed by Friend virus. Nature (Lond) 1985;314:633– 636.

280. Mucenski ML, Gilbert DJ, Taylor BA, Jenkins NA, Copeland N. Common sites of viral integration in lymphomas arising in AKXD recombinant inbred mouse. Oncogene Res 1987;2:33–48.

281. Mucenski ML, Taylor BA, Ihle JN, et al. Identification of a common ecotropic viral integration site, evi-1, in the DNA of AKXD murine myeloid tumors. Mol Cell Biol 1988;8:301–308.

282. Mueller RE, Baggio L, Kozak CA, Ball JK. A common integration locus in type B retrovirus-induced thymic lymphomas. Virology 1992;1991:628–637.

283. Mukhopadhyaya R, Wolff L. New sites of proviral integration associated with murine promonocytic leukemias and evidence for alternate modes of c-myb activation. J Virol 1992;66:6035–6044.

284. Mullins JI, Brody DS, Binari RCJ, Cotter SM. Viral transduction of c-myc gene in naturally occuring feline leukemias. Nature (Lond) 1984;308:856–858.

285. Munoz E, Courtois G, Veschambre P, Jalinnot P, Israel A. Tax induces nuclear translocation of NF-κB through dissociation of cyto-

plasmic complexes containing p105 or p100 but does not induce degradation of IκBα/MAD3. J Virol 1994;68:8035–8044.

286. Munroe DG, Peacock JW, Benchimol S. Inactivation of the cellular p53 gene is a common feature of Friend virus-induced erythroleukemia: relationship of inactivation to dominant transforming alleles. Mol Cell Biol 1990;10:3307–3313.

287. Murphy EL, Hanchard B, Figueroa JP, et al. Modeling the risk of adult T-cell leukemia/lymphoma in persons infected with human T-lymphotropic virus type I. Int J Cancer 1989;43:250–253.

288. Mushinski JF, Potter M, Bauer SR, Reddy EP. DNA rearrangement and altered RNA expression of the c-myb oncogene in mouse plasmacytoid lymphosarcomas. Science 1983;220:795–798.

289. Nair N, Davis RJ, Robinson HL. Protein tyrosine kinase activities of the EGFR and erbB proteins: correlation of oncognic activation with altered kinetics. Mol Cell Biol 1992;12:2010–2016.

290. Neel BG, Gasic GP, Rogler CE, et al. Molecular analysis of the c-myc locus normal tissue and in avian leukosis virus-induced lymphomas. J Virol 1982;44:158–166.

291. Neel BG, Hayward WS, Robinson HL, Fang J, Astrin SM. Avian leukosis virus-induced tumors have common proviral integration sites and synthesize discrete new RNAs: oncogenesis by promoter insertion. Cell 1981;23:323–334.

292. Neil JC, Hughes D, McFarlane D. Transduction and rearrangement of the myc gene by feline leukemia virus in naturally occuring T-cell leukemias. Nature (Lond) 1984;308:814–820.

293. Neiman PE, Jordan L, Weiss RA, Payne LN. Malignant lymphoma of the bursa of *Fabricius*: analysis of early transformation. Cold Spring Harbor Conference on Cell Proliferation 1980;7:519.

294. Neiman P, Wolf C, Enrietto PJ, Cooper GM. A retroviral myc gene induces preneoplastic transformation of lymphocytes in a bursal transplantation assay. Proc Natl Acad Sci U S A 1985;82:222– 226.

295. Nerenberg M, Hinrichs SH, Reynolds RK, Khoury G, Jay G. The tat gene of human T-lymphotropic virus type I induces mesenchymal tumors in transgenic mice. Science 1987;237:1324–1329.

296. Nilsen TW, Maroney PA, Goodwin RG, et al. Activation in ALV-induced erythroblastosis: novel processing and promoter insertion result in expression of an amino-truncated EGF receptor. Cell 1985; 41:719–726.

297. Noori-Daloli MR, Swift RA, Kung H-J, Crittenden LB, Witter RL. Specific integration of REV proviruses in avian bursal lymphomas. Nature (Lond) 1981;294:574–576.

298. Nusse R. Insertional mutagenesis in mouse mammary tumorigenesis. Curr Top Microbiol Immunol 1991;71:43–65.

299. Nusse R, Theunissen H, Wagenaar E, et al. The Wnt-1 (int-1) oncogene promoter and its mechanism of activation by insertion of proviral DNA of the mouse mammary tumor virus. Mol Cell Biol 1990;10:4170–4179.

300. Nusse R, van Ooyen A, Rijsewijk F, van Lohulzen M, Schuuring E, van't Veer L. Retroviral insertional mutagenesis in murine mammary cancer. Proc R Soc Lond 1985;226:3–13.

301. Nusse R, Varmus HE. Many tumors induced by the mouse mammary tumor virus contain a provirus integrated in the same region of the host genome. Cell 1982;31:991–1009.

302. O'Donnell PV, Fleissner E, Lonial H, Koehne CF, Reicin A. Early clonality and high-frequency proviral integration into the c-myc locus in AKR leukemias. J Virol 1985;55:500–503.

303. Oehler T, Pintzas A, Stumm S, Darling A, Gillespie D, Angel P. Mutation of a phosphorylation site in the DNA-binding domain os equired for redox-independent transactivation of AP1-dependent genes by v-jun. Oncogene 1993;8:1141–1147.

304. Ohtani K, Nakamura M, Saito S, et al. Identification of two distinct elements in the long terminal repeat of HTLV-I responsible for maximum gene expression. EMBO J 1987;6:389–395.

305. Osame M, Igata A, Matsumoto M, Usuku K, Izumo S, Kosaka K. HTLV-I associted myelopathy: a report of 85 cases. Ann Neurol 1987;22:116.

306. Otsu M, Hiles I, Gout I, et al. Characterization of two 85 kd proteins that associate with receptor tyrosine kinases, middle-T/pp60c-src complexes, and PI3-K. Cell 1991;65:91–104.

307. Pain B, Woods CM, Saez J, et al. EGF-R as a hemopoietic growth factor receptor: the c-erbB product is present in normal chicken erythrocyte progenitor cells and controls their self-renewal. Cell 1991; 65:37–46.

308. Park RE, HAseltine WA, Rosen CA. A nuclear factor is required for transactivation of HTLV-I gene expression. Oncogene 1988;3:275– 279.

309. Paskalis H, Felber BK, Pavlakis GN. Cis-acting sequences responsible for the transcriptional activation of human T-cell leukemia virus type I constitute a conditional enahncer. Proc Natl Acad Sci U S A 1986;83:6558–6562.

310. Paul R, Schuetze S, Kozak CA, Kozak SL, Kabat D. The Spfi-1 proviral integration site of Friend erythroleukemia encodes the ets-related transcriptional factor Pu.1. J Virol 1991;65:464–467.

311. Paul R, Schuetze S, Kozak SL, Kabat D. A common site for immortalizing proviral integrations in Friend erythroleukemia: molecular cloning and characterization. J Virol 1989;63:4958–4961.

311a. Pawson T. SH₂ and SH₃ domains in signal transduction. Adv Cancer Res 1994;64:87–110.

312. Payne GS, Bishop JM, Varmus HE. Multiple arrangements of viral DNA and activated host oncogene in bursal lymphomas. Nature (Lond) 1982;295:209–214.

313. Payne GS, Courtneidge SA, Critenden LB, Fadly AM, Bishop JM, Varmus HE. Analysis of avian leukosis virus DNA and RNA in bursal tumors: viral gene expression is not required for maintenance of the tumor state. Cell 1981;23:311–322.

314. Payne LN. Biology of avian retroviruses. In: Levy J, ed. Retroviridae. vol 1. New York: Plenum Press, 1992:299–404.

315. Pecenka V, Dvorak M, Karafiat V, et al. Avian nephoroblastomas induced by a retrovirus (MAV-2) lacking oncogene. II. Search for common sites of proviral integration in tumor DNA. Filia Biol (Praha) 1988;34:147–169.

316. Pelicci G, Lanfrancone L, Grignani F, et al. A novel transforming protein (SHC) with an SH2 domain is implicated in mitogenic signal transduction. Cell 1992;70:93–104.

317. Pelley RJ, Maihle NJ, Boerkoel C, et al. Disease tropism of c-erbB: effects of carcoxyl-terminal tyrosine and internal mutations on tissue-specific transformation. J Virol 1989;86:7164–7168.

318. Pepin N, Roulston A, Lacocte J, Lin R, Hiscott J. Subcellular redistribution of HTLV-I Tax protein by NF-κB/Rel transcription factors. Virology 1994;204:706–716.

319. Peters G, Brookes S, Smith R, Dickson C. Tumorigenesis by mouse mammary tumor virus: evidence for a common region for provirus integration in mammary tumors. Cell 1983;33:369–377.

320. Peters G, Brookes S, Smith R, Placzek M, Dickson C. The mouse homolog of the hst/k-FGF gene is adjacent to int-2 and is activated by proviral insertion in some virally induced mammary tumors. Proc Natl Acad Sci U S A 1989;86:5678–5682.

321. Peters G, Lee A, Dickson C. Conceted activation of two potential proto-oncogenes in carcinomas induced by mouse mammary tumor virus. Nature (Lond) 1984;320:628–631.

322. Pizer E, Humphries EH. RAV-1 insertional mutagenesis: disruption of the c-myb locus and development of avian B-cell lymphomas. J Virol 1989;63:1630–1640.

323. Polesz BF, Ruscetti FW, Gazdar AF, Bunn PA, Minna JD, Gallo RC. Detection and isolation of a type C retrovirus particles from fresh cultured lymphocytes of a patient with cutaneous T-cell lymphoma. Proc Natl Acad Sci U S A 1980;77:7415–7419.

324. Poirier Y, Kozak C, Jolicoeur P. Identification of a common helper provirus integration site in Abelson murine leukemia virus-induced lymphoma DNA. J Virol 1988;62:3985–3992.

325. Popovic M, Lange-Wantzin G, Sarin PS, Mann D, Gallo RC. Transformation of human umbilical cord blood T cells by human T-cell leukemia/lymphoma virus. Proc Natl Acad Sci U S A 1983;80: 5402–5406.

326. Raines MA, Lewis WG, Crittenden LB, Kung H. Activation in avian leukosis virus-induced erythroblastosis clustered integration sites and the arrangement of provirus in the c-erbB alleles. Proc Natl Acad Sci U S A 1985;82:2287–2291.

327. Raines MA, Maihle NJ, Moscovici C, Crittenden L, Kung H-J. Mechanism of c-erbB transduction: newly released transducing viruses retain poly(A) tracts of erbB transcripts and encode C-terminally intact erbB proteins. J Virol 1988;62:2437–2443.

328. Raines MA, Mahile NJ, Moscovici C, Moscovici MG, Kung H-J. Molecular characterization of three erbB transducing viruses generalized during avian leukosis virus-induced erythroleukemia: extensive internal deletion near the kinase domain acitivates the firbosarcoma and hemangioma-inducing potentials of erbB. J Virol 1988; 62:2444–2452.

329. Reicin A, Yang J-Q, Marcu KB, Fleissner E, Koehne CF, O'Donnell

PV. Deregulation of the c-myc oncogene in virus-induced thymic lymphomas of AKR/J mice. Mol Cell Biol 1986;6:4088–4092.

330. Ren R, Ye Z-S, Baltimore D. Abl protein-tyrosine kinase selects the crk adaptor as a substrate using SH3-binding sites. Genes Dev 1994;8:783–795.

331. Robbins DJ, Cheng M, Zhen E, Vanderbilt CA, Feig LA, Cobb MH. Evidence for a Ras-dependent extracellular signal-regulated protein kinase (ERK) cascade. Proc Natl Acad Sci U S A 1992;89:6924–6928.

332. Robbins DJ, Zhen E, Cheng M, Xu S, Ebert D, Cobb MH. Map kinases erk1 and erk2: pleiotropic enzymes in a ubiquitous signaling network. Adv Cancer Res 1994;63:93–116.

333. Roberts JD, Preston BD, Johnston LA, Soni A, Loeb LA, Kunkel T. Fidelity of two retroviral reverse transcriptase during DNA-dependent DNA synthesis in vitro. Mol Cell Biol 1989;9:469.

334. Robinson HL, Gagnon GC. Patterns of proviral insertion and deletion in avian leukosis virus-induced lymphomas. J Virol 1986;57: 28–36.

335. Robinson HL, Miles BD, Catalano DE, Briles WE, Crittenden LB. Susceptibility to erbB-induced erythroblastosis is a dominant trait of 15_1 chickens. J Virol 1985;55:617–622.

336. Rodriguez-Viciana P, Warne PH, Dhand R, et al. Phosphatidylinositol-3-OH kinase as a direct target of ras. Nature (Lond) 1994;370: 527–532.

337. Roelink H, Wagenaar E, Lopes da Silva S, Nusse R. Wnt-3, a gene activated by proviral insertion in mouse mammary tumors, is homologous to int-1/Wnt-1 and is normally expressed in mouse embryos and adult brain. Proc Natl Acad Sci U S A 1990;87:4519–4523.

338. Rosenblatt JD, Golde DW, Wachsman W, et al. A second HTLV-II isolate associated with atypical hairy-cell leukemia. New Engl J Med 1986;315:372–375.

339. Rosson D, Dugan D, Reddy EP. Aberrant splicing events that are induced by proviral integrations: implications for myb oncogene activation. Proc Natl Acad Sci U S A 1987;84:3137–3175.

340. Rotter V, Wolf D, Pravtcheva D, Ruddle F. Chromosomal assignment of the murine gene encoding the transformation related protein p53. Mol Cell Biol 1984;4:383–385.

341. Rous P. A sarcoma of the fowl transmissible by an agent separable from the tumor cells. J Exp Med 1911;13:397–411.

342. Rovinski B, Munroe D, Peacok M, Mowat M, Bernstein A, Benchimol S. Deletion of 5' coding sequences of the cellular p53 gene in mouse erythroleukemia: a novel mechanism of oncogene regulation. Mol Cell Biol 1987;7:847–853.

343. Rozakis-Adcock M, Fernley R, Wade J, Pawson T, Bowtell D. The SH2 and SH3 domains of mammalian Grb2 couple the EGF receptor to the Ras activator mSos1. Nature (Lond) 1993;363:83–85.

344. Rozakis-Adcock M, McGlade J, Mbamalu G, et al. Association of the Shc and Grb2/Sem5 SH2-containing proteins is implicated in activation of the Ras pathway by tyrosine kinases. Nature (Lond) 1992;360:689–692.

345. Ruddle NH, Li CB, Horne WC, et al. Mice transenic for HTLV-I LTR-tax exhibit tax expression in bone, skeletal alterations, and high bone turnover. Virology 1993;197:196–204.

346. Sakurai H, Kondo N, Tshiguro N, et al. Molecular analysis of HTLV-IpX defective human adult T-cell leukemia. Leuk Res 1992; 16:941–946.

347. Sanchez I, Hughes RT, Mayer BJ, et al. Roles of SAPK/ERK kinase-1 in the stress-activated pathway regulating transcription factor c-jun. Nature (Lond) 1994;372:794–798.

348. Saxon A, Stevens RH, Golde DW. T-lymphocyte variant of hairy-cell leukemia. Ann Intern Med 1978;88:323–326.

349. Schlessinger J. SH2/SH3 signaling proteins. Curr Opin Genet Dev 1994;4:25–30.

350. Schlessinger J, Ullrich A. Growth factor signaling by receptor tyrosine kinases. Neuron 1992;9:383–391.

351. Schwartz DE, Tizard R, Gilbert W. Nucleotide sequence of Rous sarcoma virus. Cell 1983;32:853–869.

352. Seiki M, Eddy R, Shows T, Yoshida M. Nonspecific integration of the HTLV provirus into adult T-cell leukemia cells. Nature (Lond) 1984;309:640–642.

353. Sels FT, Langer S, Schultz AS, Silver J, Sitbon M, Friedrich RW. Friend murine leukemia virus is integrated at a common site in most primary spleen tumors of erythroleukaemic animals. Oncogene 1992;7:643–652.

354. Selten G, Cuypers HT, Berns A. Proviral activation of the putative

oncogene pim-1 MuLV induced T-cell lymphomas. EMBO J 1985;4:1793–1798.

355. Selten G, Cuypers HT, Zijlstra M, Melief C, Berns A. Involvement of c-myc in MuLV-induced T cell lymphomas in mice: frequency and mechanisms of infection. EMBO J 1984;3:3215–3222.

356. Setoguchi M, Higuchi Y, Yoshida S, et al. Insertional activation of N-myc by endogenous Moloney-like murine retrovirus sequences in macrophage cell lines derived from myeloma cell line-macrophage hybrids. Mol Cell Biol 1989;9:4515–4522.

357. Settleman J, Narasimhan V, Foster LC, Weinberg RA. Molecular cloning of cDNAs encoding the GAP-associated protein p190: implications for a signaling pathway from ras to the nucleus. Cell 1992; 69:539–549.

358. Shackleford GM, MacArthur CA, Kwan HC, Varmus HE. Mouse mammary tumor virus accelerates mammary carcinogenesis in Wnt-1 transgenic mice by insertional activation of int-2/Fgf-3 and hst/Fgt-4. Proc Natl Acad Sci U S A 1993;90:740–744.

359. Sharp PA, Marciniak RA. HIV TAR: an RNA enhancer? Cell 1989; 59:229–230.

360. Shaughnessy JD Jr, Owens JD Jr, Wiener F, et al. Retroviral enhancer insertion 5' of c-myc in two translocation-negative mouse plasmacytomas upregulates c-myc expression to different extents. Oncogene 1993;8:3111–3121.

361. Shaw G, Kamen R. A conserved AU sequence from the 3' untranslated region of GM-CSF mRNA mediates selective mRNA degradation. Cell 1986;46:659–667.

362. Shen-Ong GLC, Ill HCM, Potter M, Mushinski F. Two modes of c-myb activation in virus-induced mouse myeloid tumors. Mol Cell Biol 1986;6:380–392.

363. Shen-Ong GLC, Potter M, Mushinski JF, Lavu S, Reddy EP. Activation of the c-myb locus by viral insertional mutagenesis in plasmacytoid lymphosarcomas. Science 1984;226:1077–1080.

364. Shen-Ong GLC, Wolff L. Moloney murine leukemia virus-induced myeloid tumors in adult BALB/c mice: requirement of c-myb activation but lack of v-abl involvement. J Virol 1987;61: 1067–1072.

365. Shimotohno K, Takano M, Terunsho T, Miwa M. Requirement of multiple copies of a 21-nucleotide sequence in the U3 regions of human T-cell leukemia virus type I and II long terminal repeats for transactivation of transcription. Proc Natl Acad Sci U S A 1986;83: 8112–8116.

366. Shin S, Steffen DL. Frequent activation of the lck gene by promoter insertion and aberrant splicing in murine leukemia virus-induced rat lymphomas. Oncogene 1993;8:141–149.

367. Shiramizui B, Herndier BG, Grath MS. Identification of a common clonal human immunodeficiency virus-associated lymphomas. Cancer Res 1994;54:2069–2072.

368. Shu H, Chang C, Ravi L, et al. Modulation of erbB kinase activity and oncogenic potential by single point mutations within the glycine loop of the catalytic domain. Mol Cell Biol 1994;14: 6868–6878.

369. Shu H-K, Pelley RJ, Kung H-J. Tissue-specific transformation by epidermal growth factor receptor: a single point mutation within the ATP-binding pocket of the erbB product increases its intrinsic kinase activity and activates its sarcomagenic potential. Proc Natl Acad Sci U S A 1990;87:9103–9107.

370. Silver J, Kozak C. Common proviral integration region on mouse chromosome 7 in lymphomas and myelogenous leukemias induced by Friend murine leukemia virus. J Virol 1986;57:526–533.

371. Simon MC, Smith RE, Hayward WS. Mechanisms of oncogenesis by subgroup F avian leukosis viruses. J Virol 1984;52:1–8.

372. Sinkovics JG. Kaposi's sarcoma: its "oncogenes" and growth factors. Crit Rev Oncol Hematol 1991;11:87–107.

373. Skolnik EY, Batzer A, Li N, et al. The functions of GRB2 in linking the insulin receptor to Ras signaling pathways. Science 1993;260: 1953–1955.

374. Smith MR, Greene WC. Molecular biology of the type I human T-cell leukemia virus (HTLV-I) and adult T-cell leukemia. J Clin Invest 1991;87:761–766.

375. Smith MR, Greene WC. Characterization of a novel nuclear localization signal in the HTLV-I tax transactivator protein. Virology 1992;187:316–320.

376. Sodroski J. The human T-cell leukemia virus (HTLV) transactivator (Tax) protein. Biochim Biophys Acta 1992;1114:19–29.

377. Sola B, Simon D, Mattei M-G. Fim-1, Fim-2/c-fms, and Fim-3,

three common integration sites of Friend murine leukemia virus in myeloblastic leukemias, map to mouse chromosome 13, 18, and 3, respectively. J Virol 1988;52:1–8.

378. Soret J, Dambrine G, Perbal B. Induction of nephroblastoma by myeloblastosis-associated virus type 1: state of proviral DNAs in tumor cells. J Virol 1989;63:1803–1807.

379. Speck NA, Baltimore D. Six distinct nuclear factors interact with the 75-base pair repeat of the Moloney murine leukemia virus enhancer. Mol Cell Biol 1987;7:1101–1110.

380. Spencer CA, Groudine M. Control of c-myc regulation in normal and neoplastic cells. Adv Cancer Res 1991;56:1–48.

381. Spiro C, Gliniak B, Kabat D. A tagged helper-free Freind virus causes clonal erythroblast immortality by specific proviral integration in the cellular genome. J Virol 1988;62:4129–4135.

382. Stancato LF, Chow Y-H, Hutchison KA, Perdew GH, Jove R, Pratt WB. Raf exists in a native heterocomplex with hsp90 and p50 that can be reconstituted in a cell-free system. J Biol Chem 1993;269:22157–22161.

383. Steffen D. Proviruses are adjacent to c-myc in some murine leukemia virus-induced lymphomas. Proc Natl Acad Sci U S A 1984;81:2097–2101.

384. Stewart M, Terry A, O'Hara M, Cameron E, Onions D, Neil C. Identification of myc-collaborating genes by proviral tagging in CD2-myc transgenic mice. In: Lenz J, Morse HC III, Ruscentti S, Tsichlis PN, eds. Pathogenesis of animal retroviruses. Philadelphia: Fox Chase Cancer Center, 1994:58.

385. Stewart SA, Poon B, Chen ISY. Mechanism of HTLV leukemogenesis. In: Minson A, Neil J, McCrae M, eds. Viruses and cancer. Cambridge: Cambridge University Press, 1994:189–212.

386. Stocking C, Bergholz U, Friel J, et al. Distinct classes of factor-independent mutants can be isolated after retroviral mutagenesis of a human myeloid stem cell line. Growth Factors 1993;8:197–209.

387. Stocking C, Loliger C, Kawai M, Gough N, Suciu S, Ostertag W. Identification of genes involved in growth autonomy of hematopoietic cells by analysis of factor-independent mutants. Cell 1988;53:869–879.

388. Stokoe D, Macdonald SG, Cadwallader K, Symons M, Hancock JF. Activation of raf as a result of recruitment to the plasma membrane. Science 1994;264:1463–1466.

389. Stoye JP, Moroni C, Coffin JM. Virological events leading to spontaneous AKR thymomas. J Virol 1991;65:1273–1285.

390. Sugita T, Totsuka T, Saito M, et al. Functional murine interleukin 6 receptor with the intracisternal A particle gene product at its cytoplasmic domain. J Exp Med 1990;171:2001–2009.

391. Sun S-H, Elwood J, Beraud C, Greene WC. Human T-cell leukemia virus type 1 Tax activation of NF-κB/rel involves phosphorylation and degradation of κBα and reκA (p65)-mediated induction of the c-rel gene. Mol Cell Biol 1994;14:7377–7384.

392. Suzuki T, Fujisawa J, Toita M, Yoshida M. The trans-activator Tax of human T-cell leykemia virus type I (HTLV) interacts with cAMP-responsive element (CRE) binding and CRE modulator proteins that bind to the 21-base-pair enhancer of HTLV-1. Proc Natl Acad Sci U S A 1993;90:610–614.

393. Suzuki T, Hirai H, Fujisawa J-I, Fujita T, Yoshida M. A trans-activator Tax of human T-cell leumia virus type 1 binds to NF-κB and serum response factor (SRF) and associates with enhancer DNAs of the NF-κB site and CArG box. Oncogene 1993;8:2391–2397.

394. Suzuki T, Hirai H, Yoshida M. Tax protein of HTLV-1 interacts with the Rel homology domain of NF-κB p65 and c-Rel proteins bound to the NF-κB binding site and activates transcription. Oncogene 1994;9:3099–3105.

395. Swift RA, Boerkoel C, Ridgway A, Fujita DJ, Dodgson JB, Kung H. B-lymphoma induction by reticuloendotheliosis virus: chatacterization of a mutated chicken syncytial virus provirus involved in c-myc activation. J Virol 1987;61.

396. Taira M, Yoshida M, Miagawa K, Sakamoto H, Terada M, Sugimura T. cDNA sequence of human transforming gene hst and identification of the coding sequence required for transforming activity. Proc Natl Acad Sci U S A 1987;84:2980–2984.

397. Tanaka A, Takahashi H, Yamaoka S, Nosaka T, Maki M, Hatanaka M. Oncogenic transformation by the tax gene of human T-cell leukemia virus type I in vitro. Proc Natl Acad Sci U S A 1990;87:1071–1075.

398. Tanaka S, Morishita T, Hashimoto Y, et al. C3G, a guanine nu-cleotide-releasing protein expressed ubiquitously, binds to the src homology domains of crk and Grb2/ASH proteins. Proc Natl Acad Sci U S A 1994;91:3443–3447.

399. Tanigawa T, Robb L, Green AR, Begley CG. Constitutive expression of the putative transcription factor SCL associated with proviral insertion in the myeloid leukemic cell line WEHI-3BD-. Cell Growth Differ 1994;5: 557–561.

400. Tateno M, Kondo N, Itoh T, Chubachi T, Togashi T, Yoshiki T. Rat lymphoid lines with human T-cell leukemia virus production. I. Biological and serological characterization. J Exp Med 1984;159:1105–1116.

401. Thornell A, Hallberg B, Grundstrom T. Differential protein binding in lymphocytes to a sequence in the enhancer of the mouse retrovirus SL3-3. Mol Cell Biol 1988;8:1625–1637.

402. Tohyama K, Lee K, Tashiro K, Kinashi T, Honjo T. Establishment of an interleukin-5-dependent subclone from an interleukin-3-dependent murine hemopoletic progenitor cell line, LyD9, and its malignant transformation by autocrine secretion of interleukin-5. EMBO J 1990;9:1823–1830.

403. Tornesello ML, Buonsguro FM, Beth-Giraldo E, Giraldo G. Himan immunodeficiency virus type I tat gene enhances human papillomavirus early gene expression. Intervirology 1993;36:57–64.

404. Treier M, Staszewski LM, Bohmann D. Ubiquitin-dependent c-jun degradation in vivo is mediated by the δ domain. Cell 1994;78:787–798.

405. Tremblay PJ, Kozak CA, Jolicoeur P. Identification of a novel gene, Vin-1, in murine leukemia virus-induced T-cell leukemias by provirus insertional mutagenesis. J Virol 1992;66:1344–1353.

406. Troxler DH, Parks WP, Vass WC, Scolnick EM. Isolation of a fibroblast nonproducer cell line containing the Friend strain of the spleen focus-forming virus. Virology 1977;76:602–615.

407. Trusko SP, Hoffman EK, George DL. Transcriptional activation of c-Ki-ras proto-oncogene resulting from retroviral promoter insertion. Nucl Acids Res 1989;17:9259–9265.

408. Tsatsanis C, Fulton R, Nishigaki K, et al. Genetic determinants of feline leukemia virus-induced lymphoid tumors: patterns of proviral insertion and gene rearrangement. J Virol 1994;68:8296–8303.

409. Tsichlis PN, Bear SE. Infection by mink cell focus forming (MCF) virus confers interleukin-2 (IL-2) independence to an IL-2 dependent rat T cell lymphoma line. Proc Natl Acad Sci U S A 1991;88:4611–4615.

410. Tsichlis PN, Lazo PA. Virus-host interactions and the pathogenesis of murine and human oncogenic retroviruses. Curr Top Microbiol Immunol 1991;171:95–171.

411. Tsichlis PN, Lee JS, Bear SE, et al. Activation of multiple genes by provirus integration in the Mlvi-4 locus in T-cell lymphomas induced by Moloney murine leukemia virus. J Virol 1990;64:2236–2244.

412. Tsichlis PN, Shepherd BM, Bear SE. Activation of the Mlvi-1/mis-1/prt-1 locus in Moloney murine leukemia virus-induced T-cell lymphomas. Proc Natl Acad Sci U S A 1989;86:5487–5491.

413. Tsichlis PN, Strauss PG, Hu LF. Two common regions for proviral DNA integration in MoMuLV-induced rat thymic lymphomas. Nature (Lond) 1983;302:445–449.

414. Tsichlis PN, Strauss PG, Lohse MA. Concerted DNA rearrangements in Moloney murine leukemia virus-induced thymomas: a potential synergistic relationship in oncogenesis. J Virol 1985;56:258–267.

415. Tsuchiya H, Fujii M, Tanaka Y, Tozawa H, Seiki M. Two distinct regions form a functional activation domain of the HTLV-1 trans-activator Tax1. Oncogene 1994;9:337–340.

416. Tsujimoto H, Fulton R, Nishigaki K, Matsumoto Y, Haegawa A, Tsujimoto A. A common proviral integration region, fit-1, in T-cell tumors induced by myc-containing feline leukemia viruses. Virology 1993;196:845–848.

417. Uchiyama T, Yodoi J, Sagawa K, Takatsuki K, Uchino H. Adult T-cell leukemia: clinical and hematologic features of 16 cases. Blood 1977;50:481–492.

418. Uittenbogaard MN, Armstrong AP, Chiaramello A, Nyborg JK. Human T-cell leukemia virus type I Tax protein responses gene expression through the basic helix-loop-helix family of transcription factors. J Biol Chem 1994;269:1–4.

419. van Aelst L, Barr M, Marcus S, Polverino A, Wigler M. Complex formation between RAS and RAF and other protein kinases. Proc Natl Acad Sci U S A 1993;90:6213–6217.

420. van der Geer P, Hunter T, Lindberg RA. Receptor protein-tyrosine kinases and their signal transduction pathways. Annu Rev Cell Biol 1994;10:251–337.

421. van Lohuizen M, Bern A. Tumorigenesis by slow-transforming retroviruses-an update. Biochim Biophys Acta 1990;1032:213–235.

422. van Lohuizen M, Breur M, Berns A. N-myc is frequently activated by proviral insertion in MuLV-induced T cell lymphomas. EMBO J 1989;8:133–136.

423. van Lohuizen M, Verbeek S, Krimpenfort P. Predisposition to lymphomagenesis in pim-2 transgenic mice: cooperation with c-myc and N-myc in murine leukemia virus-induced tumors. Cell 1989;56: 673–682.

424. van Lohuizen M, Verbeek S, Scheijien B, Wientjens E, Van der Gulden H, Berns A. Identification of cooperating oncogenes in Eμ-myc transgenic mice by provirus tagging. Cell 1991;65:737.

425. Varmus H. An historical overview of oncogenes. In: Weinberg R, ed. Oncogenes and molecular origins of cancer. New York: Cold Spring Harbor Laboratory Press, 1989:3–44.

425a. Varticouski L, Harrison-Findik D, Keeler ML, Susa M. Role of PI 3-kinase in mitogenesis. Biochem Biophys Acta 1994;1226:1–11.

426. Veit M, Eisel D, Pass M, Sels FT, Friedrich RW. The integration site of Fre-2 of F-MuLV is sometimes rearranged without an integrated provirus. In: Lenz J, Morse HC III, Ruscetti S, Tsichlis PN, eds. Pathogenesis of animal retroviruses. Philadelphia: Fox Chase Cancer Center, 1994:69.

427. Vijaya S, Steffen DL, Kozak C, Robinson HL. Dsi-1, a region with frequent insertions in Moloney murine leukemia virus-induced rat lympnomas. J Virol 1987;61:1164–1170.

428. Villemur R, Monczak Y, Rassart E, Kozak C, Jolicoeur P. Identification of a new common provirus integration site in gross passage A murine leukemia virus-induced mouse thymoma DNA. Mol Cell Biol 1987;7:512–522.

429. Villeneuve L, Jiang X, Turmel C, Kozak CA, Jolicoeur P. Long-range mapping of Mis-2, a common provirus integration site identified in murine leukemia virus-induced thymomas and located 160 kilobase pairs downstream of myb. J Virol 1993;67:5733–5739.

430. Villeneuve L, Rassart E, Jolicoeur P, Graham M, Adams JM. Proviral integration site mis-1 in rat thymomas corresponds to the pvt-1 translocation breakpoint in murine plasmacytomas. Mol Cell Biol 1986;6:1834–1837.

431. Vogel J, Hinrichs SH, Reynolds RK, Luciw PA, Jay G. The HIV tat gene induces derminal lesions resembling Kaposi's sarcoma in transgenic mice. Nature (Lond) 1988;335:606–611.

432. Vojtek AB, Hollenburg SM, Cooper JA. Mammalian Ras interact directly with the serine/threonine kinase Raf. Cell 1993;74:206–214.

433. Voronova AF, Sefton BF. Expression of a new tyrosine protein kinase is stimulated by retrovirus promoter insertion. Nature (Lond) 1986;319:682–685.

434. Wagner S, Green MR. HTLV-I Tax protein stimulation of DNA binding of bZIP proteins by enhancing dimerization. Science 1993;262:395–399.

435. Wang S, Nishigori C, Miyakoshi J, et al. Activation of c-mos oncogene by integration of an endogenous long terminal repeat element during transfection of genomic DNA from mouse skin tumor cells. Oncogene 1993;8:1009–1016.

436. Warne PH, Viciana PR, Downward J. Direct interaction of Ras and amino-terminal region of Raf-1 in vitro. Nature (Lond) 1993;364: 352–355.

437. Watanabe T, Seiki M, Tsujimoto H, Miyoshi I, Hayami M, Yoshida M. Sequence homology of the simian retrovirus genome with T-cell leukemia virus type I. Virology 1985;144:59–65.

438. Weinstein Y, Cleveland JL, Askew DS, Rapp UR, Ihle JN. Insertion and truncation of c-myb by murine leukemia virus in a myeloid cell line derived from cultures of normal hematopoletic cells. J Virol 1987;61:2339–2343.

439. Weinstein Y, Ihle JN, Lavu S, Reddy EP. Truncation of the c-myb gene by a retroviral integration in an interleukin 3-dependent myeloid leukemia cell line. Proc Natl Acad Sci U S A 1986;83: 5010–5014.

440. Weisman IL, Mc Grath MS. Retrovirus lymphomagenesis: relationship of normal immune receptors to malignant cell proliferation. Curr Top Microbiol Immunol 1982;98:103–112.

441. Weller I. HIV and predisposition to cancer. In: Minson A, Neil J, McCrae M, eds. Viruses and cancer. Cambridge: Cambridge University Press, 1994:293–306.

442. Westaway D, Papkoff J, Moscovici C, Varmus HE. Identification of a provirally activated c-Ha-ras oncogene in an avian nephroblastoma via a novel procedure: cDNA cloning of a chimaeric viral-host transcript. EMBO J 1986;5:301–309.

443. Westaway D, Payne G, Varmus HE. Proviral deletions and oncogene base-substitutions in insertionally mutagenized c-myc alleles may contribute to the progression of avian bursal tumors. Proc Natl Acad Sci U S A 1984;81:843–847.

444. Westwick JK, Cox AD, Der CJ, et al. Oncogenic ras activates c-jun via a separate pathway from the activation of excellular signal-regulated kinases. Proc Natl Acad Sci U S A 1994;91:6030–6034.

445. Wilks AF, Harpur AG. Cytokine signal transduction and JAK family of protein tyrosine kinases. BioEssays 1994;16:313–320.

446. Williams NG, Roberts TM. Signal transduction pathways involving the raf proto-oncogene. Cancer Metastasis Rev 1994;13:105–116.

447. Wolff L, Koller R, Davidson W. Acute myeloid leukemia induction by amphotropic murine retrovirus (4070A): clonal integrations involve c-myb in some but not all leukemias. J Virol 1991;65:3607–3616.

448. Wood KW, Sarnecki C, Roberts TM, Blenis J. ras mediates nerve growth factor receptor modulation of three signal-transducing protein kinases: MAP kinase, Raf-1 and RSK. Cell 1992;68:1041–1050.

449. Xanthoudakis S, Miao G, Wang F, Pan YC, Curran T. Redox activation of Fos-Jun DNA binding activity is modulated by a DNA repair enzyme. EMBO J 1992;11:3323–3335.

450. Yamamota T, Hihara H, Nishida T, Kawai S, Toyoshima K. A new avian erythroblastosis virus AEH-H, carries erbB gene responsible for the induction of both erythroblastosis virus and sarcomas. Cell 1983;34:225–232.

451. Yan M, Dai T, Deak JC, et al. Activation of stress-activated protein kinase by MEKK1 phosphorylation of its activator, SEK1. Nature (Lond) 1994;320:798–801.

452. Yana Y, Kobayashi S, Yasumizu R, et al. Provirus integration at the 3' region og N-myc in cell lines established from thymic lymphomas spontaneously formed in AKR mice and a [(BALB/c × B6)F1–AKR] bone marrow chimera. Jpn J Cancer Res 1991;82:176–183.

453. Ymer S, Tucker WQJ, Sanderson CJ, Hapel AJ. Constitutive synthesis of interleukin-3 by leukemia cell line WEHI-3B is due to retroviral insertion near the gene. Nature (Lond) 1985;317:255–258.

454. Yoshida T, Miyagawa K, Odagiri H, et al. Genomic, sequence of hst, a transforming gene encoding a protein homologous to fibroblast growth factors and int-2-encoded protein. Proc Natl Acad Sci U S A 1987;84:7305–7309.

455. Zack JA, Cann AJ, Lugo JP, Chen ISY. AIDS virus production from infected peripheral blood T cells following HTLV-I-induced mitogenic stimulation. Science 1988;240:1026–1029.

456. Zhang K, DeClue JE, Vass WC, Papageorge AG, McCormick F, Lowy DR. Suppression of c-ras transformation by GTPase-activating protein. Nature (Lond) 1990;346:754–756.

457. Zhang X-F, Settleman J, Kyriakis JM, et al. Normal and oncogenic p21ras proteins bind to the domain of c-raf-1. Nature (Lond) 1993; 364:308–313.

458. Zhao LJ, Giam CZ. Human T-cell lymphotropic virus type I (HTLV-I) transcriptional activator, Tax, enhances CREB binding to HTLV-I 21-base-pair repeats by protein-protein interaction. Proc Natl Acad Sci U S A 1992;89:7070–7074.

459. Zheng C-F, Guan K-L. Properties of MEKs, the kinases that phosphorylate and activate the extracellular signal-regulated kinases. J Biol Chem 1993;268:23933–23939.

Viral Pathogenesis,
edited by Neal Nathanson, et al.
Lippincott–Raven Publishers, Philadelphia © 1997

CHAPTER 12

Small DNA Tumor Viruses

Louise T. Chow and Thomas R. Broker

INTRODUCTION

Simian virus 40 (SV40) and other polyomaviruses, human adenoviruses, and animal papillomaviruses are small DNA viruses that replicate in the nucleus of permissive host cells. They gained early research prominence primarily because of their abilities to immortalize or transform mammalian cells in culture and to cause tumors in certain experimental ani-

L. T. Chow and T. R. Broker: Department of Biochemistry and Molecular Genetics, Comprehensive Cancer Center, Center for AIDS Research, The University of Alabama at Birmingham, Birmingham, Alabama 35294-0005.

mals.[157] Eventually, the human papillomaviruses garnered substantial attention after recognition of their clinical association with hyperproliferative lesions (warts, condylomata, and papillomas) and neoplasms of epithelial tissues.[360,462]

The first of the DNA tumor viruses to be discovered (in 1933) and characterized in biologic detail was the Shope cottontail rabbit (CRPV) papillomavirus, which causes benign cutaneous papillomas in cottontail rabbits, its natural host. In experimentally infected domestic rabbits, CRPV-induced papillomas often progress to carcinomas, a process accelerated by cocarcinogens. Many of the fundamental principles of viral oncogenesis, tumor promoters, and neoplastic progression were first discovered with CRPV systems.[217,462]

Mouse polyomavirus was found to cause a multitude of tumors in diverse organs if inoculated into newborn mice—hence the name, "polyoma virus." Infections in adult mice produce no symptoms. SV40 has commanded major research attention since the late 1950s, after the realization that the rhesus monkey kidney cells used for human poliovirus vaccine production harbored SV40 in the absence of obvious pathogenic effects and that millions of people had inadvertently been exposed to it.[239] The less well studied human polyomaviruses BKV and JCV are genetically related to SV40.[82] JCV has been isolated from immunosuppressed patients with progressive multifocal leukoencephalopathy, a demyelinating disease, and is trophic for oligodendrocytes in vitro.[359] BKV and JCV are both shed from infected kidney cells into the urine of immunosuppressed or pregnant patients. These infections are commonly established in early childhood. Recent investigations have found authentic SV40 in human childhood brain tumors of the choroid plexus, in ependymomas, and in a rare glioblastoma.[232] Although SV40, BKV, and JCV transform nonpermissive cells in vitro and induce tumors in newborn hamsters, infections are largely asymptomatic in the kidneys of their respective native hosts (Table 12-1).

More than 48 serotypes of human adenovirus have been isolated, with selective tropisms for the mucosal epithelia of the pharynx, conjunctiva, and intestinal tract.[176] Although none of the human adenoviruses induce human neoplasms, they can transform cells in vitro, and some serotypes have been known since the early 1960s to be moderately to strongly oncogenic in newborn hamsters because of their immature immune systems. In recent years, a high mortality rate has been reported among adenovirus-infected patients who have compromised immune systems resulting from congenital immunodeficiency, acquired immunodeficiency syndrome (AIDS), or organ transplantation.[170] Because the animal polyomaviruses and the human adenoviruses can be propagated easily in cultured cells, they have been used extensively as model systems to investigate the molecular mechanisms of replication, transcription, and transformation in vitro and of tumorigenicity in animals.

In the early 1960s, bovine papillomavirus type 1 (BPV-1), which causes fibropapillomas in cattle, was shown to transform the morphology of bovine and rodent cells in culture.[29,406] However, it attracted little attention until 1980, when there was a revisitation to the tumorigenic transformation of murine cell lines[126,248] and the demonstration that BPV-1 DNA replicates as an extrachromosomal plasmid at moderate copy number in the nuclei of transformed cells.[227,229] BPV-1 quickly became another attractive model system with which to examine the molecular mechanisms of transformation and eucaryotic DNA replication.

Human papillomaviruses (HPVs) have been recognized for decades to cause benign, hyperproliferative cutaneous warts.[462] A small number of people infected with certain HPV types develop disseminated cutaneous warts called epidermodysplasia verruciformis (EV). EV lesions can progress to invasive carcinomas in sun-exposed sites in 30% to 40% of patients. This clinical correlation was the first definitive demonstration of a human cancer virus.[295] However, because of the inability to propagate any of the human papillomaviruses in conventional cell cultures or to maintain an episomal state in the infected cells,[50,400] research on the HPVs was largely limited to pathologic and immunologic analyses of patients.

Several factors contributed to the influx of investigators into the field of HPV research. Since the late 1970s, molecular cloning of numerous types of HPV DNA from a spectrum of cutaneous and mucosal lesions (warts, dysplasias, and cervical and penile carcinomas) has emphasized the medical importance of HPVs and provided materials with which to conduct research.[110] The discovery that long-established cervical cancer cell lines (e.g., HeLa cells) that are widely used in laboratory investigations contain integrated and actively transcribed HPV DNA provided further impetus.[303,348,457] As more genotypes of HPV DNA were cloned from lesions, they in turn were used as probes for additional specimens. When more sensitive methods of detection such as in situ hybridization[386] and polymerase chain reaction (PCR) amplifica-

TABLE 12-1. *Small DNA tumor viruses, native host species and associated diseases*

Virus	Host species	Diseases
HPVs* (100 types)	Humans	Asymptomatic; warts, dysplasias, carcinomas
BPVs† (6 types)	Cattle	Asymptomatic; fibropapillomas, warts, carcinomas
CRPV	Cottontail rabbits	Papillomas, carcinomas
JCV human polyomavirus	Humans	Asymptomatic; kidney; occasional progressive multifocal leukoencephalopathy (PML) in immunosuppressed patients
BKV human polyomavirus	Humans	Asymptomatic; kidney; occasional tumors in immunosuppressed patients
SV40	Monkeys	Asymptomatic; kidney; PML in immunosuppressed macaques; childhood brain tumors in humans
Mouse polyomavirus	Mice	Asymptomatic in adult mice; tumors in multiple organs when inoculated into newborn mice
Human adenoviruses† (48 types)	Humans	Respiratory and digestive tracts; conjunctiva; pneumonia in immunosuppressed patients

HPV, human papillomavirus; BPV, bovine papillomavirus; CRPV, cottontail rabbit papillomavirus; SV40, simian virus 40.
*See Table 12-4 for the association between particular HPV types and diseases.
†Particular types have distinct tissue tropisms and are associated with various diseases.

tion[26,27,256] were developed and applied, it became evident that HPV infections are extremely widespread. Most infections are subclinical, but certain HPV types contribute centrally to the development of epithelial neoplasms at a variety of anatomic sites.[360,385,463] HPVs immortalize primary keratinocytes, transform murine cell lines in culture, and transform primary cells in collaboration with an activated *ras* oncogene.[259,319,456] Among the small DNA viruses, HPVs provide a unique opportunity to correlate pathogenesis in patients with experimentation in vitro.

From this brief history of the small DNA tumor viruses, it is easy to understand why each was highly regarded for its prototypic properties, well suited to the investigation of the underlying causes of cancers, and why each attracted large followings of dedicated investigators. Yet, no amount of hyperbole could have anticipated the important insights that have been revealed by the investigations of these small DNA tumor viruses, from the basic mechanisms of RNA transcription and processing in the late 1970s, to those of DNA replication in the past decade, to, more recently, those governing cell proliferation, oncogenesis, and apoptosis.

The oncogenicity of each of the small DNA tumor viruses can be attributed to one or more proteins (oncoproteins) that target critical host proteins, specifically p53 and the retinoblastoma susceptibility protein (pRB) and proteins related to it (Table 12-2). pRB and p53 were the first tumor suppressor genes identified, and their deletion or mutation was found in a wide variety of human cancers.[174,211] Both p53 and pRB are key control regulatory proteins governing genome stability and proliferation, differentiation, and apoptosis of mammalian cells.[197,243,371,353,433]

This chapter takes the perspective that infections in the natural host animals by the so-called small DNA tumor viruses are largely nondisruptive and self-limiting events that have evolved to achieve equilibrium between the virus and the host. Infections are primarily asymptomatic and persistent, and oncogenesis occurs at low frequency as the culmination of a long series of accidental events ultimately detrimental to the propagation of the virus. An appreciation of the viral strategies for establishment and maintenance of such benign coexistence can provide insight into the mechanisms governing cell proliferation and the consequences of dysregulation. Emphasis is placed on the HPVs, particularly the types that infect mucosal epithelia, because the virus-host interactions in vivo have been the most extensively examined among all the DNA tumor viruses.

VIRAL GENOME STRUCTURES

Each of the small DNA viruses has a nonenveloped, icosahedral protein capsid. Each contains a double-stranded chromosome. Productive infection in vitro occurs only in permissive host cells (see Table 12-1). The genome size, organization, and strategy of replication are briefly summarized here.

Polyomaviruses

The polyomaviruses have a circular genome of approximately 5200 bp that replicates in the nucleus of the host cell.[82] Viral replication is dependent on the host machinery but requires specific viral proteins to mark the origin and to initiate and sustain replication. Replication is bidirectional and semiconservative, generating theta-form intermediates. Transcripts diverge from an early promoter and a late promoter, which flank the regulatory region containing enhancers and the origin of replication. mRNAs initiated from these two promoters are polyadenylated at a convergent site located about halfway around the genome and then undergo alternative splicing.[46] Transcription of the early (E) region occurs before viral DNA replication, whereas that of the late (L) region commences after the onset of vegetative replication. The E regions of SV40, BKV, and JCV each encode a large T (tumor) antigen and a small t antigen from alternatively spliced pri-

TABLE 12-2. *Viral oncoproteins and targeted host proteins*

Virus	Viral protein	Targeted host proteins
HPV	E6	p53; ERC-55 (a calcium-binding protein)
HPV	E7	pRB, p107, p130
HPV	E5	16-kD vacuolar H+-ATPase; EGF receptor, erbB-2
BPV	E6	ERC-55
BPV	E7	Unknown
BPV-1	E5a	†16-kD vacuolar H+-ATPase; β-type PDGF receptor
BPV-1	E5b	calreticulin
SV40, BKV, JCV Polyomavirus	Large T	p53, pRB, p107, p130
Polymavirus	middle T	Src, Shc
Adenovirus	E1A	pRB, p107, p130
	E1B 55 kD	p53
	E1B 19 kD	Nip 1, 2, 3

HPV, human papillomavirus; BPV, bovine papillomavirus; SV40, simian virus; BKV, a human polyomavirus; JCV, a human polyomavirus; pRB, retinoblastoma susceptibility protein; H+-ATPase, H+-transporting adenosine triphosphatase; EGF, epidermal growth factor; PDGF, platelet-derived growth factor.

mary transcripts. The large T antigen is multifunctional and serves as a transforming protein, a transcription regulatory protein, a replication origin recognition protein, an adenosine triphosphatase (ATPase), and a helicase necessary for replication. The small t antigen inactivates host protein phosphatase-2A, thereby mobilizing the mitogen-activated protein kinase pathway and promoting cell proliferation.[84,130,255] The mouse polyomavirus additionally encodes a middle T antigen, which is the transformation protein and interacts with a number of protein tyrosine kinases, including *src* and shc. The large T antigen can immortalize primary fibroblasts, and the small t antigen increases transformation efficiency.[44] The L region encodes three capsid proteins, each derived from an alternatively spliced mRNA. With the exception of the mouse polyomavirus, the course of infection in the permissive tissues of the natural hosts has not been investigated. By in situ analysis of mouse kidneys, differentiation-dependent viral DNA replication has been observed.[8]

Adenoviruses

The adenoviruses each contain a linear double-stranded chromosome of about 36,000 bp.[362] These viruses have a very distinctive replication mechanism to assure reproduction of their termini.[419] The ends are inverted sequence duplications, and a virus-encoded terminal protein is covalently linked to each 5' end. Replication takes place in the nucleus and depends on the virus-encoded DNA polymerase, which initiates from either end by using the precursor to the terminal protein as a primer. Synthesis along a double-stranded template proceeds by a strand displacement mechanism. The displaced single strand can form a stem-loop structure upon pairing of the inverted terminal duplications. Replication then reinitiates at the hairpinned ends, which have the same terminal sequence organization as the fully duplex molecules, and the replication cycle is completed by elongation over the entire length of the single strand.

Adenovirus RNA transcripts are generated from five early promoters and from several late promoters. Some transcription units have a specific 3' end and polyadenylation site, and others terminate at alternative poly A sites. Collectively, the RNAs virtually span both DNA strands. The various primary transcripts are processed by alternative RNA splicing into families of messages that share a common 5' end or a common poly A site, or both.[46,71,73] The 13S and 12S mRNAs from the E1A region are immediate early transcripts; their synthesis can take place in the absence of protein synthesis. The E1A proteins regulate transcription of both viral and host genes through interactions with a number of host proteins.[274,288] Transcription of the E1B, E2A, E2B, E3, and E4 regions is considered to be delayed early, because synthesis commences before DNA replication but requires the activation functions of E1A. Late mRNAs are transcribed only after the onset of viral DNA replication.

Both E1A and E1B are required for cell transformation and are therefore regarded as potential oncoproteins. Notably, the E1A proteins (289 amino acids and 243 amino acids) associate with the pRB family of proteins, whereas the E1B 55-kD protein interacts with the p53 protein. The E1B 55-kD and 19-kD proteins overcome the apoptosis induced by E1A functions, and they use different mechanisms to do so.[437] The E2A and E2B regions encode three proteins required for viral DNA replication: the 72-kD single-stranded DNA binding protein, DNA polymerase, and the precursor to terminal protein.[384] The E3 region is not essential for the viral reproductive cycle in cultured cells but is involved in modulation of host immune responses in vivo.[146,441] The E4 region encodes proteins of varied functions, one of which is involved in transactivating the E2 early promoter by stabilizing the binding of the host transcription factor E2F to the E2 early promoter[292] (see Functions of pRB Proteins and E2F Proteins). The L regions encode virion and morphogenic proteins.

Papillomaviruses

Papillomaviruses contain a double-stranded, covalently closed, circular DNA genome of about 7600 to 8000 bp.[180] Sequence analyses reveal that a similar genomic organization is shared by the human and animal papillomaviruses, with all substantial open reading frames (ORFs) distributed along one of the DNA strands (Fig. 12-1). Ten percent of the genome has no obvious ORF but contains transcription regulatory sequences, one or more promoters, and the origin of DNA replication.[72,414] This segment is variously designated the upstream regulatory region (URR), the long control region, or the noncoding region. Detailed analyses of viral transcription in lesions induced by HPVs,* by BPV-1,[10] or by CRPV[287] and in cell lines containing HPV† or BPV-1[10] demonstrate that all mRNAs are indeed transcribed from the same DNA strand. Alternatively spliced mRNAs are derived from several promoters, enabling the viruses to produce more proteins than ORFs. The mRNAs are polyadenylated at the 3' end of the E region or the 3' end of the L region.

The proteins encoded by the transcripts (or deduced from their sequences) are generally analogous among the papillomaviruses. The E-region proteins comprised one or more forms of E6; E7; one or more forms of E1 and of E2; E1^E4; and zero, one, or two distinct E5 products (Table 12-3). Together, these are responsible for viral transcription regulation, viral DNA replication, and pathogenesis. The L region encodes the major L1 and minor L2 capsid proteins. The designations of the E and L regions of papillomaviruses were initially made by functional analogy to the transcription programs and gene products of SV40, polyomaviruses, and human adenoviruses, which complete their lytic infections of permissive cells in culture within 48 to 72 hours. However, the successive stages of the productive life cycle of a papillomavirus are correlated with the squamous epithelial cell differentiation program that takes place over a period of 2 or more weeks (see later discussion).

One feature that differentiates the high-risk mucosotrophic HPVs from the low-risk types (see later discussion) is the presence of one (HPV-18) or two alternative (HPV-16) splices within the E6 exon in a fraction of the transcripts. The splices not only remove parts of the E6 coding sequences but also alter the reading frame in the downstream exon such that truncated E6 proteins (termed E6* and E6**) are generated. The frameshift terminations increase the nucleotide spacing before

---

*References 66, 74, 75, 112, 286, 297, 333, 363, 372, 376, 432.
†References 11, 120, 184, 191, 208, 285, 328, 332a, 347.

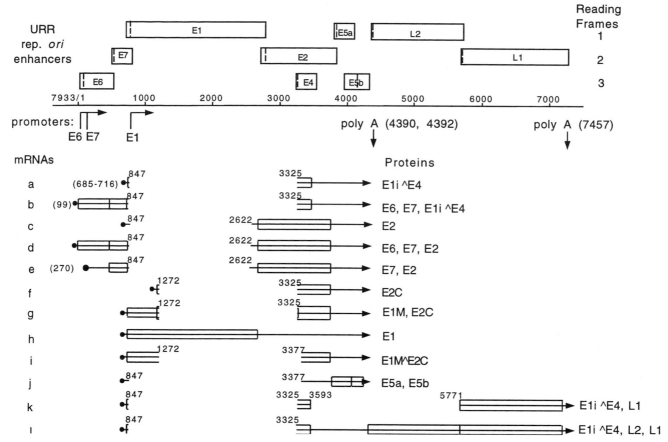

FIG. 12-1. Human papillomavirus (HPV) genome structures, transcription, and proteins. The genome organization of HPV-11 (7933 bp) is shown as representative of HPVs. The circular HPV genome was linearized in the upstream regulatory region (URR) for ease of representation. All open reading frames (ORFs), denoted by open boxes, are encoded by the same DNA strand. Dotted vertical lines signify the first AUG codon in the ORF, which is the initiation codon, except when removal of the E4 AUG by mRNA splicing occurs, as in E1i^E4. The arrows indicate direction of transcription, the arrowheads denote the polyadenylation signals, and the black dots indicate the 5' ends. Three of the 5' ends reflect the location of the promoter (*bent arrowheads*). Gaps in arrows signify spliced-out introns. The ORF contained within each message is shown as an open box over the mRNA. E5a and E5b might be translated from RNA species a through j. Proteins that are known or suspected to be encoded are listed at the right of each message. The symbol ^ represents a fusion protein derived from different ORFs brought together after mRNA splicing. The organization of other HPV types and of bovine papillomaviruses is similar and encodes many of the same proteins. The most notable feature of the high-risk HPVs is the presence of one or two alternative splices within the E6 ORF (designated E6*). The locations of promoters may also vary in individual virus types. The nucleotide positions of 5' ends, splice sites, and polyadenylation signals are indicated.

TABLE 12-3. *Human papillomavirus proteins and functions*

Protein	Function
E6	Inactivation of p53, bypassing p53-mediated G_1 arrest or apoptosis; interaction with putative calcium-binding protein p55
E6*	None identified (a result of mRNA splicing, found only in high-risk mucosotrophic viruses)
E7	Inactivation of pRB family of proteins
E1	Initiation and elongation of viral DNA replication
E2	Initiation of viral DNA replication; regulation of viral promoters
E2C	Regulation of transcription and replication
E1M^E2C	Regulation of transcription and replication
E4	Colocalization with keratin intermediate filaments; functions unknown
E5	Enhancement of signal transduction by epidermal growth factor receptor (most human or animal papillomaviruses have one or two E5 proteins; the epidermodysplasia verruciformis viruses have none)
L2	Minor capsid protein
L1	Major capsid protein

translation reinitiates at the E7 AUG codon, a consequence postulated to permit efficient E7 synthesis.[17,350,376] Nonetheless, E7 protein is clearly translated from wild-type or mutated unspliced E6-E7 messages with good efficiency in some HPV types.[65,190,326,379,403]

NATURAL HISTORY OF HOST-PAPILLOMAVIRUS INTERACTIONS

The adenoviruses, SV40, and polyomaviruses are traditionally propagated in permissive cultured cells and basically characterized through their lytic modes of infection. This investigative strategy in vitro worked quite well until efforts were made to carry out similar molecular and genetic analysis of the papillomaviruses. No member of the papillomavirus family can be grown in conventional cell cultures. This restriction led to extensive studies of papillomavirus pathogenesis in humans, the natural hosts. Such investigations in vivo provided opportunities to appreciate the natural history of DNA virus infection and to reveal new insights into the functions of the cellular proteins that the oncoproteins of the DNA tumor viruses all target. This section describes the natural sites of infection of the papillomaviruses, host cell proliferation, differentiation and apoptosis, and the induced diseases.

Diseases Associated With Papillomaviruses

Papillomaviruses infect many vertebrate animals and humans, with each virus type exhibiting stringent specificity for host species and epithelial tissue at preferred anatomic sites. Overt benign infections are manifested as warts. A small fraction of the lesions associated with certain human or animal viral types may progress to dysplasias, carcinomas in situ, and invasive cancers. Progeny viruses are produced only in warts or low-grade squamous dysplasias but not in columnar epithelia or in higher-grade dysplasias or carcinomas.

Animal Papillomaviruses

Among papillomaviruses, BPV-1 has a relatively broad cell type specificity. It infects keratinocytes and fibroblasts, causing fibropapillomas in cattle. However, productive infection takes place only in differentiated squamous epithelia,[180] as with all other human and animal papillomaviruses. BPV-4 causes epithelial hyperproliferation in the alimentary tract in cattle that can progress to cancer if the animals consume bracken ferns, which contain the carcinogen quercetin.[51] As mentioned previously, CRPV causes warts in the native host (cottontail rabbit) that occasionally progress to cancer. Warts induced in experimentally infected domestic rabbits do not produce progeny virions. These warts may regress, but progression to cancer occurs at a relatively high frequency.

Human Papillomaviruses

More than 100 genotypes of human papillomavirus have been cloned from diverse epithelial lesions.[110] Phylogenetic analyses have classified the HPVs into several major groups that correspond closely to their anatomic predilection and clinical manifestation[53] (Fig. 12-2; Table 12-4). Virus types are considered distinct if the genome exhibits more than 10% sequence divergence. The concept of virus evolution and speciation is reinforced by the absence of intertypic recombinants.

Cutaneous Viruses

Plantar and palmar warts caused by HPV-1 or -4 are benign but can be painful and debilitating. HPV-3 and -10 cause benign juvenile flat warts, and HPV-2 and -57 induce common warts. These latter four viruses have dual tropism and can also be found in the anogenital tract; they have many of the signature sequence characteristics of the mucosal group. HPV-5, -8, -47, and closely related types cause the very rare disseminated flat wart disease epidermodysplasia verruciform is (EV).[193,251,295] Many of the affected individuals have inherited deficiencies of the cell-mediated immune system (see Host Immune Responses). In sun-exposed areas such as the face and neck, EV lesions often progress to squamous carcinomas. The spread of human immunodeficiency virus (HIV) and the increasing number of organ transplantations with accompanying pharmacologic immunosuppression have led to an increase in the incidence of EV virus-associated lesions.[26,38,173]

Mucosotrophic Viruses

HPV infections are the most common venereal diseases of viral origin. The 40 or more types of HPV trophic for the mucosal epithelia lining the anogenital and aerodigestive tracts have attracted the preponderance of attention from the medical, epidemiologic, and basic research communities because they are responsible for an exceptional amount of morbidity and mortality.[461a] Subclinical infections typically extend beyond the overt lesions, and infected cells from the margin can repopulate the epithelium and reestablish the lesions after surgical removal or ablation. Reinfection by partners is very likely. Repeated physical trauma and tissue damage provoked by other sexually transmitted microbes can promote the proliferation of HPV-infected cells and elevate viral gene expression, possibly leading to reactivation of subclinical infections or progression. Moreover, the epithelial sites of infection are frequently exposed to mutagens.

On the basis of the potential for neoplastic progression, the HPVs are considered to confer either a low risk or high risk (see Table 12-4). The most common low-risk types, HPV-6 and its close relative HPV-11, typically cause benign exophytic genital warts, which rarely progress to higher-grade lesions. However, at a very low frequency, these viruses can be transmitted to newborns during delivery or to fetuses in utero, leading to a life-threatening, recurrent respiratory (laryngeal) papillomatosis.[106,369] Laser surgical ablation may be required every few weeks to few months in these patients to maintain an open airway. However, repeated laser excision and wound healing processes lead to the rapid regrowth of the papillomas. Furthermore, tracheostomy during respiratory emergency can sometimes cause the viral infection to spread down the trachea. Very rarely, infections can extend into the bronchia and

HPV Phylogenetic Relationships, Target Epithelia, Disease Manifestations, and Oncogenic Risk

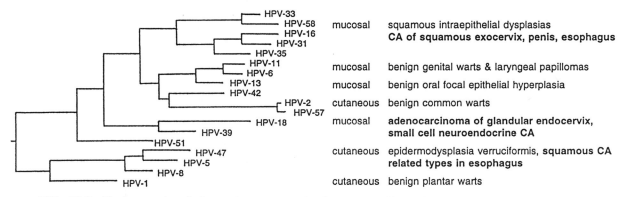

FIG. 12-2. Phylogenetic relations of representative human papillomavirus types based on the DNA sequence of the amino-terminal half of the E2 gene. The typical epithelial sites of infection and the potentials for neoplastic progression (*bold*) are indicated. (From Zhu QL, Smith TF, Lefkowitz E, Chow LT, and Broker TR. In: Nucleic Acid and protein sequence alignments of human and animal papillomaviruses constrained by functional sites. University of Alabama at Birmingham. 137 pages.)

lungs and result in pulmonary infections, pneumonia, septic cavitation, and respiratory failure.[216] This downward spread is probably caused by the lateral growth of infected cells in response to wound healing. Adults may also develop recurrent respiratory papillomatosis as a result of horizontal transmission, but the symptoms are usually less severe and require less frequent surgical intervention.

The most common high-risk types that infect the exocervix are HPV-16 (and related viruses such as HPV-35, -33, and -31), and HPV-18 (and the related types HPV-39 and -45), which cause condylomata and squamous intraepithelial lesions (SIL; see Pathologic Changes in HPV-Associated Diseases). Among sexually active women screened in numerous epidemiologic surveys, 25% to 45% of the individuals were found to be positive for HPV DNA by PCR amplification.[344] However, only about 10% of HPV-positive women exhibit overt symptoms of infection as revealed by colposcopic examination or cytologic evaluation of Papanicolaou (Pap) smears; thus, most of the infections are latent or subclinical. With time, lesions either regress or persist, with only a few percent eventually progressing to high-grade SIL, squamous carcinomas in situ, or carcinomas. In the columnar cell lining of the endocervical mucosa, adenocarcinomas in situ, invasive adenocarcinomas, or small cell neuroendocrine carcinomas can arise from infections by the high-risk HPV types.[385] Infec-

tions by HPV-18 are less common than those by HPV-16 but appear to be much more aggressive: they recur more frequently and progress faster. The high-risk viruses have also been found in up to 25% of esophageal cancers. A novel virus most closely related to the EV types has been identified in about 10% of esophageal cancers.[410]

The high-grade SIL are routinely treated by gynecologists and gynecologic oncologists by physical removal of the lesions and ablation of the metaplastic squamocolumnar (transformation) zone, from which most of the severe lesions arise. Hysterectomy is performed if lesions have progressed to carcinomas. The widely practiced Pap smear screening and treatment are the reasons for the relatively low cervical cancer incidence and death rates in developed countries. In developing countries, where early detection and treatment are not readily available, more than 500,000 new cases of cervical cancer are estimated to appear annually.[440] Many of these patients eventually die of progressive, metastatic disease; cervical cancer is the leading cause of cancer death for women younger than 35 years of age in much of the world. Males certainly harbor and transmit HPV infections, yet they usually have less severe disease, presumably because of hormonal influences; infection is less likely to be detected, because a Pap smear equivalent for men is not commonly practiced. The spectrum of disease in males ranges from benign penile and anal warts to dysplasias

TABLE 12-4. *Human papillomavirus types, anatomic sites, diseases, and risk for progression*

HPV Type	Anatomic sites	Diseases	Risk of cancer*
1, 4	Sole, palm	Plantar warts	No
2, 57	Cutaneous, genital	Common warts	No
3, 10	Cutaneous, genital	Flat warts	No
5, 8, 47, and related	Face, trunk, esophagus	Epidermodysplasia verruciformis	Very high†
6, 11	Anogenital, larynx	Benign warts	Low
16, 18, 31, and related	Anogenital, esophagus	Flat condylomata, dysplasias, carcinomas	High‡

*Immunosuppression increases rate of reactivation and risk of progression.
†30% to 40% undergo neoplastic conversion in sun-exposed areas.
‡1% to 3% progress to carcinomas.

and carcinomas; worldwide, there may be as many as 100,000 new cases of penile carcinoma annually.

Permissive Host Tissues

To understand and appreciate HPV infection and pathogenesis, it is essential to consider the permissive host tissues—the squamous epithelia—and their potential for growth and differentiation (Fig. 12-3). A normal squamous epithelium is composed of multiple layers of keratinocytes that form several morphologically distinct strata: the basal, parabasal, and spinous cells. In cutaneous skin, there are one or two additional layers of granular cells above the spinous cells, topped off with the nonliving stratum corneum, which is composed of highly crosslinked cell matrices and envelopes. Each stratum expresses distinct growth- and differentiation-stage specific host genes. The basal cells, some of which are thought to be stem cells,[196] rarely divide except during wound healing and periodic replenishment of parabasal transit amplifying cells that have exhausted their life span. Most of these cells are therefore negative for the proliferating cell nuclear antigen (PCNA), the processivity factor for DNA polymerase-δ that is necessary to support DNA replication.[105] The basal cells express the basic/acidic keratin pair K5/K14 (for keratin nomenclature, see Moll and colleagues[273]). The parabasal cells are transit amplifying cells that have committed to differentiate but still maintain the ability to complete a certain number of cell divisions.[21] Most of these cells are positive for PCNA, indicating that they are continuously cycling to generate daughter cells that move upward while undergoing terminal differentiation.[105]

Above the parabasal cells are several layers of spinous cells, as well as granular cells in the cutaneous skin. The spinous keratinocytes and granulocytes are differentiated cells that have withdrawn permanently from the cell cycle and no longer replicate their DNA; they are uniformly negative for PCNA. These interpretations are consistent with pulse-labeling experiments in which ³H-thymidine was injected into the skin of volunteers: the label was found only in the parabasal cells in skin biopsies.[162] All suprabasal cells, including the parabasal cells, no longer express K5 or K14; rather, they express K1 and K10 (or K4 and K13 in oral and

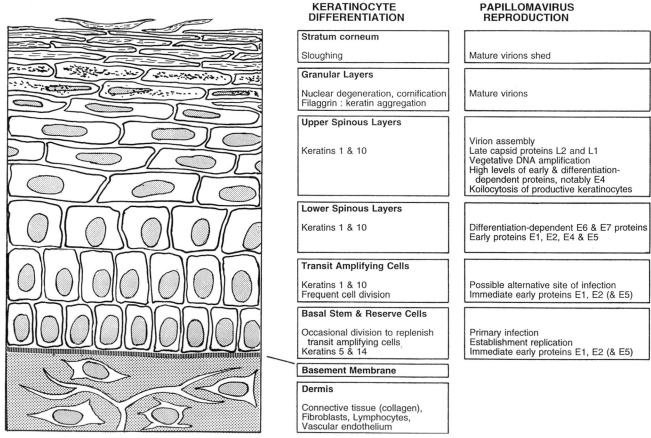

FIG. 12-3. Differentiation of normal cutaneous epithelium and viral activities in productively infected benign lesions. The various epithelial strata and the host differentiation-stage specific gene expression are indicated in the left and center panels. In cervical and laryngeal epithelia, keratins 4 and 13 replace keratins 1 and 10 in the differentiated cells. Although profilaggrin is also expressed in these two latter tissues, there are no granulocytes. Viral activities in the corresponding strata during productive infection, deduced or inferred from in situ studies, are shown on the right.

cervical squamous mucosa). The granular cells express profilaggrin, a polyprotein precursor of filaggrin, which aggregates keratins into fibrillar bundles. Lipid is also synthesized in abundance and is covalently bound to the cell envelope.[435] The cells then undergo programmed cell death and become flattened, with the RNA and DNA degraded by nucleases. The nuclear membranes break down, and the cells are converted to water-impermeable squames filled with crosslinked insoluble proteins. The continuous sheets of squame provide effective barriers to moisture exchange and to chemical and physical injury and infection, then eventually slough off. This process of orderly stratification and differentiation takes place over a period of a few days to a few weeks, depending on the body site.[162]

Under the basement membrane is the dermis, in which the fibroblasts—the principal cells—secrete collagen, elastin, fibronectin, and other matrix proteins that form the extracellular components to provide support as well as flexibility to the dermal-epidermal organ. The fibroblasts and keratinocytes secrete growth modulatory proteins, notably epidermal growth factor (EGF) and tumor growth factors α and β, which critically affect the growth and differentiation of both the dermis and the epidermis during normal maintenance and during wound healing. In addition, calcium and retinoids also affect the growth and differentiation of keratinocytes.[140]

Pathologic Changes in HPV-Associated Diseases

Histologically, a benign, clinically evident HPV infection exhibits an increased number of layers of transit amplifying cells and spinous cells, yet all the strata of a differentiated epithelium are present. This augmented thickness of the epithelium constitutes a wart (Fig. 12-4). The mucosotrophic HPVs (see later section) also can cause inverted (Schneiderian) papillomas in the nasal cavity, in which warts grow downward into the dermis instead of upward above the normal epithelium. HPV infection does not cause cell lysis or premature death, as do the other small DNA tumor viruses in vitro. Rather, infections prolong the life span of the keratinocytes by extending the interval between the time when a cell first leaves the parabasal layer and when it undergoes cornification and programmed cell death. HPV-associated papillomas and condylomata exhibit additional pathognomonic changes (see Fig. 12-4), such as koilocytosis in the upper spinous cells (characterized by an increased ratio of nuclear to cytoplasmic areas relative to uninfected cells and by a vacuole surrounding the nucleus), parakeratosis (residual nuclei in the squames), and hyperkeratosis (thickened superficial strata with delayed sloughing). These histologic features often correlate closely with high viral gene expression (see Papillomavirus DNA Replication) and viral DNA amplification. The various keratin and filaggrin genes are expressed in the morphologically appropriate strata. However, in contrast to normal epithelium, in which only the transit amplifying keratinocytes are positive for PCNA, a subset of the spinous and granular cells are also positive.[105] Yet mitotic figures are not usually found in these suprabasal cells of benign warts, and few if any aneuploid cells are detected. Polyploidy has been reported, but the topographic distribution of such cells was not specified.[365]

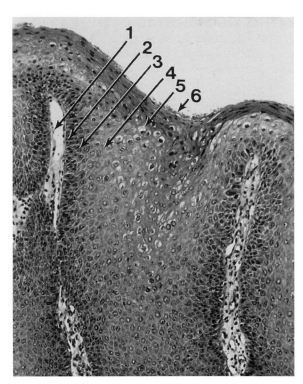

FIG. 12-4. Histologic section of a condyloma. A 3-μm section of a formalin-fixed and paraffin-embedded biopsy specimen of a vulva condyloma was stained with hematoxylin and eosin. 1, Underlying dermis with fibroblasts; 2, basal epithelial cells; 3, transit amplifying cells; 4, lower spinous cells; 5, upper spinous cells with koilocytotic changes; 6, stratum corneum (squame) with parakeratosis and hyperkeratosis.[46a]

In low-grade or high-grade SIL associated with the high-risk HPVs, the morphology is clearly distinct from either normal epithelium or condylomata in that increased layers of basal-like cells occupy suprabasal strata at the expense of the more differentiated spinous cell layers (Fig. 12-5). In carcinoma in situ, the full thickness of the epithelium is composed of basal-like proliferating cells. Infections of the glandular epithelium of the endocervix may result in dysplasias and in progressive neoplastic sequelae in which hyperchromatic basal-like cells replace the differentiated mucin-secreting cells. Through lateral proliferation, the glands become highly pleated and convoluted. In squamous cell carcinomas and adenocarcinomas, the transformed epithelial cells have penetrated through the basement membrane to invade and spread into and through the dermis. In all high-grade dysplasias and carcinomas of squamous and glandular epithelia, the expression of host proliferation- and differentiation-stage marker genes is altered.[105,105a,368] Mitotic figures are present in suprabasal cells, and aneuploid cells can be detected.[139,141]

Host Immune Responses

Extensive serologic studies in patients have demonstrated antibodies that recognize HPV virions, virus-like particles (VLP), which are experimentally produced empty particles

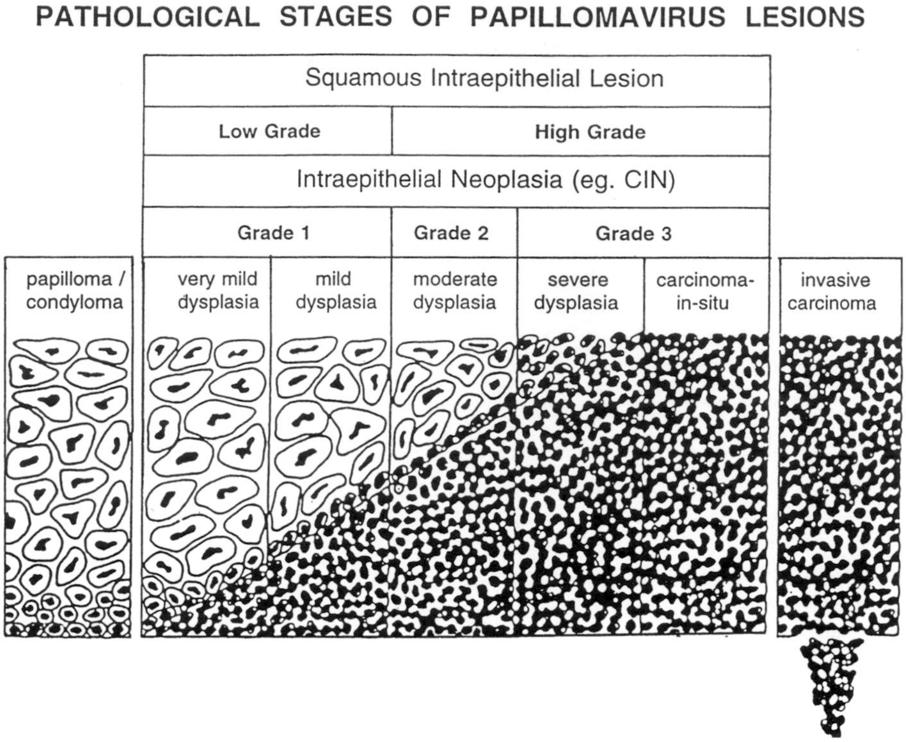

PATHOLOGICAL STAGES OF PAPILLOMAVIRUS LESIONS

Squamous Intraepithelial Lesion					
Low Grade		High Grade			
Intraepithelial Neoplasia (eg. CIN)					
	Grade 1		Grade 2	Grade 3	
papilloma / condyloma	very mild dysplasia	mild dysplasia	moderate dysplasia	severe dysplasia	carcinoma-in-situ	invasive carcinoma

FIG. 12-5. Schematic description of pathologic stages of human papillomavirus (HPV) lesions. The low-grade and high-grade squamous intraepithelial lesions (SIL) formerly were termed cervical intraepithelial neoplasia (CIN) grades I, II, and III; the correspondence is indicated. With increasing severity of the HPV-infected lesions, the differentiated cell layers decrease and the basal-like cell layers increase, until the entire epithelium is occupied by such cells in carcinoma in situ. Further progression results in invasive carcinoma, in which the cells break through the basement membrane and invade and spread in the stroma. (Adapted from Wright TC, Kurman RJ, Ferenczy A. Precancerous lesions of the cervix. In: Kurman RJ, ed. Blaustein's pathology of the female genital tract. 4th ed. New York: Springer-Verlag, 1994: 229–277).

(see Infection Processes), and many of the HPV proteins, most notably E2, E7, L1, and L2.[143,408] Although antiserum raised against HPV virions or VLP as well as patient sera can neutralize virus before infection of foreskin xenografts occurs in nude mice (see Xenografts in Athymic or SCID Mice),[76,79,332] there is no evidence that they are effective in preventing transmission or eliminating infection in humans. In one study, about 50% of cervical cancer patients demonstrated seropositivity against HPV-16 E6 and E7, compared with 5% or lower positivity in control subjects.[111,277,420] These increased serum antibodies did not provide the patients with any protection. Rather, they may reflect an increased tumor cell load. Similarly, both T cell and humoral responses to CRPV L1 and L2 proteins become elevated during progression.[353]

On the other hand, polyclonal or monoclonal antibodies raised against BPV virions or VLP, as well as hyperimmune bovine sera, can neutralize murine cell transformation in vitro by BPV-1 virus.[77,145,205,325] Furthermore, inoculation with VLP or formalin-fixed virions confers to susceptible animals protection against subsequent challenges.[25,43,398] BPV L1 and L2 proteins and native CRPV E1, E2, L1, and L2 proteins also can serve as vaccines or induce regression in animals, with variable effectiveness.[54,78,244,245,314,354] However, protection may be attributable to cell-mediated immunity rather than to humoral responses. Analyses of immune infiltrates in progressing or regressing warts in CRPV are consistent with this interpretation.[294]

In regressing human lesions, cell-mediated immunity also appears to play a major role.[408] Skin warts often resolve spontaneously without intervention. In regressing human warts, there are usually elevated levels of immune infiltrates.[1,83,327] The observations that EV patients have deficiencies of cell-mediated immunity[85,148,290] and that cancer, organ transplantation, and AIDS patients develop warts and other HPV-

associated lesions[101,144,173,195,361] are also consistent with this interpretation. Even transient immune modulation during pregnancy and physical and emotional stress can lead to short-term reactivation of subclinical infections or to more aggressive growth of warts. Normal human keratinocytes express both class I and II human leukocyte antigen (HLA) molecules. However, in HPV lesions, class I molecules are downregulated because of the loss of the transporter associated with antigen presentation.[200] There is no clear picture as to whether or how class II molecules may be affected,[408,463] but there appears to be a genetic predisposition to malignant progression. It has been reported that women with HLA-DQw3 antigen appeared to have a higher risk for squamous cell carcinoma.[431] In rabbits, there is a correlation between a restriction fragment length polymorphism of the major histocompatibility complex class II genes and regression as opposed to malignant conversion.[165]

Epitopes of HPV oncoproteins recognized by mouse cytotoxic T-cell have been investigated,[408] and vaccination with E6 or E7 proteins or peptide can prevent tumor formation in syngeneic mice injected with HPV-transformed cells or cause rejection of transplanted tumors.[59,60,131] Several T-cell determinants in the HPV-16 E6, E7, and L1 proteins have been defined with the use of human peripheral blood mononuclear cells from asymptomatic individuals.[2,396] However, it is not known whether T cells specific for these epitopes play a role in controlling infections. Interferons have been used alone or in conjunction with cryotherapy or laser surgery to treat genital and laryngeal papillomas. The effects have been variable, ranging from nonresponse and partial suppression to complete remission; recurrence is not uncommon after termination of therapy. Interferon-β and -γ appear to provide more effective long-term benefit than interferon alfa-n1.[33,238] These varied patient responses may be a reflection of heterogeneity in the makeup of their immune systems. In vitro, addition of interferon-α or -γ or leukoregulin, cytokines secreted by T lymphocytes and natural killer cells present in regressing warts, inhibited HPV-16 transcription in immortalized primary human keratinocytes (PHKs) in culture.[204,445] A potentially important observation is that HPV-infected cells produce self-limiting growth factors. HPV-16–immortalized human keratinocytes secrete tumor necrosis factor-α, which inhibits cell growth, and interleukin-6, which is an immunoregulatory cytokine with antitumor properties.[253,254] The HPV-16 enhancer-E6 promoter is downregulated by tumor necrosis factor-α and interleukin-1α.[221,222] Perhaps these complex interactions evolved between host and virus as part of the viral strategy to reach an equilibrium and establish a persistent infection.

INFECTION PROCESSES

Several obstacles have limited the study of HPV infection in vitro. First, only cutaneous HPVs generate virus particles in vivo in amounts useful for in vitro investigation, whereas the mucosotrophic HPVs produce few virions in natural warts. When HPV virions from cutaneous warts were used to infect a wide range of cultured cell types, including foreskin PHKs (the only primary human epithelial cells that are routinely available from medical clinics), viral DNA was only transiently maintained and only E-region viral mRNAs were detected, but no viruses were produced.[75,228,400] Cloned DNA was largely lost or became integrated when transfected into PHK monolayer cultures. Episomal persistence in the transfected cells is rare and of only short duration.[279] As discussed previously, BPV-1 virions or DNA can transform rodent cell lines, but no progeny viruses are produced. Because transformation requires a relatively long process of selection and growth of cells, it is not amenable to investigations of the infection process.

Consequently, little is known about the mechanism of papillomavirus infection. Recent advances in the assembly of VLP from L1 protein alone or from L1 plus L2 proteins expressed in surrogate cells* have made it possible to initiate binding, uptake, and internalization studies. The "receptor" appears to be present in a variety of cell types from many animal species.[276,324,423] Moreover, exogenously expressed viral E1 and E2 proteins can replicate viral DNA in transiently transfected cells from a variety of animal origins and tissue types.[68] Therefore, the strict species and tissue tropism of papillomaviruses probably derives from permissivity for viral gene transcription.

It is generally assumed that HPV establishes persistent infections in stem cells after the epithelium is wounded, as demonstrated after experimental infection of cattle with BPV-1 or rabbits with CRPV.[40,217] It is possible that, stimulated by wound healing and probably also by the action of the viral E5 gene product (see E5 Protein), the normally quiescent stem cells are mobilized to establish an infected cell population. After the wound healing process is complete and the dermal-epidermal organ has been restored to the maintenance state, the basal cells revert to quiescence, and most basal cells in a wart remain negative for PCNA. However, the parabasal tran-

sit amplifying cells become more proliferative, resulting in an increase in PCNA-positive cell layers, an effect probably also caused by E5 activities. The infected cells either proceed into a productive phase, culminating in the generation of progeny virions in the superficial, metabolically live cells (see next section), or the host immune surveillance keeps the viral activities in check, leading to a nonproductive, subclinical or latent infection. The lesions may regress, persist, or progress with time or with changing immune status of the patient. It is formally possible that the infections may also initiate in transit amplifying cells such that, after these infected cells exhaust their life span, the infections are "cured."

PAPILLOMAVIRUS GENE EXPRESSION IN VIVO

Over the past decade, in situ analyses have been used to examine viral transcription, DNA amplification, and protein production in a spectrum of patient specimens.[73a,385] On visual inspection of the papillomaviral transcription and replication patterns, it is immediately obvious why all attempts to propagate the viruses in vitro failed. Radioactively labeled antisense riboprobes reveal RNA transcripts. The sense-strand riboprobes detect DNA amplification after denaturation. These experiments demonstrate that both processes are tightly linked to squamous differentiation in productive infections. These numerous investigations also provide compelling evidence that HPVs are the causative agents for a wide spectrum of epithelial lesions, such as condylomata, intraepithelial neoplasias, carcinomas in situ, and invasive carcinomas. Regardless of their severity, whenever HPV RNAs are evident, there are associated pathologic changes. Conversely, in adjacent, histologically normal tissues, viral gene expression is not detected. The boundaries demarking histologically abnormal and normal tissues can be abrupt, and viral expression is fully concordant with pathologic changes.

Very low levels of HPV DNA and a subset of viral E-region transcripts can be detected in histologically normal tissues adjacent to benign lesions by Southern blot hybridization or PCR amplification,[132,257] indicative of latent virus in these tissues. As already discussed, the extremely high sensitivity of PCR has been used to reveal HPV DNA in epithelia of a high proportion of healthy individuals without any clinical symptoms. Similarly, latent CRPV infection has been demonstrated in rabbits.[3]

Physical State of HPV DNA and Patterns of HPV RNA Transcription in Benign Condylomata or Papillomas

In benign lesions, viral DNA is episomal, as shown by one- and two-dimensional Southern blot hybridizations of innumerable specimens. The levels of viral gene expression and DNA amplification in anogenital warts are extremely heterogeneous among different specimens and even among neighboring cells within a single specimen (Fig. 12-6A, B). Often, there is only a very low amount of viral RNA, with neither DNA amplification nor L1 antigen detectable. In lesions in which the infection is clearly productive, as evidenced by abundant viral mRNA, viral DNA amplification, and L1 antigen positivity, the papilloma is typically a mosaic of cells productive of viral RNAs and DNA interspersed with nonexpressing keratinocytes. Although little or no viral DNA or

---

*References 76, 159, 205, 206, 331, 339, 398, 422, 461.

RNA can be detected in the basal and parabasal cells even in productive lesions, low levels of replication and the transcription of the viral E1 and E2 genes necessary for episomal replication (see section on Papillomavirus DNA Replication) must take place so that the viral DNA is maintained during cell division. In productive infections, there is a large increase in viral transcription in the upper spinous cells; it may result from the upregulation of viral promoters during epithelial differentiation, or from an increase in DNA copy number, or both.

In situ hybridizations with exon-specific riboprobes have been performed to distinguish the expression of individual or groups of overlapping messages (see Fig. 12-1).* The probes for the E4 and E5 regions generate the highest signals, similar to signals generated by whole genomic antisense riboprobes (Fig. 12-7), because they are by far the most abundant messages and also because all other E-region messages also have a downstream exon spanning these two ORFs (see Fig. 12-1). Cytoplasmic E1 or E2 signals are relatively low and nuclear

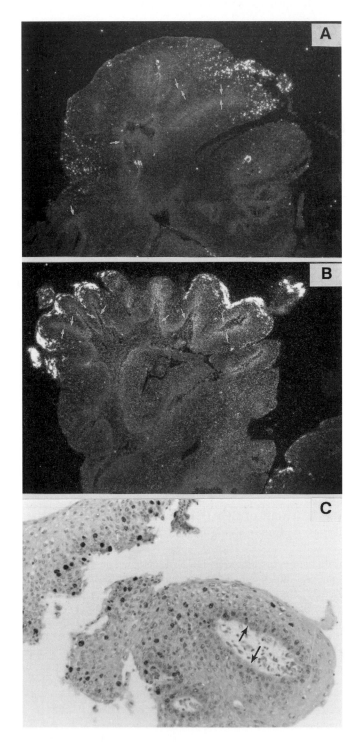

FIG. 12-6. Heterogeneity of viral DNA amplification, viral RNA expression, and host DNA replication in differentiated cells from benign laryngeal papillomas. Three cases of laryngeal papillomatosis are shown. (**A**) Human papillomavirus (HPV-11) DNA amplification was detected by in situ hybridization with sense ^{35}S-labeled whole genomic sense riboprobes after DNA in the paraffin-embedded section was denatured. Original magnification 4×, under darkfield illumination, in which the signals appear as white grains. (**B**) HPV-6 messenger RNA expression in a paraffin-embedded section was detected by antisense ^{35}S-labeled whole genomic antisense riboprobes. Original magnification 4×, under darkfield illumination. Note that viral activities are heterogenous in different parts of the papilloma. (**C**) Host DNA replication was detected after autoradiography of ^{3}H-labeled thymidine incorporation in a freshly excised laryngeal papilloma caused by HPV-6. Original magnification 40×, under darkfield illumination. Note that not only did host DNA replication take place in some basal and parabasal transit amplifying cells, as expected, but some differentiated cells in the upper spinous layers were also actively replicating their DNA. Arrows point to some of the basal and cell layers.[65] (Photomicrographs courtesy of D.C. Schmidt-Grimminger, T.R. Broker, and L.T. Chow).

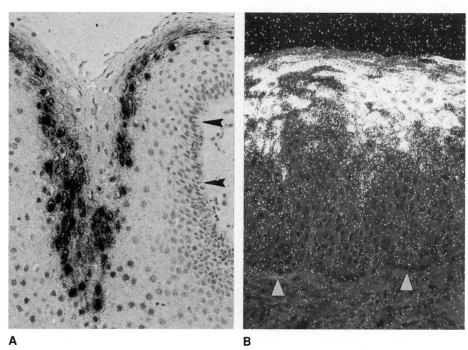

A   B

FIG. 12-7. Human papillomavirus (HPV) gene expression in a condyloma and in a low-grade squamous intraepithelial lesion (SIL). (**A**) HPV-6 gene expression in a condyloma as revealed by in situ hybridization in a 4-μm paraffin-embedded section of a formalin-fixed biopsy specimen. A ^{3}H-labeled antisense riboprobe specific for the E4-E5 exon was used, and the photomicrograph was taken with brightfield illumination. The differentiation-dependent pattern of viral expression was essentially the same as when whole genomic antisense probes were used. Arrowheads point to basal cells. (**B**) Differentiation-dependent HPV-16 gene expression in a low-grade SIL as revealed by in situ hybridization with whole genomic ^{3}H-labeled riboprobes photographed under darkfield illumination. Arrowheads point to basal cells. (Photomicrographs courtesy of M.H. Stoler, L.T. Chow, and T.R. Broker).

signals predominate, either because they are primary transcripts not yet processed or because the sequences represent residual introns spliced out of the abundant E4 and E5 messages. The relative abundance of the E6-E7 transcript is typically low, and the increase in E6-E7 signal with differentiation, if observed, is much less pronounced than that from the E4 and E5 RNAs.[65] L1 and L2 transcripts are usually found in one or two of the most superficial strata, often in only a small fraction of the cells. Moreover, few of the L1 RNA-positive cells produce the L1 antigen, suggesting an additional regulation at the posttranscriptional level. Some of the enucleated cornified squames are positive for viral DNA and L1 antigen, indicative of packaged virions. Productive cells are not lysed; rather, packets of virions are shed in the cornified envelopes as they slough off.

This differentiation-dependent pattern of viral expression also generally applies to the viral activities of BPV-1 and CRPV in productively infected papillomas.[180,459] The distribution of several specific mRNAs has been examined in bovine warts with the use of oligonucleotide probes specific for individual spliced transcripts for in situ hybridization.[19] When coupled with the information on BPV-1 RNA structures, the spatial and temporal utilization of alternative promoters and splice sites was revealed. Similar informative experiments have not yet been conducted with human specimens.

---

* References 28, 47, 95, 125, 172, 387, 388, 389.

Physical State of HPV DNA and Patterns of HPV RNA Transcription in Dysplasias and Carcinomas

In high-grade dysplasias, carcinomas in situ, and cancers, HPV DNA is often, but not always, integrated into the host chromosomes, as demonstrated by Southern blot hybridization. This conclusion has also been reached from detailed examination of viral gene expression by in situ hybridization,[96,387] which revealed distinct changes in the ability to detect amplified DNA and in the patterns of viral RNA expression (Fig. 12-8). With increasing severity of the lesions, viral DNA is less readily detected or not observable, consistent with a lack of vegetative amplification. The total viral RNA signal is usually reduced because of lack of epithelial differentiation and the absence of viral DNA amplification. In contrast to the scarce signal in the basal and parabasal cells of warts, E6-E7 gene expression is elevated in the basal-like cells of high-grade lesions and carcinomas indicating that a dysregulation of viral gene expression has occurred. The pattern and the amount of viral transcription remain constant across the boundary between carcinoma in situ and invasive cancer, suggesting that changes in the expression of host rather than viral genes are responsible for neoplastic progression (see Factors Involved in Progression).

Exon-specific probes revealed not only the dysregulation of viral gene expression but also the physical state of the viral DNA.[387] Conversely, in most cancers containing HPV-18 and in many of those associated with HPV-16, there is a relative reduction in or total absence of signals from the E4-E5 probes, and those from the E1 and E2 probes are greatly diminished or abolished. Because the polyadenylation signal and the poly A and addition site for the early genes are both located immediately downstream of the E2-E4-E5 ORFs, this pattern of viral

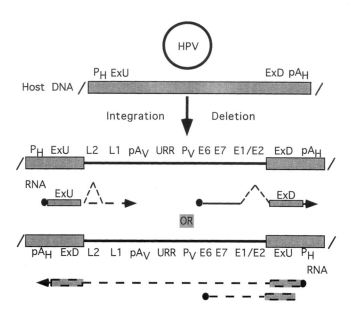

FIG. 12-8. Human papillomavirus (HPV) DNA integration and altered transcription and regulation. Viral DNA integration is probably random. However, tumors often contain integrated HPV DNA integrated in the E1-E2 region, accompanied by deletion sequences spanning part or all of E1 through L2. Cells no longer expressing the E2 or E1 gene may have a growth advantage because of the disruption of autoregulation of viral oncogenes by the E2 proteins. The diagram depicts events in which viral DNA integrates into a host gene between the host promoter (P$_H$) and upstream exon (ExU) on one side and the downstream exon (ExD) and polyadenylation site (pA$_H$) on the other side. Integration can occur in either the sense or the antisense orientation relative to P$_H$. In the sense orientation, the E6 and E7 messenger RNAs initiated from the viral promoter (P$_V$) are spliced from the E1 splice donor to host ExD and are processed by using the host polyadenylation signal. Presumably, cycling cells expressing chimeric messages with an elevated stability relative to native viral RNA have a dysregulated cell cycle control and a growth advantage. Transcripts initiated from the PH are not expected to encode the native viral L1 protein because the RNA may not traverse to the viral polyadenylation site (pA$_V$) or may not be spliced to the L1 exon, be it in frame or out of frame. When integration occurs in the opposite orientation, viral transcripts initiated may not be properly spliced or polyadenylated unless there is a fortuitous host splice acceptor and pA$_H$ in the flanking host sequence. Transcription from the P$_H$ would yield antisense viral RNA, as observed in some carcinomas. The antisense RNA would inhibit the translatability of the viral messenger RNA initiated from the P$_V$. Shaded boxes, host DNA or RNA; thick solid line, HPV DNA or RNA; dot, 5' terminus of RNA; arrowhead, 3' terminus of RNA; dashed line or box with dashed border, nonfunctional RNA; bent dashed line, RNA splicing.

transcription suggests that the viral DNA has integrated into host chromosomes in the E1 or E2 ORF with deletion of downstream sequences into the L region (see Fig. 12-8). Such integration events separate all the downstream ORFs from their promoters and dissociate the upstream transcribed regions from their polyadenylation signal. Functional E6-E7 mRNAs must then use a polyadenylation signal and 3' cleavage site from the host sequences downstream from the integration site. Such is the case in cervical carcinomas and in cell lines derived therefrom (e.g., HeLa, CaSki, SiHa).[11,347,372,376] These E6-E7-host fusion transcripts have elevated stability relative to the natural viral mRNA, and hence an increased level of the encoded oncoproteins. This mRNA stabilization is considered to be one of the factors contributing to progression of lesions in vivo and to immortalization and transformation of cells in vitro.[194]

Cytoplasmic L1 and L2 signals are usually absent from high-grade lesions because of lack of differentiation, sequence deletion, or dissociation of the coding regions from their upstream promoter in the integrants. Nuclear L1 RNA signals are observed in some HPV-18 cancers but may be attributed to transcription from host promoters situated upstream of the integrated viral genome.[387] Transcription from a host promoter across the integrated viral genome could also explain the detection of HPV antisense RNAs in some carcinomas.[171,427]

An observation that merits consideration is the apparent natural selection for neoplasms in which viral DNA is integrated within the E1 or E2 ORF. Because the family of E2 proteins can each inhibit the E6 promoter in transient transfection experiments, such an integration event could in principle result in the upregulation of the E6 promoter in proliferating cells.[69,70,117,119,330,402,405] For BPV-1, the E1 protein can also repress the promoter responsible for the transcription of the E5, E6, and E7 genes.[236,334,418] Although a direct repression of the E6 promoter by HPV E1 protein has not been demonstrated, HPV-16 and HPV-18 DNAs interrupted in the E1 or E2 gene immortalize PHKs with increased efficiency.[329,335] Exogenous expression of BPV-1 or HPV E2 proteins can repress the growth of some cervical carcinoma cells.[121,188] Yet, there is also evidence to the contrary. For instance, the rate of lesion progression in transgenic mice containing the HPV-16 E region with or without the E1 or E2 genes remains unchanged,[6] suggesting that neither E2 nor E1 protein plays a critical role in controlling the expression of the HPV oncogenes from an integrated genome in vivo. The restriction of the E6 promoter activity to the differentiated cells in epithelial raft cultures in the absence of E1 and E2 proteins also indicates that E2 proteins are not responsible for the low activities in the basal and parabasal cells[65] (see later discussion). Furthermore, the expression of E2 protein transactivates viral transcription and increases the efficiency of immortalization or transformation.[37,235,391a] These conflicting results have not been resolved but may be explained by the different levels and relative amounts of E2 or E2C proteins expressed in the different cell types, in which both the intrinsic viral promoter activity and the interactions between E2 protein and host transcription factors undoubtedly vary. Aside from the issue of the loss of E1 and E2 proteins, viral transcriptional activity from the integrated state may also vary depending on the chromosomal location, perhaps related to the local chromatin structures, state of methylation, and nearby host promoters or enhancer elements. This is best illustrated by distinct transcriptional responses of the integrated HPV-18 in different cervical carcinoma cell lines to treatment with glucocorticoid.[424]

EXPERIMENTAL SYSTEMS FOR PRODUCTIVE PAPILLOMAVIRUS INFECTION

Xenografts in Athymic or SCID Mice

A human xenograft system has been developed in which large quantities of HPV-11 and HPV-1 can be produced.[34,178,218] Neonatal foreskin or fetal skin infected with wart extracts is grafted under the renal capsule, the peritoneum, or the subcutis of athymic (nude) mice or severe combined immunodeficient (SCID) mice. Over the course of a few months, the infected human epithelia develop into internal cysts or skin warts from which abundant virions can be recovered. The infected tissues or virions purified from them can be serially passaged.

Two additional systems have also resulted in virion production or capsid protein synthesis. In the first, cells from an immortalized cell line derived from an HPV-16–containing dysplasia were grafted onto the flank of a nude mouse under an implantation chamber; the keratinocytes stratified and differentiated, and virions were detected.[382] In the second, gold pellets were coated with cloned HPV-16 DNA and impelled with a "gene gun" into human foreskin grafted onto the skin of a SCID mouse; L1 antigen was eventually detected.[41] Virus particles have not been recovered from these latter two systems. Mutagenic analyses of CRPV genes have begun by introduction of CRPV DNA into rabbit skin by scarification or the gene gun.[40]

Epithelial Raft Cultures

Epithelial raft cultures, also termed organotypic cultures, are composed of primary neonatal foreskin or adult cervical keratinocytes cultured on a dermal equivalent consisting of feeder fibroblasts and type I collagen. If the assemblies are raised to the medium-air interface for a week or more to mimic the natural environment of skin, the keratinocytes undergo orderly proliferation, stratification, and differentiation. This system was developed by cell biologists starting in the late 1970s.[7,24,214] It was first applied to papillomaviruses to examine the effects of transfected HPV-16 on epithelial differentiation.[260] The degree of differentiation achieved by PHK in vitro under different conditions has been compared with that in the native foreskin.[439]

The raft system was adapted to culture of epithelial tissue chips explanted directly ex vivo onto the dermal equivalent. When the system was set up with HPV-11–infected foreskin xenografts in nude mice, the infected keratinocytes grew out from the tissue explants as an expanding apron of cells, then stratified and differentiated over a period of 2 to 4 weeks.[118] The patterns of viral gene expression, DNA amplification, and virion assembly in vivo were recapitulated in the stratified outgrowth. Under conditions in which the outgrowth was allowed to stratify but was restricted from differentiating, viral genomes were maintained for several weeks in the keratinocytes, but

only the E4-E5 RNA could be detected readily. The E1 and E2 gene expression essential for episomal replication was inferred from the persistence of the genome. However, there was no detectible E6-E7, L2, or L1 RNA, nor was PCNA induced or viral DNA amplified. This was the first time that viral activity was experimentally modulated in vitro. Several conclusions could be drawn: first, the E1, E2, E4, and E5 mRNAs are immediate early, not dependent on epithelial differentiation or DNA amplification; second, the expression of E6-E7 genes is correlated with epithelial differentiation; and third, the absence of PCNA induction and viral DNA amplification is correlated with the lack of E6-E7 gene expression, implicating one or both genes in viral DNA amplification in the differentiated cells.

A cell line that was derived from a low-grade cervical dysplasia and contained episomal HPV-31b DNA also produced virions in raft cultures, but only if the cultures were treated with 12-O-tetradecanoylphorbol-13-acetate (TPA) or other activators of protein kinase C (e.g., synthetic diacylglycerols) that promote and accelerate terminal differentiation.[185,266] These results again demonstrate the importance of terminal differentiation in the life cycle of papillomaviruses. Initial efforts to achieve the productive program in primary keratinocyte rafts with transfected DNA have been successful with HPV-31[137] but not with HPV-11 or -16.[48] To date, it has not been possible to infect PHK in raft cultures with virions (S.C. Dollard, T.R. Broker, L.T. Chow, unpublished results).

PAPILLOMAVIRUS DNA REPLICATION

Because of the inherent limitations in studying the productive life cycle of papillomaviruses in vitro, two methods were developed to investigate the mechanisms of human and animal papillomavirus DNA replication.[72] In the first, transient replication in efficiently transfected cells was used to identify the origin of replication and the essential viral replication proteins.* In the second, cell-free replication of plasmids was achieved in mammalian cell extracts supplemented with ribonucleoside and deoxyribonucleoside triphosphate substrates and purified viral replication proteins after their expression in insect Sf9 cells or bacteria.[32,219,262,275,453] Both methods demonstrate that the full length E1 and E2 proteins and their cognate binding sites that are located in close proximity in the URR are required for efficient origin-specific replication. Thus, the papillomaviral replication origin overlaps the E6 promoter, just as in the sequence relation between the SV40 or polyomavirus origin and the early promoter elements where T antigen binds.

The E1 protein is a DNA-dependent ATPase and a DNA helicase.[42,183,356,454] It is required for both initiation and elongation of DNA synthesis.[246] The E2 protein was first identified as a transcription regulatory protein, which either activates or represses promoters containing the E2 binding sites as determined by sequence context.[163,414] E2 protein also serves multiple functions for replication initiation. It precludes nucleosome formation around the origin, thus facilitating the assembly of replication initiation complexes on the origin,[240] and stabilizes E1 protein binding to the origin.[136,250,355,453]

---

* References 67, 68, 102, 136, 152, 175, 249, 322, 399, 415, 416.

E2 also helps E1 recruit the host replication proteins to the origin, but appears not to be necessary during elongation.[246] E1M^E2C and E2C proteins repress replication.[67,246]

The large T antigen of SV40 and polyomavirus fills the same roles in viral DNA replication as do the E1 and E2 proteins of papillomaviruses.[130] For these small circular DNA tumor viruses, all the other proteins necessary to support DNA replication at the fork are supplied by the host cells, including DNA polymerase-α/primase, DNA polymerase-δ and its cofactors PCNA and RFC, RPA (single-stranded DNA binding protein), topoisomerase I, topoisomerase II, and DNA ligase.[219,383,453] The adenoviruses encode their own replication proteins: the DNA polymerase, a 72kD single-stranded DNA binding protein, and the precursor to the terminal protein, which binds to the DNA termini and serves as the primer for initiation of replication.[362,419] In contrast to the large herpesviruses and vaccinia viruses, none of these small DNA tumor viruses encodes any of the deoxyribonucleoside triphosphate synthetic or salvage enzymes necessary to supply the substrates for replication.

The requirements for DNA replication machinery and for deoxyribonucleotide synthetic enzymes do not present a problem for the polyomaviruses or the adenoviruses in cultured cells because they replicate in proliferating cells or can stimulate G_0 cells to reenter the cell cycle, a function of the viral oncoproteins. However, in vivo or in vitro papillomaviruses amplify their DNA extensively only in cells that have withdrawn from the cell cycle and are undergoing terminal differentiation. These cells are normally negative for DNA polymerase-α and for PCNA[105,283] and probably lack many of the other proteins and enzymes necessary to support DNA replication. Accordingly, it would appear that the papillomaviruses must reactivate all these host genes to support their replication, and indeed they do so in the differentiated keratinocytes of benign lesions without promoting cell division.

To this end, PCNA is induced in spinous and granular keratinocytes in productive lesions regardless of virus type.[105] Not only does viral DNA replicate in these differentiated cells, but extensive host chromosomal DNA replication also takes place[65] (see Fig. 12-6C and the section on functions of viral oncoproteins). Clearly, this ability to reactivate host DNA replication machinery can help to explain the oncogenic properties of certain HPV types in vitro and in vivo in the event that the viral oncoproteins are inappropriately expressed in cells that maintain the ability to divide (see later discussion).

BIOLOGIC ASSAYS FOR ANIMAL PAPILLOMAVIRUS ONCOPROTEINS

Transformation of Rodent Cells In Vitro and Tumorigenicity in Nude Mice

BPV-1 virions or cloned DNA transform the established murine fibroblast cell lines NIH 3T3 and C127 based on focus-formation or anchorage-independent growth in soft agar.[126,406] E6 and E5 are the responsible oncogenes (see Table 12-2).[180,390] The transformed cells are tumorigenic in nude mice, although BPV-1 normally causes only benign fibropapillomas in cattle. An efficient in vitro transformation system for CRPV in cultured rabbit skin cells has been developed.[266a]

Three CRPV oncoproteins were identified: the E7 protein and two E6 proteins translated from separate mRNAs using different in-frame AUG initiation codons. In collaboration with an activated H-ras protein[296] the E5, E6, or E7 protein of a rhesus monkey papillomavirus are also capable of transforming primary baby rat kidney cells in vitro and of tumorigenicity in nude mice.

Of the animal papillomaviruses, the BPV-1 oncoproteins have been most thoroughly investigated. The BPV-1 E6 protein is 137 amino acids long, has four CXXC motifs, and folds into two zinc finger–like domains important for the transformation activity. Unlike the HPV E6 proteins, BPV E6 apparently does not bind p53. A 55-kD calcium-binding protein, ERC-55, localized in the endoplasmic reticulum, was found to bind to BPV-1 and HPV-16 E6 proteins and was designated E6-BP.[58] The abilities of BPV-1 E6 mutations to transform rodent cells correlated with binding to this protein, which was postulated to mediate a p53-independent pathway of E6 transformation. The mechanism remains to be elucidated.

The BPV-1 E5a protein has been characterized in detail.[113,390] It is a transmembrane protein, 44 amino acids long, targeted to the plasma membrane, the Golgi apparatus, and the endoplasmic reticulum. It dimerizes through two cysteine residues and forms a ternary complex with a 16-kD pore-forming protein component of the vacuolar H+ adenosine triphosphatase (H+-ATPase) and with the β-type platelet-derived growth factor (PDGF) receptor through its transmembrane domain.[150,151,310] E5a activates the PDGF receptor in a ligand-independent manner.[122,323,378] E5a protein also interacts with a 125-kD α-adaptin–like molecule which may play a role in coated pit mediated surface receptor endocytosis, hence affecting signal transduction and transformation.[81] If cotransfected with a vector expressing the EGF or colony stimulating factor-1 receptor, BPV-1 can also activate their signal transduction pathways.[258] However, BPV-1 E5a does not transform cells via the endogenous EGF receptor.[151,289] The E5a protein is present in fibropapillomas.[49] Because epithelial cells normally do not express the PDGF receptor, the function of the E5a protein in the epidermal component of the fibropapilloma is not clear. A hydrophobic, 52-amino-acid protein encoded by the BPV-1 E5b ORF has been identified.[291] It does not transform the murine C127 cell line but does modify the processing of the endoplasmic reticulum calcium-binding protein, calreticulin (CRP55). It is intriguing that the BPV-1 E6 and E5b, and HPV E6 protein each associate with calcium-binding proteins in the endoplasmic reticulum, and that two of the three host proteins (Nip 1, 2, 3) with which the adenovirus E1B 19-kD protein and the host Bcl-2 protein interact also contain putative calcium-binding sequences.[39] The adenovirus 19-kD protein has a short sequence homology with Bcl-2, and they are functionally analogous in overcoming apoptosis triggered in response to a number of conditions.[437] In epithelial cells, high calcium concentrations trigger termination differentiation. By modulating the calcium-binding proteins, the viruses may disrupt the normal control of intracellular calcium, delaying programmed cell death to provide more time for viral reproduction.

Transgenic Animals

Transgenic mice containing 1.69 copies of the BPV-1 genome (with a duplicated E region) have been established and examined.[179] The mice developed fibromatosis, which progressed to fibrosarcomas with time or at sites of wounding. Viral transcripts were detected in pathologically affected tissues but not in normal skin, and the level of transgene transcription remained constant during progression, suggesting that mutations accumulated in critical host genes during excessive proliferation.

In a dramatic demonstration, transgenic rabbits expressing CRPV developed papillomas within a month after birth, whereas rabbits that additionally contained an activated c-Ha-ras transgene developed squamous carcinomas at birth, consistent with a multistage model of carcinogenesis.[308] The viral oncoproteins necessary for this transformation process have not been identified.[40]

BIOLOGIC ASSAYS FOR HUMAN PAPILLOMAVIRUS ONCOPROTEINS

Three HPV oncoproteins—E5, E6 and E7—have been identified through a variety of assays.[261,343,390,428,428a] The HPV E5 proteins are highly heterogeneous in sequence and in size among virus types, but each is small, hydrophobic, and known or predicted to be membrane associated. The E6 proteins are about 150 amino acids long, and the E7 proteins are approximately 100 amino acids long. Both E6 and E7 are relatively conserved among HPVs but do not share extensive homology with the BPV counterparts, except that all have CXXC motifs (four for E6, two for E7) with similar spacings and all establish zinc coordination complexes (see Binding of HPV E7 Protein to pRB Proteins).

Transformation of Rodent Cells In Vitro and Tumorigenicity In Vivo

E6 and E7 Proteins

With few exceptions, the E7 gene rather than the E6 gene of the high-risk mucosotrophic HPVs scores positive in a variety of transformation assays. If E7 is expressed from a strong heterologous promoter such as the Moloney murine leukemia virus long terminal repeat (LTR), it induces morphologic transformation or anchorage-independent growth in a number of murine cell lines.[23,313] In collaboration with activated c-Ha-ras, LTR-driven E7 expression can transform baby rat kidney epithelial cells.[22,393] If E7 is expressed from the homologous URR, transformation of primary rodent cells in collaboration with an activated c-Ha-ras or with fos additionally requires steroid hormones,[92,124,301] which stimulate the viral promoter.[149,270] Constitutive expression of c-myc confers hormone independence to transformation of primary mouse kidney cells.[89] The transformed cells are tumorigenic in both immunocompromised and immunocompetent syngeneic mice. Further attesting to the importance of these viral oncoproteins, continuous expression is required for the growth of the transformed cells in vitro and tumorigenicity in nude mice.[91,300] With few exceptions, the low-risk HPV E6-E7 regions are largely negative or at best inefficient in these assays, consistent with the small number of human cancers found to contain low-risk HPV types. In contrast to the mucosotropic HPVs, the E6 rather

than the E7 gene of the EV papillomaviruses is able to transform murine cell lines.[189,208]

E5 Proteins

Both the low-risk HPV-6 E5a and the high-risk HPV-16 E5 gene can enhance EGF-mediated signal transduction and promote anchorage-independent growth of murine fibroblast lines (see Table 12-2).[62,234,315] The HPV-16 E5 is able to induce tumorigenicity in a murine keratinocyte cell line.[237] The E5 proteins associate efficiently with the EGF receptor, its close relative erbB-2, and the PDGF receptor, as well as with the 16-kD vacuolar ATPase.[86,87,187] The mechanism of action involves prevention of the acidification of endosomes, which reduces the degradation of internalized receptor and increases its recycling to the plasma membrane.[394,395] Not surprisingly, HPV-16 E5 collaborates with HPV-16 E7 to stimulate proliferation of primary rodent epithelial cells.[36] In HPV-16–immortalized PHK that have acquired the ability to grow in the absence of EGF (see Immortalization of Human Epithelial Cells), the EGF receptor is constitutively activated.[464] In laryngeal papillomas, the abundance of the EGF receptor is elevated.[417] HPV-16 E5 also significantly reduces cell-cell communication through the gap junctions, the significance of which is not yet understood.[293]

Transgenic Mice

Mice expressing the HPV E6-E7 region under the control of a variety of strong cellular promoters have been established. The animals can develop a spectrum of conditions, depending on the promoters and the transgenes introduced.[156] High-risk HPV E6-E7 transgenes driven by promoters that are active in proliferating reserve cells tend to cause dysplasias or cancers, whereas those targeted to cells that are committed to differentiate are disposed to developing hyperplasias or warty lesions. For instance, mice expressing HPV-16 E6 and E7 from the keratin 14 promoter develop hyperplasias and dysplasias in squamous epithelium.[6] HPV-16 E6-E7 genes driven by the LTR promoters of mouse mammary tumor virus or Moloney murine leukemia virus cause cervical and vaginal dysplasias and carcinomas and testicular tumors.[213,337,338] In contrast, HPV-1 E6-E7 driven by the keratin 6 promoter induces abnormal epidermal differentiation.[409] HPV-16 or HPV-18 E6-E7 expressed from the differentiation-dependent keratin 10 promoter induces warty growth.[9,153] The fact that these mice never develop carcinomas, even in old age, indicates that expression of high-risk HPV oncoproteins differentiated cells, does not necessarily lead to dysplasias or carcinomas, an observation consistent the natural history of the virus infections and with the results obtained in epithelial raft cultures.

Transgenic mice with the HPV-16 E6 or E7 genes, or both, targeted to the eyes a promotor of the gene encoding the αA crystallin or the interstitial retinol-binding protein are most revealing of the functions of these oncoproteins and of the targeted tumor suppressor proteins, p53 and pRB.[138,154,177,226,298] Mice with E6 and E7 transgenes develop microphthalmia and cataracts with 100% penetrance, a consequence of induction of lens cell proliferation and impaired differentiation. A fraction of adult animals with high levels of viral oncogene expression eventually develop eye tumors as well as epidermal cancers. In contrast, the HPV-16 E7 transgene alone promotes lens cell proliferation and apoptosis, resulting in microphthalmia or photoreceptor cell death. However, in the background of p53$^{-/-}$ mice, the E7 transgene induces tumors. The E6 transgene alone inhibits lens fiber cell denucleation and reduces apoptosis. The SV40 large T antigen expressed from the αA crystallin promoter induces tumors in the eye,[252] while a truncated T antigen that binds only to pRB but not to p53 results in microphthalmia.[138] Transgenic mice expressing from the αA crystallin promoter the mouse polyomavirus T antigen (which immortalizes but does not transform primary cells) also have impaired eye lens cell differentiation but do not develop tumors.[155] These results demonstrate the importance and collaboration of E6 and E7 oncoproteins and, by inference, the targeted host tumor suppressor proteins in regulating cell growth, differentiation, and apoptosis, and they support the notion that the HPV (and perhaps SV40) oncoproteins potentiate the development of human cancers.

Immortalization of Human Epithelial Cells

The in vitro model system akin to HPV pathogenesis in vivo is the immortalization of primary human epithelial cells from a variety of body sites that are the normal targets for these viruses (i.e., foreskin, ectocervix, endocervix, the oral cavity, larynx, trachea, and bronchia)* and their subsequent alterations in growth properties and oncogenic transformation[114,261,461a] (see Factors Involved in Progression). To be effective in these assays, the high-risk HPV E6 and E7 genes are both required.[167,199,280,345] In contrast, using secondary mammary epithelial cells as targets, the HPV-16 E6 rather than the E7 gene has an immortalization function.[14] BPV-1 E6 and HPV-6 E6 also score positive at a much reduced efficiency.[13] The HPV E5 gene is not active in the immortalization assay.

Using the efficient method of recombinant retrovirus-mediated gene transfer, the HPV-16 E7 protein alone expressed from the retroviral promotor can immortalize PHKs, albeit at a reduced frequency.[160] Furthermore, the low-risk HPV-6 E6 or E7 protein can complement the high-risk HPV-16 E7 or E6 protein, respectively, and yield a low frequency of immortalization.[161] These results reveal that HPV-6 E6 and E7 genes do have a degree of immortalization ability, in agreement with the observation that HPV-6 and HPV-11 are occasionally found in human cancers. The HPV-8 E7 protein is also weakly positive in this complementation assay.[346]

The chromosomes of immortalized keratinocytes have restored telomere lengths, compared with the shortened telomeres in precrisis cells. The activation of telomerase is considered an important step in the immortalization process.[209,308a] The cells can still be stimulated by high Ca++ or serum to undergo a certain degree of differentiation but are not tumorigenic in nude mice. Immortalized cells also exhibit altered sensitivities to retinoic acid in growth and differentiation, as do HeLa cells.[88,265,317,366] With increasing passage in vitro or under selective culture conditions, the cells can develop altered properties such as growth factor independence, resistance to terminal differentiation, anchorage independence, and,

eventually, tumorigenicity.[186,305,318] If these cells are grafted underneath the skin of nude mice or grown as epithelial raft cultures, progressively dysplastic epithelial tissues develop.*

Acute Morphologic Transformation in Epithelial Raft Cultures

Epithelial raft cultures have been adopted to examine the immediate effects of HPV oncoprotein expression in primary human foreskin or cervical keratinocytes. The cells were acutely infected with retroviruses expressing the viral proteins under the control of the Moloney murine leukemia virus LTR.[30,161] The HPV-16 E6 virus and HPV-16 E7 virus together induced highly dysplastic morphology in the stratified raft cultures. PCNA-positive nuclei and mitotic figures were observed throughout the epithelium. Consistent with the dysplastic histology, the expression of host differentiation marker genes was substantially delayed. p53 was elevated in some of the suprabasal cells, but only if HPV-16 E6 was absent,[30] consistent with E6 protein-triggered p53 degradation (see later discussion). In contrast, analogous recombinant retroviruses expressing the low-risk HPV-6 E6 and E7 proteins were incapable of immortalizing PHK. They did not induce morphologic changes in PHK raft cultures after acute infection, nor did they induce PCNA in the suprabasal cells.[161] Epithelial cell lines derived from cervical dysplasias or squamous carcinomas also exhibited diminished abilities to differentiate, or they formed disorganized and dysplastic morphologies in raft cultures.[99,321] These experiments demonstrate convincingly that HPV-16 oncoproteins are responsible for dysplasias in vivo.

Transactivation of Adenovirus E2 Promoter

The HPV E7 proteins (and less so the HPV E6 proteins) can transactivate the adenovirus E2 promoter. This subject is discussed in detail in the section on molecular mechanisms of HPV protein functions.

FUNCTIONS OF VIRAL ONCOPROTEINS IN DIFFERENTIATED EPITHELIAL CELLS

The functions of HPV E7 protein during the infection cycle were revealed through another set of recombinant retroviruses in acute infections of PHKs in raft cultures.[65] The expression of various combinations of the high-risk HPV-18 E6 and E7 genes or cDNAs was controlled by the native URR enhancer-promoter elements so that the differentiation states of the infected cells would dictate when, where, and how abundantly the viral oncoproteins were expressed and, conversely, the experimental expression of the viral oncoproteins would not have undue influence on the course of epithelial differentiation. The cultures had unaltered differentiation profiles. All the cultures that had an intact E7 gene induced PCNA in the suprabasal differentiated cells, whereas the basal cells were not affected. ³H-thymidine incorporation indicated that many of the suprabasal spinous cells were actively replicating their

---

* References 124, 182, 299, 306, 319, 358, 413, 438, 444, 455.

* References 20, 31, 123, 260, 264, 305, 397, 430, 443.

chromosomes. The presence or absence of the E6 gene made little difference to the induction of PCNA or replication in the differentiated cells (D. Schmidt-Grimminger, S. Cheng, T. Broker, L. Chow, unpublished results). Therefore, the HPV-18 E7 protein alone is necessary and sufficient to reactivate the entire host DNA replication machinery in the differentiated cells so that the viral DNA can replicate. Extensive host chromosomal DNA replication also took place as a byproduct (see Fig. 12-6C).

The raft model system is entirely consistent with the induction of host DNA replication in differentiated spinous cells in benign papillomas.[65] The majority of the differentiated cells that are actively replicating DNA do not enter mitosis. Recent nuclear DNA content analysis suggests that a fraction of the spinous cells in vitro and in vivo are polyploid (P. van Diest, D. Schmidt-Grimminger, J. Baak, J. Walboomers, C. Meijer, L. Chow, T. Broker, unpublished results). An analogous retrovirus expressing the low-risk HPV-11 E7 gene alone from the homologous URR was able to induce PCNA in the suprabasal cells, although not as efficiently as the HPV-18 E7. The reduced efficiency may be attributed to the lower affinity of the HPV-11 E7 protein for pRB (see Binding of HPV E7 Protein to pRB Proteins). It remains to be determined whether HPV-11 E7 protein alone is able to reactivate chromosomal DNA synthesis in the differentiated cells. Mutagenic analyses in the context of episomal HPV DNA are yet to be conducted.

As discussed previously, the E2 protein can downregulate the URR enhancer-promoter in proliferating epithelial cells. The frequently observed deletion of the E2 and E1 genes from the integrated viral DNA in HPV-associated cancers has been suggested to confer a growth advantage to the cells through derepression of viral oncogene expression from the URR and through increased stability of the E6-E7 mRNAs after acquisition of a host poly A proximal sequence. Despite the absence of the E1 and E2 genes in the recombinant retroviruses, the URR promoter is relatively inactive in the basal cells of the raft cultures, as inferred from the lack of PCNA induction. Rather, it is upregulated only in the differentiated strata, as in warts that do express both E1 and E2 proteins. Therefore, the basal cells in the epithelial raft cultures have somewhat different properties from proliferating PHKs cultured in monolayers. It will be interesting to examine the effect on the expression of E6 and E7 after the introduction of the homologous E2 gene.

Although the precise functions of the E6 protein during productive infection are not evident from the raft culture experiments, one speculation is that, by binding to and inactivating p53, E6 may reduce the fraction of cells entering into premature apoptosis after p53 becomes elevated in response to E7-induced unscheduled DNA synthesis in the differentiating epithelium (Y. Jian, D. Schmidt-Grimminger, T. Broker, L. Chow, unpublished results). This issue is discussed in the next section.

MOLECULAR MECHANISMS OF HPV PROTEIN FUNCTIONS

An insight into the mechanisms by which the HPV E6 and E7 proteins function came from the realization that each of the small DNA tumor viruses encodes one or two proteins that inactivate the same host tumor suppressor proteins (see Table 12-2).[288] The adenovirus E1B 55-kD protein and the papillomavirus E6 proteins directly or indirectly interact with the p53 protein. The adenovirus E1A and papillomavirus E7 proteins bind to pRB and the related proteins p107 and p130. The SV40 and mouse polyomavirus large T antigens bind to p53 and pRB proteins. These host proteins play critical roles in regulating cell proliferation, differentiation, apoptosis, and genome stability; their inactivation by mutations is found in a wide range of human cancers. These virus-host protein interactions are essential for productive viral life cycles. The significance of these interactions in viral carcinogenesis is underscored by the observation that pRB and p53 are rarely mutated in most HPV-containing cervical carcinomas (or cell lines derived therefrom), whereas p53 mutations are found at higher frequencies in HPV-negative cervical carcinomas or cell lines.[63,94,202,220,233,341,446] In both patient lesions and cell lines derived from cervical carcinomas, E6 and E7 genes are actively transcribed. Antisense RNA to the viral oncogenes can suppress proliferation of a cervical carcinoma cell line in vitro and its oncogenicity in nude mice.[425,426]

Binding of HPV E7 Protein to pRB Proteins

There is a short domain containing the amino acid sequence LxCxE in conserved region II (CRII) of adenovirus E1A proteins which is shared by the SV40 T antigen and HPV E7 proteins[313,429] (Fig. 12-9). Each protein is able to transform established murine cells and to transactivate the adenovirus E2 early promoter through E2F sites and, to a lesser degree, an activating transcription factor (ATF) site.[247,311,392] These sequence and functional similarities quickly led to the experimental demonstration that HPV E7 proteins both bind to pRB (p105) during in vitro cotranslation.[128] pRB binding and adenovirus E2 promoter activation by the HPV E7 protein also require this conserved motif.[312] The viral oncoproteins also bind to two additional members of the pRB family, p107 and p130, by means of the same domain.[97,127] Immediately adjacent to the LxCxE pRB binding domain are casein kinase II sites, mutations of which reduce phosphorylation but do not affect pRB binding.[16,133] The amino-terminus of the E7 protein has a limited sequence homology to a region of the adenovirus E1A protein designated as conserved region I (CRI)[45,98,442] (see Fig. 12-9). The E1A CRI contributes to promoter regulation and immortalization functions by interacting with pRB family proteins, p300, and other host transcription factors.[5,274] An interaction between the E7 protein and p300 has not been demonstrated. The zinc-binding motifs near the carboxyl-terminal are important for protein stability.[312] In addition, the C-terminal two thirds of the E7 protein binds to pRB independently of CRII and is essential for displacing E2F from pRB.[181,304,447] These properties help explain why E7 protein with a C-terminal truncation is unable to reactivate host DNA replication in differentiated cells.[65]

Extensive mutagenic analyses of the HPV-16 E7 protein and domain swapping experiments have been conducted in attempt to delineate the functional domains that differentiate high-risk from low-risk HPVs.* The results that emerge are rather complex because of the different biologic and biochem-

---

* References 5, 45, 98, 129, 168, 282, 302, 336, 391, 401.

```
           37            49 // 116     121           137
            :            :    :         :             :
Ad5 E1A   HFEPPTLHE-LYDL     VP--EV--IDLTCHEAGFPPSDDEDE
SV40 Tag  REESLQLMD-LLGL     FNEE---NLFCSEEM-PSSDDDET
            :            :    :         :             :
           7             19 // 98                    117

                                                                                              pRB
           2            15              24            39/ N / 63 / N / 98 /N/   AA    AFFINITY
            :            :               :             :    :          :
HPV-18 E7  HGPKATLQDIVLHL----EPQNEI-PVDLLCHEQLSD-SEEENDE  22  CXXC  31  CXXC  3  Q (105)   HIGH
HPV-16 E7  HGDTPTLHEYMLDL----QPET----TDLYCYEQLNDSSEEEDE-  20  CXXC  29  CXXC  3  P ( 98)   HIGH
HPV-11 E7  HGRLVTLKDIVLDL----QPPD---PVGLHCYEQLEDSSEDEVDK  18  CXXC  29  CXXC  3  P ( 98)   LOW
HPV- 8 E7  IGKEVTVQDFVLKLSEI-QPEV-L-PVDLLCEEEL-PN-EQETEE  16  CXXC  29  CXXC  8  S (103)   NO

HPV- 1 E7  VGEMPALKDLVLQL----EPSV-LD-LDLYCYEEV-PPDDIEEEL  12  CXXC  29  CXXC  4  Q ( 93)   HIGH
            :            :               :             :     :          :
           2            15              23            38    52         85


HOMOLOGY*  H-----L-E  L-L       P        DL-C-EE--D SDDDDD
           R     V-D                      Q--P       EEEEE


FUNCTIONAL _____CR I_____    _____CRII_____    Zn++ BINDING MOTIFS
    DOMAIN                      pRB BINDING    CKII             pRB Binding
                                                                E2F Displacement
```

FIG. 12-9. Functional domains and sequence homology of human papillomavirus (HPV) E7, adenovirus (Ad) E1A, and simian virus 40 (SV40) T antigen (Tag). HPV-16 and HPV-18 are high-risk mucosotrophic types. HPV-11 is a low-risk mucosotrophic type. HPV-8 is a oncogenic epidermodysplasia verruciformis (EV) virus, whereas HPV-1 is a nontransforming benign cutaneous type. Gaps (-) are created for alignment. Amino acid positions are given for Ad E1A, SV40 Tag, HPV-18, and HPV-1. The last amino acid and the total number of amino acid residues (AA) for E7 proteins are provided in parentheses. The number of residues between the sequences is provided under N. The alignment also takes into consideration the E7 proteins of additional HPV types. Only fixed numbers of residues are indicated by (-) in the derived homology sequence.

ical assays used in various laboratories, including morphologic transformation of different cell lines, growth in soft agar, immortalization, tumorigenesis in nude mice in collaboration with an activated *ras* gene, promoter transactivation, pRB binding, and release of E2F.[261,343,428] In general, the pRB binding domain in CRII emerges as the most critical determinant. The affinities of E7 proteins from the high-risk HPV-16 and -18 for pRB and p107 are higher than those of the low-risk types.[80,142,168,281,336] A single amino acid in the pRB binding domain that differs between the E7 proteins of the high-risk and low-risk mucosotrophic HPVs (D24 in HPV-16 versus G in the comparable position in HPV-11; see Fig. 12-9) correlates with the affinity to pRB. However, other E7 proteins with this DLxCxE motif do not necessarily exhibit a high affinity for pRB, nor is a high affinity for pRB sufficient to explain the different properties of the various HPV E7 proteins. For example, the high-risk HPV-8 E7 protein does not appear to bind to pRB and does not transform cells in vitro[189,190] despite a perfect consensus. The benign plantar wart HPV-1 E7 protein also has this perfect binding sequence and has a relatively high affinity for pRB (see Fig. 12-9), yet it is inactive in baby rat kidney transformation[80,346] and does not cause cancer in patients. Despite being negative in immortalization or transformation assays, the low-risk mucosotrophic HPV E7 proteins are as effective in adenovirus E2 promoter transactivation as those of the high-risk HPVs. By inference, transactivation alone is not sufficient to account for immortalization and transformation potentials. Clearly, the E7 protein is multifunctional, and the correlations among protein domains,

amino acid residues, and the various biologic and biochemical assays continue to be a subject of intense research.

Functions of pRB Proteins and E2F Proteins

The pRB (p105) protein was the first tumor suppressor protein identified. The gene is deleted or mutated in many human cancers, most notably in familial and sporadic retinoblastomas.[211] Conversely, the experimental overexpression of pRB can suppress cell proliferation. p107 and p130 are two pRB-related proteins. Together, they function to control the progression of the cell cycle in response to regulation by the family of cyclin-dependent kinases (CDKs) and their respective cyclins (Fig. 12-10). At the molecular level, each member of the pRB family of proteins preferentially binds to members of the E2F family of transcription factors, which themselves form heterodimers with the DP-1 family of proteins. The underphosphorylated form of pRB sequesters E2F-1, E2F-2, and E2F-3, and these complexes act as repressors and downregulate the expression of targeted host genes that contain the E2F binding sequence in their promoters. When pRB becomes hyperphosphorylated by cyclin:CDK complexes, it dissociates from the E2F:DP-1 complex, and the targeted promoters are relieved of the negative regulation. pRB is phosphorylated mainly by CDK4 in association with cyclin D1 before the G_1-S checkpoint, and it remains phosphorylated until after the M phase, when it is dephosphorylated (see Fig. 12-10). The repression and activation of the targeted host genes are therefore cyclic. The HPV E7 and adenovirus E1A proteins and the SV40 T antigen bind to underphosphorylated pRB, preventing the association with or causing the dissociation of the E2F:DP-1 complex[56] (see Fig. 12-10).

p107 is a phosphoprotein, and the phosphorylation is also cell cycle–regulated. It forms complexes with E2F-4, cyclin A, and CDK2 in late G_1 and in S phase, whereas p130 binds E2F-5 and is abundant in G_0 cells.[433] Binding of HPV-16 E7 to p107 also leads to transactivation of the adenovirus E2 promoter.[52] The consequences of binding of the viral oncoproteins to p130 have not been explored. Because each of the pRB-like proteins binds to different E2Fs at different phases of the cell cycle, their natural functions are not redundant. This conclusion is also inferred from the fact that deletions or mutations of p107 and p130 have not been identified in cancers.

What are the genes regulated by the E2F proteins? One or more E2F consensus binding sites are known or suspected to control the transcription of cellular genes that regulate cell proliferation and cell cycle progression, such as *dihyrofolate reductase, c-myc, B-myb,* and *cdc2,* as well as *p107* and *E2F* themselves.[224,288] Introduction of E2F-1 cDNA can promote G_0 fibroblasts into S phase,[215] and the endogenous host genes induced include ribonucleotide reductase, thymidylate synthase, and DNA polymerase-α.[100]

With the use of promoter transactivation assays, a few host genes have been shown to be regulated directly by the viral oncoproteins.[224,288] For instance, the SV40 T antigen can activate the murine thymidine kinase promoter, the adenovirus E1A protein can activate *N-myc* and *DHFR,* and the HPV-16 E7 protein can activate *B-myb, cyclin A,* and *cyclin E* genes, each mediated through E2F.[225,460] In immortalized keratinocytes, the expressions of the *cdc2, cyclin A,* and *cyclin B* genes are also elevated.[381] The E7 proteins of both low-risk and high-risk HPVs also transactivate the human thymidine kinase and DNA polymerase-α promoters through a single E2F site (M.P. Sowden, T. Broker, L. Chow, unpublished results). From the observation that host DNA replication is reactivated in differentiated keratinocytes of epithelial raft cultures that express E7 alone from the URR[65] (see previous section), it is clear that pRB proteins targeted by the E7 protein control each of the genes encoding the DNA replication machinery and enzymes for deoxyribonucleoside triphosphate synthesis or salvage. At least one of the key replication genes—PCNA—does not contain an E2F site; rather, an ATF site is important for its regulation.[223] ATF and perhaps other transcription factors must also be controlled by E7, by mechanisms yet to be elucidated.[442] It is not a coincidence that the adenoviruses use E2F and ATF to control the expression of their own replication genes.[247] Clearly, the adenoviruses took advantage of host transcription factor binding proteins that orchestrate all the genes necessary for DNA replication. The viral oncoproteins that target the pRB proteins induce the DNA replication genes and drive the resting or differentiated cells into S phase (see Fig. 12-10). The high-risk HPV E7 protein can also circumvent the G_1 arrest induced by DNA damage.[103,169,367]

Association of HPV E6 Protein With p53

The SV40 T antigen, the adenovirus E1B 55-kD protein, and the E6 protein of many of the HPV genotypes can directly or indirectly bind to and inactivate the p53 protein.[84,255,343,437]

p53 is considered to be a ``guardian of the genome,'' and the loss or inactivation of p53 causes chromosomal instability.[197,243,352,371] p53 is induced after DNA damage. It is a transcription factor and in turn activates several genes, including p21(*cip1/waf1/sdi1*), *mdm2,* and *gadd45* (see Fig. 12-10). The mdm2 protein serves as a feedback control by binding to p53 and downregulating its transactivating activity.[448] The gadd45 protein interacts with PCNA and appears to function in DNA repair.[370] p21*cip1* is a universal CDK:cyclin inhibitor and is present in quaternary complexes containing cyclin:CDK:p21:PCNA.[166,450] By preventing the phosphorylation of pRB proteins by CDKs, it arrest cells in the G_1 phase, presumably to allow DNA repair before reentry into the S phase (see Fig. 12-10). In addition, p21*cip1* also interacts directly with PCNA, inhibiting processive replicative DNA synthesis and favoring repair synthesis in cell-free systems.[57,134,241]

DNA damage can also trigger apoptosis. Apoptosis, or programmed cell death, is not only a defensive mechanism through which cells that have suffered DNA damage are eliminated; it also maintains homeostasis, balancing cell proliferation and cell turnover. Expression of adenovirus E1A, HPV-16 E7, or E2F-1 in growth-arrested fibroblasts triggers both DNA replication and apoptosis. The latter response is dependent on the presence of wild-type p53. The adenovirus E1B 55-kD and 19-kD proteins and the HPV-16 E6 protein can abrogate this premature apoptosis.[215,320,436,437,449] By analogy to the observations in human fibroblasts, the HPV E6 protein may also block this p53-mediated premature apoptosis if unscheduled host DNA replication takes place in the differentiated epithelial cells in response to the HPV E7 protein (see Fig. 12-10).

There are additional effects on inactivating p53 by HPV-16 E6 in cycling cells. First, normal human fibroblasts expressing HPV-16 E6 protein alone have reduced p21*cip1* transcription. In these cells, PCNA is no longer found in complexes with cyclin:CDK:p21. The net effect is a dysregulated cell cycle control and genome instability on continuous passage.[436,451] Cells can also progress through the cell cycle even after they have suffered DNA damage.[158,203,412] The dysregulated cell cycle control would explain why human mammary epithelial cells immortalized by HPV-16 E6 are more sensitive to radiation damage than are normal mammary cells.[452] This consequence seems at first to be contradictory to the hypothesis that the E6 protein blocks p53-mediated apoptosis in differentiated cells. However, the immortalized mammary cell death is probably a result of replication of damaged chromosomes. Second, the expression of HPV E7 protein alone in differentiated keratinocytes elevates p53 protein accumulation[30,104] (Y. Jian, D. Schmidt-Grimminger, T. Broker, L. Chow, unpublished results). Through targeting p53, E6 could reduce the p53-mediated induction of p21*cip1,* which may inhibit DNA replication if present in high concentrations. Last, if it is experimentally overexpressed, p53 represses a wide range of host and viral promoters through its interaction with the TATA binding proteins,[357] and HPV E6 protein can abrogate this repression.[90,231,267] The inactivation of p53 by HPV E6 protein therefore could alleviate multiple effects detrimental to viral propagation.

p21*cip1* protein is elevated in senescent cells, and it is transcriptionally upregulated when normal human keratinocytes are induced to differentiate in vitro.[268] It may be expected that p21*cip1* would be a target for one of the viral oncoproteins so

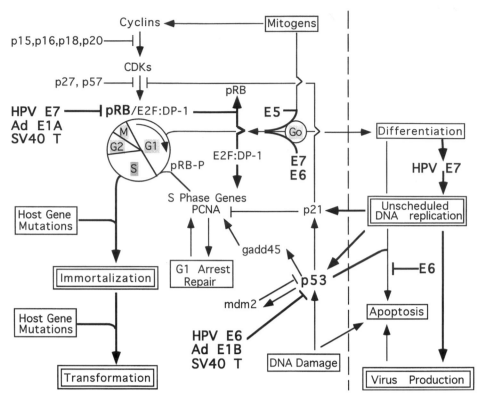

FIG. 12-10. Interplay among viral oncoproteins and host regulators of cell growth, differentiation, and apoptosis. The normal cell cycle (including G_0, G_1, S, G_2, and M phases) is shown to the left of the vertical dashed line, and cellular differentiation followed by apoptosis is shown at the right. Arrows signify induction, whereas T-bars represent inhibition. The two key host regulatory proteins are pRB and p53. pRB phosphorylation is regulated by upstream regulatory proteins: p15, p16, p18, and p20, a family of proteins that inhibit the association of cyclins with cyclin-dependent kinases (CDKs)[364]; p21*cip1*, which is a universal CDK inhibitor and may also inhibit DNA replication directly by interacting with proliferating cell nuclear antigen (PCNA); and p27 and p57, proteins that share sequence homology to p21*cip1* and are also inhibitors of cyclin:CDK complexes.[364] The protein p53, induced after DNA damage, leads to arrest G_1 arrest and DNA repair before re-entry into the cell cycle. Alternatively, cell death by apoptosis may result. On gaining entry into the epithelium after wounding, the E5 protein is likely to upregulate the signal transduction by mitogens present during healing, leading to expansion of infected stem cells and transit amplifying cells. After healing, the stem cells appear to return to quiescence; there are more layers of transit amplifying cells, but the epithelium goes on to differentiate. E7 is then upregulated to reactivate the host DNA replication machinery, deoxyribonucleoside triphosphate synthetic or salvage genes, and other S-phase genes; both host and viral DNA then replicate in the differentiated cells. In response, p53 and p21*cip1* are induced as a host defense mechanism. One of the probable functions of HPV E6 is the inactivation of p53, abrogating the consequences detrimental to virus propagation. If the viral oncoproteins E6 and E7 are inappropriately expressed in stem cells, these cells would undergo extensive cycling, resulting in mutations in host regulatory genes and genome instability. In vitro, cells can become immortalized and, in synergy with activated protooncogenes, mutagens, or the loss of other growth regulatory genes, become transformed. In patients, these consequences are manifested as high-grade lesions and carcinomas. HPV E7, human papillomavirus E7; Ad E1A, adenovirus E1A, and SV40 T, simian virus 40 T antigen.

that DNA replication capability can be restored in the differentiated cells. However, recent experiments have demonstrated that neither p53 nor p21*cip1* protein can be detected readily in suprabasal cells in neonatal foreskin or in uninfected epithelial raft cultures, although both are upregulated in raft cultures infected by HPV-18 URR E7-expressing retroviruses. p21*cip1* induction is also observed in the spinous strata of benign warts and in low-risk cervical intraepithelial neoplasias containing either low-risk or high-risk HPVs, validating the in vitro results (Y. Jian, D. Schmidt-Grimminger, X.

Wu, T. Broker, L. Chow, unpublished results). One possible explanation for these observations is that, despite the intervention of E6, a fraction of the host cells still manage to mount a defense by way of p21*cip1* protein induction against unscheduled host DNA replication in the spinous cells in response to the HPV E7 protein. This host-virus interplay (see Fig. 12-10) would explain the heterogeneity in the ability of infected cells to support high levels of viral DNA replication and gene expression as well as host DNA replication in vitro and in vivo[65,118,389] (see Fig. 12-6).

HPV E6 protein targets more than just the p53 protein. A dominant negative mutant of p53 can collaborate with HPV-16 E7 protein to immortalize PHK, although it does not have the transformation activity of wild-type HPV-16 E6.[351] The reduction in the concentration of wild-type p53 protein alone by antisense RNA does not result in growth stimulation.[192] Furthermore HPV-5, HPV-8, BPV-1, and CRPV E6 proteins do not inactivate the transactivation activity of p53.[207] Several additional host proteins that interact with the HPV-16 E6 protein have been identified,[201] but, with the exception of the 55-kD E6-BP[58] and E6-AP (see below), their identity is not known and the mechanism of action remains to be elucidated. Finally, HPV-16 and HPV-18 E6 proteins exhibit weak transcription transactivation in transient transfection assays, the significance of which is not yet understood.[109,147,350]

Mechanisms of p53 Inactivation

The high-risk HPV-16 E6 proteins incapacitate p53 by at least two mechanisms. First, they bind to p53 by association with a cellular 100-kD protein, E6-AP. Together, they function as a ubiquitin ligase for p53, resulting in ubiquitin-mediated p53 degradation and a greatly reduced halflife.[340] The ability of HPV-16 E6 mutations to target p53 for degradation correlates with their ability to overcome the DNA damage-induced growth arrest.[135] Second, inactivation of p53 does not necessarily depend on its degradation.[407] This point is amply demonstrated by the increased stability of p53 on binding to the adenovirus E1B 55-kD protein or the SV40 T antigen. The E1B 55-kD protein interferes with the transcriptional transactivation domain of p53,[458] whereas SV40 T antigen displaces p53 from its cognate DNA binding sequence.[18] The HPV E6 protein can also prevent p53 from sequence-specific binding to DNA.[230,316,407]

The association of the low-risk HPV E6 proteins with p53 and their ability to interfere with p53 transactivation are both reduced in comparison with the high-risk HPV E6 proteins, and p53 degradation in vitro is not observed.[93,230,434] However, a fusion E7-E6 protein caused the degradation of the interacting pRB in vitro regardless of whether the fusion protein contained an HPV-16 or an HPV-6 E6 moiety. These observations imply that some interaction does exist in vivo.[342] The halflife of p53 is reduced in BPV-1– or HPV-6 E6–immortalized mammary epithelial cells.[14] It is evident that there are differences among the E6 proteins, as revealed by their differential abilities to immortalize PHKs in collaboration with the high-risk E7 protein and to induce genome instability in human fibroblasts. However, regardless of whether p53 is destabilized by the E6 proteins or whether E6 also acts through p53-independent mechanisms, each E6 protein must necessarily accomplish the same tasks, because all papillomaviruses need to modulate the cellular environment conducive to reproduction in differentiating squamous epithelial tissues.

FACTORS INVOLVED IN PROGRESSION

Epidemiologic studies suggest that multiple sexual partners and infection by high-risk HPVs are the most important risk factors for development of cervical carcinomas. In addition,

carcinogens such as tobacco metabolites and betel quid and UV or radiation damage appear to play roles in the development of HPV-associated cervical and oral carcinomas.[12,55,198] Because the level of viral oncogene expression does not change significantly across the boundary between carcinoma in situ and invasive cancer, progression has been attributed to the accumulation of host cell chromosomal mutations, in agreement with a multistage models of oncogenesis[421] (see Fig. 12-10). As discussed in the section on host immune responses, immunologic factors may also influence the outcome of infection.

Somatic cell hybrids have been instrumental in demonstrating alterations in host genes in the process of carcinogenesis. HeLa cells, which contain and express integrated HPV-18 E6 and E7 genes, are tumorigenic in nude mice, whereas somatic hybrids established with normal skin fibroblasts or keratinocytes are not, indicating that one or more key negative growth regulatory genes are missing in HeLa cells. Through selective chromosome transfer, the responsible genes have been assigned to chromosome 11.[4] The reemergence of tumorigenic segregants correlated with the loss of chromosome 11.[263] In the nontumorigenic hybrid cells, the viral E6 and E7 oncogenes were downregulated, whereas in the tumorigenic segregant, viral oncogene expression once again became elevated,[35] indicative of changes of the cellular environment and, consequently, in the viral promoter activity. This cell hybrid approach has also been used to demonstrate that host genes can be classified into several complementation groups, the expressions of which are altered during immortalization of PHK and the subsequent progression in vitro.[64,272,309,349] Revertants have been isolated after introduction of cDNAs from rat embryo fibroblasts into HPV-18–transformed rat cell lines, and the loss of the cDNA is accompanied by the reacquisition of the transformed phenotype.[284] The identities of the cDNAs have not been reported.

The notion that gene products from human chromosome 11 can downregulate HPV expression also arises from a different set of experiments in human fibroblasts that have a deletion in the short arm of chromosome 11 (del-11) at a locus overlapping the Wilms' tumor suppressor gene.[404] HPV-16 can induce anchorage-independent growth in del-11 cells but not in normal diploid human fibroblasts.[373] Similarly, the del-11 cells, but not normal human fibroblasts, can be morphologically transformed by the human polyomavirus BKV.[107] Normal diploid fibroblasts can be transformed by SV40, but only if both the large T antigen and the small t antigen are present.[108] The SV40 small t antigen or the 55-kD regulatory subunit (PR55) of protein phosphatase-2A can complement HPV-16 in transforming normal diploid fibroblasts. The facts that both proteins negatively regulate protein phosphatase-2A and that PR55 is highly expressed in del-11 fibroblasts suggest that protein phosphatase-2A is the target of the tumor suppressor gene located on the chromosome 11. Interestingly, the HPV-16 URR is activated in del-11 cells or by introduction of PR55 cDNA expression vector into diploid fibroblasts.[374,375]

Additional approaches to establishing the identity of the host gene mutations associated with neoplastic progression include the investigation of the status of endogenous tumor suppressor genes, the identification of chromosomal abnormalities, the effects of introducing individual known tumor suppressor genes or oncogene expression vectors, and localization of the host chromosomal sites at which the papillomaviral DNA has integrated. pRB and p53 are usually intact in HPV-containing cervical carcinomas or cell lines derived therefrom, because the viruses already have a means to inactivate those proteins. The incidence of p53 mutations is relatively low in HPV-negative cervical cancers, but mutations tends to be detected in more advanced cases and are proposed to be a factor in metastasis.[94,233,271] Viral integration sites in the host chromosomes generally appear to be random and stable, although integration near c-myc, N-myc, or known fragile sites has been reported in some cancers or cell lines derived therefrom. c-Ha-ras and c-myc genes are activated or amplified in some cases.[114,261,463] Conversely, the introduction of Ha-ras or v-fos genes can transform the immortalized human epithelial cells to become tumorigenic in nude mice.[116,124,307] Nonrandom chromosomal abnormalities and loss of heterozygosity in several loci on chromosomes 3p, 4q, 5p, 6p, 10p, 11q, and 18q have been noted in cervical carcinomas and in HPV-immortalized cell lines.[164,212,269,278,377,380,380a]

Extensive passage of HPV-immortalized PHKs or culturing under selective conditions can result in cells with altered growth properties. Treatment with carcinogens or irradiation can speed up the process.[114,143a,242] The DCC (deleted in colon cancer) gene was altered in an HPV-18–immortalized cell line transformed by mutagenesis, whereas the introduction of wild-type DCC cDNA could suppress the malignant phenotype.[210] In such models, the viral sequences are stably maintained and expressed during progression. To date, the key negative regulatory genes in the multistage carcinogenesis pathway remain subjects of intensive investigation.

In addition to host gene alterations, the possibility that other human pathogens can function as cocarcinogens has been examined. Before HPV was recognized to play the central role in cervical neoplasia, herpes simplex viruses (HSV) were regarded as the etiologic agent. The introduction of a particular HSV DNA fragment can transform HPV-immortalized PHKs.[115] Human herpesvirus 6 was shown to activate HPV-16 gene expression in immortalized cells, and coinfections have been demonstrated in vivo.[61] These and other cohabiting microbes may also contribute to the activation of HPV gene expression by causing localized immunosuppression or wounding-and-healing cycles.

SUMMARY

Great similarities in reproductive strategies and pathogenic mechanisms have emerged from intensive research on the small DNA tumor viruses: the adenoviruses, SV40, polyomavirus, and papillomaviruses. Generally, infections by these viruses in their native host species are nondisruptive, self-limiting, or even asymptomatic. Only in nonpermissive host species or under rare circumstances do these viruses exhibit their oncogenic properties. Each virus encodes one or more proteins that target the same host tumor suppressor proteins, p53 and pRB and its related proteins. These host proteins have been independently identified to be central regulators of cell proliferation, apoptosis, and chromosome stability, and their mutations or deletions are found in a large fraction of human cancers.

Of these viruses, the virus-host interactions are best understood for HPV, both in the native human host and in experimental laboratory systems. The viruses vegetatively replicate only in cells undergoing terminal differentiation. The purposes of the viral oncoproteins are to reactivate the host DNA replication machinery in these differentiated cells in order to facilitate viral DNA replication and perhaps also to abrogate premature apoptosis that arises as a host defense mechanism against unscheduled DNA replication (see Fig. 12-10, right side). From these host-viral protein interactions, it can be inferred that, if the viral oncogenes were accidentally upregulated in stem cells that are normally quiescent, the cells would enter into the cell cycle more frequently than intended. The more frequent DNA replication, coupled with impaired host surveillance caused by reduced p53 protein, could eventually result in accumulation of mutations in additional key host regulatory genes and selected progression toward carcinomas (see Fig. 12-10, left side). These processes can be exacerbated further by deficiencies in patient immune systems and by a variety of environmental risk factors. These mechanisms also explain the ability of the oncoproteins of the other DNA tumor viruses to transform cells in vitro and to cause tumors in newborn hamsters. On the grounds that there is no need to activate host DNA replication enzymes in cycling cells to support viral replication, it is probable that these viruses are also relatively quiescent in the undifferentiated stem or reserve cells and enter into the productive phase of infection in differentiated cells in their respective native host animals.

It remains to be investigated how the differences in the interactions between the high-risk and low-risk HPV oncoproteins and host target proteins are manifested as distinct biologic properties in vivo and in vitro. Unquestionably, the search for natural and synthetic compounds that can modulate viral replication and gene expression, host proliferative responses, differentiation, apoptosis, neoplastic changes, and immune surveillance will command increasing attention in the coming years as part of the search for effective prophylactic and therapeutic modulators of diseases associated with HPVs and the other small DNA viruses.

ABBREVIATIONS

AIDS: acquired immunodeficiency syndrome
ATF: activating transcription factor
BKV: a human polyomavirus
BPV, BPV-1, BPV-4: bovine papillomaviruses
CDK, CDK2, CDK4: cyclin-dependent kinases
CRI, CRII: conserved regions I and II (of adenovirus E1A proteins, also found in T antigen and E7)
CRPV: cottontail rabbit papillomavirus
E: early (region, protein)
E#, L# = the basic designations of the early and late regions, genes, or proteins of the DNA tumor viruses. As with all the viruses, the early proteins in one form or another persist at late times, usually in elevated amounts relative to their intracellular concentrations at early times. The delayed early or intermediate proteins and the late proteins can also be seen as differentiation-dependent proteins in vivo.
EGF: epidermal growth factor
EV: epidermodysplasia verruciformis

HIV: human immunodeficiency virus
HLA: human leukocyte antigen (e.g., HLA-DQw3)
HPV, HPV-1, HPV-2, etc.: human papillomavirus types
HSV: herpes simplex virus
JCV: a human polyomavirus
L: late (region, protein)
LTR: long terminal repeat
ORF: open reading frame
Pap: Papanicolaou (smear)
PCNA: proliferating cell nuclear antigen
PCR: polymerase chain reaction
PDGF: platelet-derived growth factor
PHKs: primary human keratinocytes
PR55: the 55-kD regulatory subunit of protein phosphatase-2A
pRB: retinoblastoma susceptibility protein
SCID: severe combined immunodeficient (mice)
SIL: squamous intraepithelial lesions
SV40: simian virus 40
TPA: 12-O-tetradecanoylphorbol-13-acetate
URR: upstream regulatory region
VLP: virus-like particles

ACKNOWLEDGMENTS

Research in the authors' laboratory was supported by USPHS grants CA36200 to LTC, AI34674 to TRB, and CA43629 to Mark H. Stoler, M.D., University of Virginia and by The Council for Tobacco Research—U.S.A. #2550RA to TRB. We thank our many students, fellows, collaborators, and colleagues for their research efforts and achievements and for sharing their information and ideas.

REFERENCES

1. Aiba S, Rokugo M, Tagami H. Immunohistologic analysis of the phenomenon of spontaneous regression of numerous flat warts. Cancer 1986;58:1246–1251.
2. Altmann A, Jochmus KI, Frank R, et al. Definition of immunogenic determinants of the human papillomavirus type 16 nucleoprotein E7. Eur J Cancer 1992;28:326–333.
3. Amella CA, Lofgren LA, Ronn AM, Nouri M, Shikowitz MJ, Steinberg BM. Latent infection induced with cottontail rabbit papillomavirus: a model for human papillomavirus latency. Am J Pathol 1994;144:1167–1171.
4. Anderson MJ, Stanbridge EJ. Tumor suppressor genes studied by cell hybridization and chromosome transfer. FASEB J 1993;7:826–833.
5. Arany Z, Newsome D, Oldread E, Livingston DM, Eckner R. A family of transcriptional adaptor proteins targeted by the E1A oncoprotein. Nature 1995;374:81–84.
6. Arbeit JM, Münger K, Howley PM, Hanahan D. Progressive squamous epithelial neoplasia in K14-human papillomavirus type 16 transgenic mice. J Virol 1994;68:4358–4368.
7. Asselineau D, Prunieras M. Reconstruction of ``simplified'' skin: control of fabrication. Br J Dermatol 1984;27:219–222.
8. Atencio IA, Villarreal LP. Polyomavirus replicates in differentiating but not in proliferating tubules of adult mouse polycystic kidneys. Virology 1994;201:26–35.
9. Auewarakul P, Gissmann L, Cid AA. Targeted expression of the E6 and E7 oncogenes of human papillomavirus type 16 in the epidermis of transgenic mice elicits generalized epidermal hyperplasia involving autocrine factors. Mol Cell Biol 1994;14:8250–8258.
10. Baker CC, Cowsert LM. The genomes of papillomaviruses. In: O'Brien SJ, ed. Genetic maps: locus maps of complex genomes. 5th ed. Cold Spring Harbor, New York: Cold Spring Harbor Laboratory Press, 1990;1.121–1.128.
11. Baker CC, Phelps WC, Lindgren V, Braun MJ, Gonda MA, Howley PM. Structural and transcriptional analysis of human papillomavirus type 16 sequences in cervical carcinoma cell lines. J Virol 1987;61:962–971.
12. Balaram P, Nalinakumari KR, Abraham E, et al. Human papillomaviruses in 91 oral cancers from Indian betel quid chewers—high prevalence and multiplicity of infections. Int J Cancer 1995;61:450–454.
13. Band V, Dalal S, Delmolino L, Androphy EJ. Enhanced degradation of p53 protein in HPV-6 and BPV-1 E6-immortalized human mammary epithelial cells. EMBO J 1993;12:1847–1852.
14. Band V, DeCaprio JA, Delmolino L, Kulesa V, Sager R. Loss of p53 protein in human papillomavirus type 16 E6-immortalized human mammary epithelial cells. J Virol 1991;65:6671–6676.
15. Banks L, Edmonds C, Vousden KH. Ability of the HPV16 E7 protein to bind RB and induce DNA synthesis is not sufficient for efficient transforming activity in NIH3T3 cells. Oncogene 1990;5:1383–1389.
16. Barbosa MS, Edmonds C, Fisher C, Schiller JT, Lowy DR, Vousden KH. The region of the HPV E7 oncoprotein homologous to adenovirus E1a and SV40 large T antigen contains separate domains for Rb binding and casein kinase II phosphorylation. EMBO J 1990;9:153–160.
17. Barbosa MS, Vass WC, Lowy DR, Schiller JT. In vitro biological activities of the E6 and E7 genes vary among human papillomaviruses of different oncogenic potential. J Virol 1991;65:292–298.
18. Bargonetti J, Reynisdottir I, Friedman PN, Prives C. Site-specific binding of wild-type p53 to cellular DNA is inhibited by SV40 T antigen and mutant p53. Genes Dev 1992;6:1886–1898.
19. Barksdale SK, Baker CC. Differentiation-specific expression from the bovine papillomavirus type 1 P2443 and late promoters. J Virol 1993;67:5605–5616.
20. Barnes W, Woodworth C, Waggoner S, et al. Rapid dysplastic transformation of human genital cells by human papillomavirus type 18. Gynecol Oncol 1990;38:343–346.
21. Barrandon Y, Green H. Three clonal types of keratinocyte with different capacities for multiplication. Proc Natl Acad Sci U S A 1987;84:2302–2306.
22. Bedell MA, Jones KH, Grossman SR, Laimins LA. Identification of human papillomavirus type 18 transforming genes in immortalized and primary cells. J Virol 1989;63:1247–1255.
23. Bedell MA, Jones KH, Laimins LA. The E6-E7 region of human papillomavirus type 18 is sufficient for transformation of NIH 3T3 and rat-1 cells. J Virol 1987;61:3635–3640.
24. Bell E, Sher S, Hull B, et al. The reconstitution of living skin. J Invest Dermatol 1983;81:2s–10s.
25. Bell JA, Sundberg JP, Ghim SJ, Newsome J, Jenson AB, Schlegel R. A formalin-inactivated vaccine protects against mucosal papillomavirus infection: a canine model. Pathobiology 1994;62:194–198.
26. Berkhout RJ, Tieben LM, Smits HL, Bouwes Bavinck JN, Vermeer BJ, ter Schegget J. Nested PCR approach for detection and typing of epidermodysplasia verruciformis—associated human papillomavirus types in cutaneous cancers from renal transplant recipients. J Clin Microbiol 1995;33:690–695.
27. Bernard HU, Chan SY, Manos MM, et al. Identification and assessment of known and novel human papillomaviruses by polymerase chain reaction amplification, restriction fragment length polymorphisms, nucleotide sequence, and phylogenetic algorithms. J Infect Dis 1994;170:1077–1085.
28. Beyer-Finkler E, Stoler MH, Girardi F, Pfister H. Cell differentiation-related gene expression of human papillomavirus 33. Med Microbiol Immunol 1990;179:185–192.
29. Black PH, Hartley JW, Rowe WP, Huebner RJ. Transformation of bovine tissue culture cells by bovine papilloma virus. Nature 1963;99:1016–1018.
30. Blanton RA, Coltrera MD, Gown AM, Halbert CL, McDougall JK. Expression of the HPV16 E7 gene generates proliferation in stratified squamous cell cultures which is independent of endogenous p53 levels. Cell Growth Diff 1992;3:791–802.
31. Blanton RA, Perez RN, Merrick DT, McDougall JK. Epithelial cells immortalized by human papillomaviruses have premalignant characteristics in organotypic culture. Am J Pathol 1991;138:673–685.

32. Bonne-Andrea C, Santucci S, Clertant P. Bovine papillomavirus E1 protein can, by itself, efficiently drive multiple rounds of DNA synthesis in vitro. J Virol 1995;69:3201–3205.

33. Bonnez W, Oakes D, Bailey FA, et al. A randomized, double-blind, placebo-controlled trial of systemically administered interferon-alpha, -beta, or -gamma in combination with cryotherapy for the treatment of condyloma acuminatum. J Infect Dis 1995;171:1081–1099.

34. Bonnez W, Rose RC, Da Rin C, Borkhuis C, de Mesy Jensen KL, Reichman RC. Propagation of human papillomavirus type 11 in human xenografts using the severe combined immunodeficiency (SCID) mouse and comparison to the nude mouse model. Virology 1993;197:455–458.

35. Bosch FX, Schwarz E, Boukamp P, Fusenig NE, Bartsch D, zur Hausen H. Suppression in vivo of human papillomavirus type 18 E6-E7 gene expression in nontumorigenic HeLa X fibroblast hybrid cells. J Virol 1990;64:4743–4754.

36. Bouvard V, Matlashewski G, Gu ZM, Storey A, Banks L. The human papillomavirus type 16 E5 gene cooperates with the E7 gene to stimulate proliferation of primary cells and increases viral gene expression. Virology 1994;203:73–80.

37. Bouvard V, Storey A, Pim D, Banks L. Characterization of the human papillomavirus E2 protein: evidence of trans-activation and trans-repression in cervical keratinocytes. EMBO J 1994;13: 5451– 5459.

38. Bouwes Bavinck JN, Gissmann L, Claas FH, et al. Relation between skin cancer, humoral responses to human papillomaviruses, and HLA class II molecules in renal transplant recipients. J Immunol 1993;151:1579–1586.

39. Boyd JM, Malstrom S, Subramanian T, et al. Adenovirus E1B 19 kDa and Bcl-2 proteins interact with a common set of cellular proteins. Cell 1994;79:341–351.

40. Brandsma JL. Animal models of human-papillomavirus–associated oncogenesis. Intervirology 1994;37:189–200.

41. Brandsma JL, Brownstein DG, Xiao W, Longley BJ. Papilloma formation in human foreskin xenografts after inoculation of human papillomavirus type 16 DNA. J Virol 1995;69:2716–2721.

42. Bream GL, Ohmstede CA, Phelps WC. Characterization of human papillomavirus type 11 E1 and E2 proteins expressed in insect cells. J Virol 1993;67:2655–2663.

43. Breitburd F, Kirnbauer R, Hubbert NL, et al. Immunization with viruslike particles from cottontail rabbit papillomavirus CRPV) can protect against experimental CRPV infection. J Virol 1995;69: 3959–3963.

44. Brizuela L, Olcese LM, Courtneidge SA. Transformation by middle T antigens. Semin Virol 1994;5:381–390.

45. Brokaw JL, Yee CL, Münger K. A mutational analysis of the amino terminal domain of the human papillomavirus type 16 E7 oncoprotein. Virology 1994;205:603–607.

46. Broker TR. Animal virus RNA processing. In: Apirion D. Processing of RNA. Boca Raton, Florida: CRC Press, 1984:181—212.

46a. Broker TR, Botchan M. Papillomaviruses: retrospectives and prospectives. Cancer Cells 1986;4:17–31.

47. Broker TR, Chow LT, Chin MT, et al. A molecular portrait of human papillomavirus carcinogenesis. Cancer Cells 1989;7:197–208.

48. Brune W, Dürst M. Epithelial differentiation fails to support replication of cloned human papillomavirus type 16 DNA in transfected keratinocytes. J Invest Dermatol 1995;104:277–281.

49. Burnett S, Jareborg N, DiMaio D. Localization of bovine papillomavirus type 1 E5 protein to transformed basal keratinocytes and permissive differentiated cells in fibropapilloma tissue. Proc Natl Acad Sci U S A 1992;89:5665–5669.

50. Butel JS. Studies with human papilloma virus modeled after known papovavirus systems. J Natl Cancer Inst 1972;48:285–299.

51. Campo MS, O'Neil BW, Barron RJ, Jarrett WF. Experimental reproduction of the papilloma-carcinoma complex of the alimentary canal in cattle. Carcinogenesis 1994;15:1597–1601.

52. Carlotti F, Crawford L. Trans-activation of the adenovirus E2 promoter by human papillomavirus type 16 E7 is mediated by retinoblastoma-dependent and -independent pathways. J Gen Virol 1993; 74:2479–2486.

53. Chan SY, Delius H, Halpern AL, Bernard HU. Analysis of genomic sequences of 95 papillomavirus types: uniting typing, phylogeny, and taxonomy. J Virol 1995;69:3074–3083.

54. Chandrachud LM, Grindlay GJ, McGarvie GM, et al. Vaccination of cattle with the N-terminus of L2 is necessary and sufficient for preventing infection by bovine papillomavirus-4. Virology 1995;211: 204–208.

55. Chang KW, Chang CS, Lai KS, Chou MJ, Choo KB. High prevalence of human papillomavirus infection and possible association with betel quid chewing and smoking in oral epidermoid carcinomas in Taiwan. J Med Virol 1989;28:57–61.

56. Chellappan S, Kraus VB, Kroger B, et al. Adenovirus E1A, simian virus 40 tumor antigen, and human papillomavirus E7 protein share the capacity to disrupt the interaction between transcription factor E2F and the retinoblastoma gene product. Proc Natl Acad Sci U S A 1992;89:4549–4553.

57. Chen J, Jackson PK, Kirschner MW, Dutta A. Separate domains of p21 involved in the inhibition of Cdk kinase and PCNA. Nature 1995;374:386–388.

58. Chen JJ, Reid CE, Band V, Androphy EJ. Interaction of papillomavirus E6 oncoproteins with a putative calcium-binding protein. Science 1995;269:529–531.

59. Chen L, Mizuno MT, Singhal MC, Induction of cytotoxic T lymphocytes specific for a syngeneic tumor expressing the E6 oncoprotein of human papillomavirus type 16. J Immunol 1992;148:2617–2621.

60. Chen LP, Thomas EK, Hu SL, Hellstrom I, Hellstrom KE. Human papillomavirus type 16 nucleoprotein E7 is a tumor rejection antigen. Proc Natl Acad Sci U S A 1991;88:110–114.

61. Chen M, Popescu N, Woodworth C, et al. Human herpesvirus 6 infects cervical epithelial cells and transactivates human papillomavirus gene expression. J Virol 1994;68:1173–1178.

62. Chen SL, Mounts P. Transforming activity of E5a protein of human papillomavirus type 6 in NIH 3T3 and C127 cells. J Virol 1990; 64:3226–3233.

63. Chen TM, Chen CA, Hsieh CY, Chang DY, Chen YH, Defendi V. The state of p53 in primary human cervical carcinomas and its effects in human papillomavirus–immortalized human cervical cells. Oncogene 1993;8:1511–1518.

64. Chen TM, Pecoraro G, Defendi V. Genetic analysis of in vitro progression of human papillomavirus–transfected human cervical cells. Cancer Res 1993;53:1167–1171.

65. Cheng S, Schmidt-Grimminger DC, Murant T, Broker TR, Chow LT. Differentiation-dependent up-regulation of the human papillomavirus E7 gene reactivates cellular DNA replication in suprabasal differentiated keratinocytes. Genes Dev 1995;9:2335–2349.

66. Chiang CM, Broker TR, Chow LT. An E1M^E2C fusion protein encoded by human papillomavirus type 11 is a sequence-specific transcription repressor. J Virol 1991;65:3317–3329.

67. Chiang C-M, Dong G, Broker TR, Chow LT. Control of human papillomavirus type 11 origin replication by the E2 family of transcriptional regulatory proteins. J Virol 1992;66:5224–5231.

68. Chiang CM, Ustav M, Stenlund A, Ho TF, Broker TR, Chow LT. Viral E1 and E2 proteins support replication of homologous and heterologous papillomaviral origins. Proc Natl Acad Sci U S A 1992; 89:5799–5803.

69. Chin MT, Broker TR, Chow LT. Identification of a novel constitutive enhancer element and an associated binding protein: implications for human papillomavirus type 11 enhancer regulation. J Virol 1989;63:2967–2976.

70. Chin MT, Hirochika R, Hirochika H, Broker TR, Chow LT. Regulation of human papillomavirus type 11 enhancer and E6 promoter by activating and repressing proteins from the E2 open reading frame: functional and biochemical studies. J Virol 1988;62:2994–3002.

71. Chow LT, Broker TR. The spliced structures of adenovirus-2 fiber message and the other late mRNAs. Cell 1978;15:497–510.

72. Chow LT, Broker TR. Papillomavirus DNA replication. Intervirology 1994;37:150–158.

73. Chow, LT, Broker TR, Lewis JB. Complex splicing patterns of RNA from the early regions of adenovirus-2. J Mol Biol 1979;134: 265–304.

73a. Chow LT, Hirochika H, Nasseri M, et al. Human papillomavirus gene expression. Cancer Cells 1987;5:55–72.

74. Chow LT, Nasseri M, Wolinsky SM, Broker TR. Human papillomavirus types 6 and 11 mRNAs from genital condylomata acuminata. J Virol 1987;61:2581–2588.

75. Chow LT, Reilly SS, Broker TR, Taichman LB. Identification and mapping of human papillomavirus type 1 RNA transcripts recovered from plantar warts and infected epithelial cell cultures. J Virol 1987; 61:1913–1918.

76. Christensen ND, Hopfl R, DiAngelo SL, et al. Assembled baculovirus-expressed human papillomavirus type 11 L1 capsid protein virus-like particles are recognized by neutralizing monoclonal antibodies and induce high titres of neutralizing antibodies. J Gen Virol 1994;75:2271–2276.

77. Christensen ND, Kreider JW. Monoclonal antibody neutralization of BPV-1. Virus Res 1993;28:195–202.

78. Christensen ND, Kreider JW, Kan NC, DiAngelo SX. The open reading frame L2 of cottontail rabbit papillomavirus contains antibody-inducing neutralizing epitopes. Virology 1991;181:572–579.

79. Christensen ND, Kreider JW, Shah KV, Rando RF. Detection of human serum antibodies that neutralize infectious human papillomavirus type 11 virions. J Gen Virol 1992;73:1261–1267.

80. Ciccolini F, Di PG, Carlotti F, Crawford L, Tommasino M. Functional studies of E7 proteins from different HPV types. Oncogene 1994;9:2633–2638.

81. Cohen BD, Lowy DR, Schiller JT. The conserved C-terminal domain of the bovine papillomavirus E5 oncoprotein can associate with an alpha-adaptin–like molecule: a possible link between growth factor receptors and viral transformation. Mol Cell Biol 1993;13:6462–6468.

82. Cole, CN. Polyomavirinae: the viruses and their replication. In: Fields BN, Knipe DM, Howley PM, eds. Fields virology, 3rd ed. Philadelphia: Raven, 1996:1997–2026.

83. Coleman N, Birley HD, Renton AM, et al. Immunological events in regressing genital warts. Am J Clin Pathol 1994;102:768–774.

84. Conzen SD, Cole CN. The transforming proteins of simian virus 40. Semin Virol 1994;5:349–356.

85. Cooper KD, Androphy EJ, Lowy D, Katz SI. Antigen presentation and T-cell activation in epidermodysplasia verruciformis. J Invest Dermatol 1990;94:769–776.

86. Conrad M, Bubb VJ, Schlegel R. The human papillomavirus type 6 and 16 E5 proteins are membrane-associated proteins which associate with the 16-kilodalton pore-forming protein. J Virol 1993;67:6170–6178.

87. Conrad M, Goldstein D, Andresson T, Schlegel R. The E5 protein of HPV-6, but not HPV-16, associates efficiently with cellular growth factor receptors. Virology 1994;200:796–800.

88. Creek KE, Jenkins GR, Khan MA, et al. Retinoic acid suppresses human papillomavirus type 16 (HPV16)–mediated transformation of human keratinocytes and inhibits the expression of the HPV16 oncogenes. Adv Exp Med Biol 1994;354:19–35.

89. Crook T, Almond N, Murray A, Stanley M, Crawford L. Constitutive expression of c-myc oncogene confers hormone independence and enhanced growth-factor responsiveness on cells transformed by human papilloma virus type 16. Proc Natl Acad Sci U S A 1989;86:5713–5717.

90. Crook T, Fisher C, Masterson PJ, Vousden KH. Modulation of transcriptional regulatory properties of p53 by HPV E6. Oncogene 1994;9:1225–1230.

91. Crook T, Morgenstern JP, Crawford L, Banks L. Continued expression of HPV-16 E7 protein is required for maintenance of the transformed phenotype of cells co-transformed by HPV-16 plus EJ-ras. EMBO J 1989;8:513–519.

92. Crook T, Storey A, Almond N, Osborn K, Crawford L. Human papillomavirus type 16 cooperates with activated ras and fos oncogenes in the hormone-dependent transformation of primary mouse cells. Proc Natl Acad Sci U S A 1988;85:8820–8824.

93. Crook T, Tidy JA, Vousden KH. Degradation of p53 can be targeted by HPV E6 sequences distinct from those required for p53 binding and trans-activation. Cell 1991;67:547–556.

94. Crook T, Vousden KH. Properties of p53 mutations detected in primary and secondary cervical cancers suggest mechanisms of metastasis and involvement of environmental carcinogens. EMBO J 1992;11:3935–3940.

95. Crum CP, Nuovo G, Friedman D, Silverstein SJ. Accumulation of RNA homologous to human papillomavirus type 16 open reading frames in genital precancers. J Virol 1988;62:84–90.

96. Crum CP, Symbula M, Ward BE. Topography of early HPV 16 transcription in high-grade genital precancers. Am J Pathol 1989; 134:1183–1188.

97. Davies R, Hicks R, Crook T, Morris J, Vousden K. Human papillomavirus type 16 E7 associates with a histone H1 kinase and with p107 through sequences necessary for transformation. J Virol 1993;67:2521–2528.

98. Davies RC, Vousden KH. Functional analysis of human papillomavirus type 16 E7 by complementation with adenovirus E1A mutants. J Gen Virol 1992;73:2135–2139.

99. DeGeest K, Turyk ME, Hosken MI, Hudson JB, Laimins LA, Wilbanks GD. Growth and differentiation of human papillomavirus type 31b positive human cervical cell lines. Gynecol Oncol 1993;49:303–310.

100. DeGregori J, Kowalik T, Nevins JR. Cellular targets for activation by the E2F1 transcription factor include DNA synthesis- and G1/S-regulatory genes. Mol Cell Biol 1995;15:4215–4224.

101. de Jong Tieben LM, Berkhout RJ, Smits HL, et al. High frequency of detection of epidermodysplasia verruciformis–associated human papillomavirus DNA in biopsies from malignant and premalignant skin lesions from renal transplant recipients. J Invest Dermatol 1995;105:367–371.

102. Del Vecchio A, Romanczuk H, Howley PM, Baker CC. Transient replication of human papillomavirus DNAs. J Virol 1992;66:5949–5958.

103. Demers GW, Foster SA, Halbert CL, Galloway DA. Growth arrest by induction of p53 in DNA damaged keratinocytes is bypassed by human papillomavirus 16 E7. Proc Natl Acad Sci U S A 1994;91:4382–4386.

104. Demers GW, Halbert CL, Galloway DA. Elevated wild-type p53 protein levels in human epithelial cell lines immortalized by the human papillomavirus type 16 E7 gene. Virology 1994;198:169–174.

105. Demeter LM, Stoler MH, Broker TR, Chow LT. Induction of proliferating cell nuclear antigen in differentiated keratinocytes of human papillomavirus–infected lesions. Human Pathol 1994;25:343–348.

105a. Demeter LM, Stoler MH, Sobel ME, Broker TR, Chow LT. Expression of high affinity laminin receptor mRNA correlates with cell proliferation rather than invasion in human papillomavirus-associated genital neoplasms. Cancer Res 1992;52:1561–1567.

106. Derkay CS. Task force on recurrent respiratory papillomas. Arch Otolaryngol Head Neck Surg 1995;121:1386–1391.

107. de Ronde A, Mannens M, Slater RM, et al. Morphological transformation by early region human polyomavirus BK DNA of human fibroblasts with deletions in the short arm of one chromosome 11. J Gen Virol 1988;69:467–471.

108. de Ronde A, Sol CJA, van Strien A, ter Schegget J, van der Noordaa J. The SV40 small t antigen is essential for the morphological transformation of human fibroblasts. Virology 1989;171:260–263.

109. Desaintes C, Hallez S, Van AP, Burny A. Transcriptional activation of several heterologous promoters by the E6 protein of human papillomavirus type 16. J Virol 1992;66:325–333.

110. de Villiers EM. Human pathogenic papillomaviruses: an update. Curr Top Microbiol Immunol 1994;186:1–12.

111. Dillner J, Wiklund F, Lenner P, et al. Antibodies against linear and conformational epitopes of human papillomavirus type 16 that independently associate with incident cervical cancer. Int J Cancer 1995;60:377–382.

112. DiLorenzo TP, Steinberg BM. Differential regulation of human papillomavirus type 6 and 11 early promoters in cultured cells derived from laryngeal papillomas. J Virol 1995;69:6865–6872.

113. DiMaio D, Petti L, Hwang ES. The E5 transforming proteins of the papillomaviruses. Semin Virol 1994;5:369–380.

114. DiPaolo JA, Popescu NC, Alvarez L, Woodworth CD. Cellular and molecular alterations in human epithelial cells transformed by recombinant human papillomavirus DNA. Crit Rev Oncog 1993;4:337–360.

115. DiPaolo JA, Woodworth CD, Popescu NC, Koval DL, Lopez JV, Doniger J. HSV-2–induced tumorigenicity in HPV16-immortalized human genital keratinocytes. Virology 1990;177:777–779.

116. DiPaolo JA, Woodworth CD, Popescu NC, Notario V, Doniger J. Induction of human cervical squamous cell carcinoma by sequential transfection with human papillomavirus 16 DNA and viral Harvey ras. Oncogene 1989;4:395–399.

117. Dollard SC, Broker TR, Chow LT. Regulation of the human papillomavirus type 11 E6 promoter by viral and host transcription factors in primary human keratinocytes. J Virol 1993;67:1721–1726.

118. Dollard SC, Wilson JL, Demeter LM, et al. Production of human papillomavirus and modulation of the infectious program in epithelial raft cultures. Genes Dev 1992;6:1131–1142.

119. Dong G, Broker TR, Chow LT. Human papillomavirus type 11 E2 proteins repress the homologous E6 promoter by interfering with the

binding of host transcription factors to adjacent elements. J Virol 1994;68:1115–1127.

120. Doorbar J, Parton A, Hartley K, et al. Detection of novel splicing patterns in a HPV16-containing keratinocyte cell line. Virology 1990;178:254–262.

121. Dowhanick JJ, McBride AA, Howley PM. Suppression of cellular proliferation by the papillomavirus E2 protein. J Virol 1995;69: 7791–7799.

122. Drummond BD, Vaillancourt RR, Kazlauskas A, DiMaio D. Ligand-independent activation of the platelet-derived growth factor beta receptor: requirements for bovine papillomavirus E5-induced mitogenic signaling. Mol Cell Biol 1995;15:2570–2581.

123. Dürst M, Bosch FX, Glitz D, Schneider A, zur Hausen H. Inverse relationship between human papillomavirus (HPV) type 16 early gene expression and cell differentiation in nude mouse epithelial cysts and tumors induced by HPV-positive human cell lines. J Virol 1991;65:796–804.

124. Dürst M, Gallahan D, Jay G, Rhim JS. Glucocorticoid-enhanced neoplastic transformation of human keratinocytes by human papillomavirus type 16 and an activated ras oncogene. Virology 1989; 173:767–771.

125. Dürst M, Glitz D, Schneider A, zur Hausen H. Human papillomavirus type 16 (HPV 16) gene expression and DNA replication in cervical neoplasia: analysis by in situ hybridization. Virology 1992; 189:132–140.

126. Dvoretzky I, Shober R, Chattopadhyay SK, Lowy DR. A quantitative in vitro focus assay for bovine papilloma virus. Virology 1980;103:369–375.

127. Dyson N, Guida P, Münger K, Harlow E. Homologous sequences in adenovirus E1A and human papillomavirus E7 proteins mediate interaction with the same set of cellular proteins. J Virol 1992;66: 6893–6902.

128. Dyson N, Howley PM, Münger K, Harlow E. The human papilloma virus-16 E7 oncoprotein is able to bind to the retinoblastoma gene product. Science 1989;243:934–937.

129. Edmonds C, Vousden KH. A point mutational analysis of human papillomavirus type 16 E7 protein. J Virol 1989;63:2650–2656.

130. Fanning E, Knippers R. Structure and function of simian virus 40 large tumor antigen. Annu Rev Biochem 1992;61:55–85.

131. Feltkamp MCW, Smits HL, Vierboom MPM, et al. Vaccination with cytotoxic T lymphocyte epitope–containing peptide protects against a tumour induced by human papillomavirus type 16–transformed cells. Eur J Immunol 1993;23:2242–2249.

132. Ferenczy A, Mitao M, Nagai N, Silverstein SJ, Crum CP. Latent papillomavirus and recurring genital warts. N Engl J Med 1985;313: 784–788.

133. Firzlaff, JM, Lüscher B, Eisenman RN. Negative charge at the casein kinase II phosphorylation site is important for transformation but not for RB protein binding by the E7 protein of human papillomavirus type 16. Proc Natl Acad Sci U S A 1991;88:5187–5191.

134. Flores-Rozas H, Kelman Z, Dean FB, et al. Cdk-interacting protein 1 directly binds with proliferating cell nuclear antigen and inhibits DNA replication catalyzed by the DNA polymerase delta holoenzyme. Proc Natl Acad Sci U S A 1994;91:8655–8659.

135. Foster SA, Demers GW, Etscheid BG, Galloway DA. The ability of human papillomavirus E6 proteins to target p53 for degradation in vivo correlates with their ability to abrogate actinomycin D–induced growth arrest. J Virol 1994;68:5698–5705.

136. Frattini MG, Laimins LA. The role of the E1 and E2 proteins in the replication of human papillomavirus type 31b. Virology 1994; 204:799–804.

137. Frattini MG, Lim HB, Laimins LA. In vitro synthesis of oncogeneic human papillomaviruses requires episomal genomes for differentiation-dependent late expression. Proc Natl Acad Sci U S A 1996;93: 3062–3067.

138. Fromm L, Shawlot W, Gunning K, Butel JS, Overbeek PA. The retinoblastoma protein–binding region of simian virus 40 large T antigen alters cell cycle regulation in 20 lenses of transgenic mice. Mol Cell Biol 1994;14:6743–6754.

139. Fu YS, Reagan JW, Townsend DE, Kaufman RH, Richart RM, Wentz WB. Nuclear DNA study of vulvar intraepithelial and invasive squamous neoplasms. Obstet Gynecol 1981;57:643–652.

140. Fuchs E. Epidermal differentiation. Curr Opin Cell Biol 1990;2: 1028–1035.

141. Fujii T, Crum CP, Winkler B, Fu YS, Richart RM. Human papillomavirus infection and cervical intraepithelial neoplasia: histopathology and DNA content. Obstet Gynecol 1984;63:99–104.

142. Gage JR, Meyers C, Wettstein FO. The E7 proteins of the nononcogenic human papillomavirus type 6b (HPV-6b) and of oncogenic HPV-16 differ in retinoblastoma protein binding and other properties. J Virol 1990;64:723–730.

143. Galloway DA. Human papillomavirus vaccines: a warty problem. Infect Agents Dis 1994;3:187–193.

143a. Garrett LR, Perez RN, Smith PP, McDougall JK. Interaction of HPV-18 and nitrosomethylurea in the induction of squamous cell carcinoma. Carcinogenesis 1993;14:329–332.

144. Gassenmaier A, Fuchs P, Schell H, Pfister H. Papillomavirus DNA in warts of immunosuppressed renal allograft recipients. Arch Dermatol Res 1986;278:219–223.

145. Ghim S, Christensen ND, Kreider JW, Jenson AB. Comparison of neutralization of BPV-1 infection of C127 cells and bovine fetal skin xenografts. Int J Cancer 1991;49:285–289.

146. Ginsberg HS, Prince GA. The molecular basis of adenovirus pathogenesis. Infect Agents Dis 1994;3:1–8.

147. Gius D, Grossman S, Bedell MA, Laimins LA. Inducible and constitutive enhancer domains in the noncoding region of human papillomavirus type 18. J Virol 1988;62:665–672.

148. Glinski W, Obalek S, Jablonska S, Orth G. T cell defect in patients with epidermodysplasia verruciformis due to human papillomavirus type 3 and 5. Dermatologica 1981;162:141–147.

149. Gloss B, Bernard HU, Seedorf K, Klock G. The upstream regulatory region of the human papilloma virus-16 contains an E2 protein–independent enhancer which is specific for cervical carcinoma cells and regulated by glucocorticoid hormones. EMBO J 1987;6:3735–3743.

150. Goldstein DJ, Andresson T, Sparkowski JJ, Schlegel R. The BPV-1 E5 protein, the 16 kDa membrane pore-forming protein and the PDGF receptor exist in a complex that is dependent on hydrophobic transmembrane interactions. EMBO J 1992;11:4851–4859.

151. Goldstein DJ, Li W, Wang LM, et al. The bovine papillomavirus type 1 E5 transforming protein specifically binds and activates the beta-type receptor for the platelet-derived growth factor but not other related tyrosine kinase-containing receptors to induce cellular transformation. J Virol 1994;68:4432–4441.

152. Gopalakrishnan V, Khan SA. E1 protein of human papillomavirus type 1a is sufficient for initiation of viral DNA replication. Proc Natl Acad Sci U S A 1994;91:9597–9601.

153. Greenhalgh DA, Wang XJ, Rothnagel JA, et al. Transgenic mice expressing targeted HPV-18 E6 and E7 oncogenes in the epidermis develop verrucous lesions and spontaneous, ras-Ha–activated papillomas. Cell Growth Differ 1994;5:667–675.

154. Griep AE, Herber R, Jeon S, Lohse JK, Dubielzig RR, Lambert PF. Tumorigenicity by human papillomavirus type 16 E6 and E7 in transgenic mice correlates with alterations in epithelial cell growth and differentiation. J Virol 1993;67:1373–1384.

155. Griep AE, Kuwabara T, Lee EJ, Westphal H. Perturbed development of the mouse lens by polyomavirus large T antigen does not lead to tumor formation. Genes Dev 1989;3:1075–1085.

156. Griep AE, Lambert PF. Role of papillomavirus oncogenes in human cervical cancer: transgenic animal studies. Proc Soc Exp Biol Med 1994;206:24–34.

157. Grodzicker T, Hopkins N. Origins of contemporary DNA tumor virus research. In: Tooze J. DNA tumor viruses: molecular biology of the tumor viruses. 2nd ed. Cold Spring Harbor, New York: Cold Spring Harbor Laboratory Press, 1981:1–59.

158. Gu Z, Pim D, Labrecque S, Banks L, Matlashewski G. DNA damage induced p53 mediated transcription is inhibited by human papillomavirus type 18 E6. Oncogene 1994;9:629–633.

159. Hagensee ME, Yaegashi N, Galloway DA. Self-assembly of human papillomavirus type 1 capsids by expression of the L1 protein alone or by coexpression of the L1 and L2 capsid proteins. J Virol 1993;67:315–322.

160. Halbert CL, Demers GW, Galloway DA. The E7 gene of human papillomavirus type 16 is sufficient for immortalization of human epithelial cells. J Virol 1991;65:473–478.

161. Halbert CL, Demers GW, Galloway DA. The E6 and E7 genes of human papillomavirus type 6 have weak immortalizing activity in human epithelial cells. J Virol 1992;66:2125–2134.

162. Halprin KM. Epidermal ``turnover time''—a re-examination. Br J Dermatol 1972;86:14–19.

163. Ham J, Dostatni N, Gauthier JM, Yaniv M. The papillomavirus E2 protein: a factor with many talents. Trends Biochem Sci 1991;16: 440–444.

164. Hampton GM, Penny LA, Baergen RN, et al. Loss of heterozygosity in cervical carcinoma: subchromosomal localization of a putative tumor suppressor gene to chromosome 11q22-q24. Proc Natl Acad Sci U S A 1994;91:6953–2955.

165. Han R, Breitburd F, Marche PN, Orth G. Linkage of regression and malignant conversion of rabbit viral papillomas to MHC class II genes. Nature 1992;356:66–68.

166. Harper JW, Adami GR, Wei N, Keyomarsi K, Elledge SJ. The p21 Cdk-interacting protein Cip1 is a potent inhibitor of G1 cyclin-dependent kinases. Cell 1993;75:805–816.

167. Hawley Nelson P, Vousden KH, Hubbert NJ, Lowy DR, Schiller JT. HPV16 E6 and E7 proteins cooperate to immortalize human foreskin keratinocytes. EMBO J 1989;8:3905–3910.

168. Heck DV, Yee CL, Howley PM, Münger K. Efficiency of binding the retinoblastoma protein correlates with the transforming capacity of the E7 oncoproteins of the human papillomaviruses. Proc Natl Acad Sci U S A 1992;89:4442–4446.

169. Hickman ES, Picksley SM, Vousden KH. Cells expressing HPV16 E7 continue cell cycle progression following DNA damage induced p53 activation. Oncogene 1994;9:2177–2181.

170. Hierholzer JC. Adenoviruses in the immunocompromised host. Clin Microbiol Rev 1992;5:262–274.

171. Higgins GD, Uzelin DM, Phillips GE, Burrell CJ. Presence and distribution of human papillomavirus sense and antisense RNA transcripts in genital cancers. J Gen Virol 1991;72:885–895.

172. Higgins GD, Uzelin DM, Phillips GE, McEvoy P, Marin R, Burrell CJ. Transcription patterns of human papillomavirus type 16 in genital intraepithelial neoplasia: evidence for promoter usage within the E7 open reading frame during epithelial differentiation. J Gen Virol 1992;73:2047–2057.

173. Ho GY, Burk RD, Fleming I, Klein RS. Risk of genital human papillomavirus infection in women with human immunodificiency virus–induced immunosuppression. Int J Cancer 1994;56:788–792.

174. Hollstein M, Rice K, Greenblatt MS, et al. Database of p53 gene somatic mutations in human tumors and cell lines. Nucleic Acids Res 1994;22:3551–3555.

175. Holt SE, van Wilson G. Mutational analysis of the 18-base-pair inverted repeat element at the bovine papillomavirus origin of replication: identification of critical sequences for E1 binding and in vivo replication. J Virol 1995;69:6525–6532.

176. Horwitz MS. Adenoviruses. In: Fields BN, Knipe DM, Howley PM, eds. Fields virology. 3rd ed. Philadelphia: Raven, 1996:2149–2172.

177. Howes KA, Ransom N, Papermaster DS, Lasudry JGH, Albert DM, Windel JJ. Apoptosis or retinoblastoma: fates of photoreceptors expressing the HPV-16 E7 gene in the presence or absence of p53. Genes Dev 1994;8:1300–1310.

178. Howett MK, Kreider JW, Cockley KD. Human xenografts: a model system for human papillomvirus infection. Intervirology 1990;31: 109–115.

179. Howley PM. Tumor progression in transgenic mice containing the bovine papillomavirus genome. Basic Life Sci 1991;57:103–107.

180. Howley PM. Papillomavirinae: the viruses and their replication. In: Fields BN, Knipe DM, Howley PM, eds. Fields virology. 3rd ed. Philadelphia: Raven, 1996:2045–2076.

181. Huang PS, Patrick DR, Edwards G, et al. Protein domains governing interactions between E2F, the retinoblastoma gene product, and human papillomavirus type 16 E7 protein. Mol Cell Biol 1993; 13:953–960.

182. Hudson JB, Bedell MA, McCance DJ, Laimins LA. Immortalization and altered differentiation of human keratinocytes in vitro by the E6 and E7 open reading frames of human papillomavirus type 18. J Virol 1990;64:519–526.

183. Hughes FJ, Romanos MA. E1 protein of human papillomavirus is a DNA helicase/ATPase. Nucl Acids Res 1993;21:5817–5823.

184. Hummel M, Hudson JB, Laimins LA. Differentiation-induced and constitutive transcription of human papillomavirus type 31b in cell lines containing viral episomes. J Virol 1992;66:6070–6080.

185. Hummel M, Lim HB, Laimins LA. Human papillomavirus type 31b late gene expression is regulated through protein kinase C–mediated changes in RNA processing. J Virol 1995;69:3381–3388.

186. Hurlin PJ, Kaur P, Smith PP, Perez RN, Blanton RA, McDougall JK. Progression of human papillomavirus type 18–immortalized human keratinocytes to a malignant phenotype. Proc Natl Acad Sci U S A 1991;88:570–574.

187. Hwang ES, Nottoli T, DiMaio D. The HPV16 E5 protein: expression, detection, and stable complex formation with transmembrane proteins in COS cells. Virology 1995;211:227–233.

188. Hwang ES, Riese Dd, Settleman J, et al. Inhibition of cervical carcinoma cell line proliferation by the introduction of a bovine papillomavirus regulatory gene. J Virol 1993;67:3720–3729.

189. Iftner T, Bierfelder S, Csapo Z, Pfister H. Involvement of human papillomavirus type 8 genes E6 and E7 in transformation and replication. J Virol 1988;62:3655–3661.

190. Iftner T, Sagner G, Pfister H, Wettstein FO. The E7 protein of human papillomavirus 8 is a nonphosphorylated protein of 17 kDa and can be generated by two different mechanisms. Virology 1990;179: 428–436.

191. Inagaki Y, Tsunokowa Y, Takebe N, et al. Nucleotide sequences of cDNAs for human papillomavirus type 18 transcripts in HeLa cells. J Virol 1988;62:1640–1646.

192. Ishiwatari H, Hayasaka N, Inoue H, Yutsudo M, Hakura A. Degradation of p53 only is not sufficient for the growth stimulatory effect of human papillomavirus 16 E6 oncoprotein in human embryonic fibroblasts. J Med Virol 1994;44:243–249.

193. Jablonska S, Orth G, Jarzabek CM, et al. Twenty-one years of follow-up studies of familial epidermodysplasia verruciformis. Dermatologica 1979;158:309–327.

194. Jeon S, Lambert PF. Integration of human papillomavirus type 16 DNA into the human genome leads to increased stability of E6 and E7 mRNAs: implications for cervical carcinogenesis. Proc Natl Acad Sci U S A 1995;92:1654–1658.

195. Johnson JC, Burnett AF, Willet GD, Young MA, Doniger J. High frequency of latent and clinical human papillomavirus cervical infections in immunocompromised human immunodeficiency virus-infected women. Obstet Gynecol 1992;79:321–327.

196. Jones PH, Harper S, Watt FM. Stem cell patterning and fate in human epidermis. Cell 1995;80:83–93.

197. Kastan MB, Canman CE, Leonard CJ. p53, cell cycle control and apoptosis: implications for cancer. Cancer Metastasis Rev 1995;14: 3–15.

198. Kataja V, Syrjänen S, Yliskoski M. Risk factors associated with cervical human papillomavirus infections: a case-control study. Am J Epidemiol 1993;138:735–745.

199. Kaur P, McDougall JK, Cone R. Immortalization of primary human epithelial cells by cloned cervical carcinoma DNA containing human papillomavirus type 16 E6/E7 open reading frames. J Gen Virol 1989;70:1261–1266.

200. Keating PJ, Cromme FV, Duggan KM, et al. Frequency of down-regulation of individual HLA-A and -B alleles in cervical carcinomas in relation to TAP-1 expression. Br J Cancer 1995;72:405–411.

201. Keen N, Elston R, Crawford L. Interaction of the E6 protein of human papillomavirus with cellular proteins. Oncogene 1994;9:1493–1499.

202. Kessis TD, Slebos RJ, Han SM, et al. p53 gene mutations and MDM2 amplification are uncommon in primary carcinomas of the uterine cervix. Am J Pathol 1993;143:1398–1405.

203. Kessis TD, Slebos RJ, Nelson WG, et al. Human papillomavirus 16 E6 expression disrupts the p53-mediated cellular response to DNA damage. Proc Natl Acad Sci U S A 1993;90:3988–3992.

204. Khan, MA, Tolleson WH, Gangemi JD, Pirisi L. Inhibition of growth, transformation, and expression of human papillomavirus type 16 E7 in human keratinocytes by alpha interferons. J Virol 1993;67:3396–3403.

205. Kirnbauer R, Booy F, Cheng N, Lowy DR, Schiller JT. Papillomavirus L1 major capsid protein self-assembles into virus-like particles that are highly immunogenic. Proc Natl Acad Sci U S A 1992;89:12180–12184.

206. Kirnbauer R, Taub J, Greenstone H, et al. Efficient self-assembly of human papillomavirus type 16 L1 and L1-L2 into virus-like particles. J Virol 1993;67:6929–6936.

207. Kiyono T, Hiraiwa A, Ishii S, Takahashi T, Ishibashi M. Inhibition of p53-mediated transactivation by E6 of type 1, but not type 5, 8, or 47, human papillomavirus of cutaneous origin. J Virol 1994;68: 4656–4661.

208. Kiyono T, Nagashima K, Ishibashi M. The primary structure of major viral RNA in a rat cell line transfected with type 47 human papillomavirus DNA and the transforming activity of its cDNA and E6 gene. Virology 1989;173:551–565.

209. Klingelhutz AJ, Barber SA, Smith PP, Dyer K, McDougall JK. Restoration of telomeres in human papillomavirus–immortalized human anogenital epithelial cells. Mol Cell Biol 1994;14:961–969.

210. Klingelhutz AJ, Hedrick L, Cho KR, McDougall JK. The DCC gene suppresses the malignant phenotype of transformed human epithelial cells. Oncogene 1995;10:1581–1586.

211. Knudson AG. Antioncogenes and human cancer. Proc Natl Acad Sci U S A 1993;90:10914–10921.

212. Kohno T, Takayama H, Hamaguchi M, et al. Deletion mapping of chromosome 3p in human uterine cervical cancer. Oncogene 1993; 1825–1832.

213. Kondoh G, Nishimune Y, Nishizawa Y, Hayasaka N, Matsumoto K, Hakura A. Establishment and further characterization of a line of transgenic mice showing testicular tumorigenesis at 100% incidence. J Urol 1994;152:2151–2154.

214. Kopan R, Traska G, Fuchs E. Retinoids as important regulators of terminal differentiation: examining keratin expression in individual epidermal cells at various stages of keratinization. J Cell Biol 1987;105:427–440.

215. Kowalik TF, DeGregori J, Schwarz JK, Nevins JR. E2F1 overexpression in quiescent fibroblasts leads to induction of cellular DNA synthesis and apoptosis. J Virol 1995;69:2491–2500.

216. Kramer SS, Wehunt WD, Stocker JT, Kashima H. Pulmonary manifestations of juvenile laryngotracheal papillomatosis. Am J Roentgenol 1985;144:687–694.

217. Kreider JW, Bartlett GL. The Shope papilloma-carcinoma complex of rabbits: a model system of neoplastic progression and spontaneous regression. Adv Cancer Res 1981;35:81–110.

218. Kreider JW, Patrick SD, Cladel NM, Welsh PA. Experimental infection with human papillomavirus type 1 of human hand and foot skin. Virology 1990;177:415–417.

219. Kuo SR, Liu JS, Broker TR, Chow LT. Cell-free replication of the human papillomavirus DNA with homologous viral E1 and E2 proteins and human cell extracts. J Biol Chem 1994;269:24058–24065.

220. Kurvinen K, Tervahauta A, Syrjänen S, Chang F, Syrjänen K. The state of the p53 gene in human papillomavirus (HPV)–positive and HPV-negative genital precancer lesions and carcinomas as determined by single-strand conformation polymorphism analysis and sequencing. Anticancer Res 1994;14:177–181.

221. Kyo S, Inoue M, Hayasaka N, et al. Regulation of early gene expression of human papillomavirus type 16 by inflammatory cytokines. Virology 1994;200:130–139.

222. Kyo S, Inoue M, Nishio Y, et al. NF-IL6 represses early gene expression of human papillomavirus type 16 through binding to the noncoding region. J Virol 1993;67:1058–1066.

223. Labrie C, Morris GF, Mathews MB. A complex promoter element mediates transactivation of the human proliferating cell nuclear antigen promoter by the 243-residue adenovirus E1A oncoprotein. Mol Cell Biol 1993;13:1697–1707.

224. Lam EW, La Thangue N. DP and E2F proteins: coordinating transcription with cell cycle progression. Curr Opin Cell Biol 1994;6: 859–866.

225. Lam EW, Morris JD, Davies R, Crook T, Watson RJ, Vousden KH. HPV16 E7 oncoprotein deregulates B-myb expression: correlation with targeting of p107/E2F complexes. EMBO J 1994;13:871–878.

226. Lambert PF, Pan H, Pitot HC, Liem A, Jackson M, Griep AE. Epidermal cancer associated with expression of human papillomavirus type 16 E6 and E7 oncogenes in the skin of transgenic mice. Proc Natl Acad Sci U S A 1993;90:5583–5587.

227. Lancaster WD. Apparent lack of integration of bovine papillomavirus DNA in virus-induced equine and bovine tumor cells and virus-transformed mouse cells. Virology 1981;108:251–255.

228. LaPorta RF, Taichman LB. Human papilloma viral DNA replicates as a stable episome in cultured epidermal keratinocytes. Proc Natl Acad Sci U S A 1982;79:3393–3397.

229. Law MF, Lowy DR, Dvoretzky I, Howley PM. Mouse cells transformed by bovine papillomavirus contain only extrachromosomal viral DNA sequences. Proc Natl Acad Sci U S A 1981;78:2727–2731.

230. Lechner MS, Laimins LA. Inhibition of p53 DNA binding by human papillomavirus E6 proteins. J Virol 1994;68:4262–4273.

231. Lechner MS, Mack DH, Finicle AB, Crook T, Vousden KH, Laimins LA. Human papillomavirus E6 proteins bind p53 in vivo and abrogate p53-mediated repression of transcription. EMBO J 1992;11: 3045–3052.

232. Lednicky JA, Garcea RL, Bergsagel DJ, Butel JS. Natural simian virus 40 strains are present in human choroid plexus and ependymoma tumors. Virology 1995;212:710–717.

233. Lee YY, Wilczynski SP, Chumakov A, Chih D, Koeffler HP. Carcinoma of the vulva: HPV and p53 mutations. Oncogene 1994;9: 1655–1659.

234. Leechanachai P, Banks L, Moreau F, Matlashewski G. The E5 gene from human papillomavirus type 16 is an oncogene which enhances growth factor–mediated signal transduction to the nucleus. Oncogene 1992;7:19–25.

235. Lees E, Osborn K, Banks L, Crawford L. Transformation of primary BRK cells by human papillomavirus type 16 and EJ-ras is increased by overexpression of the viral E2 protein. J Gen Virol 1990; 71: 183–193.

236. Le Moal M, Yaniv M, Thierry F. The bovine papillomavirus type 1 (BPV1) replication protein E1 modulates transcriptional activation by interacting with BPV1 E2. J Virol 1994;68:1085–1093.

237. Leptak C, Ramon Y, Cajal S, et al. Tumorigenic transformation of murine keratinocytes by the E5 genes of bovine papillomavirus type 1 and human papillomavirus type 16. J Virol 1991;65:7078–7083.

238. Leventhal BG, Kashima HK, Mounts P, et al. Long-term response of recurrent respiratory papillomatosis to treatment with lymphoblastoid interferon alfa-N1. Papilloma Study Group. N Engl J Med 1991;325:613–617.

239. Levine, AJ. The origins of the small DNA tumor viruses. Adv Cancer Res 1994;65:141–168.

240. Li R, Botchan MR. Acidic transcription factors alleviate nucleosome-mediated repression of DNA replication of bovine papillomavirus type 1. Proc Natl Acad Sci U S A 1994;91:7051–7055.

241. Li R, Waga S, Hannon GJ, Beach D, Stillman B. Differential effects by the p21 CDK inhibitor on PCNA-dependent DNA replication and repair. Nature 1994;371:534–537.

242. Li SL, Kim MS, Cherrick HM, Doniger J, Park NH. Sequential combined tumorigenic effect of HPV-16 and chemical carcinogens. Carcinogenesis 1992;13:1981–1987.

243. Liebermann DA, Hoffman B, Steinman RA. Molecular controls of growth arrest and apoptosis: p53-dependent and independent pathways. Oncogene 1995;11:199–210.

244. Lin YL, Borenstein LA, Ahmed R, Wettstein FO. Cottontail rabbit papillomavirus L1 protein–based vaccines: protection is achieved only with a full-length, nondenatured product. J Virol 1993;67: 4154–4162.

245. Lin YL, Borenstein LA, Selvakumar R, Ahmed R, Wettstein FO. Effective vaccination against papilloma development by immunization with L1 or L2 structural protein of cottontail rabbit papillomavirus. Virology 1992;187:612–619.

246. Liu JS, Kuo SR, Broker TR, Chow LT. The functions of human papillomavirus type 11 E1, E2 and E2C proteins in cell-free DNA replication. J Biol Chem 1995;270:27283–27291.

247. Loeken MR, Brady J. The adenovirus EIIA enhancer. J Biol Chem 1989;264:6572˘2D9.

248. Lowy DR, Dvoretzky I, Shober R, Law MF, Engel L, Howley PM. In vitro tumorigenic transformation by a defined sub-genomic fragment of bovine papilloma virus DNA. Nature 1980;287:72–74.

249. Lu JZ, Sun YN, Rose RC, Bonnez W, McCance, DJ. Two E2 binding sites (E2BS) alone or one E2BS plus an A/T-rich region are minimal requirements for the replication of the human papillomavirus type 11 origin. J Virol 1993;67:7131–7139.

250. Lusky M, Hurwitz J, Seo YS. Cooperative assembly of the bovine papilloma virus E1 and E2 proteins on the replication origin requires an intact E2 binding site. J Biol Chem 1993;268:15795–15803.

251. Lutzner MA, Blanchet-Bardon C, Orth G. Clinical observations, virologic studies, and treatment trials in patients with epidermodys-

plasia verruciformis, a disease induced by specific human papillomaviruses. J Invest Dermatol 1984;83:18s–25s.

252. Mahon KA, Chepelinsky AB, Khillan JS, Overbeek PA, Piatigorsky J, Westphal H. Oncogenesis of the lens in transgenic mice. Science 1987;235:1622–1628.

253. Malejczyk J, Malejczyk M, Kock A, et al. Autocrine growth limitation of human papillomavirus type 16–harboring keratinocytes by constitutively released tumor necrosis factor-alpha. J Immunol 1992;149:2702–2708.

254. Malejczyk J, Malejczyk M, Urbanski A, et al. Constitutive release of IL6 by human papillomavirus type 16 (HPV16)–harboring keratinocytes: a mechanism augmenting the NK-cell–mediated lysis of HPV-bearing neoplastic cells. Cell Immunol 1991;136:155–164.

255. Manfredi JJ, Prives C. The transforming activity of simian virus 40 large tumor antigen. Biochim Biophys Acta 1994;1198:65–83.

256. Manos M, Ting Y, Lewis A, Wolinsky SM, Broker TR, Wright D. Detection and typing of genital human papillomaviruses using the polymerase chain reaction. Cancer Cells 1989;7:209–214.

257. Maran A, Amella CA, DiLorenzo T, Auborn KJ, Taichman LB, Steinberg BM. Human papillomavirus type 11 transcripts are present at low abundance in latently infected respiratory tissues. Virology 1995;212:285–294.

258. Martin P, Vass WC, Schiller JT, Lowy DR, Velu TJ. The bovine papillomavirus E5 transforming protein can stimulate the transforming activity of EGF and CSF-1 receptors. Cell 1989;59:21–32.

259. Matlashewski G, Schneider J, Banks L, Jones N, Murray A, Crawford L. Human papillomavirus type 16 DNA cooperates with activated ras in transforming primary cells. EMBO J 1987;6:1741–1746.

260. McCance DJ, Kopan R, Fuchs E, Laimins LA. Human papillomavirus type 16 alters human epithelial cell differentiation in vitro. Proc Natl Acad Sci U S A 1988;85:7169–7173.

261. McDougall JK. Immortalization and transformation of human cells by human papillomavirus. Curr Top Microbiol Immunol 1994;186:101–119.

262. Melendy T, Sedman J, Stenlund A. Cellular factors required for papillomavirus DNA replication. J Virol 1995;69:7857–7867.

263. Mendonca MS, Fasching CL, Srivatsan ES, Stanbridge EJ, Redpath JL. Loss of a putative tumor suppressor locus after gamma-ray–induced neoplastic transformation of HeLa x skin fibroblast human cell hybrids. Radiat Res 1995;143:34–44.

264. Merrick DT, Blanton RA, Gown AM, McDougall JK. Altered expression of proliferation and differentiation markers in human papillomavirus 16 and 18 immortalized epithelial cells grown in organotypic culture. Am J Pathol 1992;140:167–177.

265. Merrick DT, Gown AM, Halbert CL, Blanton RA, McDougall JK. Human papillomavirus-immortalized keratinocytes are resistant to the effects of retinoic acid on terminal differentiation. Cell Growth Differ 1993;4:831–840.

266. Meyers C, Frattini MG, Hudson JB, Laimins LA. Biosynthesis of human papillomavirus from a continuous cell line upon epithelial differentiation. Science 1992;257:971–973.

266a.Meyers C, Harry J, Lin YL, Wettstein FO. Identification of three transforming proteins encoded by cottontail rabbit papillomavirus. J Virol 1992;66:1655–1664.

267. Mietz JA, Unger T, Huibregtse JM, Howley PM. The transcriptional transactivation function of wild-type p53 is inhibited by SV40 large T-antigen and by HPV-16 E6 oncoprotein. EMBO J 1992;11:5013–5020.

268. Missero C, Calautti E, Eckner R, et al. Involvement of the cell-cycle inhibitor cip1/waf1 and the E1A-associated p300 protein in terminal differentiation. Proc Natl Acad Sci U S A 1995;92:5451–5455.

269. Mitra AB, Murty VVVS, Singh V, et al. Genetic alterations at 5p-15: a potential marker for progression of precancerous lesions of the uterine cervix. J Natl Cancer Inst 1995;87:742–745.

270. Mittal R, Pater A, Pater MM. Multiple human papillomavirus type 16 glucocorticoid response elements functional for transformation, transient expression, and DNA-protein interactions. J Virol 1993;67:5656–5659.

271. Miwa K, Miyamoto S, Kato H, et al. The role of p53 inactivation in human cervical cell carcinoma development. Br J Cancer 1995;71:219–226.

272. Miyasaka M, Takami Y, Inoue H, Hakura A. Rat primary embryo fibroblast cells suppress transformation by the E6 and E7 genes of human papillomavirus type 16 in somatic hybrid cells. J Virol 1991;65:479–482.

273. Moll R, Franke WW, Schiller D, Geiger B, Krepler R. The catalog of human cytokeratins: patterns of expression in normal epithelia, tumors and cultured cells. Cell 1982;31:11–24.

274. Moran E. Mammalian cell growth controls selected through protein interactions with the adenovirus E1A gene products. Semin Virol 1994;5:327–340.

275. Müller F, Seo YS, Hurwitz J. Replication of bovine papillomavirus type 1 origin–containing DNA in crude extracts with purified proteins. J Biol Chem 1994;269:17086–17994.

276. Müller M, Gissmann L, Cristiano RJ, et al. Papillomavirus capsid binding and uptake by cells from different tissues and species. J Virol 1995;69:948–954.

277. Müller M, Viscidi RP, Sun Y, et al. Antibodies to HPV-16 E6 and E7 proteins as markers for HPV-16–associated invasive cervical cancer. Virology 1992;187:508–514.

278. Mullokandov MR, Kholodilov NG, Aktin NB, Burk RD, Johnson AB, Klinger HP. Genomic alterations in cervical carcinoma: losses of chromosome heterozygosity and human papilloma virus tumor status. Cancer Res 1995;56:197–205.

279. Mungal S, Steinberg BM, Taichman LB. Replication of plasmid-derived human papillomavirus type 11 DNA in cultured keratinocytes. J Virol 1992;66:3220–3224.

280. Münger K, Phelps WC, Bubb V, Howley PM, Schlegel R. The E6 and E7 genes of the human papillomavirus type 16 together are necessary and sufficient for transformation of primary human keratinocytes. J Virol 1989;63:4417–4421.

281. Münger K, Werness BA, Dyson N, Phelps WC, Harlow E, Howley PM. Complex formation of human papillomavirus E7 proteins with the retinoblastoma tumor suppressor gene product. EMBO J 1989;8:4099–4105.

282. Münger K, Yee CJ, Phelps WC, Pietenpol JA, Moses HL, Howley PM. Biochemical and biological differences between E7 oncoproteins of the high- and low-risk human papillomavirus types are determined by amino-terminal sequences. J Virol 1991;65:3943–3948.

283. Mushika M, Miwa T, Suzuoki Y, Hayashi K, Masaki S, Kaneda T. Detection of proliferative cells in dysplasia, carcinoma in situ, and invasive carcinoma of the uterine cervix by monoclonal antibody against DNA polymerase α. Cancer 1988;61:1182–1186.

284. Nakanishi K, Yong IH, Ishiwatari H, et al. Isolation of flat revertants from human papillomavirus type 18 E6E7 transformed 3Y1 cells by transfection with a rat embryo fibroblast cDNA expression library. Cell Struct Funct 1993;18:457–465.

285. Nasseri M, Gage JR, Lörincz A, Wettstein FO. Human papillomavirus type 16 immortalized cervical keratinocytes contain transcripts encoding E6, E7, and E2 initiated at the P97 promoter and express high levels of E7. Virology 1991;184:131–140.

286. Nasseri M, Hirochika R, Broker TR, Chow LT. A human papilloma virus type 11 transcript encoding an E1-E4 protein. Virology 1987;159:433–439.

287. Nasseri M, Wettstein FO. Differences exist between viral transcripts in cottontail rabbit papillomavirus–induced benign and malignant tumors as well as non–virus-producing and virus-producing tumors. J Virol 1984;51:706–712.

288. Nevins JR, Vogt PK. Cell transformation by viruses. In: Fields BN, Knipe DM, Howley PM, eds. Fields virology. 3rd ed. Philadelphia: Lippincott-Raven, 1996:301–344.

289. Nilson LA, DiMaio D. Platelet-derived growth factor receptor can mediate tumorigenic transformation by the bovine papillomavirus E5 protein. Mol Cell Biol 1993;13:4137–4145.

290. Obalek S, Glinski W, Haftek M, Orth G, Jablonska S. Comparative studies on cell-mediated immunity in patients with different warts. Dermatologica 1980;161:73–83.

291. O'Banion MK, Winn VD, Settleman J, Young DA. Genetic definition of a new bovine papillomavirus type 1 open reading frame, E5B, that encodes a hydrophobic protein involved in altering host-cell protein processing. J Virol 1993;67:3427–3434.

292. Obert S, O'Connor RJ, Schmid S, Hearing P. The adenovirus E4-6/7 protein transactivates the E2 promoter by inducing dimerization of a heteromeric E2F complex. Mol Cell Biol 1994;14:1333–1346.

293. Oelze I, Kartenbeck J, Crusius K, Alonso A. Human papillomavirus type 16 E5 protein affects cell-cell communication in an epithelial cell line. J Virol 1995;69:4489–4494.

294. Okabayashi M, Angell MG, Budgeon LR, Kreider JW. Shope papilloma cell and leukocyte proliferation in regressing and progressing lesions. Am J Pathol 1993;142:489–496.

295. Orth G. Epidermodysplasia verruciformis. In: Salzman NP, Howley PM, eds. The papovaviridae: the papillomaviruses. New York: Plenum Press, 1986:199–243.

296. Ostrow RS, Liu Z, Schneider JF, McGlennen RC, Forslund K, Faras AJ. The products of the E5, E6, or E7 open reading frames of RhPV 1 can individually transform NIH 3T3 cells or in cotransfections with activated ras can transform primary rodent epithelial cells. Virology 1993;196:861–867.

297. Palermo-Dilts DA, Broker TR, Chow LT. Human papillomavirus type 1 produces redundant as well as polycistronic mRNAs in plantar warts. J Virol 1990;64:3144–3149.

298. Pan H, Griep AE. Altered cell cycle regulation in the lens of HPV-16 E6 or E7 transgenic mice: implications for tumor suppressor gene function in development. Genes Dev 1994;8:1285–1299.

299. Park NH, Min BM, Li SL, Huang MZ, Cherick HM, Doniger J. Immortalization of normal human oral keratinocytes with type 16 human papillomavirus. Carcinogenesis 1991;12:1627–1631.

300. Pater A, Belaguli NS, Pater MM. Glucocorticoid requirement for growth of human papillomavirus 16-transformed primary rat kidney epithelial cells: correlation of development of hormone resistance with viral RNA expression and processing. Cancer Res 1993;53: 4432–4436.

301. Pater MM, Hughes GA, Hyslop DE, Nakshatri H, Pater A. Glucocorticoid-dependent oncogenic transformation by type 16 but not type 11 human papilloma virus DNA. Nature 1988;335:832–835.

302. Pater MM, Nakshatri H, Kisaka C, Pater A. The first 124 nucleotides of the E7 coding sequences of HPV16 can render the HPV11 genome transformation competent. Virology 1992;186: 348–351.

303. Pater MM, Pater A. Human papillomavirus types 16 and 18 sequences in carcinoma cell lines of the cervix. Virology 1985; 145: 313–318.

304. Patrick DR, Oliff A, Heimbrook DC. Identification of a novel retinoblastoma gene product binding site on human papillomavirus type 16 E7 protein. J Biol Chem 1994;269:6842–6850.

305. Pecoraro G, Lee M, Morgan D, Defendi V. Evolution of in vitro transformation and tumorigenesis of HPV16 and HPV18 immortalized primary cervical epithelial cells. Am J Pathol 1991;138: 1–8.

306. Pecoraro G, Morgan D, Defendi V. Differential effects of human papillomavirus type 6, 16, and 18 DNAs on immortalization and transformation of human cervical epithelial cells. Proc Natl Acad Sci U S A 1989;86:563–567.

307. Pei XF, Meck JM, Greenhalgh D, Schlegel R. Cotransfection of HPV-18 and v-fos DNA induces tumorigenicity of primary human keratinocytes. Virology 1993;196:855–860.

308. Peng X, Olson RO, Christian CB, Lang CM, Kreider JW. Papillomas and carcinomas in transgenic rabbits carrying EJ-ras DNA and cottontail rabbit papillomavirus DNA. J Virol 1993;67:1698–1701.

309. Pereira-Smith OM, Smith JR. Genetic analysis of indefinite division in human cells: identification of four complementation groups. Proc Natl Acad Sci U S A 1988;85:6042–6946.

310. Petti L, DiMaio D. Specific interaction between the bovine papillomavirus E5 transforming protein and the beta receptor for platelet-derived growth factor in stably transformed and acutely transfected cells. J Virol 1994;68:3582–3592.

311. Phelps WC, Bagchi S, Barnes JA, et al. Analysis of trans activation by human papillomavirus type 16 E7 and adenovirus 12S E1A suggests a common mechanism. J Virol 1991;65:6922–6930.

312. Phelps WC, Münger K, Yee CL, Barnes JA, Howley PM. Structure-function analysis of the human papillomavirus type 16 E7 oncoprotein. J Virol 1992;66:2418–2427.

313. Phelps WC, Yee CL, Münger K, Howley PM. The human papillomavirus type 16 E7 gene encodes transactivation and transformation functions similar to those of adenovirus E1A. Cell 1988; 53: 539–547.

314. Pilacinski WP, Glassman DL, Glassman KF, et al. Development of a recombinant DNA vaccine against bovine papillomavirus infection in cattle. In: Howley PM, Broker TR, eds. Papillomaviruses: molecular and clinical aspects. UCLA Symp Mol Cell Biol. New York: Alan R Liss. 1985;32:257–272.

315. Pim D, Collins M, Banks L. Human papillomavirus type 16 E5 gene stimulates the transforming activity of the epidermal growth factor receptor. Oncogene 1992;7:27–32.

316. Pim D, Storey A, Thomas M, Massimi P, Banks L. Mutational analysis of HPV-18 E6 identifies domains required for p53 degradation in vitro, abolition of p53 transactivation in vivo and immortalization of primary BMK cells. Oncogene 1994;9:1869–1876.

317. Pirisi L, Batova A, Jenkins GR, Hodam JR, Creek KE. Increased sensitivity of human keratinocytes immortalized by human papillomavirus type 16 DNA to growth control by retinoids. Cancer Res 1992;52:187–193.

318. Pirisi L, Creek KE, Doniger J, DiPaolo JA. Continuous cell lines with altered growth and differentiation properties originate after transfection of primary keratinocytes with human papillomavirus type 16 DNA. Carcinogenesis 1988;9:1573–1579.

319. Pirisi L, Yasumoto S, Feller M, Doniger J, DiPaolo JA. Transformation of human fibroblasts and keratinocytes with human papillomavirus type 16 DNA. J Virol 1987;61:1061–1066.

320. Qin XQ, Livingston DM, Kaelin WJ, Adams PD. Deregulated transcription factor E2F-1 expression leads to S-phase entry and p53-mediated apoptosis. Proc Natl Acad Sci U S A 1994;91:10918–10922.

321. Rader JS, Golub TR, Hudson JB, Patel D, Bedell MA, Laimins LA. In vitro differentiation of epithelial cells from cervical neoplasias resembles in vivo lesions. Oncogene 1990;5:571–576.

322. Remm M, Brain R, Jenkins JR. The E2 binding sites determine the efficiency of replication for the origin of human papillomavirus type 18. Nucleic Acids Res 1992;20:6015–6021.

323. Riese DN, DiMaio D. An intact PDGF signaling pathway is required for efficient growth transformation of mouse C127 cells by the bovine papillomavirus E5 protein. Oncogene 1995;10:1431–1439.

324. Roden RB, Kirnbauer R, Jenson AB, Lowy DR, Schiller JT. Interaction of papillomaviruses with the cell surface. J Virol 1994a;68: 7260–7266.

325. Roden RB, Weissinger EM, Henderson DW, et al. Neutralization of bovine papillomavirus by antibodies to L1 and L2 capsid proteins. J Virol 1994b;68:7570–7574.

326. Roggenbuck B, Larsen PM, Fey SJ, Bartsch D, Gissmann L, Schwarz E. Human papillomavirus type 18 E6*, E6, and E7 protein synthesis in cell-free translation systems and comparison of E6 and E7 in vitro translation products to proteins immunoprecipitated from human epithelial cells. J Virol 1991;65:5068–5072.

327. Rogozinski TT, Jablonska S, Jarzabek-Chorzelska M. Role of cell-mediated immunity in spontaneous regression of plane warts. Int J Dermatol 1988;27:322–326.

328. Rohlfs M, Winkenbach S, Meyer S, Rupp T, Dürst M. Viral transcription in human keratinocyte cell lines immortalized by human papillomavirus type-16. Virology 1991;183:331–342.

329. Romanczuk H, Howley PM. Disruption of either the E1 or the E2 regulatory gene of human papillomavirus type 16 increases viral immortalization capacity. Proc Natl Acad Sci U S A 1992;89: 159–3163.

330. Romanczuk H, Thierry F, Howley PM. Mutational analysis of cis elements involved in E2 modulation of human papillomavirus type 16 P97 and type 18 P105 promoters. J Virol 1990;64:2849–2859.

331. Rose RC, Bonnez W, Reichman RC, Garcea RL. Expression of human papillomavirus type 11 L1 protein in insect cells: in vivo and in vitro assembly of viruslike particles. J Virol 1993;67:1936–1944.

332. Rose RC, Reichman RC, Bonnez W. Human papillomavirus (HPV) type 11 recombinant virus-like particles induce the formation of neutralizing antibodies and detect HPV-specific antibodies in human sera. J Gen Virol 1994;75:2075–209.

332a. Rotenberg MO, Chiang C-M, Ho MS, Broker TR, Chow Lt. Characterization of cDNAs of spliced HPV-11 E2 mRNA and other HPV mRNAs recovered via retrovirus-mediated gene transfer. Virology 1989;172:468–477.

333. Rotenberg MO, Chow LT, Broker TR. Characterization of rare human papillomavirus type 11 mRNAs coding for regulatory and structural proteins, using the polymerase chain reaction. Virology 1989;172:489–497.

334. Sandler AB, Vande Pol S, Spalholz BA. Repression of bovine papillomavirus type 1 transcription by the E1 replication protein. J Virol 1993;67:5079–5087.

335. Sang BC, Barbosa MS. Increased E6/E7 transcription in HPV 18-immortalized human keratinocytes results from inactivation of E2 and additional cellular events. Virology 1992;189:448–455.

336. Sang BC, Barbosa MS. Single amino acid substitutions in "low-risk" human papillomavirus (HPV) type 6 E7 protein enhance features characteristic of the "high-risk" HPV E7 oncoproteins. Proc Natl Acad Sci U S A 1992;89:8063–8067.

337. Sasagawa T, Inoue M, Inoue H, Yutsudo M, Tanizawa O, Hakura A. Induction of uterine cervical neoplasias in mice by human papillomavirus type 16 E6/E7 genes. Cancer Res 1992;52:4420–4426.

338. Sasagawa T, Kondoh G, Inoue M, Yutsudo M, Hakura A. Cervical/vaginal dysplasias of transgenic mice harbouring human papillomavirus type 16 E6-E7 genes. J Gen Virol 1994;75:3057–3065.

339. Sasagawa T, Pushko P, Steers G, et al. Synthesis and assembly of virus-like particles of human papillomaviruses type 6 and type 16 in fission yeast Schizosaccharomyces pombe. Virology 1995;206:126–135.

340. Scheffner M, Huibregtse JM, Vierstra RD, Howley PM. The HPV-16 E6 and E6-AP complex functions as a ubiquitin-protein ligase in the ubiquitination of p53. Cell 1993;75:495–505.

341. Scheffner M, Münger K, Byrne JC, Howley PM. The state of the p53 and retinoblastoma genes in human cervical carcinoma cell lines. Proc Natl Acad Sci U S A 1991;88:5523–5527.

342. Scheffner M, Münger K, Huibregtse JM, Howley PM. Targeted degradation of the retinoblastoma protein by human papillomavirus E7-E6 fusion proteins. EMBO J 1992;11:2425–2431.

343. Scheffner M, Romanczuk H, Münger K, Huibregtse JM, Mietz JA, Howley PM. Functions of human papillomavirus proteins. Curr Top Microbiol Immunol 1994;186:83–99.

344. Schiffman MH. Epidemiology of cervical human papillomavirus infections. Curr Top Microbiol Immunol 1994;186:55–81.

345. Schlegel R, Phelps WC, Zhang YL, Barbosa M. Quantitative keratinocyte assay detects two biological activities of human papillomavirus DNA and identifies viral types associated with cervical carcinoma. EMBO J 1988;7:3181–3187.

346. Schmitt A, Harry JB, Rapp B, Wettstein FO, Iftner T. Comparison of the properties of the E6 and E7 genes of low- and high-risk cutaneous papillomaviruses reveals strongly transforming and high Rb-binding activity for the E7 protein of the low-risk human papillomavirus type 1. J Virol 1994;68:7051–7059.

347. Schneider-Gädicke A, Schwarz E. Different human cervical carcinoma cell lines show similar transcription patterns of human papillomavirus type 18 early genes. EMBO J 1986;5:2285–2292.

348. Schwarz E, Freese UK, Gissmann L, Mayer W, Roggenbuck B, Stremlau A, zur Hausen H. Structure and transcription of human papillomavirus sequences in cervical carcinoma cells. Nature 1985; 314:111–114.

349. Seagon S, Dürst M. Genetic analysis of an in vitro model system for human papillomavirus type 16–associated tumorigenesis. Cancer Res 1994;54:5593–5598.

350. Sedman SA, Barbosa MS, Vass WC, et al. The full-length E6 protein of human papillomavirus type 16 has transforming and trans-activating activities and cooperates with E7 to immortalize keratinocytes in culture. J Virol 1991;65:4860–4866.

351. Sedman SA, Hubbert NL, Vass WC, Lowy DR, Schiller JT. Mutant p53 can substitute for human papillomavirus type 16 E6 in immortalization of human keratinocytes but does not have E6-associated trans-activation or transforming activity. J Virol 1992;66: 4201–4208.

352. Selivanova G, Wiman KG. p53: a cell cycle regulator activated by DNA damage. Adv Cancer Res 1995;66:143–180.

353. Selvakumar R, Borenstein LA, Lin YL, Ahmed R, Wettstein FO. T-cell response to cottontail rabbit papillomavirus structural proteins in infected rabbits. J Virol 1994;68:4043–4048.

354. Selvakumar R, Borenstein LA, Lin YL, Ahmed R, Wettstein FO. Immunization with nonstructural proteins E1 and E2 of cottontail rabbit papillomavirus stimulates regression of virus-induced papillomas. J Virol 1995;69:602–605.

355. Seo YS, Müller F, Lusky M, et al. Bovine papilloma virus (BPV)–encoded E2 protein enhances binding of E1 protein to the BPV replication origin. Proc Natl Acad Sci U S A 1993;90:2865–2869.

356. Seo YS, Müller F, Lusky M, Hurwitz J. Bovine papilloma virus (BPV)–encoded E1 protein contains multiple activities required for BPV DNA replication. Proc Natl Acad Sci U S A 1993;90:702–706.

357. Seto E, Usheva A, Zambetti GP, et al. Wild-type p53 binds to the TATA-binding protein and represses transcription. Proc Natl Acad Sci U S A 1992;89:12028–12032.

358. Sexton CJ, Proby CM, Banks L, et al. Characterization of factors involved in human papillomavirus type 16-mediated immortalization of oral keratinocytes. J Gen Virol 1993;74:755–761.

359. Shah KV. Polymaviruses. In: Fields BN, Knipe DM, Howley PM, eds. Fields virology. 3rd ed. Philadelphia: Lippincott-Raven, 1996: 2027–2044.

360. Shah KV, Howley PM. Papillomaviruses. In: Fields BN, Knipe DM, Howley PM, eds. Fields virology. 3rd ed. Philadelphia: Lippincott-Raven, 1996:2077–2110.

361. Shamanin V, Glover M, Rausch C, et al. Specific types of human papillomavirus found in benign proliferations and carcinomas of the skin in immunosuppressed patients. Cancer Res 1994;54:4610–4613.

362. Shenk T. Adenoviridae: the viruses and their replication. In: Fields BN, Knipe DM, Howley PM, eds. Fields virology. 3rd ed. Philadelphia: Lippincott-Raven, 1996:2111–2148.

363. Sherman L, Alloul N, Golan I, Dürst M, Baram A. Expression and splicing patterns of human papillomavirus type-16 mRNAs in precancerous lesions and carcinomas of the cervix, in human keratinocytes immortalized by HPV 16, and in cell lines established from cervical cancers. Int J Cancer 1992;50:356–364.

364. Sherr CJ, Roberts JM. Inhibitors of mammalian G1 cyclin-dependent kinases. Genes Dev 1995;9:1149–1163.

365. Shevchuk MM, Richart RM. DNA content of condyloma acuminatum. Cancer 1982;49:489–492.

366. Shindoh M, Sun Q, Pater A, Pater MM. Prevention of carcinoma in situ of human papillomavirus type 16–immortalized human endocervical cells by retinoic acid in organotypic raft culture. Obstet Gynecol 1995;85:721–728.

367. Slebos RJ, Lee MH, Plunkett BS, et al. p53-dependent G1 arrest involves pRB-related proteins and is disrupted by the human papillomavirus 16 E7 oncoprotein. Proc Natl Acad Sci U S A 1994; 91: 5320–5324.

368. Smedts F, Ramaekers FC, Vooijs PG. The dynamics of keratin expression in malignant transformation of cervical epithelium: a review. Obstet Gynecol 1993;82:?

369. Smith EM, Johnson SR, Cripe T, et al. Perinatal transmission and maternal risks of human papillomavirus infection. Cancer Detect Prev 1995;19:196–205.

370. Smith ML, Chen IT, Zhan Q, et al. Interaction of the p53 regulated protein gadd 45 with proliferating cell nuclear antigen. Science 1994;266:1376–1380.

371. Smith ML, Fornace AJ. Genomic instability and the role of p53 mutations in cancer cells. Curr Opin Oncol 1995;7:69–75.

372. Smits HL, Cornelissen MT, Jebbink MF, et al. Human papillomavirus type 16 transcripts expressed from viral-cellular junctions and full-length viral copies in CaSki cells and in a cervical carcinoma. Virology 1991;182:870–873.

373. Smits HL, Raadsheer E, Rood I, et al. Induction of anchorage-independent growth of human embryonic fibroblasts with a deletion in the short arm of chromosome 11 by human papillomavirus type 16 DNA. J Virol 1988;62:4538–4543.

374. Smits PH, Smits HL, Jebbink MF, ter Schegget J. The short arm of chromosome 11 likely is involved in the regulation of the human papillomavirus type 16 early enhancer-promoter and in the suppression of the transforming activity of the viral DNA. Virology 1990; 176:158–165.

375. Smits PH, Smits HL, Minnaar RP, et al. The 55 kDa regulatory subunit of protein phosphatase 2A plays a role in the activation of the HPV16 long control region in human cells with a deletion in the short arm of chromosome 11. EMBO J 1992;11:4601–4606.

376. Smotkin D, Prokoph H, Wettstein FO. Oncogenic and nononcogenic human genital papillomaviruses generate the E7 mRNA by different mechanisms. J Virol 1989;63:1441–1447.

377. Srivatsan ES, Misra BC, Venugopalan D, Wilczynski SP. Loss of alleles on chromosome 11 in cervical carcinoma. Am J Hum Genet 1991;49:868–877.

378. Stabler A, Pierce JH, Brazinski S, et al. Mutational analysis of the β-type platelet-derived growth factor receptor defines the site of inter-

action with the bovine papillomavirus type 1 E5 transforming protein. J Virol 1995;69:6507–6517.

379. Stacey SN, Jordan D, Snijders PJF, Mackett M, Walboomers JMM, Arrand JR. Translation of the human papillomavirus type 16 E7 oncoprotein from bicistronic mRNA is independent of splicing events within the E6 open reading frame. J Virol 1995;69:7023–7031.

380. Steenbergen RDM, Hermsen MAJA, Walboomers JMM, et al. Integrated human papillomavirus type 16 and loss of heterozygosity at 11q22 and 18q21 in an oral carcinoma and its derivative cell line. Cancer Res 1995;55:5465–5471.

380a. Steenbergen RDM, Walboomers JMM, Meijer CJLM, et al. Transition of human papillomavirus type 16 and 18 transfected human foreskin keratinocytes towards immortality: activation of telomerase and allele losses at 3p, 10p, 11q and/or 18q. Oncogene 1996 (in press; Fall).

381. Steinmann KE, Pei XF, Stöppler H, Schlegel R, Schlegel R. Elevated expression and activity of mitotic regulatory proteins in human papillomavirus-immortalized keratinocytes. Oncogene 1994; 9:387–394.

382. Sterling JC, Skepper JN, Stanley MA. Immunoelectron microscopical localization of human papillomavirus type 16 L1 and E4 proteins in cervical keratinocytes cultured in vivo. J Invest Dermatol 1993;100:154–158.

383. Stillman B. Smart machines at the DNA replication fork. Cell 1994;78:725–728.

384. Stillman BW, Lewis JB, Chow LT, Mathews MB, Smart JE. Identification of the gene and mRNA for the adenovirus terminal protein precursor. Cell 1981;23:497–508.

385. Stoler MH. The biology of the human papillomaviruses and their role in cervical carcinogenesis. In: Bonfiglio TA, Erozan Y, eds. Gynecologic cytopathology. Philadelphia: Lippincott-Raven, 1996 (in press).

386. Stoler MH, Broker TR. In situ hybridization detection of human papillomavirus DNAs and messenger RNAs in genital condylomas and a cervical carcinoma. Hum Pathol 1986;17:1250–1258.

387. Stoler MH, Rhodes CR, Whitbeck A, Wolinsky SM, Chow LT, Broker TR. Human papillomavirus type 16 and 18 gene expression in cervical neoplasias. Hum Pathol 1992;23:117–128.

388. Stoler MH, Whitbeck A, Wolinsky SM, et al. Infectious cycle of human papillomavirus type 11 in human foreskin xenografts in nude mice. J Virol 1990;64:3310–3318.

389. Stoler MH, Wolinsky SM, Whitbeck A, Broker TR, Chow LT. Differentiation-linked human papillomavirus types 6 and 11 transcription in genital condylomata revealed by in situ hybridization with message-specific RNA probes. Virology 1989;172:331–340.

390. Stöppler H, Stöppler MC, Schlegel R. Transforming proteins of the papillomaviruses. Intervirology 1994;37:168–179.

391. Storey A, Almond N, Osborn K, Crawford L. Mutations of the human papillomavirus type 16 E7 gene that affect transformation, transactivation and phosphorylation by the E7 protein. J Gen Virol 1990;71:965–970.

391a. Storey A, Greenfield I, Banks L, Pim D, Crook T, Crawford L, Stanley M. Lack of immortalizing activity of a human papillomavirus type 16 variant DNA with a mutation in the E2 gene isolated from normal human cervical keratinocytes. Oncogene 1992;7: 459–465.

392. Storey A, Osborn K, Crawford L. Co-transformation by human papillomavirus types 6 and 11. J Gen Virol 1990;71:165–171.

393. Storey A, Pim D, Murray A, Osborn K, Banks L, Crawford L. Comparison of the in vitro transforming activities of human papillomavirus types. EMBO J 1988;7:1815–1820.

394. Straight SW, Herman B, McCance DJ. The E5 oncoprotein of human papillomavirus type 16 inhibits the acidification of endosomes in human keratinocytes. J Virol 1995;69:3185–3192.

395. Straight SW, Hinkle PM, Jewers RJ, McCance DJ. The E5 oncoprotein of human papillomavirus type 16 transforms fibroblasts and effects the downregulation of the epidermal growth factor receptor in keratinocytes. J Virol 1993;67:4521–4532.

396. Strang G, Hickling JK, McIndoe GA, et al. Human T cell responses to human papillomavirus type 16 L1 and E6 synthetic peptides: identification of T cell determinants, HLA-DR restriction and virus type specificity. J Gen Virol 1990;71:423–431.

397. Sun Q, Tsutsumi K, Kelleher MB, Pater A, Pater MM. Squamous metaplasia of normal and carcinoma in situ of HPV 16-immortalized human endocervical cells. Cancer Res 1992;52:4254–4260.

398. Suzich JA, Ghim SJ, Palmer-Hill FJ, et al. Systemic immunization with papillomavirus L1 protein completely prevents the development of viral mucosal papillomas. Proc Natl Acad Sci U S A 1995;92:11553–11567.

399. Sverdrup F, Khan SA. Two E2 binding sites alone are sufficient to function as the minimal origin of replication of human papillomavirus type 18 DNA. J Virol 1995;69:1319–1323.

400. Taichman LB, Breitburd F, Croissant O, Orth G. The search for a culture system for papillomavirus. J Invest Dermatol 1984;83: 2s–6s.

401. Takami Y, Sasagawa T, Sudiro TM, Yutsudo M, Hakura A. Determination of the functional difference between human papillomavirus type 6 and 16 E7 proteins by their 30 N-terminal amino acid residues. Virology 1992;186:489–495.

402. Tan SH, Leong LE, Walker PA, Bernard HU. The human papillomavirus type 16 E2 transcription factor binds with low cooperativity to two flanking sites and represses the E6 promoter through displacement of Sp1 and TFIID. J Virol 1994;68:6411–6420.

403. Tan TM, Gloss B, Bernard HU, Ting RC. Mechanism of translation of the bicistronic mRNA encoding human papillomavirus type 16 E6-E7 genes. J Gen Virol 1994;75:2663–2670.

404. ter Shegget J, van der Noordaa J. Protein phosphatase 2A and the regulation of human papillomavirus gene activity. Curr Top Microbiol Immunol 1994;186:121–129.

405. Thierry F, Howley PM. Functional analysis of E2-mediated repression of the HPV18 P105 promoter. New Biologist 1991;3:90–100.

406. Thomas M, Boiron M, Tanzer J, Levy JP, Bernard J. In vitro transformation of mice cells by bovine papilloma virus. Nature 1964; 202:709.

407. Thomas M, Massimi P, Jenkins J, Banks L. HPV-18 E6 mediated inhibition of p53 DNA binding activity is independent of E6 induced degradation. Oncogene 1995;10:261–268.

408. Tindle RW, Frazer IH. Immune response to human papillomaviruses and the prospects for human papillomavirus–specific immunisation. Curr Top Microbiol Immunol 1994;186:217–253.

409. Tinsley JM, Rothnagel J, Quintanilla M, et al. Abnormalities of epidermal differentiation associated with expression of the human papillomavirus type 1 early region in transgenic mice. J Gen Virol 1992; 73:1251–1260.

410. Togawa K, Rustgi AK. A novel human papillomavirus sequence based on L1 general primers. Virus Res 1995;36:293–297.

411. Tommasino M, Adamczewski JP, Carlotti F, et al. HPV16 E7 protein associates with the protein kinase p33CDK2 and cyclin A. Oncogene 1993;8:195–202.

412. Tsang NM, Nagasawa H, Li C, Little JB. Abrogation of p53 function by transfection of HPV16 E6 gene enhances the resistance of human diploid fibroblasts to ionizing radiation. Oncogene 1995;10:2403–2408.

413. Tsutsumi K, Belaguli N, Sun Q, et al. Human papillomavirus 16 DNA immortalizes two types of normal human epithelial cells of the uterine cervix. Am J Pathol 1992;140:255–261.

414. Turek LP. The structure, function, and regulation of papillomaviral genes in infection and cervical cancer. Adv Virus Res 1994;44: 305–356.

415. Ustav M, Stenlund A. Transient replication of BPV-1 requires two viral polypeptides encoded by the E1 and E2 open reading frames. EMBO J 1991;10:449–457.

416. Ustav E, Ustav M, Szymanski P, Stenlund A. The bovine papillomavirus origin of replication requires a binding site for the E2 transcriptional activator. Proc Natl Acad Sci U S A 1993;90:898–902.

417. Vambutas A, DiLorenzo TP, Steinberg BM. Laryngeal papilloma cells have high levels of epidermal growth factor receptor and respond to epidermal growth factor by a decrease in epithelial differentiation. Cancer Res 1993;53:910–914.

418. Vande Pol S, Howley PM. Negative regulation of the bovine papillomavirus E5, E6, and E7 oncogenes by the viral E1 and E2 genes. J Virol 1995;69:395–402.

419. van der Vliet PC. Adenovirus DNA replication. Curr Top Microbiol Immunol 1995;199:1–30.

420. Viscidi RP, Sun Y, Tsuzaki B, Bosch FX, Munoz N, Shah KV. Serologic response in human papillomavirus–associated invasive cervical cancer. Int J Cancer 1993;55:780–784.

421. Vogelstein B, Kinzler KW. The multistep nature of cancer. Trends Genet 1993;9:138–141.

422. Volpers C, Schirmacher P, Streeck RE, Sapp M. Assembly of the major and the minor capsid protein of human papillomavirus type

33 into virus-like particles and tubular structures in insect cells. Virology 1994;200:504–512.

423. Volpers C, Unckell F, Schirmacher P, Streeck RE, Sapp M. Binding and internalization of human papillomavirus type 33 virus-like particles by eukaryotic cells. J Virol 1995;69:3258–3264.

424. von Knebel Doeberitz M, Bauknecht T, Bartsch D, zur Hausen H. Influence of chromosomal integration on glucocorticoid-regulated transcription of growth-stimulating papillomavirus genes E6 and E7 in cervical carcinoma cells. Proc Natl Acad Sci U S A 1991; 88:1411–1415.

425. von Knebel Doeberitz M, Oltersdorf T, Schwarz E, Gissmann L. Correlation of modified human papilloma virus early gene expression with altered growth properties in C4-1 cervical carcinoma cells. Cancer Res 1988;48:3780–3786.

426. von Knebel Doeberitz M, Rittmüller C, zur Hausen H, Dürst M. Inhibition of tumorigenicity of cervical cancer cells in nude mice by HPV E6-E7 anti-sense RNA. Int J Cancer 1992;51:831–834.

427. Vormwald DV, Fischer B, Bludau H, et al. Sense and antisense transcripts of human papillomavirus type 16 in cervical cancers. J Gen Virol 1992;73:1833–1838.

428. Vousden KH. Interactions between papillomavirus proteins and tumor suppressor gene products. Adv Cancer Res 1994;64:1–24.

428a. Vousden KH, Doniger J, DiPaolo JA, Lowy DR. The E7 open reading frame of human papillomavirus type 16 encodes a transforming gene. Oncogene Res 1988;3:167–175.

429. Vousden KH, Jat PS. Functional similarity between HPV16E7, SV40 large T and adenovirus E1a proteins. Oncogene 1989;4: 153–158.

430. Waggoner SE, Woodworth CD, Stoler MH, Barnes WA, Delgado G, DiPaolo JA. Human cervical cells immortalized in vitro with oncogenic human papillomavirus DNA differentiate dysplastically in vivo. Gynecol Oncol 1990;38:407–412.

431. Wank R, Thomssen C. High risk of squamous cell carcinomas of the cervix for women with HLA-DQw3. Nature 1991;352:723–725.

432. Ward P, Mounts P. Heterogeneity in mRNA of human papillomavirus type-6 subtypes in respiratory tract lesions. Virology 1989;168:1–12.

433. Weinberg RA. The retinoblastoma protein and cell cycle control. Cell 1995;81:323–330.

434. Werness BA, Levine AJ, Howley PM. Association of human papillomavirus types 16 and 18 E6 proteins with p53. Science 1990; 248:76–79.

435. Wertz PW, Madison KC, Downing DT. Covalently bound lipids of human stratum corneum. J Invest Dermatol 1989;92:109–111.

436. White AE, Livanos EM, Tlsty TD. Differential disruption of genomic integrity and cell cycle regulation in normal human fibroblasts by the HPV oncoproteins. Genes Dev 1994;8:666–677.

437. White E. Function of the adenovirus E1B oncogene in infected and transformed cells. Semin Virol 1994;5:341–348.

438. Willey JC, Broussoud A, Sleemi A, Bennett WP, Cerutti P, Harris CC. Immortalization of normal human bronchial epithelial cells by human papillomaviruses 16 or 18. Cancer Res 1991;51:5370–5377.

439. Wilson JL, Dollard SC, Chow LT, Broker TR. Epithelial-specific gene expression during differentiation of stratified primary human keratinocyte cultures. Cell Growth Differ 1992;3:471–483.

440. Wingo PA, Tong T, Bolden S. Cancer statistics, 1995. CA Cancer J Clin 1995;45:8–30.

441. Wold WS, Hermiston TW, Tollefson AE. Adenovirus proteins that subvert host defenses. Trends Microbiol 1994;2:437–443.

442. Wong HK, Ziff EB. The human papillomavirus type 16 E7 protein complements adenovirus type 5 E1A amino terminus–dependent transactivation of adenovirus type 5 early genes and increases ATF and Oct-1 DNA binding activity. J Virol 1996;70:332–340.

443. Woodworth CD, Cheng S, Simpson S, et al. Recombinant retroviruses encoding human papillomavirus type 18 E6 and E7 genes stimulate cellular proliferation and suppress squamous differentiation in human keratinocytes in vitro. Oncogene 1992:7:619–626.

444. Woodworth CD, Doniger J, DiPaolo JA. Immortalization of human foreskin keratinocytes by various human papillomavirus DNAs corresponds to their association with cervical carcinoma. J Virol 1989;63:159–164.

445. Woodworth CD, Lichti U, Simpson S, Evans CH, DiPaolo JA. Leukoregulin and gamma-interferon inhibit human papillomavirus type 16 gene transcription in human papillomavirus–immortalized human cervical cells. Cancer Res 1992;52:456–463.

446. Wrede D, Tidy JA, Crook T, Lane D, Vousden KH. Expression of RB and p53 proteins in HPV-positive and HPV-negative cervical carcinoma cell lines. Mol Carcinog 1991;4:171–175.

447. Wu EW, Clemens KE, Heck DV, Münger K. The human papillomavirus E7 oncoprotein and the cellular transcription factor E2F bind to separate sites on the retinoblastoma tumor suppressor protein. J Virol 1993;67:2402–2407.

448. Wu X, Bayle H, Olson D, Levine AJ. The p53-mdm2 autoregulatory feedback loop. Genes Dev 1993;7:1126–1132.

449. Wu X, Levine AJ. p53 and E2F-1 cooperate to mediate apoptosis. Proc Natl Acad Sci U S A 1994;91:3602–3606.

450. Xiong Y, Hannon GJ, Zhang H, Casso D, Kobayashi R, Beach D. p21 is a universal inhibitor of cyclin kinases. Nature 1993;366: 701–704.

451. Xiong Y, Kuppuswamy D, Li Y, et al. Alternation of cell cycle kinase complexes in human papillomavirus E6- and E7-expressing fibroblasts precedes neoplastic tranformation. J Virol 1996;70:999–1008.

452. Xu C, Meikrantz W, Schlegel R, Sager R. The human papilloma virus 16 E6 gene sensitizes human mammary epithelial cells to apoptosis induced by DNA damage. Proc Natl Acad Sci U S A 1995; 92:7829–7833.

453. Yang L, Li R, Mohr IJ, Clark R, Botchan MR. Activation of BPV-1 replication in vitro by the transcription factor E2. Nature 1991;353: 628–632.

454. Yang L, Mohr I, Fouts E, Lim DA, Nohaile M, Botchan M. The E1 protein of bovine papilloma virus 1 is an ATP-dependent DNA helicase. Proc Natl Acad Sci U S A 1993;90:5086–5090.

455. Yankaskas JR, Haizlip JE, Conrad M, et al. Papilloma virus immortalized tracheal epithelial cells retain a well-differentiated phenotype. Am J Physiol 1993;264:c1219–c1230.

456. Yasumoto S, Burkhardt AL, Doniger J, DiPaolo JA. Human papillomavirus type 16 DNA-induced malignant transformation of NIH 3T3 cells. J Virol 1986;57:572–577.

457. Yee C, Krishnan HI, Baker CC, Schlegel R, Howley PM. Presence and expression of human papillomavirus sequences in human cervical carcinoma cell lines. Am J Pathol 1985;119:361–366.

458. Yew PR, Liu X, Berk AJ. Adenovirus E1B oncoprotein tethers a transcriptional repression domain to p53. Genes Dev 1994;8: 190–202.

459. Zeltner R, Borenstein LA, Wettstein FO, Iftner T. Changes in RNA expression pattern during the malignant progression of cottontail rabbit papillomavirus–induced tumors in rabbits. J Virol 1994;68: 3620–3630.

460. Zerfass K, Schulze A, Spitkovsky D, Friedman V, Henglein B, Jansen-Durr P. Sequential activation of cyclin E and cyclin A gene expression by human papillomavirus type 16 E7 through sequences necessary for transformation. J Virol 1995;69:6389–6399.

461. Zhou J, Sun XY, Stenzel DJ, Frazer IH. Expression of vaccinia recombinant HPV 16 L1 and L2 ORF proteins in epithelial cells is sufficient for assembly of HPV virion-like particles. Virology 1991;185:251–257.

461a. zur Hausen H. Molecular pathogenesis of cancer of the cervix and its causation by specific human papillomavirus types. Curr Top Microbiol Immunol 1994;186:131–156.

462. zur Hausen H. Roots and perspectives of contemporary papillomavirus research. J Cancer Res Clin Oncol 1996;122:3–13.

463. zur Hausen H, de Villiers EM. Human papillomaviruses. Annu Rev Microbiol 1994;48:427–447.

464. Zyzak LL, MacDonald LM, Batova A, Forand R, Creek KE, Pirisi L. Increased levels and constitutive tyrosine phosphorylation of the epidermal growth factor receptor contribute to autonomous growth of human papillomavirus type 16 immortalized human keratinocytes. Cell Growth Differ 1994;5:537–547.

Viral Pathogenesis,
edited by Neal Nathanson, et al.
Lippincott–Raven Publishers, Philadelphia © 1997

CHAPTER 13

Host Susceptibility to Viral Disease

Margo A. Brinton

INTRODUCTION

Whenever populations of plants or animals are exposed to the same viral pathogen, individual variation in disease outcome is observed.[19,31,102,144,184,205] For example, by 1950 wild European rabbits had become agricultural pests in Australia and virulent myxomatosis virus was introduced to reduce the rabbit population. Rabbit mortality rates were initially 99%,[186] but 1% of the rabbits survived and bred. In areas where virulent virus was reintroduced annually, the mortality rate in rabbits decreased from 99% to 25% in 7 years.[243] In some areas, attenuated virus strains evolved, and these enhanced the selection of resistant animals. These results suggest that both host population and viral genes play important roles in achieving a balance that ensures the continued survival of the host and the virus under natural infection conditions.

Several inadvertent natural experiments in humans also indicated individual variation in virus resistance. After military personnel were inoculated with batches of yellow fever vaccine that were contaminated with hepatitis B virus, only 914 of 45,000 vaccinees developed clinical hepatitis, and only 4%

of these individuals developed severe disease.[235] Because the amount of hepatitis B virus inoculated into each vaccinee was fairly constant, the variation in the outcome of hepatitis B infection was attributed to differences in host susceptibility. Similarly, not all susceptible children who received inadequately inactivated poliovaccine in the so-called Cutter incident developed paralytic poliomyelitis.[192] About 50% of the 120,000 grade school children who received this vaccine were susceptible to poliovirus; of these, 10% to 25% became infected, as indicated by the development of mild disease symptoms or virus excretion in stool, but only 60 cases of paralytic polio occurred. This case-infection ratio is typical for poliovirus. Although it was not documented in either of these episodes exactly how many individuals received an infectious dose of virus, it may safely be concluded that there were many subclinical infections, reflecting varied host responses to similar doses of virus.

Because viruses can induce permanent impairment or death in their hosts, they have undoubtedly exerted selective pressure during the evolution of both plants and animals. Mechanisms have evolved that modulate the severity of virus-induced disease, so that some host organisms can survive viral attack. Prolonged survival of the host is advantageous to the virus as well as the host, because a virus in such a host has an increased chance of being transmitted to a new host. Host factors such as age, nutritional status, hormone status, immune

M.A. Brinton: Department of Biology, Georgia State University, Atlanta, Georgia 30303.

status, and genetic background can be important in determining the outcome of a viral infection.[12,38,41,75,178,214,227,264] Viral genes that influence virulence are also important in determining the outcome of infection (see Chap. 5).

HOST FACTORS

Certainly, the host's immune status at the time of infection as well as early defense mechanisms involving natural killer cells and interferon[280] play important roles in determining the outcome of a virus infection (see Chap. 7). However, a number of other factors can also affect the outcome of viral infections. Many instances of a correlation between the severity of a particular virus infection and the age of the host have been reported.[264] In cases in which resistance to viral infection increases with age, the greater susceptibility of younger animals in some instances is a result of the immaturity of components of the host immune system.[106,134,181] After intracranial inoculation of newborn mice with the alphavirus, Sindbis, the virus replicates predominantly in neurons and causes a fatal encephalomyelitis.[122,145,259] In contrast, weanling mice given the same virus innoculum recover after a mild encephalitis. These results suggest that age-dependent cellular factors modulate the outcome of infections with Sindbis virus. It has been reported that Sindbis virus kills cells by inducing programmed cell death (apoptosis). Expression of the oncogene, bcl-2, can block Sindbis virus-induced apoptosis.[146] The resistance of cells from older animals has been correlated with the expression of higher levels of bcl-2 in older cells than in younger in cells (see Chap. 4). A single amino acid substitution in the Sindbis virus E2 glycoprotein confers to the virus both a neurovirulent phenotype and the ability to kill cells that express bcl-2.[265]

In other instances, only older animals are susceptible to disease. The appearance of specific differentiated viral target cells has in some cases been correlated with susceptibility.[22,71,81,94,120,121,198] In humans, susceptibility to encephalitis caused by St. Louis encephalitis virus increases with age. During an outbreak of this virus in 1964 in Houston, Texas, the serologic data indicated that infection rates were similar in all age groups but disease severity was much greater in those older than 60 years of age (Table 13-1).[104,161,190] It has been postulated that because the blood-brain barrier in persons older than 60 years of age is frequently imperfect, there is an increased risk that St. Louis encephalitis virus will gain entry into the brains of older individuals.

Males are more susceptible to some types of virus infections than are females,[158,289] but infections with a number of viruses are more severe in females during pregnancy.[11,59,299] This effect has been attributed to hormones. The experimental administration of either steroid or thyroid hormones has been shown to adversely affect the outcome of infections with a number of viruses.[115,116] The host's nutritional state can also affect the severity of a virus infection. Protein malnutrition has been reported to increase the severity of measles virus, coxsackievirus, and flavivirus infections.[52,53,68,182,290] Hypercholesterolemia can also increase the severity of some virus infections.[47] Vigorous exercise has been reported to increase the severity of poliovirus infection in humans[112] and coxsackievirus infection in mice.[84] The severity of influenza is increased in chronic smokers.[127]

GENETIC RESISTANCE

Individual variation in disease resistance among domesticated plants and animals has been observed by humans since ancient times. In many instances, these differences were inheritable and were used by farmers to develop resistant strains.[19,102,144,167,184,217] Most experimental studies on genetically controlled resistance to viruses in animals have been carried out with inbred mice, although some have utilized rats.[2,105] Mice are not only easy to breed, but a number of murine genes have already been identified, and many have been mapped to specific chromosome locations.[163] An effort is currently underway to sequence the entire mouse genome, and the information generated is likely to enhance our understanding of the molecular mechanisms by which various murine genes confer virus resistance.

Murine genes have been identified that specifically modulate the outcome of infections with a number of animal viruses (Table 13-2). Genes conferring resistance to both DNA viruses and plus-strand and minus-strand RNA viruses have been found. In many instances, alleles of a single locus are responsible for the differences observed between susceptible

TABLE 13-1. *Age-specific attack rates and infection frequencies for St. Louis Encephalitis (SLE) in Houston, Texas, 1964**

Age Group	Population	Cases	Rate per 100,000	Case-Fatality Rate per 100	Percent SLE Antibody
0–9	305,000	25	8	0	41
10–19	200,000	27	13	0	29
20–29	168,000	25	15	0	38
30–39	198,000	28	14	0	36
40–49	157,000	27	17	0	26
50–59	112,000	31	28	13	38
60+	103,000	80	78	27	25

*Attack rates are shown for Harris County, Texas, which includes the city of Houston. Antibody data are from a serologic study conducted 6 months after the epidemic and are shown for one heavily infected area in the center city (percentages are based on 16 to 55 sera tested per age group).
Data from Henderson et al, 1970[104]; Luby et al, 1967[161]; and Nathanson, 1990[190].

and resistant mouse strains, but sometimes two or more loci are involved. Each of the described murine resistance genes is probably a unique gene. When tested by breeding studies, several different virus resistance loci segregated independently.[12] Also, the resistance genes that have been mapped are located on different chromosomes (see Table 13-2), and only a few of the murine resistance genes map within the major histocompatibility locus. The dominant allele of a resistance gene can code for either resistance or susceptibility, although in a few instances codominance has been observed. The resistance phenotype of some genes can be observed only in animals, whereas for others the resistance phenotype can also be observed in tissue culture cells prepared from resistant animals.

The interaction between a resistance gene and a virus is specific, because each resistance gene influences infections with only some strains of a particular virus (e.g., mouse hepatitis virus [MHV]) or with only members of a particular virus family (e.g., flaviviruses, influenza A viruses). This virus-specific characteristic distinguishes genetically controlled resistance from other types of early host-defense mechanisms that are virus-nonspecific and implies that each resistance gene product interacts with a unique event characteristic of only one group of viruses. Such an interaction could occur at the level of virus entry into the cell, viral genome uncoating, translation or translocation of viral proteins, replication of viral nucleic acids, assembly of progeny virions, development of virally-induced disease, or virus transmission between cells or between hosts. Any step in a virus life cycle that depends on a cell protein could be rendered less efficient by an alteration in that cell protein. It is possible that such a change in a host protein may not greatly affect its cellular function. Most virus resistance genes identified in mice reduce the amount of virus synthesized but do not completely inhibit virus production. However, because less virus is produced from infected cells, the spread of infection is slower, virus-induced pathology is less severe, and the induced immune response is more effective in clearing the infection.

RESISTANCE TO MOUSE HEPATITIS VIRUS

Inbred mouse strains vary in their susceptibility to different isolates of MHV. Bang and Warwick[13] showed that C3H mice were resistant but Princeton Rockefeller (PRI) mice were susceptible to a lethal infection with MHV-2. Breeding studies demonstrated that susceptibility was caused by a single dominant gene, designated *Hv-1*. Twenty backcrosses were carried out to create congenic strains of resistant and susceptible mice.[279]

Resistant adult SJL/J mice evidence no signs of infection with the MHV strains JHM, MHV-S, or A59,[14,15,16,284] whereas BALB/c mice are susceptible to all three of these viruses. Susceptibility was shown to be controlled by a single dominant gene, designated *Hv-2*. This gene was subsequently mapped to chromosome 7 and shown to be linked to the *Svp-2* locus.[131,132,133,242] In vivo susceptibility to MHV correlates with the ability of MHV to replicate in cultured macrophages or other cell types from BALB/c mice, but not from SJL/J mice.[4] The cellular receptor for MHV has recently been shown to be a biliary glycoprotein (Bgp-1a), which is a member of the murine carcinoembryonic antigen superfamily.[73,88,282] A number of isoforms of the MHV receptor protein, which result

from alternative splicing events and have either two or four immunoglobulin-like extracellular domains and intracytoplasmic tails of varying lengths, have been identified and can serve as MHV receptors.[72,296] Although these proteins are found in a wide range of tissues, including liver and intestinal epithelium, the level of expression of the various isoforms varies greatly among cultured mouse cells.[233] Resistance of SJ2 mice MHV correlates with expression of a different allele of the HV receptor called Bgp1b. The MHV receptor gene has recently been shown to map to chromosome 7 (K.V. Holmes, University of Colorado Health Sciences Center, personal communication) and is now thought to be the *Hv-1* gene.

BALB/cJ, C57BL/6J, and DBA mice are fully susceptible to virulent MHV-3 and die of fulminant hepatitis, whereas semisusceptible mice (C3H/St, C3HeB/FeJ) develop acute hepatitis, which may progress to chronic liver disease.[65,278] Resistant A/J mice develop no liver disease, although virus replicates to comparable levels in both susceptible C57B1/6 and resistant A/J mice.[65,70,164,211,293] After MHV-3 infection, disease-susceptible mice spontaneously express increased levels of a T-lymphocyte–controlled monokine with macrophage procoagulant activity, but resistant A/J mice do not.[65,147] A pathogenic role for this monokine in the development of local damage in the liver has been demonstrated.[148,165]

Recombinant inbred (RI) strains of mice were used to further analyze MHV-3 resistance. RI mouse strains are generated by inbreeding pairs of mice from the F2 generation of a mating between preexisting inbred strains.[9] Because recombination occurs during meiosis, the chromosomes of each F2 mouse consist of blocks of genetic material from both parents. By inbreeding pairs of F2 mice, heterozygosity is diluted until, by the F20 generation, strains are estimated to be 99% homozygous. The genotype of each RI strain consists of a unique assortment of parental genes that are homozygous at every locus. When RI strains derived from susceptible C57BL/6J mice and resistant A/J progenitors were infected with MHV-3, one strain was fully resistant, four were fully susceptible, and 16 were intermediate in susceptibility. In the semisusceptible mice, a range of disease from mild focal hepatitis to widespread hepatocellular necrosis was observed. This pattern best fits a two-recessive-gene model of inheritance. Neither of these two loci was linked to the H-2 complex.[65] The expression of macrophage procoagulant activity segregated in a pattern that was identical with disease susceptibility. Procoagulant activity was elevated by sevenfold in fully susceptible mice and by fourfold in semisusceptible mice. These data suggest a genetic linkage between susceptibility to liver disease in MHV-3–infected animals and the increased expression of macrophage procoagulant activity. The mouse fibrinogen-like protein has recently been shown to have MHV-induced prothrombinase activity.[208] Additional genes may be involved in susceptibility to MHV-3–induced chronic neurologic disease.[149,256,257,272,291]

RESISTANCE TO INFLUENZA A VIRUSES

Whereas the majority of inbred mouse strains are susceptible to disease caused by pneumotropic, hepatotropic, and neurotropic strains of influenza A virus, A2G mice are resistant.[156,157] Analysis of the inheritance patterns of disease

TABLE 13-2. *Mouse genetic loci that influence virus susceptibility*

Virus	Disease or effect	No. of genes or designation	Dominant trait	Maps to H-2	Investigators
DNA VIRUSES					
Herpes simplex	Encephalitis	2+	R	–	Lopez, 1975[159]; Lopez, 1980[160]
Cytomegalovirus	Replication in spleen	Cmv-1	R	– (Ch. 6)*	Chalmer, 1980[50]; Chalmer et al, 1977[51]; Grundy et al, 1981[193]; Scalzo et al, 1992[236]
	Encephalitis	1+	S	+	Chalmer, 1980[50]; Chalmer et al, 1977[51]; Grundy et al, 1981[193]; Price et al, 1990[216]
Polyoma	Tumor induction	1	R	+	Chang and Hildemann, 1964[54]; Freund et al, 1992[80]
		1	S	–	Chang and Hildemann, 1964[54]; Freund et al, 1992[80]
	Runting	1+	R	–	Chang and Hildemann, 1964[54]
Ectromelia	Mouse pox	Rmp-1	R	–	Britt and Chesebro, 1983[43]; Brownstein et al, 1991[145]; Kees and Blanden, 1976[128]
		Rmp-2	R	– (Ch. 2)	Britt and Chesebro, 1983[43]; Brownstein et al, 1991[145]; Kees and Blanden, 1976[128]
		Rmp-3	R	+ (Ch. 17)	Britt and Chesebro, 1983[43]; Brownstein et al, 1991[145]; Kees and Blanden, 1976[128]
		Rmp-4	R	–	Britt and Chesebro, 1983[43]; Brownstein et al, 1991[145]; Kees and Blanden, 1976[128]
RNA VIRUSES					
Influenza A	Pneumonia	Mx	R	– (Ch. 16)	Lindenmann, 1964[155]; Staeheli et al, 1993[250]; Staeheli et al, 1986[251]
Flavivirus	Encephalitis	Flv	R	– (Ch. 5)	Sangster et al, 1994[231]; Shi et al, 1996[239]; Webster and Clow, 1936[276]
LDV	Polioencephalitis	1+	R	–	Martinez et al, 1980[168]
EMC	Diabetes	1	R	–	Onodera et al, 1978[203]
Rabies	Encephalitis	1	R	–	Lodmell, 1983[158]
Mouse hepatitis virus	Hepatitis	Musfbp	S	–	Parr et al, 1995[208]

Virus	Function	Gene	R/S	Chromosome*	References
	Death	Hv-1	S	–	Bang and Warwick, 1960[13]
	Receptor interaction	Hv-2	S	– (Ch. 7)	Barthold et al, 1986[15]; Dveksler et al, 1993[72]; Knobler et al, 1984[133]
MURINE LEUKEMIA VIRUSES					
Ecotropic FLV	Replication	Fv-1	R	– (Ch. 4)	Jolicoeur, 1979[123]; Pincus et al, 1975[213]; Yang et al, 1980[294]
Ecotropic	Replication	CV	S	–	Teich et al, 1982[260]
Ecotropic	Replication	Akv-1	S	–	Lilly et al, 1975[153]; Rowe, 1972[226]; Teich et al, 1982[260]
Xenotropic(?)	Replication	Akv-2	S	–	Lilly et al, 1975[153]; Rowe, 1972[226]; Teich et al, 1982[260]
Xenotropic	Replication	hr.	S	–	Blank and Klyczek, 1986[28]; Greene et al, 1980[90]
Xenotropic	Replication	BXV	S	–	Teich et al, 1982[260]
Xenotropic	High replication	Nzv-1	S	–	Teich et al, 1982[260]
Xenotropic	Low replication	Nzv-2	S	–	Teich et al, 1982[260]
FLV	Focus formation	Fv-2	S	– (Ch. 9)	Kozak et al, 1993[136]; Lilly, 1970[151]; Wettstein and Blank, 1982[282]
FLV	Suppressed lymphocyte proliferation	Fv-3	—	–	Kumar and Bennett, 1976[138]
FLV	Replication of helper	Fv-4	R	– (Ch. 12)	Odaka et al, 1981[197]; Teich et al, 1982[260]
FLV	Anemia or polycythemia	Fv-5	—	–	Teich et al, 1982[260]
FLV	Generation of recombinants	Fv-6	R	–	Teich et al, 1982[260]
FLV	Recovery from splenomegaly	Rfv-1	R/S	+	Britt and Chesebro, 1980[42]; Britt and Chesebro, 1983[43]; Chesebro et al, 1990[56]; Chesebro and Wehrly, 1978[57]
FLV	Recovery from splenomegaly	Rfv-2	R/S	+	Chesebro and Wehrly, 1978[57]; Miyazawa et al, 1992[179]; Miyazawa et al, 1992[180]
FLV	Recovery from splenomegaly	Rfv-3	R	–	Chesebro et al, 1974[58]; Doig and Chesebro, 1979[67]
GLV	Recovery from leukemia	Rgv-1	R	+	Aoki et al, 1966[3]; Blank and Klyczek, 1986[28]
GLV	Recovery from leukemia	Rgv-2	R	–	Blank and Klyczek, 1986[28]; Teich et al, 1982[260]
WM 1504 E	Slow disease of CNS	2	R	–	Oldstone et al, 1980[199]

R, resistance; S, susceptibility; LDV, lactate dehydrogenase elevating virus; EMC encephalomyocarditis virus; FLV, Friend leukemia virus; GLV, Gross leukemia virus.
*Chromosome number (modified from Brinton et al, 1984[38]).

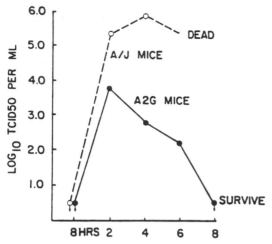

Fig. 13-1. Comparison of the growth of neurotropic influenza virus (A$_o$/WSN) in the brains of adult susceptible A/J and resistant A2G mice. The virus inoculum (70 times the median lethal dose [LD50]) was given by the intracerebral route. All of the A/J mice died from the infection, whereas 100% of the A2G mice survived. Although similar amounts of virus were required to initiate infection in the two strains of mice, the amount of virus produced in A2G brain tissue was always at least 100-fold less than the amount produced in A/J tissue. (Data from Fiske RA, Klein PA. Effect of immunosuppression on the genetic resistance of A2G mice to neurovirulent influenza virus. Infect Immun 1975;11:576–586.)

susceptibility among F1 and F2 progeny produced from a mating between resistant A2G and susceptible A/J mice showed that resistance to influenza A viruses is controlled by a single autosomal dominant allele, designated *Mx* (for myxovirus).[95,157] Although comparable amounts of virus are required to initiate infection in A2G and A/J mice, the amount of virus produced in A2G tissues is always at least 100 times lower (Fig. 13-1) than in the tissues of A/J mice.[76] Brain parenchyma cells from A2G mice bound influenza virions as efficiently as cells from suscep-

tible (A/J) animals, indicating that cells from resistant animals contain receptors for influenza A virus.

Induction of Mx Expression Depends on Interferon

Data from three types of experiments indicate that the immune system does not play a role in the phenotypic expression of resistance to influenza A virus. Immunosuppression by cyclophosphamide treatment or x-irradiation did not alter the resistance of A2G mice to intracerebral inoculation of the neurotropic influenza A virus strain, WSN, nor did it increase the level of virus replication in the brains of treated A2G mice.[76] A2G mice that had been thymectomized either as newborns or adults and were unable to mount an immune response to influenza virus were also resistant to intracerebral inoculation of WSN. Seventy-five percent of the F2 progeny of crosses between A2G and nude mice were resistant to influenza virus–induced disease despite their T-cell deficiency.[98]

The first clue to understanding the virus resistance phenotype induced by the *Mx* allele came from studies with cultured peritoneal macrophages. A2G macrophages produced low yields of influenza A virus if infected during the first 2 weeks in culture, whereas A2G macrophages infected after 2 weeks in culture efficiently replicated influenza A virus. This alteration in susceptibility was correlated with the disappearance of interferon.[96] Subsequently, injection of antiinterferon antibody was shown to render A2G mice susceptible to challenge with a lethal dose of influenza A virus (Table 13-3). Virus titers in the tissues of A2G mice or F1 (A2G × A/J) hybrid mice given antiinterferon antibody were equal to those observed in susceptible A/J mice. Interferon had not initially been thought to play a role in A2G resistance to influenza virus–induced disease, because the interferon levels in the brains of infected A2G mice were three to five times lower than in the brains of infected A/J mice. This is not unexpected, because the amount of interferon induced by a virus infection usually correlates closely with the level of virus replication.[191] Apparently, it was the antiviral effect of the interferon in A2G mice rather than the amount of interferon present that was important for the expression of the influenza A virus resistance phenotype.

TABLE 13-3. *Abrogation of resistance to hepatotropic influenza virus in mice by antiinterferon serum (AIF)*

Mouse strain	Genotype	Treatment*	Mortality	Log$_{10}$ EID50 No. per milliliter of blood
A/J	r/r	None	4/4	6.0
		AIF	4/4	6.0
A2G	R/R	None	0/4	3.7
		AIF	4/4	6.3
F1	R/r	None	0/4	3.5
		AIF	4/4	6.5

R, resistant; r, susceptible; EID50, egg median infectious dose.

*Mice were treated with AIF just before intraperitoneal infection with 10^4 LD50 of influenza A/Turkey/England 63. Blood pooled from five mice was titrated 2 days after infection.

Data from Haller O, Arnheiter H, Lindenmann J, Gresser I. Host gene influences sensitivity to interferon action selectively for influenza virus. Nature 1980;283:660–662.

Further experiments with cultured A2G macrophages linked the phenotypic expression of resistance to influenza A virus to the presence of interferon type 1, a mixture of α- and β-interferon, rather than to γ-interferon.[97,248] Smaller amounts of interferon were required to protect 2-week-old A2G peritoneal macrophage cultures than susceptible A/J cultures from influenza A infection. However, this difference in sensitivity to the antiviral effect of interferon was limited to influenza A viruses, because A2G and A/J macrophages, hepatocytes, and brain cells showed identical antiviral responses after interferon treatment if infected with other types of viruses.[5,96,97]

Identification of the Mx Gene Product

Interferon is an important cell regulatory protein that affects cell growth, cell differentiation, and the immune response to viruses.[212,228] Interferon treatment of animal cells can result in increased expression of almost 50 different cellular genes. Biochemical functions for almost two dozen of these have been identified.[228] Interferon also causes decreased expression of a limited number of cellular genes, including c-myc, the μ chain of immunoglobulin M, and collagen.[262]

A 72.5-kD protein that was detected by two-dimensional gel electrophoresis in cytoplasmic extracts from interferon-treated A2G cells was not detected in extracts from interferon-treated A/J cells.[111] Further, when the A2G Mx allele was backcrossed into a number of different susceptible murine genetic backgrounds, interferon inducibility of the 72.5-kD protein cosegregated with the influenza resistance phenotype of the Mx allele, confirming an association between the presence of this protein and resistance to influenza A virus infection. Because susceptible cells did not appear to produce the 72.5-kD protein, susceptible cells were designated Mx−, and resistant cells were designated Mx+. Polyclonal and monoclonal antibodies were produced to the 72.5-kD Mx protein by immunization of Mx− mice with extracts of congenic Mx+ cells that had been stimulated with interferon.[244] With these antibodies, the Mx protein was detected in the nuclei of interferon-treated cultured Mx+ cells[69] as well as in the nuclei of cells in tissue sections from interferon-treated A2G mice.[292]

To determine whether resistance to influenza resulted solely from the expression of the Mx protein or whether additional interferon-induced proteins were also required, the Mx+ gene was cloned and sequenced.[247] Poly A+ RNA from interferon-treated Mx+ cells was size-fractionated on a methylmercury agarose gel, and the RNA in each fraction was used in in vitro translation reactions. The products of these reactions were then precipitated with anti-Mx antibody. The Mx protein was found in fractions that contained an mRNA of about 3 kb. The mRNA in these fractions was then copied into cDNA and cloned. The resulting cDNA library was screened by differential colony hybridization using cDNA probes made from 3-kb mRNA fractionated from either interferon-treated Mx+ cells or interferon-treated Mx− cells. Two of 10,000 clones screened hybridized only to the probe from the Mx+ cells.[247] The mouse Mx protein is composed of 631 amino acids and is expressed from a 3.5-kb mRNA. No homology was found between any proteins in the databases and the Mx protein. If Mx− NIH 3T3 cells were transformed with Mx+ cDNA, they constitutively expressed the 72.5-kD Mx protein and displayed resistance to influenza

A virus.[247] Southern blot analysis showed that Mx− inbred mouse strains contained deleted forms of the Mx allele. The Mx+ gene (redesignated as Mx1) and the Mx− gene (redesignated Mx2) shared a high degree of sequence similarity. In cells from some inbred mouse strains, the Mx2 gene did not respond to interferon and no Mx2 mRNA was detected, whereas other mouse strains synthesized Mx2 mRNA in response to interferon treatment.[252] However, the levels of Mx2 mRNA produced were 15-fold lower than in interferon-treated Mx+ cells, possibly because of a decreased stability of the mutant mRNA.

Three distinct patterns of restriction fragment length polymorphism were observed in Mx− mice. Further analysis showed that most Mx− mice contained a large deletion in the coding region of the Mx gene. Sometimes this deletion was 423 nucleotides in length and included exons 9, 10, and 11, but often the deletion was longer and included sequences flanking these three exons.[245] In CBA/J and two other Mx− strains, a point mutation was present at position 1378 that converted the lysine codon to a termination codon (Fig. 13-2).

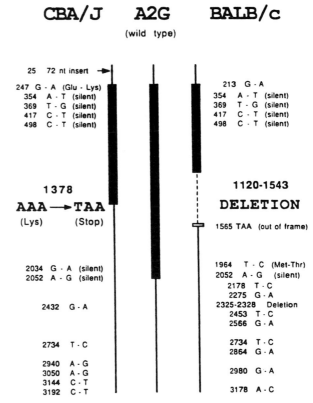

Fig. 13-2. Comparison of the complementary DNAs (cDNAs) for the Mx gene from influenza-resistant A2G mice and susceptible BALB/c and CBA/J mice. The changes found in the CBA/J cDNA are listed on the left and those in the BALB/c cDNA on the right. All strains of susceptible (Mx) mice contain either a deletion or a point mutation that truncates the coding region of the Mx protein. None of the susceptible mice produces an Mx protein that confers resistance to influenza virus. (Data from Staeheli P, Grob R, Meier E, et al. Influenza virus-susceptible mice carry Mx genes with a large deletion or a nonsense mutation. Mol Cell Biol 1988;8:4518–4523.)

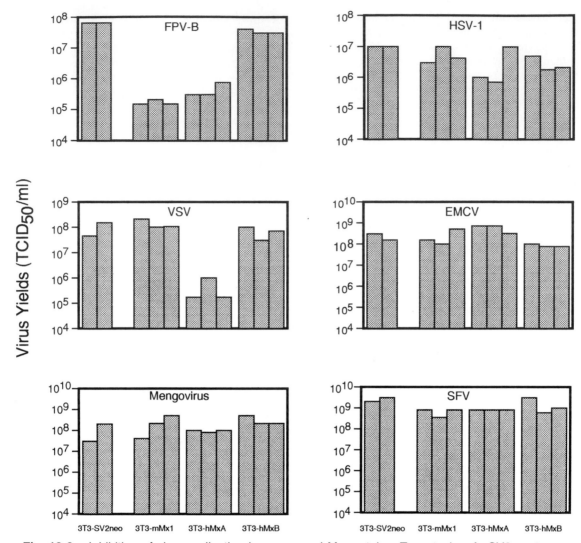

Fig. 13-3. Inhibition of virus replication by expressed Mx proteins. Two stocks of pSV2neo-transfected 3T3 (influenza A–susceptible) mouse cells or individual clonal lines of 3T3-mMx1, 3T3-hMxA, or 3T3-hMxB cells were infected with 1 plaque-forming unit per cell of either influenza A virus (FPV-B), vesicular stomatitis virus (VSV), Mengo virus, Semliki Forest virus (SFV), encephalomyocarditis virus (EMCV), or herpes simplex virus, type 1 (HSV-1). The virus titers in the culture fluids were assayed 24 hours after infection. Only the mouse Mx1 and the human MxA inhibited influenza virus replication. The human MxA protein also inhibited the replication of the rhabdovirus, VSV. The replication of the other viruses was unaffected by the expression of the Mx proteins. $TCID_{50}$, median tissue culture infectious dose; mMX1, the mouse Mx protein that confers influenza resistance; hMxA and hMxB, two different human homologs of the mouse Mx1 protein; pSV2neo, control plasmid expressing a marker gene that was cotransfected with the various *Mx* gene plasmids. (Data from Pavlovic J, Zürcher T, Haller O, Staeheli P. Resistance to influenza virus and vesicular stomatitis virus conferred by expression of human MxA protein. J Virol 1990;64:3370–3375.)

However, the expected truncated translation products from the various *Mx−* genes were not detected in cells or tissues of interferon-treated mice.[245] Correction of the point mutation that created the premature stop codon by site-directed mutagenesis resulted in the expression of an 80-kD cytoplasmic protein in transfected NIH 3T3 cells that cross-reacted with *Mx1* antibodies.[301] This Mx2 protein conferred a high degree of resistance to the rhabdovirus, vesicular stomatitis virus (VSV), but conferred no resistance to influenza A virus.

Mx Homologs Found in Other Species

Homologs of the Mx protein have been detected in every mammalian species analyzed to date. The expression of Mx proteins can be induced not only by α- and β-interferon but also by double-stranded RNA and by some viruses.[86,114] Mx genes have also been found in birds[20] and fish.[253] Often, a small family of interferon-inducible *Mx* genes are present. All of the Mx proteins have molecular masses of about 70 to 80 kD. The N-terminal regions of the various Mx proteins show a high degree of sequence conservation, suggesting the presence of a functional domain in this region. In contrast, the sequences of the C-terminal regions of the Mx proteins vary considerably.[1]

Mouse Mx protein antibody detected an 80-kD homolog in human cells that was also induced by α- and β- interferon but not by γ-interferon. However, unlike the mouse Mx protein, which localizes in the nucleus, the human protein (designed MxA) was found in the cytoplasm.[246] Subsequently, human cells were found to express two interferon-induced proteins with homology to the mouse Mx protein, MxA and MxB.[210] Both human Mx proteins accumulated in the cytoplasm. In interferon-treated diploid human embryonic lung cells, the MxA protein represented 0.5% to 1% of the total cytosolic protein.[108] Expression of human MxA in transfected mouse NIH 3T3 cells conferred an influenza A–resistant phenotype but had no effect on the replication of two picornaviruses, an alpha togavirus, or herpes simplex virus type 1. MxA also conferred resistance to VSV. In contrast, NIH 3T3 cells transfected with the human MxB gene were not resistant to either influenza or VSV (Fig. 13-3). A Gluto-Arg substitution at amino acid residue 645 in the MxA protein produced a mutant protein that still had antiviral activity to influenza virus but no longer had antiviral activity to VSV.[300] This evidence suggests that a domain near the carboxyl-terminal end is responsible for the VSV-specific antiviral activity and that the influenza and VSV antiviral activities are distinct and are controlled by separate domains in the MxA protein. Analysis of the localization and antiviral activity of 14 mutant Mx1 proteins with mutations in different regions indicated that multiple domains of the Mx protein, not just the C-terminal region, are required for antiviral activity and the characteristic focal nuclear distribution of this protein.[83]

The Mx proteins of humans and most other mammals normally localize in the cytoplasm,[209] whereas the Mx proteins of mice,[69] rats,[172,173] hamsters, and guinea pigs[109] accumulate in the nucleus (Fig. 13-4). Analysis of transiently expressed Mx1 proteins with various carboxyl-terminal truncations suggests that nuclear localization of this protein is mediated by an SV40 T antigen–like nuclear targeting signal.[193] Mouse Mx1 proteins with mutations in the C-terminal nuclear localization signal accumulated in the cytoplasm but conferred no antiviral activity against influenza A virus in that location.[193] In contrast, MxA proteins to which a nuclear targeting signal was added accumulated in the nucleus and retained their anti-influenza activity.[193]

Recent studies have shown that murine *Mx1*-mediated resistance extends to two tickborne orthomyxoviruses, Thogoto and Dhori, that infect humans, livestock, and rodents in Africa, Asia, and Europe.[79] Human MxA confers resistance in mice to Thogoto virus but not to Dhori virus.[261]

Mapping of the *Mx* Gene

Forty-eight known murine genetic markers were analyzed by classic breeding studies for possible linkage to the *Mx* gene. Although these markers were widely distributed over the mouse chromosomes and represented almost the entire mouse genome except for chromosome 16, no linkage to the *Mx* gene was observed.[251] The availability of mouse-hamster somatic cell hybrids as well as a cDNA probe for the *Mx* gene[251] offered an alternative means for mapping the chromosome location of *Mx*. The mouse-hamster hybrids were made from the BALB/c cell line Meth A and the Chinese hamster cell line E36. Genomic Southern blots performed on *Eco* RI–digested liver DNA from *Mx*− BALB/c mice detected three major fragments of 2.5, 4, and 10 kb when probed with a 1.65-kb Bam HI fragment of the *Mx* gene.[251] In contrast, the *Mx* probe only weakly detected several fragments of *Eco* RI–digested hamster E36 cell DNA.[251] In only three of nine hybrid cell lines were both mouse-specific and hamster-specific hybridization fragments detected with the *Mx* probe. One of these cell lines contained only mouse chromosomes 16 and X. Analysis of the concordance of the *Mx* gene signal with particular chromosomes revealed unambiguously that the *Mx* gene mapped to mouse chromosome 16 (Table 13-4).[251]

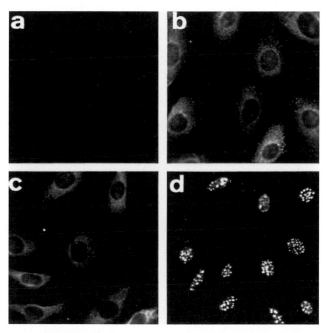

Fig. 13-4. Localization of expressed Mx proteins in transfected Swiss 3T3 cells by direct immunofluorescence. The Mx1 protein of mice accumulates in the nucleus, whereas both of the Mx proteins of humans accumulate in the cytoplasm. (**A**) Control 3T3-SV2neo cells immunostained with mouse antiserum to a β-galactosidase–MxA fusion protein. The control plasmid pSV2neo expresses a marker gene that was cotransfected with the various *Mx* gene plasmids. (**B**) A clone of 3T3 cells expressing human MxB stained with the same antibody as in **A**. (**C**) A clone of 3T3 cells expressing human MxB stained with mouse antiserum to a β-galactosidase–MxB fusion protein. (**D**) A clone of 3T3 cells expressing mouse Mx1 stained with rabbit antiserum to a synthetic peptide consisting of the 16 C-terminal amino acids of mouse Mx1. (Data from Pavlovic J, Zürcher T, Haller O, Staeheli P. Resistance to influenza virus and vesicular stomatitis virus conferred by expression of human MxA protein. J Virol 1990;64:3370–3375.)

TABLE 13-4. *Cosegregation of* Mx *and chromosome 16 in hamster-mouse hybrid cell lines**

Mouse chromosome	Concordance (No. hybrids)		Disconcordance (No. hybrids)		% Concordance
	+/+	-/-	+/-	-/+	
1	0	3	3	3	33
2	2	3	3	1	55
3	0	4	2	3	44
4	0	4	2	3	44
5	1	6	0	2	77
6	0	3	2	2	43†
7	1	3	3	2	44
8	0	4	2	2	50†
9	0	4	2	3	44
10	1	5	1	2	66
11	0	5	1	3	55
12	2	2	4	1	44
13	1	3	3	2	44
14	1	4	2	2	55
15	2	4	2	1	66
16	3	6	0	0	100
17	1	3	3	2	44
18	1	4	2	2	55
19	2	3	3	1	55
X	2	1	5	1	33

*For example, the first line is read as follows: no hybrids contain chromosome 1 and *Mx* (+/+), three hybrids lack chromosome 1 and also lack *Mx* (-/-), three hybrids contain chromosome 1 but lack *Mx* (+/-), and three hybrids lack chromosome 1 but contain *Mx* (-/+). The results indicate that the *Mx* gene is located on chromosome 16.

†Rearranged chromosomes 6 and 8 found in some hybrid cell lines were not included in the calculations.

Data from Staeheli P, Prautcheva D, Lundin L-G, et al. Interferon-regulated influenza virus resistance gene *Mx* is located on mouse chromosome 16. J Virol 1986;58:967–969.

With human cells, the *Mx* genes have been mapped to human chromosome 21.[139]

Characteristics of the Mx Protein

Purification of Mx proteins under nondenaturing conditions has been difficult because they tend to form insoluble aggregates. This difficulty has been partially overcome with buffers containing glycerol, nonionic detergents, or polyethylene glycol.[174] Crosslinking experiments suggest that Mx proteins form trimers in vivo. A leucine-zipper motif located near the C-terminal end is thought to mediate Mx protein oligomerization.[174] Large amounts of histidine-tagged recombinant Mx protein have been purified successfully under nondenaturing conditions after expression in *Escherichia coli*.[250]

Analysis of the sequences of the cloned *Mx* genes revealed an N-terminal tripartite sequence motif[64] commonly found in proteins that bind and hydrolyze guanosine triphosphate (GTP; Fig. 13-5). Subsequently, both the mouse Mx1 and human MxA proteins were shown to have GTPase activity. The rates of GTP hydrolysis carried out by purified Mx proteins have been estimated to range from 10 to 100 molecules per minute.[108,187] GTP binding to the Mx protein has been demonstrated by ultraviolet (UV) light–induced crosslinking experiments.[187] Compared with most GTPases, the Mx proteins require a relatively high concentration of substrate for a maximum rate of GTP hydrolysis, have relatively low binding affinities for GTP and guanosine diphosphate (GDP), and in vitro can carry out multiple rounds of GTP hydrolysis in the absence of guanine-nucleotide-exchange factors or GTPase-activating proteins.[250]

The Mx proteins show some similarity to the yeast proteins, VPS1 and MGM1,[219,295] to rat dynamin,[196] and to the gene product of the *shibire* gene of *Drosophila melanogaster*.[55] Each of these proteins contains a tripartite GTP-binding consensus motif located in the N-terminal region (see Fig. 13-5) that shares significant sequence homology with the GTP-binding domain in Mx proteins. Also, each of these proteins displays a very high intrinsic GTP hydrolysis rate and can carry out multiple cycles of GTP hydrolysis in the absence of accessory factors. The 80-kD VPS1 protein displays a punctate cytoplasmic distribution and is thought to be associated with the Golgi apparatus and involved in vacuolar protein sorting.[271] The MGM1 protein is involved in maintaining the yeast mitochondrial genome.[125] Rat dynamin is a microtubule-

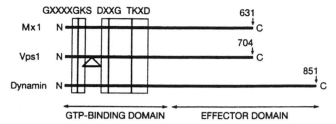

Fig. 13-5. A schematic drawing of the functionally important regions of mouse Mx1, yeast VPS1, and rat dynamin. The regions of highest homology among the three proteins are boxed. The vertical bars within these boxes indicate the relative positions of the three parts of the sequence motif commonly found in proteins that bind or hydrolyze guanosine triphosphate (GTP). The conserved amino acids of this motif are shown at the top of the drawing. (Data from Dever TE, Glynias MJ, Merrich WC. GTP-binding domain: three consensus sequence elements with distinct spacing. Proc Natl Acad Sci U S A 1987;84:1814–1818; and Staeheli P, Pitossi F, Pavlovic J. Mx proteins: GTPases with antiviral activity. Trends Cell Biol 1993;3:268–272.)

associated protein that may be involved in the initial stages of endocytosis.[195,268] The C-terminal region of dynamin appears to mediate its association with an unidentified component of the endocytotic machinery. The *Drosophila shibire* gene product is a homolog of mammalian dynamin and is involved in the formation of coated and noncoated vesicles at the plasma membrane.[55,129,269] Although the Mx, VPS1, and dynamin proteins are very similar in the organization of their functional domains, with the N-terminal domain providing GTP-binding and -hydrolysis activity and the C-terminal domain probably mediating association with another cell component, these proteins each carry out unique functions and cannot complement each other.[250] The Mx protein is the only one of these proteins whose synthesis is regulated by interferon.

Mechanism of Mx Resistance

Although the gene product of the murine *Mx* gene has been identified and characterized and its antiinfluenza activity has been well established, the mechanism by which the Mx protein interferes with influenza virus replication is not yet well understood. The RNA genome of influenza virus is single-stranded, segmented, and of negative polarity. Influenza virions enter a cell by means of receptor-mediated endocytosis and are uncoated in the cytoplasm. The released viral nucleocapsids then migrate to the nucleus, where the viral genome RNAs are transcribed into mRNAs by the virion-associated RNA-dependent RNA polymerase, a process known as primary transcription. Primary transcription involves the "stealing" of 5' capped sequences from cellular pre-mRNAs. Replication of the genome to complementary positive strands, and replication of these in turn to new genome RNAs, occurs only after viral proteins translated from the viral mRNAs have returned to the nucleus. The newly synthesized genome RNAs form complexes with viral proteins, and these migrate to the cytoplasm, where they are

packaged into virions by a process involving budding through the plasma membrane.[130]

The Mx1 protein does not interfere with the attachment, entry, or uncoating steps of the influenza virus replication cycle, nor with transport of the nucleocapsids to the nucleus.[44,110,177] However, the concentrations of the primary transcripts encoding the three viral polymerase proteins, PB1, PB2, and PA, were reduced by 50-fold or more in infected cells expressing the Mx1 protein. The accumulation of the other viral mRNAs was also inhibited, but to a lesser degree.[137,209] Both the mouse Mx1 protein and the human MxA protein inhibit influenza virus replication, even though these two proteins localize to different regions of the cell; the human MxA protein accumulates in the cytoplasm, whereas the murine Mx1 protein accumulates in the nucleus.[209] In cells expressing cytoplasmic MxA protein, all of the viral mRNAs accumulated at normal levels in the nucleus and were polyadenylated and translationally active in an in vitro translation system. However, even though the viral mRNAs were efficiently transported to the cytoplasm, viral protein synthesis was strongly inhibited and the reduction in viral protein synthesis resulted in a significant decrease in the synthesis of progeny genome RNA. The MxA protein could interfere with either the transport of viral mRNAs within the cytoplasm, the translation of viral mRNAs, or the translocation of viral proteins from the cytoplasm to the nucleus.[209] MxA probably does not inhibit protein synthesis, because influenza virus proteins were efficiently translated after MxA-expressing cells were transfected with plasmid vectors encoding influenza proteins.[209] However, the observation that mutant MxA protein, which accumulated in the nucleus because of an added nuclear transport signal, inhibits influenza A virus primary transcription, as does the Mx1 protein, suggests a common mechanism of inhibition by MxA in both the cytoplasmic and nuclear locations.[300] Although the MxA protein also inhibits VSV at the primary transcription step, this activity maps to a different region of the MxA protein than the influenza inhibitory activity, and it therefore seems likely that the mechanisms of inhibition of VSV and influenza primary transcription by Mx are distinct.[249]

To determine whether the GTPase activity of Mx proteins is required for their antiviral activity, mutations were introduced into the conserved N-terminal consensus sequences (see Fig. 13-5) of the mouse Mx1 and human MxA proteins. A strict correlation was observed between the GTPase activity of these proteins in vitro and their antiviral activity in transfected 3T3 cells,[250] indicating that Mx proteins exert their antiviral effect through a GTP/GDP-dependent mechanism. Because all of the mutants lost both their ability to bind to GTP and their ability to hydrolyze it, it is possible that the binding of GTP to the Mx protein may cause a conformational change necessary for its activity.

One study, which showed that the inhibitory effect of the Mx1 protein on influenza virus replication could be overcome by overexpression of the three viral polymerase proteins, PB1, PB2, and PA, and, to a lesser extent, by the PB2 protein alone, suggests that the Mx1 protein interacts with a component of the influenza viral polymerase complex.[113] Mx1 may form a complex with PB2, preventing it from binding to the other polymerase components or to the template RNA. Alternatively, Mx may compete with the PB2 protein for its normal site on the viral polymerase complex.[250] Cell proteins have recently been reported that may play important roles during influenza virus replication. The cell NPI-1 protein can bind to the influenza A virus nucleocapsid protein and may function by tethering viral RNPs to nuclear membranes.[202] Two cell proteins that bind to influenza virus polymerase components and may function as part of the influenza virus polymerase complex have been reported.[201] Further analysis of the components and functions of the influenza virus polymerase complex is necessary before the precise mechanism by which the Mx protein inhibits influenza mRNA synthesis can be described.

Although it is not known what cellular function Mx proteins provide, it is likely that they do provide a cellular function, because a number of the Mx proteins identified have no antiviral activity. If Mx proteins functioned by altering protein trafficking in the host cell, they could be expected to be active against a broad spectrum of viruses, but this is not the case. Instead, some of the Mx proteins have mutations that enable them to interact with a polymerase component or RNA of influenza A virus and, in some cases, also with a component of VSV in addition to or instead of their normal cellular targets, which may be a fortuitous activity.[6] Because the synthesis of the Mx protein is controlled by interferon in all vertebrates, its cellular function is apparently needed only transiently. Since interferon is an important cellular regulatory protein that affects a variety of cell processes, ranging from cell growth and differentiation to the regulation of the immune response to viruses,[212,228] the control of Mx synthesis by interferon does not imply that this protein functions solely in an antiviral capacity.

Development of Influenza-Resistant Animals

Both chickens and pigs are susceptible to influenza virus epidemics. As a means of improving the disease resistance of economically important farm animals, the production of murine Mx1 transgenic pigs was attempted. Although two transgenic pig lines that expressed interferon-inducible mouse Mx1 mRNA were established, none of the transgenic animals expressed detectable levels of Mx1 protein, possibly because of a spontaneous mutation in the coding region.[185] All attempts to produce transgenic pigs constitutively expressing Mx1 were unsuccessful. It was possible to produce transgenic mice that constitutively expressed the Mx1 protein, but the level of resistance achieved in these animals was at best two thirds of that seen in A2G mice after interferon induction. A2G mice efficiently express Mx1 in all organs of the body. In contrast, constitutive expression of Mx1 in transgenic mice was organ restricted and did not provide an increased level of virus resistance.[135] Also, constitutive Mx1 protein synthesis was suppressed in transgenic mice after a few months, suggesting that constitutive expression was not well tolerated.[135] To successfully develop transgenic influenza-resistant farm animals, it will probably be necessary to use an endogenous Mx promotor that is tightly regulated during embryonic development. Ideally, this promotor should produce high levels of Mx protein when induced by interferon, irrespective of its chromosomal integration site.

RESISTANCE TO FLAVIVIRUSES

Studies conducted in the early 1920s[273] demonstrated that individuals within a stock of randomly bred mice varied greatly in their susceptibility to *Bacillus enteriditis* and louping ill virus. By selection and inbreeding, bacteria-resistant and bacteria-susceptible strains as well as virus-resistant and virus-susceptible mouse strains were developed.[274] Bacterial and viral resistance segregated independently.[275] The virus resistance phenotype was inherited as a simple autosomal dominant allele.[162,275] Mice that were resistant to louping ill virus were subsequently shown to be resistant to mosquito-borne St. Louis encephalitis virus[275] and to tickborne Russian spring-summer virus[49] as well. It was not known until 10 years later that all of these viruses are flaviviruses.[225] Subsequently, mice carrying this virus resistance gene were reported to be resistant to six additional flaviviruses.[62,118,230] Although this resistance is active against both mosquito-borne and tickborne flaviviruses, it does not extend to other types of viruses.

Genetically controlled resistance to the flavivirus, yellow fever virus (YFV), was independently observed among randomly bred Rockefeller Institute mice,[234] in randomly bred "Det" mice,[162] and in PRI mice.[224,223] A dominant allele conferring resistance to flaviviruses was also identified in wild mice by backcrossing wild mice from Maryland and California in the United States (Table 13-5)[62] and from Australia[230] with susceptible C3H/He mice. All commonly used inbred laboratory mouse strains are susceptible to flavivirus infection, but most of these were developed from a small number of progenitors and represent only a selected pool of murine alleles. The *Flv^r* gene from the donor strain PRI was introduced onto the C3H/He background to produce the congenic inbred C3H/RV strain by a standard backcross protocol consisting

TABLE 13-5. *Resistance of wild* Mus musculus *to yellow fever virus (YFV)**

Type of mouse	Number tested	% Mortality
Wild (Maryland)†	10	20
Wild (Soledad, CA)‡	5	0
Wild (LaPuenta, CA)‡	5	0
Wild (Devonshire, CA)‡	5	0
C3H/RV	34	0
C3H/He	38	100
F1 (Wild x C3H/He)	91	45
F2 (F1 x C3H/He)§	41	17

*Mice were injected intracerebrally with 0.03 mL of undiluted 17D-YFV vaccine. Some individuals in each of the wild populations tested had a dominant gene for flavivirus resistance.

†Third and fourth generation randomly bred wild mice.

‡Location where mice were trapped.

§The F2 animals were from matings with F1 animals that had survived challenge with YFV.

Data from Darnell MB, Koprowski H, Lagerspetz K. Genetically determined resistance to infection with group B arboviruses. I. Distribution of the resistance gene among various mouse populations and characteristics of gene expression in vivo. J Infect Dis 1974;129:240–247.

TABLE 13-6. *Resistance of inbred mouse strains to challenge with Murray Valley encephalitis (MVE) and yellow fever (YF) viruses*

Mouse strain	Virus strain used for challenge*	% Mortality (no. dead/no. infected)	No. days to death (mean ± SEM)
CASA/Rk	MVE virus OR2	15 (2/13)	17, 20†
	YF virus 17D	0 (0/14)	—
CAST/Ei	MVE virus OR2	0 (0/5)	—
	YF virus 17D	0 (0/3)	—
MOLD/Rk	MVE virus OR2	100 (20/20)	9.9 ± 0.3
	YF virus 17D	4 (1/26)	16
C3H/HeJ	MVE virus OR2	100 (9/9)	7.9 ± 0.4
	YF virus 17D	85 (11/13)	13.6 ± 0.6
C3H/RV	MVE virus OR2	0 (0/14)	—
	YF virus 17D	0 (0/12)	—

*Adult mice were infected intracerebrally with virus doses of 10^3 intracerebral LD50 for C3H/HeJ mice. The CASA/Rk, CAST/Ei and C3H/RV mice were resistant to flaviviruses.
†The number of days to death for each mouse is shown.
Data from Sangster MY, Heliams DB, Mackenzie JS, Shellam GR. Genetic studies of flavivirus resistance in inbred strains derived from wild mice: evidence for a new resistance allele at the flavivirus resistance locus (*Flv*). J Virol 1993;67:340–347.

of nine backcross generations and selection at each generation for the resistance phenotype.[91] Three additional inbred flavivirus-resistant mouse strains, CASA/Rk, CAST/Ei, and MOLD/Rk, have recently been established from wild Australian mice that displayed a flavivirus resistance phenotype (Table 13-6).[229] Whereas flavivirus resistance in CASA/Rk and CAST/Ei mice is conferred by a single autosomal dominant allele that is essentially identical to the *Flv^r* allele of C3H/RV, the intermediate resistance phenotype observed in the MOLD/Rk strain is conferred by a different allele at the *Flv* locus, designated *Flv^mr* to indicate minor resistance to flavivirus infection.[229]

Chromosomal Mapping of the Resistance Gene

During studies to map the murine gene that controls natural resistance to *Rickettsia tsutsugamushi*, which causes experimental scrub typhus in mice, the C3H/HeJ strain and the flavivirus resistant congenic strain, C3H/RV, were shown to carry different alleles, *Ric^s* and *Ric^r*, respectively, at the *Ric* locus on chromosome 5.[92,119] A second difference between congenic C3H/RV and C3H/HeJ mice was subsequently identified at the chromosome 5 *rd* locus, which is tightly linked to the *Ric* locus.[92,163] The C3H/RV mice carry the wild-type *rd* allele, whereas the C3H/HeJ mice carry the recessive, defective allele of this gene, which causes retinal degeneration.[32,141] Retinal degeneration is caused by a defect in the β subunit of the rod photoreceptor cGMP-phosphodiesterase,[32] and this defect can be detected histologically. Because the C3H/RV mice are congenic with C3H/HeJ mice and were selected for flavivirus resistance, the observed differences between C3H/HeJ and congenic C3H/RV mice at the two loci, *rd* and *Ric*, on chromosome 5 suggests that these genes are linked to the flavivirus resistance gene *Flv^r*. To confirm the chromosome 5 lo-

cation of the *Flv* gene, three-point backcross linkage analyses were performed to define the map position of *Flv^r* relative to four chromosome 5 markers, *Pgm-1*, *Eta-1* (a locus synonymous with *Ric*), *rd*, and *Gus-s*.[231,238] The results indicated a gene order of *Pgm-1–Eta-1–rd–Flv–Gus-s* (Table 13-7). The region on mouse chromosome 5 to which the *Flv* gene maps contains homologs of genes located on human chromosomes 7 and 12.[163] Recently the Flv gene has been fine-mapped using 12 microsatellite markers to a 0.9 cm segment.[265a]

Data from the 1981 dengue hemorrhagic fever (dengue shock syndrome) epidemic in Cuba suggest the existence of a flavivirus resistance gene among black Cubans.[99] Human resistance to yellow fever in areas of Africa where this virus is endemic has also been reported.[226]

TABLE 13-7. *Recombination analysis of pairs of chromosome 5 markers to map the location of the flavivirus resistance gene, Flv*

Locus pair	No. Recombinants/ Sample Size	Percent recombination ± SEM
Pgm-1, Flv	46/164	28.0 ± 3.5
Pgm-1, Gus-s	71/164	43.3 ± 3.9
Flv, Gus-s	25/164	15.2 ± 2.8

*The data indicate a gene order of *Pgm-1–Flv–Gus-S*.
Data from Sangster MY, Urosevic N, Mansfield JP, et al. Mapping the *Flv* locus controlling resistance to flaviviruses on mouse chromosome 5. J Virol 1994;68:448–452, and Shallem GR, Urosevic N, Sangster MY, et al. Characterization of allelic forms at the retinal degeneration (*rd*) and β-glucuronidase (*Gus*) loci for the mapping of the flavivirus resistance (*Flv*) gene on mouse chromosome 5. Mouse Genome 1993;91:572–574.

Characteristics of Flavivirus Replication in Resistant Mice

Flaviviruses can replicate in mice that possess the *Flv* allele, but virus titers in the tissues of resistant mice are lower (by 1000- to 10,000-fold) than in susceptible mice (Fig. 13-6). Also, the spread of infection in resistant mice is slower,[62,88] and the host immune response is able to clear the infection, often before observable disease symptoms can develop. Factors such as the age of the host, the degree of virulence of the infecting flavivirus, the route of infection, and immunosuppression can alter the outcome of a flavivirus infection in resistant mice. For example, although C3H/RV mice are completely resistant to an intracerebral inoculation of undiluted 17D-YFV vaccine and C3H/He mice all die from the same inoculation, C3H/RV mice can be killed by an intracerebral inoculation of a more virulent flavivirus such as West Nile encephalitis virus (WNV). However, the minimal lethal dose of WNV required for the C3H/RV mice is 10 to 100 times higher than that for the congenic susceptible C3H/He mice, death in the C3H/RV mice is delayed by at least 3 days, and the peak brain titers in the C3H/RV mice are 10,000-fold lower than those in the brains of C3H/He mice.[62,100,267] Resistance to flavivirus infection develops postnatally in C3H/RV mice, reaching adult levels by about 4 weeks of age, coincident with the maturation of the immune system. Studies by Bhatt and Jacoby[23] showed that both antiviral antibody and T cells are important for clearing flavivirus infections. These results suggest that although a normally functioning immune system is required for the survival of flavivirus-infected resistant animals, the immune system is not specifically involved in the action of the gene product of the flavivirus resistance allele, which acts by reducing the yield of virus produced. In contrast to Mx-controlled resistance to influenza A viruses, flavivirus resistance is not mediated by interferon induction, because no change was observed in the flavivirus resistance of C3H/RV animals after injection of antiinterferon antibody (Table 13-8).[37]

Characteristics of Flavivirus Replication in Resistant Cell Cultures

Comparable numbers of cells in cultures obtained from the tissues of resistant and susceptible mice can be infected by flaviviruses, as demonstrated by the presence of virus-specific immunofluorescence,[61] indicating that this resistance phenotype is not controlled at the receptor level. Cell cultures from resistant mice consistently produce lower yields of virus than do cultures from susceptible mice.[266,277] Whereas peak brain virus titers in resistant and susceptible mice differ by 10^4 or more, cell culture titers differ by 10^2 to 10^{3}.[35,61] The tissue from which cell cultures are prepared does not appear to be important, because primary brain, kidney, macrophage, and embryo fibroblast cultures (as well as SV40-transformed embryo fibroblast cultures) from resistant animals all produce reduced yields of flaviviruses.[61,266,277]

Flaviviruses are spherical, enveloped, and about 50 nm in diameter. The viral genome RNA is single-stranded and of positive polarity.[1] The entire flavivirus replication cycle takes place in the perinuclear region of the cytoplasm. Comparison of the various stages of the flavivirus replication cycle within resistant C3H/RV and susceptible C3H/He cells showed that the synthesis of progeny genome RNA was specifically limited, although the amounts of replicative form/replicative intermediate RNA synthesized in the two types of cells was similar (Fig. 13-7).[34,35] This observation

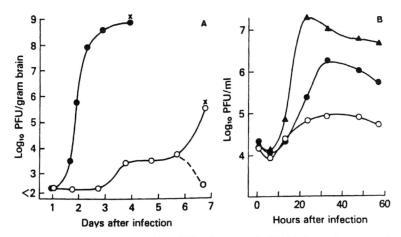

Fig. 13-6. Replication of the flavivirus, West Nile virus, strain E101, in resistant and susceptible animals and cell cultures. (**A**) Adult susceptible C3H/He (●) and resistant C3H/RV (○) mice were injected intracerebrally with $10^{5.5}$ plaque-forming units (PFU) of virus. All of the C3H/He mice died by day 5 (x=moribund), but only 50% of the C3H/RV mice died by day 8. If virus is given by the intraperitoneal route, 100% of the C3H/He mice die and all of the C3H/RV mice survive. Virus titers increased somewhat on day 7 in C3H/RV mice that were moribund (X) and decreased in recovering animals (*dashed line*). (**B**) Cultures of resistant C3H/RV primary mouse embryo fibroblasts (○), susceptible C3H/He primary embryo fibroblasts (●), and baby hamster kidney cells (BHK 21/Wl2; ▲) were infected with virus at a multiplicity of 10 PFU/cell. Virus titers were assayed by plaque assay in BHK cells. (Data from Brinton MA. Replication of flaviviruses. In: Schlesinger S, Schlesinger MJ, eds. The togaviridae and flaviviridae. New York: Plenum, 1986:327– 374.)

TABLE 13-8. *Effect of antibody to mouse interferon on the expression of flavivirus resistance in mice.* *

Mouse strain	Genotype	Treatment	Mortality	Log$_{10}$ virus titer (PFU per brain)
C3H/He	r/r	NSG	4/4	5.7
		AIF	4/4	6.5
C3H/RV	R/R	NSG	0/4	2.4
		AIF	0/4	2.8

R, resistant; r, susceptible.

*Mice were injected with 10$^{3.7}$ plaque-forming units of yellow fever virus (17-D strain) by the intracerebral route. Sheep normal serum globulin (NSG) or sheep antimouse interferon globulin (AIF) was diluted 1 to 3 with phosphate-buffered saline, and 0.1 mL was injected intravenously just before virus was injected. The results indicate that antiinterferon antibody did not abrogate flavivirus resistance.

Data from Brinton MA, Arnheiter H, Haller O. Interferon independence of genetically controlled resistance to flaviviruses. Infect Immun 1982;36:284–288.

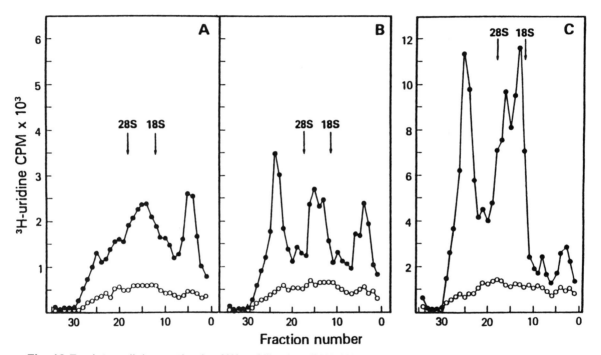

Fig. 13-7. Intracellular synthesis of West Nile virus RNA (**A**) in resistant C3H/RV embryo fibroblasts, (**B**) in susceptible C3H/He embryo fibroblasts, and (**C**) in baby hamster kidney cells (BHK 21/Wl2). RNA synthesized in the cytoplasm of infected cells between 24 and 25.5 hours after infection was labeled with ^{3}H-uridine in the presence of actinomycin D, harvested from cells, and sedimented through a sodium dodecylsulfate (SDS)-sucrose gradient. The positions of 28S and 18S ribosomal RNA markers were estimated from absorbance profiles. RNA patterns for infected (•—•) and uninfected (○—○) cultures are shown. The leftmost peak contains nascent genome plus-strand RNA. The middle peak contains replicative form/replicative intermediate (RF/RI) RNA. The RF/RI peak is broader, but of about the same magnitude, in the C3H/RV cells as compared to the C3H/He cells. However, the amount of nascent plus-strand RNA synthesized is significantly reduced in C3H/RV cells. CPM, counts per minute. (Data from reference 34.)

suggests that the product of the flavivirus resistance gene functions at the level of viral RNA synthesis. Infectious virus could no longer be detected after three serial passages of WNV in resistant C3H/RV cells, whereas virus titers remained high during passage in C3H/He cells (Fig. 13-8). The low titers of virus produced by C3H/RV cells could be amplified by a single passage in C3H/He cells.

Flavivirus defective interfering particles were produced in both C3H/He and C3H/RV cells during serial high multiplicity passage of WNV, but they interfered more efficiently with standard virus replication in resistant cells than in susceptible cells (Table 13-9),[35,61] probably because of the reduced amount of standard flavivirus produced by resistant cells. In

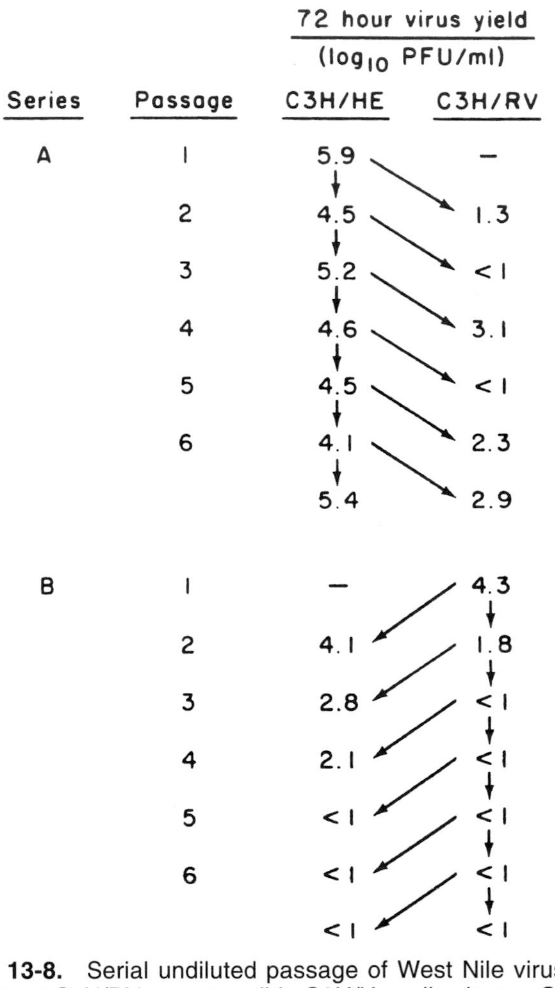

Fig. 13-8. Serial undiluted passage of West Nile virus in resistant C3H/RV or susceptible C3H/He cell cultures. Cells were initially infected with virus that had been sequentially plaque-purified six times at a multiplicity of 10 plaque-forming units (PFU) per cell. Culture media were harvested 3 days after infection. Half of the virus from each passage was transferred to a fresh culture of the same cell type, and the other half was transferred to a fresh culture of the other cell type, as indicated by the arrows. Susceptible C3H/He cells supported extended serial passage of West Nile virus, but resistant C3H/RV cells did not. (Data from Brinton MA. Analysis of extracellular West Nile virus particles produced by cell cultures from genetically resistant and susceptible mice indicates enhanced amplification of DI particles by resistant cultures. J Virol 1983;46:860–870.)

vivo, defective interfering Banzi virus activity was detected in the spleens and brains of both C3H/RV and C3H/He mice, but this activity appeared later and was of a lower titer in C3H/He mice than in C3H/RV mice.[241] Previous experimental evidence suggests that differences in the efficiency of generation and amplification of defective particles observed with the same virus in different types of cells can be regulated by host cell factors at the level of RNA synthesis.[107,126,142,237]

Mechanism of Flavivirus Resistance

Host cell proteins have been identified as components of positive- and negative-strand RNA virus replication complexes.[17,18,103,140,201] For instance, the Qβ phage replicase complex consists of four proteins, only one of which, the RNA-dependent RNA polymerase, is virally encoded. The other three proteins are host-encoded proteins and have been identified as the cellular S1 ribosomal protein and two cellular translation elongation factors, EF-Tu and EF-Ts.[24,140] However, only a few instances has it been possible to purify functionally active viral replication complexes composed of viral and cellular proteins.[18,103,140] Host proteins have also been shown to bind specifically to cis-acting elements located at the 3' ends of the genome RNAs and antigenome RNAs of a number of animal RNA viruses by competition gel shift assays.* Although some proteins recognize RNA in a sequence-specific manner,[169] others require the presence of secondary or tertiary RNA structures.[60] The 3' ends of the minus- and plus-strand RNAs of a particular virus usually bind to unique sets of cell proteins.[26,188,189] These data suggest that host proteins are intimately involved in viral RNA transcription initiated from both plus- and minus-strand templates. In cells infected with the plus-strand RNA viruses, the viral plus and minus strands are synthesized disproportionately; approximately 10 to 100 times more plus-strand RNA than minus-strand RNA is produced. The interaction of cellular proteins with the 3' terminal structures of the viral RNAs may be involved in regulating the rate of viral RNA transcription. However, the precise functional contributions of the various cell proteins that have been shown to bind to viral RNAs during viral replication remain to be elucidated.

The flavivirus genome is the only animal plus-strand RNA virus genome without a 3' poly A tract; it terminates instead with CU_{OH}.[281] Stable secondary structures are located at both the 3' and 5' terminal ends of the flavivirus genome RNA.[36,39] Comparative analyses of these structures in the genomes of different flaviviruses indicated that their sizes and shapes are highly conserved among flaviviruses, even though most of the sequence comprising them is not.[36,40] Recent data suggest that conserved tertiary structures may be present at the 3' ends of both the plus- and minus-strand flavivirus RNAs.[239,239a] With the use of WNV synthetic plus- and minus-strand 3' RNAs as probes in UV light–induced crosslinking and northwestern blotting assays, two baby hamster kidney cell proteins (56- and 84-kD) that bind specifically to the 3' end of the WNV plus-strand RNA, three cell proteins (42-, 50-, and 60-kD) that bind specifically to the 3' end of the WNV minus-strand RNA, and one cell protein (105-kD) that binds to both the WNV

---

*References 82, 117, 143, 188, 189, 206, 207, 263, 285.

TABLE 13-9. *Assay of interference with standard West Nile virus (WNV) by C3H/He- or C3H/RV-passaged WNV**

| | Virus yield ($\log_{10}$ PFU/mL) at 48 h after infection | |
Virus source	C3H/RV Cells	C3H/He cells
Standard WNV	5.6	6.3
C3H/He-WNV	5.2	5.9
C3H/He-WNV + standard WNV	5.4	6.4
C3H/RV-WNV	3.5	4.6
C3H/RV-WNV + standard WNV	4.7	5.7

*Multiplicities of infection (moi) were as follows: standard WNV, 0.1; C3H/He - WNV, 4; C3H/RV-WNV, 0.06. Standard WNV was sequentially plaque-purified six times. C3H/He and C3H/RV cells were infected with WNV at an moi of 10 and progeny virus was pelleted from the tissue culture fluid 48 h after infection and resuspended at 10% of the original concentration. The results indicate that virus produced by C3H/RV cells contains detectable homologous interfering activity.

Data from Brinton MA. Analysis of extracellular West Nile virus (WNV) particles produced by cell cultures from genetically resistant and susceptible mice indicates enhanced amplification of DI particles by resistant cultures. J Virol 1983;46:860–870.

plus- and minus-strand 3' RNAs have been detected.[26,239] Viral proteins were not detected with the viral 3' probes by either gel shift or UV light–induced crosslinking assays. For some of the positive-strand RNA viruses, the interaction of cellular proteins with the viral template RNA may be the first step in the assembly of active replication complexes. This initial interaction between cell proteins and viral RNA may result in conformational changes in both components. If this is the case, the viral polymerases may be able to recognize their templates only after the 3' ends of the templates have bound to the appropriate cell proteins.

No difference was found in the numbers or molecular mass of the proteins that bound to either the plus- or minus-strand 3' RNA WNV probes in resistant C3H/RV and susceptible C3H/He mouse cells, indicating that both resistant and susceptible cells express each of the WNV RNA binding proteins and that none of these proteins contains a detectable deletion. However, further analysis showed that although there were no differences in the binding affinities of any of the C3H/RV and C3H/He proteins that bound to the WNV plus-strand 3' RNA, one of the gel mobility shift complexes formed between proteins from the resistant cells and the WNV minus-strand 3' RNA had a longer halflife than did the comparable complex from susceptible C3H/He cells.[239] These results suggest that a mutation in one of the C3H/RV proteins that binds to the WNV minus-strand 3' RNA has increased the binding affinity of this protein for the viral RNA. Because it would be expected that proteins involved in the formation of a viral RNA transcription initiation complex would bind to the 3' end of a viral template RNA in a reversible manner, the effect of a mutant cell protein that binds more tightly to the viral RNA would be to delay the progression of the replication complex and thus preferentially reduce the efficiency of progeny plus-strand RNA transcription initiation. A further understanding of the mechanism of flavivirus resistance will be obtained only after the products of the alleles of the *Flv* locus have been successfully cloned and characterized.

Because the same set of baby hamster kidney cell proteins were detected with 3' plus-strand RNA probes made from four divergent flaviviruses, WNV, YFV, tickborne encephalitis virus (TBE), and dengue-2 virus[26] (J.L. Blackwell, M.A. Brinton, unpublished data), and because the 3' terminal viral RNA structures are highly conserved among flaviviruses, it is expected that all flaviviruses use the same group of cell proteins for replication. Also, because flaviviruses replicate in nature in a very wide variety of hosts (insects, amphibians, mammals, birds), it is expected that the host proteins or protein domains used by flaviviruses during their RNA replication cycle are highly conserved.

RESISTANCE TO MURINE LEUKEMIA VIRUSES

The expression of host genes affects various stages of the induction of erythroleukemia by Friend murine leukemia virus, of leukemia by Gross virus, and of spontaneous thymic lymphoma in AKR and C58 mice.[28] Many of these genes and their phenotypic effects are listed in Table 13-2. The host genes that influence the development of virus-induced lymphoid malignancies fall into two groups, those that control a virus replication step and those that affect the immune response to the virus or to virus-induced cell surface antigens. These two groups of genes may act in concert to determine whether a particular infection will lead to the development of leukemia. Genes that confer resistance to retrovirus replication have been described both at the level of virus cell receptor interactions and at the level of intracellular replication processes. Although only host genes affecting the development of leukemia are discussed here, retrovirus-encoded oncogenes also play an important role in the induction of leukemia[25,87,150] (see Chaps. 11 and 26).

Characteristics of Resistance Controlled by the *Fv-1* Locus

The *Fv-1* gene confers resistance to the induction of erythroleukemia in Friend leukemia virus–infected mice.[123] Restriction by *Fv-1* does not completely inhibit formation of virus-induced foci but reduces it by 1000-fold. *Fv-1* resistance can be overcome with higher multiplicities of virus.[154,213] The *Fv-1* gene has been mapped to mouse chromosome 4.[123] Stocks of Friend leukemia virus contain two components, a replication-competent helper virus (F-MuLV) and a defective, transforming, spleen-focus-forming virus (SFFV). The genomes of replication-competent retroviruses encode three polyproteins, *gag* (virion core proteins), *pol* (viral replicative proteins), and *env* (virion envelope glycoproteins). The F-MuLV component affected by the Fv-1 gene product maps to a portion of the capsid region of *gag*.[204,218] The *b* allele of *Fv-1* restricts the replication of *N*-tropic viruses, whereas the *n* allele restricts replication of *B*-tropic viruses. Heterozygous *Fv-1^{n/b}* (NB-type) mice are resistant to both *N*- and *B*-tropic viruses, indicating that resistance is dominant.

Infected *Fv-1*–resistant cells contain significantly less integrated provirus DNA and circular viral DNA than do susceptible cells, even though the total levels of unintegrated viral DNA are the same. Also, there is no difference in the rate of degradation of viral DNA in resistant cells.[124,294] How the intracellular interaction of the Fv-1 gene products with a region of a viral core protein results in a specific restriction of *N*- or *B*-tropic retroviruses is not known. It has been reported that four different endogenous xenotropic murine leukemia viruses, *Xmv-8*, *Xmv-9*, *Xmv-14*, and *Xmv-44*, are linked to the *Fv-1^b* gene.[77] However, it is not clear whether any of these loci affect the function of the *Fv-1* gene.

Characteristics of Resistance Controlled by the *Fv-2* Locus

Fv-2, a second host gene that downregulates virus production, inhibits the replication of SFFV and blocks foci formation and mitogenesis of SFFV-infected cells.[30,254] The effect of the *Fv-2* gene is observed only in erythroprogenitor cells of homozygous *Fv-2* mice.[74,151,200] Most inbred mouse strains are homozygous for the allele *Fv-2^s*, which confers susceptibility to Friend leukemia virus. Expression of the *Fv-2^r* allele is limited to C57 and C58 mice. Susceptibility is dominant in *Fv-2^r/Fv-2^s* F1 mice. The *Fv-2* gene has been mapped to mouse chromosome 9 and is closely linked to the H-7 locus.[151,282]

The *Fv-2* gene is involved in controlling the normal development of hematopoietic cells.[258] The recombinant *env* gene of SFFV produces a gp52 that stimulates proliferation of an early erythroid progenitor cell by binding to its erythropoietin receptor (Epo-k) and inducing erythropoietin (EPO)-independent proliferation.[222,297] The mitogenic effect of SFFV is blocked in mice homozygous for the Fv-2^r resistance gene. A negative regulatory protein has been purified from the bone marrow of Fv-2^r/Fv-2^r mice that downregulates cell DNA synthesis in the early erythroid progenitor cell, and has been designated late burst-forming unit–erythroid (BFU-E). This downregulation decreases the number of target cells available for Friend virus infection.[7]

Several host-range adapted Friend virus variants, BB6, BSB, RBV, and EYAB6, which can produce Friend virus–like disease in *Fv-2^r/Fv-2^r* mice, have been produced.[85,255] The disease in *Fv-2^r/Fv-2^r* mice is similar to classic Friend virus disease but has a longer latency period. Whereas massive splen-

omegaly and polycythemia develop in SFFV-infected Fv-2^s mice by 14 to 21 days after infection, massive splenomegaly occurs only after 4 to 6 months in either Fv-2^s or Fv-2^r mice infected with the BB6 variant. The *env* genes of these variant viruses were sequenced, and the biologically relevant regions were compared to comparable regions in the wild-type *env* gene.[85,166,255] The 3' region of the SFFV *env* gene contains a 585-bp deletion that fuses the regions encoding gp70 and p15E. In each of the host-range variant viruses, the size of this deletion was increased to about 744-bp.[166] This additional deletion truncates the membrane-proximal extracellular domain of the encoded glycoprotein. Retrovirus vectors expressing either the wild-type SFFV or variant BB6 env proteins had no effect on interleukin 3–dependent BaF3 hematopoietic cells, but both caused growth factor independency in BaF3 cells expressing recombinant Epo receptors on their surface. Because both wild-type and variant *env* glycoproteins formed detectable complexes with Epo receptors, it was clear that both SFFV and BB6 glycoproteins could specifically activate these receptors. In addition, in *Fv-2^ss/Fv-2^rr* chimeric mice only Fv-2^ss erythroblasts proliferated after Friend virus infection.[21,240]

The Epo receptor is known to associate with a number of accessory proteins,[48,170,298] and some of these proteins can be displaced by the SFFV *env* glycoprotein.[48] It has been hypothesized that *Fv-2*–encoded proteins associate with the Epo receptor and function to control its activation by various ligands, such as the Epo and SFFV *env* glycoproteins.[136] Additional studies are required to identify the *Fv-2*–encoded proteins and to understand at the molecular level how a host gene controls the activity of an oncogenic protein.

Genetic Control of Immune Responses to Retroviruses

The mouse major histocompatibility complex (MHC) contains genes that control both the humoral and cellular immune responses to viruses. Immunosuppression has been shown to increase the susceptibility of mice to retrovirus infection and virus-induced tumors.[101,175,286] A few of the identified retrovirus resistance genes that are known to be linked to the murine MHC locus appear to have intracellular effects on retrovirus replication in vivo and in vitro rather than on the immune response.[28,78,287,288] Two H-2–linked resistance genes, *Rfv-1* and *Rgv-1*, do affect immune system function and influence the rate of spontaneous recovery from Friend virus-induced splenomegaly in congenic mice of the (C57BL/10 × A) F1 background given low doses of virus.[56] The *Rfv-1* gene has been mapped to the H-2D region and has been shown to control cellular immune responses against leukemia cells.[42,43] Although both susceptible and resistant mouse strains can mount a cellular immune response against F-MuLV–infected cells, the response in susceptible mice is slower and of a lower magnitude.[27,43,176,215] H-2D^b class I molecules can be incorporated into Friend virus particles, but H-2D^k molecules are not. However, it is not known whether or not this phenomenon is related to resistance to virus-induced tumor growth in H-2^b mice.[29,46]

The *Rfv-2* gene maps to the Qa/TLa region of the mouse MHC.[180] A large number of class I–like genes are located in the Q and TL regions of the mouse MHC. Although it has been suggested that some of these nonconventional class I molecules can function as restriction elements for TCR-γ/δ T cells, their role in immune responses to viruses is not known. *Rfv-2* controls resistance to Friend virus only in animals that contain susceptible *Rfv-1* alleles. Because the effect of the *Rfv-2ˢ* allele can be overcome by a mutation in the D-L gene region of H-2, it is thought to map to that region.[180] It is possible that the D-L genes and the Q/TL genes function in similar ways to influence resistance to Friend virus infection. The *Rfv-2* gene was shown to be physically and functionally distinct from an I-A–linked immune response gene that controls the responsiveness of T helper cells to the F-MuLV envelope glycoprotein.[179] This I-A–linked gene influences the rate of spontaneous recovery from erythroleukemia induced by a low dose of Friend virus[56,179] and influences class switching of F-MuLV–neutralizing antibodies from immunoglobulin M to immunoglobulin G in Friend virus–infected mice.[179]

Another H-2–linked gene, *Rgv-1*, maps near the H-2 I region of the MHC and appears to be a classic immune response gene. This gene controls resistance to Gross virus disease. Resistance is defined as recovery from Gross virus–induced splenomegaly.[3,150,152] Antibodies to Gross virus–induced antigens are detected in resistant homozygous H-2ᵇ mice but not in susceptible homozygous H-2ᵏ mice.[3,232] However, it is possible that the decreased serum antibody levels in susceptible H-2ᵏ mice result from H-2 control of increased virus production, which in turn leads to virus-induced immunosuppression.[194] It is also possible that the tumor cells growing in the susceptible mice may absorb the antibodies and thereby reduce the serum antibody titers.[28]

Even though the *Rfv-3* gene is not linked to H-2, this gene influences the immune response to Friend virus.[58,67] The *Rfv-3* gene controls serum levels of anti–Friend virus antibodies. These antibodies decrease both the amount of viral antigen expressed on the surfaces of Friend virus–infected cells and the amount of infectious virus released.[58] However, high-titer anti–Friend virus antibodies alone are not sufficient to mediate recovery from Friend virus–induced leukemia. Appropriate H-2–linked genes must also be present.[58,67]

GENETIC DETERMINANTS OF VIRUS SUSCEPTIBILITY IN HUMANS

After the development of human histocompatibility (HLA) tests,[8] large numbers of individuals were typed for class I and class II antigens as part of organ transplant donor searches. As data accumulated, the typing laboratories began to look for correlations between HLA type and the incidence of certain diseases. Some striking correlations were observed, and numerous reviews were published on these studies.[10,41,63,89,171,183,270] Because few of the well-described mouse virus resistance loci map to the H-2 region, and even fewer map to the I region of H-2, there are as yet few data to support the hypothesis that variation in the immune response of individual humans is what determines differences in virus susceptibility.

Also, the human homolog of the influenza A virus resistance gene (*Mx*) clearly does not map to the HLA locus. As additional mouse virus resistance genes are sequenced, probes can be generated to search for additional human homologs.

The Human Genome Project should generate sequence information on additional genetic markers that will be very useful in future studies of virus resistance genes in humans because it will be possible to type individual humans at many non-HLA loci.

Investigators are beginning to understand the molecular basis of some virus resistance phenotypes in plants and mice.[33,66,167,250,283] Some of the most extensively studied murine virus resistance genes have already been discussed as specific examples of the types of interactions that can occur between the products of host resistance genes and viral molecular events. It is possible that the large amount of information obtained on the genes controlling virus-induced leukemogenesis in mice may be helpful in identifying homologous human genes that control resistance in humans to T-lymphotropic virus (HTLV-1).

Epidemiologic data suggests that there are host genes that control resistance to human immunodeficiency virus (HIV) in humans.[220] As part of a recent conference cosponsored by the National Institutes of Health, "Immunologic and Host Genetic Resistance to HIV Infection and Disease," so-called resistant individuals were classified into three groups. The first group consisted of individuals who had been exposed to HIV but had not been infected. Among hemophiliacs, 100% of those receiving the highest doses of contaminated factor VIII became infected with HIV, but only about half of those who received lower doses became infected. This suggests that individuals vary in the dose of virus they require for infection. Some individuals in this group, who are seronegative and nonviremic as demonstrated by both polymerase chain reaction and viral culture assays, display T-cell proliferation in response to HIV peptides, indicating exposure to HIV.

A second group consisted of individuals infected with HIV who had stable CD4+ T-cell counts higher than 200 cells/μL. Although all HIV-positive individuals display an initial CD4+ cell decline from 1000 to 500 cells/μL, in about 15% of patients the CD4+ cell levels stabilize or rise slightly. These individuals show strong cellular and humoral responses to a variety of epitopes, including highly conserved HIV epitopes. The individuals in the third group had CD4+ cell counts below 200 cells/μL but had not developed symptoms of stage IV acquired immunodeficiency syndrome. A higher level of CD4+ function in these patients may account for their lack of disease.

Although the data are currently inadequate to prove that host genes are responsible for some of the individual variation in HIV disease, the characteristics of these three groups of individuals are similar in many respects to those of various inbred mouse strains that contain identified genes controlling either the extent of virus replication or the host's immune response to viral antigens and virus-infected cells. Also, a recent study reported correlation between HLA profiles and the predicted time from HIV-1 infection to the onset of AIDS.[136a]

ABBREVIATIONS

AIF: antiinterferon serum
Bgp-1ᵃ: a biliary glycoprotein
EMC: encephalomyocarditis virus
F-MuLV: the replication-competent helper virus component of Friend murine leukemia virus complex

GDP: guanosine diphosphate
GLV: Gross leukemia virus
GTP: guanosine triphosphate
HIV: human immunodeficiency virus
HLA: human leukocyte (MHC) antigen
HTLV-1: human T-lymphotropic virus
LDV: lactate dehydrogenase elevating virus
MHC: major histocompatibility complex
MHV, MHV-2, MHV-3: mouse hepatitis virus
MVE: Murray Valley encephalitis (virus)
PRI: Princeton Rockefeller (mice)
RI: recombinant inbred (mouse strains)
SFFV: the spleen-focus-forming virus component of Friend murine leukemia virus complex
UV: ultraviolet (light)
WNV: West Nile encephalitis virus
YFV: yellow fever virus

ACKNOWLEDGMENTS

The author wishes to thank H.L. Robinson and K.V. Holmes for critical comments on portions of this chapter, S. Methven and A. Black for bibliographic assistance, H. Heath and R. Simmons for graphic assistance, and P. Brooks for typing the manuscript.

REFERENCES

1. Aebi M, Fäh J, Hurt N, et al. cDNA structures and regulation of two interferon-induced human Mx proteins. Mol Cell Biol 1989; 9:5062–5072.
2. Anderson GW Jr, Rosebrock JA, Johnson AJ, Jennings GB, Peters CJ. Infection of inbred rat strains with Rift Valley fever virus: development of a congenic resistant strain and observations on age-dependence of resistance. Am J Trop Med Hyg 1991;44:475–480.
3. Aoki T, Boyse EA, Old LJ. Occurrence of natural antibody to the G (Gross) leukemia antigen in mice. Cancer Res 1966;26:1415–1419.
4. Arnheiter H, Baechi T, Haller O. Adult mouse hepatocytes in primary monolayer culture express genetic resistance to mouse hepatitis virus. J Immunol 1982;129:1275–1281.
5. Arnheiter H, Haller O, Lindenmann J. Host gene influence on interferon action in adult mouse hepatocytes: specificity for influenza virus. Virology 1980;103:11–20.
6. Arnheiter H, Meier E. Mx proteins: antiviral proteins by chance or by necessity. New Biologist 1990;2:851–857.
7. Axelrad AA, Croizat HJ, Eskinazi D. A washable macromolecule from Fv-2^{rr} marrow negatively regulates DNA synthesis in erythropoietic progenitor cells BFU-E. Cell 1981;26:233–244.
8. Bach FH, van Rood JJ. The major histocompatibility complex: genetics and biology. N Engl J Med 1976;295:806–813,872–878, 927–936.
9. Bailey DW. Recombinant inbred strains: an aid to finding identity, linkage and function of histocompatability and other genes. Transplantation 1971;11:325–327.
10. Bais WB, Chase GA. Genetic implications of HLA and disease associations. Transplant Proc 1977;9:531–542.
11. Baker D, Plotkin S. Enhancement of vaginal infection in mice by herpes simplex virus type II with progesterone. Proc Soc Exp Biol Med 1978;158:131–134.
12. Bang F. Genetics of resistance of animals to viruses. I. Introduction and studies in mice. Adv Virus Res 1978;23:269–348.
13. Bang F, Warwick A. Mouse macrophages as host cells for the mouse hepatitis virus and the genetic basis of their susceptibility. Proc Natl Acad Sci U S A 1960;46:1065–1075.
14. Barthold SW. Host age and genotypic effects on enterotropic mouse hepatitis virus infection. Lab Anim Sci 1987;37:36–40.
15. Barthold SW, Beck DS, Smith AL. Mouse hepatitis virus nasoen-
16. Barthold SW, Smith AL. Mouse hepatitis virus strain-related patterns of tissue tropism in suckling mice. Arch Virol 1984;81: 103–112.
17. Barton DJ, Black EP, Flanegan JB. Complete replication of poliovirus in vitro: preinitiation RNA replication complexes require soluble factors for the synthesis of Vpg-linked RNA. J Virol 1995; 69 5516–5527.
18. Barton DJ, Sawicki SG, Sawicki DI. Solubilization and immunoprecipitation of alphavirus replication complexes. J Virol 1991;65: 1496–1506.
19. Baulcombe D. Strategies for virus resistance in plants. Trends Genet 1989;5:56–60.
20. Bazzigher L, Schwarz A, Staeheli P. No enhanced influenza virus resistance of murine and avain cells expressing cloned duck Mx protein. Virology 1993;195:100–112.
21. Behringer RR, Dewey MJ. Cellular site and mode of *Fv-2* gene action. Cell 1985;40:441–447.
22. Beushausen S, Dales S. In vivo and in vitro models of demyelinating disease. XXI. Relationship between differentiation of rat oligodendrocytes and control of JHMV replication. Adv Exp Med Biol 1987;218:239–254.
23. Bhatt PN, Jacoby RO. Genetic resistance to lethal flavivirus encephalitis II. Effect of immunosuppression. J Infect Dis 1976;134: 166–173.
24. Biebricker CK, Eigan M. Kinetics of RNA replication of Qβ replicase. In: Domingo E, Holland JJ, Ahlquist P, eds. RNA genetics. Vol. 1. Boca Raton, Florida: CRC Press, 1988:1–18.
25. Bishop JM. Viral oncogenes. Cell 1985;42:23–38.
26. Blackwell JL, Brinton MA. BHK cell proteins that bind to the 3' stem-loop structure of the West Nile virus genome RNA. J Virol 1995;69:5650–5658.
27. Blank KJ, Freedman H, Lilly F. T-lymphocyte response to Friend virus–induced tumor cell lines in mice of strains congenic at H-2. Nature 1978;260:250–252.
28. Blank KJ, Klyczek KK. Host genetic control of retrovirus-induced leukemogenesis in the mouse: direct genetic and epistatic effects. J Leukoc Biol 1986;40:479–490.
29. Blank KJ, Lilly F. Construction of a DBA/2.Fv-2^r congenic strain: apparent lethality of the homozygous *Fv-2^r* genotype. J Natl Cancer Inst 1978;59:1335–1336.
30. Blank KJ, Steeves RA, Lilly F. The *Fv-2^r* resistance gene in mice: its effect on spleen colony formation by Friend virus-transforming cells. J Natl Cancer Inst 1976;57:925–930.
31. Blumberg BS. Inherited susceptibility to disease. Arch Environ Health 1961;3:612–636.
32. Bowes C, Li T, Danciger M, Baxter LC, Applebury ML, Farber DB. Retinal degeneration in the *rd* mouse is caused by a defect in the beta subunit of rod cGMP-phosphodiesterase. Nature 1990;347: 677– 680.
33. Boyle JF, Weismiller DG, Holmes KV. Genetic resistance to mouse hepatitis virus correlates with absence of virus-binding activity on target tissues. J Virol 1987;61:185–189.
34. Brinton MA. Isolation of a replication efficient mutant of West Nile virus from a persistently infected genetically resistant mouse cell culture. J Virol 1981;39:413–421.
35. Brinton MA. Analysis of extracellular West Nile virus (WNV) particles produced by cell cultures from genetically resistant and susceptible mice indicates enhanced amplification of DI particles by resistant cultures. J Virol 1983;46:860–870.
36. Brinton MA. Replication of flaviviruses. In: Schlesinger S, Schlesinger MJ, eds. The togaviridae and flaviviridae. New York: Plenum, 1986:327–374.
37. Brinton MA, Arnheiter H, Haller O. Interferon independence of genetically controlled resistance to flaviviruses. Infect Immun 1982; 36:284–288.
38. Brinton M, Blank K, Nathanson N. Host genes that influence susceptibility to viral diseases. In: Notkins AL, Oldstone MBA, eds. Concepts in viral pathogenesis. New York: Springer-Verlag, 1984: 71–78.
39. Brinton MA, Dispoto JH. Sequence and secondary structure analysis of the 5'-terminal region of flavivirus genome RNA. Virology 1988;162:290–299.

40. Brinton MA, Fernandez AV, Dispoto JH. The 3'-nucleotides of flavivirus genome RNA form a conserved secondary structure. Virology 1986;153:113–121.

41. Brinton M, Nathanson N (1981). Genetic determinants of virus susceptibility: epidemiologic implications of murine models. Epidemiol Rev 1981;3:115–139.

42. Britt WJ, Chesebro B. H-2D (Rfv-1) gene influence on recovery from Friend virus leukemia is mediated by nonleukemic cells of the spleen and bone marrow. J Exp Med 1980;152:1795–1804.

43. Britt WJ, Chesebro B. H-2D control of recovery from Friend virus leukemia: H-2D region influences the kinetics of the T lymphocyte response to Friend virus. J Exp Med 1983;157:1736–1745.

44. Broni B, Julkunen I, Condra JH, Davies M-E, Berry MJ, Krug RM. Parental influenza virion nucleocapsids are efficiently transported into the nuclei of murine cells expressing the nuclear interferon-induced Mx protein. J Virol 1990;64:6335–6340.

45. Brownstein DG, Bhatt PN, Gras L, Jacoby RO. Chromosomal locations and gonadal dependence of genes that mediate resistance to ectromelia (mousepox) virus-induced mortality. J Virol 1991;65:1946–951.

46. Bubbers JE, Lilly F. Selective incorporation of H-2 antigenic determinants into Friend virus particles. Nature 1977;266:458–459.

47. Campbell A, Lorio R, Madge G, Kaplan A. Dietary hepatic cholesterol elevation: effects on coxsackievirus B5 infection and inflammation. Infect Immun 1982;37:307–317.

48. Casadevall N, Lacombe C, Muller O, Gisselbrecht S, Mayeux P. Multimeric structure of the membrane erythropoietin receptor of murine erythroleukemia cells (Friend cells): cross-linking of erythropoietin with the spleen focus-forming virus envelope protein. J Biol Chem 1991;266:16015–16020.

49. Casals J, Schneider H. Natural resistance and susceptibility to RSSE in mice. Proc Soc Exp Biol Med 1943;54:201–202.

50. Chalmer J. Genetic resistance to murine cytomegalovirus infection. In: Skamene E, Kongshavn PAL, Landy M, eds. Genetic control of natural resistance to infection and malignancy. New York: Academic Press, 1980:283–291.

51. Chalmer J, Mackenzie J, Stanley NF. Resistance to murine cytomegalovirus linked to the major histocompatability complex of the mouse. J Gen Virol 1977;37:107–114.

52. Chandra R. Nutritional deficiency and susceptibility to infection. Bull World Health Organ 1979;57:167–177.

53. Chandra R. Nutrition, immunity, and infection: present knowledge and future directions. Lancet 1983;1:688–691.

54. Chang SS, Hildemann WH. Inheritance of susceptibility to polyoma virus in mice. J Natl Cancer Inst 1964;33:303–313.

55. Chen MS, Obar RA, Schroeder CC, et al. Multiple forms of dynamin are encoded by shibire, a Drosophila gene involved in endocytosis. Nature 1991;351:583–586.

56. Chesebro B, Miyazawa M, Britt WJ. Host genetic control of spontaneous and induced immunity to Friend murine retrovirus infection. Annu Rev Immunol 1990;8:477–499.

57. Chesebro B, Wehrly K. Rfv-1 and Rfv-2: two H-2 associated genes that influence recovery from Friend leukemia virus–induced splenomegaly. J Immunol 1978;120:1081–1085.

58. Chesebro B, Wehrly K, Stimpfling JH. Host genetic control of recovery from Friend leukemia virus–induced splenomegaly: Mapping of a gene within the major histocompatibility complex. J Exp Med 1974;140:1457–1467.

59. Christie A, Allan A, Aref M, Muntasser I. Pregnancy hepatitis in Libya. Lancet 1976;2:827–829.

60. Dam ET, Pleij K, Draper D. Structural and functional aspects of RNA pseudoknots. Biochemistry 1992;31:11665–11676.

61. Darnell MB, Koprowski H. Genetically determined resistance to infection with group B arboviruses. II. Increased production of interfering particles in cell cultures from resistant mice. J Infect Dis 1974;129:248–256.

62. Darnell MB, Koprowski H, Lagerspetz K. Genetically determined resistance to infection with group B arboviruses. I. Distribution of the resistance gene among various mouse populations and characteristics of gene expression in vivo. J Infect Dis 1974;129:240–247.

63. Dausset J, Hors J. Some contributions of the MLA-complex to the genetics of human diseases. Transplant Rev 1975;22:44–74.

64. Dever TE, Glynias MJ, Merrich WC. GTP-binding domain: three consensus sequence elements with distinct spacing. Proc Natl Acad Sci U S A 1987;84:1814–1818.

65. Dindzans V, MacPhee P, Fung LS, Leibowitz JL, Levy GA. The immune response to mouse hepatitis virus: expression of monocyte procoagulant activity and plasminogen activator during infection in vivo. J Immunol 1985;135:4189–4197.

66. Dinesh-Kumar SP, Whitham S, Choi D, Hehl R, Corr C, Baker B. Transposon tagging of tobacco mosaic virus resistance gene N: its possible role in the TMV-N–mediated signal transduction pathway. Proc Natl Acad Sci U S A 1995;92:4175–4180.

67. Doig D, Chesebro B. Anti-Friend virus antibody is associated with recovery from anemia and loss of viral leukemia cell surface antigens mice. J Exp Med 1979;150:10–19.

68. Dover A, Escobar J, Duenas A, Leal E. Pneumonia associated with measles. JAMA 1975;234:612–614.

69. Dreiding P, Staeheli P, Haller O. Interferon-induced protein Mx accumulates in nuclei of mouse cells expressing resistance to influenza viruses. Virology 1985;140:192–196.

70. Dupuy C, Lafforet-Cresteil D, Dupuy JM. Genetic study of MHV-3 infection in mice: in vitro replication of virus in macrophages. In: Skamene E, Kongshavn PAL, Landy M, eds. Genetic control of natural resistance to infection and malignancy. New York: Academic Press, 1980:241.

71. Dutko F, Oldstone MBA. Cytomegalovirus causes a latent infection in undifferentiated cells and is activated by induction of cell differentiation. J Exp Med 1981;154:1636–1651.

72. Dveksler GS, Dieffenbach CW, Cardellichio CB, et al. Several members of the mouse carcinoembryonic antigen-related glycoprotein family are functional receptors for the coronavirus mouse hepatitis virus-A59. J Virol 1993;67:1–8.

73. Dveksler GS, Pensiero MN, Cardellichio CB, et al. Cloning of the mouse hepatitis virus (MHV) receptor: expression in human and hamster cell lines confers susceptibility to MHV. J Virol 1991;65:6881–6891.

74. Evans LH, Duesberg PH, Scolnick EM. Replication of spleen focus-forming Friend virus in fibroblasts from C57BL mice that are genetically resistant to spleen focus formation. Virology 1980;101:534–539.

75. Fenner F. The biology of animal viruses. Orlando: Academic Press, 1968:475–613.

76. Fiske RA, Klein PA. Effect of immunosuppression on the genetic resistance of A2G mice to neurovirulent influenza virus. Infect Immun 1975;11:576–586.

77. Frankel WN, Stoye JP, Taylor BA, Coffin JM. Genetic analysis of endogenous xenotropic murine leukemia viruses: association with two common mouse mutations and the viral restriction locus Fv-1. J Virol 1989;63:1763–1774.

78. Freeman HA, Lilly F, Strand M, August JT. Variation in viral gene expression in Friend virus–transformed cell lines congenic with respect to the H-2 locus. Cell 1979;13:33–40.

79. Frese M, Kochs G, Meier-Dieter U, Siebler J, Haller O. Human MxA protein inhibits tick-borne Thogoto virus but not Dhori virus. J Virol 1995;69:3904–3909.

80. Freund R, Dubensky T, Bronson R, Sotnikov A, Carroll J, Benjamin T. Polyoma tumorigenesis in mice: evidence for dominant resistance and dominant susceptibility genes of the host. Virology 1992;191:724–731.

81. Fujimura FK, Silbert PE, Eckhart W, Linney E. Polyomavirus infection of retinoic acid–induced differentiated teratocarcinoma cells. J Virol 1981;39:306–312.

82. Furuya T, Lai MMC. Three different cellular proteins bind to complementary sites on the 5'-end–positive and 3'-end–negative strands of mouse hepatitis virus RNA. J Virol 1993;67:7215–7222.

83. Garber EA, Hrenink DL, Scheidel LM, van der Ploeg LHT. Mutations in murine Mx1: effects on localization and antiviral activity. Virology 1993;194:715–723.

84. Gatmaitan B, Chason J, Lerner A. Augmentation of the virulence of murine coxsackie-virus B-3 myocardiopathy by exercise. J Exp Med 1970;131:1121–1136.

85. Geib RW, Seaward MB, Stevens ML, Cho C-L, Majumdar M. RB virus: a strain of Friend virus that produces a "Friend-virus–like" disease in Fv-2rr mice. Virus Res 1989;14:161–174.

86. Goetschy JF, Zeller H, Content J, Horisberger MA. Regulation of the interferon-inducible IFI-78K gene, the human equivalent of the

murine *Mx* gene, by interferons, double-stranded RNA, certain cytokines, and viruses. J Virol 1989;63:2616–2622.

87. Goff SP. The genetics of murine leukemia viruses. Curr Top Microbiol Immunol 1984;112:45–71.

88. Goodman GT, Koprowski H. Macrophages as a cellular expression of inherited natural resistance. Proc Natl Acad Sci U S A 1962;48:160–165.

89. Grayston JT, Payne FJ. Summary of a workshop on the major histocompatibility complex in infectious disease epidemiology. J Infect Dis 1979;139:246–249.

90. Greene N, Hiai H, Elder JH, et al. Expression of leukemogenic recombinant viruses associated with a recessive gene in HRS/J mice. J Exp Med 1980;152:249–256.

91. Groschel D, Koprowski H. Development of a virus-resistant inbred mouse strain for the study of innate resistance to arbo B viruses. Arch Ges Virusforsch 1965;17:379–391.

92. Groves MG, Rosenstreich DL, Taylor BA, Osterman JV. Host defenses in experimental scrub typhus: mapping the gene that controls natural resistance in mice. J Immunol 1980;125:1395–1399.

93. Grundy J, Mackenzie J, Stanley N. Influence of H-2 and non–H-2 linked genes on resistance to murine cytomegalovirus infection. Infect Immun 1981;32:277–286.

94. Guetta E, Ron D, Tal J. Developmental-dependent replication of minute virus of mice in differentiated mouse testicular lines. J Gen Virol 1986;67:2549–2554.

95. Haller O. Inborn resistance of mice to orthomyxoviruses. In: Haller O, ed. Natural resistance to tumors and viruses. Berlin: Springer-Verlag, 1981:25–52.

96. Haller O, Arnheiter H, Gresser I, Lindenmann J. Genetically determined, interferon-dependent resistance to influenza virus in mice. J Exp Med 1979;149:601–602.

97. Haller O, Arnheiter H, Lindenmann J, Gresser I. Host gene influences sensitivity to interferon action selectively for influenza virus. Nature 1980;283:660–662.

98. Haller O, Lindenmann J. Athymic (nude) mice express gene for myxovirus resistance. Nature 1974;250:679–680.

99. Halstead SB. The XXth century dengue pandemic: need of surveillance and research. World Health Stat Q 1992;45:292–298.

100. Hanson B, Koprowski H. Interferon-mediated natural resistance of mice to arbo B virus infection. Microbios 1969;1B:51–68.

101. Haran-Ghera N, Rubio N, Leef F, Goldstein G. Characteristics of preleukemia cells induced in mice. Cell Immunol 1978;37:308–314.

102. Hartmann W. Evaluation of "major genes" affecting disease resistance in poultry in respect to their potential for commercial breeding. Recent Adv Avian Immunol Res 1989:221–231.

103. Hayes RJ, Buck KW. Complete replication of a eukaryotic virus RNA in vitro by a purified RNA-dependent RNA polymerase. Cell 1990;63:363–368.

104. Henderson BF, Pigford CA, Work T, Wende RD. Serologic survey for St. Louis encephalitis and other group B arbovirus antibodies in residents of Houston, Texas. Am J Epidemiol 1970;91:87–98.

105. Herzog S, Frese K, Rott R. Studies on the genetic control of resistance of black hooded rats to Borna disease. J Gen Virol 1991;72:535–540.

106. Hirsch MS, Zisman B, Allison AC. Macrophages and age-dependent resistance to herpes simplex virus in mice. J Immunol 1970;104:1160–1165.

107. Holland JJ, Villarreal LP, Breindl M. Factors involved in the generation and replication of rhabdovirus defective T particles. J Virol 1976;17:805–815.

108. Horisberger MA. Interferon-induced human protein MxA is a GTPase which binds transiently to cellular proteins. J Virol 1992;66:4705–4709.

109. Horisberger MA, Gunst MC. Interferon-induced proteins: identification of Mx proteins in various mammalian species. Virology 1991;180:185–190.

110. Horisberger MA, Haller O, Arnheiter H. Interferon-dependent genetic resistance to influenza virus in mice: virus replication in macrophages is inhibited at an early step. J Gen Virol 1980;50:205–210.

111. Horisberger MA, Staeheli P, Haller O. Interferon induces a unique protein in mouse cells bearing a gene for resistance to influenza virus. Proc Natl Acad Sci U S A 1983;80:1910–1914.

112. Horstmann D. Acute poliomyelitis: relation of physical activity at the time of onset to the course of the disease. JAMA 1950;142:236–241.

113. Huang T, Pavlovic J, Staeheli P, Krystal M. Overexpression of the influenza virus polymerase can titrate out inhibition by the murine Mx1 protein. J Virol 1992;66:4154–4160.

114. Hug H, Costas M, Staeheli P, Aebi M, Weissmann C. Organization of the murine *Mx* gene and characterization of its interferon- and virus-inducible promotor. Mol Cell Biol 1988;8:3065–3079.

115. Hurst E, Melvin P, Thorpe J. The influence of cortisone, ACTH, thryoxine, and thiouracil on equine encephalomyelitis in the mouse and on its treatment with mepacrine. J Comp Pathol 1960;70:361–373.

116. Imam I, Hammon W. Susceptibility of hamsters to peripherally inoculated Japanese B and St. Louis viruses following cortisone, x-ray, trauma. Proc Soc Exp Biol Med 1957;95:6–11.

117. Jacobson SJ, Konings DAM, Sarnow P. Biochemical and genetic evidence for a pseudoknot structure at the 3' terminus of the poliovirus RNA genome and its role in viral RNA amplification. J Virol 1993;67:2961–2971.

118. Jacoby RO, Bhatt PN. Genetic resistance to lethal flavivirus encephalitis. I. Infection of congenic mice with Banzi virus. J Infect Dis 1976;134:158–165.

119. Jerrells TR, Osterman JV. Host defenses in experimental scrub typhus: inflammatory response of congenic C3H mice differing at the *Ric* gene. Infect Immun 1981;31:1014–1022.

120. Johnson RT. The pathogenesis of herpes virus encephalitis. II. A cellular basis for the development of resistance with age. J Exp Med 1964;120:359–374.

121. Johnson RT. Selective vulnerability of neural cells to viral infection. Brain 1980;103:447–472.

122. Johnson RT, McFarland HF, Levy SE. Age-dependent resistance to viral encephalitis: studies of infections due to Sindbis virus in mice. J Infect Dis 1972;125:257–262.

123. Jolicoeur P. The *Fv-1* gene of the mouse and its control of murine leukemia virus replication. Curr Topics Microbiol Immunol 1979;86:67–122.

124. Jolicoeur P, Rassart E. Effect of *Fv-1* gene product on synthesis of linear and supercoiled viral DNA in cells infected with murine leukemia virus. J Virol 1980;33:183–195.

125. Jones BA, Fangman WL. Mitochondrial DNA maintenance in yeast requires a protein containing a region related to the GTP-binding domain of dynamin. Genes Dev 1992;6:380–389.

126. Kang CY, Allen R. Host function–dependent induction of defective interfering particles of vesicular stomatitis virus. J Virol 1978;25:202–206.

127. Kark J, Lubiush M, Rannon L. Cigarette smoking as a risk factor for epidemic A (H₁N₁) influenza in young men. N Engl J Med 1982;307:1042–1046.

128. Kees U, Blanden RV. A single genetic element in H-2K affects mouse T-cell antiviral function in poxvirus infection. J Exp Med 1976;143:450–455.

129. Kessell I, Holst B, Roth TF. Membranous intermediates in endocytosis are labile, as shown in a temperature-sensitive mutant. Proc Natl Acad Sci U S A 1989;86:4968–4972.

130. Kingsbury DW. Orthomyxoviridae and their replication. In: Fields BN, Knipe DM. Virology. 2nd ed. New York: Raven Press, 1990:527–541.

131. Knobler RL, Haspel MV, Oldstone MBA. Mouse hepatitis virus type 4 (JHM strain)–induced fatal central nervous system disease. I. Genetic control and the murine neuron as the susceptible site of disease. J Exp Med 1981;153:832–843.

132. Knobler RL, Linthicum DS, Cohn M. Host genetic regulation of acute MHV-4 viral encephalomyelitis and acute experimental autoimmune encephalomyelitis in (BALB/cKe X SJL/J) recombinant-inbred mice. J Neuroimmunol 1985;8:15–28.

133. Knobler RL, Taylor BA, Woddell MK, Beamer WG, Oldstone MBA. Host genetic control of mouse hepatitis virus type-4 (JHM strain) replication. II. The gene locus for susceptibility is linked to the Svp-2 locus on mouse chromosome 7. Exp Clin Immunogenet 1984;1:217–222.

134. Kohl S, Loo L. Protection of neonatal mice against herpes simplex virus infection: probable antibody-dependent cellular cytotoxity. J Immunol 1982;129:370–376.

135. Kolb E, Laine E, Strehler D, Staeheli P. Resistance to influenza virus infection of Mx transgenic mice expressing Mx protein under the control of two constitutive promotors. J Virol 1992;66:1709–1716.

136. Kozak SL, Hoatlin ME, Ferro FE, Jr, Majumdar MK, Geib RW, Fox MT, Kabat D. A Friend virus mutant that overcomes Fv-2^{rr} host resistance encodes a small glycoprotein that dimerizes, is processed to cell surfaces, and specifically activates erythropoietin receptors. J Virol 1993;67:2611–2620.

136a. Kislow RA, Garrington M, Apple R, et al. Influence of combinations of human major histocompatibility complex genes on the course of HIV-1 infection. Nature Medicine 1996;2:405–411.

137. Krug RM, Shaw M, Broni B, Shapiro G, Haller O. Inhibition of influenza viral mRNA synthesis in cells expressing the interferon-induced Mx gene product. J Virol 1985;56:201–206.

138. Kumar V, Bennett M. Mechanisms of genetic resistance to Friend virus leukemia in mice. II. Resistance of mitogen-responsive lymphocytes mediated by marrow-dependent cells. J Exp Med 1976;143:713–727.

139. Lalley PA, Davisson MT, Graves JAM, et al. Report of the committee on comparative mapping: human gene mapping 10. Cytogenet Cell Genet 1989;51:503–532.

140. Landers TA, Blumenthal T, Weber K. Function and structure in ribonucleic acid phage Qβ ribonucleic acid replicase. J Biol Chem 1974;249:5801–5808.

141. LaVail MM, Sidman RL. C57BL/6 mice with inherited retinal degeneration. Arch Ophthalmol 1974;91:394–400.

142. Lazzarini, RA, Keene JD, Schubert M. The origins of defective interfering particles of the negative-strand RNA viruses. Cell 1981;26:145–154.

143. Leopardi R, Hukkanen V, Vainionpää R, Salmi AA. Cell proteins bind to sites within the 3' noncoding region of the positive-strand leader sequence of measles virus RNA. J Virol 1993;67:785–790.

144. Levin HA. Disease resistance and immune response genes in cattle: strategies for their detection and evidence of their existence. J Dairy Sci 1989;72:1334–1348.

145. Levine B, Harwick JM, Trapp BD, Crawford TO, Bollinger RC, Griffin DE. Antibody-mediated clearance of aphavirus infection from neurons. Science 1991;254:856–860.

146. Levine B, Huang Q, Isaacs JT, Reed JC, Griffin DE, Hardwick JM. Conversion of lytic to persistent alphavirus infection by the bcl-2 cellular onogene. Nature 1993;361:739–742.

147. Levy GA, Leibowitz JL, Edgington TS. Induction of monocyte procoagulant activity by murine hepatitis virus type 3 (MHV-3) parallels disease susceptibility in mice. J Exp Med 1981;154:1150–1163.

148. Levy GA, MacPhee PJ, Fung LS, Fisher MM, Rappaport AM. The effect of mouse hepatitis virus infection on the microcirculation of the liver. Hepatology 1983;3:964–973.

149. Levy-LeBlond E, Oth D, Dupuy JM. Genetic study of mouse sensitivity to MHV-3 infection: influence of the H-2 complex. J Immunol 1979;122:1359–1362.

150. Lilly F. The histocompatibility-2 locus and susceptibility to tumor induction. J Natl Cancer Inst 1966;22:631–642.

151. Lilly F. Fv-2: identification and location of a second gene governing the spleen focus response to Friend leukemia virus in mice. J Natl Cancer Inst 1970;45:163–169.

152. Lilly F, Boyse EA, Old LJ. Genetic basis of susceptibility to viral leukemogenesis. Lancet 1964;2:1207–1209.

153. Lilly F, Duran-Reynolds ML, Rowe WP. Correlation of early murine leukemia virus titer and H-2 type with spontaneous leukemia in mice of the BALB/ c × AKR cross: a genetic analysis. J Exp Med 1975;141:882–889.

154. Lilly F, Pincus T. Genetic control of murine viral leukemogenesis. Adv Cancer Res 1973;17:231–277.

155. Lindenmann J. Inheritance of resistance to influenza virus in mice. Proc Soc Exp Biol 1964;116:506–509.

156. Lindenmann J, Klein PA. Further studies on the resistance of mice to myxoviruses. Infect Immun 1966;11:1–11.

157. Lindenmann J, Lance CA, Hobson D. The resistance of A2G mice to myxoviruses. J Immunol 1963;90:942–951.

158. Lodmell DL. Genetic control of resistance to street rabies virus in mice. J Exp Med 1983;157:451–460.

159. Lopez C. Genetics of natural resistance to herpes virus infections in mice. Nature 1975;258:152–153.

160. Lopez C. Resistance to HSV-1 in the mouse in governed by two major independently segregating, non H-2 loci. Immunogenetics 1980;11:87–92.

161. Luby JP, Miller G, Gardner P, Pigford CA, Henderson BE, Eddius D. The epidemiology of St. Louis encephalitis in Houston, Texas. Am J Epidemiol 1967;86:584–597.

162. Lynch CJ, Hughes TP. The inheritance of susceptibility to yellow fever encephalitis in mice. Genetics 1936;21:104–112.

163. Lyon MF, Kirby MC. Mouse chromosome atlas. Mouse Genome 1993;91:40–80.

164. MacNaughton MR, Patterson S. Mouse hepatitis virus strain 3 infection of C57, A/Sn, and A/J strain mice and their macrophages. Arch Virol 1980;66:71–75.

165. MacPhee PJ, Dindzans V, Fung LS, Levy GA. Acute and chronic changes in the microcirculation of the liver of inbred mice following infection with mouse hepatitis virus type 3. Hepatology 1985;5:649–660.

166. Majumdar MK, Cho CL, Fox MT, et al. Mutations in the env gene of Friend spleen focus-forming virus overcome Fv-2^r–mediated resistance to Friend virus-induced erythroleukemia. J Virol 1992;66:3652–3660.

167. Mansky LM, Hill JH. Molecular basis for virus disease resistance in plants. Arch Virol 1993;131:1–16.

168. Martinez D, Brinton MA, Tachovsky TG, Phelps AH. Identification of lactate dehydrogenase–elevating virus as the etiologic agent of the genetically restricted age-dependent polioencephalitis of mice. Infect Immun 1980;27:979–987.

169. Mattaj IW. RNA recognition: a family matter? Cell 1993;73:837–838.

170. Mayeux P, Casadevall N, Lacombe C, Muller O, Tambourin P. Solubilization and hydrodynamic characteristics of the erythropoietin receptor. Eur J Biochem 1990;194:271–278.

171. McDevitt HD, Bodmer WF. ML-A, immune response genes and disease. Lancet 1974;1:1269–1275.

172. Meier E, Fäh J, Grob MS, End R, Staeheli P, Haller O. A family of interferon-induced Mx-related mRNAs encodes cytoplasmic and nuclear proteins in rat cells. J Virol 1988;62:2386–2393.

173. Meier E, Kunz G, Haller O, Arnheiter H. Activity of rat Mx proteins against a rhabdovirus. J Virol 1990;64:6263–6269.

174. Melen K, Ronni T, Broni B, Krug RM, von Bonsdorff CH, Julkunen I. Interferon-induced Mx proteins form oligomers and contain a putative leucine zipper. J Biol Chem 1992;267:25898–25907.

175. Meruelo D. A role for elevated H-2 antigen expression in resistance to neoplasia caused by radiation induced leukemia virus. J Exp Med 1979;149:898–909.

176. Meruelo D, Nimelstein SH, Jones PP, Liberman M, McDevitt HO. Increased synthesis and expression of H-2 antigens on thymocytes as a result of radiation leukemia virus infection: a possible mechanism for H-2-linked control of virus-induced neoplasia. J Exp Med 1978;147:470–487.

177. Meyer T, Horisberger. Combined action of mouse α and β interferons in influenza virus–infected macrophages carrying the resistance gene Mx. J Virol 1984;49:709–716.

178. Mims CA, White DO. Viral pathogenesis and immunology. Oxford: Blackwell Scientific, 1984.

179. Miyazawa M, Nishio J, Wehrly K, Chesebro B. Influence of MHC genes on spontaneous recovery from Friend retrovirus induced leukemia. J Immunol 1992;148:644–647.

180. Miyazawa M, Nishio J, Wehrly K, David CS, Chesebro B. Spontaneous recovery from Friend retrovirus-induced leukemia: Mapping of the Rfv-2 gene in the Q/TL region of mouse MHC. J Immunol 1992;148:1964–1967.

181. Morgensen S. Role of macrophages in natural resistance to virus infection. Microbiol Rev 1979;43:1–26.

182. Morely D. The severe measles of West Africa. Proc R Soc Med 1969;57:846–849.

183. Morris PJ. Histocompatibility systems, immune response and disease in man. Contemp Top Immunobiol 1974;23:141–164.

184. Müeller M, Brem G. Disease resistance in farm animals. Experientia 1991;47:923–934.

185. Müeller M, Winnacker EL, Brem G. Molecular cloning of porcine

Mx cDNAs: new members of a family of interferon-inducible proteins with homology to GTP-binding proteins. J Interferon Res 1992;12:119–129.

186. Myers KM, Marshall ID, Fenner F. Studies in the epidemiology of infectious myxomatosis of rabbits. III. Observations on two succeeding epizootics in Australian wild rabbits on Riverine Plain of southeastern Australia, 1951–1953. J Hyg 1954;52:337–360.

187. Nakayama M, Nagata K, Kato A, Ishihama A. Interferon-inducible mouse Mx1 protein that confers resistance to influenza virus is GTPase. J Biol Chem 1991;266:21404–21408.

188. Nakhasi HL, Cao XQ, Rouault TA, Lui TY. Specific binding of host cell proteins to the 3'-terminal stem-loop structure of rubella virus negative-strand RNA. J Virol 1991;65:5961–5967.

189. Nakhasi HL, Rouault TA, Haile DJ, Lui TY, Klausner RD. Specific high-affinity binding of host cell proteins to the 3' region of rubella virus RNA. New Biologist 1990;2:255–264.

190. Nathanson N. Epidemiology. In: Fields BN, Knipe DM, eds. Virology. 2nd ed. New York: Raven Press, 1990:267–294.

191. Nathanson N, Cole GA. Immunosuppression and experimental infection of the nervous system. Adv Virus Res 1970;16:397–448.

192. Nathanson N, Langmuir A. The Cutter incident: poliomyelitis following formaldehyde-inactivated poliovirus vaccination in the United States during the spring of 1955. Am J Hyg 1963;78:16–81.

193. Noteborn M, Arnheiter H, Richter-Mann L, Browning H, Weissmann C. Transport of the murine Mx protein into the nucleus is dependent on the basic carboxy-terminal sequence. J Interferon Res 1987;7:657–669.

194. Notkins AL, Mergenhagen SE, Howard RJ. Effect of virus infection on the function of the immune system. Ann Rev Microbiol 1970;24:525–538.

195. Obar RA, Collins CA, Hammarback JA, Shpetner HS, Vallee RB. Molecular cloning of the microtubule-associated mechanochemical enzyme dynamin reveals homology with a new family of GTP-binding proteins. Nature 1990;347:256–261.

196. Obar RA, Shpetner HS, Vallee RB. Dynamin: a microtubule-associated GTP-binding protein. J Cell Sci 1991;14:S143–S145.

197. Odaka T, Ikeda H, Yoshikura H, Moriwaki K, Suzuki S. Fv-4: gene controlling resistance to NB-tropic Friend murine leukemia virus. Distribution in wild mice, introduction into genetic background of BALB/c mice, and mapping of chromosomes. J Natl Cancer Inst 1981;67:1123–1127.

198. Oldstone MBA, Ahmed R, Buchmeier M, Blount P, Tishon A. Perturbation of differentiated functions during viral infection in vivo. I. Relationship of lymphocytic choriomeningitis virus and host strains to growth hormone deficiency. Virology 1985;142:158–174.

199. Oldstone MBA, Jensen F, Dixon FJ, Lampert PW. Pathogenesis of the slow disease of the central nervous system associated with wild mouse virus. II. Role of virus and host gene products. Virology 1980;107:180–193.

200. Okada T. Inheritance of susceptibility to Friend mouse leukemia virus. VII. Establishment of a resistant strain. Int J Cancer 1970;6:18–23.

201. O'Neill RE, Palese P. Cis-acting signals and trans-acting factors involved in influenza virus RNA synthesis. Infect Agents Dis 1994;3:77–84.

202. O'Neill RE, Palese P. NP1-1, the human homologue of SRP-1, interacts with influenza virus nucleoprotein. Virology 1995;206:116–125.

203. Onodera T, Yoon JW, Brown KS, Notkins AL. Virus-induced diabetes mellitus: evidence for a single locus controlling susceptibility. Nature 1978;274:693–696.

204. Ou CY, Boone LR, Koh CK, Tennant RW, Yang WK. Nucleotide sequences of gag-pol regions that determine the Fv-1 host range property of BALB/c N-tropic and B-tropic murine leukemia viruses. J Virol 1983;48:779–784.

205. Panum P. Observations made during the epidemic of measles on the Faroe Islands in the year 1846. Hatcher AS, translator. Reprint published by American Public Health Association, New York, 1940.

206. Pardigon N, Lenches E, Strauss JH. Multiple binding sites for cellular proteins in the 3' end of Sindbis alphavirus minus-sense RNA. J Virol 1993;67:5003–5011.

207. Pardigon N, Strauss JH. Cellular proteins bind to the 3' end of Sindbis virus minus-strand RNA. J Virol 1992;66:1007–1015.

208. Parr RL, Fung L, Reneker J, Myers-Mason N, Leibowitz JL, Levy G. Association of mouse fibrinogen-like protein with murine hepatitis virus-induced prothrombinase activity. J Virol 1995;69:5033–5038.

209. Pavlovic J, Haller O, Staeheli P. Human and mouse Mx proteins inhibit different steps of the influenza virus multiplication cycle. J Virol 1992;66:2564–2569.

210. Pavlovic J, Zürcher T, Haller O, Staeheli P. Resistance to influenza virus and vesicular stomatitis virus conferred by expression of human MxA protein. J Virol 1990;64:3370–3375.

211. Pereira CA, Steffan AM, Kirn A. Interaction between mouse hepatitis viruses and primary cultures of Kupffer and endothelial liver cells from resistant and susceptible inbred mouse strains. J Gen Virol 1984;65:1617–1620.

212. Pestka S, Langer JA, Zoon KC, Samuel CE. Interferons and their actions. Annu Rev Biochem 1987;56:727–777.

213. Pincus T, Hartley JW, Rowe WP. A major genetic locus affecting resistance to infection with murine leukemia viruses. IV. Dose-response relationships in Fv-1 sensitive and resistant cell cultures. Virology 1975;65:333–342.

214. Pincus T, Snyder HW. Genetic control of resistance to viral infection in mice. In: Viral immunology and immunopathology. New York: Academic Press, 1975:167.

215. Plata F, Lilly F. Viral specificity of H-2 restricted T killer cells directed against syngeneic tumors induced by Gross, Friend, or Rauscher leukemia virus. J Exp Med 1979;150:1174–1186.

216. Price P, Gibbons AI, Shellam GR. H-2 class I loci determine sensitivity to MCMV in macrophages and fibroblasts. Immunogenetics 1990;32:20–26.

217. Purchase HG, Gilmour DG, Romero CH, Okazaki W. Post-infection genetic resistance to avian lymphoid leukosis resides in B target cell. Nature 1977;270:61–62.

218. Rommelaere J, Donis-Keller H, Hopkins N. RNA sequencing provides evidence for allelism of determinants of the N-, B-, or NB-tropism of murine leukemia viruses. Cell 1979;16:43–50.

219. Rothman JH, Raymond CK, Gilbert T, O'Hara PJ and Stevens TH. A putative GTP binding protein homologous to interferon-inducible Mx proteins performs an essential function in yeast protein sorting. Cell 1990;61:1063–1074.

220. Rowe PM. Resistance to HIV infection. Lancet 1993;341:624.

221. Rowe WP. Studies of genetic transmission of murine leukemia virus by AKR mice. I. Crosses with Fv-1 strains of mice. J Exp Med 1972;136:1272–1285.

222. Ruscetti SK, Janesch NJ, Chakraborti A, Sawyer ST, Hankins WD. Friend spleen focus-forming virus induces factor independence in an erythropoietin-dependent erythroleukemia cell line. J Virol 1990;63:1057–1062.

223. Sabin AB. Genetic, hormonal and age factors in natural resistance to certain viruses. Ann N Y Acad Sci 1952;54:936–944.

224. Sabin AB. Nature of inherited resistance to viruses affecting the nervous system. Proc Natl Acad Sci U S A 1952;38:540–546.

225. Sabin AB. Relationships between arthropod-borne viruses based on antigenic analysis, growth requirements, and selective biochemical inactivation. Ann N Y Acad Sci 1953;56:580–582.

226. Sabin AB. Genetic factors affecting susceptibility and resistance to virus diseases of the nervous system. Res Publ Assoc Res Nerv Ment Dis 1954;33:57–67.

227. Sabin A, Olitsky P. Influence of host factors on neuroinvasiveness of vesicular stomatitis virus. J Exp Med 1937;66:15–34,35–57;67:201–208,229–249.

228. Samuel CE. Mechanisms of the antiviral actions of interferons. Prog Nucleic Acids Res Mol Biol 1988;35:27–72.

229. Sangster MY, Heliams DB, Mackenzie JS, Shellam GR. Genetic studies of flavivirus resistance in inbred strains derived from wild mice: evidence for a new resistance allele at the flavivirus resistance locus (Flv). J Virol 1993;67:340–347.

230. Sangster MY, Shellam GR. Genetically controlled resistance to flaviviruses within the house mouse complex of species. Curr Top Microbiol Immunol 1986;127:313–318.

231. Sangster MY, Urosevic N, Mansfield JP, Mackenzie JS, Shellam GR. Mapping the Flv locus controlling resistance to flaviviruses on mouse chromosome 5. J Virol 1994;68:448–452.

232. Sato H, Boyse EA, Aoki T, Iritani C, Old LJ. Leukemia-associated transplantation antigens related to murine leukemia viruses. The X.1 system: immune response controlled by a locus linked to H-2. J Exp Med 1973;138:593–606.

233. Sawicki SG, Lu J-H, Holmes KV. Persistent infection of cultured cells with mouse hepatitis virus (MHV) results from the epigenetic expression of the MHV receptor. J Virol 1995;69:5535–5543.

234. Sawyer WA, Lloyd W. The use of mice in tests of immunity against yellow fever. J Exp Med 1931;54:533–555.

235. Sawyer W, Meyer K, Eaton M, Bauer J, Putnam P, Schwentker F. Jaundice in army personnel in the western region of the United States and its relation to vaccination against yellow fever. Am J Hyg 1944;39:337–430.

236. Scalzo AA, Fitzgerald NA, Wallace CR, et al. The effect of the *Cmv-1* resistance gene, which is linked to the natural killer cell gene complex, is mediated by natural killer cells. J Immunol 1992; 149:581–589.

237. Schubert M, Keene JD, Lazzarini RA. A specific internal RNA polymerase recognition site of VSV RNA is involved in the generation of DI particles. Cell 1979;18:749–57.

238. Shallem GR, Urosevic N, Sangster MY, Mansfield JP, Mackenzie JS. Characterization of allelic forms at the retinal degeneration (*rd*) and β-glucuronidase (*Gus*) loci for the mapping of the flavivirus resistance (*Flv*) gene on mouse chromosome 5. Mouse Genome 1993;91:572–574.

239. Shi PY, Li W, Brinton MA. Cell proteins bind specifically to the 3' stem-loop structure of West Nile virus minus-strand RNA. J Virol 1996;70 (in press).

239a. Shi PY, Brinton MA, Veal JM, et al. Evidence for the existence of a pseudoknot structure at the 3' terminus of the flavivirus genomic RNA. Biochemistry 1996;35:4222–4230.

240. Silver J, Teich N. Expression of resistance to Friend virus-stimulated erythropoiesis in bone marrow chimeras containing Fv-2ʳ and Fv-2ˢ bone marrow. J Exp Med 1981;154:126–137.

241. Smith AL. Genetic resistance to lethal flavivirus encephalitis: effect of host age and immune status and route of inoculation on production of interfering Banzi virus in vivo. Am J Trop Med Hyg 1981;30:1319–1323.

242. Smith MS, Click RE, Plagemann PGW. Control of MHV replication in macrophages by a recessive gene on chromosome 7. J Immunol 1984;133:428–432.

243. Sobey WR. Selection of resistance to myxomatosis in domestic rabbits (*Oryctolagus cuniculus*). J Hyg 1969;67:743–754.

244. Staeheli P, Dreiding P, Haller O, Lindenmann J. Polyclonal and monoclonal antibodies to the interferon-inducible protein Mx of influenza virus-resistant mice. J Biol Chem 1985;260:1821–1825.

245. Staeheli P, Grob R, Meier E, Sutcliffe JC, Haller O. Influenza virus-susceptible mice carry MX genes with a large deletion or a nonsense mutation. Mol Cell Biol 1988;8:4518–4523.

246. Staeheli P, Haller O. Interferon-induced human protein with homology to protein Mx of influenza virus-resistant mice. Mol Cell Biol 1985;5:2150–2153.

247. Staeheli P, Haller O, Boll W, Lindenmann J, Weissmann C. Mx protein: constitutive expression in 3T3 cells transformed with cloned Mx cDNA confers selective resistance to influenza virus. Cell 1986; 44:147–158.

248. Staeheli P, Horisberger MA, Haller O. Mx-dependent resistance to influenza viruses is induced by mouse interferons α and β but not γ. Virology 1983;132:456–461.

249. Staeheli P, Pavlovic J. Inhibition of vesicular stomatitis virus messenger RNA synthesis by human MxA protein. J Virol 1991;65: 4498–4501.

250. Staeheli P, Pitossi F, Pavlovic J. Mx proteins: GTPases with antiviral activity. Trends Cell Biol 1993;3:268–272.

251. Staeheli P, Pravtcheva D, Lundin L-G, et al. Interferon-regulated influenza virus resistance gene Mx is located on mouse chromosome 16. J Virol 1986;58:967–969.

252. Staeheli P, Sutcliffe JG. Identification of a second interferon-regulated murine Mx gene. Mol Cell Biol 1988;8:4524–4528.

253. Staeheli P, Yu Y-X, Grob R, Haller O. A double-stranded RNA inducible fish gene homologous to the murine influenza virus resistance gene Mx. Mol Cell Biol 1989;9:3117–3121.

254. Steeves RA, Bubbers JE, Plata F, Lilly F (1978). Origin of spleen colonies generated by Friend virus–infected cells in mice. Cancer Res 1978;38:2729–2733.

255. Steeves RA, Mirand EA, Bulba A, Trudel PJ. Spleen foci and polycythemia in C57BL mice infected with host-adapted Friend leukemia virus complex. Int J Cancer 1970;5:346–356.

256. Stohlman SA, Frelinger JA. Resistance to fatal central nervous system disease by mouse hepatitis virus, strain JHM. I. Genetic analysis. Immunogenetics 1978;6:277–281.

257. Stohlman SA, Frelinger JA. Genetic control of resistance of mouse hepatitis virus, strain JHM, induced encephalomyelitis. In: Skamene E, Kongshavn PAL, Landy M, eds. Genetic control of natural resistance to infection and malignancy. New York: Academic Press, 1980:247–253.

258. Suzuki S, Axelrad AA. *Fv-2* locus controls the proportion of erythropoietic progenitor cells (BFU-E) synthesizing DNA in normal mice. Cell 1980;19:225–236.

259. Taylor RM, Hurlbut HS, Work TH, Kingston JR, Frothingham TE. Sindbis virus: a newly recognized arthropod-transmitted virus. Am J Trop Med Hyg 1955;4:844–862.

260. Teich N, Wyke J, Mak T, Bernstein A, Hardy W. Pathogenesis of retrovirus-induced disease. In: Weiss R, Teich N, Varmus H, Coffin J, eds. Molecular biology of tumor viruses: RNA tumor viruses. 2nd ed. Cold Spring Harbor, New York: Cold Spring Harbor Laboratory, 1982:785–998.

261. Thimme R, Frese M, Kochs G, Haller O. *Mx*1 but not *Mx*A confers resistance against tickborne Dhori virus in mice. Virology 1995;211: 296–301.

262. Thomis DC, Samuel CE. Mechanism of interferon action: alpha and gamma interferons differentially affect mRNA levels of the catalytic subunit of protein kinase A and protein *Mx* in human cells. J Virol 1992;66:2519–2522.

263. Todd S, Nguyen JHC, Semler BL. RNA-protein interactions directed by the 3' end of human rhinovirus genomic RNA. J Virol 1995;69:3605–3614.

264. Tyler KL, Fields BN. Pathogenesis of viral infections. In: Fields BN, Knipe DM. Virology. 2nd ed. New York: Raven Press, 1990: 191–239.

265. Ubol S, Tucker PC, Griffin DE, Hardwick JM. Neurovirulent strains of alphavirus induce apoptosis in *bcl-2*–expressing cells: role of a single amino acid change in the E2 glycoprotein. Proc Natl Acad Sci U S A 1994;91:5202–5206.

265a. Urosevic N, Mansfield JP, Mackenzie JS, Shellam GR. Low resolution mapping around the flavivirus resistance locus (Flv) on mouse chromosome 5. Mammalian Genome 1995;6:454–458.

266. Vainio T. Virus and hereditary resistance in vitro. I. Behavior of West Nile (E-101) virus in the cultures prepared from genetically resistant and susceptible strains of mice. Ann Med Exp Biol Fenn 1963;41:1–24.

267. Vainio T, Gavatkin R, Koprowski H. Production of interferon by brains of genetically resistant and susceptible mice infected with West Nile virus. Virology 1961;14:385–387.

268. Vallee RB, Herskovits JS, Aghajanian JG, Burgess CC, Shpetner HS. Dynamin, a GTPase involved in the initial stages of endocytosis. Ciba Found Symp 1993;176:185–197.

269. van der Blick AM, Meyerowitz EM. Dynamin-like protein encoded by the *Drosophila shibire* gene associated with vesicular traffic. Nature 1991;351:411–414.

270. van Rood JJ, van Hooff JP, Keuning JJ. Disease predisposition, immune responsiveness and the fine structure of the HLA-A supergene. Transplant Rev 1975;22:75–104.

271. Vater CA, Raymond CK, Ekena K, Howaldstevenson I, Stevens TH. The VPS1 protein, a homolog of dynamin required for vacuolar protein sorting in *Saccharomyces cerevisiae*, is a GTPase with two functionally separable domains. J Cell Biol 1992;119:773–786.

272. Virelizier JL, Dayan AD, Allison AC. Neuropathological effects of persistent infection of mice by mouse hepatitis virus. Infect Immun 1975;12:1127–1140.

273. Webster LT. Microbic virulence and host susceptibility in mouse typhoid infection. J Exp Med 1923;37:231–244.

274. Webster LT. Inherited and acquired factors in resistance to infection. I. Development of resistant and susceptible lines of mice through selective breeding. J Exp Med 1933;57:793–817.

275. Webster LT. Inheritance of resistance of mice to enteric bacterial and neurotropic virus infections. J Exp Med 1937;65:261–286.

276. Webster LT, Clow AD. Experimental encephalitis (St. Louis type) in mice with high inborn resistance. J Exp Med 1936;63:827–846.

277. Webster LT, Johnson MS. Comparative virulence of St. Louis encephalitis virus cultured with brain tissue from innately susceptible and innately resistant mice. J Exp Med 1941;74:489–494.

278. Wege H, Siddell S, ter Meulen V. The biology and pathogenesis of coronaviruses. Curr Top Microbiol Immunol 1982;99:165–200.
279. Weiser W, Vellisto I, Bang FB. Congenic strains of mice susceptible and resistant to mouse hepatitis virus. Proc Soc Exp Biol Med 1976;152:499–502.
280. Welsh RM. Natural cell-mediated immunity during viral infections. In: Haller O, ed. Natural resistance to tumors and viruses. Berlin: Springer-Verlag, 1981:25–52.
281. Wengler G, Wengler G. Terminal sequences of the genome and replicative-form RNA of the flavivirus West Nile virus: absence of poly (A) and possible role in RNA replication. Virology 1981;113:544–555.
282. Wettstein P, Blank KJ. Use of H-2; H-7 congenic mice to study H-2 mediated resistance to Friend leukemia virus. J Immunol 1982;129:358–361.
283. Williams RK, Jiang G-S, Holmes KV. Receptor for mouse hepatitis virus is a member of the carcinoembryonic antigen family of glycoproteins. Proc Natl Acad Sci U S A 1991;88:5533–5536.
284. Wilson GAR, Dales S. In vivo and in vitro models of demyelinating disease: efficiency of virus spread and formation of infectious centers among glial cells is genetically determined by murine host. J Virol 1988;62:3371–3377.
285. Wilusz J, Kurilla MG, Keene JD. A host protein (La) binds to a unique species of minus-sense leader RNA during replication of vesicular stomatitis virus. Proc Natl Acad Sci 1983;80:5827–5831.
286. Wolfe JH, Blank KJ. Identification of a variant of Gross leukemia virus that induces disease in mice inoculated as adults. J Exp Med 1983;158:629–634.
287. Wolfe JH, Blank KJ, Pincus T. Variation in RNA tumor virus expression in H-2–congenic leukemia cell line. Immunogenetics 1981;12:187–190.
288. Wolfe JH, Blankenhorn EP, Blank KJ. Variation in p30-related proteins in Gross virus–induced tumor cell lines derived from H-2 congenic mice. J Virol 1984;49:14–19.
289. Wong C, Woodruff JJ, Woodruff JF. Generation of cytotoxic T lymphocytes during coxsackievirus B_3 infection. III. Role of sex. J Immunol 1977;119:591–597.
290. Woodruff J. The influence of quantitated post-weaning undernutrition on coxsackievirus B_3 infection of adult mice. J Infect Dis 1970;121:164–181.
291. Woyciechowska JL, Trapp BD, Patrick DH, et al. Acute and subacute demyelination induced by mouse hepatitis virus strain A59 in C3H mice. J Exp Pathol 1984;1:295–306.
292. Wüthrich R, Staeheli P, Haller O. Monoclonal antibodies detect protein Mx in lung cells of interferon-treated influenza virus resistant mice. In: Kirchner H, Schellekens H, eds. The biology of the interferon system. Rotterdam: Elsevier, 1985:317–323.
293. Yamada A, Taguchi F, Fujiwara K. T lymphocyte dependent difference in susceptibility between DDD and C3H mice to mouse hepatitis virus, MHV-3. Jpn J Exp Med 1979;49:413–421.
294. Yang WK, Kiggans JO, Yang DM, et al. Synthesis and circularization of N- and B-tropic retroviral DNA in Fv-1 permissive and restrictive mouse cells. Proc Natl Acad Sci U S A 1980;77:2994–2998.
295. Yeh E, Driscoll R, Coltrera M, Olins A, Bloom K. A dynamin-like protein encoded by the yeast sporulation gene SP015. Nature 1991;34:713–715.
296. Yokomori K, Lai MMC. Mouse hepatitis virus utilizes two carcinoembryonic antigens as alternative receptors. J Virol 1992;66:6194–6199.
297. Yoshimura A, D'Andrea AD, Lodish HF. Friend spleen focus-forming virus glycoprotein gp55 interacts with Epo-R in the endoplasmic reticulum and affects receptor metabolism. Proc Natl Acad Sci U S A 1990;87:4139–4143.
298. Yoshimura A, Lodish HF. In vitro phosphorylation of the erythropoietin receptor and an associated protein, pp130. Mol Cell Biol 1992;12:706–715.
299. Young E, Gomez C. Enhancement of herpes virus type 2 infections in pregnant mice. Proc Soc Exp Biol Med 1979;160:416–420.
300. Zürcher T, Pavlovic J, Staeheli P. Mechanism of human MxA protein action: variants with changed antiviral properties. EMBO J 1992;11:1657–1661.
301. Zürcher T, Pavlovic J, Staeheli P. Mouse Mx2 protein inhibits vesicular stomatitis virus but not influenza virus. Virology 1992;187:796–800.

Viral Pathogenesis,
edited by Neal Nathanson, et al.
Lippincott–Raven Publishers, Philadelphia © 1997

CHAPTER 14

Vector Biology in Arboviral Pathogenesis

Scott C. Weaver

INTRODUCTION

Arthropod-borne viruses (arboviruses) comprise a taxonomically diverse group of animal viruses that replicate within and are transmitted biologically by arthropod vectors. Vectors of arboviruses are primarily insects (class Insecta) in the order Diptera, most notably mosquitoes (*Culicidae*), sandflies (*Psychodidae*) and biting midges or "no-see-ums" (*Ceratopogonidae*).[98] Black flies (*Simuliidae*) have also been shown to transmit an arbovirus (vesicular stomatitis virus) and may be important epizootic vectors.[35] The other major group of arbovirus vectors are ticks and mites in the subclass Acari (class Arachnida). Although some arboviruses may be maintained in nature by vertical (transovarial) transmission alone, most rely on horizontal transmission among vertebrate hosts by their arthropod vectors. Arboviruses therefore differ ecologically from animal viruses that rely on direct spread among vertebrate hosts. This fundamental difference has important

implications regarding the epidemiology and evolution of arboviruses and the control of diseases that they cause.

The most recent catalog of arboviruses contains more than 500 members, including 100 known to infect humans and 40 that infect livestock.[98] The most important human and animal arboviral pathogens are RNA viruses in the families *Togaviridae, Flaviviridae, Bunyaviridae, Reoviridae,* and *Rhabdoviridae*; only one DNA arbovirus (African swine fever virus) has been described. RNA genomes, which are highly plastic and adaptable,[82] may be favored for arthropod-borne transmission because of the requirement for alternate replication in vertebrate and invertebrate hosts.[12]

Human arboviral diseases are classified generally into systemic febrile illnesses, encephalitides, and hemorrhagic fevers; veterinary arboviral diseases are more diverse but also include encephalitis and hemorrhagic syndromes[17] (see later discussion). Most tickborne viruses are encephalitic.[178] The most severe arboviral epidemics and epizootics have been caused by togaviruses, alphaviruses, flaviviruses, and bunyaviruses. Yellow fever virus, a flavivirus and the first virus for which arthropod transmission was demonstrated (by Walter Reed and colleagues in 1900),[140] causes sporadic, seasonal epidemics, which were first recognized during the 17th cen-

S.C. Weaver: Department of Biology, University of California, San Diego, La Jolla, California 92093-0116; present address: Center for Tropical Diseases, Department of Pathology, University of Texas Medical Branch, Galveston, Texas 77555-0609.

tury. Despite improvements in mosquito control and the availability of an effective, live attenuated vaccine, yellow fever virus continues to cause epidemics in tropical Latin America and Africa.[120,140] Dengue, first recognized as a viral disease in 1907, continues to affect hundreds of thousands of people each year in tropical locations around the world.[141] The alphavirus Ross River virus has caused arthritic epidemics in the Pacific involving up to 69% of the population of some islands,[101] and Venezuelan equine encephalomyelitis (VEE) virus has caused massive encephalitic outbreaks among equids and humans in the Americas since the 1920s.[215] Despite an effective equine vaccine, epizootic VEE viruses continued to emerge during 1995.[162] Although most bunyaviruses cause less severe human disease than alphaviruses and flaviviruses, Rift Valley fever virus causes severe morbidity and mortality in domestic animals.[128] This virus reemerged during 1993, after a 12-year absence, to cause a new epidemic/epizootic in Africa.[2] These recent outbreaks suggest that arboviral diseases will continue to occur throughout the world, underscoring the need for maintenance of research and control measures.

TRANSMISSION OF ARBOVIRUSES BY ARTHROPOD VECTORS

Transmission Cycles of Arboviruses

Transmission cycles of arthropod-borne viruses vary widely as to the hosts involved (both vertebrate and vector) and the complexity of the cycle. Some of the most important arboviruses, such as those causing dengue and yellow fever, infect only primates, with sylvan and urban cycles involving primarily nonhuman primates and humans, respectively. Different mosquito vectors transmit these viruses in the two cycles, with *Aedes aegypti*, a peridomestic mosquito, the predominant vector in urban settings.[69,140] Some alphavirus transmission cycles are more complex, with distinct enzootic and epidemic/epizootic forms. For example, most antigenic subtypes and varieties of VEE virus occur in sylvatic, enzootic transmission cycles involving small mammalian hosts and mosquitoes in the subgenus *Culex (Melanoconion)*[215] (Fig. 14-1). Epizootics occur periodically when one of these equine-avirulent enzootic viruses, the ID antigenic variety that occurs in northern South America and Panama, mutates to become an equine-virulent, variety IABC phenotype.[222] These epidemic/epizootic forms produce high-titered viremias in a variety of large mammalian hosts and can therefore be transmitted by numerous mammalophilic mosquitoes. The IABC VEE viruses can spread rapidly through large mammalian populations, causing massive outbreaks with high mortality rates, especially in equine populations.[215]

Transmission cycles of some tickborne viruses are even more complicated as a result of the complex, seasonal life cycles of tick vectors and the different vertebrate hosts used by the various tick life stages (see later discussion). For example, the Kyasanur Forest disease virus, a flavivirus, is transmitted primarily by the forest-dwelling tick, *Hemaphysalis spinigera*, among a variety of mammals in India (Fig. 14-2). Transstadial transmission among ticks and infestation of

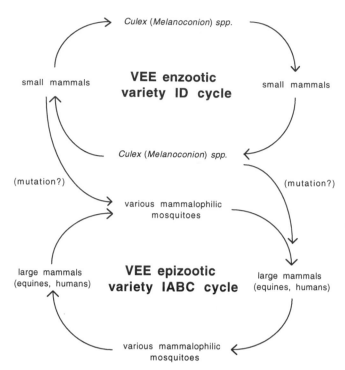

FIG. 14-1. Transmission cycles of antigenic varieties of Venezuelan equine encephalomyelitis (VEE) viruses. Enzootic cycles in Panama and northern South America involve *Culex (Melanoconion)* spp mosquitoes and small mammalian hosts.[44,215] Epizootics occur when equine-avirulent ID viruses mutate to generate equine-virulent IABC viruses. These epizootic viruses emerge from enzootic transmission foci and cause high-titered viremias in horses and other large mammals, resulting in encephalitic outbreaks involving a variety of mammalophilic mosquito vectors.[222]

viremic hosts by multiple ticks contribute to virus amplification and epizootics. Monkeys and porcupines appear to be important amplifying hosts, and the movement of cattle into enzootic habitats may contribute to epidemic transmission when tick-infested cattle return to villages. Nymphal ticks, which exist primarily during the winter and spring (the dry season), are believed to be responsible for most human transmission.[5]

The Life History of Arthropod Vectors

Because the majority of arboviruses use mosquito hosts,[98] the emphasis here is on mosquito biology at the expense of other important arthropod taxa. For more thorough treatments of other vectors, see reviews describing the biology of sandflies,[117] biting midges,[79,104] black flies,[34] and ticks.[79,104,178]

Like other insects, mosquitoes undergo complex life histories including metamorphosis.[29,79] After embryonic development, eggs hatch and four larval stages (instars) follow in an aquatic environment. Eggs of some *Aedes* mosquitoes undergo diapause (a period of arrested development) under appropriate conditions. Mosquito larvae occur only in aquatic habitats protected from wind and waves, because most species

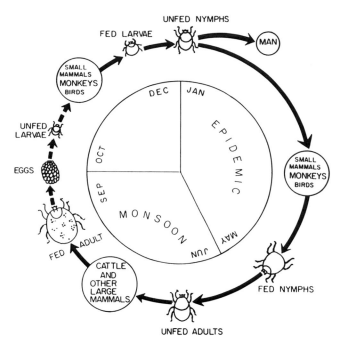

FIG. 14-2. Natural transmission cycle of Kyasanur Forest disease (KFD) virus. The virus is transmitted by nymphs and adults of the forest-dwelling tick, *Hemaphysalis spinigera*, among a variety of mammals and birds. This tick is a three-host species: adults feed primarily on large mammals, whereas larvae and nymphs feed mainly on small mammals, including monkeys, porcupines, and squirrels. Nymphal ticks, which exist primarily during the winter and spring (the dry season), are believed to be responsible for most human transmission. Monkeys and porcupines appear to be important amplifying hosts and sources of larval and nymphal infection. The movement of cattle into enzootic habitats may contribute to epidemic transmission when tick-infested cattle return to villages. Transstadial transmission among *H spinigera* and infestation of viremic hosts by multiple ticks also contribute to virus amplification and epizootics. Maintenance mechanisms during the monsoon season are unknown; *H spinigera* are not abundant, and infected adults are not known to transmit KFD virus transovarially. Ixodid ticks, which are more abundant during the monsoon, may maintain the virus during this period. (Courtesy of Kalyan Banerjee, National Institute of Virology, Pune, India.)

breath air while suspended from the water surface. Exceptions include larvae of the genera *Mansonia* and *Coquillettidia*, which have siphons specially adapted for piercing aquatic plants to acquire air. Most mosquito larvae filter feed on a variety of microorganisms and particulate material or browse on microorganisms attached to solid surfaces. However, larvae of mosquitoes in the genus *Toxorhynchites* are predacious on other mosquito larvae, and the adults do not feed on blood.[29,79] Larvae of several species in the subgenus *Psorophora* (*Psorophora ciliata*, *Psorophora howardii*) are also predaceous, but the adult females are hematophagous.

After three molts to larval instar 4, a final molt results in the mosquito pupal stage. The total time spent in the larval and pupal stages varies widely with mosquito species, tempera-

ture, and food availability, but it is typically on the order of a few days to several weeks. During the pupal stage, mosquitoes undergo metamorphosis from aquatic larvae to adults.[29] Some larval organs are destroyed and replaced by adult structures, but others persist to the adult stage. After their development is complete, adult mosquitoes split the pupal cuticle and climb to the water surface. Males of a given brood usually emerge before females.

Female mosquitoes of many species are refractory to mating until a few days after emergence. Mating often occurs in male swarms into which females enter during dawn and dusk hours. Females usually mate only once and store enough sperm to fertilize many egg batches. Male mosquitoes do not feed on blood and tend to be short lived, usually surviving only about 1 week. The survival of females varies widely: those of tropical species usually live only days to weeks, whereas females of temperate species may survive up to several months, and some hibernate or estivate. However, high mortality rates in nature limit survival of most individuals to only a fraction of their potential longevity.[143] Dispersal of adults varies widely, with some species such as *A aegypti* typically remaining within 0.5 km of their breeding site. However, other mosquitoes, especially salt marsh species, migrate for days soon after emergence, traveling tens of kilometers.[79,104]

In tropical locations, mosquitoes breed almost continuously throughout the year, fluctuating in numbers mainly with rainy and dry seasons. In temperate regions, breeding is limited to warmer seasons, and inseminated females of some species hibernate after developing their fat body (instead of eggs) in response to a blood meal. Other species survive the winter as larvae in water not subject to complete freezing or as eggs.[79,104]

Most other insect vectors in the order Diptera have life cycles similar to those of mosquitoes, including an egg, a variable number of larval instars, a pupal stage, and an adult stage.[79,104] Black fly larvae occur only in running water,[34,79] and sandflies are completely terrestrial.[117] Sandfly eggs are laid in moist soil, and the four larval instars develop slowly, feeding on decomposing organic matter. Biting midges in the genus *Culicoides* (no-see-ums) have aquatic or semiaquatic larvae that burrow into the substrate and require weeks to years to develop to the adult stage. Sandflies and biting midges are weak fliers with limited dispersal capabilities; this leads to local concentrations and focal transmission of viruses and other pathogens. Many species of black flies are exceptionally strong fliers and disperse long distances, particularly along rivers and streams; others actively orient into weather fronts, by which they may be carried hundreds of miles.

Ticks that serve as arbovirus vectors are classified in the families *Argasidae* (soft ticks) and *Ixodidae* (hard ticks). Hard ticks have a hard dorsal scutum and are usually free ranging, whereas soft ticks are leathery in appearance and are primarily lair ectoparasites. Ticks differ from insect vectors, and they vary widely among species in their life histories.[79,104,178] However, all ticks are terrestrial and pass through egg, larval, nymphal, and adult stages. Species vary in the length of the life cycle, requiring several months to years to complete all four stages. Ixodid ticks lay eggs in one batch, often numbering in the thousands, whereas argasids lay several, smaller clutches. Six-legged, terrestrial larvae hatch from eggs laid by engorged females and often climb vegetation to attach to vertebrate hosts passing by. Subsequently, one to five eight-legged nymphal stages occur. After a molt to the adult stage, mating occurs. Both female and male ticks, as well as larval, nymphal, and adult stages, feed on blood. Argasid ticks feed quickly, completing a blood meal in minutes, whereas ixodid ticks attach firmly to the host and feed slowly for several days or weeks. Many ticks consume several hundred microliters of blood, increasing their body weight by about 200-fold. In argasids, there is little sexual dimorphism; male ixodid ticks have a large dorsal scutum, whereas that of females is small.

Tick molting usually, but not always, occurs off of the vertebrate host. One-host ticks complete all feeding and molting on the same host, whereas different life stages of two- or three-host ticks use two or more different vertebrate hosts. The longevity of ticks can be remarkable, with some species surviving starvation for up to 16 years. Ecologically, ticks can be divided into those that occupy open habitats such as forests, savannas, and meadows (exophilic) and those that remain in closer association with vertebrate hosts, occupying secluded enclosures such as caves or nests (nidicolous).[178]

The Gonotrophic Cycle of Arthropod Vectors

The gonotrophic cycle of blood-feeding arthropods is the series of events, beginning with host seeking and ending with egg laying (oviposition), that is required for reproduction by most species.[13] Because arboviruses capitalize on obligate blood feeding by most vectors, the gonotrophic cycle is critical to the transmission of these pathogens.

Most female mosquitoes require one or more blood meals to produce eggs, although a few species, termed autogenous, rely on nutritional reserves from the larval stages for production of their first egg batch. Females of most species also rely on plant sugars as an energy source, whereas males feed exclusively on plant juices, lacking mouthparts adapted for blood feeding. In locations lacking sugar sources, female mosquitoes may also take additional blood meals to satisfy their energetic needs.[50] Anautogenous mosquitoes in the genera *Aedes* and *Culex* usually require one or more full blood meals to undergo oogenesis. However, if a blood meal is interrupted, two or more partial meals may occur before egg development can proceed.

Host Seeking

Blood feeding by mosquitoes and other biting flies usually follows an endogenous circadian rhythm that varies widely among species. Most feed during crepuscular (dawn and evening) or nocturnal hours.[79,104] Mosquitoes and many other blood-feeding insects locate potential vertebrate hosts by sensing carbon dioxide and body odors, orienting upwind to their source. At closer range, increases in air temperature caused by homeothermic hosts also serve as cues. After engorgement, during blood digestion and egg development, host seeking is inhibited in some *Aedes* mosquitoes but not in certain anopheline species.[106]

Most mosquitoes show some degree of specificity in selection of hosts, the mechanism of which is not understood. Many species feed primarily on mammals or birds, although a few

feed mainly on amphibians, reptiles, or even fish.[29] Host specificity can be important in the maintenance of some arbovirus transmission cycles. For example, *Culiseta melanura*, the enzootic mosquito vector of eastern equine encephalomyelitis (EEE) virus in North America, feeds almost exclusively on passerine birds, the primary vertebrate amplifying hosts of the virus.[177] Most populations of *A aegypti*, the principal urban vector of dengue viruses, are highly peridomestic. Vectors of some other arboviruses have more catholic feeding preferences yet maintain efficient transmission because of intrinsic susceptibility, large population size, longevity, and other factors regulating vector competence (see later discussion).

Blood Feeding and Digestion

Mosquitoes and other solenophagous (vessel-feeding) vectors acquire blood by penetrating a peripheral blood vessel with their elongate probosces. Many other arthropod vectors, including sandflies, black flies, biting midges, and ticks, are telmophagous (pool feeding); they lacerate vessels and ingest blood from the resultant pool.[79]

The mosquito proboscis is composed of a sheath-like outer labium that encloses six inner needlelike stylets.[29,104] The stylets function collectively as a fascicle and penetrate the vertebrate epidermis and dermis, forming a channel for the deposition of mosquito saliva and for imbibing blood after a blood vessel is pierced. During a mosquito's exploratory probing phase, when the fascicle repeatedly penetrates the dermis in search of a suitable blood vessel, saliva is discharged into the host before a venule or arteriole is penetrated; introduction of arboviruses within saliva also appears to be extravascular.[212] Salivation within blood vessels has rarely been observed. Mosquito probing can result in laceration of blood vessels and hemorrhages, providing hematomas as an alternative source of blood. During probing, the mosquito detects the presence of blood by its adenosine diphosphate (ADP) and adenosine triphosphate (ATP) content.[29,104]

The saliva of blood-feeding arthropods has several general functions, including lubrication of the stylets during probing and feeding. It is also the source of vertebrate allergens, which elicit immune reactions that interfere with blood feeding by some arthropods. Mosquito saliva contains enzymes for digesting sugars obtained from plant secretions and several compounds that facilitate blood vessel location and delay hemostasis.[25,156] Salivary apyrases block ADP-dependent platelet aggregation, thereby disrupting hemostasis, and tachykinin-like vasodilators increase blood availability. Similar pharmacologic activities have been identified in the saliva of other hematophagous arthropods, including ticks[99,158,159] sandflies,[116,161] and black flies.[33,36,37,93]

Mosquito blood feeding success is usually greatest in highly vascularized tissues.[160] Blood is sucked by the cibarial and pharyngeal muscular pumps and usually passes into the abdominal midgut of engorged mosquitoes, although small amounts may also be deposited in the thoracic diverticula and later regurgitated into the thoracic midgut[199] (Figs. 14-3 through 14-5). Most mosquitoes, sandflies, biting midges, and black flies feed to repletion in less than 10 minutes. These insects consume several times their own mass in blood (several microliters of blood for mosquitoes, less for smaller flies).

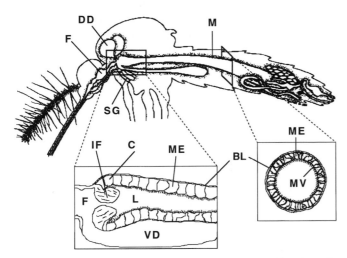

FIG. 14-3. Mosquito internal anatomy. BL, basal lamina; C, cardial midgut; DD, dorsal diverticulum; F, foregut; IF, intussuscepted foregut; L, lumen; M, midgut; ME, midgut epithelium; MV, microvilli or brush border; SG, salivary glands; VD, ventral diverticulum. (Modified from Weaver SC, Scott TW, Lorenz LH, Lerdthusnee K, Romoser WS. Togavirus-associated pathologic changes in the midgut of a natural mosquito vector. J Virol 1988;62:2083–2090.)

However, because of antimosquito defensive behavior by vertebrate hosts, mosquitoes sometimes imbibe only a fraction of the maximum blood meal volume.[107] If several partial blood meals are taken during a short period, the potential for mechanical transmission by contaminated mouthparts, as well as biologic transmission to several hosts by previously infected vectors, is enhanced. Partial blood meals separated by several days can also result in biologic transmission without the completion of a gonotrophic cycle.[139] Termination of blood feeding is initiated by stretch receptors activated by distention of the abdominal midgut.[29]

Ixodid ticks usually remain attached to their hosts for several days to weeks and therefore must circumvent hemostatic mechanisms as well as slower-acting host immune defenses. This is accomplished by secretion of apyrases, anticoagulants, and vasodilators (prostaglandins) in the saliva; immunosuppressive (anticomplement), antihistamine, and anaphylatoxin-destroying activities have also been detected.[157] Many species of hard ticks also secrete a salivary cement that anchors their mouthparts to the skin during prolonged engorgement, while their mass increases by up to 100-fold.[99] Salivary antigens apparently result in the development of acquired immunity to repeated tick infestations. At the site of attachment, the skin of sensitized animals accumulates large numbers of leukocytes and develops hyperplasia and erythema, disrupting tick feeding.[178] Argasid ticks are intermittent blood feeders and rarely attach to the host for long periods.

In the mosquito alimentary tract, blood digestion occurs primarily within the abdominal or posterior midgut (see Fig. 14-3). Ingested blood first passes through the pharyngeal pump and the cuticle-lined foregut. From there, most blood passes through a cardiac valve at the anterior end of the thoracic midgut and proceeds into the larger, bulbous abdominal midgut or stomach. At the posterior end of the midgut is a py-

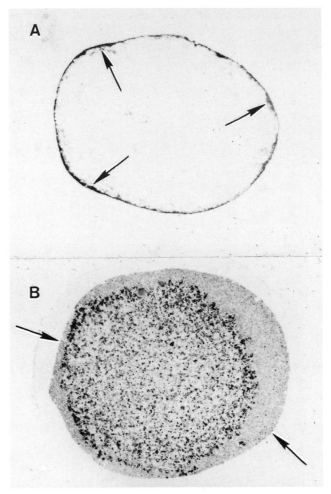

FIG. 14-4. Transverse abdominal sections of *Culex tarsalis* 30 to 90 minutes after infection with western equine encephalomyelitis virus. **(A)** Concentration of radiolabeled virus, detected autoradiographically by silver grains (*arrows*) in a thin band adjacent to the midgut epithelium after engorgement on a viremic chick. **(B)** Concentration of virus within the central portion of the midgut lumen after feeding on a suspension of purified virus, washed red blood cells, and 1.0% sucrose. Note low concentration of virus in the midgut periphery, adjacent to the epithelium (*arrows*). Brightfield microscopy (mosquito tissues are invisible), original magnification 40×. (From Weaver SC, Lorenz LH, Scott TW. Distribution of western equine encephalitis virus in the alimentary tract of *Culex tarsalis* (Diptera: Culicidae) following natural vs. artificial blood meals. J Med Entomol 1993;30:391–397.)

loric valve, which leads into the cuticle-lined hindgut. The midgut is composed of a single layer of epithelial cells surrounded by a basal lamina and a network of circular and longitudinal muscle cells (see Fig. 14-3). The majority of midgut cells are columnar digestive cells that become flattened during midgut distention after engorgement. Situated basally are undifferentiated regenerative cells that presumably replace digestive cells. A small number of peptidergic endocrine cells are also present throughout the midgut.[29]

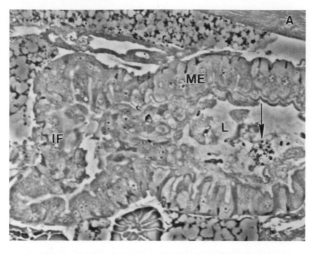

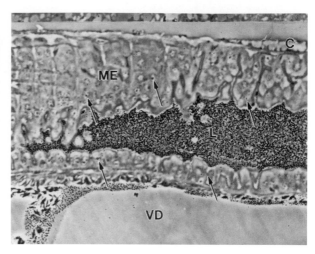

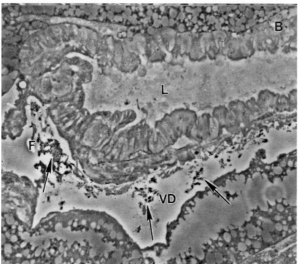

FIG. 14-5. Sagittal thoracic sections of *Culex tarsalis* 30 to 90 minutes after infection with western equine encephalomyelitis virus. (**A**) Small amounts of radiolabeled virus are detected autoradiographically by silver grains (*arrow*) within the lumen (L) of the thoracic midgut after engorgement on a viremic chick. IF, intussuscepted foregut. (**B**) Small amounts of virus (*arrows*) within the ventral diverticulum (VD) and foregut (F) after engorgement on a viremic chick. (**C**) Large amounts of virus within the thoracic midgut lumen (L) and ventral diverticulum (VD) after feeding on a suspension of purified virus, washed red blood cells, and 2.5% sucrose. Arrows show virus within the cytoplasm of midgut epithelial (ME) cells. Phase contrast, original magnification 200×. (From Weaver SC, Lorenz LH, Scott TW. Distribution of western equine encephalitis virus in the alimentary tract of *Culex tarsalis* (Diptera: Culicidae) following natural vs. artificial blood meals. J Med Entomol 1993;30:391–397.

The columnar digestive cells of the abdominal midgut of mosquitoes are believed to be the principal cells involved in blood digestion. The apical cell membrane contains a brush border of microvilli, with a high concentration of mitochondria in the adjacent apical cytoplasm. The luminal microvillar surface has little ionic content in *Culex tarsalis*, but the basolateral membranes and basal lamina are negatively charged.[88,89] Apically, continuous junctions (zonula continua) separate digestive cells; gap and septate junctions occur more basally, along with desmosomes and hemidesmosomes.[29] The nucleus lies basally, and a deeply convoluted basolateral plasma membrane separates the cytoplasm from the underlying basal lamina (see Fig. 14-3). The basal lamina is composed of a meshed network of collagen fibers in sheet-like arrays and surrounds the entire midgut. Pores of approximately 20 nm have been measured within individual laminar sheets, although the basal lamina of *C tarsalis* is only marginally permeable to colloidal thorium of diameter 5 to 8 nm,[87] a size smaller than that of any arbovirus. The thickness of the basal lamina varies in *Aedes triseriatus* according to the size of the mosquito, reflecting larval nourishment.[67]

Blood digestion in the mosquito, normally completed in a few days, is accomplished by several enzymes, including trypsin, chymotrypsin, aminopeptidases, esterases, and li-

pases. The pH of the blood meal has been reported to be 7.5 to 7.9 within the first hour after engorgement but is unknown later, after digestive enzyme secretion begins.[29] Of the endopeptidases, trypsin appears to predominate within the midgut lumen, whereas most aminopeptidase activity is membrane-bound on epithelial microvilli.[29] Trypsin synthesis in *A aegypti* appears to be at least partially regulated by transcription; trypsin cannot be detected within 15 minutes of blood feeding, but it is found in the secretory pathway and midgut lumen within 8 to 12 hours after engorgement. Aminopeptidase activity is present in the midgut before blood feeding and peaks about 24 hours after engorgement, when most activity is luminal.[29] Presumably, attachment of arboviruses to the midgut epithelium occurs soon after engorgement and is not affected to a great extent by secretion of digestive enzymes.[230] However, attachment of La Crosse virus to the midgut of *A triseriatus* mosquitoes may depend on proteolytic cleavage of viral glycoproteins by midgut enzymes present before peak synthesis occurs[119,121] (see later discussion).

The peritrophic matrix or membrane, a chitinous substance secreted by adult mosquito midgut epithelial cells, surrounds the blood meal and may serve to prevent mechanical damage by digested blood products.[29] Peritrophic matrix secretion begins in *A aegypti* midguts within a few hours of blood feeding, and a discrete layer is formed around the blood meal within 12 hours[152]; similar timing has been reported in *C tarsalis*[91] and *C melanura*.[228] If a mosquito takes two or more partial blood meals separated by many hours or days, the second meal surrounds the first and is separated from it by the first peritrophic matrix; on histologic examination, this structure is an indicator of multiple blood meals.[165] Mature peritrophic matrices are about 1 to 5 μm in thickness and laminar or fibrillar in structure. The matrix is retained in some mosquito species even after remnants of the blood meal are voided.[164]

Ovarian Development and Oviposition

Egg development in anautogenous mosquitoes and other dipteran vectors occurs in response to blood feeding, and eggs mature synchronously in a single batch during each gonotrophic cycle. Vitellogenesis, or egg yolk protein synthesis, uses amino acids derived from the digested blood meal and occurs within fat body trophocytes of adult female mosquitoes. Follicles within the ovaries are the sites of egg development; each includes an oocyte and several nurse cells, surrounded by a follicular epithelium. Before blood feeding, groups of sister follicles separate synchronously from the germaria and oocytes become competent to take up vitellogenin, the precursor of the egg yolk.[29] Vitellogenin molecules are secreted into the hemolymph from fat body trophocyte secretory granules and diffuse into the oocytes through the follicular epithelium, entering cells by receptor-mediated endocytosis. On entry into oocytes, vitellogenin crystallizes to form vitellin, increasing oocyte volume more than 100-fold. The chorion, part of the eggshell, is secreted by the follicular epithelium.

Spermatozoa stored in the spermathecae of inseminated mosquitoes fertilize mosquito oocytes during ovulation, and embryonation proceeds immediately after oviposition. Gravid mosquitoes lay their eggs in suitable locations based on many physical and chemical stimuli. *Culex* and *Culiseta* mosquitoes deposit their eggs, usually 50 to 500 at a time, on the surface of shallow, quiet bodies of water in raft-like clusters; *Aedes* and *Psorophora* species lay their eggs singly on surfaces subject to periodic flooding. At the time of oviposition, the eggs are soft and white; sclerotization or tanning begins within minutes and results in the dark color and hardness characteristic of mature mosquito eggs. *Culex* and *Culiseta* eggs usually hatch soon after oviposition on the water surface, but only a portion of *Aedes* eggs hatch during each flooding. Eggs of many *Aedes* mosquitoes survive the winter in temperate regions, and several species are known to survive several years if maintained with adequate moisture.[79] Within hours of oviposition, mosquitoes commence another gonotrophic cycle, beginning with host seeking.[29]

Susceptibility of Arthropods to Infection by Arboviruses

The vector competence of an arthropod reflects "the combined effect of all the physiologic and ecologic factors of vector, host, pathogen, and environment that determine the vector status of members of a given arthropod population."[126] The occurrence of arboviral outbreaks associated with relatively insusceptible vectors[135] underscores the fact that susceptibility to infection is but one factor determining a vector's role in transmission. Other aspects of vector competency, such as host preference and longevity, can have a profound influence on the vector's role in virus transmission. However, susceptibility to and ability to transmit a virus can be critical epidemiologic factors and therefore have received considerable attention.

The ability of arthropods to become infected with and transmit an arbovirus (Table 14-1) is affected by both intrinsic (genetic) and extrinsic factors.[24,42,73,75] The first evidence of a genetic component regulating vector susceptibility to an arbovirus came from studies showing differences in infection rates by dengue,[70] chikungunya,[196] and western equine encephalomyelitis (WEE) viruses[77] among different populations of mosquito vectors. Tesh[190] also demonstrated differences in rates of transovarial transmission of San Angelo and Kunjin viruses by the mosquito, *Aedes albopictus*. Later work also showed differences in oral susceptibility to yellow fever,[186] West Nile encephalitis,[80] and bluetongue[96] viruses among vector populations.

Jones and Foster[95] first demonstrated a genetic basis for midgut susceptibility to bluetongue virus by selecting strains of the biting midge, *Culicoides variipennis*, that were resistant or susceptible after oral infection. Similar results were obtained with *C tarsalis* mosquitoes and WEE virus,[74] *A albopictus* and dengue-2 virus,[70] *Culex tritaeniorhynchus* and West Nile virus,[80] and *A aegypti* and yellow fever virus.[214] A single genetic locus has been shown to control oral susceptibility of *C variipennis* midges to bluetongue virus.[185] The resistance of a strain of *A aegypti* mosquitoes to disseminated oral infection by several flaviviruses also appears to be regulated by a single major gene or closely linked genes.[133] Presumptive genetic changes accompanying colonization of vectors also lead to changes in infection and transmission rates of several arboviruses.[63,118,129]

The genetic makeup of several arboviruses can also affect their ability to be transmitted by mosquito vectors[73] (see Table 14-1). Beaty and colleagues[9] first identified the portion of an arboviral genome (the middle-sized or M segment of La Crosse virus) that determines its ability to infect a vector (*A triseriatus*). Different serotypes of bluetongue virus have been found to vary in their ability to infect a single population of *C variipennis* midges,[96] and closely related antigenic subtypes and varieties of VEE virus differ dramatically in their ability to infect and be transmitted by a given *Culex* (*Melanoconion*) mosquito vector.[173,227] Similar results have been obtained for different strains of yellow fever, St. Louis encephalitis (SLE), and dengue viruses.[73] A single amino acid substitution in the E2 surface glycoprotein of the VEE virus was shown to decrease its ability to replicate and disseminate in *A aegypti* mosquitoes.[236] The ability of vectors to transmit live attenuated arbovirus vaccine strains, as opposed to their parent viruses, can also differ, and the genetic and phenotypic stability exhibited by live attenuated vaccine strains is of obvious epidemiologic importance.[73]

Despite decades of study, the viral- and vector-specific factors that regulate arbovirus vector specificity and the nature of their interactions remain poorly understood. The almost uniform susceptibility of many vectors to intrathoracic infection by small amounts of arboviruses suggests that the initial virus-midgut cell interaction is the critical one regulating vector

TABLE 14-1. *Examples of Arbovirus-Vector Specificity*

Vector	Arbovirus	Log$_{10}$ blood meal titer*	Percentage infected	Reference
Aedes albopictus, Philippine	Dengue-4	7.3	5	70
Aedes albopictus, Malaysian	Dengue-4	7.3	68	70
Aedes aegypti, Nigerian	Yellow fever	8.0	10	133
Aedes aegypti, Puerto Rican	Yellow fever	8.0	90	133
Aedes aegypti, Nigerian	Dengue-2	5.8	0	133
Aedes aegypti, Puerto Rican	Dengue-2	5.8	57	133
Culex tarsalis Knight's Landing	WEE	6.1	95	74
Culex tarsalis WR (lab selected)	WEE	6.1	0	74
Culicoides variipennis, Maple Spr., KY	Bluetongue	>6	0	96
Culicoides variipennis, McAllen, TX	Bluetongue	>6	68	96
Culex (Melanoconion) taeniopus	VEE, variety IE	<2.7	100	171
Culex (Melanoconion) taeniopus	VEE, varieties IAB, IC, ID, II, III, IV	>5	0–40	172,173
Aedes aegypti	VEE strain TC-83	7.3	38†	236
Aedes aegypti	VEE 1A3B variant‡	7.3	0†	236

VEE, Venezuelan equine encephalitis; WEE, western equine encephalitis.
*Plaque forming units (PFU) or 50% infectious doses (ID50) per milliliter of blood ingested
†Infections disseminated beyond the midgut
‡monoclonal antibody-resistant variant differing from the TC-83 strain by one amino acid in the E2 glycoprotein

specificity (see later discussion). Now that genetic tools are available to approach the molecular determinants of these interactions, particularly receptor-ligand interactions (see later discussion), this topic should be a fertile area of future arbovirus research.

The role of host-parasite evolution in the regulation of arbovirus vector specificity also deserves more attention (see later discussion). The extreme sensitivity of many primary mosquito vectors to infection with many arboviruses suggests that these viruses may adapt specifically to certain vectors that maintain appropriate host contacts and other ecologic requirements for efficient transmission. However, natural evolutionary adaptation has not been thoroughly investigated or documented. Numerous studies of the susceptibility of mosquitoes and other vectors to infection with allopatric arboviruses (those that do not circulate within the vector's geographic range) have yielded a wide range of susceptibilities, including examples of allopatric virus infection thresholds equal to or lower than those seen in some natural virus-vector interactions.[201] This suggests that chance preadaptation may also be involved in successful arbovirus introductions and emergence of new arboviral diseases.

Oral Infection of Arthropod Vectors

Mechanisms of arthropod infection and transmission of arboviruses have been studied intensively since transmission cycles were elucidated during the first half of this century, and they have been the subject of many comprehensive reviews.[23,42,73,75,114,127,138,142,201] The focus here is on basic concepts and recent findings.

Although a few animal viruses (e.g., myxoma virus[60]) are disseminated among vertebrates solely by mechanical transmission, without multiplication in a vector, arboviruses are transmitted biologically, requiring replication in an arthropod.

Replication occurs after an infectious blood meal is taken from a viremic vertebrate host. A large body of evidence indicates that arboviruses replicate first in the alimentary tract of their vectors. Consistent with this hypothesis, bypass of alimentary tract replication by injection of arboviruses into the hemocoel of mosquito vectors usually reduces the incubation time required for transmission.[73]

Because the foregut and hindgut of the vector are lined with cuticle and are presumably impervious to viruses, initial infection is believed to occur in the midgut epithelium.[23,24,42,75,114,127,138,142] The posterior or abdominal midgut has been presumed to be the site of initial epithelial cell infection because most of the blood imbibed by mosquitoes is directed there for digestion (see previous discussion). However, studies have shown that a small portion of blood,[58] along with EEE and WEE viruses from artificial or natural blood meals,[224,230] is deposited into the thoracic diverticula and anterior midgut of mosquitoes (see Fig. 14-5). Rift Valley fever virus appears to replicate in the thoracic midgut of *Culex pipiens* early after an infectious blood meal, and this be a site of early virus dissemination to other tissues[166] (Fig. 14-6).

In the posterior or abdominal portion of the mosquito midgut, blood cells become concentrated centrally and serum is expressed to the periphery soon after feeding. This results in concentration of ingested virus adjacent to the epithelium[230] (see Fig. 14-4A). However, if mosquitoes are infected experimentally with artificial blood meals that do not clot in the midgut, this concentration does not occur[224] (see Fig. 14-4B); this probably explains the reduced susceptibility of mosquitoes to infection with arboviruses introduced in artificial blood meals.[150,202] Viruses presumably enter midgut cells within minutes or a few hours, before secretion of the chitinous peritrophic matrix,[91,224,230] and replicate within the epithelium before systemic infection ensues. Most of the entry of virus into abdominal midgut cells may occur before secretion of large amounts of digestive enzymes, while the luminal

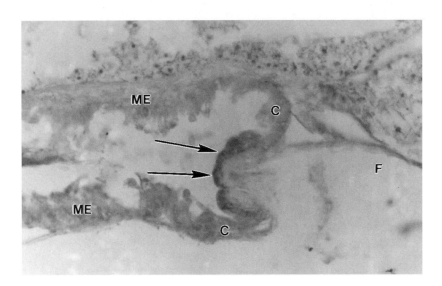

FIG. 14-6. Immunoperoxidase staining of thoracic alimentary tract of *Culex pipiens* after infection with Rift Valley Fever virus. Note viral antigen within the intussuscepted foregut (*arrows*) adjacent to the anterior midgut. Original magnification 200×. C, cardial midgut; F, foregut; ME, midgut epithelium. (Micrograph courtesy of William S. Romoser, Ohio University.)

pH is still slightly alkaline (see previous discussion). Penetration could occur later in the thoracic portion of the midgut, where no peritrophic matrix is produced.

Mechanisms of entry into arthropod cells are poorly understood for most arboviruses. Infection of the mosquito midgut by La Crosse virus has received the most attention. Initial studies indicated a role for the G1 viral glycoprotein in infection of *A triseriatus* mosquitoes.[184] More recent work suggests that the G2 glycoprotein plays an important role in attachment to midgut cells. Proteolytic removal of protein G1 apparently exposes G2 to specific cellular receptors on midgut epithelial cells.[119] Proteolytic treatment of bluetongue virus also increases infectivity in *C variipennis* midges,[130] suggesting a similar mechanism of midgut infection. The La Crosse virus G1 protein also serves as the attachment protein for vertebrate cells and possibly for some nonalimentary mosquito tissues.[121] The high-affinity laminin receptor serves as a receptor for Sindbis virus in C6/36 mosquito cells and vertebrate cells in vitro,[216] but its presence has not yet been investigated in vivo in mosquitoes. A related 32-kD protein, which also binds laminin and crossreacts immunologically with the high-affinity laminin receptor, serves as a receptor for VEE virus on C6/36 cells (George Ludwig, United States Army Medical Research Institute of Infectious Diseases, personal communication May, 1994). WEE virus appears to fuse and penetrate microvillar membranes of *C tarsalis* mosquitoes within 3 hours of an infectious blood meal[90]; it binds specifically to isolated microvillar membranes, with higher affinity for membranes recovered from susceptible than from refractory mosquitoes.[86]

Initial infection of tick midguts by arboviruses probably differs fundamentally from that of insects, because ticks are heterophagous, digesting the blood meal intracellularly.[145]

Arbovirus Replication and Dissemination Within Vectors

The time between ingestion of an infectious blood meal and transmission of an arbovirus is referred to as the extrinsic incubation period. The early stage of extrinsic incubation in

many vectors is characterized by an "eclipse phase," during which titers of virus within the blood meal decline before detectable viral replication occurs.[24,35,73,75,92,130] The eclipse phase usually lasts 1 to 4 days, depending on the quantity of virus imbibed, the vector species, and the temperature of incubation. Declines in infectious titers are presumably caused by inactivation within the proteolytic midgut environment and disassembly of virions entering epithelial cells.[73]

Initial replication of arboviruses can usually be detected in the vector midgut by infectious assay,[71,175] electron microscopy,[90,218,229] or antigen detection[11,92,111,134] within hours to a few days after oral infection. Electron micrographs reveal that alphaviruses[90,218,229] and vesicular stomatitis virus[233] bud primarily from the basolateral membranes of infected epithelial cells and often accumulate in large numbers between these cells and the surrounding basal lamina (Fig. 14-7). In contrast, mature SLE virions are first seen within the endoplasmic reticulum and nuclear envelope of *C pipiens* midgut cells and mature within cytoplasmic vacuoles.[234] The distribution of infected cells within the midgut varies considerably, with some viruses primarily infecting cells in the most posterior portion during early stages of extrinsic incubation.[47,111] After initial infection, at a time when only a fraction of epithelial cells show signs of viral replication, most arboviruses replicate widely throughout the abdominal midgut.[229,234] However, SLE virus infects only a small fraction of mosquito midgut cells.[234] Some viruses, such as Japanese encephalitis[47] and Rift Valley fever[166,167] viruses, also replicate in the anterior, thoracic region of the midgut, whereas others such as dengue-2 virus,[111] do not appear to spread into this region of the alimentary tract. The proximity of the thoracic midgut to mosquito salivary glands (see Fig. 14-3) suggests that viral amplification there could affect transmission.

Dugbe virus infection of *Amblyomma variegatum* ticks has been studied with the use of organ titration, in situ antigen and RNA detection, and electron microscopy.[16] About 10% of gut digestive cells are antigen positive 24 hours after oral infection. The percentage of infected gut cells increases to about 40% after a noninfectious blood meal as a result of cell proliferation.

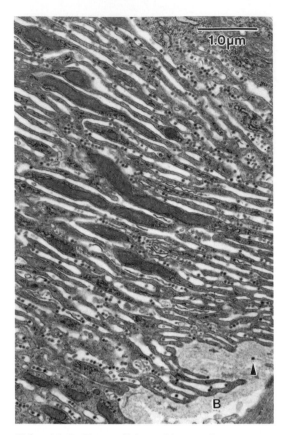

FIG. 14-7. Extracellular virions of eastern equine encephalomyelitis adjacent to the basolateral membrane of an abdominal midgut cell of the mosquito vector, *Culiseta melanura*, 3 days after an infectious blood meal. Note also a virion (*arrowhead*) within the basal lamina (B). (From Weaver SC, Scott TW, Lorenz LH. Patterns of eastern equine encephalomyelitis virus infection in *Culiseta melanura*. J Med Entomol 1990;27:878–891.)

Although two studies have revealed evidence of spread of mosquito-borne viruses through neural pathways,[115,132] most appear to disseminate through the hemolymph in a stepwise manner.[73,114,130] The mechanism by which arboviruses cross the basal lamina to enter the hemocoel of mosquitoes is unknown. However, infection of the midgut by a variety of arboviruses after intrathoracic inoculation suggests that penetration of the basal lamina does occur. Although the pore size of the basal lamina appears to be too small for penetration of any arbovirus (see previous discussion), visualization of arboviruses within the basal lamina[229,234] (see Fig. 14-7) suggests that some sort of dynamic interaction must occur during penetration. Basal laminae surround several mosquito organs that appear to be important for dissemination and transmission of arboviruses, such as the fat body, epidermis, and salivary glands (see later discussion). Improved understanding of the interactions of virions with this structure is essential to elucidation of the mechanisms of arbovirus transmission.

Reports of rapid appearance of arboviruses in the hemocoel before replication and dissemination from the midgut[15,58,132,218,224,230] presumably reflect disruptions or leaks in the midgut occurring during blood engorgement (see later discussion). Rough handling of engorged mosquitoes does not increase the numbers of mosquitoes with early signs of virus spread, suggesting that midgut disruptions accompany normal blood feeding.[58]

Once present in the hemocoel of a vector, an arbovirus has direct access to a variety of tissues and organs, including the fat body, ovaries and salivary glands (see Fig. 14-3). Fat body (Fig. 14-8) and epidermis appear to be important sites of replication by several arboviruses, whereas neural tissues are variably involved in mosquito and midge infections.[4,11,26,47,92,111,115,218,229] Rift Valley fever virus disseminates sporadically but rapidly to the intussuscepted foregut of infected mosquitoes and then to fat body, salivary glands, epidermis, and neural and endocrine tissues.[167] Because some arboviruses can be detected in salivary glands at the same time that replication is first detected in other nonalimentary tissues such as fat body, it is unknown whether amplification in these tissues is necessary for biologic transmission.[73] In adult *A variegatum* ticks infected transstadially from infected nymphs, Dugbe virus replicates primarily in the epidermis, hemocytes, and phagocytic gut digestive cells.[16] Because virus within tick hemolymph is associated entirely with hemocytes, spread to organs including the salivary glands may be mediated by hemocytes. Blood feeding by tick vectors appears to enhance viral replication and transmission by stimu-

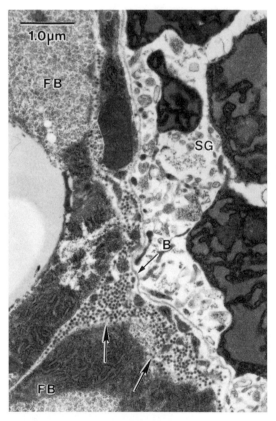

FIG. 14-8. Fat body (FB) and salivary gland (SG) cells in the thorax of *Culiseta melanura* 2 days after infection with eastern equine encephalomyelitis virus. Note the large number of virions (*arrows*) in the fat body adjacent to the basal lamina (B). (From Weaver SC, Scott TW, Lorenz LH. Patterns of eastern equine encephalomyelitis virus infection in *Culiseta melanura*. J Med Entomol 1990;27:878–891.)

lating proliferation of salivary gland and reproductive tissues.[45]

Some alphaviruses disseminate rapidly within their mosquito vectors and can be transmitted within 3 to 4 days of an infectious blood meal.[6,175] Vesicular stomatitis virus can also be transmitted by infected sandflies 3 days after a viremic blood meal.[193] Flaviviruses, bunyaviruses, and orbiviruses usually require longer times of extrinsic incubation.[73,75,130]

Arboviruses must first traverse the salivary gland basal lamina before infecting acinar secretory cells. This event may depend on the hemolymph titer, which would explain the salivary gland infection barrier exhibited by mosquitoes with low titers (see later discussion). Alphaviruses and vesicular stomatitis nucleocapsids form in the cytoplasm of infected acinar cells and mature by budding (Fig. 14-9). In *A triseriatus* salivary glands, EEE virus budding is random, virions maturing on both the apical and basal plasma membrane and into cytoplasmic vesicles. However, maturation of EEE virus in salivary gland cells of *C melanura* mosquitoes[229] and of vesicular stomatitis virus in *Lutzomyia shannoni* sandflies[233] appears to occur by budding exclusively from apical membranes into the salivary matrix. This could represent adaptation of these viruses for maximal transmission by their natural vectors. (*A triseriatus* is not an enzootic vector of EEE virus.)

As in midgut cells, dengue[179] and SLE[234] viruses mature in the rough endoplasmic reticulum of mosquito salivary acinar cells. Later, secretory membranes fuse with the plasma membrane to release virions into the apical cavities. SLE virus also enters the saliva after the apical plasma membrane is disrupted, releasing cytoplasmic contents. This process does not damage acinar cells.[234] During later stages of salivary gland infection by several arboviruses, the majority of acinar cells show signs of infection, and apical cavities are often filled with virions.[229,234] Different arboviruses appear to have differing affinities for the three lobes of each mosquito salivary gland; most viruses replicate first, and often exclusively, within the lateral lobes.[73]

Dugbe virus does not appear in salivary gland cells of *A variegatum* ticks until after the start of feeding, when small foci of antigen appear.[16] Continued feeding may stimulate viral replication. Antigen but no detectable RNA occurs throughout the salivary glands after 10 to 12 days of feeding.

Titers of arboviruses within vectors usually peak within a few days to 1 week of an infectious blood meal and then decline over time, decreasing about tenfold[75] (Fig. 14-10). Selection of high- and low-virus-producing *C tarsalis* mosquitoes indicates that their ability to suppress replication of WEE virus is genetically controlled.[73,108] Declines in titer are also observed in mosquito cell cultures infected with alphaviruses, and they appear to be caused by an antiviral protein that blocks RNA synthesis.[123]

Because most larval, nymphal, and adult stages of ixodid ticks feed on a single host, tickborne arboviruses require

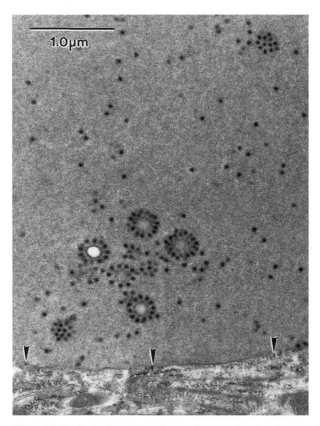

FIG. 14-9. Apical cavity of a salivary gland acinar cell 3 days after infection with eastern equine encephalomyelitis virus. Note circular arrays of virions surrounding fingerlike cytoplasmic extensions into the apical cavity. Cytoplasmic nucleocapsids are seen lining the plasma membrane (*arrows*). (From Weaver SC, Scott TW, Lorenz LH. Patterns of eastern equine encephalomyelitis virus infection in *Culiseta melanura*. J Med Entomol 1990;27:878–891.)

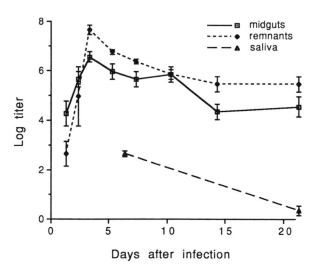

FIG. 14-10. Titers of eastern equine encephalomyelitis virus, expressed as median tissue culture infective dose (TCID50) per tissue or organ, in midguts, remnants (tissues remaining after dissection of midguts), and saliva samples taken from *Culiseta melanura* after oral infection with 10[7.6] to 10[7.8] TCID50 per milliliter of blood. Vertical bars indicate standard errors. Saliva samples were not taken before day 6. (Data from Weaver SC, Scott TW, Lorenz LH. Patterns of eastern equine encephalomyelitis virus infection in *Culiseta melanura*. J Med Entomol 1990;27:878–891.)

transstadial transmission from one instar to the next for horizontal, oral transmission to occur. Histolytic enzymes that accompany tissue replacement during metamorphosis affect replication of some but not all tickborne viruses.[145] The primary means of transstadial transmission of Dugbe virus in *A variegatum* ticks appears to be infected hemocytes, and the amounts of Dugbe virus decrease during molting.[16] The lack of transstadial transmission of Dugbe virus from *Rhipicephalus appendiculatus* nymphal ticks apparently prevents this species, which is susceptible to oral infection, from serving as a natural vector.[180]

Horizontal Transmission of Arboviruses

Horizontal transmission of arboviruses to susceptible vertebrates occurs because infected vectors salivate during blood feeding.[23,24,42,75,114,127,138,142,145] The titers of virus in vector saliva vary widely with the time of extrinsic incubation, the blood meal titer, and the virus and vector studied, with most estimates in the range of a few to 10^5 infectious particles in a volume of a few μm^3 inoculated during feeding.[73] Titers within mosquito saliva usually decline over time after 1 or 2 weeks of infection, resulting in decreased transmission rates.[24,155,229] Most mosquito saliva and virus appears to be deposited extravascularly within the host during the search for a suitable blood vessel.[212]

A unique phenomenon of nonviremic transmission has been described for tickborne viruses, in which tick-to-tick transmission occurs during cofeeding on a vertebrate without detectable viremia.[94,145] Tick salivary components appear to potentiate this form of transmission, which is termed salivary activated transmission. The nonviremic transmission mode selects for avirulence in vertebrates, ensuring that hosts remain alive for the duration of tick feeding.[145]

Barriers to Arbovirus Infection and Dissemination Within Vectors

The failure of arboviruses to infect, disseminate within, or be transmitted by arthropods has been attributed to several barriers. All of these barriers vary widely with the species or strain of both virus and vector and with the temperature of incubation.[73]

A midgut infection barrier apparently prevents initial viral replication in vector midguts after ingestion of a viremic blood meal with a titer below the infection threshold.[73,75,130,145,201] The relatively uniform susceptibility of mosquitoes to intrathoracic infection with small amounts of arboviruses implies that this barrier operates at the level of initial alimentary tract infection. Most studies also indicate that this barrier is dose dependent, high blood meal titers overcoming insusceptibility in somewhat refractory species. Evidence of a possible mechanism for the midgut infection barrier comes from studies demonstrating that WEE virus binds poorly to midgut microvillar membranes of some insusceptible mosquitoes, suggesting a lack of WEE-specific receptors.[86] However, other work indicates that the infection barrier may also be related to the ability of mosquitoes to modulate virus replication within infected cells.[73]

The failure of infected mosquitoes to transmit an arbovirus can also reflect one of several dissemination barriers. Some viruses replicate in the vector midgut but fail to disseminate to other tissues, including the salivary glands, and therefore are not transmitted.[73,75] This phenomenon has been termed a midgut escape barrier, and it is often dose dependent. The time and temperature of extrinsic incubation appear to have variable effects on the midgut escape barrier in different arbovirus-mosquito interactions.[73] Differences in the thickness of mosquito midgut basal laminae exhibiting the midgut escape barrier to La Crosse virus suggest that it is a physical barrier that can be modified by nutritional deprivation of mosquito larvae.[67] Lower viral titers in midguts of mosquitoes[108,226] and midges[130] exhibiting nondisseminated infections (i.e., those confined to the midgut) suggest that a factor that modulates arbovirus titers after initial midgut infection may be responsible for both susceptibility to oral infection and escape from infected midguts. However, midgut titers of *C pipiens* mosquitoes exhibiting the escape barrier to Rift Valley fever virus do not differ significantly from those with disseminated infections,[58,207] implying that viral replication in the midgut is not the only factor regulating escape into the hemocoel.

A salivary gland infection barrier, which apparently prevents infection of acinar cells, has also been identified.[73,110,151] Low viral titers within nonalimentary tissues of mosquitoes exhibiting the salivary infection barrier suggest that it is related to the failure of the virus to replicate to a threshold hemolymph titer after it disseminates from the midgut.[109] A salivary gland escape barrier is also exhibited by mosquitoes with virus in their salivary glands that fail to transmit by bite.[9,65,97] In some but not all virus-vector interactions, this barrier may be related to modulation of viral replication in the salivary glands, which results in a reduction in saliva titers and transmission rates over time (see Fig. 14-10).

Mechanical Transmission of Arboviruses

Several animal viruses, not considered arthropod-borne because they do not replicate in vectors, rely to some extent on mechanical transmission by contaminated mouthparts of blood-feeding insects and ticks. The most notable example is myxoma virus, which is transmitted mechanically by mosquitoes among rabbits.[60] Another poxvirus, avian or fowl pox virus, is also transmitted mechanically by mosquitoes and causes serious economic effects on poultry production. Encephalomyocarditis virus, also transmitted by mosquitoes, infects a variety of wild and domestic animals, and equine infectious anemia and hog cholera viruses may be transmitted mechanically by tabanid flies.[79]

Mechanical transmission is not thought to contribute greatly to the maintenance cycles of most arboviruses. However, arboviral outbreaks may occasionally be caused or augmented by mechanical transmission. For example, during one Colombian epizootic of VEE, black flies were incriminated as mechanical vectors.[170] The potential for mechanical transmission should be considered for any virus exhibiting appropriate stability and reaching high titers in the blood of infected vertebrates.

Vertical Transmission of Arboviruses

Vertical or transovarial transmission occurs when an arbovirus is passed from an infected adult female to her offspring within the embryo. Vertical transmission of an arbovirus (yellow fever virus) was first reported by Marchoux and Simond in 1905.[124] However, others were unable to confirm this finding during the early 20th century. Transovarial transmission was recognized for many years among tickborne viruses[85] and was later demonstrated for sandfly-borne[194] and mosquito-borne[217] viruses. Since the early 1970s, vertical transmission has been demonstrated in laboratory studies with a large number of bunyaviruses, rhabdoviruses, alphaviruses, and reoviruses that infect mosquitoes and sandflies.[201] Field isolations of additional arboviruses from vector larvae or adult males suggest that vertical transmission is even more widespread in nature.[30,31,49,62,191]

Relatively little is known concerning mechanisms of transovarial transmission. Transmission presumably occurs when an arbovirus present in vector hemolymph penetrates the ovarian and ovariole sheaths, infecting the follicular epithelium. From there, the virus can infect oocytes in an early stage of development, before the chorion is produced. However, the mechanism by which arboviruses enter the germ cells of vectors remains speculative.

San Angelo virus is first observed in the ovarian sheath, oviduct, ovariole sheath, and interstitial cells of vertically infected *A albopictus* mosquitoes within 12 hours of adult emergence; it later appears in the follicular epithelium, nurse cells, and oocytes.[195] After blood feeding, large amounts of antigen are seen in the follicular epithelium and within mature oocytes.

Transovarial transmission usually involves only the second and subsequent egg batches after an infectious blood meal, because oogenesis begins soon after engorgement and dissemination of arboviruses to the ovaries usually occurs after chorion development. Embryos within mosquito eggs remain infected for up to 19 months, allowing virus survival during overwintering of temperate organisms or interruption of transmission cycles during dry seasons. Many vertically transmitted viruses persist in the vector through larval and pupal stages to the adult and can be transmitted horizontally by bite, even after several consecutive transovarial infection cycles without vertebrate infection.[201]

Like oral infection, the efficiency or vertical transmission of arboviruses can vary with the virus and vector strains involved.[201] The rate of transovarial transmission (percentage of females transmitting virus to one or more progeny) can reach 98% for La Crosse virus in *A triseriatus* mosquitoes.[136] However, some mosquito species that transmit vertically at high rates have low filial infection rates (percentage of offspring infected). For example, 67% of *Aedes trivittatus* transmitted trivittatus virus to their offspring, yet only 11% of progeny were infected.[28] Rates of transovarial transmission by mosquitoes tend to be highest with California serogroup and phlebovirus members of the family *Bunyaviridae* and lower with most flaviviruses and Rhabdoviruses.[32,191] However, *Aedes mediovittatus* mosquitoes transmit dengue viruses at rates up to 95%, with filial infection rates of about 20%.[61] Vertical transmission has been reported (at low frequency) for only two alphaviruses, Ross River virus[100] and WEE virus.[62] How-

ever, negative results of laboratory transmission trials may warrant reevaluation with more sensitive methods of virus detection, such as reverse transcription–polymerase chain reaction amplification of viral RNA.

Although many tickborne viruses can be transmitted vertically, rates are usually low.[145] However, nonviremic transmission can amplify transovarially transmitted viruses, suggesting that vertical transmission may be critical to maintenance transmission cycles in nature.[112]

The relative contributions of vertical versus horizontal transmission of arboviruses has been the subject of experimental and theoretical work. As pointed out by Turell,[201] if a virus is transmitted to only 20% of an infected mosquito's progeny, horizontal transmission must provide a fivefold increase in mosquito infection rates for an arbovirus to be maintained in nature. This estimate assumes a naturally low survival rate of mosquitoes (infected or uninfected), whereby population numbers are stable and vertical transmission rates of 100% are required for virus maintenance in the absence of horizontal transmission. The lower rates of vertical transmission to first ovarian cycle progeny and the possible deleterious effects on infected progeny imply that the contribution of horizontal transmission must be even higher. For many arboviruses (including flaviviruses and alphaviruses) that have vertical transmission rates of 1% or less, horizontal transmission cycles must increase vector infection rates by more than 100-fold for virus maintenance. It therefore seems unlikely that most arboviruses can be maintained for long periods by transovarial transmission alone.[201]

A possible exception to the requirement for horizontal transmission is found among several arboviruses, including vesiculoviruses and phleboviruses transmitted by sandflies[192] and San Angelo[198] and California encephalitis[209] viruses transmitted by mosquitoes, that infect the germ lines of their vectors. Because these viruses exhibit high, sustained rates of stabilized vertical transmission, even to progeny of the first ovarian cycle, they may be maintained for many generations even in the absence of horizontal transmission.[191]

Venereal or sexual transmission of arboviruses can occur if eggs are inseminated immediately before oviposition and has also been demonstrated during experimental infections. La Crosse virus is transmitted from transovarially infected males to females at rates of about 50% in *A triseriatus* mosquitoes.[149] However, oral and transovarial transmission rates from venereally infected females are only about 25%, suggesting that venereal transmission makes only a small contribution to La Crosse virus maintenance in nature. Sindbis virus is transmitted venereally by *Aedes australis*,[146] as is Japanese encephalitis virus by *C tritaeniorhynchus*[168] and SLE virus by several mosquito species.[144] Toscana virus is transmitted venereally by *Phlebotomus pernicious* sandflies,[197] and African swine fever virus is transmitted sexually by orally-infected *Ornithodoros moubata* ticks.

Extrinsic Factors Affecting the Ability of Vectors to Transmit Viruses

Several extrinsic factors have been shown to have important influences on the ability of arthropods to transmit arboviruses. Titers of viruses in the blood meal can have consid-

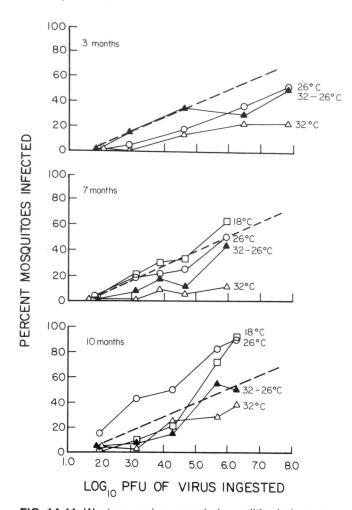

FIG. 14-11. Western equine encephalomyelitis viral susceptibility profiles obtained with different subcolonies of the Chico strain of *Culex tarsalis* that were reared and maintained under three or four different temperature regimens (18°C, 26°C, 32°C, or 26°C to 32°C) for 3, 7, or 10 months before infection. All mosquitoes were maintained at 24°C after oral infection. The broken lines indicate the susceptibility profile of the parental females at the time the subcolonies were initiated. (From Hardy JL, Meyer RP, Presser SB, Milby MM. Temporal variations in the susceptibility of a semi-isolated population of *Culex tarsalis* to peroral infection with western equine encephalomyelitis and St. Louis encephalitis viruses. Am J Trop Med Hyg 1990;42:500–511.)

erable effects on infection and transmission rates. Early work established the concept of an infection threshold titer, below which arboviruses fail to infect vectors.[24] Thresholds vary widely with the vector species (or even population) and the virus strain examined.[75] Low infection thresholds may represent evolutionary adaptation of viruses to primary vector species, although appropriate studies have not been carried out to test this assumption.

The temperature at which mosquito larvae develop and the ambient temperature at which adult mosquitoes are held during arbovirus infection and replication can significantly affect their susceptibility and ability to transmit viruses (Fig. 14-11). In general, the temperature at which mosquitoes are incubated after experimental oral infection is inversely related to the

time required for transmission by bite.[73,122,155,201,203,205,210] Studies simulating natural diurnal temperature variation have usually yielded results similar to those of studies using an intermediate, constant temperature.[73,122,203,210] There appears to be a "zero-development" temperature below which some arboviruses fail to replicate detectably within their vectors.[201,210] However, some arboviruses remain viable, and normal replication and dissemination usually ensue after temperatures are raised to appropriate levels. This may allow arboviruses to persist within overwintering adult female mosquitoes, with horizontal transmission occurring after temperatures rise in the spring or summer.[73]

Different temperatures of extrinsic incubation can have different effects on arbovirus infection and transmission rates.[201] Infection rates are correlated positively with temperatures of incubation for some arbovirus-vector systems, such as Rift Valley fever virus in *C pipiens* mosquitoes. In contrast, WEE virus infection rates (but not transmission rates) in *C tarsalis* are inversely related to incubation temperatures. Higher temperatures of extrinsic incubation may stimulate genetically controlled factors that suppress WEE viral replication in mosquitoes.[73,201] For other interactions, such as Rift Valley fever virus infection of *Aedes taeniorhynchus* mosquitoes, temperature has little or no effect on mosquito infection rates.[201] Although larval nutrition does not appear to influence susceptibility of *Culex annulirostris* mosquitoes to infection with Murray Valley encephalitis virus,[102] the temperature at which mosquito larvae develop can affect the susceptibility of adults to arbovirus infection. Lower laboratory rearing temperatures usually enhance infection rates,[103,131,205] and ambient air temperature also appears to influence susceptibility of natural mosquito populations of *C tarsalis* to infection with arboviruses.[76]

Developmental temperatures of vertically infected mosquito larvae can also affect rates of transstadial transmission to adult mosquitoes.[78] In some cases, virus persists to the adult stage only in larvae reared at low temperatures,[201] but in other experiments, no effect of temperature has been observed.[197] If global warming increases average temperatures in regions in which arboviruses circulate, epidemics may occur in previously unaffected areas because of differences in virus replication and dissemination within vectors as well as differences in mortality rates among vector populations.[154]

The presence of antibodies in artificial blood meals[150] or the completion of engorgement on an immune host after a partial infectious meal[147] can reduce infection of mosquito vectors with La Crosse virus. The nutritional status of the vector can also influence its ability to become infected and transmit an arbovirus. Small mosquitoes that are nutritionally deprived as larvae are more efficient vectors of Japanese encephalitis[187] and La Crosse viruses.[67] These differences in vector competence may be epidemiologically important, because field populations are probably nutritionally deprived in comparison with laboratory colonies, from which experimental data are usually derived.[187]

Effects of Vector Transmission on Virus Evolution

Arthropod-borne viruses often exhibit remarkable genetic stability during experimental[3,14] and natural[19,43,105,163,200] transmission cycles. All arboviruses for which estimates of evolutionary rates can be made appear to evolve on the order often to 100 times more slowly than most single-host vertebrate RNA viruses.[225] This is not to say that arboviruses evolve slowly in comparison with organisms that have DNA-based genomes, which exhibit mutation frequencies roughly a million times lower.[48,84,181] Some arboviruses appear to diversify very rapidly. For example, alphaviruses appear to have evolved from a common ancestor during the last few thousand years.[223] The *Bunyaviridae* and *Flaviviridae* families and the alphavirus genus are among the most diverse animal virus taxa.[8,21,22]

Several hypotheses have been proposed to explain the relative genetic conservation of arboviruses.[225] Conservation does not appear to be caused by differences in mutation rates, because natural populations of at least one arbovirus, EEE virus, exhibit mutation frequencies similar to those of faster-evolving, single-host RNA viruses.[220] Another theory maintains that rates of arbovirus evolution are limited by multiple, differing selective constraints imposed by the requirement for both arthropod and vertebrate infection during the alternating-host transmission cycles.[180,219,225] Experimental transmission cycles, including alternate replication in vertebrates and vectors, promote genetic[3] and phenotypic[189] conservation. However, rapid genetic changes accompany serial passage of some alphaviruses in single-host cell types. For example, EEE virus underwent the equivalent of roughly 40 years of natural evolution during only 100 serial passages in BHK or C6/36 cells (SCW, unpublished observations). These results are consistent with the idea that alternation between phylogenetically divergent hosts imposes strict selection for arbovirus phenotypes able to replicate efficiently in both arthropods and vertebrates.

Several characteristics of arthropod vector infection may be expected to provide a greater opportunity for viral evolution than replication in vertebrate hosts.[12] These include persistence of arboviruses in orally and transovarially infected vectors, which may enhance opportunities for mutation, recombination, or reassortment of segmented arbovirus genomes. Reassortment has been demonstrated during Rift valley fever virus infection of *C pipiens*,[211] bluetongue infection of *C variipennis*,[169] and bunyavirus infection of *A triseriatus*.[10] During experimental mixed infections, all possible La Crosse and Tahyna reassortant viruses were detected, and reassortants occurred at high frequency.[27] Long-lived vectors such as ticks may be especially conducive to reassortment during dual infections,[12] and reassortment of Thogoto virus has been demonstrated in its vector, *R appendiculatus*.[39]

Persistent infection of arthropod vectors does not necessarily promote mutational change of arboviruses. EEE virus recovered from *C melanura* mosquitoes after 35 days of persistent infection showed no genetic change from virus present in the blood meal (SCW, unpublished observations). Dual infection of arthropods feeding on two or more hosts infected with different arboviruses (or on dually infected hosts) may occasionally provide the opportunity for generation of novel, recombinant, unsegmented genomes such as WEE virus.[72] However, interference to superinfection with related arboviruses[7,38,73,183,211] may limit such opportunities to either multiple (i.e., interrupted) blood meals within a short period (probably hours) or engorgement on dually infected vertebrate hosts. The detection of natural, dual EEE virus infections within avian but not mosquito hosts may reflect this limitation.[220]

The high degree of diversity within arthropod vector taxa, especially mosquitoes, may provide opportunities for diversification of arboviruses through long-term coevolution (codiversification) with vectors[51] or by host switching.[219,221,222] Alphaviruses such as VEE, which use diverse mosquito vector taxa (the *Culex* subgenus), tend to be more diverse than viruses such as the North American EEE and WEE viruses, which are transmitted by taxa (*Culiseta* and *Culex*) that are species-poor in North America.[225] Phylogenetic studies of alphaviruses have indicated that host switching often results in allopatric and sometimes sympatric diversification. For example, EEE virus presumably switched from *Culex* (*Melanoconion*) mosquitoes to *C melanura* when it was introduced into North America about one thousand years ago,[221] and Everglades virus presumably adopted *Culex cedecei* as its mosquito vector on more recent introduction into Florida from South or Central America.[222] Available evidence suggests that Fort Morgan and Buggy Creek viruses originated in North America after host switching from mosquitoes to swallow bugs (*Oeciacus vicarius*), probably a sympatric event (SCW, unpublished observations).

Arbovirus diversity may also be related to the degree of vertebrate host mobility, because mosquitoes and other vectors tend to have limited dispersal. For example, alphaviruses such as Sindbis, WEE, and North American EEE viruses that use avian hosts tend to be less diverse than VEE and South or Central American EEE viruses that infect small mammals with limited mobility.[221] Many human viruses that do not rely on vectors but spread instead by host-to-host contact are also less isolated geographically than highly focal zoonotic arboviruses such as enzootic VEE serotypes.

VIRULENCE OF ARBOVIRUSES FOR VERTEBRATE AND ARTHROPOD HOSTS

Pathogenic Effects of Arboviruses on Vertebrate Hosts

Arboviruses vary widely in their effects on vertebrate hosts, and some produce extreme illnesses in humans and others. For example, many New World alphaviruses are encephalitic in humans and equids, with severe morbidity and high mortality rates, and the Old World Ross River and chikungunya alphaviruses cause severe arthralgia.[153] New World bunyaviruses such as La Crosse virus also cause human encephalitis, and Rift Valley fever virus causes high mortality in domestic animals in Africa.[128] The yellow fever and dengue flaviviruses both cause severe human illnesses with significant mortality, and many tickborne viruses, such as tickborne encephalitis and Crimean-Congo hemorrhagic fever viruses, are extremely virulent human and veterinary pathogens.[17]

Some of the most severe arboviral diseases occur in hosts that do not normally participate in maintenance transmission cycles. For example, EEE, VEE, and WEE viruses cause high rates of encephalitis in equids during epizootics but less disease in avian and small mammalian enzootic amplifying hosts. Equids are believed to be deadend hosts for EEE virus in North America because they develop only low-titer viremia, insufficient in magnitude for infection of most mosquito vectors.[177] Equids infected with epizootic VEE viruses produce viremias capable of infecting mosquito vectors, but these epizootic viruses circulate only transiently until the supply of susceptible large mammalian hosts is exhausted.[215] These examples suggest that the most extreme examples of arbovirus virulence for vertebrate hosts may not reflect evolutionary adaptation (see later discussion). However, diseases in other unnatural hosts can be mild, indicating that the effects of arboviruses on hosts not normally involved in transmission cycles are unpredictable and probably reflect chance tissue tropisms and replication efficiency.

Pathogenic Effects of Arboviruses on Arthropod Hosts

For many years, arboviruses were thought to have no detrimental effects on their arthropod vectors. However, evidence has accumulated since the 1980s that many viruses have deleterious effects on infected vectors. Rift Valley fever virus infection decreases the survival rate of *C pipiens* mosquitoes[59] and also reduces blood feeding success and fecundity.[208] Environmental stress, in the form of carbohydrate deprivation, can alter the effect of Rift Valley fever virus on survival of infected *C pipiens*.[46] La Crosse virus infection also reduces the ability of *A triseriatus* to obtain blood meals.[66] Although most tickborne viruses appear to cause no detrimental effects on their vectors,[145] African swine fever virus has been shown to increase the mortality rate of infected ticks, including nymphs of *Ornithodoros coriaceus*,[68] third instar *Ornithodoros puertoricensis*,[52] adult female *O moubata* and *Ornithodoros serraticus,* and several stages of *Ornithodoros marocanus*.[53] Tick mortality can lead to clearance of African swine fever virus from colonies.[81]

Other arboviruses, including yellow fever, Kunjin, San Angelo, and California encephalitis viruses, delay larval development of transovarially infected mosquito vectors and also increase mortality rates.[201] Direct inoculation of mosquito larvae with EEE, chikungunya, and Rift Valley fever viruses also causes increased mortality.[204] However, La Crosse virus causes no detectable deleterious effects on transovarially infected mosquitoes.[148] Flaviviruses are not known to cause any deleterious effects on their insect or tick vectors.[120]

A mutualistic relationship may be necessary to sustain an arbovirus by vertical transmission alone, without a horizontal transmission component[114] (see later discussion). Oral infection of mosquitoes with some arboviruses leads to more severe effects than transovarial transmission, consistent with this hypothesis. Resistance to oral superinfection by related arboviruses, exhibited by vertically infected mosquitoes, could protect the vector and allow for the evolution of mutualism.[151]

Pathologic lesions have also been detected within tissues of mosquitoes infected with several alphaviruses. Semliki Forest virus causes cytopathic changes in the salivary glands of infected *A aegypti*,[113,137] although this mosquito is not known to be a natural vector of this virus. Both EEE[232] and WEE[90,232] viruses cause cytopathic changes in midgut epithelial cells of their natural mosquito vectors (Figs. 14-12 and 14-13). Infection with high-titered blood meals results in sloughing of epithelial cells into the midgut lumen, which may decrease viral loads and modulate the infection. Midgut lesions sometimes compromise the integrity of the abdominal midgut, allowing blood meal components and virus direct access to the hemocoel[231,232] (see Fig. 14-12). These pathologic changes may en-

hance viral dissemination to the salivary glands, providing some selective advantage for mosquito virulence (see later discussion). The lack of arbovirus-induced pathologic lesions outside the midgut of most mosquito vectors may reflect modulation of viral replication during later stages of infection. However, salivary glands produce large amounts of virus without apparent cytopathology.[229,234]

Evolution of Arbovirus Virulence

Because viruses are obligate intracellular parasites, their evolution can be considered in the same manner as other host-parasite interactions. Until recently, host-parasite relations were believed to evolve toward commensalism (i.e., attenuation of the parasite and resistance of the host). This view relied on the assumption that virulent pathogens are subject to extinction if host populations are diminished drastically because of parasite-associated mortality.[20] This theory considers only selection of populations (group or interdemic selection), whereby the survival of genetically similar individuals infecting a given host is favored over survival of groups in other hosts.[235] Because faster-replicating, more virulent genotypes outcompete less virulent forms during mixed infections, regardless of their effect on the host, group selection is maximized if genetic diversity *among* parasite populations is high but operates inefficiently if populations *within* a given host are heterogeneous. However, group selection disregards selection pressures acting on individuals or genes within a population. Also, the role of group selection in virus evolution is controversial, and Mayr[125] has argued that viruses are subject only to individual selection because they lack group properties such as altruism or social facilitation. Therefore, the selective advantage of a viral population cannot differ from the mean advantage of its individuals, and selection for attenuation of a virus, exemplified by myxoma virus in Australia,[60] really reflects individual selection.

More recently, alternative views of host-parasite evolution have challenged the idea that highly evolved relations are always commensal. Considering selection at the level of individual pathogens or genes, virulent genotypes can be favored if they are associated with an increase in transmission frequency to new hosts. This hypothesis has been presented mathematically[1] as a simple equation for the reproductive rate (R_0) of a parasite:

$$R_0 = \frac{\beta(\alpha, N)N}{\alpha + \mu + \nu(\alpha)}$$

where β is the transmission rate, N is the parasite population size, α is the mortality rate of infected hosts, μ is the uninfected host mortality rate, and ν is the infected host recovery rate. If the transmission rate is independent of the mortality rate of infected hosts, parasite reproduction (and fitness) are maximized by minimizing host mortality, or attenuation. However, if virulence is associated with increased transmission (i.e., they are not independent), attenuation is not always selected. In other words, competing evolutionary forces may act on individual genomes or genotypes (individual selection toward virulence) and on parasite populations (group selection toward attenuation).

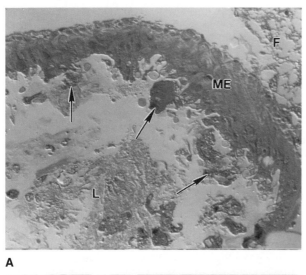

A

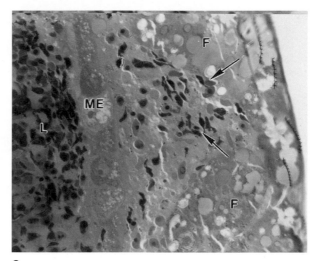

C

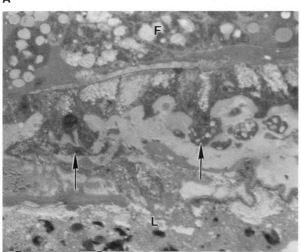

B

FIG. 14-12. Light micrographs of *Culex tarsalis* abdominal midguts 1 to 3 days after infection with western equine encephalomyelitis virus. (**A**) Detached epithelial cells (*arrows*) within the lumen (L). Original magnification 100×. (**B**) Vacuolated epithelial cells (*arrows*) extending into the lumen. Original magnification 400×. (**C**) Chicken blood cells from the blood meal (*arrows*) within the hemocoel adjacent to the fat body (F). Original magnification 400×. ME, midgut epithelium. (From Weaver SC, Scott TW, Lorenz LH. Pathologic changes in the midgut of *Culex tarsalis* following infection with western equine encephalomyelitis virus. Am J Trop Med Hyg 1992;47: 691–701.)

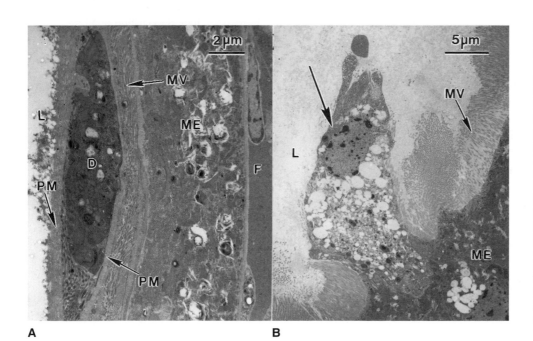

A   B

FIG. 14-13. Electron micrographs of *Culex tarsalis* abdominal midguts 1 to 2 days after infection with western equine encephalomyelitis virus. (**A**) Detached, dense, infected epithelial cell (D) within the lumen (L). Note peritrophic membrane or matrix (PM) surrounding this cell. Original magnification 7500×. (**B**) Highly vacuolated epithelial cell (*arrow*) extending through the epithelial microvilli (MV) into the lumen (L). Original magnification 3100×. F, fat body; ME, midgut epithelium. (From Weaver SC, Scott TW, Lorenz LH. Pathologic changes in the midgut of *Culex tarsalis* following infection with western equine encephalomyelitis irus. Am J Trop Med Hyg 1992; 47: 691–701.)

Parasite virulence must also be considered from the perspective of the host; ideally, the host would suffer no loss of fitness if infected by a parasite. If the host incurs some cost related to its defense against the parasite, fitness must be affected to some degree. If the cost to the host of parasite infection is exceeded by the cost of defensive mechanisms, the parasite can be tolerated with only a small net cost to the host. Therefore, if parasite selection favors higher virulence, an equilibrium level should be reached that lies somewhere between the optima of parasite and host.[54]

As discussed previously, heterogeneity *within* versus *among* populations of pathogens can affect the ability of group selection to operate. The limited information available on genetic diversity within arbovirus populations suggests that heterogeneity may be more common in vertebrate hosts than in mosquitoes because multiple mosquito bites occasionally result in dual infections of vertebrate hosts. Phylogenetically distinct genotypes of EEE virus were found in two of three unpassaged avian isolates examined, whereas dual infections were not detected in five mosquito isolates.[220] These results suggest that group selection may operate more efficiently during arbovirus replication within vertebrate hosts than in invertebrate hosts. Furthermore, the high mutation rates and resultant quasispecies populations characteristic of RNA viruses,[83] including arboviruses,[220] may also limit opportunities for group selection by restricting phenotypic homogeneity within groups.

The fundamentally different roles played by vertebrate and arthropod hosts during natural transmission cycles suggest dramatically different evolutionary pressures on arbovirus virulence. Because vectors can transmit viruses efficiently only if their mobility and host contacts remain high, group selection would be expected to strongly influence arbovirus virulence for arthropod hosts.[54,56] The relatively mild pathogenic changes and slight fitness declines observed after vector infection (see previous discussion) are consistent with this prediction. The reduced susceptibility of *A triseriatus* mosquitoes from regions of enzootic La Crosse virus transmission, compared with populations not exposed to the virus, also implies that selection for insusceptibility occurs in nature.[64] However, the midgut pathology that accompanies infection of mosquitoes by EEE[232] and WEE viruses[90,231] may facilitate dissemination and transmission of virulent genotypes, suggesting that individual selection also occurs in the vector. Individual selection for vector-virulent, rapidly replicating viruses may be expected to operate optimally during epidemic/epizootic conditions, when large numbers of susceptible hosts are available for only a limited time and competition to quickly infect those hosts is high.

Theoretically, the strongest group selection for vector attenuation should occur among arboviruses that are transmitted vertically to offspring. If transovarially infected vectors exhibit decreased fitness associated with infection (see previous discussion), and infection thereby interferes directly with vector reproductive success and transmission of virus to offspring, a parasite population cannot be maintained exclusively by vertical and uniparental transmission. However, with the addition of horizontal transmission, some virulence can be tolerated.[54]

Some work indicates that transovarially infected mosquitoes avoid the detrimental effects that accompany oral infec-

tion[148] (see previous discussion). Supporting this view, Ewald and Schubert[57] have argued that mosquito-borne viruses that are vertically transmitted at high rates are more benign in their mosquito hosts than are viruses undergoing little or no transovarial transmission. Experimental work has shown that bacteriophages maintained primarily by vertical transmission (from infected bacteria to their progeny) evolve toward attenuation, whereas horizontal transmission favors higher virulence.[18] Homologous interference that prevents arbovirus superinfection may provide vertically infected mosquitoes with a selective advantage, allowing for mutualism between transovarially transmitted arboviruses and their vectors[114] (see previous discussion). This could theoretically eliminate the requirement for horizontal transmission in arbovirus maintenance cycles.

In contrast, high replication rates and pathogenicity within vertebrate hosts may be advantageous for many vector-borne pathogens (Fig. 14-14). This prediction is supported by the higher average vertebrate virulence exhibited by vector-borne parasites (including arboviruses) in comparison with those not transmitted by vectors.[54] Because vertebrate host mobility is not required for arbovirus transmission by mobile insect vectors, group and individual selection may both favor viruses that replicate to high titers, maximizing their potential to infect engorging vectors. Febrile responses could also favor vector-borne transmission, because most vectors are attracted by body heat.[29,79] Waterborne enteric bacterial pathogens also appear to be more virulent than those transmitted directly by host contact; transport by contaminated water can be considered analogous to vector-borne transmission and should favor the evolution of virulence for the same reasons described previously.[55] Furthermore, pathogenic effects associated with increased vertebrate attractiveness or decreased defensive behavior against biting insects should enhance transmission and be favored during arbovirus evolution.[54,56] Although vertebrates infected with nonviral parasites are known to exhibit reduced antimosquito defensive behavior,[40,41,213] results of experiments examining the ability of mosquitoes to obtain blood meals from viremic versus uninfected hosts have been mixed. Infection of vertebrate hosts with three different North American arboviruses had little or no effect on mosquito attraction[176] or feeding success.[174] However, Rift Valley fever virus infection of lambs did increase blood feeding success by mosquito vectors, presumably because of elevated temperature and carbon dioxide output as well as reduced antimosquito behavior.[206]

An exception to evolution of arbovirus virulence for vertebrate hosts may be found in tickborne viruses that undergo nonviremic transmission (see previous discussion). Nuttall and colleagues[145] have suggested that this form of transmission may select for vertebrate avirulence, ensuring that hosts remain alive during the long periods required for ixodid ticks to feed to repletion. Ticks also exhibit limited mobility in comparison with flying insect vectors, and they rely on vertebrate movement for host encounters. Tickborne viruses may therefore be under selective pressure for reduced virulence to maintain mobility of vertebrate hosts and ensure efficient transmission.

In general, the evolutionary concepts discussed here predict arbovirus evolution toward attenuation in vectors and virulence in vertebrate hosts, based on the assumption of indepen-

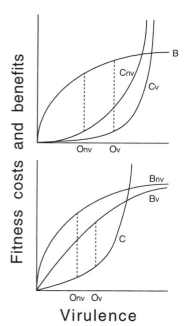

FIG. 14-14. Optimal levels of virulence for vector-borne (v) versus nonvector-borne (nv) pathogens in their vertebrate hosts. Increased virulence is assumed to result from increased replication within the vertebrate and subsequent enhanced transmissibility. Fitness costs (C) result from decreased transmission to new hosts because of excessive deleterious effects on the vertebrate. Fitness benefits (B) result from the increased probability of transmission of fast-replicating (virulent) genotypes to a new vertebrate, at the expense of slower-replicating forms. Benefit curves plateau as the probability of complete exclusion of less virulent forms approaches 1. Dotted lines indicate virulence optima (maximum net pathogen fitness, or maximal difference between benefit and cost) of vector-borne (Ov) and nonvector-borne (Onv) pathogens in vertebrate hosts.

For illustrative purposes, the benefit curve is assumed to be the same for both v and nv pathogens in the upper graph. Cv rises later (at higher virulence levels) than Cnv because vectors transmit pathogens efficiently even if vertebrate hosts are ill and severely immobilized; decreased defensive behavior of infected vertebrates may even enhance vector feeding. Cost curves rise more steeply as virulence levels increase to the point at which infected hosts die before transmission can occur. For illustrative purposes, the cost curve is assumed to be the same for both v and nv pathogens in the lower graph. Bv rises more slowly than Bnv because systemic infection, presumably associated with increased virulence, is usually required for infection of vectors, whereas nv pathogens such as respiratory or enteric viruses can be transmitted after localized replication alone. In each graph, Ov exceeds Onv. (Modified from Ewald PW. Host-parasite relations, vectors, and the evolution of disease severity. Ann Rev Ecol Syst 1983;14:465–485.)

dent evolution in the two hosts. However, this assumption may be unrealistic because arboviruses must alternate frequently between hosts, which presumably limits their ability to adapt optimally to either. Arboviruses probably evolve toward compromise fitness levels in their two hosts, and this may limit their adaptation and evolutionary rates.[225] The lack

of complete independence of evolutionary forces operating within vertebrate and vector hosts is also inferred from experimental studies with Ross River virus. When the virus was passaged serially in mice alone, virulence increased.[188] However, alternate passages between mosquitoes and mice resulted in stable virulence levels comparable to those in field strains.[189] These results suggest that replication in vectors may suppress the evolution of vertebrate virulence by arboviruses, in comparison with levels that may be achieved by efficient mechanical transmission.

ACKNOWLEDGMENTS

I thank Alan Barrett, Ed Cupp, John Holland, George Ludwig, Fred Murphy, Neal Nathanson, and Michael Turell for reviewing the manuscript and offering helpful suggestions. My research is supported by NIH grants AI 10984 and AI 14627. The literature review for this chapter was completed in May 1994.

ABBREVIATIONS

ADP: adenosine diphosphate
DNA: deoxyribonucleic acid
EEE: eastern equine encephalomyelitis
KFD: Kyasanur Forest disease
RNA: ribonucleic acid
SLE: St. Louis encephalitis
TCID50: median tissue culture infective dose
VEE: Venezuelan equine encephalomyelitis
WEE: western equine encephalomyelitis

REFERENCES

1. Anderson RM, May RM. Infectious diseases of humans: dynamics and control. Oxford: Oxford University Press, 1991:656.
2. Arthur RR, el-Sharkawy MS, Cope SE, et al. Recurrence of Rift Valley fever in Egypt. Lancet 1993;342:1140–1150.
3. Baldridge GD, Beaty BJ, Hewlett MJ. Genomic stability of LaCrosse virus during vertical and horizontal transmission. Arch Virol 1989;108:89–99.
4. Ballinger ME, Rice CM, Miller BR. Detection of yellow fever virus nucleic acid in infected mosquitoes by RNA:RNA in situ hybridization. Mol Cell Probes 1988;2:331–338.
5. Banerjee K. Kyasanur Forest disease. In: Monath TP, ed. The arboviruses: epidemiology and ecology. Vol 3. Boca Raton, Florida: CRC Press, 1988:93–116.
6. Barnett HC. The transmission of western equine encephalitis virus by the mosquito *Culex tarsalis* Coq. Am J Trop Med Hyg 1956; 5:86–98.
7. Beaty BJ, Bishop DHL, Gay M, Fuller F. Interference between bunyaviruses in *Aedes triseriatus* mosquitoes. Virology 1983;127:83.
8. Beaty BJ, Calisher CH. Bunyaviridae: natural history. Curr Top Microbiol Immunol 1991;169:27–78.
9. Beaty BJ, Holterman M, Tabachnick W, et al. Molecular basis of bunyavirus transmission by mosquitoes: role of the middle-sized RNA segment. Science 1981;211:1433–1435.
10. Beaty BJ, Sundin DR, Chandler LJ, Bishop DH. Evolution of bunyavirus by genome reassortment in dually infected mosquitoes (*Aedes triseriatus*). Science 1985;230:548–550.
11. Beaty BJ, Thompson WH. Tropisms of La Crosse virus in *Aedes triseriatus* (Diptera: Culicidae) following infective blood meals. J Med Entomol 1978;14:499–503.
12. Beaty BJ, Trent DW, Roehrig JT. Virus variation and evolution: mechanisms and epidemiological significance. In: Monath TP, ed.

The arboviruses: epidemiology and ecology. Vol 1. Boca Raton, Florida: CRC Press, 1988:59–85.

13. Beklemishev WN. Gonotrophic rhythm as a basic principle of the biology of Anopheles. Voprosy Fiziologii Ekologii Malyariinogo Komara 1940;1:3–22.

14. Bilsel PA, Tesh RB, Nichol ST. RNA genome stability of Toscana virus during serial transovarial transmission in the sandfly *Phlebotomous perniciosus*. Virus Res 1988;11:87–94.

15. Boorman J. Observations on the amount of virus present in the hemolymph of *A. aegypti* infected with Semliki Forest virus. Trans R Soc Trop Med Hyg 1960;54:362–365.

16. Booth TF, Steele GM, Marriott AC, Nuttall PA. Dissemination, replication, and trans-stadial persistence of Dugbe virus (Nairovirus, Bunyaviridae) in the tick vector, *Amblyomma variegatum*. Am J Trop Med Hyg 1991;45:146–157.

17. Bres P. Impact of arboviruses on human and animal health. In: Monath TP, ed. The arboviruses: epidemiology and ecology. Vol 1. Boca Raton, Florida: CRC Press, 1988:1–18.

18. Bull JJ, Molineux IJ, Rice WR. Selection of benevolence in a host-parasite system. Evolution 1991;45:875–882.

19. Burness AT, Pardoe I, Faragher SG, Vrati S, Dalgarno L. Genetic stability of Ross River virus during epidemic spread in nonimmune humans. Virology 1988;167:639–643.

20. Burnet M. White DO. Natural history of infectious disease. Cambridge: Cambridge University Press, 1972:278.

21. Calisher CH, Karabatsos N. Arbovirus serogroups: definition and geographic distribution. In: Monath TP, ed. The arboviruses: epidemiology and ecology. Vol 1. Boca Raton, Florida: CRC Press, 1988:19–57.

22. Calisher CH, Karabatsos N, Dalrymple JM, et al. Antigenic relationships between flaviviruses as determined by cross-neutralization tests with polyclonal antisera. J Gen Virol 1989;70:37–43.

23. Chamberlain RW. Epidemiology of arthropod-borne togaviruses: the role of arthropods as hosts and vectors and of vertebrate hosts in natural transmission cycles. In: Schlesinger RW, eds. The togaviruses. New York: Academic Press, 1980: 175–227.

24. Chamberlain RW, Sudia WD. Mechanisms of transmission of viruses by mosquitoes. Annu Rev Entomol 1961;61: 371–390.

25. Champagne DE, Ribeiro JM. Sialokinin I and II: vasodilatory tachykinins from the yellow fever mosquito *Aedes aegypti*. Proc Natl Acad Sci U S A 1994;91:138–142.

26. Chandler LJ, Ballinger ME, Jones RH, Beaty BJ. The virogenesis of bluetongue virus in *Culicoides variipennis*. In: Barber TL, Joachim MM, eds. Bluetongue and related orbiviruses. New York: Liss, 1985:245–253.

27. Chandler LJ, Hogge G, Endres M, et al. Reassortment of La Crosse and Tahyna bunyaviruses in *Aedes triseriatus* mosquitoes. Virus Res 1991;20:181–191.

28. Christensen BM, Rowley WA, Wong YW, Dorsey DC, Hausler WJ. Laboratory studies of transovarial transmission of trivittatus virus by *Aedes trivittatus*. Am J Trop Med Hyg 1978;27:184.

29. Clements AN. The biology of mosquitoes. London: Chapman and Hall, 1992:509.

30. Comer JA, Corn JL, Stallknecht DE, Landgraf JG, Nettles VF. Titers of vesicular stomatitis virus, New Jersey serotype, in naturally infected male and female *Lutzomyia shannoni* (Diptera: Psychodidae) in Georgia. J Med Entomol 1992;29:368–370.

31. Comer JA, Tesh RB. Phlebotomine sandflies as vectors of vesiculoviruses: a review. Parassitologia 1991;33:143–150.

32. Comer JA, Tesh RB, Modi GB, Corn JL, Nettles VF. Vesicular stomatitis virus, New Jersey serotype: replication in and transmission by *Lutzomyia shannoni* (Diptera: Psychodidae). Am J Trop Med Hyg 1990;42:483–490.

33. Cross ML, Cupp MS, Cupp EW, Galloway AL, Enriquez FJ. Modulation of murine immunological responses by salivary gland extract of *Simulium vittatum* (Diptera: Simuliidae). J Med Entomol 1993; 30:928–935.

34. Cupp EW, Gordon AE. Notes on the systematics, distribution and bionomics of black flies (Diptera: Simuliidae) in the northeastern United States. Search Agric 1983;1–75.

35. Cupp EW, Mare CJ, Cupp MS, Ramberg FB. Biological transmission of vesicular stomatitis virus (New Jersey) by *Simulium vittatum* (Diptera: Simuliidae). J Med Entomol 1992;29:137–140.

36. Cupp MS, Cupp EW, Ramberg FB. Salivary gland apyrase in black flies (*Simulium vittatum*). J Insect Physiol 1993; 39:817–821.

37. Cupp MS, Ribeiro JMC, Cupp EW. Vasodilative activity in black fly salivary glands. Am J Trop Med Hyg 1994;50: 241–246.

38. Davey MW, Mahon RJ, Gibbs AJ. Togavirus interference in *Culex annulirostris* mosquitoes. J Gen Virol 1979;42: 641–643.

39. Davies CR, Jones LD, Green BM, Nuttall PA. In vivo reassortment of Thogoto virus (a tick-borne influenza-like virus) following oral infection of *Rhipicephalus appendiculatus* ticks. J Gen Virol 1987; 68:2331–2338.

40. Day JF, Ebert KM, Edman JD. Feeding patterns of mosquitoes (Diptera: Culicidae) simulataneously exposed to malarious and healthy mice, including a method for separating blood meals from conspecific hosts. J Med Entomol 1983;20: 120–127.

41. Day JF, Edman JD. Malaria renders mice susceptible to mosquito feeding when gametocytes are most infective. J Parasitol 1983;69: 163–170.

42. DeFoliart GR, Grimstad PR, Watts DM. Advances in mosquito-borne arbovirus/vector research. Annu Rev Entomol 1987;32:479–505.

43. Deubel V, Pailliez JP, Cornet M, et al. Homogeneity among Senegalese strains of yellow fever virus. Am J Trop Med Hyg 1985;34: 976–983.

44. Dickerman RW, Cupp EW, Groot H, et al. Venezuelan equine encephalomyelitis virus activity in northern Colombia during April and May 1983. PAHO Bulletin 1986;20:276–283.

45. Dickson DL, Turell MJ. Replication and tissue tropisms of Crimean-Congo hemorrhagic fever virus in experimentally infected adult *Hyalomma truncatum* (Acari: Ixodidae). J Med Entomol 1992;29: 767–773.

46. Dohm DJ, Romoser WS, Turell MJ, Linthicum KJ. Impact of stressful conditions on the survival of *Culex pipiens* exposed to Rift Valley fever virus. J Am Mosq Control Assoc 1991;7:621–623.

47. Doi R. Studies on the mode of development of Japanese encephalitis virus in some groups of mosquitoes by the fluorescent antibody technique. J Exp Med 1970;40:101–115.

48. Domingo E, Holland JJ. Mutation rates and rapid evolution of RNA viruses. In: Morse SS, ed. Evolutionary biology of viruses. New York: Raven Press, 1994:161–184.

49. Dutary BE, Petersen JL, Peralta PH, Tesh RB. Transovarial transmission of Gamboa virus in a tropical mosquito, *Aedeomyia squamipennis*. Am J Trop Med Hyg 1989;40: 108–113.

50. Edman JD, Strickman D, Kittsyspong P, Scott TW. Female *Aedes aegypti* (Diptera: Culicidae) in Thailand rarely feed on sugar. J Med Entomol 1992;29:1035–1038.

51. Eldridge B. Evolutionary relationships among California serogroup viruses (Bunyaviridae) and *Aedes* mosquitoes (Diptera: Culicidae). J Med Entomol 1990;27:738–749.

52. Endris RG, Haslett TM, Hess WR. African swine fever virus infection in the soft tick, *Ornithodoros (Alectorobius) puertoricensis* (Acari: Argasidae). J Med Entomol 1992;29:990–994.

53. Endris RG, Hess WR, Caiado JM. African swine fever virus infection in the Iberian soft tick, *Ornithodoros (Pavlovskyella) marocanus* (Acari: Argasidae). J Med Entomol 1992;29:874–878.

54. Ewald PW. Host-parasite relations, vectors, and the evolution of disease severity. Annu Rev Ecol Syst 1983;14: 465–485.

55. Ewald PW. Waterborne transmission and the evolution of virulence among gastrointestinal bacteria. Epidemiol Infect 1991;106:83–119.

56. Ewald PW. Evolution of infectious disease. New York: Oxford University Press, 1994:83–119.

57. Ewald PW, Schubert J. Vertical and vector-borne transmission of insect endocytobionts and the evolution of benignity. In: Schwemmler W, Gassner G, eds. Insect endocytobiosis: morphology, physiology, genetics, evolution. Boca Raton, Florida: CRC Press, 1989:21–35.

58. Faran ME, Romoser WS, Routier RG, Bailey CL. The distribution of Rift Valley fever virus in the mosquito *Culex pipiens* as revealed by viral titration of dissected organs and tissues. Am J Trop Med Hyg 1988;39:206–213.

59. Faran ME, Turell MJ, Romoser WS, et al. Reduced survival of adult *Culex pipiens* infected with Rift Valley fever virus. Am J Trop Med Hyg 1987;37:403–409.

60. Fenner F, Myers K. Myxoma virus and myxomatosis in retrospect: the first quarter century of a new disease. In: Kurstak E, Maramorosh

K, eds. Viruses and environment. New York: Academic Press, 1978: 539–570.

61. Freier JE, Rosen L. Vertical transmission of dengue viruses by *Aedes mediovittatus*. Am J Trop Med Hyg 1988;39: 218–222.

62. Fulhorst CF, Hardy JL, Eldridge BF, Presser SB, Reeves WC. Natural vertical transmission of western equine encephalomyelitis virus in mosquitoes. Science 1994;263: 676–678.

63. Gargan TP, Bailey CL, Higbee GA, Gad A, Said SE. The effect of laboratory colonization on the vector-pathogen interactions of Egyptian *Culex pipiens* and Rift Valley fever virus. Am J Trop Med Hyg 1983;32:1154.

64. Grimstad PR, Craig GB Jr, Ross QE, Yuill TM. *Aedes triseriatus* and La Crosse virus. Geographic variation in vector susceptibility and ability to transmit. Am J Trop Med Hyg 1977;26:990–996.

65. Grimstad PR, Paulson SL, Craig GB Jr. Vector competence of *Aedes hendersoni* Cockerell (Diptera: Culicidae) for La Crosse virus and evidence for a salivary gland escape barrier. J Med Entomol 1985;22:447–453.

66. Grimstad PR, Ross QE, Craig GB Jr. *Aedes triseriatus* (Diptera: Culicidae) and La Crosse virus. II. Modification of mosquito feeding behavior by virus infection. J Med Entomol 1980;17:1–7.

67. Grimstad PR, Walker ED. *Aedes triseriatus* (Diptera: Culicidae) and La Crosse virus. IV. Nutritional deprivation of larvae affects the adult barriers to infection and transmission. J Med Entomol 1991; 28:378–386.

68. Groocock CM, Hess WR, Gladney WJ. Experimental transmission of African swine fever virus by *Ornithodoros coriaceus*, an argasid tick indigenous to the United States. Am J Vet Res 1980;41: 591–594.

69. Gubler DJ. Dengue. In: Monath TP, ed. The arboviruses: epidemiology and ecology. Vol 2. Boca Raton, Florida: CRC Press, 1988:223–260.

70. Gubler DJ, Rosen L. Variations among geographic strains of *Aedes albopictus* in susceptibility to infection with dengue viruses. Am J Trop Med Hyg 1976;25:318–325.

71. Gubler DJ, Rosen L. Quantitative aspects of replication of Dengue viruses in *Aedes albopictus* (Diptera: Culicidae) after oral and parenteral infection. J Med Entomol 1977;13: 469–472.

72. Hahn CS, Lustig S, Strauss EG, Strauss JH. Western equine encephalitis virus is a recombinant virus. Proc Natl Acad Sci U S A 1988;85:5997–6001.

73. Hardy JL. Susceptibility and resistance of vector mosquitoes. In: Monath TP, ed. The arboviruses: epidemiology and ecology. Vol 1. Boca Raton, Florida: CRC Press, 1988: 87–126.

74. Hardy JL, Apperson G, Asman SM, Reeves WC. Selection of a strain of *Culex tarsalis* highly resistant to infection following ingestion of western equine encephalomyeltis virus. Am J Trop Med Hyg 1978;27:313–321.

75. Hardy JL, Houk EJ, Kramer LD, Reeves WC. Intrinsic factors affecting vector competence of mosquitoes for arboviruses. Annu Rev Entomol 1983;28:229–262.

76. Hardy JL, Meyer RP, Presser SB, Milby MM. Temporal variations in the susceptibility of a semi-isolated population of *Culex tarsalis* to peroral infection with western equine encephalomyelitis and St. Louis encephalitis viruses. Am J Trop Med Hyg 1990;42:500–511.

77. Hardy JL, Reeves WC, Sjogren RD. Variations in the susceptibility of field and laboratory populations of *Culex tarsalis* to experimental infection with western equine encephalomyeltis virus. Am J Epidemiol 1976;103:498–505.

78. Hardy JL, Rosen L, Reeves WC, Scrivani RP, Presser SB. Experimental transovarial transmission of St. Louis encephalitis virus by *Culex* and *Aedes* mosquitoes. Am J Trop Med Hyg 1984;33:166–175.

79. Harwood RF, James MT. Entomology in human and animal health. New York: Macmillan, 1979:548.

80. Hayes CG, Baker RH, Baqar S, Ahmed T. Genetic variation for West Nile virus susceptibility in *Culex tritaeniorhynchus*. Am J Trop Med Hyg 1984;33:715–724.

81. Hess WR, Endris RG, Lousa A, Caiado JM. Clearance of African swine fever virus from infected tick (Acari) colonies. J Med Entomol 1989;26:314–317.

82. Holland JJ, de la Torre JC, Clarke DK, Duarte E. Quantitation of relative fitness and great adaptability of clonal populations of RNA viruses. J Virol 1991;65:2960–2967.

83. Holland JJ, de la Torre JC, Steinhauer D. RNA virus populations as quasispecies. Curr Top Microbiol Immunol 1992;176:1–20.

84. Holland JJ, Spindler K, Horodyski F, et al. Rapid evolution of RNA genomes. Science 1982;215:1577–1585.

85. Hoogstraal H. Ticks in relationship to human diseases caused by viruses. Annu Rev Entomol 1966;11:261.

86. Houk EJ, Arcus YM, Hardy JL, Kramer LD. Binding of western equine encephalomyelitis virus to brush border fragments isolated from mesenteronal epithelial cells of mosquitoes. Virus Res 1990; 17:105–117.

87. Houk EJ, Hardy JL, Chiles RE. Permeability of the midgut basal lamina in the mosquito, *Culex tarsalis* Coquillett (Insecta: Diptera). Acta Trop (Basel) 1981;38:163–171.

88. Houk EJ, Hardy JL, Chiles RE. Histochemical staining of the complex carbohydrates of the midgut of the mosquito, *Culex tarsalis* Coquillett. Insect Biochem 1986;16:667–675.

89. Houk EJ, Hardy JL, Chiles RE. Mesenteronal epithelial cell surface charge of the mosquito, *Culex tarsalis* Coquillett (Diptera: Culicidae): Binding of colloidal iron hydroxide, native ferritin and cationized ferritin. J Submicrosc Cytol 1986;18:385–396.

90. Houk EJ, Kramer LD, Hardy JL, Chiles RE. Western equine encephalomyelitis virus: in vivo infection and morphogenesis in mosquito mesenteronal epithelial cells. Virus Res 1985;2:123–138.

91. Houk EJ, Obie F, Hardy JL. Peritrophic membrane formation and the midgut barrier to arboviral infection in the mosquito, *Culex tarsalis* Coquillett (Insecta, Diptera). Acta Trop (Basel) 1979;36:39–45.

92. Jackson AC, Bowen JC, Downe AER. Experimental infection of *Aedes aegypti* (Diptera: Culicidae) by the oral route with Sindbis virus. J Med Entomol 1993;30:332–337.

93. Jacobs JW, Cupp EW, Sardana M, Friedman PA. Isolation and characterization of a coagulation factor Xa inhibitor from black fly salivary glands. Thromb Haemost 1990;64: 235–238.

94. Jones LD, Hodgson E, Nuttall PA. Enhancement of virus transmission by tick salivary glands. J Gen Virol 1989; 70:1895–1898.

95. Jones RH, Foster NM. Oral infection of *Culicoides variipennis* with bluetongue virus: development of susceptible and resistant lines from a colony population. J Med Entomol 1974;11:316–323.

96. Jones RH, Foster NM. Heterogeneity of *Culicoides variipennis* field populations to oral infection with bluetongue virus. Am J Trop Med Hyg 1978;27:178–183.

97. Jupp PG. *Culex theileri* and Sindbis virus: salivary gland infection in relation to transmission. J Am Mosq Control Assoc 1985;1:374.

98. Karabatsos N. International catalog of arboviruses including certain other viruses of vertebrates. San Antonio, Texas: American Society of Tropical Medicine and Hygiene, 1985;1147.

99. Kaufman WR. Tick-host interaction: a synthesis of current concepts. Parasitology Today 1989;5:47–56.

100. Kay BH. Three modes of transmission of Ross River virus by *Aedes vigilax* (Skuse). Aust J Exp Biol Med Sci 1982; 60:339–344.

101. Kay BH, Aaskov JG. Ross River virus (epidemic polyarthritis). In: Monath TP, ed. The arboviruses: epidemiology and ecology. Vol 4. Boca Raton, Florida: CRC Press, 1988: 93–112.

102. Kay BH, Edman JD, Fanning ID, Mottram P. Larval diet and the vector competence of *Culex annulirostris* (Diptera: Culicidae) for Murray Valley encephalitis virus. J Med Entomol 1989;26:487–488.

103. Kay BH, Fanning ID, Mottram P. Rearing temperature influences flavivirus vector competence of mosquitoes. Med Vet Entomol 1989;3:415–422.

104. Kettle DS. Medical and veterinary entomology. Wallingford, Oxon, UK: CAB International, 1990:658.

105. Kinney RM, Tsuchiya KR, Sneider JM, Trent DW. Molecular evidence for the origin of the widespread Venezuelan equine encephalitis epizootic of 1969–1972. J Gen Virol 1992;73:3301–3305.

106. Klowden MJ, Briegel H. Mosquito gonotrophic cycle and multiple feeding potential: contrasts between *Anopheles* and *Aedes* (Diptera: Culicidae). J Med Entomol 1994;31: 618–622.

107. Klowden MJ, Lea AO. Effect of defensive host behavior on the blood meal size and feeding success of natural populations of mosquitoes. J Med Entomol 1979;15:514–517.

108. Kramer LD, Hardy JL, Houk EJ, Presser SB. Characterization of the mesenteronal infection with western equine encephalomyelitis virus in an incompetent strain of *Culex tarsalis*. Am J Trop Med Hyg 1989;41:241–250.

109. Kramer LD, Hardy JL, Presser SB. Effect of temperature of extrinsic incubation on the vector competence of *Culex tarsalis* for western equine encephalomyelitis virus. Am J Trop Med Hyg 1983; 32:1130–1139.

110. Kramer LD, Hardy JL, Presser SB, Houk EJ. Dissemination barriers for western equine encephalomyelitis virus in *Culex tarsalis* infected after ingestion of low viral doses. Am J Trop Med Hyg 1981;30:190–197.

111. Kuberski T. Fluorescent antibody studies on the development of dengue-2 virus in *Aedes albopictus* (Diptera: Culicidae). J Med Entomol 1979;16:343–349.

112. Labuda M, Danielova V, Jones LD, Nuttall PA. Amplification of tick-borne encephalitis virus infection during co-feeding of ticks. Med Vet Entomol 1993;7:339–342.

113. Lam KSK, Marshall ID. Dual infections of *Aedes aegypti* with arboviruses. II. Salivary gland damage by Semliki Forest virus in relation to dual infections. Am J Trop Med Hyg 1968;17:637–644.

114. Leake CJ. Arbovirus-mosquito interactions and vector specificity. Parasitology Today 1992;8:123–128.

115. Leake CJ, Johnson RT. The pathogenesis of Japanese encephalitis virus in *Culex tritaeniorhynchus* mosquitoes. Trans R Soc Trop Med Hyg 1987;81:681–685.

116. Lerner EA, Ribeiro JM, Nelson RJ, Lerner MR. Isolation of maxadilan, a potent vasodilatory peptide from the salivary glands of the sand fly *Lutzomyia longipalpis*. J Biol Chem 1991;266:11234–11236.

117. Lewis JD. The biology of *Phlebotomidae* in relation to leishmaniasis. Annu Rev Entomol 1974;19:363–384.

118. Lorenz L, Beaty BJ, Aitken THG, Wallis GP, Tabachnick WJ. The effect of colonization upon *Aedes aegypti* susceptibility to oral infection with yellow fever virus. Am J Trop Med Hyg 1984;33:690.

119. Ludwig GV, Cristensen BM, Yuill TM, Schultz KT. Enzyme processing of La Crosse virus glycoprotein G1: a bunyavirus-vector infection model. Virology 1989;171:108– 113.

120. Ludwig GV, Iacono-Connors LC. Insect-transmitted vertebrate viruses: Flaviviridae. In Vitro Cell Dev Biol 1993;29A:296–309.

121. Ludwig GV, Israel BA, Cristensen BM, Yuill TM, Schultz KT. Role of La Crosse virus glycoproteins in attachment of virus to host cells. Virology 1991;181:564–571.

122. Lundstrom JO, Turell MJ, Niklasson B. Effect of environmental temperature on the vector competence of *Culex pipiens* and *Cx. torrentium* for Ockelbo virus. Am J Trop Med Hyg 1990;43:534–542.

123. Luo T, Brown DT. A 55-kDa protein induced in *Aedes albopictus* (mosquito) cells by antiviral protein. Virology 1994;200:200–206.

124. Marchoux E, Simond P-L. La transmission hereditaire du virus se la fievre jaune chez le *Stegomyia fasciata*. C R Soc Biol (Paris) 1905;59:259–260.

125. Mayr E. Myxoma and group selection. Biol Zentbl 1990;109:453–457.

126. McKelvey JJ, Eldridge BF, Maramorosch K. Vectors of disease agents. New York: Praeger, 1981:229.

127. McLintock J. Mosquito-virus relationships of American encephalitides. Annu Rev Entomol 1978;23:17–37.

128. Meegan JM, Bailey CL. Rift Valley fever virus. In: Monath TP, ed. The arboviruses: epidemiology and ecology. Vol 4. Boca Raton, Florida: CRC Press, 1988:51–76.

129. Meegan JM, Khalil GM, Hoogstraal H, Adhan FK. Experimental transmission and field isolation studies implicating *Culex pipiens* as a vector of Rift Valley fever virus in Egypt. Am J Trop Med Hyg 1980;29:1405.

130. Mellor PS. The replication of bluetongue virus in *Culicoides* vectors. Curr Topics Microbiol Immunol 1990;162: 143–161.

131. Meyer RP. Estimations of vectorial capacity: pathogen extrinsic incubation and vector competence. Bull Soc Vector Ecol 1989;14: 60–66.

132. Miles JAR, Pillai JS, Maguire T. Multiplication of Whataroa virus in mosquitoes. J Med Entomol 1973;10:176– 185.

133. Miller BR, Mitchell CJ. Selection of a flavivirus-refractory strain of the yellow fever mosquito *Aedes aegypti*. Am J Trop Med Hyg 1991;45:399–407.

134. Miller BR, Mitchell CJ, Ballinger ME. Replication, tissue tropisms and transmission of yellow fever virus in *Aedes albopictus*. Trans R Soc Trop Med Hyg 1989;83: 252–255.

135. Miller BR, Monath TP, Tabachnick WJ, Ezike VI. Epidemic yellow fever caused by an incompetent mosquito vector. Trop Med Parasitol 1989;40:396–399.

136. Miller BR, DeFoliart GR, Yuill TM. Vertical transmission of La Crosse virus (California encephalitis group): transovarial and filial infection rates in *Aedes triseriatus* (Diptera: Culicidae). J Med Entomol 1977;14:437.

137. Mims CA, Day MF, Marshall ID. Cytopathic effects of Semliki Forest virus in the mosquito, *Aedes aegypti*. Am J Trop Med Hyg 1966;15:775–784.

138. Mitchell CJ. Mosquito vector competence and arboviruses. Curr Top Vector Res 1983;

139. Mitchell CJ, Bowen GS, Monath TP, Cropp CB, Kerschner J. St. Louis encephalitis virus transmission following multiple feeding of *Culex pipiens pipiens* (Diptera: Culicidae) during a single gonotrophic cycle. J Med Entomol 1979;16: 254–258.

140. Monath TP. Yellow fever. In: Monath TP, ed. The arboviruses: epidemiology and ecology. Vol 5. Boca Raton, Florida: CRC Press, 1988:139–241.

141. Monath TP. Dengue: the risk to developed and developing countries. Proc Natl Acad Sci U S A 1994;91: 2395–2400.

142. Murphy FA, Whitfield SG, Sudia WD, Chamberlain RW. Interactions of vector with vertebrate pathogenic viruses. In: Maramorosch K, Shope RE, eds. Invertebrate immunity. New York: Academic Press, 1975:25–48.

143. Nasci RS, Edman JD. *Culiseta melanura* (Diptera: Culicidae): population structure and nectar feeding in a freshwater swamp and surrounding areas in southeastern Massachusetts, USA. J Med Entomol 1984;21:567–572.

144. Nayer JK, Rosen L, Knight JW. Experimental vertical transmission of Saint Louis encephalitis virus by Florida mosquitoes. Am J Trop Med Hyg 1986;35:1296–1301.

145. Nuttall PA, Jones LD, Labuda M, Kaufman WR. Adaptations of arboviruses to ticks. J Med Entomol 1994; 31:1–9.

146. Ovenden JR, Mahon RH. Venereal transmission of Sindbis virus between individuals of *Aedes australis* (Diptera: Culicidae). J Med Entomol 1984;21:292–295.

147. Patrican LA, Bailey CL. Ingestion of immune bloodmeals and infection of *Aedes fowleri*, *Aedes mcintoshi*, and *Culex pipiens* with Rift Valley fever virus. Am J Trop Med Hyg 1989;40:534–540.

148. Patrican LA, DeFoliart GR. Lack of adverse effect of transovarially acquired La Crosse virus infection on the reproductive capacity of *Aedes triseriatus* (Diptera: Culicidae). J Med Entomol 1985;22: 604–611.

149. Patrican LA, DeFoliart GR. *Aedes triseriatus* and La Crosse virus: similar venereal infection rates in females given the first bloodmeal immediately before mating or several days after mating. Am J Trop Med Hyg 1987;36:648–652.

150. Patrican LA, DeFoliart GR, Yuill TM. Oral infection and transmission of La Crosse virus by an enzootic strain of *Aedes triseriatus* feeding on chipmunks with a range of viremia levels. Am J Trop Med Hyg 1985;34:992–998.

151. Paulson SL, Grimstad PR, G B Craig J. Midgut and salivary gland barriers to LaCrosse virus dissemination in mosquitoes of the *Aedes triseriatus* group. Med Vet Entomol 1989;3:113–123.

152. Perrone JB, Spielman A. Time and site of assembly of the peritrophic membrane of the mosquito *Aedes aegypti*. Cell Tissue Res 1988;252:473–478.

153. Peters CJ, Dalrymple JM. Alphaviruses. In: Fields BN, Knipe DM, eds. Virology, 2nd ed. New York: Raven Press, 1990:713–761.

154. Reeves WC, Hardy JL, Reisen WK, Milby MM. Potential effect of global warming on mosquito-borne arboviruses. J Med Entomol 1994;31:323–332.

155. Reisen WK, Meyer RP, Presser SB, Hardy JL. Effect of temperature on the transmission of western equine encephalomyelitis and St. Louis encephalitis viruses by *Culex tarsalis* (Diptera: Culicidae). J Med Entomol 1993;30: 151–160.

156. Ribeiro JMC. Role of saliva in blood-feeding by arthropods. Annu Rev Entomol 1987;32:1–7.

157. Ribeiro JM. Role of saliva in tick/host interactions. Exp Appl Acarol 1989;7:15–20.

158. Ribeiro JM, Endris TM, Endris R. Saliva of the soft tick, *Ornithodoros moubata*, contains anti-platelet and apyrase activities. Comp Biochem Physiol 1991;100:109–112.

159. Ribeiro JM, Evans PM, MacSwain JL, Sauer J. *Amblyomma ameri-*

canum: characterization of salivary prostaglandins E2 and F2 alpha by RP-HPLC/bioassay and gas chromatography–mass spectrometry. Exp Parasitol 1992;74: 112–116.

160. Ribeiro JMC, Rossignol PA, Spielman A. Role of saliva in blood vessel location. J Exp Biol 1984;108:1–7.

161. Ribeiro JMC, Vachereau A, Modi GB, Tesh RB. A novel vasodilatory peptide from the salivary glands of the sand fly, *Lutzomyia longipalpus*. Science 1989;243:212–214.

162. Rico-Hesse R, Weaver SC, Siger JD, Medina G, Salas RA. Emergence of a new epidemic/epizootic Venezuelan equine encephalitis virus in South America. Proc Natl Acad Sci U S A 1995;92: 5278–5281.

163. Roehrig JT, Hunt AR, Chang G-J, et al. Identification of monoclonal antibodies capable of differentiating antigenic varieties of eastern equine encephalitis viruses. Am J Trop Med Hyg 1990;42 : 394–398.

164. Romoser WS, Cody E. The formation and fate of the peritrophic membrane in adult *Culex nigripalpus* (Diptera: Culicidae). J Med Entomol 1975;12:371–378.

165. Romoser WS, Edman JD, Lorenz LH, Scott TW. Histological parameters useful in the identification of multiple bloodmeals in mosquitoes. Am J Trop Med Hyg 1989; 41:737–742.

166. Romoser WS, Faran ME, Bailey CL. Newly recognized route of arbovirus dissemination from the mosquito (Diptera: Culicidae) midgut. J Med Entomol 1987;24:431– 432.

167. Romoser WS, Faran ME, Bailey CL, Lerdthusnee K. An immunocytochemical study of the distribution of Rift Valley fever virus in the mosquito *Culex pipiens*. Am J Trop Med Hyg 1992;46:489–501.

168. Rosen L, Lien JC, Shroyer DA, Baker RH, Lu LC. Experimental vertical transmission of Japanese encephalitis virus by *Culex tritaeniorhynchus* and other mosquitoes. Am J Trop Med Hyg 1989; 40:548–556.

169. Samal SK, el-Hussein A, Holbrook FR, Beaty BJ, Ramig RF. Mixed infection of *Culicoides variipennis* with bluetongue virus serotypes 10 and 17: evidence for high frequency reassortment in the vector. J Gen Virol 1987;68: 2319–2329.

170. Sanmartin C, Mackenzie RB, Trapido H, et al. Encefalitis equina Venezolana en Colombia, 1967. Bol Oficina Sanit Panam 1967; 74:108.

171. Scherer WF, Cupp EW, Lok JB, Brenner RJ, Ordonez JV. Intestinal threshold of an enzootic strain of Venezuelan equine encephalomyelitis virus in *Culex (Melanoconion) taeniopus* mosquitoes and its implication to vector competency and vertebrate amplifying hosts. Am J Trop Med Hyg 1981;30:862–869.

172. Scherer WF, Weaver SC, Taylor CA, Cupp EW. Vector incompetency: its implications in the disappearance of epizootic Venezuelan equine encephalomyelitis virus from Middle America. J Med Entomol 1986;23:23–29.

173. Scherer WF, Weaver SC, Taylor CA, et al. Vector competence of *Culex (Melanoconion) taeniopus* for allopatric and epizootic Venezuelan equine encephalomyelitis viruses. Am J Trop Med Hyg 1987;36:194–197.

174. Scott TW, Edman JD, Lorenz LH, Hubbard JL. The role of vector-host interactions in disease transmission. Misc Publ Entomol Soc Am 1988;68:9–17.

175. Scott TW, Hildreth SW, Beaty BJ. The distribution and development of eastern equine encephalitis virus in its enzootic mosquito vector, *Culiseta melanura*. Am J Trop Med Hyg 1984;33:300–310.

176. Scott TW, Edman JD, Lorenz LH, Hubbard JL. The role of vector–host interactions in disease transmission. Misc Publ Entomol Soc Am 1988;68:9–17.

177. Scott TW, Weaver SC. Eastern equine encephalomyelitis virus: epidemiology and evolution of mosquito transmission. Adv Virus Res 1989;37:277–328.

178. Sonenshine DE. Biology of ticks. New York: Oxford University Press, 1991.

179. Sriurairatna S, Bhamarapravati N. Replication of dengue-2 virus in *Aedes albopictus* mosquitoes. Am J Trop Med Hyg 1977;26: 1199–1205.

180. Steele GM, Nuttall PA. Difference in vector competence of two species of sympatric ticks, *Amblyomma variegatum* and *Rhipicephalus appendiculatus*, for Dugbe virus (Nairovirus, *Bunyaviridae*). Virus Res 1989;14:73–84.

181. Steinhauer DA, Holland JJ. Rapid evolution of RNA viruses. Annu Rev Microbiol 1987;41:409–433.

182. Strauss JH, Strauss EG. The alphaviruses: gene expression, replication, and evolution. Microbiol Rev 1994;58: 491–562.

183. Sundin DR, Beaty BJ. Interference to oral superinfection of *Aedes triseriatus* infected with La Crosse virus. Am J Trop Med Hyg 1988;38:428–432.

184. Sundin DR, Beaty BJ, Nathanson N, Gonzalez-Scarano F. A G1 glycoprotein epitope of La Crosse virus: a determinant of infection of *Aedes triseriatus*. Science 1987;235: 591–593.

185. Tabachnick WJ. Genetic control of oral susceptibility to infection of *Culicoides variipennis* with bluetongue virus. Am J Trop Med Hyg 1991;45:666–671.

186. Tabachnick WJ, Wallis GP, Aitken TH, Miller BR, Amato GD, et al. Oral infection of *Aedes aegypti* with yellow fever virus: geographic variation and genetic considerations. Am J Trop Med Hyg 1985; 34:1219–1224.

187. Takahashi M. The effects of environmental and physiological conditions of *Culex tritaeniorhynchus* on the pattern of transmission of Japanese encephalitis virus. J Med Entomol 1976;13:275.

188. Taylor WP, Marshall ID. Adaptation studies with Ross River virus: laboratory mice and cell cultures. J Gen Virol 1975;28:59–72.

189. Taylor WP, Marshall ID. Adaptation studies with Ross River virus: retention of field level virulence. J Gen Virol 1975;28:73–83.

190. Tesh RB. Experimental studies on transovarial transmission of Kunjin and San Angelo viruses in mosquitoes. Am J Trop Med Hyg 1980;23:1153–1160.

191. Tesh RB. Transovarial transmission of arboviruses in their invertebrate vectors. Curr Top Vector Res 1984;2:57–76.

192. Tesh RB, Chaniotis BN. Transovarial transmission of viruses by phlebotomine sandflies. Ann N Y Acad Sci 1975;266:125–134.

193. Tesh RB, Chaniotis BN, Johnson KM. Vesicular stomatitis virus, Indiana serotype: multiplication in and transmission by experimentally infected phlebotomine sandflies (*Lutzomyia trapidoi*). Am J Epidemiol 1971;93:491–495.

194. Tesh RB, Chaniotis BN, Johnson KM. Vesicular stomatitis virus (Indiana serotype): transovarial transmission by phlebotomine sandflies. Science 1972;175:1477.

195. Tesh RB, Cornet M. The location of San Angelo virus in developing ovaries of transovarially infected *Aedes albopictus* mosquitoes as revealed by fluorescent antibody technique. Am J Trop Med Hyg 1981;30:212–218.

196. Tesh RB, Gubler DJ, Rosen L. Variation among geographic strains of *Aedes albopictus* in susceptibility to infection with chikungunya virus. Am J Trop Med Hyg 1976; 25:1153–1160.

197. Tesh RB, Lubroth J, Guzman H. Simulation of arbovirus overwintering: survival of Toscana virus (*Bunyaviridae:* Phlebovirus) in its natural vector *Phlebotomus perniciosus*. Am J Trop Med Hyg 1992;47:574–581.

198. Tesh RB, Shroyer DA. The mechanism of arbovirus transovarial transmission in mosquitoes: San Angelo virus in *Aedes albopictus*. Am J Trop Med Hyg 1980;29:1394.

199. Trembley HL. The distribution of certain liquids in the esophageal diverticula and stomach of mosquitoes. Am J Trop Med Hyg 1952;1:693–710.

200. Trent DW, Grant JA. Comparison of New World alphaviruses in the western equine encephalomyelitis complex by immunochemical and oligonucleotide fingerprint techniques. J Gen Virol 1980; 47: 261–282.

201. Turell MJ. Horizontal and vertical transmission of viruses by insect and tick vectors. In: Monath TP, ed. The arboviruses: epidemiology and ecology. Vol 1. Boca Raton, Florida: CRC Press, 1988:127–152.

202. Turell MJ. Reduced Rift Valley fever infection rates in mosquitoes associated with pledget feedings. Am J Trop Med Hyg 1988; 39:597–602.

203. Turell MJ. Effect of environmental temperature on the vector competence of *Aedes fowleri* for Rift Valley fever virus. Res Virol 1989;140:147–154.

204. Turell MJ. Virus-dependent mortality in Rift Valley fever, eastern equine encephalomyelitis, and chikungunya virus-inoculated mosquito (Diptera: Culicidae) larvae. J Med Entomol 1992;29:792–795.

205. Turell MJ. Effect of environmental temperature on the vector competence of *Aedes taeniorhynchus* for Rift Valley fever and Venezuelan equine encephalitis viruses. Am J Trop Med Hyg 1993;49: 672–676.

206. Turell MJ, Bailey CL, Rossi CA. Increased mosquito feeding on Rift

Valley fever virus-infected lambs. Am J Trop Med Hyg 1984; 33:1232–1238.

207. Turell MJ, Gargan TP, Bailey CL. Replication and dissemination of Rift Valley fever virus in *Culex pipiens*. Am J Trop Med Hyg 1984;33:176–181.

208. Turell MJ, Gargan TP, Bailey CL. *Culex pipiens* (Diptera: Culicidae) morbidity and mortality associated with Rift Valley fever virus infection. J Med Entomol 1985; 22:332–337.

209. Turell MJ, Hardy JL, Reeves WC. Stabilized infection of California encephalitis virus in *Aedes dorsalis* and its implications for viral maintenance in nature. Am J Trop Med Hyg 1982;31:1252.

210. Turell MJ, Lundstrom JO. Effect of environmental temperature on the vector competence of *Aedes aegypti* and *Ae. taeniorhynchus* for Ockelbo virus. Am J Trop Med Hyg 1990;43:543–550.

211. Turell MJ, Saluzzo JF, Tamariello RF, Smith JF. Generation and transmission of Rift Valley fever viral reassortants by the mosquito, *Culex pipiens*. J Gen Virol 1990;71:2307–2312.

212. Turell MJ, Spielman A. Nonvascular delivery of Rift Valley fever virus by infected mosquitoes. Am J Trop Med Hyg 1992;47: 190–194.

213. Waage JK, Nondo J. Host behavior and mosquito feeding success: an experimental study. Trans R Soc Trop Med Hyg 1982;76:119–122.

214. Wallis GP, Aitken TH, Beaty BJ, et al. Selection for susceptibility and refractoriness of *Aedes aegypti* to oral infection with yellow fever virus. Am J Trop Med Hyg 1985; 34:1225–1231.

215. Walton TE, Grayson MA. Venezuelan equine encephalomyelitis. In: Monath TP, ed. The arboviruses: epidemiology and ecology. Vol 5. Boca Raton, Florida: CRC Press, 1988:59–85.

216. Wang K-S, Kuhn RJ, Strauss EG, Ou S, Strauss JH. High-affinity laminin receptor is a receptor for sindbis virus in mammalian cells. J Virology 1992;66:4992–5001.

217. Watts DM, Pantuwatana S, DeFoliart GR, Yuill TM, Thompson WH. Transovarial transmission of La Crosse virus (California encephalitis group) in the mosquito, *Aedes triseriatus*. Science 1973;180: 1140.

218. Weaver SC. Electron microscopic analysis of infection patterns for Venezuelan equine encephalomyelitis virus in the mosquito vector, *Culex (Melanoconion) taeniopus*. Am J Trop Med Hyg 1986; 35:624–631.

219. Weaver SC. Evolution of alphaviruses. In: Gibbs AJ, Calisher CH, Garcia-Arenal F, eds. Molecular basis of virus evolution. Cambridge: Cambridge University Press, 1995:501–530.

220. Weaver SC, Bellew LA, Gousset LA, et al. Diversity within natural populations of eastern equine encephalomyelitis virus. Virology 1993;195:700–709.

221. Weaver SC, Bellew LA, Hagenbaugh A, et al. Evolution of alphaviruses in the eastern equine encephalomyelitis complex. J Virol 1994;68:158–169.

222. Weaver SC, Bellew LA, Rico-Hesse R. Phylogenetic analysis of alphaviruses in the Venezuelan equine encephalitis complex and iden-

tification of the source of epizootic viruses. Virology 1992;191: 282–290.

223. Weaver SC, Hagenbaugh A, Bellew LA, et al. A comparison of the nucleotide sequences of eastern and western equine encephalomyelitis viruses with those of other alphaviruses and related RNA viruses. Virology 1993;197: 375–390.

224. Weaver SC, Lorenz LH, Scott TW. Distribution of western equine encephalitis virus in the alimentary tract of *Culex tarsalis* (Diptera: Culicidae) following natural vs. artificial blood meals. J Med Entomol 1993;30:391–397.

225. Weaver SC, Rico-Hesse R, Scott TW. Genetic diversity and slow rates of evolution in New World alphaviruses. Curr Top Microbiol Immunol 1992;176:99–117.

226. Weaver SC, Scherer WF, Cupp EW, Castello DA. Barriers to dissemination of Venezuelan encephalitis viruses in the Middle American enzootic vector mosquito, *Culex (Melanoconion) taeniopus*. Am J Trop Med Hyg 1984;33: 953–960.

227. Weaver SC, Scherer WF, Taylor CA, Castello DA, Cupp EW. Laboratory vector competence of *Culex (Melanoconion) cedecei* for sympatric and allopatric Venezuelan equine encephalomyelitis viruses. Am J Trop Med Hyg 1986;35:619–623.

228. Weaver SC, Scott TW. Peritrophic membrane formation and cellular turnover in the midgut of *Culiseta melanura* (Diptera: Culicidae). J Med Entomol 1990;27:864–873.

229. Weaver SC, Scott TW, Lorenz LH. Patterns of eastern equine encephalomyelitis virus infection in *Culiseta melanura*. J Med Entomol 1990;27:878–891.

230. Weaver SC, Scott TW, Lorenz LH. Detection of eastern equine encephalomyelitis virus deposition in *Culiseta melanura* following ingestion of radiolabeled virus in blood meals. Am J Trop Med Hyg 1991;44:250–259.

231. Weaver SC, Scott TW, Lorenz LH. Pathologic changes in the midgut of *Culex tarsalis* following infection with western equine encephalomyelitis virus. Am J Trop Med Hyg 1992;47:691–701.

232. Weaver SC, Scott TW, Lorenz LH, Lerdthusnee K, Romoser WS. Togavirus-associated pathologic changes in the midgut of a natural mosquito vector. J Virol 1988;62:2083–2090.

233. Weaver SC, Tesh RB, Guzman H. Ultrastructural aspects of replication of the New Jersey serotype of vesicular stomatitis virus in a suspected sandfly vector, *Lutzomyia shannoni*. Am J Trop Med Hyg 1992;46:201–210.

234. Whitfield SG, Murphy FA, Sudia WD. St. Louis encephalitis virus: an ultrastructural of infection in a mosquito vector. Virology 1971;56:70–87.

235. Wilson DS. The natural selection of populations and communities. Menlo Park, California: Benjamin Cummings, 1980:186.

236. Woodward TM, Miller BR, Beaty BJ, Trent DW, Roehrig JT. A single amino acid change in the E2 glycoprotein of Venezuelan equine encephalitis virus affects replication and dissemination in *Aedes aegypti* mosquitoes. J Gen Virol 1991;72:2431–2435.

Viral Pathogenesis,
edited by Neal Nathanson, et al.
Lippincott–Raven Publishers, Philadelphia © 1997

CHAPTER 15

Evolution of Viral Diseases

Neal Nathanson and Frederick A. Murphy

INTRODUCTION

The evolution of viral diseases is distinct from, although related to, the evolution of viruses in general. The emergence of a viral disease can in some instances reflect evolutionary change in the causal agent, but more often emergence occurs in the absence of any such change. It is other factors, external to the virus, that most commonly drive the emergence of new diseases and the reemergence of old diseases. To emphasize this distinction between the evolution of viruses and the evolution of viral diseases, we use the terms emergence, endemicity, epidemicity, and control primarily to refer to the diseases, not the viruses.[62] The body of this chapter traces the evolutionary progression of exemplary viral diseases and the waxing and waning in disease incidence, mainly from epidemiologic and natural history perspectives. We then summarize the dynamic mechanisms that drive evolution, with respect to the influence of change in the virus, the host, the host population, and the environment. The approach we have taken is one advocated by Stephen Jay Gould[25]:

> The beauty of nature lies in detail; the message in generality. Optimal appreciation demands both, and I know no better tactic than the illustration of exciting principles by well-chosen particulars.

N. Nathanson: University of Pennsylvania Medical Center, Philadelphia, Pennsylvania 19104.

F. A. Murphy: School of Veterinary Medicine, University of California, Davis, California 95616.

EMERGENCE OF NEW VIRAL DISEASES

The emergence of a new viral disease can occur for several reasons, including (1) initial recognition of a previously unrecognized disease, (2) an increase in the ratio of cases to infections, (3) an increase in the number of infections, and (4) an increase in transmission. Each of these mechanisms is explored in the following discussion.[36,38,55–57,62]

Initial Recognition

In some instances, the presence of a viral infection (and the virus itself) is not recognized as a specific nosologic entity until it emerges as a new disease. Recognition may be triggered through a variety of circumstances, such as the occurrence of a specific outbreak that leads to intensive investigation or the isolation of the agent and subsequent development of laboratory methods (e.g., the polymerase chain reaction) that permit a specific etiologic diagnosis. New diseases that are clinically unique, such as Hantavirus pulmonary syndrome and bovine spongiform encephalopathy (BSE), are more likely to be recognized early than diseases that closely resemble well-established clinical entities, such as novel diarrheas and pneumonias.

One example of emergence resulting from recognition is California encephalitis, which is caused by the La Crosse virus.[27,29] La Crosse virus was first isolated from a 4-year-old child with encephalitis who was hospitalized and died in La Crosse, Wisconsin, in 1960; the isolation was made 4 years later from stored brain tissue.[85] Using this isolate as a source of antigen, retrospective serologic surveys of cases diagnosed as "viral encephalitis, undetermined etiology" indicated that La Crosse virus was the cause of many of these cases in the upper Mississippi valley of the United States.[84] Since that time, La Crosse encephalitis has been reported each year from a large area of the midwestern United States, at an average annual incidence of about 75 cases, with no evidence of increasing occurrence over the last 25 years (Fig. 15-1).

Was recognition of La Crosse encephalitis in the mid-1960s a result of the sudden introduction or evolutionary progression of the virus? Evidence now suggests that La Crosse infection had been present for many years before the recognition of the disease. A major serologic survey was conducted in Indiana on blood samples collected in 1978 and 1979.[26] When the presence of antibody was plotted by age, its prevalence increased incrementally from 0% at birth to almost 30% among those older than 70 years of age. This is consistent with an endemic infection that had been occurring regularly for many decades. In this instance, recognition was triggered by the isolation of the etiologic agent and the development of serologic methods to identify the cause of a set of cases of "encephalitis, undetermined etiology."

The emergence of Hantavirus pulmonary syndrome was appreciated only recently even though there is now evidence that it has long been endemic in its rodent reservoir hosts.[31,64,65,67] In May 1993, a cluster of cases of acute respiratory disease was reported in the southwestern region of the United States, and within a short time cases were found in eight states. Clinical signs included a prodrome of fever, myalgia, headache, and cough, followed by acute pulmonary congestion, edema, transudation, and interstitial infiltration leading to hypoxia, shock, and, in many cases, death. Testing of patients' sera showed evidence of an antibody response against several known Hantaviruses. Using that lead, primers were designed from sequences

of known Hantaviruses, and reverse transcriptase polymerase chain reaction was used to amplify viral RNA from autopsy tissues. It was immediately shown that the amplified fragments were derived from a previously unknown Hantavirus. The same methods, applied to rodents collected in the areas in which patients lived, showed that the primary reservoir host of the newly recognized virus was *Peromyscus maniculatus*, the deer mouse. This virus, like other Hantaviruses, does not cause disease in its reservoir rodent hosts, but virus is shed in urine, saliva, and feces for long periods, probably throughout the life of the host. Human infection occurs by inhalation of aerosols or dust containing dried infected rodent urine, saliva, or excreta.

It is now clear that this newly recognized virus (actually a set of closely related variant viruses), now designated Sin Nombre virus, is endemic in the large area of the western region of the United States inhabited by *Peromyscus* species. The virus was recognized in 1993 because of the number and clustering of human cases, which in turn was probably caused by a great increase in rodent numbers after two especially wet winters and a consequently great increase in availability of seeds of the piñon pine and other rodent food. In this instance, an important virus remained hidden and the disease it causes emerged only after environmental conditions favored an outbreak and consequent intensive investigation.

Increase in Ratio of Cases to Infections

An important mechanism for the emergence of new viral diseases, particularly in epidemic form, is an increase in the ratio of cases to infections. Sporadic cases of an illness may escape attention altogether or may not be considered important, even if there have been very large numbers of infections. An increase in the ratio of cases to infections can call attention to the infection and the virus in the absence of any increase in the number of infections. Two mechanisms can produce an increase in the ratio of cases to infections: (1) host resistance can be altered without any change in the virulence of the virus, or (2) the virus may increase in virulence without any change in host resistance. In rare instances, both host resistance and viral virulence change coincidentally.

Altered Host Resistance

It is likely that poliomyelitis has occurred as a sporadic disease since ancient times.[71] During the 18th century and the first half of the 19th century, a number of individual cases and a few clusters of cases were reported. About 1870, poliomyelitis burst on the scene in the form of epidemics of "infantile paralysis." The first scattered outbreaks were in rural areas of the northern United States and Sweden. Such outbreaks soon became more common, and from about 1905 onward, epidemics were reported annually in the United States (Fig. 15-2). This pattern of emergence of poliomyelitis as an epidemic disease has been repeated many times since, first in developed and then in developing countries. It is still going on in some parts of the world, such as India, even as the global program for eradication of the disease is proceeding. Paul and Horstmann have reviewed the history of poliomyelitis in an authoritative and fascinating monograph.[71]

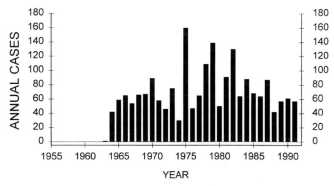

FIG. 15-1. Incidence of La Crosse viral encephalitis in the United States, 1963 through 1991, based on reports to the Centers for Disease Control and Prevention. Incidence has remained essentially constant during this period, suggesting that the emergence of this disease represented recognition of the nosologic entity that followed the isolation of the agent and development of a diagnostic serologic test. (Data from Griot C, Tselis A, Tsai TF, Gonzalez-Scarano F, Nathanson N. Bunyavirus diseases. In: Stroop WG, McKendall RR, eds. Handbook of neurovirology. New York: Marcel Dekker, 1994:439–454.)

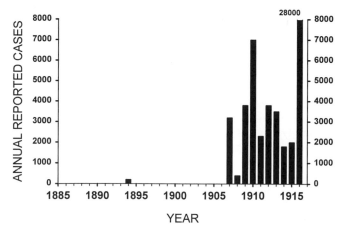

FIG. 15-2. The appearance of epidemic poliomyelitis in the United States, 1885 to 1916. This graph shows the dramatic appearance of poliomyelitis as an epidemic disease. The figure is based on reported cases, most of which were paralytic, during an era when reporting was estimated at about 50%. (Data from Lavinder CH, Freeman SW, Frost WH. Epidemiologic studies of poliomyelitis in New York City and the northeastern United States during the year 1916. Washington: United States Public Health Service, 1918.)

TABLE 15-1. *Poliomyelitis attack rates and age distribution, European and Moroccan populations of Casablanca, 1947–1953.**

Parameter	European	Moroccan
Population	125,000	530,000
Paralytic cases	117	25
Annual attack rate (per 100,000)	13.4	0.7
1953 cases by age (y)		
0–1	8	9
2–9	15	2
10–39	5	—

*Table shows that the incidence of clinical poliomyelitis was much higher and the age distribution older in the European population than in the native population in a single city, where it may be presumed that the same strains of poliovirus were circulating. This observation is consistent with the view that the emergence of epidemic poliomyelitis was related to the age of initial infection, which in turn altered the ratio of cases to infections.

Data from Paul J, Horstmann D. A survey of poliomyelitis virus antibodies in French Morocco. Am J Trop Med Hyg 1955;4:512–524.

What accounts for this emergence of epidemic poliomyelitis? There is no evidence that it was caused by the appearance of a virus strain of increased virulence. Evidence against strain variation comes from several sources, but one of the most convincing is a study conducted in Casablanca, Morocco, in the 1950s. At that time, there was a substantial European population in the city, and this population experienced a poliomyelitis attack rate about 20-fold that of the native Moroccan population (Table 15-1). Furthermore, the cases among Europeans were in children and teenagers, but almost all the cases among Moroccans were in very young infants. Although it can be assumed that the same wild polioviruses were circulating in both populations in the city, the age of victims was very different.

Clues to the explanation of this kind of difference in clinical attack rate were provided by serologic surveys, also conducted in the early 1950s, in Cairo and Miami. In Cairo, poliomyelitis was very rare; in Miami there were regular outbreaks of disease.[70] Poliovirus infection was ubiquitous in Cairo, and essentially the whole population acquired antibody in early childhood. In contrast, in Miami, infection was often delayed until the teenage years or later, although cumulative infection prevalence later approached 100%. As in Casablanca, the age distribution of cases matched the serologic profile.

These data suggest that there was a correlation between age at the time of poliovirus infection and risk of paralytic disease. Because the early epidemics were almost exclusively concentrated in children younger than 5 years of age (hence the name infantile paralysis), the explanation must be sought in variables occurring within the first 5 years of life. It is well established that the case:infection ratio for poliomyelitis is about 1:100 to 1:200, and it is possible that the ratio varies greatly with age. However, the available data bearing on this point indicate that the case:infection ratio was only a few times lower in infants than in children 1 to 4 years of age,[53] a difference not great enough to explain the dramatic emergence of epidemic poliomyelitis.

Another serologic study done in Casablanca provides a potential explanation (Fig. 15-3). The age-specific antibody profile in native Moroccans indicates that many infants become infected while they are still protected by maternal antibody. Even so, the data probably underestimate the proportion of infants who retain passive antibody until the time of exposure, because neutralizing antibody was measured at a serum dilution of 1:10, which is about 10 times the level needed to provide protection against paralysis.[5]

Synthesizing all these observations, Nathanson and Martin[61] proposed that the appearance of epidemic poliomyelitis was caused, paradoxically, by improvements in public sanitation and in personal hygiene, which led to a reduction in virus transmission. A delay in the age of initial infection, beyond the age at which infants were protected by passively acquired maternal antibody, is postulated to have increased the risk of clinical disease. An intrinsically lower case:infection ratio in infancy than in early childhood may represent a secondary contributing factor.

Increased Viral Virulence

In some instances, mutation of an existing virus strain may be the cause of increased virulence and transmissibility. This may result in an increase in the ratio of cases of clinical disease to infections. A familiar example is the introduction of new influenza virus reassortants, bearing new hemagglutinin or neuraminidase genes, into a host population. The host population may be immunologically naive to the reassortant virus, with epidemic consequences.[89]

One dramatic example was the epidemic of avian influenza that devastated the poultry industry of Pennsylvania in the early 1980s. In April 1983, a new strain of influenza virus

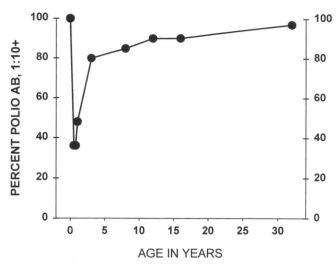

FIG. 15-3. Age-specific proportion of native Moroccans with type 1 poliovirus neutralizing antibody at a 1:10 titer or greater, Casablanca, 1953. The profile shows that many infants acquired infection and active immunity while they were still under the protection of passive maternal antibody. The actual proportion was probably greater than shown, because antibody titers less than 1:10 were not measured. (Data from Paul J, Horstmann D. A survey of poliomyelitis virus antibodies in French Morocco. Am J Trop Med Hyg 1955; 4:512–524.)

(H5N2) appeared in commercial flocks of chickens in Pennsylvania; it produced low mortality and did not cause great concern. Suddenly, in October 1983, this virus began to produce outbreaks with a mortality rate of 80% and began to spread in epidemic fashion to flocks in neighboring states. During the succeeding few months, the epidemic was controlled only by draconian measures involving destruction of infected flocks; in the end, the control program involved the destruction of 15 million birds and a cost of almost $100 million. The virus isolated during the epidemic exhibited a markedly increased virulence compared with isolates from the spring of 1983. Elegant laboratory studies[88] showed that a single point mutation in the hemagglutinin of the original virus enormously enhanced its virulence and initiated the epidemic. The mutation increased the cleavability of the viral hemagglutinin by cellular proteases, which in turn led to a broader cellular host range and higher viral titers, thereby enhancing viral virulence and transmissibility. A similar sequence of events occurred in Mexico in 1995.[90] It is rare to be able to capture such a vivid snapshot of the emergence of epidemic disease, but this example indicates that an epidemic can be caused by a viral mutation, even one that is very limited in extent.

Increase in the Number of Infections

A major increase in the incidence of infections can produce an epidemic of a known disease or an emergence of a previously unrecognized nosologic entity. Such an increase in the incidence of infections may have any of several underlying causes: (1) viral reinvasion of an isolated population from which the virus has been absent for some time, (2) viral inva-

sion across a previously uncrossed species barrier, and (3) an increased rate of virus transmission.

Viral Invasion or Reinvasion of an Isolated Population

Iceland is an island sufficiently distant from other population centers so that its animal and human populations are not constantly exposed to viruses that regularly circulate in mainland populations. As a result, certain viruses have disappeared from Iceland, only to cause dramatic outbreaks after reintroduction. Three examples illustrate this situation.

Measles requires a human population of more than 500,000 for its perpetuation; it tends to fade out in smaller populations.[3,94] The population of Iceland is about 250,000, and measles has periodically disappeared, only to be reintroduced as striking epidemics that last 1 to 2 years and then fade away (Fig. 15-4). Canine distemper, the morbillivirus of dogs, has shown a similar epidemic pattern. Distemper is usually absent from Iceland, and immunization of dogs is not practiced. However, during the 20th century, the virus has been introduced three times, each time by the importation of a dog that had not been properly quarantined, and each time causing a devastating epidemic (with losses of up to 90% of infected animals), which was controlled only by the most stringent measures.[63] Finally, maedi/visna, an endemic lentivirus disease of sheep, was introduced into Iceland in the 1930s by the importation of sheep from Germany; it subsequently spread through more than half the sheep population of the island. The result was an emergence in epidemic form of respiratory and neurologic diseases that occur at a relatively low incidence in other sheep-raising countries.[28,60,68] The epidemic was controlled only by dividing the island into many sectors, sequentially destroying all animals in each affected sector, and restocking from an uninfected part of the country. This heroic control program, which extended from 1949 through 1965, probably represents the only successful eradication of a lentivirus from a host population.[68]

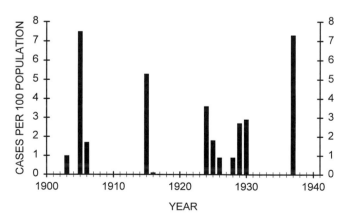

FIG. 15-4. Reported cases of measles in Iceland, 1900 to 1940. This display shows the recurrent epidemics of measles, each of which was followed by fadeout of the disease. (Data from Tauxe [unpublished] and from Nathanson N. Epidemiology. In: Fields BN, Knipe DM, eds. Virology. New York: Raven Press, 1990:267–292.)

Crossing the Species Barrier

Periodically, a virus crosses the species barrier and becomes a new virus—that is, one new to the invaded species. Epidemiologically, such events can be divided into three important categories: (1) invasions in which there is no further spread by individual contact, the new species acting as a deadend host; (2) invasions in which there is limited propagation in the new host species and the infection dies out after a few generations of spread; and (3) invasions in which the virus spreads freely in its new host species, with devastating consequences. In general, viruses respect the species barrier, and some genetic evolution is probably required for full adaptation to a new host species. The term species barrier is a relative one, and experience suggests that viruses are more likely to cross between species that are closely related than between widely disparate species. The emergences of canine parvovirus disease (caused by a virus crossing from cats to dogs) and acquired immunodeficiency syndrome (AIDS; caused by a crossing from subhuman primates to humans) exemplify this point.

Invasion of a New Species With no Further Spread in the New Host Population

There are a considerable number of zoonotic viruses[19] that can be transmitted to humans, who then become deadend hosts. Many of these viruses are arthropod-borne, including alphaviruses such as the Venezuelan, eastern, and western equine encephalitis viruses; flaviviruses such as Murray Valley, Japanese B, and St. Louis encephalitis viruses; and bunyaviruses such as La Crosse virus and Rift Valley fever virus. In other instances, viruses are transmitted directly to humans from zoonotic reservoirs by fomites. Examples include bunyaviruses such as the Hantaan, Seoul, and Sin Nombre viruses and arenaviruses such as the Machupo (Bolivian hemorrhagic fever) and Junin (Argentine hemorrhagic fever) viruses. Historically, each of these viruses has been responsible for the emergence of a new human disease.

BSE is a scrapie-like prion disease of cattle[91,93] that has occurred primarily in the United Kingdom. BSE is a newly recognized entity, and it is questionable whether it ever occurred before the recent epidemic. The first cases of BSE probably began in England in April 1985, but it was not until November 1986 that the disease was officially recognized. The epidemic curve through April 1995 is shown in Figure 15-5; at the peak of the epidemic there were more than 10,000 cases reported per quarter.

What was the cause of this dramatic epidemic? An exhaustive search[92] for possible causal events that may have occurred in the early 1980s focused on meat and bone meal (MBM), which is used as a supplemental nutrient for most cattle, particularly for dairy cattle. MBM is produced in many rendering plants in England and is usually distributed locally. These plants process abattoir waste that contains the carcasses of ruminants, including sheep. Scrapie has been endemic in sheep in the United Kingdom for centuries, and the agent is present in high titer in sheep brain and spleen. The rendering plants used heat treatment, milling, and solvent extraction to produce two main products, tallow (fat) and MBM (a dry

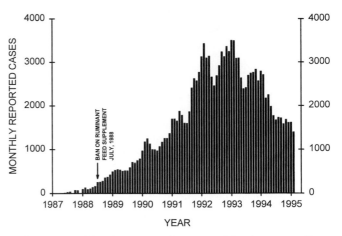

FIG. 15-5. Epidemic curve of cases of bovine spongiform encephalopathy (BSE) by month and year of onset of clinical signs. The dramatic appearance and increase of BSE is shown in this graph. (Data from Wilesmith JW. Bovine spongiform encephalopathy: epidemiological factors associated with the emergence of an important new animal pathogen in Great Britain. Semin Virol 1994;5: 179–187.)

powder); the fact that this harsh process inactivated any scrapie agent present in the sheep tissues was unappreciated. Because of the increasing cost of petroleum products, solvent extraction began to be abandoned in 1977; by 1982, only 10% of MBM produced in England was made by this method. Work with experimental scrapie in mice had established that the agent is sensitive to fat solvents, and the importance of the termination of solvent extraction as a risk factor was suggested by the low rate of BSE in Scotland, where solvent extraction continued to be used. In July 1988, in an attempt to terminate the epidemic, the British Ministry of Agriculture prohibited the inclusion of ruminant tissues in nutritional supplements destined for cattle.

The hypothesis that the BSE epidemic was caused by contamination of MBM supplements with scrapie-infected sheep tissues leaves unanswered another question: Why did the epidemic of BSE occur in the United Kingdom, whereas other cattle raising countries experienced only a few scattered cases? One explanation[93] is that there were several requirements for the occurrence of the BSE outbreak, all of which came together only in the United Kingdom. These were (1) a large sheep population relative to other ruminants, so that sheep contributed a substantial proportion of the raw material used in rendering; (2) a fairly high endemic level of scrapie in sheep; (3) intensive feeding of MBM mainly to dairy cattle; and (4) changes in the rendering process, including cessation of solvent extraction, which reduced the inactivation of the scrapie agent during the production of MBM.

The epidemic peaked in early 1993 and has fallen substantially since (see Fig. 15-5). If it is assumed that transmission of BSE ceased in late 1988 (allowing 6 months after the ban for exhaustion of supplies of food supplements in the distribution chain) and that the average incubation period is about 5 years, then the epidemic would be predicted to wane rapidly after 1993. The accuracy of this prediction will become clearer over the next 5 years.

*Invasion of a New Species With Limited Spread
in the New Host Population*

There are a few viruses that are endemic in reservoir species but that, if transmitted to humans, spread from person to person for only a few generations. Examples are Crimean-Congo hemorrhagic fever virus, a tickborne bunyavirus; Lassa virus, an arenavirus endemic in *Mastomys natalensis* rats; Ebola virus, a filovirus whose reservoir remains unknown; and equine morbillivirus, whose origin is yet to be discovered.[2,7,16,33,45–47,73,77,78,86]

In each instance, the virus also appears to be transmitted by fomites, and secondary cases occur mainly among hospital personnel and family members who come in close contact with acutely ill patients. Cases may also occur in persons exposed to syringes and needles previously used on infected patients. As a corollary, hospital outbreaks can usually be terminated by institution of adequate isolation procedures.

*Invasion of a New Species With Unlimited Propagation
in the New Host Population*

There are many ways in which new diseases can emerge, but none is as ominous as the emergence of a new disease in the absence of any change in host or environment, simply by mutational events in the virus and selective events stabilizing the mutant in the host population. These are the least frequent but most significant instances of the crossing of the species barrier.

Canine parvovirus disease emerged with explosive impact in 1978 and spread worldwide in the succeeding 2 years.[69] The disease is most devastating in the fetus and newborn; it is most damaging in lymphoid tissues, heart tissue, and intestinal tissues, resulting in leukopenia, anemia, diarrhea, myocarditis, and often death. The virus is shed in the feces and is extremely resistant in the environment; this characteristic favors transport by inanimate objects even in the presence of strict animal quarantine. The emergence of this disease was an absolutely new occurrence; retrospective serologic surveys of dogs have shown that the virus was not present earlier in that species.

The genetic source of this emergence seems clear: canine parvovirus originated as a mutant of feline panleukopenia virus, an ancient and important pathogen of cats. Viral genome sequence analyses were used to determine this relation; the line of descent from the feline virus to the canine virus started in 1974 and involved only three or four changes in the DNA of the feline virus.[69] An ancestral virus that changes as abruptly as feline panleukopenia virus did when it mutated to yield canine parvovirus has the potential to cause a virgin-soil pandemic in its new, nonimmune host population. Concern has been raised about the risk of further changes in the canine parvovirus (or another parvovirus) that would allow replication in humans. The fact that human parvovirus B19 has some of the same biologic qualities as the animal parvoviruses, including a capacity to cause important damage to the fetus, adds to this concern.

Although the origins of the human immunodeficiency viruses, HIV-1 and HIV-2, will probably always remain cryptic, there is strong circumstantial evidence that AIDS was initiated by the entry of HIV into a previously uninfected population. It appears that, after the initial crossing of the species barrier, mutation and selection continued, with the virus eventually evolving into the deadly pathogen we know today. Fragmentary data suggest that HIV-1 first appeared extensively in humans in Africa in the mid-1970s.[76] It is well documented that HIV-1 began to spread widely in the United States and Europe beginning about 1978[35] and in Asia in the mid-1980s. In each case, after its initial introduction the virus has spread rapidly; there do not seem to be any further barriers to the movement of the virus after it is introduced into a risk group.

As to the source of HIV-1 and HIV-2, the leading hypothesis is that these viruses were derived from one or several viruses of subhuman primates indigenous to the African continent.[1,13] This hypothesis rests mainly on four observations. First, surveys have shown that certain African primates are endemically infected with HIV-like lentiviruses, the simian immunodeficiency viruses (SIVs). Second, genetic comparisons of viruses isolated from endemically infected primates indicate a relation of these viruses with certain isolates of HIV-1 and HIV-2. Third, there is a geographic overlap between the range of some of these endemically infected primate species and areas in which HIV initially appeared.[62] Finally, there has always been close contact between human and monkey populations in these regions.

The most striking support for this four-pronged argument comes from studies of the epidemiology and natural history of HIV-2. This virus initially appeared among humans in West Africa and has been disseminated to the rest of Africa, Europe, and North America.[80] The region where HIV-2 first appeared overlaps closely the range of *Cercocebus atys*, a subspecies of the sooty mangabey. Surveys of wild *C atys* indicate that at least 10% are endemically infected with a lentivirus, SIV_{SM}, which is virtually indistinguishable from HIV-2.[14,21,22,44]

Another monkey species, *Cercopithecus aethiops,* the African green monkey, ranges over most of sub-Saharan Africa, including the areas of central Africa in which HIV-1 has its highest seroprevalence. It is estimated that 20% to 50% of African green monkeys are infected with a lentivirus, SIV_{AGM}, but this virus is only distantly related to HIV-1 (about 60% amino acid identity), whereas SIV_{SM} exhibits about an 80% identity to HIV-2.[13,14]

If HIV-1 and HIV-2 were derived from viruses of subhuman primates, it will probably never be possible to document the exact time and location of the original crossings of the species barrier. It is possible that HIV invaded the human population some time ago and did not spread widely until disruptions of the fabric of African society promoted its dissemination. What is better established is that HIV-1 did not spread widely in humans in Africa until the late 1970s and that HIV-2 was detected in West Africa only in the mid-1980s.[23,40,76] From these sites, HIV-1 spread to Europe and the United States in the late 1970s, and HIV-2 spread to the same areas in the late 1980s.[80] Whatever the secret that allowed the initial invasion of the human species by these viruses, there has been seemingly unlimited propagation of the viruses in their new host ever since.

Increase in Transmission

The transmissibility of a given virus can vary dramatically in different subpopulations and circumstances. An increase in transmission may an important contributory factor in the emergence of a viral disease, although it is rarely the only cause of emergence.

Tomato spotted wilt was first recognized as a disease of tomatoes in Australia in 1915. In 1927, the disease was shown to be transmitted by thrips, a large family of very small insects. In 1930, the disease was shown to be caused by a virus, tomato spotted wilt virus, but only recently was the virus classified as a bunyavirus (on the basis of its genomic structure).[11,24] Over the past 50 years, a number of diseases of agriculturally important vegetable and fruit crops have been shown to be caused by tomato spotted wilt virus (tospovirus), but it was only in the 1980s that these diseases emerged as a global problem, affecting more than 500 plant species and causing massive damage.[24] The spread of disease appears to have been associated with the spread of the western flower thrip (*Frankliniella occidentalis*), a particularly efficient vector. It is postulated[24] that the spread of the virus and vector have been caused by increases in the intercontinental shipment of vegetables and fruits, together with the mass cultivation of plants that has accompanied the development of international agribusiness. Tospovirus diseases appear to represent emergence of a viral disease on a global basis as the result of increased transmission. It is also postulated on the basis of sequence homologies[24] that tospoviruses may have evolved quite recently from an ancestral bunyavirus of animals.

AIDS provides another salient example of the importance of increased transmission in the emergence of viral disease. Serologic studies[66] suggest that HIV infection may have been present for one or more decades before AIDS emerged in Africa in the 1970s as a newly recognized clinical entity. AIDS was present in certain villages as an infrequent infection, poorly transmitted under the conditions of rural life. After the infection moved to the cities along with a massive urbanization movement and gained entry into the rapidly growing, sexually active urban populations (in which multiple partners and prostitution were common), its spread was vastly accelerated, leading to the devastating epidemic that is now ongoing in many countries of Africa. Serial serologic studies in one rural area showed a prevalence of antibodies to HIV that remained constant (less than 1%) over a 10-year interval,[66] while at about the same time in Kinshasa, Zaire, the prevalence of HIV antibodies in female prostitutes rose from less than 10% to 80%.[76] In parallel fashion, HIV infections in the Indian subcontinent and in southeast Asia have expanded very rapidly in urban subpopulations where conditions favor spread of sexually transmitted diseases.

WANING AND DISAPPEARANCE OF VIRAL DISEASES

Just as virus diseases emerge, so they may wane and sometimes disappear. In contrast to emergence, the waning of a viral disease frequently reflects deliberate human intervention in an attempt to control the problem. The preeminent approach to control is preexposure immunization, which has been successfully used to reduce the incidence of many viral diseases (see Chap. 16). Development of vaccines is currently a very active field, and immunization will bring a number of additional viral diseases under control in the next decades. Several other approaches to control of virus transmission have been used less frequently but have successfully contained some viral diseases; these include provision of safe food, clean water, and sanitary sewage treatment and control of zoonotic reservoirs or vector populations. Finally, as exemplified by smallpox, regional elimination and global eradication are the ultimate methods to achieve disease control. Such successful human intervention into the natural history of a pathogenic virus represents an evolutionary outcome that, from our anthropocentric perspective, is most satisfying.

Vaccines

Viral vaccine development is one of the great successes of modern biomedical research; the advance of vaccine usage represents a parallel success of public health and preventive medicine. Attenuated live virus vaccines, inactivated virus vaccines, and subunit vaccines are currently in use, and many novel kinds of vaccines derived from recombinant DNA technology are on the horizon (see Chap. 16). In all cases, the goal is that the immunized individual will, on subsequent exposure to wild virus, undergo a limited infection that is detectable only by an anamnestic immune response. Most important for the topic at hand, immunized individuals cannot serve as links in the infection chain. If a sufficient proportion of the population are immunized, opportunities for transmission may be so reduced that the wild virus can no longer be perpetuated.

Two notable examples of vaccine-mediated disease control in the United States are shown in Figures 15-6 and 15-7. Poliomyelitis represents a success that exceeded the expectations of even the most sanguine vaccinologists at the time of vaccine introduction in the 1950s and 1960s. It appears[58] that by the early 1970s wild polioviruses had ceased to circulate in the United States, even though there was a residual population of nonimmunized, susceptible children and young adults, estimated at many millions. On analysis, it seems that this cessation was caused by the dieout of poliovirus during the seasonal trough when viral transmission was naturally very low (Fig. 15-8). Other than one introduction of wild poliovirus in 1979, into a nonimmunized subpopulation that did not participate in vaccination programs, wild poliovirus has not circulated in the United States in more than 20 years. Poliovirus has now been eradicated from the western hemisphere,[10] again by the use of repeated mass immunization. The World Health Organization has made global eradication of wild poliovirus a goal with a target date of 2001 (see Eradication).

Measles has also been successfully controlled by vaccination; disease incidence has been reduced by 100- to 1000-fold compared with the prevaccine era (see Fig. 15-7). At least 3,000,000 cases of measles are estimated to have occurred in the United States each year before the introduction of vaccine; in recent years, fewer than 3000 cases have been reported. In contrast to poliovirus, the measles virus has eluded elimina-

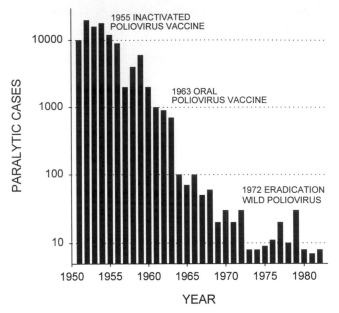

FIG. 15-6. Reported cases of paralytic poliomyelitis in the United States, 1951 through 1982. This figure illustrates the course of the decline of poliomyelitis after introduction of inactivated poliovirus vaccine in 1955 and oral poliovirus vaccine in 1963. Elimination was achieved in 1972, and cases reported after 1973 are either vaccine-associated or imported, with the exception of an outbreak in 1979 in the unvaccinated Amish population. (Data from Poliomyelitis incidence in the United States. MMWR Morb Mortal Wkly Rep 1982;30:12–17, and Nathanson N. Epidemiologic aspects of poliomyelitis eradication. Rev Infect Dis 1984;6:S308–S312.)

tion of measles virus in the United States is within reach but will be difficult to achieve until the virus is better controlled in South America, Europe, and Africa.

Control of Transmission

Some very important viral diseases are controlled by means other than the use of vaccines. Systems for the provision of safe food, clean water, sanitary sewage removal and treatment, and organized mosquito control are the pillars of public health programs and, indeed, have been used to measure the status of societal development. Such disease control programs are extremely diverse.

A dramatic example of disease control has been the use of rodenticides to control epidemics of Bolivian hemorrhagic fever. Reduction of the local population of the murine reservoir host, *Callomys callosus,* has greatly reduced transmission to humans of the etiologic agent of this disease, Machupo virus.[34] A very different strategy has been necessary to control rabies in wildlife. For many years, fox rabies control in Europe involved population reduction by bounty hunting and poisoning, but increasing objection from conservationists and newer control strategies (e.g., bait-delivered vaccination of foxes) have rendered fox killing obsolete. In the case of arboviruses, vector control measures have been very successful in preventing disease. One historic example is the eradication of *Aedes aegypti* from Cuba in 1902, with consequent elimination of yellow fever.[82] This was done by a government-organized program to eliminate mosquito breeding habitats.

In contrast to these active intervention strategies, passive changes reducing mosquito exposure also have been effective. The incidence of St. Louis encephalitis acquired during episodes of mosquito activity has been lessened by the increasing use of screening, closed house foundations, and especially air conditioning (leading to closure of all windows). It has even been said that the advent of television has been a factor reducing exposure to mosquito vectors, because its presence has attracted spectators indoors into closed, air-conditioned rooms.[41]

tion, probably because of its greater transmissibility. However, application of molecular epidemiology indicates that there is little indigenous measles virus remaining in the United States and that most recent outbreaks can be traced to foreign importations (W. Bellini, PhD, Centers for Disease Control, Atlanta, GA, personal communication, 1995). It appears that elimina-

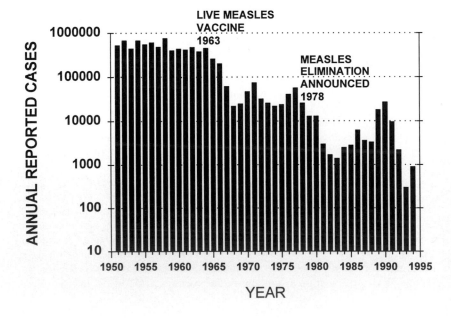

FIG. 15-7. Reported cases of measles in the United States, 1951 through 1993. This figure illustrates the decline in cases after the introduction of live measles vaccine in 1963. Measles was underreported before the introduction of the vaccine; an estimated 3,000,000 cases were occurring each year at that time. Reporting has been much more complete in recent years because of the small number of cases and the effort to contain any outbreaks. The vaccine has probably reduced the number of cases by about 1000-fold, to a level of no more than 3000 cases per year. (Data from R. Bernier, Centers for Disease Control, Atlanta, GA, personal communication, 1995, and references 8, 9, 50–52, 58, 83, and 94.)

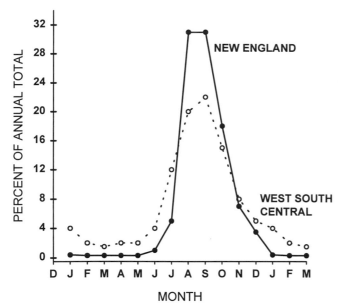

Fig. 15-8. Seasonal distribution of poliomyelitis in the New England and West South Central regions of the United States, based on cumulative reports for paralytic and non-paralytic cases, 1942 through 1951. In New England, more than 30% of annual cases occurred in each of the peak months of August and September, whereas fewer than 1% occurred in each of the trough months of February through May. (Data from Serfling RE, Sherman IL. Poliomyelitis distribution in the United States. Public Health Rep 1953;68: 453–466.)

Again, the behavior of the human population can be more important in the evolution of a disease than any ecologic or virologic factor. On occasion, epidemic animal diseases have been controlled by slaughter and restocking with animals known to be free of the virus. As previously described, this strategy was successfully used to eradicate maedi/visna virus from Iceland[68]

and to control avian influenza in Pennsylvania and surrounding states in 1983.[88] This approach is still the fail-safe tactic kept in readiness for the elimination of foot-and-mouth disease whenever it is introduced into cattle in the developed world. In that case, the slaughter of animals is extensive in magnitude and is combined with massive disinfection of contaminated premises.

Control in the case of many other categories of viral diseases involves specialized measures. For example, sexually transmitted viral diseases, viral diseases associated with day care, childhood diseases transmitted in the community that are not vaccine-preventable, and iatrogenic diseases all require specific, complex control methods. Even among the iatrogenically transmitted viral diseases, different strategies are required for dealing with diseases associated with immunosuppressive therapy, diseases associated with organ transplantation (including xeno-transplantation), diseases associated with blood banking, and diseases associated with kidney dialysis. In this regard, one notable success has been the elimination of bloodborne viruses by screening of blood and heating of blood products. This has markedly reduced the transmission of hepatitis B and has virtually eliminated the transmission of HIV to transfusion recipients in the United States (Fig. 15-9).

Eradication

The eradication of smallpox, the first and only example of global elimination, is an historic milestone in the control of viral diseases that has been documented in a fascinating monograph by Fenner and colleagues.[18] The conquest of smallpox, and current attempts to eliminate poliomyelitis and measles have helped to formulate the requirements for any successful eradication program. These may be summarized as follows:

1. *The causative virus must be confined to a single host species, such as humans or an important domestic animal species, and not maintained in a zoonotic reservoir.* By this

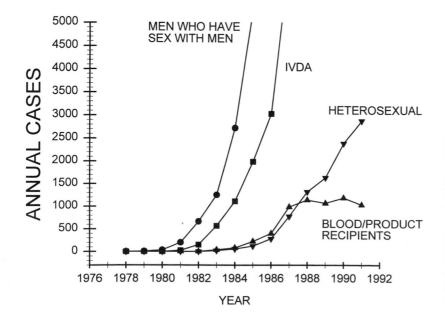

FIG. 15-9. Annual incidence of AIDS in the United States for four risk groups, 1978 to 1991. Cases are shown for recipients of blood transfusions and blood products, men who have sex with men, intravenous drug users (IVDA), and heterosexual women and men. The subepidemics in different groups progressed at different rates during the early phases of the AIDS epidemic. The incidence among recipients of blood products began to plateau in 1988 owing to screening of blood that began in 1985. (Data from references 6 and 62.)

criterion, varicella-zoster, rubella, mumps, and hepatitis A could be considered as candidates for elimination or eradication (although each suffers from other negative characteristics), but yellow fever, because of its zoonotic reservoirs in South America and Africa, would not be an appropriate candidate. Likewise, human influenza, which is maintained in avian and porcine reservoirs, would be an unlikely candidate for elimination or eradication.

2. *There must be a successful vaccine, so that immunologically naive individuals can be eliminated as potential links in the virus transmission chain.* On this point, poliomyelitis, measles, and hepatitis B could today be considered as candidates for elimination, but respiratory syncytial disease and herpesvirus diseases could not. Viruses that exists in a large number of different serotypes or that undergo frequent changes in their antigenic composition also would not yield readily to an immunization-based eradication strategy.

3. *The virus must spread slowly enough so that a search and containment strategy can be successfully applied.* Smallpox was eliminated only after it was recognized that it was not necessary to apply mass immunization to the whole population. Instead, it was possible to control the disease by identifying and controlling local outbreaks and using vaccine to create a ring of immune hosts around each nidus of infection. Measles tests elimination strategies because of its high transmissibility, which results in frequent reintroductions into regions in which indigenous circulation of the virus has been eliminated.

4. *The disease must be of sufficient importance as a cause of human or animal illness to justify the major investment of resources required to mount a global control program.* This is often a social and political matter of public will combined with a pragmatic willingness to devote hard-earned resources.

Currently, the foremost human disease target for eradication is poliomyelitis, which already has been eliminated from the western hemisphere. The disease and its etiologic agent meet all of the foregoing criteria. In the last few years, remarkable progress toward its elimination has been made. The World Health Organization is redoubling its efforts in remaining foci in India, Russia and countries of the Commonwealth of Independent States, and other countries in Asia and Africa.[75] Measles also meets many of the criteria except for its greater transmissibility, but it is too early to predict whether a global effort at elimination is practical. Another important viral disease is hepatitis B, which is the cause of major morbidity and mortality globally. However, any hepatitis B elimination program will require a very long-term effort because of the large population of persistently infected persons, who represent a reservoir that disappears only with the turnover of a whole generation.

As the ultimate terminal step in the natural history of a viral disease, only eradication of a virus can obviate all worries about unpredictable future dangers along the path of viral evolutionary progression. Very few viral pathogens have disappeared without human intervention (among them O'nyongnyong virus and horsepox virus), and we cannot expect the successful viruses, the common pathogens of humans and animals, to succumb spontaneously or to yield easily to human eradication schemes. Controlling the end game is as difficult in regard to viral disease evolution as it is when chess masters compete.

MECHANISMS IN THE EVOLUTION OF VIRAL DISEASES

In the foregoing sections, we have documented the various stages in the evolution of viral diseases, from initial emergence through potential control, regional elimination, and global eradication. The dynamic mechanisms that drive the evolution of viral diseases may be grouped under four controlling rubrics: those centered on the virus, the host, the host population, and the environment.

The Virus

In nature, viruses undergo an infinitely long series of replication cycles as they are transmitted from host to host. During this process, spontaneous mutants are continually generated, some of which have biologic properties that are different from those of the parent virus from which they arise. The in vivo environment brings pressures to bear which favor the selection of certain of these biologic variants, primarily because of their preferential ability to be serially transmitted. Properties that have been shown to be important in the survival and perpetuation of various viruses in nature include the following:

1. *Capacity to replicate rapidly.* In many cases, the most virulent strains of a virus can be shown to replicate faster than more temperate strains. For example, enteropathic strains of mouse hepatitis virus replicate and are shed very quickly compared with more temperate laboratory-passaged strains. However, if replication is too rapid, it can be self-defeating for the virus; extremely rapid viral growth may not allow time enough for transmission before the host is removed as a virus source by death or morbidity.[17]

2. *Capacity to replicate to high titer.* Very high vertebrate host viremia titer is employed by arthropod-borne viruses (e.g, Venezuelan equine encephalitis virus) to favor infection of the next arthropod. The same viruses produce very high titers in the salivary glands of their arthropod hosts so as to favor infection of the next vertebrate host. Although such high titers can be associated with silent infections in natural vertebrate hosts (e.g., reservoir host birds), the evolution of this capacity for growing to very high titer often seems to be associated with capacity to produce disease in the vertebrate host.

3. *Capacity to replicate in certain key tissues.* This quality is often important for the completion of the transmission cycle. The evolution of viral tropisms and the employment of specific host cell receptors that underpins all specific tropisms together define many clinical signs and disease patterns. For example, the employment of the acetylcholine receptor at neuromuscular end organs is a key to the pathogenesis and unique transmission pattern of rabies virus. In addition, the ability of a virus to grow in immunologically sequestered sites (e.g., brain, kidney) protected by basement membranes, myelin sheaths, and other structures pro-

vides great survival advantage. If a virus replicates in a sequestered site, there is often little stimulation of the immune response, and immune mediators often have poor capability of getting to infected target cells; examples include rabies in nerves and salivary glands and arenaviruses in salivary glands and the urinary system.

4. *Capacity to be shed quickly or for long periods of time.* In the simplest viral cycle of entry and transmission, all aspects of infection take place at the same superficial target site. For example, parainfluenzavirus infection involves airway epithelial cells almost exclusively. This infection pattern does not stimulate vigorous host response until after transmission has already been accomplished. The capacity for chronic shedding offers even better opportunity for virus survival and entrenchment; in maedi/visna virus infection, for example, persistence is so sustained that disease control has required slaughter of animals and repopulation over large areas. Recrudescence and intermittent shedding add additional advantages to the virus (e.g., varicella-zoster and shingles).

5. *Capacity to elude host defenses.* The defenses presented by antibody, cytolytic T cells, interferon, and other host responses may be thwarted by characteristics of the virus. Some viruses (particularly those with large genomes) possess genes that encode proteins that interfere with specific antiviral activities[49]; these are discussed elsewhere in this book (see Chaps. 5, 6 and 22). Although the origin of such viral genes is unclear, some may have been captured from the host genome by recombination. Presumably, these genes have been incorporated into the viral genome because of the selective advantage that they confer on the virus. The capacity to initiate an infection that leads to immunologic tolerance or to infection of germ line cells represents an extreme survival advantage. Circumvention of the immune response (e.g., lymphocytic choriomeningitis virus infection in the mouse, bovine viral diarrhea virus infection in calves, mouse endogenous retrovirus infections), or even partial immunosuppression (e.g., HIV infection in humans, feline immunodeficiency virus infection in cats), is a very effective survival strategy for the virus.

6. *Capacity to survive after being shed into the external environment.* All things being equal, a virus that is environmentally stable must have a survival advantage. For example, canine parvovirus, an extremely stable virus, was transported around the world within 2 years of its emergence, mostly by carriage on human shoes and clothing. Alternatively, a virus that employs vertical transmission (e.g., congenital rubella) can survive without ever confronting the external environment.

Successful viruses employ one or several of these strategies, and the diversity of viruses and virus infection patterns underlines the truism that there are many potential tactics whereby a virus can survive.

The Host

In many ways, the influence of the host on the evolution of disease is more pervasive and persistent than that of the virus. The host brings a much more complex genome to the battle (see Chap. 13). The primordial struggle between virus and host involves a faceoff between the qualities of the virus that are crucial for its transmission and survival, which have been described, and the countering qualities of the host, which are usually categorized as follows: (1) specific host genes that influence susceptibility or resistance, (2) nonspecific responses such as interferon, (3) acquired resistance (e.g., macrophages, the cellular and humoral immune responses), and (4) physiologic factors affecting resistance (e.g., age, nutritional status, hormonal effects especially in pregnancy).

Certain viruses have taken advantage of weak links in the immune system; an example is HIV, which attacks the central cell in the immune response system, the CD4+ lymphocyte. Similarly, hepatitis B has the ability to induce immune-mediated liver disease and immune tolerance, which is associated with late-developing hepatocellular carcinoma. However, in most cases, a finely titrated immune response is evoked that is efficacious and is critical to host survival.

Just as in vivo passage may select for viruses with the ability to be better transmitted, so serial passage may select for hosts with a genetic capacity to survive infection. Studies with inbred mice have identified a large repertoire of genes that confer survival value on the host (see Chap. 13). Most of these genes are specific for a single family of viruses, although a few map to the major histocompatibility locus and encode proteins that influence host immune responses to multiple antigens. Alternatively, linebreeding and inbreeding have been used to develop classic strains of mice that are exquisitely sensitive to certain viruses; these strains have been used for many years to isolate arboviruses, rabies virus, and picornaviruses. Although the origin of most resistance alleles is unknown, their analogs in nature may carry survival value and be subject to positive selection.

The Host Population

Population parameters influence viral diseases and their evolution in several ways. Most of the examples used to make specific points in this chapter pertain primarily to the influence of the host population on the evolution of disease. There are numerous qualities of populations that affect disease evolution, including community age distribution, gender distribution, educational status, subpopulation size and density, vaccination rate and immune status, economic and nutritional status, sanitation status, water supply status, exposure to potential vectors, and the like. All such community-based parameters influence the risk of disease, the key parameters being determined by the biologic characteristics of the specific disease.

Most viral infections are maintained by person-to-person transmission, which depends on the density of susceptible individuals who can serve as links in the transmission chain. The density of susceptible hosts is equal to the population density multiplied by the proportion of the population that is susceptible. If this density is below a critical threshold, the virus may not be serially propagated, which is exemplified by the spontaneous disappearance of measles from populations of fewer than 500,000 persons (see Fig. 15-4). This phenomenon has led to the speculation that human measles virus emerged from some animal morbillivirus only with the rise of civilizations producing population aggregates of sufficient size to maintain the virus.[4] The importance of density of susceptible hosts is also illustrated by the success of immunization programs such as the poliomyelitis vaccination program in the United States, which eliminated wild poliovirus even though herd immunity was not overwhelming (see Fig. 15-6).

Of all population parameters, age must be most important in the evolution of most viral diseases. Age at time of infection, coupled with the turnover rate of the population, affects many disease and infection attributes, including those driving transmission. In dense urban tropical populations, for example, many viruses spread very rapidly so that initial infections occur at a very early age. This may be associated with either a low ratio of cases to infections (e.g., poliomyelitis) or a high ratio of disease to infections (e.g., rotavirus disease, measles). As the average age at time of infection increases because of improved public health or personal hygiene factors, disease incidence may evolve to become more or less common or severe. In any event, population attributes have had an important influence on the evolution of many viral diseases.

Coevolution of Virus and Host

The best-documented example of coincident change in host and virus leading to the emergence of a variant disease involves the rabbit and myxoma virus. (The overall pathogenesis of poxviruses is described in detail in Chapter 22.)

Myxomatosis, caused by the poxvirus, myxoma virus, occurs naturally as a mild infection of rabbits in South America and California (*Sylvilagus* spp.); in these hosts, it produces a skin tumor from which virus is transmitted mechanically by biting insects. However, in European rabbits, myxoma virus causes a lethal infection, a finding that led to its use for biologic control of wild European rabbits in Australia. The wild European rabbit was introduced into Australia in 1859 for sporting purposes and rapidly spread over the southern part of the continent, where it became the major animal pest of the agricultural and pastoral industries. Myxoma virus from South America was successfully introduced into this rabbit population in 1950; when originally liberated, the virus produced case-fatality rates of more than 99%. This highly virulent virus was readily transmitted by mosquitoes. Farmers carried out "inoculation campaigns" to introduce virulent myxoma virus into wild rabbit populations.

It may have been predicted that the disease and with it the virus would disappear at the end of each summer, because of the greatly diminished numbers of susceptible rabbits and the greatly lowered opportunity for transmission by mosquitoes during the winter. This must often have occurred in localized areas, but it did not happen over the continent as a whole. The ability of virus to survive the winter conferred a great selective advantage on viral mutants of reduced lethality, because during this period, when mosquito numbers were low, rabbits infected by such mutants survived in an infectious condition for weeks instead of a few days. Within 3 years, such mutants became the dominant strains throughout Australia (Table 15-2). Although some inoculation campaigns produced localized, highly lethal outbreaks, in general the viruses that spread through the rabbit populations each year were the attenuated strains, because the prolonged illness produced in their hosts provided a greater opportunity for mosquito transmission. The original, highly lethal virus was progressively replaced by a heterogeneous collection of strains of lower virulence, most of them still virulent enough to kill 70% to 90% of genetically unselected rabbits.

Rabbits that recover from myxomatosis are immune to reinfection. However, because most wild rabbits have a life span of less than a year, herd immunity is not as important in the epidemiology of myxomatosis as it is in infections of longer-lived species. Selection for genetically more resistant animals operated from the outset. In areas in which repeated outbreaks occurred, the genetic resistance of surviving rabbits increased progressively (Table 15-3). The early appearance of viral strains of lower virulence, which allowed 10% of genetically unselected rabbits to recover, was an important factor in allowing the number of genetically resistant rabbits to increase.

TABLE 15-2. *Virulence of field isolates of myxoma virus, 1951–1981**

	Virulence grade					
	I	II	III	IV	V	
Fatality rate (%)	>99	95–99	70–95	50–70	<50	
Mean survival time (d)	<13	14–16	17–28	29–50	NA	Number of samples
Percentage of isolates by year						
1950–51	100	0.0	0.0	0.0	0.0	1
1952–55	13	20	53	13	0.0	60
1955–58	0.7	5	55	24	15	432
1959–63	1.7	11	61	22	5	449
1964–66	0.7	0.3	64	34	1.3	306
1967–69	0.0	0.0	62	36	1.7	229
1970–74	0.6	5	74	21	0.0	174
1975–81	1.9	3	67	28	0.0	212

*Myxoma virus was successfully introduced into the wild rabbit population in December 1950. The introduced strain was highly virulent and caused epidemics with very high mortality. However, with the passage of time, field isolates exhibited reduced virulence. It is noteworthy that strains of moderate virulence became dominant, probably because strains of lowest virulence were less transmissible and because strains of maximum virulence killed rabbits very quickly.

NA, not applicable.

Data from Fenner F. Biological control as exemplified by smallpox eradication and myxomatosis. Proc R Soc Lond B Biol Sci 1983;218:259–285.

TABLE 15-3. *The susceptibility of nonimmune wild rabbits after successive epidemics of myxomatosis in Lake Urana, Australia.**

No. Epidemics	Fatality rate (%)	Severe disease (including fatalities, %)	Moderate disease (%)	Mild disease (%)
0	90	93	5	2
2	88	95	5	0
3	80	93	5	2
4	50	61	26	12
5	53	75	14	11
7	30	54	16	30

*Rabbits were challenged with a virus of grade III (intermediate) virulence.
Data from Fenner F. Biological control as exemplified by smallpox eradication and myxomatosis. Proc R Soc Lond B Biol Sci 1983;218:259–285.

In areas in which annual outbreaks occurred, the genetic resistance of the rabbits changed such that the case-fatality rate after infection under laboratory conditions with a particular strain of virus fell from 90% to 25% within 7 years. Subsequently, in areas in which there were frequent outbreaks of myxomatosis, somewhat more virulent strains of myxoma virus became dominant, because they produced the kind of disease that was best transmitted in populations of genetically resistant rabbits. The ultimate balance struck between myxoma virus and Australian rabbits involved adaptations of both virus and host populations, reaching a dynamic equilibrium that finds rabbits still greatly reduced compared with their premyxomatosis numbers but too numerous for the wishes of farmers and conservationists.

This is the classic example of coevolution of virus and host, and it has had considerable influence on thinking about evolution of viruses and viral disease. The example of myxomatosis has been generalized to suggest that, during a long association of a virus with a host population, both virus and host evolve in a manner similar to that described for myxomatosis. Sometimes this has been interpreted to predict that the result of coevolution is a benign relation between host and pathogen in which mortality in the natural host is very low. However, the experience with myxomatosis suggests that coevolution may lead to a steady state in which a virus continues to cause severe disease and significant mortality.

Consistent with this view are observations on well-known viruses of humans or animals. For instance, as shown in Table 15-4, strains of smallpox virus could be divided into two groups with different mortality rates.[18] Variola major was an ancient disease that killed up to 30% of those who contract it. Variola minor, with a mortality of about 1%, was first recognized in southern Africa and Florida at the end of the 19th century. In Africa, both diseases coexisted, with no evidence that variola minor was replacing the more severe disease. Similarly, field isolates of human poliovirus differ markedly in their neurovirulence, yet there is no evidence of natural selection for strains of lower virulence.[61] Yellow fever virus sustains its high virulence for humans even after many years of maintenance in an urban cycle.[82] Rabies virus is highly lethal for all of its hosts, both animal and human. Finally, HIV appears to be associated with a very high mortality rate, although it is too early to determine whether there will be any selection for strains of reduced virulence.[39]

It may be postulated that those properties of a virus that determine its ability to be perpetuated in a host population are

TABLE 15-4. *Fatality rates from variola major and variola minor**

Country	No. cases	No. deaths	Case-fatality rate (%)
VARIOLA MAJOR			
India	23546	4103	17
Pakistan	17491	1646	9
Indonesia	11966	930	8
West Africa	5628	540	10
VARIOLA MINOR			
Brazil	9854	75	0.8
Ethiopia	54991	838	1.5
Sudan	3019	35	1.2
Somalia	3022	12	0.4

*Country reports submitted between 1965 and 1977, before certification of eradication of smallpox.
Data from Fenner F, Henderson DA, Arita I, Jezek Z, Ladnyi ID. Smallpox and its eradication. Geneva: World Health Organization, 1988.

the major determinants of natural selection. Because most acute viruses are transmitted for very short periods of time, followed by self-sterilization and lifelong immunity, it may be relatively unimportant whether the host survives the acute infection, so long as death is not extraordinarily swift. Fenner[17] postulated that, for myxoma virus, strains of intermediate virulence replaced strains of highest virulence because the latter killed so rapidly that they were less well transmitted than strains of intermediate virulence. However, strains of low virulence also were not as effectively transmitted and did not become predominant. High lethality may, in certain circumstances, actually confer a survival advantage. For instance, in rabies, high lethality may be essential to perpetuation of the virus in certain wildlife populations, because a sublethal immunizing rabies infection would create a subpopulation of resistant hosts that would not be able to transmit the virus. The effectiveness of rabies immunization in controlling wildlife rabies[87] testifies that this is not just a hypothetical possibility. Persistent infections such as HIV or hepatitis B, although they may eventually kill the host (by AIDS or hepatocellular carcinoma, respectively), have such long incubation periods (about 10 years or 30 years, respectively) that there is adequate time for transmission anywhere along the infection chain.

Environment and Ecosystem

Environmental factors play an important role in the evolution of many viral diseases, and their effects depend on the particular mode of transmission. Furthermore, as Figure 15-10 indicates, changes in the global environment and its multiple ecosystems are occurring at an ever-accelerating tempo. Some of the environmental factors noted here may best be understood through the illustrative vignettes that follow.

Environmental variables are particularly important in the evolution of zoonotic viral diseases, whether the virus is transmitted to humans directly from a reservoir population or indirectly by an arthropod vector. In both situations, a complex and delicate web of factors determines the probability that humans become infected, and this probability is sensitive to a variety of ecologic changes. The arthropod-borne viruses are excellent examples of emergence, epidemicity, endemicity, and entrenchment following on human environmental manipulation and natural environmental change. Changes in breeding areas, in vector density, and in human exposure to vectors are all determined by the ecosystem in which vectors and humans coexist. Population movements and the intrusion of humans and domestic animals into new arthropod habitats have resulted in many new, emergent disease episodes. The classic example was the emergence of yellow fever after susceptible humans entered the Central American jungle to build the Panama Canal.[82]

Ecologic factors also pertain to unique and isolated environments. Remote econiches, such as islands, that are free of particular species of reservoir hosts and vectors are often particularly vulnerable to an introduced virus. For example, the initial spread of Ross River virus among the Pacific islands in the 1980s from its original niche in Australia caused virgin-soil epidemics of arthritis-myalgia syndrome in Fiji and Samoa.

Deforestation has been the key to the exposure of farmers and domestic animals to new arthropods. In recent years, the occurrence of Mayaro virus disease among Brazilian woodcutters as they cleared the Amazonian forest is a case in point (J. Dalrymple, U.S. Army Medical Research Institute for Infectious Diseases, Frederick, MD, personal communication, 1985). Increased long-distance travel (see Fig. 15-10) has facilitated the carriage of exotic arthropod vectors around the world. The introduction of the Asian mosquito, *Aedes albopictus*, to the United States in the water contained in used tires illustrates this phenomenon. Long-distance livestock transportation has enhanced the spread of viruses and arthropods (especially ticks) around the world. The introduction of African swine fever virus from Africa into Portugal (1957), Spain (1960), and South America (1960s and 1970s) is

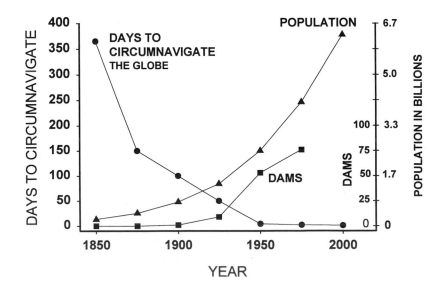

FIG. 15-10. Many global changes over the last 150 years have enhanced the probability of the emergence of new viral diseases of humans and animals. This chart depicts three examples of such trends. The rise in the human population has been accompanied by a massive increase in large urban populations, markedly increasing the risk of epidemic spread of infection. Dramatic reductions in the time required to travel long distances has increased the possibility of global transport of infectious agents over short periods of time. The rise in the number of large dams (>75 m) built in the United States between 1880 and 1975 exemplifies increases in manmade manipulation of the environment. (Data from references 43, 48, 57, and 81.

thought to have occurred in this way, and it is just a matter of time until this virus makes further international forays.

Environmental pollution and uncontrolled urbanization are contributing to many new, emergent disease episodes. Arthropod vectors breeding in accumulations of water (e.g., tin cans, old tires) and sewage-laden water are a worldwide problem. Environmental chemical toxicants (e.g., herbicides, pesticides, residues) can also affect vector-virus relations directly or indirectly. For example, mosquito resistance to all licensed insecticides in parts of California is a known direct effect of unsound mosquito abatement programs; this resistance may also have been augmented indirectly by uncontrolled pesticide use.

The increasing use of irrigation and the expanding reuse of water are becoming very important factors in virus disease emergence. The problem with primitive water and irrigation systems, which are developed without attention to arthropod control, is exemplified in the emergence of Japanese encephalitis in new areas of Southeast Asia.

Finally, global warming, which affects sea level, estuarine wetlands, swamps, and human habitation patterns, may be affecting vector-virus relations throughout the tropics.

One example of the effect of environmental factors on the evolution of viral disease is dengue. Dengue is one of the most rapidly emerging diseases in the tropical parts of the world, with millions of cases occurring each year. Puerto Rico had five dengue epidemics in the first 75 years of this century but has had six epidemics in the past 12 years.[12,32] Record numbers of cases have occurred elsewhere in the Americas, and Brazil, Bolivia, Paraguay, Ecuador, Nicaragua, and Cuba have experienced their first major dengue epidemics in more than 50 years. These epidemics have involved multiple virus types; of the four dengue virus types, three are now circulating in the Caribbean region. These are the circumstances that have led to dengue hemorrhagic fever, the lethal end of the dengue disease spectrum. Dengue hemorrhagic fever first occurred in the Americas in 1981; since then, 11 countries have reported cases, and since 1990, more than 3000 cases have been reported each year.

Why is dengue emerging or reemerging, especially in the Americas? The answer is simple: urban mosquito habitats are expanding for the vector mosquito, A aegypti. Mosquito density is increasing, and mosquito control is failing. This is occurring not just in the least developed countries but in many developed countries, including the southern region of the United States. In all countries, financial resources for public health are severely limited and must be prioritized. Priority lists are political in nature and tend to emphasize everyday troubles, not episodic problems. Too often, mosquito control, which is very expensive, falls off the priority list. Meanwhile, mosquito control is becoming more expensive as older, cheaper chemicals lose effectiveness or are banned as damaging to the environment and must be replaced by more expensive chemicals. As mosquito control fails, dengue follows quickly.

While A aegypti control has been declining, a new dengue virus vector, A albopictus, the Asian tiger mosquito, has been imported from southeast Asia into many of the same urban areas of the western hemisphere.[20,54] Larvae of this mosquito are carried in the water contained within the very large numbers of used tires that are moved in international trade. If the two Aedes species occupy the same area, they complement each other, A aegypti occupying its traditional niche within houses and A albopictus concentrating in nearby brush and vegetation.

An even more frightening scenario associated with failing mosquito control is the possible reemergence of yellow fever virus, which is transmitted by the same mosquito vector as dengue, A aegypti.[55,56] Where dengue occurs, the conditions are appropriate for yellow fever, lacking only importation of the virus by means of an infected person or an infected mosquito. It is one of the mysteries of tropical medicine that yellow fever has not occurred more often in circumstances in which vector density and a susceptible human population coexist. No one knows where, when, or even if yellow fever virus will reemerge in the kind of epidemics that were the scourge of tropical and subtropical cities of the Western hemisphere and Africa throughout the 17th, 18th, and 19th centuries.[82]

A final example is provided by St. Louis encephalitis. In the United States, most outbreaks of this disease occur in years when rainfall leads to an increase in the population of mosquito vectors such as Culex pipiens. Environmental factors such as screening, air conditioning, and closed basements (which decrease human exposure to mosquitoes) can markedly decrease risk.[41] A classic example is the original outbreak of encephalitis in St. Louis in 1933: disease occurred in only one of four institutions in St. Louis county, because of the lack of screening in that one building (Table 15-5).

Summary and Conclusions

Nothing in biology makes sense, except in the light of evolution.

T. Dobzhansky, 1973[15]

TABLE 15-5. *Attack rates of St. Louis encephalitis in four institutions, Suburban St. Louis 1933.*

Institution	Population	Cases	Rate per 100,000	Screening
Mental hospital	400	0	—	Yes
Hospital for the insane	4000	0	—	Yes
Isolation hospital*	500	0	—	Yes
Almshouse (infirmary)	1200	13	10,800	No

*The isolation hospital cared for 300 patients with St. Louis encephalitis but no cases occurred among the staff (estimated at 500).

Data from Lumsden LL. St. Louis encephalitis in 1933: Observations on epidemiological features. Public Health Rep 1958;73:340–353.

The study of viral disease evolution brings together a wide variety of disciplines, ranging from viral genetics to global epidemiology. Evolutionary phenomena do not exist separately in nature; they exist as a seamless cloth of interrelated, interdependent parameters that characterize the biology of the virus, the host, the host population, and the environment. Understanding some of the mechanisms involved in the evolution of viral disease may furnish insights to help researchers assess, interpret, prevent, and control future episodes of viral disease.

Specific examples from nature, some of which have been used as illustrations in the body of this chapter, provide a potential key to understanding the principles that guide the evolution of viral diseases. However, the examples lead to more questions than answers, and many of the questions are open-ended. For instance, it is not known why both DNA and RNA viruses have been responsible for major recent instances of viral disease evolution and disease emergence despite the fact that the latter group can evolve, genotypically, more than a million times faster than the former. Likewise, some very similar, phylogenetically related viruses, such as the retroviruses, have evolved quite different modes of transmission and mechanisms of disease. Retroviruses can initiate diseases as disparate as sarcoma, leukemia, anemia, immunosuppression, pulmonary interstitial pneumonia, transverse myelitis, and demyelination. Different members of a single virus family can be transmitted by mosquito bite, by sexual contact, by a respiratory route, and by fecal-oral transfer. What then is the common ground in regard to the role of the virus in the natural history and evolution of disease? Clearly, understanding the evolution of viral disease remains a continuing challenge for the future.

ACKNOWLEDGMENTS

This review was initially inspired by discussions on emerging infectious diseases with Frank Fenner, Ashley Haase, Richard Krause, Donald Krogstad, and Thomas Monath at a workshop sponsored by the National Institute of Allergy and Infectious Diseases in Hamilton, Montana, July, 1991. The ideas were revised in the course of preparation of several reviews on the subject.[56,57,62] We thank Frank Fenner and Helen Davies for reading this chapter.

ABBREVIATIONS

AIDS: acquired immunodeficiency syndrome
BSE: bovine spongiform encephalopathy
HIV-1, HIV-2: human immunodeficiency viruses
MBM: meat and bone meal
SIV, SIV_{AGM}, SIV_{SM}: simian immunodeficiency viruses

REFERENCES

1. Allan JS. Viral evolution and AIDS. J N I H Res 1992;4:51–54.
2. Baron RC, McCormick JC, Zubeir OA. Ebola virus disease in southern Sudan: hospital dissemination and intrafamilial spread. Bull W H O 1981;61:997–1003.
3. Bartlett MS. Measles periodicity and community size. J R Stat Soc 1957;120:48–70.
4. Black FL. Infectious diseases in primitive societies. Science 1975; 187:515–518.
5. Bodian D. Experimental studies on passive immunization. II. The prophylactic effect of human gamma globulin on paralytic poliomyelitis in cynomolgus monkeys after virus feeding. Am J Hyg 1952;56: 78–89.
6. Brookmeyer R. Reconstruction and future trends of the AIDS epidemic in the United States. Science 1991;253:37–42.
7. Burney MI, Ghafoor A, Saleen M, Webb PA, Casals J. Nosocomial outbreak of viral hemorrhagic fever caused by Crimean hemorrhagic fever–Congo virus in Pakistan, January 1976. Am J Trop Med Hyg 1980;29:941–947.
8. Cases of specific notifiable diseases in the United States. MMWR Morb Mortal Wkly Rep 1983;31:704.
9. Cases of specific notifiable diseases: United States, weeks ending December 27, 1986. MMWR Morb Mortal Wkly Rep 1988;36:842.
10. Certification of poliomyelitis eradication: the Americas, 1994. MMWR Morb Mortal Wkly Rep 1994;43:720–722.
11. de Haan P, Wagemakers L, Peters D, Goldbach R. The S RNA segment of tomato spotted wilt virus has an ambisense character. J Gen Virol 1990;71:10001–10007.
12. Dengue and dengue hemorrhagic fever: guidelines for prevention and control. Washington DC: Pan American Health Organization, 1994: 12–13.
13. Desrosiers RC. A finger on the missing link. Nature 1990;345: 288–289.
14. Desrosiers RC, Daniel MD, Li Y. HIV-related lentiviruses of nonhuman primates. AIDS Res Hum Retroviruses 1989;5:465–471.
15. Dobzhansky T. Nothing in biology makes sense except in the light of evolution. American Biology Teacher 1973;35:125–129.
16. Ebola haemorrhagic fever in Zaire, 1976: report of an international commission. Bull W H O 1978;56:271–293.
17. Fenner F. Biological control as exemplified by smallpox eradication and myxomatosis. Proc R Soc Lond Series B Biol Sci 1983;218: 259–285.
18. Fenner F, Henderson DA, Arita I, Jezek Z, Ladnyi ID. Smallpox and its eradication. Geneva: World Health Organization, 1988.
19. Fields BN, Knipe DM. Virology. 2nd ed. New York: Raven Press, 1990.
20. Francy DB, Karabatsos N, Wesson DM, et al. A new arbovirus from *Aedes albopictus*, an Asian mosquito established in the United States. Science 1990;250:1738–1740.
21. Fultz PN, McClure HM, Anderson DC, Swenson RB, Anand R, Srinivasan A. Isolation of a T-lymphocytotropic retrovirus from naturally infected sooty mangabey monkeys (*Cercocebus atys*). Proc Natl Acad Sci U S A 1986;83:5286–5290.
22. Gao F, Yue L, White AT, et al. Human infection by genetically diverse SIVsm-related HIV-2 in West Africa. Nature 1992;358:495–499.
23. Getchell JP, Hicks DR, Srinivasan A, et al. Human immunodeficiency virus isolated from a serum sample collected in 1976 in central Africa. J Infect Dis 1987;156:833–837.
24. Goldbach R, Peters D. Possible causes of the emergence of tospovirus diseases. Semin Virol 1994;5:113–120.
25. Gould SJ. Wonderful life. New York: WW Norton, 1989.
26. Grimstad PR, Barrrett RL, Humphrey RL, Sinsko MJ. Serologic evidence for widespread infection with La Crosse and St. Louis encephalitis viruses in the Indiana human population. Am J Epidemiol 1984;119:913–930.
27. Griot C, Tselis A, Tsai TF, Gonzalez-Scarano F, Nathanson N. Bunyavirus diseases. In: Stroop WG, McKendall RR, eds. Handbook of neurovirology. New York: Marcel Dekker, 1994:439–454.
28. Gudnadottir M. Visna-maedi in sheep. Prog Med Virol 1974;18: 336–349.
29. Henderson BE, Coleman PH. The growing importance of California arboviruses in the etiology of human disease. Prog Med Virol 1971; 13:404–461.
30. HIV/AIDS surveillance report. Atlanta: Centers for Disease Control, 1992.
31. Hughes HM, Peters CJ, Cohen ML, Mahy BWJ. Hantavirus pulmonary syndrome: an emerging virus disease. Science 1993;262: 850–851.
32. Imported dengue: United States, 1993–1994. MMWR Morb Mortal Wkly Rep 1995;44:353–356.
33. Jarhling PB, Geisbert TW, Dalgard DW. Preliminary report: isolation of Ebola virus from monkeys imported to USA. Lancet 1990;335: 502–505.
34. Johnson KM, Halstead SB, Cohen SN. Hemorrhagic fevers of southeast Asia and South America: comparative appraisal. Prog Med Virol 1967;9:105–158.

35. Kaslow RA, Francis DP. The epidemiology of AIDS. Oxford: Oxford University Press, 1989.
36. Krause RM. The origin of plagues: old and new. Science 1995;257: 1073–1078.
37. Lavinder CH, Freeman SW, Frost WH. Epidemiologic studies of poliomyelitis in New York City and the northeastern United States during the year 1916. Washington: United States Public Health Service, 1918.
38. Lederberg J, Shope RE, Oaks S. Emerging infections: microbial threats to health in the United States. Washington, DC: US National Academy of Sciences Press, 1992.
39. Levy JA. HIV and the pathogenesis of AIDS. Washington, DC: ASM Press, 1994.
40. Levy JA, Pan L-Z, Beth-Giraldo E, et al. Absence of antibodies to human immunodeficiency virus in sera from Africa prior to 1975. Proc Natl Acad Sci U S A 1986;83:7935–7937.
41. Luby JP, Miller G, Gardner P, Pigford CA, Henderson BA, Eddins D. The epidemiology of St. Louis encephalitis in Houston, Texas. Am J Epidemiol 1967;86:584–597.
42. Lumsden LL. St. Louis encephalitis in 1933: Observations on epidemiological features. Public Health Rep 1958;73:340–353.
43. Mandzhavidze NF, Mamradze GP. The high dams of the world. Springfield, VA: United States Department of Commerce, Clearinghouse for Federal Scientific and Technical Information, 1966.
44. Marx PA, Li Y, Lerche NW, et al. Isolation of a simian immunodeficiency virus related to human immunodeficiency virus type 2 from a West African pet sooty mangabey. J Virol 1991;65:4480–4485.
45. McCormick JB. Epidemiology and control of Lassa fever. Curr Top Microbiol Immunol 1987;134:69–78.
46. McCormick JB. Arena viruses. In Fields BN, Knipe DM, eds. Virology. 2nd ed. New York: Raven Press, 1990:1245–1267.
47. McCormick JB, Bauer SP, Elliott LH, Webb PA, Johnson KM. Biologic differences between strains of Ebola virus from Zaire and Sudan. J Infect Dis 1983;147:264–267.
48. McEvedy C, Jones R. Atlas of world population history. London: Penguin Books, 1978.
49. McFadden G, Graham K. Modulation of cytokine networks by poxvirus: the myxoma virus model. Semin Virol 1994;5:421–429.
50. Measles: United States, 1987. MMWR Morb Mortal Wkly Rep 1988; 37:527–531.
51. Measles incidence: United States, 1912–1994. Atlanta: Centers for Disease Control, 1995.
52. Measles surveillance report, 1977–1981. Atlanta: Centers for Disease Control, 1981:11.
53. Melnick JL, Ledinko N. Development of neutralizing antibodies against the three types of poliomyelitis virus during an epidemic period. Am J Hyg 1953;58:207–222.
54. Mitchell CJ, Mieblyski ML, Smith CG, et al. Isolation of eastern equine encephalitis virus from Aedes albopictus in Florida. Science 1992;257:526–527.
55. Morse SS. Emerging viruses. New York: Oxford University Press, 1993.
56. Murphy FA. New, emerging, and reemerging infectious diseases. Adv Virus Res 1993;43:1–52.
57. Murphy FA, Nathanson N. The emergence of new virus diseases: an overview. Semin Virol 1994;5:87–102.
58. Nathanson N. Epidemiologic aspects of poliomyelitis eradication. Rev Infect Dis 1984;6:S308–S312.
59. Nathanson N. Epidemiology. In Fields BN, Knipe DM, eds. Virology. 2nd ed. New York: Raven Press, 1990:267–292.
60. Nathanson N, Georgsson G, Palsson PA, Najjar JA, Lutley R, Petursson G. Experimental visna in Icelandic sheep: the prototype lentiviral infection. Rev Infect Dis 1985;7:75–82.
61. Nathanson N, Martin JR. The epidemiology of poliomyelitis: enigmas surrounding its appearance, epidemicity, and disappearance. Am J Epidemiol 1979;110:672–692.
62. Nathanson N, McGann KA, Wilesmith JW, Desrosiers RC, Brookmeyer R. The evolution of virus diseases: their emergence, epidemicity, and control. Virus Res 1993;29:3–20.
63. Nathanson N, Palsson PA, Gudmundsson G. Multiple sclerosis and canine distemper in Iceland. Lancet 1978;2:1127–1129.
64. News and comment. Hantavirus outbreak yields to PCR. Science 1993;262:832–836.
65. Nichol ST, Spiropoulou CF, Morzunov S, et al. Genetic identification of a hantavirus associated with an outbreak of acute respiratory illness. Science 1993;262:914–917.
66. Nzilamni N, De Cock KM, Foethai DM, et al. The prevalence of infection with human immunodeficiency virus over a 10-year period in rural Zaire. N Engl J Med 1988;318:276–279.
67. Outbreak of acute illness: southwestern United States, 1993. MMWR Morb Mortal Wkly Rep 1993;42:421–424.
68. Palsson PA. Maedi and visna in sheep. In Kimberlin RA, ed. Slow virus diseases of animals and man. Amsterdam: North-Holland, 1976: 17–44.
69. Parrish CR. The emergence and evolution of canine parvovirus: an example of recent host range mutation. Semin Virol 1994;5:121–132.
70. Paul J. Epidemiology of poliomyelitis. In: Poliomyelitis. Geneva: World Health Organization, 1955:9–30.
71. Paul J. A history of poliomyelitis. New Haven: Yale University Press, 1971.
72. Paul J, Horstmann D. A survey of poliomyelitis virus antibodies in French Morocco. Am J Trop Med Hyg 1955;4:512–524.
73. Peters CJ, Sanchez A, Rollin PE, Ksiazek TG, Murphy FA. Filoviridae: Marburg and Ebola viruses. In: Fields BN, Knipe DM, Howley PM, eds. Fields virology. 3rd ed. New York: Raven Press, 1996:1161–1176.
74. Poliomyelitis incidence in the United States. MMWR Morb Mortal Wkly Rep 1982;30:12–17.
75. Progress toward poliomyelitis eradication: People's Republic of China. MMWR Morb Mortal Wkly Rep 1994;43:857–859.
76. Quinn TC, Mann J. HIV-1 infection and AIDS in Africa. In: Kaslow RA, Francis DP, eds. The epidemiology of AIDS. Oxford: Oxford University Press, 1989:194–220.
77. Sanchez A, Ksiazek TG, Rollin PE, et al. Reemergence of Ebola virus in Africa. Emerging Infectious Diseases 1995;1:96–97.
78. Selvey LA, Wells RM, McCormack JG, et al. Infection of humans and horses by a newly described morbillivirus. Med J Aust 1995; 162: 642–645.
79. Serfling RE, Sherman IL. Poliomyelitis distribution in the United States. Public Health Rep 1953;68:453–466.
80. Smallman-Raynor M, Cliff A. The spread of human immunodeficiency virus type 2 into Europe: a geographic analysis. Intl J Epidemiol 1991;20:480–489.
81. Statistical yearbook, 1990–1991. New York: United Nations Statistical Office, 1993.
82. Strode GK, Bugher JC, Kerr JA, et al. Yellow fever. New York: McGraw-Hill, 1951.
83. Summary of notifiable diseases, United States, 1986. MMWR Morb Mortal Wkly Rep 1987;35:1–55.
84. Thompson WH, Evans AS. California encephalitis virus studies in Wisconsin. Am J Epid 1965;81:230–242.
85. Thompson WH, Kalfayan B, Anslow RO. Isolation of California encephalitis virus from a fatal human illness. Am J Epidemiol 1965; 81:245–253.
86. van Eeden PJ, Joubert JR, van de Wal BW, King JB, de Kock A, Gorenewald JH. A nosocomial outbreak of Crimean-Congo hemorrhagic fever at Tygerberg Hospital. S Afr Med J 1985;68:711–717.
87. Wandeler A. Oral immunization of wildlife. In Baer GM, ed. The natural history of rabies. Orlando: CRC Press, 1991:486–503.
88. Webster RG, Kawaoka Y, Bean WJ Jr. Molecular changes in A/chicken/Pennsylvania/83 (H5N2) influenza virus associated with acquisition of virulence. Virology 1986;149:165–173.
89. Webster RG, Murphy BR. Orthomyxoviruses. In Fields BN, Knipe DM, eds. Virology. 2nd ed. New York: Raven Press, 1990:1099–1154.
90. Weutrich B. Playing chicken with an epidemic. Science 1995;267: 1594
91. Wilesmith JW. Bovine spongiform encephalopathy: epidemiological factors associated with the emergence of an important new animal pathogen in Great Britain. Semin Virol 1994;5:179–187.
92. Wilesmith JW, Ryan JBM, Atkinson MJ. Bovine spongiform encephalopathy: epidemiology studies on the origin. Vet Record 1991; 128:199–202.
93. Wilesmith JW, Wells GAH. Bovine spongiform encephalopathy. Curr Top Microbiol Immunology 1991;172:21–38.
94. Yorke JA, Nathanson N, Piangiani G, Martin JR. Seasonality and the requirements for perpetuation and eradication of viruses in populations. Am J Epidemiol 1979;109:103–123.

Viral Pathogenesis,
edited by Neal Nathanson, et al.
Lippincott–Raven Publishers, Philadelphia © 1997

CHAPTER 16

Viral Vaccines

Gordon Ada

INTRODUCTION

The experiment of Edward Jenner in 1796, in which he inoculated young James Phipps with cowpox and the boy subsequently failed to develop disease after challenge with smallpox, is credited with marking the beginning of the modern day

G. Ada: Division of Cell Biology, John Curtin School of Medical Research, Australian National University, Canberra City, ACT, 2601, Australia.

practice of immunization.[60] In honor of Jenner, Pasteur coined the term vaccination in 1880 to describe the general practice of prior immunization to protect against disease caused by exposure to the wild-type infectious agent. This term entered the language even though some vaccines (e.g., rabies) are administered to people already infected by the agent. In contrast, the term vaccinology has only recently been adopted (and not universally) to describe vaccine development and usage.

Pasteur, the first great experimental immunologist, discovered a means of changing the properties of live microbes so that their potential for causing disease (virulence) was greatly reduced, a process which became known as attenuation. The rabies virus, which is highly virulent for humans, was attenuated by serial passage in a less susceptible host, the rabbit (1885). The first yellow fever virus vaccine was produced from mouse brain in the mid-1930s. Also in the 1930s, the ability to propagate some viruses in the allantoic or amniotic cavities of the chick embryo led first to the development of the 17D strain of yellow fever (attenuated) virus and shortly afterward to the influenza virus (inactivated) vaccine.

The ability to grow viruses in tissue culture, which was achieved in minced tissues in the 1920s but developed mainly after World War II, particularly by Enders and colleagues with polio virus,[57] transformed the scene. This became the preferred way to propagate viruses, and its application led to many of the viral vaccines in use today[6] (Table 16-1). Some of our most successful vaccines are attenuated strains of viruses.

It was the study of bacterial preparations rather than viruses that led to two early immunologic findings of fundamental importance for vaccinology, both by the English scientist, Glenny. He first noted the difference in the rate of antibody response to diphtheria toxin in nonimmune compared with immune animals.[68] The principles of primary versus secondary antibody responses which Burnet later proposed in his clonal selection theory could be explained only on a cellular basis. Second, Glenny and colleagues noted that the brief antibody response to soluble antigens was related to the rapid loss of antigen from the injection site. More than 50 years ago, they pioneered the use of alum-precipitated bacterial toxoids as a means of slowing the release of toxoid from the injection site and its subsequent loss from the body.[67]

One of the greatest public health achievements in history was the Smallpox Eradication Campaign of the World Health Organization (WHO), which was initiated in 1966 and concluded successfully in 1977, when the last case of endemic smallpox was detected.[60] The world was declared free of smallpox 3 years later. In 1985, the director of the Pan American Health Organization proposed an initiative to eradicate the indigenous transmission of wild-type poliovirus from the Americas by the year 1990. This was extended by the World Health Assembly to achieve global eradication by the year 2000. The success of the program in the Americas after 1990 was spectacular, the record for more than 2 years of absence of indigenous poliomyelitis in the region being spoilt only by introduction of the disease from Europe into Canada by nonimmunized members of a small religious group. However, the global eradication of poliomyelitis represents a much greater challenge than the elimination of smallpox.[3]

THE NATURE OF VACCINES

The history of vaccine development has some very dark episodes, and many dedicated researchers have died as a result

TABLE 16-1. *Conventional human viral vaccines in use or in late-stage clinical trials in the United States**

Current vaccines	Candidate vaccines under trial
LIVE ATTENUATED VIRUS VACCINES	
Vaccinia	Varicella-zoster†
Polio (OPV)	Cytomegalovirus
Measles	Hepatitis A
Mumps	Influenza A (cold-adapted)
Rubella	Influenza B (cold-adapted)
Adenovirus	Dengue
	Rotavirus
	Parainfluenza type B
	Japanese encephalitis
COMBINATION VACCINES	
Measles, mumps, rubella (MMR)	
INACTIVATED WHOLE VIRUS VACCINES	
Influenza	Hepatitis A†
Rabies	
Japanese encephalitis	
Polio (IPV)	
VIRAL PROTEIN SUBUNIT VACCINES	
Hepatitis B	
Influenza A	

*The development and properties of these vaccines are described in detail in Plotkin SA, Mortimer EA. Vaccines. 2nd ed. Philadelphia: WB Saunders, 1994.

†Licensed for use in other countries.

From Ada GL. Vaccines. In: Paul WE, ed. Fundamental immunology. 3rd ed. New York: Raven Press, 1994;1309–1352.

of exposure to infectious agents during their studies.[188] Over many years, a procedure evolved and was refined for testing the two basic requirements of a vaccine, safety and efficacy, along the following lines (modified from Ada[2]):

1. Isolation and characterization of the infectious agent
2. Growth of the organism in bulk in a suitable system
3. Establishment of conditions for attenuation and for inactivation, or determination or isolation of the protective antigens of the agent
4. Immunization of a susceptible nonhuman host to determine safety and conditions for inducing a protective response after challenge
5. Animal experiments to eliminate the risk of teratogenicity
6. Initiation of clinical trials (for specialized pediatric use, studies may first be done in adults, then in immune children, and finally in nonimmune children)
   Phase I. Safety and limited immunogenicity
   Phase II. More extensive analyses of these two parameters in larger, sometimes more diverse groups
   Phase III. Efficacy studies in a population in an endemic region
7. Postregistration surveillance.

Table 16-1 lists the viral vaccines registered for use in many industrial countries and those in the later stages of clinical assessment before registration. There are three types: live attenuated viruses, inactivated whole viruses, and subunit preparations.

Live Attenuated Virus Vaccines

Most of the infections targeted by the vaccines listed in Table 16-1 are acute, with the majority of those infected recovering within 1 or 2 weeks, provided the infectious dose is not too high. The immune response resulting from vaccination with these preparations should mimic that seen after infection by the corresponding wild-type agents in regard to both type and duration. For instance, one or two administrations of vaccinia (smallpox vaccine), yellow fever vaccine, or measles vaccine leads to decades-long specific immunity in most recipients. The elimination of polio from the Americas followed successive administrations of oral (attenuated) polio vaccine. Such preparations are relatively inexpensive because the amount of virus administered is very low; the accumulating viral progeny induce the subsequent immune response. The live attenuated preparations in current use have been so successful in general that this approach continues to be widely used for development of new vaccines (see Table 16-1, column 2).

Four general approaches have been used to develop attenuated virus vaccines. The first is the Jennerian approach, in which a virus that is a natural pathogen in another host is used as a human vaccine. Apart from smallpox, examples are bovine parainfluenza in humans and turkey herpes virus administered to chickens to prevent Marek's disease. A more recent example is the use of avipox viruses, and particularly canarypox, in humans[37] (see later discussion).

The measles, yellow fever, and polio vaccines typify the second approach—extensive passaging of the virus in nonhuman cells in culture. However, this may result in the selection of mutants that are antigenically different from the original strain and possibly less protective in humans.[159] This approach attempts, on an ad hoc basis, to balance the loss of virulence with maintenance of immunogenicity. The attempt is not always completely successful, as illustrated by the reversion to virulence of the type 3 poliovirus strain (see Safety Aspects of Vaccines).

The third approach is the use of naturally-occurring attenuated human viruses. One example is the type 2 poliovirus strain. More recently, rotavirus strains potentially suitable for vaccine use have been recovered from human nurseries after extended outbreaks of infection in which some infected children showed little sign of disease.

The fourth approach is to select virus mutants that grow only poorly at temperatures higher than 37°C. In the case of influenza virus, such temperature-sensitive mutants were found to grow well in the upper respiratory tract, but proved to be genetically unstable. However, prolonged cultivation of the virus at progressively lower temperatures produced cold-adapted (*ca*) strains, which grew at 25°C and were shown to have mutations in four of the internal genes. Such preparations have so far been shown to be genetically stable.[38]

An unusual approach is to administer a live virulent virus by a route that does not result in disease. United States Armed Forces recruits take orally a live adenovirus vaccine in an enteric-coated capsule, which is used mainly to protect the virus from gastric acidity. Although it is grown in tissue culture, there are no markers of attenuation for this virus; nevertheless, its oral administration has been shown to be both safe and protective.[157]

A variety of other approaches involving deletions or mutations are being tried. Perhaps the most successful of these to date is the deletion of 18 open reading frames from the Copenhagen strain of vaccinia virus, including six genes involved in nucleotide metabolism, to form a preparation called NY-VAC.[174] It retains strong immunogenicity but is virtually nonpathogenic. The selective deletion of specific DNA sequences, pioneered with poxviruses,[33] is an attractive approach for other viruses because it offers the prospect of a selective and reproducible means of producing adequately attenuated viruses. This approach has already been tried with some success with the simian immunodeficiency virus (SIV).[48] However, there is widespread concern about using this approach with viruses that incorporate their genetic material into the host cell genome at some stage during the infectious process and especially as part of the replication cycle. Lentiviruses and hepadnaviruses (hepatitis B) are in this category.

There are potential disadvantages to the use of attenuated live virus vaccines. These include the risk of contamination with adventitious agents, reversion to virulence (e.g., type 3 poliovirus strain), administration to immunocompromised people, possible interference if other live viruses are administered at or near the same time, and finally, the instability of some preparations (e.g., polio vaccines) at higher temperatures.

Inactivated Whole Virus Vaccines

Inactivation of whole virus, frequently by exposure to formalin, is also a well-established procedure for vaccine development. The four such vaccines listed in Table 16-1 are administered parenterally, and the main immunoglobulin (Ig) induced is IgG. Inactivated poliovirus (IPV) vaccine, Japanese encephalitis vaccine, and rabies virus vaccine (produced in diploid cells) are safe and effective at preventing disease, even though IPV does not prevent a mucosal infection. The influenza virus vaccine is less effective (approx. 70%), but this is considered to be mainly a result of the continuous antigenic drift to which this virus is subject. These preparations are relatively heat stable and safe, but compared with live virus vaccines, a greater antigenic dose is required and sometimes several administrations. Furthermore, such vaccines frequently do not induce all the types of immune responses resulting after immunization with live viruses, notably a cytotoxic T lymphocyte (CTL) response.

Viral Protein Subunit Vaccines

For most viruses, the reaction of antibody with one or more of the surface protein (glycoprotein) antigens neutralizes infectivity. Because for many years the generation of neutralizing antibody was considered to be the major protective function of a vaccine, it seemed reasonable that a vaccine composed only of these components would be both very safe and effective. The two examples given in Table 16-1 are likely to be the forerunners of many later products.

The surface antigen (HBsAg) of the hepatitis B virus is secreted from infected cells and occurs in the blood of infected people as 22-nm particles. The first hepatitis B vaccine was made of these particles, which were harvested from the blood of infected people and carefully disinfected to inactivate any infectious virus. It proved to be quite safe and about 85% effective, the remaining recipients being either nonresponders or poor responders.[54] When it is given to newborn babies, hyperimmune serum is added to increase the efficacy, because the latter protects during the period needed for the immune response to be generated by the vaccine.[20] In the industrialized world, this vaccine has largely been replaced by a product made using recombinant DNA (rDNA) technology to become the first genetically engineered vaccine.[84] In these countries, a course of injections of either product is expensive. However, the success of the product has greatly influenced later approaches to development of other vaccines.

The surface antigens of the influenza virus, hemagglutinin (HA), which is recognized by neutralizing antibody, and neuraminidase, can readily be stripped from the virus and are used as a subunit preparation. The preparation is less reactogenic than whole virus, especially in young children, and is considered to be just as effective as inactivated whole virus.[94]

SAFETY ASPECTS OF VACCINES

Before registration of a vaccine, all available data are reviewed by regulatory authorities. The information available at that time should reveal safety hazards that occur with frequencies of up to perhaps 1 in 10,000, depending on the size and nature of the population involved in the phase III trials. There are examples of untoward severe side effects occurring at very low frequencies (1 in 50,000 or more) that were detected only

during immunosurveillance after registration of the vaccine. Their frequencies were so low that it was difficult to prove beyond reasonable doubt that they were a consequence of vaccination. An example is the occurrence of the Guillain-Barré syndrome after the swine influenza vaccination program in 1976 and 1977.

Recently, adverse events associated with the use of childhood vaccines, and particularly the evidence bearing on causality and specific adverse health outcomes mainly within the United States, have been evaluated by an expert committee for the Institute of Medicine.[179] The possibility of adverse neurologic events after vaccination has fuelled much of the concern about vaccine safety. The disorders included both demyelinating diseases (e.g., acute disseminated encephalomyelitis, multiple sclerosis, focal lesions, Guillain-Barré syndrome) and nondemyelinating diseases such as encephalopathy, subacute sclerosing panencephalitis, residual seizure disorder, and sensorineural deafness and neuropathy. Immunologic reactions to vaccination included anaphylaxis, autoimmune reactions, Arthus reaction, and delayed-type hypersensitivity (DTH). Adverse effects after immunization with measles, mumps, polio, and hepatitis B vaccines were studied.

In most cases, the evidence was considered inadequate to either accept or reject a causal relation between measles and mumps vaccine and encephalitis or encephalopathy. For example, in uncontrolled studies, the calculated rate of these effects per million doses of vaccine varied from 1 to 11. However, the evidence suggested a causal relation between the trivalent measles, mumps, rubella (MMR) vaccine (but not the monovalent preparations) and thrombocytopenia, and also between MMR or the measles vaccine and anaphylaxis. Because of these effects, there was a causal relation between MMR vaccine and death, although the risk was considered to be extraordinarily low. Natural measles infection induces an immunosuppressive state from which the great majority of children recover. The Institute of Medicine document[179] records only two cases of immunosuppression in immunocompromised children after vaccination with measles vaccine.

The WHO Expanded Programme of Immunization published a comparison of the incidence of side effects after natural infection compared with those after immunization. The findings for measles, summarized in Table 16-2, indicate the remarkable safety of the standard vaccine compared with infection by wild-type virus.[65]

In the case of oral polio vaccine (OPV), there was a clear relation with paralytic and nonparalytic polio (1 case per 520,000 first doses administered), and the vaccine could lead to vaccine strain infection in contacts. The type 1 strain of virus contains 57 separate base substitutions, of which 21 code for amino acid changes that are scattered throughout the genome. In practice, this virus rarely if ever reverts to virulence. In contrast, type 3 does revert. By comparing three strains of type 3 virus, it was found that attenuation produced at most ten point mutations, of which only three resulted in amino acid substitutions. It has been found that a backmutation at amino acid position 472 in type 3 poliovirus correlates with reversion to neurovirulence.[57a,170]

A causal relation was also found between OPV and Guillain-Barré syndrome. In both cases, the risk of death was again considered to be extraordinarily low. In the case of hep-

TABLE 16-2. *Estimated rates of serious adverse reactions after measles immunization compared with complications of natural infection and background rate of illness*

Rates per 100,000	Adverse reactions				
	Encephalitis	SSPE*	Pneumonia	Convulsions	Death
Natural infection	50–400	0.5–2.0	3800–7300	500–1000	10–10,000
Vaccination	0.1	0.05–0.1	—	0.02–190	0.02–0.3
Background levels*	0.1–0.3	—	—	30	—

SSPE, subacute sclerosing panencephalitis.
*In a normal population of the same age group.
Modified from Galaska AM, Lauer BA, Henderson RH, Keja J. Indications and contraindications for vaccines used in the Expanded Programme of Immunization. Bull World Health Organ 1984;62: 357–366.

atitis B vaccine, the evidence established a causal relation with anaphylaxis.

A recent experience provides an example of the care that must be taken before a vaccine is released for general use, particularly in third world countries.[77] One factor contributing to the 1 to 2 million deaths from measles that occur each year is the variable time gap (3 to 4 months) between the waning of maternally-derived antimeasles antibody in infants in some developing countries and immunization with the live attenuated Schwartz measles vaccine at 9 months (which does not immunize in the presence of specific antibody). To lessen this window of opportunity for infection by wild-type virus, high-titer vaccines were developed. After their administration to 5- and 6-month-old infants in several countries induced satisfactory immune responses, their general use was authorized by WHO in 1989. Within a short time, there were reports of a higher than expected mortality rate, particularly among young girls in populations at the lower end of the socioeconomic scale, and this led to the withdrawal of these vaccines from use.

Some of the vaccines listed in Table 16-1 are inactivated whole virus preparations. However, inactivation of a virus to destroy infectivity should not be regarded as guaranteeing a safe product. In at least two cases, measles and respiratory syncytial virus (RSV), immunization with formalin-inactivated preparations sensitized the recipients to severe reactions when they were later exposed to the wild-type agent.[188] Examination showed that the severe reactions had characteristics of both Arthus reaction (antibody-mediated) and DTH, caused in the first instance to changes in the properties of one or more viral surface antigens by exposure to formalin.

EFFICACY OF VACCINES

The efficacy of vaccines is primarily assessed by their ability to prevent disease on subsequent exposure of the vaccinated person to the wild-type agent. After methods for the quantitative estimation of specific antibody became available, the practice of estimating seroconversion (i.e., the neutralization titer, or the quantitative difference in antibody that specifically prevents infection of susceptible cells in vitro) was widely adopted. With experience, the neutralization titer could be used to predict the efficacy of specific vaccines (e.g.,

influenza). Particularly in those cases in which great antigenic variation occurred, such a correlation was not always observed, and it was slowly realized that cell-mediated immune (CMI) responses, which may not parallel the antibody response, could also be helpful.[9] If there has been preexposure to the same virus, a more rapid and enhanced (secondary) immune response after vaccination could also indicate efficacy.

From an epidemiologic viewpoint, the efficacy of vaccination can be assessed by recording the number of cases that occur during the period when vaccination is progressively introduced. In 1979, there were about 2000 cases of disease caused by poliovirus infection in Brazil. Two years later, after the introduction of special vaccination days, this figure had dropped by more than 90%. By mid-1994, no cases of indigenous poliomyelitis had been reported in the Americas for more than 2 years.[3]

A comparison of whooping cough notifications in England and Wales from 1940 through 1992 is even more revealing. The number of cases per annum before the 1950s, when vaccination was begun, ranged from 60,000 to 170,000. During the mid-1970s, when vaccine uptake had reached more than 80% of the population, this figure ranged from less than 1000 to 10,000. During the next 10 years, at least in part because of a media scare about side reactions after vaccination, the coverage dropped to 30%, and cases rose to 20,000 to 60,000 per year. After an intensive public health campaign, vaccination uptake rose to about 90% by 1992, and the number of cases fell to fewer than 5000 per year.

Occasionally, during vaccine development, misleading efficacy data about a candidate product may be obtained. Early results indicated that monkeys immunized with inactivated SIV were protected from challenge with the homologous live virus.[171] This result, obtained in several laboratories, raised hope that it should be relatively straightforward to make a safe and effective vaccine against human immunodeficiency virus (HIV). It was then realized that the virus used both for immunization and for challenge of the monkeys had been grown in a human cell line. When the immunizing and challenge viruses were grown in monkey cells, protection was not observed. Lentiviruses such as SIV and HIV have since been shown to incorporate into their surface membranes a number of cellular membrane-associated components, including major histocompatibility complex (MHC) antigens.[11] The probable explanation for the earlier protection is that the monkeys mounted a host-versus-graft reaction to the human MHC antigens in the SIV particles, and this protected against the subsequent challenge virus. The possibility has been raised whether a vaccine to HIV should in part be directed against foreign MHC antigens. Immunization of an uninfected female with MHC antigens from a single infected male may facilitate protection from infection by that male.

RELEVANT COMPONENTS OF THE IMMUNE SYSTEM

The immune response is composed of two main parts, the nonadaptive and the adaptive systems. Two properties distinguish the systems: specificity and memory. These properties characterize one class of cells, the lymphocytes. Reactions not involving this cell type form the nonadaptive system.

The Nonadaptive System

Components of the nonadaptive system include a number of cell types, such as natural killer (NK) cells, neutrophils, polymorphonuclear cells, and eosinophils, together with a number of soluble factors, including complement and cytokines such as interferon-α (IFN-α) and IFN-β. Although some of these responses (e.g., NK cells) may show some selectivity in their activity, none is specific, and there is no evidence to date of a memory effect. Because of this, vaccines for prophylaxis are not designed specifically to stimulate these responses.

The Adaptive System

The only cell type that displays both specificity and memory is the lymphocyte, of which there are two classes: B cells and T cells. B cells have IgM and IgD receptors for antigen on their surface. Activation of B cells may occur after an encounter with an antigen. If the antigen (e.g., a polysaccharide) is not processed by an antigen-presenting cell (APC) and T cells are not activated, it may bind to receptors having the appropriate specificity on B cells and activate those cells, which then secrete mainly IgM antibodies of that specificity. More often, a T cell, which has been activated by exposure to an antigen after processing by the APC, may provide "help" for the B cell that has been exposed to the same antigen. The activated B cell may initially produce IgM antibodies, but after close contact between the T and B cells and under the influence of cytokines produced by the T cell, it switches to the production of IgG, IgA, or IgE antibodies. T cells may have not only this regulatory role (THs, or helper T lymphocytes) and suppressor activity (CTLs) but may also have effector roles, mediating DTH responses or cytotoxic activity of CTLs. Recently, it has been found that there are two types of TH cells, called TH1 and TH2, which differ in the profiles of the cytokines they secrete. It is thought that they derive from a common precursor cell, designated TH0, and that the influence of certain cytokines on this cell determines whether TH1 or TH2 cells are preferentially produced. Interleukin-4 (IL-4)

favors TH2 cell production, whereas IL-12 favors TH1 cell production.

All of these responses are adaptive, because after stimulation by antigen, replication and differentiation of T and B cells occurs. Affinity maturation of the antibody produced by B cells occurs over time. The T-cell responses are usually referred to as CMI responses, whereas the B-cell response is referred to as a humoral response.

Antibody recognizes a shape defined by continuous or discontinuous sequences of amino acids or sugars (called epitopes), either free in solution or at a cell surface. T-cell receptors (TCRs) also recognize a shape, but this is defined by a complex formed between the MHC antigen of the native cell plus a peptide derived by degradation of a protein (self or foreign) within that cell, the complex being expressed at the surface of the APC. In this case, the peptide component is often referred to as a determinant. There are two main classes of such complexes. Peptides derived from the processing in lysosomes of exogenous (noninfectious) antigens associate with class II MHC antigens and are recognized by TH cells; hence, these responses are called class II MHC–restricted. The responding T cell is characterized by a membrane marker, the CD4 molecule, which is expressed adjacent to the TCR and helps to stabilize it. Peptides derived from endogenous proteins (self proteins or viral proteins being synthesized in the cell cytoplasm) associate with class I MHC molecules, and the complexes are recognized by CTLs; these responses are called class I MHC–restricted. The responding T cell is characterized by the CD8 molecule, which also has the role of stabilizing the TCR on these cells. In this latter case, the peptide determinant is not only very restricted in length, being usually a nonapeptide, but also has a motif, so that certain amino acids preferentially occupy certain positions in the cleft of the MHC molecule.

As well as having specific receptors for antigens, T and B cells and APCs also communicate with each other in two other ways. One is by the secretion of cytokines, which act over a very short range. T cells in particular are both major producers of and responders to cytokines. Some similarities and differences between the major effector T cells in this respect are summarized in Table 16-3. Sometimes, CTLs and TH1 cells are grouped together under the heading of TH1-like cells. Although there are clear similarities in the pattern of secreted cytokines, there are also major differences between them, such as mediation of DTH reactivity (which involves many different cytokines) and conditions for their generation, a point of particular importance for vaccine development. Activation of naive T cells by APCs requires one additional condition, the expression of costimulator molecules and other cell surface proteins on the APC and their recognition by ligands on the T cell. The most important costimulator molecule on an APC is B7, and the corresponding ligand on the T cell is CD28. APCs that possess all of these characteristics are sometimes referred to as professional APCs. The importance of these different components is seen clearly in current efforts to develop effective vaccines against certain tumors (see later discussion).

Figure 16-1 summarizes the nature and sequence of events that result in the production of regulatory T cells (TH2s) or effector T cells (TH1s, CTLs) after the processing of antigen

TABLE 16-3. *Some characteristics of TH1 and TH2 cells and cytotoxic T lymphocytes*

REGULATORY FUNCTIONS (CD4+ TH2 CELLS)
Secrete IL-3, -4, -5, -6, -10, and -13 and TNF-α
Provide help for production of IgG, IgA, and IgE

REGULATORY/EFFECTOR FUNCTIONS (CD4+ TH1 CELLS)
Provide help for Ig2a antibody (mice), IgG1 (humans)
May provide help for CTL generation (not mandatory)
Secrete IL-2, -3; IFN-γ and TNF-α, TNF-β
Primary cells* usually do not lyse infected cells, but cultured or cloned cells may do so
Main mediator of DTH reactivity (little evidence that DTH activity helps to clear viral infections)

EFFECTOR FUNCTIONS (CD8+ CTLs)
Secrete IL-2, IFN-γ, and TNF-β
Primary cells may lyse infected cells shortly after infection
Poor mediator of DTH reactivity

CTL, cytotoxic T lymphocyte; DTH, delayed-type hypersensitivity; IFN, interferon; Ig, immunoglobulin; IL, interleukin; TH, helper T lymphocyte; TNF, tumor necrosis factor.
*Cells taken directly from the infected host without further culture in the presence of specific antigen.

(either an infectious agent such as a virus or a noninfectious preparation) in an APC.

Figure 16-2 summarizes the events that lead to the activation and differentiation of B cells. The B cell receptors may recognize a particular epitope on a single protein molecule or repeating epitopes on a protein polymer; this means that they may bind part or presumably all of an intact virus particle. The complex is then endocytosed and degraded, and class II MHC–peptide complexes are expressed at the cell surface. This activity induces the expression of costimulator molecules on the B cell, which in turn switch on the expression of the corresponding ligand on those T cells (mainly TH2) whose receptors have already recognized the MHC–peptide complex expressed by the B cell. This double recognition event induces both the expression of other T cell membrane markers (e.g., CD40) and the secretion of particular cytokines. The subsequent expression of the ligand for CD40 on the B cell enhances the already tight and intimate connection between the

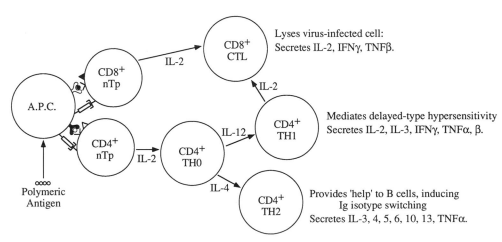

FIG. 16-1. Antigen presentation and T-cell activation. APC, antigen-presenting cell; nTp, naive precursor cells; TH0, early activated CD4+ T cell; ILs, interleukins; INFγ, interferon-γ; TH1, TH2, CTLs, regulatory/effector T cells; TNFa,β, tumor necrosis factors.
⚥ and ♥, class I and II major histocompatibility complex (MHC) antigens; ○,● peptides from degraded antigen bound to MHC molecules; ∨, T-cell receptor; CD4,△, and CD8,▲, T-cell differentiation antigens; ▯, costimulator molecules on APC; ⊔, ligand on T cell recognizing costimulator molecules.

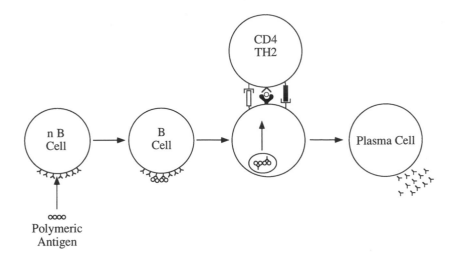

FIG. 16-2. Antigen presentation and B-cell activation. nB cell, naive B cell; ϒ, immunoglobulin receptors or secreted antibodies; ♥, class II major histocompatibility complex with bound peptide; ⊐, costimulator molecule on activated B cell; ⌄, T-cell receptor; ↳, ligand on T cell binding to costimulator molecule; ▬, CD40 differentiation antigen expressed on helper T cell; ⊣, ligand on activated B cell specific for CD40.

T and B cells. This and the local abundance of interleukins leads to B-cell differentiation, immunoglobulin isotype switching, and finally conversion to a plasma cell, whose role is to secrete large amounts of immunoglobulin of the chosen specificity.

Although a knowledge of the interaction between T and B cells is required to understand the immune response after vaccination or infection, the subject has become extraordinarily complex. A 1993 review by Schwartz[163] summarizes current knowledge of this interaction as it occurs both in vitro and in vivo.

STAGES IN VIRAL INFECTIONS

In general two situations may exist: (1) infection of a naive individual who has not previously been exposed to the particular infectious agent or (2) exposure of an individual who has been previously infected or immunized to the homologous or a related infectious agent.

Acute Infections of Naive Individuals

Provided the infectious dose is sublethal, acute infections are defined as infections from which the great majority of people recover within a short period, usually one or a few weeks, because their immune system has controlled and then cleared the infection. It is convenient to divide the cycle into four stages: the entry of the virus, limiting the rate of replication of the virus, control (reduction) of replication, and clearance of the virus. In model systems (e.g., influenza virus replicating in the murine lung after intranasal inoculation[9]), the sequence of appearance of immune responses is as follows: specific CD4+ T cells (1 to 3 days), CD8+ T cells (3 to 5 days), antibody-secreting cells (ASCs) producing IgM (5 to 10 days), and other immunoglobulin isotypes (10 days or longer). Whereas effector CTLs cannot be recovered from the lung after about 14 days, ASCs (predominantly IgG secre-

tors), are present for at least 20 months after the infection.[9] This sequence in shown in Figure 16-3A for three parameters—presence of infectious virus (curve A), of CTLs (curve B), and of specific ASCs (curve C) after infection. It is assumed that the titer of neutralizing antibody follows a pattern similar to curve C.

Initial Infection by Virus and its Prevention

Although some viruses infect by means of a vector (arboviruses) or through injury such as abrasions or sores on the skin (pox and papilloma), most infect by a mucosal route. In most cases, free virus is responsible, but lentiviruses can also be transmitted by infected cells.

A variety of effects can limit the access of a virus to susceptible cells. Cilia in the lung air passages can sweep particles toward the throat, where they may be swallowed. Complement can lyse some enveloped viruses[112] and so reduce the infectious dose. But the only mechanism that has the potential for completely preventing infection is the continuing presence of specific neutralizing antibody, as a result of either a prior infection by the homologous virus or by immunization. Most vaccines probably do not generate a sufficiently high titer of neutralizing antibody to give sterilizing immunity; it is more likely that the infecting virus titer is reduced to such a low level that the host's own immune system can cope with the remainder as a subclinical infection. The host thus may benefit from both the vaccination and a natural infection. In some cases (e.g., HIV, hepatitis B), sterilizing immunity would be advantageous, because in these infections, viral DNA or complementary DNA (cDNA) is incorporated into the host cell's genome. Such cells remain infected until they die or are destroyed. Some idea of the potential difficulty of inducing sterilizing immunity is given by experiments of Parker Small and colleagues.[145] Mice were transfused with hyperimmune antiinfluenza serum (IgG). After intranasal challenge with virus, the mice were protected from disease, but on investigation, many cells lining the respiratory tract mucosa were shown to be infected (i.e., the mice

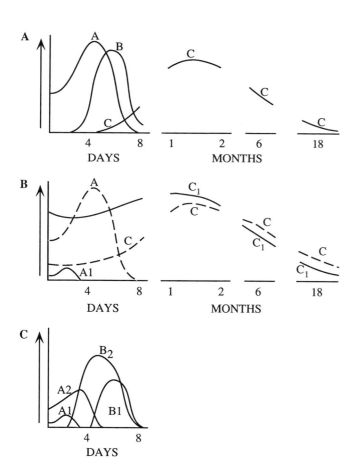

FIG. 16-3. Viral replication and two immune responses, by antibody-secreting cells (ASCs) and cytotoxic T lymphocytes (CTLs), in primary and secondary acute viral infection. The curves are based on experiments with influenza virus infections in mouse lungs (see Fig. 16-4). (**A**) Primary infection in naive mice. Curve A, viral titers; curve B, CTL levels; curve C, ASC levels. (**B**) Curves A and C as in **A**. After a second exposure to the homologous virus, curve A1 represents replication of escaping, nonantibody-neutralized virus, and curve C1 represents antibody titers at the time of and subsequent to the infectious challenge. (**C**) Viral replication (curve A1) and CTL activity (curve B1) after a second exposure to the homologous virus, as in **B**. If the challenge virus shares many T cell determinants but no epitopes recognized by neutralizing antibody with the first virus, curve A2 represents viral replication in the lung and curve B2 the more rapid and higher CTL activity.

had tracheitis). In a second set of experiments,[150] mice were transfused with antibody from a hybridoma expressing poly-IgA specific for influenza HA. In vivo, this was converted to secretory IgA and secreted into the lumen of the respiratory tract; on exposure to the same virus, most but not all mice in the experiment showed no sign of infection of cells lining the mucosa. Furthermore, in mice convalescent from a respiratory influenza virus infection, treatment with anti-α antisera but not anti-u or anti-γ antisera destroyed the resistance to a second infection of mucosal cells with the homologous virus.[151]

Exposure to infected cells, as during sexual intercourse or by needlesticking, presents a different problem. In the case of HIV, two situations may exist.[8] A cell may be latently infected and not be synthesizing any viral proteins, or the cell may be actively secreting infectious virus particles. In both cases, usually the MHC haplotype of the invading cells is recognized as foreign by the recipient, and a strong CMI response (a host-versus-graft reaction) is mounted and destroys the invading cells. Although there remains the possibility that within a few days some donor cells could migrate to a privileged site, this is unlikely because the host-versus-graft immune response is both rapid and strong. Destruction of virus-secreting cells may add slightly to the load of infecting free virus. This mechanism may not be sufficiently effective in the case of perinatal infections.

Neutralization of Infectivity

Neutralizing epitopes are known for a number of viruses. In the case of influenza, five sites on the HA molecules were identified (1) by analysis of sequence changes in mutants derived under immune selection in the presence of neutralizing monoclonal antibodies (MAbs), (2) by analysis of the three-dimensional structure of trimeric HA molecules, and (3) by a comparison of sequences from related epidemic and mutant strains.[187] The sequences at these sites are mainly nonlinear (discontinuous). Panels of neutralizing MAbs specific for four of these sites were mixed with denatured HA, monomeric HA, and trimeric HA (the form in which it exists in the virus). None bound to the denatured HA, and at three of the four sites they bound preferentially to the trimer. For one site, they bound equally well to monomer and trimer.[128]

In a few known situations, the epitope is continuous and may be mimicked by short peptides. An early recognized example was a short peptide from the VP1 protein of foot-and-mouth disease virus; antibody raised to a conjugate of this peptide with keyhole limpet hemocyanin protein could neutralize viral infectivity.[27] Similarly, the V3 loop, the principal neutralizing domain of gp120 of the HIV, is a linear sequence of about 33 amino acids in a disulfide-bonded loop.[125] In both of these cases, however, it has been shown that a mutation at a single amino acid site outside the loop affects the conformation of the linear neutralizing epitope so that it no longer binds some previously neutralizing MAbs.[125,139]

If the specificity of neutralizing antibody after immunization or infection matches that of a challenge virus, Figure 16-3B shows the effect on virus replication (curve A1) and neutralizing antibody titers (curve C1). If the antigenic specificities are very different, as occurs for example between H1N1 and H2N2 strains of influenza virus, the pattern of viral replication and neutralizing antibody production (Fig. 16-3B, curves A and C) resembles those seen in Figure 16-3A.

Slowing the Rate of Replication

In the nonimmune host, the generation of lymphocyte-based responses may take between several days (influenza) and several months (HIV). During this time, nonspecific responses may slow the rate and extent of replication. A mild influenza virus infection in humans may be confined to the upper respiratory tract. The inflammatory response that occurs during a mild influenza infection in the ferret consists mainly of polymorphonuclear cells which are extruded onto the mucosal surface at the site of the infection.[173a] There is a correlation between the extent of fever and the rate of decline of viral titers in the nose; suppression of the fever results in a delay of viral clearance.[87] If mice are pretreated with *Corynebacterium parvum* before intranasal infection with influenza virus, lower viral titers and lower mortality rates occur, and these differences correlate with an increased IFN-α titer, increased NK cell activity, and increased numbers of activated macrophages in the lung.[107] Mice bearing the Mx gene have an enhanced sensitivity to IFN-α, and this results in a greater resistance to influenza virus infection.[76a]

Differences between strains of mice that are susceptible or resistant to cytomegalovirus can be seen within 2 to 3 days and are in part a function of activity of NK cells.[167] Treatment of mice with anti-asialoGM$_1$ antibody, which depletes NK cells, enhances the growth of several viruses, including cytomegalovirus.[32]

Although a prophylactic vaccine may stimulate these responses, the beneficial effect would probably be minimal unless the live viral challenge occurred shortly thereafter. With the increasing interest in immunotherapy of already infected people (e.g., those infected with HIV), it may be possible to obtain information on the benefit of such responses in controlling an already-established infection.

Recovery From and Clearance of Infection

Role of Nonadaptive Responses

Nonadaptive responses may contribute to clearance of an infection, but I am unaware of any evidence that these responses can clear an infection in the absence of B- and T-lymphocyte responses in model systems. For example, athymic (nu+/nu+) mice infected with influenza virus experience a persistent lung infection even though they develop IgM antibodies and have elevated NK-cell activity and activated macrophages.[193]

Role of Antibodies

Antibody specific for viral antigens expressed on the infected cell surface can contribute to recovery in one of two ways: by lysis of the infected cell in association with complement (the classic pathway) or by antibody-dependent cell-mediated cytotoxicity. The cells involved include NK cells, monocytes, and neutrophils.[81] Studies have shown that antibody may modify the disease process, both in human influenza infections[169] and in animal models. Passive transfer of immune serum to mice early after infection reduced lung virus titers,[191] and, in infected nude mice, passively-administered antibody prevented virus dissemination. However, the effect

was transient because virus shedding occurred as the antibody titer waned.[18]

Two examples have shown that antibody may clear particular infections. Some MAbs to the fusion protein of RSV were found not only to protect against infection but also to clear an established RSV infection. At 6 days after infection (the time of maximum lung viral titers), MAbs were capable of clearing the infection within 6 hours of administration.[175] Of the activities measured, the only biologic property that correlated with this ability was prevention of syncytia formation by the virus.[175] It seems likely that bound antibodies were endocytosed into the infected cell and were able to prevent viral formation. In the second example, MAbs or hyperimmune serum specific for Sindbis virus were able to clear this virus from infected neurones in mice, even if administered some days after the original infection.[73] This latter work is of additional interest because neurones are one of the few cell types in the body that do not express (or express at very low levels) class I MHC molecules, and it was thought that CTLs would not be able to contain and clear such infections (see later discussion).

Effector T cells are the major mechanisms for RSV clearance in infected calves.[175] Also, because children with Bruton's sex-linked agammaglobulinemia who become infected with some viruses such as influenza or measles[69,106] recover and clear the infection, it is most likely that specific antibody is not essential for recovery in many acute viral infections. To judge from the two cases mentioned, immunotherapy that uses highly specific MAbs may become an effective means to clear such infections, particularly in infants hospitalized with an RSV infection. Such treatment should be highly beneficial because it should result in little inflammation.[175] In contrast, effector T cells may cause considerable inflammation because of the action of liberated cytokines. A second question of considerable importance is whether any method of immunization acceptable for human use and administered by a parenteral or mucosal route can raise antibody of sufficiently high titer and affinity to clear either of these infections; this has yet to be tested.

Role of Effector T Cells

CD8+ Cells

There is now general agreement that effector T cells are the major mechanism for clearance of viruses causing acute infections, whether they are primary or secondary infections. CD8+ CTLs have been referred to as auditors that unceasingly monitor molecular events in the body's cells: "Without this constant vigilance, the body would be out of business very quickly."[66] Persistent or lethal infections usually occur because the virus outwits or overwhelms the T-cell response (see later discussion). The role of CTLs has been studied in many model systems, often by transfer of primary, cultured, or cloned cell preparations[82]; major reductions in viral titers and sometimes prevention of death, if a lethal dose of virus had been administered, have been obtained.[7]

CTLs exert their antiviral effect in two ways. One is by the liberation of certain cytokines, especially IFN-γ. With the use of vaccinia virus as a vector of genes coding for cytokines such as IFN-γ or IL-2, it has been shown that IFN-γ can clear the viral infection in athymic mice in the absence of effector T cells.[148] It may be that the amount of cytokine produced in this way is substantially greater than the amount produced during a normal infection. Another function of IFN-γ is to upregulate class I MHC expression on potential target cells, thus making them more susceptible to CTL-mediated lysis.

A second potential activity of CTLs in vivo is the lysis of virus-infected cells. Although there has been no evidence to contradict the belief that CTLs are cytotoxic in vivo, as they were initially shown to be in vitro,[120] it is only recently that very persuasive data has been obtained to support the occurrence of CTL-mediated lysis of virus-infected cells in vivo. In one investigation, mice were depleted of both CD4+ T cells, so that they could not make antibody, and CD8+ T cells, so that they could not form CTLs. They were then infected with lymphocytic choriomeningitis virus (LCMV). On transfer of LCMV-specific CTLs to the infected mice, the internal nucleoprotein of LCMV rapidly appeared in the sera. (The formation of antinucleoprotein antibody after infection would normally block detection of this protein). Because LCMV is noncytopathic, the nucleoprotein appeared to be released as a direct result of the lysis of infected cells by the transferred CTLs.[96a]

The lytic activity of CTLs is caused mainly by the exocytosis of perforin-containing granules that cause lesions in the membranes, resulting in the lysis of target cells.[182] Purified perforin has been shown to lyse cells in a calcium-dependent fashion and may also have a role in DNA fragmentation. In one approach, perforin antisense oligonucleotides were found to partially inhibit cell lysis by CTLs.[10] More direct evidence was provided by the observation that perforin knockout mice failed to clear an LCMV infection, even though the mice showed no defects in lymphocyte migration, MHC class II–disparate allograft rejection, or cytokine secretion.[93] Presumably, the level of IFN-γ produced in these mice was insufficient to clear the viral infection. The demonstration that lysis occurs in vivo is of special importance because it has been shown that an infected cell may become susceptible to lysis by CTLs long before intact virus particles are formed and released.[89]

A few cell types, notably sperm and neurones, express little if any class I MHC antigens and therefore potentially could provide a sanctuary or reservoir for certain viruses.[73] However, it has been shown[180] that virus in infected neurones can be cleared by transfer of virus-specific CTLs. In mice in which neurones were persistently infected with LCMV, transfer of CTLs cleared virus from more than 99.9% of infected cells. However, the neurones were not lysed, suggesting that clearance occurred by another mechanism, possibly secretion of cytokines (IFN-γ) from the CTLs.

Clones of CTLs specific for influenza virus HA that are cytotoxic in vitro but differ in their in vivo activity have been described.[105,177] One clone, which secreted IFN-γ and expressed DTH activity, was able to reduce viral titers in vivo; another clone, which neither secreted IFN-γ nor mediated DTH, failed to reduce viral titers in vivo. Whether the need to secrete lymphokines to reduce titers of viruses exists for viruses other than influenza in vivo remains to be established.

Figure 16-3C illustrates the generation of CTLs in secondary viral infections. If preexisting antibody (from a primary infection or immunization) neutralizes most incoming virus, the subsequent replication of escaped virus may be so small (curve A1) that less CTL activity is induced, as indicated by curve B1 (compared with curve B, Fig. 16-3A). If the incoming virus is not neutralized and the two viruses share few or no CTL determinants, then the extent of viral replication and the CTL response are similar to the curves in Figure 16-3A. However, if the two viruses share many CTL determinants but no epitopes inducing neutralizing antibody, there is a rapid and enhanced CTL response (Fig. 16-3C, curve B2). This has the effect of reducing the extent of viral replication (Fig. 16-3C, curve A2) that would otherwise occur (Fig. 16-3A, curve A). (An example of this situation is described in the section on immunologic memory.)

CD4+ Cells

Cytotoxic Activity. Cultured or cloned CD4+ effector T cells specific for some viruses (e.g., influenza, Epstein-Barr, HIV) may be cytotoxic in vitro,[106a,114,134] but there are very few reports demonstrating that primary CD4+ T cells (i.e., as they occur in vivo) are cytotoxic. One report[101] claims not only that CD4+ T cells from HIV-infected people have this property but that there are as many such cells present as CD8+ CTLs. This finding is in sharp contrast to many other reports showing that only CD8+ T cells from HIV-infected people are cytotoxic. However, primary CD4+ T cells in infected β$_2$-microglobulin–deficient mice clearly have this property,[121a] as though in the absence of CD8+ CTLs primary CD4+ T cells could develop this activity, perhaps as a compensatory mechanism. A potential hazard of such a response is that activated B cells may be lysed by these cells before antibody is secreted. Indeed, one investigation reported a great decrease in specific IgG production in such mice during a viral infection.[170] Although knockout mice, in which selected genes are deleted, have been and continue to be extraordinarily useful experimental models, the pattern of effector mechanisms they reveal may differ from that displayed by normal mice. It seems that in some cases, alternative mechanisms may compensate to varying extents if a major response is lacking.

CD4+ TH1 Versus TH2 Cells. The role of TH1 cells in viral infections is currently a topic of great interest. There is increasing evidence that during HIV infection a predominance of TH1-type cells is characteristic of those cases in which the virus is being controlled (i.e., long-term survivors); there is also a considerable amount of supportive evidence from in vitro studies (reviewed by Clerici and Berzofsky[39]). It is well known that measles infections are characterized by a period of selective but transient suppression from which most children recover; it has recently been shown[74] that this suppression is characterized by a functional impairment of CMI-type responses and an increase in the production of IL-4 and IL-10 (characteristic of TH2 responses), resulting in a strong antibody response. This is usually self-limiting, but in some patients in whom the infection becomes severe or fatal, the depression of CMI responses persists.[83a] Some in vitro responses suggest that TH1-type cytokines such as IL-2, IFN-γ, and TNF can upregulate a viral infection such as HIV.[58]

In contrast, TH2 helper T cells can sometimes be critically important, especially in those situations in which particular immunoglobulin isotypes are required, such as secretory IgA in mucosal immunity or IgE in some parasitic infections.

TH1 Cells and DTH Activity. CD4+ T cells are clearly the main mediators of DTH activity,[101a] because CD8+ CTLs frequently display little or no DTH activity (e.g., CTLs specific for herpes virus[129]). Although this response has been shown to be important in some bacterial infections, there is surprisingly little direct evidence (e.g., by cell transfer) that it is a protective response in a viral infection. In fact, contrary results have been obtained[103] (see later discussion). The profile of other cytokines secreted by TH1 cells is similar to that of CD8+ CTLs, so they would be expected to contribute to the recovery phase of a viral infection. The pattern of cytokines observed in HIV infections does suggest that a preponderance of TH1-like cells favors a delayed progression toward acquired immunodeficiency syndrome (AIDS).[166]

An observation of potentially great interest is that in several systems, administration of small amounts of an antigen favors induction of TH1 rather than TH2 cells (see review by Bodmer and colleagues[29]).

T Cell–Mediated Immunopathology

T cells not only require lymphokines for their activation, but they are also major producers of lymphokines, which in turn mediate many of their activities. It was early shown that unless a cloned CD8+ CTL specific for influenza virus HA secreted IFN-γ, it was ineffective in reducing viral titers when administered in vivo.[106,177] Similarly, although the presence of cyclosporin did not affect the activity of influenza virus–specific CTLs in lysing target cells in vitro or the migration of those cells to the mouse lung, the CTLs failed to reduce lung virus titers in cyclosporin-treated mice, suggesting an important role of secreted lymphokines in this system.[160]

Lymphokines have been described as the major mediators of inflammation, and many examples could be given in support of this concept. For CD8+ CTLs, one interesting example is LCMV infections. LCMV, when administered by most parenteral routes to mice, does replicate, but the infection is cleared and CTLs are the major mechanism involved.[199] In contrast, mice infected intracerebrally with low doses of LCMV may develop a fatal choriomeningitis[52] that is dependent on the induction of virus-specific CTLs.[40] T cell–deficient mice do not get the disease, which can, however, be adoptively transferred by cloned CTLs.[19] Whether disease develops in normal mice may be a finely balanced determination; it depends on the contribution of many factors, including the dose and strain of virus, the genetic background of the mouse strain, and the extent to which immunosuppression may occur. This system has been exploited[132a] to show that preimmunization with a live vector containing the gene coding for a single LCMV antigen, which resulted in a low and restricted CTL response, accentuated the pathology and resulted in premature death; in contrast, preimmunization with intact LCMV, which induced a more rapid and stronger CTL response (because of the more numerous CTL determinants), protected against death. Based on this result, it was suggested that the use as vaccines of preparations containing only a few CTL determinants may have detrimental results.

If primary CD4+ T cells are noncytolytic, then an important activity that would result in significant immunopathology is their mediation of DTH activity. This is illustrated in two experiments. In one,[103] enriched preparations of influenza virus–specific secondary effector cells were adoptively transferred to mice 24 hours after intranasal inoculation of virus. Class II MHC–restricted cells failed to reduce lung viral titers within 5 days after transfer and, in fact, resulted in a higher mortality rate than occurred in the control animals. The transferred cells increased the cellular infiltration into the lungs, an effect that was very marked in athymic recipients. In contrast, transfer of class I MHC–restricted cells reduced viral titers, protected the mice from death, and decreased the level of cellular infiltration in normal mice (producing a slight increase in athymic mice), even though it was shown in other experiments that this preparation could mediate some DTH. In the second experiment,[129] the corneal stromata of normal mice and of mice in which CD4+ or CD8+ T cells had been selectively depleted were infected with herpes simplex virus, and the resulting inflammatory responses (stromal keratitis) were measured. CD8+ T cell–depleted mice developed antibody, DTH, and a more rapid stromal keratitis; CD4+ T cell–depleted mice developed little antibody and DTH reactivity but normal CTL responses. The results implicated CD4+ cells as principally involved in stromal keratitis immunopathology.

The extent of pathology caused by effector T cells is largely a function of the extent of the infection, as illustrated in the experiment reported in Table 16-4.[108] Mice were inoculated intranasally with a *ca* strain or the parental strain of influenza virus. The degree of lung consolidation, the lung weights, the NK cell and cytotoxic macrophage activities, the DTH and CTL responses, and the lung viral titers were measured at various times between 6 and 12 days after infection. At inocula of five times the median tissue culture infective dose (5.0 TCID50) of both viruses, the sizes of the CTL and DTH responses were similar in the two groups. Yet, the pathologic damage, as indicated by the extent of lung consolidation and the increase in lung weight, was greatly different; this difference relates to the extent of viral replication (and hence the number of infected cells), which differed by up to a thousandfold at day 6.

A vaccine should aim not only to minimize the extent of the initial infection (neutralization of virus by antibody is the principal mechanism) but also to rapidly clear any residual infection. The data described and other evidence[51] clearly show that CD8+ CTLs are the major effector population for viral clearance. If a large pool of memory CTLs generated by the vaccine can be activated rapidly after a wild-type virus challenge occurs, destruction of the relatively small number of infected cells should cause minimum pathology.

Generation of Immunologic Memory

Particularly where antigenic variation is minimal, many infections and some live attenuated vaccines induce long-lived protection against the wild-type virus.[28,43] Because in general ASCs[111], effector T cells, and antibody itself have short halflives (days to weeks), the continuing presence of antibody must be a result of the continuing generation of memory B cells and their recruitment to form ASCs.

There are a number of markers that are used to differentiate memory B or T cells from naive cells (reviewed by Gray and

TABLE 16-4. *Responses of mice after intranasal inoculation with the parental strain or a cold-adapted (ca) strain of influenza virus, A/Ann Arbor/6/60**

Virus	TCID50 inoculum	Lung consolidation (%)[†]	Lung weight (g)	^{51}Cr release[‡]		DTH[§]	
				100:1	50:1	100:1	50:1
Parent	5.0	35	0.27	70.2	3.4	16.4	5.3
Ca variant	5.0	<5	0.14	71	3.1	14.8	3.9

^{51}Cr, chromium = 51; DTH, delayed-type hypersensitivity; TCID50, median tissue culture infective dose.

*Responses were measured at day 9 after virus administration. At day 6, the TCID50 values were 4.2 and 0.02 for the parental strain, and <2.0 for the ca strain; at day 9, no virus was recovered from either group. Normal lung weight is 0.15 g.

†Consolidation measured between day 6 and day 12 after infection varied from 20% to 60% for parental virus, and from <5% to 15% for the ca strain.

‡Measured at effector-target ratios of 100:1 and 50:1.

§Mean increase in footpad thickness. The same virus was used to both sensitize for and elicit DTH reactions in individual mice.

Sprent[72]). With the former, one difference is the expression of receptors of different immunoglobulin isotypes (after isotype switching), such as IgG, IgE, or IgA. A number of markers have been identified on T cells, and some of them are expressed in greater amounts on memory T cells. Furthermore, the conditions for activating memory T cells are less restrictive than for naive T cells. However, there are two properties that differentiate memory B from memory T cells: (1) receptor isotype switching occurs with B cells but not with T cells, and (2) the B-cell but not the T-cell receptor undergoes affinity maturation.

The number of memory cells compared with naive, competent cells present after an infection or vaccination can be quantitated using plaque assays (ASCs) or limit dilution analyses (effector T cells). In the case of a murine lung influenza virus infection, the frequency of antigen-specific CD8+ T cells that can be stimulated in vitro by the antigen to become effector CTLs increases 20- to 100-fold by 2 weeks after infection begins.[5] In contrast, the level of B cells that, on stimulation, can become specific ASCs reaches peak frequencies (100- to 1000-fold higher than control levels) about 3 months after infection.[9]

Formation, Persistence, and Recruitment of Memory B Cells

Several possible explanations for how memory B cells are formed, maintained, and recruited have been proposed[6,36]:

1. Persistence of the infectious agent. Although this happens in many chronic infections (e.g., HIV) and viral RNA has been shown to persist in a nonproductive form in the brains of alphavirus-infected mice,[104] persistence of viral RNA has been shown not to occur after murine influenza infections,[55] so this mechanism cannot be a general explanation.
2. Stimulation by crossreacting antigens. This is also unlikely because, in the case of vaccinia virus, the only other poxvirus that replicates in humans is monkeypox. Human infections by this virus are very rare.
3. Idiotype-antiidiotype antibody networks. There are many examples of such networks but few reports of effects over

very long periods. This mechanism may contribute to the effect, but it is unlikely to be the main mechanism.
4. Persistence of (noninfectious) antigen. This effect is very well documented and has recently been extensively reviewed.[36]

It was found about 30 years ago[131] that, within a few days after injection of radiolabeled antigen, some antigen in the form of antigen-antibody complexes localized in primary lymphoid follicles in the draining lymph nodes and spleen. The complexes were bound by virtue of receptors for Fc and complement on the surface of follicular dendritic cells. Since then, the following points have been established[4,36]:

1. Antigen can persist for a very long period at this site, in an apparently undegraded state, so that it retains its antigenic properties.
2. Treatment of mice with cobra venom, which disrupts the complement cycle, abolishes both localization in the spleen and B cell priming for a secondary response. This finding led to the conclusion that this antigen trapping was necessary for formation of memory B cells.
3. Two pathways of B cell maturation occur—one that leads to a primary response and a second that results in clonal expansion in the follicles, leading to the formation of germinal centers and the development of memory B cells.
4. Somatic mutation leading to affinity maturation of the antibody response characterizes cells in the second pathway.
5. Antigen-antibody complexes may bud off from the follicular dendritic cells to form iccosomes (immune complex–coated bodies), which are taken up by memory B cells and processed; then, with T cell help, the B cells differentiate to become ASCs.
6. Over time, a combination of somatic mutation and steadily dwindling amounts of retained antigen favors the progressive selection of B cells with higher-affinity receptors, leading in turn to the production of antibody of high affinity.

This localization of antigen has been aptly referred to as "a library of past antigenic experiences."[71] In order to persist on follicular dendritic cells for years and retain its native conformation, the antigen must resist degradation (e.g., by proteases). Because many high-affinity antiviral antibodies recognize discontinuous epitopes, the antigen must persist as aggregates, or even sometimes as apparently intact viral particles, as has been shown with HIV.[137] It is most probable that live attenuated viruses are effective vaccines because, among other things, (1) antigen in its native conformation is produced and persists for long periods, and (2) a large pool of memory B cells is generated.

Formation and Persistence of Memory T Cells

The situation with memory T cells is not so clearcut. There is general agreement that a pool of memory CTLs is formed. There is disagreement on two points: (1) the length of the halflife of these cells and (2) whether persistence of antigen is required for persistence of these cells. Lack of space precludes a detailed discussion of these points, but several papers[17,55] support the belief that the halflife of these cells is at least many months, if not a year or more. The first experiments seemed to show that persistence of antigen was required if memory CTLs were to persist,[71] although the form in which such antigen may persist was unclear. More recent experiments indicate convincingly that retention of antigen is not necessary for persistence of memory T cells.[85,99,121]

Role of Memory T Cells

A major role of memory B cells is to provide a continuing supply of specific antibody to prevent or greatly decrease infection by the challenge virus. In such a case, the level of newly-induced immune responses, including CTL activity generated in the challenged host, is very small and possibly undetectable because the extent of infection is so small. However, if important (neutralizing) B cell epitopes of the challenge virus are antigenically distinct from those of the immunizing virus but the viruses share common T cell (including CTL) determinants, then CTLs rapidly appear after challenge. The general effect is described in Figure 16-3C and is readily demonstrable with murine influenza virus infections, using three antigenically distinct types: H1N1, H2N2, and H3N2. In one report, one of two groups of mice was infected with A/Jap virus (H2N2). Some weeks later, both groups of mice were inoculated intranasally with A/WSN virus (H1N1). The levels of infectious A/WSN virus and of CTL activity (assayed on target cells infected with A/Port Chalmers virus, H3N2) in the lungs were measured on days 3, 4, 5, and 7 (Fig. 16-4).[190a] Although there is very little cross-neutralizing activity of antibodies between H1 and H2 molecules, the level of virus in the preprimed mice was lower at 3 days compared with the level in the control animals, and this level further decreased sharply by day 5, coinciding with the early and rapid increase in CTL activity in this group of mice. To judge from other related experiments,[192] and Table 16-4, it can be predicted that, had a lethal dose of A/Jap virus been used in this experiment, the more rapid (by 1 to 2 days) CTL response in the primed mice would have decreased the extent of immunopathology and may have protected them from death.

A major rationale for adopting a viral vaccination protocol that induces memory CTL formation is the role of these cells

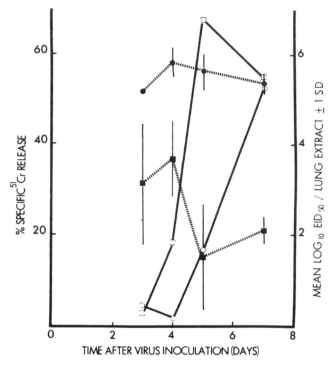

FIG. 16-4. Effect of prepriming in vivo on the time of appearance and magnitude of the cross-reactive cytotoxic T-lymphocyte (CTL) response to influenza viruses. Solid lines indicate cross-reactive CTL activity recovered from the lungs of mice preinfected with A/JAP (H2N2) virus (*open squares*) and from naive mice (*open circles*) after a challenge infection with A/WSN (H1N1) virus. CTL activity was measured on target cells infected with A/Port Chalmers (H3N2) virus. Dotted lines show virus levels in the lungs of preprimed mice (*filled squares*) or naive mice (*filled circles*) after challenge. Each point represents the mean $\log_{10}$ EID50 per lung extract from three lungs, and vertical lines represent ± 1 standard deviation from these values. EID50, 50% egg infectious dose.

in acting as an enhanced safety net, should preexisting antibody fail to reduce the viral load to such a low level that the normal rate of CTL generation is sufficient to cope with the escaped virus.

IMMUNE EVASION

Antigenic Variation

B Cell Epitopes

Amino acid sequence variation in important B cell epitopes is perhaps the most common example of immune evasion used by viruses that cause acute as well as persistent infections. In the case of DNA viruses, which have highly effective repair mechanisms to overcome spontaneous mutations, variation may be reflected by the existence of a number of different serotypes (e.g., hepatitis B virus). In the case of bacteria, this has been overcome by including many of the regionally important serotypes in one vaccine, the 23-valent pneumococcal vaccine.

Replication of RNA is error prone because it is not subject to the same repair mechanisms that operate during DNA replication.[86] RNA viruses are more likely to demonstrate antigenic drift—which is caused by the accumulation of mutations in particular regions of some of the viral antigens. The classic example is influenza virus, in which mutations are found in about 10% of the HA molecule. Mutants may emerge under the immune pressure of antibody specific for the parental virus. The ability to evade preexisting antibody may be greatly enhanced by the occurrence of antigenic shift—that is, the recombination of RNA segments that may occur if the virus has a segmented genome.[122] In the case of influenza virus vaccines, the effect of antigenic drift is largely controlled by the annual production of vaccine with the antigenic specificity of the most recently isolated prevalent strains. Fortunately, antigenic shift occurs much less frequently.

The additional steps involved in the replication of retroviruses, such as the need for a reverse transcriptase that is especially error prone,[98] can lead to an even greater prevalence and accumulation of mutations. For instance, not only has more than 30% of the amino acid sequence in the envelope antigen of HIV been found to vary, but, in the V3 loop of the antigen, more than 10 different amino acids can occupy some individual residue sites.[123]

It is not clear why some RNA viruses such as measles seem to remain for the most part antigenically constant, whereas others such as polio occur as several subtypes, each of which shows only limited antigen drift, and still others, such as influenza and HIV, show marked drift.

T Cell Determinants

Particularly in persistent infections, antigenic drift in T cell determinants should also be expected to occur. Escape by a virus from CTL control was first shown with LCMV in a transgenic mouse model.[142] The high prevalence of amino acid sequence variation makes HIV a good candidate for production of CTL escape mutants.[110] Many CTL determinants have been identified in the major antigens of HIV.[130] Escape mutants were found in several determinants in the gag protein presented by human leukocyte antigen B8 (HLA-B8); in contrast, the response directed by HLA-B27 was found to be more stable.[130] Mutations that allow escape of infected cells from CTL lysis could be a factor contributing to the final escape of HIV from the immune response. Should this turn out to be a critical event, then vaccines composed of only one or two viral antigens, in contrast to whole virus, may have a lesser chance of inducing protective CTL-based immunity. An important factor however, would be the rate at which mutations occurred in different CTL determinants.

Other Mechanisms

Antibodies

Antibody may result in immune enhancement by facilitating uptake of viral-antibody complexes by receptors for Fc or complement into cells that support viral replication. The classic case is dengue virus infection, in which immune enhancement is thought to lead to hemorrhagic shock. Immune enhancement has been shown with HIV in vitro, especially with serum from patients with AIDS-related complex or AIDS,[155] but the extent to which this contributes to viral escape from control in vivo is not clear. The finding that epitopes recognized by enhancing antibodies sometimes differ from neutralizing epitopes[156] is of potential importance for HIV vaccine development.

T Cells

In a primary infection (in the absence of preexisting specific antibody), viral persistence occurs primarily because of the ability to evade the T-cell response. This may take different forms. A variety of viruses, including vesicular stomatitis virus,[83] SV40,[152] herpes simplex virus,[91] adenovirus,[135a] and pseudorabies,[111] can induce the downregulation of MHC antigens in various ways, for example by a viral protein that binds to the MHC molecule (adenovirus[34]) or interferes with the stability of the MHC molecule (cytomegalovirus[21]). In vivo in mice, cytomegalovirus can induce suppression of CTL formation; suppression is released if cells in the draining lymph nodes are cultivated in vitro with a cytokine such as IL-2.[169a] Transfer of CTLs that recognize early or intermediate viral antigens mediates protective immunity,[149] as has been shown with other viruses.

In the case of such infections, a protective vaccine should aim to induce high protective antibody levels and a large pool of memory CTL cells, which, on early stimulation, should lyse infected cells early during the replication cycle, before their numbers become sufficient to cause the major suppressive effects seen in natural infections. This is based on the current indications that the requirements for activation of memory T cells are less stringent than those for naive T cells. It is probable that the highly effective adenovirus vaccine acts in this way.

Potentially more difficult to control are situations in which important cells of the immune system become infected, such as CD4+ T cells and dendritic cells in the case of HIV.[105] Many people infected with HIV develop remarkably strong and continuing CTL responses,[105] which, however, fail to control the infection. It was early proposed[1] that progeny of the invading virus were able to reach immunologic sanctuaries before the immune system responded adequately. It is known that once viremia occurs after infection, HIV can be recovered from distant sites such as the central nervous system and semen. In one case, HIV-1 was detected in the brain within 2 weeks of infection.[49] The aim of a vaccine is clearly to inactivate free virus and destroy infected cells in those regions draining the infection site before widespread dispersion occurs.

MOLECULAR MIMICRY AND AUTOIMMUNITY

Very extensive databanks of amino acid sequences have shown that the antigens of many pathogens and normal host proteins share some amino acid sequences. These have mainly been revealed through the use of MAbs,[133] but it is expected to occur at the T-cell level as well. In one case in which a peptide from a viral antigen shared 60% homology with myelin basic protein, immunization with the viral peptide induced pathologic lesions in the brain.[63] (The homology needs to be partial, not complete, in order to induce immunity). The prevalence of molecular mimicry is so high that infection with any virus would be expected to induce some autoimmunity. Viral infections have been implicated in at least eight different diseases with an autoimmune etiology.[4] To my knowledge, standard vaccination practices have not resulted in the development of autoimmune disease.[179]

As shown by amino acid sequence analogies or serology, different regions of HIV proteins, but especially env, have been found to share amino acid homology with at least 12 different normal host proteins, including HLA, IL-2, and immunoglobulins. Autoantibodies to a wide range of different cells and proteins have also been detected in HIV infection (see Tables 30 and 31 in Levy[104]). This autoimmunity is considered by many to be a significant contributing factor to the pathogenesis of this infection. So common are these sequence analogies in the env protein in particular that it becomes impractical to delete many sequences from a vaccine candidate. For example, homology has been reported between the pentapeptide sequence at the crown of the V3 loop, the principal neutralizing domain of HIV, and some variable regions of human immunoglobulin.[184]

Some viral infections (e.g., HIV, Epstein-Barr virus) can result in polyclonal B cell proliferation and excess antibody production, including autoantibodies. It is possible that certain cytokines (IL-6, TNF-α) are involved in this process.[104]

OPTIMIZING THE PROSPECTS FOR SUCCESSFUL VACCINATION

Successful vaccination involves two levels of consideration—one of a general nature, of importance in most cases, and a second that applies to particular circumstances.

General Requirements

Four general requirements for successful vaccination can be formulated, based primarily but not entirely on our understanding of the reasons why live attenuated virus vaccines in particular are usually highly effective[5]:

1. Activation of APCs, which involves the processing of antigens by either the lysosomal or the cytoplasmic route, expression of costimulatory factors at the cell surface, and probably also the secretion of cytokines.
2. Activation, replication, and differentiation of T and B lymphocytes to generate large pools of memory cells of both types.
3. Generation of effector T and B cells to sufficient peptide determinants and epitopes, respectively, preferably (if possible) from conserved regions of the viral antigens. This is both to limit the effects of antigen variation and, in the case of T cells, to minimize the effects of MHC antigen polymorphism in an outbred population.
4. Long-term persistence of conformationally-intact antigen, preferably as aggregates of antigen complexed with anti-

body, to allow the continuing formation of memory B cells, followed by their recruitment to form ASCs. This is to ensure the continuing production of viral-specific antibody of increasingly higher affinity.

Routes of Immunization

With the exceptions mainly of vector-borne viruses and those that can infect the body through breaks in the skin (e.g., poxviruses), most viruses infect through a mucosal surface. Yet, the majority of current viral vaccines are administered parenterally. Two exceptions are the live poliovirus and adenovirus vaccines, which illustrate two points: (1) immunization at the site of natural infection (poliovirus) can be remarkably effective, and (2) immunization through one mucosal surface can protect at another mucosal site. The adenovirus vaccine is administered orally in an enteric-coated capsule and protects against a respiratory infection. This protective effect is transmitted through the common mucosal system. Similarly, preparations to protect against a respiratory infection have been administered both to humans and to animals through the respiratory tract.

Studies on the gut-associated lymphoid tissue and the different conditions that influence the development of immunity or tolerance are far too extensive to review here. In contrast, much less is known about conditions for generating long-lasting immunity in the eye or in the genitourinary system and the rectum. Although sexually transmitted diseases have been with us since time immemorial, the advent of antibiotics largely controlled bacterial infections, and viral infections were considered not life-threatening. The HIV pandemic, reinforced by the association of human papillomavirus with cervical cancer and the spread of genital herpes, has forever changed that view.

Although the rectal mucosa is rich in associated lymphoid tissue,[97] there are relatively few reports of developing this route for immunization.[61a] In contrast, the female reproductive tract is not well endowed with accessory lymphoid tissue, and although immune responses to locally deposited noninfectious preparations occur, they are in general weak and short-lived.[138,113] Two factors may be important. First, there is evidence for neuroendocrinal regulation of mucosal immunity, particularly at this site.[25] Second, it is known that the production by a small proportion of women of antisperm antibodies results in infertility, so that in order to reproduce the species, females should not readily mount an immune response to sperm (a noninfectious particle). A paucity of lymphoid tissue adjacent to the mucosal epithelium could be one way to achieve this situation. In contrast, intravaginal administration of an attenuated virus (herpesvirus type 2) to mice was rapidly followed by an immune response that protected against challenge by the virulent organism administered by the same route. Here, it was shown that effector T cells, including CTLs, migrated from the draining lymph nodes (where the virus replicated) to the infected genital tissue. Adoptive transfer of CTLs (but not B cells) was protective.[109]

Will immunization by other mucosal routes confer protection in the female reproductive tract? Is this tract part of the common mucosal system? There are several reports that administration of antigens orally, especially the beta subunit of cholera toxin (CT-*B*), leads to the presence of antibody in vaginal washes.[190] In another case, apparently complete protection against chlamydial infection in the lung and genital tract occurred after oral administration of live chlamydial organisms in mice.[47] However, the relative paucity of encouraging findings suggests that use of this route by itself may not be an effective approach. Several recent reports[78,101,179] suggest that vaccines intended for protection at the vaginal mucosa may best be administered by the rectal route. Immunization with a recombinant SIV p27 gag protein expressed as a hybrid Ty virus particle and conjugated with CT-*B* at the vaginal or rectal sites, gave good IgA responses, especially if it was augmented by an oral boost.[100,179]

Another approach is to immunize at nonmucosal sites in the subserous and presacral spaces in the pelvic area, and this has resulted in higher and better-sustained IgA titers in the vaginal washings.[138] It is likely that these responses were initiated and generated in the iliac and lumbar lymph nodes that drain the reproductive tract. It was subsequently shown[95] that immunization with the SIV construct and alum[95,179] at a subcutaneous site adjacent to the lymph nodes draining the genitourinary region (GURALT immunization) resulted in mucosal secretory IgA and IgG antibody formation, serum antibody production, and T cell proliferatve responses. It is not known whether this effect can also be augmented by oral administration of the candidate vaccine.

The prospects for finding practical and effective ways to generate long-lasting responses in the genitourinary region now look more promising. At the same time, some progress is being made toward immunization against chlamydial eye infection to prevent trachoma.

Immunopotentiation

Although first used more than 50 years ago,[67] alum remains the only adjuvant licensed for general medical use. The development of other adjuvants led to Freund's complete adjuvant,[15] composed of whole mycobacteria and mineral oil, which is much more potent but so granulomagenic that it is unsuitable for human use (and, in some countries, for animal use). This, in turn, led to a search for the active components of such complex preparations and, finally, to the isolation of the muramyl dipeptides and some bacterial cell wall components. This search for effective but safe adjuvants was intensified after subunit preparations of microorganisms became prospects as candidate vaccines for many diseases.

A formulated adjuvant can have three roles. One role is to act simply as a depot so that the antigen is released over time. More recently, this role has been largely subsumed by devices such as controlled-release formulations composed of neutral, biodegradable materials.[118]

A second role occurs when a formulation is used that targets appropriate cells, particularly APCs and lymphocytes. Three categories of formulations have been described.[124] The first is covalently-linked (or mixed) antigen-immunostimulant complexes; an example is the complexing of antigen with CT-*B*

TABLE 16-5. *Activities of some immunostimulants in adjuvant for formulations*

Product	Formulation	Immune response (enhancement/ induction)	Cytokine profile
Alum	As Alhydrogel	Most Ig classes, poor DTH	TH2>TH1
FCA	Without emulsion	Most Ig classes, strong DTH	TH1>TH2
MDP derivatives	Free	Selected Ig classes, poor DTH	TH2>TH1
	As emulsion	Selected Ig classes, improved DTH	TH1/TH2
LPS		Most Ig classes, strong DTH	TH1>TH2
MPL		Selected Ig classes, strong DTH	TH1>TH2
CT-*B*	Mixed with or conjugated	Strong IgA	TH2>TH1
Inulin	With alum (Algammulin)	Most Ig classes, good DTH, CTLs	TH1/TH2
Quil A, QS21.	Free or as ISCOMS	Selected Ig classes Selected Ig classes, good DTH, CTLs	TH1>TH2

FCA, Freund's complete adjuvant; MDP, muramyl dipeptide; LPS, lipopolysaccharide; MPL, monophosphoryl lipid; CT-*B*, the beta subunit of cholera toxin; QS21, an isolated fraction of saponin; ISCOMS, immunostimulating complexes.

Modified from Ada GL. Vaccines. In: Paul WE, ed. Fundamental immunology. 3rd ed. New York: Raven Press, 1994:1309–1352; and Cooper PD. The selective induction of different immune response by vaccine adjuvants. In: Ada GL, ed. Strategies in vaccine design. Austin: RG Landes, 1994:125–158.

subunit, which is an efficient immunostimulant for mucosal immunity because it binds to ganglioside GM$_1$ receptors on cells.[87] Second is encapsulation of the antigen into formulations such as liposomes or gels. For example, liposomes readily disperse to draining lymph nodes, where they can interact with APCs. Finally, emulsions of antigen and immunostimulant with oil droplets can be used, commonly with Arlacel A as a stabilizer. Emulsions of metabolizable oils in water are now emerging as efficient formulations,[178] because they also promote rapid dispersion to lymph nodes.[124]

The third and critical role is performed by the immunostimulant itself, which, on contact with the target cell, may induce cytokine production and secretion, expression of cellular receptors for the cytokines, and efficient processing of antigen in APCs.

The use of stimulants may achieve two desirable effects. One is a general enhancement of the immune response; the second is a qualitative change in the type of immune response generated. Other, less specific responses may contribute to unacceptable adverse effects such as local necrosis, granuloma formation, hypersensitivity, and fever.[44,118] Such unwanted responses can often be lessened if the immunostimulant has a short halflife in vivo. A great range of substances display immunostimulating activity,[6,44,124] and it is impracticable to comment on all of these in this chapter. Table 16-5 summarizes both some data and interpretations (in part from Cooper[44] and from Myers and Gustafson[124]) concerning the activities of various preparations that are either in clinical evaluation or in experimental investigation. All provide enhancement of selected or most immunoglobulin subclasses. Some give no enhancement of DTH responses, and their effects therefore mimic those of a TH2-type response. Others may considerably enhance DTH responses, and two induce CTL responses,[129a] leading to an interpretation that TH1 responses are strongly enhanced.

Much of the recent work in this area is consistent with the interpretation that the principal role of immunostimulators is to induce the production and secretion of cytokines and the expression of their receptors. Some cytokines have profound effects on the final immune response. IL-5 (expressed by infection with a recombinant viral vector) enhances specific mucosal IgA responses in vivo.[146] In addition, infection of mice with a recombinant virus expressing IL-4, a cytokine which strongly favors TH2-type responses, substantially suppressed the generation of CTLs and led to a delayed clearance of the virus.[165] In contrast, IL-12 has been shown to favor TH1 responses. The time may now be close at hand when certain cytokines will be used in vaccine preparations to induce selective immune responses. For instance, *Leishmania major* infection in BALB/c mice results in a predominantly TH2 response, with serious disease and eventually death. By immunizing mice with a preparation of leishmanial antigens and IL-12, antigen-specific CD4+ TH+ cells were generated, and the mice became resistant to challenge with the live organisms.[12]

MAJOR ADVANCES IN THE DESIGN OF VACCINES

Although a number of new approaches have been described for the development of vaccines against infectious diseases,

TABLE 16-6. *New approaches to vaccine development*

Synthesis of oligonucleotides: important peptide sequences, either B cell epitopes or T cell determinants, linked together or conjugated to carrier proteins to form the immunogen

Application of recombinant DNA (rDNA) technology

Transfection of cells with rDNA coding for viral proteins—bacterial cells, yeast cells, or mammalian cells (primary cells, cell strains, or cell lines)

Recombinant (chimeric) live vectors: incorporation of DNA or complementary DNA coding for viral antigens into the genome of other viruses or bacteria, some of which are the basis of current vaccines

"Naked" DNA: DNA coding for viral proteins, in the form of a plasmid, injected directly into cells

two general approaches stand out (Table 16-6). One is the synthesis and linkage of oligopeptides representing desired amino acid sequences (B cell epitopes, T cell determinants) from relevant antigens. The second depends on the ability to manipulate DNA coding for proteins (glycoproteins) of the infectious agent. Three approaches involving rDNA are briefly discussed: transfection of cells with DNA coding for one or more antigens; construction of recombinant live vectors, either viruses or bacteria, containing DNA coding for antigens; and direct administration of DNA (in the form of a plasmid) containing coding for the antigens of interest. The latter two approaches have an advantage in not requiring additional immunopotentiation.

Oligopeptide-Based Approaches

Ever since Sela[164] showed almost 30 years ago that antibody could be raised against synthetic oligopeptides constructed in different ways, and the later realization that neutralizing antibody and T cells were directed to only small segments of one or a few viral antigens, there has been continuing interest in developing oligopeptide-based vaccines. In principle, such preparations have some very attractive advantages, but there are also some potential disadvantages (Table 16-7).

Major constraints to this approach include the extent of antigenic variation in a protective viral antigen, the probable need for multiple epitopes or determinants to compensate for MHC polymorphism, and the finding that many B cell epitopes in viral antigens are not only conformational but probably also discontinuous (i.e., are formed by different segments of the same or adjacent molecules).[16,128] But there are examples in the viral, bacterial, parasitic, and hormonal areas of investigation[6] in which at least one important B cell epitope is clearly linear. Viral examples[31] include HIV (the env antigen), foot-and-mouth disease virus (the VP1 antigen), and hepatitis B virus (the surface antigen).

There are several sites in the HIV gp120 that are important for neutralization of viral infectivity. The V3 loop, often called the immunodominant neutralizing domain of HIV-1, is linear and immunogenic. The loop contains about 33 amino acid residues. Although the amino acid sequence GPGR, which forms the crown of the loop, is largely conserved, as

TABLE 16-7. *Perceived advantages and disadvantages in the production and use of peptide-based vaccines*

PERCEIVED ADVANTAGES

1. Chemically well-defined product
2. High-temperature, chemical, and biologic stability
3. No infectious agent (or nucleic acid genome) present in final product or during production
4. Ability to include only those sequences representing protective B cell epitopes and T cell determinants
5. Ability to largely, if not entirely, eliminate sequences with undesirable properties, such as suppressor activity, molecular mimicry with host sequences (risk of autoimmune disease), and induction of infection-enhancing antibody responses. In certain cases, administration of a peptide-based preparation may be the most effective way to avoid the risk of autoimmune disease.
6. Ability to conjugate with other components (hydrophobic transmembrane peptide sequences, lipid tails) so that class I as well as class II MHC–restricted responses are generated
7. Ability to conjugate with a carrier protein that is a rich source of T cell determinants
8. Ability to produce as particles, as multiple antigenic peptides or other forms
9. Ability to encapsulate with biodegradable microspheres or capsules to give potentially long-term immune responses after a single administration

PERCEIVED DISADVANTAGES

1. Particularly in the case of viruses (e.g., influenza, polio), not only are important B cell epitopes discontinuous, but adjacent molecules contribute; there is no general way to synthesize a corresponding B cell epitope.
2. Even if a B cell epitope is linear, single amino acid mutations outside the sequence can affect the antigenic specificity of the epitope, presumably by conformational changes.
3. The need in some cases to include several B cell epitopes and T cell determinants may make this approach impracticable.
4. One or more peptide bonds that, in the protein, may be protected by conformational constraints or sugar side chains, may make the corresponding peptide more susceptible to proteolysis.
5. A potent adjuvant, capable of causing undesirable side effects, may be required to induce a sufficient immune response.
6. Depending on the manufacturing process used (chemical versus biological synthesis), the manufacturing costs may make the product unaffordable for some countries.

Modified from Ada GL. Vaccines. In: Paul WE, ed. Fundamental immunology. 3rd ed. New York: Raven Press, 1994: 1309–1352.

many as 11 different amino acids can occupy some individual residue sites on the flanks of the loop. Apart from the neutralizing epitope, the loop contains both a TH and a CTL determinant.[95] Although it is linear, the loop has a preferred conformation, because a single mutation in a site downstream from the loop can affect the binding of some MAbs to the loop sequence.[125] A number of other TH and CTL determinants in gp120 have also been identified.[24]

Three families of constructs have been made and are in clinical trials. The T1-SP10 construct contain a 16-residue helper T cell determinant, joined by the amino terminal to a peptide sequence from the V3 loop.[136] HIV-IIIB and HIV-MN constructs elicited high-titer, type-specific neutralizing antibodies[79,136] as well as CD8+ CTL responses.[80] A panel of hybrid peptides containing clusters of helper T cell determinants fused to a V3 loop segment derived from HIV-IIIB has been made. One construct, PCLUS6-18, produced responses in all four haplotypes of mice tested and high neutralizing antibody titers that were partially crossreactive.[13] After a single admin-

istration with the adjuvant QS21, several constructs elicited memory CD8+ CTLs.[168] Additional experimentation should further elucidate optimum conditions for linking peptide epitopes and determinants to obtain improved responses.

Another approach that looks particularly promising is to construct multiantigenic peptides. It is known that repetition of epitopes enhances the immunogenicity of a protein preparation,[55] and this can also apply to linked peptides.[31] Eight V3 peptides of HIV-IIIB, including the conserved GPGR at the apex of the V3 loop together with a sequence upstream of the loop, were linked by the amino terminals of a heptalysine core.[186] The resulting octamer was used to immunize guinea pigs. After two administrations in alum, high and long-persisting neutralizing titers were obtained. Their specificity broadened over time to include neutralization (but to lower titers) of MN and RF_2 strains. By mixing preparations of different epitope specificities, it should be possible to prepare cocktails of octamers that largely match the specificity profiles in different regions.

Peptides may be modified so that they prime for CTL responses. One way is to covalently attach a lipophilic tail, such as tripalmitoyl-glycerylcysteinyl-seryl-serine, to the peptide.[50] Another is to select an appropriate adjuvant (see Table 16-5). In each case, the net result may be insertion of the complexes into the plasma membrane, with subsequent facilitation of processing by the cytoplasmic pathway.

Although no peptide-based vaccine is yet licensed for general medical use, it seems only a matter of time before this occurs.

Approaches Based on Recombinant DNA Technology

The discovery of bacteriophage-mediated transduction in 1952[198] indicated the potential of viruses as tools for moving foreign genetic material from one cell to another. With the advent of rDNA technology, infectious vectors could be engineered to have particular properties, which in turn would help to answer specific questions. Two approaches have evolved. A plasmid can be constructed and used to transfect a cell, leading to expression of the incorporated DNA. Or an infectious virus can be used as a vector to replicate inside the cell. Both of these approaches can serve as means to determine the importance of individual gene products of disease agents in protective immune responses or to produce large amounts of particular gene products. The former approach is discussed first.

Transfection of Cells

Three types of cell systems have been used for transfection: prokaryotic cells (e.g., *Escherichia coli*), lower eukaryotic cells (e.g., yeast), and mammalian cells, either as primary cells, cell strains, or cell lines.

Prokaryotes

Two modes of expression have been used in *E coli*, either expression as a fusion protein (i.e., the new polypeptide is fused to an existing bacterial protein such as β-galactosidase), or expression as a "native" protein. Some bacterial proteins, such as the pilus antigens of *E coli*, have been made in this way, but direct expression of the HA gene of influenza virus or of the HBsAg resulted in unsatisfactory products. Because proteins produced in this way are not glycosylated, this approach is probably inadequate for glycoproteins and possibly for mammalian viral proteins in general.

Lower Eukaryotes

Yeast (*Saccharomyces cerevisiae*) has several advantages as an expression system, and much is known about its genetics. Yeast components as impurities in a product are unlikely to be a concern because exposure to yeast is commonplace, and a yeast-derived product could be produced by bulk fermentation. Though glycosylation occurs, the pattern is different from that seen in mammalian cells. HBsAg, the first genetically engineered human vaccine, is produced by transfected yeast. It is treated by thiocyanate and formaldehyde to obtain and fix an optimum conformation.[84] Both complete and anchor-deficient influenza virus HA molecules in a glycosylated form have been made in this way, and the products reacted with MAbs to the native molecule.[127] However, an HIV gp120 made in this way failed to bind to CD4, the receptor on TH cells for HIV attachment, and hence was regarded as denatured, because this binding is strictly conformation dependent.[1894]

Mammalian Cells

Although cultured mammalian cells are used for the production of some viral vaccines (e.g., poliovirus in primary monkey kidney cells, rubella and rabies viral vaccines in cells that have a finite capacity to replicate), there remains some concern about the production of vaccines in cells that have the capacity to replicate indefinitely. However, as experience is gained, they are being used more extensively. For example, genetically modified Chinese hamster ovary cells are used as substrates for the production of HIV gp120.[22,23] One product made in this way[76] gave antibody with higher neutralization titers than a comparable product made in yeast, and, after repeated immunization, more crossreactive antibody.

Recombinant Live Vectors of Foreign DNA

The second approach has additional advantages to those already outlined. Because many attenuated live virus vaccines in particular have been highly successful, there is a great potential for making genetic recombinants of some of these viruses, to be used as vaccines to control diseases for which no vaccines exist. Incorporation of the genes coding for different cytokines would also provide the opportunity to study the effects of individual cytokines on the immune response to the candidate immunogens.

TABLE 16-8. *Infectious agents in use or proposed as vectors of nucleic acids from other sources*

Viruses—animal
  Vaccinia*
  ORF
  Herpes
  Varicella
  Adenovirus*
  Papillomavirus
  SV40
  Poliovirus*
  Influenza
Viruses—avipox
  Fowlpox
  Canarypox*
Bacteria
  Salmonella spp
  Bacille Calmette-Guérin
  Escherichia coli

*Examples of these agents as vectors are presented in the text.

Table 16-8 contains a list of infectious agents either in use or proposed as vectors of nucleic acids from other sources. Far more work has been carried out with poxviruses, especially vaccinia, than with any other vector, for reasons such as the large capacity for insertion of foreign DNA, the existence of promoters that allow gene expression either early or late in the replication cycle, a broad host range, and the availability of different viral strains used during the smallpox eradication campaign.[26]

Recombinant Poxviruses

Many nucleotide sequences near both ends of the viral genome are nonessential for viral growth and can be deleted, making room for the insertion of foreign DNA. Different promoters allow early, intermediate, or late expression of the inserted gene, and this can have selective effects, such as the induction of CTL activity to some determinants. In the case of the influenza virus nucleoprotein determinants, CTLs specific for the sequence 50-63, but not for the sequence 365-379, could recognize late-expressed nucleoprotein. This defect in late presentation could be overcome by increasing the rate of degradation of the expressed antigen in the cell.[181] Similarly, whereas antibody levels to early- and late-expressed herpesvirus glycoprotein D were indistinguishable, DTH and T-cell proliferation to the late-expressed antigen were reduced.[185] The early expression of T-cell determinants appears to optimize the effector T-cell response well before infectious viral particles are assembled and secreted.

Construction of recombinant vaccinia viruses has become an extraordinarily useful technique. Viruses that have served as sources of DNA or cDNA coding for different antigens include rabies, hepatitis B, herpes, cytomegalovirus, Epstein-Barr, influenza, parainfluenza, measles, dengue, Japanese encephalitis, Lassa fever, RSV, and HIV/SIV.[43,45] Immunization of mammals, especially rodents, with most of these preparations has resulted in antibody production, T-cell proliferation, and CTL memory. Solid protection against the wild-type agent has frequently been demonstrated. Two examples are given here.

First, a vaccinia-rabies glycoprotein construct has been used to protect foxes from rabies infection.[140] The vaccine was administered as bait for oral consumption and has undergone successful field trials. The local eradication of fox (and possibly other wild-type) rabies may be achieved if the following criteria are met: a potent, safe, and thermostable vaccine; an efficient bait system; a practical and sure method of bait dispersal; and an effective spatial and temporal pattern of bait distribution. Second, a construct containing the HA or fusion proteins (or both) of rinderpest virus has elicited neutralizing antibodies and protected cattle from a severe challenge.[195] This virus is a major pathogen of cattle, particularly in Africa, and it has been suggested that this vaccine may offer the prospect of rinderpest eradication in the future.[194]

In contrast, immunization of chimpanzees, the animal model closest to humans, with hepatitis B[119] and RSV[41] constructs has not yielded such impressive protection, and this has dimmed some of the enthusiasm for this vector for human use. It remains, however, a potent way to produce viral antigens in their natural conformational state, especially since a two-step procedure has been described that results in higher yields of the foreign antigen.[62]

A potential problem with the use of current smallpox vaccine strains as vectors for human vaccination is the level of complications observed during the eradication campaign.[59] This has stimulated three different approaches to overcome this disadvantage. First is the production of recombinants containing DNA coding for interleukins, the first example of which was the inclusion of the gene for IL-2. When such constructs were administered to athymic (nu−/nu−) mice,[61,147] the treated mice survived the vaccinia virus infection even though all mice receiving the control vaccinia died. It was later shown that the expression of IL-2 induced the expression of IFN-γ, a potent antiviral agent.[148] Although this approach may not be used widely as a means of indirectly attenuating viral virulence, it is proving valuable for defining the roles of different cytokines in modulating infection by the vector.

In contrast to the classic methods for viral attenuation, vaccinia virus can now be reproducibly attenuated by the specific deletion of certain genes without diminishing its potential as a vector of foreign genes. This remarkable development has been reviewed elsewhere.[26] One preparation, NYVAC,[174] was constructed by deleting 18 open reading frames, including six genes involved in nucleotide metabolism, from the Copenhagen vaccine strain.

The third approach is the use of avipox virus strains that undergo abortive replication in mammalian cells. The inability of this virus to productively replicate in humans should make it very safe to use as a vector. Infection of mammalian cells with a recombinant fowlpox containing genes coding for the gag/pol proteins of SIV resulted in the secretion of lentivirus-like particles.[90] A canarypox virus (ALVAC) construct containing the rabies virus glycoprotein has been shown to be as effective as the donor rabies virus in conferring protection against rabies.[176] When a similar preparation was administered in a phase I trial to human volunteers, it generated protective levels of antirabies antibody that were only slightly less in titer to those given by the diploid cell vaccine. A single booster dose at 6 months induced a similar recall response in volunteers primed with either vaccine.[37] This result suggests that the level of neutralizing antibody to the vector itself after a primary immunization is so low that it would not prevent an effective response to a second immunization with a different ALVAC recombinant, a very useful property for a vector to possess. ALVAC constructs containing the genes coding for one or more antigens of HIV are currently in clinical trials.[90]

Recombinant Adenoviruses

Human adenoviruses offer several advantages as a vector. Serotypes Ad4 and Ad7, the strains present in the safe and effective human vaccine (see Table 16-1), have been adapted as potential vectors and can accommodate up to 7 kb of foreign DNA. In addition, the virus is readily grown in mammalian cell tissue culture, a high copy number of the viral DNA is present in the infected cell, and the viral genome possesses several strong promoters. Oral administration of the recombinant should provide mucosal immunity against the donor of the inserted DNA. Recombinant constructs have been made with genes from hepatitis B (HBsAg[1117,196]), measles (HA[14]), herpes simplex virus (glycoprotein B[97]), and HIV/gp160.[126]

Adenovirus may become very important as a vector for mediating gene therapy at different sites.[46] For example, in in vivo experiments, constructs containing the gene for 1-antitrypsin successfully delivered the inserted gene to rat lung epithelial cells,[156] and one containing a β-galactosidase (as a reporter gene) delivered the latter to muscle cells.[144a]

Recombinant Polioviruses

The success of OPV in providing effective protection at a mucosal surface raised the possibility that it could be used as a vector for foreign genes.[16] Intertypic hybrid viral particles were constructed, in which short amino acid sequences (approximately 15 amino acids in length) from type 2 or type 3 polioviruses were grafted into the highly-exposed B-C loop of VP1 (antigenic site 1) of the very safe type 1 virus. It then became feasible to graft amino acid sequences (B cell epitopes) from other viruses into this same site. However, this approach was severely limited by the small size of the fragment that could successfully be inserted without compromising the infectivity of the recombinant virus.

A more recent approach has been to replace the VP2 and VP3 genes within the capsid precursor protein, P1, by the in-frame insertion of foreign genes. This recombinant virus can successfully be encapsidated if P1 is provided in trans by a recombinant vaccinia helper virus.[144] On infection, the minireplicons so formed expressed HIV-1 *gag* and *pol*. Because these structures do not productively replicate, it remains to be seen whether such structures are sufficiently immunogenic when administered by either a mucosal or a parenteral route.

DNA Vaccines

The discovery that DNA itself can function as a vaccine and induce protective responses has generated great interest. Injection of plasmids containing the DNA sequence coding for a viral antigen directly into muscle can lead to the persistent production of specific antibody and CTLs. Injection of cDNA encoding the influenza nucleoprotein that contains CTL determinants recognized by all strains was shown to result in the long-lived (for many months) production of CTLs that gave cross-protection against lethal disease.[183] Mice immunized in this way with a plasmid containing the influenza HA resisted a lethal challenge of virus of the same subtype.[151a] In an extension of this work, it was shown[64] that the DNA could be administered by different routes, including a mucosal (respiratory) route. Particularly impressive was the demonstration that by the use of a gene gun, DNA-coated, microscopic gold beads (300 to 600 plasmids per bead) could be injected into the abdominal epidermis, whence other cells, probably Langerhans dendritic cells, carried the particles to the draining lymph nodes. Delivery by gene gun is far more efficient than injection of the DNA in saline. In preliminary experiments with plasmids containing DNA coding for HIV *env, pol,* or *env+pol,* high titers of neutralizing antibody have been achieved.[153]

IMMUNOTHERAPY

Most vaccines were designed for the prevention of disease on subsequent exposure to the wild-type agent. Specific neutralizing antibody was the first line of defense, reducing the load of challenge infectious virus to the extent that the host's own immune response could cope with nonneutralized virus without disease occurring. The two situations in which vaccine was knowingly administered to those already exposed to the wild-type agent were hepatitis B in newborn infants and rabies. In the former case, administration with specific immune serum enhances the level of protection.

The advent of HIV/AIDS changed this outlook. Here was an infectious disease that persisted for many years without outward signs of morbidity but resulted finally in death for most exposed people. Salk[158] first suggested immunizing asymptomatic people with the intention of clearing the infection or delaying progress toward disease, and others soon followed.[197,154] It has now become a significant field of endeavor, with many groups participating.[42] Using initially the rate of decrease of CD4+ T cells as a marker of effective immunization, some early results suggested that immunization stabilized the CD4+ T-cell count. A measurement of viral burden (in blood) was later added as a more general indicator of efficacy. However, although there is clearly a much higher level of infection in lymph nodes compared with blood, this is difficult to measure routinely, so it may take a considerable time to establish how effective this type of intervention may be.

There are three types of immune responses that are potentially beneficial in HIV infection:

1. Increased proliferative T-cell responses, particularly to determinants either not or only poorly recognized during natural infection. This has been observed in some cases.[42,150] It is thought that this in turn may lead to an increase in other effector responses (antibody, CTLs), resulting in greater protection.
2. The generation of higher levels of protective antibody. The evidence that this may be helpful is not strong (see later discussion). It may depend on the extent to which the new antibody is more crossreactive compared with existing antibody.
3. The generation of higher levels and more broadly crossreacting CTL responses.{/NL}

It is not difficult to produce arguments suggesting that these approaches may do little more than either offer temporary respite or perhaps be counterproductive. First, it has been pointed out[162] that increases in the number of activated CD4+ T cells after immunization may lead to greater opportunities for HIV infection and hence viral spread. Second, there are several reports of transfer of human immune serum or hyperimmune animal immunoglobulin to asymptomatic HIV-infected persons[135] with some apparently beneficial effects, but presumably this would favor over time the emergence of resistant, mutant strains, which could persist even if additional transfusions were carried out. Trials are in progress to transfuse immune sera to HIV-infected mothers in the hope that this will reduce the risk of perinatal viral transmission. This approach could be more successful, because the critical period during which viral load should be reduced is relatively short.

Third, there is encouraging but circumstantial evidence that CTLs hold viral levels in check for long periods. Should asymptomatic HIV patients progressing toward AIDS-related complex or AIDS receive injections of homologous CTLs at a time when the natural response is deteriorating? Trials are in progress to study the feasibility of storing peripheral blood lymphocytes of recently infected asymptomatic patients and, when appropriate, stimulating aliquots containing the CTL precursors in vitro for reinjection to the donor. Finally, in view of the correlation between slow progression to disease and CD4+ TH1 response,[166] an additional approach may be to immunize asymptomatic patients in a way that favors a TH1-type T cell response.

VIRUS-ASSOCIATED TUMORS

The term immunosurveillance was introduced to describe the concept of resistance to the development of tumor by an immunologic mechanism.[35] However, nude (athymic, nu−/nu−) mice were usually found to be no more susceptible to spontaneous tumors than their normal littermates.[116] Similarly, common cancers do not occur with greater than normal frequency among immunodeficient people with AIDS[75] or among immunosuppressed recipients of allografts.[141] Therefore, the common tumors do not seem to be controlled by immune responses. In contrast, recent observations suggest that at least some tumors grow and persist because they have developed ways to evade an immune response that may otherwise be mounted against them.[29]

The experience with virally-induced or virus-associated tumors is quite the opposite and is more consistent with the concept of immunosurveillance.[161] The DNA viruses, SV40 and polyomavirus, may induce tumors in animals. CTLs specifically recognize fragments from the SV40 T antigen in association with class I MHC and so control the virus-infected cells.[132] The early antigens of adenovirus, E1A and E1B, are transcribed in both normal and transformed cells, and the antigens so produced are required for maintenance of the transformed phenotype. Adenovirus downregulates the expression of the class I MHC molecule at the infected cell surface.[135a] This makes transformed cells less susceptible to CTLs, thus providing a mechanism for the tumor to avoid immunosurveillance.

At least three DNA viruses are associated with human cancer. Primary liver cancer may occur after infection with hepatitis B virus. The availability since the early 1980s of a vaccine to prevent this infection is expected to lower the incidence of this cancer. This effect will take some time to become evident, because the vaccine has only recently become available in regions (particularly Asia) where the prevalence of this cancer is high. Some strains of human papillomaviruses are associated with cervical cancer, and Epstein-Barr virus infection is associated with endemic Burkitt's lymphoma and nasopharyngeal carcinoma. Only one RNA virus, human T-cell lymphotropic virus (HTLV-1), is known to be associated with a human cancer, endemic adult T-cell leukemia. Vaccines are not yet available against these oncogenic viruses.

SUMMARY AND CONCLUSIONS

Role of Different Immune Responses

Table 16-9 summarizes the role of different effector populations (or their products) after vaccination against viral infections. Binding of antibody to particular epitopes is the only effector mechanism that can specifically prevent or greatly limit an initial infection. Preformed antibody can be a major means of limiting and reducing an infection. Under special circumstances, it may clear an intracellular infection, but it is doubtful whether this ever occurs in a natural infection, and it may be difficult to find an immunization schedule that induces the formation of antibody of sufficiently high titer and affinity to achieve clearance.

CMI responses have the major role to play in reducing and clearing viral infections. In experimental (unmodified) animal models, CD8+ CTLs have been shown to clear several different acute infections. It is uncertain whether CD4+ TH1 cells can achieve this result in the absence of CTLs, although the findings to date strongly suggest that TH1 cells can at least limit viral infections. Although certain interleukins may favor production of one or the other cell type, one of the difficulties facing attempts to elucidate further the role of both TH1 and TH2 cells is that there is currently no way of physically separating them.

Most live attenuated virus vaccines induce both a strong humoral and a CMI response. How may this be achieved with noninfectious viral vaccines? Use of an adjuvant (see Table 16-5) that enhances both responses may be satisfactory. But if there is a need for a strong secretory IgA response as well as a strong TH1/CTL response, which would seem to be the case with sexually transmitted diseases and especially with HIV, an

TABLE 16-9. *Roles of different immune responses during viral infections*

Response	Prevent infection	Limit infection	Reduce infection	Clear infection
Nonadaptive*	—	++	+	—
Adaptive				
Antibody	+++	+++	+++	+/—
CD4+, TH1	—	++	++	++?
CD8+, CTLs	—	+/++	+++	+++

*Not possessing memory or specificity.

+++, major mechanism; ++, important mechanism; +, has some effect; +/− only a few positive examples; −, no effect.

alternative approach may be to administer the preparation simultaneously by two routes—a mucosal route for an adjuvant that preferentially stimulates secretory IgA responses, and a parenteral route for an adjuvant that enhances both TH1 and CTL responses.

Mixed Vaccine Formulations

An additional possibility, suggested by recent work on HIV candidate vaccines, is the use of different formulations of a vaccine preparation for priming as opposed to boosting the immune response. This was suggested by the finding that immunization of vaccinia-naive volunteers with an HIV gp160–vaccinia virus construct followed by boosting with a recombinant gp160 preparation gave higher anti-gp160 antibody titers than use of either preparation for both priming and boosting.[70] In an extension of this work,[56] it was found that after the priming immunization alone, there were persistent (>1 year) T-cell proliferative responses and production of IFN-γ. After boosting at this late time point, specific T-cell proliferative responses, IFN-γ production, and CTL activity occurred, and these activities persisted for more than 15 months. The concept that different ways of presenting a given antigen may favor priming versus boosting of the response is relatively new. It seems to depend on the efficacy of induction of T cell memory by the priming immunization. Use of such a finding could be a valuable approach, especially in cases such as HIV, in which the antibody responses to the current candidate vaccines have usually been poor.

Combination Vaccines

Currently, MMR live attenuated virus vaccines are administered as a mixture. The success of such a cocktail depends on establishing that interference among the viruses is not a problem (i.e., that each replicates sufficiently well to induce an adequate immune response).

The current WHO Expanded Programme of Immunization schedule for the administration of childhood vaccines, including those against polio and measles viruses and shortly also against hepatitis B, involves in developing countries up to six visits by health workers. Additional vaccines to combat childhood diseases will probably be added to the list in due course. There is great pressure to reduce this number of visits.[53] One approach is to use biodegradable, controlled-release preparations[118] to minimize repeated administrations of subunit and possibly peptide-based vaccines. Two of the new technologies described here also offer special opportunities for simplifying the administration of protein-based vaccines. The first is the use of live vectors. The different poxvirus preparations offer particular opportunities. Either DNA coding for several foreign proteins can be incorporated into a single virion, or different chimeric preparations using the same vector can be included in a single formulation. In either case, the formulation could be tailored to suit particular regional needs. Potentially, the technique of vaccinating with mixtures of different naked DNA plasmid constructs coding for different antigens would seem to offer a similar flexibility.

ABBREVIATIONS

AIDS: acquired immunodeficiency syndrome
APC: antigen-presenting cell
ASC: antibody-secreting cell
ca: cold-adapted [strain of influenza virus]
CMI: cell-mediated immunity
CT-*B*: the beta subunit of cholera toxin
CTL: cytotoxic T lymphocyte
DTH: delayed-type hypersensitivity
HA: hemagglutinin
HBsAg: surface antigen of hepatitis B virus
HIV: human immunodeficiency virus
HLA, HLA-B8, HLA-B27: human leukocyte antigens
HTLV-1: human T-cell lymphotropic virus
IFN, IFN-α, IFN-β, IFN-γ: interferons
IgA, IgD, IgE, IgG, IgM: immunoglobulins
IL-2, IL-4, IL-5, IL-6, IL-10, IL-12: interleukins
IPV: inactivated poliovirus [vaccine]
LCMV: lymphocytic choriomeningitis virus
MAb: monoclonal antibody
MHC: major histocompatibility complex
MMR: measles, mumps, rubella [vaccine]
NK: natural killer [cell]
NP: nucleoprotein
OPV: oral polio vaccine
rDNA: recombinant DNA
RSV: respiratory syncytial virus
SIV: simian immunodeficiency virus
SSPE: subacute sclerosing panencephalitis
SV40: simian virus 40
TCR: T-cell receptor
TH: helper T lymphocyte
TNF-α, TNF-β: tumor necrosis factors
WHO: World Health Organization

REFERENCES

1. Ada GL. Prospects for HIV vaccines. J AIDS 1988;1:295–303.
2. Ada GL. The immune response to antigens: the immunological principles of vaccination. Lancet 1990;335:523–526.
3. Ada GL. Vaccination in third world countries. Curr Opin Immunol 1993;5:683–686.
4. Ada GL. Immune response: general features. In: Webster RG, Granoff A, eds. Encyclopedia of virology. Vol 2. New York: Academic Press, 1994:698–703.
5. Ada GL. Vaccination strategies to control infections: an overview. In: Ada GL, ed. Strategies in vaccine design. Austin: RG Landes, 1994;2–16.
6. Ada GL. Vaccines. In: Paul WE, ed. Fundamental immunology. 3rd ed. New York: Raven Press, 1994:1309–1352.
7. Ada GL. Vaccines and immune response. In: Webster RG, Granoff A, eds. Encyclopedia of virology. Vol 3. New York: Academic Press, 1994:1503–1507.
8. Ada GL, Blanden RV, Mullbacher A. HIV: to vaccinate or not to vaccinate. Nature 1992;359:572.
9. Ada GL, Jones PD. The immune response to influenza virus. Curr Top Microbiol Immunol 1986;128:1–54.
10. Acha-Orbea H, Scarpellino L, Hertig S. et al. Inhibition of lymphocyte-mediated cytotoxicity by perforin anti-sense oligonucleotides. EMBO J 1990;9:3815–3819.
11. Adler LO, Bess JW, Sowder RC II, et al. Cellular proteins bound to immunodeficiency viruses: implications for pathogenesis and vaccines. Science 1992;258:1935–1938.

12. Afonso LCC, Scharton TM, Vieira LQ, et al. The adjuvant effect of interleukin-12 in a vaccine against *Leishmania major*. Science 1994;263:235–237.

13. Ahlers JD, Pendelton CD, Dunlop N, et al. Construction of an HIV-1 peptide vaccine containing a multideterminant helper peptide linked to a V3 loop peptide 18 inducing strong neutralizing antibody responses in mice of multiple MHC haplotypes after two immunizations. J Immunol 1993;150:5647–5665.

14. Alkhatib G, Briedis DJ. High-level eucaryotic in vivo expression of biologically active measles virus hemagglutinin by using an adenovirus type 5 helper-free vector system. J Virol 1988;62:2718–2827.

15. Allison AC, Byars NE. Adjuvants for a new generation of vaccines. In: Woodrow GC, Levine MM, eds. New generation vaccines. New York: Marcel Dekker, 1990:129–140.

16. Almond JW, Burke KL. Poliovirus as a vector for the presentation of foreign antigens. Semin Virol 1990;1:11–20.

17. Ashman RB. Persistence of cell-mediated immunity to influenza A virus in mice. Immunology 1982;47:165–168.

18. Askonas BA, McMichael AJ, Webster RG. The immune response to influenza virus infection and the problem of protection against infection. In: Beare, ed. Basic and applied influenza virus research. Boca Raton, FL: CRC Press, 1982:159–188.

19. Baenziger J, Hengartner H, Zinkernagel RM, Cole GA. Induction or prevention of immunopathological disease by cloned cytotoxic T cell lines specific for lymphocytic choriomeningitis virus. Eur J Immunol 1986;16:387–393.

20. Beasley RP, Hwang LY, Lee G C-Y. Prevention of perinatally transmitted hepatitis B virus infections with hepatitis B immune globulin and hepatitis B vaccine. Lancet 1983;2:1099–1102.

21. Beersma MFC, Bijlmakers MJE, Ploegh HL. Human cytomegalovirus down-regulates HLA class 1 expression by reducing the stability of class 1 H chains. J Immunol 1993;151:4455–4464.

22. Bermann PW, Gregory TJ, Riddle L, et al. Protection of chimpanzees from infection by HIV-1 after vaccination with recombinant glycoprotein gp120 but not gp160. Nature 1990;345:622–625.

23. Bermann PW, Mathews TJ, Riddle L, et al. Neutralization of multiple laboratory and clinical isolates of human immunodeficiency virus type-1 (HIV-1) by antisera raised against gp120 from the MN isolate of HIV-1. J Virol 1992;66:4464–4469.

24. Berzofsky JA, Pendelton CD, Clerici M, et al. Construction of peptides encompassing multideterminant clusters of HIV envelope to induce in vitro T-cell responses in mice and humans of multiple MHC types. J Clin Invest 1991;88:876–885.

25. Bienenstock J, Croitoru K, Ernst PB, et al. Neuroendocrine regulation of mucosal immunity. Immunol Invest 1989;18:69–76.

26. Binns MM, Smith GL, eds. Recombinant poxviruses. Boca Raton, FL: CRC Press, 1992:1–343.

27. Bittle JL, Houghten RA, Alexander H, et al. Protection against foot and mouth disease by immunization with a chemically synthesized peptide predicted from the viral nucleotide seqence. Nature 1982; 298:30–33.

28. Black FL, Rosen L. Patterns of measles antibodies in residents of Tahiti and their stability in the absence of re-exposure. J Immunol 1962;88:725–731.

29. Bodmer WF, Browning MJ, Krausa P, et al. Tumor escape from immune response by variation in HLA expression and other mechanisms. Ann N Y Acad Sci 1993;690:42–49.

30. Bretscher PA. Requirements and basis for efficacious vaccination by a low dose regimen against intracellular pathogens uniquely susceptible to a cell-mediated attack. In: Ada GL, ed. Strategies in vaccine design. Austin: RG Landes, 1994:99–112.

31. Brown F. The potential of peptides as vaccines. Semin Virol 1990; 1:67–74.

32. Bukowski JF, Woder BA, Welch RM. Pathogenesis of murine cytomegalovirus infection in natural killer cell-depleted mice. J Virol 1984;52:119–128.

33. Buller ML. Rational designs for attenuated live virus vaccines. In: Ada GL, ed. Strategies in vaccine design. Austin: RG Landes, 1994: 159–178.

34. Burgert H-G, Kvist S. The E3/19K protein of adenovirus type 2 binds to the domains of histocompatibility antigens required for CTL recognition. EMBO J 1987;6:2016–2019.

35. Burnet FM. The concept of immunological surveillance. Prog Exp Tumor Res 1970;13:1–27.

36. Burton GF, Kapasi ZF, Szakal AK, Tew JG. The generation and maintenance of antibody and B cell memory: the role of retained antigen and follicular dendritic cells. In: Ada GL, ed. Strategies in vaccine design. Austin: RG Landes, 1994:35–50.

37. Cadoz M, Strady A, Meigner B, et al. Immunization with canary pox virus expressing rabies glycoprotein. Lancet 1992;339:1429–1432.

38. Chanock RM, Murphey BR, Collins PL, et al. Live viral vaccines for respiratory and enteric tract disorders. Vaccine 1988;6:129–133.

39. Clerici M, Lucey DR, Berzofsky JA, et al. Restoration of HIV-specific cell–mediated immune responses by interleukin 12 in vitro. Science 1993;262:1721–1724.

40. Cole GA, Nathanson N, Prendergast RA. Requirements for theta-bearing cells in lymphocytic choriomeningitis virus–induced central nervous system disease. Nature 1972;238:335–338.

41. Collins PL, Purcell RH, London WT, et al. Evaluation in chimpanzees of vaccinia virus recombinants that express the surface glycoproteins of human respiratory syncytial virus. Vaccine 1990;8: 164–168.

42. Conference on Advances in AIDS Vaccine Development: National Cooperative Vaccine Development Groups, Alexandria, October 1993.

43. Cooney EL, Collier AC, Greenberg PD, et al. Safety and immunological response to a recombinant vaccinia virus vaccine expressing HIV-1 glycoprotein Lancet 1991;337:567–572.

44. Cooper PD. The selective induction of different immune response by vaccine adjuvants. In: Ada GL, ed. Strategies in vaccine design. Austin: RG Landes, 1994:125–158.

45. Cox WI, Tartaglia J, Paoletti E. Poxvirus recombinants as live vaccines. In: Binns M, Smith GL, eds. Recombinant poxviruses. Boca Raton, FL: CRC Press, 1992:123–162.

46. Cristiano RJ, Smith LC, Kay MA, et al. Hepatic gene therapy: efficient gene delivery and expression in primary hepatocytes utilizing a conjugated adenovirus-DNA complex. Proc Nat Acad Sci U S A 1993;90:11548–11552.

47. Cui Z-D, Tristram D, LaScolea LJ, et al. Induction of antibody response to *Chlamydia trachomatis* in the genital tract by oral administration. Infect Immun 1991;59:1465–1469.

48. Daniel MD, Kirchoff F, Czajak SC, et al. Protective effects of a live attenuated SIV vaccine with a deletion in the *nef* gene. Science 1992;258:1938–1941.

49. Davis LE, Hjelle Bl, Miller VE, et al. Early viral brain invasion in iatrogenic human immunodeficiency virus infection. Neurology 1992;42:1736–1739.

50. Deres K, Schild H, Weismuller K-H, et al. In vivo priming of virus-specific cytotoxic T lymphocytes with synthetic lipopeptide vaccine. Nature 1989;342:561–564.

51. Doherty PC. Virus infections in mice with targeted gene disruptions. Curr Opin Immunol 1993;5:479–483.

52. Doherty PC, Zinkernagel RM. T cell-mediated pathology in viral infections. Transplant Rev 1974;19:89–120.

53. Douglas RG. The children's vaccine initiative: will it work? J Infect Dis 1993;168:269–274.

54. Egea E, Iglesias A, Salazar M, et al. The cellular basis for lack of antibody response to hepatitis B vaccine in humans J Exp Med 1991;173:531–538.

55. Eichelberger MC, Wang M, Allan W, et al. Influenza virus RNA in the lung and lymphoid tissue of immunologically intact and CD4-depleted mice. J Gen Virol 1991;72:1695–1698.

56. El-Daher N, Keefer MC, Reichman RC, et al. Persisting immunodeficiency virus type 1 gp160-specific human T lymphocyte responses including CD8+ cytotoxic activity after receipt of envelope vaccines. J Infect Dis 1993;168:306–313.

57. Enders JF, Weller TM, Robbins FC. Cultivation of the Lansing strain of poliomyelitis virus in cultures of various human embryonic tissues. Science 1949;109:85–87.

57a.Evans DMA, Dunn G, Minor PD, et al. Increased neurovirulence associated with a single nucleotide change in a noncoding region of the Sabin type 3 polio vaccine genome. Nature 1985;314:548–550.

58. Fauci AS. Multifactorial nature of human immunodeficiency virus disease: implications for therapy. Science 1993;262:1011–1018.

59. Fenner F. Viral vectors for vaccines. In: Bell R, Torrigiani G, eds. New approaches for vaccine development. Basel: Schwabe, 1984: 187–192.

60. Fenner FJ, Henderson DA, Arita I, Jezek Z, Ladnyi ID. Smallpox and its eradication. Geneva:World Health Organization, 1988.
61. Flexner H, Hugin A, Moss B. Prevention of vaccinia virus infection in immunodeficient mice by vector-directed IL-2 expression. Nature 1987;330:259–262.
61a.Forrest BD, Shearman DJC, LaBrooy JT. Specific immune responses in humans following rectal delivery of live typhoid vaccine. Vaccine 1990;8:209–212.
62. Fuerst TR, Earl PL, Moss B. Use of a hybrid vaccinia virus T7 RNA polymerase system for expression of target genes. Mol Cell Biol 1987;7:2538–2544.
63. Fujinami R, Oldstone MBA. Amino acid homology between the encephalitogenic site of myelin basic protein and virus: mechanism for autoimmunity. Science 1985;230:1043–1045.
64. Fynan EF, Webster RG, Fuller DH et al. DNA vaccines: protective immunizations by parenteral, mucosal, and gene-gun inoculations. Proc Nat Acad Sci U S A 1993;90:11478–11482.
65. Galaska AM, Lauer BA, Henderson RH, Keja J. Indications and contraindications for vaccines used in the Expanded Programme of Immunization. Bull World Health Organ 1984;62:357–366.
66. Geisow MJ. Unravelling the mysteries of molecular audit: MHC class I restriction. Tibtech 1991;9:403–404.
67. Glenny AT, Pope GC, Waddington H, Wallace U. Immunological notes 23: the antigenic value of toxoid precipitated with potassium alum. J Pathol Bacteriol 1926;29:38–39.
68. Glenny AT, Sudmerson NJ. Notes on production of immunity to diphtheria toxin. J Hygiene 1921;20:176–220.
69. Good RA, Zak SJ. Disturbances in gamma globulin synthesis as "experiments of nature." Pediatrics 1956;18:109–149.
70. Graham BS, Matthews TJ, Belshe RB, et al. Augmentation of human immunodeficiency virus type 1 neutralizing antibody by priming with gp160 recombinant vaccinia and boosting with rgp160 in vaccinia naive adults. J Infect Dis 1993;167:533–537.
71. Gray D, Skarvall HB. B cell memory is shortlived in the absence of antigen. Nature 1988;336:70–72.
72. Gray D, Sprent J, eds. Immunological memory. Curr Top Microbiol Immunol 1990;159:1–141.
73. Griffin DE, Levine B, Tyor WB, Irani DN. The immune response in viral encephalitis. Semin Immunol 1992;4:111–119.
74. Griffin DE, Ward BJ. Differential CD4 T cell activation in measles. J Infect Dis 1993;168:275–281.
75. Groopman JE. Neoplasms in the acquired immune deficiency syndrome: the multidisciplinary approach to treatment. Semin Oncol 1987;14:1–6.
76. Haigwood NL, Nara PL, Brooks E, et al. Native but not denatured recombinant human immunodeficiency virus type 1 gp120 generates broad spectrum neutralizing antibodies in baboons. J Virol 1992;66:172–182.
76a.Haller O. Inborn resistant of mice to orthomyxoviruses. Curr Top Microbiol Immunol 1981;92:25–52.
77. Halsey NA. Increased mortality following high titer measles vaccines: too much of a good thing. Pediatr Infect Dis J 1993; 12: 462–465.
78. Haneberg B, Kendall D, Amerongen HM, et al. Induction of specific immunoglobulin A in the small intestine, colon-rectum, and vagina measured by a new method for collection of secretions from local mucosal surfaces. Infect Immun 1994;62:15–23.
79. Hart MK, Palker TJ, Matthews TJ, et al. Synthetic peptides containing T and B cell epitopes from human immunodeficiency virus envelope gp120 induce anti-HIV proliferative responses and high titers of neutralizing antibodies in rhesus monkeys. J Immunol 1990;145:2677–2685.
80. Hart MK, Weinhold KJ, Scearce RM, et al. Priming of anti-human immunodeficiency virus (HIV) CD8+ cytotoxic T cells in vivo by carrier-free HIV synthetic peptides. Proc Nat Acad Sci U S A 1991; 88:9448–9452.
81. Hashimoto G, Wright PF, Karzon DT. Antibody-dependent cell-mediated cytotoxicity against influenza virus–infected cells. J Infect Dis 1983;148:785–794.
82. Hayder H, Blanden RV. Role of CD8+ T cells in viral infections. In: Ada GL, ed. Strategies in vaccine design. Austin: RG Landes, 1994: 69–82.
83. Hecht TT, Summers DF. Effect of vesicular stomatitis virus infection on the histocompatibility antigens of L cells. J Virol 1972;10: 578–585.
83a.Hilleman MR. The dilemmas of HIV vaccine and therapy: possible clues from comparative pathogenesis with measles. AIDS Res Hum Retrovir 1992;8:1743–1747.
84. Hilleman MR. Vaccine perspectives from the vantage of hepatitis B. Vaccine Res 1992;1:1–15.
85. Hiu S, Hyland L, Ryan KW, Portner A, Doherty PC. Virus-specific CD8+ T-cell memory determined by clonal burst size. Nature 1994;369:652–654.
86. Holland J, Spindler K, Horodyski F, et al. Rapid evolution of RNA genomes. Science 1982;215:1577–1585.
87. Holmgren J, Lycke N, Czerkinsky C. Cholera toxin and cholera B subunit as oral-mucosal adjuvant and antigen vector systems. Vaccine 1993;11:1179–1184.
88. Hussein RH, Sweet C, Collie MH, Smith H. Elevation of nasal viral levels by suppression of fever in ferrets infected with influenza viruses of differing virulence. J Infect Dis 1982;145:520–524.
89. Jackson DC, Ada GL, Tha Hla R. Cytotoxic T cells recognize very early, minor changes in ectromelia virus–infected target cells. Aust J Exp Biol Med Sci 1976;54:349–363.
90. Jenkins S, Gritz L, Fedor CH, et al. Formation of lentivirus particles by mammalian cells infected with recombinant fowlpox virus. AIDS Res Hum Retroviruses 1991;7:991–998.
91. Jennings SR, Rice PL, Kloszewski ED, et al. Effect of herpes simplex virus types 1 and 2 on the surface expression of class 1 major histocompatibity complex antigens on infected cells. J Virol 1985; 56:757–766.
92. Johnson DC, Ghosh-Choudhury G, Smiley JR, et al. Abundant expression of herpes simplex virus glycoprotein gB using an adenovirus vector. Virology 1988;164:1–14.
93. Kagi D, Ledermann B, Burki K. et al. Cytotoxicity mediated by T cells and natura killer cells is greatly impaired in perforin-deficient mice. Nature 1994;369:31–36.
94. Kapikian AZ, Mitchell RH, Chanock RM, Shvedoff RA, Stewart CE. An epidemiological study of altered reactivity to respiratory syncytial (RS) virus infection in children previously vaccinated with an inactivated virus vaccine. Am J Epidemiol 1969;89:405–421.
95. Karzon D. Preventive vaccines. In: Broder S, Merigan TC, Bolognesi D, eds. Textbook of AIDS Medicine. Baltimore: Williams & Wilkins, 1994;667–692.
96. Kundu SK, Merigan TC. Equivalent recognition of HIV proteins, env, gag and pol, by CD4+ and CD8+ cytotoxic T lymphocytes. AIDS 1992;6:643–649.
96a.Kyburz D, Speiser DE, Battegay M, et al. Lysisi of infected cells in vivo by antiviral cytotoxic T cells demonstrated by release of cell internal viral proteins. Eur J Immunol. 1993;23:1540–1545.
97. Langman JM, Rowland R. The number and distribution of lymphoid follicles in the human large intestine. J Anat 1986;194:189–195.
98. Larder BA, Kemp SD, Purifoy DJM. Infectious potential of human immunodeficiency virus type 1 reverse transcriptase mutants with altered inhibitor sensitivity. Proc Nat Acad Sci U S A 1989;86: 4803–4807.
99. Lau LL, Jamieson BD, Somasundaram T, Ahmed R. Cytotoxic T cell memory without antigen. Nature 1994;369:648–651.
100. Lehner T, Bergmeier LA, Panagiotidi C, et al. Induction of mucosal and systemic immunity to a recombinant simian immunodeficiency viral protein. Science 1992;258:1365–1369.
101. Lehner T, Brookes R, Klavinskis L, et al. T cell and antibody responses induced by mucosal or associated lymphoid tissue immunization of macaques with SIV vaccines. J Cell Biochem Suppl 18B 1994:157(Abst J 409).
101a.Leung KN, Ada GL. The effect of helper T cells on the primary in vitro production of delayed type hypersensitivity to influenza virus. J Exp Med 1981;153:1029–1053.
102. Leung KN, Ada GL. Different functions of subsets of effector T cells in murine influenza virus infection. Cell Immunol 1982;67: 312–324.
103. Levine B, Griffin DE. Persistance of viral RNA in mouse brain following recovery from acute alphavirus encephalitis. J Virol 1992; 66:6429–6435.
104. Levy JA. Pathogenesis of human immunodeficiency virus infection. Microbiol Rev 1993;57:183–289.
105. Lin YL, Askonas BA. Biological properties of an influenza A virus-specific killer T cell clone. J Exp Med 1981;154:225–234.

106. Lipsey AI, Kahn MJ, Bolande RJ. Pathological variants of congenital hypogammaglobulininemia: an analysis of three patients dying of measles. Pediatrics 1967;39:659–674.

106a. Luchacher AE, Morrison LA, Braciale VA, et al. Expression of specific cytolytic activity by H-2 I-region restricted influenza-specific T lymphocyte clones. J Exp Med 1985;162:171–187.

107. Mak NK, Schiltknecht E, Ada GL. Protection of mice against influenza virus infection: enhancement of non-specific cellular responses by *Corynebacterium parvum*. Cell Immunol 1983;78:314–324.

108. Mak N-K, Zhang Y-H, Ada GL, Tannock GA. Humoral and cellular responses of mice to infection with a cold-adapted influenza A virus variant. Infect Immun 1982;38:218–225.

109. McDermott LR, Goldsmith CH, Rosenthal KL, Brais LJ. T lymphocytes in genital lymph nodes protect mice from intravaginal infection with herpes simplex virus type 2. J Infect Dis 1989;159:460–466.

110. McMichael A, Gotch F. The role of cytotoxic T lymphocytes in HIV infection. In: Neu HC, Levy JA, Weiss RA, eds. Focus on HIV. Edinburgh: Churchill Livingstone, 1993:135–148.

111. Mellencamp MW, O'Brien PCM, Stevenson JR. Pseudorabies virus–induced suppression of major histocompatibility complex class I antigen expression. Virology 1991;65:3365–3368.

112. Miller CJ, Alexander NJ, McChesney MB. Vaccines to prevent sexually transmitted diseases: the challenge of generating protective immunity at genital mucosal surfaces. In: Ada GL, ed. Strategies in vaccine design. Austin: RG Landes, 1994:194–212.

113. Miller JJ III. An autoradiograph study of plasma cell and lymphocyte survival in rat popliteal lymph nodes. J Immunol 1964;92:673–676.

114. Mims CA, White DO. Viral pathogenesis and immunology. Oxford: Blackwell Scientific, 1984.

115. Misko IS, Pope JH, Hutter R, et al. HLA-DR-antigen-associated restriction of EBV-specific cytotoxic T cell clones. Int J Cancer 1984;33:239–243.

116. Moller G, ed. Experiments and the concept of immunological surveillance. Transplant Rev 1976;28:1–97.

117. Molnar-Kimber KL, Davis AR, Jarocki-Witek V, et al. Characterization and assembly of hepatitis B envelope proteins expressed by recombinant adenoviruses. UCLA Symp Mol Cell Biol 1987;70:173–187.

118. Morris W, Steinhoff MC, Russell PK. Potential of polymer microencapsulation technology for vaccine innovation. Vaccine 1994;12:5–11.

119. Moss B, Smith GL, Gerin JL, Purcell RH. Live recombinant vaccinia virus protects chimpanzees against hepatitis B. Nature 1984;311:67–71.

120. Mullbacher A. The long-term maintenance of cytotoxic T cell memory does not require persistence of antigen. J Exp Med 1994;179:317–321.

121. Mullbacher A, Ada GL. How do cytotoxic T cells work in vivo? Microb Pathog 1987;3:315–318.

121a. Muller D, Koller BH, Whitton JL, et al. LCMV-specific class II–restricted cytotoxic T cells in β2-microglobulin deficient mice. Science 1992;255:1576–1577.

122. Murphey BR, Webster RG. Orthomyxoviruses. In: Fields BN, ed. Virology. 2nd ed. New York: Raven Press, 1990:1091–1154.

123. Myers G. Analysis: protein information summary. In: Myers G, Berzofsky JA, Korber B, Smith RF, Pavlakis G, eds. Human retroviruses and AIDS, 1991: a compilation and analysis of nucleic acid and amino acid sequences. Los Alamos, NM: Los Alamos National Laboratory, 1991:iii–4.

124. Myers KR, Gustafson GL. Adjuvants for human vaccine usage: a rational design. In: Cryz SJ, ed. Vaccines and immunotherapy. New York: Pergamon Press, 1991:404–411.

125. Nara PL, Smit L, Dunlop N, et al. Emergence of viruses resistant to neutralization by V3 specific antibodies in experimental human immunodeficiency virus type IIIB infection of chimpanzees. J Virol 1990;64:3779–3791.

126. Natuk RJ, Chanda PK, Lubeck MD, et al. Adenovirus-human immunodeficiency virus (HIV) envelope recombinant vaccines elicit high-titered HIV-neutralizing antibodies in the dog model. Proc Nat Acad Sci U S A 1992;89:7777–7781.

127. Nayak DP, Jabbar MA. Expression of influenza viral hemagglutinin (HA) in yeast. In: Kendall AP, Patriaca PA, eds. *Saccharomyces cerevisiae*. New York: Alan R Liss, 1986:357–373.

128. Nestorowicz A, Laver G, Jackson DC. Antigenic determinants of influenza virus hemagglutinin: X. A comparison of the physical and antigenic properties of the monomeric and trimeric forms. J Gen Virol 1985;65:1687–1695.

129. Newell CK, Martin S, Sendele D, Mercadal CM, Rouse BT. Herpes simplex virus-induced stromal keratitis: role of T lymphocyte subsets in immunopathology. J Virol 1989;63:769–755.

129a. Newman MJ, Munroe KJ, Anderson CA, et al. Induction of antigen-specific killer T lymphocyte responses using subunit SIV_{mac251} *gag* and *env* vaccines containing QS21 saponin adjuvant. AIDS Res Hum Retroviruses 1994;10:853–860.

130. Nixon DF, Brodilen K, Ogg G, Brodilen P-A. Cellular and humoral antigenic epitopes on HIV and SIV. Immunology 1992;76:515–534.

131. Nossal GJV, Ada GL. Antigens, lymphoid cells and the immune response. New York: Academic Press, 1971:1–324.

132. O'Connell KA, Gooding LR. Cloned cytotoxic T lymphocytes recognize cells expressing dicrete fragments of the SV40 tumor antigen. J Immunol 18984;132:953–958.

132a. Oehen S, Hengartner H, Zinkernagel RM. Vaccination for disease. Science 1991;251:195–198.

133. Oldstone MBA, Schwimmbeck P, Dyrberg T, Fujinami R. Mimicry by virus of host molecules: implications for autoimmune disease. Prog Immunol 1986;6:787–798.

134. Orentas RJ, Hildreth JF, Obeh E, et al. Induction of human CD4 cytotoxic T cells specific for HIV-infected cells by a gp160 subunit vaccine. Science 1990;248:1234–1237.

135. Osther K, Wiik A, Black F, et al. PASSHIV-1 treatment of patients with HIV infection: a preliminary report of a phase I trial of hyperimmune porcine immunoglobulin to HIV-1. AIDS 1992;6:1457–1464.

135a. Paabo S, Severinsson L, Andersson M, et al. Adenovirus proteins and MHC expression. Adv Cancer Res 1989;52:151–163.

136. Palker TJ, Matthews TJ, Langois A, et al. Polyvalent human immunodeficiency virus synthetic immunogen comprised of envelope gp120 T helper cell sites and B cell neutralization epitopes. J Immunol 1989;142:3612–3619.

137. Pantaleo G, Graziosi C, Demarest JF, et al. HIV infection is active and progressive in lymphoid tissue during the clinically latent stage of disease. Nature 1993;362:355–358.

138. Parr EL, Parr MB. Local immunization for anti-fertility immunity. In: Griffin PD, Johnson PM, eds. Local immunity in reproductive tract tissues. Oxford: Oxford University Press, 1993;441–458.

139. Parry N, Fox G, Rowlands D, et al. Structural and serological evidence for a novel method of antigenic variation in foot and mouth disease virus. Nature 1990;347:569–572.

140. Pastoret P-P, Brochier B, Blancou J, et al. Development and deliberate release of a vaccinia-rabies recombinant virus for the oral vaccination of foxes against rabies. In: Binns M, Smith GL, eds. Recombinant poxviruses. Boca Raton, FL: CRC Press, 1992:163–206.

141. Penn I. Tumors of the immunocompromised patient. Annu Rev Med 1988;39:373–385.

142. Pircher H, Moskophidis D, Rohrer U, et al. Viral escape by selection of cytotoxic T cell resistant virus variant in vivo. Nature 1990;346:629–633.

143. Plotkin SA, Mortimer EA. Vaccines. 2nd ed. Philadelphia: WB Saunders, 1994:1–995.

144. Porter DC, Ansardi DC, Choi WS, Morrow CD. Encapsidation of genetically engineered poliovirus minireplicons which express human immunodeficiency virus type 1 gag and pol proteins upon infection. J Virol 1993;67:3712–3719.

144a. Quantum B, Perricaudet LD, Tajbakhsh S, Mandel J-L. Adenovirus as an expression vector in muscle cells in vivo. Proc Nat Acad Sci U S A 1992;89:2581–2584.

145. Ramphal R, Cogliano RE, Shands JW, Small PA. Serum antibody prevents lethal murine influenza pneumonitis but not tracheitis. Infect Immun 1979;25:992–996.

146. Ramsay AJ, Kohonen-Corish M. Interleukin-5 expressed by a recombinant virus vector enhances specific mucosal IgA responses in vivo. Eur J Immunol 1993;23:3141–3145.

147. Ramshaw IA, Andrew ME, Phillips SM, et al. Recovery of immunodeficient mice from a vaccinia virus/IL-2 recombinant infection. Nature 1987;329:545–546.

148. Ramshaw I, Ruby J, Ramsey A, Ada G, Karupiah G. Expression of cytokines by recombinant vaccinia viruses: a model for studying

cytokines in virus infections in vivo. Immunol Rev 1992;127: 157–182.

149. Reddehase MJ, Mutter W, Munch K, et al. CD8+ T lymphocytes specific for murine cytomegalovirus immediate-early antigens mediate protective immunity. J Virol 1987;61:3102–3108.

150. Redfield RR, Birx DL, Ketter N, et al. A phase I evaluation of the safety and immunogenicity of vaccination with recombinant gp160 in patients with early human immunodeficiency virus infection. N Engl J Med 1991;324:1677–1684.

150a.Renegar KB, Small PA. Passive transfer of local immunity to influenza virus infection by IgA antibody. J Immunol 1991;146:1972–1978.

151. Renegar KB, Small PA. Immunoglobulin A mediates murine anti-influenza virus immunity. J Virol 1992;65:2146–2148.

151a.Robinson HL, Hunt LA, Webster RG. Protection against a lethal influenza virus challenge by immunization with a hemagglutinin-expressing plasmid DNA. Vaccine 1993;11:957–959.

152. Robinson HL, Fynan EF, Lu S, et al. Gene vaccines: a new approach to immunization. J Cell Biochem 1994;18B:J5.

153. Robinson WE, Gorny MK, Xu J-Y, et al. Two immunodominant domains of gp41 bind antibodies which enhance human immunodeficiency virus type 1 infection in vitro. J Virol 1991;65:4169–4176.

154. Robinson WE, Montifiore DC, Mitchell WM. Antibody-dependent enhancement of human immunodeficiency virus type 1 infection. Lancet 1988;1:790–794.

155. Rogers MJ, Gooding LR, Margulies DH, Evans GA. Analysis of a defect in the H2 genes of SV40 transformed C3H fibroblasts that do not express H-2Kk. J Immunol 1983;130:2418–2422.

156. Rosenfeld MA, Siegfried W, Yoshimura K, et al. Adenovirus-mediated transfer of a recombinant 1-anti-trypsin gene to the lung epithelium in vivo. Science 252:431–434.

157. Rubin BA, Rorke LB. Adenovirus vaccines. In: Plotkin SA, Mortimer EA, eds. Vaccines. Philadelphia: WB Saunders, 1988:492–512.

158. Salk J. Prospects for the control of AIDS by immunizing seropositive individuals. Nature 1987;327:473–476.

159. Schild GC, Oxford JS, DeJong JC, Webster RG. Evidence for host cell selection of influenza virus antigenic determinants. Nature 1983;303:706–709.

160. Schiltknecht E, Ada GL. Influenza virus specific T cells fail to reduce lung viral titers in cyclosporin-treated infected mice. Scand J Immunol 1985;22:99–103.

161. Schreiber H. Tumor immunology In: Paul WE, ed. Fundamental immunology. 3rd ed. New York: Raven Press, 1993:1143–1178.

162. Schwartz DH. Potential pitfalls on the road to an effective HIV vaccine. Immunol Today 1994;15:54–57.

163. Schwartz RH. Costimulation of T lymphocytes: the role of CD28, CTLA-4 and B7/BB1 in interleukin-2 production and immunotherapy. Cell 1993;71:1065–1068.

164. Sela M. Immunological studies with synthetic polypeptides. Adv Immunol 1966;5:29–129.

165. Sharma DP, Ramsey AJ, Ramshaw IA. Interleukin-4 expression enhances the pathogenicity of vaccinia virus and suppresses cytotoxic T lymphocyte responses. J Exp Med 1994 (submitted).

166. Shearer GM, Clerici M. CD4+ functional T cell subsets: their roles in infections and vaccine development. In: Ada GL, ed. Strategies in vaccine design. Austin: RG Landes, 1994:113–124.

167. Shellam GR, Grundy JE, Harnett GB, Allen JE. Natural killer cells. Prog Immunol 1986;6:1209–1217.

168. Shirae M, Pendelton CD, Ahlers J, et al. Helper CTL determinant linkage required for priming of anti-HIV CD8+CTL with peptide vaccine constructs. J Immunol 1994 (in press).

169. Shvartsman YS, Zykov MP. Secretory influenza immunity. Adv Immunol 1976;22:291–300.

169a.Sinikas VG, Ashman RB, Blanden RV. The cytotoxic response to murine cytomegalovirus: II. In vitro requirements for generation of cytotoxic T cells. J Gen Virol 1985;66:757–765.

170. Spriggs MK, Koller BH, Sato T, et al. B2-microglobulin- CD8+ T cell-deficient mice survive inoculation with high doses of vaccinia virus and exhibit altered IgG responses. Proc Nat Acad Sci U S A 1992;89:6070–6074.

171. Stanway G, Hughes PJ, Mountford RC, et al. Comparison of the compete nucleotide sequence of the genomes of the neurovirulent Ps/Leon/37 and its attenuated Sabin vaccine derivative P3/Leon/12a,b. Proc Natl Acad Sci U S A 1983;81:1539–1543.

172. Stott J, Kitchen PA, Page M, et al. Anti-cell antibody in macaques. Nature 1991;353:393.

173. Stratton KR, Howe CJ, Johnston RB. Adverse events associated with childhood vaccines: evidence bearing on causality. Washington, DC: Institute of Medicine, National Academy Press, 1994: 1–464.

173a.Sweet C, Smith H. Pathogenicity of influenza viruses. Microbiol Rev 1980;44:303–330.

174. Tartaglia J, Perkus ME, Taylor J, et al. NYVAC: a highly attenuated strain of vaccinia virus. Virology 1992;188:217–232.

175. Taylor G. The role of antibody in controlling and/or clearing virus infections. In: Ada GL, ed. Strategies in vaccine design. Austin: RG Landes, 1994:17–34.

176. Taylor J, Trimarch C, Weinberg R. Efficacy studies on a canarypox-rabies recombinant virus. Vaccine 1991;9:190–196.

177. Taylor PM, Askonas BA. Diversity in the biological properties of anti-influenza cytotoxic T cell clones. Eur J Immunol 1983; 13: 707–711.

178. ten Hagen TLM, Sulzer AJ, Kidd MR, et al. Role of adjuvants in the modulation of antibody isotype, specificity, and induction of protection by whole blood-stage Plasmodium yoelli vaccines. J Immunol 1993;151:7077–7085.

179. Thompson C. Commentary: a slippery defence against HIV. Lancet 1993;342:1500.

180. Tishon A, Eddleston M, de la Torre JC, Oldstone MBA. Cytotoxic T lymphocytes cleanse viral gene products from individually infected neurones and lymphocytes in mice persistently infected with lymphocytic choriomeningitis virus. Virology 1993;197:463–467.

181. Townsend A, Bastin J, Gould K, et al. Defective presentation to class I restricted cytotoxic lymphocytes in vaccinia-infected cells is overcome by enhanced degradation of antigen. J Exp Med 1988; 168:1211–1214.

182. Tschopp J, Nabholz M. Perforin-mediated target cell lysis by cytolytic T lymphocytes. Annu Rev Immunol 1990;8:279–302.

183. Ulmer JB, Donnelly JJ, Parker SE, et al. Heterologous protection against influenza by injection of DNA encoding a viral protein. Science 1993;259:1745–1749.

184. Veljkovic V, Metlas R. Potentially negative effects of AIDS vaccines based on recombinant viruses carrying HIV-1 derived envelope gene. Vaccine 1993;11:291–292.

185. Wachsman M, Aurelian L, Smith CC, et al. Regulation of expression of herpes simplex virus (HSV) glycoprotyein D in vaccinia recombinants affects their ability to protect from cutaneous HSV-2 disease. J Infect Dis 1989;159:625–634.

186. Wang CY, Looney DJ, Li ML, et al. Long-term high-titer neutralizing activity induced by octameric synthetic HIV antigen. Science 1991;254:285–288.

187. Wiley DC, Wilson IA, Skehel JJ. Structural identification of the antibody-binding sites of Hong Kong influenza hemagglutinin and their involvement in antigenic variation. Nature 1981;289: 373–378.

188. Wilson GS. The hazards of immunization. London: Athlone Press, 1967.

189. Wintsch J, Chaignat C-L, Braun DG, et al. Safety and immunogenicity of a genetically engineered human immunodeficiency virus vaccine. J Infect Dis 1991;163:219–225.

190. Wu H-Y, Russell MW. Induction of mucosal immunity by intranasal application of a streptococcal surface protein antigen with the cholera toxin B subunit. Infect Immun 1993;61:314–322.

190a.Yap KL, Ada GL. The recovery of mice from influenza A virus infection: adoptive transfer of immunity with influenza virus–specific cytotoxic T lymphocytes recognizing a common virion antigen. Scand J Immunol 1978;8:413–420.

191. Yap KL, Ada GL. The effect of specific antibody on the generation of cytotoxic T lymphocytes and the recovery of mice from influenza virus infection. Scand J Immunol 1979;10:325–332.

192. Yap KL, Ada GL, McKenzie IFC. Transfer of specific cytotoxic T lymphocytes protects mice inoculated with influenza virus. Nature 1978;273:238–239.

193. Yap KL, Braciale TJ, Ada GL. Role of T cell function in recovery from influenza virus infection. Cell Immunol 1979;103:341–351.

194. Yilma TD. Prospects for the total eradication of rinderpest. Vaccine 1989;7:484–485.
195. Yilma TD, Hsu D, Jones L, et al. Protection of cattle against rinderpest with vaccinia virus recombinants expressing the HA or F gene. Science 1988;242:1058–1061.
196. Yuasa T, Kajino K, Saito I, Miyamura T. Preferential expression of the large hepatitis B surface antigen gene by an adenovirus-hepatitis B virus recombinant. J Gen Virol 1991;72:1927–1934.
197. Zagury D, Bernard J, Cheynier R, et al. A group-specific anamnestic reaction against HIV-1 induced by a candidate vaccine against AIDS. Nature 1988;332:344–346.
198. Zinder ND, Lederberg J. Genetic change in *Salmonella*. J Bacteriol 1952;64:679–685.
199. Zinkernagel RM, Welsh RM. H-2 compatibility requirement for virus-specific T cell–mediated effector functions in vivo: 1. Specificity of T cells conferring antiviral protection against lymphocytic choriomeningitis virus is associated with H-2K and H-2D. J Immunol 1976;117:1495–1499.

Viral Pathogenesis,
edited by Neal Nathanson, et al.
Lippincott–Raven Publishers, Philadelphia © 1997

CHAPTER 17

Antiviral Agents

Martin S. Hirsch, Joan C. Kaplan, and Richard T. D'Aquila

INTRODUCTION

In the continuing battle between invading viruses and host responses, interposition of specific antiviral drugs should ideally tilt the balance in favor of the host. Progress during the past two decades has led to the discovery and characterization of molecules required for virus replication and to the development of antiviral agents to inhibit them. The genetic agility of some viruses, however, has enabled them to counter antiviral inhibition and in certain cases to regain advantage over the host.

The course of viral infections is governed by complex interactions between the virus and the host immune system. Pathogenesis is also related to the virulence of the virus and the titer and site of inoculation. Most infections resolve in the absence of antiviral intervention because of the natural host immune response to the virus. Others, particularly with members of the herpes group, resolve but become latent with periodic clinical and subclinical activations. In both these types of interaction between virus and host, antiviral agents may have a role in facilitating healing but are of secondary importance to a protective immune response, except in specific circumstances. Individuals infected with human immunodeficiency virus type 1 (HIV-1) may experience a third type of host–virus interaction. Both humoral and cell-mediated responses develop against HIV-1 antigens and are temporarily protective. Primary HIV-1

M. S. Hirsch: Infectious Disease Unit, Massachusetts General Hospital, Harvard Medical School, Boston, Massachusetts 02114.

J. C. Kaplan and R. T. D'Aquila: Infectious Disease Unit, Massachusetts General Hospital, Charlestown, Massachusetts 02129.

infection is generally followed by a dramatic decrease in virus load, presumably mediated by the host immune response. This suggests that at least a partial, transient limitation of disease progression occurs. The virus continues to replicate in lymph nodes and possibly other sites, however, which leads to increased virus burden. Antiviral agents directed against HIV-1 can interrupt the pathogenic process, although the impact of anti-HIV chemotherapy is complex and temporary. The outcome depends on many factors, including drug specificity, pharmacokinetics and toxicity, the immune status of the host, virus burden, and selection of drug-resistant viruses. If both antiviral agents and immune factors work together to restrict disease progression, it should be advantageous to initiate antiviral treatment early in the course of infection while the immune system is still intact and before an excessive increase in viral load has developed. For chronic infections, this approach necessitates development of relatively nontoxic drugs that can be tolerated for prolonged periods, that do not readily induce resistance, and that do not have adverse effects on the immune system.

Drug-resistant virus mutants are often selected during antiviral therapy, especially if there is a high virus load, viral genetic diversity is extensive, and antiviral therapy takes place over a long period (e.g., HIV-1). Selection of drug-resistant variants suggests effective chemotherapeutic inhibition of a mutable gene product and, in some cases (e.g., influenza M2 protein), permits delineation of the role of a particular gene product in pathogenesis. The emergence of drug-resistant variants may also enable the virus to counter attempts to restrict its replication and to increase its overall pathogenicity. This may depend on the immune competence of the host in whom drug resistance develops. In some immunocompromised individuals, drug-resistant virus variants are associated with recurrence of disease manifestations, (e.g., acyclovir, resistant herpesvirus in transplant recipients or patients with acquired immunodeficiency syndrome [AIDS]). Drug-resistant variants are not always pathogenic, which is determined by the mechanism underlying development of the drug resistance phenotype or the degree of immune capability. For example, some types of acyclovir-resistant herpes simplex viruses do not cause significant problems in an intact host. In contrast, zidovudine-resistant HIV-1 can trigger disease progression during therapy, although such mutants may arise more slowly in individuals with relatively intact immune responses and lower virus burdens. These issues often present clinicians with difficult decisions as to when to initiate therapy to maximize clinical benefit, to minimize virus replication and resistance development, and to prevent toxicity. The current debate about when to initiate zidovudine therapy in HIV-1 infection is an example of this conundrum.[181,336]

This chapter explores strategies for use of antiviral drugs, considers steps involved in the development and testing of clinically useful agents, and reviews mechanisms of action of and preclinical and clinical information about available and promising drugs. The pathogenic effects of drug-resistant viruses also are considered. Interferons and other agents that act primarily on host immune responses (e.g., cytokine inhibitors) are reviewed elsewhere. The emphasis is on human viral disease, the area in which the greatest therapeutic progress has been made, and on the three virus groups (in-fluenza, herpes, and HIV) for which useful drugs have been developed.

DRUG DISCOVERY, PRECLINICAL DEVELOPMENT, AND CLINICAL TRIALS

Antiviral agents have been discovered and characterized in increasingly sophisticated ways. The most straightforward approach involves screening compounds for their ability to interfere with virus replication in cell culture. Such assays must include controls for cellular toxicity to avoid the selection of compounds that inhibit virus replication only indirectly because of their toxic effects on host cells. Theoretically, the best targets for antiviral attack are molecules that serve a function unique to the virus, with no analogous counterpart in host cells. To identify the virus-specific molecule with which a putative antiviral agent interacts, it is important to characterize viruses in terms of particle and genome structure, to define specific biochemical events that occur in infected cells, and to analyze the genetics of antiviral resistance.

Once a particular virus-specific target has been identified, empiric, mechanism-based screening assays can be developed. The particular virus function, such as an enzyme activity, can be assayed and compounds screened for interference with this function in vitro. The proof that a replicative function is virus specific and localized to a particular viral gene has frequently been aided by characterization of viruses resistant to an inhibitor. If resistance is due to a mutation in a viral gene, the inhibitor is likely to have a direct effect on the function of that virus protein.[53,176]

Regardless of how an antiviral agent is discovered and its in vitro activity optimized, demonstrating in vitro activity of a drug against a virus is far removed from establishing its clinical efficacy, which follows only after laborious preclinical study and carefully controlled patient trials. Most drugs with antiviral activity in vitro fail somewhere along the path between discovery and licensure. Nevertheless, demonstration of activity against virus replication is a crucial first step. Cell culture tests should use a variety of cell types, including primary human host cells, several multiplicities of virus inoculum, and various virus preparations, including clinical isolates. The genetic diversity of viruses mandates that such attempts be made in order to discern the range of potential effectiveness in early preclinical studies; laboratory strains of virus may not accurately represent the true in vivo situation. Once sufficient in vitro data have suggested that further testing is warranted, appropriate animal models are studied to evaluate routes of administration, absorption and bioavailability after oral administration, pharmacokinetics and excretion mechanisms, capacity to reach infected tissues in adequate concentrations, stability in body fluids, and toxicity.

Human trials may begin once sufficient in vitro and animal studies have been performed to suggest clinical utility. The first step is phase I trials, in which graduated, escalating doses of a drug are administered to a limited number of individuals to establish pharmacokinetic and excretion patterns and maximum tolerated doses. Conclusions about drug efficacy must not be based on early phase I trials or anecdotal case reports, however, particularly in disorders with a variable natural course.

If promising results about the bioavailability and toxicity of an antiviral agent are obtained, one can proceed to more complex, large-scale, controlled clinical trials. Before beginning clinical trials, several parameters must be adequately defined: entry requirements for target populations, proper endpoints, adequate sample sizes, appropriate treatment and monitoring schedules, and mechanisms for randomization and analysis.[303] Blind trials are often used to reduce analytical bias. In double-blind studies, neither the patient nor the investigator knows the randomization group until the code is broken. If there is no established therapy for a particular infection, one group of individuals is often given a placebo. Once an agent has been established as an effective form of antiviral treatment (e.g., acyclovir in herpes encephalitis or zidovudine in AIDS), it should be used as the standard with which new agents are compared.

INFLUENZA VIRUS

Influenza viruses, members of the Orthomyxovirus class, contain a single-stranded, negative-sense RNA genome organized into eight individual segments. These RNA molecules are transcribed separately and packaged into viral ribonucleoprotein particles (vRNPs) in association with the matrix (M1) and nucleocapsid proteins (Fig. 17-1). Influenza virions attach to cells by an interaction between the viral hemagglutinin[HA] and sialic acid (neuraminic acid) residues on cell surface sialoglycolipid or sialoglycoprotein receptors. Virus particles enter cellular endosomes by receptor-mediated endocytosis.[243] Low endosomal pH (pH 5.0) causes a conformational change in HA[41] and converts it to an irreversibly denatured form with extended amino terminal alpha helices.[41,88,357] This change exposes the hydrophobic amino terminal sequence of HA that mediates fusion of the viral and endosomal membranes.[41,357] Virus membrane fusion with the endosomal membrane allows entry of the vRNP–M1 complex into the cytoplasm of the infected cell. After entering into the cytoplasm, the M1 protein is removed from the complex (see Fig. 17-1)[174] and the vRNPs enter the nucleus to initiate replication and transcription.[245,246] Newly synthesized viral RNA molecules are assembled into preformed nucleocapsids before leaving the nucleus and migrating through the trans-Golgi network for assembly with viral envelope proteins at the cell surface.

The M2 protein is a nonglycosylated integral membrane protein[437], expressed on the surface of infected cells[215] and to a limited extent in virions[438], whose transmembrane domain is highly conserved for all human and avian strains of influenza A virus. It can function as an ion channel for hydrogen ions.[304] It has been proposed that this channel permits proton flux from the endosome into the interior of the virion before virus envelope–endosome membrane fusion takes place.[304] Acidification of the virion interior may induce changes in the conformation of the virus nucleocapsid protein and prime it for disruption of the vRNP-M1 complex (see Fig. 17-1).[246] The M2 ion channel may also allow protons to flow out of the normally mildly acidic trans-Golgi compartment to increase the lumenal pH so that acid-induced conformational changes of HA are prevented during virion assembly and egress from the infected cell.[174,304]

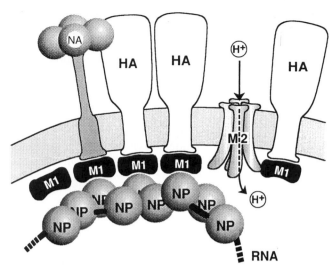

Fig. 17-1. Molecular interactions between structural components of influenza virus relevant to the mechanism of action of amantadine and rimantadine. Amantadine and rimantadine bind to M2 and block its function as a proton channel. Proton flow is depicted moving into the virion. Point mutations in the transmembrane domain of M2 render influenza virus resistant to inhibition by amantadine and rimantadine. NP, nucleoprotein; HA, hemagglutinin; NA, neuraminidase (sialidase); RNA, one segment of influenza virus genomic RNA. (Reprinted with permission from Helenius A. Unpacking the incoming influenza virus. Cell 1992; 69:577–578.)

Amantadine and Rimantadine

Mechanism of Action

Amantadine and rimantadine specifically inhibit influenza A virus. The mechanisms of action vary according to influenza A virus subtype. Most human strains are inhibited early in infection after attachment (penetration or uncoating),[36] whereas certain avian strains are also inhibited later in replication during virus maturation.[382] Amantadine is the one-amino derivative of adamantane, a complex ten-carbon compound with a cage-like structure, and rimantadine is a nearly identical methyl derivative of amantadine that differs only in some pharmacologic properties. Both drugs inhibit in vitro replication of influenza A viruses at concentrations achievable in vivo.[9,358] At these concentrations, neither drug inhibits influenza B viruses, which can also cause serious human disease.

Amantadine and rimantadine act by abolishing the ion channel activity of the M2 protein.[95,414] As a result, the M1 protein does not dissociate from the vRNP-M1 complex when the virus enters the cytoplasm, and this prevents transport of the vRNPs to the nucleus.[245] In addition to this effect of amantadine at an early stage of infection, the drug has a second late effect on some subtypes of influenza A virus whose HAs undergo fusion-promoting conformational changes at a relatively high pH. In the presence of amantadine, the intralumenal pH of the trans-Golgi compartment is decreased so the HA undergoes a premature, acid-induced conformational change thought to be detrimental to the release of infectious virus particles.[50,153,330] Studies with fowl plague virus indicate that the M2 protein regulates the pH of intracellular compartments, thereby stabilizing HA in its native (pH-neutral) form.[289,388]

Pharmacology, Toxicity, and Clinical Trials

Both amantadine and rimantadine are available in oral formulations. Despite their similar structures, they differ significantly in pharmacokinetic patterns. Amantadine achieves peak plasma levels 2 to 4 hours after oral dosing, and more than 90% is recovered unchanged in the urine.[367,397] Excretion is by both renal tubular secretion and glomerular filtration. Adequate antiviral levels are achieved in lung, nasal mucus, saliva, and cerebrospinal fluid. In elderly subjects, plasma concentrations average 50% higher and elimination takes longer, so dose reductions may be necessary. Dosage adjustments are also required in patients with impaired renal function.

Rimantadine is also well absorbed orally (>90%) but achieves slightly lower plasma levels than does amantadine. Plasma half-life for rimantadine is approximately twice that for amantadine, and rimantadine may be more concentrated in respiratory secretions.[87] The drug is extensively metabolized and is excreted primarily by renal mechanisms. Less than 10% of rimantadine is excreted unchanged, with most of it being excreted as hydroxylated and glucuronidated metabolites.[172]

The most common adverse effects related to amantadine use are minor central nervous system complaints (nervousness, lightheadedness, insomnia, difficulty concentrating) that often resolve despite continued administration of drug. More serious neurotoxic reactions (seizures, delirium) can occur in patients with disordered renal function, in whom higher plasma levels are attained.[190] Rimantadine has qualitatively similar toxicity, but at 200 mg/day, the frequency of adverse effects is much less.[87] When matched for drug levels achieved in plasma, amantadine and rimantadine do not appear to differ significantly in their neurologic toxic effects.[171]

Several placebo-controlled, blinded studies have demonstrated that amantadine is an effective prophylaxis against naturally occurring influenza A infections.[87,145,273,303,309,365] Protection against clinical disease has generally ranged from 50% to 90%, but efficacy in preventing laboratory-documented infection is lower, indicating that some infected and treated individuals have subclinical infection. Prophylaxis has been demonstrated against a variety of influenza A strains in adults and children, family contacts, and hospitalized patients. Rimantadine is similarly effective in preventing influenza A virus infections.[35,90,355]

Both amantadine and rimantadine are useful therapeutic agents for uncomplicated influenza A virus infections if treatment is initiated within 48 hours of symptom onset.[144,205,395] Duration of fever and systemic complaints are reduced by approximately 50% and peripheral airway function is improved compared with placebo.[231] Comparative trials of amantadine and rimantadine have shown no major differences in their therapeutic effects in uncomplicated influenza.[87,404] For influenza pneumonia, the major life-threatening complication of this infection, results of controlled trials of either drug have not yet been reported.

In recent years, expert groups assembled by the US Public Health Service and the World Health Organization have made recommendations for use of these agents.[2,282,430] Populations at high risk for influenza complications include those with cardiopulmonary disease, the immunocompromised, and the elderly. Although influenza vaccines are recommended as seasonal prophylaxis, amantadine or rimantadine can be considered as alternatives if the vaccine is contraindicated because of allergy or significant immunodeficiency, if the epidemic strain is different from the vaccine strain, or if vaccination has been neglected until the epidemic is present. Amantadine is often recommended as an adjunct to late immunization.[91] Initiation of chemoprophylaxis depends on knowledge of the epidemic strain since influenza B viruses are not susceptible. Amantadine or rimantadine treatment should be continued for the duration of expected exposure, generally 4 to 8 weeks in a given community or 10 days for healthy contacts in a family postexposure setting. Early treatment of uncomplicated clinical disease is warranted in high-risk groups, as well as in healthy individuals in whom shortening of illness by 1 or 2 days may be important (e.g., health care workers, police). Treatment for 5 to 10 days or for 48 hours after resolution of symptoms is usually recommended.

Resistance

The mechanisms of action for amantadine and rimantadine have been elucidated with the aid of amantadine-resistant influenza virus mutants that have been selected both in vivo and in vitro and demonstrate cross-resistance to rimantadine.[20,346] The M2 protein is encoded by a spliced RNA from RNA segment 7.[214] Sequencing RNA segment 7 of amantadine- and rimantadine-resistant mutants has demonstrated that nucleotide changes conferring the resistant phenotype lie within the locus encoding the transmembrane portion of M2.[20,166,167] Single nucleotide changes have been demonstrated at residues 26, 27, 30, 31, and 34, with mutations in codon 31 being the most common.[20,166,167] These amino acid residues are thought to line the ion channel and form a drug-binding site. Most resistant isolates have a single amino acid change, although mixed virus populations have been described with independent resistance mutations.[18,20] Identical mutations in M2 are responsible for abolishing susceptibility to both the early and late effects of amantadine. Amantadine- and rimantidine-resistant viruses emerge rapidly during drug passage in vitro and within a few days of initiating therapy in vivo and seem to be genetically stable.[169,170]

Although epidemic strains of influenza A virus remain susceptible to amantadine and rimantadine, cross-resistant mutants emerge rapidly during treatment.[159,169] By days 5 to 7 of therapy, 16% to 45% of isolates from treated patients may be resistant,[159,169] and under conditions of close family contact, transmission of resistant isolates and secondary illness can occur. It is unclear whether resistant mutants can be perpetuated in the absence of these drugs or whether they are at a competitive disadvantage to wild-type virus.[272] Naturally occurring resistant strains have not been found, except when linked epidemiologically to patients treated with amantadine or rimantadine, which suggests that resistance does not confer a selective advantage to the virus in the absence of drug therapy.

HERPESVIRUSES

Acyclovir, Ganciclovir, and Related Agents

Mechanism of Action

Acyclovir (9-[(2-hydroxyethoxy) methyl] guanine, Zovirax) is a guanosine analog with an acyclic side chain at the 9 position (Fig. 17-2). It is a specific inhibitor of herpes simplex virus (HSV)-1, HSV-2, and varicella-zoster virus (VZV) replication with little toxicity for host cells.[23,99,343] It is less effective against Epstein-Barr virus (EBV), cytomegalovirus

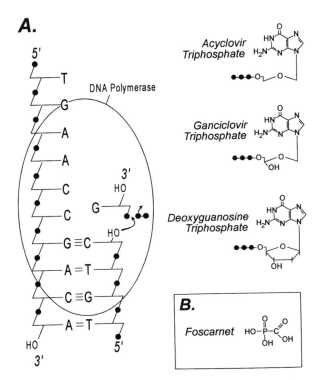

A.

Acyclovir Triphosphate

Ganciclovir Triphosphate

Deoxyguanosine Triphosphate

DNA Polymerase

B.

Foscarnet

Fig. 17-2. Inhibitors of the polymerization reaction of herpesvirus DNA polymerase between a nucleoside triphosphate and the 3'-hydroxyl end of an elongating DNA primer strand. (A) As catalyzed by a DNA polymerase, the 3'-hydroxyl group of the deoxyribose ring reacts with the innermost phosphate of an incoming deoxynucleoside triphosphate to form a covalent phosphodiester bond. This growing DNA chain is extended by incorporation of a nucleoside monophosphate moiety with displacement of pyrophosphate. Deoxyguanosine triphosphate (dGTP) depicted on the left is shown in greater detail on the right, as are acyclovir triphosphate and ganciclovir triphosphate, structural analogs of dGTP that lack a deoxyribose ring. Phosphate groups are represented as closed circles. (Depiction of polymerase and growing DNA chain, modified from Watson JD, Hopkins NH, Roberts JW, Steitz JA, Weiner AM. Molecular biology of the gene. Menlo Park, California: Benjamin/Cummings, 1987:287.) (B) The pyrophosphate analog foscarnet is illustrated here. It is thought to bind to herpesvirus and other polymerases and interfere with binding of the pyrophosphate moiety cleaved from an incoming deoxynucleoside triphosphate.

(CMV), and human herpesvirus virus type 6 (HHV-6) in cell culture.[38,78] Ganciclovir (9-[1,3-dihydroxy-2-propoxy]methyl-guanine [DHPG]), is an acyclic analog of guanosine that is closely related structurally to acyclovir. It shows much greater inhibition than acyclovir against CMV[239,394] and HHV-6 in vitro[38] and also has activity against acyclovir-susceptible herpesviruses.[49,117,134,239] Ganciclovir is more toxic than acyclovir both in cell culture and in vivo.

Acyclovir is transported into cells by the nucleoside transporter that also transports guanine.[240] It requires a virus-encoded thymidine kinase (TK) for efficient intracellular activation, which accounts in part for its selectivity.[99,143] HSV, varicella-zoster virus (VZV), and EBV encode TKs that catalyze the phosphorylation of acyclovir to acyclovir monophosphate (ACVMP), as well as of thymidine and some other nucleoside analogs to their respective monophosphates.[60,85,203,232] Acyclovir therefore competes with thymidine for the viral TK. After this key initial phosphorylation step, ACVMP is converted by cellular kinases to acyclovir diphosphate (ACVDP) and triphosphate (ACVTP), the metabolically active form of acyclovir.[265,266] In uninfected cells, the cytoplasmic 5'-nucleotidase catalyzes the formation of such low levels of ACVMP[201] that the amount of ACVTP produced in HSV-infected cells may be 40- to 100-fold greater than levels in uninfected cells.[98,139,143,200] ACVTP inhibits HSV DNA polymerase much more effectively than it does cellular DNA polymerases.[82,141]

ACVTP competes with deoxyguanosine triphosphate (dGTP) for the viral DNA polymerase, and ACVMP is preferentially incorporated into elongating DNA chains[99,141] (see Fig. 17-2). This 3'-terminal ACVMP is not excised from the primer template by the 3',5'-exonuclease activity that is an integral component of herpesvirus DNA polymerases.[82] As a result, elongation of the DNA chain ceases because its terminus lacks the 3'-hydroxyl group on the 2'-deoxyribose sugar that is required for reaction with the next incoming nucleoside triphosphate[142,255] (see Fig. 17-2). Therefore, ACVTP is referred to as an obligate chain terminator.[313] Compared with the HSV and VZV polymerases, the cellular DNA polymerases that have been studied have relatively poor affinity for ACVTP, and little ACVMP is incorporated into host cell DNA.[141]

An additional mechanism for acyclovir inhibition of herpesvirus replication has been demonstrated with purified HSV-1 DNA polymerase in vitro. ACVTP causes a time-dependent inactivation of HSV-1 polymerase activity that cannot be explained by termination of primer extension[142] and that occurs only in the presence of primer-template and all four deoxynucleoside triphosphates (dNTPs).[142,313] Binding of the next dNTP encoded for incorporation into elongating DNA immediately after ACVMP is necessary to prevent the polymerase from dissociating and moving to an alternative, extendable primer-template.[313] This is an example of induced substrate inhibition in which an inactive, "dead-end" complex is formed between viral polymerase, ACVMP-terminated primer-template and the next specific dNTP encoded by the template. Induced substrate inhibition of the HSV-1 polymerase is less marked with other obligate chain terminators.[313] This mechanism appeared to be selective for the HSV-1 polymerase in that ACTVP was not found to inhibit a major host cell polymerase (HeLa cell polymerase-α) in a time-dependent manner.[141,312]

In summary, the markedly selective action of acyclovir against HSV-1, HSV-2, and VZV is a consequence of several enzymatic reactions, each of which is unique to virus replication: specific activation (phosphorylation) by a virus-induced TK, selective inhibition of the viral DNA polymerase by ACVTP acting as a competitor with the natural substrate, dGTP, termination of viral DNA chain growth by incorporation of ACVMP, and inactivation of the viral DNA polymerase following ACVMP incorporation in the presence of dNTPs.[314] The relative degree of potency of acyclovir in inhibiting replication of different herpesviruses in cell culture (HSV-1 > HSV-2 > VZV) seems to be explained by some of these enzymatic events.

Ganciclovir is more toxic than acyclovir but acts by similar mechanisms. Its active form, ganciclovir-triphosphate (GCVTP), selectively inhibits herpesvirus DNA polymerase.[240] In HSV-infected cells, ganciclovir is converted to ganciclovir monophosphate (GCVMP) by the same virus-specific TK that phosphorylates acyclovir.[11,48,117,362] Ganciclovir is an even more efficient substrate than acyclovir for the herpes TK, and nearly 10-fold more GCVTP than ACVTP is produced in HSV-1–infected cells.[11,25] Although CMV does not encode an enzyme related to the HSV and VZV TKs,[110] at least 10-fold more GCVTP accumulates in CMV-infected cells than in uninfected cells.[25,134] Conversion of GCVMP to the diphosphate and triphosphate forms is catalyzed by cellular guanylate and phosphoglycerate kinases,[26,361] and, once formed, GCVTP persists in cells long after ganciclovir has been removed.[25,362]

The initial phosphorylation of ganciclovir to GCVMP is the crucial step in its activation, and the mechanism underlying the increased accumulation of GCVMP in CMV-infected cells has been explained by genetic and biochemical studies.[233,385] Despite CMV induction of cellular nucleoside kinases, some of which phosphorylate ganciclovir to a slight degree,[134] the assumption that GCVMP formation is due to a CMV-induced cellular enzyme has been challenged by the characterization of a ganciclovir-resistant CMV mutant.[24] Ganciclovir resistance was transferable by DNA fragments cloned from the UL97 open reading frame of this mutant, and recombinant ganciclovir-resistant viruses that had acquired the mutant UL97 fragment did not anabolize ganciclovir.[385] A recombinant-expressed, wild-type CMV protein produced from the UL97 open reading frame had ganciclovir kinase activity.[233]

The protein encoded by the UL97 open reading frame of CMV has homology to protein kinases but differs from consensus protein kinase motifs at those positions that also vary in bacterial aminoglycoside phosphotransferases and in other enzymes that transfer phosphates to sugar hydroxyl groups.[45] The acyclic sugar-like substituent of ganciclovir is phosphorylated at the position corresponding to the 5'-hydroxyl of the 2'-deoxyribose ring (see Fig. 17-2). Although conservation of the UL97 open reading frame in other herpesviruses, including HHV-6, implies an important role for its gene product in virus replication, its physiologic function remains to be determined, and it is not yet clear if it is essential for CMV replication. The mutation in the ganciclovir-resistant mutant deletes residues implicated in substrate binding to a homologous protein kinase and raises the possibility that this mutant enzyme may retain catalytic activity but have altered substrate specificity.[385]

GCVTP is a better substrate for herpesvirus polymerases than for host cell polymerases; it competes with dGTP for polymerase binding and inhibits polymerization after binding.[134,239,312,320] In contrast to ACVTP, which lacks a 3'-hydroxyl group necessary for phosphodiester bond formation with an incoming nucleoside triphosphate, ganciclovir possesses a hydroxyl group corresponding to the 3'-hydroxyl of the 2'-deoxyribose ring, which may allow further extension and internal incorporation of GCVMP into elongating DNA chains (see Fig. 17-2). GCVTP is defined as a nonobligate chain terminator and the rate of virus DNA chain elongation is decreased in its presence.[48,132,240,374] Incorporation of GCVMP into the terminus of elongating DNA leads to chain termination in vitro.[312,320] In studies of the HSV polymerase in vitro using defined primer templates, the V_{max} for incorporation of the nucleotide after GCVMP incorporation was decreased and the K_m for the second nucleotide following GCVMP incorporation was increased, which effectively resulted in chain termination.[312] In the presence of ganciclovir, only short fragments of viral DNA accumulate in CMV-infected cells.[163,164] Although these observations are consistent with chain termination, it is not known whether GCVMP or a natural deoxynucleoside monophosphate is present at the 3' terminus of these short fragments. Given the cellular toxicity of ganciclovir, it is of interest that in one in vitro system, the kinetic constants for continued incorporation into GCVMP-terminated DNA by HeLa polymerase-α were more favorable than those of HSV polymerase.[312] This suggests that with high enough dNTP levels, GCVMP may be internalized into elongating cellular DNA. In contrast to ACVTP, GCVTP does not cause induced substrate inhibition of HSV DNA polymerase in vitro.[312]

Mechanistically Related Agents

Several other strategies are under study to improve inhibitory activity against VZV, CMV, and even acyclovir-resistant HSV by increasing oral bioavailability, intracellular phosphorylation, and half-life of the active anabolite of acyclovir or related compounds. Valaciclovir[308] and famciclovir[405] have recently been approved for use in the USA; other compounds under study include bromovinyl arabinosyluracil (BV-araU),[80] and certain phosphonomethylether derivatives, including 3-hydroxy-2-phosphonylmethoxypropyl-cytosine (HPMPC) and 3-hydroxy-2-phosphonylmethoxypropyl-adenine.[81]

Efforts have been made to improve the antiviral effect of acyclovir by causing a decrease in intracellular levels of dGTP that competes with ACVTP for binding to the viral DNA polymerase in infected cells. HSV and VZV both code for ribonucleotide reductases that catalyze the reduction of ribonucleotides to deoxynucleotides,[97,369] which results in high intracellular concentrations of dGTP. Conversely, inhibitors of the herpesvirus-specific ribonucleotide reductase, such as A110U, cause a decrease in the intracellular levels of dGTP, which potentiates ACVTP activity against herpesvirus polymerases in vitro.[368] Combination therapy with acyclovir and A110U has been found to increase intracellular ACVTP levels about 10-fold, and synergistic inhibition of HSV-1, HSV-2, and VZV replication has been demonstrated in cell culture with a combination of acyclovir and A110U.[368]

Pharmacology, Toxicity, and Clinical Trials of Acyclovir

Acyclovir is available in topical, oral, and parenteral preparations. After intravenous administration of 0.5 to 15.0 mg/kg, the serum half-life of acyclovir is 2 to 4 hours. Peak plasma levels achieved after an intravenous dose of 5 mg/kg are 30 to 40μ M, whereas after oral administration of 200 mg, peak levels of 1.4 to 4.0μ M (mean, 2.5μ M) are reached after 1 to 2 hours.[226,403,420] The inhibitory doses for HSV range from 0.1 to 1.6μ M, whereas those for VZV are 3 to 4μ M.[19,79] Thus, oral doses to treat VZV are usually three- to four-fold higher than those for HSV. The drug is widely distributed, and cerebrospinal fluid levels are about half those of plasma levels.[420] Acyclovir is excreted mainly by the kidney, primarily by glomerular filtration and partially by tubular secretion.[226] Dose reductions and interval prolongations are suggested in patients with renal insufficiency. Hemodialysis removes about 60% of acyclovir.[227]

Acyclovir is a remarkably nontoxic drug. The major toxicity of parenteral acyclovir has been renal dysfunction, which is uncommon.[21,422] High-dose (>5 mg/kg) intravenous administration in the presence of dehydration and preexisting renal insufficiency can result in crystallization of acyclovir in renal tubules and in reversible elevations in serum creatinine.[301] Central nervous system abnormalities, including delirium, tremors, and coma, have been described but rarely.[113]

Because long-term oral suppression of HSV recurrences is often used, it is necessary to monitor carefully for carcinogenic effects. There is no substantial evidence that acyclovir is a carcinogen in either animals or humans. At extremely high doses, acyclovir may be a radiosensitizer.[89] At therapeutic concentrations, no effects on the immune system or hematopoietic precursor cells have been observed.[254,296,378] The safety of acyclovir during pregnancy has not been definitively established, but preliminary data are reassuring.[135] In animals, most studies indicate that the drug is not a significant teratogen.[274] It does cross the placenta, however, and a registry of acyclovir in pregnancy has been established.[7]

Herpes Simplex Infections

Two placebo-controlled trials have compared acyclovir and vidarabine (see later) in patients with HSV encephalitis.[359,418] Both studies show substantially reduced mortality in acyclovir recipients. Moreover, at 6-month follow-up, 14% of vidarabine recipients were functioning normally, compared with 38% of acyclovir recipients.

A similar comparison between vidarabine and acyclovir was conducted in infants with neonatal herpesvirus infection.[419] The overall mortality rates, adverse effects, and laboratory toxicities were similar in the two treatment groups for infants with encephalitis or disseminated infection. Most pediatricians would nevertheless choose acyclovir over vidarabine for initial therapy of neonatal herpesvirus infections.

Acyclovir has been compared with placebo for both the prophylaxis and therapy of mucocutaneous herpes simplex virus infections in immunosuppressed hosts. Saral and colleagues reported a double-blind trial of intravenous prophylactic acyclovir in bone marrow transplant recipients seropositive for HSV.[340] Culture-positive lesions developed in seven of ten placebo recipients but in none of ten acyclovir recipients. Once acyclovir was discontinued, herpes infections developed in seven patients, five of whom had symptoms, indicating no effect of acyclovir on latent virus. These studies have been confirmed and extended in several other trials among bone marrow and renal transplant recipients[338] and in patients undergoing chemotherapy for acute leukemia.[339] In a randomized double-blind trial of intravenous acyclovir for treatment of established, culture-proven HSV infections after bone marrow transplantation,[409] patients received either intravenous acyclovir or placebo for 7 days. Thirteen of 17 patients given acyclovir had therapeutic responses, compared with two of 17 given placebo. Acyclovir-treated patients also had shorter durations of virus-positive cultures. No effect on latency was observed; 16 of the 17 acyclovir-treated patients reactivated infection after termination of therapy. Similar controlled-treatment studies have been performed in heart transplant recipients and other immunosuppressed patients.[263] Intravenous acyclovir shortened periods of virus shedding, lesion pain, and times to scabbing and healing. Oral acyclovir therapy (400μg five times daily for 10 days) also significantly shortens the duration of viral shedding, new lesion formation, pain, and healing and compares favorably with results obtained with intravenous therapy.[350]

The optimal therapy for individual patients varies. Small, isolated mucocutaneous lesions can be treated with topical acyclovir but for more extensive infections, with or without systemic manifestations, oral or intravenous therapy is recommended. In immunologically intact individuals, topical acyclovir therapy does not appear to be effective for HSV-1 orolabial infections,[372] possibly because of poor penetration. Oral acyclovir reduces the duration of pain and healing slightly when therapy is begun during the erythematous or prodromal stages of infection,[373] but it cannot be recommended for routine treatment of herpes labialis.[422] Oral acyclovir has a short-term suppressive benefit in otherwise healthy patients at high risk for reactivation secondary to trigeminal ganglion surgery,[342] alpine skiing,[370] or experimental ultraviolet light exposure.[369] For long-term suppression in frequently recurrent herpes labialis, oral acyclovir can reduce viral shedding (71%) and recurrences (41% to 53%) compared with placebo.[327]

The most widespread use of acyclovir against HSV is for genital disease. Topical, intravenous, and oral formulations are all useful in primary genital herpes infections. Acyclovir as a 5% ointment in a polyethylene glycol base was evaluated in a double-blind, placebo-controlled trial among 77 patients with first episodes of genital herpes and 111 patients with recurrent episodes.[67] Topical acyclovir or placebo was applied four times a day for 7 days. In acyclovir-treated patients with first-episode primary genital herpes, the mean duration of viral shedding was reduced by acyclovir from 7 to 4.1 days, and the time to complete crusting was reduced from 10.5 to 7.1 days. Acyclovir also reduced viral shedding in men with recurrent herpes but only by about 1 day. Acyclovir did not facilitate healing in women with recurrent infection or delay recurrences in either sex. A second controlled trial in 88 patients with recurrent herpes genitalis demonstrated similar small effects of acyclovir (e.g., shortened virus shedding in men), but no other significant differences between acyclovir and placebo groups.[318] In this study, patients were treated within 48 hours of the onset of lesions, and ointments were administered six times a day.

Intravenous acyclovir has more dramatic effects on the course of primary genital herpes infection, shortening median healing times, duration of new lesion formation, vesicle persistence, duration of symptoms, and times of virus shedding.[267] None of the oral acyclovir recipients with initial or recurrent genital disease had new lesion formation, whereas 43% of placebo recipients had new lesions.[285] Times to crusting and healing, viral shedding, and duration of pain were also substantially shortened by oral acyclovir. A second trial of oral acyclovir in initial-episode genital herpes continued treatment for 10 days rather than 5[34] and showed clinical and virologic benefits in both men and women. Subsequent recurrences were unaffected. The issue of when to initiate therapy has also been studied.[319] In one trial, treatment was begun by physicians within 48 hours of the onset of lesions; in another, therapy was initiated by patients at the onset of lesions. In both studies, the duration of virus shedding and times to crusting and healing were shortened in acyclovir recipients. Patient-initiated therapy resulted in the most rapid healing and cessation of viral shedding.

The question of long-term prophylaxis or suppression of frequently recurrent genital herpes by oral acyclovir has also been addressed. Various regimens have been effective for up to 3 years.[197,202,250,261,270,276] The upper limit of recommended duration for acyclovir suppression is unresolved, although treatment interruption every 12 months to reassess the need for continued suppression has been recommended.[379] Breakthrough recurrence on suppressive therapy usually cannot be correlated with the emergence of acyclovir-resistant virus strains, although recurrences due to resistant HSV have been described.[210]

Varicella-Zoster Infections

Intravenous acyclovir therapy (1500 $\mu g/m^2$/day) of herpes zoster in immunocompromised adults retarded the spread of cutaneous lesions in patients with either localized or disseminated cutaneous zoster at entry compared with placebo.[13] In addition, acyclovir significantly reduced the frequency of development of visceral zoster. Effects of the drug on localized healing, pain, and viral shedding were relatively small but generally suggested benefit. In immunocompromised children with VZV, intravenous acyclovir has also proved safe and effective.[286,305] When begun early in the course of disease, acyclovir therapy can significantly retard clinical deterioration compared with placebo; although a 5-day course of therapy is generally sufficient, rare recurrences can develop on discontinuation of therapy. Acyclovir has also been directly compared with vidarabine infusion. In immunocompromised patients with VZV, acyclovir was more effective than vidarabine in preventing complications, shortening periods of virus positivity, diminishing pain, and facilitating healing.[349] Patients with disseminated herpes zoster who received acyclovir were discharged from the hospital more promptly than were vidarabine recipients.[423] Thus, intravenous acyclovir is considered the agent of choice for both varicella and herpes zoster among immunocompromised patients.

Early therapy with oral acyclovir can reduce the duration and severity of chickenpox in healthy children,[96] adolescents,[15] and adults.[412] In children, the benefits are modest and must be weighed against the cost, potential toxicity, possible induction of resistance, and unknown long-term effects on host immunity, viral latency, and reactivation. In older individuals, in whom complications such as pneumonia are common, therapy is probably warranted.[158]

Herpes zoster may lead to significant morbidity, particularly in the elderly. Intravenous acyclovir in doses of 15 to 30 mg/kg/day for 5 days, when compared with placebo, resulted in reduced acute pain, time to healing, and viral shedding.[17,300,302,394] Because intravenous therapy is often impractical for such patients, placebo-controlled trials of oral acyclovir have also been conducted. Using oral doses of 600 to 800 mg five times a day, significant reductions in acute pain and skin healing were demonstrated if patients were enrolled within 48 to 72 hours of rash onset.[187,299] Lower doses have been less effective.[187,299]

Epstein-Barr Virus and Cytomegalovirus

Cytomegalovirus and EBV are less sensitive to acyclovir than is HSV. Nevertheless, some clinical trials have suggested benefit for prophylactic acyclovir in reducing clinical CMV disease in the setting of renal or bone marrow transplantation.[14,262] In contrast, the high-dose oral acyclovir was ineffective prophylaxis against CMV disease in liver transplant recipients.[355]

Intravenous or oral acyclovir may reduce pharyngeal shedding of EBV but does not alter the course of infectious mononucleosis.[4,5,401] Oral hairy leukoplakia, an EBV-associated condition primarily affecting individuals infected with HIV-1, may respond to acyclovir.[321]

Pharmacology, Toxicity, and Clinical Trials of Ganciclovir

Current ganciclovir formulations have limited oral bioavailability (13%), necessitating intravenous administration for sustained therapeutic levels. After administration of intravenous doses of 7.5 mg/kg, peak serum levels of ganciclovir range between 18 and 24 μM, with cerebrospinal fluid levels of 2 to 3 μM; the half-life of ganciclovir is 3 to 4 hours.[130,366] Serum concentrations are dose related and surpass the median effective dose for CMV (0.04 to 11 μM). Renal excretion is the major route of elimination, and doses must be reduced during renal impairment. Ganciclovir has a narrow therapeutic/toxic ratio and often causes reversible neutropenia or thrombocytopenia. CMV retinitis, esophagitis, colitis, polyradiculopathy, and pneumonia may be amenable to therapy in some situations.

Ganciclovir was first shown to reverse ongoing CMV retinitis in a patient with AIDS in 1985.[114] About 90% of patients with CMV retinitis improve or stabilize on ganciclovir therapy,[35,61,248,381] although prolonged maintenance is required. Up to 80% of responders experience relapse if therapy is discontinued,[35,61,248] and many do so despite maintenance therapy. Responses in gastrointestinal CMV infection vary, with response rates ranging from 75% to 83%.[35,83] Other placebo-controlled trials in AIDS patients and bone marrow transplant recipients have shown only marginal benefit.[84,317]

CMV interstitial pneumonia is a major cause of morbidity and mortality in bone marrow transplant recipients. Although ganciclovir as a single agent has shown little benefit, combinations of ganciclovir with intravenous immune globulin have shown promise, with survival rates improving to 31% to 70%.[234,316] CMV causes a progressive disabling polyradiculopathy in immunocompromised individuals, particularly those with AIDS, and some benefit from ganciclovir has been suggested in this setting.[264]

Because CMV is a major pathogen in immunocompromised hosts, several trials have evaluated ganciclovir as a prophylactic or suppressive agent for prevention of disease manifestations during periods of maximal risk. Studies have been conducted in bone marrow transplant recipients,[151,344,433] as well as in those receiving liver,[235,355] heart,[260] kidney,[178] and lung,[12] transplants. In CMV-seropositive bone marrow transplant recipients, ganciclovir therapy, begun either at the time of engraftment or when surveillance cultures become positive for CMV, suppresses both CMV excretion and disease for up to 120 days after transplantation. Similarly, among CMV-seropositive organ transplant recipients, what has been called preemptive therapy during periods of maximal immunosuppression (e.g., patients receiving antilymphocyte or OKT3 antibodies) reduces the frequency and severity of CMV disease. Reductions in CMV disease were from 33% to 52% in untreated patients to 9% to 14% in ganciclovir-treated recipients of kidneys, hearts, and livers.[178,235,260] Short course (1-week) parenteral ganciclovir also proved more effective in reducing CMV disease in liver transplant recipients than high-dose acyclovir (4% versus 29%, respectively).[355] In contrast, the combination of ganciclovir and immune globulin failed to prevent CMV disease in CMV-seronegative recipients of lung transplants from CMV-seropositive donors.[12] Oral ganciclovir (3 gm/day) can be used for maintenance suppression of CMV retinitis once induction with intravenous ganciclovir is completed.

Resistance

Acyclovir-Resistant Herpes Simplex Virus and Varicella-Zoster Virus

Resistance of HSV to acyclovir develops readily in vitro and also occurs in vivo.[58,70,102,107,119,345] Mutations conferring acyclovir resistance can be in the tk gene or polymerase (pol) gene or both.[58,70,345] These mutations have been demonstrated before drug exposure in laboratory stocks of virus and clinical isolates at a fairly high frequency (10^{-4} to 10^{-3}).[51,295] The DNA polymerase differs from the TK in being essential for virus replication in dividing cells. Other cellular enzymes that may be limiting in nondividing (e.g., neural) cells can substitute for the viral TK in dividing cells, presumably to synthesize the dNTPs required for both cellular and viral DNA synthesis.

Most acyclovir-resistant HSV isolates are TK mutants, and a single point mutation in the tk gene is sufficient to cause resistance.[77,204] Double mutants with mutations in tk and pol can

also be selected. There are three classes of tk mutation that confer the resistance phenotype[53]:

1. TK-negative mutants, in which enzyme activity is abolished and phosphorylation of acyclovir does not occur[143]
2. TK-partial mutants, in which enzyme activity is decreased but not abolished
3. TK-altered mutants, which express enzymes with altered substrate specificity. There is little or no change in the ability of such mutants to phosphorylate thymidine, but they do not phosphorylate acyclovir.[76,100,220,222]

Another mechanism of acyclovir resistance in HSV involves pol mutations that alter the DNA polymerase so it can synthesize viral DNA in the presence of high concentrations of ACVTP.[63,138,207,249,333] Most of these mutations cluster in conserved regions of pol that have homologies to other DNA polymerases[63,147,189,224] and that are located in or near conserved regions I, II, III, V, VII, and A.[53,90,147,189,206,224,241] It does not seem that any particular conserved region is uniquely involved with a specific enzymatic function, such as dNTP substrate recognition or pyrophosphate binding. Rather, it appears that functional domains are formed by folding of the polymerase protein so that regions of the polypeptide encoded in disparate, noncontiguous parts of the primary sequence are physically approximated.[147] Studies of tertiary protein structure and detailed enzymologic analyses are necessary, in addition to molecular genetic data, to identify the role in enzyme function served by the specific residues altered by mutation. Mapping acyclovir resistance mutations to these conserved regions suggests that ACVTP selectively inhibits herpes but not cellular polymerases because of relatively subtle differences in key functional domains. The herpes DNA polymerase catalytic function need not be impaired for acyclovir resistance to occur.

Different types of TK mutants each share patterns of cross-resistance with other agents. They may be resistant to ganciclovir, famciclovir, or other compounds that also require phosphorylation by TK yet retain in vitro susceptibility to agents like foscarnet that do not. Many polymerase mutations selected during acyclovir therapy can also cause resistance to ganciclovir, vidarabine (ara A), and foscarnet.[55,63,333] Double mutants in both tk and pol may be cross-resistant to all available clinical agents, and mixed populations of virus that include some pol mutants may have a greater degree of acyclovir resistance than expected from the net composition of the pool. Although the replication of both wild-type and acyclovir-resistant viruses can be inhibited in a cell coinfected with a mixture of TK-deficient and wild-type HSV, acyclovir has little effect on virus replication in cells coinfected with a mixture of wild-type and altered pol mutant HSVs.[58]

There are differences in the degree of pathogenicity of various acyclovir-resistant mutants as measured by their ability to kill mice after intracerebral inoculation or to reactivate from latency. In such mouse models, TK-deficient mutants are generally less pathogenic than wild-type virus.[121] TK-negative mutants do not reactivate from latent infections in mice unless rescued by superinfecting TK-positive virus.[57,97,392,431] TK-altered mutants are somewhat attenuated for pathogenicity,[76] as are most polymerase mutants,[52] but less so than TK-negative mutants. Heterogeneity of virus isolates is an important factor in pathogenesis and resistance. Pathogenesis studies have been conducted in mice infected with defined mixtures of acyclovir-resistant (TK-deficient or TK-altered) and acyclovir-sensitive (TK-positive) HSV.[101,118,120] After passage in acyclovir-treated mice, heterogeneous mixtures of virus were selected that were both more pathogenic and more resistant than mixtures of input virus. A predominance of TK-altered mutants in a mixture could be associated with progressive disease.[101] The ability of acyclovir-sensitive and acyclovir-resistant viruses to complement one another for pathogenicity and acyclovir resistance in vivo is an increasingly impotant issue[391,393] in view of the heterogeneity of HSV clinical isolates.[295]

Acyclovir-resistant isolates of HSV have been obtained from immunocompromised individuals, especially AIDS patients.[333,334,352,408] Clinical acyclovir resistance is mostly associated with TK deficiency.[107] Less commonly, acyclovir-resistant clinical isolates are TK-altered mutants, including those with altered substrate specificity.[76,100,210] Occasionally, a clinical isolate is resistant to acyclovir because of a mutation in the HSV DNA polymerase.[63,333] Genetic heterogeneity in both pol and tk can occur in HSV isolates from acyclovir-treated patients.[100,333]

Acyclovir-resistant VZV isolates have been recovered from immunocompromised transplant recipients and AIDS patients.[191,230,293,334,389] Although a single VZV isolate has been reported to have acyclovir resistance resulting from a pol mutation,[377] all other acyclovir-resistant VZV isolates described have had mutations in TK.[341,389]

Ganciclovir-Resistant Cytomegalovirus

As expected from the genetic mechanisms of acyclovir resistance in HSV and VZV, ganciclovir-resistant CMV can contain mutations in either the CMV UL97 gene that encodes a ganciclovir kinase or the CMV pol gene that encodes the polymerase inhibited by GCVTP. However, all four laboratory strains of ganciclovir-resistant CMV characterized thus far have contained mutations in both genes, which is in contrast to the apparently rare occurrence of mutations in both tk and pol in acyclovir-resistant HSV and VZV.[236,383] Studies have suggested that part of the resistance of these CMV mutants is due to decreased ganciclovir kinase activity, and some of the phenotype is attributable to pol gene mutation. Each of the four doubly mutant CMVs retained susceptibility to foscarnet but were cross-resistant to HPMPC and HPMPA.[236,383] Ganciclovir resistance mutations in the CMV pol genes are widely separated from each other in the primary gene sequence, and some map to conserved regions in HSV that are different from those containing mutations that confer acyclovir resistance.[236,383]

Ganciclovir-resistant clinical isolates of CMV cause progressive disease in severely immunocompromised patients during ganciclovir therapy[104] and may be present in heterogeneous virus populations in infected humans before starting therapy.[104,390] A fairly high prevalence (8%) of urinary excretion of ganciclovir-resistant CMV was seen in 72 AIDS patients receiving ganciclovir for more than 3 months,[93] although no ganciclovir-resistant isolates were found among 42

solid organ transplant recipients receiving shorter courses of ganciclovir or acyclovir therapy.[27] Each ganciclovir-resistant isolate was associated with treatment failure, but clinical deterioration was also seen among patients who excreted ganciclovir-susceptible CMV.[93] The mechanism of resistance in clinical isolates commonly involves decreased phosphorylation of ganciclovir.[377] However, only one of nine isolates with reduced ganciclovir kinase activity had its DNA polymerase activity assessed for GCVTP susceptibility in vitro.[377] Another report described a ganciclovir-resistant isolate that phosphorylated ganciclovir to wild-type levels and that, because of minimal resistance to foscarnet, may have been a pol mutant.[390] It is not clear how frequently pol mutations contribute to ganciclovir resistance in clinical isolates, either alone or in conjunction with a ganciclovir kinase mutation.

Foscarnet

Mechanism of Action

Foscarnet (trisodium phosphonoformate) (see Fig. 17-2B) is a nonnucleoside derivative with activity against the polymerases of herpes[242,287] and hepatitis B viruses.[177] It also inhibits retrovirus reverse transcriptases in vitro, including that of HIV-1.[146,337,386] Foscarnet is a pyrophosphate analog that is a noncompetitive inhibitor of the viral polymerase.[175] It does not require intracellular activation but evidently inhibits DNA polymerase directly by interacting with the pyrophosphate-binding site to block binding of the pyrophosphate moiety that is cleaved from a dNTP during DNA synthesis. Foscarnet is not incorporated into viral DNA, and it inhibits viral polymerases at lower concentrations than are required to inhibit host cell polymerases.[47,79]

Pharmacology, Toxicity, and Clinical Trials

Foscarnet is cleared rapidly from the blood after intravenous administration but is not metabolized. About 10% to 30% of the dose accumulates in bone, the remainder being excreted unchanged in urine.[287] The drug is not orally bioavailable, and intravenous administration is required because of its highly alkaline pH. The disposition of foscarnet appears to be triphasic, with mean half-lives of 0.45, 3.3, and 18 hours.[356] Infusions of 60 mg/kg three times a day produce peak and trough serum levels of 557 and 155 μM/L, respectively[192]; concentrations in cerebrospinal fluid are approximately 27% of serum concentrations.[310]

Because of poor solubility, large fluid volumes are required for foscarnet administration. Nephrotoxicity is the most common adverse event. Metabolic abnormalities (hypocalcemia, hypomagnesemia, hyperphosphatemia) occur because foscarnet binds to ionized calcium in plasma. Seizures and anemia can also be drug related, and neuropathy, penile ulcers, and nephrogenic diabetes insipidus have been described.[402]

In uncontrolled trials, 14 to 21 days of intravenous foscarnet therapy stabilized or improved CMV retinitis in more than 90% of patients,[193,230,413] including those intolerant of ganciclovir or infected with ganciclovir-resistant isolates. Foscarnet offered a slight survival advantage when compared with ganciclovir for initial treatment of CMV retinitis in AIDS patients, possibly because of anti-HIV activity[131,315,337] or because of the use of concomitant medications with anti-HIV activity.[180] The actual effects of the two drugs on the retinitis were equivalent.[381]

Foscarnet has also shown activity against acyclovir-resistant mucocutaneous HSV and VZV infections in patients with AIDS.[334,334a] A decrease in indirect measurements of HIV-1 replication in vivo has been reported in studies of HIV-1–infected patients receiving foscarnet.[131,315]

Resistance

The isolation of HSV and CMV strains with pol mutations conferring resistance to pyrophosphate analogs suggests that foscarnet and the related analog, phosphonoacetic acid, are specific inhibitors of the HSV and CMV polymerases.[51,74,386] Foscarnet-resistant viruses have been found at lower frequencies in laboratory strains of CMV than of HSV[386] although foscarnet-resistant clinical isolates of both HSV and CMV have been detected after foscarnet use.[22,333] The mechanism of resistance to foscarnet involves alteration in binding to the polymerase, but it is not clear how much overlap exists between the nucleoside triphosphate/ACVTP/GCVTP- and pyrophosphate-binding sites. Laboratory-derived foscarnet-resistant pol mutants of HSV have generally been slightly resistant to acyclovir,[147,189] and seven of ten foscarnet-resistant HSV-2 isolates from AIDS patients, emerging during foscarnet therapy for acyclovir-resistant HSV, were susceptible enough to acyclovir to permit its use clinically.[335] Ganciclovir-resistant CMV laboratory strains have not been resistant to foscarnet, nor have foscarnet-resistant CMV laboratory strains been resistant to ganciclovir.[24,236,383,384] However, some clinical CMV isolates from immunocompromised patients have been resistant to both ganciclovir and foscarnet.[208,390]

Other Anti-Herpesvirus Agents

Vidarabine

Mechanism of Action

Vidarabine (adenine arabinoside [ara A], α-β-D-arabinofuranosyl adenine) is a purine nucleoside analog with some activity versus all members of the human herpesvirus group, but it is less effective against CMV or EBV than against HSV or VZV. It also inhibits certain animal herpesviruses, poxviruses, rhabdoviruses, and retroviruses.[92] Vidarabine inhibits viral DNA synthesis at concentrations below those required to inhibit host cell DNA synthesis[351] and may have multiple sites of action within an infected cell. It is phosphorylated to the active triphosphate form, ara ATP, by cellular kinases rather than by a virus-induced TK, so it is capable of inhibiting TK-deficient HSV mutants resistant to acyclovir.[219] Mechanisms that have proposed to explain the inhibition of HSV replication by vidarabine include the following:

- Selective inhibition of the viral DNA polymerase by ara-ATP due to competitive inhibition for the normal substrate, dATP[278]
- Inhibition of virus-induced ribonucleotide reductase by either ara ATP or ara ADP, which reduces the dATP pool and ultimately inhibits DNA synthesis[59,217]
- Selective incorporation of ara AMP into viral DNA, causing a decrease in the rate of primer elongation and chain termination

This last mechanism was suggested by some investigators,[277] but others observed random incorporation of ara AMP into internal linkages in both viral and cellular DNAs.

Pharmacology, Toxicity, and Clinical Trials

Vidarabine is readily deaminated in vivo to arabinosyl hypoxanthine, which has less antiviral activity than the parent compound. The plasma half-life is 3 to 4 hours, and nearly 60% of a dose is recovered in the urine, principally as arabinosyl hypoxanthine. Vidarabine is widely distributed in the body, with levels in cerebrospinal fluid 30% to 50% those in serum.[417] Vidarabine is relatively insoluble, and its intravenous administration requires a large fluid load.

The most common adverse effects of intravenous vidarabine therapy are gastrointestinal (nausea, vomiting, and diarrhea) and neurologic (tremors, paresthesias, ataxia, and seizures).[328,332] Preexisting neurologic, hepatic, or renal disease may predispose patients to vidarabine neurotoxicity, as may the concomitant use of allopurinol.[136] At high doses, megaloblastic anemia, leukopenia, and thrombocytopenia may occur. Inappropriate secretion of antidiuretic hormone has also been described.[311] In some experimental models, vidarabine has teratogenic, mutagenic, and carcinogenic properties. Its use in pregnant women and infants should be limited to those with life-threatening illnesses who are refractory to treatment with less toxic agents.

Placebo-controlled trials showed vidarabine to be beneficial in the treatment of HSV encephalitis,[426,428] neonatal HSV infection,[425] varicella and zoster in immunocompromised patients,[421,424,427] and mucocutaneous HSV infection in immunocompromised hosts.[429] Subsequent trials, however, demonstrated acyclovir to be more effective, less toxic, or both for these conditions.[422] Foscarnet has also shown greater efficacy and less toxicity than vidarabine as an alternative drug when resistance to acyclovir occurs.[334] Topical vidarabine remains useful for the management of superficial dendritic or geographic HSV keratitis.[68,298]

Resistance

Proof that the HSV-specific DNA polymerase is a selective target of vidarabine has been the isolation of vidarabine-resistant strains with mutations linked to the pol gene.[51,56] Several vidarabine-resistant mutants specified altered DNA polymerases that were less susceptible than wild-type enzyme to ara ATP.[16,56] Vidarabine resistance was subsequently mapped to a 0.8-kilobase pair region within the pol gene.[54,129] These data suggest that at least some of vidarabine's action is directed against the viral DNA polymerase. Most HSV mutations conferring resistance to vidarabine cluster in the same region of pol as do the acyclovir resistance mutations.[148] Vidarabine-resistant mutants share a pattern of cross-resistance with other agents, such as acyclovir.[55]

Idoxuridine and Trifluridine

Idoxuridine (5'-iodo-2'-deoxyuridine [IdU]) and trifluridine (trifluorothymidine [TFT]) are nucleoside analogs that are converted to triphosphates that are both inhibitors and substrate analogs for herpesvirus polymerases, which they inhibit more effectively than host cell polymerases.[173,307] IdU and TFT are not selectively activated but are phosphorylated by both virus-induced and cellular kinases.[307] In herpesvirus-infected cells with increased kinase activities, more IdU is converted to the monophosphate form than in uninfected cells. TFT monophosphate is a potent inhibitor of thymidylate synthetase.[173]

Ophthalmic preparations are licensed in the United States for topical treatment of HSV keratitis. IdU was synthesized in 1959[306] and shown to be effective in treating ocular HSV infections.[198] Although intravenous IdU was initially promoted as an inhibitor of HSV encephalitis, subsequent trials showed it to be neither safe nor effective for this condition.[29] Thus, IdU is not used as a systemic antiviral drug. TFT is also licensed for treatment of HSV keratitis and corneal ulcers.[68] Although it inhibits CMV replication in vitro,[432] TFT is not used clinically for this purpose. TFT has been studied as a topical treatment for acyclovir-resistant chronic mucocutaneous genital HSV lesions in HIV-infected patients, either alone[279] or in combination with interferon-α.[22] Preliminary clinical reports appear promising, but the frequency of complete healing remains to be determined.

HUMAN IMMUNODEFICIENCY VIRUS TYPE I

A number of virus-mediated steps in the HIV-1 replication cycle (Fig. 17-3) have been targeted for chemotherapeutic inhibition. The first step in the infectious cycle of HIV-1 is attachment of its envelope glycoprotein to a specific receptor on the cell surface, whose major component is CD4. This binding can be blocked by monoclonal antibodies to CD4 or by rsCD4, a recombinant, soluble, truncated form of the CD4 molecule.[126,363] To inhibit clinical isolates of HIV-1, however, much higher levels of rsCD4 are required than for laboratory strains,[75,275] and clinical trials have not shown any virologic or clinical effectiveness of rsCD4 or its derivatives.[183,195,347] Once the virus is internalized and uncoated, reverse transcription takes place in the cytoplasm within a preintegration complex of viral, and possibly cellular, proteins. This conversion of a single-stranded RNA genome to double-stranded DNA involves both DNA polymerization and RNase H enzymatic activities of the HIV-1 reverse transcriptase and is the source of most of the extensive genetic heterogeneity of HIV-1. The DNA polymerization portion of this process is the target of many agents in clinical use and many of those in development. While reverse transcription is occurring, a cellular factor may specifically bind a nuclear localization signal within the HIV-1 matrix protein to actively transport the viral preintegration complex into the nucleus.[37] Unlike other retroviruses, which do not integrate into cellular DNA until nuclear membrane integrity is disrupted during mitosis, HIV-1 proviral DNA can be formed by the viral integrase that inserts viral genetic material into host chromosomal DNA of nondividing, terminally differentiated monocyte/macrophages and of CD4+ T lymphocytes arrested in G_2 and S phase.[229,416] Inhibition of any of the replication steps up to this point prevents establishment of a productive infection.

Virus replication in cells that already contain integrated HIV-1 proviral DNA can be inhibited only by targeting steps late in the replication cycle. Integrated HIV-1 DNA is transcribed by host cell RNA polymerase II, but the process is modulated by viral regulatory signals recognized by cellular transcription factors like NF-κB[280] as well as virus-specific regulatory gene products. The mRNA and genomic RNA transcripts are spliced, capped, polyadenylated, and transported to the cytoplasm, where they are translated into viral proteins. On some HIV-1 mRNAs, ribosomes shift reading frames to bypass a translational stop codon at the end of the gag open reading frame; this frame shifting leads to an abundance of gag precursor polypeptide and a smaller amount of read-through gag-pol precursor polypeptide. Posttranslational processing includes myristylation and glycosylation; the glycosylation inhibitors castanospermine and deoxynojirimycin inhibit replication in vitro.[155,411] HIV-1 regulatory gene products, including tat, rev, and nef, modulate virus protein synthesis by acting at transcriptional or posttranscriptional levels. Inhibitors of tat function have been identified by mechanism-based screening[186] but seem to act through cellular proteins and have been disappointing in clinical trials. Viral structural proteins, replicative enzymes, and genomic RNA are assembled, associated with envelope glycoproteins, and released by budding from the plasma membrane where viral glycoproteins have congregated. Processing of HIV-1 proteins within budding virions includes specific cleavage of the gag-pol and gag precursor polypeptides by protease into mature forms, which are necessary to render the virion capable of reinitiating the infectious cycle when it encounters a susceptible host cell. Three HIV-1 protease inhibitors have been approved in the United States, and others under study.

Zidovudine and Other Nucleoside Derivatives

Mechanism of Action

Zidovudine (3-azido-3'-deoxythymidine, azidothymidine [AZT], Retrovir) is a synthetic pyrimidine analog that differs from thymidine only in having an azido substituent instead of a hydroxyl group at the 3' position of the deoxyribose ring. It was initially developed as an anticancer agent[185] and was subsequently found to inhibit the reverse transcriptase of Friend leukemia virus.[291] Soon after the identification of a human retrovirus as the etiologic agent of AIDS, zidovudine was shown to have anti-HIV activity in vitro.[268]

The active form of zidovudine, AZT triphosphate (AZTTP), is a competitive inhibitor of the reverse transcriptase. AZTTP not only binds better to HIV-1 reverse transcriptase than its natural substrate, dTTP, but also functions as an alternate substrate for enzyme.[46,376] AZTTP has been shown to have a 100-fold greater affinity for reverse transcriptase than for cellular DNA polymerases α or β.[137,140] The intracellular concentration of AZTTP is greater than the K_i value for the HIV reverse transcriptase but is less than K_i values for cellular polymerases α and β.[140] AZTTP may be incorporated as AZT monophosphate (AZTMP) into growing DNA chains, which leads to premature chain termination.[376] The incorporated AZTMP does not provide a 3'-hydroxyl group to form a phosphodiester bond with the incoming nucleotide, so chain elongation is terminated, specifically at thymidine residues.[140,376] Viral DNA synthesis is halted because the reverse transcriptase cannot excise the incorporated analog.

Zidovudine selectivity is due to the preferential interaction of AZTTP with the reverse transcriptase.[140,376] Phosphorylation of zidovudine to its active form, AZTTP, is accomplished by cellular enzymes.[140,268] Zidovudine is an efficient substrate for the cellular TK, which converts it to AZTMP in both infected and uninfected cells. AZTMP accumulates in cells because of slow phosphorylation to AZTDP by host cell thymidylate kinase, which is the rate-limiting step in AZTTP formation. AZTMP is a competitive inhibitor of thymidylate kinase and reduces the conversion of dTMP to dTDP, which leads to decreased production of dTTP. Conversion of AZTDP to AZTTP is thought to be catalyzed by the cellular nucleoside diphosphate kinase.[137] Phosphorylation of AZT may be more efficient in some cell types (e.g., CD4+ T lymphocytes) than in others (e.g., resting monocyte/macrophages). It has been speculated that other metabolites of AZT may also be involved in its mechanism of action. Ribavirin has been shown to antagonize the in vitro anti–HIV-1 activity of zidovudine by inhibiting its phosphorylation.[407] Ganciclovir has also been reported to antagonize zidovudine action in vitro.[258]

Other nucleoside analogs, including didanosine (2',3'-dideoxyinosine [ddI] and zalcitabine (2',3'-dideoxycytidine [ddC]), also have activity against HIV-1.[268] Didanosine was developed as a prodrug of dideoxyadenosine (ddA) and avoids the nephrotoxicity of orally administered ddA[415]; it is converted to ddA after absorption. The only mechanism of action identified for didanosine and zalcitabine is the same as that described for AZT—competition with the natural nucleoside triphosphate substrate and chain termination after incorporation of the inhibitor. Both ddA and ddC are phosphorylated by cellular enzymes to ddA triphosphate and ddC triphosphate that compete for reverse transcriptase binding with either deoxyadenosine triphosphate or deoxycytidine triphosphate, respectively.

Molecular mechanisms underlying the complex process of reverse transcription require further definition to extend our understanding of mechanisms of action of reverse transcriptase inhibitors. Modeling of the three-dimensional structure of the HIV-1 reverse transcriptase, based on x-ray diffraction of cocrystals of enzyme with either an inhibitor (nevirapine)[209] or DNA monoclonal antibody Fab fragment,[10] is a first step toward a comprehensive correlation of reverse transcriptase structure with function (Fig. 17-4A). To accomplish such crystallographic studies, it was necessary to produce large amounts of purified enzyme by cloning the pol gene and expressing it to high levels in bacteria.[73,225] Initial studies have clarified differences in folding of each subunit of the reverse transcriptase heterodimer that help to form specific active sites and have indicated similarities with other polymerases in motifs that are essential for certain functions: primer-template binding, DNA polymerization, and RNase H activity The model also suggests that one subdomain of p66 (the "thumb") may move when primer-template translocates after incorporation of a nucleoside monophosphate onto the primer terminus. Another subdomain of p66 (the "fingers") may contact and orient the template strand (see Fig. 17-4A,B).[209] Further characterization of reverse transcriptases complexed with other inhibitors, substrates, and inhibitor-terminated primer-templates, is neces-

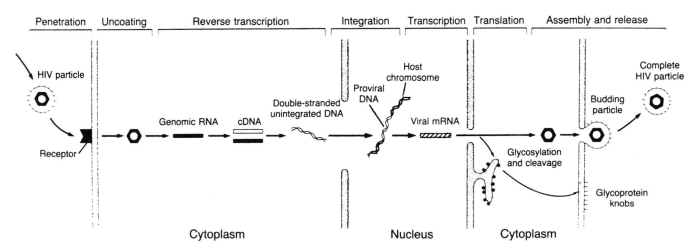

Fig. 17-3. Replicative cycle of human immunodeficiency virus-1 (HIV-1), indicating potential sites of action for HIV-1 inhibitors. cDNA, complementary DNA; mRNA, messenger RNA. (Reprinted with permission from Hirsch MS, D'Aquila RT. Therapy for human immunodeficiency virus infection. N Engl J Med 1993;325:1686–1695.)

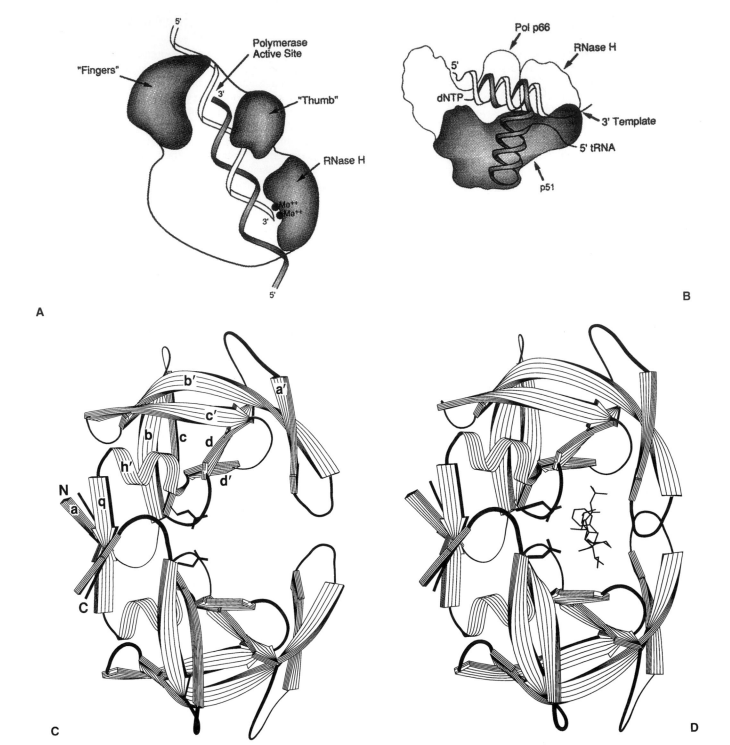

Fig. 17-4. Schematic drawings of the structures of the human immunodeficiency virus-1 (HIV-1) reverse transcriptase (RT) and protease. (A, B) HIV-1 RT heterodimer with different primer-templates modeled into the structure. In A, the RT heterodimer (p66/p51) is shown as it may hypothetically bind an RNA-DNA hybrid. This suggests how the RNA genomic template strand (white) may be progressively cleaved at the RNase H active site (in the p51 subunit) in concert with elongation of the DNA primer/product strand (black) at the polymerase active site (between the "fingers" and "thumb" subdomains of the p66 subunit). In B, a hypothetical complex between a tRNA-primed RNA template and the RT heterodimer (p66/p51) is shown. It is hypothesized that the p51 subunit may bind the anticodon and dihydrouridine stems and loops of the physiologic primer tRNA. (A and B reprinted with permission from Kohlstaedt LA, Wang J, Friedman JM, Rice PA, Steitz TA. Crystal structure at 3.5 resolution of HIV-1 reverse transcriptase complexed with an inhibitor. Science 1992;256:1783–1790.) (C, D) HIV-1 protease homodimer chain tracing. In C, apoenzyme is pictured with letters labeling the beta-strands of one subunit. In D, enzyme is depicted as complexed with a peptidomimetic inhibitor. (C and D reprinted with permission from Wlodawer A, Erickson JW. Structure-based inhibitors of HIV-1 protease. Annu Rev Biochem 1993;62:543–585.)

sary to further define reverse transcriptase functions and to allow for inhibitor design based on the structure of the enzyme and its mechanisms of action.

Pharmacology, Toxicity, and Clinical Trials

After oral dosing, zidovudine is rapidly absorbed, with peak serum concentrations occurring at 30 to 90 minutes. Chronic dosing of 250 mg every 4 hours in phase II studies[125,322] resulted in peak and trough concentrations of 0.62 and 0.16 μg/mL, respectively. Because zidovudine is metabolized primarily by glucuronidation, drugs that inhibit this step (e.g., probenicid) can increase its half-life. The drug penetrates the blood-brain barrier, producing effective antiviral concentrations within the CSF.

The major toxicity of zidovudine is on bone marrow cells, with macrocytic anemia and granulocytopenia as common occurrences. The mechanisms of these toxic effects are uncertain. Rare instances of pancytopenia with hypocellular marrow have been described.[150] Nausea, myalgia, insomnia, fever, rash, nail pigmentation, and severe headaches may also be observed.[322] An apparently rare syndrome of lactic acidosis, which may occur in association with severe hepatomegaly with steatosis, has been described in zidovudine-treated, HIV-1–infected patients.[133] Although the etiology of this syndrome is not known, it has also been observed with other nucleosides; it has been speculated that chronic nucleoside inhibition of mitochondrial DNA synthesis may be involved in the etiology.

From February 1986 to the end of June 1986, 282 patients with advanced HIV infection were enrolled in a clinical trial at 12 different centers in the United States.[125,322] One hundred forty-five patients received an oral dose of 250 mg of zidovudine every 4 hours, and 137 patients received placebo. By September 1986, it was apparent that differences in survival had emerged, and the study was terminated by an independent data safety monitoring board. Nineteen patients in the placebo group had died, compared with only one who received zidovudine. Furthermore, there was a significant difference in opportunistic infections in patients who received placebo (45 infections) compared with zidovudine recipients (24 infections). Patients who received zidovudine generally gained weight, whereas placebo recipients lost weight. Karnofsky scores of functional capability also improved in zidovudine recipients but did not improve in the placebo groups. Individuals who received zidovudine generally showed an increase in CD4+ cells, although this effect was lost after 5 months in patients with AIDS. Because of these results, zidovudine was licensed in 1987 for patients with symptomatic HIV infections and fewer than 200 CD4+ lymphocytes/μL in peripheral blood. The decreased mortality rates for patients receiving zidovudine were also seen during extended follow-up of the originally enrolled patients through 21 months of therapy.[179] In subsequent trials, lower doses of zidovudine (1200 mg daily for 1 month followed by 600 mg daily) were equivalent in efficacy to high doses (1500 mg daily) in patients with advanced HIV infection and were associated with far less toxicity.[123]

Beginning zidovudine therapy before the onset of AIDS delays the progression of disease, as manifested by the delayed onset of opportunistic infections, neurologic disease, and tumors.[124,162] In two trials that together enrolled more than 2000 patients with early or no symptoms of HIV infection and CD4+ cell counts below 500/μL, AIDS developed earlier in the patients receiving placebo than in those treated with zidovudine. The rates of progression were similar in patients treated with 1500 mg daily and in those treated with a lower dose (500 mg daily), although hematologic toxicity occurred more frequently in the former (11.8% and 2.9%, respectively).

Another study compared early and late zidovudine therapy (1500 mg daily) in 338 symptomatic patients with 200 to 500 CD4+ cells/μL.[162] The patients in the late-treatment group received placebo until their CD4+ counts fell below 200/μL or until AIDS was diagnosed. During a mean follow-up of more than 2 years, AIDS developed in 28 patients in the early-therapy group compared with 48 in the late-therapy group (P = .02). However, the number of deaths was similar in the two groups (23 and 20 deaths, respectively), with a 3-year survival rate of approximately 80% in both. Results of a large European trial comparing early and late zidovudine therapy in asymptomatic subjects[65] also suggested that survival of HIV-1–infected patients was equivalent whether zidovudine therapy was begun early or late in the course of infection.

In children with HIV infection, zidovudine therapy is also associated with weight gain and improvement in cognitive function and both virologic and immunologic markers.[256] Doses of 180 mg/m² every 6 hours are recommended for children older than 3 months of age who have clinical or laboratory evidence of progressive HIV infection. Anemia and leukopenia are the major side effects of zidovudine in children, as they are in adults.

Zidovudine is well tolerated during pregnancy and does not cause fetal distress, malformation, or premature birth.[368] Transmission of HIV-1 from mother to newborn can be reduced by zidovudine.[283] Pregnant women with CD4+ counts above 200/μL who had not previously received zidovudine were enrolled into a placebo-controlled trial of AZT between 1991 and 1993. Women received study drug between their 14th and 34th weeks of pregnancy. Within 24 hours of birth and for 6 weeks thereafter, newborns also received the same blinded medication as their mothers. Of 364 newborns tested, 53 had HIV infection, of whom 40 (25.5%) were placebo recipients and 13 (8.3%) were AZT recipients. Zidovudine's role in occupational post-exposure prophylaxis has been shown in case control studies.[44a]

Resistance

Viruses resistant to AZT were first identified in isolates from patients treated with AZT for at least 6 months.[221] HIV-1 also develops resistance to AZT with in vitro serial passage in subinhibitory drug concentrations.[218] Specific substitutions in reverse transcriptase codons 41, 67, 70, 215, and 219 accumulate sequentially and lead to increasing degrees of resistance.[199,223] The highest level of resistance, whch is associated with four or five of these subtitutions, is at least a 100-fold increase in 50% inhibitory concentration (IC50) of AZT. Clinical isolates from patients undergoing prolonged AZT therapy can have varied levels of resistance; many retain full susceptibility even after years of therapy. The likelihood of isolating an AZT-resistant virus increases with duration of therapy and advancing disease.[323] Resistant variants have been found at some low frequently in virus populations in vivo before antiretroviral exposure.[269,281a] If antiretroviral therapy is terminated, zidovudine-resistant virus is slowly replaced by more susceptible HIV-1.[216]

The biochemical mechanisms by which the mutant reverse transcriptase confers AZT resistance to the virus require further definition. Substitutions at the base of the reverse transcriptase p66 thumb subdomain close to the polymerase active site (i.e., either in codon 215[244] or in both codons 215 and 219[109]) decrease AZTTP binding to purified reverse transcriptase enzyme in vitro. However, mutant enzyme with mutations that confer high-level resistance to the virus can be inhibited just as readily as wild-type enzyme by AZTTP in vitro.[109,212] The structural model of the HIV-1 reverse transcriptase suggests that in such highly resistant virus, not all residues that have been altered by mutation cluster in a potential dNTP-binding site near the polymerase active site[209] but that some (e.g., amino acids 41, 67, and 70 in the fingers subdomain) are physically distant and may affect reverse transcriptase function in other ways. Presumably, in vitro polymerase assays do not fully reflect reverse transcriptase enzyme function in the infected cell.

AZT-resistant virus is cross-resistant only to other HIV reverse transcriptase inhibitors that contain a 3'-azido substituent, such as 3'-azido-2',3'-dideoxyuridine.[221] Cloned mutant viruses that differ from wild-type only in that they possess specific AZT resistance mutations are not cross-resistant to didanosine, zalcitabine, or didehydrodeoxythymidine.[221] However, two clinical isolates with an AZT-resistant phenotype have been found to be cross-resistant to d4T.[326] Others have reported a direct correlation between AZT IC50s and didanosine or zalcitabine IC50s of isolates from AZT-treated patients.[251] The genetic bases for these latter two phenomena remain to be elucidated.

AZT-resistant virus has been transmitted by both documented[8] and presumed[127] parenteral exposure to HIV-1–infected blood. It has also been isolated from a patient with primary HIV-1 infection acquired by homosexual contact.[105] High-level zidovudine resistance has been associated with more rapid clinical progression during therapy than occurs in patients with AZT-susceptible isolates,[72,211,271,288,398] which suggests that AZT-resistant virus is pathogenic. This association persists even when controlling for other factors that predict clinical deterioration.[72,194a,271] One report correlated a high circulating virus load with the presence of one of the AZT resistance mutations.[211] Therapeutic failure is complex and multifactorial; patients can deteriorate an AZT therapy even while harboring AZT-susceptible virus.

Didanosine

Pharmacology, Toxicity, and Clinical Trials

Didanosine is acid labile. Current preparations include buffered chewable tablets and a powder for suspension with antacid. Its oral bioavailability varies, and the buffered didanosine may interfere with the absorption of other drugs that depend on gastric acidity, such as dapsone and ketoconazole. Although the plasma half-life is short (30 minutes), the intracellular half-life is prolonged ($\geq$12 hours), which allows for dosing regimens twice daily. The cerebrospinal fluid/plasma ratio for didanosine is 0.2, lower than for zidovudine.[436] Peripheral neuropathy is the principal dose-limiting side effect and occurs in 13% to 34% of patients taking didanosine at or below recommended doses. The neuropathy is characterized by distal numbness, tingling, or pain and occurs more often in patients with a history of neuropathy or previous neurotoxic drug therapy. Pancreatitis, ranging from mild abdominal pain and elevated serum amylase concentrations to fatal disease, occurs in 5% to 10% of patients. Patients with renal impairment or previous pancreatitis may be at a higher risk of pancreatitis.

Didanosine was initially approved for use in patients with advanced HIV infection who were intolerant to zidovudine treatment or in whom such treatment had been unsuccessful. The results of several trials[86,181,196,371] support the concept that a switch from zidovudine to didanosine may be beneficial in patients with advanced disease after a certain period of zidovudine therapy, although the optimal time for the change is unclear. Moreover, recent clinical trials in adults and children suggest that diclanosine, either as monotherapy or in combination with zidovudine, is preferable to zidovudine as initial therapy.[162a]

Resistance

The mechanism of didanosine inhibition of reverse transcriptase has been described previously, and its specificity for the HIV-1 reverse transcriptase is supported by studies of didanosine-resistant viruses that emerge after months of didanosine therapy. Substitutions in reverse transcriptase amino acids 74,[109,375] 184,[156] and 65[440] confer a minimal increase in IC50 relative to viruses isolated from drug-naive individuals; the substitution at codon 74 appears to be most common. Didanosine resistance mutations decrease inhibition of reverse transcriptase enzymatic activity by ddATP, the active metabolite of didanosine.[109,156,244,440] One report indicates that the codon 74 mutation in the fingers subdomain of the reverse transcriptase p66 subunit contacts the RNA template strand and reorients the terminus of the growing DNA chain downstream in the active site so that binding of ddATP is decreased but binding of the natural substrate (dATP) is unimpaired.[30] Cross-resistance occurs between didanosine and zalcitabine. The clinical significance of didanosine-resistant viruses has not yet been defined.

Zalcitabine

Pharmacology, Toxicity, and Clinical Trials

Zalcitabine is orally bioavailable (87%), with a plasma half-life of 20 minutes and an intracellular half-life as active triphosphate of 2.6 hours.[32] Its cerebrospinal fluid/plasma ratio is approximately 0.2.[436] The major toxicity is peripheral neuropathy (17% to 31%), which is related to both the cumulative and daily dose. Rash and stomatitis commonly occur 2 to 6 weeks after onset of therapy but usually subside despite continued therapy.

Zalcitabine has been studied both as monotherapy and in combination with zidovudine. A 1-year interim analysis of a trial in patients with baseline CD4+ counts below 200 cells/μL and less than 3 months of previous zidovudine therapy demonstrated poorer survival of patients taking zalcitabine than of those taking zidovudine.[122] In another trial, the efficacy of zalcitabine was equivalent to that of didanosine in patients in whom zidovudine therapy had been unsuccessful or who could no longer tolerate zidovudine.[1]

Resistance

Viruses resistant to zalcitabine, another chain-terminating nucleoside analog, have not been studied extensively. Mutations in reverse transcriptase codon 69[128] or 65[440] are responsible for zalcitabine resistance of HIV-1 in cell culture. The codon 65 mutation also causes the reverse transcriptase to be resistant to zalcitabine triphosphate inhibition in vitro. Cross-resistance to didanosine has been observed for reverse transcriptase codon 65 and 74 mutants.

Other HIV-1 Reverse Transcriptase Inhibitors

Stavudine (2'3' didehydro-3'-deoxythymidine [d4T]) is a pyrimidine nucleoside with inhibitory activity against HIV-1 reverse transcriptase. It has good oral bioavailability and antiviral activity against both zidovudine-sensitive and zidovudine-resistant viruses.[94,221] Phase I trials have demonstrated biologic activity against HIV-1 (decreased serum p24 antigen, increased or stable CD4+ cell counts) at doses below those that cause a sensory peripheral neuropathy.[33] More than 14,000 patients have received this drug worldwide, and stavudine has been approved in the United States for patients who have failed therapy with zidovudine and didanosine or zalcitabine.

Lamivudine, also known as 3TC, is the (−) enantiomer of the cytosine analog 2′-deoxy-3′-thiacytidine. It has good oral bioavailability and low toxicity. Resistance of HIV-1 develops rapidly, related to a single amino acid substitution at codon 184 of reverse transcriptase. However, when this mutation is introduced into virions with zidovudine resistance, those virions frequently regain susceptibility to zidovudine.[224a] Lamivudine is approved for use in combination with Zidovudine in the United States.

Another class of agent directed against the HIV-1 reverse transcriptase, frequently called nonnucleoside reverse transcriptase inhibitors, are also known as HIV-1–specific reverse transcriptase inhibitors.[71] This class includes compounds with diverse chemical structures that are unrelated to nucleosides, such as nevirapine, TIBO compounds, ateverdine, delavirdine and L697,661, as well as a few agents that are derived from nucleosides, such as TSAO and HEPT compounds. All of these inhibitors are uncompetitive with respect to substrates or primer-template and potently inhibit HIV-1 reverse transcrip-

tase in vitro with minimal cellular toxicity. They are extremely specific for HIV-1 reverse transcriptase and have no activity against the highly related HIV-2 reverse transcriptase. Structural modeling of the reverse transcriptase indicates that these compounds bind, with small differences, to a hydrophobic pocket of the p66 subunit near the active site. They may indirectly affect residues in the polymerase active site or impair mobility of the thumb subdomain.

Resistant viruses can have one or more mutations that alter the reverse transcriptase–binding pocket, and they emerge rapidly in vitro. Clinical trials have also shown a rapid development of resistant virus in many patients for most compounds in this class. Development of resistance correlated with loss of antiviral suppression, which is the best evidence that drug-resistant HIV-1 can cause virologic failure of antiretroviral therapy.[331] Clinical trials have shown that these agent may be useful in combination therapy,[71a] and one of these agents, nevirapine is now approved for use in the United States. Structural information concerning their reverse transcriptase binding site may aid in modifying such compounds so that it may be more difficult for mutations to disrupt binding.

Inhibitors of Other HIV-1 Enzymes

Many inhibitors of the HIV-1 protease are now in development and three have been approved in the United States. The posttranslational cleavage of gag and gag-pol polypeptides by HIV-1 protease is essential for virion assembly and maturation within budding virions. If this function is blocked by an inactivating mutation or an inhibitor, immature, noninfectious virus particles bud from infected cell membranes.[208,257] Protease inhibitors are the first agents described that appear to be capable of blocking late stages of the viral replicative cycle in vivo. They may also impair an early preintegration event that depends on cleavage of nucleocapsid protein within the virion.[281] The HIV-1 protease is a homodimer in which the two subunits are related by a twofold (C2) axis of symmetry, and a single peptide-binding active site formed at the subunit interface (see Fig. 17-4C). Its three-dimensional structure is known,[434] and its functional mechanism is similar to that of previously characterized aspartyl proteases.

The use of structure-based, rational design of antiviral agents is becoming increasingly important. Preclinical studies of protease inhibitors are guided by structural and biochemical data and have led to promising new design principles and synthetic strategies. Crystallographic analyses of protease complexed with inhibitors have elucidated interactions between enzyme and inhibitor and have been used to improve the potency and specificity of lead compounds (see Fig. 17-4D).[434] Most inhibitors are peptidomimetic, are difficult to synthesize, and often have poor bioavailability. Although the active site of the enzyme is fairly symmetric, not all inhibitors are symmetric. The flexibility of the peptidomimetic inhibitor backbones appears to facilitate binding to the enzyme.

Highly specific nonpeptide protease inhibitors have also been designed.[213,317a] Because it had been observed that a structural water molecule was necessary for tight binding of peptidomimetic inhibitors to the enzyme active site, a three-dimensional pharmacophore was designed to incorporate the binding features of this water molecule. The pharmacophore was used to search databases of three-dimensional molecular structures, and a six-membered ring was found that could position a mimic of the structural water molecule into the protease active site. Using this six-membered ring structure as a guide, nonpeptide molecules were synthesized to optimize binding.[213]

Protease inhibitor–resistant virus has been selected by laboratory passage in the presence of protease inhibitor. These variants showed a twofold to tenfold increase in IC50, with substitutions in amino acids 8, 46, and 82.[182,292] In one case, a substitution at residue 8 decreased favorable interactions between the enzyme and the terminal portion of the inhibitor and impaired the replicative capacity of the virus. This was seen only in the presence of a compensating drug-selected substitution at residue 46, which returned virus replication to normal levels.[182] Each of these residues approximates the active site where substrates and inhibitors bind. Preliminary reports from early clinical trials of protease inhibitor monotherapy suggest that a more complex pattern of mutations may be selected in vivo by some of these drugs.[65a,270a] Indinavir- and ritonavir-selected viruses appear to share cross-resistance to the alternate drug and a proportion of viruses from patients treated with indinavir have isolates that are also cross-resistant to saquinavir. Saquinavir-resistant mutants isolated from patients treated with saquinavir have one or two specific substitutions in residues contributing to the active site and cross-resistance appears to extend less commonly to indinavir or ritonavir.[343a] An understanding of drug resistance may be furthered by analyzing inhibitor-enzyme complexes at the molecular level. It is already possible to design second-generation HIV-1 protease inhibitors that are modified in positions where the first-generation parent congener interacts with the substituted residue that confers protease resistance.[324]

The HIV-1 integrase has also been studied as a target for inhibitors, but this work is still at an early stage. The integration reaction has been dissected into two biochemical steps: site-specific cleavage of DNA and strand transfer.[406] Inhibitors of integrase enzymatic activity in vitro have been identified by screening a small number of preselected compounds,[116] and an assay suitable for large-scale random screening has been described.[69] It remains to be seen whether compounds identified by such biochemical assays will inhibit virus replication in vivo. The structure of integrase has not yet been fully determined crystallographically, but the structure of the catalytic core domain has been reported.[96a]

Drug Combinations

Monotherapy with available nucleosides has had only limited success against HIV infection. Combination antiretroviral therapy is receiving considerable attention for several reasons[39,252]:

1. Two or more drugs may offer additive to synergistic anti-HIV activity leading to better efficacy.
2. Toxicity may be reduced if doses of individual drugs can be reduced.
3. Broadened coverage against potentially resistant viruses could be achieved.

4. Different cellular and tissue reservoirs can be targeted, as well as cells at different levels of activation.

Agents may be targeted either to different stages or to the same stage in the viral replication cycle, and combinations of drugs have been used either simultaneously or in alternation.[39]

Small pilot trials of either two or three drug combinations have provided promising data suggesting superiority of combinations over monotherapy.[39,62,112,259,360,436] Recently, definitive results of several large combination trials have become available indicating that two-drug combinations are of greater benefit than zidovudine monotherapy at various stages of disease.[162a,181a] Moreover, three-drug combinations may be better than two-drug combinations in controlled trials recently completed.[71a,181a]

OTHER VIRUSES

Respiratory Syncytial Virus

Ribavirin (α-β-D ribofuranosyl-1,2,4-triazole-3-carboxamide), a synthetic purine nucleoside derivative resembling guanosine and inosine, has been used to treat a number of virus infections, including respiratory syncytial virus (RSV), which is a negative-strand RNA virus.[353] Ribavirin is phosphorylated intracellularly to 5'-monophosphate, 5'-diphosphate, and 5'-triphosphate forms.[354] Although virtually no mechanistic studies have been done with RSV, the effect of ribavirin on replication of other negative-strand RNA viruses like vesicular stomatitis virus[396] and La Crosse virus,[42] a bunyavirus, have been studied at the molecular level. Several theories have been proposed to explain the molecular mode of action of ribavirin[296]:

1. Ribavirin-5'-monophosphate inhibits cellular inosine-5'-monophosphate dehydrogenase activity, thereby depleting intracellular pools of GTP. In fact, some of the antiviral effects of ribavirin in vitro can be reversed by the addition of guanosine.[238,380]
2. Ribavirin-5'-triphosphate interferes with 5'-capping of mRNAs by inhibiting host cell guanylyl transferase activity. Synthesis of RNA with abnormal or missing 5'-cap structures would lead to inefficient translation of viral transcripts.[152]
3. Phosphorylated ribavirin compounds have direct inhibitory effects on viral RNA-dependent RNA polymerase activity. This has been demonstrated for the polymerases of influenza virus[106,435] and vesicular stomatitis virus.[396] A similar polymerase has been described in La Crosse virions.[297]

These theories may not be mutually exclusive in explaining the complex and unclear mechanism of action of ribavirin.

Ribavirin is licensed in the United States for treatment of RSV infection by small particle (1 to 2 μm) aerosol. After aerosol administration, its half-life in lower respiratory secretions is about 2 hours.[40] Concentrations in respiratory secretions after aerosol administration may be 100 times higher than those in blood. Aerosol ribavirin has not been associated with significant toxicity, although reticulocytosis, rash, and conjunctivitis have been observed. A small percentage of health care workers exposed to aerosolized ribavirin have had reversible mucous membrane irritation, primarily eye irritation in contact lens wearers.[194]

In one study of nonhuman primates, ribavirin was not teratogenic, and no such effects have been reported in humans after 7 years of using aerosolized ribavirin against RSV, although it is teratogenic in most rodent species tested.[115] Ribavirin is also mutagenic, embryotoxic, and possibly carcinogenic. Pregnant women are advised not to care directly for any patients receiving aerosolized ribavirin.[31,165,325] Exposure to health care workers can be reduced by using a ventilator or a vacuum hood exhaust system.[31]

Most cases of RSV infection in children are mild and self-limiting and do not require antiviral treatment. In 1983, two groups reported that ribavirin aerosol was beneficial to infants hospitalized with RSV-induced lower respiratory tract disease, bronchiolitis, and pneumonia. Patients who were treated with ribavirin in these controlled studies had fewer lower respiratory tract signs and more rapid improvement in arterial oxygen saturation, viral shedding, and clinical status.[161,387] Other studies, including a trial among previously healthy mechanically ventilated infants, have confirmed its safety and efficacy,[364] although some researchers consider the benefits to be marginal.[410] In 1993, the Committee on Infectious Diseases of the American Academy of Pediatrics recommended ribavirin aerosol treatment for infants hospitalized with RSV lower respiratory tract disease who are (1) at high risk for a severe or complicated course because of underlying conditions such as complicated congenital heart disease, bronchopulmonary dysplasia, cystic fibrosis or other chronic lung disease, prematurity, or immunodeficiency; (2) severely ill with RSV, or (3) mechanically ventilated.[160] In addition, it was stated that ribavirin treatment should be considered for infants hospitalized with RSV who are younger than 6 weeks of age or have other underlying diseases.[160]

Viruses Causing Hemorrhagic Fever Syndromes

Systemic ribavirin has been used to treat severe hemorrhagic fever syndromes[6] caused by an arenavirus (Lassa fever) and by a bunyavirus (Hantaan virus). The primary adverse effects of systemic ribavirin are hematologic. Transient anemia due to rapid extravascular clearance of erythrocytes or bone marrow suppression with resultant hyperbilirubinemia has been described.[149]

Often fatal, Lassa fever is spread from urine of infected rodents in endemic areas such as West Africa. After weeks of fever and nonspecific systemic complaints, hemorrhage occurs, largely in the gastrointestinal tract. Death can result from hypovolemic shock. Compared with historical controls, ribavirin treatment reduced the mortality rate from 55% to 5% in patients with a poor prognosis if begun within 6 days of onset of fever; the fatality rate was 26% if treatment was begun after 7 days of fever.[253] Oral ribavirin has also been used for prophylaxis of high-risk nosocomial contacts.[184] Ribavirin had some beneficial virologic effect in advanced Argentine hemorrhagic fever caused by Junin virus, another arenavirus, although the mortality rate was not reduced.[103]

Hemorrhagic fever with renal syndrome is a clinical entity in Asia caused by Hantaan virus, a bunyavirus in the Hantavirus genus. The virus is transmitted from rodent urine in endemic areas, and human-to-human spread has not been documented. The mortality rate is 5% to 10% and is generally limited to patients who progress through sequential febrile and hypotensive phases to an oliguric phase. Ribavirin, which has potent in vitro activity against Hantaan virus, reduced the proportion of patients entering the oliguric phase and experiencing hemorrhage and significantly reduced mortality as adjusted for baseline risk estimators.[188]

An outbreak in the United States with unique pathophysiologic features, including prominent, progressive adult respiratory distress syndrome and limited renal involvement, led to the recognition of a Hantavirus pulmonary syndrome,[44] caused by a novel Hantavirus, tentatively called Sin Nombre virus.[284] The agent is spread by urine from the deer mouse (*Peromyscus maniculatus*), a rodent with widespread range in the United States. The syndrome has a tenfold higher case-fatality rate than other Hantavirus diseases (as of December 31, 1993, 60% of reported cases had died). Intravenous ribavirin was made available (through the Centers for Disease Control and Prevention) as an investigational agent during this outbreak. However, it has not proven effective, perhaps because it may not be possible to start ribavirin therapy early enough.[43]

Rhinovirus

Human rhinoviruses are the major causative agents of the common cold, and most of the 102 recognized serotypes use a single cellular receptor, ICAM-1. Crystallographic studies of one serotype led to the proposal that a deep canyon on the virion surface is involved in a specific interaction with this major cellular receptor.[329] The three-dimensional structure of the virus-receptor complex has also been obtained.[290] A number of strategies have been used to design inhibitors that might prevent or ameliorate the common cold.[3,64] Virus receptor antagonists include anti–ICAM-1 monoclonal antibodies[64] and immunoadhesins composed of ICAM-1 domains arrayed on immunoglobulin constant regions that are intended to bind free human rhinovirus virions.[247] Chemotherapeutic agents have also been found that bind to human rhinoviruses and interfere with receptor binding and uncoating.[3,348,439] Another important issue is drug delivery to the site of virus attachment to the cellular receptor (i.e., nasal secretions).[157,168,399] All these approaches are undergoing preclinical and clinical testing.

SUMMARY AND CONCLUSIONS

The ultimate aim of antiviral therapy is to find regimens and strategies that provide either cure of an acute infection or long-term virus suppression in chronic infections, with limited toxicity to the host. Because crucial factors in restricting viral pathogenesis include virus burden and the status of the host immune response, it should be preferable to treat early in the course of chronic infection, possibly before symptoms occur. To achieve this, it is necessary to design and develop potent, specific, and relatively nontoxic antiviral agents that can be tolerated for prolonged periods and that can penetrate appropriate virus reservoirs in the host. Advances in protein crystallography and computer-assisted drug design, together with detailed analyses of enzyme mechanism at the molecular level, will continue to guide the development of drugs directed against specific viral targets. Another approach for optimizing antiviral effects may be to passively or actively bolster the antiviral immune response at the time of administering antiviral drugs. Certain immunomodulating cytokines (e.g., interleukin-2, interferon-γ) can also supplement the effects of virus-specific drugs. Antiviral strategies must address the important issue of drug resistance to prevent the emergence of resistant virus mutants that may correlate with failure of therapy and cause resurgent disease progression despite continuing treatment. It is likely that combination therapy will be one approach to slow the emergence of drug-resistant viruses in chronic virus infections such as HIV-1.

ABBREVIATIONS

ACVDP: acyclovir diphosphate
ACVMP: acyclovir monophosphate
ACVTP: acyclovir triphosphate
AIDS: acquired immunodeficiency syndrome
ara A: adenine arabinoside
AZT: azidothymidine
AZTDP: azidothymidine diphosphate
AZTMP: azidothymidine monophosphate
AZTTP: azidothymidine triphosphate
CMV: cytomegalovirus
dGTP: deoguanosine triphosphate
dNTP: deoxynucleoside triphosphate
EBV: Epstein-Barr virus
GCVMD: ganciclovir monophosphate
GCVTP: ganciclovir triphosphate
HA: hemagglutinin
HHV: human herpesvirus virus
HIV: human immunodeficiency virus
HPMDA: 3-hydroxy-2-phosphonylmethoxypropyl-adenine
HPMDC: 3-hydroxy-2-phosphonylmethoxypropyl-cytosine
HSV: herpes simplex virus
IC50: 50% inhibitory concentration
IdU: idoxuridine
M: matrix
RSV: respiratory syncytial virus
TFT: trifluorothymidine
TK: thymidine kinase
vRNP: viral ribonucleoprotein particle
VZV: varicella-zoster virus

REFERENCES

1. Abrams D, Goldman A, Launer C, et al. A comparative trial of didanosine or zalcitabine in patients with human immunodeficiency virus infection. N Engl J Med 1994;330:657–662.
2. Advisory Committee on Immunization Practices. Prevention and control of influenza. MMWR 1986;35:317–325.
3. al Nakib W, Tyrrell DA. Drugs against rhinoviruses. J Antimicrob Chemother 1992;30:115–117.
4. Anderson J, Britten S, Ernberg J, et al. Effect of acyclovir on infectious mononucleosis: a double-blind, placebo-controlled study. J Infect Dis 1986;153:283–290.
5. Anderson J, Ernberg I. Management of Epstein-Barr virus infection. Am J Med 1988;85:107–115.
6. Andrei G, De Clercq E. Molecular approaches for the treatment of hemorrhagic fever virus infections. Antiviral Res 1993;22:45–75.
7. Andrews ER, Tilson HH, Hurn BAL, Cordero JF. Acyclovir in pregnancy registry. Am J Med 1988;85:123–128.
8. Anonymous. Clinical practice: HIV seroconversion after occupational exposure despite early prophylactic zidovudine therapy. Lancet 1993;341:1077–1078.
9. Aoki FY, Stirer HG, Sitar DS, Boudreault A, Ogilvie RI. Prophylactic amantadine dose and plasma concentration-effect relationship in healthy adults. Clin Pharmacol Ther 1985;37:128–136.
10. Arnold E, Jacobo MA, Nanni RG, et al. Structure of HIV-1 reverse transcriptase/DNA complex at 7 A resolution showing active site locations. Nature 1992;357:85–89.
11. Ashton WT, Karkas JD, Dield AK, Tolman RL. Activation by thymidine kinase and potent antiherpetic activity of 2'-nor-'2-deoxyguanosine (2'NDG). Biochem Biophys Res Commun 1982;108:1716–1721.
12. Bailey TC, Trulock EP, Ettinger NA, Storch GA, Cooper JD, Powderly WG. Failure of prophylactic ganciclovir to prevent cytomegalovirus disease in recipients of lung transplants. J Infect Dis 1992;165:548–552.
13. Balfour HH, Bean B, Laskin OL, et al. Acyclovir halts progression of herpes zoster in immunocompromised patients. N Engl J Med 1983;308:1448–1453.
14. Balfour HH, Chase BA, Stapleton JT, Simmons RL, Fryd DS. A randomized, placebo-controlled trial of oral acyclovir for the prevention of cytomegalovirus disease in recipients of renal allografts. N Engl J Med 1989;320:1381–1387.
15. Balfour HH, Rotbart HA, Feldman S, et al. Acyclovir treatment in varicella in otherwise healthy adolescents. J Pediatr 1992;120:627–633.
16. Bastow KF, Derse DD, Cheng Y-C. Susceptibility of phosphonoformic acid–resistant herpes simplex virus variants to arabinosylnucleosides and aphidicolin. Antimicrob Agents Chemother 1983;23:914–917.
17. Bean B, Braun C, Balfour HHJ. Acyclovir therapy for acute herpes zoster. Lancet 1982;2:118–121.
18. Bean WJ, Threlkeld SC, Webster RG. Biologic potential of amantadine-resistant influenza A virus in an avian model. J Infect Dis 1989;159:1050–1056.
19. Belshe RB, Hay AJ. Drug resistance and mechanisms of action of influenza A viruses. J Res Dis Supp 1989;10:S52–S61.
20. Belshe RB, Smith MH, Hall CB, Betts R, Hay AJ. Genetic basis of resistance to rimantadine emerging during treatment of influenza virus infection. J Virol 1988;62:1508–1512.
21. Bianchetti MG, Roduit C, Oetiker OH. Acyclovir-induced renal failure: course and risk factors. Pediatr Nephrol 1991;5:238–239.
22. Birch CJ, Tachedjian G, Doherty RR, Hayes K, Gust ID. Altered sensitivities to antiviral drugs of herpes simplex virus isolates from a patient with the acquired immunodeficiency syndrome. J Infect Dis 1990;162:731–734.
23. Biron KK, Elion GB. In vitro susceptibility of varicella-zoster virus to acyclovir. Antimicrob Agents Chemother 1980;18:443–447.
24. Biron KK, Fyfe JA, Stanat SC, et al. A human cytomegalovirus mutant resistant to the nucleoside analog 9{[2-hydroxyl-1-(hydroxymethyl)ethoxy]methyl} guanine (BW B759U) induces reduced levels of BW B759U triphosphate. Proc Natl Acad Sci U S A 1986;83:8769–8773.
25. Biron KK, Stanat SC, Sorrell JB, et al. Metabolic activation of the nucleoside analog 9-{[2-hydroxy-1-(hydroxymethyl) ethoxy] methyl]} guanine in human diploid fibroblasts infected with human cytomegalovirus. Proc Natl Acad Sci U S A 1985;82:2473–2477.
26. Boehme RE. Phosphorylation of the antiviral precursor 9-(1,3-dihydroxyl-2-propoxymethyl) guanine monophosphate by guanylate kinase isozymes. J Biol Chem 1984;259:12346–12349.

27. Boivin G, Erice A, Crane DD, Dunn DL, Balfour HHJ. Acyclovir susceptibilities of herpes simplex virus strains isolated from solid organ transplant recipients after acyclovir or ganciclovir prophylaxis. Antimicrob Agents Chemother 1993;37:357–359.

28. Boivin G, Erice A, Crane DD, Dunn DL, Balfour HHJ. Ganciclovir susceptibilities of cytomegalovirus (CMV) isolates from solid organ transplant recipients with CMV viremia after antiviral prophylaxis. J Infect Dis 1993;168:332–335.

29. Boston Interhospital Virus Study Group and the NIAID-Sponsored Cooperative Antiviral Clinical Study. Failure of high dose 5-iodo-2'-deoxyuridine in the therapy of herpes simplex virus encephalitis. N Engl J Med 1975;292:599–603.

30. Boyer PL, Tantillo C, Jacobo-Molina A, et al. The sensitivity of wild-type human immunodeficiency virus reverse transcriptase to dideoxynucleosides depends on template length; the sensitivity of drug-resistant mutants does not. Proc Natl Acad Sci USA 1994;91:4882–4886.

31. Bradley JS, Connor JD, Compogiannis LS, Eiger LL. Exposure of health care workers to ribavirin during therapy for respiratory syncytial virus infections. Antimicrob Agents Chemother 1990;34:668–670.

32. Broder S. Pharmacodynamics of 2',3'-dideoxycytidine: an inhibitor of human immunodeficiency virus. Am J Med 1990;88 (Suppl 5B):2S–7S.

33. Browne MJ, Mayer KH, Chafee SBD, et al. 2',3'-didehydro-3'-deoxythymidine (d4T) in patients with AIDS or AIDS-related complex: a phase I trial. J Infect Dis 1993;167:21–29.

34. Bryson YJ, Dillon M, Lovett M, et al. Treatment of first episodes of genital herpes simplex virus infection with oral acyclovir: a randomized double-blind controlled trial in normal subjects. N Engl J Med 1982;308:916–921.

35. Buhles WCJ, Mastro BJ, Tinker AJ, Strand V, Koretz SH, Group SCGS. Ganciclovir treatment of life or sight-threatening cytomegalovirus infection: experience in 314 immunocompromised patients. Rev Inf Dis 1988;10:S495–S504.

36. Bukrinskaya AG, Vorkunova NK, Kornilayeva RA, Narman-Betova RA, Vorkunova GK. Influenza virus uncoating in infected cells and effect of rimantadine. J Gen Virol 1982;60:49–59.

37. Bukrinsky MI, Haggerty S, Dempsey MP, et al. A nuclear localization signal within HIV-1 matrix protein that governs infection of non-dividing cells. Nature 1993;365:666–669.

38. Burns WH, Sandford GR. Susceptibility of human herpesvirus 6 to antivirals in vitro. J Infect Dis 1990;162:634–637.

39. Caliendo AM, Hirsch MS. Combination therapy for infection due to human immunodeficiency virus type I. Clin Infect Dis 1994;18:516–524.

40. Canonico PG, Kende M, Huggins JW. The toxicology and pharmacology of ribavirin in experimental animals. In: Smith RA, Knight V, Smith JAD, eds. Clinical application of ribavirin. Orlando: Academic Press, 1994:65–77.

41. Carr CM, Kim PS. A spring-loaded mechanism for the conformational change of influenza hemagglutinin. Cell 1993;73:823–832.

42. Cassidy LF, Patterson JL. Mechanism of La Crosse virus inhibition by ribavirin. Antimicrob Agents Chemother 1989;33:2009–2011.

43. CDC. Update: hantavirus pulmonary syndrome—United States, 1993. MMWR 1993;42:816–20.

44. CDC. Hantavirus pulmonary syndrome, United States 1993. JAMA 1994;271:498.

44a. CDC. Case-control study of HIV seroconversion in health-care workers after percutaneous exposure to HIV-infected blood-France, United Kingdom, and United States, January 1988-August 1994. MMWR 1995;44:929–933.

45. Chee MS, Lawrence GL, Barrell BG. Alpha-, beta- and gamma-herpesviruses encode a putative phosphotransferase. J Gen Virol 1989;70:1151–1160.

46. Cheng Y-C, Dutschman GE, Bastow KW, Sarngadharan MG, Ting RYC. Human immunodeficiency virus reverse transcriptase: general properties and its interactions with nucleoside triphosphate analogs. J Biol Chem 1987;262:2187–2189.

47. Cheng Y-C, Grill S, Derse D, Chen J-Y. Mode of action of PFA as an anti–herpes simplex agent. Biochim Biophys Acta 1981;652:90–98.

48. Cheng Y-C, Grill SP, Dutschman GE, Nakayama K, Bastow KF. Metabolism of 9-(1,3-dihydroxy-2-propoxymethyl)guanine, a new anti–herpes virus compound, in herpes simplex virus–infected cells. J Biol Chem 1983;258:12460–12464.

49. Cheng Y-C, Huang E-S, Lin J-C, et al. Unique spectrum of activity of 9-(1,3-dihydroxy-2-propoxymethyl)-guanine against herpes viruses in vitro and its mode of action against herpes simplex virus type 1. Proc Natl Acad Sci U S A 1983;80:2767–2770.

50. Ciampor F, Bayley PM, Nermut MV, Hirst EMA, Sugrue RJ, Hay AJ. Evidence that the amantadine-induced, M2-mediated conversion of influenza A virus hemagglutinin to the low pH conformation occurs in an acidic trans Golgi compartment. Virology 1992;188:14–24.

51. Coen DM. General aspects of virus drug resistance with special reference to herpes simplex virus. J Antimicrob Chemother 1986;18 (Suppl B):1–10.

52. Coen DM. Antiviral drug resistance. Ann N Y Acad Sci 1990;616:224–237.

53. Coen DM. The implications of resistance to antiviral agents for herpesvirus drug targets and drug therapy. Antiviral Res 1991;15:287–300.

54. Coen DM, Aschman DP, Gelep PT, Retondo MJ, Weller SK, Schaffer PA. Fine mapping and molecular cloning of mutations in the herpes simplex virus DNA polymerase locus. J Virol 1984;49:236–247.

55. Coen DM, Fleming HE, Leslie LK, Retondo SK. Sensitivity of arabinosyladenine-resistant mutants of herpes simplex virus to other antiviral drugs and mapping of drug hypersensitivity mutations to the DNA polymerase locus. J Virol 1985;53:477–488.

56. Coen DM, Furman PA, Gelep PT, Schaffer PA. Mutations in the herpes simplex virus DNA polymerase gene can confer resistance to 9-β-D-arabinofuranosyladenine. J Virol 1982;41:909–918.

57. Coen DM, Kosz-Vnenchak M, Jacobson JG, et al. Thymidine kinase negative herpes simplex virus mutants establish latency in mouse trigeminal ganglia but do not reactivate. Proc Natl Acad Sci U S A 1989;86:4736–4740.

58. Coen DM, Schaffer PA. Two distinct loci confer resistance to acycloguanosine in herpes simplex type 1. Proc Natl Acad Sci U S A 1980;77:2265–2269.

59. Cohen GM. Ribonucleotide reductase activity of synchronized KB cells infected with herpes simplex virus. J Virol 1972;9:408–418.

60. Colby BM, Furman PA, Shaw JE, Elion GB, Pagano JS. Phosphorylation of acyclovir [9-(2-hydroxyethoxymethyl)guanine] in Epstein-Barr virus–infected lymphoblastoid cell lines. J Virol 1981;38:606–611.

61. Collaborative DHPG Treatment Study Group. Treatment of serious cytomegalovirus infections with 9-(1,3-dihydroxy-2-propoxymethyl) guanine in patients with AIDS and other immunodeficiencies. N Engl J Med 1986;314:801–805.

62. Collier AC, Coombs RW, Fischl MA, et al. Combination therapy with zidovudine and didanosine compared with zidovudine alone in HIV-1 infection. Ann Intern Med 1993;119:786–793.

63. Collins P, Larder BA, Oliver NM, Kemp S, Smith IW, Darby G. Characterization of a DNA polymerase mutant of herpes simplex virus from a severely compromised patient receiving acyclovir. J Gen Virol 1989;70:375–382.

64. Colonno RJ. Virus receptors: the Achilles' heel of human rhinoviruses. In: Block T, et al, eds. Innovations in antiviral development and the detection of virus infection. New York: Plenum Press, 1992:61–70.

65. Concorde Coordinating Committee. Concorde: MRC/ANRS randomized double-blind controlled trial of immediate and deferred zidovudine in symptom-free HIV infection. Lancet 1994;343:871–881.

65a. Condra JH, Schleif WA, Blahy OM, et al. In vivo emergence of HIV-1 variants resistant to multiple protease inhibitors. Nature 1995;374:569–571.

66. Cooper DA, Gatell J, Kroon S, et al. Zidovudine in persons with asymptomatic HIV infection and CD4+ cell counts greater than 400 per cubic millimeter. N Engl J Med 1993;329:297–303.

67. Corey L, Nahmias AJ, Guinan ME, Benedetti JK, Critchlow CW, Holmes KK. A trial of topical acyclovir in genital herpes simplex virus infections. N Engl J Med 1982;306:1313–1319.

68. Coster DJ, Jones BR, McGill JJ. Treatment of amoeboid herpetic ulcers with adenine arabinoside or trifluorothymidine. Br J Ophthalmol 1979;63:418–421.

69. Craigie R, Mizuuchi K, Bushman FD, Engelman A. A rapid in vitro assay for HIV DNA integration. Nucleic Acids Res 1991;19:2729–2734.

70. Crumpacker CS, Schnipper LE, Marlowe SI, Kowalsky PN, Hershey BJ, Levin MJ. Resistance to antiviral drugs of herpes simplex virus isolated from a patient treated with acyclovir. N Engl J Med 1982;306:343–346.

71. D'Aquila RT. HIV-1 drug resistance: molecular pathogenesis and laboratory monitoring. Clin Lab Med 1994;14:1–30.

71a. D'Aquila RT, Hughes MD, Johnson VA, et al. Nevirapine, zidovudine, and didanosine compared with zidovudine and didanosine in patients with HIV-1 infection. Ann Intern Med 1996;124:1019–1030.

72. D'Aquila RT, Johnson VA, Welles SL, et al. Zidovudine resistance and human immunodeficiency virus type 1 disease progression during antiretroviral therapy. Ann Intern Med 1995;122:401–408.

73. D'Aquila RT, Summers WC. HIV-1 reverse transcriptase/RNase H: high level expression in *Escherichia coli* from a plasmid constructed using the polymerase chain reaction. J AIDS 1989;2:579–587.

74. D'Aquila RT, Summers WC. Physical mapping of the human cytomegalovirus DNA polymerase gene: DNA-mediated transfer of a genetic marker for an HCMV gene. Virology 1989;171:312–316.

75. Daar ES, Li X-L, Moudgil T, Ho DD. High concentrations of recombinant soluble CD4 are required to neutralize primary human immunodeficiency virus type 1 isolates. Proc Natl Acad Sci U S A 1990;87:6574–6578.

76. Darby G, Field HJ, Salisbury SA. Altered substrate specificity of herpes simplex virus thymidine kinase confers acyclovir-resistance. Nature 1981;289:81–83.

77. Darby G, Larder BA, Inglis MM. Evidence that the "active center" of the herpes simplex virus thymidine kinase involves an interaction between three distinct regions of the polypeptide. J Gen Virol 1986;67:753–758.

78. Datta AK, Colby BM, Shaw JE, Pagano JS. Acyclovir inhibition of Epstein-Barr virus replication. Proc Natl Acad Sci U S A 1980;77:5163–5166.

79. Datta AK, Hood RE. Mechanism of inhibition of EBV replication by phosphonoformic acid. Virology 1981;114:52–59.

80. De Clercq E. Biochemical aspects of the selective antiherpes activity of nucleoside analogues. Biochem Pharmacol 1984;33:2159–2169.

81. De Clercq E, Holy A, Rosenberg I, Sakuma T, Balzarini J, Madugal PC. A novel selective broad spectrum anti-DNA virus agent. Nature 1986;323:464–467.

82. Derse D, Cheng Y-C, Furman PA, St. Clair MH, Elion GB. Inhibition of purified human and herpes simplex virus–induced DNA polymerases by 9-(2-hydroxyethoxymethyl)guanine triphosphate: effects on primer-template function. J Biol Chem 1981;256:11447–11451.

83. Dietrich DT, A. C, LaFleur F, Worrell C. Ganciclovir treatment of gastrointestinal infections caused by cytomegalovirus in patients with AIDS. Rev Infect Dis 1988;10:S532–537.

84. Dietrich DT, Kotler DP, Busch DF, et al. Ganciclovir treatment of cytomegalovirus colitis in AIDS: a randomized, double-blind, placebo-controlled multicenter study. J Infect Dis 1993;167:278–282.

85. Doberson MJ, Jerkofsky M, Geer S. Enzymatic basis for the selective inhibition of varicella-zoster virus by 5-halogenated analogues of deoxycytidine. J Virol 1976;20:478–486.

86. Dolin R, Amato DA, Fischl MA, et al. Zidovudine compared to didanosine in patients with advanced HIV-1 infection and little or no previous experience with zidovudine. Arch Intern Med 1995;155:961–974.

87. Dolin R, Reichman RC, Madore HP, Maynard R, Linton PN, Webber-Jones JA. A controlled trial of amantadine and rimantadine in the prophylaxis of influenza A infection. N Engl J Med 1982;307:580–584.

88. Doms RW, Helenius A, White J. Membrane fusion activity of the influenza virus hemagglutinin: the low pH-induced conformational change. J Biol Chem 1985;260:2973–2981.

89. Dorsky DI, Crumpacker CS. Drugs five years later. Ann Intern Med 1987;107:859–874.

90. Dorsky DI, Plourde C. Resistance to antiviral inhibitors caused by the mutation S889A in the highly conserved 885-GDTDS motif of the herpes simplex virus type 1 DNA polymerase. Virology 1993;195:831–835.

91. Douglas RGJ. Prophylaxis and treatment of influenza. N Engl J Med 1990;322:443–450.

92. Drach JC. Purine nucleoside analogs as antiviral agents. In: DeClercq E, Walker RT, eds. Targets for the design of antiviral agents. New York: Plenum Press, 1984.

93. Drew WL, Miner RC, Busch DF, et al. Prevalence of resistance in patients receiving ganciclovir for serious cytomegalovirus infection. J Infect Dis 1991;163:716–719.

94. Dudley MN, Graham KK, Kaul S, et al. Pharmacokinetics of stavudine in patients with AIDS or AIDS-related complex. J Infect Dis 1992;166:99–104.

95. Duff KC, Ashley RH. The transmembrane domain of influenza A M2 protein forms amantadine-sensitive proton channels in planar lipid bilayers. Virology 1992;190:485–489.

96. Dunkle LM, Arvin AM, Whitley RJ, et al. A controlled trial of acyclovir for chickenpox in normal children. N Engl J Med 1991;325:1539–1544.

96a. Dyda F, Hickman AB, Jenkins TM, et al. Crystal structure of the catalytic domain of HIV-1 integrase: similarity to other polynucleotidyl transferases. Science 1994;266:1981–1986.

97. Efstathiou S, Kemp S, Darby G, et al. The role of herpes simplex virus type 1 thymidine kinase in pathogenesis. J Gen Virol 1989;70:869–879.

98. Elion GB. Mechanism of action and selectivity of acyclovir. Am J Med 1982;73:7–13.

99. Elion GB, Furman PA, Fyfe JA, de Miranda P, Beauchamp L, Schaeffer HJ. Selectivity of action of an antiherpetic agent, 9-(2-hydroxyethoxymethyl) guanine. Proc Natl Acad Sci U S A 1977;74:5716–5720.

100. Ellis MN, Keller PM, Fyfe JA, et al. Clinical isolate of herpes simplex virus type 2 that induces a thymidine kinase with altered substrate specificity. Antimicrob Agents Chemother 1987;31:1117–1125.

101. Ellis MN, Waters R, Hill EL, Lobe DC, Selleseth DW, Barry DW. Orofacial infection of athymic mice with defined mixtures of acyclovir-susceptible and acyclovir-resistant herpes simplex virus type 1. Antimicrob Agents Chemother 1989;33:304–310.

102. Englund JA, Zimmerman ME, Swierkosz EM, Goodman JL, Scholl DR, Balfour HH. Herpes simplex virus resistant to acyclovir. Ann Intern Med 1990;112:416–422.

103. Enria D, Maiztegui JI. Antiviral treatment of Argentine hemorrhagic fever. Antiviral Res 1994;23:23–31.

104. Erice A, Chou S, Biron KK, Stanat SC, Balfour HH, Jordan MC. Progressive disease due to ganciclovir-resistant cytomegalovirus in immunocompromised patients. N Engl J Med 1989;320:289–293.

105. Erice A, Mayers DL, Strike DG, et al. Brief report: primary infection with zidovudine-resistant human immunodeficiency virus type 1. N Engl J Med 1993;328:1163–1165.

106. Eriksson B, Helgstrand E, Johnson NG, et al. Inhibition of influenza virus ribonucleic acid polymerase by ribavirin triphosphate. Antimicrob Agents Chemother 1977;11:946–951.

107. Erlich KS, Mills J, Chatis P, et al. Acyclovir-resistant herpes simplex virus infections in patients with the acquired immunodeficiency virus syndrome. N Engl J Med 1989;320:293–296.

108. Erlich KS, Mills J, Chatis P, et al. Foscarnet therapy for severe acyclovir-resistant herpes simplex virus type-2 infections in patients with the acquired immunodeficiency syndrome (AIDS): an uncontrolled trial. Ann Intern Med 1989;110:710–713.

109. Eron JJ, Chow Y-K, Caliendo AM, et al. Pol mutations conferring zidovudine and didanosine resistance with different effects in vitro yield multiply resistant human immunodeficiency virus type 1 isolates in vivo. Antimicrob Agents Chemother 1993;37:1480–1487.

110. Estes JE, Huang E-S. Stimulation of cellular thymidine kinase by human cytomegalovirus. J Virol 1977;24:13–21.

111. Executive Summary. AIDS Clinical Trials Group of the NIAID. ACTG 155. May 23, 1993.

112. Collier AC, Coombs R, Schoenfeld D, et al. Treatment of human immunodeficiency virus infection with saquinavir, zidovudine and zalcitabine. N Engl J Med 1996;334:1011–1017.

113. Feldman S, Rodman J, Gregory B. Excessive serum concentrations of acyclovir and neurotoxicity. J Infect Dis 1988;157:385–388.

114. Felsenstein D, D'Amico DJ, Hirsch MS, et al. Treatment of cytomegalovirus retinitis with 9-[2-hydroxy-1(hydroxyethyl)ethoxymethyl] guanine (BWB759U). Ann Intern Med 1985;103:377–380.

115. Fernandez H, Banks G, Smith R. Ribavirin: A clinical overview. Eur J Epidemiol 1986;2:1–14.

116. Fesen MR, Kohn KW, Leteurtre F, Pommier Y. Inhibitors of human immunodeficiency virus integrase. Proc Natl Acad Sci U S A 1993; 90:2399–2403.

117. Field AK, Davies ME, Dewitt C, et al. 9-{[2-hydroxy-1-(hydroxymethyl)ethoxymethyl} guanine: a selective inhibitor of herpes group virus replication. Proc Natl Acad Sci U S A 1983;80:4139–4143.

118. Field HJ. Development of clinical resistance to acyclovir in herpes simplex virus–infected mice receiving oral therapy. Antimicrob Agents Chemother 1982;21:744–752.

119. Field HJ, Darby G, Wildy P. Isolation and characterization of acyclovir-resistant mutants of herpes simplex virus. J Gen Virol 1980; 49:115–124.

120. Field HJ, Lay E. Characterization of latent infections in mice inoculated with herpes simplex virus which is clinically resistant to acyclovir. Antiviral Res 1984;4:43–52.

121. Field HJ, Wildy P. The pathogenicity of thymidine kinase deficient mutants of herpes simplex virus in mice. J Hygeine 1978;81:267–277.

122. Fischl MA, Olsen RM, Follansbee SE, et al. Zalcitabine compared with zidovudine in patients with advanced HIV-1 infection who received previous zidovudine therapy. Ann Intern Med 1993;118:762–769.

123. Fischl MA, Parker CB, Pettinelli C, et al. A randomized controlled trial of a reduced daily dose of zidovudine in patients with the acquired immunodeficiency syndrome. N Engl J Med 1990;323:1009–1014.

124. Fischl MA, Richman DD, Hansen N, et al. The safety and efficacy of zidovudine (AZT) in the treatment of subjects with mildly symptomatic human immunodeficiency virus type 1 (HIV) infection. Ann Intern Med 1990;112:727–737.

125. Fischl MA, Richman GG, Grieco MH, et al. The efficacy of azidothymidine (AZT) in the treatment of subjects with AIDS and AIDS-related complex: a double-blind placebo-controlled trial. N Engl J Med 1987;317:185–191.

126. Fisher RA, Bertonis JM, Meier W, et al. HIV infection is blocked in vitro by recombinant soluble CD4. Nature 1988;331:76–78.

127. Fitzgibbon JE, Gaur S, Frenkel LD, Laraque F, Edlin BR, Dubin DT. Transmission from one child to another of human immunodeficiency virus type 1 with a zidovudine-resistance mutation. N Engl J Med 1993;329:1835–1841.

128. Fitzgibbon JE, Howell RE, Haberzettl CA, Sperber SJ, Gocke DJ, Dubin DT. Human immunodeficiency virus type 1 pol gene mutations which cause decreased susceptibility to 2',3'-dideoxycytidine. Antimicrob Agents Chemother 1992;36:153–157.

129. Fleming HEJ, Coen DM. Herpes simplex virus mutants resistant to arabinosyl adenine in the presence of deoxycoformycin. Antimicrob Agents Chemother 1984;26:382–387.

130. Fletcher C, Sawchuk R, Chinnock B, de Miranda P, Balfour HH. Human pharmacokinetics of the antiviral drug DHPG. Clin Pharmacol Ther 1986;40:281–286.

131. Fletcher CV, Collier AC, Rhame FS, et al. Foscarnet for suppression of human immunodeficiency virus replication. Antimicrob Agents Chemother 1994;38:604–607.

132. Frank KB, Chiou J-F, Cheng Y-C. Interaction of herpes simplex virus-induced DNA polymerase with 9-(1,3-dihydroxy-2-propoxymethyl) guanine triphosphate. J Biol Chem 1984;259:1566–1569.

133. Freiman JP, Helfert KE, Hamrell MR, Stein DS. Hepatomegaly with severe steatosis in HIV-seropositive patients. AIDS 1993;7:379–385.

134. Freitas VR, Smee DF, Chernow M, Boehme R, Matthews TR. Activity of 9-(1,3-dihydroxy-2-propoxymethyl)guanine compared with that of acyclovir against human monkey and rodent cytomegaloviruses. Antimicrob Agents Chemother 1985;28:240–245.

135. Frenkel LM, Brown ZA, Bryson YJ, et al. Pharmacokinetics of acyclovir in the term human pregnancy and neonate. Am J Obstet Gynecol 1991;164:569–576.

136. Friedman HM, Grasela T. Adenine arabinoside and allopurinol—possible adverse drug interaction. N Engl J Med 1981;304:423.

137. Furman PA, Barry DW. Spectrum of antiviral activity and mechanism of action of zidovudine. Am J Med 1988;85(Suppl 2A):176–181.

138. Furman PA, Coen DM, St. Clair MH, Schaffer PA. Acyclovir-resistant mutants of herpes simplex virus type 1 express altered DNA polymerase or reduced acyclovir phosphorylating activities. J Virol 1981;40:936–941.

139. Furman PA, de Miranda F, St. Clair MH, Elion GB. Metabolism of acyclovir in virus-infected and uninfected cells. Antimicrob Agents Chemother 1981;20:518–524.

140. Furman PA, Fyfe JA, St. Clair MH, et al. Phosphorylation of 3'-azido-3'-deoxythymidine and selective interaction of the 5'-triphosphate with HIV reverse transcriptase. Proc Natl Acad Sci U S A 1986;83:8333–8337.

141. Furman PA, St. Clair MH, Fyfe JA, Rideout JL, Keller PM, Elion GB. Inhibition of herpes simplex virus-induced DNA polymerase activity and viral DNA replication by 9-(2-hydroxyethoxymethyl) guanine and its triphosphate. J Virol 1979;32:72–77.

142. Furman PA, St. Clair MH, Spector T. Acyclovir triphosphate is a suicide inactivator of the herpes simplex virus DNA polymerase. J Biol Chem 1984;259:9575–9579.

143. Fyfe JA, Keller PM, Furman PA, Miller RL, Elion GB. Thymidine kinase from herpes simplex virus phosphorylates the new antiviral compound 9-(2-hydroxyethoxymethyl)guanine. J Biol Chem 1978; 253:8721–8727.

144. Galbraith AW, Oxford JS, Schild GC, Potter CW, Watson GI. Therapeutic effect of 1-adamantanamine hydrochloride in naturally occurring influenza A2/Hong Kong infection. Lancet 1971;2:113–115.

145. Galbraith AW, Oxford JS, Schild GC, Watson GI. Protective effect of 1-adamantanamine hydrochloride on influenza A2 infections in the family environment. Lancet 1969;2:1026–1028.

146. Gaub J, Pederson C, Poulson AG, et al. The effect of foscarnet (phosphonoformate) on human immunodeficiency virus isolation. AIDS 1987;1:27–33.

147. Gibbs JS, Chiou HC, Bastow KF, Cheng Y-C, Coen DM. Identification of amino acids in herpes simplex virus DNA polymerase involved in substrate and drug recognition. Proc Natl Acad Sci U S A 1988;85:6672–6676.

148. Gibbs JS, Chiou HC, Hall JD, et al. Sequence and mapping analyses of the herpes simplex virus DNA polymerase gene product predict a C-terminal substrate binding domain. Proc Natl Acad Sci U S A 1985;82:7969–7973.

149. Gilbert BE, Knight V. Biochemistry and clinical application of ribavirin. Antimicrob Agents Chemother 1986;30:201–205.

150. Gill PS, Rarick M, Brynes RK, Causey D, Loureiro C, Levine AM. Azidothymidine associated with bone marrow failure in the acquired immunodeficiency syndrome (AIDS). Ann Intern Med 1987;107:502–505.

151. Goodrich JM, Bowden RA, Fisher L, Keller C, Schoch G, Meyers JD. Ganciclovir prophylaxis to prevent cytomegalovirus disease after allogeneic marrow transplant. Ann Intern Med 1993;118:173–178.

152. Goswami BB, Borek E, Sharma OK, Fujitaki J, Smith RA. The broad spectrum antiviral agent ribavirin inhibits capping of mRNA. Biochem Biophy Res Commun 1979;89:830–836.

153. Grambas S, Hay AJ. Maturation of influenza A virus hemagglutinin: estimates of the pH encountered during transport and its regulation by the M2 protein. Virology 1992;190:11–18.

154. Groothuis JR, Simoes EA, Levin MJ, et al. Prophylactic administration of respiratory syncytial virus immune globulin to high-risk infants and young children: the Respiratory Syncytial Virus Immune Globulin Study Group. N Engl J Med 1993;329:1524–1530.

155. Gruters RA, Neefjes JJ, Tersmette M, et al. Interference with HIV-induced syncytium formation and viral infectivity by inhibitors of trimming glucosidase. Nature 1987;330:74–77.

156. Gu Z, Gao Q, Li X, Parniak MA, Wainberg MA. Novel mutation in the human immunodeficiency virus type 1 reverse transcriptase gene that encodes cross- resistance to 2',3'-dideoxyinosine and 2',3'-dideoxycytidine. J Virol 1992;66:7128–7135.

156a. Gulick R, Mellors J, Havlir D, et al. Potent and sustained antiretroviral activity of indinavir in combination with zidovudine and lamivudine. 3rd Conference on Retroviruses & Opportunistic Infections, Washington, 1996:162.

157. Gwaltney MJ, Jr. Combined antiviral and antimediator treatment of rhinovirus colds. J Infect Dis 1992;166:776–782.

158. Haake DA, Zakowski PC, Haake DL, Bryson YJ. Early treatment with acyclovir for varicella pneumonia in otherwise healthy adults:

retrospective controlled study and review. Rev Infect Dis 1990;12: 788–798.

159. Hall CB, Doli R, Gala GL, et al. Children with influenza A infection: treatment with rimantadine. Pediatrics 1987;80:275–282.

160. Hall CB, Granoff DM, Gromisch DS, et al. American Academy of Pediatrics Committee on Infectious Diseases: use of ribavirin in the treatment of respiratory syncytial virus infection. Pediatrics 1993; 92:501–504.

161. Hall CB, McBride JT, Walsh EE, et al. Aerosolized ribavirin treatment of infants with respiratory syncytial viral infection: a randomized double-blind study. N Engl J Med 1983;308:1443–1447.

162. Hamilton JD, Hartigan PM, Simberkoff MS, et al. A controlled trial of early versus late treatment with zidovudine in symptomatic human immunodeficiency virus infection. N Engl J Med 1992;326: 437–443.

162a. Hammer SM, Katzenstein D, Hughes M, et al. Nucleoside monotherapy versus combination therapy in HIV-infected adults: a randomized, double blind, placebo-controlled trial in persons with CD4 cell counts between 200-500 per cubic millimeter; submitted.

163. Hamzeh FM, Lietman PS. Intranuclear accumulation of subgenomic noninfectious human cytomegalovirus DNA in infected cells in the presence of ganciclovir. Antimicrob Agents Chemother 1991;35: 1818–1823.

164. Hamzeh FM, Lietman PS, Gibson W, Hayward GS. Identification of the lytic origin of DNA replication in human cytomegalovirus by a novel approach utilizing ganciclovir-induced chain termination. J Virol 1990;64:6184–6195.

165. Harrison RJ, Bellows J, Rempel D, Rudolph L, Kizer KW. Assessing exposures of health-care personnel to aerosols of ribavirin-California. MMWR 1988;37:560–562.

166. Hay AJ, Wolstenholme AJ, Skehel JJ, Smith MH. The molecular basis of the specific anti-influenza action of amantadine. EMBO J 1985;4:3021–3024.

167. Hay AJ, Zambon HC, Wolstein-Holme AJ, Skehel JJ, Smith MH. Molecular basis of resistance of influenza A viruses to amantadine. J Antimicrob Chemother 1986;18(Suppl B):19–29.

168. Hayden FG, Andries K, Janssen PA. Safety and efficacy of intranasal pirodavir (R77975) in experimental rhinovirus infection. Antimicrob Agents Chemother 1992;36:727–732.

169. Hayden FG, Belshe RB, Clover RD, Hay AJ, Oakes MG, Soo W. Emergence and apparent transmission of rimantadine-resistant influenza A virus in families. N Engl J Med 1989;321:1696–1702.

170. Hayden FG, Hay AJ. Emergence and transmission of drug-resistant influenza A viruses. Curr Top Microbiol Immunol 1992;176:119–130.

171. Hayden FG, Hoffman HE, Spyker DA. Differences in side effects of amantadine hydrochloride and rimantadine hydrochloride relate to differences in pharmacokinetics. Antimicrob Agents Chemother 1983;23:458–464.

172. Hayden FG, Minocha A, Spyker DA, Hoffman HE. Comparative single-dose pharmacokinetics of amantadine hydrochloride and rimantadine hydrochloride in young and elderly adults. Antimicrob Agents Chemother 1985;28:216–221.

173. Heidelberger C, King D. Trifluorothymidine. Pharmacol Ther 1979; 6:427–442.

174. Helenius A. Unpacking the incoming influenza virus. Cell 1992; 69:577–578.

175. Helgstrand E, Erikkson B, Johansson NG, et al. Trisodium phosphonoformate, a new antiviral compound. Science 1978;201:819–821.

176. Herrmann ECJ, Herrman JA. A working hypothesis: virus resistance development as an indicator of specific antiviral activity. Ann N Y Acad Sci 1977;284:632–637.

177. Hess G, Arnold W, Meyer Zum Buschenfelde KH. Inhibition of hepatitis B virus DNA polymerase by phosphonoformate: studies on its mode of action. J Med Virol 1980;5:309–316.

178. Hibberd PL, Tolkoff-Rubin NE, Conti D, et al. Preemptive ganciclovier therapy to prevent cytomegalovirus disease in cytomegalovirus antibody-positive renal transplant receipients. Am Int Med 1995;123:18–26.

179. Hirsch MS. AIDS-commentary: azidothymidine. J Infect Dis 1988; 157:427–431.

180. Hirsch MS. The treatment of cytomegalovirus in AIDS: more than meets the eye. N Engl J Med 1992;326:264–265.

181. Hirsch MS, D'Aquila RT. Therapy for human immunodeficiency virus infection. N Engl J Med 1993;325:1686–1695.

181a. Hirsch MS, Yeni P. A bend in the read-implications of ACTG 175 and delta trials. Antiviral Therapy 1996;1:6–8.

182. Ho DD, Toyoshima T, Mo H, et al. Characterization of human immunodeficiency virus type 1 variants with increased resistance to a C_2-symmetric protease inhibitor. J Virol 1994;68:2016–2020.

183. Hodges TI, Kahn JO, Kaplan LD, et al. Phase I study of recombinant human CD4–immunoglobulin G therapy of patients with AIDS and AIDS-related complex. Antimicrob Agents Chemother 1991;35: 2580–2586.

184. Holmes GP, McCormick JB, Trock SC, et al. Lassa fever in the United States: investigation of a case and new guidelines for management. N Engl J Med 1990;323:1120–1123.

185. Horwitz JP, Chua J, Noel M. The mononesylates of 1-(2'-deoxy-beta-D-lyxofuranosyl) thymidine. J Organ Chem 1964;29:2076–2078.

186. Hsu M-C, Schutt AD, Holly M, et al. Inhibition of HIV replication in acute and chronic infections in vitro by a tat antagonist. Science 1991;254:1799–1802.

187. Huff JC, Bean B, Balfour HHJ, et al. Therapy of herpes zoster with oral acyclovir. Am J Med 1988;85:84–89.

188. Huggins JW, Hsiang CM, Cosgriff TM, et al. Prospective, double-blind, concurrent, placebo-controlled clinical trial of intravenous ribavirin therapy of hemorrhagic fever with renal syndrome. J Infect Dis 1991;164:1119–1127.

189. Hwang CBC, Ruffner KL, Coen DM. A point mutation within a distinct conserved region of the herpes simplex virus DNA polymerase gene confers drug resistance. J Virol 1992;66:1774–1776.

190. Ing TS, Dougirdas JT, Soung LS, et al. Toxic effects of amantadine in patients with renal failure. Can Med Assoc J 1979;120: 695–697.

191. Jacobson MA, Berger TG, Fikrig S, et al. Acyclovir-resistant varicella zoster virus infection after chronic oral acyclovir therapy in patients with the acquired immunodeficiency syndrome (AIDS). Ann Intern Med 1990;112:187–191.

192. Jacobson MA, Crow S, et al. Effect of foscarnet therapy on infection with human immunodeficiency virus in patients with AIDS. J Infect Dis 1988;158:862–865.

193. Jacobson MA, Drew WL, Feinberg J, et al. Foscarnet therapy for ganciclovir-resistant cytomegalovirus retinitis in patients with AIDS. J Infect Dis 1991;163:1348–1351.

194. Janai HK, Marks MI, Zaleska M, Stutman HR. Ribavirin: adverse drug reactions, 1986 to 1988. Pediatr Infect Dis J 1990;9:209–211.

194a. Japour AJ, Welles S, D'Acquila RT, et al. Prevalence and clinical significance of zidovudine resistance mutations in human immunodeficiency virus isolated from patients following long-term zidovudine treatment. J Infect Dis 1995;171:1172–1179.

195. Kahn JO, Allan JD, Hodges TL, et al. The safety and pharmacokinetics of recombinant soluble CD4 (rCD4) in subjects with the acquired immunodeficiency syndrome (AIDS) and AIDS-related complex. Ann Intern Med 1990;112:254–261.

196. Kahn JO, Lagakos SW, Richman DD, et al. A controlled trial comparing continued zidovudine with didanosine in human immunodeficiency virus infection. N Engl J Med 1992;327:581–587.

197. Kaplowitz LG, Baker D, Gelb L, et al. Prolonged continuous acyclovir treatment of normal adults with frequently recurring genital herpes simplex virus infection. JAMA 1991;265:747–751.

198. Kaufman HE, Martola EL, Dohlman CI. Use of 5-iodo-2'-deoxyuridine (IDU) in treatment of herpes simplex keratitis. Arch Ophthalmol 1962;68:235–239.

199. Kellam P, Boucher CAB, Larder BA. Fifth mutation in human immunodeficiency virus type 1 reverse transcriptase contributes to the development of high-level resistance to zidovudine. Proc Natl Acad Sci U S A 1992;89:1934–1938.

200. Keller PM, Fyfe JA, Beauchamp L, et al. Enzymatic phosphorylation of acyclic nucleoside analogs and correlations with antiherpetic activities. Biochem Pharmacol 1981;30:3071–3077.

201. Keller PM, McKee SA, Fyfe SA. Cytoplasmic 5'-nucleotidase catalyzes acyclovir phosphorylation. J Biol Chem 1985;260:8664–8667.

202. Kinghorn GR. Long-term suppression with oral acyclovir of recurrent herpes simplex virus infections in otherwise healthy patients. Am J Med 1988;85:26–29.

203. Kit S, Dubbs DR. Acquisition of thymidine kinase activity by herpes simplex infected mouse fibroblast cells. Biochem Biophys Res Commun 1963;11:55–59.

204. Kit S, Sheppard M, Ichimura H, et al. Nucleotide sequence changes in thymidine kinase gene of herpes simplex virus type 2 clones from an isolate of a patient treated with acyclovir. Antimicrob Agents Chemother 1987;31:1483–1490.

205. Knight V, Fedson D, Baldini J, Douglas RJ, Couch RB. Amantadine therapy of epidemic influenza A2 (Hong Kong). Infect Immunol 1970;1:200–204.

206. Knopf CW. Nucleotide sequence of the DNA polymerase of herpes simplex virus type 1 strain Angelotti. Nucleic Acids Res 1986;14:8225–8226.

207. Knopf CW, Weisshart K. The herpes simplex virus DNA polymerase: analysis of the functional domains. Biochim Biophys Acta 1988;951:13475–13491.

208. Kohl NE, Emini EA, Schleif WA, et al. Active human immunodeficiency virus protease is required for viral infectivity. Proc Natl Acad Sci U S A 1988;85:4686–4690.

209. Kohlstaedt LA, Wang J, Friedman JM, Rice PA, Steitz TA. Crystal structure at 3.5 A resolution of HIV-1 reverse transcriptase complexed with an inhibitor. Science 1992;256:1783–1790.

210. Kost RG, Hill EL, Tigges M, Straus SE. Brief report: recurrent acyclovir-resistant genital herpes in an immunocompetent patient. N Engl J Med 1993;329:1777–1782.

211. Kozal MJ, Shafer RW, Winters MA, Katzenstein DA, Merigan TC. A mutation in human immunodeficiency virus reverse transcriptase and decline in CD4 lymphocyte numbers in longterm zidovudine recipients. J Infect Dis 1993;167:526–532.

212. Lacey SF, Reardon JE, Furfine ES, et al. Biochemical studies of the reverse transcriptase and RNase H activities from human immunodeficiency virus strains resistant to 3'-azido-3'-deoxythymidine. J Biol Chem 1992;267:15789–15794.

213. Lam PYS, Jadhav PK, Eyermann CJ, et al. Rational design of potent, bioavailable, nonpeptide cyclic ureas as HIV protease inhibitors. Science 1994;263:380–384.

214. Lamb RA, Lai C-J, Choppin PW. Sequences of mRNAs derived from genome RNA segment 7 of influenza virus: colinear and interrupted mRNAs code for overlapping proteins. Proc Natl Acad Sci U S A 1981;78:4170–4174.

215. Lamb RA, Zebedee SL, Richardson CD. Influenza virus M2 protein is an integral membrane protein expressed on the infected cell surface. Cell 1985;40:627–633.

216. Land S, McGavin K, Birch C, Lucas R. Reversion from zidovudine resistance to sensitivity on cessation of treatment. Lancet 1991;338:830–831.

217. Langelier Y, Buttin G. Characterization of ribonucleotide reductase induction in BHK-21/C13 Syrian hamster cell line upon infection by herpes simplex virus (HSV). J Gen Virol 1981;57:21–31.

218. Larder BA, Coates KE, Kemp SD. Zidovudine-resistant human immunodeficiency virus selected by passage in cell culture. J Virol 1991;65:5232–5236.

219. Larder BA, Darby G. Susceptibility to other antiherpes drugs of pathogenic variants of herpes simplex virus selected for resistance to acyclovir. Antimicrob Agents Chemother 1986;28:894–898.

220. Larder BA, Darby G, Cheng Y-C. Characterization of abnormal thymidine kinase induced by drug resistant strains of herpes simplex type 1. J Gen Virol 1983;64:523–532.

221. Larder BA, Darby G, Richman DD. HIV with reduced sensitivity to zidovudine (AZT) isolated during prolonged therapy. Science 1989;243:1731–1734.

222. Larder BA, Derse D, Cheng Y-C, Darby G. Properties of purified enzymes induced by pathogenic drug-resistant mutants of herpes simplex virus: evidence for virus variants expressing normal DNA polymerase and altered thymidine kinase. J Biol Chem 1983;258:2027–2033.

223. Larder BA, Kemp SD. Multiple mutations in HIV-1 reverse transcriptase confer high-level resistance to zidovudine (AZT). Science 1989;246:1155–1158.

224. Larder BA, Kemp SD, Darby G. Related functional domains in virus DNA polymerases. EMBO J 1987;6:169–175.

224a. Larder BA, Kemp SD, Harrigan PR. Potential mechanism for sustained antiviral efficacy of AZT-3TC combination therapy. Science 1996;269:696–699.

225. Larder BA, Purifoy DJM, Powell KI, Darby GK. AIDS virus reverse transcriptase defined by high level expression on E. coli. EMBO J 1987;6:3133–3137.

226. Laskin OL, Longstreth JA, Saral R, de Miranda P, Keeney R, Lietman PS. Pharmacokinetics and tolerance of acyclovir, a new anti–herpes virus agent, in humans. Antimicrob Agents Chemother 1982;21:393–398.

227. Laskin OL, Longstreth JA, Whelton A, et al. Acyclovir kinetics in end stage renal failure. Clin Pharmacol Ther 1982;31:594–601.

228. LeHoang P, Girard B, Robinet M, et al. Foscarnet in the treatment of cytomegalovirus retinitis in acquired immunodeficiency syndrome. Ophthalmology 1989;96:865–873.

229. Lewis P, Hensel M, Emerman M. Human immunodeficiency virus infection of cells arrested in the cell cycle. EMBO J 1992;11:3053–3058.

230. Linnemann CCJ, Biron KK, Hoppenjans WG, Solinger AM. Emergence of acyclovir-resistant varicella zoster virus in an AIDS patient on prolonged acyclovir therapy. AIDS 1990;4:577–579.

231. Little JW, Hall WJ, Douglas Jr RG, Hyde RW, Speers DM. Amantadine effect on peripheral airway abnormalities in influenza. Ann Intern Med 1976;85:177–182.

232. Littler E, Arrand JR. Characterization of the Epstein-Barr virus–encoded thymidine kinase expressed in heterologous eucaryotic and procaryotic systems. J Virol 1988;62:3892–3895.

233. Littler E, Stuart AD, Chee MS. Human cytomegalovirus UL97 open reading frame encodes a protein that phosphorylates the antiviral analogue ganciclovir. Nature 1992;358:160–162.

234. Ljungman P, Englehard D, Link H, et al. Treatment of interstitial pneumonitis due to cytomegalovirus with ganciclovir and intravenous immune globulin: experience of European bone marrow transplant group. Clin Infect Dis 1992;15:831–835.

235. Lumbreras C, Otero JR, Herrero JA, et al. Ganciclovir prophylaxis decreases frequency and severity of cytomegalovirus disease in seropositive liver transplant recipients treated with OKT3 monoclonal antibodies. Antimicrob Agents Chemother 1993;37:2490–2492.

236. Lurain NS, Thompson KD, Holmes EW, Read GS. Point mutations in the DNA polymerase gene of human cytomegalovirus that result in resistance to antiviral agents. J Virol 1992;66:7146–7152.

237. Mahony WB, Domin BA, McConnell RT, Zimmerman TP. Acyclovir transport into human erythrocytes. J Biol Chem 1988;263:9285–9291.

238. Malinoski F, Stollar V. Inhibitors of IMP dehydrogenase prevent Sindbis virus replication and reduce GTP levels in Aedes albopictus cells. Virology 1981;110:281–291.

239. Mar E-C, Cheng Y-C, Huang E-S. Effect of 9-(1,3-dihydroxy-2-propoxymethyl) guanine on human cytomegalovirus replication in vitro. Antimicrob Agents Chemother 1983;24:518–521.

240. Mar E-C, Chiou JF, Cheng Y-C, Huang E-S. Inhibition of cellular DNA polymerase-α and human cytomegaloviral induced DNA polymerase by the triphosphates of 9-(2-hydroxyethoxymethyl) guanine and 9-(1,3-dihydroxy-2-propoxymethyl) guanine. J Virol 1985;53:776–780.

241. Marcy AI, Hwang CBC, Ruffner KL, Coen DM. Engineered herpes simplex virus DNA polymerase point mutants: the most highly conserved region shared among α-like DNA polymerases is involved in substrate recognition. J Virol 1990;64:5883–5890.

242. Margalith M, Manor D, Usidi V, Goldblum N. Phosphonoformate inhibits synthesis of Epstein-Barr virus (EBV) capsid antigen and transformation of human cord blood lymphocytes by EBV. Virology 1980;102:226–230.

243. Marsh M, Helenius A. Virus entry into animal cells. Adv Virus Res 1989;36:107–151.

244. Martin JL, Wilson JE, Haynes RL, Furman PA. Mechanism of resistance of human immunodeficiency virus type 1 to 2', 3'-dideoxyinosine. Proc Natl Acad Sci U S A 1993;90:6135–6139.

245. Martin K, Helenius A. Nuclear transport of influenza virus ribonucleoproteins: the viral matrix protein (M1) promotes export and inhibits import. Cell 1991;67:117–130.

246. Martin K, Helenius A. Transport of incoming influenza virus nucleocapsids into the nucleus. J Virol 1991;65:232–244.

247. Martin S, Casasnovas JM, Staunton DE, Springer TA. Efficient neutralization and disruption of rhinovirus by chimeric ICAM-1/immunoglobulin molecules. J Virol 1993;67:3561–3568.

248. Masur H, Lane CH, Palestine A, et al. Effect of 9-(1,3-dihydroxy-α-propoxymethyl)guanine for cytomegalovirus infection in patients with the acquired immunodeficiency syndrome. Ann Intern Med 1986;104:41–44.

248a. Mathez D, De Truchis P, Gorin J, et al. Ritonavir, AZT, and ddC as a triple combination in AIDS patients. 3rd Conference on Retroviruses and Opportunistic Infections, Washington, DC 1996:106.

249. Matthews JT, Carroll RD, Stevens JT, Haffey ML. In vitro mutagenesis of the herpes simplex virus type 1 DNA polymerase gene results in altered drug sensitivity of the enzyme. J Virol 1989;63:4913–4918.

250. Mattison HR, Reichman RC, Benedetti J, et al. Double-blind, placebo-controlled trial comparing long-term suppressive with short-term oral acyclovir therapy for management of recurrent genital herpes. Am J Med 1988;85:20–25.

251. Mayers D, Wagner KF, Chung RCY, et al. Drug susceptibilities of HIV isolates from patients receiving serial dideoxynucleoside therapy with ZDV, ddI and ddC. Second International HIV Drug Resistance Workshop, Noordwijk, The Netherlands, 1993:47.

252. Mazzulli T, Hirsch MS. Combination therapy for HIV-1 infection. In: Mills J, Corey L, eds. New directions in antiviral therapy. New York: Elsevier, 1993:385–414.

253. McCormick JB, King IJ, Webb PA, et al. Lassa fever: Effective therapy with ribavirin. N Engl J Med 1986;314:20–26.

254. McGuffin RW, Shiota FM, Meyers JD. Lack of toxicity of acyclovir to granulocyte progenitor cells. Antimicrob Agents Chemother 1980;18:471–473.

255. McGuirt PV, Shaw JE, Elion GB, Furman PA. Identification of small DNA fragments synthesized in herpes simplex virus–infected cells in the presence of acyclovir. Antimicrob Agents Chemother 1984;25:507–509.

256. McKinney REJ, Maha MA, Conner EM, et al. A multicenter trial of oral zidovudine in children with advanced immunodeficiency virus disease. N Engl J Med 1991;324:1018–1025.

257. McQuade TJ, Tomasselli AG, Liu L, et al. A synthetic HIV-1 protease inhibitor with antiviral activity arrests HIV-like particle maturation. Science 1990;247:454–456.

258. Medina DJ, Hsiung GD, Mellors JW. Ganciclovir antagonizes the anti-human immunodeficiency virus type 1 activity of zidovudine and didanosine in vitro. Antimicrob Agents Chemother 1992;36:1127–1130.

259. Meng TC, Fischl MA, Boota AM, et al. Combination therapy with zidovudine and dideoxycytidine in patients with advanced human immunodeficiency virus infection: a phase I/II study. Ann Intern Med 1992;116:13–20.

260. Merigan TC, Renlund DG, Keay S, et al. A controlled trial of ganciclovir to prevent cytomegalovirus disease after heart transplantation. N Engl J Med 1992;326:1182–1186.

261. Mertz GJ, Eron L, Kaufman R, et al. Prolonged continuous versus intermittent oral acyclovir treatment in normal adults with frequently recurring genital herpes simplex virus infection. Am J Med 1988;85:14–19.

262. Meyers JD, Reed EC, Shepp DH. Acyclovir for prevention of cytomegalovirus infection and disease after allogeneic marrow transplantation. N Engl J Med 1988;318:70–75.

263. Meyers JD, Wade JC, Mitchell CD, et al. Multicenter collaborative trial of intravenous acyclovir for treatment of mucocutaneous herpes simplex virus infection in the immunocompromised host. Am J Med 1982;73:229–235.

264. Miller RG, Storey JR, Greco CM. Ganciclovir in the treatment of progressive AIDS-related polyradiculopathy. Neurology 1990;40:569–574.

265. Miller WH, Miller RL. Phosphorylation of acyclovir monophosphate by GMP kinase. J Biol Chem 1980;255:7204–7207.

266. Miller WH, Miller RL. Phosphorylation of acyclovir diphosphate by cellular enzymes. Biochem Pharmacol 1982;31:3879–3884.

267. Mindel A, Adler MW, Sutherland S, Fiddian AP. Intravenous acyclovir treatment for primary genital herpes. Lancet 1982;1:697–700.

268. Mitsuya H, Weinhold KJ, Furman PA, et al. 3'-Azido-3'-deoxythymidine (BWA509U): An antiviral agent that inhibits the infectivity and cytopathic effect of human T-lymphotropic virus type III/lymphadenopathy-associated virus in vitro. Proc Natl Acad Sci U S A 1985;82:7096–7100.

269. Mohri H, Singh MK, Ching WTW, Ho DD. Quantitation of zidovudine-resistant human immunodeficiency virus type 1 in the blood of treated and untreated patients. Proc Natl Acad Sci U S A 1993;90:25–29.

270. Molin L, Ruhnek-Forsbeck M, Svennerholm B. One year acyclovir suppression of frequently recurring genital herpes: a study of efficacy safety, virus sensitivity and antibody response. Scan J Inf 1991;S78:33–39.

270a. Molla A, Bouche C, Kornyeva M, et al. Evolution of resistance to the protease inhibitor ritonavir (ABT-538) in HIV infected patients. Fourth International Workshop on HIV Drug Resistance, Sardinia, Italy, 1995.

271. Montaner JSG, Singer J, Schecter MT, et al. Clinical correlates of in vitro HIV-1 resistance to zidovudine: results of the Multicentre Canadian AZT Trial. AIDS 1993;7:189–196.

272. Monto AS, Arden NH. Implications of viral resistance to amantadine in control of influenza A. Clin Infect Dis 1992;7:362–367.

273. Monto AS, Gunn RA, Bandyk MG, King CL. Prevention of Russian influenza by amantadine. JAMA 1979;241:1003–1007.

274. Moore JL, Szczech GM, Rodwell DE, Kapp RWJ, de Miranda P, Tucker WEJ. Preclinical toxicity studies with acyclovir: teratologic, reproductive, and neonatal tests. Fundam Appl Toxicol 1983;3:560–568.

275. Moore JP, McKeating JA, Huang Y, Ashkenazi A, Ho DD. Virions of primary human immunodeficiency virus type 1 isolates resistant to soluble CD4 (sCD4) neutralization differ in sCD4 binding and glycoprotein gp120 retention from sCD4-sensitive isolates. J Virol 1992;66:235–243.

276. Mostow SR, Mayfield JL, Marr JJ, Drucker JL. Suppression of recurrent genital herpes by single daily dosages of acyclovir. Am J Med 1988;85:30–33.

277. Muller WEG, Zahn RK, Beyer R, Falke D. 9-beta-D-arabinofuranosyladenine as a tool to study herpes simplex virus DNA replication in vitro. Virology 1977;76:787–796.

278. Muller WEG, Zahn RK, Bittlengmaier K, Falke D. Inhibition of herpes DNA synthesis by 9-beta-D-arabinofuranosyl-adenine in cellular and cell-free systems. Ann N Y Acad Sci 1977;284:34–48.

279. Murphy M, Morley A, Eglin RP, Monteiro E. Topical trifluridine for mucocutaneous acyclovir-resistant herpes simplex II in an AIDS patient. Lancet 1992;340:1040.

280. Nabel G, Baltimore D. An inducible transcription factor activates expression of human immunodeficiency virus in T cells. Nature 1987;326:711–713.

281. Nagy K, Young M, Baboonian C, Merson J, Whittle P, Oroszlan S. Antiviral activity of human immunodeficiency virus type 1 protease inhibitors in a single cycle of infection: evidence for a role of protease in the early phase. J Virol 1994;68:757–765.

281a. Najera I, Holguin A, Quinones-Mateu ME, et al. Pol gene quasispecies of human immunodeficiency virus: mutations associated with drug resistance in virus from patients undergoing no drug therapy. J Virol 1995;69:23–31.

282. NIAID Consensus Conference. Amantadine: does it have a role in the prevention and treatment of influenza? Ann Intern Med 1980;92:256–258.

283. NIAID News. ACTG 076 press release. February 21, 1994.

284. Nichol ST, Spiropoulou CF, Morzunov S, et al. Genetic identification of a hantavirus associated with an outbreak of acute respiratory illness. Science 1993;262:914–917.

285. Nilsen AE, Aasen T, Halsos AM, et al. Efficacy of oral acyclovir in the treatment of initial and recurrent genital herpes. Lancet 1982;2:571–573.

286. Nyerges G, Meszner Z, Gyarmati E, Kerpel-Fronius S. Acyclovir prevents dissemination of varicella in immunocompromised children. J Infect Dis 1988;157:309–313.

287. Oberg B. Antiviral effects of phosphonoformate (PFA, Foscarnet sodium). Pharmacol Ther 1983;19:387–415.

288. Ogino MT, Dankner WM, Spector SA. Development and significance of zidovudine resistance in children infected with human immunodeficiency virus. J Pediatr 1993;123:1–8.

289. Ohuchi M, Cramer A, Vey M, Ohuchi R, Garten W, Klenk H-D. Rescue of vector-expressed fowl plague virus hemagglutinin in biologically active form by acidotropic agents and coexpressed M2 protein. J Virol 1994;68:920–926.

290. Olson NH, Kolatkar PR, Oliveira MA, et al. Structure of a human rhinovirus complexed with its receptor molecule. Proc Natl Acad Sci U S A 1993;90:507–511.

291. Ostertag W, Roesler G, Krieg CJ, et al. Induction of endogenous virus and of thymidine kinase by bromodeoxyuridine in cell cultures transformed by Friend virus. Proc Natl Acad Sci U S A 1974;71: 4980–4985.

292. Otto MJ, Garber S, Winslow DL, et al. In vitro isolation and identification of human immunodeficiency virus (HIV) variants with reduced sensitivity to C-2 symmetrical inhibitors of HIV type 1 protease. Proc Natl Acad Sci U S A 1993;90:7543–7547.

293. Pahwa S, Biron K, Lim W, et al. Continuous varicella-zoster infection associated with acyclovir resistance in a child with AIDS. JAMA 1988;260:2879–2882.

294. Parker LM, Lipton JM, Binder N, Crawford EL, Kudisch M, Levin MJ. Effect of acyclovir and interferon on human hematopoietic progenitor cells. Antimicrob Agents and Chemother 1982;21:146–150.

295. Parris DS, Harrington JE. Herpes simplex virus variants resistant to high concentrations of acyclovir exist in clinical isolates. Antimicrob Agents Chemother 1982;22:71–77.

296. Patterson JL, Fernandez-Larsson R. Molecular mechanisms of action of ribavirin. Rev Infect Dis 1990;12:1139–1146.

297. Patterson JL, Holloway B, Kolakofsky D. La Crosse virus contains a primer-stimulated RNA polymerase and a methylated cap-dependent endonuclease. J Virol 1984;52:215–222.

298. Pavan-Langston D, Buchanan RA. Vidarabine therapy of simple and IDU-complicated herpetic keratitis. Trans Am Acad Ophthalmol Otolaryngol 1976;81:OP813–OP825.

299. Pelling JC, Drach JC, Shipman C. Internucleotide incorporation of arabinosyl adenine into herpes simplex and mammalian cell DNA. Virology 1981;109:323–335.

300. Peterslund NA. Management of varicella zoster in immunocompetent hosts. Am J Med 1988;85:74–78.

301. Peterslund NA, Black FT, Tauris P. Impaired renal function after bolus injections of acyclovir. Lancet 1983;1:243–244.

302. Peterslund NA, Ipsen J, Schonheyder H, Seyer-Hansen K, Esmann V, Juhl H. Acyclovir in herpes zoster. Lancet 1981;2:827–830.

303. Peto R, Pike MC, Armitage P, et al. Design and analysis of randomized clinical trials requiring prolonged observation of each patient. I. Introduction and design. Br J Cancer 1976;34:585–612.

304. Pinto LH, Holsinger LJ, Lamb RA. Influenza virus M2 protein has ion channel activity. Cell 1992;69:517–528.

305. Prober CG, Kirk LE, Keeney RE. Acyclovir therapy of chickenpox in immunosuppressed children: a collaborative study. J Pediatr 1982;101:622–625.

306. Prusoff WH. Synthesis and biological activation of iododeoxy-uridine, an analog of thymidine. Biochim Biophys Acta 1959;32:295–296.

307. Prusoff WH, Mancini WR, Lin TS, Lee JJ, Siegel SZ, Otto MJ. Physical and biological consequences of incorporation of antiviral agents into virus DNA. Antiviral Res 1984;4:303–315.

308. Purifoy DJ, Beauchamp LM, de Miranda P, et al. Review of research leading to new anti-herpesvirus agents in clinical development: valaciclovir hydrochloride (256U, the L-valyl ester of acyclovir) and 882C, a specific agent for varicella zoster virus. J Med Virol 1993;1:139–145.

309. Quarles JM, Couch RB, Cate TR, Goswick CB. Comparison of amantadine and rimantadine for prevention of type A (Russian) influenza. Antiviral Res 1981;1:149–155.

310. Raffi F, Taburet AM, Ghaleh B, Huart A, Singlas E. Penetration of foscarnet into cerebrospinal fluid of AIDS patients. Antimicrob Agents Chemother 1993;37:1777–1780.

311. Ramos E, Timmons RF, Schimpff SC. Inappropriate anti-diuretic hormone following adenine arabinoside administration. Antimicrob Agents Chemother 1979;15:142–144.

312. Reardon JE. Herpes simplex virus type 1 and human DNA polymerase interactions with 2'-deoxyguanosine 5'-triphosphate analogues: kinetics of incorporation into DNA and induction of inhibition. J Biol Chem 1989;264:19039–19044.

313. Reardon JE, Spector T. Herpes simplex virus type 1 DNA polymerase: mechanism of inhibition by acyclovir triphosphate. J Biol Chem 1989;264:7405–7411.

314. Reardon JE, Spector T. Acyclovir: mechanism of antiviral action and potentiation by ribonucleotide reductase inhibitors. Adv Pharmacol 1992;22:1–27.

315. Reddy MM, Grieco MH, McKinley GF, et al. Effect of foscarnet therapy on human immunodeficiency virus p24 antigen levels in AIDS patients with cytomegalovirus retinitis. J Infect Dis 1992; 166:607–610.

316. Reed EC, Bowdan RA, Kandiker PS, Lilleby KE, Meyers JD. Treatment of cytomegalovirus pneumonia with ganciclovir and intravenous cytomegalovirus immunoglobulin in patients with bone marrow transplants. Ann Intern Med 1988;109:783–788.

317. Reed EC, Wolford JL, Kopecky KJ, et al. Ganciclovir for the treatment of cytomegalovirus gastroenteritis in bone marrow transplant patients: a randomized placebo-controlled trial. Ann Intern Med 1990;112:505–510.

317a.Reich SH, Melnick M, Davies JFI, et al. Protein structure-based design of potent orally bioavailable, nonpeptide inhibitors of human immunodeficiency virus protease. Proc Natl Acad Sci USA 1995; 92:3298–3302.

318. Reichman RC, Badger GJ, Guinan ME, et al. Topically administered acyclovir in the treatment of recurrent herpes simplex genitalis. J Infect Dis 1983;147:336–340.

319. Reichman RC, Badger GJ, Mertz GJ. Treatment of recurrent genital herpes simplex infections with oral acyclovir: a controlled trial. JAMA 1984;251:2103–2107.

320. Reid R, Mar E-C, Huang E-S, Topal MD. Insertion and extension of acyclic, dideoxy, and ara nucleotides by herpesviridae, human alpha and human beta polymerases: a unique inhibition mechanism for 9-(1,3-dihydroxy-2-propoxymethyl)guanine triphosphate. J Biol Chem 1988;263:3898–3904.

321. Resnick L, Herbst JS, Ablashi DV, et al. Regression of oral hairy leukoplakia after orally administered acyclovir therapy. JAMA 1988;259:384–388.

322. Richman DD, Fischl MA, Grieco MH, et al. The toxicity of azidothymidine (AZT) in the treatment of patients with AIDS and AIDS-related complex: a double-blind, placebo-controlled trial. N Engl J Med 1987;317:192–197.

323. Richman DD, Grimes JM, Lagakos SW. Effect of stage of disease and drug dose on zidovudine susceptibilities of isolates of human immunodeficiency virus. J AIDS 1990;3:743–746.

324. Robins T, Vasavononda S, Blohm S, et al. Isolation and characterization of HIV-1 mutants resistant to HIV-1 protease inhibitors. First National Conference on Human Retroviruses and Related Infections, Washington, DC, 1993:101.

325. Rodriguez WJ, Dang Bui RH, Connor JD, et al. Environmental exposure of primary care personnel to ribavirin aerosol when supervising treatment of infants with respiratory syncytial virus infections. Antimicrob Agents Chemother 1987;31:1143–1146.

326. Rooke R, Parniak MA, Tremblay M, et al. Biological comparison of wild-type and zidovudine-resistant isolates of human immunodeficiency virus type 1 from the same subjects: susceptibility and resistance to other drugs. Antimicrob Agents Chemother 1991;35:988–991.

327. Rooney JF, Straus SE, Mannix ML, et al. Oral acyclovir to suppress frequently recurrent herpes labialis: double-blind, placebo-controlled trial. Ann Intern Med 1993;118:268–272.

328. Ross AH, Balakrishnan C. Toxicity of adenine arabinoside in humans. J Infect Dis 1976;133:A192–A198.

329. Rossman MG, Arnold E, Erickson JW, et al. Structure of a human cold virus and functional relationship to other picornaviruses. Nature 1985;317:624–627.

330. Ruigrok RWH, Hirst EMA, Hay AJ. The specific inhibition of influenza A virus maturation by amantadine: an electron microscopic examination. J Gen Virol 1991;72:191–194.

331. Saag MS, Emini EA, Laskin OL, et al. A short-term clinical evaluation of L-697,661, a non-nucleoside inhibitor of HIV-1 reverse transcriptase: L-697,661 Working Group. N Engl J Med 1993;329: 1065–1072.

332. Sacks SL, Smith JL, Pollard RB. Toxicity of vidarabine. JAMA 1979;241:28–29.

333. Sacks SL, Wanklin RJ, Reece DE, Hicks KA, Tyler KL, Coen DM. Progressive esophagitis from acyclovir-resistant herpes simplex: clinical roles for DNA polymerase mutants and viral heterogeneity? Ann Intern Med 1989;111:893–899.

334. Safrin S, Berger TG, Gilson I, et al. Foscarnet therapy in five patients with the AIDS and acyclovir-resistant varicella-zoster virus infection. Ann Intern Med 1991;115:19–21.

334a. Safrin S, Crumpacker C, Chatis P, et al. A controlled trial comparing foscarnet with vidarabine for acyclovir-resistant mucocutaneous herpes simplex in the acquired immunodeficiency syndrome. N Engl J Med 1991;325:551–555.

335. Safrin S, Kemmerly S, Plotkin B, et al. Foscarnet-resistant herpes simplex virus infection in patients with AIDS. J Infect Dis 1994;169:193–196.

336. Sande M, Carpenter CCJ, Cobbs GC, et al. Antiretroviral therapy for adult HIV-infected patients: recommendations from a state-of-the-art conference. JAMA 1993;270:2583–2589.

337. Sandstrom EG, Kaplan JC, Byington RE, Hirsch MS. Inhibition of human T-lymphotropic virus type III in vitro by phosphonoformate. Lancet 1985;1:1480–1482.

338. Saral R. Management of mucocutaneous herpes simplex infections in immunocompromised patients. Am J Med 1988;85:57–60.

339. Saral R, Ambinder RF, Burns WH. Acyclovir prophylaxis against herpes simplex virus infection in patients with leukemia: a randomized, double-blind controlled trial in bone-marrow-transplant recipients. Ann Intern Med 1983;99:773–776.

340. Saral R, Burns WH, Laskin OL, Santos GW, Lietman PS. Acyclovir prophylaxis of herpes-simplex virus infections: a randomized double-blind controlled trial in bone-marrow transplant recipients. N Engl J Med 1981;305:63–67.

341. Sawyer MH, Inchauspe G, Biron KK, Waters DJ, Straus SE, Ostrove JM. Molecular analysis of the pyrimidine deoxyribonucleoside kinase gene of wild-type and acyclovir-resistant strain of varicella-zoster virus. J Gen Virol 1988;69:2585–2593.

342. Schadelin J, Schilt HV, Rohner M. Preventive therapy of herpes labialis associated with trigeminal surgery. Am J Med 1988;85 (Suppl 2A):46–48.

343. Schaeffer HJ, Beauchamp L, de Miranda P, Elion GB, Bauer DJ, Collins P. 9-(2-hydroxyethoxymethyl)guanine activity against viruses of the herpes group. Nature 1978;272:583–585.

343a. Schapiro JM, Winters MA, Stewart F, et al. The effects of high-dose saquinavir on viral load and CD4+ T cell-counts in HIV-infected patients. Ann Int Med 1996;124:1039–1050.

344. Schmidt GM, Horak DA, Niland JC, et al. A randomized, controlled trial of prophylactic ganciclovir for cytomegalovirus pulmonary infection in recipients of allogeneic bone marrow transplants. N Engl J Med 1991;324:1005–1011.

345. Schnipper LE, Crumpacker CS. Resistance of herpes simplex virus to acyclovir: Role of thymidine kinase and DNA polymerase loci. Proc Natl Acad Sci U S A 1980;77:2270–2273.

346. Scholtissek E, Faulkner GP. Amantadine-resistant and sensitive influenza A strains and recombinants. J Gen Virol 1979;44:807–815.

347. Schooley RT, Merigan TC, Gaut P, et al. Recombinant soluble CD4 therapy in patients with the acquired immunodeficiency syndrome (AIDS) and AIDS-related complex: a phase I–II escalating dosage trial. Ann Intern Med 1990;112:247–253.

348. Shepard DA, Heinz BA, Rueckert RR. WIN 52035-2 inhibits both attachment and eclipse of human rhinovirus 14. J Virol 1993;67:2245–2254.

349. Shepp DH, Dandliker PS, Meyers JD. Treatment of varicella-zoster infection in severely immunocompromised patients: a randomized comparison of acyclovir and vidarabine. N Engl J Med 1986;314:208–212.

350. Shepp DH, Newton BA, Dandliker PS, Flournoy M, Meyers JD. Oral acyclovir therapy for mucocutaneous herpes simplex virus infections in immunocompromised marrow transplant recipients. Ann Intern Med 1985;102:783–785.

351. Shipman C, Smith S, Carlson RH, Drach JC. Antiviral activity of arabinosyladenine and arabinosylhypoxanthine in herpes simplex virus infected KB cells: selective inhibition of viral DNA synthesis in synchronized suspension cultures. Antimicrob Agents Chemother 1976;9:120–127.

352. Sibrack CD, Gutman LT, Wilfert CM, et al. Pathogenicity of acyclovir-resistant herpes simplex virus type 1 from an immunodeficient child. J Infect Dis 1982;146:673–680.

353. Sidwell RW, Huffman JH, Khare GP, Allen LB. Broad-spectrum antiviral activity of Virazole: 1-β-D-ribofuranosyl-1,2,4-triazole-3-carboxamide. Science 1972;177:705–706.

354. Sidwell RW, Robins RK, Hillyard JW. Ribavirin: an antiviral agent. Pharmacol Ther 1979;6:123–146.

355. Singh N, Yu VL, Mieles L, Wagener MM, Miner RC, Gayowski T. High-dose acyclovir compared with short-course preemptive ganciclovir therapy to prevent cytomegalovirus disease in liver transplant recipients. A randomized trial. Ann Intern Med 1994;120:375–381.

356. Sjovall J, Karlsson A, Ogenstad S, Sandstrom EG, Saarimaki M. Pharmacokinetics and absorption of foscarnet after intravenous and oral administration to patients with human immunodeficiency virus. Clin Pharmacol Ther 1988;44:65–73.

357. Skehel JJ, Bayley P, Brown E, et al. Changes in the conformation of influenza virus hemagglutinin at the pH optimum of virus-mediated membrane fusion. Proc Natl Acad Sci U S A 1982;79:968–972.

358. Skehel JJ, Hay AJ, Armstrong JA. On the mechanism of inhibition of influenza virus replication by amantadine hydrochloride. J Gen Virol 1978;38:97–110.

359. Skoldenberg B, Alestig K, Burman L. Acyclovir versus vidarabine in herpes simplex encephalitis: randomized multicenter study in consecutive Swedish patients. Lancet 1984;2:707–711.

360. Skowron G, Bozzette SA, Lim L, et al. Alternating and intermittent regimens of zidovudine and dideoxycytidine in patients with AIDS or AIDS-related complex. Ann Intern Med 1993;118:321–330.

361. Smee DF. Interaction of 9-(1,3-dihydroxy-2-propoxymethyl) guanine with cytosol and mitochondrial deoxyguanosine kinases: possible role in anti-cytomegalovirus activity. Mol Cell Biochem 1985;69:75–81.

362. Smee DF, Boehme R, Chernow M, Binko BP, Matthews DR. Intracellular metabolism and enzymatic phosphorylation of 9-(1,3-dihydroxy-2-propoxymethyl) guanine and acyclovir in herpes simplex virus–infected and uninfected cells. Biochem Pharmacol 1985;34:1049–1056.

363. Smith DN, Byrn RA, Masters SA, Gregory T, Groopman JE, Capon DJ. Blocking of HIV-1 infectivity by a soluble, secreted form of the CD4 antigen. Science 1987;238:1704–1707.

364. Smith DW, Frankel LR, Mathers LH, et al. A controlled trial of aerosolized ribavirin in infants receiving mechanical ventilation for severe respiratory syncytial virus infection. N Engl J Med 1991;325:24–29.

365. Smorodintsev AA, Zlydnikov DM, Kiseleva AM, Romanov JA, Kazantsev AP. VI. Evaluation of amantadine in artifically induced A2 and B influenza. JAMA 1970;213:1448–1454.

366. Sommadosi JP, Bevan R, Ling T, et al. Clinical pharmacokinetics of ganciclovir in patients with normal and impaired renal function. Rev Infect Dis 1988;10:5507–5514.

367. Soung LS, Ing TS, Davgirdas JT, et al. Amantadine hydrochloride pharmacokinetics in hemodialysis patients. Ann Intern Med 1980;93:46–49.

368. Sperling RS, Stratton P, O'Sullivan M, et al. A survey of zidovudine use in pregnant women with human immunodeficiency virus infection. N Engl J Med 1992;326:857–861.

369. Spruance SL, Freeman DJ, Stewart JCB, et al. The natural history of ultraviolet radiation induced herpes simplex labialis and response to therapy with peroral and topical formulations of acyclovir. J Infect Dis 1991;163:728–734.

370. Spruance SL, Hamill ML, Hoge WS, Davis GL, Mills J. Acyclovir prevents reactivation of herpes simplex labialis in skiers. JAMA 1988;260:1557–1599.

371. Spruance SL, Pavia AT, Peterson D, et al. Didanosine compared with continuation of zidovudine in HIV-infected patients with signs of clinical deterioration while receiving zidovudine: a randomized, double-blind clinical trial. Ann Intern Med 1994;120:360–368.

372. Spruance SL, Schnipper LE, Overall JC, et al. Treatment of herpes simplex labialis with topical acyclovir in polyethylene glycol. J Infect Dis 1982;146:85–90.

373. Spruance SL, Stewart JCB, Rowe NH, McKeough MB, Wenerstrom G, Freeman OJ. Treatment of recurrent herpes simplex labialis with oral acyclovir. J Infect Dis 1990;161:185–190.

374. St. Clair MH, Lambe CV, Furman PA. Inhibition by ganciclovir of cell growth and DNA synthesis of cells biochemically transformed with herpes virus genetic information. Antimicrob Agents Chemother 1987;31:844–849.

375. St. Clair MH, Martin JL, Tudor-Williams G, et al. Resistance to ddI and sensitivity to AZT induced by a mutation in HIV-1 reverse transcriptase. Science 1991;253:1557–1559.

376. St. Clair MH, Richards CA, Spector T, et al. 3'-Azido-3'-deoxythymidine triphosphate as an inhibitor and substrate of purified human immunodeficiency virus reverse transcriptase. Antimicrob Agents Chemother 1987;31:1972–1977.

377. Stanat SC, Reardon JE, Erice A, Jordan MC, Drew WL. Ganciclovir-resistant cytomegalovirus clinical isolates: mode of resistance to ganciclovir. Antimicrob Agents Chemother 1991;35:2191–2197.

378. Steele RW, Marmer DJ, Keeney RE. Comparative in vitro immunotoxicity of acyclovir and other antiviral agents. Infect Immun 1980;28:957–962.

379. Strauss SE, Croen KD, Sawyer MH, et al. Acyclovir suppression of frequently recurring genital herpes: efficacy and diminishing need during successive years of treatment. JAMA 1988;260:2227–2230.

380. Streeter DG, Witkowski JT, Khare GP, et al. Mechanism of action of 1-β-D-ribofuranosyl-1,2,4-triazole-3-carboxamide (virazole) a new broad-spectrum antiviral agent. Proc Natl Acad Sci U S A 1973; 70:1174–1178.

381. Studies of Ocular Complications of AIDS Research Group in Collaboration with the AIDS Clinical Trials Group. Mortality in patients with the acquired immunodeficiency syndrome treated with either foscarnet or ganciclovir for cytomegalovirus retinitis. N Engl J Med 1992;326:213–220.

382. Sugrue RJ, Bahadur G, Zambon MC, Hall-Smith M, Douglas AR, Hay AJ. Specific structural alteration of the influenza hemagglutinin by amantadine. EMBO J 1990;9:3469–3476.

383. Sullivan V, Biron KK, Talarico C, et al. A point mutation in the human cytomegalovirus DNA polymerase gene confers resistance to ganciclovir and phosphonylmethoxyalkyl derivatives. Antimicrob Agents Chemother 1993;37:19–25.

384. Sullivan V, Coen DM. Isolation of foscarnet-resistant human cytomegalovirus patterns of resistance and sensitivity to other antiviral drugs. J Infect Dis 1991;164:781–784.

385. Sullivan V, Talarico C, Stanat SC, Davis M, Coen DM, Biron KK. A protein kinase homologue controls phosphorylation of ganciclovir in human cytomegalovirus-infected cells. Nature 1992;358:162–164.

386. Sundquist B, Oberg B. Phosphonoformate inhibits reverse transcriptase. J Gen Virol 1979;45:273–281.

387. Taber LH, Knight V, Gilbert BE, et al. Ribavirin aerosol treatment of bronchiolitis associated with respiratory syncytial virus infection in infants. Pediatrics 1983;72:613–618.

388. Takeuchi K, Lamb RA. Influenza virus M2 protein ion channel activity stabilizes the native form of fowl plague virus hemagglutinin during intracellular transport. J Virol 1994;68:911–919.

389. Talarico CL, Phelps WC, Biron KK. Analysis of the thymidine kinase genes from acyclovir-resistant mutants of varicella-zoster virus isolated from patients with AIDS. J Virol 1993;67:1024–1033.

390. Tatarowicz WA, Lurain NS, Thompson KD. A ganciclovir-resistant clinical isolate of human cytomegalovirus exhibiting cross-resistance to other DNA polymerase inhibitors. J Infect Dis 1992;166: 904–907.

391. Tenser RB, Edris WA. Trigeminal ganglion infection by thymidine kinase-negative mutants of herpes simplex virus after in vivo complementation. J Virol 1987;61:2171–2174.

392. Tenser RB, Jones JC, Ressel SJ. Acute and latent infection by thymidine kinase mutants of herpes simplex virus type-2. J Infect Dis 1985;151:548–550.

393. Tenser RB, Ressel S, Dunstan ME. Herpes simplex virus thymidine kinase expression in trigeminal ganglion infection: correlation of enzyme activity with ganglion virus titer and evidence of in vivo complementation. Virology 1981;112:328–341.

394. Tocci MV, Livelli TJ, Perry HC, Crumpacker CS, Field AK. Effects of the nucleoside analog 2'-nor-2'-deoxyguanosine on human cytomegalovirus replication. Antimicrob Agents Chemother 1984;25: 247–252.

395. Togo Y, Hornick RB, Felitti VJ, et al. Evaluation of therapeutic efficacy of amantadine in patients with naturally occurring A2 influenza. JAMA 1970;211:1149–1156.

396. Toltzis P, O'Connell K, Patterson JL. Effect of phosphorylated ribavirin on vesicular stomatitis virus transcription. Antimicrob Agents Chemother 1988;32:492–497.

397. Tominack RL, Hayden FG. Rimantadine hydrochloride and amantadine hydrochloride use in influenza A virus infection. Infect Dis Clin North Am 1978;1:459–478.

398. Tudor-Williams G, St. Clair M, McKinney RE, et al. HIV-1 sensitivity to zidovudine and clinical outcome in children. Lancet 1992;339:15–19.

399. Turner RB, Dutko FJ, Goldstein NH, Lockwood G, Hayden FG. Efficacy of oral WIN 54954 for prophylaxis of experimental rhinovirus infection. Antimicrob Agents Chemother 1993;37:297–300.

400. Van den Broek PJ, Van der Meer JWM, Mulder JD, Versteeg J, Mattie H. Limited value of acyclovir in the treatment of uncomplicated herpes zoster. Infection 1987;12:338–341.

401. Van der Horst C, Joncas J, Ahronheim G, et al. Lack of effect of peroral acyclovir for the treatment of acute infectious mononucleosis. J Infect Dis 1991;164:788–792.

402. Van Der Pijl JW, Frissen PHJ, Reiss P, et al. Foscarnet and penile ulceration. Lancet 1990;335:286.

403. Van Dyke RB, Connor JD, Wyborny C, Hintz M, Keeney RE. Pharmacokinetics of orally administered acyclovir in patients with herpes progenitalis. Am J Med 1982;73:172–175.

404. Van Voris LP, Betts RF, Hayden PG, Christmas WA, Douglas RGJ. Successful treatment of influenza A/USSR/77 HINI. JAMA 1981; 245:1128–1131.

405. Vere-Hodge RA. Famciclovir and penciclovir. The mode of action of famciclovir including its conversion to penciclovir. Antiviral Chem Chemother 1993;4:67–84.

406. Vink C, Pasterk RHA. The human immunodeficiency virus integrase protein. Trends Genet 1993;9:433–437.

407. Vogt MW, Hartshorn KL, Furman PA, et al. Ribavirin antagonizes the effect of azidothymidine on HIV replication. Science 1987;235: 1376–1379.

408. Wade JC, McLaren C, Meyers JD. Frequency and significance of acyclovir-resistant herpes simplex virus isolated from marrow transplant patients receiving multiple courses of treatment with acyclovir. J Infect Dis 1983;148:1077–1082.

409. Wade JC, Newton B, McLaren C, Flournoy N, Keeney RE, Meyers JD. Intravenous acyclovir to treat mucocutaneous herpes simplex virus infection after marrow transplantation. Ann Intern Med 1982; 96:265–269.

410. Wald ER, Dashefsky B, Green M. In re ribavirin: a case of premature adjudication. J Pediatr 1988;112:154–158.

411. Walker BD, Kowalski M, Goh WC, et al. Inhibition of human immunodeficiency virus syncytium formation and virus replication by castanospermine. Nature 1987;84:8120–8124.

412. Wallace MR, Bowler WA, Murray NB, Brodine SK, Oldfield ECI. Treatment of adult varicella with oral acyclovir: a randomized, placebo-controlled trial. Ann Intern Med 1992;117:358–363.

413. Walmsley SL, Chew E, Read SE, et al. Treatment of cytomegalovirus retinitis with trisodium phosphonoformate hexahydrate (foscarnet). J Infect Dis 1988;157:569–572.

414. Wang CW, Takeuchi K, Pinto LH, Lamb RA. Ion channel activity of influenza A virus M2 protein: characterization of the amantadine block. J Virol 1993;67:5585–5594.

415. Warner WL. Toxicology and pharmacology of adenosine in animals and man. Transfusion 1977;17:326–332.

416. Weinberg JB, Mathews TJ, Cullen BR, Malim MH. Productive human immunodeficiency virus type 1 (HIV-1) infection of nonproliferating human monocytes. J Exp Med 1991;174:1477–1482.

417. Whitley RJ, Alford C, Hess F, Buchanan R. A preliminary review of its pharmacology and properties and therapeutic use. Drugs 1980;20:267–282.

418. Whitley RJ, Alford CA, Hirsch MS, et al. Vidarabine versus acyclovir therapy in herpes simplex encephalitis. N Engl J Med 1986; 314:144–149.

419. Whitley RJ, Arvin A, Prober C, et al. A controlled trial comparing vidarabine with acyclovir in neonatal herpes simplex virus infection. N Engl J Med 1991;324:444–449.

420. Whitley RJ, Blum MR, Barton N, de Miranda P. Pharmacokinetics of acyclovir in humans following intravenous administration. Am J Med 1982;73:165–171.

421. Whitley RJ, Chien LT, Dolin R, Galasso GJ, Alford CAJ, Group TCS. Adenine arabinoside therapy of herpes zoster in the immunosuppressed. N Engl J Med 1976;294:1193–1199.

422. Whitley RJ, Gnann JW, Jr. Acyclovir: a decade later. N Engl J Med 1992;327:782–789.
423. Whitley RJ, Gnann JWJ, Hinthorn D, et al. Disseminated herpes zoster in the immunocompromised host: a comparative trial of acyclovir and vidarabine. J Infect Dis 1992;165:450–455.
424. Whitley RJ, Hilty M, Haynes R, et al. Vidarabine therapy of varicella in immunosuppressed patients. J Pediatr 1982;101:125–131.
425. Whitley RJ, Nahmias AJ, Soong S-J, Galaso GG, Fleming CL, Alford CA. Vidarabine therapy of neonatal herpes simplex virus infection. Pediatrics 1980;66:495–501.
426. Whitley RJ, Soong S-J, Dolin R, et al. Adenine arabinoside therapy of biopsy-proven herpes simplex encephalitis. N Engl J Med 1977; 297:289–294.
427. Whitley RJ, Soong S-J, Dolin R, et al. Early vidarabine therapy to control the complications of herpes zoster in immunosuppressed patients. N Engl J Med 1982;307:971–975.
428. Whitley RJ, Soong S-J, Hirsch MS, et al. Herpes simplex encephalitis. N Engl J Med 1981;304:313–318.
429. Whitley RJ, Spruance S, Hayden PG, et al. Vidarabine therapy for mucocutaneous herpes simplex infections in the immunocompromised host. J Infect Dis 1984;149:1–8.
430. WHO. Current status of amantadine and rimantadine as anti-influenza A agents. Bull WHO 1985;63:51.
431. Wilcox CL, Crnic LS, Pizer LI. Replication, latent infection and reactivation in a neuronal culture with a herpes simplex virus thymidine kinase-negative mutant. Virology 1992;187:348–352.
432. Wingard J, Stuart RK, Saral R, Burns WH. Activity of trifluorothymidine against cytomegalovirus. Antimicrob Agents Chemother 1981; 20:286–290.
433. Winston DJ, Ho WG, Bartoni K, et al. Ganciclovir prophylaxis of cytomegalovirus infection and disease in allogeneic bone marrow transplant recipients: results of a placebo-controlled, double-blind trial. Ann Intern Med 1993;118:179–184.
434. Wlodawer A, Erickson JW. Structure-based inhibitors of HIV-1 protease. Ann Rev Biochem 1993;62:543–585.
435. Wray SK, Gilbert BE, Knight V. Effect of ribavirin triphosphate on primer generation and elongation during influenza virus transcription in vitro. Antiviral Res 1985;5:39–48.
436. Yarchoan R, Mitsuya H, Myers CE, Broder S. Clinical pharmacology of 3'-azido-2',3'-dideoxythymidine (zidovudine) and related dideoxynucleosides. N Engl J Med 1989;321:726–738.
437. Zebedee SJ, Richardson CD, Lamb RA. Characterization of influenza virus M2 integral membrane protein and expression at the infected cell surface from cloned cDNA. J Virol 1985;56:502–511.
438. Zebedee SL, Lamb RA. Influenza A virus M2 protein: monoclonal antibody restriction of virus growth and detection of M2 in virions. J Virol 1988;62:2762–2772.
439. Zhang A, Nanni RG, Li T, et al. Structure determination of antiviral compound SCH 38057 complexed with human rhinovirus 14. J Mol Biol 1993;230:857–867.
440. Zhang D, Caliendo AM, Eron JJ, et al. Resistance to 2',3'-dideoxycytidine conferred by a mutation in codon 65 of the human immunodeficiency virus type 1 reverse transcriptase. Antimicrob Agents Chemother 1994;38:282–287.

PART **II**

Experimental Pathogenesis

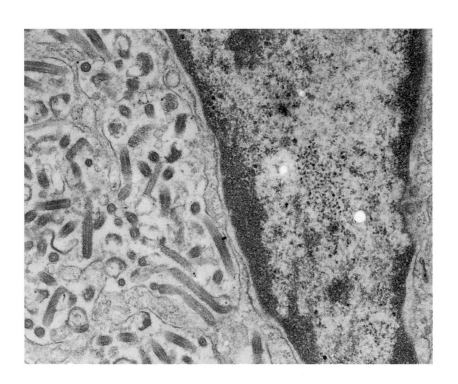

Viral Pathogenesis,
edited by Neal Nathanson, et al.
Lippincott–Raven Publishers, Philadelphia © 1997

CHAPTER 18

An Atlas of Viral Disease Pathogenesis

Frederick A. Murphy and Neal Nathanson

INTRODUCTION

This book examines the subject of viral disease pathogenesis comprehensively from three principle perspectives: from

F. A. Murphy: School of Veterinary Medicine, University of California, Davis, Davis, California 95616.
N. Nathanson: Departent of Microbiology, School of Medicine, University of Pennsylvania, Philadelphia, Pennsylvania 19104-6076.

the perspective of basic concepts of virus entry, spread, tissue damage and host response; from the perspective of classic integrative experimental models; and from the perspective of major organ systems and important disease syndromes that affect them. This chapter adds another perspective: the morphologic perspective.

The morphologic perspective demands that we try to understand what we see and forces us to ask more and more questions when we do not understand what we see. Additionally, even though the methods of viral disease pathogenesis in most cases present static images of cells and tissues frozen in time by our favorite fixatives, the morphologic perspective allows us to mentally transform static data into dynamic images. It allows us to understand and conceptualize in time as well as space. Understanding the dynamic development of disease defines our purpose in studying viral disease pathogenesis.

The morphologic perspective may also remind us of the human ability to see beauty in all of the structures of living organisms at all levels of magnification, but it may also remind us of a different, terrible beauty seen when living cells, tissues, and organisms are damaged and destroyed by viral infection. If the eternal argument over black and white versus color photography were to be extended from Ansel Adams versus Eliot Porter to viral disease pathogenesis, one could argue whether the most beautiful books on the laboratory shelf are the black and white ultrastructural pathology atlases or the color light microscopic histopathologic atlases. Somewhere on the same shelf would also be the atlases of virus structure—there is great beauty in illustrations of these ultimate examples of genetic economy, genetic parasitism—there is great beauty in the structures of their protective coats and great beauty in the functional efficiency of their ligands (which bring them to their target cell receptors) and their enzymatic arsenals (which, once inside their target cell, assure them success in completing their replication and transmission cycles).

There are other books on the laboratory shelf that illustrate the mindset of the pathologist-virologist: those dealing with histologic techniques. The sheer mass of these books suggests that the pathologist-virologist has never been satisfied with the information content of images. It has never been enough to minimally record pathologic changes as observed; the tradition of the pathologist-virologist has been to record as much detail as possible. Technologic advances are adding useful images at an exponential pace. Higher resolution microscopy (e.g., thin-section electron microscopy, negative-contrast electron microscopy, scanning electron microscopy), quantitative microscopy (e.g., microscopic morphometry, scanning microdensitometry), microscopic tomography (e.g., confocal microscopy, other tomographic approaches), freeze-fracture microscopy, electron probe microscopy, scanning-tunneling microscopy, immunofluorescence, immunohistochemistry, in situ hybridization, and in situ PCR greatly extend the scope and scale of images and image analysis. Fortunately, the development of these technologies has coincided with the development of computer-based image acquisition, storage, and analysis.

Historically, pathogenesis research has always had a morphologic perspective. At first, images were used to record gross pathologic observations, dissections, and other adaptations from the science of anatomy, and these images took the form of drawings, engravings, and even paintings, many rivaling the best artwork of the time. Later, with the invention of the microscope by van Leeuwenhoek and the grinding of improved lenses by Amici, images recorded histopathologic observations of incredible diversity; again, the images took the form of artwork, some even more beautiful and certainly more intriguing than those recording structures and phenomena visible to the unaided human eye. Older editions of histopathology books capture a wide sampling of such artwork. This chapter focuses on the photographic record—mostly the photomicrographic record.

It has been difficult to decide which sources to use for the images presented in this chapter. In the end, we decided to personalize our choices, thereby to some extent avoiding the difficulty of looking very far back and very far forward. Our approach is organized according to "Mims-ian" themes.[24] It touches on the basic ingredients of viral infection, virus entry, virus trafficking, virus growth, damage in target organs and tissues, and virus shedding. The subject is worthy of much more breadth and depth and many more examples and lessons than it was possible to include here.

VIRUS ENTRY

Infection in an Arthropod Vector Leading to Transmission Through Bite

Consideration of the nature of virus entry must start with an understanding of the source of the virus. The arboviruses (arthropod-borne viruses) infect their arthropod vector hosts after entry in a viremic blood-meal. Vertebrate host viremia high enough to lead to infection of the arthropod host is one of the hallmarks of arbovirus transmission—after all, the arthropod blood-meal represents a very small volume. The virus usually infects the midgut epithelium of the arthropod and grows its way through to the hemolymph and other visceral organs. Progressive infection leads to invasion of the salivary glands, where these viruses grow very well. The virus titer in the saliva of the arthropod host must be high enough to lead to infection of the next vertebrate host; the arthropod injects only microliter volumes of saliva into its vertebrate host as it probes for its blood-meal. Arbovirus transmission cycles are very effective in nature—so effective that these viruses include some of the great epidemic pathogens of humans and animals.

Figure 18-1 depicts St. Louis encephalitis virus virions accumulating in the salivary gland of *Culex pipiens pipiens* at 25 days postinfection. Paracrystalline arrays of virions are concentrated in the salivary space at the margins of apical diverticula of salivary gland epithelial cells. From this site, virions are ready to be injected into the vertebrate host when the mosquito takes its next blood-meal. As in most natural virus-mosquito pairings, there is no cytopathology associated with this infection.

Figure 18-2 depicts at higher magnification one of the paracrystalline arrays seen in Figure 18-1; this array, if the same size in its third dimension, contains more than 50,000 virions.[29,31,39,41,61]

Infection in a Reservoir Host Leading to Transmission Through Bite

The entry of rabies virus is virtually unique—it is transmitted through the bite of a rabid animal. This requires infection of the limbic system of the brain, driving the animal to fury, while infection of the salivary gland produces highly infectious saliva. In reservoir hosts, virus titers in saliva at the time of peak transmissibility may reach 10^6 infectious units per milliliter.

Figure 18-3 depicts rabies virions budding (*arrowhead*) from the lateral canalicular plasma membrane of two mucogenic epithelial cells in the submandibular salivary gland of a rabid fox. This site of budding is delivering virus into an intracellular canaliculus, which represents the farthest upstream channel of the salivary duct system.

Figure 18-4 depicts the accumulation of rabies virions downstream in the major salivary duct of this gland in the same fox. As illustrated, extraordinary numbers of virions can accumulate at this site.[6,44]

Invasion Through Olfactory Nerve Endings

As a potential site of virus entry, one of the most unprotected endings of the nervous system is the olfactory end organ in the nares. In this organ, the sensory projections of olfactory neurons are directly exposed to the body surface, and their axonal endings are embedded in the olfactory bulb of the brain itself. Rabies virus, and in some circumstances other viruses, is able to invade these neuronal sensory projections at this site and thereby gain direct access to the brain. This is the likely route of entry of neurotropic viruses that are infectious by aerosolization (e.g., rabies virus transmission in bat caves) and is also the likely route of entry in certain laboratory accidents.

Figure 18-5 depicts rabies virus, vampire bat strain, in neurons of the olfactory end organ of a hamster at 5 days postinfection.[49,51]

VIRUS TRAFFICKING

Viremia

From the site of initial infection, many viruses are shed into the vascular system either directly or via lymphatics. There are numerous examples of the correlation between viremia titer and severity of infection in ultimate target organs—the more virus trafficking in the bloodstream and capillary bed of the ultimate target organs, the more cells will become infected, and the more damage will be caused.

Figure 18-6 depicts one of the highest titering viremias ever recognized, that of Rift Valley fever virus. In a mouse moribund at 4 days postinfection, large numbers of virions are seen in a single plane of section through a small capillary in the brain. This represents an extraordinarily high virus burden. In the course of many studies carried out over many years, we have never seen anything like this concentration of virions within the lumen of a vessel.

VIRUS SHEDDING

Intestinal Infection

Viral infection in two organ systems illustrate the simplest connection between virus entry and virus shedding: the intestinal and respiratory systems. Entry into the body of viruses destined to infect the gastrointestinal tract usually starts with contaminated food, water, hands, and other fomites. Virus must survive the acidic conditions of the stomach and the al-

kaline conditions and presence of enzymes and bile salts in the small intestine before reaching the epithelial cells of the intestine, which are invaded directly. These harsh environmental conditions in the digestive system must destroy large numbers of virions continuously, but in nature, there are physiologic circumstances in which pH extremes are buffered (e.g., in infants by milk; in adults by normal intermittent gastric alkalosis) so that enough virus is protected and can go on to cause infection. In fact, the previous generalization that viral enteric pathogens must be stable (i.e., acid and bile salt resistant), as are the enteroviruses, reoviruses, rotaviruses, parvoviruses, and adenoviruses, is now known to be inaccurate. Important pathogens that are sensitive to low pH and intestinal enzymes and bile salts include enteric coronaviruses, pestiviruses, toroviruses, and paramyxoviruses; the latter are particularly important in birds. In the intestinal tract, entry and shedding involve the same cells—epithelial cells immediately exposed and infected by invading virus. Most viruses that infect intestinal epithelium exhibit common pathogenetic characteristics such as rapid growth and high yield, all aimed at completing the fecal-oral transmission cycle before host immune defenses intervene.

Figure 18-7 depicts one of the most explosive models of virus diarrhea available for study—the disease was first attributed to a virus called lethal intestinal virus of infant mice, which is now known to be an enterotropic strain of mouse hepatitis virus. The small intestine and colon of this 10-day-old mouse, which was moribund when euthanized, are flaccidly distended and contain watery, yellowish contents. The pathophysiologic effects of viral diarrhea are a consequence of rapid infection and destruction of epithelial cells and their replacement by immature, transitional cells that cannot carry out normal absorptive, resorptive, and enzyme secretory functions. Glucose-coupled sodium transport is impaired, disaccharidase (lactase, sucrase) activities are diminished, and in some cases, adenylate cyclase and cAMP levels are increased, the latter causing hypersecretion of water and chlorides. The osmotic disequilibrium is most severe in infants because of the normal presence of high concentrations of milk lactose in the intestinal lumen. Osmotic equilibrium returns when the regenerating intestinal epithelium matures sufficiently to produce lactase and to absorb the hexoses produced by the enzyme's action. Although the pathophysiologic mechanism of diarrhea is similar whatever the etiologic virus, there are differences in clinical and epidemiologic manifestations of disease caused by each of the important groups of diarrhea viruses: rotaviruses, caliciviruses (Norwalk-like viruses), coronaviruses, and toroviruses. The topography and course of destruction of intestinal villus epithelium also varies between viral pathogens.

Figure 18-8 depicts a cross section of the jejunum of a 10-day-old mouse infected with enterotropic mouse hepatitis virus. Villi are blunted and club-shaped, and there is massive syncytium formation, seen as large clumps of nuclei in epithelial cells. This status gives way to cytonecrosis and massive desquamation of epithelium. Infection is nearly always lethal.[2,17,18,32,37]

Perpetuation of enteropathogenic viruses is favored by an explosive infection causing diarrhea and a burst of virus shedding rather than a smoldering infection. Nearly all such infections are localized to the intestinal epithelium and, to a lesser extent, to cells of the lamina propria. The failure to penetrate further may represent an evolutionary progression that maximizes shedding capacity and transmissibility without destroying the host population. For example, the diarrheal feces of mice infected with enterotropic mouse hepatitis virus contains extraordinary numbers of virions, and the intestinal epithelium is totally destroyed by the infection, yet very little damage is seen in underlying tissues, and no lesions are seen in other organs.

Figure 18-9 depicts the intestinal lumen of a mouse infected with mouse hepatitis virus at a stage when epithelial cell destruction is rampant. Some virus that has matured by way of budding on intracytoplasmic membranes is shed from intact cells by exocytosis, but most virus is shed during cell disruption.

Figure 18-10 depicts the luminal margin of an intestinal epithelial cell of the mouse in Figure 18-9; characteristically, some virions shed into the extracellular space are readsorbed to the plasma membrane of the same and adjacent cells.[2,17,18,32,37]

Airway Infection

The shedding of viruses from the respiratory tract would seem to be a straightforward matter—the cellular surfaces of the respiratory tract are constantly at risk from airborne and fomite-borne pathogens. The frequency and diversity of clinical respiratory infection episodes are only the tip of the iceberg in relation to the number of viral assaults occurring in the close-contact environment of contemporary life. It is estimated that viruses are the cause of more than 90% of upper respiratory infections, and the average number of infections per person is more than six per year. The entry and shedding of most respiratory pathogens involve the same cells: airway epithelial cells immediately exposed and infected by invading virus. Different viruses are considered to favor different levels in the respiratory tract from the nasal turbinates to the alveoli, but in experimental models there is more overlap than is usually appreciated. Studies over the years in many species indicated that droplets of different sizes lodge at different levels of the respiratory tree. Of course, in nature, virus-laden droplets vary widely in size, and whether an infection is first established in the upper, middle, or lower respiratory tract is determined by many factors other than droplet size, most importantly, the tropism of the virus. For example, whatever the droplet size in which it is delivered, in a high proportion of the population at risk, influenza virus causes tracheitis, bronchitis, and only to a lesser extent, alveolar infection and pneumonia.

As viruses are delivered to the respiratory system, they face two physiologic barriers. One is the mucus film that covers the upper tract epithelium and may contain antibody and glycoprotein viral inhibitors. When intact, this mucus layer serves to prevent contact between virus and cell surfaces. However, it has been shown with influenza viruses, parainfluenza viruses, and other viruses that initial sialidase-mediated invasion and destruction of just a few epithelial cells can initiate a lesion that, with the consequent influx of inflammatory cells and transudated fluid, can progressively damage the mucous protective layer and lay bare more and more epithelial cells. A second physiologic barrier in the airways is the flushing action of beating cilia; inhaled particles, including virus

particles, are normally carried by the mucous flow generated by cilial action to the pharynx, where they are swallowed. However, one of the first effects of virus infection of airway epithelium is cessation of cilial action. This also allows infection to spread from cell to cell. In experimental animals, this spread has been shown to occur by contiguous expansion from multifocal initial infection sites; often the progression leads to infection of virtually every columnar (differentiated) epithelial cell at a particular airway level. The result is complete denuding of large areas of epithelial surfaces, leading to accumulation in the airways of transudates, exudates, inflammatory infiltrates, and necrotic epithelial cell debris. There may be edema, hyperemia, and congestion, which add to the local state of anoxia and acidosis.

Figure 18-11 depicts infection of tracheal epithelial cells of an adult mouse by parainfluenza virus 1 (Sendai virus) at 60 hours postinfection.

Figure 18-12 depicts infection of a bronchiole of the mouse in Figure 18-11. In this experimental model, virtually every epithelial cell in the trachea, bronchi, and bronchioles was infected at this stage; later, these cells became necrotic and sloughed, filling the airways with debris and contributing to respiratory distress. In animals that survive, at this stage of infection airways are lined by a layer of flat, undifferentiated, basal epithelial cells, which are resistant to further progression of the infection. These cells lack viral receptors and probably are temporarily protected by interferons. By the time these cells differentiate into ciliated and mucus-secreting columnar epithelial cells, the evolving host immune response protects them from continuing rounds of infection.[24,25,32,37]

Salivary Gland Infection

Virus shedding from salivary gland epithelium into saliva offers certain advantages to the virus. Shedding may continue for a longer time than is the case with shedding from airway or intestinal epithelium. Shedding continues after the immune response is initiated because of the immunologically sequestered status of the salivary gland epithelium and the directional shedding of virus only on apical plasma membranes directly into salivary space. This is the pattern of shedding of the Hantaviruses, including Sin Nombre virus, the causative agent of Hantavirus pulmonary syndrome, and of the arenaviruses, including Lassa virus.

Figure 18-13 depicts the submandibular salivary gland of a cotton rat (Sigmodon hispidus) infected with the arenavirus Tamiami virus at 24 days postinfection. This is a natural host-virus pairing and reflects a key element in the natural history of this virus. Viral antigen fills the cytoplasm of most of these serous epithelial cells.

Figure 18-14 depicts the submandibular salivary gland of the rodent Calomys callosus infected with another arenavirus, Machupo virus, the causative agent of Bolivian hemorrhagic fever, at 24 days postinfection. Again, large numbers of virions are seen in this intercellular canaliculus between two mucous epithelial cells. C callosus is the natural host of Machupo virus; therefore, the productivity of the infection in this site reflects a key element in the transmission pattern of this virus in nature.[22,35,63]

Urinary Tract Infection

Virus shedding may continue in the urine long after the immune response is initiated because of the immunologically sequestered status of the renal tubular epithelium, kidney calyx epithelium, and urinary duct epithelium, each outside a substantial basement lamina, and because of the directional shedding of virus only on apical plasma membranes directly into urinary space. Virus shedding in urine represents one of the most persistent shedding patterns known.

Figure 18-15 depicts the kidney calyx of a cotton rat (*S hispidus*) infected with Tamiami virus at 30 days postinfection. Viral antigen fills the cytoplasm of epithelial cells but not deeper tissues.

Figure 18-16 depicts the bladder of a cotton rat (*S hispidus*) from the same study as in Figure 18-15 at 60 days postinfection. Again, viral antigen is localized in epithelial cells at a time when neutralizing antibody is being produced. In this natural host-virus pairing, long-term shedding in urine represents a key element in the perpetuation of the virus in its niche. The extreme of this kind of infection is lymphocytic choriomeningitis virus infection in the mouse, in which, in mice infected congenitally, infection continues in the kidneys and bladder, and animals shed virus in their urine for their entire lifetime.[30,34,35,63]

Genital Tract Infection

Virus shedding that contributes to sexually transmitted viral diseases originates in several different sites according to the virus. Human papillomaviruses are transmitted sexually, usually from chronic-persistent infection sites in the skin and mucous membranes of the penis, vagina, and rectum.

Figure 18-17 depicts a biopsy specimen from a person with anorectal papillomatosis. Papillomavirus infection of the anorectal epithelium is evidenced by pyknotic nuclei containing intranuclear inclusions. The etiologic link between infection by certain human papillomaviruses and esophageal, cervical, penile, and anorectal carcinoma has been greatly strengthened in the past few years. In this regard, the smoking gun has been the demonstration of papillomavirus DNA in the right places at the right times.

Figure 18-18 depicts a biopsy specimen from a person with anorectal carcinoma. Papillomavirus infection of neoplastic anorectal epithelial cells is evidenced by the presence of papillomavirus DNA in nuclear inclusions in some of the cells. Carefully constructed controls assure the specificity of this localization in the nucleus of tumor cells.

VIRUS INFECTION IN THE MUSCULOSKELETAL SYSTEM

Striated Muscle

Many different organs and tissues are used by particular viruses as their secondary sites of amplification—amplification that yields the virus that is used in transmission to the next host. These sites of infection are usually associated with major clinical signs and symptoms and major pathologic changes. In many cases, this phase of infection is thought to be rather nondiscriminating—that is, it often seems that many or most organs and tissues become involved. However, this is not true—this phase of infection is as specific as earlier phases, it is just not understood as well. Most of the alphaviruses employ striated muscle as the major site of their secondary amplifying infection. These viruses are often the cause of clinical myalgia, often called breakbone fever in clinical settings.

Figures 18-19 and 18-20 depict Ross River virus infection in striated muscle of the mouse, a major site of replication that contributes greatly to the viremia needed to infect mosquitoes and complete the life cycle of this virus. Figure 18-19 depicts the quadriceps muscle of a 13-day-old uninfected control mouse. Figure 18-20 depicts the same muscle of a mouse of the same age that had been infected with Ross River virus 12 days earlier. Muscle architecture is completely effaced by necrosis of virtually all myocytes.

Figure 18-21 depicts Semliki Forest virus infection of striated muscle of a young mouse. The muscle microarchitecture is severely damaged; contractile elements are disarrayed, and virions are budding from intracytoplasmic and plasma membranes. Even if such events are much more localized in human infections, they can easily explain clinical signs of severe myalgia.[26,38]

Musculoskeletal Connective Tissue

The same important group of alphaviruses that employ striated muscle as the site of their secondary amplifying infection also infect contiguous connective tissue, including fibroblastic cells associated with cartilage, tendons, muscle insertions, and periosteum. In addition to clinical myalgia, these viruses also cause arthralgia and arthritis, the other hallmarks of these breakbone fever and polyarthritis syndromes. The viruses associated with the polyarthritis syndrome include chikungunya, Mayaro, Sindbis, and Ross River viruses, and to a lesser extent Venezuelan equine encephalitis (VEE) virus.

Figure 18-22 depicts Semliki Forest virus infection of paravertebral periosteum of a young mouse. The connective tissue of this periosteal muscle insertion is undergoing massive necrotic change.[41,46]

Musculoskeletal Tissue

Coxsackieviruses are another important group of viruses that employ striated muscle as the site of secondary amplifying infection. These viruses also cause clinical myalgia.

Figure 18-23 depicts coxsackievirus B3 infection of striated muscle of a young mouse. So much virus is synthesized in this site that virions form paracrystalline arrays. In association with this site of virus replication and intracytoplasmic accumulation of virions, the contractile elements of the host muscle cell become completely disarrayed. Later in the course of this infection in mice, myocyte necrosis is overwhelming.[13,15]

Another arbovirus that relies on replication in striated muscle to produce the viremia required to transmit infection to its mosquito host is La Crosse virus, the cause of California encephalitis, a significant pediatric encephalitis in the midwestern United States. Early in infection, this virus replicates mainly in striated muscle tissue, and the plasma viremia is presumably produced by virus shed from this site.

Figure 18-24 depicts viral antigen in a group of striated muscle cells of a suckling mouse injected with LaCrosse virus 3 days earlier by the subcutaneous route.[21]

In the case of rabies and the rabies-like viruses (genus *Lyssavirus*), early virus amplification may be crucial for providing the amount of virus necessary to infect sensory and motor nerve endings, thereby initiating the centripetal neural transit that brings virus to the central nervous system.

Figure 18-25 depicts street rabies virus infection of striated muscle in the limb of a young hamster inoculated distally in the limb 2 days earlier. This was the first site of infection detected in this model system; similar observations indicating the importance of early striated muscle infection were made with 12 different street rabies viruses and 3 rabies-like viruses.

Figure 18-26 depicts Mokola virus (a rabies-like virus) infection of striated muscle in the limb of a young hamster inoculated distally in the limb 2 days earlier. One virion is seen budding from the sarcoplasmic reticulum (*upper right*). This infection cannot be too efficient; unlike rabies infection in the salivary gland, infection in striated muscle cells is characterized by virus budding mostly on intracytoplasmic membranes. There is no cytopathology that would release this virus from within muscle cells; however, a small amount of virus does bud from plasma membranes and is shed into extracellular spaces in close proximity to unprotected nerve endings.[45,49,51]

VIRUS INFECTION IN THE LIVER

Focal infection of the liver is a feature of several acute viral diseases; viruses infecting the liver usually do so by way of the blood. Because the reticuloendothelial cells (Kupffer cells and less-differentiated endothelial cells) lining the liver sinusoids form a functionally complete barrier between blood and hepatic cells, no virus has access to hepatic cells except through this barrier.[24] Virus uptake by or passage between these cells is a necessary first step in infection of the liver. The types of virus–Kupffer cell interactions in the liver can be classified as follows:

No uptake by macrophages. This has been described for a few viruses, such as lymphocytic choriomeningitis virus in congenitally infected mice; this certainly favors persistence of viremia.

Uptake and destruction in macrophages. This is the fate of most viruses circulating in the plasma. If viremia is to be maintained, there must be extensive seeding of virus into the blood to make up for clearance by macrophages, especially Kupffer cells.

Uptake and passive transfer from macrophages to hepatic cells. Circulating virions may be taken up by Kupffer cells but fail to establish infection; however, they may be passively carried across Kupffer and endothelial cells and pre-

sented to adjacent hepatic cells. If the virus cannot then grow in hepatic cells, infection goes no further, although sometimes such viruses are excreted into the bile. Viruses that infect hepatic cells, however, have an opportunity to cause hepatitis despite their inability to infect macrophages. This is so for certain arthropod-borne viruses such as Rift Valley fever virus and is probably the case for hepatitis A and hepatitis B viruses as well.

Uptake and growth in macrophages, endothelial cells, or both. When this occurs, progeny virus particles are released in proximity to hepatic cells, and hepatitis again becomes a possibility. Liver infection in smallpox, ectromelia, and yellow fever probably involves this pathway.

In the adult mouse, vesicular stomatitis viruses (VSV-IND, VSV-NJ) cause severe hepatitis. Because this infection is so predictable, it is a good model for studying the progression of infection from Kupffer cells to the hepatic parenchyma.

Figure 18-27 depicts VSV-IND in the liver of an infected mouse at 36 hours postinfection. At this stage, infection of Kupffer cells has progressed to yield large amounts of virus. Virions are most concentrated in the perisinusoidal space of Disse (i.e., the space between Kupffer cells and endothelial cells and parenchymal cells), where they are in a perfect position to invade underlying hepatocytes.[40]

Infection of mice with wild-type lymphocytic choriomeningitis virus strains is characterized by a florid hepatitis with an exuberant cell-mediated immune response. In these mice, infection progresses rapidly, and death follows the immunopathologic consequences of that infection.

Figure 18-28 depicts lymphocytic choriomeningitis virus (WE strain, the laboratory strain most like wild-type virus) in the liver of an adult mouse at 6 day postinfection. Viral antigen fills the cytoplasm of hepatocytes in this infection site, which then becomes a target for the immunopathologic host response. As is typical in immunofluorescence or immunoperoxidase localization of viral antigen in liver, the infection (or lack of infection) of Kupffer cells cannot be discerned against the background of intense hepatocellular infection.[3,19,20,58,60]

The progression of focal infection from Kupffer cells to hepatocytes causes a disruption of the normal flow of blood through the liver's sinusoidal network. This nascent infarction results in focal anoxia in this organ, which has a high metabolic rate and high oxygen demand and exacerbates pathologic changes caused by the infection.

Figure 18-29 depicts an early focus of infection caused by the arenavirus Pichinde virus in the liver of a hamster at 4 days postinfection. To measure sinusoidal patency, 30 minutes before the hamster was sacrificed, colloidal carbon was inoculated intracardially. The colloidal carbon appears bright red with the filter system used. In normal animals, carbon is phagocytosed by all Kupffer cells, producing a very even pattern outlining the sinusoidal architecture of the organ. However, in this infected animal, carbon has been excluded from the area in and around this focus of Pichinde virus infection, indicative of restricted or ablated sinusoidal blood flow.[33]

Of all of Mims' important observations about the pathogenesis of viral liver infections, one stands out as most striking. In mice inoculated intravenously with large doses of Rift Valley fever virus and examined histopathologically in serial fashion, at 6 hours postinfection, intact, infected hepatocytes had lost their intercellular attachments and floated free in the circulation. Mims noted that this was the only instance ever described other than in massive compressive trauma (e.g., automobile accidents) where emboli of hepatocytes could be found lodged in brain and lung vessels. Shortly thereafter, focal or total liver necrosis supervened.[24]

Figure 18-30 depicts Rift Valley fever virus budding on intracytoplasmic membranes of a hepatocyte of a mouse that was moribund at 4 days postinfection. This extraordinary concentration of virions is observed in hepatocytes throughout the liver of mice at this stage of infection. One piece of evidence of the extremely rapid course of this infection is the number of nascent budding virions seen in this single plane of section; arrowheads depict only some of the profiles of budding virions.

In the course of a Lassa fever epidemic in Sierra Leone in 1972, a liver biopsy was obtained from a moribund patient, and the pathogenesis of the infection was correlated with the pathologic changes observed. **Figure 18-31** depicts focal hepatocellular damage ranging from slight vacuolization to frank necrosis; the necrotic cells are intact and have been left in place. There is a paucity of inflammatory infiltration. **Figure 18-32** depicts the same liver biopsy prepared for thin-section electron microscopy. Very large numbers of virions are observed at the margins of hepatocytes undergoing necrotic changes. Lesions in animals infected with the prototype arenavirus, lymphocytic choriomeningitis virus, were known to be immunopathologic in nature and not a direct consequence of target cell infection. The fact that in this human infection hepatocellular damage was directly attributable to acute virus infection led further investigations toward antiviral treatment regimens (e.g., immune globulin, ribavirin) rather than immunomodulatory treatment regimens.[30,34,56,59,62]

Histopathologic changes in fatal human Marburg and Ebola (filovirus) hemorrhagic fever cases include focal necroses of liver, lymphatic organs, lungs, kidneys, testes, and ovaries. Most dramatic are the focal necrotic lesions in the liver; hepatocytes often exhibit eosinophilic hyaline change and contain large eosinophilic inclusion bodies. Characteristically, there are very few inflammatory cells associated with these changes, probably because they develop so rapidly.

Figure 18-33 depicts the liver of a human patient who died of Marburg hemorrhagic fever 6 days after onset of symptoms; there is widespread hyaline necrosis of hepatocytes.

Figure 18-34 depicts the liver of a patient who died of Ebola hemorrhagic fever in Zaire in 1976; hepatocellular necrosis is associated with the production of very prominent eosinophilic intracytoplasmic inclusion bodies; by electron microscopy of this and other liver specimens from Ebola virus victims, it was found that inclusion bodies are composed of extraordinary masses of preformed viral nucleocapsids.

Figure 18-35 depicts the liver of a *Cercopithecus aethiops* (African green) monkey inoculated with Marburg virus and sacrificed at day 7 postinfection when clinically ill. This image depicts an area where hepatocytes are still intact; at this site, virions fill the intercellular space as a result of budding from plasma membranes.

Figure 18-36 depicts liver from the same animal as in Figure 18-35 but from a focal area where hepatocytes had undergone further necrotic changes; here, cellular architecture is totally effaced, and intercellular spaces contain incredible numbers of virions intermixed with cellular debris. It is hard to think of an instance in which an infected host organ is replaced by more viral mass—that is, virions and viral constituent materials such as those that constitute inclusion bodies—than monkey liver in a filovirus infection.[22,23,36,43,48,53]

VIRUS INFECTION IN ENDOCRINE AND EXOCRINE ORGANS

Adrenal Cortex

Viral infections of the adrenal gland, notably the adrenal cortex, have been described over many years, but in most cases, observations were not tied to any particular pathophysiologic changes or clinical manifestations. More recently, the concept of disease caused by viral effects on cellular luxury functions has been advanced by Oldstone and colleagues, and this has stimulated a reexamination of the importance of viral infection in tissues involved in physiologic homeostasis, growth, and regulation. Oldstone has defined luxury functions of cells as distinct from those necessary for cell survival, growth, and division—that is, functions that primarily support a whole organ or the whole individual rather than the cell itself.[24] Of course, the epithelial cells of the endocrine organs are at the center of this concept, and virtually every endocrine tissue has been considered in regard to functional loss or change following infection. In several instances, correlations have been found between infection, abnormal hormonal levels, and crucial hormonal effects.

Figure 18-37 depicts the adrenal cortex of a cotton rat (*S hispidus*) inoculated with Tamiami virus and sacrificed at 60 days postinfection. In this plane of section, viral antigen fills the cytoplasm of virtually every cell of the zona fasciculata, which is the site of cortisol and aldosterone synthesis.[35,63]

Thyroid Gland

Traditionally, viral thyroiditis has been identified as the etiology of all sorts of clinical presentations involving that gland. Mumps virus has been identified as a cause of acute thyroiditis, and in a few instances, other viruses have been etiologically associated with thyroid inflammation; however, in most cases, the diagnosis of viral thyroiditis has been a poor substitute for a diagnosis of "acute thyroid inflammation, etiology unknown."

Figure 18-38 depicts the thyroid gland of a cotton rat (*S hispidus*) inoculated with Tamiami virus and sacrificed at 60 days postinfection. Viral antigen fills the cytoplasm of many follicular epithelial cells, but none is present in colloid or parafollicular cells. Seemingly, either all or none of the cells of individual follicles are infected.[35,63]

Pancreas

Classic studies of coxsackievirus pancreatitis in mice by Pappenheimer and colleagues in the 1950s initiated the idea that viruses may play an etiologic role in acute-onset juvenile diabetes mellitus.[24] This idea was strengthened by pathogenetic studies of encephalomyocarditis virus infection in mice by Craighead and colleagues in the 1970s, in which virus was precisely localized in the b cells of the islets of Langerhans of experimentally infected mice.[12] Other viral infections have also been incriminated as the cause of acute pancreatitis; mumps virus stands out in this regard. Despite the appearance of many papers on this subject over the years, the true importance of viral infections in human pancreatitis and diabetes mellitus remains unresolved.

Figure 18-39 depicts the cytoplasm of an exocrine acinar cell in the pancreas of a mouse infected with Rocio virus, a highly pathogenic flavivirus from Brazil. Virions are visible in the lumen of the well-developed endoplasmic reticulum of this cell. This infection resulted in the localization of virions within zymogen granules in acinar cells and eventually in infection of b cells in the islets of Langerhans. Terminally, there was massive necrosis of the pancreatic parenchyma.[12,13,15]

VIRUS INFECTION IN THE HEMATOPOIETIC AND LYMPHORETICULAR SYSTEMS

Hematopoietic Tissue

Every cell in the hematopoietic and lymphopoietic lineages could be used to demonstrate an important effect of virus infection in these organ systems. The lessons from pathogenetic studies in experimental animals dealing with hematopoietic and lymphoreticular cell infections are complex and are intertwined with immune response and other crucial host function abnormalities. In most instances, these interactions are not fully understood. There is a massive body of literature that deals with this subject; nevertheless, only one example is presented here.[63]

Figure 18-40 depicts part of the cytoplasm of a megakaryocyte in the spleen of a cotton rat (*S hispidus*) inoculated with Tamiami virus and sacrificed at 9 days postinfection. At this time, virtually every one of these cells in the bone marrow and in the splenic red pulp was found to contain a high concentration of viral antigen spread throughout its cytoplasm. This infection was very productive; substantial numbers of typical arenavirus particles are present in the platelet demarcation channels of this infected megakaryocyte. As in other sites with extensive intercellular channeling of extravascular fluid, there were no focal accumulations of released virions. No virus association with formed platelets was observed. Although Tamiami virus infection persists for an extremely long time in the cotton rat, the natural host of the virus, there was no evidence of any platelet-mediated effects that might represent an experimental animal analog of the hemorrhagic fevers caused by several arenaviruses in humans.[32,35,63]

Lymphoreticular Tissue

Any pathogenetic sequence of infection is a dynamic process that requires continuing virus production to replace virus lost by normal host phagocytic and immunologic activities. In this regard, two of the most effective infection sites from the standpoint of an invading virus are the reticuloendothelial and lymphoid tissues. The infection and destruction of these tissues assures the virus protection from phagocytic removal and from inflammatory-immunologic inactivation. Some of the most destructive and lethal viruses exhibit this tropism.

Figure 18-41 depicts the spleen of a hamster inoculated with the arenavirus Pichinde virus at 4 days postinfection. Thirty minutes before the hamster was sacrificed, colloidal carbon was inoculated intracardially. The colloidal carbon, which fluoresces bright red with the filter system used, has filled the sinuses of the red pulp and outlines clearly the margins of the white pulp. At this early stage of infection, viral antigen is present only in dendritic macrophages in the marginal zone of the white pulp; the extensions of a few infected macrophages are seen intruding into the lymphoid center of this white pulp profile. This represents the initial site of invasion of this organ, probably as a result of normal phagocytic activity of these cells. Later, virus shed from these cells infects the lymphoid cells of the splenic white pulp, especially cells of the periarteriolar sheath.

Figure 18-42 illustrates a somewhat later stage in this pathogenetic sequence of infection as it unfolds in the lymph nodes. This figure depicts a mesenteric lymph node of a hamster inoculated with Pichinde virus and sacrificed at 8 days postinfection, when infection has spread from the dendritic macrophages to lymphocytes. In lymph nodes, macrophages are concentrated at the margins of subcapsular sinuses; from here, infection has spread to involve most of the lymphocytes of this follicular profile. This progression from initial macrophage infection to amplified infection of lymphoid cells was easily seen because of the long progressive course of infection and torpid development of the immune response in this experimental animal model.[33]

Many encounters between viruses and elements of reticuloendothelial and lymphoid tissues are subtle and can be most thoroughly studied by nonmorphologic means using isolated cells. However, such studies usually turn our attention to the host immune aspects of these encounters rather than to the infectious agent. In contrast, when the pathology and pathogenesis of these encounters are studied in situ, it is often seen that the outcome can be devastating. VEE virus infection in hamsters stands out as a useful model, because there is a precise chronologic and topographic progression of virus infection and destruction in these tissues. In thymus, spleen, lymph nodes, bone marrow, and Peyer's patches, there is early productive infection of reticular cells (dendritic macrophages and less differentiated reticular cells) and later infection and severe cytonecrosis of lymphoid and myeloid cells that leads to the acute death of all infected animals.

Figure 18-43 depicts splenic white pulp of a hamster inoculated with VEE virus type IAB at 30 hours postinfection. There is frank necrosis of dendritic macrophages in the marginal zone of the white pulp and the beginnings of the focal progression to necrosis of lymphoid cells of the periarteriolar sheath. The phagocytosis of virus by splenic macrophages is expected to trigger the afferent limb of the immune response; antigenic materials are presented to neighboring lymphocytes, and the immune response is initiated. However, when the initiation of this cascade is prevented by acute cytonecrosis of these macrophages, subsequent immunologically specific events are obviated.

Figure 18-44 depicts thymic cortex of a hamster inoculated with VEE virus 36 hours postinfection. The dendritic reticulum cells are already undergoing necrotic changes as a result of infection (virus particles can be seen in surrounding extracellular space), but surrounding lymphoid cells still appear normal.

Figure 18-45 depicts a small monofollicular lymph node of a hamster inoculated with VEE virus at day 3 postinfection. Whereas at day 2 lymph node necrosis was localized in cortical areas of lymph nodes (areas rich in marginal sinus macrophages), by day 3 necrosis involves whole follicles. Most lymphocytes have been lysed, and there is frank hemorrhage into the necrotic follicle.

Figure 18-46 depicts thymic cortex of a hamster inoculated with VEE virus at 3 days postinfection. Virus particles are seen budding on the plasma membrane of a lymphocyte, which is still intact.

Figure 18-47 depicts femoral bone marrow of a hamster inoculated with VEE virus at 3 days postinfection. Seemingly, every cell is undergoing necrosis.

Figure 18-48 depicts a Peyer's patch at 4 days postinfection, at which time the hamster is moribund; the lymphoid center of this Peyer's patch is totally necrotic, and the local integrity of the intestinal wall is about to break down. This might be thought of as the basis for sepsis, except that these animals do not live long enough for this to be an important pathogenetic event. This precise progression in the pathogenesis of VEE infection in the hamster is rapid, efficient, extremely destructive, and dependent on the sensitivity to infection of reticuloendothelial, lymphoid, and hematopoietic cells. This model seems to represent an exaggeration in magnitude of a phenomenon that is becoming more and more appreciated; for example, it is now recognized that this same progression is operative in the early stages of HIV infection in humans.[32,37,57]

VIRUS INVASION OF THE NERVOUS SYSTEM

The Hematogenous Pathway

Many neurotropic viruses take a hematogenous pathway to the brain; such viruses usually require substantial replication at extraneural sites to generate the high and persisting viremia needed to deliver virus to the margins of the central nervous system. Virus in the lumen of blood vessels moves through the central nervous system; there, it faces the obstacle of the blood-brain barrier. This anatomic and functional barrier made up of capillary endothelial cells with tight junctions, vascular basement lamina, and choroid plexus and ependymal epithelia with tight junctions, has been well characterized, but little is known about how most viruses cross this barrier and gain entrance into the parenchyma of the central nervous system. Studies using inert particles the same size as viruses have shown that there is no absolute hindrance to direct movement across capillary walls, yet some small viruses seem to penetrate and others do not. Some viruses are able to infect the endothelium and other layers of blood vessels and grow across the barrier; studies, however, have not led to any generalizations, because experimental results have not been consistent,

and early events of endothelial infection have not been readily discernible.

The Peripheral Nerve Pathway

The neural pathway to the central nervous system is used by herpesviruses and rabies virus. This pathway involves virus penetration of the peripheral nervous system and virus replication and genome transit in the axoplasm of nerve fibers, with or without myelin sheath infection. This pathway offers the invading virus maximum sequestration from host defense mechanisms and maximum opportunity for the establishment of persistent or slowly progressive infection.

Virus Infection in Nerve Endings

The most common site of rabies virus entry as a result of the bite of a rabid animal is deep in limb tissues, where muscle constitutes most of the cellular mass. Figures 18-25 and 18-26 depict the role of striated muscle cells in amplifying entering virus for a more effective assault on the peripheral nervous system in this site. Given the nature of the myelin sheath protecting peripheral nerves, it seems likely that the site of entry of peripheral nerves is their relatively unprotected specialized endings. Deep in muscles, the most common motor nerve endings are motor end plates, and the most common sensory nerve endings are neuromuscular and neurotendinal spindles. Productive virus infection of the modified muscle cells of neuromuscular spindles brings virus into close contact with the many unprotected intertwined sensory nerve endings of these proprioceptive organs.

Figure 18-49 depicts a cross section of a neuromuscular spindle deep in a limb muscle of a hamster inoculated with street rabies virus distally in the same limb 2 days earlier. Viral antigen fills the cytoplasm of the modified muscle cells and the sensory nerve leading away from this end organ, but there is no evidence of infection of any other tissues in this site.

Figure 18-50 depicts an unprotected nerve ending in contact with a modified muscle cell in a spindle of a hamster infected with Mokola virus; three virions (two in cross section, one in oblique section) are present at this site, where the plasma membrane of the nerve ending has no protective sheath.[16,45,49,50,51]

Virus Infection in Nerve Endings in the Taste Buds

Figure 18-51 depicts a papilliform taste bud on the tongue of a hamster infected with rabies virus street virus isolate from a bat. Unprotected sensory nerve endings exist at all sites where rabies virus is known to enter. This image represents late infection in a moribund animal in which centrifugal passage has brought infection to this end organ, but the likelihood that the same route would be used in centripetal passage points to the importance of all sensory nerve endings in skin, mucous membranes, and specialized epithelial surfaces as potential sites for virus entry. In this image, viral antigen virtually outlines the plexus-like or basket-like architecture of the sensory innervation of this taste bud.[49,50]

Virus Infection in Peripheral Nerves

When rabies virus adsorbs to the plasma membrane of a peripheral nerve neuronal axon, the viral genome (as viral nucleocapsid or ribonucleoprotein [RNP]) enters the axoplasm and starts to move centripetally at a rather slow, steady pace. With fixed rabies virus strains, following footpad inoculation, limb amputation as late as 10 hours later can prevent central nervous system infection; with street virus strains, amputation may be effective much later. Centripetal passage is not a wave front effect with massive virus buildup distally and decreasing amounts occurring centrally; instead, peripheral nerve infection appears constant along long nerve fiber profiles. This is the result of the passive transport of viral RNP within the cytosol of neuronal processes at a rate similar to slow axoplasmic flow—about 5 cm/24 hours. Study of early events in viral disease pathogenesis requires much more patience and time for observation, and micrographs illustrating the earliest infection events are less dramatic than those in later stages of infection, but the ability to relate the dynamics of pathogenetic processes makes the effort worthwhile.

Figure 18-52 depicts the sciatic nerve of a hamster that had been inoculated distally in the hind limb with rabies virus, vampire bat isolate, 5 days earlier. Infection has progressed to involve nearly all of the nerve fibers in this large nerve. Antigen is distributed evenly along the course of the nerve fibers, rather like strings of pearls. Along the course of its centripetal passage in peripheral nerve axoplasm, the rabies virus genome does replicate and initiate the synthesis of viral proteins. This amplification of the genome is probably necessary given the modest half-life of viral RNA (RNP) in the milieu of cytosol at body temperature. In any case, viral genomic RNA is replicated and transcribed, viral proteins are translated, and virion synthesis occurs by budding on host cell membranes. Because intracytoplasmic membranes in axons are concentrated at nodes of Ranvier, virus replication is concentrated at these sites, thereby explaining the string-of-pearls appearance of viral antigen along nerve fibers.

Figure 18-53 depicts the sciatic nerve of a hamster inoculated with Mokola virus intramuscularly distally in the leg 5 days earlier. Virions are budding from intracytoplasmic membranes at this node of Ranvier.

Figure 18-54 depicts the same node of Ranvier as in Figure 18-53 at higher magnification; early virion budding is evident, and in the same site there is the beginning of an accumulation of excess viral nucleocapsid material (i.e., the beginning of Negri body formation). Between nodes, some viral budding does occur on the plasma membrane of the axon; virus formed in this way is trapped under the surrounding myelin sheath. One conclusion from these observations is that very little rabies virus is released as an antigenic stimulus during the early stages of street rabies virus infection.[49–51]

Virus Infection in Ganglia

Rabies virus genome in its centripetal transit in sensory nerves makes a diversion into neuronal cell bodies in dorsal root ganglia. Whether this diversion and viral replication and amplification in the perikaryon of ganglionic neurons is necessary is not known, but the continuity of the axoplasmic compartment is not interrupted by its junction with the stalk of the cell body, so perhaps viral genome moves directly past this site. Infection of neuronal cell bodies in ganglia may contribute to horizontal spread of infection; the cell bodies of ganglionic neurons are not as isolated from each other as are their myelinated processes.

Figure 18-55 depicts a lumbar dorsal root ganglion of a hamster inoculated with rabies virus, vampire bat strain, intramuscularly distally in the leg at 48 hours postinfection. Against a background of barely visible uninfected ganglionic neurons, a single neuron is seen to be infected.

Figure 18-56 depicts the same ganglion from a hamster inoculated with the same virus at 6 days postinfection. Nearly every neuronal cell body contains large amounts of antigen, some condensing into Negri bodies. Even when infection is massive in terms of antigen load and amount of virus seen by thin-section electron microscopy, street rabies virus strains cause little or no cytopathology.

Figure 18-57 depicts a submaxillary sensory ganglion of a dog inoculated with a street rabies virus isolate and sacrificed at the onset of clinical signs at 26 days postinfection. Every neuron is heavily infected, because are many of the nerve fiber profiles in the section, but no damage is evident, and there is no inflammatory infiltration. Images such as Figure 18-57 raise the question of what is the nature of the neuronal damage or dysfunction that accounts for the lethality of rabies virus infection?[7,49,50]

VIRUS INFECTION IN THE CENTRAL NERVOUS SYSTEM

In most cases, central nervous system infection seems to be a dead end in the natural history of viruses; that is, shedding and transmission of most neurotropic viruses do not depend on pathogenetic events in the nervous system. For example, in the encephalitis caused by measles virus and its late manifestation, subacute sclerosing panencephalitis, and in the encephalitides caused by paramyxoviruses, coronaviruses, and parvoviruses in many species, virus may be recovered from brain tissue long after the acute phase of infection, but only by methods such as co-cultivation and explant culture and never under circumstances in which transmission might occur. Togavirus, flavivirus, and bunyavirus encephalitides represent dead ends also; in these cases, it is the extraneural sites of virus replication that generate the viremia and thereby sustain transmission by allowing the infection of the next arthropod host. The exceptions to this generalization are important, however. Varicella zoster virus and herpes simplex virus depend on delivery of virus from cranial and spinal sensory ganglia to epithelial sites. Epithelial shedding, which follows on recrudescent virus emergence from ganglia, is important because it offers the opportunity for transmission long after primary lesions have resolved. There are other examples in which virus that is seemingly trapped in the nervous system may become a source for transmission. For example, in Kuru, transmission of the agent has occurred via cannibalism, and in Creutzfeldt-Jakob disease, transmission of the agent has occurred through diagnostic electrodes and human dural patches used in surgical trauma repair. Transmission of rabies and other neurotropic viruses to humans has occurred by way of corneal transplants and through laboratory aerosolization of animal brain material. It seems anomalous that neurotropism should be the outstanding characteristic of so many of the most notorious pathogens of humans and animals and yet be the pathogenetic characteristic least related to virus perpetuation in nature. The irreparable damage that is of such grave consequence to the host is of such little consequence to the virus.

Virus Infection in the Brain

Following entry into the central nervous system, the localization and dynamics of progression of a virus is often precise and uniform. In the case of rabies, the ascending progression is rapid and almost entirely limited to neurons. The ascending wave front of this infection has been demonstrated by sequential immunohistochemical and infectivity studies. Precise and consistent topographic localization of rabies virus infection in the brain is the most likely explanation for the specific signs and symptoms at various stages of clinical illness in humans and animals. Richard Johnson stated this very well: "the greater localization to limbic system with relative sparing of neocortex provides a fascinating clinicopathologic correlate with the alertness, loss of natural timidity, aberrant sexual behavior and aggressiveness that may occur in clinical rabies. No other virus is so diabolically adapted to selective neuronal populations that it can drive the host in fury to transmit the virus to another host animal."[30]

Figure 18-58 depicts the brain of a dog infected with a street rabies virus isolate and sacrificed at the onset of clinical signs 26 days postinfection. Neuronal cell bodies and processes are heavily infected, but the neuropil appears normal, and there is no inflammatory infiltration.[7]

The hallmark of rabies encephalitis is the occurrence of Negri bodies in the cytoplasm of neurons. Late in infection, these inclusion bodies are largest in the largest neurons, such as in the pyramidal cells in the hippocampus, the ganglionic neurons of the pontine nuclei, and the Purkinje cells of the cerebellum. Small inclusions occur in small neurons with the least cytoplasmic volume, such as in the olfactory bulb and the granule cell layer of the cerebellum. Because of this trait, studies of the topography of rabies infection, whether done by serial immunofluorescence, immunoperoxidase, or histopathology with special stains, is inherently biased toward sites where large antigen aggregates form. Negri body size is also affected by virus strain, host species, and of course by the stage of infection, and each variable adds to the overall bias of such studies.

Figure 18-59 depicts the cytoplasm of a neuron of a hamster inoculated with Lagos bat virus (a rabies-like virus). This image represents the earliest stage of Negri body formation. Individual strands of viral nucleocapsid, which are synthesized in great excess, can be seen. Aggregation of viral nucleocapsids displaces cytoplasmic organelles, which otherwise appear unaffected by the infection.

Figure 18-60 depicts a neuron at a later stage of development; viral nucleocapsid strands have condensed and have trapped some normal cytoplasmic material, forming the typi-

cal Negri body profile. Virions are evident budding from adjacent endoplasmic reticulum membranes.[50]

Inflammatory Lesions in the Neuroparenchyma

The most obvious histologic sign of acute viral encephalitis or poliomyelitis is the inflammatory response to infection. This response presumably reflects a host's defensive effort to contain the infection and to clear the virus, as well as to remove cellular debris resulting from virus-initiated destruction. Destruction is initiated by several different mechanisms, including antigen-specific recruitment of T lymphocytes, cytokines, and the response to tissue necrosis. Inflammation is not seen until 1 or 2 weeks after the initiation of the central nervous system phase of the infection; therefore, it may be minimal or absent in the most fulminant infections, in which death occurs prior to elicitation of a full-blown inflammatory response. Additionally, inflammation is often less severe in very young or newborn animals, who often experience overwhelming infections.

Figures 18-61 and 18-62 depict exuberant inflammation in sheep infected intracerebrally with visna-maedi virus, strain 1514, and sacrificed 6 weeks later with signs of weakness. Typically, visna-maedi produces a nonlethal subacute encephalitis permitting development of a full-blown inflammatory response. Figure 18-61 illustrates a large perivascular cuff of mononuclear cells in the forebrain, and Figure 18-62 depicts the central canal and surrounding gray matter with a severe diffuse infiltration of mononuclear cells plus a number of perivascular cuffs.[54]

Although by usual methods of microscopic examination (i.e., light and transmission electron microscopy) the intercellular spaces of the neuropil appear completely collapsed, they are patent and offer a free conduit for host defense cells and inflammatory mediators, which are delivered from the vascular bed in response to damage; however, often, this is too little too late.

Figure 18-63 depicts the massive neuropil destruction characteristic of Eastern equine encephalitis virus infection in mice, horses, and in some cases, humans. It is taken from a serial study of the development of encephalitis in adult mice and represents the last stage of infection at 60 hours postinfection when the mouse was moribund. The progression from the point when there was no visible intercellular space and no cellular changes involved two parallel events: there was a progressive development of intercellular (interstitial) edema and a progressive development of intracytoplasmic neuronal vacuolization, each contributing to the Swiss-cheese appearance of the brain late in the course of this encephalitis. There was also progressive neuronal lysis, but probably because of the swiftness of the progression, there was none of the perivascular and perineuronal inflammatory infiltration that is seen in horses and humans infected with the same virus. Eastern equine encephalitis is one of the most dramatically destructive encephalitides ever encountered.[32,46,47]

Most viral encephalitides that progress to cause the death of the host are evidenced histopathologically at the level of resolution of the light microscope by rather bland changes. However, the extent of neuronal damage seen at the level of resolution of the electron microscope (i.e., thin-section transmission electron microscopy) is generally much greater. Evidence of viral replication in neurons does not directly explain neuronal dysfunction, but in experimental animal models of acute encephalitides, it is clear that the normal structure-function paradigm is grossly upset by viral replicative events, as well as host defense events.

Figure 18-64 depicts the cytoplasm of a neuron in the brain of a mouse infected with Eastern equine encephalitis virus, a member species of the genus Alphavirus, family *Togaviridae*, at 36 hours postinfection. At this time, virus titer in the brain reached 10^{11} median infectious dose (ID50) per gram of tissue. The cytoplasm is filled with preformed nucleocapsids localized on newly formed intracytoplasmic membranes. Later, neuronal cytolysis became spectacular, leaving only fluid-filled spaces and large numbers of virions intermixed with cellular debris.

Figures 18-65 and 18-66 depict the cytoplasm of neurons of mice infected with Russian spring-summer encephalitis virus and St. Louis encephalitis virus, member species of the genus Flavivirus, family *Flaviviridae*), at 5 days postinfection. At this time, virus titer in the brain reached 10^8 and 10^{10} ID50/g of tissue, respectively. The perikaryonic cytoplasm of these neurons are filled with masses of newly synthesized endoplasmic reticulum membrane. Virions are present within the lumina of this endoplasmic reticulum. In Figure 18-66, the masses of new endoplasmic reticulum membranes are characteristically folded into precise three-dimensional arrays, further adding to the displacement of normal cytoplasmic organelles. At terminal stages of flavivirus encephalitides, most neurons remain intact, although they usually appear dense and basophilic as a consequence of their large burden of newly formed intracytoplasmic membrane.[39,41,42,46,47]

Certain viruses are traditionally associated with encephalomyelitis, whereas others are not. One would not expect oncogenic retroviruses to be neuronotropic and the cause of encephalitis. There is one exception, however: the murine retrovirus WM-E, isolated from wild *Mus musculus* in California by Gardner and colleagues.[8] WM-E virus is a typical mammalian type C virus that is transmitted in the wild from mother to offspring in milk and establishes a persistent productive infection throughout the life of its host. The incubation period of the neurologic disease ranges from a few weeks to more than 1 year, and the disease is marked by tremors, progressive hindlimb paralysis, and neurogenic atrophy of limb muscles. As studied by Portis and colleagues by light and electron microscopy, there is progressive loss of motor neurons in the ventral gray matter of the spinal cord and nuclei of the brain stem and cerebellum, as well as microglial proliferation and astrocytosis, but there is no inflammatory infiltration. Neurons, and to a lesser extent glial cells, undergo a vacuolar degeneration somewhat similar in appearance to that caused by spongiform encephalopathy agents. There is also an infection of vascular endothelial cells in the central nervous system with impressive arrays of mature virions often filling subendothelial spaces. The disease is a direct consequence of virus infection of neurons; it is not an outcome of an immunopathologic reaction.[55]

Figure 18-67 depicts immature WM-E virions budding aberrantly into intracytoplasmic vesicles (endoplasmic reticulum) and mature virions accumulating within the lumen of these organelles in the cytoplasm of a neuron in the brain of a mouse.[8,55]

Virus Infection Leading to Hydrocephalus

Hydrocephalus in mice and hamsters infected with reoviruses, mumps virus, and coxsackieviruses has been used as an experimental model for many years. In Ross River virus infection of mice, extraneural infection usually predominates (see Figs. 18-19 and 18-20), but when experimental conditions are adjusted so that there is long-term survival (e.g., a less pathogenic virus strain, older mice, intracerebral route of inoculation), hydrocephalus is common.

Figure 18-68 depicts a hydrocephalic mouse (*left*) and an uninnoculated control (*right*) at 35 days postinfection, when virus had disappeared from the brain. This condition evolved slowly, but at the stage illustrated, there is almost complete replacement of the cerebral cortex with fluid. Nevertheless, there were no clinical signs of neurologic deficiency, and the basal ganglia, medulla, and spinal cord were unaffected. Mice like this one survive for more than 1.5 years.[38] As Mims noted, "life in a cage places few demands on the mouse, but affected mice may have serious defects in learning, ability to seek food, and other behavior traits vital for life in the wild."

The pathogenetic events leading to hydrocephalus start with infection of ependymal epithelial cells, especially in the aqueduct of Sylvius. In Ross River virus infection in mice, initial evidence of ependymal infection was detected by frozen-section immunofluorescence at day 3 following intracerebral inoculation. Viral antigen had disappeared from this site by day 7, but damage continued to evolve. In contrast, in lymphocytic choriomeningitis virus infection of adult mice, the infection and damage of ependyma is progressive and unremitting until death, usually at day 6 or 7 postinfection. This clinical course can be extended, by use of diazepam to prevent the seizures that cause death of infected animals from respiratory arrest, for example, but the ependymal infection continues to progress, and subependymal tissue is also invaded and damaged. Thus, in each of these two different experimental models of aqueductal pathology, there is no evidence of incipient repair and no evidence of any return to normal cerebrospinal fluid flow.

Figure 18-69 depicts the aqueduct of Sylvius of a mouse that was inoculated intracerebrally with Ross River virus, strain NB 5092, 8 days postinfection. Epithelial damage is substantial, and necrosis extends into subependymal tissues. The lumen of the aqueduct can still be seen, but incipient stenosis is present.

Figure 18-70 depicts the aqueduct of Sylvius of a mouse inoculated with lymphocytic choriomeningitis virus and treated daily through the course of the infection with diazepam. This mouse lived several days longer than it would have if not treated with this anticonvulsive drug; the infection continued to progress so that in this plane of section, every aqueductal epithelial cell is infected, and many subependymal cells are infected as well.[3,26,38,58,60]

Following the aqueductal stenosis that leads to hydrocephalus, the osmotic equilibrium of the brain parenchyma is maintained while fluid accumulates slowly and pressure-effect damage evolves. The major consequence is rarefaction and thinning, first of the basal layers, and then of the outer layers of the cerebral cortex. In Ross River virus infected mice, fluid accumulation in lateral ventricles was evident by day 18 postinfection and progressed thereafter.

Figure 18-71 depicts the rarefaction of the basal zone of the cerebral cortex (i.e., porencephaly) adjacent to the distended lateral ventricle in a mouse injected with Ross River virus (strain NB 5092), 18 days postinfection. The unaffected choroid plexus floats free in the hydrocephalic ventricle (*bottom*). By 35 days postinfection, the cortex was often virtually missing, with only a few cells left between the meninges and the residual ventricular ependyma.[26,38]

In Ross River virus–infected mice, the slowly evolving effects of intraventricular fluid pressure, leading to ablation of the cerebral cortex, continues inexorably. The subsequent effect of this pressure build-up is exophthalmus and herniation of the brain into foramina of the skull.

Figure 18-72 depicts the cerebellum of a mouse infected with Ross River virus, 35 days postinfection. The posterior lobe of the otherwise intact cerebellum is herniated through the foramen magnum, and there is a conification of the cerebellum similar to that found in the Arnold-Chiari type II malformation in human hydrocephalus.[26]

Virus Infection Leading to Cerebellar Hypoplasia

Lymphocytic choriomeningitis virus Armstrong E-350 strain, when injected intracerebrally into newborn rats, produces a fulminant infection of the external granule cells of the cerebellum, leading to their destruction and consequent hypoplasia of the cerebellum. This is known to be an immune-mediated process, because infected rats can be protected against the lesion by treatment with antithymocyte serum. This lesion contrasts with the disease produced in mice by this virus, partly because when mice are infected with the Armstrong E-350 strain at birth, they fail to raise an effective immune response and become lifelong virus carriers. This points out the complex interactions between the virus and its host that determine the nature of disease, which is dependent in part on species-specific differences in the immune response and other host defenses.

Figure 18-73 depicts perfused and dissected brains of 4-day-old rats infected with lymphocytic choriomeningitis virus, Armstrong E-350 strain, by intracerebral injection. These animals were anesthetized and sacrificed by perfusion at 21 days of age. The figure on the left depicts a sham-injected animal; the figure on the right depicts a virus-injected animal showing almost complete hypoplasia of the cerebellum.[27,28]

Virus-Induced Hemorrhage in the Central Nervous System

Viruses can also produce unexpected lesions in the central nervous system. Rat virus, a parvovirus that replicates almost exclusively in dividing cells because it lacks the enzymes to replicate its DNA genome, infects endothelial cells lining capillaries in the brain. Through a complex mechanism, probably involving disseminated intravascular coagulopathy, infection leads to multiple, focal, bland hemorrhages throughout the brain and spinal cord; why hemorrhage is not seen in other tissues is unclear.

Figure 18-74 depicts the brain of a rat infected with rat virus illustrating the characteristic hemorrhage in the white matter of the cerebellum using a special procedure that stains the erythrocytes red and the neuroparenchyma blue.[1,4]

Virus-Induced Demyelination

A number of viruses produce persistent infection of the central nervous system, often causing chronic disease as a result. One important type of lesion associated with some persistent viral infections of the nervous system is primary demyelination, in which the axons remain intact, but the myelin sheaths surrounding them are destroyed. This can be the result of a direct lytic infection of oligodendroglia, which produce myelin, or of an indirect immunologic attack on the myelin itself. The latter mechanism is thought to be involved in the demyelinating lesions associated with lentivirus infections such as visna-maedi of sheep and HIV encephalopathy of humans.

Figure 18-75 depicts the spinal cord of a sheep injected intracerebrally with strain 1514 of visna virus and sacrificed 6 years later, several months after it developed evidence of chronic lameness. This electron micrograph of the white matter shows a number of intact axons that have completely lost their sheaths; for comparison, a few myelinated axons are seen in the field, as is one thin myelin sheath representing remyelination. There is no evidence of inflammatory cells in this field, although they may be seen in areas of chronic demyelination.[9,52]

VIRUS INFECTION IN THE SURFACE STRUCTURES OF THE CENTRAL NERVOUS SYSTEM

Virus Infection in the Ependyma

A classic example of the exquisite specificity of virus tropism is the affinity of lymphocytic choriomeningitis virus for all the brain surfaces: the ependyma, choroid plexus, and meninges. When virus is spread through the cerebrospinal fluid, it has the opportunity to infect every epithelial cell over large areas of surface.

Figure 18-76 depicts the lateral ventricle of a mouse infected with lymphocytic choriomeningitis virus, 4 days postinfection. Every ependymal cell in this plane of section is infected, but there is no infection of any subependymal cells; this is the hallmark manifestation of acute lymphocytic choriomeningitis virus infection in the immunocompetent adult mouse. Orange fluorescence is glycogen within a few subependymal cells.[3,19,20,30,34,58,60]

Virus Infection in the Choroid Plexus

Viruses such as lymphocytic choriomeningitis virus that infect the choroid plexus exert part of their pathophysiologic effects by causing acute imbalances in the osmotic and ionic equilibrium status of the brain parenchyma. In this infection, the choroid plexus is also a key target for the exuberant T-cell–mediated immunopathologic attack that further damages the osmotic integrity of the brain and causes lethal convulsions.

Figure 18-77 depicts the choroid plexus in a lateral ventricle of a 3-week-old mouse inoculated with lymphocytic choriomeningitis virus strain WE, day 6 postinfection. Viral antigen fills the cytoplasm of choroid plexus epithelial cells; virions and viral antigen on the free surface of these cells are the specific targets for the immunopathologic host response.[3,19,20,30,34,58,60]

Based on immunofluorescence studies showing viral antigen in ependyma and choroid plexus epithelial cells at sites of T-cell infiltration in murine lymphocytic choriomeningitis virus infection in mice, it was presumed that these cells were the targets of the immunopathologic response that is the classic hallmark of the infection. The discovery, by thin-section electron microscopy, of virions enmeshed in the microvillous surface projections of choroid plexus epithelial cells elucidated the precise nature and localization of target antigens.

Figure 18-78 depicts the microvillous luminal border of a choroid plexus epithelial cell of a 3-week-old ICR mouse infected with lymphocytic choriomeningitis virus WE strain, 6 days postinfection. Virions are entrapped after having budded from this convoluted plasma membrane. These virions and nascent budding particles were clearly the precise target of the lethal cell-mediated immunopathologic host response; this was evidenced late in infection by the close apposition of many lymphocytes to these microvillous surfaces.[34,30,58,60]

Virus Infection in the Meninges

During an intracerebral injection, the virus inoculum is forced partly into the subarachnoid space and ventricles, partly into the neuroparenchyma, and partly into the circulation. This provides an opportunity for viruses that are capable of replicating in the leptomeninges, ependyma, or choroid plexus to produce infections of these external tissues. Lymphocytic choriomeningitis and other arenaviruses appear to have this tropism and can produce widespread infection of these surface structures.

Figures 18-79 and 18-80 depict an adult mouse infected intracerebrally with lymphocytic choriomeningitis virus, Armstrong E-350 strain, and sacrificed 6 days later when moribund with choriomeningitis. Figure 18-79 demonstrates a very focal leptomeningitis with no involvement of the underlying neuroparenchyma, and Figure 18-80 shows that the infection was, in fact, confined to the leptomeninges and did not spread to the parenchyma of the brain.[5,10,11]

The pathologic manifestations of acute lymphocytic choriomeningitis virus infection in the adult mouse, as described in several preceding figures, are so unique that it might be said they are pathognomonic. The lesions are so uniform in presentation and so different from lesions in other viral infections of mice that one would expect an observation of exuberant lymphocytic choriomeningitis to be diagnostic, certain to be confirmed by any virus-specific diagnostic method. However, as valuable as histopathology can be in diagnostic virology,

it is subject to the exceptions inherent in any nonspecific method.

Figure 18-81 depicts the meninges of an adult mouse inoculated intracerebrally with Quaranfil virus strain Ar 1113, 7 days postinfection. This florid meningitis resembles strikingly that of lymphocytic choriomeningitis virus. Quaranfil is an unclassified virus, first isolated from ticks (*Argas arboreus*), cattle egrets (*Bubulcus ibis*), and pigeons (*Columba livia*) in Egypt. Images produced using thin-section electron microscopy have been somewhat confusing; despite high-quality images of well-preserved virions, it is not certain whether Quaranfil virions most closely resemble an arenavirus or a bunyavirus. RNA sequencing and protein characterization have yet to be completed for Quaranfil virus. With the incomplete state of knowledge concerning this virus, this histopathologic image of an exuberant lymphocytic choriomeningitis becomes an important piece of information. Because bunyaviruses are not known to cause this kind of lesion, the working hypothesis to be tested by further molecular biologic studies should be that Quaranfil virus is either a new arenavirus (it has been tested against all known arenaviruses) or a novel virus, the prototype of a new taxon.

Virus Infection in the Retina: An Extension of the Central Nervous System

Extensions of the central nervous system that are closest to the brain are commonly infected by way of centrifugal transit of virus in the terminal stages of central nervous system infection. The retinal involvement in the late stages of herpesvirus encephalitis is well known, and there is indirect evidence that many more neurotropic viruses make their way to the eye as well.

Figure 18-82 depicts St. Louis encephalitis virus infection in the ganglion cell layer at the surface of the retina of a mouse, 5 days postinfection. Viral antigen fills the cytoplasm of these neurons, and there is some spread from these cells into the rod and cone layers.

Figure 18-83 depicts ganglionic neurons in the retina of a mouse infected with the same virus, also 5 days postinfection. Virions in large numbers are contained in and around the unique intracytoplasmic membranous masses that are characteristic of flavivirus-infected cells. This kind of retinal infection is a common occurrence in many togavirus and flavivirus infections in experimental rodent models, but it has not been well documented in appropriate pathogenesis studies.[12,14,42]

Virus Infection in the Tactile Hair Root: Centrifugal Spread From the Central to the Peripheral Nervous System

In the introduction to this chapter, it is noted that the morphologic perspective may serve to remind us of the terrible beauty of living cells, tissues, and organs as they are invaded, infected, and damaged by viruses.

Figure 18-84 represents this terrible beauty. It depicts a cross section of a tactile hair (a whisker) of a hamster infected with Mokola virus, a rabies-like virus, 5 days postinfection. At this time, centrifugal transit of viral RNA (as viral nucleocapsid or RNP) from the central nervous system leads to infection in many nerve endings and heavily innervated glandular epithelial cells. The elaborate sensory innervation of this tactile hair is outlined by its immunofluorescent viral antigen content. Sensory nerve endings are inserted in radial array into the middle layer of the dermal root sheath of the tactile hair. The cortical substance and cuticle of the hair shaft exhibit autofluorescence, and the root sheath has taken up the rhodamine counterstain, but viral antigen is localized only in the nerve endings that serve the precise proprioceptive tactile function of these structures. This may not be the most important target of rabies virus infection, but it certainly is one of the most beautiful and interesting.[49–51]

ABBREVIATIONS

ID50: median infectious dose
RNP: ribonucleoprotein
VEE: Venezuelan equine encephalitis
VSV: vesicular stomatitis virus

ACKNOWLEDGMENT

Frederick A. Murphy wishes to express his thanks to his colleagues who contributed to this atlas. This project has served as a nice reminder of 14 years of pathogenetic research in the Viral Pathology Branch, Division of Viral and Rickettsial Diseases, National Center for Infectious Diseases, Centers for Disease Control and Prevention, Atlanta, Georgia. Throughout this time, every project involved the efforts of Sylvia Whitfield and Alyne Harrison. Many people were involved at various times: G. William Gary, Jr., Sally P. Bauer, Mary Flemister, Martin S. Hirsch, Bernard N. Fields, Thomas P. Monath, Pekka E. Halonen, Ernest C. Borden, Washington C. Winn, Jr., David H. Walker, Owyle Tomori, Patricia A. Webb, and Karl M. Johnson. Other collaborators from many places are cited in the references. These were wonderful years, brought back to life by these images.

Neal Nathanson wishes to express his thanks to his colleagues who contributed to this atlas and to his understanding of viral pathogenesis, including Richard Baringer, Ernest Borden, Gerald Cole, Adnan El Dadah, Gudmundur Georgsson, Donald Gilden, Francisco Gonzalez-Scarano, Christian Griot, Robert Janssen, Andrew Monjan, Pall Palsson, Andrew Pekosz, and Gudmundur Petursson.

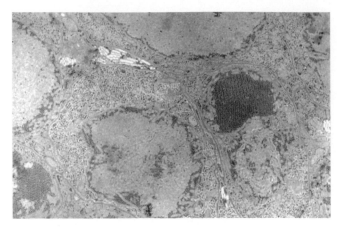

FIG. 18-1. St. Louis encephalitis virus infection in the salivary gland of a *Culex pipiens* mosquito. Thin-section electron microscopy. Uranyl acetate and lead citrate stain; original magnification ×12,000.

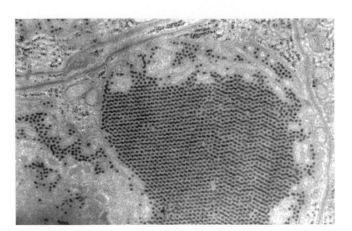

FIG. 18-2. St. Louis encephalitis virus infection in the salivary gland of a *Culex pipiens* mosquito. Thin-section electron microscopy. Uranyl acetate and lead citrate stain; original magnification ×46,000.

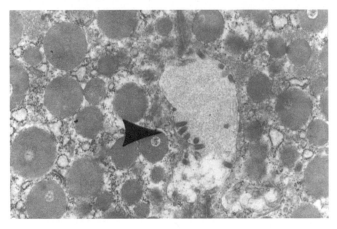

FIG. 18-3. Rabies virus infection in mucogenic epithelium in the salivary gland of a fox. Thin-section electron microscopy. Uranyl acetate and lead citrate stain; original magnification ×25,000.

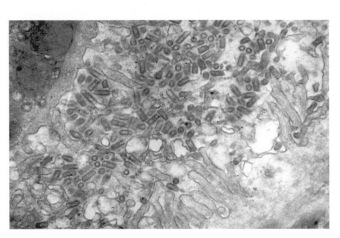

FIG. 18-4. Rabies virus particles in the salivary duct of a fox. Thin-section electron microscopy. Uranyl acetate and lead citrate stain; original magnification ×55,000.

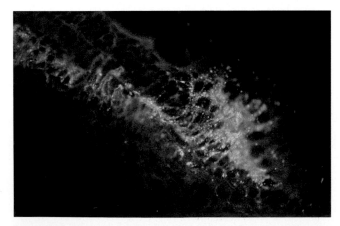

FIG. 18-5. Rabies virus infection in the olfactory end organ of a hamster. Polyethylene glycol–embedded frozen section. Immunofluorescence, FITC-conjugated goat antirabies globulin; original magnification ×500.

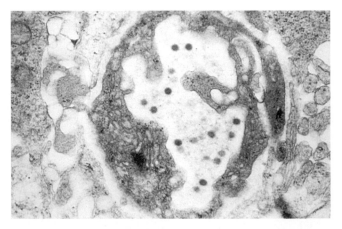

FIG. 18-6. Rift Valley fever virus particles within the lumen of a capillary of a mouse. Thin-section electron microscopy. Uranyl acetate and lead citrate stain; original magnification ×40,000. (Courtesy of J.M. Dalrymple, U.S. Army Medical Research Institute of Infectious Diseases, Ft. Detrick, MD, and F.A. Murphy.)

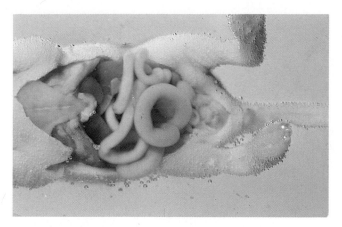

FIG. 18-7. Enterotropic mouse hepatitis virus infection in the intestine of a mouse. Gross photograph of animal submerged in water. Original magnification ×0.5.

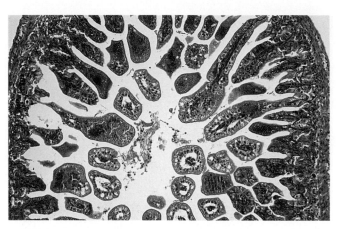

FIG. 18-8. Enterotropic mouse hepatitis virus infection in the intestine of a mouse. Paraffin section. Hematoxylin and eosin stain; original magnification ×200.

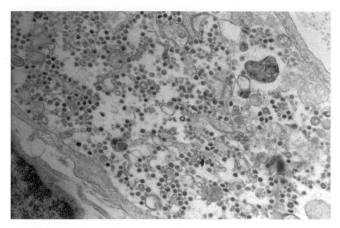

FIG. 18-9. Enterotropic mouse hepatitis virus infection in the intestine of a mouse. Thin-section electron microscopy. Uranyl acetate and lead citrate stain; original magnification ×30,000.

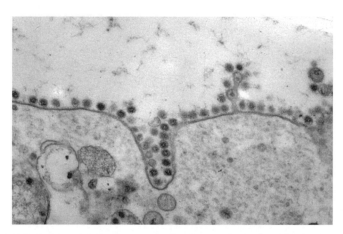

FIG. 18-10. Enterotropic mouse hepatitis virus infection in the intestine of a mouse. Thin-section electron microscopy. Uranyl acetate and lead citrate stain; original magnification ×80,000.

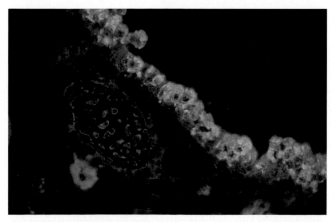

FIG. 18-11. Parainfluenza virus 1 infection in the trachea of a mouse. Paraffin section, including rapid formalin fixation, paraffin embedment, and deparaffinization. Immunofluorescence, FITC-conjugated goat anti-parainfluenza virus 1 globulin; original magnification × 500.

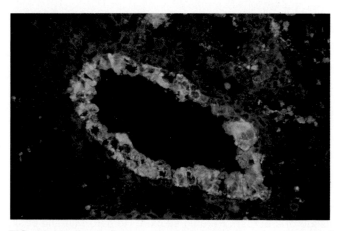

FIG. 18-12. Parainfluenza virus 1 infection in a bronchiole of a mouse. Paraffin section, including rapid formation fixation, paraffin embedment, and deparaffinization. Immunofluorescene, FITC-conjugated goat anti-parainfluenza virus 1 globulin; original magnification × 600.

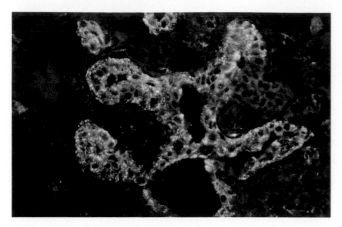

FIG. 18-13. Tamiami virus infection in the salivary gland of its reservoir host, the cotton rat (*Sigmodon hispidus*). Polyethylene glycol–embedded frozen section. Immunofluorescence, FITC-conjugated mouse (ascitic fluid) anti–Tamiami virus globulin; original magnification ×300.

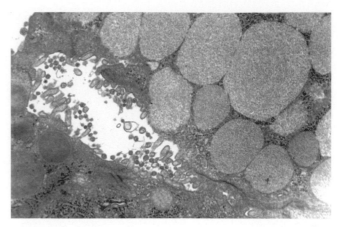

FIG. 18-14. Machupo virus infection in the salivary gland of its reservoir host, *Calomys callosus*. Thin-section electron microscopy. Uranyl acetate and lead citrate stain; original magnification ×30,000.

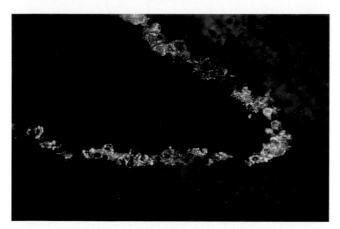

FIG. 18-15. Tamiami virus infection in the kidney calyx of a cotton rat (*Sigmodon hispidus*). Polyethylene glycol–embedded frozen section. Immunofluorescence, FITC-conjugated mouse (ascitic fluid) anti–Tamiami virus globulin; original magnification ×200.

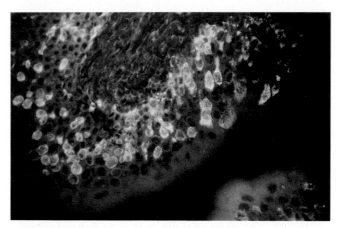

FIG. 18-16. Tamiami virus infection in the bladder of a cotton rat (*Sigmodon hispidus*). Polyethylene glycol–embedded frozen section. Immunofluorescence, FITC-conjugated mouse (ascitic fluid) anti–Tamiami virus globulin; original magnification ×300.

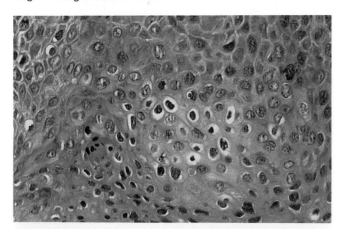

FIG. 18-17. Human papillomavirus infection in anorectal tissue of a human. Paraffin section. Hematoxylin and eosin stain; original magnification ×400.

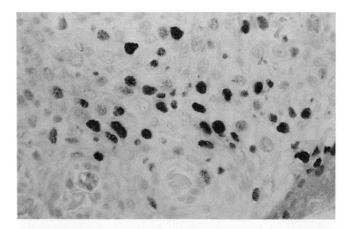

FIG. 18-18. Human papillomavirus infection in anorectal carcinoma tissue of a human. Paraffin section. In situ hybridization using a human papillomavirus DNA as probe and biotin-avidin-alkaline phosphatase detection system; original magnification ×400. (Courtesy of S. Zaki, Division of Viral and Rickettsial Diseases, Centers for Disease Control and Prevention, Atlanta, GA.)

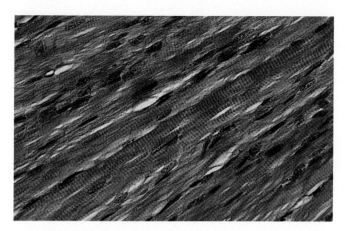

FIG. 18-19. Ross River virus infection in striated muscle of a mouse (uninfected control). Paraffin section. Trichrome stain; original magnification ×200.

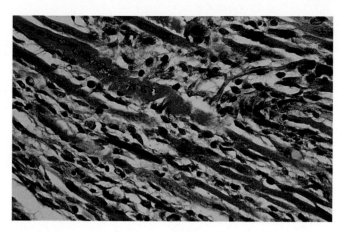

FIG. 18-20. Ross River virus infection in striated muscle of a mouse. Paraffin section. Trichrome stain; original magnification ×200.

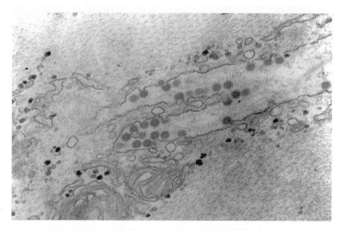

FIG. 18-21. Semliki Forest virus infection in striated muscle of a mouse. Thin-section electron microscopy. Uranyl acetate and lead citrate stain; original magnification ×40,000.

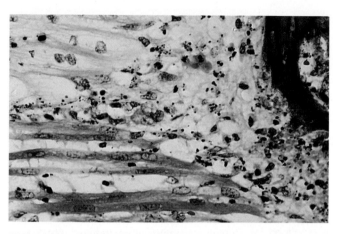

FIG. 18-22. Semliki Forest virus infection in musculoskeletal connective tissue of a mouse. Paraffin section. Hematoxylin and eosin stain; original magnification ×300.

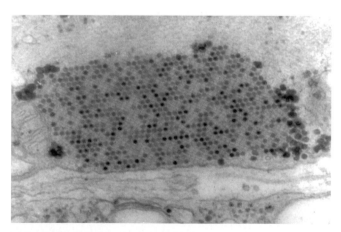

FIG. 18-23. Coxsackievirus B3 infection in musculoskeletal tissue of a mouse. Thin-section electron microscopy. Uranyl acetate and lead citrate stain; original magnification ×30,000.

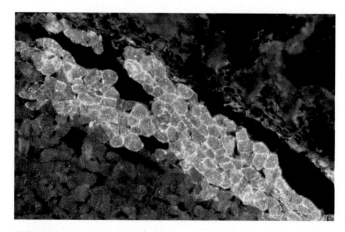

FIG. 18-24. La Crosse virus infection in musculoskeletal tissue of a mouse. Frozen section. Immunofluorescence, using FITC-conjugated rabbit anti–La Crosse virus globulin counterstained with Evans blue; original magnification ×200.

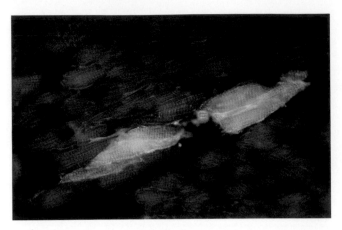

FIG. 18-25. Rabies virus infection in striated muscle tissue of a hamster. Polyethylene glycol–embedded frozen section. Immunofluorescence, FITC-conjugated goat antirabies globulin; original magnification ×500.

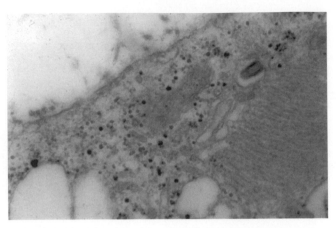

FIG. 18-26. Rabies-like virus (Mokola) infection in striated muscle tissue of a hamster. Thin-section electron microscopy. Uranyl acetate and lead citrate stain; original magnification ×40,000.

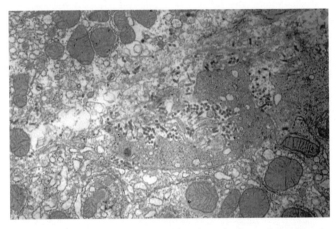

FIG. 18-27. Vesicular stomatitis virus Indiana infection in the liver of a mouse. Thin-section electron microscopy. Uranyl acetate and lead citrate stain; original magnification ×30,000.

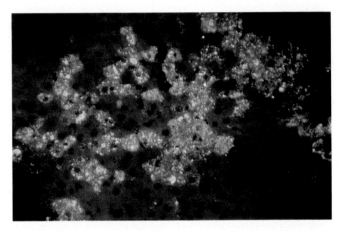

FIG. 18-28. Lymphocytic choriomeningitis virus infection in the liver of a mouse. Polyethylene glycol–embedded frozen section. Immunofluorescence, FITC-conjugated mouse (ascitic fluid) anti–lymphocytic choriomeningitis virus globulin; original magnification ×300.

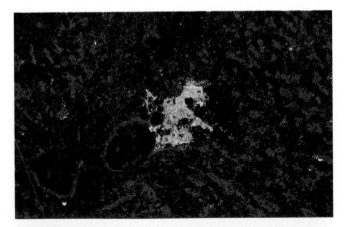

FIG. 18-29. Pichinde virus infection in the liver of hamster. Polyethylene glycol–embedded frozen section. Immunofluorescence, FITC-conjugated hamster anti–Pichinde virus globulin. The filter system makes the colloidal carbon appear red. Original magnification ×300.

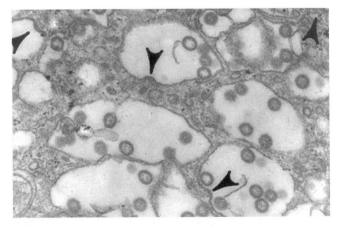

FIG. 18-30. Rift Valley fever virus infection in the liver of a mouse. Thin-section electron microscopy. Uranyl acetate and lead citrate stain; original magnification ×50,000. (Courtesy of J.M. Dalrymple, U.S. Army Medical Research Institute of Infectious Diseases, Ft. Detrick, MD, and F.A. Murphy.)

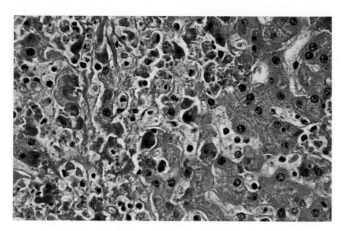

FIG. 18-31. Lassa virus infection in the liver of a human. Plastic-embedded 1 μ section. Hematoxylin and eosin stain; original magnification ×300.

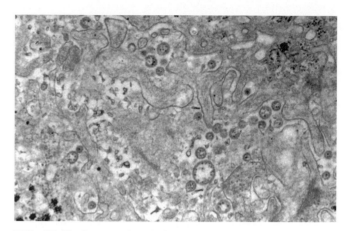

FIG. 18-32. Lassa virus infection in the liver of a human. Thin-section electron microscopy. Uranyl acetate and lead citrate stain; original magnification ×50,000

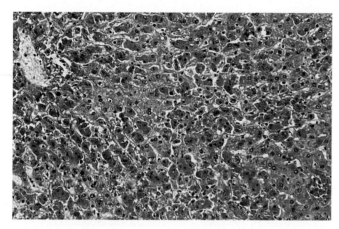

FIG. 18-33. Marburg virus infection in the liver of a human. Paraffin-embedded section. Hematoxylin and eosin stain; original magnification ×300.

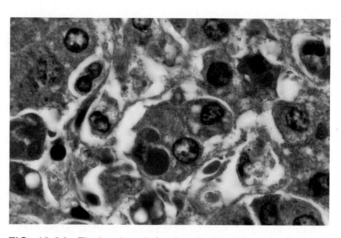

FIG. 18-34. Ebola virus infection in the liver of a human. Paraffin-embedded section. Hematoxylin and eosin stain; original magnification ×700.

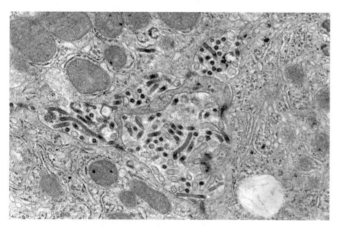

FIG. 18-35. Marburg virus infection in the liver of an African green monkey (*Cercopithecus aethiops*). Thin-section electron microscopy. Uranyl acetate and lead citrate stain; original magnification ×50,000.

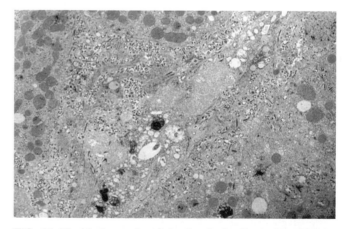

FIG. 18-36. Marburg virus infection in the liver of an African green monkey (*Cercopithecus aethiops*). Thin-section electron microscopy. Uranyl acetate and lead citrate stain; original magnification ×30,000.

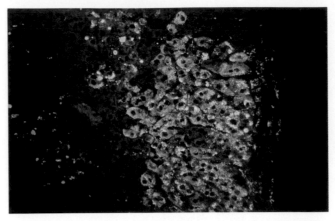

FIG. 18-37. Tamiami virus infection in the adrenal cortex of a cotton rat (*Sigmodon hispidus*). Polyethylene glycol–embedded frozen section. Immunofluorescence, FITC-conjugated mouse (ascitic fluid) anti–Tamiami virus globulin; original magnification ×300.

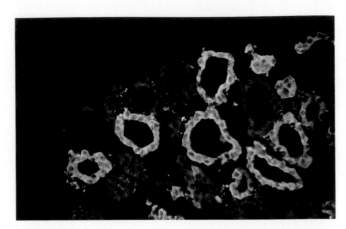

FIG. 18-38. Tamiami virus infection in the thyroid gland of a cotton rat (*Sigmodon hispidus*). Polyethylene glycol–embedded frozen section. Immunofluorescence, FITC-conjugated mouse (ascitic fluid) anti–Tamiami virus globulin; original magnification ×300.

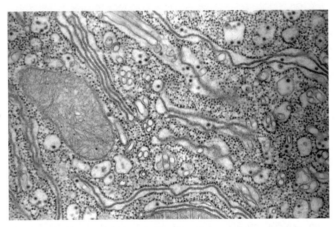

FIG. 18-39. Rocio virus infection in the exocrine pancreas of a mouse. Thin-section electron microscopy. Uranyl acetate and lead citrate stain; original magnification ×40,000.

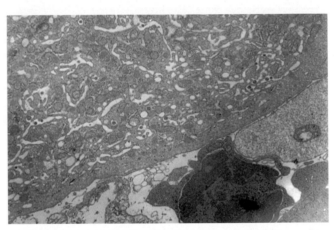

FIG. 18-40. Tamiami virus infection in a megakaryocyte of a cotton rat (*Sigmodon hispidus*). Thin-section electron microscopy. Uranyl acetate and lead citrate stain; original magnification ×40,000.

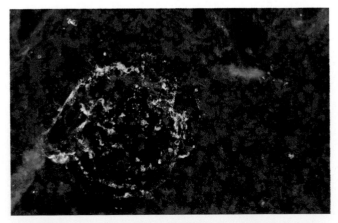

FIG. 18-41. Pichinde virus infection in the spleen of a hamster. Polyethylene glycol–embedded frozen section. Immunofluorescence, FITC-conjugated hamster anti–Pichinde virus globulin. The filter system makes the colloidal carbon appear red. Original magnification ×300.

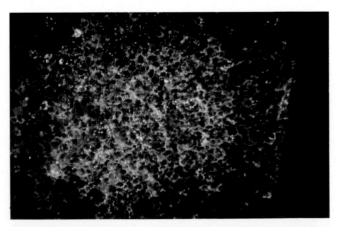

FIG. 18-42. Pichinde virus infection in a lymph node of a hamster. Polyethylene glycol–embedded frozen section. Immunofluorescence, FITC-conjugated hamster anti–Pichinde virus globulin; original magnification ×300.

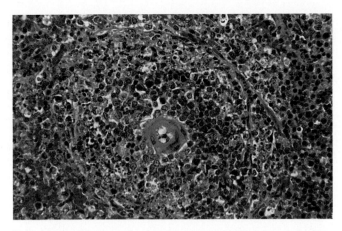

FIG. 18-43. Venezuelan equine encephalitis virus infection in the spleen of a hamster. Paraffin-embedded section. Hematoxylin and eosin stain; original magnification ×600.

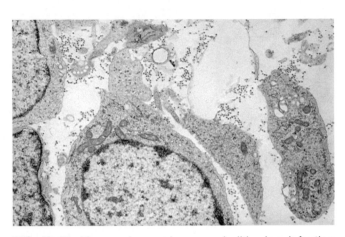

FIG. 18-44. Venezuelan equine encephalitis virus infection in the thymus of a hamster. Thin-section electron microscopy. Uranyl acetate and lead citrate stain; original magnification ×25,000.

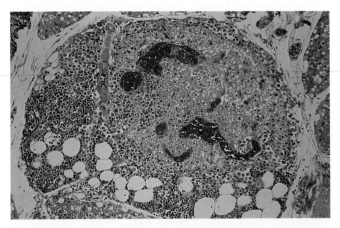

FIG. 18-45. Venezuelan equine encephalitis virus infection in a lymph node of a hamster. Paraffin-embedded section. Hematoxylin and eosin stain; original magnification ×250.

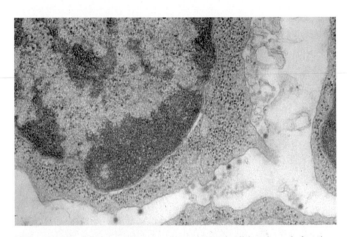

FIG. 18-46. Venezuelan equine encephalitis virus infection in the thymus of a hamster. Thin-section electron microscopy. Uranyl acetate and lead citrate stain; original magnification ×50,000.

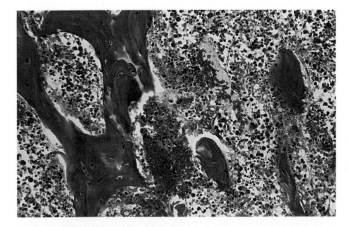

FIG. 18-47. Venezuelan equine encephalitis virus infection in bone marrow of a hamster. Paraffin-embedded section. Hematoxylin and eosin stain; original magnification ×400.

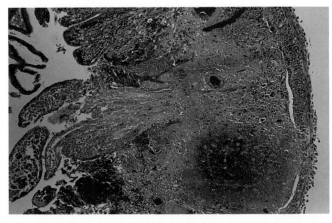

FIG. 18-48. Venezuelan equine encephalitis virus infection in a Peyer's patch of a hamster. Paraffin-embedded section. Hematoxylin and eosin stain; original magnification ×250.

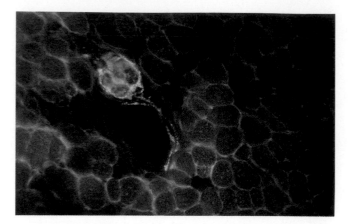

FIG. 18-49. Rabies virus infection in a neuromuscular spindle within striated muscle of a hamster. Polyethylene glycol–embedded frozen section. Immunofluorescence, FITC-conjugated goat antirabies globulin; original magnification ×400.

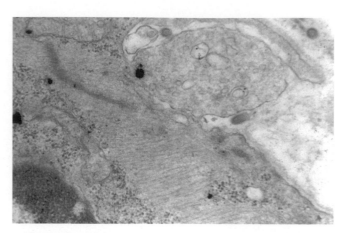

FIG. 18-50. Rabies virus particles in a neuromuscular spindle of a hamster. Thin-section electron microscopy. Uranyl acetate and lead citrate stain; original magnification ×50,000.

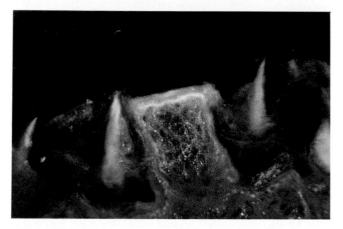

FIG. 18-51. Rabies virus infection in nerve endings in a taste bud of a hamster. Polyethylene glycol–embedded frozen section. Immunofluorescence, FITC-conjugated goat antirabies globulin; original magnification ×600.

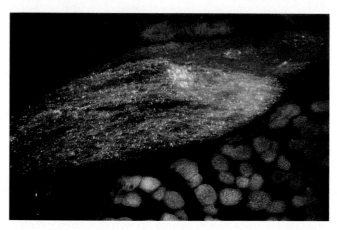

FIG. 18-52. Rabies virus infection in a peripheral nerve of a hamster. Polyethylene glycol–embedded frozen section. Immunofluorescence, FITC-conjugated goat antirabies globulin; original magnification ×400.

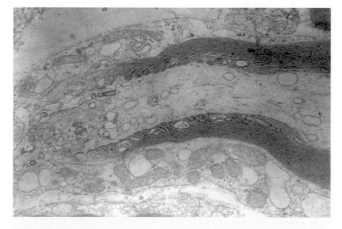

FIG. 18-53. Rabies-like virus (Mokola) infection in a peripheral nerve of a hamster. Thin-section electron microscopy. Uranyl acetate and lead citrate stain; original magnification ×50,000.

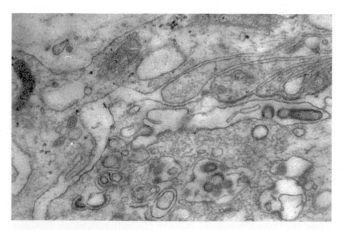

FIG. 18-54. Rabies-like virus (Mokola) infection in a peripheral nerve of a hamster. Thin-section electron microscopy. Uranyl acetate and lead citrate stain; original magnification ×90,000.

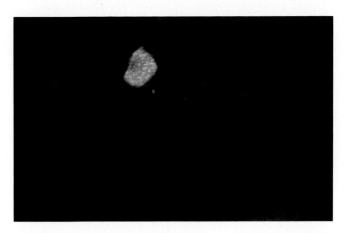

FIG. 18-55. Rabies virus infection in a dorsal root ganglion of a hamster. Polyethylene glycol–embedded frozen section. Immunofluorescence, FITC-conjugated goat antirabies globulin; original magnification ×300.

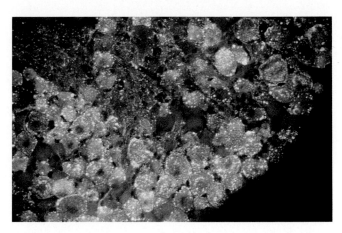

FIG. 18-56. Rabies virus infection in a dorsal root ganglion of a hamster. Polyethylene glycol–embedded frozen section. Immunofluorescence, FITC-conjugated goat antirabies globulin; original magnification ×300.

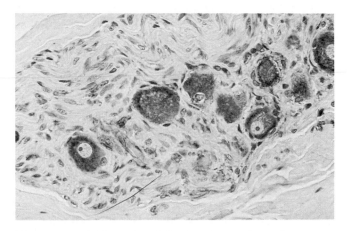

FIG. 18-57. Rabies virus infection in a submaxillary ganglion of a dog. Paraffin section. Avidin-biotin immunoperoxidase technique, mouse monoclonal antirabies globulin, biotinylated antimouse globulin, avidin-biotin peroxidase, and counterstain; original magnification ×500.

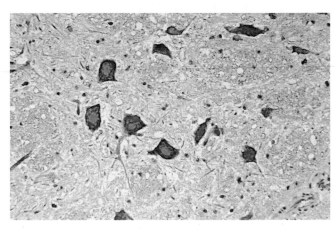

FIG. 18-58. Rabies virus infection in the brain of a dog. Paraffin section. Avidin-biotin immunoperoxidase technique, with mouse monoclonal antirabies globulin, biotinylated antimouse globulin, avidin-biotin peroxidase, and counterstain; original magnification ×300.

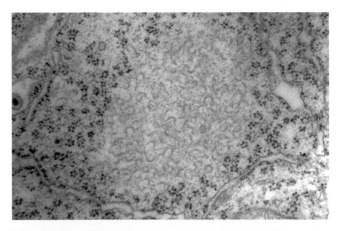

FIG. 18-59. Rabies-like virus (Lagos bat) infection in the brain of a hamster. Thin-section electron microscopy. Uranyl acetate and lead citrate stain; original magnification ×75,000.

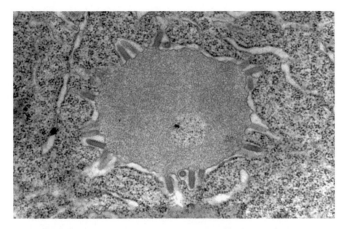

FIG. 18-60. Rabies-like virus (Lagos bat) infection in the brain of a hamster. Thin-section electron microscopy. Uranyl acetate and lead citrate stain; original magnification ×60,000.

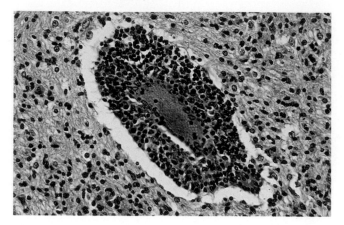

FIG. 18-61. Visna-maedi virus infection with inflammation in the brain of a sheep. Paraffin-embedded section. Hematoxylin and eosin stain; original magnification ×100.

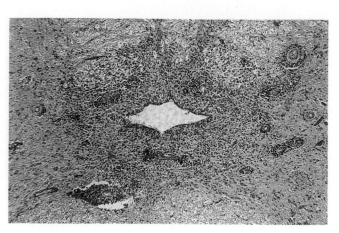

FIG. 18-62. Visna-maedi virus infection with inflammation in the brain of a sheep. Paraffin-embedded section. Hematoxylin and eosin stain; original magnification ×25.

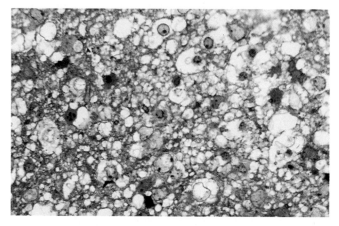

FIG. 18-63. Eastern equine encephalitis virus infection in the brain of a mouse. Plastic-embedded 1-mm section. Azure-eosin stain; original magnification ×500.

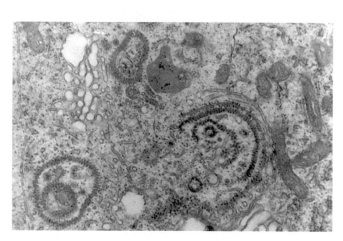

FIG. 18-64. Eastern equine encephalitis virus infection in the brain of a mouse. Thin-section electron microscopy. Uranyl acetate and lead citrate stain; original magnification ×60,000.

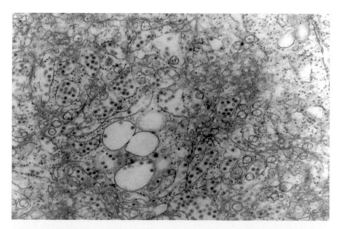

FIG. 18-65. Russian spring-summer encephalitis virus infection in the brain of a mouse. Thin-section electron microscopy. Uranyl acetate and lead citrate stain; original magnification ×65,000.

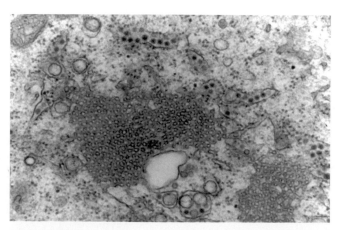

FIG. 18-66. St. Louis encephalitis virus infection in the brain of a mouse. Thin-section electron microscopy. Uranyl acetate and lead citrate stain; original magnification ×70,000.

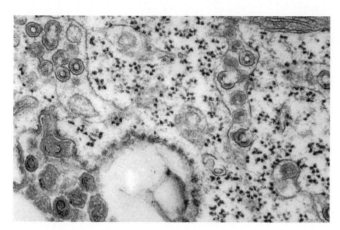

FIG. 18-67. Mammalian type C retrovirus (WM-E) infection in the brain of a mouse. Thin-section electron microscopy. Uranyl acetate and lead citrate stain; original magnification ×60,000.

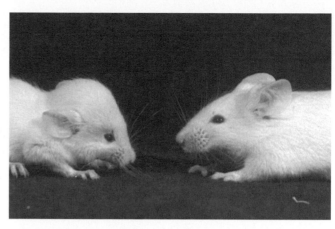

FIG. 18-68. Ross River virus infection leading to hydrocephalus in a mouse (left, infected; right, control). Gross photograph of animals; original magnification ×0.5

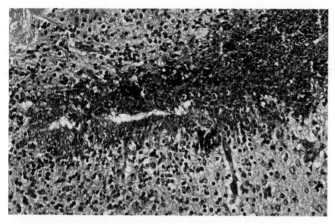

FIG. 18-69. Ross River virus infection leading to hydrocephalus in a mouse. Paraffin-embedded section. Hematoxylin and eosin stain; original magnification ×600.

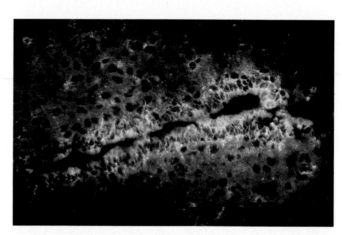

FIG. 18-70. Lymphocytic choriomeningitis virus infection leading to hydrocephalus in a mouse. Polyethylene glycol–embedded frozen section. Immunofluorescence technique using FITC-conjugated mouse (ascitic fluid) anti–lymphocytic choriomeningitis virus globulin; original magnification ×600.

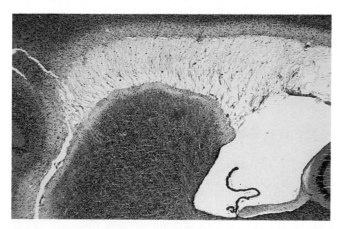

FIG. 18-71. Ross River virus infection leading to cerebral porencephaly and hydrocephalus in a mouse. Paraffin-embedded section. Hematoxylin and eosin stain; original magnification ×600.

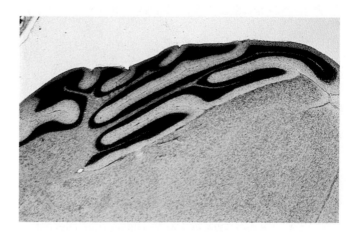

FIG. 18-72. Ross River virus infection leading to hydrocephalus and cerebellar herniation through the foramen magnum in a mouse. Paraffin-embedded section. Hematoxylin and eosin stain; original magnification ×200.

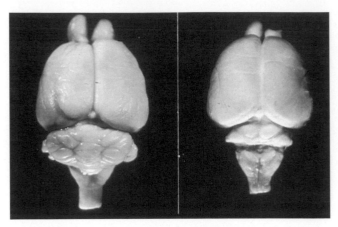

FG. 18-73. Lymphocytic choriomeningitis virus infection leading to cerebellar hypoplasia in a rat. Gross photograph of rat brains. *Left,* Sham-injected animal. *Right,* LCM virus–injected animal. Original magnifications ×5.

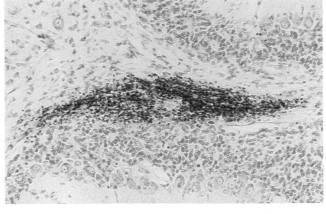

FIG. 18-74. Rat virus (parvovirus) infection leading to hemorrhage in the central nervous system of a rat. Paraffin section stained to reveal hemorrhagic lesions; first stained with Biebrich scarlet, then with Giemsa, and finally with fast green. Original magnification ×250.

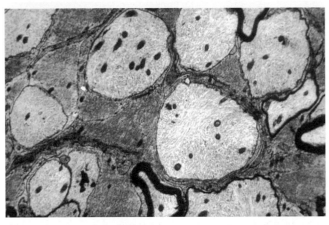

FIG. 18-75. Visna-maedi virus infection leading to demyelination in the spinal cord of a sheep. Thin-section electron microscopy. Uranyl acetate and lead citrate stain; original magnification ×100.

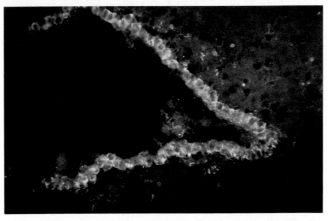

FIG. 18-76. Lymphocytic choriomeningitis virus infection in the ependyma of a mouse. Polyethylene glycol–embedded frozen section. Immunofluorescence, FITC-conjugated mouse (ascitic fluid) anti–lymphocytic choriomeningitis virus globulin; original magnification ×300.

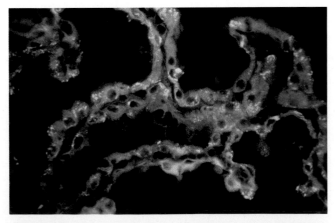

FIG. 18-77. Lymphocytic choriomeningitis virus infection in the choroid plexus of a mouse. Polyethylene glycol–embedded frozen section. Immunofluorescence, FITC-conjugated mouse (ascitic fluid) anti–lymphocytic choriomeningitis virus globulin; original magnification ×500.

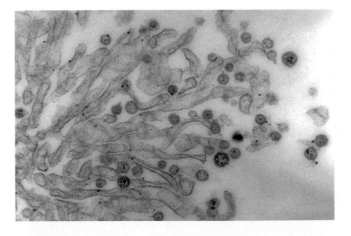

FIG. 18-78. Lymphocytic choriomeningitis virus infection in the choroid plexus of a mouse. Thin-section electron microscopy. Uranyl acetate and lead citrate stain; original magnification ×25,000.

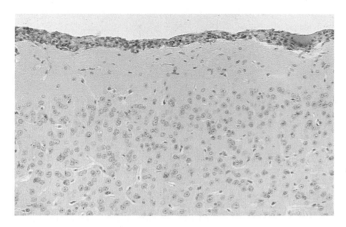

FIG. 18-79. Lymphocytic choriomeningitis virus infection in the meninges of a mouse. Paraffin section. Hematoxylin and eosin stain; original magnification ×280.

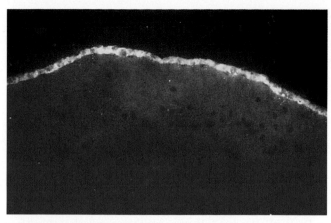

FIG. 18-80. Lymphocytic choriomeningitis virus infection in the meninges of a mouse. Frozen section. Immunofluorescence, using FITC-conjugated anti–lymphocytic choriomeningitis virus globulin with Evans blue counterstain; original magnification ×280.

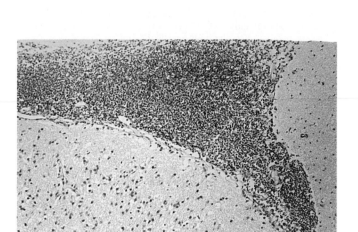

FIG. 18-81. Quaranfil virus infection in the meninges of an adult mouse. Paraffin section. Hematoxylin and eosin stain; original magnification ×200. (Courtesy of C.H. Calisher, Division of Vector-Borne Viral Diseases, Centers for Disease Control and Prevention, Ft. Collins, CO, and F.A. Murphy.)

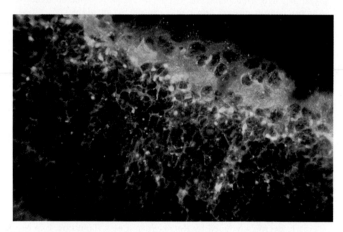

FIG. 18-82. St. Louis encephalitis virus infection in the retina of a mouse. Polyethylene glycol–embedded frozen section. Immunofluorescence, FITC-conjugated mouse (ascitic fluid) anti–St. Louis encephalitis virus globulin; original magnification ×500.

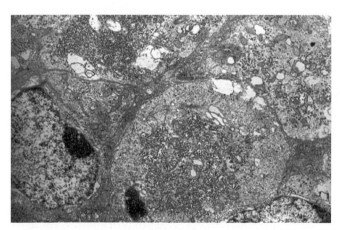

FIG. 18-83. St. Louis encephalitis virus infection in the retina of a mouse. Thin-section electron microscopy. Uranyl acetate and lead citrate stain; original magnification ×25,000.

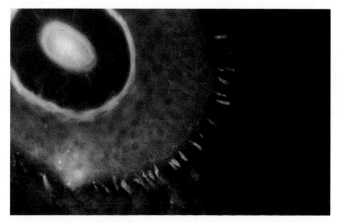

FIG. 18-84. Rabies-like virus (Mokola) infection in the nerve endings in a tactile hair root of a hamster. Polyethylene glycol–embedded frozen section. Immunofluorescence, FITC-conjugated mouse (ascitic fluid) anti–Mokola virus globulin; original magnification ×400.

REFERENCES

1. Baringer JR, Nathanson N. Parvovirus hemorrhagic encephalopathy of rats. Electron microscopic observations of the vascular lesions. Lab Invest 1972;27:514–522.
2. Broderson JR, Murphy FA, Hierholzer JC. Lethal enteritis in infant mice caused by mouse hepatitis virus. Lab Animal Sci 1976;26: 824–825.
3. Camenga D, Walker DH, Murphy FA. Anticonvulsant prolongation of lymphocytic choriomeningitis survival. I. Diazepam effects on lcm virus infection. J Neuropathol Exp Neurol 1977;36:9–20.
4. Cole GA, Nathanson N, Rivet H. Viral hemorrhagic encephalopathy of rats. II. Pathogenesis of central nervous system lesions. Am J Epidemiol 1970;91:339–350.
5. Cole GA, Gilden GH, Monjan AA, Nathanson N. Lymphocytic choriomeningitis virus: pathogenesis of acute central nervous system disease. Fed Proc 1971;30:1831–1841.
6. Dierks RE, Murphy FA, Harrison AK. Extra-neural rabies virus infection: virus development in fox salivary gland. Am J Pathol 1969; 54:251–273.
7. Fekadu M, Greer PW, Chandler FW, Sanderlin DW. Use of avidin-biotin peroxidase system to detect rabies antigen in formalin-fixed paraffin-embedded tissues. J Virol Methods 1988;19:91–96.
8. Gardner MB, Henderson BE, Officer JE, et al. A spontaneous lower motor neuron disease apparently caused by an indigenous type-C RNA virus in wild mice. J Natl Cancer Inst 1973;51:1243–1254.
9. Georgsson G, Martin JR, Klein J, Palsson PA, Nathanson N, Petursson G. Primary demyelination in visna. An ultrastructural study of Icelandic sheep with clinical signs following experimental infection. Acta Histopathol 1982;57:171–178.
10. Gilden DH, Cole GA, Monjan AA, Nathanson N. Immunopathogenesis of acute central nervous system disease produced by lymphocytic choriomeningitis virus. I. Cyclophosphamide-mediated induction of the virus carrier state in adult mice. J Exp Med 1972;135:860–873.
11. Gilden DH, Cole GA, Nathanson N. Immunopathogenesis of acute central nervous system disease produced by lymphocytic choriomeningitis virus. II. Adoptive immunization of virus carriers. J Exp Med 1972;135:874–889.
12. Harrison AK, Bauer SP, Murphy FA. Viral pancreatitis: ultrastructural pathologic effects of coxsackie B3 virus on newborn mouse pancreas. Exp Mol Pathol 1972;17:206–219.
13. Harrison AK, Murphy FA, Gardner JJ, Bauer SP. Myocardial and pancreatic necrosis induced by Rocio virus, a new flavivirus. Exp Mol Pathol 1980;32:102–113.
14. Harrison AK, Murphy FA, Gardner JJ. Visceral target organs in systemic St. Louis encephalitis virus infection of hamsters. Exp Mol Pathol 1982;37:292–304.
15. Harrison AK, Murphy FA, Gary, GW Jr. Ultrastructural pathology of coxsackie A4 virus infection of mouse striated muscle. Exp Mol Pathol 1971;14:30–42.
16. Harrison AK, Murphy FA. Lyssavirus infection of muscle spindles and motor end plates in striated muscle of hamsters. Arch Virol 1978;57:167–175.
17. Hierholzer JC, Broderson JR, Murphy FA. A new strain of mouse hepatitis virus as the cause of lethal enteritis (LIVIM infection) in infant mice. Infect Immun 1979;24:508–522.
18. Hierholzer JC, Murphy FA, Dowdle WR. Lethal enteritis of infant mice (LIVIM) caused by a mouse hepatitis virus. Proceedings, Fourth International Congress of Virology. Wageningen, The Netherlands: Centre for Agricultural Publishing, 1978.
19. Hirsch MS, Murphy FA. Effects of anti-lymphoid sera on viral infections. Lancet 1969;2:37–40.
20. Hirsch MS, Murphy FA, Hicklin MD. Immunopathology of lymphocytic choriomeningitis virus infection of newborn mice: anti-thymocyte sera effects on glomerulonephritis and wasting disease. J Exp Med 1968;127:757–766.
21. Janssen R, Gonzalez-Scarano F, Nathanson N. Mechanisms of bunyavirus virulence: comparative pathogenesis of a virulent strain of La Crosse and an avirulent strain of Tahyna virus. Lab Invest 1984;50:447–455.
22. Johnson KM, Webb PA, Justines G, Murphy FA. Ecology of hemorrhagic fever viruses: arenavirus biology and the Marburg-Ebola riddle. In: Bachmann P, ed. Third Munich Symposium on Microbiology: natural history of emerging and re-emerging viral zoonoses. Munich: UNI-Druck, 1978.
23. Kissling RE, Murphy FA, Henderson BE. Marburg virus. Ann N Y Acad Sci 1970;174:932–945.
24. Mims CA, Dimmock NJ, Nash A, Stephen J. Mims pathogenesis of infectious disease. 4th ed. London: Academic Press, 1995.
25. Mims CA, Murphy FA. Parainfluenza virus (Sendai) infection in macrophages, ependyma, choroid plexus, vascular endothelium and respiratory tract of mice. Am J Pathol 1973;70:315–328.
26. Mims CA, Murphy FA, Taylor WP, Marshall ID. The pathogenesis of Ross River virus infection in mice. I. Hydrocephalus and porencephaly. J Infect Dis 1973;127:121–128.
27. Monjan AA, Cole GA, Nathanson N. Pathogenesis of cerebellar hypoplasia produced by lymphocytic choriomeningitis virus infection of neonatal rats: protective effect of immunosuppression with anti-lymphoid serum. Infect Immun 1974;10:499–502.
28. Monjan AA, Gilden DH, Cole GA, Nathanson N. Cerebellar hypoplasia in neonatal rats caused by lymphocytic choriomeningitis virus. Science 1971;171:194–196.
29. Murphy FA. Cellular resistance to arbovirus infections. Ann N Y Acad Sci 1975;266:197–203.
30. Murphy FA. Rabies pathogenesis: brief review. Arch Virol 1977;54:279–297.
31. Murphy FA. Pathology of Ebola virus infection. In: Pattyn SR, ed. International colloquium on Ebola virus infection and other hemorrhagic fevers. Amsterdam: Elsevier/North Holland Biomedical Press, 1978:43–60.
32. Murphy FA. Viral pathogenetic mechanisms. In: Bachmann P, ed. Fourth Munich Symposium on Microbiology: mechanisms of viral pathogenesis. Munich: UNI-Druck, 1979.
33. Murphy FA. St. Louis encephalitis virus: morphology and morphogenesis. In: Monath TP, ed. St. Louis encephalitis. New York: CC Thomas, 1980:65–103.
34. Murphy FA. Togavirus morphology and morphogenesis. In: Schlesinger RW, ed. Togaviruses. New York: Academic Press, 1980:241–316.
35. Murphy FA. Pathogenesis of viral diseases of veterinary importance. In: Della Porta AJ, ed. Virus diseases of veterinary importance in Southeast Asia and the Western Pacific. Sydney: Academic Press, 1985.
36. Murphy FA, Bauer SP. Early street rabies virus infection in striated muscle. Intervirology 1975;3:256–268.
37. Murphy FA, Bauer SP, Harrison AK, Winn WC Jr. Comparative pathogenesis of rabies and rabies-like viruses: viral infection and transit from inoculation site to the central nervous system. Lab Invest 1973;28:361–375.
38. Murphy FA, Buchmeier MJ, Rawls WE. The reticuloendothelium as the target in a virus infection: Pichinde virus pathogenesis in two strains of hamsters. Lab Invest 1977;37:502–515.
39. Murphy FA, Dierks RE, Harrison AK. Extra-neural rabies virus infection. Proceedings, First International Congress for Virology, international virology I. Basel: Karger, 1969.
40. Murphy FA, Harrison AK, Bauer SP. Experimental vesicular stomatitis virus infection: ultrastructural pathology. Exp Mol Pathol 1975;23:426–440.
41. Murphy FA, Harrison AK, Collin WK. The role of extraneural arbovirus infection in the pathogenesis of encephalitis: an electron microscopic study of Semliki Forest virus infection of mice. Lab Invest 1970;22:318–328.
42. Murphy FA, Harrison AK, Gary GW Jr, Whitfield SG, Forrester FT. St. Louis encephalitis virus infection of mice: electron microscopic studies of central nervous system. Lab Invest 1968;19:652–667.
43. Murphy FA, Harrison AK, Winn WC Jr, Bauer SP. Comparative pathogenesis of rabies and rabies-like viruses: infection of the central nervous system and centrifugal spread of virus to peripheral tissues. Lab Invest 1973;29:1–16.
44. Murphy FA, Kiley MS, Fisher-Hoch S. Filoviridae. In: Fields BN, Knipe DM, eds. Virology, 2nd ed. New York: Raven Press, 1990:933–942.
45. Murphy FA, Simpson DIH, Whitfield SG, Zlotnik I, Carter GB. Marburg virus infection in monkeys: ultrastructural studies. Lab Invest 1971;24:279–291.
46. Murphy FA, Taylor WP, Mims CA, Marshall ID. The pathogenesis of Ross River virus infection in mice. I. Muscle, heart, and brown fat lesions. J Infect Dis 1973;127:129–138.

46a. Murphy FA, van der Groen G, Whitfield SG, Lange JV. Ebola and Marburg virus morphology and taxonomy. In: Pattyn SR, ed. International colloquium on Ebola virus infection and other hemorrhagic fevers. Amsterdam: Elsevier/North Holland Biomedical Press, 1978: 61–82.

47. Murphy FA, Whitfield SG. Eastern equine encephalitis virus infection: electron microscopic studies of mouse central nervous system. Exp Mol Pathol 1970;13:289–291.

48. Murphy FA, Whitfield SG. Morphology and morphogenesis of the arenaviruses. Bull World Health Organ 1975;52:409–419.

49. Murphy FA, Whitfield SG, Sudia WD. Interactions of vector with vertebrate pathogenic viruses. In: Maramorosch K, ed. Invertebrate immunity: mechanisms of invertebrate vector/parasite relations. New York: Academic Press, 1975:25–48.

50. Murphy FA, Whitfield SG, Webb PA, Johnson KM. Ultrastructural studies of arenaviruses. In: Lehmann-Grube F, ed. Lymphocytic choriomeningitis and other arenaviruses. Berlin: Springer-Verlag, 1973:273–285.

51. Murphy FA, Winn WC Jr, Walker DH, Flemister MR, Whitfield SG. Early lymphoreticular viral tropism and viral antigen persistence: Tamiami virus infection in the cotton rat. Lab Invest 1976;34: 125–140.

52. Nathanson N, Georgsson G, Palsson PA, Najjar JA, Lutley R, Petursson G. Experimental visna virus in Icelandic sheep: the prototype lentiviral infection. Rev Infect Dis 1985;7:75–82.

53. Peters CJ, Sanchez A, Rollin PE, Ksiazek TG, Murphy FA. Filoviridae: Marburg and Ebola viruses. In: Fields BN, Knipe DM, Howley PM, eds. Virology, 3rd ed. New York: Lippincott-Raven Publishers, 1996:1161–1176.

54. Petursson G, Nathanson N, Georgsson G, Panitch H, Palsson PA. Pathogenesis of visna. II. Sequential virologic, serologic, and pathologic studies. Lab Invest 1976;35:402–412.

55. Portis JL. Neurovirulent retrovirus of wild mice. In: Notkins AL, Oldstone MBA, eds. Concepts in viral pathogenesis, 3rd ed. New York: Springer-Verlag, 1989:247–252.

56. Walker DH, Camenga D, Whitfield SG, Murphy FA. Anticonvulsant prolongation of lymphocytic choriomeningitis survival. I. Ultrastructural observations on pathogenetic events. J Neuropathol Exp Neurol 1977;36:21–40.

57. Walker DH, Harrison AK, Murphy K, Flemister MR, Murphy FA. Lymphoreticular and myeloid pathogenesis of Venezuelan equine encephalitis in hamsters. Am J Pathol 1976;84:351–370.

58. Walker DH, Murphy FA, Whitfield SG, Bauer SP. Lymphocytic choriomeningitis: ultrastructural pathology. Exp Mol Pathol 1975;23: 245–265.

59. Walker DH, Wulff H, Lange JV, Murphy FA. Comparative pathology of Lassa virus infection in monkeys, guinea pigs, and Mastomys natalensis. Bull World Health Organ 1975;52:523–534.

60. Walker DH, Wulff H, Murphy FA. Experimental Lassa virus infection in the squirrel monkey. Am J Pathol 1975;80:261–278.

61. Whitfield SG, Murphy FA, Sudia WD. St. Louis encephalitis virus: an ultrastructural study of infection in a mosquito vector. Virology 1973;56:70–87.

62. Winn WC Jr, Monath TP, Murphy FA, Whitfield SG. Lassa virus hepatitis: observations on a fatal case from the 1972 Sierra Leone epidemic. Arch Pathol 1975;99:599–604.

63. Winn WC Jr, Murphy FA. Tamiami virus in mice and cotton rats. In: Arenaviral Infections of Public Health Importance. Bull World Health Organ 1975;52:501–506.

Viral Pathogenesis,
edited by Neal Nathanson, et al.
Lippincott–Raven Publishers, Philadelphia © 1997

CHAPTER 19

Methods in Viral Pathogenesis

Tissues and Organs

Ashley T. Haase

INTRODUCTION

Viral infections follow a course with discrete stages defined by critical virus-host interactions that determine outcome (see Chap. 3 and Haase[26]). In the usual course of events, viruses gain entry to their hosts, multiply at that site and spread through the bloodstream and lymphatics to reach organ systems, where further replication may cause sufficient pathologic damage to result in severe disease or death. More frequently, however, innate and specific immune defenses limit viral replication, spread, and adverse pathologic consequences to such an extent that infection is clinically inapparent or is manifest as an acute, self-limited illness. Human immunodeficiency virus (HIV) infection is an especially important contemporary example of a class of persistent and slowly progressive viral infections in which host defenses fail to eradicate virus and infected cells; after several years, acquired immunodeficiency syndrome (AIDS) ensues from the immune depletion associated with infection.[22]

The enduring questions in viral pathogenesis[26] follow from this conceptual framework: (1) In the course of viral infection, where does a virus go? (2) How does it get there? (3) If there is injury to an organ system, what is the mechanism? (4) If infection is persistent, how does the virus elude host defenses?

Experimental approaches to these questions have evolved from tracing the trail of histopathologic changes left by a virus, to quantitative assays of infectious virus in tissue culture, to modern methods of measuring viral genomes, messenger ribonucleic acids (mRNAs), and proteins.[26,66] This chapter focuses on these techniques; the succeeding chapters focus on classic and newer methods of investigation of viral pathogenesis in animal models.

PLAUSIBILITY CRITERIA IN PATHOGENESIS

The initial objective in pathogenesis studies is descriptive. The further and more fundamental objective is to understand the mechanisms that govern the infectious process, including the localization of viruses to specific cells and tissues, organ damage, oncogenesis, and persistence. Theories about pathogenetic mechanisms should generate testable hypotheses that satisfy plausibility criteria. For theories of virally induced organ damage, these can be briefly summarized as "the right number of the right cells in the right place at the right time"[26] (Table 19-1).

Many of the technologic advances in experimental viral pathogenesis have been driven by the need for greater sensitivity and sampling power to understand subtle virus-host cell interactions in persistent infections. The illustrations described in this chapter have been chosen to exemplify experimental

---

A. T. Haase: Department of Microbiology, University of Minnesota, Minneapolis, Minnesota 55455.

TABLE 19-1. *Plausibility criteria for pathogenetic mechanisms*

1. Is there evidence of viral infection in an appropriate cell type to plausibly account for the pathologic changes in an organ system?
2. Is there evidence that a sufficient number of cells (or quantity of a cell product) is involved in the infectious process?
3. Is there a plausible mechanism to relate infection to injury or death of cells?
4. Is there a plausible temporal and spatial relation between infection and organ damage?
5. For persistent viral infections in vivo, is there experimental evidence that supports an account of how immune surveillance mechanisms have been evaded?

approaches that decisively address pathogenetic mechanisms and fulfill plausibility criteria.

POPULATION VERSUS SINGLE-CELL AND WHOLE-MOUNT ASSAYS

Viral nucleic acids and proteins can be detected in material extracted from tissues (population analysis), in sections of tissues (single-cell analysis), or in whole organs or animals (whole-mount analysis) by a variety of methods. Table 19-2 summarizes for viral nucleic acids the kinds of information, advantages, and questions that can be answered with the various assays.[3,28] (Methods to isolate, detect, and characterize viral nucleic acids by hybridization, recombinant DNA techniques, and sequencing are well described by Maniatis and colleagues[39]; the polymerase chain reaction [PCR] and application of amplification methods are described by Mullis and colleagues.[44]) In general, population analyses are more suitable for fully characterizing virus and viral subcomponents, particularly in situations in which infected cells are well represented in the population. The single-cell and whole-mount assays, on the other hand, are useful if only a small fraction of the cells in a tissue are infected, which is the usual situation in vivo. The single-cell approaches are also more likely to provide the kinds of information required by the plausibility criteria set forth in Table 19-1. For these reasons, this chapter is largely devoted to methods applicable to studies of individual infected cells in vivo.

MOLECULAR ANATOMY OF VIRAL REPLICATION IN VIVO

Immunofluorescent, cytochemical, and in situ hybridization methods are the single-cell techniques that are particularly useful in determining unambiguously the number and types of infected cells, the relation of infection to histopathologic alterations in tissues, and viral gene expression in vivo. In both direct (Fig. 19-1A) and indirect (Fig. 19-1B) methods, antibody or nucleic acid probes specific for viral antigen or for nucleic acids, respectively, are reacted with their targets in a tissue section to generate a signal localized to infected cells. Cellular morphology is usually preserved, so examination of the section often reveals both the number and types of infected cells. Quantitation of the signal (see later discussion) provides an estimate of the number of copies of viral proteins, genomes, or transcripts in the cell.

RADIOACTIVE VERSUS NONRADIOACTIVE METHODS

Virus-specific antibodies or nucleic acid probes can be labeled by incorporation or attachment of radioactive or nonradioactive reporter molecules such as fluorochromes or enzymes. Bound radioactive probes are then detected by radioautography, fluorochrome-labeled probes by fluorescence, and enzyme-labeled probes by reaction with substrates that stain the cell.[9,25,35,62,67] In direct methods, the probe bears the label. In the most widely used indirect methods, the antiviral antibody or nucleic acid bound to its target is recognized by a second antibody or avidin, which is labeled. Alternatively, a third molecule carries the reporter label (see Fig. 19-1B). Currently, both direct and indirect methods, using either radioactive or nonradioactive labels, detect and localize viral components with good sensitivity and morphologic resolution. The nonradioactive methods often excel at localization. For optimal sensitivity, ^{35}S-labeled probes are widely used because of their high specific activity and efficiency in forming silver grains in radioautographic emulsion, which makes it possible to detect a few copies of viral genomes or transcripts in cells with reasonable resolution (signal localized within a few microns of its source).[28]

Quantitative assays for viral antigens in single cells have also been developed, based on similar principles. Antigen content can be estimated in immunocytochemically stained cells by computer-assisted microdensitometry[68]; or, more simply, tissue sections are reacted sequentially with primary antibody, biotinylated secondary antibody, and ^{35}S-labeled streptavidin. After emulsion radioautography, silver grains are enumerated and related to antigen concentration by comparison with the signal generated by a known number of viral particles adsorbed to the cell or produced at different stages of the viral life cycle.[10]

QUANTITATION AND RESTRICTED VIRAL GENE EXPRESSION IN PERSISTENT INFECTION

The relative abundance of viral genomes (DNA or RNA) and mRNAs can be estimated semiquantitatively by densito-

TABLE 19-2. *Comparison of population, single-cell, and whole-mount assays for viral nucleic acids*

Category	Assay	Information	Comment
Population	Hybridization (dot, Southern, and Northern blots)	Detection	Limits of detection (<1 pg) insufficient to study infection if only a small fraction of the cells in a tissue are infected and contain only a few copies of viral nucleic acid per cell.
	Cloning and sequencing	Characterization Size Conformation Replicative form Integration Restriction map Sequences Transcript class	Main advantage of population assays. Provides information on the size, state and nature of viral DNA and RNA (e.g., whether DNA is extrachromosomal or integrated, contains mutations or deletions, size and nature of transcripts (e.g., spliced or unspliced).
	Polymerase chain reaction		Increases sensitivity by several orders of magnitude.
Isolated populations	Separation of cells by type (e.g., fluorescence-activated cell sorter to separate CD4+ lymphocytes from peripheral blood mononuclear cells		Bridging technology that provides information on the number and type of infected cells. Limitation is the extent to which a cell type can be purified free of contaminants.
Single cell	In situ hybridization	Detection	Detects viral genomes and transcripts in the range of a few copies per cell of a 2–10 kb target in small numbers of cells in tissues.
		Quantitation	Provides estimates of the number of infected cells in tissues and the levels of viral gene expression.
		Characterization Replicative forms Genomes Transcript	Distinguishes viral DNA and RNA, ss and ds classes, expression of specific genes, unspliced and spliced mRNAs.
		Tissue distribution	Main advantage: spatial distribution of infected cells vis-a-vis pathologic changes provides insight into mechanisms of lesion formation.
	In situ hybridization coupled to immunocytochemical demonstration of viral or cellular antigens	Identify types of infected cells	Unequivocal definition of viral tropisms; host range and reservoirs; extent of infection vis-a-vis pathologic changes in tissues or organ system.
		Colocalize viral and host genes and gene products	Relation of viral gene expression to cellular factors and number.
	In situ polymerase chain reaction	Detection of viral and host nucleic acids in individual cells	Sensitivity increased to detection of single copies of viral genomes in individual cells.
			Possible to estimate the number of infected cells vis-a-vis pathologic change, size of reservoir of infected cells in tissues and organ systems.
		Characterization Viral genomes Transcripts	Can investigate viral replication in vivo in individual cells with low levels of viral nucleic acids.
			Detection of viral and host transcripts expressed at low levels provides insight into relation between infection to expression of host genes.
		Tissue distribution	Increased sampling power.
Whole animal or whole organ	Whole animal or whole organ sections	Detection Characterization	Distribution of infected cells in whole animal or organ.
		Determination of tissue distribution of viral genomes, viral and host transcripts in whole animal or organ	Determination of viral tropisms, spread, reservoirs, clearance.
	Macroscopic-microscopic Hybridization topography		Adds single cell resolution.

Direct Methods for Detection of Viral Nucleic Acids and Proteins in Cells and Tissues

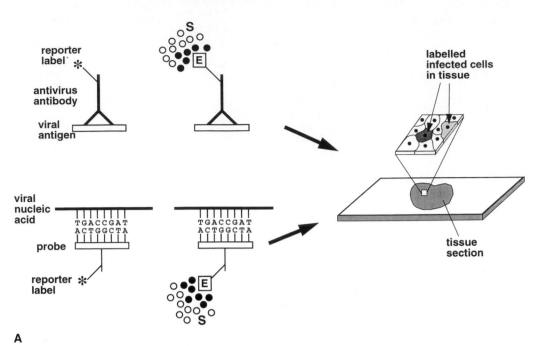

Indirect Methods for Detection of Viral Nucleic Acids and Proteins in Cells and Tissues

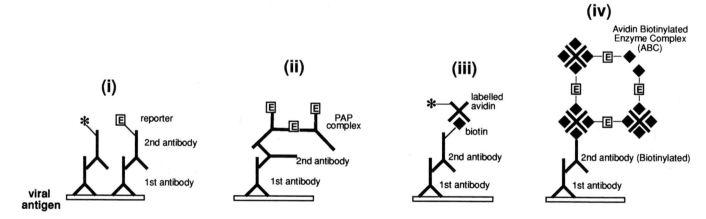

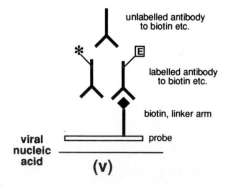

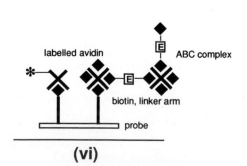

B

FIG. 19-1.

metric scanning of immunocytochemical reactions or radioautographs.[37,68] With radioactive probes, the relative number of copies of viral nucleic acid in a cell can be measured more precisely by enumeration of silver grains within a cell in the developed radioautograph.[28] The grain count can be converted to copy number by calculations based on the specific activity of the probe, efficiency of hybridization and formation of silver grains, and exposure time. This conversion can be validated over a range of copy numbers by independent measurement of copy numbers in a population of infected cells and the average number of silver grains in individual cells in the population, as shown in Figure 19-2.

Quantitative approaches to analysis of viral gene expression in cells in tissues were first developed in studies of the mechanisms of persistence of visna virus, a retrovirus in the subfamily of lentiviruses that cause slow and persistent infection in animals, including primates and humans (e.g., HIV).[27] Comparison of the abundance of viral RNA (as a measure of gene expression) in cells in culture, where infection is productive (Fig. 19-3A), with gene expression in infected cells in the nervous systems of sheep (Fig. 19-3B) demonstrated lower levels of gene expression in vivo (Fig. 19-3C).[7]{FIG3} The restriction in lentiviral gene expression in vivo is evidence in support of the hypothesis that cells infected with lentiviruses escape detection and destruction by immune surveillance because of constraints on viral gene expression.[27]

USE OF POLYMERASE CHAIN REACTION TO ASSESS VIRAL LATENCY, HOST RANGE, AND GENE EXPRESSION AT LOW LEVELS

In the experiments just described, in situ hybridization was sufficiently sensitive to identify infected cells with low levels of viral gene expression. However, truly latently infected cells (operationally defined as those with a single copy of the viral genome [provirus] and no detectable viral RNA) cannot be assessed because the limit of detection of proviruses by in situ hybridization (10 kb) is about two copies per cell. The development and application of in situ amplification methods based on PCR[44] is the subject of this and the following section on double-label methods.

With in situ PCR[2,11,19,31,36,38,48,49,50,53,57] the individual cell is used as its own reaction vessel (Fig. 19-4A). PCR reagents and primers are added to fixed and permeabilized cells, and then the cells in suspension or on slides are cycled (Fig. 19-4B). In direct in situ PCR, biotin- or digoxygenin-labeled nucleotides are incorporated and detected at the conclusion of the amplification cycles by immunocytochemistry. With indirect in situ PCR, the products are detected by in situ hybridization. The success of all of the current methods is dependent on finding the right set of conditions to amplify and retain products in the cell (Fig. 19-4C), by optimizing conditions for fixation and

(text continues on page 474)

FIG. 19-1. **(A)** Direct methods for detection of viral nucleic acids and proteins in cells in tissue sections employ probes to which labels have been attached or incorporated. The reporter molecules may be radioactive or nonradioactive labels (*) such as fluorescein, or enzymes (E) such as alkaline phosphatase or horseradish peroxidase. The probes are antibodies to viral antigens, or they are cDNA, cRNA, or oligonucleotide probes with sequences complementary to the viral target. The cellular localization of the target is revealed by immunofluorescence, by radioautography, or by immunocytochemistry after addition of substrate, S (*open circles*), which is converted to a colored product (*filled circles*). Details of the methods for isolation and labeling of monoclonal antibodies, cloning of nucleic acid probes, and synthesis of oligonucleotide probes are described elsewhere.[39,62] Probes for in situ hybridization can be labeled with [35S], [3H], [125I], [32P], or [32P] by incorporation of precursors into double-stranded DNA by nick translation or random priming or into single-stranded cRNA riboprobes.[8,25,29,35,70] Oligonucleotide probes can be labeled by incorporation of radioactive precursors into homopolymeric or heteropolymeric tails with terminal transferase.[69] Enzymes are incorporated into the probes through reactions with modified bases. For example, during automated synthesis of an oligonucleotide probe, a modified base with a linker arm and terminal primary amino group is introduced. Subsequent reaction with a bifunctional reagent crosslinks the base to alkaline phosphatase.[35]

(B) In indirect methods of detection of viral antigens, antibody to the antigen may be detected by several means: (i) a second antibody is used that carries a radioactive or nonradioactive label (*) such as fluorescein, or an enzyme (E); (ii) a second antibody is used that also binds a peroxidase-antiperoxidase (PAP) complex; (iii) in detection systems based on avidin or streptavidin, the second antibody is biotinylated and the avidin is labeled; or (iv) the avidin is complexed with biotin and enzyme (ABC). In indirect methods for detection of viral nucleic acids, the probe is labeled with digoxygenin or biotin, and the signal is generated by reacting the probe with labeled antibody to biotin or digoxygenin (v) or with labeled avidin or ABC complex (vi). Further amplification can be achieved with unlabeled antibody to biotin and the indirect methods shown (i through iv). Digoxygenin or biotin with linker arms can be incorporated into probes as described for radioactive labeling with the use of digoxygenin-dUTP or biotin-dUTP. Biotin can also be linked to probes by irradiation with strong light of the probe and photobiotin, which has a photoactivatable group bound to biotin through a linker arm. The secondary reagents such as those used in the ABC system are available commercially. (Modified from Kiyama H, Emson PC, Tohyama M. Recent progress in the use of the technique of non-radioactive in situ hybridization histochemistry: new tools for molecular neurobiology. Neurosci Res 1990;9:1–21.)

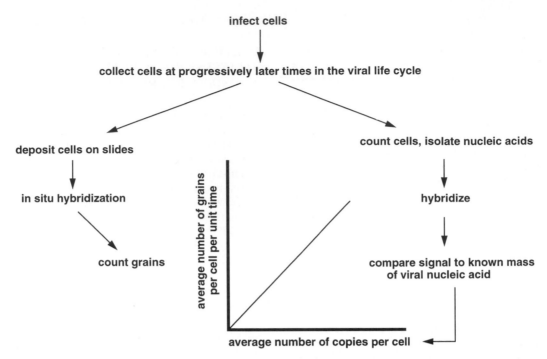

FIG. 19-2. Quantitative in situ hybridization involves determination of the relation between the number of silver grains per cell and the number of copies per cell of viral nucleic acid. Cells are infected at a high multiplicity of infection to ensure uniform infection. As the life cycle progresses, and viral genomes are reproduced and mRNAs are synthesized, aliquots of the culture are removed. The cells are counted, and DNA and RNA are isolated from one portion of the aliquot; the remaining cells are deposited on slides and hybridized in situ to detect viral DNA or RNA. After hybridization and radioautography, the average number of silver grains per cell (minus background in uninfected cultures) is determined and expressed per unit of time of exposure (usually min^{-1}). The nucleic acids isolated from the known number of cells in the population are hybridized, usually by a solid-phase procedure (e.g., dot-blot, Northern blot), to a labeled, virus-specific probe. The signal generated is measured densitometrically and compared with known masses of cloned viral nucleic acids. From this comparison, the average copy number of viral DNA or RNA per cell can be ascertained. This number is plotted against average grain count and used to convert grain counts to copy numbers in infected cells in tissue sections and cultures. (From Haase AT. Analysis of viral infections by in situ hybridization. In: Valentino K, Roberts J, Barchas J, eds. In situ hybridization: applications to neurobiology. Fairlawn, NJ: Oxford University Press, 1987:197–219.)

FIG. 19-3. Viral gene expression in productive infections in vitro and in persistent infections in vivo. **(A)** Viral gene expression in vitro. Quantitative in situ hybridization for viral DNA and RNA was developed originally[7] for studies of the pathogenesis of slow infections caused by visna virus, a retrovirus in the subfamily of lentiviruses. In permissive cultured cells infected at a multiplicity of infection (moi) of 3, 30 to 50 copies of viral RNA are introduced into each cell. Reverse transcription and superinfection produce 200 to 300 copies of primarily extrachromosomal DNA and about 5000 copies of viral RNA per cell by the end of the lentiviral life cycle. This tissue culture system is particularly well suited to determine the relation of silver grains to copy numbers over a wide range of concentrations of viral DNA or viral RNA. Some representative microscopic fields are shown: infected cells with a few copies of viral DNA 3 hours after infection and with 30 copies at 30 hours, and infected cells with a few copies of viral RNA 7 hours after infection and more than 1000 copies at 30 hours. The radioautographic exposure before development for the 3- and 30-hour time points were 13 and 8 days, respectively, for DNA; for RNA, the exposure times were 6 days for the 7-hour and 1 day for the 30-hour time point. (From Haase AT. Analysis of viral infections by in situ hybridization. In: Valentino K, Roberts J, Barchas J, eds. In situ hybridization: applications to neurobiology. Fairlawn, NJ: Oxford University Press, 1987:197–219.)

(B) Viral gene expression in vivo. In the nervous systems of chronically infected sheep, the level of viral gene expression is reduced compared with infection in vitro. Arrows point to three cells with visna virus RNA adjoining a blood vessel (bv) with a perivascular cuff (pvc) of inflammatory cells. The 50 copies of viral RNA estimated to be present per cell is one to two orders of magnitude less than the average copy number in a productively infected cell in culture.

(C) A comparison of gene expression in vitro and in vivo. The left panel depicts frequency distributions of viral RNA copy number in infected cells in culture; the right panel is an averaged distribution of infected cells in the brains of three persistently infected sheep. (Modified from Brahic M, Stowring L, Ventura P, Haase AT. Gene expression in visna virus infection in sheep. Nature 1981;292:240–242.)

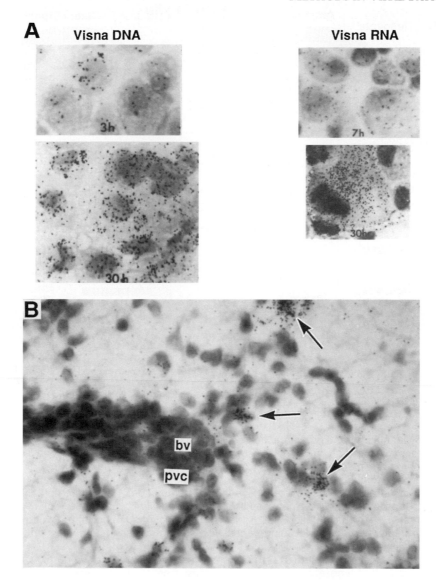

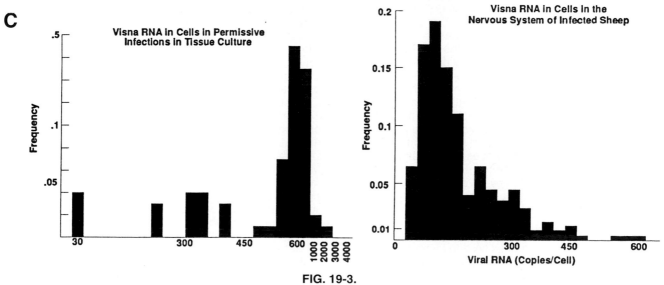

FIG. 19-3.

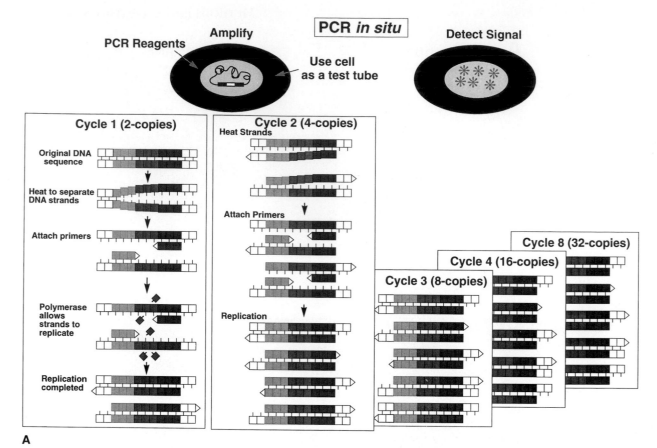

FIG. 19-4. In situ polymerase chain reaction (PCR). (**A**) Principles of the method. The cell is used as a reaction vessel to amplify target sequences, illustrated here as a single copy of a provirus such as the human immunodeficiency virus (▭) integrated into the DNA of the cell (🧬). The exponential increase in target is shown through eight cycles of denaturation, annealing of primers (▭▷), and extension and incorporation of nucleotides (▬); the different shades from white to black represent the bases A, G, C, and T, and the lines between the primers and DNA represent template pairing of complementary bases. After amplification, the products are detected (*) either directly or indirectly, as described in **B**. (Modified from Amplification of nucleic acid sequences: the choices multiply. J NIH Res 1991;3(2):81–94.)

(**B**) Procedures. In situ PCR methods are currently in a state of active development, but most of the protocols in use at this time are depicted in the figure. Target nucleic acid sequences have been amplified in suspended cells,[2,31,57] in cells deposited on slides cut to fit thermocycling tubes,[33] and in sections of frozen tissues[33] or tissues fixed in aldehyde or nonaldehyde fixatives and adhered to slides.[19,36,38,48,61] In most cases, the specimens are permeabilized by proteolytic digestion or detergents before addition of the PCR reaction mixture. In direct in situ PCR, and in situ PCR in which product retention probably depends on ballasting (see **C**), biotin or digoxygenin oligonucleotides are used in the reaction. To prevent evaporation during thermocycling, either the cells and reaction mix under a coverslip are covered with mineral oil, or the reaction mix is sealed (e.g., with nail polish). After thermocycling, the cells or sections are washed, the cells are deposited on slides if they were in suspension, and the amplified products are detected either directly or indirectly by in situ hybridization with radioactive or nonradioactive probes. Direct detection methods may be subject to higher backgrounds and artifacts.[38] It is essential to provide controls, for example by omitting primers or enzyme or by hybridizing probes to a nonamplified region or a different virus. To detect viral RNA genomes or viral or host messenger RNAs with increased sensitivity by amplification, the RNA is converted to complementary DNA by reverse transcription (RT) before amplification. An immunocytochemical step to mark cells by type or colocalize a viral or host gene product may also precede or follow amplification.

(**C**) Strategies. The success of in situ PCR depends on optimizing conditions to amplify and retain products in individual cells. In addition to optimizing fixation, permeabilization, and reaction conditions,[19,48] two general strategies have been employed to satisfy the antithetical requirements of in situ PCR, in which amplification in the fixed cell is most efficient for small products but retention increases with product size. One solution is to create larger products from smaller ones[11,31] (overlapping products). In the first cycles of amplification, the products of multiple primers (*filled rectangles, open circles*) are short but can anneal (*short vertical lines*) at the overlapping ends to generate transiently larger products that are retained. In later cycles, after the primers are exhausted, the intermediate products are used as primers. Elongation and displacement synthesis yields long, covalently-linked products. In the ballasted product strategy, incorporation of bulky groups into short products decreases diffusion of the products. (Modified from Haase AT, Retzel EF, Staskus KA. Amplification and detection of lentiviral DNA inside cells. Proc Natl Acad Sci U S A 1990;87:4971–4975.)

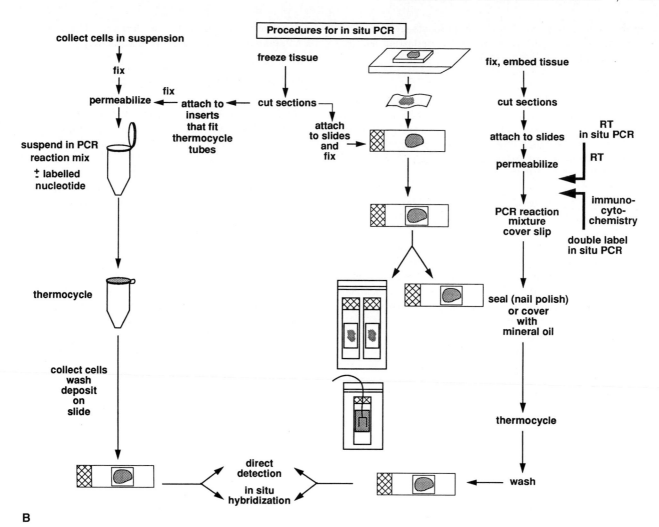

In Situ PCR: Strategies to Efficiently Amplify and Retain Products

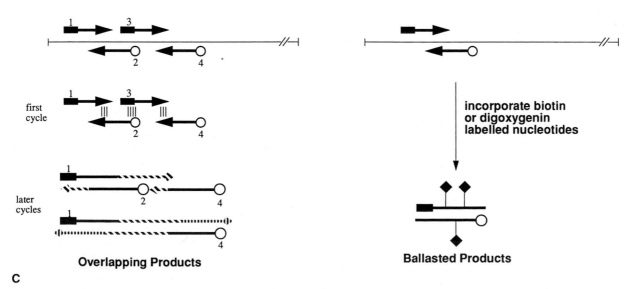

FIG. 19-4. *Continued.*

permeabilization; on generating larger products from smaller ones in the course of the reaction; or on ballasting shorter products with biotin or digoxygenin.

The in situ PCR technique was originally developed and applied in investigations of the persistence of visna virus.[31,61] These studies provided the first direct experimental proof of a reservoir of latently infected cells[61] and established bronchiolar epithelium as the cell type infected by visna virus (Fig. 19-5). In situ PCR has now provided direct evidence of latency in HIV infections, as well as an extended host range,[2,20,21,54,57] described in more detail in the section on double-label methods. Latent herpes simplex virus also has been shown by in situ PCR to reside in a variety of previously unrecognized host cells.[42]

By coupling in situ PCR to reverse transcription, it is now possible to detect RNA viruses or viral or host mRNAs even if the concentration of RNA in the cell is too low to be detected by conventional in situ hybridization.[19,33,52] Furthermore, expression of a host gene held to be responsible for tissue damage can now be detected in the region of injury with much greater confidence. Tumor necrosis factor-α (TNF-α), for example, has been hypothesized to play a role in the neuropathology of HIV infection, and accordingly the number and location of cells expressing TNF-α should be correlated with anatomic regions of infection and encephalitis. The low abundancy of transcripts and the problems of tissue preservation and fixation make this a difficult question to address with standard in situ hybridization methods. With reverse transcription PCR in situ, TNF mRNA has been demonstrated in microglial cells in the nervous system in the predicted spatial relation to infection and inflammation.[51]

In situ PCR can also be preceded or followed by immunocytochemistry with reagents that identify cells by type or colocalize viral and host gene products. These double-label techniques are described in the next section.

DOUBLE-LABEL TECHNIQUES

Plausibility criteria for pathogenetic mechanisms require evidence that a sufficient number of cells of a particular type in a particular anatomic location are infected to account for the pathology. It is often possible to satisfy this criterion by detecting signal in cells recognizable by their morphology,[25,29] but in other instances morphology alone does not suffice to identify unambiguously which cell types have been infected. Double-label techniques, which couple the sensitivity of in situ detection of nucleic acids with immunocytochemical marking of cells or gene products, were devised to solve this problem.

As originally described,[6] immunocytochemistry with peroxidase-specific antibodies and diaminobenzidene (DAB) as substrate deposited an insoluble product at cellular sites of accumulation of a viral protein. The DAB precipitate was shown to withstand the subsequent in situ hybridization with a radioactive virus probe so that, in the developed radioautographs, viral RNA and protein could be analyzed simultaneously in brown-stained cells with large numbers of silver grains.

Ensuing developments[5,9,23,32,46,47,55,65] of diverse methods to simultaneously detect two or more genomes, genes, or gene products in individual cells or to identify viral nucleic acids in specific cell types are summarized in Fig. 19-6. These double-label methods have been used to investigate the pathogenesis of a number of chronic viral infections—for example, the persistent infection of the central nervous system (CNS) by a murine picornavirus, Theiler's murine encephalomyelitis virus

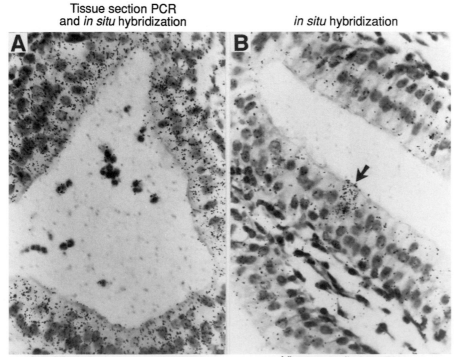

Tissue section PCR and *in situ* hybridization

A

Amplified visna-maedi virus DNA in bronchiolar epithelium

***in situ* hybridization**

B

Visna-maedi virus RNA in bronchiolar epithelium

FIG. 19-5. (**A**) Photograph of the developed radioautograph after in situ PCR and hybridization demonstrating maedi/visna virus in bronchiolar epithelial cells in the lung of an infected sheep. The cells probably harbor only a single copy of viral DNA, because no signal was detectable by conventional in situ hybridization. (**B**) With in situ PCR, the large number of black silver grains over the cells provide direct visual evidence of infection. In subjacent sections, only a rare cell (*arrow*) contains viral RNA, experimental proof of the transcriptionally silent nature of infection. (From Staskus KA, Couch L, Bitterman P, et al. In situ amplification of visna virus DNA in tissue sections reveals a reservoir of latently infected cells. Microb Pathog 1991;11:67–76.)

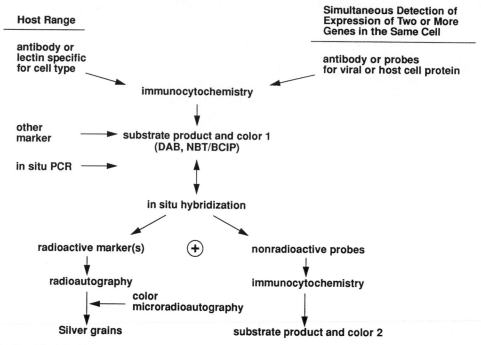

FIG. 19-6. Double-label immunocytochemistry and in situ hybridization procedures. To detect expression of two genes in the same cell, one gene product can be detected by immunocytochemistry and the other by in situ hybridization with a radioactive probe and radioautography. After development, a brown (diaminobenzidine [DAB]) or blue (nitroblue tetrazolium chloride/bromochloroindolyl phosphate, [NBT/BCIP]) stain identifies one gene product and silver grains identify the other. Expression of two genes can also be detected with a nonradioactive probe by using peroxidase and alkaline phosphatase and the two substrates in the antibody and hybridization steps.[7,23,43,63] Alternatively, two different RNAs (e.g., viral genomes) can be detected in the same cell with probes labeled with ^{3}H and ^{35}S and differentiated by color microradioautography in a two-layer emulsion in which only the ^{35}S decay is recorded in the upper layer.[32] Radioactive and nonradioactive probes can also be combined ($\oplus$) to simultaneously detect the following combinations: two genomes or expression of two or three genes (e.g., two mRNAs in the same cell) with probes labeled with biotin or digoxygenin and ^{35}S[55]; two viral DNAs in the same cell (e.g., herpes simplex and human papillomavirus or cytomegalovirus) with biotinylated and haptenized (acetylaminofluorine, digoxygenin) probes[43]; two mRNAs and one protein with a radioactive and two nonradioactive probes labeled with peroxidase and alkaline phosphatase[65]; or three fluorescent labels on three probes derivatized with three haptens.[46] The order of the steps can also be reversed ⇕, with in situ hybridization and radioautography performed first. After development, in a second hybridization step, a biotinylated oligonucleotide probe penetrates a permeabilized emulsion and is detected by immunocytochemistry.[9,47] For very stable antigens, the immunocytochemical step can also follow in situ hybridization with a radioactive probe and radioautography.[5] For studies of host range, antibodies or lectins specific for cell type and immunocytochemistry are used to mark the cell before detection of viral genomes, genes, or proteins as described for simultaneous detection of two or more genes. Other insoluble markers may be used to identify cell type (e.g., ferritin for activated microglia[71]). In situ PCR can also be used to amplify target sequences in marked cells.[21,51,57]

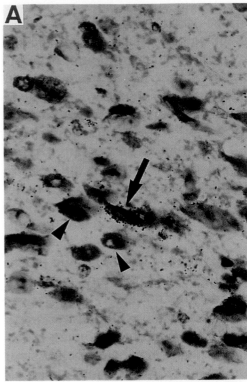

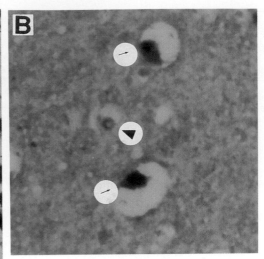

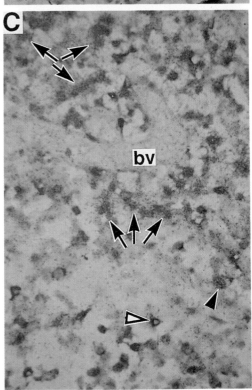

FIG. 19-7. Double-label in situ techniques, viral host range, and extent of infection of cell subsets. (**A**) Theiler's murine encephalomyelitis virus (TMEV). The arrow points to an infected, brown-stained oligodendrocyte with large numbers of silver grains indicating viral RNA; arrowheads point to uninfected oligodendrocytes with few grains. (Modified from Aubert C, Chamorro M, Brahic M. Identification of Theiler's virus infected cells in the central nervous system of the mouse during demyelinating disease. Microb Pathog 1987;3:319–326.) (**B**) Human immunodeficiency virus (HIV). After in situ polymerase chain reaction (PCR), HIV DNA was detected by immunocytochemistry with nitroblue tetrazolium chloride/bromochloroindolyl phosphate (NBT/BCIP) as substrate; the nuclei of positive cells are blue. Antibodies to neuron-specific enolase and immunocytochemistry, with fast red as chromogen, stains neurons red and reveals evidence of infection in neurons (*small arrows*) but not oligodendrocytes. Large arrowhead points to a cell with the small halo and scant cytoplasm typical of oligodendrocytes. (Modified from Nuovo GJ, Gallery F, MacConnell P, Braun A. In situ detection of polymerase chain reaction–amplified HIV-1 nucleic acids and tumor necrosis factor-α RNA in the central nervous system. Am J Pathol 1994;144:659–666.) (**C**) HIV DNA in CD4+ lymphocytes in lymphoid tissue has been identified by in situ PCR, after immunocytochemistry with antibodies that use diaminobenzidine (DAB) as substrate and stain the CD4+ subset of T lymphocytes brown. In the developed radioautograph, epipolarized illumination imparts a greenish hue to the silver grains over the nuclei of cells with HIV DNA. A brown-stained cell with greenish nucleus indicates infection of a CD4+ cell. The large number of infected CD4+ lymphocytes identified in this way and evident in the figure reflect the scope of infection and size of the viral reservoir at early stages of HIV infection. Arrows point to CD4+ T cells containing HIV DNA; the solid arrowhead indicates single HIV DNA + cell, and the open arrowhead indicates single HIV DNA − cell. bv, blood vessel.(Modified from Embretson J, Zupancic M, Ribas JL, et al. Massive covert infection of helper T lymphocytes and macrophages by HIV during the incubation period of AIDS. Nature 1993;362:359–362.)

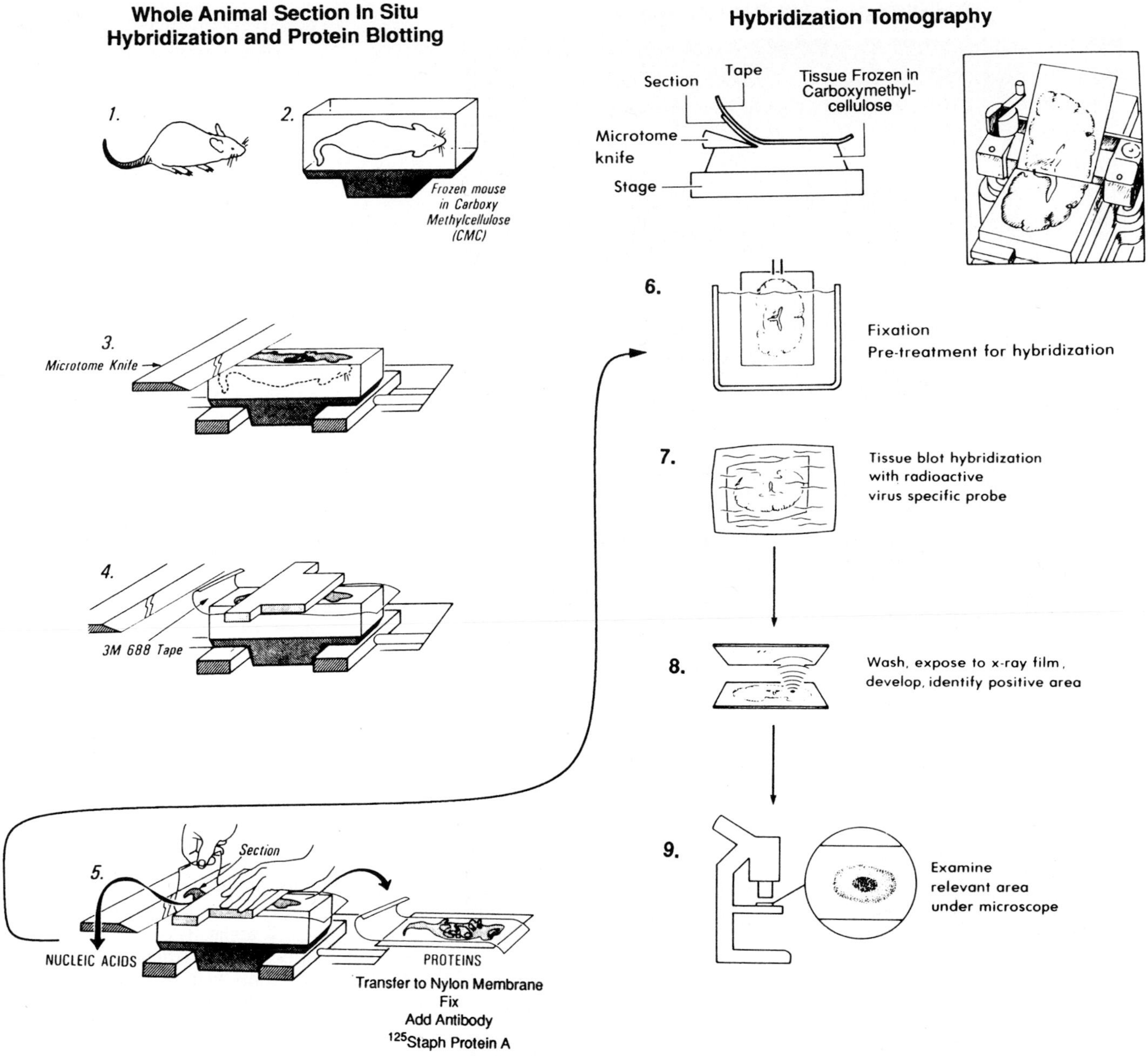

Whole Animal Section In Situ Hybridization and Protein Blotting

Hybridization Tomography

FIG. 19-8. Major steps and principles of whole-animal and organ methods to detect and quantitate viral or host cell nucleic acids and proteins. Whole organs or animals are frozen in carboxymethylcellulose, and sections are cut and transferred to tape (steps 1 through 5). For nucleic acid detection, the sections are air-dried, fixed, and pretreated for hybridization with specific probes labeled with ^{32}P or with ^{125}I and ^{35}S (steps 6 and 7). After washing and film radioautography, the developed film reveals the anatomic location of cells with the nucleic acid (step 8). For single-cell resolution, the tissue blot is coated with emulsion, exposed, and developed. The positive area identified by film radioautography is used as a guide to the area to examine microscopically (step 9). For proteins, after transfer to nylon membrane, fixation, and sequential addition of blocking buffers, antibody and ^{125}I-labeled staphylococcal protein A, the membrane is washed and exposed to film. The quantitative distribution of viral antigen is determined by laser scanning densitometry of the radioautograph. (see Fig. 19-9A). (Modified from Haase AT, Gantz D, Blum H, et al. Combined macroscopic and microscopic detection of viral genes in tissues. Virology 1985;140:201–206, and Lipkin WI, Villarreal LP, Oldstone MBA. Whole animal section in situ hybridization and protein blotting: new tools in molecular analysis of animal models for human disease. Curr Top Microbiol Immunol 1989;143:33–54.)

Quantification of LCMV Antigens

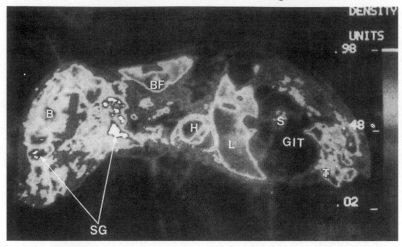

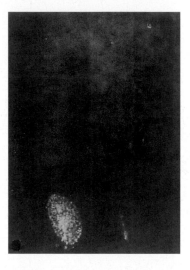

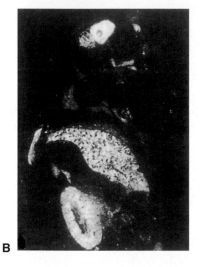

LCMV
persistent
infection

transfer immune cells →

Clearance

GSHV   RV   LCMV

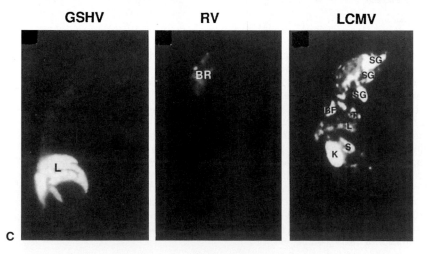

FIG. 19-9. Quantitative assessment of viral nucleic acids in studies of viral persistence, clearance, and host range. (**A**) The distribution of lymphocytic choriomeningitis virus (LCMV) antigen in a persistently infected mouse. B, brain; BF, brown fat; GIT, gastrointestinal tract; H, heart; L, liver; S, spleen; SG, salivary glands; T, testis. The relative concentration of antigen was determined by densitometry (scale at right), with white representing the highest concentration. (**B**) Two months after adaptive transfer of LCMV immune splenocytes, there is extensive clearing of LCMV in many organ systems, with residual antigens in the kidney and central nervous system. (**C**) Distribution of viral nucleic acids of ground squirrel hepatitis virus (GSHV), rabies virus (RV), and LCMV. The highest concentrations of GSHV and RV RNA are found in liver (L) and brain (BR), respectively, in contrast to the multiple-organ distribution of LCMV. BF, brown fat; K, kidney; L, liver; S, spleen; SG, salivary gland; T, testis. (From Lipkin WI, Villarreal LP, Oldstone MBA. Whole animal section in situ hybridization and protein blotting: new tools in molecular analysis of animal models for human disease. Curr Top Microbiol Immunol 1989;143:33–54.)

(TMEV). Infection by some strains of TMEV leads to paralysis as a consequence of primary demyelination. TMEV has been shown to infect oligodendrocytes, the cells that provide the myelin sheaths of nerves in the CNS, by a method that identifies these cells with antibodies to an oligodendrocyte-specific antigen and infected cells by in situ hybridization with a radioactive virus-specific probe[1] (Fig. 19-7). Infection also affects myelin metabolism, as shown by double-label studies of proteolipid mRNA levels in uninfected and infected cells, identified by detection of viral antigens by immunocytochemistry.[56] Similarly, double-label methods have been used to investigate the host range and state of viral gene expression of lentiviruses,[63,71] herpetic viruses,[24,41] and hepatitis B virus.[4]

The combination of in situ PCR with in situ hybridization and immunocytochemistry is illustrated in Figures 19-7B and 19-7C. This powerful approach has provided new insight into the host range of HIV and possible mechanisms of persistence, immune depletion, and neurologic disease. The discovery of a large reservoir of CD4+ lymphocytes with HIV DNA but little if any detectable RNA[21] again suggests that HIV, like animal lentiviruses,[27] eludes host defenses by establishing covert infections. At the same time, the large number of infected CD4+ lymphocytes with the potentials for activation of viral gene expression and elimination by host defenses or other mechanisms is consistent with immune depletion related to infection. In a straightforward way, this observation satisfies the plausibility criterion for disease causation, by infection of an appropriate number of an appropriate type of cells. The discovery, with these methods, of increasing numbers of infected cells in the CNS in later stages of infection, in concert with increasing pathologic changes and neurologic disease, also satisfies the criterion on extent of infection; and the identification

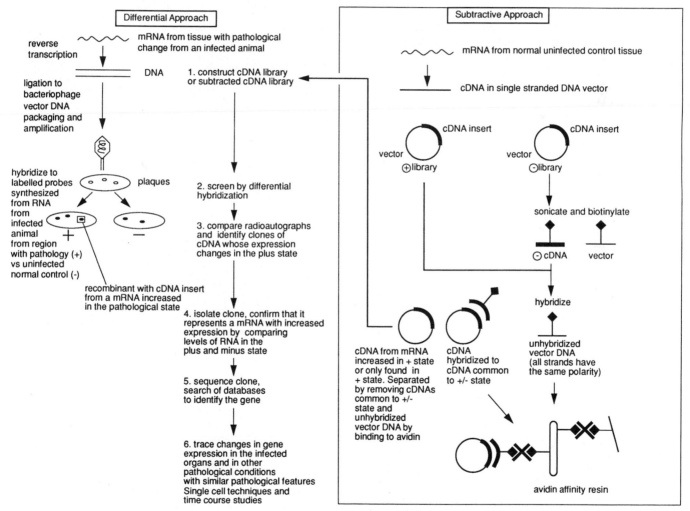

Fig. 19-10. Plus-minus differential and subtractive hybridization screening of cDNA libraries to identify modulated genes. The representation of low-abundancy mRNAs in the libraries can be increased by subtractive approaches, as shown in the inset. After subtractive hybridization, the single-stranded DNA in the vector with cDNAs enriched in the positive (+) state is converted to double-stranded DNA and used to transform *Escherichia coli* to generate the subtracted library, which is screened differentially. Steps 3 through 6 are the same for both approaches. With undefined RNAs that can be obtained only in small amounts, the polymerase chain reaction can be used to amplify the cDNAs for cloning. (Modified from Diedrich J, Wietgrefe S, Haase A, Duguid J, Carp RI. Identifying and mapping changes in gene expression involved in the neuropathology of scrapie and Alzheimer's disease. Curr Top Microbiol Immunol 1991;172:259–274.)

of HIV in neurons extends the host range of the virus to a cell type whose injury could clearly account for the pathologic changes and dysfunction that have been described.[51]

WHOLE-ANIMAL AND ORGAN METHODS

Whole-mount techniques[17,30,37] carry forward the themes of how to determine viral tropism, extent of infection and virus spread, and clearance, but from a broader perspective with greater sampling power. This approach improves the chance of finding small foci of infected cells that are sparsely distributed in tissues. If film and emulsion radioautography are combined to identify the foci of infected cells and the cells are then examined by light microscopy, the greater sampling power of this approach is achieved at single-cell resolution.[30]

The major steps, principles, and some applications of these methods are illustrated in Figures 19-8 and 19-9. By mapping and quantification of the location of viral genes and proteins, the course of infection can be followed and the response to experimental manipulation determined.[37] For example, in persistent lymphocytic choriomeningitis virus infection, adaptive transfer of immune cells clears virus from many organ systems, with residual virus in the kidney, in immune complexes, and in the CNS, where it is cleared more slowly without evidence of inflammation or neuronal injury. It may be that neurons express so little class I major histocompatibility complex products that cytotoxic T lymphocytes cannot recognize infected neurons. As shown in Figure 19-9C, whole-mount techniques also provide a visually compelling overview of the organ tropisms of DNA and RNA viruses.

DIFFERENTIAL AND SUBSTANTIVE HYBRIDIZATION

How can new hypotheses be formulated to explain pathogenetic processes without the requirement for prior incrimination of a particular molecule or process? One approach is to find, by plus-minus hybridization screening, genes whose expression is modulated in the pathologic state. After sequencing is done to identify a candidate gene, a change in its expression can be mapped to determine whether that change bears a plausible temporal and spatial relation to the pathologic lesions (Fig. 19-10). Finally, if two pathologic conditions share common features, the second condition can be examined for changes in expression of the newly identified genes as part of a search for convergent pathologic mechanisms.[16,18]

As an example, scrapie, a transmissible disease caused by unconventional agents called prions (see Chap. 37), and the human neurodegenerative dementing disorder called Alzheimer's disease (AD) share pathologic features such as astrogliosis and the deposition of amyloid proteins in the CNS. Investigation of scrapie by the plus-minus hybridization approach revealed that activation of a number of genes in the neuropathologic lesions followed closely on the formation of amyloid protein, the abnormal isoform of the prion protein (PrPSc). Both PrPSc accumulation and gene modification were expressed in activated astrocytes in areas of the brain in which the neuropathologic changes were most extensive.[13–15]

Among the modulated genes that have been identified in scrapie are several that may represent a programmed response

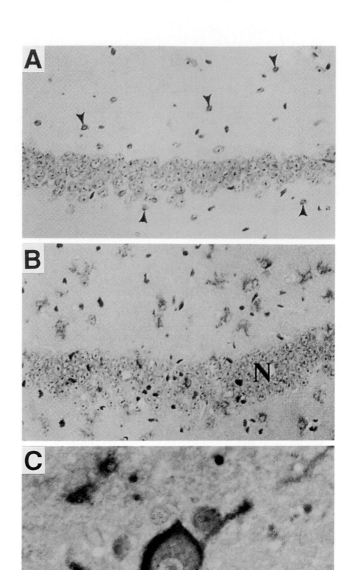

FIG. 19-11. Increased expression of apolipoprotein E (apoE) in astrocytes and around neurons in scrapie and Alzheimer's disease (AD). ApoE was identified by plus-minus hybridization screening and comparative sequence analysis as a gene whose expression is modulated in scrapie infection. To map the altered pattern of expression, sections of hippocampus from uninfected control mice (**A**) or scrapie-infected animals (**B**), or sections of cerebral cortex from an AD patient (**C**), were reacted with antibody to apoE, and antibody-antigen complexes were identified immunocytochemically. Most of the cells in the infected animals with increased expression of apoE are astrocytes (indicated by *arrowheads* in **A** for control animals) on either side of a layer of neurons (N). In AD, apoE also increases. The figure shows accumulation of apoE protein around the cell body of a neuron and in association with neuronal processes (**C**). (Modified from Diedrich JF, Minnigan M, Carp RI, et al. Neuropathological changes in scrapie and Alzheimer's disease are associated with increased expression of apolipoprotein E and cathepsin D in astrocytes. J Virol 1991;65:4759–4768.)

to neuronal injury induced by amyloid. Chaperonins (hsp70 and ab crystallin), proteases (cathepsin D), and glial fibrillary acidic protein may be induced, respectively, to renature, digest, and transport the abnormal proteins.[13–18] Neuronal growth factors such as transferrin are also upregulated, and apolipoprotein E (apoE) increases (see Fig. 19-11), possibly to function in lipid transport and membrane transport, as it does in peripheral nerve injury and regeneration.[34]

Similar approaches in AD, undertaken to identify molecules involved in the pathologic process and to discover convergent pathogenetic mechanisms, have shown increased expression of many of the same astrocyte genes, including that for apoE, in both AD and scrapie.[15] The association of apoE with neuronal processes is consistent with a role in maintaining membrane homeostasis or with the recent hypothesis that interactions of isoforms of apoE with the β amyloid protein of AD may be critical determinants of solubility or aggregation.[12,40,45,58–60,64] In any case, the independent identification of the potential importance of apoE in amyloidogenic processes illustrates the power of the plus-minus hybridization approach in pointing to potentially important roles of unsuspected molecules and processes in pathologic conditions.

SUMMARY AND CONCLUSIONS

The major events and stages in viral infection can now be investigated with a variety of molecular techniques that measure the concentrations and map the distribution of viral genes and proteins in cells, tissues, organs, and even whole animals. In this way, viral tropisms and gene expression and the extent and localization of infection can be defined with great precision. The predominantly single-cell techniques described in this chapter, coupled with amplification of viral genes, also provide unprecedented levels of sensitivity and insight into the subtlest kinds of viral-host cell interactions in latent or covert infections. With plus-minus hybridization screening, genes that are activated or repressed in infection can be identified and the change in expression mapped anatomically. In this way, previously unrecognized genes can be implicated, leading to new hypotheses about pathogenetic processes and mechanisms. Collectively, the experimental approaches described provide the investigator with the requisite capabilities to answer many of the central questions in viral pathogenesis with a new level of rigor.

ABBREVIATIONS

AD: Alzheimer's disease
AIDS: acquired immunodeficiency syndrome
apoE: apolipoprotein E
CNS: central nervous system
DAB: diaminobenzidene
GSHV: ground squirrel hepatitis virus
HIV: human immunodeficiency virus
LCMV: lymphocytic choriomeningitis virus
moi: multiplicity of infection
mRNAs: messenger ribonucleic acids
NBT/BCIP: nitroblue tetrazolium chloride/bromochloroindolyl phosphate
PrPSc: the abnormal isoform of the prion protein
Theiler's murine encephalomyelitis virus (TMEV)
TNF-α: tumor necrosis factor-a

REFERENCES

1. Aubert C, Chamorro M, Brahic M. Identification of Theiler's virus infected cells in the central nervous system of the mouse during demyelinating disease. Microb Pathog 1987;3:319–326.
2. Bagasra O, Hauptman SP, Lischner HW, Sachs M, Pomerantz RJ. Detection of human immunodeficiency virus type 1 provirus in mononuclear cells by in situ polymerase chain reaction. N Engl J Med 1992;326:1385–1391.
3. Blum HE, Figus A, Haase AT, Vyas GN. Laboratory diagnosis of hepatitis B virus infection by nucleic acid hybridization analyses and immunohistologic detection of gene products. Dev Biol Stand 1985;59:125–139.
4. Blum HE, Haase AT, Vyas GN. Molecular pathogenesis of hepatitis B virus infection: simultaneous detection of viral DNA and antigens in paraffin-embedded liver sections. Lancet 1984;8406:771–775.
5. Brahic M, Haase AT. Double-label techniques of in situ hybridization and immunocytochemistry. Curr Top Microbiol Immunol 1989;143:9–20.
6. Brahic M, Haase AT, Cash E. Simultaneous in situ detection of viral RNA and antigens. Proc Natl Acad Sci U S A 1984;81:5445–5448.
7. Brahic M, Stowring L, Ventura P, Haase AT. Gene expression in visna virus infection in sheep. Nature 1981;292:240–242.
8. Bresser J, Evinger-Hodges MJ. Comparison and optimization of in situ hybridization procedures yielding rapid, sensitive mRNA detections. Genet Anal Tech Appl 1987;4:89–104.
9. Bugnon C, Bahjaoui M, Fellmann D. A simple method for coupling in situ hybridization and immunocytochemistry: application to the study of peptidergic neurons. J Histochem Cytochem 1991;39:859–862.
10. Cash E, Chamorro M, Brahic M. Quantitation, with a new assay, of Theiler's virus capsid protein in the central nervous system of mice. J Virol 1986;60:558–563.
11. Chiu KP, Cohen SH, Morris DW, Jordan GW. Intracellular amplification of proviral DNA in tissue sections using the polymerase chain reaction. J Histochem Cytochem 1992;40:333–341.
12. Corder EH, Saunders AM, Strittmatter WJ, et al. Gene dose of apolipoprotein E type 4 allele and the risk of Alzheimer's disease in late onset families. Science 1993;261:921–923.
13. Diedrich JF, Carp RI, Haase AT. Increased expression of heat shock protein, transferrin, and β_2-microglobulin in astrocytes during scrapie. Microb Pathog 1993;15:1–6.
14. Diedrich JF, Duguid JR, Haase AT. The role of astrocytes in the neuropathology of scrapie and Alzheimer's disease. Semin Virol 1991;2:233–238.
15. Diedrich JF, Minnigan M, Carp RI, et al. Neuropathological changes in scrapie and Alzheimer's disease are associated with increased expression of apolipoprotein E and cathepsin D in astrocytes. J Virol 1991;65:4759–4768.
16. Diedrich J, Wietgrefe S, Haase A, Duguid J, Carp RI. Identifying and mapping changes in gene expression involved in the neuropathology of scrapie and Alzheimer's disease. Curr Top Microbiol Immunol 1991;172:259–274.
17. Dubensky TW, Murphy FA, Villarreal LP. The detection of DNA and RNA virus genomes in the organ systems of whole mice: patterns of mouse organ infection by polyomavirus. J Virol 1984;50:779–783.
18. Duguid JR, Bohmont CW, Liu N, Tourtellote WW. Changes in brain gene expression shared by scrapie and Alzheimer's disease. Proc Natl Acad Sci U S A 1989;86:7260–7264.
19. Embretson J, Staskus K, Retzel E, Haase AT, Bitterman P. PCR amplification of viral DNA and viral host cell mRNAs in situ. In: Mullis KB, Ferré F, Gibbs RA, eds. The polymerase chain reaction. Boston: Birkhäuser, 1994:55–64.
20. Embretson J, Zupancic M, Beneke J, et al. Analysis of human immunodeficiency virus–infected tissues by amplification and in situ hybridization reveals latent and permissive infections at single-cell resolution. Proc Natl Acad Sci U S A 1993;90:357–361.
21. Embretson J, Zupancic M, Ribas JL, et al. Massive covert infection of helper T lymphocytes and macrophages by HIV during the incubation period of AIDS. Nature 1993;362:359–362.
22. Fauci AS. Multifactorial nature of human immunodeficiency virus disease: implications for therapy. Science 1993;262:1011–1018.
23. Gendelman HE, Moench TR, Narayan O, Griffin DE, Clements JE. A double labeling technique for performing immunocytochemistry and in situ hybridization in virus infected cell cultures and tissues. J Virol Methods 1985;11:93–103.

24. Gentilomi G, Musiani M, Zerbini M, Gibellini D, Gallinella G, Venturoli S. Double in situ hybridization for detection of herpes simplex virus and cytomegalovirus DNA using non-radioactive probes. J Histochem Cytochem 1992;40:421–425.

25. Haase AT. Analysis of viral infections by in situ hybridization. In: Valentino K, Roberts J, Barchas J, eds. In situ hybridization: applications to neurobiology. Fairlawn, NJ: Oxford University Press, 1987: 197–219.

26. Haase AT. Preface. Curr Top Microbiol Immunol 1989;143:vii–x.

27. Haase AT. The role of active and covert infections in lentivirus pathogenesis. Ann N Y Acad Sci 1994;724:75–86.

28. Haase AT, Blum H, Stowring L, Geballe A, Brahic M, Jensen R. Hybridization analysis of viral infection at the single-cell level. In: Nakamura RM, ed. Clinical laboratory molecular analyses. Orlando: Grune & Stratton, 1985:247–256.

29. Haase AT, Brahic M, Stowring L, Blum H. Detection of viral nucleic acids by in situ hybridization. In: Maramorosch K, Koprowski H, eds. Methods in virology. New York: Academic Press, 1984;189–226.

30. Haase AT, Gantz D, Blum H, et al. Combined macroscopic and microscopic detection of viral genes in tissues. Virology 1985;140:201–206.

31. Haase AT, Retzel EF, Staskus KA. Amplification and detection of lentiviral DNA inside cells. Proc Natl Acad Sci U S A 1990;87:4971–4975.

32. Haase AT, Walker D, Stowring L, et al. Detection of two viral genomes in single cells by double-label hybridization in situ and color microradioautoradiography. Science 1985;227:189–192.

33. Heniford BW, Shum-Siu A, Leonberger M, Hendler FJ. Variation in cellular EGF receptor mRNA expression demonstrated by in situ reverse transcriptase polymerase chain reaction. Nucl Acids Res 1993; 21:3159–3166.

34. Ignatius MJ, Gebicke-Haerter P, Pitas RE, Shooter EM. Apolipoprotein E in nerve injury and repair. In: Seil FJ, Herbert E, Carlson BM, eds. Progress in brain research. Vol 71. New York: Elsevier, 1987: 177–184.

35. Kiyama H, Emson PC, Tohyama M. Recent progress in the use of the technique of non-radioactive in situ hybridization histochemistry: new tools for molecular neurobiology. Neurosci Res 1990;9:1–21.

36. Komminoth P, Long AA. In-situ polymerase chain reaction: an overview of methods, applications, and limitations of a new molecular technique. Virchows Arch B Cell Pathol Incl Mol Patho 1993; 64:67–73.

37. Lipkin WI, Villarreal LP, Oldstone MBA. Whole animal section in situ hybridization and protein blotting: new tools in molecular analysis of animal models for human disease. Curr Top Microbiol Immunol 1989;143:33–54.

38. Long AA, Komminoth P, Lee E, Wolfe HJ. Comparison of indirect and direct in-situ polymerase chain reaction in cell preparations and tissue sections. Histochemistry 1993;99:151–162.

39. Maniatis T, Fritsch EF, Sambrook J. Molecular cloning. New York: Cold Spring Harbor Laboratory, 1982. Laboratory manual.

40. Mayeux R, Stern Y, Ottman R, et al. The apolipoprotein e4 allele in patients with Alzheimer's disease. Ann Neurol 1993;34:752–754.

41. Mercer JA, Wiley CA, Spector DH. Pathogenesis of murine cytomegalovirus infection: identification of infected cells in the spleen during acute and latent infections. J Virol 1988;62:987–997.

42. Mitchell WJ, Gressens P, Martin JR, DeSanto R. Herpes simplex virus type 1 DNA persistence, progressive disease and transgenic immediate early gene promoter activity in chronic corneal infections in mice. J Gen Virol 1994;75:1201–1210.

43. Mullink H, Walboomers JMM, Raap AK, Meyer CJLM. Two colour DNA in situ hybridization for the detection of two viral genomes using non-radioactive probes. Histochemistry 1989;91:195–198.

44. Mullis KB, Ferré F, Gibbs RA, eds. The polymerase chain reaction. Boston: BirkhÑuser, 1994.

45. Nathan BP, Bellosta S, Sanan DA, Weisgraber KH, Mahley RW, Pitas RE. Differential effects of apolipoproteins E3 and E4 on neuronal growth in vitro. Science 1994;264:850–852.

46. Nederlof PM, Robinson D, Abuknesha R, et al. Three-color fluorescence in situ hybridization for the simultaneous detection of multiple nucleic acid sequences. Cytometry 1989;10:20–27.

47. Normand E, Bloch B. Simultaneous detection of two messenger RNAs in the central nervous system: a simple two-step in situ hybridization procedure using a combination of radioactive and non-radioactive probes. J Histochem Cytochem 1991;39:1575–1578.

48. Nuovo, GJ. PCR in situ hybridization: protocols and applications. New York: Raven Press, 1992.

49. Nuovo GJ, Gallery F, Hom R, MacConnell P, Bloch W. Importance of different variables for enhancing in situ detection of PCR-amplified DNA. PCR Methods Appl 1993;2:305–312.

50. Nuovo GJ, Gallery F, MacConnell P, Becker J, Bloch W. An improved technique for the detection of DNA by in situ hybridization after PCR-amplification. Am J Pathol 1991;139:1239–1244.

51. Nuovo GJ, Gallery F, MacConnell P, Braun A. In situ detection of polymerase chain reaction–amplified HIV-1 nucleic acids and tumor necrosis factor-a RNA in the central nervous system. Am J Pathol 1994;144:659–666.

52. Nuovo GJ, Gorgone GA, MacConnell P, Margiotta M, Gorevic PD. In situ localization of PCR-amplified human and viral cDNAs. PCR Methods Appl 1992;2:117–123.

53. Nuovo GJ, MacConnell P, Forde A, DeIvenne P. Detection of human papillomavirus DNA in formalin fixed tissues by in situ hybridization after amplification by the polymerase chain reaction. Am J Pathol 1991;139:847–854.

54. Nuovo GJ, Margiotta M, MacConnell P, Becker J. Rapid in situ detection of PCR-amplified HIV-1 DNA. Diagn Mol Pathol 1992;1:98–102.

55. Ozden S, Aubert C, Gonzalez-Dunia D, Brahic M. Simultaneous in situ detection of two mRNAs in the same cell using riboprobes labeled with biotin and 35S. J Histochem Cytochem 1990;38:917–922.

56. Ozden S, Aubert C, Gonzalez-Dunia D, Brahic M. In situ analysis of proteolipid protein gene transcripts during persistent Theiler's virus infection. J Histochem Cytochem 1991;39:1305–1309.

57. Patterson BK, Till M, Otto P, et al. Detection of HIV-1 DNA and messenger RNA in individual cells by PCR-driven in situ hybridization and flow cytometry. Science 1993;260:976–979.

58. Sanan DA, Weisgraber KH, Russell SJ, et al. Apolipoprotein E associates with β amyloid peptide of Alzheimer's disease to form novel monofibrils. J Clin Invest 1994;94:860–869.

59. Saunders AM, Schmader K, Breitner JCS, et al. Apolipoprotein E E4 allele distributions in late-onset Alzheimer's disease and in other amyloid-forming diseases. Lancet 1993;342:710–711.

60. Schmechel DE, Saunders AM, Strittmatter WJ, et al. Increased amyloid β-peptide deposition in cerebral cortex as a consequence of apolipoprotein E genotype in late-onset Alzheimer disease. Proc Natl Acad Sci USA 1993;90:9649–9653.

61. Staskus KA, Couch L, Bitterman P, et al. In situ amplification of visna virus DNA in tissue sections reveals a reservoir of latently infected cells. Microb Pathog 1991;11:67–76.

62. Sternberger LA. Immunocytochemistry. 2nd ed. New York: John Wiley & Sons, 1979.

63. Stowring L, Haase AT, Petursson G, et al. Detection of visna virus antigens and RNA in glial cells in foci of demyelination. Virology 1985;141:311–318.

64. Strittmatter WJ, Saunders AM, Schmechel D, et al. Apolipoprotein E: high avidity binding to β-amyloid and increased frequency of type 4 allele in late-onset familial Alzheimer disease. Proc Natl Acad Sci U S A 1993;90:1977–1981.

65. Trembleau A, Roche D, Calas A. Combination of non-radioactive and radioactive in situ hybridization with immunohistochemistry: a new method allowing the simultaneous detection of two mRNAs and one antigen in the same brain tissue section. J Histochem Cytochem 1993;41:489–498.

66. Tyler KL, Fields BN. Pathogenesis of neurotropic viral infections. In: McKendall RR, ed. Handbook of clinical neurology (viral disease). Amsterdam: Elsevier, 1989;12:25–49.

67. Unger ER, Brigati DJ. Colorimetric in-situ hybridization in clinical virology: development of automated technology. Curr Top Microbiol Immunol 1989;143:21–31.

68. Van Noorden CJF, Jonges GN. Quantification of the histochemical reaction for alkaline phosphatase activity using the indoxyl-tetranitro BT method. Histochem J 1987;19:94–102.

69. Watson SJ, Sherman TG, Kelsey JE, Burke S, Akil H. Anatomical localization of mRNA: in situ hybridization of neuropeptide systems. In: Valentino KL, Eberwine JH, Barchas JD, eds. In situ hybridization (applications to neurobiology). New York: Oxford University Press, 1987;126–145.

70. Wilcox JN. Fundamental principles of in situ hybridization. J Histochem Cytochem 1993;41:1725–1733.

71. Yashioka M, Shapshak P, Sun NCJ, et al. Simultaneous detection of ferritin and HIV-1 in reactive microglia. Acta Neuropathol (Berl) 1992;84:297–306.

Viral Pathogenesis,
edited by Neal Nathanson, et al.
Lippincott–Raven Publishers, Philadelphia © 1997

CHAPTER 20

Methods in Viral Pathogenesis

Animals

Abigail L. Smith and Stephen W. Barthold

INTRODUCTION

Experimental infection of laboratory animals under controlled conditions provides a wealth of information about the pathogenesis of specific virus infections. This chapter describes the classic methods that have been used for such studies and discusses some of the important variables to be considered in their design and interpretation. The other chapters in this section complement this chapter and provide an atlas of viral pathogenesis and pathology, the methods used for the assay of viral genes and gene products at a single cell level, and an overview of transgenic and knockout animals, which have made a new group of methods available for pathogenesis studies.

INFORMATION DERIVED FROM PATHOGENESIS STUDIES

Pathogenesis experiments can reveal many important details about the sequential aspects of virus infections. The mode of entry and primary site or sites of virus replication can be deduced if a presumed natural route of inoculation is used and tissues are assayed at an appropriately early interval. For

A. L. Smith: Section of Comparative Medicine and Department of Epidemiology and Public Health, Yale University School of Medicine, New Haven, CT 06520-8016.
S.W. Barthold: Section of Comparative Medicine, Yale University School of Medicine, New Haven, CT 06520-8016.

instance, mouse hepatitis virus (MHV), strain JHM, and herpes simplex virus were shown by combined application of infectivity assays and immunochemistry to replicate first (within 48 hours of inoculation) in the nasal epithelium after intranasal inoculation of susceptible mice.[5,7,8,67,93,173,192] Similarly, as shown by infectivity and morphologic assays in vivo and by muscle-nerve organ cultures, rabies virus replicates in muscle cells proximal to the inoculation site before nerve entry.[130,204]

Secondary sites of virus replication can be identified either grossly at the organ level or, with appropriate methods such as immunohistochemistry or electron microscopy, at the cellular level. The mode of dissemination from the primary site of replication can also be assessed. Olfactory receptors extend into and beyond the olfactory epithelium, providing direct communication of nerve fibers with the external environment.[96,97] Therefore, infection of the brain can occur by direct extension along olfactory tracts.[5,7,8,67,93,173] Classic studies with rabies virus confirmed neural dissemination by demonstrating that limb amputation and nerve severing spared animals inoculated in extremities from disease.[3,66,94,134,135] In the case of polytropic MHV strains, infection of the brain can occur either by olfactory-neural pathways or hematogenously in susceptible mice.[8] Viruses spread by the hematogenous route may or may not be cell associated. Colorado tick fever virus and at least some parvoviruses may be found in association with erythrocytes[139] (P.J. Tattersall, Yale University, personal communication, 1988), and MHV may be associated with leukocytes.[11] It may be predicted that any virus capable of agglutinating erythrocytes or infecting leukocytes of the natural host could disseminate in this way.

Although pathogenesis studies do not definitively identify modes of transmission, the organ distribution of virus can reveal clues about possible routes of excretion. For example, a low-passage isolate of rat parvovirus that causes persistent infection of rats inoculated as infants may be found in the kidney[90,142] and, during the persistent phase, in the lung,[60,90] suggesting that excretion through the urinary tract and by aerosols may have important transmission potential. Replication of enterotropic MHV strains may be restricted to the intestine,[6,12,14] suggesting that transmission must occur by fecal-oral means.

METHODS

Establishing Median Infectious Dose Versus Median Lethal Dose

Before pathogenesis studies are undertaken, it is important to define virus concentration. In most cases, this can be determined with the use of cultured cells; however, it may be equally or more relevant to determine the dose in relation to the live animal, because animals and cell cultures can have vastly different sensitivity levels. For instance, the mouse is several orders of magnitude more sensitive than cell culture for detection of infectious MHV.[47]

It is also critical that the same criterion be used throughout a series of experiments. The median infectious dose (ID50) based on seroconversion is liable to be more sensitive than an

ID50 based on disease development or a median lethal dose (LD50). Determinations of ID50 and LD50 should be made with animals of the same genotype and age as those planned for use in pathogenesis experiments. This is particularly important if inbred animals are to be used, because genetically determined resistance can impact heavily on results. For instance, higher doses of several viruses are required to infect C57BL/6 mice than other mouse strains.[24,26] Age-dependent resistance to infection or disease has been reported for many viruses and may play a critical role for some, such as parvovirus, MHV, and reovirus.[8,13] In the case of parvovirus, it is thought that infant animals have a larger pool of dividing cells and factors present during S phase that are required for parvovirus replication. Rat parvovirus, for instance, kills a proportion of infant rats but not weanling rats, and higher virus doses are required to infect weanling rats.[89] Because the virus causes persistent infection in rats surviving inoculation as infants,[90,142] it is crucial to use a dose that does not kill all inoculated rats if persistence is to be studied.

Tables 20-1 and 20-2 illustrate calculation of titers as median dose or as plaque-forming units (PFU) or focus-forming units (FFU).

Morphologic Approaches

Morphologic analysis adds an important dimension to infectious disease studies. At the crudest level, animals can be monitored for clinical signs that provide clues about anatomic sites of virus-induced tissue effects. Enterotropic viruses may be expected to cause diarrhea, neurotropic ones neurologic signs, and pneumotropic ones dyspnea. At the next level, organs can be examined for gross pathology. Changes are apt to depend heavily on virus strain–related virulence, stage of infection, and susceptibility of the host. During acute disseminated infection with polytropic MHV strains in susceptible mice, white foci can be seen on the surface of the liver (Fig. 20-1), and spleen and lymph node size may be altered. Rat parvovirus infection in infant rats can cause cerebellar hypoplasia, severe hepatic necrosis, and jaundice.[89] Recovered rats can have fibrotic, nodular livers.[89]

Although clinical signs and gross organ weight, size, or characteristics may be useful indices of effect, they seldom provide the depth of insight that microscopic analysis can provide in pathogenesis experiments. At the very least, light microscopy confirms and extends gross findings. The white foci seen grossly on the liver during acute MHV infection are areas of necrosis, syncytium formation, and inflammation (Fig. 20-2). The quality of such lesions varies according to stage of infection and host response. Changes too subtle to be detected grossly become evident on histosections. These may include leukocyte infiltrates, tissue proliferative responses, or other events that occur in the course of most viral infections. Microscopic analysis permits accurate correlation of sites and degree of virus replication or virus-induced tissue damage with cell type, sites of replication, excretion, and persistence. For example, both respiratory and enterotropic strains of MHV replicate in intestine, but light microscopy reveals that respiratory (polytropic) MHV strains replicate principally in gut-associated lymphoid tissue, whereas enterotropic MHV

TABLE 20-1. *Reed and Muench calculation of 50% end point, illustrated with sample data (quantal assay)*

Log of virus dilution	Infected test units*	Cumulative infected (x)	Cumulative uninfected (y)	Ratio x/(x+y)	Percent infected
−3	8/8	14	0	14/14	100
−4	5/8	6	3	6/9	67
−5	1/8	1	10	1/11	9
−6	0/8	0	18	0/18	0

The logarithmic proportion between the two closest dilutions is calculated as follows:

$$\frac{(\% \text{ positive above } 50\%) - 50\%}{(\% \text{ positive above } 50\%) - (\% \text{ positive below } 50\%)} = \text{proportionate distance with the data shown,}$$

$$\frac{67-50}{67-9} = 0.3.$$

The 50% end point (or dilution that will infect 50% of the inoculated test units) is therefore $10^{-4.3}$.

*Infected test units may be wells with cytopathic effect (TCID50), dead animals (LD50), infected eggs (EID50) or animals with pneumonia (PD50).

After Reed LJ, Muench H. A simple method of estimating fifty percent endpoints. Am J Hyg 1938; 27:493–497.

TABLE 20-2. *Lorenz and Bogel calculation of plaque-forming units (PFU) or focus-forming units (FFU), illustrated with sample data*

Log of virus dilution (d)	Number of replicates (k)	Number of plaques (n_1, n_2, n_3)	Sum of plaques ($n_1 + n_2 + n_3$)
−3	3	47, 52, 49	148
−4	3	4, 3, 4	11
−5	3	0, 0, 1	1
−6	3	0, 0, 0	0
Total (N)			160

$$\text{PFU per inoculum} = x = \frac{N}{\Sigma k \cdot d}$$

$$\begin{aligned}\Sigma k \cdot d &= 3 \times 10^{-3} + 3 \times 10^{-4} + 3 \times 10^{-5} + 3 \times 10^{-6} \\ &= 3 \times 10^{-6}(10^3 + 10^2 + 10^1 + 10^0) \\ &= 3 \times 10^{-6} \times 1111 \\ &= 3333 \times 10^{-6}\end{aligned}$$

$$\text{Then, } x = \frac{160}{3333 \times 10^{-6}} = 0.048 \times 10^6 = 4.8 \times 10^4$$

The standard deviation, $s(x) = \frac{x}{\Sigma k \cdot d}$. In the example,

$$s(x) = \frac{4.8 \times 10^4}{3333 \times 10^{-6}} = 0.0014 \times 10^{10} = 0.0374 \times 10^5 = 0.374 \times 10^4$$

The estimated number of PFU per inoculum volume (assume 100 µL) of undiluted suspension is

$$x \pm s(x) = 4.8(\pm 0.4) \times 10^4 \text{ per inoculum, or } 4.8(\pm 0.4) \times 10^5 \text{ PFU/mL.}$$

After Lorenz RJ, Bogel K. Calculation of titers and their significance. In: Kaplan M, Koprowski H, eds. Laboratory techniques in rabies. Geneva: World Health Organization, 1973:321–335.

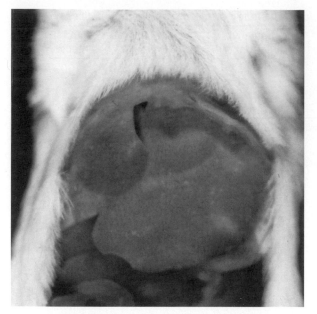

FIG. 20-1. BALB/c (susceptible) mouse infected with respiratory (polytropic) mouse hepatitis virus, strain JHM. The liver has multiple, randomly distributed white spots, which represent foci of necrotizing hepatitis. Original magnification 2.5×.

strains replicate principally in enterocytes.[6,8,14] Histopathology, histochemistry, immunohistochemistry, and nucleic acid analysis can be used alone or in combination in pathogenesis experiments. Many investigators are reluctant to avail themselves of the benefits of microscopic analysis because it re-

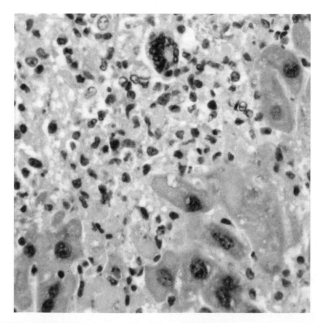

FIG. 20-2. Liver of a mouse with mouse hepatitis virus (MHV). There is focal necrosis of hepatic parenchyma and leukocytic infiltration with formation of a syncytium (*top*), typical of MHV infection. Hematoxylin and eosin stain, original magnification 300×.

quires technical and professional expertise for proper evaluation and interpretation. Nevertheless, seeking collaborative morphologic expertise is sound practice and greatly enhances the depth and quality of virus-related research.

Preparation of Tissues for Microscopic Analysis

The reader is referred to any histology reference text for in-depth coverage of histologic techniques and principles. No one preparative method is universal for all purposes. Optimal tissue processing must be performed with the purpose in mind. Tissue fixation is a critical step in this process. An optimal fixative would preserve the tissue, its antigens, and its nucleic acids without alteration. No such fixative exists, because the very act of fixation stops autolysis by inactivating chemical processes through denaturation. There are a number of fixatives, which work in a variety of ways, including aldehydes, oxidizing agents, precipitating agents (alcohols and acids), physical methods (heat or microwave), and others that work by unknown mechanisms, such as picric acid. Each method and type of fixation results in some form of compromise, because proteins, carbohydrates, lipids, and nucleic acids become denatured or modified in different ways and to different degrees.

Formalin, neutral-buffered to approximate tissue pH, is the most widely used fixative for histology, because it is inexpensive and effective and does not require postfixation processing. Generally, formalin-fixed tissue is suitable for routine histology, immunohistochemistry, and nucleic acid hybridization. Protein crosslinking aldehyde fixatives such as formalin are superior to precipitating fixatives for nucleic acid studies because they facilitate retention of nucleic acids. Electron microscopy requires stronger crosslinking fixatives such as glutaraldehyde, which may destroy antigenicity and render nucleic acids inaccessible because of their excessive crosslinking properties. Under certain circumstances, other fixatives may be selected. For example, Bouin's fixative, which contains a mixture of fixative types, including formalin, acetic acid, and picric acid, may be chosen to accentuate nuclear morphology, and it is often suitable for immunohistochemistry.

Choice of fixative is probably most critical for immunohistochemistry. Some antigens are better preserved than others after fixation, and a fixative must be selected that allows retention of antigenicity for the particular antigen under study. Formalin is usually suitable, but some antigens may be better preserved with protein-precipitating fixatives. Antigens and nucleic acids can often be enhanced by treating tissue sections with proteases, which digest some of the crosslinked protein to permit reagent access, or with microwaves.[21,167] Immunohistochemical detection of MHV antigen is best in tissue fixed with formalin instead of Bouin's fixative, and it is enhanced by protease treatment.[21] Protein crosslinking fixatives sometimes destroy antigenic epitopes, so an alternative fixative such as periodate-lysine-paraformaldehyde (PLP),[120] which crosslinks carbohydrates and only modestly crosslinks proteins, may be superior for some labile antigens and for nucleic acids.[58] Some antigens are too labile for any fixative and require application of immunohistochemical stains before fixation (Fig. 20-3). If all else fails, frozen sections can be used without fixation, but histomorphology is significantly compromised. Osseous or mineralized tissue must be decalcified before sectioning, and this is accomplished with acid or ethylenediamine tetraacetic acid (EDTA) decalcifying solutions. Acid solutions are effective at decalcification but may sufficiently denature proteins so as to preclude immunohistochemical analysis or alter nucleic acids.

The process of tissue fixation must be performed properly, with the fixative permitted to penetrate the tissue. Immersion-fixation in formalin requires that tissues not exceed 0.5 cm in thickness, and the ratio of fixative volume to tissue volume must be 10 : 1. Glutaraldehyde and PLP penetrate tissues poorly, so tissue sections should not exceed 1 mm in thickness. Other fixatives may requires postfixation processing; for example, Bouin's-fixed tissues are placed through graded alcohols. Most fixed tissues for light microscopy are embedded in paraffin, but tissues for electron microscopy require a harder substrate, such as plastic resin. Immunohistochemistry with resin-embedded tissue is possible but more difficult. To circumvent this problem, tissues can be perfused or treated with immunohistochemical labels such as colloidal gold or ferritin, in vivo or in vitro, before fixation and embedding.[29]

Optimal organ fixation may require direct perfusion of fixative. Intratracheal perfusion of lungs is required for accurate evaluation of pulmonary parenchymal changes or distribution of virus antigen or nucleic acid. With alveoli thus expanded to their normal volume, cell tropism can be discerned more readily (Fig. 20-4). Intestine requires immediate fixation to arrest the rapid autolysis inherent to this tissue. This is accomplished in large species by opening segments of bowel, flushing digesta from the mucosa, then immersing the organ in fixative. In rodents, intraluminal perfusion of fixative by syringe and needle at periodic intervals along the bowel, followed by immersion of the organ into fixative, is effective. Murine rotavirus has a tropism for the most terminally differentiated enterocytes on villus tips. There are very small numbers of such cell targets in the adult mouse, and they are among the first to degenerate postmortem. Because of the very subtle morphologic changes induced by infection, gut tissue must be fixed carefully and immediately.[166] Furthermore, the intestinal tract must be viewed as multiple organs (duodenum, jejunum, ileum, cecum, proximal colon, and distal colon), each with different function and susceptibility to viruses. Virus tropism for intestine is remarkably segmental. For example, enterotropic MHV replicates preferentially in the cecum and proximal colon,[6] whereas murine rotavirus replicates preferentially in the small intestine.[166]

Tissues can also be perfused intravascularly for different purposes. Perfusion of vessels with saline before perfusion with fixative allows optimal morphologic analysis of vascular-related pathology and optimal and rapid fixation of tissues such as brain. Perfusion can also be used as a means of introducing reagents for immunohistochemistry before fixation. Vascular perfusion is usually accomplished while the animal is deeply anesthetized by introducing solutions into the arterial circulation, allowing egress through the venous vasculature. Cannulation of the abdominal aorta and vena cava, carotid artery and jugular vein, or appropriate chambers of the heart are options used for vascular perfusion.

Histochemistry provides a plethora of stains for differentially visualizing various tissue elements for morphologic analysis,

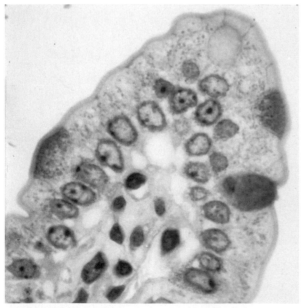

FIG. 20-3. Mouse encephalomyelitis virus antigen, labeled by immunoperoxidase, in the apical cytoplasm of two enterocytes. This antigen is labile to fixatives, so the intestine was immunoperoxidase-labeled before fixation to determine virus cell tropism and distribution in the intestine. Original magnification 500×.

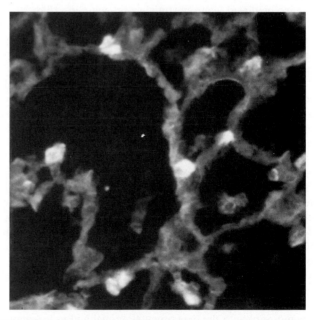

FIG. 20-4. Pulmonary parenchyma of a mouse infected with Sendai virus. The lung has been properly perfused with fixative, allowing expansion of alveoli for better visualization of target cell distribution. Sendai virus selectively infects type 2 pneumocytes, which are visualized by an immunofluorescent label. Original magnification 300×.

and selection of stains is largely a personal choice. Hematoxylin and eosin is the most commonly applied stain for routine tissue morphology, but stains can also be used to enhance virus inclusion bodies, such as Feulgen stains for DNA. Counterstains are used in combination with immunohistochemistry and nucleic acid hybridization to enhance visualization of perspective and orientation of virus antigen or nucleic acid within a tissue. Immunohistochemistry and nucleic acid hybridization can be performed with a variety of markers, including radioisotopic labels and so-called cold labels such as fluorescein, peroxidase, or alkaline phosphatase. The simultaneous combination of histochemistry, immunohistochemistry, and nucleic acid hybridization with different labels permits elegant and informative multiple-labeling in pathogenesis experiments at the microscopic level.

Morphologic Observations and Their Interpretation

Virus effects on host tissues are remarkably varied and depend on both the agent and the host. Effects can be reflected as morphologic and functional changes in the host and can be caused by the direct effect of the virus or by host response to the virus. Cytolytic viruses, such as MHV, can cause direct tissue damage, resulting in foci of necrosis in sites of virus replication. Some viruses can induce characteristic markers of infection, such as syncytium formation (see Fig. 20-2), intranuclear inclusion bodies (Fig. 20-5), or intracytoplasmic inclusion bodies (Fig. 20-6). These features, coupled with tissue specificity of a particular virus, can be highly pathognomonic and can serve as accurate diagnostic markers. Some viruses have minimal direct cytolytic effect on their target tissue but elicit a vigorous host immune response that results in tissue damage. For example, infection of immunocompetent mice with Sendai virus causes immune-mediated acute necrotizing bronchiolitis (Fig. 20-7), which is absent in Sendai virus–infected immunodeficient mice (Fig. 20-8). The necrotizing bronchiolitis of Sendai virus is typical and diagnostic of this infection in mice and rats, but it is host-mediated.[26]

Conversely, some viruses induce minimal or no detectable morphologic changes. This may result from low virulence of agents that can be potentially cytolytic, as is the case with a newly recognized murine parvovirus.[178] Likewise, mice can be infected by lymphocytic choriomeningitis virus (LCMV), with extensive virus infection and replication in multiple tissues, in the absence of overt disease or microscopic lesions. This occurs in immunologically tolerant mice infected in utero or as neonates with LCMV. Conversely, if LCMV is inoculated into immunocompetent adult mice, there is a notable host cellular response, including lymphocytic choriomeningitis (Fig. 20-9). However, the absence of pathology does not necessarily translate into a lack of functional impact.[101] LCMV, in the absence of direct or immune-mediated cell damage, may modify cell function sufficiently to cause metabolic effects (e.g., endocrinopathy).[137,138,205]

Familiarity with the experimental animal and use of appropriate controls avoids potential pitfalls in morphology-based experiments. Accurate assessment of virus-induced damage requires knowledge of normal tissue morphology and of the idiosyncrasies of the species being used in pathogenesis studies. Extramedullary hematopoiesis, including the presence of

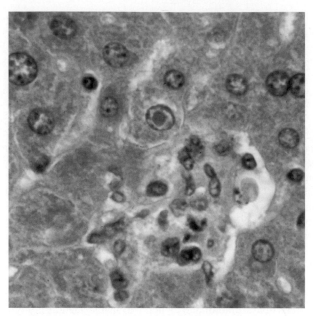

FIG. 20-5. Liver of a mouse infected with murine cytomegalovirus, showing focal necrosis, inflammation, and an intranuclear inclusion body in a hepatocyte. Hematoxylin and eosin stain, original magnification 300×.

megakaryocytes, is normal in the spleen of adult mice and rats (Fig. 20-10). Extramedullary hematopoiesis can also be found in the liver of adult rodents with chronic inflammatory disease. Myeloid cells in sinusoids and portal tissue may be misconstrued as inflammatory change, and megakaryocytes may be misinterpreted as virus-induced syncytia (Fig. 20-11). Hepato-

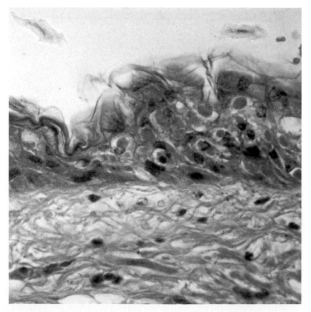

FIG. 20-6. Skin of a mouse infected with ectromelia virus, a pox virus. There are multiple intracytoplasmic inclusion bodies in epidermal cells. Hematoxylin and eosin stain, original magnification 300×.

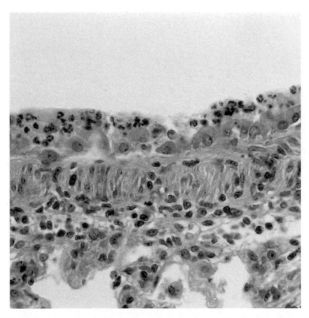

FIG. 20-7. Bronchiole of an immunocompetent mouse infected with Sendai virus, showing early epithelial necrosis, which is a host immune-mediated event and a characteristic of Sendai virus pneumonia in rodents. Hematoxylin and eosin stain, original magnification 200×.

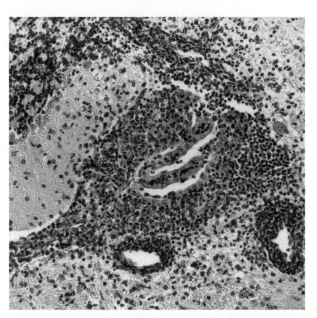

FIG. 20-9. Lymphocytic meningitis in the brain of an adult, immunocompetent mouse infected with lymphocytic choriomeningitis virus. Immunocompetent mice respond immunologically to the presence of this noncytolytic virus with infiltration of lymphocytes, resulting in development of disease and mortality. Mice exposed in utero or as neonates are immunologically tolerant to the virus; they and immunodeficient mice do not elicit such a response and do not develop these lymphocytic infiltrates or disease. Hematoxylin and eosin stain, original magnification 150×.

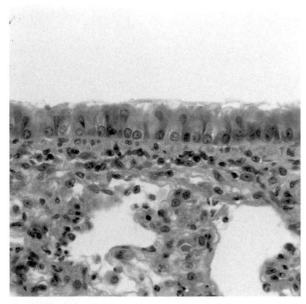

FIG. 20-8. Bronchiole of a SCID mouse, infected with Sendai virus at the same time as the mouse depicted in Figure 20-7. Note absence of immune-mediated bronchiolar necrosis in this immunodeficient animal. Hematoxylin and eosin stain, original magnification 200×.

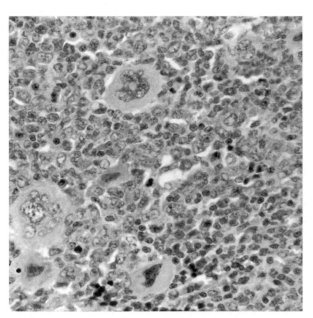

FIG. 20-10. Megakaryocytes (large multinucleate cells) in splenic red pulp of a normal adult mouse. Splenic hematopoiesis with prominent megakaryocytes is normal for this and several other rodent species, but it can be misconstrued as abnormal. Hematoxylin and eosin stain, original magnification 300×.

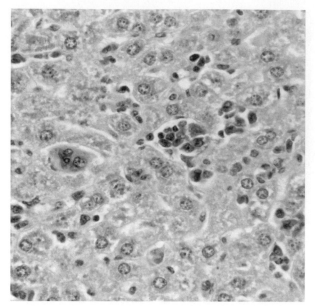

FIG. 20-11. Extramedullary myelopoiesis and megakaryocyte in hepatic sinusoids of an adult mouse with a chronic bacterial infection. Hepatic extramedullary hematopoiesis normally ceases at about weaning age in rodents but can occur in adults in response to disease. The cellular elements, including megakaryocytes, must not be misconstrued as hepatitis or syncytia (see Figs. 20-2 and 20-5). Hematoxylin and eosin stain, original magnification 300×.

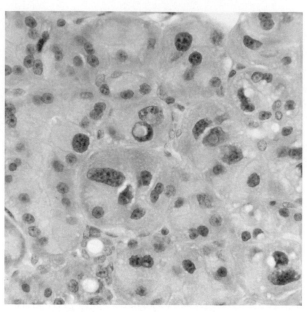

FIG. 20-13. Exorbital lacrimal gland of a normal rat. Note the marked variation in nuclear size and the intranuclear invagination of cytoplasm. Such changes can be mistaken for lesions caused by cytomegalovirus or other agents. Hematoxylin and eosin stain, original magnification 300×.

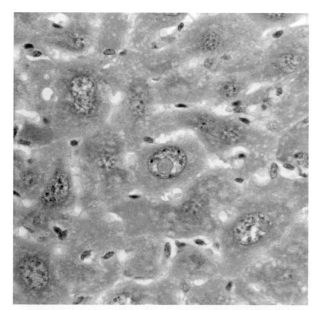

FIG. 20-12. Intranuclear invagination of cytoplasm in a mouse hepatocyte, a normal finding in rodent livers. Note that the inclusion is surrounded by a well-defined membrane. These invaginations and intracytoplasmic eosinophilic bodies, which often increase in a variety of disease states, can be misconstrued as viral inclusions (see Fig. 20-5). Hematoxylin and eosin stain, original magnification 500×.

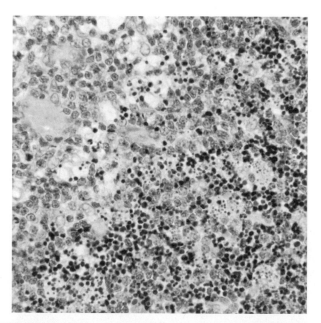

FIG. 20-14. Severe stress-induced acute necrosis (apoptosis) of lymphocytes in the thymic corticomedullary junction. This is a common response of rodents to a variety of stressors and can be misinterpreted as a specific virus effect. Hematoxylin and eosin stain, original magnification 200×.

cytes of rodents frequently possess intranuclear invaginations of cytoplasm, mimicking intranuclear viral inclusions (Fig. 20-12). Eosinophilic intracytoplasmic inclusions are also commonly found in normal rodent livers. These structures become more common in aged or diseased rodents. The exorbital lacrimal glands of rats possess striking karymegaly, intranuclear cytoplasmic invaginations, and other anomalies that resemble cytomegalovirus-induced changes (Fig. 20-13). Aged pathogen-free rodents typically develop lymphoplasmacytic infiltrates in a variety of organs, which may erroneously be blamed on an infecting virus. A variety of stressors, such as dehydration or infection with an experimental virus, can induce massive acute lymphocytic necrosis in lymphoid organs of rodents, particularly the thymus (Fig. 20-14).

Tissues can also be examined at the ultrastructural level, but this approach is usually reserved for tissues supporting high-level virus replication. Electron microscopy is highly focused and relatively insensitive, so it cannot be applied easily to tissues with minimal viral disease or containing little virus. However, sensitivity can be improved and the search for infected cells made easier with the use of immunoelectron microscopy.[29]

Virus Recovery and Quantification

Detection of Virus

A number of methods exist for detecting infectious virus in animal tissues. The most commonly applied involve inoculation of animals or permissive cells, usually continuous cell lines. Historically, intracerebral inoculation of suckling mice was the standard method for recovering numerous viruses, most notably arboviruses and ecologically related viruses. More recently, as animals have become more expensive to purchase and use and as pressures to reduce the use of animals in research have intensified, cell culture substrates have largely replaced mouse-based assays. In some cases, however, animals remain the standard because they are so much more sensitive than cell cultures.[8,48]

Virus recovery can be facilitated in some instances by the use of less conventional methods. For instance, during persistent rat parvovirus infection, virus cannot be recovered by tissue trituration and inoculation of permissive cells or rats; however, explantation of kidney, lung, and spleen fragments, followed by inoculation of permissive cells with explant lysates, has revealed that most infected rats have virus in one or more tissues.[142] Whether explantation simply represents an amplification step or whether the multiple medium changes required as the cells grow out dilute neutralizing antibody is not known. The disadvantage of this technique is that it does not permit quantification of virus in infected tissue. A similar approach, with or without cocultivation on permissive cells, has been required to detect herpes virus in latently infected ganglia.[133,185,186] Although more costly in time and labor than continuous cell lines, use of primary cells or tissue explants may be required for recovery of certain viruses (Figs. 20-15 and 20-16).

Detection of some viruses requires what at first seem to be rather peculiar approaches. For example, there is no conventional assay system for lactate dehydrogenase elevating virus

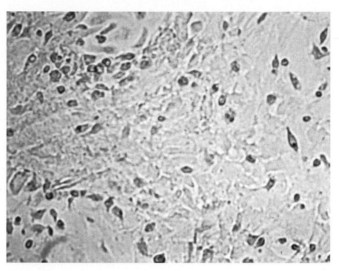

FIG. 20-15. Normal mouse lung explant after 9 days in culture. Phase contrast, original magnification 200×.

(LDV). Detection of LDV is performed by assaying plasma for lactate dehydrogenase 72 hours after inoculation of the mouse.[30,190] Because normal lactate dehydrogenase levels vary dramatically from mouse to mouse,[52] care must be taken when interpreting the results of these assays.

Quantification of Virus

Virus quantification can also be performed with the use of animals or cultured cells. In either case, virus titers can be expressed as median infectious doses, commonly LD50 or ID50

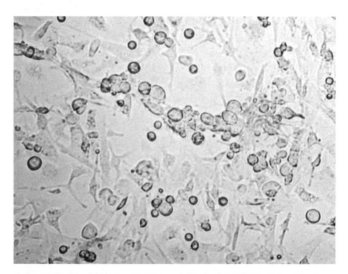

FIG. 20-16. Mouse lung explant infected for 3 days with murine cytomegalovirus, Smith strain. Note large, rounded, refractile cells. Phase contrast, original magnification 200×.

for animal-based assays, and median tissue culture infectious dose (TCID50) for culture-based assays.[153] Results are based on proportions of animals or cultures infected at varying doses of inoculum, as illustrated in Table 20-1. Noncytopathic viruses can be assayed with the use of immunofluorescence or enzyme immunoassays.[170,179,180] Somewhat more quantitative results may be obtained by using plaque assays or fluorescent focus assays, the results of which are expressed as PFU or FFU, respectively (see Table 20-2). A further advantage of the plaque assay is that virus clones representing homogenous populations can be selected. Virus recovery and quantification permit assessment of virus at the organ level and may ideally be combined with antigen localization or other methods that can be interpreted at the cellular level.

Molecular approaches to detection and quantification, reviewed in Chapter 19, include Northern and Southern blots, quantitative and reverse transcriptase polymerase chain reaction, and in situ hybridization. Results should be interpreted with caution, however, because they may not correlate with infectivity, and gene targets may vary with stage of infection, agent, and host. The use of strand-specific probes for hybridization can, for some agents, reveal sites of replication as opposed to sites of sequestration.

Localization of Viral Antigen

Immunohistochemistry, using serum containing virus antibody, monoclonal antibodies, or ascitic fluid, can reveal information about the proportion of cells infected within an organ or tissue suspension and the precise cell types infected. Several factors, aside from virus and host factors, influence the sensitivity of immunohistochemistry, including type and duration of fixation (see Morphologic Approaches).

Early studies used immunofluorescence staining of cryostat-sectioned frozen tissues. This technique may still be required for highly labile antigens, but the approach does not support the accurate structural analysis required by most morphologists, and preparations require immediate examination. The technique has been modified and adapted for use in fixed and paraffin-embedded tissue, permitting examination of archival material. Both fluorescent and enzyme-linked markers can now be used with fixed tissues. Fluorescent markers are used less often, because they still require immediate examination and because tissue morphology is not clear, but sometimes they provide spectacular visualization of viral antigens in tissue. Enzyme-based markers are usually preferred; the preparations are permanent, and reaction product can be enhanced with metallic salts. Commercial kits are readily available. With appropriate counterstains such as hematoxylin, enzyme immunohistochemical preparations also provide accurate morphologic analysis of tissues relative to viral antigen distribution.

Double-label techniques, in combination with light microscopy, have been used with increasing frequency in viral pathogenesis studies. This approach takes the guesswork out of identifying cell types supporting replication by permitting immunologic identification of cells. For instance, antibody to factor VIII identifies endothelial cells, a major target of rodent parvoviruses.[58] Antibodies to a multitude of immune cell surface markers are commercially available. These permit fine identification of lymphocytes that can support virus replication. The study of host cell receptors for viruses has also been facilitated by double-label techniques.[29]

Characterization of Host Immune Response to Virus Infection

Successful infection can be confirmed by a variety of serologic assays. In general, indirect fluorescent antibody tests and enzyme-linked immunosorbent assays (ELISA) have replaced the traditional complement fixation and hemagglutination inhibition tests. Assays of neutralizing antibody, although somewhat cumbersome and clearly more expensive and time-consuming than the others mentioned, have more biologic relevance. Testing the ability of passively administered antibody-containing serum to protect a challenged host is an even more stringent assay of humoral biologic function. An extension of that test has been achieved by experimentally addressing the role of maternal antibody in protection. Studies of maternal antibody have revealed that immunity to polytropic MHV strains is virus strain–specific, whereas immunity to enterotropic MHV isolates is less so.[9,82]

Several approaches have been used to address the role of cell-mediated immunity in virus infections. These include cytotoxicity assays that identify functional cytotoxic T cells or natural killer cells, cell transfers, and deletion experiments. Cellular immunologists measure effector T cell functions in several ways, including target cell killing, macrophage activation, B cell activation, and lymphokine production.[91] Bioassays for cytotoxic function assess both effector cell specificity and function. The simplest and most rapid assay has been adapted for use in viral pathogenesis studies. Briefly, live virus-infected target cells are exposed to radioactively labeled sodium chromate, washed free of unincorporated label, and cultured with varying numbers of effector cells that are of the same haplotype as the target cells. Labeled cells that are killed release radioactive chromate, which can be measured in supernatant culture medium. Natural killer cells can be assayed by a similar protocol; however, natural killer cells selectively kill target cells with low major histocompatibility complex class I expression.[91] In both cytotoxic T cell and natural killer cell bioassays, a dose-response relation is expected—that is, higher effector-target ratios yield a greater proportion of lysed target cells until a plateau is reached.

In addition to stimulating an immune response, some virus infections may alter host immune responsiveness. The question of immune modulation can be addressed in vivo and in vitro. For instance, several virus infections have been shown to alter the predominant isotype of antibody produced in response to protein antigens.[43,44,174] Some virus infections can alter the ability of the host to reject allogeneic skin grafts[45] or tumors.[157] In vitro assays of immune function that may be altered during virus infection include proliferative responses to mitogens or allogeneic cell stimulation,[40,49,50,175,181] cytokine assays,[50,175] and immunologic detection of activation markers, such as the interleukin-2 receptor.

VARIABLES TO CONSIDER WHEN PLANNING A PATHOGENESIS STUDY

Host Variables

Species

The choice of host species must be based on considerations that are both scientific and pragmatic. These include the established host range of the virus of interest. However, the issue of cost and public perception may also play a role. Rodents are much less expensive to procure and maintain than larger species. In addition, there are increasing pressures on the scientific community to reduce or eliminate research using pet species and primates.

It is not unusual for viral pathogenesis studies to be undertaken with the absolute goal of developing an animal model for a human disease. Sundberg[191] has summarized the desired features of such models, suggesting that they ideally should reproduce the disease of interest, be readily available and easily transported, be a polytocous species (one producing multiple offspring in a single birth) if a genetic component is to be studied, be of a convenient size (small enough to be easily housed and husbanded, yet large enough to tolerate multiple samplings), and survive long enough to permit thorough study of the disease. If rodents provide an appropriate model, they are the hosts of choice, because specific pathogen-free, genetically defined rodents permit study under very strictly defined and reproducible conditions. However, some viruses exhibit remarkable host specificity, so expensive or exotic species may be required for study. In other cases, use of artificial routes of inoculation has overcome species barriers.[75,182,200]

Because rodents are used for more than 90% of animal-based research in the United States, this chapter is largely devoted to pathogenesis studies in those species.

Genotype

On occasion, pathogenesis studies requiring the use of inbred rodents are performed in species other than mice[62]; however, this is unusual, because mice afford the greatest diversity of genotypes and are the best characterized species genetically and immunologically. Having established the species, most likely a mouse, in which to perform the experiments, the researcher is faced with the fact that there are literally hundreds of stocks and strains commercially available. Among the first decisions is whether to use random-bred or inbred animals. At this point, the investigator should reflect seriously on the goal of the research and do some long-range planning. There are no right or wrong answers; however, some thoughtful reflection and discussions with colleagues may eliminate the need to backtrack and repeat experiments needlessly. Is the goal of the studies to develop an animal model for human disease? If so, random-bred animals more accurately reflect the human condition, and they are also less expensive to purchase. On the other hand, if it is at all likely that cell transfer studies or genetic or immunologic analysis will ultimately be required, then the use of inbred animals is essential. If the choice is to use inbred animals, is anything known about genetically determined resistance? Is the infection to be studied in both a susceptible and a resistant host, with a long-range goal of understanding the basis of resistance? For those systems in which nothing is known about genetically determined resistance or susceptibility, infections may be studied in inbred mice known to be most distantly related.[195]

The development of virus-resistant homozygous inbred mouse strains that are congenic with a virus-susceptible parent has provided a great deal of insight into factors contributing to genetically determined resistance.[19,47,71,207] A flavivirus genetic resistance model based on congenic C3H mouse stocks revealed resistance to be a result, at least in part, of generation of interfering virus.[19,47,169,177] Recombinant inbred strains of mice have provided a tool to acquire more precise information about linkage. They have been used to study host responses to several viruses, including ectromelia[23] and murine coronavirus.[105] Recombinant inbred strains derived from BALB/c (susceptible) and STS/A (moderately resistant) mice suggested that both acute and late disease after infection with the MHV-JHM coronavirus are under polygenic control.[105]

Some generalizations or predictions can be made regarding how selected strains of inbred mice will respond to virus infections. As shown in Table 20-3, C57BL/6 mice tend to be phenotypically resistant to many viruses, whereas BALB/c, A, and C3H strains of mice tend to be moderately to very susceptible. Different stocks or sublines of a single mouse strain may exhibit subtle differences in response to infection.[171] Occasionally, in vitro correlates can be developed using cells or tissues from mice that display genetically determined resistance and susceptibility. Such was the case in the classic studies by Bang and Warwick,[4] who showed that macrophages from susceptible mice were destroyed by virus infection, whereas those from resistant mice retained normal morphology after exposure to MHV-2 in vitro. The genetics of in vivo infection could also be modeled in vitro using macrophages from parental and backcross mice.[4] Collins and colleagues[38] developed a similar in vitro correlate for MHV-JHM using glial cells from susceptible and resistant mouse strains.

The basis of susceptibility or resistance to virus infections may be more or less complex. In general, it is safe to assume that the basis is multifactorial (see Chap. 13). In the case of MHV-JHM, inbred mice that were susceptible to lethal infection produced systemic interferon-α (IFN-α) and IFN-β later than random-bred mice that were resistant.[61] Administration of exogenous interferons to the susceptible genotype conferred significant protection.[61] In contrast, interferon response kinetics of SJL (resistant) and C3H (susceptible) mice after infection with MHV-JHM did not appear to explain the disparate phenotypes of these mice.[147]

There are occasional instances in which two or several genotypes of mice are susceptible to lethal infection, but pathology may vary among mouse strains given the same dose of virus by a single route. As an example, MVM(i) infects neonatal DBA/2, BALB/c, SWR, SJL, CBA, and C3H mice with lethal outcome. DBA/2 mice die from intestinal hemorrhage, but all the other genotypes die with renal papillary hemorrhage.[25]

The relatively recent ability to manipulate the mouse genome, either by introduction of genetic material to relatively targeted tissues or by inactivation of selected genes,

TABLE 20-3. *Susceptibility of commonly used inbred mouse strains to virus-induced disease*

Virus	Mouse strain						References
	DBA/2	C3H	A	BALB	C57BL/6	SJL	
Ectromelia virus	S	—	S	S	R	—	87, 202
Herpes simplex virus, type 1	—	s	S	—	R	—	183
LDV	—	—	—	—	R	—	100
MVM(i)	S*	S*	—	S*	R*	—	25
MHV-3	—	—	R	—	s	—	53, 115
MHV-JHM	S	S	S	S	r	R	8, 102, 181, 188
MHV-Y	—	—	—	S	—	S	6
MCMV	—	R	—	S	—	—	121
Rabies virus (street strain)	r	—	S	r	—	R	111
Sendai virus	S	—	—	s	R	—	26, 141

S, very susceptible with some lethality; R, very resistant with no lethality; s, semisusceptible, clinical signs with complete recovery; r, semiresistant, a small proportion of mice die from infection; LDV, lactate dehydrogenase elevating virus; MVM, minute virus of mice; MHV, mouse hepatitis virus; MCMV, murine cytomegalovirus.
*Neonatal mice; mice >24 h old do not develop clinical signs.

has been used to advantage by virologists to study the role of particular immune cell types and cytokines in viral pathogenesis. These animals complement and extend naturally occurring mutants as tools for dissecting pathogenesis (see Chap. 21).

Age

As mentioned, age-dependent resistance to infection or disease is a phenomenon observed for many virus infections (Table 20-4). It can occur gradually over the course of weeks.[8] In contrast, age-dependent resistance to mortality induced by the immunosuppressive strain of minute virus of mice, the oncogenic effect of polyomavirus, or the thymic necrosis caused by mouse thymic virus develops within 48 hours of birth. LCMV is lethal if it is given intracerebrally to immunologically competent adult mice, but not if it is inoculated into infant mice. The choice of neonate, infant, weanling, or fully mature adult for research involves questions such as, Do inoculated neonates or infants have a high mortality rate? If so, do the animals die so quickly that the infection cannot adequately be studied? and Are fully mature animals susceptible to infection?

Age-related susceptibility to disease caused by enterotropic viruses may be mediated by enterocyte kinetics.[6] However, age-related susceptibility to infection and disease is often related to immunologic or lymphoreticular maturity; infant mice are not immunologically competent until after 2 weeks of age and not fully competent until after 6 weeks of age.

Protection of C3H mice that were susceptible to lethal MHV-JHM infection by virtue of age could be attained by ex-

TABLE 20-4. *Susceptibility of mice of varying ages to virus infection or disease*

Virus	Host Genotype	Route of Inoculation	Host age								References
			Neonate (<24 h)		Infant		Weanling		Adult		
			I	D	I	D	I	D	I	D	
Reovirus	Random-bred	Oral	+	+	+	+	NA	NA	—	—	13
MHV-Y	BALB/c	Oral	+	+	+	+	+	—	+	—	6, 12
	SJL	Oral	+	+	+	+	+	—	+	—	6, 12
MHV-JHM	BALB/c	Intranasal	+	+	+	+	+	+	+	±	8
	SJL	Intranasal	+	+	+	+	±	—	±	—	8
	C3H	Intraperitoneal	NA	NA	+	+	+	—	NA	NA	149
MHV-S	C3H	Intraperitoneal	NA	NA	+	+	+	—	NA	NA	193
EDIM virus	Most	Oral	+	+	+	+*		—*	+	—	166
MAdV-1	Random-bred	Intraperitoneal	+	+	+	±	NA	NA	+	—	209
K virus		Oral	+	NA	+	±†	+	NA	+	NA	69

I, infection; D, disease; NA, not applicable; MHV, mouse hepatitis virus (coronavirus); EDIM, epizootic diarrhea of infant mice (rotavirus); MAdV, mouse adenovirus; K virus (papovavirus);+, infection or disease occurs uniformly; −, infection or disease does not occur, ±, infection or disease occurs in less than 100% of inoculated mice.
*Diarrhea occurs in mice inoculated at 7 days of age, but not 14 days of age.
†Fatal infection in 4-day-old mice; clinically silent infection in 8-day-old mice.

posure to maternal antibody or by transfer of spleen cells from adult immune donors, but not from adult naive donors.[149] A common finding is the requirement of larger doses of virus necessary for infection or induction of lethal disease as the mice age.[144,173] Older mice may also support virus replication in a reduced spectrum of tissues than do infants,[69] or virus may spread less efficiently in older animals.[95]

There are several model systems in which viruses with the capacity to cause persistent infection are less likely to do so with increasing age of the host. In the case of Theiler's mouse encephalomyelitis virus, strain BeAn 8386, persistence could be established after intracerebral inoculation of 1-, 3-, 9-, or 40-week-old CD-1 mice, but virus was isolated with lower frequency and titers were lower in the last two groups.[184] Mice older than 3 weeks at the time of inoculation also had a lower incidence of clinically evident demyelinating disease.[184] In a more natural model, oronasal exposure of infant rats to rat parvovirus resulted in persistent infection of essentially all survivors, whereas oronasal inoculation of weanling rats resulted in acute, self-limiting infection.[89,90,142]

The capacity of an infected host to transmit infection or the pattern of transmission may also depend on age at exposure. For instance, the SR-11 strain of Hantavirus, which is antigenically distinct from the prototype ROK 76-118 strain, can be transmitted by rats inoculated at less than 48 hours of age, but not by rats inoculated as weanlings.[126] A newly recognized parvovirus of laboratory mice is shed intermittently for at least 6 weeks by random-bred mice inoculated as infants, whereas contact transmission by mice inoculated as weanlings occurred for 1 month and transmission was continuous, not intermittent.[178] Age at infection may also dictate how selective or generalized immunosuppressive sequelae may be.[196]

Sex

Host sex can affect the course of some virus infections in a number of ways (Table 20-5). Although female Swiss mice are more resistant than males to intraperitoneal infection with encephalomyocarditis virus (EMCV), this difference was not observed in weanlings, castrated adults, or intracerebrally inoculated adults. Administration of testosterone to female mice rendered them equal to males in susceptibility.[64] Administration of antibody to mouse IFN-α and IFN-β negated the sex dependence of EMCV infection.[151] In addition, spleen cell cultures from female Swiss mice showed increased Ia antigen expression at 24 hours after infection, compared with cultures from male mice.[118] Treatment with monoclonal anti–mouse IFN-γ eliminated the upregulation of Ia antigen expression, and female cells produced this cytokine earlier and in greater concentration than did male cells. Treatment of cell donors with antibody to the natural killer (NK) cell antigen, asialoGM$_1$, abolished the early production of IFN-γ by female cells.[118]

In studies designed to address mechanisms of sex-related differences in response to coxsackievirus B3 (CVB3) infection, primed male BALB spleen cell cytotoxicity against virus-infected myofibers was strong at 4 to 7 days after infection.[85] Female spleen cells reacted weakly against both infected and uninfected myofibers.[85] This finding correlated with the tendency of males to develop clinical myocarditis and pericarditis. Early, unrestricted killing by both male and female cells was attributable to NK cells, and males, but not females, mounted a cytotoxic T lymphocyte (CTL) response.[94] Host age as well as hormone treatment modulated disease severity and virus concentration in the heart.[113,114] More recent studies have revealed that male and female mice respond differently to CVB3 infection, with males mounting a predominant TH1 CD4+ T-cell response and females mounting a TH2 CD4+ T-cell response.[87] This was supported by sex-related differential isotype responses and cytokine production. Responses could be altered by treatment of male mice with estradiol or of female mice with testosterone before infection, suggesting that sex hormones have a direct or indirect effect on CD4+ T-cell responses.

Host Microbial Status

The microbial status of the experimental animals should be evaluated in all pathogenesis studies. If the study virus is one that occurs naturally in the experimental host, then the host could already have been infected and acquired immunity before experimental challenge. For instance, MHV-immune mice could have become infected with a heterotypic strain of MHV,[9,80] the most common virus infecting laboratory mice worldwide. Another complication introduced by concurrent infections with extraneous agents is that some viruses may alter the response of the host to the experimental infection. Strains of MHV have been shown to cause dramatic reduction of immune function after experimental inoculation or natural infection.[35,41,45,49,50,175,181] Antigen-presenting cell function is also independently affected among mice infected by a natural route with MHV-JHM.[49] A recently identified mouse parvovirus replicates in cultured T cell clones and suppresses T cell function in vivo[119] (MD McKisic and ALS, unpublished observations) in the absence of discernible pathology.[178] Mice are susceptible to infection with several viruses that have yet to be examined for effects on functional parameters. Therefore, it is essential to use animals that are specific pathogen-free if they are available. Animals used for experimental pathogenesis studies should be screened for indigenous pathogens before and after experimental infection to avoid possible misinterpretation of results.[176]

Virus Variables

Virus Strain or Isolate

Strain variation in virulence, organotropism, cell tropism, and other behavior is a well-established feature of many viruses. Antigenically and genetically similar isolates can have markedly divergent tissue tropisms. Therefore, it is important that the investigator consider the biologic properties of the virus strain selected for study. Among the biologic properties that can influence the outcome of experimental infection are tropism and virulence. In addition, it is important to consider whether the virus stock is genetically a mixed population or has been cloned with the application of biologic or molecular methods. Finally, it is important to be sure that

TABLE 20-5. *Effect of host sex on viral pathogenesis*

Virus*	Host genotype	Manipulation	Effect	References
EMCV	Susceptible inbred	None	Females have less severe disease (diabetes) than males	17
EMCV	Swiss	None	Females more resistant than males to intraperitoneal infection	151
EMCV	DBA/2 males	Castration	Less severe hypoglycemia than intact males	17
EMCV	Swiss females	Exogenous testosterone	Equivalent of males in susceptibility to intraperitoneal infection	64
EMCV, D variant	(NZBxNZW)F1	None	Males more susceptible than females to infection	212
EMCV, D variant	(NZBxNZW)F1	Castration	Susceptibility reduced compared to intact males	212
CVB3	BALB/c	None	Mortality, cardiac necrosis greater for males than females	84
CVB3	BALB/c males	Castration	Reduced mortality compared with untreated males	84
Ectromelia virus	A strain	None	Males have shorter survival time than females	202
Ectromelia virus	C57BL/6, DBA/2	None	Genetic analysis revealed resistance is controlled by gonad-dependent and -independent genes	22–24
TMEV	C57, SJL, SWR	None	Males more susceptible than females to virus-induced demyelination	99

EMCV, encephalomyocarditis virus; CVB3, coxsackievirus B3; TMEV, Theiler's mouse encephalomyelitis virus.
*All but ectromelia (poxvirus) are picornaviruses.

the virus stock is not contaminated by an unknown and unwanted passenger agent, either viral or microbial. Failure to consider these issues has led to many confusing or misinterpreted studies.

As an example of virus variation, murine coronaviruses (e.g., MHV) provide an illuminating illustration. A virus designated MHV-S/CDC was isolated during an epizootic of lethal enteritis in newborn mice and was shown to be most closely related antigenically to MHV-S, a prototypic polytropic MHV strain that is not enterotropic.[7,74] It is now clear that MHV strains possess two patterns of biologic behavior: an enterotropic pattern[14] and a polytropic pattern, in which virus replicates in nasal epithelium and then disseminates to multiple organs in susceptible hosts.[5,8] To date, there is no known distinguishing antigenic or genetic marker among MHV strains that predicts or determines biologic behavior.

Virus Dose

The quantity of virus to which an animal is exposed may or may not affect the outcome of infection. An idealized dose-response outcome is shown in Table 20-6. Clinical disease or mortality is likely to occur at higher doses, whereas infection

may occur at doses several orders lower than that required for disease induction. An additional point illustrated in Table 20-6 is that survival time may be inversely related to virus dose. There are, of course, many variations in host response, including situations in which the LD50 and ID50 are essentially identical[48] and those in which high-dose inoculation is nonlethal because of the presence of interfering virus in the inoculum.[169]

Route of Inoculation

Decisions regarding route of inoculation are based on several factors, one of the most important being whether the experiment is designed to simulate the natural situation. For instance, arthropod-borne viruses are frequently inoculated subcutaneously to simulate the bite of a mosquito, and enterotropic viruses are inoculated orally or by lavage. Neurotropic viruses usually enter through the skin, the barrier of which is breached by a bite, or by aerosols or the gastrointestinal tract.[65,127]

It may be of some interest to compare natural routes with parenteral injection to determine the spectrum of organs susceptible to infection when mucosal barriers are by-

TABLE 20-6. *Effect of virus dose on mouse infection, disease, and survival time**

Virus dilution	N	Mortality	Seroconversion	ADD†
10^{-2}	8	8	—	6.2 ± 0.5
10^{-3}	8	6	2	7.5 ± 0.4
10^{-4}	8	2	6	8.5 ± 1.0
10^{-5}	8	0	8	—
10^{-6}	8	0	4	—
10^{-7}	8	0	0	—

*LD50 (based on mortality data) = $10^{3.5}$ per inoculum; ID50 (based on seroconversion) = $10^{6.5}$ per inoculum
†Average days to death ± standard deviation.

passed. LDV is a common contaminant of murine transplantable tumors,[39] but its natural mode of transmission within mouse colonies, if it is indeed transmitted by other than needle injection, is unknown. Cafruny and Hovinen[30] examined the infectivity of the virus for adult random-bred mice after administration by several routes. Infection rates were very high among mice inoculated intraperitoneally or in the cartilage of the tail. In contrast, infection was 4 million times less efficient when virus was administered in the drinking water and 2000 times less efficient after inoculation into the rectum.[30] Efficiencies of oral, vaginal, and ocular inoculations were intermediate between the latter two routes. They postulated that mucosal barriers to LDV infection are formidable and that transmission probably occurs through contamination of open wounds or, perhaps, by vertical means.[30] Other illustrations of route-dependent outcome of infections, emphasizing murine coronaviruses, are shown in Table 20-7.

The natural route of exposure probably involves nasal epithelium, but experimental intranasal inoculation results in artificial infection of the posterior depths of the nasal cavities, where olfactory epithelium is most abundant.

Useful indices of neurovirulence and neuroinvasiveness, based on routes of inoculation, may be found in the bunyavirus literature.[56,92] Neurovirulence is expressed as the ratio of PFU to median lethal dose after intracerebral inoculation.[56] Neuroinvasiveness is similarly expressed after host inoculation by a peripheral route.[92]

PATHOGENESIS EXPERIMENTS IN IMMUNOSUPPRESSED OR GENETICALLY IMMUNODEFICIENT HOSTS

There now exist several models of immunosuppression, some complementary to or confirmatory of others. Chemi-

TABLE 20-7. *Effect of route of inoculation on outcome of virus infection*

Virus	Route	Host age	Host genotype	Outcome	Reference
MHV-2	IP, IV, or IC	Any	(DDD × BALB/c)F1	Acute hepatitis	77
	SC, IN, or PO	Infant	(DDD × BALB/c)F1	Death	77
		≥3 wk	(DDD × BALB/c)F1	Survival	77
MHV-2, -3	IC, IP, or IV	4 wk	Random-bred	<1 PFU killed 50% of mice	76
	IN	4 wk	Random-bred	5 $\log_{10}$ PFU required to kill 50% of mice	76
MHV-JHM, -NuA	IC	4 wk	Random-bred	<1 PFU killed 50% of mice	76
	IP, IV, or IN	4 wk	Random-bred	$4 \times 10^3 - 2 \times 10^6$ PFU required to kill 50% of mice	76
MHV-A59,-Nu66, NuU,-S, -1	IC, IP, IV, or IN	4 wk	Random-bred	Very high doses required to kill 50% of mice	76
MHV-A59	IG, IN, IC, or IP	Young adult	C57BL/6	All developed hepatitis, but higher dose required for disease development after IG or IN inoculation	106
Polytropic MHV	PO	Any	Susceptible	Multisystemic infection excluding brain	S.W. Barthold (unpublished)
	IN	Any	Susceptible	Multisystemic infection with encephalitis	5, 7, 8, 67

MHV, mouse hepatitis virus (coronavirus); IP, intraperitoneal; IV, intravenous; IC, intracerebral; SC, subcutaneous; IN, intranasal; PO, oral; IG, intragastric; PFU, plaque-forming units.

cally-induced immunosuppression offers a quick way to screen various arms of the immune system for roles in spread, clearance, persistence, and so on. Although relatively inexpensive, some of the commonly used chemicals have effects beyond those that may be of interest. For instance, some doses of cyclophosphamide can affect T-cell responses as well as B-cell responses.[169] Investigators have, therefore, become increasingly reliant on the use of mouse mutants to clarify the roles of different immune cells in pathogenesis. The three most commonly used mouse mutants with immunodeficiency are described in this section. However, numerous other mutations of interest have been identified and catalogued.[68,156] Immune cell depletion by injection of antibody to cell surface markers has gained in popularity as hybridoma technology has become more commonplace. Also available now are several knockout mice that can be used to confirm and extend results with mutant or depleted mice. These animals tend to be used sparingly because they are very expensive to produce and maintain in a specific pathogen-free state.

Chemical Immunosuppression

Treatment of animals with cyclophosphamide, corticosteroids, or cyclosporins during the course of viral infection usually leads to more severe disease. For example, intranasal infection of BALB/c mice with murine cytomegalovirus (MCMV) normally yields virus replication in the lung without consistent histopathology. In contrast, mice given a single dose of cyclophosphamide 24 hours after virus inoculation developed interstitial pneumonia 10 to 14 days later.[163] Another study in which mice were given hydrocortisone for 2 days after MCMV infection revealed inhibition of NK cell responses that correlated with enhanced virus replication in spleen and lung and increased susceptibility to lethal infection.[152] Cyclosporin A treatment reduced delayed-type hypersensitivity responses to MCMV in both resistant and susceptible mouse strains to levels seen in control (uninfected) mice.[107] Administration of cyclosporin A had little effect on the susceptibility of susceptible B10 (H-2^b) and resistant B10.BR (H-2^k) mice to the virus. However, cyclosporin A increased the susceptibility of susceptible BALB/c mice (H-2^d) by 100-fold and that of resistant BALB.K mice (H-2^k) by 15-fold.[107]

The effects of immunosuppression may vary depending on timing relative to infection. Virus concentrations in livers of mice given a single dose of cyclophosphamide 2 days before MHV-JHM infection were 5 $\log_{10}$ lower than titers in sham-treated mice but were unaffected if cyclophosphamide was given 2 days after inoculation of the virus.[10] The authors hypothesized that early drug treatment depleted a subset of leukocytes critical to viremic dissemination of virus.

Genetically Immunodeficient Hosts

Athymic Rodents

Wasting disease is a common consequence of virus infection in athymic or nude mice; however, as shown in Table 20-8, athymic mice are capable of clearing some viruses and do not always exhibit clinical signs.

No clinical signs were observed after intraperitoneal inoculation of K papovavirus into athymic mice, in contrast to the fatal outcome in infant or cyclophosphamide-treated mice.[125] The athymic mice mounted a weak immunoglobulin (IgM) response. Transfer of primed cells from athymic mice conferred protection that was apparently mediated by B cells.[125] The role of B cells in papovavirus protection was further confirmed in a study involving high-dose intracerebral inoculation of K virus into athymic mice.[70] Mice in that study developed both IgM and IgG responses and were found capable of limiting systemic virus dissemination but not local progression. Chronically infected athymic mice also sustained infection of renal tubular epithelial cells, a cell type not previously associated with K virus.[70]

No clinical disease was observed after subcutaneous inoculation of avirulent Venezuelan encephalitis virus (VEV) into athymic and BALB/c mice, and viremias were of similar duration and magnitude.[108] In contrast, virulent VEV killed athymic mice earlier despite similar virus concentrations in brain and blood of athymic and normal BALB/c mice.[108] Intraperitoneal inoculation of athymic and euthymic mice with dengue virus resulted in longer survival times in the athymic mice but similar mortality rates.[82] Athymic mice produced only IgM, in contrast to the IgG switch seen with euthymic mice. The initial finding of relatively higher dengue virus concentrations in hearts of athymic mice was confirmed[81] with similar titers in other tissues of immunocompetent and athymic mice.

The herpesvirus, mouse thymic virus, infects and kills developing T cells in the thymus of infant mice and causes a persistent infection with regular shedding in salivary secretions. Only about 20% of athymic mice infected as young adults with mouse thymic virus shed virus in saliva,[128] confirming the preferential T cell tropism (or even T cell requirement) of this virus. Another mouse herpesvirus, MCMV, has been studied in athymic mice in order to evaluate antiviral drug efficacy.[33] Most untreated athymic mice developed polytropic infection and died within 3 weeks after inoculation. Administration of acyclovir starting 1 day after infection resulted in dramatically reduced lesion scores and complete protection from mortality.[33] Another study emphasized adrenal involvement after MCMV infection of athymic mice and protection by acyclovir administered in drinking water.[165]

Beige Mice

The *beige* mouse mutation yields a phenotype similar to that of Chediak-Higashi syndrome of humans, a recessive mutation resulting in lowered resistance to infection because of dysfunction of NK cells, CTLs, and granulocytes.[15] Experiments using beige mice must be interpreted with some caution, because, in addition to impaired NK cell function, these mice generate CTLs with reduced lytic capacity but in expanded numbers.[15] Viruses that have been studied in beige mice include but are not limited to Sindbis virus,[78] MHV,[123] MCMV,[140] and Theiler's mouse encephalomyelitis virus.[143] Virus infection of beige mice frequently yields exacerbated

TABLE 20-8. *Use of athymic rodents in viral pathogenesis studies*

Virus	Mutant host	Outcome	Reference
MAdV-1	Athymic mice	Wasting, duodenal hemorrhage	211
Polyoma virus	Athymic mice	Wasting, demyelinating disease, hind-leg paralysis	116, 162
MHV	Athymic mice	Wasting, production of neutralizing antibody, expression of T cell markers on thymus-derived cells	14, 57, 161, 194
PVM	Athymic mice	"Terminal emaciation"; absence of necrotizing bronchiolitis characteristically seen in immunocompetent mice	154, 205
LCMV	Athymic mice	Chronic, subclinical infection; zoonotic hazard	54
Sindbis virus	Athymic mice	Clinical outcome and central nervous system clearance identical to response of immuno-competent mice	79
Sendai virus	Athymic rats	Persistent infection; extensive interstitial necrosis	34
SDAV	Athymic rats	Persistent infection; chronic inflammation; viral antigen in abnormal sites (renal pelvis, urinary bladder); low-level seroconversion	206
Papovavirus	Athymic rats	Wasting, sialoadenitis	203
Rat parvovirus	Athymic rats	Subclinical persistent infection with low-level virus-specific IgG production	59, 60

MAdV, mouse adenovirus; MHV, mouse hepatitis virus (coronavirus); PVM, pneumonia virus of mice (pneumovirus); LCMV, lymphocytic choriomeningitis virus (arenavirus); SDAV, sialodacryoadenitis virus (coronavirus).

infection without altered tissue distribution; however, Sindbis virus infection was not changed in comparison to its presentation in fully immunocompetent mice.[78]

Mice With Severe Combined Immunodeficiency

The murine severe combined immunodeficiency (*SCID*) mutation was recognized in 1980 by Bosma and colleagues at the Fox Chase Cancer Center and has served as a model for human severe combined immunodeficiency, first recognized in 1950.[16] The mouse mutation arose in C.B-17 mice that are congenic with BALB/cAn mice, differing only at the IgH locus on chromosome 12.[2,46,168] Mice of several genotypes now bear the SCID mutation, which is on chromosome 16. T-cell development is arrested at 14 to 15 days gestational age, and 98% of T cells are CD4− and CD8−. A small fraction of cells do express CD2 and CD3. B cells are arrested at the pro-B stage, before the expression of cytoplasmic or surface immunoglobulin. Myeloid and erythroid lineages are unaffected, and these mice have normal or elevated NK cell function.[2,104] The B- and T-cell deficiencies can be corrected by grafting bone marrow or fetal liver cells from normal BALB/c mice into adult C.B-17 SCID mice.[16] Full reconstitution requires sublethal irradiation before cell transfer. There is a very large literature concentrating on viral pathogenesis in SCID mice, and the ability to produce xenogeneic chimeric mice has permitted the study of human agents for which no small animal models had previously been available.

A problem that has received increasing attention is the fact that SCID mice tend to be "leaky"; that is, a proportion have detectable, or even normal, levels of serum immunoglobulin.[136] The SCID mutation has been introduced into several inbred mouse strains, and 79% of C.B-17 SCID mice were shown to have detectable serum IgG, whereas only 15% of C3H SCID mice had serum IgG.[136] In addition, higher proportions of aged C.B-17 SCID mice had IgG, whereas a similar increase was not seen among aged C3H mice. Because of the incomplete penetrance or "leakiness" of the SCID mutation and the fact that the mutation is not lymphoid specific but affects a general DNA repair pathway, there is concern that these mice may not be the optimal model for study of human disease.[73] The SCID mutation has been combined with other immunodeficiency mutations in attempts to improve the model. One such combination on which there is increasing emphasis is the SCID/beige mouse, which lacks functional B, T, and NK cells.[73] Only 3% of these mice are reportedly leaky.[73] RAG-1 and RAG-2 knockout mice, which completely lack functional B and T cells and have a 10- to 100-fold decrease in absolute cell numbers in spleen and thymus, may replace SCID mice as model immunodeficient rodents.[73]

Despite its shortcomings, the SCID mouse has clarified the role of virus, as opposed to the immune response itself, in the pathology of several infections. For instance, coxsackievirus B3 was reported to cause severe cardiomyocyte injury in SCID mice,[36,37] leading to the conclusion that the effect is direct and not immune mediated. The general finding in most studies comparing virus infections in SCID and normal mice has been that infection is either persistent or fatal in the immunocompromised hosts. LDV causes persistent infection of both immunocompetent and SCID mice.[20] Infection of *Pneumocystis carinii*–free SCID mice with pneumonia virus of mice resulted in mild clinical signs (ruffled fur) at 2 months, despite very high lung virus titers.[18] In contrast, SCID mice chronically infected with *P carinii* died 1 month after infection with pneumonia virus of mice, apparently the result of exacerbated *P carinii* disease.[18,158]

As with virus infections of athymic rodents, infections of SCID mice tend to be chronic or persistent. Several studies have addressed the role of immune cells or subsets thereof in protection of SCID mice against virus infection, disease, or mortality (Table 20-9). SCID mice have also provided models for some human diseases (see Table 20-9). For example, intraperitoneal inoculation of C.B-17 SCID mice with mouse adenovirus-1 yielded a model for Reye's syndrome that included the mitochondrial swelling and microvesicular fatty degenerative liver changes that are hallmarks of this disease in children.[150]

SCID mice engrafted with xenogeneic tissues have been used to study the pathogenesis of many virus infections, most commonly human herpesviruses and human immunodeficiency virus (HIV). SCID mice implanted with human fetal liver and thymus support human T-cell and B-cell differentiation, including a transient wave of human CD4+ and CD8+ T cells and human IgG production.[117] Human tonsil cells or peripheral blood lymphocytes from donors who were seronegative for Epstein-Barr virus (EBV) were implanted in C.B-17 SCID mice that were then injected with EBV. These mice developed an aggressive lymphoproliferative disorder of human B-cell origin within 19 to 33 days.[31] In other studies, SCID mice have been implanted with tonsillar mononuclear cells or peripheral blood lymphocytes from EBV-seropositive donors.[131,159] Twenty-nine percent of mice receiving tonsillar tissue developed tumors of human origin that had the appearance of large cell lymphomas and contained EBV genome and antigen.[136] Peripheral blood lymphocytes from seropositive donors also resulted in B-cell tumors that did not resemble Burkitt's lymphoma.[159]

Human cytomegalovirus (HCMV) pathogenesis has also been studied and antiviral drug efficiency evaluated in SCID mice bearing human fetal thymus and liver implants.[124] Virus-positive cells were localized to thymic medulla, and HCMV antigen was found in epithelial but not hematopoietic cells. Gangcyclovir treatment resulted in decreased HCMV replication.[124]

SCID mice implanted with human fetal thymus or lymph node cells supported replication of HIV-1, with infection more apparent in medulla than in cortical areas.[132] In a study comparing the pathogenesis of macrophage-tropic and T-cell–tropic HIV isolates in SCID mice implanted with human peripheral blood lymphocytes, it was noted that the former virus resulted in loss of CD4+ T cells, whereas the latter did not.[129] Subsequently, attempts have been made to reproduce features of the AIDS dementia complex using SCID mice inoculated intracerebrally with human peripheral blood mononuclear cells; either the cells were preinfected with HIV or the mice were inoculated intracerebrally with HIV 1 day later.[198] Thirteen of 33 mice contained recoverable infectious virus and p24 antigen detected by immunohistochemistry. Despite

TABLE 20-9. *Viral pathogenesis studies in mice bearing the severe combined immunodeficiency (SCID) mutation*

Virus	Manipulation	Outcome	Reference
Reovirus 1 or 3	None	Pantropic infection with mortality 4–6 weeks after oral inoculation	63
Reovirus 1 or 3	Transfer of Peyer's patch cells	Protection	63
EDIM virus	None	Subclinical chronic infection and virus excretion	155
EDIM virus	Transfer of immune CD8+ T cells	Viral clearance, the duration of which depended of route of immunization	51
HSV-1	None	Pantropic infection with death less than 3 weeks after intracutaneous infection; immunocompetent mice support replication only locally and in central nervous system	122
HSV-1	Transfer of immune spleen cells	Protection	122
Sindbis virus	None	Persistent infection of brain and spinal cord following intracerebral inoculation	110
Sindbis virus	Transfer of hyperimmune virus-specific antibody	Viral clearance	110
Sindbis virus	Transfer of sensitized T cells	No effect (i.e., persistent central nervous system infection)	110
Rhesus monkey rotavirus	None	Fourfold increase in prevalence of hepatitis after oral inoculation (compared with immunocompetent mice)	199
Sendai virus	None	Uniformly lethal infection with viral antigen persisting in respiratory tract	145, 146
MHV	None	High morbidity and mortality	146
PVM	None	High morbidity and mortality	42, 146

EDIM, epizootic diarrhea of infant mice (rotavirus); HSV, herpes simplex virus; MHV, mouse hepatitis virus (coronavirus); PVM, pneumonia virus of mice (pneumovirus).

the variability of the model, this is an encouraging step toward reproduction of HIV-associated encephalopathy.

Cell Depletion by Serotherapy

The roles of various lymphoid cells in viral pathogenesis have been studied in mice depleted of cells by administration of antibodies to specific cell surface markers. This approach, using antibody to a neutral glycosphingolipid, asialoGM$_1$, has shown that NK cells play a critical role in MHV, MCMV, herpes simplex virus-1, vaccinia virus, and ectromelia virus infections, but no overwhelming role in either acute or persistent LCMV infection.[27,28,72,88] When an effect has been shown, it usually has consisted of infectability with lower virus doses, increased mortality, or enhanced virus titers in target organs.[27,28,72,88] In the case of an enterotropic isolate of MHV, treatment with anti-asialoGM$_1$ enhanced persistence of virus in the intestine.[32] This effect was caused by an NK-like cell that constituted a small subpopulation of intraepithelial leukocytes. Studies that have used anti-asialoGM$_1$ should be interpreted with caution, however, because treatment also diminishes virus-specific CTL activity by 60% to 95%.[187] Another antibody, anti-NK1.1, is being used with increasing frequency because it is more specific for NK cells, but it can be used only in mouse strains that have NK cells bearing this marker.[208] Use of this antibody supported a role for NK cells in infections with MCMV and Pichinde virus, but not MHV or LCMV.[160,164,201,208]

The relative roles of T-cell subsets in viral pathogenesis have been studied using three complementary approaches. These include, in order of development, adoptive transfer of cells enriched in vitro, in vivo depletion using monoclonal antibodies specific for surface molecules, and knockout mice (see Chap. 21). Mice depleted of CD4+ T cells were capable of clearing influenza A virus from the respiratory tract.[1] Similarly, Sendai virus clearance from mouse lung was relatively unaffected in CD4+ T cell–depleted mice, whereas clearance was delayed among CD8+ T cell–depleted mice.[83] Simultaneous depletion led to delayed Sendai virus clearance and death; however, most mice depleted of only CD8+ T cells survived the infection. In contrast, clearance of MHV-JHM from the central nervous system after intracerebral inoculation was shown to depend on the presence of both CD4+ and CD8+ T cells,[210] although clearance of MHV-JHM from intracerebrally inoculated rats required only CD4+ T cells.[103] CD4+ T cell–depleted mice infected with vaccinia or LCMV had CTL activities that were fivefold to 15-fold reduced compared with controls,[109] and this function was partly corrected by administration of recombinant interleukin-2. Intraperitoneal inoculation of BALB/c mice with Semliki Forest virus, strain A7,[74] resulted in primary demyelination that was dependent on activated T cells. Depletion of CD4+ T cells in this model yielded increased virus replication and demyelination, whereas CD8+ T-cell depletion reduced CNS inflammation and eliminated demyelination.[189]

In another neurotropic virus model system, depletion of CD4+ T cells reversed the resistance of SJL and BALB/c mice and inhibited production of neutralizing antibody to street rabies virus infection after intraperitoneal inoculation,

whereas CD8+ T-cell depletion had no detectable effect on the infection.[148] In another model in which the contribution of CD8+ T cells had usually been thought to be essential, MCMV was eliminated with normal kinetics by mice depleted of CD8+ T cells.[95,98] A murine gammaherpesvirus originally isolated from wild bank voles in Europe required CD8+ T cells for BALB/c mice to recover, but CD4+ T cells were shown to be a major component of the splenomegaly that is a hallmark of the infection.[55]

SUMMARY

Although by no means exhaustive, this chapter is intended to make the reader aware of the many virus and host factors that can influence the outcome of pathogenesis experiments, sometimes in unexpected ways. The methods described yield information that complements and extends data obtained with the use of molecular tools and genetically modified hosts, which are described in Chapters 19 and 21.

ACKNOWLEDGEMENTS

Preparation of this chapter was supported in part by NIH grants RR04507 and RR00393. The assistance of Valeria Krizsan with manuscript preparation is greatly appreciated.

ABBREVIATIONS

CTL: cytotoxic T lymphocyte
EBV: Epstein-Barr virus
EDTA: ethylenediamine tetraacetic acid
ELISA: enzyme-linked immunosorbent assay
FFU: focus-forming units
HCMV: human cytomegalovirus
HIV: human immunodeficiency virus
ID50: median infectious dose
IFN-α, IFN-β, IFN-γ: interferons
IgG, IgM: immunoglobulins
LCMV: lymphocytic choriomeningitis virus
LD50: median lethal dose
LDV: lactate dehydrogenase elevating virus
MCMV: murine cytomegalovirus
MHV-JHM: mouse hepatitis virus, strain JHM
PFU: plaque-forming units
PLP: periodate-lysine-paraformaldehyde
TCID50: median tissue culture infectious dose
VEV: Venezuelan encephalitis virus

REFERENCES

1. Allen W, Tabi ZS, Cleary A, Doherty PC. Cellular events in the lymph node and lung of mice with influenza. Consequences of depleting CD4+ T cells. J Immunol 1990;144:3980–3986.
2. Ansel JD, Bancroft GJ. The biology of the SCID mutation. Immunol Today 1989;10:322–325.
3. Baer GM, Cleary WF. A model in mice for the pathogenesis and treatment of rabies. J Infect Dis 1972;125:520–527.

4. Bang FB, Warwick A. Mouse macrophages as host cells for the mouse hepatitis virus and the genetic basis of their susceptibility. Proc Natl Acad Sci U S A 1960;46:1065–1075.

5. Barthold SW, Beck DS, Smith AL. Mouse hepatitis virus nasoencephalopathy is dependent upon virus strain and host genotype. Arch Virol 1986;91:247–256.

6. Barthold SW, Beck DS, Smith AL. Enterotropic coronavirus (mouse hepatitis virus) in mice: influence of host age and strain on infection and disease. Lab Anim Sci 1993;43:276–284.

7. Barthold SW, Smith AL. Mouse hepatitis virus S in weanling Swiss mice following intranasal inoculation. Lab Anim Sci 1983;33:355–360.

8. Barthold SW, Smith AL. Response of genetically susceptible and resistant mice to intranasal inoculation with mouse hepatitis virus JHM. Virus Res 1987;7:225–239.

9. Barthold SW, Smith AL. Virus strain specificity of challenge immunity to coronavirus. Arch Virol 1989;104:187–196.

10. Barthold SW, Smith AL. Duration of mouse hepatitis virus infection: studies in immunocompetent and chemically immunosuppressed mice. Lab Anim Sci 1990;40:133–137.

11. Barthold, SW, Smith AL. Viremic dissemination of mouse hepatitis virus JHM following intranasal inoculation of mice. Arch Virol 1992;122:35–44.

12. Barthold SW, Smith AL. Role of host age and genotype in murine enterotropic coronavirus infection. In: Laude H, Vautherot JF, eds. Coronaviruses: molecular biology and pathogenesis. New York: Plenum, 1993:371–376.

13. Barthold SW, Smith AL, Bhatt PN. Infectivity, disease patterns, and serologic profiles of reovirus serotypes 1, 2, and 3 in infant and weanling mice. Lab Anim Sci 1993;43:425–430.

14. Barthold SW, Smith AL, Povar ML. Enterotropic mouse hepatitis virus infection in nude mice. Lab Anim Sci 1985;35:613–618.

15. Biron CA, Pedersen KF, Welsh RM. Aberrant T cells in beige mutant mice. J Immunol 1987;138:2050–2056.

16. Bosma MJ. The scid mutation: occurrence and effect. Curr Top Microbiol Immunol 1989;152:3–9.

17. Boucher DW, Hayashi K, Rosenthal J, Notkins AL. Virus-induced diabetes mellitus. III. Influence of the sex and strain of the host. J Infect Dis 1975;131:462–466.

18. Bray MV, Barthold SW, Sidman CL, Roths J, Smith AL. Exacerbation of Pneumocystis carinii pneumonia in immunodeficient (scid) mice by concurrent infection with a pneumovirus. Infect Immunol 1993;61:1586–1588.

19. Brinton MA. Analysis of extracellular West Nile virus particles produced by cell cultures from genetically resistant and susceptible mice indicates enhanced amplification of defective interfering particles by resistant cultures. J Virol 1983;46:860–870.

20. Broen JB, Bradley DS, Powell KM, Cafruny WA. Regulation of maternal-fetal virus transmission in immunologically reconstituted SCID mice infected with lactate dehydrogenase-elevating virus. Viral Immunol 1992;5:133–140.

21. Brownstein DG, Barthold SW. Mouse hepatitis virus immunofluorescence in formalin- or Bouin's-fixed tissues using trypsin digestion. Lab Anim Sci 1982;32:37–39.

22. Brownstein DG, Bhatt PN, Gras L, Budris T. Serial backcross analysis of genetic resistance to mousepox, using marker loci for Rmp-2 and Rmp-3. J Virol 1992;66:7073–7079.

23. Brownstein DG, Bhatt PN, Gras L, Jacoby RO. Chromosomal locations and gonadal dependence of genes that mediate resistance to ectromelia (mousepox) virus-induced mortality. J Virol 1991;65:1946–1951.

24. Brownstein DG, Bhatt PN, Jacoby RO. Mousepox in inbred mice innately resistant or susceptible to lethal infection with ectromelia virus. V. Genetics of resistance to the Moscow strain. Arch Virol 1989;107:35–41.

25. Brownstein DG, Smith AL, Jacoby RO, Johnson EA, Hansen G, Tattersall P. Pathogenesis of infection with a virulent allotropic variant of minute virus of mice and regulation by host genotype. Lab Invest 1991;65:357–364.

26. Brownstein DG, Smith AL, Johnson EA. Sendai virus infection in genetically resistant and susceptible mice. Am J Pathol 1981;105:156–163.

27. Bukowski JF, Woda BA, Habu S, Okumura K, Welsh RM. Natural killer cell depletion enhances virus synthesis and virus-induced hepatitis in vivo. J Immunol 1983;131:1531–1538.

28. Bukowski JF, Woda BA, Welsh RM. Pathogenesis of murine cytomegalovirus infection in natural killer cell-depleted mice. J Virol 1984;52:119–128.

29. Burrage TG, Tignor GH, Smith AL. Rabies virus binding at neuromuscular junctions. Virus Res 1985;2:273–289.

30. Cafruny WA, Hovinen DE. The relationship between route of infection and minimum infectious dose: studies with lactate dehydrogenase-elevating virus. J Virol Methods 1988;20:265–268.

31. Cannon MJ, Pisa P, Fox RI, Cooper NR. Epstein-Barr virus induces aggressive lymphoproliferative disorders of human B cell origin in SCID/hu chimeric mice. J Clin Invest 1990;85:1333–1337.

32. Carman PS, Ernst PB, Rosenthal KL, Clark DA, Befus AD, Bienenstock J. Intraepithelial leukocytes contain a unique subpopulation of NK-like cytotoxic cells active in the defense of gut epithelium to enteric murine coronavirus. J Immunol 1986;136:1548–1553.

33. Carthew P. Therapeutic effect of acyclovir (Zovirax™) on the pathogenesis of chronic murine cytomegalovirus infection in the immunodeficient nude mouse. Br J Exp Path 1982;63:625–632.

34. Carthew P, Sparrow S. Sendai virus in nude and germ-free rats. Res Vet Sci 1980;29:289–292.

35. Casebolt DB, Spalding DM, Schoeb TR, Lindsey JR. Suppression of immune response induction in Peyer's patch lymphoid cells from mice infected with mouse hepatitis virus. Cell Immunol 1987;109:97–103.

36. Chow LH. Studies of virus-induced myocardial injury in mice: value of the scid mutation on different genetic backgrounds and combined with other mutations. Lab Anim Sci 1993;43:133–135.

37. Chow LH, Beisel KW, McManus BM. Enteroviral infection of mice with severe combined immunodeficiency: evidence for direct viral pathogenesis of myocardial injury. Lab Invest 1992;66:24–31.

38. Collins AR, Tunison LA, Knobler RL. Mouse hepatitis virus tpe 4 infection of primary glial cultures from genetically susceptible and resistant mice. Infect Immun 1983;40:1192–1197.

39. Collins MJ Jr, Parker JC. Murine virus contaminants of leukemia viruses and transplantable tumors. J Natl Cancer Inst 1972;49:1139–1143.

40. Compton SR, Barthold SW, Smith AL. The cellular and molecular pathogenesis of coronaviruses. Lab Anim Sci 1993;43:15–28.

41. Cook-Mills JM, Munshi HG, Perlman RL, Chambers DA. Mouse hepatitis virus infection suppresses modulation of mouse spleen T-cell activation. Immunology 1992;75:542–545.

42. Copps JS, Percy DH, Croy BA, MacInnis JI, Stirtzinger T. Comparison of lesions in the respiratory tract of scid and scid/bg mice infected with pneumonia virus of mice (PVM). Lab Anim Sci 1993;43:163–164.

43. Coutelier J-P, van der Logt JTM, Heessen FWA, Vink A, van Snick J. Virally induced modulation of murine IgG antibody subclasses. J Exp Med 1988;168:2373–2378.

44. Coutelier J-P, van der Logt JTM, Heessen FWA, Warnier G, van Snick J. IgG 2a restriction of murine antibodies elicited by viral infections. J Exp Med 1987;165:64–69.

45. Cray C, Mateo MO, Altman NH. In vitro and long-term in vivo immune dysfunction after infection of BALB/c mice with mouse hepatitis virus strain A59. Lab Anim Sci 1993;43:169–174.

46. Custer RP, Bosma GC, Bosma MJ. Severe combined immunodeficiency (SCID) in the mouse: pathology, reconstitution, neoplasms. Am J Pathol 1985;120:464–477.

47. Darnell MB, Koprowski H. Genetically determined resistance to infection with group B arboviruses. II. Increased production of interfering particles in cell cultures from resistant mice. J Infect Dis 1974;129:248–256.

48. de Souza MS, Smith AL. Comparison of isolation in cell culture with conventional and modified mouse antibody production tests for detection of murine viruses. J Clin Microbiol 1989;27:185–187.

49. de Souza MS, Smith AL. Characterization of accessory cell function during acute infection of BALB/cByJ mice with mouse hepatitis virus (MHV), strain JHM. Lab Anim Sci 1991;41:112–118.

50. de Souza MS, Smith AL, Bottomly K. Infection of BALB/cByJ mice with the JHM strain of mouse hepatitis virus alters in vitro splenic T cell proliferation and cytokine production. Lab Anim Sci 1991;41:99–105.

51. Dharakui T, Rott IU, Greenberg HB. Recovery from chronic rotavirus infection in mice with severe combined immunodeficiency: virus clearance mediated by adoptive transfer of immune CD8+ T lymphocytes. J Virol 1990;64:4375–4382.

52. Dillberger JE, Monroy P, Altman NH. The effect of three bleeding techniques on lactic dehydrogenase levels in mice: implications for lactic dehydrogenase virus bioassay. Lab Anim Sci 1987;37:356–359.

53. Dupuy JM, Levey-Leblond E, Le Prevost C. Immunopathology of mouse hepatitis virus type 3 infection. II. Effect of immunosuppression in resistant mice. J Immunol 1975;114:226–230.

54. Dykewicz CA, Dato VM, Fisher-Hoch SP, et al. Lymphocytic choriomeningitis outbreak associated with nude mice in a research institute. JAMA 1992;267:1349–1353.

55. Ehtisham S, Sunil-Chandra NP, Nash AA. Pathogenesis of murine gammaherpesvirus infection in mice deficient in CD4 and CD8 T cells. J Virol 1993;67:5247–5252.

56. Endres MJ, Valsamakis A, Gonzalez-Scarano F, Nathanson N. Neuroattenuated bunyavirus variant: derivation, characterization, and revertant clones. J Virol 1990;64:1927–1933.

57. Fujiwara K. Persistent mouse hepatitis virus infection in nude mice. Jpn J Exp Med 1988;58:115–121.

58. Gaertner DJ, Jacoby RO, Johnson EA, Paturzo FX, Smith AL, Brandsma JL. Characterization of acute rat parvovirus infection by in situ hybridization. Virus Res 1993;28:1–18.

59. Gaertner DJ, Jacoby RO, Paturzo FX, Johnson EA, Brandsma JL, Smith AL. Modulation of lethal and persistent rat parvovirus infection by antibody. Arch Virol 1991;118:1–9.

60. Gaertner DJ, Jacoby RO, Smith AL, Ardito RB, Paturzo FX. Persistence of rat parvovirus in athymic rats. Arch Virol 1989;105:259–268.

61. Garlinghouse LE Jr, Smith AL. Responses of mice susceptible or resistant to lethal infection with mouse hepatitis viurs, strain JHM, after exposure by a natural route. Lab Anim Sci 1985;35:469–472.

62. Genovesi EV, Johnson AJ, Peters CJ. Susceptibility and resistance of inbred strains of Syrian golden hamsters (*Mesocricetus auratus*) to wasting disease caused by lymphocytic choriomeningitis virus: pathogenesis of lethal and non-lethal infections. J Gen Virol 1988;69:2209–2220.

63. George A, Kost SI, Witzleben CL, Cebra JJ, Rubin DH. Reovirus-induced liver disease in severe combined immunodeficient (SCID) mice: a model for the study of viral infection, pathogenesis, and clearance. J Exp Med 1990;171:929–934.

64. Giron DJ, Patterson RR. Effect of steroid hormones on virus-induced diabetes mellitus. Infect Immun 1982;37:820–822.

65. Gonzales-Scarano F, Tyler KL. Molecular pathogenesis of neurotropic viral infections. Ann Neurol 1987;22:565–574.

66. Goodpasture EW. A study of rabies with reference to neural transmission of the virus in rabbits and the structure and significance of Negri bodies. Am J Path 1925;1:547–582.

67. Goto N, Hirano N, Aiuchi M, Hayashi T, Fujiwara K. Nasoencephalopathy of mice infected intranasally with a mouse hepatitis virus, JHM strain. Jpn J Exp Med 1977;47:59–70.

68. Green MC, Witham BA, eds. Handbook on genetically standardized JAX mice. 4th ed. Bar Harbor, Maine: The Jackson Laboratory, 1991.

69. Greenlee JE. Effect of host age on experimental K virus infection in mice. Infect Immun 1981;33:297–3.

70. Greenlee JE. Chronic infection of nude mice by murine K papovavirus. J Gen Virol 1986;67:1109–1114.

71. Groschel D, Koprowski H. Development of virus-resistant inbred mouse strain for the study of innate resistance to arbo B viruses. Arch Gesamte Virusforsch 1965;17:379–391.

72. Habu S, Akamatsu K-I, Tamaoki N, Okumura K. In vivo significance of NK cell on resistance against virus (HSV-1) infections in mice. J Immunol 1984;133:2743–2747.

73. Hendrickson EA. The SCID mouse: relevance as an animal model system for studying human disease. Am J Pathol 1993;143:1511–1522.

74. Hierholzer JC, Broderson JR, Murphy FA. New strain of mouse hepatitis virus as the cause of lethal enteritis in infant mice. Infect Immun 1979;24:508–522.

75. Hirano N, Goto N, Ogawa T, Ono K, Murakami T, Fujiwara K. Hydrocephalus in suckling rats infected intracerebrally with mouse hepatitis virus, MHV-A59. Microbiol Immunol 1980;24:825–834.

76. Hirano N, Murakami T, Fujiwara K, Matumoto M. Comparison of mouse hepatitis virus strains for pathogenicity in weanling mice infected by various routes. Arch Virol 1981;70:69–73.

77. Hirano N, Takenaka S, Fujiwara K. Pathogenicity of mouse hepatitis virus for mice depending upon host age and route of infection. Jpn J Exp Med 1975;45:285–292.

78. Hirsch RL. Natural killer cells appear to play no role in the recovery of mice from Sindbis virus infection. Immunology 1981;43:81–89.

79. Hirsch RL, Griffin DE. The pathogenesis of Sindbis virus infection in athymic nude mice. J Immunol 1979;123:1215–1218.

80. Homberger FR, Barthold SW, Smith AL. Duration and strain-specificity of immunity to enterotropic mouse hepatitis virus. Lab Anim Sci 1992;42:347–351.

81. Hotta H, Murakami I, Miyasaki K, Takeda Y. Localization of Dengue virus in nude mice. Microbiol Immunol 1981;25:89–93.

82. Hotta H, Murakami I, Miyasaki K, Takeda Y, Shirane H, Hotta S. Inoculation of Dengue virus into nude mice. J Gen Virol 1981;52:71–76.

83. Hou S, Doherty PC, Zijlstra M, Jaenisch R, Katz JM. Delayed clearance of Sendai virus in mice lacking class I MHC-restricted CD8 + T cell. J Immunol 1992;149:1319–1325.

84. Huber SA, Job LP, Auld KR. Influence of sex hormones on Coxsackie B-3 virus infection in Balb/c mice. Cell Immunol 1982;67:173–189.

85. Huber SA, Job LP, Woodruff JF. Sex-related differences in the pattern of coxsackievirus B-3–induced immune spleen cell cytotoxicity against virus-infected myofibers. Infect Immun 1981;32:68–73.

86. Huber SA, Pfaeffle B. Differential Th$_1$ and Th$_2$ cell responses in male and female BALB/c mice infected with coxsackievirus group B type 3. J Virol 1994;68:5126–5132.

87. Jacoby RO, Bhatt PN. Mousepox in inbred mice innately resistant or susceptible to lethal infection with ectromelia virus. II. Pathogenesis. Lab Anim Sci 1987;37:16–22.

88. Jacoby RO, Bhatt PN, Brownstein DG. Evidence that NK cells and interferon are required for genetic resistance to lethal infection with ectromelia virus. Arch Virol 1989;108:49–58.

89. Jacoby RO, Bhatt PN, Gaertner DJ, Smith AL, Johnson EA. The pathogenesis of rat virus infection in infant and juvenile rats after oronasal infection. Arch Virol 1987;95:251–270.

90. Jacoby RO, Johnson EA, Paturzo FX, Gaertner DJ, Brandsma JL, Smith AL. Persistent rat virus infection in individually housed rats. Arch Virol 1991;117:193–205.

91. Janeway CA, Travers P. Immunobiology: the immune system in health and disease. New York: Garland, 1994.

92. Janssen RS, Nathanson N, Endres MJ, Gonzalez-Scarano F. Virulence of LaCrosse virus is under polygenic control. J Virol 1986;59:1–7.

93. Johnson RT. The pathogenesis of herpes virus encephalitis. I. Virus pathways to the nervous system of suckling mice demonstrated by fluorescent antibody staining. J Exp Med 1964;119:343–356.

94. Johnson RT. The pathogenesis of experimental rabies. In: Nogano Y, Davenport FM, eds. Rabies. Baltimore: University Park Press, 1969;59–75.

95. Johnson RT, McFarland HF, Levy SE. Age-dependent resistance to viral encephalitis: studies of infections due to Sindbis virus in mice. J Infect Dis 1972;125:257–262.

96. Johnson RT, Mims CA. Pathogenesis of viral infections of the nervous system. N Engl J Med 1968;278:23–30.

97. Johnson RT, Mims CA. Pathogenesis of viral infections of the nervous system. N Engl J Med 1968;278:84–92.

98. Jonjic S, Pavic I, Lucin P, Rukavina D, Koszinowski UH. Efficacious control of cytomegalovirus infection after long-term depletion of CD8 + T lymphocytes. J Virol 1990;64:5457–5464.

99. Kappel CA, Melvold RW, Kim BS. Influence of sex on susceptibility in the Theiler's murine encephalomyelitis virus model for multiple sclerosis. J Neuroimmunol 1990;29:15–19.

100. Kascsak RJ, Carp RI, Donnenfeld H, Bartfeld H. Kinetics of replication of latate dehydrogenase-elevating virus in age-dependent polioencephalomyelitis. Intervirology 1983;19:6–15.

101. Klavinskis LS, Oldstone MB. Lymphocytic choriomeningitis virus selectively alters differentiated but not housekeeping functions: block in expression of growth hormone gene is at the level of transcriptional initiation. Virology 1989;168:232–235.

102. Knobler RL, Haspel MV, Oldstone MBA. Mouse hepatitis virus type 4 (JHM strain)-induced fatal central nervous system disease. I. Genetic control and the murine neuron as the susceptible site of disease. J Exp Med 1981;153:832–843.

103. Korner H, Schliephake A, Winter J, et al. Nucleocapsid or spike protein-specific CD4+ T lymphocytes protect against coronavirus-induced encephalomyelitis in the absence of CD8+ T cells. J Immunol 1991;147:2317–2323.

104. Kumar V, Hackett J Jr, Tutt MM, et al. Natural killer cells and their precursors in mice with severe combined immunodeficiency. Curr Top Microbiol Immunol 1989;152:47–52.

105. Kyuwa S, Yamaguchi K, Toyoda Y, Fujiwara K, Hilgers J. Acute and late disease induced by murine coronavirus, strain JHM, in a series of recombinant inbred strains between BALB/cHeA and STS/A mice. Microb Pathog 1992;12:95–104.

106. Lavi E, Gilden DH, Highkin MK, Weiss SR. The organ tropism of mouse hepatitis virus A59 in mice is dependent on dose and route of inoculation. Lab Anim Sci 1986;36:130–135.

107. Lawson CM, Hodgkin PD, Shellam GR. The effect of cyclosporin on major histocompatibility complex-linked resistance to murine cytomegalovirus. J Gen Virol 1989;70:1253–1259.

108. LeBlanc PA, Scherer WF, Sussdorf DH. Infections of congenitally athymic (nude) and normal mice with avirulent and virulent strains of Venezuelan encephalitis virus. Infect Immun 1978;21:779–785.

109. Leist TP, Kohler M, Zinkernagel RM. Impaired generation of antiviral cytotoxicity against lymphocytic choriomeningitis and vaccinia virus in mice treated with CD4-specific monoclonal antibody. Scand J Immunol 1989;30:679–686.

110. Levine B, Hardwick JM, Trapp BD, Crawford TO, Bollinger RC, Griffin DE. Antibody-mediated clearance of alphavirus infection from neurons. Science 1991;254:856–860.

111. Lodmell DL, Ewalt LC. Pathogenesis of street rabies virus infections in resistant and susceptible strains of mice. J Virol 1985;55:788–795.

112. Lorenz RJ, Bogel K. Calculation of titers and their significance. In: Kaplan M, Koprowski H, eds. Laboratory techniques in rabies. Geneva: World Health Organization, 1973:321–335.

113. Lyden DC, Olszewski J, Feran M, Job LP, Huber SA. Coxsackievirus B-3–induced myocarditis: effect of sex steroids on viremia and infectivity of cardiocytes. Am J Pathol 1987;126:432–438.

114. Lyden D, Olszewski J, Huber S. Variation in susceptibility of Balb/c mice to coxsackievirus group B type 3-induced myocarditis with age. Cellular Immunol 1987;105:332–339.

115. Macnaughton MR, Patterson S. Mouse hepatitis virus strain 3 infection of C57, A/Sn and A/J strain mice and their macrophages. Arch Virol 1980;66:71–75.

116. McCance DJ, Sebesteny A, Griffin BE, Balkwill F, Tilly R, Gregson NA. A paralytic disease in nude mice associated with polyoma virus infection. J Gen Virol 1983;64:57–67.

117. McCune JM, Namikawa R, Kaneshima H, Shultz LD, Lieberman M, Weissman IL. The SCID-hu mouse: murine model for the analysis of human hematolymphoid differentiation and function. Science 1988;241:1632–1639.

118. McFarland HI, Bigley NJ. Sex-dependent, early cytokine production by NK-like spleen cells following infection with the D variant of encephalomyocarditis virus (EMCV-D). Viral Immunol 1989;2:205–214.

119. McKisic, MD, Lancki DW, Otto G, et al. Identification and propagation of a putative immunosuppressive orphan parvovirus in cloned T cells. J Immunol 1993;150:419–428.

120. McLean IW, Makane PK. Periodate-lysine-paraformaldehyde fixative: a new fixative for immunoelectron microscopy. J Histochem Cytochem 1974;22:1077–1083.

121. Mercer JA, Spector DH. Pathogenesis of acute murine cytomegalovirus infection in resistant and susceptible strains of mice. J Virol 1986;57:497–504.

122. Minagawa H, Sakuma S, Mohri S, Mori R, Watanabe T. Herpes simplex virus type 1 infection in mice with severe combined immunodeficiency (SCID). Arch Virol 1988;103:73–82.

123. Minagawa H, Takenaka A, Mohri S, Mori R. Protective effect of recombinant murine interferon beta against mouse hepatitis virus infection. Antiviral Res 1987;8:85–95.

124. Mocarski ES, Bonyhadi M, Salimi S, McCune JM, Kaneshima H. Human cytomegalovirus in a SCID-hu mouse: thymic epithelial cells are prominent targets of viral replication. Proc Natl Acad Sci U S A 1993;90:104–108.

125. Mokhtarian F, Shah KV. Pathogenesis of K papovavirus infection in athymic nude mice. Infect Immun 1983;41:434–436.

126. Morita CH, Matsuura Y, Morikawa SH, Kitamura T. Age-dependent transmission of hemorrhagic fever with renal syndrome (HFRS) virus in rats. Arch Virol 1985;85:145–149.

127. Morrison LA, Fields BN. Parallel mechanisms in neuropathogenesis of enteric virus infections. J Virol 1991;65:2767–2772.

128. Morse SS. Mouse thymic virus (MTLV; murid herpesvirus 3) infection in athymic nude mice: evidence for a T lymphocyte requirement. Virology 1988;163:255–258.

129. Mosier DE, Gulizia, RJ, MacIsaac PD, Torbett BE, Levy JA. Rapid loss of CD4+ T cells in human-PBL–SCID mice by noncytopathic HIV isolates. Science 1993;260:689–692.

130. Murphy, FA. The pathogenesis and pathology of rabies virus infection. Ann Inst Pasteur/Virol 1985;136E:373–386.

131. Nadal D, Albini B, Schlapfer E, Bernstein JM, Ogra PL. Role of Epstein-Barr virus and interleukin 6 in the development of lymphomas of human origin in SCID mice engrafted with human tonsillar mononuclear cells. J Gen Virol 1992;73:113–121.

132. Namikawa R, Kaneshima H, Lieberman M, Weissman IL, McCune JM. Infection of the SCID-hu mouse by HIV-1. Science 1988;242:1684–1686.

133. Nesburn AB, Cook ML, Stevens JG. Latent herpes simplex virus: isolation from rabbit trigeminal ganglia between episodes of recurrent ocular infection. Arch Ophthal 1972;88:412–417.

134. Nicolau S, Meteiesco E. Septinevrites a virus rabique des rue: preuves de la marche centrifuge du virus dans les nerfs peripheriques des lapins. Compt Rend Acad Sci 1928;186:1072–1074.

135. Nicolau S, Serbanescu V. Septinevrite experimentale a virus rabique fixe dans l'organisme du lapin. Compt Rend Soc Biol 1928;99:294–297.

136. Nonoyama S, Smith FO, Bernstein ID, Ochs HD. Strain-dependent leakiness of mice with severe combined immune deficiency. J Immunol 1993;150:3817–3824.

137. Oldstone MB, Ahmed R, Buchmeier MJ, Blount P, Tishon A. Perturbation of differentiated functions during viral infection in vivo. I. Relationship of lymphocytic choriomeningitis virus and host strains to growth hormone deficiency. Virology 1985;142:158–174.

138. Oldstone MB, Sinha YN, Blount P, et al. Virus-induced alterations in homeostasis: alteration in differentiated functions of infected cells in vivo. Science 1982;218:1125–1127.

139. Oshiro LS, Dondero DV, Emmons RW, Lennette EH. The development of Colorado tick fever virus within cells of the haemopoietic system. J Gen Virol 1978;39:73–79.

140. Papadimitriou JM, Shellam GR, Allan JE. The effect of the beige mutation on infection with murine cytomegalovirus: Histopathologic studies. Am J Pathol 1982;108:299–309.

141. Parker JC, Whiteman MD, Richter CB. Susceptibility of inbred and outbred mouse strains to Sendai virus and prevalence in infection in laboratory rodents. Infect Immun 1978;19:123–130.

142. Paturzo FX, Jacoby RO, Bhatt PN, Smith AL, Gaertner DJ, Ardito RB. Persistence of rat virus in seropositive rats as detected by explant culture. Arch Virol 1987;95:137–142.

143. Paya CV, Patick AK, Leibson PJ, Rodriguez M. Role of natural killer cells as immune effectors in encephalitis and demyelination induced by Theiler's virus. J Immunol 1989;143:95–102.

144. Pearson J, Mims CA. Selective vulnerability of neural cells and age-related susceptibility to OC43 virus in mice. Arch Virol 1983;77:109–118.

145. Percy DH, Auger DC, Croy BA. Signs and lesions of experimental Sendai virus infection in two genetically distinct strains of SCID/beige mouse. Vet Pathol 1994;31:67–73.

146. Percy DH, Barta JR. Spontaneous and experimental infections in scid and scid/beige mice. Lab Anim Sci 1993;43:127–132.

147. Pereira CA, Mercier G, Oth D, Dupuy JM. Induction of natural killer cells and interferon during mouse hepatitis virus infection of resistant and susceptible inbred mouse strains. Immunobiology 1984;166:35–44.

148. Perry LL, Lodmell DL. Role of CD4+ and CD8+ T cells in murine resistance to street rabies virus. J Virol 1991;65:3429–3434.

149. Pickel K, Muller MA, ter Meulen V. Analysis of age-dependent resistance to murine coronavirus JHM infection in mice. Infect Immun 1981;34:648–654.

150. Pirofski L, Horwitz MS, Scharff MD, Factor SM. Murine adenovirus infection of SCID mice induces hepatic lesions that resemble human Reye syndrome. Proc Natl Acad Sci U S A 1991;88: 4358–4362.

151. Pozzetto B, Gresser I. Role of sex and early interferon production in the susceptibility of mice to encephalomyocarditis virus. J Gen Virol 1985;66:701–709.

152. Quinnan GV Jr, Manischewitz JF, Kirmani N. Involvement of natural killer cells in the pathogenesis of murine cytomegalovirus interstitial pneumonitis and the immune response to infection. J Gen Virol 1982;58:173–180.

153. Reed LJ, Muench H. A simple method of estimating fifty percent endpoints. Am J Hyg 1938;27:493–497.

154. Richter CB, Thigpen JE, Richter CS, Mackenzie JM Jr. Fatal pneumonia with terminal emaciation in nude mice caused by pneumonia virus of mice. Lab Anim Sci 1988;38:255–261.

155. Riepenhoff-Talty M, Dharakul T, Kowalski E, Michalak S, Ogra PL. Persistent rotavirus infection in mice with severe combined immunodeficiency. J Virol 1987;61:3345–3348.

156. Rihova B, Vetvicka A, eds. Immunologic disorders of mice. Boca Raton, Florida: CRC Press, 1991.

157. Rommelaere J, Cornelis JJ. Antineoplastic activity of parvoviruses. J Virol Methods 1991;33:233–251.

158. Roths, JB, Smith AL, Sidman CL. Lethal exacerbation of *Pneumocystis carinii* pneumonia in severe combined immunodeficiency mice after infection by pneumonia virus of mice. J Exp Med 1993; 177:1193–1198.

159. Rowe M, Young LS, Crocker J, Stokes H, Henderson S, Rickinson AB. Epstein-Barr virus (EBV)–associated lymphoproliferative disease in the *SCID* mouse model: implications for the pathogenesis of EBV-positive lymphomas in man. J Exp Med 1991;173:147–158.

160. Scalzo AA, Fitzgerald NA, Wallace CR, et al. The effect of the Cmv-1 resistance gene, which is linked to the natural killer cell gene complex, is mediated by natural killer cells. J Imunol 1992;149: 581–589.

161. Scheid MP, Goldstein G, Boyse EA. Differentiation of T cells in nude mice. Science 1975;190:1211–1213.

162. Sebesteny A, Tilly R, Balkwill F, Trevan D. Demyelination and wasting associated with polyomavirus infection in nude (*nu/nu*) mice. Lab Anim 1980;14:337–345.

163. Selgrade MK, Nedrud JG, Collier AM, Gardner DE. Effects of cell source, mouse strain and immunosuppressive treatment on production of virulent and attenuated murine cytomegalovirus. Infect Immun 1981;33:840–847.

164. Shanley JD. In vivo administration of monoclonal antibody to the NK 1.1 antigen of natural killer cells: Effect on acute murine cytomegalovirus infection. J Med Virol 1990;30:58–60.

165. Shanley JD, Pesanti EL. Murine cytomegalovirus adrenalitis in athymic nude mice. Arch Virol 1986;88:27–35.

166. Sheridan JF, Vonderfecht S. Mouse rotavirus. In: Bhatt PN, Jacoby RO, Morse HC III, New AE, eds. Viral and mycoplasmal infections of laboratory rodents: effects on biomedical research. New York: Academic Press, 1986:217–243.

167. Shi S-R, Key ME, Kalra KL. Antigen retrieval in formalin-fixed, paraffin-embedded tissues: an enhancement method for immunohistochemical staining based on microwave oven heating of tissue sections. J Histochem Cytochem 1991;39:741–748.

168. Shultz LD, Sidman CL. Genetically determined murine models of immunodeficiency. Annu Rev Immunol 1987;5:367–403.

169. Smith AL. Genetic resistance to lethal flavivirus encephalitis: effect of host age and immune status and route of inoculation on production of interfering Banzi virus in vivo. Am J Trop Med Hyg 1981; 30:1319–1323.

170. Smith AL. An enzyme immunoassay for identification and quantification of infectious murine parvovirus in cultured cells. J Virol Methods 1985;11:321–327.

171. Smith AL. Splenic T cell function of BALB/cAnN (AnN) and BALB/cByJ (ByJ) mice after infection with mouse hepatitis virus, strain JHM (MHV-JHM). FASEB J 1988;2:A905.

172. Smith AL, Barthold SW. Factors influencing susceptibility of laboratory rodents to infection with mouse adenovirus strains K87 and FL. Arch Virol 1987;95:143–148.

173. Smith AL, Barthold SW, Beck DS. Intranasally administered alpha/beta interferon prevents extension of mouse hepatitis virus, strain JHM, into the brains of BALB/cByJ mice. Antiviral Res 1987; 8:239–246.

174. Smith AL, Barthold SW, de Souza MS, Bottomly K. The role of gamma interferon in infection of susceptible mice with murine coronavirus, MHV-JHM. Arch Virol 1991;121:89–100.

175. Smith AL, Bottomly K, Winograd DF. Altered splenic T cell function of BALB/cByJ mice infected with mouse hepatitis virus or Sendai virus. J Immunol 1987;138:3426–3430.

176. Smith AL, Casals J, Main AJ. Antigenic characterization of Tettnang virus: complications caused by passage of the virus in mice from a colony enzootically infected with mouse hepatitis virus. Am J Trop Med Hyg 1983;32:1172–1176.

177. Smith AL, Jacoby RO, Bhatt PN. Genetic resistance to lethal flavivirus infection: detection of interfering virus produced in vivo. In: Skamene E, Kongshavn PAL, Landy M, eds. Genetic control of resistance to infection and malignancy. New York: Academic Press, 1980;305–312.

178. Smith AL, Jacoby RO, Johnson EA, Paturzo F, Bhatt PN. In vivo studies with an "orphan" parvovirus of mice. Lab Anim Sci 1993; 43:175–182.

179. Smith AL, Tignor GH, Emmons RW, Woodie JD. Isolation of field rabies virus strains in CER and murine neuroblastoma cells. Intervirology 1978;9:359–361.

180. Smith AL, Tignor GH, Mifune K, Motohashi T. Isolation and assay of rabies serogroup viruses in CER cells. Intervirology 1977;8: 92–99.

181. Smith AL, Winograd DF, de Souza MS. In vitro splenic T cell responses of diverse mouse genotypes after oronasal exposure to mouse hepatitis virus, strain JHM. Lab Anim Sci 1991;41: 106–111.

182. Sorensen O, Dugre R, Percy D, Dales S. In vivo and in vitro models of demyelinating disease: endogenous factors influencing demyelinating disease caused by mouse hepatitis virus in rats and mice. Infect Immun 1982;37:1248–1260.

183. Sprecher E, Becker Y. Herpes simplex virus type 1 pathogenicity in footpad and ear skin of mice depends on Langerhans cell density, mouse genetics, and virus strain. J Virol 1987;61:2515–2522.

184. Steiner CM, Rozhon EJ, Lipton HL. Relationship between host age and persistence of Theiler's virus in the central nervous system of mice. Infect Immun 1984;43:432–434.

185. Stevens JG, Cook ML. Latent herpes simplex virus in spinal ganglia of mice. Science 1971;173:843–845.

186. Stevens JG, Cook ML, Jordan MC. Reactivation of latent herpes simplex virus after pneumococcal pneumonia in mice. Infect Immun 1975;11:635–639.

187. Stitz L, Baenziger J, Pircher H, Hengartner H, Zinkernagel RM. Effect of rabbit anti-asialo Gm1 treatment in vivo or with anti-asialo Gm1 plus complement in vitro on cytotoxic T cell activities. J Immunol 1986;136:4674–4680.

188. Stohlman SA, Frelinger JA. Resistance to fatal central nervous system disease by mouse hepatitis virus, strain JHM. Immunogenetics 1978;6:277–281.

189. Subak-Sharpe I, Dyson H, Fazakerley J. In vivo depletion of CD8+ T cells prevents lesions of demyelination in Semliki Forest virus infection. J Virol 1993;67:7629–7633.

190. Subcommittee on rodent viral and mycoplasmal infections (American Committee on Laboratory Animal Diseases).Special topic overview: detection methods for the identification of rodent viral and mycoplasmal infections. Lab Anim Sci 1991;41:199–225.

191. Sundberg JP. Conceptual evaluation of inbred laboratory mouse models as tools for the study of diseases in other species. Lab Anim 1992;21:48–51.

192. Taguchi F, Goto Y, Aiuchi M, Hayashi T, Fujiwara K. Pathogenesis of mouse hepatitis virus infection; the role of nasal epithelial cells as a primary target of low-virulence virus, MHV-S. Microbiol Immunol 1979;23:249–262.

193. Taguchi F, Yamada A, Fujiwara K. Factors involved in the age-dependent resistance of mice infected with low-virulence mouse hepatitis virus. Arch Virol 1979;62:333–340.

194. Tamura T, Taguchi F, Ueda K, Fujiwara K. Persistent infection with mouse hepatitis virus of low virulence in nude mice. Microbiol Immunol 1977;21:683–691.

195. Taylor BA. Genetic relationships between inbred strains of mice. J Hered 1972;68:83–86.

196. Tishon A, Borrow P, Evans C, Oldstone MBA. Virus-induced immunosuppression. 1. Age at infection relates to a selective or generalized defect. Virology 1993;195:397–405.

197. Tishon A, Oldstone MB. Perturbation of differentiated functions during viral infection in vivo: in vivo relationship of host genes and lymphocytic choriomeningitis virus to growth hormone deficiency. Am J Pathol 1990;137:965–969.

198. Tyor WR, Power C, Gendelman HE, Markham RB. A model of human immunodeficiency virus encephalitis in *scid* mice. Proc Natl Acad Sci U S A 1993;90:8658–8662.
199. Uhnoo I, Riepenhoff-Talty M, Dharakul T, et al. Extramucosal spread and development of hepatitis in immunodeficient and normal mice infected with rhesus rotavirus. J Virol 1990;64:361–368.
200. van Berlo MF, Warringa R, Wolswijk G, Lopes-Cardozo M. Vulnerability of rat and mouse brain cells to murine hepatitis virus (JHM-strain): studies in vivo and in vitro. Glia 1989;2:85–93.
201. Vargas-Cortes M, O'Donnell CL, Maciaszek JW, Welsh RM. Generation of "natural killer cell-escape" variants of pichinde virus during acute and persistent infections. J Virol 1992;66:2532–2535.
202. Wallace GD, Buller RML, Morse HC III. Genetic determinants of resistance to ectromelia (mousepox) virus-induced mortality. J Virol 1985;55:890–891.
203. Ward JM, Lock A, Collins MJ Jr, Gonda MA, Reynolds CW. Papovaviral sialoadenitis in athymic nude rats. Laboratory Anim 1984; 18:84–89.
204. Watson H, Tignor GH, Smith AL. Entry of rabies virus into the peripheral nerves of mice. J Gen Virol 1981;56:371–382.
205. Weir EC, Brownstein DG, Smith AL, Johnson EA. Respiratory disease and wasting in athymic mice infected with pneumonia virus of mice. Lab Anim Sci 1988;38:133–137.
206. Weir EC, Jacoby RO, Paturzo FX, Johnson EA, Ardito RB. Persistence of sialodacryoadenitis virus in athymic rats. Lab Anim Sci 1990;40:138–143.
207. Weiser W, Vellisto I, Bang FB. Congenic strains of mice susceptible and resistant to mouse hepatitis virus. Proc Soc Exp Biol Med 1976;152:499–502.
208. Welsh RM, Dundon PL, Eynon EE, Brubaker JO, Koo GC, O'Donnell GL. Demonstration of the antiviral role of natural killer cells in vivo with a natural killer cell-specific monoclonal antibody (NK 1.1). Nat Immun Cell Growth Regul 1990;9:112–120.
209. Wigand R. Age and susceptibility of Swiss mice for mouse adenovirus, strain FL. Arch Virol 1980;64:349–357.
210. Williamson JSP, Stohlman SA. Effective clearance of mouse hepatitis virus from the central nervous system requires both CD4+ and CD8+ T cells. J Virol 1990;64:4589–4592.
211. Winters AL, Brown HK. Duodenal lesions associated with adenovirus infection in athymic "nude" mice. Proc Soc Exp Biol Med 1979;164:280–286.
212. Yoon JW, Melez KA, Smathers PA, Archer JA, Steinberg AD. Virus-induced diabetes in autoimmune New Zealand mice. Diabetes 1983; 32:755–759.

Viral Pathogenesis,
edited by Neal Nathanson, et al.
Lippincott–Raven Publishers, Philadelphia © 1997

CHAPTER 21

Methods in Viral Pathogenesis

Transgenic and Genetically Deficient Mice

Glenn F. Rall and Michael B. A. Oldstone

G. F. Rall: Division of Virology, The Fox Chase Cancer Center,
Philadelphia, Pennsylvania 19111.
M. B. A. Oldstone: Division of Virology, Department of Neuropharmacology, The Scripps Research Institute, La Jolla, California 92037.

INTRODUCTION

General Concepts and Uses of Transgenic and Knockout Mice

Targeted manipulation of the germ line of the laboratory mouse has proven to be one of the most powerful biologic tools developed in the last decade. Transgenic mice and mice with targeted gene deletions introduced by homologous recombination (known as knockout mice) have provided unique insights into many areas of biology, including development, gene regulation, and the identification, characterization, and regulation of oncogenes. Furthermore, the manipulation of individual genes in vivo has shed light on the complex cellular interactions among dynamic systems, including the immune system, the central nervous system (CNS), and the endocrine system. In principle, there are no limitations to the overexpression or deletion of any murine-encoded gene or the expression of any nonmurine (e.g., human) gene in mice.

There are clear advantages that have made the inbred laboratory mouse particularly suitable for genome manipulation studies. The mouse is a robust, easily managed animal with extensively characterized physiologic systems, many of which parallel the equivalent system in humans. The relatively short murine gestation cycle (approximately 20 days), coupled with a high fecundity, allows for rapid expansion of genetically modified mice. Further, the average 2-year lifespan of the laboratory mouse provides a reasonable window to assess the development of chronic or progressive diseases that model human illnesses. Finally, practical issues such as the size, cost, and temperament of the laboratory mouse make it an attractive host for experimental studies.

The basis of transgenic technology is the juxtaposition of a coding sequence to be expressed (the transgene) with specific regulatory elements that dictate cell tropism and temporal expression at the transcriptional level. The regulatory sequence consists of a promoter, often coupled to additional regulatory elements that confer tissue or developmental specificity to the promoter. The transcriptional regulatory sequence can be derived either from the authentic promoter of the transgene or from a gene with a transcriptional profile different than that of the transgene. In either case, when integrated into the host cell genome, the transgene is transcribed according to the specificity dictated by the regulatory elements with which it is coupled.

Gene knockout achieves a targeted disruption of the coding sequence of a host cell gene. The gene interruption is usually accomplished by insertion of a marker gene whose protein product allows easy selection, such as the gene conferring neomycin resistance. The interrupted host gene can no longer be expressed; it is replaced by the marker gene, which is used to select modified stem cells and which can subsequently be used as a molecular tag for the analysis of progeny litters.

Virology has benefited greatly from advances in mouse genetic manipulation. Transgenic models have complemented our understanding of the mechanisms of viral infection and the identification of gene products required for viral replication and have led to the characterization of genes mediating disease or conferring immunity. Examples include the expression of cellular molecules that are necessary for viral infection, such as receptor molecules for polioviruses; the identification of the oncogenic properties of viral gene products, such as tax of human T-cell lymphotropic virus type 1 (HTLV-1) and tat of human immunodeficiency virus (HIV-1); and the study of pathogenic viruses and their gene products that ordinarily do not infect mice, such as the correlation of hepatitis B virus (HBV) expression in the liver with hepatitis and hepatocellular carcinoma and HIV-1 gp120 expression with resultant pathology in the CNS.

In addition, transgenic and knockout studies have contributed to our understanding of the host response to viral challenges. Specific expression of mediators of the immune response, such as interleukin-6 (IL-6), interferon-γ (IFN-γ), tumor necrosis factor-α (TNF-α), TNF-β, or B7 molecules, or deletion of these mediators (cytokine knockout mice) or of immune cell populations (CD4 and CD8 knockout mice) have helped to clarify how specific cells of the immune response and their mediators influence viral infections.

For this chapter, examples of transgenic and knockout paradigms were selected that demonstrate the influence these technologies have had on the study of viral pathogenesis. The goal is not to catalog every model system developed but rather, by highlighting aspects of viral pathogenesis that have benefited from these in vivo methodologies, to show how transgenic and knockout mouse models have influenced virology and to demonstrate the potential for future advances. The chapter concludes with a brief discussion of recent advances in plant virus pathogenesis and nonmurine transgenic models, to indicate the prospective usefulness of these methodologies to the study of viral pathogenesis.

Gene Expression In Vivo: Advantages and Disadvantages

Transgenic Constructs

A standard transgenic construct consists of a transcriptional regulatory region, including a promoter and other sequences responsible for tissue-specific or development-specific transcriptional control, coupled to a coding sequence to be expressed[52] (Fig. 21-1). In general, the regulatory and promoter elements that drive transgene transcription can be grouped into three categories: the authentic promoter of the gene to be expressed, a tissue-specific promoter that directs transgene expression to a particular tissue or cell type in vivo, and inducible promoters, in which the activity of the promoter sequence can be manipulated to upregulate transcription in vivo.

The authentic promoter is used most frequently to correlate specific viral protein expression with tissue tropism of the virus. For example, expression of the simian virus 40 (SV40) large T antigen under the control of its own promoter and enhancer allowed Levine and colleagues[86] to detect large T expression in the choroid plexus of transgenic animals, overlapping with the occurrence of SV40-mediated tumors at this site.

Alternatively, tissue-specific promoters restrict transgene expression to an individual cell type or group of cells, allowing the assessment of the pathogenic role of a viral product in a cell type of interest. Analysis of the contribution of an individual gene product to specific tissue damage (e.g., the role of the HIV-1 envelope protein, gp120, in neurodegeneration) can then be addressed. Chisari and colleagues[21] have used this approach successfully to model liver-specific HBV expression and HBV-induced disease by expressing components of the HBV genome under the control of the albumin promoter, which directs transcription to hepatocytes.

Inducible promoters, such as the metallothionein promoter, contain regulatory elements that can experimentally be induced to upmodulate transcription of the adjacent coding sequence, allowing the investigator some control regarding when the transgene is expressed. The metallothionein promoter, used by Brinster and colleagues[13] in conjunction with the herpesvirus thymidine kinase (*tk*) gene, was among the first transgenes expressed in mice by pronuclear injection. Injection of heavy metal ions such as cadmium, zinc, or copper[37,57] into the transgenic mice activates the metallothionein promoter, increasing transcription of the adjacent transgene.

Despite the successes in directing transgene expression, not all constructs are capable of driving expression, and not all genomic integration events lead to the anticipated transcription and expression of the transgene. Potential pitfalls exist both in the design of the construct and in events that occur after microinjection into the oocyte. For example, many tissue-specific promoters are "leaky," allowing transcription in cell types other than in the target cell or tissue. This is probably caused by a lack of the necessary regulatory elements needed to produce a restricted tissue expression or is due to the site of integration within the mouse genome. For example, β-globin, which is expressed predominantly in erythrocytes, is regulated by a complex series of enhancers that dictate cell-specific expression.[153] Transcription mediated by the β-globin promoter in the absence of these enhancers results in a loss of tissue specificity. In designing transgenes, it is important to realize that key enhancer elements, perhaps located far from the promoter region adjacent to the coding sequence or within the coding region itself, may be critical for tissue specificity. It is for this reason that many tissue-specific promoter systems have been initially coupled to the lacZ gene (or similar indicator systems) to confirm tissue-restricted expression (see later discussion).

In addition, linear transgene constructs are microinjected into the pronucleus of fertilized oocytes with the expectation that the DNA fragment will integrate into the genome within the first cycles of cell division. Although the amount of DNA injected can be controlled, the number of copies integrated, the site of integration within the mouse genome, and the developmental stage at which the linear transgene construct integrates cannot. The inability to control these variables poses a

Transgenic Methodology

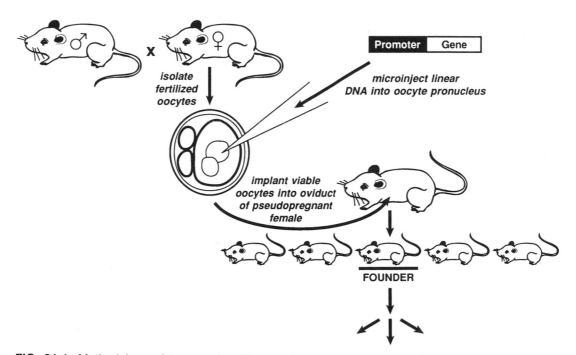

FIG. 21-1. Methodology of transgenics. The common approach to the development of transgenic mice and lineages is shown. Fertilized oocytes are removed from female mice that were mated 24 hours earlier with a male. The linear transgene, consisting of a gene to be expressed and transcriptional regulatory sequences, is microinjected into the pronuclei of the oocytes, and viable eggs are implanted into a pseudopregnant foster mother previously mated with a vasectomized male. Pups born are assayed for the presence of the transgene by tail biopsy and DNA screening, and positive founder mice are bred to establish lineages.

number of potential problems. Because integration is random, one concern is that the transgene will integrate within the open reading frame of an essential gene. Subsequent changes in the transgenic mouse's biology or metabolism therefore, may be caused by insertional gene inactivation rather than effects of transgene expression if heterozygous expression of the essential gene from the other allele is insufficient. Appropriate molecular characterization can rule out this possibility: clear identification of transgene RNA and protein in the target tissue should correlate tissue expression with phenotype. Furthermore, at least two lines of transgenic mice displaying similar phenotypes should be identified to eliminate the possibility of unintentional gene inactivation, since the likelihood of a transgene integrating at an identical locus in two independently microinjected oocytes is negligible.

An additional, although costly, control of value is the parallel establishment of transgenic mice in which a different gene product is expressed under the control of the same promoter. This would demonstrate that an observed phenotype is transgene-specific rather than a consequence of nonspecific transgene expression. For example, it is possible that expression of any foreign (viral) gene may cause generalized cell sickness independent of the function of that gene product or that over-expression of a coding sequence from a specific promoter may result in accumulation of the transgene product, leading to a storage disease.

Furthermore, genome integration may occur at varying times after microinjection, causing the progeny founder mice to be a genetic mosaic for the transgene. Ideally, the transgene integrates at the single-cell stage, resulting in heterozygous expression in all diploid cells. In this instance, half of the gametes are transgenic, and subsequent breeding of these founder mice results in approximately equal numbers of transgenic and nontransgenic offspring. However, if integration occurs after the oocyte has divided, fewer gametes (and therefore fewer progeny) are transgenic. Tail biopsy DNA screening of F_1 litters identifies mosaic founders.

Finally, many promoters are developmentally regulated and have complex expression patterns that can change over the lifetime of the host. Therefore, the expression profile of a transgene may differ significantly during the development of an animal from an embryo to a mature adult. Quantitative screening of messenger RNA (mRNA) levels (addressed in the next section) throughout the stages of development can identify developmentally altered patterns of transcription.

Knockout Constructs

Deletion of endogenous genes has been accomplished primarily by manipulation of embryonic stem (ES) cells, because

Gene Targeting

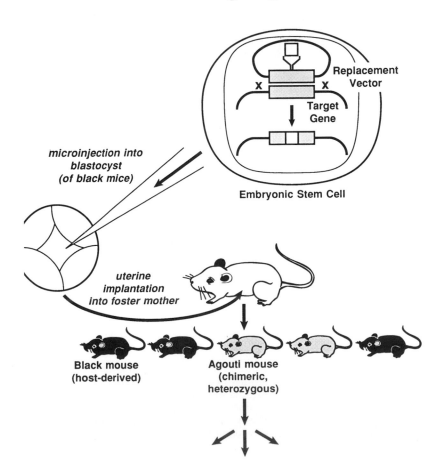

FIG. 21-2. Gene targeting and establishment of knockout mice. The common approach to the development of knockout mice is shown. A replacement vector that contains a targeted coding sequence (*gray box*), interrupted by a marker gene (*white box*), is introduced into embryonic stem (ES) cells. Recombination between the flanking sequences of the vector and the ES cell genome results in the replacement of the wild-type sequence with the interrupted coding sequence, and recombinants are selected by the expression of the marker gene. The recombinant ES cells are injected into blastocysts of black mice, and the blastocysts are then implanted into the uteri of pseudopregnant foster mothers. Mice born are either black (normal mice) or agouti, the hair color reflecting the influence of the ES cells on the development of the mouse. Agouti heterozygous chimeric mice are intercrossed to establish homozygous knockout mice.

they can easily be maintained and manipulated in vitro, then reintroduced into the murine blastocyst. The basic strategy of knockout constructs is to disrupt the targeted gene by insertion of a marker gene within the targeted coding sequence. The gene conferring resistance to the antibiotic neomycin is most often used because it allows for easy drug selection of recombinants in vitro. The replacement vector, consisting of the interrupted target gene plus flanking sequences (Fig. 21-2), is introduced into the ES cell; recombination between the endogenous gene and the interrupted construct occurs in a small percentage of cells. ES cell clones containing the interrupted target gene are selected and introduced into the murine blastocyst, and heterozygous founder mice are identified. The identification is usually by coat color, because introduction of the ES cell into a blastocyst that would normally give rise to a black mouse results in an agouti (tan or brown) color. Interbreeding of heterozygous mice results in homozygous mice in which the gene of interest has been deleted, or knocked out, on both chromosomes.[93]

An important advance that has made this technology possible is the development of plasmid DNA vectors that allow manipulation of genomic sequences by homologous recombination. Replacement of a sequence of DNA; introduction of insertions, deletions, or both; and introduction of point mutations are possible, all predicated on the design of the vector.[59,93,137,144]

One disadvantage of the use of ES cells in the derivation of knockout mice is the variability in cloning efficiency and success of incorporation of ES cells into the maturing blastocyst. Another disadvantage of knockout technology is more philosophic. Frequently, homozygous deletion of a presumed critical gene has had no detectable phenotype in the mouse, suggesting that complex organisms like the mouse have significant genetic redundancy, so that loss of function of one gene product can be compensated by other, unmodified gene products. Hence, phenotypes observed in knockout mice may underestimate the importance of a specific gene and may be more of a reflection of how well the developing mouse can accommodate the loss.

Nevertheless, many knockout models have established definitive roles for deleted genes, and the field of ES genetic manipulation and introduction of permanent modifications in the mouse genome is currently experiencing rapid and powerful advances. For example, strategies are being developed that target gene inactivation in specific cell types rather than in the whole animal[55] or that produce gene deletion in adult mice, obviating the concern of developmental redundancy.[83] These new advances in the establishment of knockout mice create new avenues for understanding the role of individual gene products in the prevention or precipitation of disease as a consequence of viral infection.

METHODOLOGIC APPROACHES

This review describes recent advances in viral pathogenesis brought about by the use of transgenic and knockout methodologies. For the detailed experimental strategies needed to create such genetically manipulated mice, the reader is referred to the work of Hogan and associates[62] and Wasserman and DePamphilis[162]. This brief overview is intended to provide a familiarity with the terms and procedures required to establish genetically modified mouse lineages.

Technology of Transgenics

Microinjection of cloned DNA into the pronucleus of a fertilized mouse oocyte has been the most widely used approach to introduce foreign DNA into cells in order to generate transgenic mice. Typically, microinjected DNA molecules arrange in a head-to-tail array and integrate into the host genome, using random chromosome breaks as integration sites. These breaks are possibly caused by repair enzymes induced by the free ends of the injected DNA molecules. Other methods to introduce foreign DNA into the genomes of mice exist, including the use of retroviruses and retroviral vectors. This review focuses on transgenic models generated by standard pronuclear injection of foreign DNA.

Construct Preparation

Figure 21-1 highlights the essential stages in the establishment of a transgenic mouse. The transgenic clone is constructed by standard molecular procedures, usually involving the subcloning of the gene of interest into a plasmid vector containing the regulatory region. Based on exhaustive studies using various promoter-transgene chimeras,[12,26,118] it is generally agreed that the use of a genomic clone of a transgene (in most cases, one that contains introns) is preferred, because the splicing opportunities increase transcriptional efficiency in vivo compared with the use of a complementary DNA (cDNA) clone. In the case of nonspliced transgenes or the unavailability of a full-length genomic clone, a heterologous splice site at the 5' end of an intron-less transgene also increases mRNA levels in transgenic mice, suggesting that mRNA splicing and export from the nucleus may be linked events.

The transgene construct, consisting of the gene to be expressed driven by the regulatory region of choice, is freed from plasmid sequences by restriction endonuclease digestion, because these extraneous plasmid sequences are potentially recombinogenic and could interfere with transgene expression. The linearized, purified construct is then dialyzed against the buffer used for the microinjection at a concentration of 2 to 10 ng of DNA per microliter (for a transgene averaging 5 to 10 kb in length).

In some experimental paradigms, the major histocompatibility complex (MHC) background of the transgenic mice is important because of variation among mouse strains in susceptibility to viral infections, or because the immunologic background may be important in generating an immune response to a particular viral gene or virus. In general, microinjection into hybrid oocytes is more efficient than microinjection into inbred strains because of hybrid vigor. After the hybrid founders are identified, repeated breeding to inbred normal mice of the desired strain results in pure inbred transgenic progeny after approximately eight to ten generations. For some purposes, fewer backcrosses may be necessary. For example, in breeding C57BL/6 × BALB/c hybrid mice to inbred BALB/c mice over successive generations, the immune response of these mice, measured in cytotoxic T lymphocyte (CTL) chromium release assays, is completely restricted to the BALB/c MHC after four generations[114] (Rall and Oldstone, unpublished observations).

Microinjection and Identification of Founder Mice

A female mated with a male the day before microinjection is used as a source of fertilized oocytes. The oviduct of the sacrificed female is removed, and the fertilized eggs are isolated. With the use of fine pulled pipettes, the transgene-carrying solution is microinjected into the pronucleus of the fertilized oocytes until the pronucleus visibly swells. After microinjection, the surviving oocytes are implanted into the oviducts of pseudopregnant foster mothers. These females have been mated with vasectomized males, and, although not pregnant, have initiated a hormone cascade that supports the implanted oocytes.

Progeny mice resulting from this microinjection are allowed to suckle on the foster mother and are separated by sex 3 to 5 weeks after birth. Mice become sexually mature at 5 to 6 weeks and should be separated before that time, because mating between siblings presents difficulties in breeding to establish lineages. Small tail biopsies are taken, and DNA is purified by proteinase K digestion followed by phenol-chloroform separation of nucleic acid from protein. The DNA is then analyzed either by Southern blot (principally for copy number determination) or by a slot blot device and subsequently hybridized with a labeled DNA fragment that differentiates transgenic mice from nontransgenic littermates. In addition, many laboratories use polymerase chain reaction (PCR) to identify transgenic pups, a nonradioactive, rapid method that usually does not require extensive purification of genomic DNA.

Each positive mouse identified at this stage is termed a founder mouse and represents the product of an unique microinjection and integration site. The founders are bred with normal mice (of the MHC haplotype of choice), and resultant progeny are screened as has been described. F_1 progeny that are transgenic by DNA analysis can then be used either as breeders or to characterize the RNA and protein expression of the transgene. Mice can be bred to homozygosity by mating transgenic mice from the same lineage to one another.

Detection of RNA Expression in Transgenic Tissues and Cells

To detect the presence of mRNA, tissues are removed from the transgenic animal, and either total or polyadenylated RNA is isolated. Identification of mRNA can be accomplished by either Northern hybridization, reverse transcriptase PCR (RT-PCR), or in situ hybridization. If the mRNA is highly expressed and bears no homology to endogenous mouse transcripts, Northern hybridization is a valid approach. The major benefit of Northern hybridization over the other strategies is the ability to quantitate the amount of mRNA (relative to known mRNAs) of the transgene. However, because the sequences of many genes expressed in transgenic animals are similar to those of endogenous transcripts, detection of a specific transgene message may be difficult.

An alternative approach is the use of RT-PCR. Primers can be designed that are specific for the transgene and that yield different-sized products based on whether the input nucleic acid is spliced mRNA, unspliced RNA, or contaminating DNA in the preparation. Primers that are designed to span an intron yield amplified fragments that differ by the size of the intron. Likewise, deletion of reverse transcriptase from the reverse transcription step determines whether RNA or DNA was the original substrate in the PCR reaction. PCR amplification of a pure sample generates a product only if the RNA has been converted to an RNA-cDNA duplex by reverse transcriptase. Because PCR is not normally quantitative, the primary disadvantage of this approach is the inability to determine the relative amount of transcript present in the tissue. Quantitative PCR approaches are available but require an internal standard with which to compare the transgenic RNA.

In situ RNA hybridization also allows testing of tissues and cells for transgene specificity. Because the hybridization is done on tissue sections, the cell types expressing the transgene are identifiable and the analysis is quantitative insofar as the number of expressing cells (compared with nonexpressing cells) can be determined. However, the procedure does not indicate the number of RNA copies present in transgenic cells. Usually, in situ hybridization is useful and informative after tissues that express the transgene are identified by either Northern blot or PCR.

Regardless of the method used, an extensive organ survey should be performed on each line to determine the potential tissue leakiness of the promoter and of nonspecificity caused by the integration site.

Identification of Protein Expression in Transgenic Tissues and Cells

The approach used to detect protein expression depends on whether the transgene is cell associated or secreted. In general, cell-associated proteins (e.g., MHC molecules, viral glycoproteins) can be identified by immunohistochemistry with the use of antibodies specific for the transgene, coupled to an enzyme (e.g., peroxidase) or a chromagen (e.g., fluorescein), to determine the cell type that is expressing the protein. Soluble proteins, such as cytokines, may also be identified by immunohistochemistry, although the chance of washing the transgene away before fixation is high. Therefore, Western blot procedures are more appropriate for secreted transgenes. Finally, functional assays, in which the transgene protein product is detected based on its activity, are particularly appropriate for cytokines or potential viral receptors.

In general, the methodology used to detect protein expression varies according to the transgene and the tissue in which it is expressed. Standard methods, such as immunohistochemistry and Western blot, are the most well established and direct approaches. However, less routine alternatives may be helpful in identifying protein expression if more standard methods prove unsuccessful. For example, identification of the class I MHC molecule D[b] on transgenic neurons was accomplished by isolation of embryonic hippocampal neurons and subsequent culture of these cells on coverslips precoated with a monoclonal antibody to the D[b] molecule.[115,133] Only transgenic neurons adhered, and the transgene product was correctly folded because the antibody used was conformation dependent.

Transgene products that are easily detected are useful in determining the tissue or developmental specificity of a promoter construct. The lacZ gene of *Escherichia coli*, the most widely used of the marker genes, is particularly useful because its product, β-galactosidase (β-gal), is readily detected in tissue sections by a simple enzyme reaction that produces a blue precipitate and does not have a biologic effect on most tissues in which it is expressed.[1] A potential biologic function of the β-gal protein should not be completely dismissed, however; one study of both lacZ and chloramphenicol acetyl transferase as marker genes for the same promoter suggested that the lacZ sequence may negatively influence transcription.[116]

Technology of Knockouts

ES cells are established in vitro from explanted blastocysts and retain their normal karyotype in culture. Genes can be efficiently introduced into ES cells by transfection or by retrovirus-mediated transduction, and ES cell clones selected for the presence of the interrupted target gene retain their pluripotent character.

Introduction of DNA Into Embryonic Stem Cells

Although many methods of introducing vector DNA into ES cells exist, including calcium phosphate precipitation, microinjection, and retroviral infection, the predominant approach has been the use of electroporation. This technique transduces large numbers of cells, and subsequent recombination events result in single-copy insertions of vector DNA.[151] In many ES transduction systems, the introduced replacement vector contains the targeted gene interrupted by the neomycin resistance gene, and surviving cells are identified by their ability to grow in media containing the antibiotic neomycin. The vector is constructed to promote recombination between the vector and the ES cell genome by flanking the indicator gene with sequences that are homologous to the gene to be deleted (see Fig. 21-2). The structure of the mutated gene in targeted ES cell clones and the progeny of germ line chimeras is confirmed by Southern blot analysis.

ES cell clones containing the interrupted target are injected into a maturing blastocyst from a mouse of black coat color. The blastocysts are surgically returned to the uterus of a pseudopregnant foster mother, and founder mice are identified by coat color. The ES-derived component is agouti; that is, the black hairs contain trace yellow tinges, which cause the mice to appear tan or brown, distinguishing them from normal black progeny. The founder mice, heterozygous for the gene deletion, are used to establish heterozygous F$_1$ progeny. These mice, if intercrossed, produce offspring with the homozygous deleted genotype (i.e., knockout mice).

Distinguishing Between Heterozygotes and Homozygotes

Standard slot blot approaches that are useful in identifying transgenic mice are not suitable for distinguishing between heterozygous and homozygous knockout mice, because both are positive for the marker gene used as a probe. PCR is the simplest way to distinguish between the two types. Routinely, two sets of primers are used to amplify the marker gene and the target gene. PCR amplification of tail DNA derived from progeny mice gives rise either to a targeted gene band only (normal mice), a marker gene band only (homozygous knockout mice), or both bands (heterozygous knockout mice).

Tissue-Specific Knockout Approaches

A major advantage in transgenic technology has been the characterization of promoters that directly express transgenes in specific tissues or cells. This approach has recently become available for knockout mice.[55]

In the standard manner of establishing knockout models, the recombination event resulting in the gene deletion occurs at the single-cell stage, and, therefore, the gene is deleted from all tissues of the adult animal. The absence of tissue-specific gene knockouts has been problematic, because proteins that play a specific role in development and those for which deletion from the entire animal is lethal could not be studied by knockout technology.

Gu and coauthors[55] have designed an approach in which a gene is knocked out in a tissue-specific manner. The procedure, outlined in Figure 21-3, uses the bacteriophage recombinase, *cre,* to align specific sequences, the loxP sites, and delete the intervening sequences. Two genetically engineered mice are constructed, one that expresses the *cre* protein in a tissue-specific manner and another in which the gene to be deleted is cloned between two loxP sequences. Doubly transgenic mice, then, have a *cre*-mediated deletion only in tissues in which the bacteriophage recombinase is expressed.

Development and Tissue-Specific Knockout Approaches

Using an IFN-responsive promoter to control the expression of cre recombinase, Kuhn and coworkers[83] have recently developed a knockout model in which a gene is inducibly deleted from the genome in adult mice. The approach was to use the IFN-α or IFN-β inducible promoter of the mouse Mx1 gene to control the expression of a cre recombinase transgene. On treatment with IFN, the Mx promoter is induced, and cre recombinase is synthesized, which mediates the deletion of

Targeted Knockout

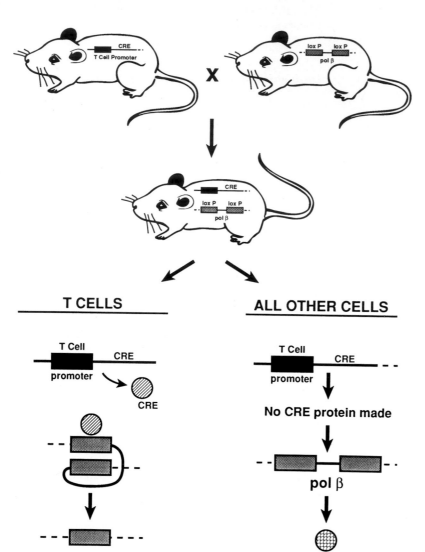

FIG. 21-3. Targeted deletion of genes in knockout mice. An example of tissue-specific gene targeting is depicted. The Cre enzyme, which deletes sequences between loxP sites, was expressed in T lymphocytes of transgenic mice. These mice were crossed with mice that contained a portion of the polymerase-beta (pol β) gene flanked by loxP sites. In the doubly transgenic mice, Cre protein expression was restricted to T cells, mediating the deletion of the pol β sequence only in T cells. Modified from Science 265:26.

the genetic sequence (the targeted gene) that resides between two loxP sites. Because the IFN can be administered at any time during development or adulthood, the concern about developmental compensatory mechanisms is eliminated.

TRANSGENIC STUDIES IN VIROLOGY: SELECTED MODELS

Cell-Specific Expression of Viral Proteins Under the Control of the Authentic Viral Promoter

Expression of viral gene products under the control of their authentic promoters has led to a number of critical findings. Reviewed here are three such examples: (1) the identification

of the *tax* gene of HTLV-1 and the *tat* gene of HIV-1 as oncogenic, correlating independent expression of those genes with oncogenesis; (2) the finding that SV40 large T antigen expression in transgenic mice causes tumor formation by binding and disabling the tumor suppressor gene, *p53*; and (3) the mapping of the tropism of the human cytomegalovirus (HCMV) immediate early promoter using lacZ as a marker gene.

Discovery of HTLV-1 Tax and HIV-1 Tat as Oncogenes

HTLV-1 is the causative agent of adult T-cell leukemia, after a latency period that may range up to 40 years.[108] An unusual property of this virus is that transformed cells contain single genomic copies of the virus but do not express viral proteins. One of the transactivating viral genes, *tax* (formerly "*tat*" in the literature), encodes a protein that results in transactivation of viral gene expression and regulates the expression of cellular genes important for cell growth and inflammation. Transgenic mice expressing the HTLV-1 tax protein under the control of the HTLV-1 long terminal repeat (LTR) were constructed, and the cell types permissive for the viral promoter were studied.[109] By derivation of transgenic mice in which the transcription of the *tax* gene was controlled by the authentic viral promoter, the expression and function of this gene could be studied in the absence of a viral infection.

Founder mice developed fibroblastic tumors at multiple sites between 13 and 17 weeks of age, establishing tax of HTLV-1 as an oncogenic protein and HTLV-1 as a transforming virus. The tumors clustered around sites of previous wounding.[14] As in the HTLV-1 virus, the transgenic LTR was suppressed after transformation. Transcriptional studies of tumor cell lines derived from these mice revealed a novel mechanism of suppression, which explains the tendency of this virus to remain latent.[163] Binding of upstream transcription factors maintain the LTR in an open conformation, whereas a downstream suppressor factor prevents transcription.[14,163] Latency is regulated by a balance between these two opposing factors.

The HTLV-1 tax transgenic mice have also shown that tax can activate multiple transcription pathways, either directly or indirectly. One of these pathways is through NF-κB, a potent transcription factor involved in the activation of a number of inflammatory genes expressed in macrophages and lymphocytes.[75] The in vivo depletion of NF-κB by antisense oligodeoxynucleotides inhibited the growth of late stage tax-induced tumors; however, antisense oligodeoxynucleotides directed against the *tax* transgene did not (Fig. 21-4). This suggests that tax may transform cells by a hit-and-run mechanism: at late stages, tax activates NF-κB, which then is responsible for the maintenance of the malignant phenotype.[75,76] However, tax expression itself at late stages is dispensable.

The consequence of expression of the transactivating protein from another T lymphotropic virus, HIV-1, the causative agent of acquired immunodeficiency syndrome (AIDS), was also studied by transgenic technology.[159] In addition to the immunodeficiency and neurologic complications associated with HIV-1 infection, malignancies have been described in individuals infected with HIV-1, including Kaposi's sarcoma and non-Hodgkin's lymphoma. When the HIV-1 *tat* gene was expressed in mice under the control of its own regulatory region (the viral LTR), skin lesions and liver adenomas developed in older mice,[158] indicating that HIV-1 could play a direct or indirect role in cancer in AIDS patients.

It has been demonstrated that the LTR-tat transgenic mice express the *tat* gene in the epidermal portion of the skin and that tat transcription can be markedly induced by ultraviolet light at a variety of wavelengths, including those attainable in outdoor sunlight exposure.[157] The effect of ultraviolet light in this system may be to transiently increase the transcriptional level of tat in cell types in which it is already being expressed at nominal levels. Upregulation may then affect the proliferation of specific cells in the dermis, leading to the development of tumors.

Inactivation of Tumor Suppression by Expression of SV40 T Antigen

Tumor formation is a complex process involving the activation and expression of oncogenes and the inactivation of tumor suppressor genes. Several diverse cancers appear to select for mutations in both alleles of the tumor suppressors retinoblastoma (Rb) and p53. In vitro transfection with either of these genes suppresses the ability of a tumorigenic cell line to produce tumors in nude mice, indicating that the wild type *Rb* and *p53* genes negatively regulate cell growth.[95,146] As a consequence, mutations in these genes may eliminate their ability to suppress cell division.

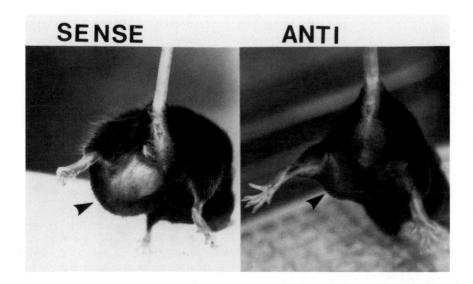

SENSE   ANTI

FIG. 21-4. Transgenic model of human T-cell leukemia virus type 1 (HTLV-1) tax gene product: effect of in vivo antisense oligonucleotide treatment on HTLV-1 tax in tumor-bearing mice. Transgenic mice expressing HTLV-1 tax under its own viral promoter (the long terminal repeat) develop tumors.[109] In vivo administration of antisense, but not sense, oligodeoxynucleotides targeting the transcription factor NF-κB to mice bearing late-stage, tax-induced tumors reduces the size of the tumor. After tumors were established, the oligodeoxynucleotides were administered in three doses over 10 days.[75] (Courtesy of Michael Nerenberg, The Scripps Research Institute.)

The SV40 large tumor antigen, or T antigen, is responsible for virtually all of this virus' ability to transform cells or produce tumors in animals.[86] The large and small SV40 tumor oncogenes, placed under the control of tissue-specific enhancer-promoter elements in transgenic mice, most often produce tumors in targeted, differentiated tissues. For example, transgenic mice expressing the large T oncogene under the control of the insulin gene promoter in the beta cells of the pancreas develop pancreatic tumors.[58] Similar results were found using the crystalline gene promoter in the lens[91] and the albumin gene promoter in the liver,[117] among others. However, when the large T antigen is put under the control of its own enhancer-promoter, expression and tumor formation are most commonly found in the choroid plexus within the brain.[156] These mice express T antigen solely in the brain by 2 weeks after birth, and the lag period between detection of T antigen and tumor development has prompted speculation that other events, such as activation of a second oncogene, may be required for tumor progression.

To better understand how T antigen induces tumorigenesis, a variety of oncogenes were studied by mRNA expression in tissue sections, and only one, *p53*, was shown to be elevated more than fivefold in multiple tumors of the choroid plexus.[94] Furthermore, immunoprecipitation with anti-p53 monoclonal antibodies detected p53-SV40 large T complexes, consistent with in vitro work which showed an interaction of the large T antigen with a protein of molecular weight 53,000 in SV40-transformed mouse cells.[84] If the binding of SV40 large T antigen to p53 inactivates the ability of p53 to suppress tumor cell division, then SV40-induced tumors expressing T antigen should contain a wild-type p53 gene and protein, reflecting the absence of a need to select for mutant p53 forms. Monoclonal antibodies specific for the wild-type form of the p53 protein reacted with p53 in these extracts, whereas a monoclonal antibody specific for mutant forms did not. Further, direct sequencing detected only wild-type sequences,[100] strongly supporting the hypothesis that T antigen inactivates the tumor-suppressing activity of wild-type p53. This eliminates the need to select for mutations at the p53 locus, and suggests that tumorigenesis is mediated, in part, through the activity and function of p53 in SV40-induced tumors.

Tropism of the Immediate Early Protein of Human Cytomegalovirus Using β-Galactosidase as a Marker

HCMV, a member of the herpesvirus family, has a complex transcriptional profile in which expression of early viral genes activates the transcription and translation of viral gene products expressed later in infection. Humans are the only known reservoir for HCMV, and therefore the determinants responsible for host and tissue restriction are not approachable by in vivo methodologies.

The HCMV major immediate early promoter (MIEP) is one of the first promoters to activate on infection; it regulates the expression of a series of immediate early proteins that determines the productive state of the virus. Because MIEP activity is highly dependent on cellular transcription factors, promoter function may determine tissue specificity in HCMV infection. To address this possibility, transgenic mice were established in which the lacZ marker gene was driven by the MIEP. The en-

hancer domain of the MIEP targeted expression in 19 of the 29 organs examined; however, promoter activity within these tissues was restricted to specific cell types.[5b] LacZ expression was seen predominately in highly differentiated cells, including retinal cells of the eye, ductile cells of the salivary gland, exocrine cells of the pancreas, and neuronal cells of the hippocampus. β-gal expression, indicative of the activity of the MIEP, paralleled expression in tissues naturally infected with HCMV in vivo.

Embryonic expression of this promoter in transgenic mice has also been addressed.[5a] At embryonic day 8.5 to 9.5, there is panactivation of the MIEP, with a majority of the developing embryonic tissues expressing the lacZ transgene (Fig. 21-5A). However, by embryonic day 10.5, expression is restricted to specific tissues, including the aortic endothelia, somites, and the fourth ventricle of the brain, which gives rise to the cerebellum (Fig. 21-5C). There is a correlation between the tissues targeted in these developing transgenic mice (e.g., the developing cerebellum) and the congenital defects associated with HCMV infection (e.g., CNS malformations).

Creation of Animals Models to Study Viral Pathogenesis

For many viruses, small animal models of infection do not exist because of the restricted host tropism of the virus. Poliovirus, HBV, and HIV-1 are all serious human pathogens for which no small animal model of infection is available. Presented here are three approaches to dissect issues of viral entry, replication, pathogenesis, and immunity using transgenic mouse technology. Each of these models has been used to address pathogenesis in a different manner. First, development of mice expressing the viral receptor for poliovirus rendered transgenic mice susceptible to infection with nonmouse adapted virulent and attenuated strains of virus. Second, expression of all or part of the HBV genome under the control of HBV regulatory sequences or under liver-specific promoter control has created transgenic models with viral expression similar to that of the human virus infection. This has allowed an assessment of HBV virulence and the precise determination of viral epitopes seen by the immune response. Finally, expression of a single gene product of HIV-1 in the CNS of mice resulted in neuropathology similar to the neuronal degeneration seen in patients with AIDS dementia complex, demonstrating the central role played by that viral protein in neuropathology.

Expression of Viral Receptor in a Host Devoid of Such Molecules: Human Poliovirus Receptor Transgenic Mice

Poliovirus causes an acute disease of the CNS that has largely been controlled by vaccines developed in the 1950s. The live attenuated Sabin vaccine strains of poliovirus were derived by multiple passage of neurovirulent viruses in primates and cultured primate cells.[141] To identify the viral sequences responsible for the attenuation phenotype in the vaccine strains and thereby understand how the virulent virus causes disease, it was necessary to develop an appropriate an-

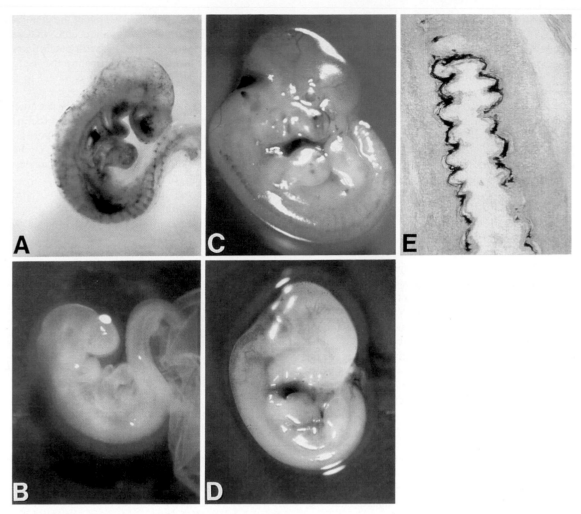

FIG. 21-5. Expression of lacZ in transgenic tissues from mice in which the β-galactosidase (β-gal) gene is driven by the human cytomegalovirus (HCMV) major immediate early promoter (MIEP). Embryonic mice either transgenic for the MIEP-lacZ transgene (**A** and **C**) or nontransgenic (**B** and **D**) are shown at embryonic days 8.5 (**A** and **B**) and 9.5 (**C** and **D**), stained to detect the presence of β-gal. Note that the expression at day 8.5 is throughout the embryo, whereas expression at day 9.5 is restricted to specific tissues. (**E**) Aortic endothelial cells from an adult transgenic mouse that were stained to detect the expression of β-gal. Other data with Marek's disease in birds, murine CMV in mice, and HCMV in humans has suggested involvement of herpesviruses in atherosclerosis. (Courtesy of Peter Ghazal, The Scripps Research Institute, and Jay Nelson, Oregon Health Sciences University.)

imal model. Although monkeys are the best natural experimental models for poliovirus infection, the expense of acquiring and maintaining them makes their use impractical.

To circumvent this difficulty, transgenic mouse lines expressing the human cellular receptor for poliovirus (PVR) under the transcriptional control of the authentic human promoter were established.[77,135] Poliovirus initiates infection by binding to a cellular receptor that is a member of the immunoglobulin superfamily of proteins[98,131]; the host range restriction of poliovirus infection in cultured cells is determined at the level of the cellular receptor. Accordingly, transgenic mice expressing PVR were susceptible to poliovirus infection, and poliovirus replicated in neurons of the CNS, giving rise to poliomyelitis (Fig. 21-6). These mice have subsequently been

used to dissect aspects of poliovirus cell tropism, trafficking to the CNS, and identification of neurovirulence determinants within the virus.

In the primate host, poliovirus infection is characterized by a restricted tissue tropism; the virus replicates only in the pharynx, gut, and neurons within certain regions of the CNS, despite its presence in many organs during the viremic phase of infection.[140] Because the basis for the restricted tropism of poliovirus is not known, it was of interest to determine whether transgenic PVR mice could be used to study poliovirus tropism. PVR gene expression and susceptibility to viral infection were examined by in situ hybridization.[136] Although many tissues expressed the PVR, only some cell types (neurons and skeletal muscle) were susceptible to viral infection, indicating that tissue tropism is not governed solely by expression of the PVR gene nor by accessibility of virus to cells (see Fig. 21-6). The basis for the restriction of replication in tissues that express the PVR is not known, but it appears to involve post-entry steps in replication.

Transgenic PVR mice have also been used to assess viral trafficking to the CNS. Initially, the virus replicates in the oropharnyx and the gut, resulting in a transient viremia. In approximately 1% of human infections, the virus invades the CNS, replicates in motor neurons, and produces paralytic poliomyelitis. Two possibilities of how the virus gains access to the CNS exist: entry from blood across the blood-brain barrier or peripheral nerve transport by axonal processes.[102] Multiple lines of evidence using PVR transgenic mice have indicated that spread into the CNS is along nerve pathways: the median lethal dose (LD50) for intramuscular or intracerebral injection routes is similar, showing that poliovirus may follow a direct pathway to the CNS after intramuscular injection. Further, after intramuscular injection, poliovirus spreads gradually to the CNS, replicating first in the inferior segment of the spinal cord, then in the superior spinal cord, and ultimately in the brain. Finally, development of CNS disease after hind limb inoculation is blocked by sciatic nerve axotomy. Based on these findings, Ren and Racaniello[136] proposed an alternative strategy for the pathogenesis of poliovirus in humans: ingested poliovirus initially replicates in the alimentary tract, possibly in epithelial cells lining the gut. Replication leads to release of virus and corresponding viremia. Disseminated virus then replicates in skeletal muscle cells, enters peripheral nerve cells, and spreads to the CNS by retrograde transport along axonal processes.

The identification of neurovirulence determinants of polioviruses has been aided by PVR transgenic mice. Infection of transgenic mice with a variety of recombinant viruses derived from virulent and avirulent strains mapped viral segments within the 5′ proximal region of the genome that appear to be responsible for poliovirus-induced CNS disease.[64] These neurovirulent sequences overlap with determinants identified after infection of monkeys, reaffirming the usefulness of the PVR transgenic mouse as a suitable model to assess poliovirus pathogenesis.

The establishment of transgenic mice that are able to serve as hosts for poliomyelitis infection allows the in vivo dissection of the various stages of the viral life cycle and the subsequent immune response,[92] and this model may be used in the future to test the efficacy of therapeutic strategies to block viral infection.

However, reconstitution of a viral receptor may not always be sufficient to allow for a viral infection. For example, transgenic mice expressing the HIV-1 receptor, CD4, are not infectable with HIV-1, either because of a lack of a cell surface coreceptor or, more likely, because of a block in replication that occurs after the virus has entered the cell.

Expression of Viral Components in a Host That Ordinarily is Not Infected by the Virus

Transgenic Mouse Model for Study of Hepatitis B Virus Pathogenesis

HBV causes acute and chronic hepatocellular injury and hepatocellular carcinoma. The mechanisms of disease and malignancy are poorly understood, in large part because of the absence of appropriate tissue culture and animal models to study stages of these processes. The immune response to HBV gene products is responsible both for clearance of virus and for liver disease.[22] Transgenic models of HBV infection have expanded our understanding of the consequence of viral infection and the immune response to the infection, elucidating some of the interactions of virus and host that may determine the outcome of infection.[21] Transgenic mice that express HBV sequences under the control of an HBV promoter (the preS1) and under the control of non-HBV, liver-specific promoters (the metallothionein and albumin promoters) have been established.

Transgene constructs containing HBV-derived regulatory sequences have resulted in mice that preferentially express HBV transcripts in hepatocytes of the liver and proximal convoluted tubules of the kidney; in some lineages, other tissues also contain viral transcripts.[2,5,18,42] Although the HBV genome may contain cis-acting regulatory elements that enhance transcription in the liver and kidney, the fairly widespread tissue distribution of transgenic HBV RNAs under HBV-specific transcriptional control suggests that the tropism of the virus to the liver in the natural infection may reflect multiple limitations to viral entry, replication, and gene expression.

Analysis of independent transgenic mouse lineages demonstrates that HBV gene expression is also regulated at multiple levels. Several groups have documented that a lack of HBV expression is associated with hypermethylation of the transgene sequences,[3,164] consistent with findings that correlate upregulation of HBV gene expression with demethylation of HBV sequences during embryonic development.[123] Nevertheless, expression of integrated viral DNA requires other factors in addition to the methylation status of the integrated DNA. In

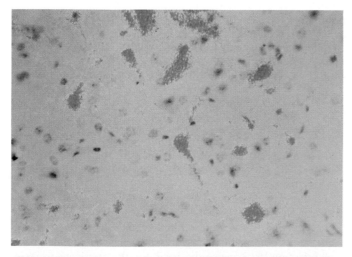

FIG. 21-6. Expression of poliomyelitis virus receptor (PVR) RNA in spinal cord of transgenic mice. A transverse tissue section through the spinal cord of a mouse transgenic for the PVR was hybridized with a ³⁵S antisense PVR RNA probe. Silver grains were visualized by polarized light epiluminescence microscopy and appear blue-green.[136] (Courtesy of Vincent Racaniello, Columbia University.)

transgenic mice and during chronic HBV infection, genomic flanking sequences, chromatin structure, and exposure to cellular and viral binding proteins may act cooperatively to regulate viral replication.

One of the unique characteristics of HBV infection is its relative prevalence (more than fivefold greater) in male compared with female humans. Several groups have reported enhanced HBV envelope expression in male transgenic mice.[5,24,34,43] Because castration causes a decline in expression that is reversible by administration of androgens, transgenic mice have confirmed the hypothesis that sex hormones may also function to regulate HBV transcription.

The most immediate histologic consequence of the overexpression of the large HBV envelope protein from a liver-specific regulatory promoter (either metallothionein, which is inducible, or the albumin promoter, which gives constitutively high RNA expression in the liver) is an expansion of the endoplasmic reticulum of the hepatocyte,[24] which results from an accumulation of HBV surface antigen (HBsAg) filaments. As a consequence, many hepatocytes develop severe and protracted hepatocellular injury, which initiates a programmed

response within the liver that eventually leads to neoplasia (Fig. 21-7).[23,25] These experiments are noteworthy for two reasons: like the HTLV-1 tax model, they demonstrate that the expression of a single viral gene, in the absence of a viral infection, can result in malignancy. Furthermore, prolonged cellular injury (mediated by the accumulation of the transgene) induces a proliferative response that encourages random mutations throughout the cellular genome, some of which program the cell for unrestricted growth.[21] Hepatocellular carcinoma in human HBV infection therefore may be caused by secondary events unrelated to the integration or expression of HBV sequences, with the acquisition of these events predicated on the extent of liver damage.

The HBV transgenic mouse model has also been useful in the characterization of the pathogenic potential of the HBV-specific CTL response. The importance of CTLs in human HBV infections had been addressed, but before the establishment of HBV transgenic mice it was not possible to demonstrate CTL participation in liver disease. Using a transgenic line that did not spontaneously develop liver disease, adoptive transfer of anti-HBsAg primed spleen cells or HBsAg-specific

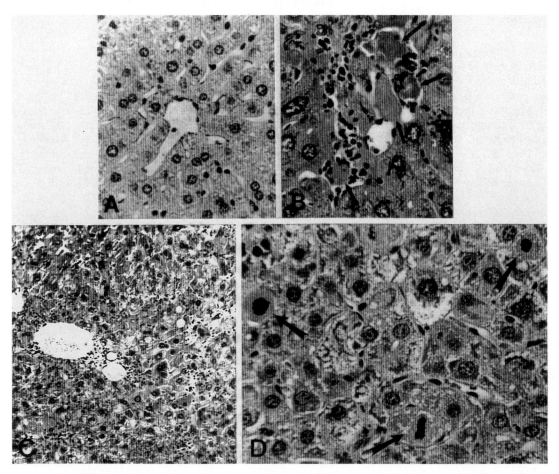

FIG. 21-7. Hepatocellular carcinoma and inflammation induced in transgenic mice expressing the hepatitis B virus (HBV) surface antigen. Shown are photomicrographs of sections taken from non-transgenic mice (**A**) and mice transgenic for the HBV envelope (**B** through **D**) after adoptive transfer of HBV envelope–primed splenocytes. Both lymphocytic infiltration (**B** and **C**) and dense areas of mitosis, characteristic of hepatocellular carcinoma (**D**), can be seen. (Courtesy of Frank Chisari, The Scripps Research Institute.)

antibody resulted in liver disease.[101] Injury occurred several days after adoptive transfer of primed splenocytes and was characterized by widespread liver necrosis and cellular infiltrates, resembling chronic hepatitis. Liver injury was mediated by CD8+ T lymphocytes, and establishment of CD8+ T-lymphocyte clones allowed fine mapping of an HBV epitope between residues 21 and 40 of the major envelope protein.[101] These cells caused liver cell injury when transferred into transgenic mice, indicating that endogenously synthesized HBV envelope antigens are expressed in the context of class I MHC on the hepatocyte. Despite a severe necroinflammatory disease after CTL transfer, suppression of viral gene expression and replication was mediated by IFN-γ and TNF-α and did not involve cell death.[22,56]

Studies with transgenic mice expressing all or part of the HBV genome have established that HBV-induced liver disease is a consequence of the direct effect of virus-induced cytotoxicity (specifically, aberrant overexpression of the large envelope protein), which induces random mutations in the genome, and as a result of immune reactivity to viral envelope antigens expressed on infected hepatocytes.

Transgenic Mouse Model Mimicking HIV-1 Central Nervous System Disease

During the course of HIV-1 infection, some individuals develop neurologic complications that, in their most severe form, can culminate in dementia and paralysis. As many as two thirds of HIV-1–positive patients may suffer from some form of neurologic damage, which can include psychomotor dysfunction, memory impairment, and behavioral abnormalities. This neurodegenerative condition, known as HIV-1–associated cognitive-motor complex, (or AIDS dementia complex in its most severe form), can occur independently of superinfection with opportunistic pathogens and in the absence of HIV-1 infection of neurons.[87,88]

The condition is characterized by neuronal degeneration and loss, glial activation, increased numbers of perivascular macrophages,[15] alterations of the blood-brain barrier,[122,125] and possible loss of oligodendrocytes.[40] Damage is greatest in the white matter tracts and cerebral cortex. In the cortex, neuronal loss can be as great as 18% to 38%.[41,73,96] The discrepancy between the severity of impairment and the inability to demonstrate neuronal HIV-1 infection has led to the hypothesis that diffusible factors of either viral or host origin, arising as a consequence of HIV-1 infection, may be the causative agents of the neuropathologic changes.[40,150] Cytokines, excitatory amino acids, antibodies to the HIV gp41 that crossreact with CNS cells, and either the full-length or fragmented envelope protein of HIV-1, gp120, have been implicated in the production of CNS damage.[60,154]

With the use of mixed brain cell culture systems, it has been shown that gp120 contributes to neurotoxicity[8,11,36] and that gp120-induced neuronal injury can be blocked by antagonists of the N-methyl-D-aspartate subtype of glutamate receptors[89] and by calcium channel antagonists.[36] In addition, HIV-infected macrophages secrete a neurotoxin whose action can also be prevented by N-methyl-D-aspartate antagonists.[50,145]

Intracerebroventricular injection of gp120 into adult rats[51] and systemic injection of gp120 into neonatal rats[61] resulted in dystrophic neurites and behavioral changes, demonstrating a potential neurotoxic effect of the gp120 molecule in vivo. To dissect the cause of HIV-1–induced CNS damage, transgenic mice expressing soluble gp120 under the control of the astrocyte-specific glial fibrillary acidic protein (*GFAP*) gene were established.[152] Mice expressing gp120 had a spectrum of neurologic abnormalities, including neuronal and glial changes mimicking those seen in HIV-1–infected individuals. The severity of dendritic vacuolization, loss of dendritic processes, and decrease in synaptic density correlated with the brain level of gp120 mRNA, providing in vivo evidence for a role of gp120 in HIV-1–associated nervous system damage (Fig. 21-8). To further analyze the pathogenesis of gp120-induced neurotoxicity and to assess the potential neuroprotective function of human amyloid precursor proteins (hAPP), hAPP was expressed in neurons of bigenic gp120/hAPP mice. Results indicated that hAPP can be neuroprotective, because the bigenic mice showed significantly less neuronal loss than mice expressing gp120 alone. These data suggest that molecules that mimic hAPP may be useful in the prevention or treatment of HIV-1 CNS damage.[103]

Focal Expression of Host Proteins That Influence Pathogenesis: Prion Protein Expression in the Central Nervous System

Prions are pathogens that differ from bacteria, fungi, parasites, viroids, and viruses, with respect to both their structure and the diseases that they cause. Kuru, Cruetzfeldt-Jacob disease, and Gerstmann-Sträussler-Scheinker syndrome (GSS) are all human neurodegenerative diseases caused by prions which are transmissible to laboratory animals.[49,126] In addition to the human disorders, maladies of animals are included in the family of prion diseases, including scrapie of sheep and goats, bovine spongiform encephalopathy (mad cow disease), transmissible mink encephalopathy, and chronic wasting disease of captive mule deer and elk.[20,126]

Prion diseases are mediated by changes in protein conformation: the prion protein (PrP), encoded by the host genome, undergoes posttranslational conformational modifications that do not include changes in the primary amino acid sequence of the protein.[126,127] The altered protein (PrPSc) can then influence the conformation of unmodified cellular proteins (PrPc), transmitting the disease from host to host. Transgenic models have allowed several aspects of prion disease to be studied, including prion synthesis, control of incubation times, determinants of neuropathology, and the genetic mechanisms of disease that result in varying incubation times when prions are transmitted between species.[127]

If scrapie prions from one species are passaged into another species, the incubation time required for the disease to manifest lengthens, a phenomenon referred to as the species barrier.[120] To determine whether this barrier is a result of differences in the primary structure of the prion protein among different species, transgenic mice were established that contained a hamster genomic fragment which included the coding sequence for the Syrian hamster PrP. The PrP genes of Syrian hamsters and mice encode proteins differing by at least 14 residues. Incubation times in hamster prion-expressing transgenic mice inoculated with mouse scrapie prions were pro-

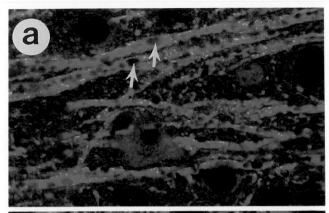

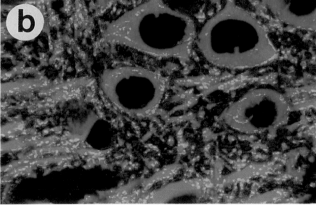

FIG. 21-8. Effects of gp120 expression in the central nervous system of transgenic mice. Astroglial expression of gp120 mRNA and associated neuronal damage in glial fibrillary acidic protein (GFAP)–gp120 transgenic mice. Laser confocal images of neocortical sections show neuronal cell bodies and dendrites (*green*) and presynaptic terminal boutons (*red*) from a high expressor of GFAP-gp120 (**A**) and from a nontransgenic mouse (**B**). Arrows indicate vacuolization of neuronal processes.[152] (Courtesy of Lennart Mucke, The Scripps Research Institute.)

longed, compared with times in nontransgenic control mice inoculated with mouse prions,[128] suggesting that expression of the hamster-specific transgene impeded the synthesis of mouse prions and reinforced the basis of the species barrier. Inoculation of transgenic mice with hamster prions produced high levels of hamster prions, whereas inoculation with mouse prions gave rise to exclusively mouse prions in the transgenic mice. Furthermore, the neuropathology in transgenic mice receiving either hamster or mouse prions differed and correlated with the distribution of spongiform changes and formation of PrP amyloid plaques seen in infected hamsters and mice, respectively. Collectively, these findings argue that the origin of the prion inoculum determines the outcome of synthesis and disease within transgenic mice that are capable of supporting the replication of either prion. Recent studies[64] have reported the establishment of transgenic mice in which a chimeric mouse and human PrP was expressed. All of these mice developed CNS disease within 200 days of inoculation with brain homogenates from Creutzfeldt-Jakob patients, whereas only about 10% of transgenic mice expressing the human PrP had developed disease by more than 500 days after inoculation.

These studies suggest that other species-specific factors, such as chaperone proteins, are involved in prion replication.

Mutations in the human PrP gene have been associated with a variety of inherited prion diseases,[48] supporting the hypothesis that cumulative changes in the PrP protein can lead to CNS degeneration. To test this concept, transgenic mice were developed that expressed a form of mouse PrP which was mutated at position 101 in the protein sequence, the same position that has been associated with GSS in humans.[65,147] These mice spontaneously developed disease between 7 and 39 weeks of age, initiating a course of degeneration usually resulting in animal death. The brains of these mice possessed features of spongiform degeneration, amyloid plaque formation, and astrogliosis, indicating that the mutation at position 101 is responsible for de novo prion synthesis and the murine disease, and, by extension, may participate in GSS disease of humans.

Focal Expression of a Viral Gene to Study Pathogenesis: Virus-Induced Autoimmune Disease

In the model systems that have been described, viruses or viral products directly responsible for human diseases were used to determine mechanisms of viral pathogenesis by means of transgenic technology. However, transgenic models employing viruses that are not directly implicated in human diseases have also been established to understand the pathogenic mechanisms of human diseases. In the following example, a murine virus, lymphocytic choriomeningitis virus (LCMV), and its gene products were used to study the human disease, insulin-dependent diabetes mellitus (IDDM). These reports do not imply that LCMV is a causative agent of IDDM but rather show, using a well-established murine viral model, how an antiviral immune response to a viral transgene expressed in the beta cells of the islets of Langerhans can produce many of the clinical and pathologic symptoms of the human disease.

IDDM, also known as type 1 diabetes or juvenile-onset diabetes, results from the destruction of the insulin-producing beta cells in the islets of Langerhans in the pancreas.[155] The disease is characterized by high blood glucose levels, low blood insulin levels, and mononuclear cell infiltration into the islets. The destruction of the islets usually occurs over a prolonged period and eventually results in the onset of clinical diabetes. The cause of the disease is not known, although host genes, T-cell responses, and viral infections have all been implicated in this and other autoimmune diseases.[38,113]

Viruses have been linked with IDDM from a variety of lines of evidence. Virus isolated from a patient with acute-onset diabetes was able to induce diabetes in normal mice.[166] Several systemic viral infections can destroy islets and cause immune cell infiltration, and many of these viruses also infect and replicate in islet cells in vitro.[68,110] Further, a number of viral infections have been associated with IDDM or abnormal glucose tolerance, including rubella, mumps, and coxsackievirus.[110] Finally, both RNA and DNA viruses are capable of initiating antiviral responses that crossreact with insulin and other nonviral molecules in or on islet cells, potentially precipitating autoimmunity.[113]

In order to assess what role, if any, viruses play in the autoimmune response and to better understand immunologic issues of tolerance in vivo, two groups[112,114] created transgenic mice in which the LCMV glycoprotein or nucleoprotein was expressed in pancreatic beta cells under the control of the rat insulin promoter. The protein expression of the transgene alone rarely produced IDDM over the animal's lifetime (fewer than 5% of more than 300 transgenic mice spontaneously developed diabetes). However, if transgenic animals were infected with LCMV, a lymphocytic infiltrate that was restricted to the islet cells of more than 90% of transgenic mice occurred, yielding the canonical signs of IDDM, including hyperglycemia, hypoinsulinemia, and mononuclear cell infiltration. The onset of diabetes occurred with varying kinetics: Ohashi and colleagues[112] documented increased blood glucose levels 9 to 11 days after infection, whereas Oldstone and associates[114] showed that diabetes occurred 2 to 6 months after infection. Rate of onset correlated with a lack of thymic expression of the transgene in the fast-onset mice and with thymic expression in those mice with the slower onset of IDDM.[161] Although CD8+ antiviral (self) CTLs alone were responsible for fast islet injury, the slow-onset IDDM required CD4 help.[111,112] Further, by breeding transgenic mice to different MHC class I haplotypes, a difference in the kinetics of the severity of disease was noted.[160]

Thus, by expressing a viral protein (in this case, a protein perceived by the host immune system as self) within a restricted cell type and subsequently challenging the animal with a viral infection, an immune response was raised in which CTL generated against the infecting virus also responded to the viral transgene (Fig. 21-9). According to this scenario, two possible explanations exist. A viral infection that initiates a CTL immune response to a viral epitope that is similar or identical to a host protein may result in an anti-self (i.e., autoimmune) response. Alternatively, a virus with a tropism for beta cells in the islets of Langerhans may persistently infect those cells after a congenital in utero or early life infection. A novel immune response induced later in juvenile or adult life by a virus with determinants that are immunologically crossreactive could then lead to an immune response directed at the beta cells until their destruction ultimately causes the clinical manifestations of IDDM.

Transgenic models have also been established in which expression of a transgene in the beta cells can directly result in diabetes. The influenza hemagglutinin gene was expressed in the beta cells of pancreatic islets and resulted in hyperglycemia, which was a direct consequence of lymphocyte-mediated destruction of pancreatic beta cells in the absence of an influenza superinfection.[139] Only a fraction of the transgenic animals developed the disease, and the onset of illness was extremely variable, suggesting that multiple factors, both genetic and environmental, may influence the development of IDDM.

GENE DYSFUNCTION (KNOCKOUT) STUDIES IN VIROLOGY

Deletion of Cells of the Immune System That Respond to an Infecting Virus

Helper and cytotoxic subsets of T lymphocytes can be broadly distinguished by their surface expression of either the CD4 or CD8 glycoproteins, respectively.[46] These molecules assist in mediating related functions for the two types of T cells. On the outside of the cell, CD8 has been shown to bind a

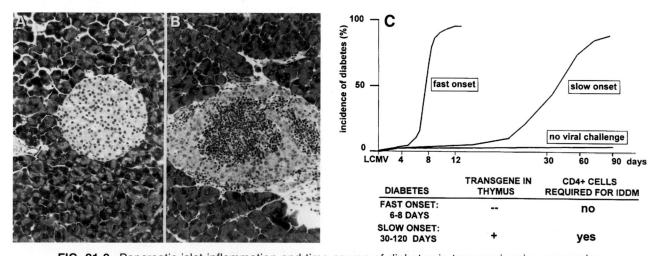

FIG. 21-9. Pancreatic islet inflammation and time course of diabetes in transgenic mice expressing viral genes and challenged with a viral infection. Photomicrograph of an islet of Langerhans in the pancreas of a nontransgenic mouse (**A**) and a transgenic mouse (**B**) expressing the nucleoprotein of lymphocytic choriomeningitis virus (LCMV) under the control of the rat insulin promoter (RIP), after infection with LCMV. Panel **C** diagrams the kinetics of diabetes for both the slow and fast onset of insulin-dependent diabetes mellitus (IDDM) in RIP-LCMV transgenic mice after viral challenge. Panel **C** further indicates the role of CD4+ cells in generating the disease and of thymic expression in determining the speed of disease onset.[114,161] (Courtesy of Matthias von Herrath, The Scripps Research Institute.)

nonpolymorphic region of the alpha 3 domain of the MHC class I molecule.[142,143] Similarly, the CD4 molecule engages an analogous region on the MHC class II beta chain,[80] an src-related tyrosine kinase essential for T-cell signaling. Both of these molecules bind antigen-presenting structures with their ectodomains and are coupled to a major T-cell signaling component with their endodomains.

The development and function of most T cells are dependent on the function of the CD4 or CD8 molecule, because antibodies to these molecules block in vitro and in vivo immune responses. However, antibody-mediated CD4 or CD8 depletion in vivo is rarely complete and therefore cannot completely address the role of these molecules (and these cell types) in the development of the immune system. To fully understand the developmental and regulatory roles of these molecules and the cells on which they are expressed, site-specific recombination in ES cells has been used to create CD4 and CD8 knockout mice.

Class II MHC Knockout Mice: A Deficiency in CD4 T Cells

Mice lacking CD4+ T lymphocytes have been established by two approaches: deletion of MHC class II sequences[19,31,52] and direct mutagenesis of the CD4 sequence.[132]

By disruption of an MHC class II gene in ES cells, mice were generated that lack cell surface expression of class II molecules.[31] These MHC class II–deficient mice were found to be depleted of mature CD4+ T cells, and, despite having normal or elevated serum levels of immunoglobulin (IgM), were unable to make IgG antibodies to T cell–dependent protein antigens. Two-color fluorescence-activated cell sorter (FACS) analysis revealed that although the population of CD4+/CD8− cells in these mice was significantly lower than in normal littermates (0.6% versus 10%), the proportions of progenitor CD4+/CD8+ cells in both mice were equivalent, indicating that expression of CD4 during T-cell maturation in the thymus does not require the presence of class II molecules but that progression from the double-positive stage to the single-positive CD4+/CD8− stage does.

To address the role of CD4+ T lymphocytes in viral infections (and the potential autoimmune response that follows as a consequence of the antiviral response), the class II knockout mice were bred to mice transgenic for the LCMV glycoprotein expressed constitutively in the beta cells in the pancreatic islets of Langerhans (described in the previous section). Mice that express the glycoprotein in the pancreas but lack class II molecules and CD4+ mature T lymphocytes respond normally to LCMV challenge: both knockout mice and mice with intact immune responses develop the hyperglycemia that precedes diabetes in this model. Infiltration in the CD4 knockout mice are of CD8+ T lymphocytes only. These results show that CD4+ T cells and class II MHC molecules are not required for the response to the viral infection that leads to rapid-onset IDDM in the transgenic mice.

Mice with a targeted disruption of the CD4 gene were also established and, as predicted, CD4 expression on the surface of lymphocytes was absent.[132] In addition, the major soluble mediators produced by CD4 T cells, including IL-2, were greatly reduced in unchallenged mice. The CD4-deficient

mice mounted poor responses to sheep erythrocytes, indicating that antibody production in these mice was negligible.

To investigate the participation of CD4 help in the clearance of viral infection and its role in the establishment of persistent viral infections, CD4 knockout mice were infected with varying doses of LCMV intraperitoneally.[6] CD4-deficient mice were able to clear a low dose (2×10^2 plaque-forming units) acute infection by mounting an effective CTL response. However, infection with a high dose of virus (2×10^6 plaque-forming units) resulted in an exhaustion of specific antiviral CTL, causing an incomplete clearance of virus and leading to a persistent infection in the mice. Normal mice, on the other hand, efficiently cleared the virus and developed antiviral memory CTL. Therefore, the absence of CD4+ T-cell help may enhance the establishment of a persistent viral infection.

β₂-Microglobulin Knockout Mice: A Deficiency in Class I MHC Expression and in CD8 T Cells

MHC-encoded class I molecules play a critical role in the protective immune response to viral infections. The primary role of the class I MHC molecules is to present antigens, processed intracellularly into small (9 to 11 amino acids) peptides, on the cell surface in a manner recognizable to the T-cell receptor of CTL.[166] Class I MHC molecules are composed of a membrane-spanning chain (the heavy chain) of approximately 45 kD and a nonmembrane-associated light chain, β₂-microglobulin, of approximately 12 kD. The heavy chain of the class I MHC molecule is highly polymorphic. In contrast, the light chain is encoded by a single gene and is therefore not variable in the class I molecule. Expression of β₂-microglobulin is necessary for normal cellular expression of the class I molecule,[67] and, given the high degree of variability within class I heavy-chain genes in the mouse, it was more reasonable to construct class I MHC knockout mice by engineering mutations in the β₂-microglobulin gene than in the heavy chain. Two groups initially established the β₂-microglobulin–deficient mice, yielding mice with class I MHC deficiency.[79,134,169,170]

Despite a severe deficiency in the cell surface expression of class I MHC molecules, the β₂-microglobulin knockout mice showed no developmental difficulties, lived to normal ages, and were fertile.[78] Adult mice were subjected to an array of procedures to determine how a loss of class I MHC antigen-presenting capacity would impact on the immune response to a variety of grafts, susceptibility to natural killer (NK) cells, lymphocyte development, and viral infections. The results from nonvirologic studies are extensively summarized in a review by Raulet.[134]

Briefly, immunologic studies of the class I MHC knockout mice indicated that they suffered from a number of alterations, including a deficiency in CD8+ T lymphocytes, impairment in NK cell activity, and a potential deficiency in a subset of gamma-delta cells that recognize class I MHC molecules. Given these defects, it may be predicted that the immune response of these animals to viral infections would be significantly impaired, because CD8+ T lymphocytes play a critical role in immunity to most viral infections. The results of antibody-mediated CD8+ cell depletion studies have confirmed their importance in the clearance of viral infections.[71] The response of the class I MHC knockout mice to three viral infections—LCMV, influenza, and Theiler's murine encephalomyelitis virus (TMEV)—are reviewed. Several of these studies remain controversial, perhaps emphasizing the issue of genomic plasticity in these knockout models.

Intracerebral infection of normal mice with LCMV leads to a choriomeningeal encephalitis, which results in the death of the animal within 6 to 8 days after infection. The disease in mice is mediated predominately by CD8+ T lymphocytes. Intracerebral infection of β_2-microglobulin knockout mice with LCMV led to a less severe disease than in control animals,[35,104,130] characterized by meningitis, wasting, and some mortality. These studies indicate that CD4+ T cells can mediate a milder form of LCMV disease in the β_2-microglobulin knockout mouse. The possibility that the illness seen in these animals is caused by the presence of CD4+ CTLs has been suggested.[104]

The ability of class I–deficient mice to clear an acute, nonlethal LCMV challenge points to some of the difficulties in the use of knockout mice with different derivations. Lehmann-Grube and colleagues[85] showed that class I–deficient mice infected intravenously did not clear the virus, and significant titers were detected in these mice 3 months after infection. By contrast, Fung-Leung and associates[47] showed that mice harboring a mutant form of CD8, which also results in a decreased presence of class I MHC molecules on the surfaces of target cells, did clear virus, leading the authors to speculate that CD4+ T cells alone can clear an acute LCMV infection. The disparity in findings may be caused by different functional abilities of the CD4+ cells in each knockout mouse[134] or by the presence of CD8+ cells in the studies by Fung-Leung and colleagues.

Both normal and β_2-microglobulin–deficient mice challenged with an intranasal influenza infection were able to clear the infection within 10 to 13 days after infection.[39] In previous studies employing antibody-mediated depletion of CD8+ or CD4+ lymphocytes, it was found that elimination of either subset did not impair the ability of mice to clear the infection; however, depletion of both CD4 and CD8 cells resulted in a fatal infection. It appears, then, that either lymphocyte population can clear the virus, but at least one must be present. The virus used in these studies was weakly virulent, which may impact on the efficiency of clearance by an impaired immune response. In a separate study by Bender and associates,[7] the kinetics of clearance of a weakly virulent influenza strain (A/Port Chalmers/1/73 [H3N2]) in β_2-microglobulin–deficient mice was delayed compared with clearance in normal mice. When challenged with the more virulent A/Puerto Rico/8/34 strain, 90% of the β_2-microglobulin deficient mice died, compared with 20% of the normal littermates, implying that class I MHC expression may be dispensable in weakly virulent viral challenges but essential in more serious infections.

TMEV is a murine picornavirus that infects the CNS and results in a chronic demyelinating disease.[9] It has been suggested that the lesions in TMEV-induced demyelination are caused by immunopathologic reactions mediated by CD8+ T cells.[17] Mice of the H-2^b MHC haplotype are normally resistant to TMEV infection and are able to clear the virus within 25 days after infection. In contrast, all β_2-microglobulin

knockout mice on the H-2^b background had viral antigens detectable more than 50 days after infection and developed demyelinating plaques, although these mice, unlike nude mice, did not die as a consequence of the persistent viral infection.[44,129,138] These studies suggest that CD8+ T cells are not responsible for the demyelinating lesions in TMEV-infected mice and that the presence of an intact CD4 immune component in the absence of a CD8 immune response is able to prevent mice from succumbing to a lethal infection.

Deletion of Effector Molecules Made During Immune Responses to Viral Infections

Knockout of Perforin

Although cell contact–dependent cytolytic activity is the functional hallmark of CD8+ and NK cells in vitro, the relative contributions of released cytotoxic granules, secretion of soluble factors (e.g., serine esterases, TNF), and apoptotic cell death are not known. To dissect these various factors, a number of knockout mice have been established, including mice deficient in the synthesis of perforin.

Perforin is a molecule expressed in the cytoplasmic granules of both CTL and NK cells, and its transfer into target cells results in lysis. Further, perforin release has been noted at sites of CTL-induced injury of virally infected targets.[167,168] To test the role of perforin directly, perforin-deficient mice were generated[69]; such mice were viable and fertile and had normal numbers of CD8 and NK cells. However, antiviral class I MHC–dependent CTL activity and MHC-independent NK cell activity were absent in these mice. As a result, these mice were unable to clear an acute infection with LCMV and had a reduced capacity to control the growth of fibrosarcoma tumor cells, despite normal levels of CTL activation. Although normal and heterozygous mice had eliminated virus from all tissues by day 8 after infection, homozygous perforin-deficient mice still had high titers of virus in spleen, liver, brain, and kidney. Eventually, these mice succumbed to the viral infection, initially evidenced by wasting and ultimately by death of the animal. These results demonstrate that pore formation by perforin is a major mechanism for the antiviral cytotoxicity mediated by CTL and NK cells.

Knockout of Interferon-γ

IFN-γ, a cytokine secreted by activated T cells, NK cells, and macrophages, has a wide range of immunomodulatory effects on several cell types and antiviral activity in vitro and in vivo.[32] The direct antiviral activity attributed to the IFN family involves the inhibition of viral replication by impaired accumulation of viral-specific mRNA and proteins. To gain a better understanding of the role of IFN-γ in the development and function of the immune system as well as its antiviral effect in vivo, mice were developed that had a targeted mutation of the IFN-γ gene.[32] These mice developed normally and were healthy in the absence of pathogens. However, they had impaired production of macrophage antimicrobial products and reduced expression of macrophage MHC class II antigens.

IFN-γ was shown not to be necessary for either recovery from experimental influenza infection or in vivo effector activity of influenza-specific CD4+ or CD8+ CTLs, which are cytolytic in vitro and protect in vivo.[53] The absence of IFN-γ led to increased production of influenza-specific IgG1, IL-4, and IL-5 in the knockout mice, compared with wild-type littermate control animals, but there was no difference in the development of an effective CTL response between IFN-γ–deficient and wild-type animals in response to viral infection. The data indicate that although IFN-γ may be dispensable for intracellular organisms such as viruses, it seems to play a crucial role in protective cellular immunity to tuberculosis infection.[29]

Other Knockout Models of Potential Relevance to Viral Pathogenesis

Different viruses may result in different effects in mice with targeted disruptions of specific genes. Many of the knockout models presently available have only recently been established, and the animals have not been tested for their ability to respond to a variety of viral infections. Not only should these experiments tell us about the role of the specific deleted gene product, but they may also shed light on the mechanism of pathogenesis of the virus. Recently established knockout mice with deletions in adhesion molecules,[148] transcriptional regulators of IFNs,[97] recombination activation genes (RAG1 and RAG2, which control T- and B-cell rearrangements),[149] and cytokines such as IL-6[81] and IL-4[70] may be valuable tools to understand the antiviral immune response (Table 21-1).

Additionally, knockout mice can be used to complement transgenic mice. For example, Bueler and colleagues have knocked out the prion protein in mice[16] and have found that these mice were normal physiologically and behaviorally, were resistant to scrapie infection, and failed to propagate prions. These investigators are now positioned to reconstitute scrapie disease by mating such mice with mice expressing murine or hamster prion under the control of cell-specific promoters. Similar strategies for making double- and triple-transgenic mice to allow focal expression of specific viral or host proteins in selected cells (e.g., beta cells in the pancreas, oligodendrocytes, astrocytes) are also possible.

APPROACHES TO VIRAL PATHOGENESIS IN NONMURINE MODELS

In the past decade, manipulation of the mouse genome has afforded the opportunity to determine the contribution of individual gene products in vivo. Transgenic and knockout technologies have also been used with systems other than the mouse, and these efforts, although perhaps comprising a minority of the total transgenic and knockout models developed, represent interesting pathways for gene therapy and homologous recombination studies.

Nonmurine Animal Transgenic Models

Most gene transfer experiments in farm animals have been carried out with the ultimate goal of producing larger or higher-quality offspring.[10] The issue of disease resistance has been addressed with the introduction of immunoglobulin gene constructs and specific viral resistance genes into animals other than mice.[90,106]

The Mx1 (myxovirus-resistance) system of some mouse strains is a rare example of single-locus disease resistance to

TABLE 21-1. *Knockout models that may be used to address issues of viral pathogenesis*

Targeted gene	References
Class I major histocompatibility complex	
β_2-microglobulin	Zijlstra et al., 1989[170]; Koller and Smithies, 1989[79]
CD8	Fung-Leung et al., 1991[47]
Class II major histocompatibility complex	
A^b_β	Grusby et al., 1991[54]; Cosgrove et al., 1991[31]
CD4	Rahemtulla et al., 1991[132]; Killeen et al., 1993[74]
Perforin	Kagi et al., 1994[69]
Interferon-gamma	Dalton et al., 1993[32]
CD28	Shahinian et al., 1993[148]
Interferon response factors 1 and 2	Matsuyama et al., 1993[97]
RAG1/RAG2	Mombaerts et al., 1992[99]; Shinkai et al., 1992[149]
Cytokines	
Interleukin-4	Kanagawa et al., 1993[70]
Interleukin-6	Kopf et al., 1994[81]
Interleukin-10	Kuhn et al., 1993[83]
Prion protein	Bueler, et al., 1993[16]

viruses such as influenza. If transgenic mice of a background normally susceptible to influenza infections are made to express the Mx1 gene,[4] these animals exhibit minimal viral spread and survive infection. Mx homologs have been found in all eucaryotic organisms tested,[106] and the antiviral effect of Mx proteins appears to act at the level of inhibition of viral mRNA or protein synthesis.[82,121]

The possibility of improving porcine resistance to influenza virus infections was addressed by the establishment of pigs transgenic for the Mx1 gene. The gene, under the transcriptional control of the IFN-γ–inducible Mx1 promoter, was incorporated into the germ line of piglets, and a number of founder animals expressed transgene mRNA levels in response to exogenous IFN.[105] The improvement of disease resistance in animals raised for human consumption has immediate benefits from an agricultural perspective. These studies allow the field of viral pathogenesis to move from the inbred, pathogen-protected world of the laboratory mouse to the more relevant issues of animal disease resistance in natural settings.

In other studies, transgenic sheep were constructed that expressed envelope genes of visna virus under the control of the visna LTR, in order to investigate the function of the *env* gene in lentivirus pathogenesis in the natural host. Visna virus is a prototype of the ovine lentiviruses, which cause encephalitis, arthritis, and pneumonia in sheep worldwide.[28] Transgenic lambs expressed the *env* gene on differentiated macrophages, paralleling infection of target cells. This established a model to study the role of the lentivirus envelope in preventing infection or modulating disease subsequent to viral challenge in the natural host.[28]

Transgenic Plant Virus Pathogenesis

Transgenic plants carrying nucleotide sequences derived from plant viruses can exhibit increased resistance to viral disease. Many sequences tested to date confer either resistance to infection or suppression of virus-induced disease. Viral genes used in transgenic studies are either structural (including coat proteins) or nonstructural, such as replicases and the movement proteins.[45]

In 1986, Powell and colleagues[124] described experiments in which tobacco plants transgenic for the coat protein of tobacco mosaic virus (TMV) were produced. These plants were found to have an increased resistance to TMV infection, prompting the development of other transgenic plants that expressed single viral genes. Although many of these plants do demonstrate higher levels of resistance to viral infection, it is unlikely that a single, common mechanism of resistance exists in all transgenic models studied.

In the TMV system, a number of factors may contribute to viral resistance; these include an action on the early events of infection, because the number of infection sites is lower in transgenic plants compared with nontransgenic controls.[107] All plant models predict that the transgene-derived protein is the resistance-conferring entity and that plants expressing higher levels of the transgene have a higher resistance to viral infection. An important potential method of viral resistance is indicated by the fact that accumulation of RNA, rather than protein, is responsible for the resistance seen in some plants. In cases in which specific alterations were made in the coding sequence that prevented translation, antiviral resistance was as efficient as in the protein-competent forms.[33,72]

How plant viruses move from the original site of infection to the surrounding cells and systemically invade the plant to cause disease is another important question in plant virus pathogenesis. Plant viruses encode movement proteins, which are nonstructural proteins essential for infection that do not affect viral replication or encapsidation.[66] The best studied movement protein is that of TMV, whose movement protein is a nucleic acid binding protein. Viral RNA, bound to the movement protein, is compacted and directed to the plasmodesmata, where the viral RNA is extruded from the cell wall.[27] Despite a lack of sequence similarity among plant viruses, movement proteins encode similar functions, as demonstrated by transgenic plants expressing a defective mutant of TMV movement protein, which impacted on the ability of other plant viruses to accumulate.[30] Recent findings using transgenic plants have demonstrated ways in which plant viruses can alter cellular connections within a host plant to mediate viral trafficking and result in disease. The movement proteins BL1 and BR1 of a prototype geminivirus (squash leaf curl virus) were expressed in transgenic plants, and BL1 (but not BR1) was sufficient to produce disease symptoms similar to those of the viral disease in the absence of a viral infection.[119] Furthermore, BL1 cofractionated with the cell wall, reaffirming the role of these proteins in geminivirus movement within a plant host.

Although the mechanisms of plant resistance and disease are only beginning to be understood, the field of plant virus pathogenesis and the usefulness of transgenic plant approaches to understanding of these viral infections will no doubt be a major focus of viral pathogenesis in the coming years.

SAFETY CONSIDERATIONS

Transgenic mice have been particularly useful in the establishment of mouse models for viruses that infect only humans or nonhuman primates, including poliovirus, measles, HBV, and HIV-1. Whereas common laboratory mice are naturally nonpermissive for infection with a pathogenic virus because of the lack of one or more essential human proteins such as the viral receptors, transgenic mice expressing such molecules may be susceptible to infection. Two major concerns exist. Transgenic, infected animals may theoretically shed and transmit infectious virus to humans exposed to the animals in the laboratory, and infected animals may escape from the laboratory and breed with wild mice, establishing a potential wild reservoir for a pathogenic human virus.

Although they are powerful experimental tools, transgenic mice that can serve as reservoirs for human viral pathogens pose obvious public health hazards. Although the risk of these potential hazards does not outweigh their scientific benefit, consideration must be given to provision of appropriate safety precautions (Table 21-2).

TABLE 21-2. *Partial list of recommendations concerning the maintenance and transport of transgenic animals susceptible to pathogenic human viruses*

Extensive characterization of the natural history of the viral infection in the transgenic animals, including routes of infection, size of inoculum required to establish infection, and tissues affected by the infection.

Detailed registry of transgenic animals, with information regarding date of birth, transportation details, and disposal of infected mice.

Tight security and limited access to transgenic animals and infected suites.

Enforcement of laboratory practices appropriate for the virus, including containment facilities, employee training, and routine inspections of such facilities.

Protective immunization, if possible, for exposed workers.

Strict enforcement of local and international laws regarding transport of animals among facilities and the use of barrier cages that exclude transmission of infectious virus.

Development of a subline of transgenic animals that contain a lethal mutation in the absence of a particular drug or food additive, or castration of male mice distributed for collaborative purposes.

ACKNOWLEDGMENTS

The authors acknowledge the assistance of Roger Beachy of The Scripps Research Institute for advice on the transgenic plant discussion; Jenny Price of The Scripps Transgenic Microinjection Facility, Claire Evans, Marc Horwitz, Mari Manchester, and Stephanie Toggas for reviewing the manuscript; Jody Anderson, Amy Goddard, and Sarah Costello for excellent secretarial aid; and Monica Hambalko and Ed Rockenstein.

Supported by a Fellowship from the J. D. and Ida Leiper Foundation and NIH Training Grant MH19185 (GFR), and in part, by NIH grants #AIO9484, NS12428, and AG04342, and MH19185 (MBAO).

ABBREVIATIONS

AIDS: acquired immunodeficiency syndrome
β-gal: β-galactosidase
cDNA: complementary DNA
CNS: central nervous system
CTL: cytotoxic T lymphocyte
ES: embryonic stem (cell)
FACS: fluorescence-activated cell sorter (analysis)
GSS: Gerstmann-Sträussler-Scheinker syndrome
hAPP: human amyloid precursor proteins
HBsAg: surface antigen of HBV
HBV: hepatitis B virus
HCMV: human cytomegalovirus
HIV: human immunodeficiency virus
HTLV-1: human T-cell lymphotropic virus type 1
IDDM: insulin-dependent diabetes mellitus
IFN, IFN-α, IFN-β, IFN-γ: interferons
IgG, IgG1, IgM: immunoglobulins
IL-2, IL-4, IL-5, IL-6: interleukins
LCMV: lymphocytic choriomeningitis virus
LD50: median lethal dose
LTR: long terminal repeat
MHC: major histocompatibility complex
MIEP: major immediate early promoter (of HCMV)
mRNA: messenger RNA
NF-κB: a transcription factor
NK: natural killer (cell)

PCR: polymerase chain reaction
PrP: prion protein
PrPc: unmodified cellular prion
PrPSc: altered prion protein (in scrapie)
PVR: human poliovirus receptor
RT-PCR: reverse transcriptase polymerase chain reaction
SV40: simian virus 40
TMEV: Theiler's murine encephalomyelitis virus
TMV: tobacco mosaic virus
TNF, TNF-α, TNF-β: tumor necrosis factors

REFERENCES

1. Allen N, Cran D, Barton S, Hettle S, Reik W, Surami M. Transgenes as probes for active chromosomal domains in mouse development. Nature 1988;333:852.
2. Araki K, Miyazaki J, Hino O, et al. Expression and replication of hepatitis B virus genome in transgenic mice. Proc Natl Acad Sci U S A 1989;86:207.
3. Araki K, Miyazaki J, Tsurimoto T, et al. Demethylation by 5-azacytidine results in the expression of hepatitis B virus surface antigen in transgenic mice. Jpn J Cancer 1989;80:295.
4. Arnheiter H, Skuntz S, Noteborn M, Chang S, Meier E. Transgenic mice with intracellular immunity to influenza virus. Cell 1990; 62:51.
5. Babinet C, Farza H, Morello D, Hadchouel M, Pourcel C. Specific expression of hepatitis B surface antigen (HBsAg) in transgenic mice. Science 1985;230:1160.
5a. Baskar JF, Smith PP, Ciment GS, et al. Developmental analysis of the cytomegalovirus enhancer in transgenic animals. J Virol 1996; 70:3215.
5b. Baskar JF, Smith PP, Nalaver G, et al. The enhancer domain of the human cytomegalovirus major immediate early promoter determines cell type-specific expression in transgenic mice. J Virol 1996; 70:3207.
6. Battegay M, Moskophidis D, Rahemtulla A, Hengartner H, Mak T, Zinkernagel R. Enhanced establishment of a virus carrier state in adult CD4+ T cell-deficient mice. J Virol 1994;68:4700.
7. Bender B, Croghan T, Zhang L, Small P. Transgenic mice lacking class I major histocompatibility complex–restricted T cells have delayed viral clearance and increased mortality after influenza virus challenge. J Exp Med 1992;175:1143.
8. Benos D, Hahn B, Bubien J, et al. Envelope glycoprotein gp120 of human immunodeficiency virus type 1 alters ion transport in astrocytes: implications for AIDS dementia complex. Proc Natl Acad Sci U S A 1994;91:494.

9. Brahic M, Stroop W, Baringer J. Theiler's virus persists in glial cells during demyelinating disease. Cell 1981;26:123.

10. Brenig B, Brem G. Principles of genetic manipulation in livestock. Dev Anim Vet Sci 1991;25:1.

11. Brenneman D, Westbrook G, Fitzgerald S, et al. Neuronal cell killing by the envelope protein of HIV and its prevention by vasoactive intestinal peptide. Nature 1988;335:639.

12. Brinster R, Allen J, Behringer R, Gelinas R, Palmiter R. Introns increase transcriptional efficiency in transgenic mice. Proc Natl Acad Sci U S A 1988;85:836.

13. Brinster R, Chen H, Trumbauer M, Senear A, Warren R, Palmiter R. Somatic expression of herpes thymidine kinase in mice following injection of a fusion gene into eggs. Cell 1981;27:223.

14. Brown D, Xu X, Kitajima I, et al. Genomic footprinting of the HTLV-1 LTR in a transgenic mouse tumorigenesis model. Transgene 1994 (in press).

15. Budka H. Neuropathology of human immunodeficiency virus infection. Brain Pathol 1991;1:163.

16. Bueler H, Aguzzi A, Sailer A, et al. Mice devoid of PrP are resistant to scrapie. Cell 1993;73:1339.

17. Bureau J, Manotagutelli X, Lefebrve S, Guenet J, Pla M, Brahic M. The interaction of two groups of murine genes determines the persistence of Theiler's virus in the central nervous system. J Virol 1992;66:4698.

18. Burk R, DeLoia J, ElAwady M, Gearhart J. Tissue preferential expression of the hepatitis B virus (HBV) surface antigen gene in two lines of HBV transgenic mice. J Virol 1988;62:649.

19. Cardell S, Merkenschlager M, Bodmer H, et al. The immune system of mice lacking conventional MHC class II molecules. Adv Immunol 1994;55:423.

20. Chesebro B. Spongiform encephalopathies: the transmissible agents. In: Fields B, Knipe D, eds. Virology. 2nd ed. New York: Raven Press, 1990.

21. Chisari F. Analysis of hepadnavirus gene expression biology and pathogenesis in the transgenic mouse. Curr Top Microbiol Immunol 1991;68:85.

22. Chisari F, Ferrari C. Hepatitis B virus immunopathogenesis. Annu Rev Immunol 1995;13:29.

23. Chisari F, Ferrari C, Mondelli M. Hepatitis B virus structure and biology. Microb Pathog 1989;6:311.

24. Chisari F, Filippi P, Buras J, et al. Structural and pathological effects of synthesis of hepatitis B virus large envelope polypeptide in transgenic mice. Proc Natl Acad Sci U S A 1987;84:6909.

25. Chisari F, Klopchin K, Moriyama T, et al. Molecular pathogenesis of hepatocellular carcinoma in hepatitis B virus transgenic mice. Cell 1989;58:1145.

26. Choi T, Huang M, Gorman C, Jaenisch R. A generic intron increases gene expression in transgenic mice. Mol Cell Biol 1991;11:3070.

27. Citovsky V, Wong M, Shaw A, Prasad B, Zambryski P. Visualization and characterization of tobacco mosaic virus movement protein binding to single-stranded nucleic acids. Plant Cell 1992;4:397.

28. Clement J, Wall R, Narayan O, et al. Development of transgenic sheep that express the visna virus envelope gene. Virology 1994; 200:370.

29. Cooper A, Dalton D, Stewart T, Griffin J, Russell D, Orme I. Disseminated tuberculosis in interferon gamma gene disrupted mice. J Exp Med 1993;178:2243.

30. Cooper B, Lapidot M, Heick J, Dodds J, Beachy R. A defective movement protein of TMV in transgenic plants confers resistance to multiple viruses whereas the functional analog increases susceptibility. Virology 1995;206:307.

31. Cosgrove D, Gray D, Dierich A, et al. Mice lacking MHC class II molecules. Cell 1991;66:1051.

32. Dalton D, Pitts-Meek S, Keshav S, Figari I, Bradley A, Stewart T. Multiple defects of immune cell function in mice with disrupted interferon-gamma genes. Science 1993;259:1739.

33. DeHaan P, Gielen J, Prins M, Wijkamp I, Van Schepen A. Characterization of RNA-mediated resistance to tomato spotted wilt virus in transgenic tobacco plants. Biotechnology 1992;65:221.

34. DeLoia J, Burk R, Gearhart J. Developmental regulation of hepatitis B surface antigen expression in two lines of hepatitis B virus transgenic mice. J Virol 1989;63:4069.

35. Doherty P, Hou S, Southern P. Lymphocytic choriomeningitis virus induces a chronic wasting disease in mice lacking class I major histocompatibility complex glycoproteins. J Neuroimmunol 1993;46: 11.

36. Dreyer E, Kaiser P, Offerman J. Lipton S. HIV-1 coat protein neurotoxicity prevented by calcium channel agonists. Science 1990; 248:364.

37. Durnam D, Palmiter R. Transcriptional regulation of the mouse metallothionein-1 gene by heavy metals. J Biol Chem 1981;256: 5712.

38. Dyrberg T, ed. The role of viruses and the immune system in diabetes mellitus. Curr Top Microbiol Immunol 1990;156.

39. Eichelberger M, Allan W, Zijlstra M, Jaenisch R, Doherty P. Clearance of influenza virus respiratory infections in mice lacking class I major histocompatibility complex restricted CD8+ T cells. J Exp Med 1991;174:875.

40. Epstein L, Gendelman H. Human immunodeficiency virus type I infection of the nervous system: pathogenetic mechanisms. Ann Neurol 1993;33:429.

41. Esiri M, Morris C, Millard P. Fate of oligodendrocytes in HIV-1 infection. AIDS 1991;5:1081.

42. Farza H, Hadchouel M, Scotto J, Tiollais P, Babinet C, Pourcel C. Replication and gene expression of hepatitis B virus in a transgenic mouse that contains the complete viral genome. J Virol 1988;62: 4144.

43. Farza H, Salmon A, Hadchoeul M, Moreau J. Hepatitis B surface antigen gene expression is regulated by sex steroids and glucocorticoids in transgenic mice. Proc Natl Acad Sci U S A 1987;84:1187.

44. Fiette L, Aubert C, Brahic M, Rossi C. Theiler's virus infection of beta-2 microglobulin deficient mice. J Virol 1993;67:589.

45. Fitchen J, Beachy R. Genetically engineered protection against viruses in transgenic plants. Annu Rev Microbiol 1993;47:739.

46. Fowlkes B, Pardoll D. Molecular and cellular events of T cell development. Adv Immunol 1989;44:207.

47. Fung-Leung W, Kundig T, Zinkernagel R, Mak T. Immune response against lymphocytic choriomeningitis virus infection in mice without CD8 expression. J Exp Med 1991;174:1425.

48. Gabizon R, Rosenmann M, Meiner Z, et al. Mutation and polymorphism of the prion protein gene in Libyan Jews with Creutzfeldt Jakob disease. Am J Hum Genet 1993;53:828.

49. Gajdusek C. Unconventional viruses causing subacute spongiform encephalopathies. In: Fields B, ed. Virology. New York: Raven Press, 1985:1519.

50. Giulian D, Vaca K, Noonan C. Secretion of neurotoxins by mononuclear phagocytes infected with HIV-1. Science 1990;250:1593.

51. Glowa J, Panlillo L, Brenneman D, Gozes I, Fridkin M, Hill J. Learning impairment following intracerebral administration of the HIV envelope protein gp120 or a VIP antagonist. Brain Res 1992; 570:49.

52. Gordon J. Production of transgenic mice. In: Wassarman P, DePamphilis M, eds. Methods in enzymology. Vol 225. San Diego: Academic Press, 1993:747.

53. Graham M, Dalton D, Giltinan D, Braciale V, Stewart T, Braciale T. Response to influenza infection in mice with a targeted disruption in the interferon gamma gene. J Exp Med 1993;178:1725.

54. Grusby M, Johnson R, Papiaoannou V, Glimcher L. Depletion of CD4+ T cells in major histocompatibility complex class II–deficient mice. Science 1991;250:1417.

55. Gu H, Marth J, Orban P, Mossmann H, Rajewsky K. Depletion of a DNA polymerase beta gene segment in T cells using cell type specific gene targeting. Science 1994;265:103.

56. Guidotti L, Ando K, Hobbs M, et al. Cytotoxic T lymphocytes inhibit hepatitis B virus gene expression by a non cytolytic mechanism in transgenic mice. Proc Natl Acad Sci U S A 1994;91:3764.

57. Hamer D. Metallothionein. Annu Rev Biochem 1986;55:913.

58. Hanahan D. Heritable formation of pancreatic beta cell tumors in transgenic mice expressing recombinant insulin-simian virus 40 oncogenes. Nature 1985;315:115.

59. Hergueux J, Bodmer H, Cardell S, et al. Knockout mice: a new tool for transplantation immunologists. Transplant Proc 1993;25:30.

60. Heyes M, Brew B, Martin A, et al. Quinolinic acid in cerebrospinal fluid and serum from HIV-1 infection: relationship to clinical and neurological status. Ann Neurol 1991;29:202.

61. Hill J, Mervis R, Avidor R, Moody T, Brenneman D. HIV envelope protein induced neuronal damage and retardation of behavioral development in rat neonates. Brain Res 1993;603:222.

62. Hogan B, Constantini F, Lacy E. Manipulating the mouse genome. New York: Cold Spring Harbor, 1986.
63. Horie H, Koike S, Kurata T, et al. Transgenic mice carrying the human poliovirus receptor: new animal model for study of poliovirus neurovirulence. J Virol 1994;68:681.
64. Hsaio K, Groth D, Scott M, et al. Serial transmission in rodents of neurodegeneration from transgenic mice expressing mutant prion protein. Proc Natl Acad Sci U S A 1994;91:9126.
65. Hsaio K, Scott M, Foster D, Groth D, DeArmond S, Prusiner S. Spontaneous neurodegeneration in transgenic mice with mutant prion protein of Gerstmann-Straussler-Scheinker syndrome. Science 1990;250:1587.
66. Hull R. The movement of viruses within plants. Semin Virol 1991;2:89.
67. Hyman R, Stallings V. Coordinate change in phenotype in a mouse cell line selected for CD8 expression. Immunogenetics 1992;36:149.
68. Jenson A, Rosenberg H. Multiple viruses in diabetes mellitus. Prog Med Virol 1984;29:197.
69. Kagi D, Ledermann B, Burki K, et al. Cytotoxicity mediated by T cells and natural killer cells is greatly impaired in perforin-deficient mice. Nature 1994;369:31.
70. Kanagawa O, Vaupel B, Gayama S, Koehler G, Kopf M. Resistance of mice deficient in IL-4 to retrovirus-induced immunodeficiency syndrome (MAIDS). Science 1993;262:240.
71. Kast W, Bronkhurst A, de Waal L, Melief C. Cooperation between cytotoxic and helper T lymphocytes in protection against lethal Sendai virus infection: protection by T cells is MHC-restricted and MHC-regulated. A model for MHC disease associations. J Exp Med 1986;164:723.
72. Kawchuk L, Martin R, McPherson J. Sense and anti-sense RNA-mediated resistance to potato leafroll virus in Russett Burbank potato plants. Mol Plant Microbe Interact 1991;4:227.
73. Ketzler S, Weis S, Haug H, Budka H. Loss of neurons in the frontal cortex in AIDS brains. Acta Neuropathol 1990;80:92.
74. Killeen N, Sawada S, Littman D. Regulated expression of human CD4 rescues helper T cell development in mice lacking expression of endogenous CD4. EMBO J 1993;12:1547.
75. Kitajima I, Shinohara T, Bilakovics J, Brown D, Xu X, Nerenberg M. Ablation of transplanted HTLV-1 tax-transformed tumors in mice by antisense inhibition of NF-κB. Science 1992;258:1792.
76. Kitajima I, Shinohara T, Minor T, Bibbs L, Bilakovics J, Nerenberg M. Human T cell leukemia virus type 1 tax transformation is associated with increased uptake of oligodeoxynucleotides in vitro and in vivo. J Biol Chem 1992;267:25881.
77. Koike S, Taya C, Kurata T, et al. Transgenic mice susceptible to poliovirus. Proc Natl Acad Sci U S A 1991;88:951.
78. Koller B, Marrack P, Kappler J, Smithies O. Normal development of mice deficient in beta-2-microglobulin, MHC class I proteins, and CD8+ T cells. Science 1990;248:1227.
79. Koller B, Smithies O. Inactivating the beta-2-microglobulin locus in mouse embryonic stem cells by homologous recombination. Proc Natl Acad Sci U S A 1989;86:8932.
80. Konig R, Huang L, Germain R. MHC class II interaction with CD4 mediated by a region analogous to the MHC class I binding site for CD8. Nature 1992;356:796.
81. Kopf M, Baumann H, Freer G, et al. Impaired immune and acute-phase responses in interleukin-6 deficient mice. Nature 1994;368:339.
82. Krug R, Shaw M, Broni B, Shapiro G, Haller O. Inhibition of influenza viral mRNA synthesis in cells expressing the interferon-induced Mx gene product. J Virol 1985;56:201.
83. Kuhn R, Schwenk F, Aguet M, Rajewsky K. Inducible gene targeting in mice. Science 1995;269:1427.
84. Lane D, Crawford L. T antigen is bound to a host protein in SV40-transformed cells. Nature 1979;278:261.
85. Lehmann-Grube F, Lohler J, Utermoehlen O, Gegin C. Antiviral immune responses of lymphocytic choriomeningitis virus-infected mice lacking CD8+ T lymphocytes because of a disruption of the beta-2-microglobulin gene. J Virol 1993;67:332.
86. Levine A. The tumor suppressor genes. Annu Rev Biochem 1993;62:623.
87. Lipton S. Models of neuronal injury in AIDS: another role for the NMDA receptor? Trends Neurosci 1992;15:75.
88. Lipton S. Calcium channel antagonists in the prevention of neurotoxicity. Adv Pharmacol 1991;22:271.
89. Lipton S, Sucher N, Kaiser P, Dreyer E. Synergistic effects of HIV coat protein and NMDA receptor-mediated neurotoxicity. Neuron 1991;7:111.
90. Lo D, Pursel V, Linton P, et al. Expression of a mouse IgA by transgenic mice, pigs and sheep. Eur J Immunol 1991;21:1001.
91. Mahon K, Chepelinsky A, Khillian J, Overbeek P, Piatigorsky J, Westphal H. Oncogenesis of the lens in transgenic mice. Science 1987;235:1622.
92. Mahon B, Katrak K, Nomoto A, Macadem A, Minor P, Mills K. Polio virus specific CD4+ Th1 clones with both cytotoxic and helper activity mediate protective humoral immunity against a lethal poliovirus infection in transgenic mice expressing the human poliovirus receptor. J Exp Med 1995;181:1285.
93. Mansour S, Thomas K, Capecchi M. Gene targeting in murine embryonic stem cells: introduction of specific alterations into the mammalian genome. Nature 1988;336:348.
94. Marks J, Lin J, Hinds P, Miller D, Levine A. Cellular gene expression in papillomas of the choroid plexus from transgenic mice that express the simian virus 40 large T antigen. J Virol 1989;63:790.
95. Martinez J, Georgoff I, Martinez J, Levine A. Cellular localization and cell cycle regulation by a temperature sensitive p53 protein. Genes Dev 1991;5:151.
96. Masliah E, Achim C, Ge N, De Theresa R, Wiley C. Cellular neuropathology in HIV-1 encephalitis. Res Publ Assoc Res Nerv Ment Dis 1994;72:119.
97. Matsuyama T, Kimura T, Kitagawa M, et al. Targeted disruption of IRF-1 and IRF-2 results in abnormal type I IFN gene induction and aberrant lymphocyte development. Cell 1993;75:83.
98. Mendelsohn C, Wimmer E, Racaniello V. Cellular receptor for poliovirus: molecular cloning, nucleotide sequence, and expression of a new member of the immunoglobulin superfamily. Cell 1989;56:855.
99. Mombaerts P, Iacomini J, Johnson R, Herrup K, Tonegawa S, Papaioannou V. RAG-1 deficient mice have no mature B and T lymphocytes. Cell 1992;68:869–877.
100. Moore M, Teresky A, Levine A, Seiberg M. p53 mutations are not selected for in simian virus 40 T antigen induced tumors from transgenic mice. J Virol 1992;66:641.
101. Moriyama T, Guilhot S, Klopchin K, et al. Immunobiology and pathogenesis of hepatocellular injury in hepatitis B virus transgenic mice. Science 1990;248:361.
102. Morrison L, Fields B. Parallel mechanisms in the neuropathogenesis of enteric virus infections. J Virol 1991;65:2767.
103. Mucke L, Abraham C, Ruppe M, et al. Protection against HIV-1 gp120-induced brain damage by neuronal expression of human amyloid precursor protein. J Exp Med 1995;181:1551.
104. Muller D, Koller B, Whitton J, LaPan K, Brigman K, Frelinger J. LCMV-specific class II restricted cytotoxic T cells in beta-2-microglobulin deficient mice. Science 1992;255:1576.
105. Muller M, Brenig B, Winnacker E, Brem G. Transgenic pigs carrying cDNA copies encoding the murine Mx1 protein which confers resistence to influenza virus infection. Gene 1992;121:263.
106. Muller M, Winnacker E, Brem G. Molecular cloning of porcine Mx cDNAs: new members of a family of interferon-inducible proteins with homology to GTP-binding proteins. J Interferon Res 1992;12:119.
107. Nelson R, Powell Abel P, Beachy R. Lesions and virus accumulation in inoculated transgenic tobacco plants expressing the coat protein of tobacco mosaic virus. Virology 1987;158:126.
108. Nerenberg M. Biological and molecular aspects of HTLV-1 associated diseases. In: Roos R, ed. Molecular neurovirology. Totowa, New Jersey: Humana Press, 1992:225.
109. Nerenberg M, Hinrichs S, Reynolds R, Khoury G, Jay G. The tat gene of human T lymphotropic virus type I induces mesenchymal tumors in transgenic mice. Science 1987;237:1324.
110. Notkins A, Yoon J. Virus-induced diabetes mellitus. In: Notkins A, Oldstone M, eds. Concepts in viral pathogenesis. New York: Springer-Verlag, 1984:241.
111. Ohashi P, Oehen S, Aichele P, et al. Induction of diabetes is influenced by the infectious virus and local expression of MHC class I and tumor necrosis factor. J Immunol 1993;150:5185.

112. Ohashi P, Oehen S, Buerki K, et al. Ablation of "tolerance" and induction of diabetes by virus infection in viral antigen transgenic mice. Cell 1991;65:305.

113. Oldstone M. Molecular mimicry and autoimmune disease. Cell 1987;50:819.

114. Oldstone M, Nerenberg M, Southern P, Price J, Lewicki H. Virus infection triggers insulin-dependent diabetes mellitus in a transgenic model: role of anti-self (virus) immune response. Cell 1991;65:319.

115. O'Malley M, MacLeish P. Induction of class I MHC antigens on adult primate retinal neurons. J Neuroimmunol 1993;43:45.

116. Paldi A, DeHour L, Jami J. Cis effect of lacZ sequences in transgenic mice. Transgenic Res 1993;2:325.

117. Palmiter R, Brinster R. Germ line transformation of mice. Annu Rev Genet 1986;20:465.

118. Palmiter R, Sandgren E, Avarbock M, Allen D, Brinster R. Heterologous introns can enhance expression of transgenes in mice. Proc Natl Acad Sci U S A 1991;88:478.

119. Pascal E, Goodlove P, Wu L, Lazarowitz S. Transgenic tobacco plants expressing the geminivirus BL1 protein exhibit symptoms of viral disease. Plant Cell 1993;5:795.

120. Pattison J. Experiments with scrapie with special reference to the nature of the agent and the pathology of the disease. In: Gadjusek C, Gibbs C, Alpers M, eds. Slow, latent and temperant virus infections. Washington, DC: US Government Printing Office, 1965:249.

121. Pavlovic J, Haller O, Staeheli P. Human and mouse Mx proteins inhibit different steps of the influenza virus multiplication cycle. J Virol 1992;66:2564.

122. Petito C, Cash K. Blood brain abnormalities in the acquired immunodeficiency syndrome: immunohistochemical localization of serum proteins in post-mortem brain. Ann Neurol 1992;32:658.

123. Pourcel C. Souris transgeniques pour le genome du virus de l'hepatite B. Medecine/Sciences 1989;5:626.

124. Powell P, Nelson R, Hoffman N, et al. Delay of disease development in transgenic plants that express the tobacco mosaic virus coat protein gene. Science 1986;232:738.

125. Power C, Kong P, Crawford T, et al. Cerebral white matter changes in acquired immunodeficiency syndrome dementia: alterations of the blood-brain barrier. Ann Neurol 1993;34:339.

126. Prusiner S. Molecular biology of prion diseases. Science 1991; 252:1515.

127. Prusiner S. Transgenetics and cell biology of prion diseases: investigations of PrPSc synthesis and diversity. Br Med Bull 1993;49:873.

128. Prusiner S, Scott M, Foster D, et al. Transgenetic studies implicate interactions between homologous PrP isoforms in scrapie prion replication. Cell 1990;63:673.

129. Pullen A, Miller S, Dal Canto M, Kim B. Class I deficient resistant mice intracerebrally inoculated with Theiler's virus show an increased T cell response to viral antigens and susceptibility to demyelination. Eur J Immunol 1993;23:2287.

130. Quinn D, Zajac A, Frelinger J, Muller D. Transfer of lymphocytic choriomeningitis disease in beta-2-microglobulin deficient mice by CD4+ T cells. Int Immunol 1993;5:1193.

131. Racaniello V, Ren R, Bouchard M. Poliovirus attenuation and pathogenesis in a transgenic mouse model for poliomyelitis. In: Brown, F, Lewis B. Poliovirus attenuation: molecular mechanisms and practical aspects. Basel: Karger, 1993:109.

132. Rahemtulla A, Fung-Leung W, Schilham M, et al. Normal development and function of CD8+ cells but markedly decreased helper cell activity in mice lacking CD4. Nature 1991;353:180.

133. Rall G, Mucke L, Oldstone M. Consequences of cytotoxic T lymphocyte interaction with major histocompatibility complex class 1-expressing neurons in vivo. J Exp Med 1995;182:1201–1212.

134. Raulet D. MHC class I deficient mice. Adv Immunol 1994;55:381.

135. Ren R, Constantini F, Gorgacz E, Lee J, Racaniello V. Transgenic mice expressing a human poliovirus receptor: a new model for poliomyelitis. Cell 1990;63:353.

136. Ren R, Racaniello V. Human poliovirus receptor gene expression and poliovirus tissue tropism in transgenic mice. J Virol 1992; 66:296.

137. Robertson E. Using embryonic stem cells to introduce mutations into the mouse germ line. Biol Reprod 1991;44:238.

138. Rodriguez M, Dunkel A, Thiemann R, Leibowitz J, Zijlstra M, Jaenisch R. Abrogation of resistance to Theiler's virus-induced demyelination in H-2b mice deficient in beta-2-microglobulin. J Immunol 1993;151:266.

139. Roman L, Simons L, Hammer R, Sambrook J, Gething M. The expression of influenza hemagglutinin in the pancratic beta cells of transgenic mice results in autoimmune diabetes. Cell 1990;61: 383.

140. Sabin A. Pathogenesis of poliomyelitis: reappraisal in light of new data. Science 1956;123:1151.

141. Sabin A. Oral poliovirus vaccine: history of its development and prospects for eradication of poliomyelitis. JAMA 1965;194:130.

142. Salter R, Benjamin R, Wesley P, et al. A binding site for the T cell co-receptor CD8 on the alpha 3 domain of HLA-A2. Nature 1990; 345:41.

143. Salter R, Norment A, Chen B, et al. Polymorphism in the alpha 3 domain of HLA-A molecules affects binding to CD8. Nature 1989; 338:345.

144. Sauer B. Manipulation of transgenes by site-specific recombination: use of cre recombinase. In: Wassarman P, DePamphilis M. Methods in enzymology. Vol 225. San Diego: Academic Press, 1993:890.

145. Savio T, Levi G. Neurotoxicity of HIV coat protein gp120, NMDA receptors, and protein kinase C: a study with rat cerebellar granule cell cultures. J Neurosci Res 1993;34:265.

146. Scheffner M, Munger K, Byrne J, Howley P. The state of the p53 and retinoblastoma genes in human cervical carcinoma cell lines. Proc Natl Acad Sci U S A 1991;88:5523.

147. Scott M, Foster D, Mirenda C, et al. Transgenic mice expressing hamster prion protein produce species-specific scrapie infectivity and amyloid plaques. Cell 1989;59:847.

148. Shahinian A, Pfeffer K, Lee K, et al. Differential T cell costimulatory requirements in CD28-deficient mice. Science 1993;261:609.

149. Shinkai Y, Rathbun G, Lam K, et al. RAG-2 deficient mice lack mature lymphocytes owing to the inability to initiate V(D)J rearrangement. Cell 1992;68:855.

150. Spencer D, Price R. Human immunodeficiency virus and the central nervous system. Annu Rev Microbiol 1992;46:655.

151. Thomas K, Cappechi M. Site directed mutagenesis by gene targeting in mouse embryo-derived stem cells. Cell 1987;51:503.

152. Toggas S, Masliah E, Rockenstein E, Rall G, Abraham C, Mucke L. Central nervous system damage produced by expression of the HIV-1 coat protein gp120 in transgenic mice. Nature 1994;367:188.

153. Townes T, Lilngrel J, Chen H, Brinster R, Palmiter R. Erythroid specific expression of human beta-globin genes in transgenic mice. EMBO J 1985;4:1715.

154. Tyor W, Glass J, Becker P. Cytokine expression in the brain during AIDS. Ann Neurol 1992;31:349.

155. Unger R, Foster D. Diabetes mellitus. In: Wilson J, Foster D, eds. Williams textbook of endocrinology. 7th ed. Philadelphia: WB Saunders, 1985:1018.

156. Van Dyke T, Finlay C, Miller D, Marks J, Lozano G, Levine A. Relationship between simian virus 40 large tumor antigen expression and tumor formation in transgenic mice. J Virol 1987;61:2029.

157. Vogel J, Cepeda M, Tschachler E, Napolitano L, Jay G. UV inactivation of human immunodeficiency virus gene expression in transgenic mice. J Virol 1992;66:1.

158. Vogel J, Hinrichs S, Napolitano L, Ngo L, Jay G. Liver cancer in transgenic mice carrying the human immunodeficiency virus tat gene. Cancer Res 1991;51:6686.

159. Vogel J, Hinrichs S, Reynolds R, Luciw P, Jay G. The HIV tat gene induces dermal lesions resembling Kaposi's sarcoma in transgenic mice. Nature 1988;335:606.

160. von Herrath M, Allison J, Miller J, Oldstone M. Focal expression of IL-2 does not break unresponsiveness to "self" (viral) antigen expressed in beta cells but enhances development of autoimmune disease (diabetes) after initiation of an anti-self immune response. J Clin Invest 1995;95:477.

161. von Herrath M, Docker J, Oldstone M. How virus-induced rapid or slow onset insulin-dependent diabetes mellitus in a transgenic model occurs. Immunity 1994;1:231.

162. Wassarman P, DePamphilis M, eds. Methods in enzymology. Vol 225. San Diego: Academic Press, 1994.

163. Xu X, Brown D, Kitajima I, Bilakovics J, Fey L, Nerenberg M. Transcriptional suppression of HTLV-1 occurs by an unconven-

tional interaction of a CREB factor with the R region. Mol Cell Biol 1994;14:5371.

164. Yamamura K, Tsurimoto T, Ebihara T, et al. Methylation of hepatitis B virus DNA and liver-specific suppression of RNA production in transgenic mice. Jpn J Cancer Res 1987;78:681.

165. Yewdell J, Bennick J. Cell biology of antigen processing and presentation to major histocompatibility complex class I molecule restricted T lymphocytes. Adv Immunol 1992;52:1.

166. Yoon J, Austin M, Onodera T, Notkins A. Virus-induced diabetes mellitus: isolation of a virus from the pancreas of a child with diabetic ketoacidosis. N Engl J Med 1979;300:1173.

167. Young J, Hengartner H, Podack E, Cohn Z. Purification and charac-

terization of a cytolytic pore-forming protein from granules of cloned lymphocytes with natural killer activity. Cell 1986;44: 849.

168. Young L, Klavinskis L, Oldstone M, Young J. In vivo expression of perforin by CD8+ lymphocytes during an acute viral infection. J Exp Med 1989;169:2159.

169. Zijlstra M, Bix M, Simister N, Loring J, Raulet D, Jaenisch R. Beta-2-microglobulin deficient mice lack CD4−/CD8+ cytolytic T cells. Nature 1990;344:742.

170. Zijlstra M, Li E, Sajjadi F, Subramani S, Jaenisch R. Germ line transmission of a disrupted beta 2 microglobulin gene produced by homologous recombination in embryonic stem cells. Nature 1989; 342: 435.

PART III

Classic Models of Viral Pathogenesis

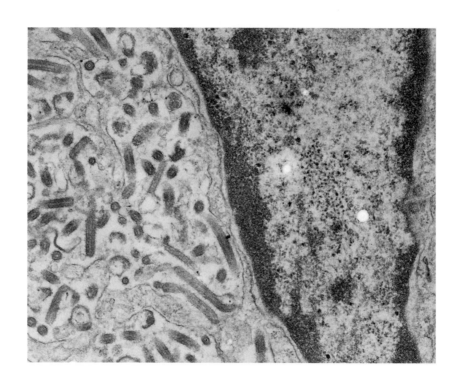

Viral Pathogenesis,
edited by Neal Nathanson, et al.
Lippincott–Raven Publishers, Philadelphia © 1997

CHAPTER 22

Mousepox

Frank Fenner and R. Mark L. Buller

INTRODUCTION

Animal viruses have three types of life cycle: the replication cycle within the cell, the cycle between entry into and exit from the body of an individual animal, and the cycle between animals within populations. The first, viral replication, is described at length, for all families of viruses, in standard texts of virology.[66] The last-mentioned cycle constitutes the subject matter of epidemiology.[49] Here we are concerned with the virus life cycle within the body of an individual animal—that is, the pathogenesis of infection.

Ectromelia virus was discovered in England in 1930 as the cause of a severe and often fatal disease of laboratory mice, which was subsequently named mousepox. Mousepox has been studied for half a century as a model of the pathogenesis of acute exanthematous diseases. In the late 1940s and 1950s, experiments in Australia on the kinetics of virus spread during infection of susceptible mice with ectromelia virus led to the concept of a primary and secondary viremia, which probably also occurs in the acute exanthematous diseases of humans. During the 1970s, the mousepox model was used to determine the role of cell-mediated immunity in recovery from infection, emphasizing the importance of the T lymphocytes and macrophages. More recently, since 1980, the part played by host genotype in the production of disease has been examined by investigators in the United States, and genetic determinants of disease susceptibility and resistance are in the process of being mapped. The latter half of the 1990s should see mousepox being used as an ideal model for the elucidation of the molecular pathogenesis of a generalized infection caused by a large and complex virus.

F. Fenner: The John Curtin School of Medical Research, The Australian National University, Mills Road, Canberra, Australia, 0200.
R. M. L. Buller: Department of Molecular Microbiology and Immunology, Saint Louis University Medical Center, St Louis, Missouri 63110.

Discovery of the Virus

The disease now called mousepox was first described in 1930 by Marchal,[93] working at the National Institute for Medical Research at Hampstead, England. She noted that a disease characterized by swelling and later amputation of a foot and by increased mortality had been occurring in their breeding stocks of mice during the previous few years. It was named infectious ectromelia because of the observed loss of a foot— *ectromelia*, defined as congenital absence or marked imperfection of one or more of the limbs, and *infectious*, to differentiate it from the congenital disease. However, Marchal recognized that it was a generalized disease, with lesions in the spleen and liver as well as the foot.

Geographic Distribution of Enzootic Mousepox

After its discovery as a disease of laboratory mice in England, mousepox was recognized as an enzootic disease in many laboratory mouse colonies in Europe, Japan, and China,[60] but its natural reservoir was unknown. Mousepox-like lesions have been described in wild mice and voles in Germany,[74] but the cause of this disease was not adequately investigated, and no further studies have been reported. Because laboratory mouse colonies in the United States appeared to be free of the disease for several years after its discovery in England and its recognition in other European countries, restrictions were placed on the importation or interstate movement of ectromelia virus or materials infected with the virus.[122]

Despite of these regulations, the virus has been introduced into the United States on several occasions. The first recognized outbreaks occurred at Yale University between 1951 and 1953, after which a committee of the National Institutes of Health reinforced the quarantine exclusion and advised research workers using mice to be especially careful about inadvertent introduction of the virus from overseas in mice or mouse tissues or cells.[122] A few other accidental introductions occurred, some of which resulted in epizootics among laboratory mice.[17,68,137,138] In addition, in the Yale Arbovirus Research Unit,[8,123] ectromelia virus was demonstrated on several occasions in imported material from mice suspected of being infected with other viruses.[40] Dr. B.A. Briody, who had worked at the Walter and Eliza Hall Institute in 1946 when work was in progress there on mousepox, contributed to the definitive diagnosis of the outbreak at Yale University,[128] and in 1956 he set up the Mouse Pox Service Laboratory. He contributed substantially to the surveillance of mouse colonies in the United States until his death in 1976.[17,18,19] In 1979 and 1980, there were disastrous outbreaks of mousepox in several laboratories in the United States,[102] which led to a commitment from the National Institutes of Health to undertake investigation of the disease in microbiologically secure laboratories.

Characterization of Ectromelia Virus

Because Marchal was unable to grow any bacteria from the livers of mice dying from acute infectious ectromelia and had also demonstrated that infection could be transmitted by material that had been passed through Pasteur-Chamberland L2, Mandler, and Berkefeld N filters, she concluded that the disease was caused by a filterable virus. Shortly after this, her colleagues Barnard and Elford[5] calculated the diameter of the virus to be between 100 and 150 nm by filtration and demonstrated particles about the same size by darkfield and ultraviolet photomicroscopy (see Inclusion Bodies), commenting that these particles were much the same size as those described earlier for the viruses of fowlpox and molluscum contagiosum.

The American pathologist E.W. Goodpasture first demonstrated that viruses could be grown on the chorioallantoic membrane of the developing chick embryo.[139] Australian virologist F.M. Burnet, who in 1932 and 1933 was working at the National Institute of Medical Research at Hampstead, adapted Goodpasture's technique so that it could be used for the assay of viruses by pock counting in a manner analogous to the plaque assay of bacteriophages,[32] and he demonstrated that ectromelia virus and antibodies to it could be titrated in this way.[35] After hemagglutination by influenza virus was discovered by Hirst in 1942,[77] Burnet and his colleagues in Melbourne investigated this phenomenon in depth, and also tested a number of other viruses to see whether they would agglutinate chicken red blood cells. Among these was vaccinia virus, which Nagler[101] demonstrated would agglutinate certain chicken red blood cells. Soon after this, Burnet[33] demonstrated not only that ectromelia virus agglutinated the same limited range of chicken red blood cells as did vaccinia virus, but that ectromelia virus hemagglutination could be inhibited by antivaccinia serum. Crossprotection tests demonstrated that ectromelia virus was a member of the vaccinia-variola group of poxviruses; it was included in the first official description of that group[61] and remains a member of the genus *Orthopoxvirus*.

Experimental Epidemiology Using Ectromelia Virus

Marchal's discovery of ectromelia virus in 1930 was immediately exploited by W.W.C. Topley and colleagues in their classic work on experimental epidemiology, adding a viral disease to their earlier studies with mouse typhoid and mouse pasteurellosis.[73] These studies demonstrated that under conditions of natural spread infectious ectromelia had a high mortality and that animals that survived in an infected herd for several weeks appeared to be immune. As has been described, in 1945 Burnet had demonstrated the immunologic relation between vaccinia and ectromelia viruses. Later that year, as Director of the Walter and Eliza Hall Institute of Medical Research, he recruited one of the authors (F.F.) to undertake experimental epidemiologic studies in the new knowledge that ectromelia virus was a member of the vaccinia-variola virus group.

Pathogenesis of Mousepox

Early studies showed that prior inoculation with vaccinia virus conferred substantial immunity to mousepox,[50] that the most important route of natural infection was through minute abrasions of the skin,[51] and that virus was eliminated from infected mice in the feces, urine, saliva, conjunctival discharge, and lesions in the skin, the latter two being the principal sources of environmental contamination.[52] In the course of this work, it was noticed that many mice that did not die of acute hepatitis developed a generalized rash,[51,54] and, by analogy with the terms smallpox and variola virus, the name mousepox was proposed for the disease and ectromelia virus for the infectious agent.[52]

In the 1940s, there was little understanding of what occurred during the long incubation period of generalized infectious diseases such as typhoid fever, smallpox, chickenpox, and measles—the incubation period, like the eclipse phase in the viral replication cycle, was a black box. Studies of mouse typhoid as a model of typhoid fever[107] had shown that after ingestion of a small dose of bacteria there was a stepwise infection of the intestine, then local lymph nodes, then liver and spleen, and then peripheral lymph nodes, but there was no suitable laboratory model for the viral exanthems. The observation that ectromelia virus, which was related to smallpox virus, produced a generalized pustular rash in a convenient laboratory animal prompted investigation of how the virus spreads in the body during the incubation period.[53,56]

At the time, the only method of viral assay was by titration of infectivity; assays were usually carried out in groups of susceptible animals, but mouse inoculation on the scale required for these experiments was exorbitantly laborious and expensive. Plaque assay of animal viruses was not introduced until 1952,[44,45] but pock-counting on the chorioallantoic membrane had been developed during the early 1930s,[32] and was applicable to ectromelia virus.[35] Experiments by Fenner,[53] later confirmed by Mims,[95] showed that pock-counting was about one tenth as sensitive as assay by mouse inoculation, but the ratio was consistent and the method reasonably accurate. Experiments were undertaken which led to a description of the way in which virus spreads in the body during the incubation period of mousepox,[53] and the results were generalized to explain the pathogenesis of the acute exanthems of humans.[56] Further experiments on the spread of ectromelia virus through the body, exploiting immunofluorescence techniques, were carried out at the John Curtin School of Medical Research by C.A. Mims[95–98] and his student J.R. Roberts.[113–115]

Immune Response in Mousepox

Studies in mice inoculated with vaccinia virus and challenged with ectromelia virus showed that heterologous immunity was not as protective as homologous immunity; passive immunization experiments showed similar differences. G.B. Mackaness, who was associated with the John Curtin School of Medical Research from 1948 to 1963, conducted pioneering research on cell-mediated immunity in a model bacterial infection of mice, listeriosis.[90] In 1963, he was joined by a research student, R.V. Blanden, who returned to the John Curtin School of Medical Research in Canberra in 1968 to study the immune response to mousepox. Here, he carried out classic experiments that demonstrated the importance of cell-mediated immunity in the process of recovery from this generalized viral infection.[10–13]

Mousepox in Inbred Strains of Mice

In the late 1950s, K. Schell,[117,118] working in Canberra, investigated the basis of genetic resistance to mousepox in inbred and outbred mice. After the outbreaks in the United States in 1979 and 1980, there was considerable concern in that country about inapparent infections in some inbred strains and dissatisfaction with existing diagnostic and screening methods for the disease. Special microbiologically secure laboratories were set up at the National Institutes of Health and experiments were begun by G.D. Wallace and P.N. Bhatt in 1980. One of the authors (R.M.L.B.) was appointed in 1982 to accelerate the work at the National Institutes of Health and worked there until 1994, when he moved to Saint Louis University. This research effort led to (1) the development of an enzyme-linked immunosorbent assay for the rapid screening of mouse sera for orthopoxvirus antibodies,[26] (2) the description of the kinetics of ectromelia virus transmission and the clinical response in infected C57BL/6, BALB/c, and AKR mice,[133] and (3) preliminary studies into the genetics resistance to severe mousepox.[31,134]

SPREAD OF ECTROMELIA VIRUS THROUGHOUT THE BODY

Virus Entry

Mice can be infected with a small dose of ectromelia virus inoculated intradermally, subcutaneously, intranasally, intravenously, intraperitoneally, or intracerebrally; oral infection usually requires a larger dose.[51] Infection can apparently occur through the intact conjunctiva but not through intact skin. In natural infections, ectromelia virus usually enters the body of the host through minute abrasions of the skin, from virus-contaminated bedding or other sources (including, potentially, the hands of laboratory attendants). It usually produces a primary lesion at the site of entry (Fig. 22-1B, C), which begins as a small macule that becomes papular and then scabs and heals. In closed epidemics in which 15 male outbred mice infected with a virulent strain of virus were introduced into a group of 100 normal male mice housed in a series of five interconnected Topley cages, careful daily examination of each mouse revealed primary lesions in 72 of 97 contact mice. Most of the mice that did not develop a primary lesion died of acute hepatitis before a primary lesion could be detected.[55]

During episodes of cannibalism, which sometimes occurred in closed colonies of mice,[51] entry probably occurred through lesions of the mucous membrane of the mouth, or through the conjunctiva or the gastric mucous membrane. Although Fenner thought that the oral route was probably unimportant except after cannibalism, Gledhill[71] showed that genetically susceptible mice could always be infected per os with large doses of virus, and some could be infected by even quite small doses. Although it was not clear from Gledhill's work whether per os infection bypassed any possible lesions of the oral mucosa, Wallace and Buller[133] were able to infect mice through a soft plastic cannula that had been carefully inserted down the esophagus into the stomach.

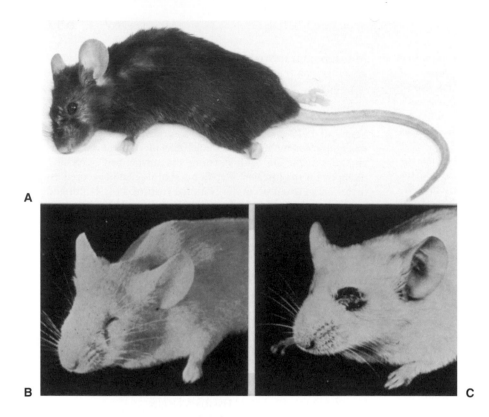

FIG. 22-1. (**A**) Mouse that had recovered from natural infection with mousepox, showing amputation of the left hind foot (the lesion that prompted Marchal to call the disease "infectious ectromelia") and scars of an earlier, generalized rash. (**B**) Primary lesion of mousepox on the left eyebrow of a naturally infected mouse 8 days after infection. (**C**) Same mouse as in **B**, 14 days after infection. (From Fenner F. Mousepox. In: Foster HL, Small JD, Fox JG, eds. The Mouse in Biomedical Research. Vol 2: Diseases. New York: Academic Press, 1982:209–230.)

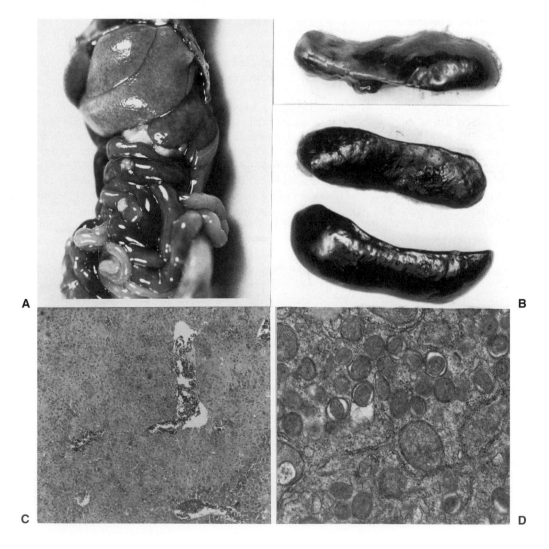

FIG. 22-2. Pathology of mousepox. (**A**) Swelling and necrosis of the liver and spleen, enlarged Peyer's patches, and hemorrhagic small intestine in a susceptible mouse killed when moribund from acute disease. (**B**) Scarring of the spleen, one of the most reliable postmortem signs of previous mousepox in recovered mice. (**C**) Section of liver, showing extensive irregular necrosis, with little inflammatory reaction. (**D**) Electron micrograph of liver cell, showing many scattered virions in the cytoplasm. A-type inclusion bodies do not develop in the liver. (**A** from Allen AM, Clarke GL, Ganaway JR, Lock A, Werner RM. Pathology and diagnosis of mousepox. Lab Anim Sci 1981; 31:599–608; **B** through **D** from Fenner F. Mousepox. In: Foster HL, Small JD, Fox JG, eds. The Mouse in Biomedical Research. Vol 2: Diseases. New York: Academic Press, 1982:209–230.)

Mice can also be infected by the inhalation of aerosols,[46,113] but the clinical and pathologic picture after aerosol infection or inhalation of small volumes of viral suspensions does not resemble that seen in natural infections.[46,51] Epidemiologic observations in a breeding colony in England,[60] during experimental studies over a period of 30 years in Australia, and in the 1979—1980 outbreak at the National Institutes of Health[135] also suggest that respiratory infection is not an important mode of natural spread, at least between mouse cages. However, droplet transmission of virus excreted from the oropharynx is by far the most important route of transmission in smallpox.[63]

Using immunofluorescent staining of appropriate sections of stripped epidermis, Roberts[114] investigated the histopathogenesis of cutaneous infections. Preliminary experiments confirmed that infection does not occur through intact skin; efficient infection requires introduction of virus into the dermis. The first cells infected are either dermal cells or cells in the malpighian layer of the epidermis, and spread occurs mostly in the dermis. Edema of the lesion is caused by an increase in capillary permeability, which begins by the third day after infection. The epidermal hyperplasia that accompanies development of the primary lesion occurs in an annulus of cells just beyond the margin of the infected cells. This hyperplastic response accompanying epidermal lesion development is a hallmark of poxvirus infections and, with analogy to other orthopoxviruses, is caused in part by a virus-encoded protein that is a functional homolog of epidermal growth factor.[27,28]

Roberts[113] also examined the pulmonary lesions produced after exposure of mice to infective aerosols. The first infected cells are either alveolar macrophages or mucosal cells of the upper or lower respiratory tract, to which infection is confined until the third day, when viral antigen is found in free macrophages in the draining lymph nodes. Mice infected by aerosol expel virus from their noses, occasionally as early as 2 to 3 days after infection and regularly by the sixth day—that is, before an exanthem (or enanthem) develops.

From Local to Systemic Infection

Marchal[93] had observed that ectromelia virus often produced an initial lesion in the foot. Sometimes the mouse recovered, with or without amputation of the affected foot (Fig. 22-1A); sometimes there were similar lesions on the tail, around the mouth, or on other parts of the skin; she commented that such mice, with a generalized disease, invariably died with severe lesions in the liver and spleen (Fig. 22-2). Subsequently, Fenner[51,52,54] observed that infected mice sometimes die of acute liver disease without developing a primary lesion. More commonly, a primary skin lesion develops, and the mice either die of acute liver disease or develop a generalized cutaneous eruption (Fig. 22-3) and then either die during the second or third week after infection, or recover.

The procedure adopted for studying the systemic spread of virus[53] was straightforward; the results were later confirmed and extended by Mims,[95–97] using immunofluorescence to identify infected cells. Large numbers of outbred mice (the only strain available in Australia at that time) were inoculated in the footpad (i.e., subcutaneously) with a small dose of virus, to mimic infection by the natural route. (In retrospect, it

may have been preferable to infect by gentle scarification of the dorsum of the foot). At daily intervals, two mice were sacrificed, serum was assayed for antibody, and blood and various organs (inoculated foot, skin from the belly, regional lymph node, spleen, and liver) were removed and assayed for their viral content.[53] The results of these assays (Fig. 22-4) were interpreted as described here and shown in Fig. 22-5.[56]

Infection with ectromelia virus takes place by the introduction of a few virus particles into the skin, and within a few hours virus can be detected in the regional lymph node. Virus multiplies in lymphatic endothelial cells as well as in macrophages and lymphoid cells in the node. Virus leaving the afferent lymphatics enters the thoracic duct and thence the bloodstream to give a primary viremia. On first entering the blood, virus is rapidly removed by macrophages lining the sinusoids of the liver, spleen, and bone marrow. Studies by Mims,[96] using immunofluorescence as well as infectivity assays, showed that after intravenous injection of a large dose of ectromelia virus, 90% of the inoculated virus was taken up by the Kupffer

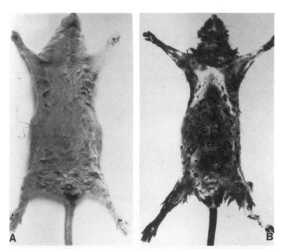

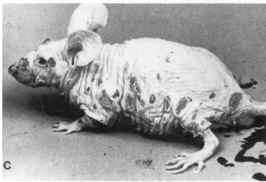

FIG. 22-3. The rash of mousepox as it appears 14 days after infection. (**A**) Normal mouse of a susceptible strain. (**B**) Normal mouse after depilation to reveal the rash. (**C**) A naturally infected hairless mutant mouse (not athymic). (**A** and **B** from Fenner F. Mousepox. In: Foster HL, Small JD, Fox JG, eds. The Mouse in Biomedical Research. Vol 2: Diseases. New York: Academic Press, 1982:209–230; **C** from Deerberg F, Kästner W, Pittermann W, Schwanzer V. Nachweis einer Ektromelie–Enzootie bei haarlosen Mäusen. Dtsch Tierärztl Wochenschr 1973;80:78–81.)

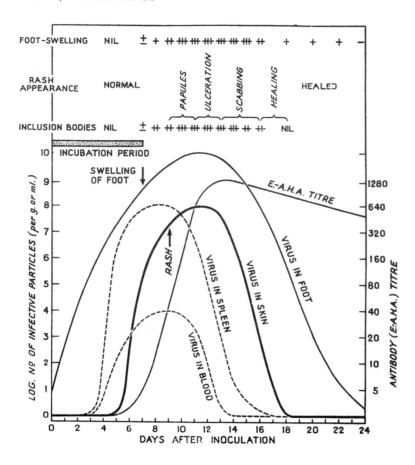

FIG. 22-4. Curves showing the concentration of virus in the foot, spleen, blood, and skin of mice inoculated in the foot with a small dose of virulent ectromelia virus. Development and disappearance of primary footpad lesion and rash are shown at top, as is the occurrence of inclusion bodies in skin distant from the inoculation site (stained by Mann's stain.) E-AHA, ectromelia antihemagglutinin antibody. (From Fenner F. The pathogenesis of the acute exanthems. An interpretation based on experimental investigations with mousepox (infectious ectromelia of mice). Lancet 1948;2:915–920.)

cells of the liver. Infection of the parenchymal cells of the liver and lymphoid cells of the spleen produces high titers of virus in these organs, with spillover into the bloodstream (secondary viremia). The virus in the blood is cell-associated, primarily in monocytes.[96,97] The prolonged secondary viremia leads to infection of other internal organs (e.g., intestine, pancreas, salivary glands) and to focal infection of the skin.

Immunofluorescence studies with cowpox virus[99] helped in the interpretation of the development of the rash of mousepox. After localization in small blood vessels of the dermis, cowpox virus infects endothelial and perivascular cells, then spreads to dermal fibroblasts and histiocytes, finally reaching the epidermis, producing focal necrosis in the epidermal cells. There is focal necrosis at the sites of infection in the liver and spleen, and if death from liver failure occurs before the eighth day there are no visible skin lesions. Nevertheless, in such animals the virus content of the skin is high, and sections of the skin shows a focal distribution of infected cells containing inclusion bodies. By the ninth day after the initial infection, at a time when the immune response has developed, edema of the infected skin cells leads to the development of pale macules, which rapidly become papular and then ulcerated, with liberation of large amounts of virus into the environment. Bilateral conjunctivitis (part of the secondary rash) is often observed before the skin lesions appear, and also in some fatal cases in which no rash is seen. The conjunctival discharge from such animals is highly infectious; there is also an enanthem, with

ulcers on the tongue and buccal mucosa.[52] Serum antibody is demonstrable on the eighth day and in survivors rises to a high level by the 14th day.

The suggestion that this pattern, with variations in relation to the site of entry and the internal organs within which multiplication occurs before the secondary viremia, applies to other generalized viral infections that produce a rash[56] was confirmed by later studies with rabbitpox in rabbits,[7] myxomatosis in rabbits,[65] and smallpox in monkeys.[76] Grose[75] suggested that although the route of infection is different (droplet infection of the upper respiratory tract), the pathogenesis of chickenpox follows the same basic pattern, with the additional feature that virus ascends the sensory nerve tracts to localize and become latent in certain sensory nerve ganglia.

The foregoing studies were carried out with a highly virulent strain of virus (Moscow) in outbred, highly susceptible mice. Subsequently, Fenner[58] showed that with an attenuated virus strain (Hampstead egg), the delay between footpad inoculation and appearance of virus in the internal organs is some 2 days longer, and attenuated strains also grow more slowly in the liver and spleen. Using immunofluorescence after intravenous inoculation of these two strains, Roberts[115] showed that the differential growth results from the lower efficiency with which the attenuated virus successfully infects Kupffer cells. Once the virus is established in the parenchymal cells of the liver, both strains grow equally well. The key role of the Kupffer cells is also demonstrated by the fact that if ec-

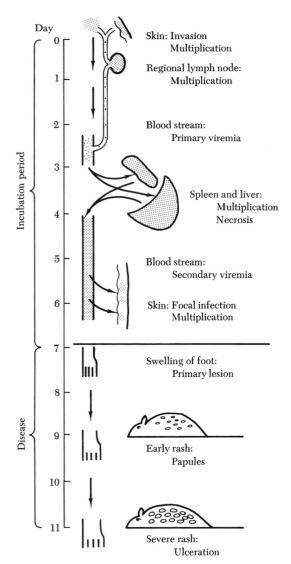

Day

0 — Skin: Invasion
Multiplication

1 — Regional lymph node:
Multiplication

2 — Blood stream:
Primary viremia

3 —

4 — Spleen and liver:
Multiplication
Necrosis

5 — Blood stream:
Secondary viremia

6 — Skin: Focal infection
Multiplication

7 —

Swelling of foot:
Primary lesion

8 —

9 — Early rash:
Papules

10 —

11 — Severe rash:
Ulceration

Incubation period

Disease

FIG. 22-5. Diagram illustrating the spread of ectromelia virus through the body. This concept has served as a model for the spread of virus through the body in many systemic viral infections (diseases of domestic animals[62] and human diseases[136]). (From Fenner F. The pathogenesis of the acute exanthems. An interpretation based on experimental investigations with mousepox (infectious ectromelia of mice). Lancet 1948;2:915–920.)

tromelia virus is mixed with antibody-containing serum and the mixture inoculated intravenously, the complex localizes in the Kupffer cells but the virus is digested.[97] The early protective effect of the Kupffer cells can be abolished by pretreatment of the mice with carrageenan.[129]

Shedding

The primary lesion and lesions of the secondary rash are the principal routes of shedding of virus, and contamination of the environment by such virus is probably the principal method of transmission.[52] Virus is also occasionally excreted in the feces and urine of mice infected through the skin. Some mice infected by the oral route excrete ectromelia virus in their feces for weeks after infection, and such mice often have virus-containing lesions at the base of the tail.[71] Wallace and Buller[132] confirmed the excretion of ectromelia virus in the feces of both susceptible (BALB/c) and resistant (C57BL) strains of mice for about 6 weeks after intragastric inoculation, as well as transmission to contact mice for up to 5 weeks. Because the C57BL mice are essentially asymptomatic throughout the course of the infection, such animals can constitute a hidden source of infection.

VIRUS-CELL INTERACTIONS

Replication of Ectromelia Virus

Little work has been done on the replication cycle of ectromelia virus; basically, it is very similar to that of vaccinia virus, the prototype *Orthopoxvirus*, which has been studied in considerable detail (Fig. 22-6).[100] Replication occurs in the cytoplasm and can be demonstrated in enucleated cells. After fusion of the virion with the plasma membrane or by endocytosis, the viral core is released into the cytoplasm. Transcription is initiated by a virion-associated transcriptase, and functional capped and polyadenylated mRNAs are produced within minutes after infection. The polypeptides produced by translation of these mRNAs complete the uncoating of the core; transcription of about 100 genes, distributed throughout the genome, occurs before viral DNA synthesis begins. Early proteins include enzymes for DNA metabolism and intermediate gene transcription as well as functions important for modification of the metabolism of the infected cell and modulation of the host's response to infection (see later discussion).

With the onset of DNA replication 2 to 5 hours after infection, there is a dramatic shift in gene expression and almost the entire genome is transcribed, but transcripts from the early genes (i.e., those transcribed before DNA replication begins) are not translated. Virion formation occurs in circumscribed areas of the cytoplasm (basophilic B-type inclusion bodies; see later discussion). Spherical immature particles can be visualized by electron microscopy; their outer bilayer becomes the outer membrane of the virion, and the core and lateral bodies differentiate within it. Some of these mature particles move to the vicinity of the Golgi complex, acquire an envelope, and are released from the cell by exocytosis. This virus is critical for cell-to-cell spread and virulence in vivo. However, most particles are not enveloped and are released by cell disruption. Both enveloped and nonenveloped particles are infectious. Ectromelia virus, like vaccinia virus, is cytocidal, but infected cells of most tissues (but not liver cells) produce eosinophilic A-type inclusion bodies (see later discussion), which are not found in vaccinia virus-infected cells.

Recent experiments have begun to unravel some of the molecular biologic aspects of ectromelia virus-cell interactions, especially as these relate to host range in cultured cells and the A-type inclusion bodies.

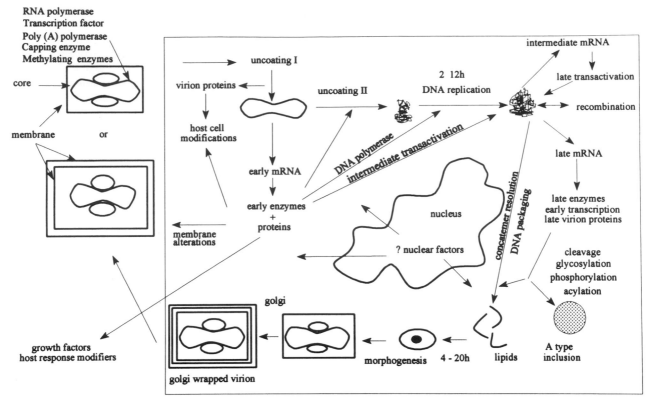

FIG. 22-6. Diagram illustrating the replication cycle of orthopoxvirus. The replication cycle of ectromelia virus is very similar except that with most strains (in most organs) the mature virions occur within inclusion bodies (see FIG. 22-8). (Modified from Moss B. Poxviridae and their replication. In: Fields BN, Knipe DM, Howley PM, eds. Fields virology. 3rd ed. New York: Raven Press, 1994;6: 2638.)

Molecular Biologic Aspects of Virus-Cell Interactions

The ectromelia virus genome is colinear with the genomes of the other orthopoxviruses and has a highly conserved central region (Fig. 22-7).[48,91] By analogy to vaccinia virus, this central region contains the virus genes involved in the production of progeny virions, whereas genes in the terminal regions of the genome are nonessential for replication in vitro and probably encode functions important in virus pathogenesis. Even in the more variable terminal regions of the genome, ectromelia virus shares extensive genetic homology with vaccinia virus, as indicated by greater than 90% predicted amino acid identity at the protein level of the products of the p16, p28, and K1L host range (*hr*) genes (see Fig. 22-7).[38,119] The ectromelia virus genome is approximately 20 kbp larger than the vaccinia virus counterpart, and a portion of this DNA represents sequences unique to ectromelia virus,[48] which possibly encode functions specific to ectromelia virus pathogenesis in the mouse.

Expression of the ectromelia virus genome appears to be identical to that of vaccinia virus, with early and late proteins.[37] Early ectromelia virus gene transcription probably involves the same transcriptional regulatory signals as vaccinia virus, with a 16-bp, A-rich critical region for the initiation of transcription approximately 30 bp upstream of the translational initiator codon and an mRNA transcription termination sequence TTTTTNT near the translational stop codon of the

gene.[37,38] Ectromelia virus genes can be expressed faithfully in vaccinia virus, and this relation is reciprocal.[38]

Because one important parameter in determining ectromelia virus pathogenesis is the range of cells and tissues in the mouse that are permissive for virus replication, a class of virus genes that govern tissue culture host range deserves comment. Unlike other viruses, in which a virion ligand has a major role in determining which cells are productively infected, poxviruses attach to, and penetrate into, most cells tested. The tissue culture host range of orthopoxviruses is governed in part by a series of unrelated genes which are required for the continued expression of the virus genome after infection. To date, three host-range genes with overlapping specificities have been identified for orthopoxviruses: the Chinese hamster ovary host range gene (CHO*hr*),[125] the K1L*hr* gene,[70] and the C7L*hr* gene.[111] Studies in a limited number of cell lines have determined a functional host-range hierarchy: CHO*hr* (Chinese hamster ovary, rabbit, human, and pig) > K1L*hr* (rabbit, human, and pig) > C7L*hr* (human and pig).[111] Seeking a genetic basis for the failure of ectromelia virus to productively infect animal species other than the mouse, and its poor replication in the majority of cell lines from the hamster and rabbit, Chen and colleagues[37,38] examined the structure and function of the CHO*hr*, K1L*hr*, and C7L*hr* genes. They found the CHO*hr* gene to be fragmented into five open reading frames and to be nonfunctional by marker rescue experiments, whereas the K1L and C7L genes were partially active, supporting ectromelia

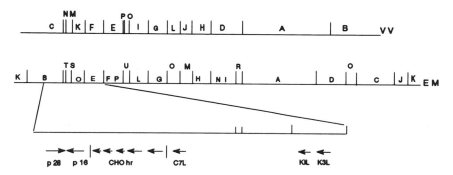

FIG. 22-7. Schematic representation of the sequenced region of the ectromelia virus (EM) genome in comparison with the vaccinia virus (VV) genome. (Hin*dIII* map of the genome of vaccinia virus WR strain from DeFilippes FM. Restriction enzyme mapping of vaccinia virus DNA. J Virol 1982;43:136–149. Hin*dIII* map of ectromelia virus DNA from Mackett M, Archard LC. Conservation and variation in orthopoxvirus genome structure. J Gen Virol 1979;45:683–701, with modifications from Senkevich TG, Muravnik GL, Chernos VI. Search for unique sequences in ectromelia virus genome by criss-cross hybridizations with DNA of other orthopoxviruses. Mol Gen Mikrobiol Virusol 1992;9–10: 13–15.)

virus replication but in a more limited number of cell lines than their vaccinia virus counterparts. Complete inactivation of the K1L gene had no apparent effect on ectromelia virus pathogenesis in the A/J and C57BL/6J mouse strains tested, but this did not rule out its importance in other inbred or outbred strains of mice. Although the loss of function of the ectromelia virus *hr* genes can explain the limited tissue culture host range of ec-

tromelia virus, it does not explain the narrow species tropism in vivo or the pattern of virus replication in tissues of susceptible mouse strains: an ectromelia virus CHO*hr*+ recombinant (but not wild-type ectromelia virus) replicated well in Chinese hamster ovary, RK-13 (rabbit kidney), and MRC-5 (human embryonic lung) cells, yet failed to produce lesions after infection of the rat and Syrian hamster (W. Chen, R.M.L. Buller, un-

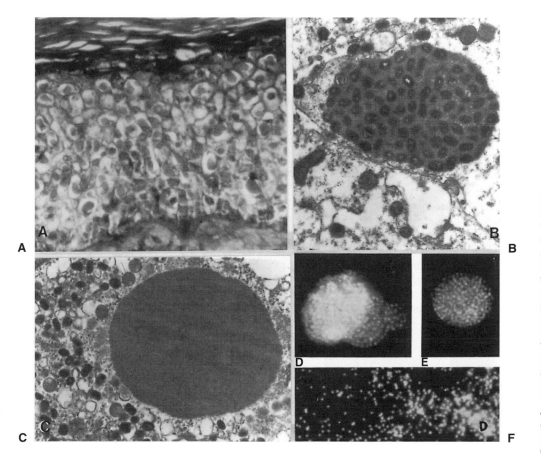

FIG. 22-8. A-type inclusion bodies in the cytoplasm of cells infected with ectromelia virus. (**A**) Section of skin, stained with Mann's stain. (**B** and **C**) Electron micrographs of inclusion bodies with occluded virions (V+) or lacking virions (V-). (Courtesy of Dr. Y. Ichihashi, Institute for Virus Research, Kyoto University.) (**D** and **E**) Virions within inclusion bodies. Darkfield illumination, original magnification 1250×. (**F**) Virions released from macerated inclusion body. Darkfield illumination, original magnification 1250×. (**D** through **F**, from Barnard JE, Elford WJ. The causative organism in infectious ectromelia. Proc R Soc Lond B Biol Sci 1931; 09:360–380.)

published results). This occurred in spite of the fact that the CHO*hr* gene supports orthopoxvirus replication in a broader range of cell types than either the K1L or C7L genes, suggesting that there are other genes involved in ectromelia virus host range in vivo.

Inclusion Bodies in Cells Infected With Ectromelia Virus

Marchal[93] was struck by the large eosinophilic cytoplasmic inclusion bodies found in virus-infected cells in most tissues and organs (but not in liver cells), and Barnard and Elford,[5] using darkfield microscopy, showed that such inclusion bodies were packed with virus particles (Fig. 22-8*D* through *F*). Subsequent investigations showed that there are two types of cytoplasmic inclusion bodies in most cells infected with ectromelia virus: those what Japanese investigators[86] have called A-type inclusion bodies (ATIs), which appear late in infection and are eosinophilic, and the basophilic B-type inclusion bodies, which are present in all poxvirus-infected cells (including those infected with vaccinia virus) from an early stage after infection and are the sites of viral replication. With most strains of ectromelia virus (e.g., the original Hampstead strain), ATIs contain large numbers of virus particles (see Fig. 22-8*B,D* through *F*), such strains are designated V+.[80] Virions are completely absent from the ATIs of some other strains (e.g., Ishibashi strain), which are designated V− (see Fig. 22-8*C*). The factor necessary for inclusion of virions into ATIs, designated VO, is present on the surface of the virion, into which it is incorporated a short time before occlusion takes place.[121] If cells are infected with mixed V+ and V− strains, only V+ inclusion bodies are found; however the ATIs contain virions of both types. With cowpox and raccoonpox viruses (and probably with ectromelia virus), the dominant and probably the only protein in V− ATIs is a 160-Kb protein that is produced late and in great abundance.[110] The WR strain of vaccinia virus also encodes the gene for this protein, but it is fragmented and ATIs are not produced during infection.[3]

IMMUNE RESPONSES

In experiments on the spread of virus in the body, Fenner[53] tested for humoral antibodies by the hemagglutination inhibition test and for cell-mediated immunity by the accelerated footpad reaction to the injection of a large dose of virus. Antibody was first detected on the seventh day after footpad inoculation of the virulent strain and on the ninth day after inoculation of the more slowly progressive attenuated strain, in both cases reaching a peak by the 14th day. A slightly accelerated delayed-type hypersensitivity reaction was first seen after inoculations made 7 days after the primary infection, and a strong reaction was always found by the 14th day.

Active Immunity

Early investigations showed that mice that had recovered from mousepox are immune to reinfection.[73,93] This immunity declines slowly, but even a year after the first infection, replication of virus after footpad inoculation is confined to the local skin lesion and only very rarely can virus be isolated from the spleen.[59] When replication occurs, the foot becomes swollen and the antibody titer usually rises. Long-continued experimental epidemics have demonstrated the epidemiologic importance of this durable immunity. In only 3 out of 168 mice that had recovered from mousepox did any sign of reinfection or recurrence occur, and in none of these did it proceed beyond a local lesion in the foot.[55]

Prior infection with an orthopoxvirus provides some protection against infection with any other orthopoxvirus. Before restriction mapping of the viral DNA became available, crossprotection in a suitable animal was the definitive test for the allocation of a virus to a genus.[34,64] Fenner[57] followed the growth of virus in various organs after footpad inoculation in mice that had recently recovered from infection with either ectromelia virus or vaccinia virus. In mice that had recovered from an attack of mousepox, there was a delayed-type hypersensitivity response to doses of 10^6 times the median infectious dose (ID50) or more. There was limited replication in the foot in most mice tested after challenge with a small dose; assay of the spleen between the 4th and the 12th days was positive in only 1 of 18 animals, and viremia was never detected. In other words, prior infection with ectromelia virus was almost completely effective in suppressing invasion. Active immunization with vaccinia virus provided much less protection (Fig. 22-9*B*). The level of ectromelia virus in the inoculated foot was reduced about 50-fold compared with control mice; invasion of the spleen occurred in most mice, but the titer reached only 10^2 rather than 10^8 times the ID50; viremia was rarely detected; and the skin distant from the inoculation site was infected in very few animals. There is no measurable change in antibody levels of ectromelia hemagglutinin after homologous immunization, but in mice infected with vaccinia virus there is a substantial rise in titer and a reversal of the ectromelia-vaccinia hemagglutinin titer from the seventh day after infection. This reversal of titer is a useful index of infection with ectromelia virus in mice that have previously been vaccinated with vaccinia virus.

Passive Immunity

It has long been believed that the humoral component of the immune response plays an important role in both protection against orthopoxvirus infections and recovery from established infections. The early protective effect of antibodies is most clearly demonstrated by passive immunization, which has been studied in mousepox both by the inoculation of antisera and by testing of suckling mice. Subsequent studies (see later discussion) have shown that cell-mediated immunity is much more important than the humoral response in the recovery process.

Using the same protocol as in actively immunized mice, Fenner[57] followed the growth of virus in various organs after footpad inoculation of mice that had been inoculated intraperitoneally with 1 mL of mouse antiectromelia serum or antivaccinia serum so that before challenge inoculation their serum ectromelia antihemagglutinin titers were 80 and 20, re-

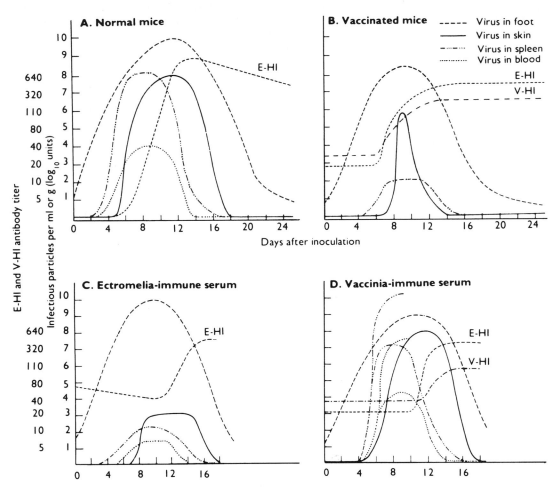

FIG. 22-9. Spread of ectromelia virus through the organs of mice. (**A**) Normal unprotected mice. (**B** through **D**) Mice protected by infection 14 days earlier with vaccinia virus (**B**), by passive immunization with ectromelia-immune mouse serum (**C**), or by vaccinia-immune mouse serum (**D**). E-HI and V-HI, hemagglutinin-inhibiting antibodies to ectromelia and vaccinia antigens, respectively. (From Fenner F. Studies in mousepox (infectious ectromelia in mice). IV. Quantitative investigations on the spread of virus through the host in actively and passively immunized animals. Aust J Exp Biol Med Sci 1949;27:1–17.)

spectively, with vaccinia antihemagglutinin titer 40 in both cases. The growth curves after inoculation of the virulent Moscow strain are shown in Figures 22-9C and D. Passive immunization with antivaccinia serum was almost without effect on the progress of the infection; the growth curves in various organs were little different from those found in normal mice, and several deaths occurred on the ninth day in both passively immunized and control mice. On the other hand, homologous antiserum gave much greater protection; although replication in the inoculated foot was similar to that in controls, the growth curves in the spleen and skin, as well as the viremia, were much lower.

The route of passage of antibody in natural passive immunity was demonstrated in mice that were borne by mothers that had recovered from mousepox and suckled by immune or normal mothers.[54] Serum assays of newborn and full-term young delivered by cesarean section showed that some antibody is transmitted through the placenta but much more in the colostrum and milk. Challenge footpad inoculation at 14 days of age showed that mice borne by either normal or immune mothers that have suckled on immune mothers survive infection with small doses of virus, whereas the offspring of immune mothers that have suckled on normal mothers all die at the same time as the controls.

Cell-Mediated Immunity in Recovery From Mousepox

Early experiments by Blanden[10] showed that subcutaneous inoculation of rabbit antimouse thymocyte serum depletes thymus-dependent areas of lymphoid tissue and selectively depresses blood lymphocyte counts but does not affect the function of Kupffer cells and other macrophages. All C57BL mice given two doses of antimouse thymocyte serum before subcutaneous inoculation with the Moscow strain of ectromelia virus died, with high titers of virus in the liver and spleen, whereas only 20% of control mice died. The deaths occurred before neutralizing antibody or delayed-type hypersensitivity could be detected, but the interferon (IFN) levels were higher in the treated mice than in the controls. When the Hampstead egg attenuated strain of ectromelia virus was used, there was a much higher mortality rate and level of virus in liver and spleen in mice treated with antimouse thymocyte serum; although the levels of neutralizing antibody were similar, there was a much depressed delayed-type hypersensitivity reaction. Other experiments[11,12] showed that immune spleen cells transfer highly efficient antiviral activity, which is virus-specific, whereas passively administered IFN or antibody are ineffective. Anti-theta treatment deleted effector activity from immune cell populations, whereas elimination of B cells and macrophages had no effect, showing that the essential effector cells are T lymphocytes. Cell-mediated immunity appears to operate by promoting the invasion of foci of infection in target organs by inflammatory cells. The results of cell transfer experiments suggest that specifically sensitized T cells first enter the foci as a consequence of antigen recognition and trigger this invasion by the secretion of cytokines. The elimination of infectious virus then depends on its phagocytosis and destruction by mononuclear phagocytes that are attracted to the foci, probably by cytokines elaborated by T cells.[13]

The development of the understanding of T-cell function led to refinements in both experimentation and interpretation. Shortly after the discovery of major histocompatibility complex restriction in the same laboratory by Zinkernagel and Doherty,[140] Blanden and colleagues[15] confirmed that the efficient transfer of antiviral activity in vivo and the activity of cytotoxic T cells in vitro required that the donors and recipients share the same *H-2* gene complex. With the use of an in vitro assay, the cytotoxic T-cell response showed similar kinetics, with a peak response 5 to 6 days after infection, coinciding with a decline of virus titer in the spleen.[16] After intravenous inoculation of graded doses of ectromelia virus, spleen titers increased logarithmically for 2 days, then declined to undetectable levels by day 5. Memory T cells appeared in the spleen within 12 to 14 days after primary infection, reaching a plateau at 5 to 6 weeks and persisting for at least 16 months.[69]

The weight of the experimental evidence supported an essential role of cell-mediated immunity in the clearance of ectromelia virus infectivity from liver and spleen, commencing 5 to 7 days after footpad infection; however, it was not known whether CD8+ cytotoxic T cells were also an early component in the host response to ectromelia virus infection. Accordingly, O'Neill and Brenan[105] examined C57BL/6 mice after inoculation in the footpad and detected cytotoxic T-cell precursors and cytotoxic T cells in the popliteal lymph node by 2 and 4 days after infection, respectively. A subsequent study found this early induction of cytotoxic T cells to be under *H-2* control.[101] Together, these studies are consistent with the importance of cytotoxic T cells in the early host immune response to infection.

More recently, the importance of the CD4+ and CD8+ T-cell subsets in the recovery of C57BL/6 mice from mousepox has been examined using both monoclonal antibody therapy and gene knockout mouse strains. In agreement with the early work of Blanden, Buller and colleagues[29] showed that infected C57BL/6 mice lacking both T-cell subsets and those lacking only CD8+ T cells were unable to generate a virus-specific cytotoxic T-cell response and suffered uniformly fatal mousepox.

C57BL/6 mice lacking only the CD4+ T cells did not succumb to lethal mousepox and were shown to generate a virus-specific cytotoxic T-cell response, although the magnitude of the response appeared to depend on experimental conditions. Although CD4+ T cell—deficient mice did not experience higher rates of fatal mousepox than intact control mice, these mice were unable to clear virus from spleen, liver, and lung tissues, and high levels of virus infectivity were still detected in skin 26 days after infection, when the experiment was terminated (G. Karupiah and RMLB, Laboratory of Viral Diseases, NIAID, NIH, 1993). This suggests that there is a tissue-dependent differential importance of CD4+ T cells in the clearance of ectromelia virus. A similar finding has been reported for CD4+ T cell—deficient C57BL/6 mice infected with murine cytomegalovirus.[83]

Role of Interferons in Resistance to Mousepox

Although the foregoing experiments emphasized the overwhelming importance of cell-mediated immunity in recovery from mousepox, certain nonimmunologic factors have been shown to be important in resistance. Jacoby and colleagues[83] found that in the highly resistant C57BL strain, both NK cells and INF-α and INF-β, which are activated during the first 3 to 4 days of infection, are critical for survival. It was subsequently confirmed that although INF-α and INF-β play an important role, INF-γ is even more important.[84] Treatment of ectromelia virus—infected C57BL/6 mice with anti–INF-γ antibody transforms a mild, inapparent infection into a severe, rapidly progressive disease with 100% mortality and a mean survival time of 7 to 7.2 days, the same as that of infected, untreated susceptible A/J mice but shorter than the 9.5 days observed for infected, untreated mice with the severe combined immunodeficiency mutation (strain C.B-17), which lacks B and T cells. These results are consistent with the hypothesis that IFN-γ plays an early role in host defense and is the critical effector cytokine in cytotoxic T-cell—mediated virus clearance during the latter portion of the recovery process. Potential sources of IFN-γ during infection are NK cells and T cells expressing the T-cell receptor gd or ab. The importance of IFNs in recovery from mousepox was unanticipated, because of the high resistance shown by ectromelia virus replication in L929 cells to INFs-α, -β, or -γ at concentrations up to 500 U (W. Chen and RMLB, Laboratory of Viral Diseases, NIAID, NIH, 1993).

Although INF-γ has been shown to be important in the in vivo clearance of other viruses, including murine cytomegalovirus[89] and herpes simplex virus type 1,[128] the mechanism involved has not been elucidated. In the case of ectromelia virus, the results cannot be explained entirely through IFN-γ effects on cell-mediated immunity or induction of the antiviral P1/eIF-2 kinase or 2',5'-oligoA synthetase pathways; rather, the data suggest the existence of a distinct IFN-γ—induced antiviral mechanism that is not present in all cell lineages. Karupiah and colleagues[85] found an IFN-γ—induced antiviral pathway in mouse RAW264.7 macrophage-like cells and primary mouse macrophages, but not in L929 or 293 human renal epithelial cells; subsequent experiments identified nitric oxide as the antiviral mediator. This study supports four conclusions.

First, the activity of nitric oxide synthase is both necessary and sufficient for a substantial antiviral effect of IFN-γ in vitro. Second, although nitric oxide synthase has many potential enzymatic actions, provision of nitric oxide alone is sufficient to inhibit viral replication. Third, nitric oxide probably has an in vivo role in IFN-γ–mediated host clearance of ectromelia virus. Finally, the replication of other DNA-containing viruses, such as herpes simplex virus type 1 and vaccinia virus, is also sensitive to nitric oxide.

GENETIC AND PHYSIOLOGIC RESISTANCE

Resistance of Different Mouse Genotypes

Early experiments and experience with mousepox involved outbred, highly susceptible mice. However, in an outbreak in Buffalo, New York, in 1954 and 1955, case-fatality rates among different inbred strains of mice differed greatly; in some strains, the disease produced obvious signs and a high mortality, but in other strains it was subclinical.[20] Noting that mice of the C57BL strain were highly resistant, Schell[117,118] compared the responses to ectromelia virus in susceptible outbred and C57BL mice. He found no differences in the infectivity end points in the two strains after footpad inoculation or natural infection, but the titer of virus in the footpad of C57BL mice ceased to rise 6 days after infection, and the highest titers in the blood and internal organs were 2 to 3 $\log_{10}$ units lower than in the susceptible mice. Cultured cells from each strain were equally susceptible to infection, but neutralizing antibody, delayed-type hypersensitivity, and active immunity were demonstrable 1 to 2 days earlier in the C57BL mice.

The variation in genetic resistance to mousepox among mouse strains cannot be explained solely on the basis of induction of cell-mediated immunity. Using C57BL/10 strains congenic for the various *H-2* haplotypes of mouse strains susceptible to severe mousepox, O'Neill and colleagues[105] found only minor differences in disease severity attributable to the *H-2* haplotypes. This and additional studies by Blanden and colleagues[14,104] supported the existence of at least one major resistance gene not linked to *H-2*.

Further analysis of different recombinant *H-2* haplotypes in the presence of the C57BL background gene have shown that the C57BL/10.A(5R) mouse strain has a median lethal dose (LD50) that is 100- to 10,000-fold lower than that of other C57BL/10 *H-2* congenics.[14] In spite of the induction of a strong virus-specific cytotoxic T-cell response, C57BL/10.A(5R) mice died, but without the severe liver necrosis found in A/J mice, much later (9 to 14 days after infection), and with large necrotic foci in the spleen, perhaps because in these mice a splenocyte subpopulation allowed efficient viral replication but displayed insufficient class I major histocompatibility complex antigen on the cell surface for efficient recognition by cytotoxic T cells.

After the concern arising out of the 1979—1980 outbreaks of mousepox in the United States, comparisons between mice of different genotypes were greatly expanded by workers at the National Institutes of Health[132] and at Yale University.[9] Both groups found that all mouse strains tested were equally susceptible to infection by footpad inoculation (Table 22-1), but the outcome was usually lethal in some strains and subclinical in others. Further experiments were carried out with BALB/c and A/J mice, as prototypes of genetically highly susceptible strains, and with C57BL/6, as a highly resistant strain. The disease in BALB/c mice infected by footpad inoculation or in contact experiments closely resembled that in outbred mice, as described by Fenner, but rashes were rarely seen, although conjunctivitis was common in nonfatal cases.[9] About 30% of BALB/c mice survived infection induced by gastric inoculation with a soft plastic tube and developed chronic, severe scabbing of the tail and feet and conjunctivitis.[132] Immunohistochemical studies revealed, in addition to the sites of replication previously identified, focal areas of infection in bone marrow, ovary, uterus, Peyer's patches, and adjacent intestinal epithelium, nasal turbinates, and oral mucosa.[81] Infection of the skin, nasal turbinates, oral mucosa, and small intestine were regarded as being important for transmission to contact mice.

The disease in A/J mice inoculated into the footpad with the Moscow strain of ectromelia virus is even more severe than that seen in BALB/c mice; virus spreads to the spleen and liver within 3 days after infection and produces almost confluent necrosis of the popliteal node by 4 days and liver by 7 days after infection. Infected mice showed a rapid onset of disease signs (i.e., ataxis, hunched posture, and ruffled fur) approximately 24 hours before death, which occurred 7 and 8 days after infection, before the formation of the primary lesion. Ermolaeva and colleagues[47] found the LD50 for the A/J mouse to be fivefold lower than that for the BALB/c mouse, and O'Neill and Blanden[104] found it to be 100-fold lower. The relative LD50 values reported for these two mouse strains by these workers differ from those reported in Table 22-1, possibly because of sex and BALB/c substrain differences.[25]

In contrast, the only sign of disease in C57BL/6 mice was swelling of the foot. Although virus was not detected in the blood on days 3 through 9, transient viremia must have occurred, because serial histologic and immunohistochemical examination of the internal organs showed that there were a few necrotic foci in the liver, around which mononuclear cells

TABLE 22-1. *Comparison of infectivity and lethality of ectromelia virus in inbred strains of mice**

Mouse strain	Lethality (LD50)†	Infectivity (ID50)‡
C57BL/6J	1.0	7.0
AKR/J	1.0	—
BALB/cByJ	6.9	7.1
DBA/2J	6.2	6.2
A.By/SNJ	6.3	7.0
C3H/HeJ	7.1	7.2

*NIH-79 strain of ectromelia virus, titer $10^{6.3}$ plaque-forming units per mL in BS-C-1 cells. Mice were inoculated with 0.05 mL by the footpad route. Only male mice 6 to 10 weeks of age were used in this study.
†Expressed as negative log base 10.
‡Infection defined by positive enzyme-linked immunosorbent assay.
From Wallace GD, Buller RML. Kinetics of ectromelia virus (mousepox) transmission and clinical response in C57BL/6J, BALB/cByJ and AKR/J inbred mice. Lab Anim Sci 1985;35:41—46.

accumulated. Small quantities of viral antigen and small areas of necrosis were also seen in the bone marrow and nasal mucosa, but not in the spleen.[81]

Kinetic studies following the spread of ectromelia virus from the footpad site of inoculation to the spleen and liver in BALB/c mice revealed earlier detectable virus replication and higher virus infectivity levels in tested tissues than in C57BL/6 mice.[105] The lower viral levels in C57BL/6 mice correlated with an earlier and stronger nonspecific and virus-specific cytotoxic T-cell response,[106] and a similar correlation was observed among resistant and susceptible C57BL/10 congenic mouse strains.[103] However, with the use of *H-2*-compatible radiation chimeras, it was shown that the major resistance genes in C57BL/6 mice did not operate through radiosensitive lymphoid cells (i.e., stem cells, T cells, B cells, or tissue macrophages).

Genetics of Resistance

The number of resistance genes detected in breeding experiments depends on the route of inoculation of the virus and the genotypes of the crossed parents. In crosses between the disease-resistant C57BL strain and susceptible outbred mice, Schell[118] demonstrated that resistance to footpad challenge is dominant and appears to be largely determined by a single, autosomal gene. Similar results were obtained by Ermolaeva and colleagues[47] using a C57BL/6 × susceptible A strain cross; they also determined that resistance was not linked to coat color. This gene was provisionally termed *Rmp-1* (*r*esistance to *m*ouse*p*ox) by Wallace and colleagues, who extended these studies to crosses between the C57BL/6 and BALB/c or DBA/2 strains and found resistance to be dominant, polygenic, and with a sexual dimorphism.[25,134] Analysis of the *H-2* haplotypes of ectromelia virus-infected progeny of a A/J × (C57BL/10J × A/J) F1 backcross showed that *Rmp-1* segregated independently of the *H-2* gene complex and therefore is not located on chromosome 17.[14] More recently, Brownstein and colleagues[23,24] continued the analysis of the C57BL/6 × DBA/2 cross and determined that resistance in male mice was mediated by three unlinked genes: two gonad-dependent genes, which they named *Rmp-2* and *Rmp-3,* and an unmapped gonad-independent gene (presumably *Rmp-1*), which alone was fully protective. Serial backcross analysis confirmed significant linkage of *Rmp-2* to the *Hc* locus on chromosome 2, which encodes the gene for the fifth component of complement, and of *Rmp-3* to the *H-2* complex on chromosome 17. Evidence was also provided for the existence of a fourth resistance gene, *Rmp-4*.[22] A recent study supports an early role for at least one of the *Rmp* genes in the genetic control of ectromelia virus replication.[21]

Physiologic Determinants of Resistance

If mouse genotype is held constant, a number of physiologic factors affect the host response, and thereby the lethality of the infection. Two factors that have been studied are age[59] and exposure to low temperature.[116] In contrast to the resistance of 8-week-old mice, both suckling and year-old mice are highly susceptible to the attenuated Hampstead egg-passaged strain. After footpad inoculation of 10^2 times the ID50, survivors were 5 out of 19 suckling mice, 19 out of 20 8-week-old mice, and 1 out of 16 56-week-old mice. In closed epidemics, the aged mice suffered 19 deaths among 50 mice, and the 8-week-old mice only 2 out of 50. The increased susceptibility of the suckling mice, but not that of the aged mice, is associated with much more rapid progress of the infection and shorter survival times, possibly because of less protection by immature phagocytic cells in the reticuloendothelial system.

VIRUS VIRULENCE

Determination of the virulence of ectromelia virus, defined in terms of the potential of a virus strain for producing a fatal infection in its natural host (the mouse) in natural or simulated infections, depends on strict definition of mouse genotype; physiologic parameters such as age, sex, pregnancy, and concurrent infection with other viruses; and environmental factors. Virtually all strains of ectromelia virus isolated from naturally infected laboratory mice are highly virulent for outbred or susceptible inbred strains of mice, although there are small differences in the virulence of different strains. Serial passage on the chorioallantoic membrane[58] and in chick embryo fibroblasts[92,133] results in substantial attenuation.

Roberts[115] compared the virulence in susceptible outbred mice of the Hampstead mouse-passaged strain (by footpad inoculation 1 LD50=10 ID50) and the attenuated egg-passaged derivative (1 LD50>10^7 ID50). After intravenous inoculation, even 100 times the footpad ID50 of the egg-passaged strain failed to infect, whereas 1 ID50 of the mouse-passaged strain was infectious. Infectivity titrations of the livers after intravenous inoculation with 10^7 times the footpad ID50 of each viral strain showed that the egg-passaged strain grows more slowly; immunofluorescence studies showed that this is a result of its lower infectivity and level of replication in Kupffer cells. Once in the parenchymal cells of the liver, both strains grow equally well. This lower virulence for phagocytic reticuloendothelial cells probably operates at each step in the sequence of tissue infections that characterizes natural infections with ectromelia virus.

Virulence and Infectivity

In early studies, Andrewes and Elford[4] found that the Hampstead (mouse-passaged) strain was much less infectious, as defined by its rate of spread, than the Moscow (mouse-passaged) strain. Closed epidemic experiments[54] showed that the attenuated Hampstead egg strain was associated with a lower mortality rate and a longer incubation period than the highly virulent Moscow strain and was also much less infectious. Subsequently, by comparing two nonattenuated strains and the attenuated derivative of one of these strains in closed epidemics, Fenner[58] found that virulence and infectivity could vary independently; the Moscow strain was highly virulent and highly infectious, the Hampstead mouse-passaged strain was highly virulent but less infectious, and the Hampstead egg-passaged strain was of low virulence and low infectivity (Table 22-2).

TABLE 22-2. *Lack of correlation between virulence and infectivity of three strains of ectromelia virus*

Assay of infectivity or virulence	Strain of virus		
	Moscow (mouse-passaged)	Hampstead (mouse-passaged)	Hampstead (egg-passaged)
Chorioallantoic membrane assay (pocks/mL)	$10^{8.5}$	$10^{8.4}$	$10^{8.3}$
Footpad inoculation assay with 0.05 mL of 10^{-6} dilution (dead/total)	19/20	16/20	1/20
Fomite exposure* (infected/total)	27/48	3/48	5/48

*Six mice per cage exposed for 24 hours in cages in which 40 g of sawdust litter had been sprayed with 2 mL of undiluted virus suspension.

Modified from Fenner F. Studies in mousepox (infectious ectromelia in mice). VI. A comparison of the virulence and infectivity of three strains of ectromelia virus. Aust J Exp Biol Med Sci 1949;27:31–43.

Molecular Determinants of Virulence

By analogy with the other orthopoxviruses, ectromelia virus virulence genes can be expected to fall into at least three categories. First, there are the genes that are involved in stimulating host synthesis of macromolecules in resting cells. In vaccinia virus, enzymes for nucleic acid metabolism, such as thymidine kinase,[30] ribonucleotide reductase,[39] thymidylate kinase,[78] DNA ligase,[87] and vaccinia growth factor,[27,28] fall into this class. Second, there are a large number of virus-encoded functions involved in the production of extracellular enveloped virus which, in vivo, are probably essential for cell-to-cell spread of virus, induction of a generalized infection, and transmission from animal to animal. In vaccinia virus, at least four genes have been identified in the formation of this type of virion.[124] Finally, a third class of virus genes encodes functions that target the host responses to infection and perhaps extend the time for virus replication and transmission before clearance by the immune system. To date, the identified poxvirus host response modifier (*hrm*) genes predominantly modulate the innate host response mechanisms, such as IFNs, complement, and inflammatory cells (Fig. 22-10). Not all poxvirus species encode the same repertoire of *hrm* genes. In the case of vaccinia virus strain Copenhagen, the genes with homology to the virus tumor necrosis factor receptor appear to be nonfunctional, and the *crm A* gene is fragmented, even though these genes are important in the pathogenesis of myxoma virus and cowpox virus infections, respectively.[67,72,109,130] Similarly, vaccinia complement control protein is present in vaccinia virus,[79,88] but not in swinepox virus.[94] This suggests that each poxvirus, through coevolution with its host, has developed a unique pattern of virulence genes.

Study of the ectromelia virus—encoded virulence genes is still in its infancy; however, screening of ectromelia virus—infected cell lysates and culture supernatants and DNA sequence analysis of ectromelia virus genomic DNA have detected the products of the *hrm* genes described in Figure 22-10, except for the genes encoding the vIL-1R and veIF-2α homologs. The vIL-1R could not be found through competition binding assays using radiolabeled mouse interleukin-1β under conditions that could detect vIL-1R in vaccinia virus culture supernatants (M.K. Spriggs, R.M.L. Buller, unpub-

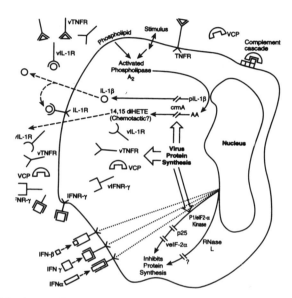

FIG. 22-10. Poxvirus host response modifier (*hrm*) genes. Comparison of translated poxvirus DNA sequences with the protein gene bank has led to the identification and study of virus genes that modulate the host's responses to infection. These *hrm* genes are predominantly directed against the innate and inflammatory responses to infection. Vaccinia complement control protein (VCP) blocks the antibody-dependent classic and alternate complement pathways.[79,88] Cytokine response modifier A (crmA) blocks the conversion of precursor interleukin-1-beta (pIL-1β) to mature IL-1β[112] and inhibits the production of a 14,15-dihydroxyeicosatetraenoic acid (14,15-diHETE) molecule from arachidonic acid (AA).[108] Secreted virus IL-1β receptor homolog (vIL-1R) binds mouse IL-1β and blocks IL-1β function in vitro.[1,126] Secreted virus tumor necrosis factor receptor homolog (vTNFR) binds TNF and is a virulence factor for myxoma virus.[130] Secreted virus interferon-gamma receptor homolog (vIFNR-γ) binds specifically to IFN-γ and blocks IFN-γ–mediated protection of L929 cells from vesicular stomatitis virus replication.[131] In addition, p25, a double-stranded RNA-binding protein previously called specific kinase inhibitory factor (SKIF), blocks activation of the interferon-induced P1/eIF-2α kinase,[36] and virus eIF-2α homolog (veIF-2α) protects eIF-2α from phosphorylation by the interferon-induced P1/eIF2-2α kinase.[6,41]

lished data). The gene encoding the veIF-2α homolog appears to be nonfunctional, because there are numerous substitutions and deletions along its 241-nucleotide length, and the insertion of a T at nucleotide 89 resulted in a switch in reading frames and a stop codon after amino acid 31. The lack of a functional veIF-2α homolog may suggest that there is an additional gene that functions in its absence or that the p25 (specific kinase inhibitory factor) is able to compensate for the loss of veIF-2α. The work of Beattie and colleagues[6] argues against the latter possibility, because a vaccinia virus mutant lacking the veIF-2α homolog was approximately 100-fold more sensitive to the antiviral effect of α/β IFN (Lee Biomolecular Research Laboratories, Inc., San Diego, CA) than wild-type vaccinia virus.

Recently, Senkevich and colleagues,[119] identified a p28 gene from the left-hand end of the ectromelia virus genome (see Fig. 22-7) which was of crucial importance for virulence in A/J mice. Ectromelia virus p28− mutant and wild-type ectromelia virus replicated to identical levels of infectivity in tested cell lines. Whereas low doses of wild-type ectromelia virus in the footpad induced signs of morbidity by 7 days and uniform mortality with a mean survival time of 9.7 days (LD50=0.25 plaque-forming units per mouse), infections with the p28− mutant at doses up to 2.5×10^5 plaque-forming units resulted in no mortality and very little morbidity. More recent in vitro studies showed that the p28− mutant infection of resting peritoneal macrophages from the A/J mouse was abortive, suggesting a role for p28 in virus replication, at least in this cell type (Senkevich, Wolk, and Buller, personal communication).

The prominent feature of the p28 protein of ectromelia virus is the presence of a zinc finger-like motif (C_3HC_4) in the C-terminus and the ability of this region of the molecule to bind zinc ion (Zn^{++}).[120] The C-terminal domain is completely conserved among the viral proteins of ectromelia, cowpox, and variola viruses but are fragmented in the WR strain of vaccinia virus and completely deleted in the Copenhagen strain. The conserved motif—the so-called RING finger—is typical of a family of proteins of diverse evolutionary origin, some of which have important roles in transcription, differentiation, oncogenesis, DNA repair, or site-specific recombination. A role for p28 in the regulation of virus or host cell gene expression would be consistent with the activities of other members of this family of proteins.

THE FUTURE: MOLECULAR PATHOGENESIS USING MOUSEPOX AS A MODEL

Future studies of pathogenesis, as of so many other aspects of infectious diseases, require a synthesis of the molecular biologic attributes of viruses and host cells with observations at the level of the whole animal. Already, with the prototype orthopoxvirus, vaccinia virus, a number of genes have been identified that encode proteins that are similar to a number of regulatory proteins found in vertebrate cells, including lymphokines, other cytokines, epidermal growth factor, and receptors for IFNs and interleukins.

Ectromelia virus is ideal for elucidating the relevance of such virus-encoded proteins, because selected mutations can easily be introduced into the viral genome and because the course of events in a naturally acquired infection of the mouse can readily be reproduced experimentally. Further, strains of virus of high and low virulence are available for study. Clearly, an early priority would be to sequence the viral genome, but before the availability of the complete sequence, a start could be made by studying genes homologous to those that produce interesting products in cells infected with vaccinia or myxoma viruses.

The mouse is the optimal host in which to study pathogenesis because so much is known of its genetics and immunology. Inbred strains of mice of high and low genetic resistance to ectromelia virus are available, and recent advances in genetics have enabled the targeted disruption of specific genes of the mouse chromosome. The experience with gene targeting suggests that most of the genes specific to cytokines and cells of the immune system can be mutated, thus permitting the elucidation of their role in the immune response to a pathogen such as ectromelia virus. These mutant mouse strains will be invaluable tools toward further understanding of the molecular and cellular basis of ectromelia virus pathogenesis.

ABBREVIATIONS

ATI: A-type inclusion body
CHO*hr*: Chinese hamster ovary host range gene
ID50: median infectious dose
INF, INF-α, INF-β, INF-γ: interferons
LD50: median lethal dose

REFERENCES

1. Alcami A, Smith GL. A soluble receptor for interleukin-1b encoded by vaccinia virus: a novel mechanism of virus modulation of the host responses to infection. Cell 1992;71:153–160.
2. Allen AM, Clarke GL, Ganaway JR, Lock A, Werner RM. Pathology and diagnosis of mousepox. Lab Anim Sci 1981;31:599–608.
3. Amegadzie BY, Sisler JR, Moss B. Frame-shift mutations within the vaccinia virus A-type inclusion protein gene. Virology 1992;166:777–782.
4. Andrewes CH, Elford WJ. Infectious ectromelia: experiments on interference and immunization. Br J Exp Path 1947;28:278–285.
5. Barnard JE, Elford WJ. The causative organism in infectious ectromelia. Proc R Soc Lond B Biol Sci 1931;109:360–380.
6. Beattie E, Tartaglia J, Paoletti E. Vaccinia virus-encoded eIF-2a homolog abrogates the antiviral effect of interferon. Virology 1991;183:419–422.
7. Bedson HS, Duckworth MJ. Rabbitpox: an experimental study of the pathways of infection in rabbits. J Pathol Bacteriol 1963;85:1–20.
8. Bhatt PN, Downs WG, Buckley SM, Casals J, Shope RM, Jonas AM. Mousepox epizootic in an experimental and a barrier mouse colony at Yale University. Lab Anim Sci 1981;31:560–564.
9. Bhatt PN, Jacoby RO. Mousepox in inbred mice innately resistant or susceptible to lethal infection with ectromelia virus. I. Clinical responses. Lab Anim Sci 1987;37:11–15.
10. Blanden RV. Mechanisms of recovery from a generalized viral infection: mousepox. I. The effects of anti-thymocyte serum. J Exp Med 1970;132:1035–1054.
11. Blanden RV. Mechanisms of recovery from a generalized viral infection: mousepox. II. Passive transfer of recovery mechanisms with immune lymphoid cells. J Exp Med 1971;133:1074–1089.
12. Blanden RV. Mechanisms of recovery from a generalized viral infection: mousepox. III. Regression of infectious foci. J Exp Med 1971;133:1090–1104.

13. Blanden RV. T cell response to viral and bacterial infections. Transplant Rev 1974;19:56–88.

14. Blanden RV, Deak BD, McDevitt HO. Strategies in virus-host interactions. In: Blanden RV, ed. Immunology of virus diseases. First Frank and Bobbie Fenner Conference on Medical Research. Canberra: John Curtin School of Medical Research, 1989:125–138

15. Blanden RV, Doherty PC, Dunlop MBC, Gardner ID, Zinkernagel RM, David CS. Genes required for cytotoxicity against virus-infected target cells in *K* and *D* regions of H-2 complex. Nature 1975;254:269–270.

16. Blanden RV, Gardner ID. The cell-mediated immune response to ectromelia virus infection. I. Kinetics and characteristics of the primary effector T cell response in vivo. Cell Immunol 1976;22:271–282.

17. Briody BA. Mouse pox (ectromelia) in the United States. Lab Anim Care 1955;6:1–8.

18. Briody, BA. Response of mice to ectromelia and vaccinia viruses. Bacteriol Rev 1959;23:61–95.

19. Briody BA. The natural history of mousepox. Monogr Natl Cancer Inst 1966;20:105–116.

20. Briody BA, Hauschka TS, Mirand EA. The role of genotype in resistance to an epizootic of mouse pox (ectromelia). Am J Hyg 1956;63:59–68.

21. Brownstein DG, Bhatt PN, Gras L. Ectromelia virus replication in major target organs of innately resistant and susceptible mice after intravenous infection. Arch Virol 1993;129:65–75.

22. Brownstein DG, Bhatt PN, Gras L, Budris T. Serial backcross analysis of genetic resistance to mousepox, using marker loci for *Rmp-2* and *Rmp-3*. J Virol 1992;66:7073–7079.

23. Brownstein DG, Bhatt PN, Gras L, Jacoby RO. Chromosomal locations and gonadal dependence of genes that mediate resistance to ectromelia (mousepox) virus-induced mortality. J Virol 1991;65:1946–1951.

24. Brownstein D, Bhatt PN, Jacoby RO. Mousepox in inbred mice innately resistant or susceptible to lethal infection with ectromelia virus. V. Genetics of resistance to the Moscow strain. Arch Virol 1989;107:35–41.

25. Buller RML. The BALB/c mouse as a model to study orthopoxviruses. Curr Topics Microbiol Immunol 1985;122:148–153.

26. Buller RML, Bhatt PN, Wallace GD. Evaluation of an enzyme-linked immunosorbent assay for the detection of ectromelia (mousepox) antibody. J Clin Microbiol 1983;18:1220–1225.

27. Buller RML, Chakrabarti S, Cooper JA, Twardzik DR, Moss B. Deletion of the vaccinia virus growth factor gene reduces virus virulence. J Virol 1988;62:866–874.

28. Buller RML, Chakrabarti S, Moss B, Fredrickson T. Cell proliferative response to vaccinia virus is mediated by VGF. Virology 1988;164:182–192.

29. Buller RML, Holmes KL, Hügin A, Fredrickson TN, Morse HC III. Induction of cytotoxic T cell responses in vivo in the absence of CD4 helper cells. Nature 1987;328:77–79.

30. Buller RML, Smith GL, Cremer K, Notkins AL, Moss B. Decreased virulence of recombinant vaccinia virus expression vectors is associated with a thymidine kinase negative phenotype. Nature 1985;317:813–815.

31. Buller RML, Wallace GD, Morse HC III. Genetics of innate resistance to ectromelia virus (mousepox) in inbred strains of mice. In: Skamene E, ed. Genetic control of host resistance to infection and malignancy. New York: Alan R Liss 1985:187–193.

32. Burnet FM. The use of the developing egg in virus research. Medical Research Council Special Report Series No. 220. London, His Majesty's Stationery Office, 1936;27–30.

33. Burnet FM. An unexpected relationship between the viruses of vaccinia and infectious ectromelia of mice. Nature 1945;155:543.

34. Burnet FM, Boake WC. The relationship between the virus of infectious ectromelia of mice and vaccinia virus. J Immunol 1946;53:1–13.

35. Burnet FM, Lush D. The propagation of the virus of infectious ectromelia of mice in the developing egg. J Pathol Bact 1936;43:105–120.

36. Chang H-W, Watson JC, Jacobs BL. The E3L gene of vaccinia virus encodes an inhibitor of the interferon-induced, double-stranded, RNA-dependent protein kinase. Proc Natl Acad Sci U S A 1992;89:4825–4829.

37. Chen W, Drillien R, Spehner D, Buller RML. Restricted replication of ectromelia virus in cell culture correlates with mutations in virus-encoded host range gene. Virology 1992;187:433–442.

38. Chen W, Drillien R, Spehner D, Buller RML. In vitro and in vivo study of the ectromelia virus homolog of the vaccinia virus K1L host range gene. Virology 1993;196:682–693.

39. Child SJ, Palumbo GJ, Buller RML, Hruby DE. Insertional inactivation of the large subunit of ribonucleotide reductase encoded by vaccinia virus is associated with reduced virulence in vivo. Virology 1990;174:625–629.

40. Dalldorf G, Gifford R. Recognition of mouse ectromelia. Proc Soc Exp Biol Med 1955;88:290–292.

41. Davies MV, Chang H-W, Jacobs BL, Kaufman RJ. The E3L and K3L vaccinia virus gene products stimulate translation through inhibition of the double-stranded RNA-dependent protein kinase by different mechanisms. J Virol 1993;67:1688–1692.

42. Deerberg F, Kästner W, Pittermann W, Schwanzer V. Nachweis einer Ektromelie-Enzootie bei haarlosen Mäusen. Dtsch Tierarztl Wochenschr 1973;80:78–81.

43. DeFilippes FM. Restriction enzyme mapping of vaccinia virus DNA. J Virol 1982;43:136–149.

44. Dulbecco R. Production of plaques in monolayer tissue cultures by single particles of an animal virus. Proc Nat Acad Sci U S A 1952;38:747–752.

45. Dulbecco R. The plaque technique and the development of quantitative animal virology. In: Cairns J, Stent GS, Watson JD. eds. Phage and the origins of molecular biology. Cold Spring Harbor, Cold Spring Harbor Laboratory of Quantitative Biology, 1966:287–291.

46. Edward DGff, Elford WJ, Laidlaw P. Studies in air-borne virus infections: experimental technique and preliminary observations on influenza and infectious ectromelia. J Hyg 1943;43:1–10.

47. Ermolaeva SN, Blandova ZK, Dushkin VA. Genetic study on susceptibility of different mouse lines to ectromelia virus. Sov Genet (USA) 1972;8:161–163.

48. Esposito JJ, Knight JC. Orthopoxvirus DNA: a comparison of restriction profiles and maps. Virology 1985;143:230–251.

49. Evans AS, ed. Viral Infections of humans: epidemiology and control. 3rd ed. New York: Plenum Medical, 1989.

50. Fenner F. Studies in infectious ectromelia in mice. I. Immunization of mice against ectromelia with living vaccinia virus. Aust J Exp Biol Med Sci 1947;25:257–274.

51. Fenner F. Studies in infectious ectromelia in mice. II. Natural transmission: the portal of entry of the virus. Aust J Exp Biol Med Sci 1947;25:275–282.

52. Fenner F. Studies in infectious ectromelia in mice (mouse-pox). III. Natural transmission: elimination of the virus. Aust J Exp Biol Med Sci 1947;25:327–335.

53. Fenner F. The clinical features and pathogenesis of mouse-pox (infectious ectromelia of mice). J Pathol Bacteriol 1948;60:529–552.

54. Fenner F. The epizootic behaviour of mouse-pox (infectious ectromelia). Br J Exp Pathol 1948;29:69–91.

55. Fenner F. The epizootic behaviour of mousepox (infectious ectromelia of mice). II. The course of events in long-continued epidemics. J Hyg 1948;46:385–393.

56. Fenner F. The pathogenesis of the acute exanthems: an interpretation based on experimental investigations with mousepox (infectious ectromelia of mice). Lancet 1948;2:915–920.

57. Fenner F. Studies in mousepox (infectious ectromelia in mice). IV. Quantitative investigations on the spread of virus through the host in actively and passively immunized animals. Aust J Exp Biol Med Sci 1949;27:1–17.

58. Fenner F. Studies in mousepox (infectious ectromelia in mice). VI. A comparison of the virulence and infectivity of three strains of ectromelia virus. Aust J Exp Biol Med Sci 1949;27:31–43.

59. Fenner F. Studies in mousepox (infectious ectromelia in mice). VII. The effect of the age of the host upon the response to infection. Aust J Exp Biol Med Sci 1949;27:45–53.

60. Fenner F. Mousepox. In: Foster HL, Small JD, Fox JG, eds. The mouse in biomedical research. Vol 2: Diseases. New York: Academic Press, 1982:209–230.

61. Fenner F, Burnet FM. A short description of the poxvirus group (vaccinia and related viruses). Virology 1957;4:305–314.

62. Fenner F, Gibbs EPJ, Murphy FA, Rott R, Studdert MJ, White DO. Veterinary virology. 2nd ed. San Diego: Academic Press, 1993.

63. Fenner F, Henderson DA, Arita I, Jezek Z, Ladnyi ID. Smallpox and its eradication. Geneva: World Health Organization, 1988.
64. Fenner F, Wittek R, Dumbell KR. The orthopoxviruses, San Diego: Academic Press, 1989.
65. Fenner F, Woodroofe GM. The pathogenesis of infectious myxomatosis: the mechanism of infection and the immunological response in the European rabbit (*Oryctolagus cuniculus*). Br J Exp Pathol 1953;34:400–411.
66. Fields BN, Knipe DM, Howley PM, eds. Fields virology. 3rd ed. New York: Raven Press, 1994.
67. Fredrickson TN, Sechler JMG, Palumbo GJ, Buller RML. Acute inflammatory response to cowpox virus infection of the chorioallantoic membrane of the chick embryo. Virology 1992;187:693–704.
68. Flynn RJ. The diagnosis and control of ectromelia infection in mice. Lab Anim Care 1963;13:130–136.
69. Gardner ID, Blanden RV. The cell-mediated immune response to ectromelia virus infection. II. Secondary response in vitro and kinetics of memory T cell production in vivo. Cell Immunol 1976;22:283–296.
70. Gillard S, Spehner D, Drillien R, Kirn A. Localization and sequence of a vaccinia virus gene required for multiplication in human cells. Proc Natl Acad Sci U S A 1986;83:5573–5577.
71. Gledhill AW. Latent ectromelia. Nature 1962;196:298.
72. Goebel SJ, Johnson GP, Perkus ME, Davies SW, Winslow JP, Paoletti E. The complete DNA sequence of vaccinia virus. Virology 1990;179:247–266.
73. Greenwood M, Hill AB, Topley WWC, Wilson J. Experimental epidemiology. Medical Research Council Special Report Series No. 209. London, His Majesty's Stationery Office, 1936:64–129.
74. Gröppel K-H. The occurrence of ectromelia (mousepox) in wild mice. Arch Exp Veterinarmed 1962;16:243–278.
75. Grose C. Variation on a theme by Fenner: the pathogenesis of chickenpox. Pediatrics 1981;68:735–737.
76. Hahon N. Smallpox and related poxvirus infections in the simian host. Bacteriol Rev 1961;25:459–476.
77. Hirst GK. The agglutination of red cells by allantoic fluid of chick embryos infected with influenza virus. Science 1941;94:22–23.
78. Hughes SJ, Johnston LH, deCarlos A, Smith GL. Vaccinia virus encodes an active thymidylate kinase that complements a cdc8 mutant of *Saccharomyces cerevisiae*. J Biol Chem 1991;266:20103–20109.
79. Isaacs SV, Kotwal GJ, Moss B. Vaccinia virus complement control protein prevents antibody-dependent complement-enhanced neutralization of infectivity and contributes to virulence. Proc Natl Acad Sci U S A 1992;89:628–632.
80. Ishihashi Y, Matsumoto S, Dales S. Biogenesis of poxviruses: role of A-type inclusions and host cell membranes in virus dissemination. Virology 1971;46:507–532.
81. Jacoby RO, Bhatt PN. Mousepox in inbred mice innately resistant or susceptible to lethal infection with ectromelia virus. II. Pathogenesis. Lab Anim Sci 1987;37:16–22.
82. Jacoby RO, Bhatt PN, Brownstein DG. Evidence that NK cells and interferon are required for genetic resistance to lethal infection with ectromelia virus. Arch Virol 1989;108:49–58.
83. Jonjib S, Mutter W, Weiland F, Reddehase MJ, Koszinowski UH. Site-restricted persistent cytomegalovirus infection after selective long-term depletion of CD4+ T lymphocytes. J Exp Med 1989;169:1199–1212.
84. Karupiah G, Fredrickson TN, Holmes KL, Khairallah LH, Buller RML. Importance of interferons in recovery from mousepox. J Virol 1993;67:8214–8226.
85. Karupiah G, Xie Q-W, Buller RML, Nathan C, Duarte C, MacMicking JD. Inhibition of viral replication by interferon-g-induced nitric oxide synthase. Science 1993;261:1445–1448.
86. Kato S, Takahashi M, Kameyama S, Kamahora J. A study on the morphological and cyto-immunological relationship between the inclusions of variola, cow pox, rabbit pox, vaccinia (variola origin) and vaccinia IHD and a consideration of the term "Guarnieri" body. Biken's J 1959; 2:253–263.
87. Kerr SM, Johnston LH, Odell M, Smith GL. Vaccinia DNA ligase complements *Saccharomyces cerevisiae* cdc9, localizes in cytoplasmic factories and affects virulence and virus sensitivity to DNA damaging agents. EMBO J 1991;10:4343–4350.
88. Kotwal GJ, Moss B. Vaccinia virus encodes a secretory polypeptide structurally related to complement control proteins. Nature 1988;335:176–181.
89. Lucin P, Pravic I, Polic B, Jonjic S, Koszinowski UH. γ-Interferon-dependent clearance of cytomegalovirus infection in salivary glands. J Virol 1992;66:1977–1984.
90. Mackaness GB. The influence of immunologically committed lymphoid cells on macrophage activity in vivo. J Exp Med 1969;129:973–992.
91. Mackett M, Archard LC. Conservation and variation in orthopoxvirus genome structure. J Gen Virol 1979;45:683–701.
92. Mahnel H. Attenuierung von Mausepocken (Ektromelie)-Virus. Zbl Vet Med 1983;B30:701–707.
93. Marchal J. Infectious ectromelia. A hitherto undescribed virus disease of mice. J Pathol Bacteriol 1930;33:713–728.
94. Massung RF, Jayarama V, Moyer RW. DNA sequence analysis of conserved and unique regions of swinepox virus: identification of genetic elements supporting phenotypic observations including a novel G protein-coupled receptor homologue. Virology 1993;197:511–528.
95. Mims CA. The response of mice to large intravenous injections of ectromelia virus. I. The fate of injected virus. Br J Exp Pathol 1959;40:533–542.
96. Mims CA. The response of mice to large intravenous injections of ectromelia virus. II. The growth of virus in the liver. Br J Exp Pathol 1959;40:543–550.
97. Mims CA. Aspects of the pathogenesis of virus diseases. Bacteriol Rev 1964;28:30–71.
98. Mims CA. Pathogenesis of rashes in virus diseases. Bacteriol Rev 1966;30:739–760.
99. Mims CA. The response of mice to the intravenous injection of cowpox virus. Br J Exp Pathol 1968;49:24–32.
100. Moss B. *Poxviridae*: the viruses and their replication. In: Fields BN, Knipe DM, Howley PM, eds. Fields virology. 3rd ed. New York: Raven Press, 1996:2637–2671.
101. Nagler FPO. Application of Hirst's phenomenon to the titration of vaccinia virus and vaccinia immune serum. Med J Aust 1942;1:281–283.
102. New AE (Chairman). Ectromelia (mousepox) in the United States. Proceedings of a seminar presented at the 31st Annual Meeting of the American Association for Laboratory Animal Science. Lab Anim Sci 1981;31:551–635.
103. O'Neill HC. Resistance to ectromelia virus infection in mice: analysis of H-2-linked gene effects. Arch Virol 1991;118:253–259.
104. O'Neill HC, Blanden RV. Mechanisms determining innate resistance to ectromelia virus infection in C57BL mice. Infect Immun 1983;41:1391–1394.
105. O'Neill HC, Blanden RV, O'Neill TJ. *H-2*--linked control of resistance to ectromelia virus infection in B10 congenic mice. Immunogenetics 1983;18:255–265.
106. O'Neill HC, Brenan M. A role for early cytotoxic T cells in resistance to ectromelia virus infection in mice. J Gen Virol 1987;68:2669–73.
107. Ørskov J. Der Bakterielle Infektionsmechanismus. Acta Pathol Microbiol Scand 1932;Suppl 11:10–58.
108. Palumbo GJ, Glasgow WC, Buller RML. Poxvirus-induced alteration of arachidonate metabolism. Proc Natl Acad Sci U S A 1993;90:2020–2024.
109. Palumbo GJ, Pickup DJ, Fredrickson TN, McIntyre LJ, Buller RML. Inhibition of an inflammatory response is mediated by a 38kDa protein of cowpox virus. Virology 1989;172:262–273.
110. Patel DD, Pickup DJ, Joklik WK. Isolation of cowpox virus A-type inclusions and characterization of their major protein component. Virology 1986;149:174–189.
111. Perkus ME, Goebel SJ, Davis SW, et al. Vaccinia virus host range genes. Virology 1990;179:276–286.
112. Ray CA, Black RA, Koronheim SR, et al. Viral inhibition of inflammation: cowpox virus encodes an inhibitor of the interleukin-1b converting enzyme. Cell 1992;69:597–604.
113. Roberts JA. Histopathogenesis of mousepox. I. Respiratory infection. Br J Exp Pathol 1962;43:451–461.
114. Roberts JA. Histopathogenesis of mousepox. II. Cutaneous infection. Br J Exp Pathol 1962;43:462–468.

115. Roberts JA. Histopathogenesis of mousepox. III. Ectromelia virulence. Br J Exp Pathol 1963;44:465–472.

116. Roberts JA. Enhancement of the virulence of attenuated ectromelia virus in mice maintained in a cold environment. Aust J Exp Biol Med Sci 1964;42:657–666.

117. Schell K. Studies on the innate resistance of mice to infection with mouse-pox. I. Resistance and antibody production. Aust J Exp Biol Med Sci 1960;38:271–288.

118. Schell K. Studies on the innate resistance of mice to infection with mouse-pox. II. Route of inoculation and resistance: and some observations on the inheritance of resistance. Aust J Exp Biol Med Sci 1960;38:289–299.

119. Senkevich TG, Koonin EV, Buller RML. A poxvirus protein with a RING zinc finger motif is of crucial importance for virulence. Virology 1994;198:118–128.

120. Senkevich TG, Muravnik GL, Chernos VI. Search for unique sequences in ectromelia virus genome by criss-cross hybridizations with DNA of other orthopoxviruses. Mol Gen Mikrobiol Virusol 1992;9-10:13–15.

121. Shida H, Tanabe K, Matsumoto S. Mechanism of virus inclusion into A-type inclusion during poxvirus infection. Virology 1977;76: 217–233.

122. Shope RE. Report of committee on infectious ectromelia of mice (mouse pox). J Nat Cancer Inst 1954;15:405–408.

123. Shope RE. Infectious disease research. In: Bhatt PN, Jacoby RO, Morse HC, New AE, eds. Viral and mycoplasmal infections of laboratory rodents: effects on biomedical research. Orlando: Academic Press, 1986:679–687.

124. Smith GL. Vaccinia virus glycoproteins and immune evasion. J Gen Virol 1993;74:1725–1740.

125. Spehner DS, Gillard S, Drillien R, Kirn A. A cowpox virus gene required for multiplication in Chinese hamster ovary cells. J Virol 1988;62:1297–1304.

126. Spriggs MK, Hruby DE, Maliszewski CR, Pickup DJ, Sims JE, Buller RML, van Slyke J. Vaccinia and cowpox viruses encode a novel, secreted interleukin-1 binding protein. Cell 1992;71:145–152.

127. Stanton GJ, Jordan C, Hart A. Nondetectable levels of interferon-g is a critical host defense during the first day of herpes simplex infection. Microbiol Pathol 1987;3:179–183.

128. Trentin JJ, Briody BA. An outbreak of mouse-pox (infectious ectromelia) in the United States. II. Definitive diagnosis. Science 1953;117:227–228.

129. Tsuru S, Kitani H, Seno M, Abe M, Zinnaka Y, Nomoto K. Mechanism of protection during the early phase of a generalized viral infection. I. Contribution of phagocytes to protection against ectromelia virus. J Gen Virol 1983;64:2021–2026.

130. Upton C, Macen JL, Schreiber M, McFadden G. Myxoma virus expresses a secreted protein with homology to the tumor necrosis factor receptor gene family that contributes to viral virulence. Virology 1991;184:370–382.

131. Upton C, Mossman K, McFadden G. Encoding of a homolog of the interferon-g receptor by myxoma virus. Science 1992;258: 1369–1372.

132. Wallace GD, Buller RML. Kinetics of ectromelia virus (mousepox) transmission and clinical response in C57BL/6J, BALB/cByJ and AKR/J inbred mice. Lab Anim Sci 1985;35:41–46.

133. Wallace GD, Buller RML. Ectromelia virus (mousepox): biology, epizootiology, prevention and control In: Bhatt PN, Jacoby RO, Morse HC, New AE, eds. Viral and mycoplasmal infections of laboratory rodents: effects on biomedical research. Orlando: Academic Press, 1986:539–556.

134. Wallace GD, Buller RML, Morse HC III. Genetic determinants of resistance to ectromelia (mousepox) virus-induced mortality. J Virol 1985;55:890–891.

135. Wallace GD, Werner RM, Golway PL, Alling DW, George DA. Epizootiology of an outbreak of mousepox at the National Institutes of Health. Lab Anim Sci 1981; 31:609–615.

136. White DO, Fenner F. Medical virology. 4th ed. San Diego: Academic Press, 1994.

137. Whitney Jr RA. Ectromelia in mouse colonies. Science 1974;184: 609.

138. Whitney Jr RA, Small JD, New AE. Mousepox–National Institutes of Health experiences. Lab Anim Sci 1981;31:570–573.

139. Woodruff AM, Goodpasture EW. Susceptibility of chorioallantoic membrane of chick embryos to infection with fowl-pox virus. Am J Pathol 1931;7:209–222.

140. Zinkernagel RM, Doherty PC. Immunological surveillance against altered self components by sensitized T lymphocytes in lymphocytic choriomeningitis. Nature 1974;251:547–548.

BIBLIOGRAPHY

Buller RML, Potter M, Wallace GD. Variable resistance to ectromelia (mousepox) virus among genera of *Mus*. Curr Top Microbiol Immunol 1986;127:319–322.

Fenner F. Mouse-pox (infectious ectromelia of mice): a review. J Immunol 1949;63:341–373.

Viral Pathogenesis,
edited by Neal Nathanson, et al.
Lippincott–Raven Publishers, Philadelphia © 1997

CHAPTER 23

Poliovirus

Philip D. Minor

INTRODUCTION

The earliest documentary evidence of disease caused by a virus infection is believed to be a funerary stele (Fig. 23-1) from 18th dynasty Egypt (1580–1350 BC). It depicts the priest Rom with the withered limb and dropped foot typical of paralytic poliomyelitis, the most serious and obvious consequence of infection with poliovirus. Despite its antiquity, however, recognizable descriptions of poliomyelitis are uncommon before the late 19th and early 20th century, and it is generally agreed that the disease was not a major health concern until it began to occur in epidemics at the turn of the century. Transmission of the virus to monkeys was first reported by Landsteiner and Popper in 1909,[38] and many of the epidemiologic and pathogenic features of poliomyelitis were described as a result of studies of the first large outbreaks in the world (in Sweden) by Wickman in 1905[66] and by Kling and colleagues in 1912.[33] The history of poliomyelitis before 1970 has been documented in a classic book by Paul.[66]

Much of the work on poliomyelitis was carried out before the development of tissue culture systems, making progress dependent on the use of animals, particularly primates, in numbers that are extraordinary by modern standards. The studies culminated in the development of two vaccines of very high safety and efficacy, one a killed preparation given by injection (inactivated polio vaccine, or IPV), the other a live attenuated virus preparation given by mouth (oral polio vaccine, or OPV). The effect of these vaccines on the incidence of the disease in the United States is presented in Figure 23-2, which shows that by 1979 poliomyelitis had an incidence at least 1000-fold less than in the prevaccine era. The success in both developed and developing countries has been such that the World Health Organization has declared its aim of eliminating poliomyelitis attributable to wild-type virus infections from the world by the year 2000. Considerable progress has been made toward this goal; for example, at the time of writing, no case of poliomyelitis attributable to an indigenous strain had been reported in the entirety of the Americas since 1991.

THE VIRUS

The molecular biologic aspects of the virus relevant to pathogenesis are reviewed in greater depth later in this chapter. Polioviruses are members of the picornavirus family and are the archetypal members of the enterovirus genus. Picornaviruses are about 27 nm in diameter, nonenveloped,

P. D. Minor: National Institute for Biological Standards and Control, South Mimms, Herts, United Kingdom EN6 3QG.

and contain a positive-stranded RNA genome; members of the family cause a variety of diseases of animals and humans.[52]

Polioviruses can be classified antigenically into three serotypes, designated types 1, 2, and 3; infection of either animals or humans with one serotype does not confer solid protection against another. The serotypes were established by a collaborative study involving cross-protection experiments in primates in the 1940s; currently, they are differentiated by serologic in vitro tests. There is very limited cross-reaction of biologically active neutralizing antibodies between the serotypes, although type 1 virus can be neutralized to some extent by antibody raised against type 2, including certain monoclonal antibodies.[65,93] No fourth serotype has been convincingly identified, although candidates have occasionally been put forward.[18] In general, in unvaccinated populations paralytic poliomyelitis is most commonly associated with infection with a type 1 strain; type 3 occurs less frequently and type 2 least often. The three serotypes circulate with comparable frequencies, as shown by the similar age at which a given population seroconverts to each serotype,[15] implying an intrinsic general difference in virulence. It is conceivable that serotype 4 exists but is of such low virulence that it does not cause poliomyelitis. However, all three known poliovirus serotypes use the same specific receptor to enter the host cell, and this molecule is not used by any other known picornavirus.[43,55,62] Serotype 4 therefore would have to be a picornavirus that uses a different receptor site and does not cause poliomyelitis, which stretches the definition of poliovirus severely. Other viruses in the enterovirus genus include the coxsackie A and B viruses, echoviruses, and enteroviruses; a total of 68 members are recognized.[52]

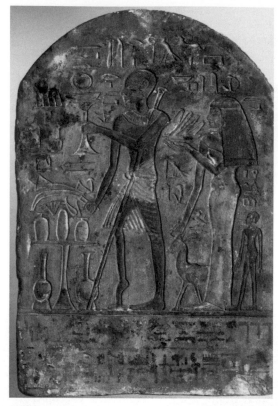

FIG. 23-1. Funerary stele of the priest Rom from 18th dynasty Egypt (1580–1350 BC) showing the withered limb and dropped foot typical of paralytic poliomyelitis. (Photograph courtesy of Dr. Jørgensen, Ny Carlsberg Glyptotek, Copenhagen, Denmark.)

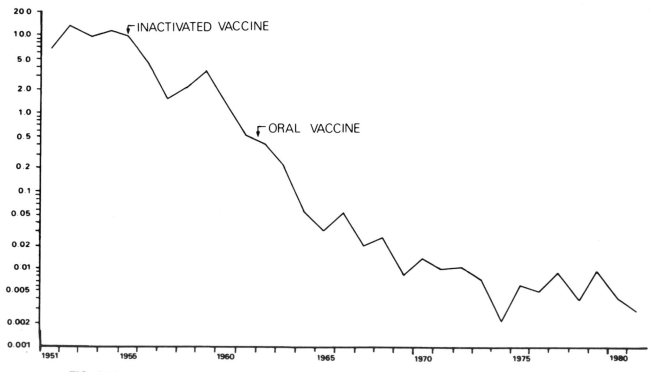

FIG. 23-2. Incidence of poliomyelitis in the United States from 1951 to 1980 in cases per 100,000 population, showing the effects of the introductions of inactivated vaccine and live oral poliovaccine. (From Minor PD. The molecular biology of poliovaccines. J Gen Virol 1992;73:3065–3077.)

In tissue culture systems, only cells derived from Old World primates or humans are naturally susceptible to infection with poliovirus, although a variety of cells can be rendered susceptible by transfection and stable integration of DNA encoding the human or primate receptor sites.[50,68] Humans are believed to be the only natural host of the virus, which makes elimination by vaccination theoretically possible. However, chimpanzees and certain Old World monkeys (especially cynomolgous and bonnet monkeys) are susceptible to oral infection, and chimpanzees and many Old World monkey species, including rhesus monkeys, may be infected by intravenous, intramuscular, or subcutaneous injection. If virus is directly inoculated into the central nervous system (CNS) by either the intracerebral or intraspinal route, certain rodents, including mice, hamsters, and cotton rats, can be infected by particular strains, notably (but not exclusively) of serotype 2. The failure to infect cells from these species in vitro remains unexplained at present. Based on studies in animals, on the epidemiology of the disease (including numbers of infections per paralytic case), and on infection of animals and humans with vaccine strains, it is believed that the susceptibility of the human gut to infection is highest, followed by that of the chimpanzee, and then the monkey, whereas the susceptibility of the CNS to infection is greatest for the monkey and least for the human. The chimpanzee is of intermediate susceptibility.[77]

Poliovirus is regarded today as a primarily enteric virus that occasionally invades the CNS, although certain aspects of its pathogenesis are still uncertain. The issues that must be considered include the clinical aspects of the disease, the sites in which infectious virus may be found, the transmission of the virus from the gut to other sites, and the mechanism by which poliovirus gains access to the CNS.

CLINICAL ASPECTS OF THE DISEASE

Clinical Consequences of Infection With Poliovirus

Although paralytic poliomyelitis is the most familiar of the clinical consequences of infection with poliovirus, it is in fact a rare complication, occurring at a rate of 1 case per 75 to 1000 infections.[9] Clinical signs associated with poliovirus infection are divided into the minor illness, which occurs 3 to 4 days after exposure, and the major illness, which may occur 8 to 30 days after exposure. The symptoms of the minor illness include malaise, fever, and sore throat and are typical of a systemic viral infection. If the symptoms resolve without further difficulty, as is frequently the case, the infected individual is said to have suffered abortive poliomyelitis. Alternatively, the minor illness can be the forerunner of the major illness, which occurs after the virus has invaded the CNS. The major illness may take the form of an aseptic meningitis, including headache and vomiting, which is termed nonparalytic poliomyelitis. However, in a minority of patients paralytic poliomyelitis develops, to varying degrees of severity depending on the area of the CNS affected and the extent of damage to neuronal tissue. In some cases, only the motor neurons of the spine are affected; paralysis is then typically more prominent in the lower rather than the upper limbs and is hemilateral rather than bilateral. Bulbar poliomyelitis derives its name from the medulla oblongata or bulb; it is characterized by paralysis of the cranial nerves, especially those of the pharynx. Bulbar poliomyelitis is the more life-threatening form, because it affects the reflexes required for breathing. Polioencephalitis involving the brain itself is also recognized. It is estimated that 5% to 10% of persons with paralytic poliomyelitis die, 10% recover with no sequelae, and about 80% survive with some residual paralysis. An illustrative example of the distribution in an American epidemic is given later. The idealized sequence of clinical events is summarized in Figure 23-3 and strongly suggests that virus multiplies in extraneural and neural sites, more or less in sequence, and with different effects. The link between the minor and major illnesses, which is not necessarily obvious, was proposed in the 1920s.[66]

In addition to the immediate effect, postpolio syndrome has been identified in survivors of paralytic poliomyelitis many years after the disease was acquired.[57] It is characterized by loss of residual function in the affected limb, and it has been suggested that this is caused by reactivation of virus that has remained latent since the original attack. Although there is little evidence for this as a mechanism for the syndrome, latency of certain picornaviruses has been reported.[99] An alternative

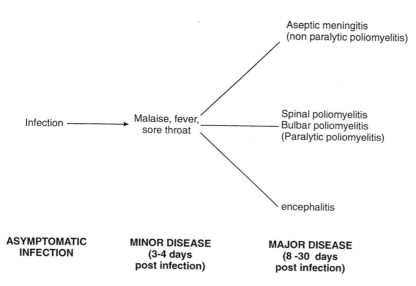

FIG. 23-3. Idealized scheme of course of infection with poliovirus.

explanation is anatomic, based on the assumption that, after the original infection, surviving neurons are to some extent able to compensate for those that have been destroyed and in so doing restore function to the affected area. As further neurons are lost with age, however, the ability to compensate declines, and the condition of the limb deteriorates.

As mentioned previously, poliomyelitis was not recognized as a major public health problem before its emergence in epidemic form, when the number of cases increased dramatically. This is usually explained in terms of a delay in first exposure to virus because of improved sanitation, coupled with increasing susceptibility to disease with age. However, after the virus appears in a community, there is a trend toward increasing age of new patients but not increasing numbers of patients; this implies that the frequency of disease after infection and therefore the pathogenesis of the disease does not dramatically alter with age.[60]

Histopathology of Paralytic Poliomyelitis

Poliomyelitis gets its name from πολιοζ, meaning "gray," and μθελοοζ, "marrow," indicating that the disease involves the destruction of neurons located in the gray matter of the anterior horn of the spinal cord. Kussmaul is credited by Paul[66] with naming the paralytic form of the disease poliomyelitis anterior acuta. Although there have been reports of infection of glial cells resulting in death of neurons,[87] the histopathologic evidence overwhelmingly supports the view that the virus replicates in the neurons themselves; in experimental models, viral antigens and genomic material are both detectable specifically in the neurons.[10] After infection of the neuron, a number of cytologic changes take place, including chromatolysis with whole or partial disappearance of the Nissl granules, nuclear abnormalities, and shrunken or pyknotic cytoplasm. Secondary to neuronal destruction, there is an inflammatory reaction involving perivascular cuffing and infiltration of the gray matter with polymorphonuclear cells, microglial cells, and lymphocytes.

Neuronal damage is highly selective. In experimental infections of monkeys and in infections of humans so far as can be determined, although most of the brain stem centers are involved—including the reticular formation, the vestibular nuclei, the roof nuclei of the cerebellum, and the nuclei of the cranial nerves—other areas of the brain, including the olfactory, visual, and auditory centers, are entirely unaffected. The cerebral cortex is unaffected even if directly inoculated with virus.[7] The cervical and lumbar spinal cord are highly susceptible to damage, but the thoracic cord which separates them is not. It is particularly striking that neuronal destruction is concentrated on the motor and not the sensory neurons. Virus replication in extraneural sites is not associated with any noticeable histopathology. The highly selective nature of the damage after infection has not yet been satisfactorily explained, although it is one of the most striking features of the disease.

DISTRIBUTION OF VIRUS IN THE INFECTED INDIVIDUAL

In 1912, Kling and associates[33] demonstrated the presence of poliovirus in washings from the small intestine in three out of six patients with fatal poliomyelitis, as well as in washings from the mouth and nose and from the trachea, and in material obtained from the CNS. (Until the development of tissue culture systems in the 1950s, all studies detected poliovirus by transmission to primates.) These findings were largely ignored for the next 30 years.

Kessel and coworkers[32] reported the distribution of poliovirus in autopsies, patients, and contacts studied between 1934 and 1940. The results are summarized in Table 23-1 and illustrate the restricted distribution of virus in infected individuals. Virus was found in spinal cord and medulla, colon contents, and tonsil-adenoid material in autopsy specimens, with isolation from the olfactory bulb in only one of the 11 fatal cases examined. No other material gave infectious virus in titers high enough to be detected. The low rate of isolation from the olfactory bulb was of particular interest, because it suggested that this was not a major site of virus replication, in contrast to the model of pathogenesis favored at the time (see later discussion). In view of later work, it is also notable that lymphoid tissue other than tonsils and adenoids was not infectious, including the single sample of Peyer's patches examined. In living patients, virus was isolated only from stools, and virus was isolated from the stool of an asymptomatic contact in one case.

Sabin and Ward[82] reported a detailed examination of material from fatal cases of poliomyelitis; more than 200 rhesus monkeys were used in this study, and the results of seven cases are summarized in Table 23-2. In no case was virus detected in the olfactory bulbs, although it was detected in other CNS material. In one case, there was evidence of poliovirus in lymph nodes and other material, but the most frequently detected nonneural locations of the virus were the alimentary tract and its contents and the pharyngeal mucosa and tonsils. All of the patients examined had virus infectivity in the colon In 1951, Wenner and Rabe[96] reported studies of lymphatic tissues in nine patients with fatal poliomyelitis, all of whom had evidence of virus infectivity in the CNS. Six of the nine had infectious virus in one or more of the axillary, inguinal, or mesenteric lymph nodes; none had virus in the pancreas. It is not clear why these workers detected virus at a higher rate than others, but the involvement of lymphoid tissue is regarded as highly significant in some current views of polio pathogenesis.

TRANSMISSION OF VIRUS FROM THE GUT

Effect of Passive Antibody on Development of Poliomyelitis

Early studies attempted to assess the potential effect of immune serum from human donors on poliomyelitis after development of CNS symptoms. The significance of the minor illness was not yet generally acknowledged, and the attempt to intervene at the stage of the major illness was reasonable, although ineffective. A major trial of highly potent gammaglobulin from the American Red Cross was conducted in 1952 to assess the ability of antibodies to give prophylactic protection from poliomyelitis.[19] The trial was based in two centers, one in Texas, and the other involving Nebraska and Iowa. The incidence and distribution of poliomyelitis cases differed in the two centers during the period of the study. In Texas, the total number of reported cases was 718 (82 per 100,000) of which 16.1% involved bulbar polio, 1% encephalitic polio, 50.7% nonbulbar paralytic polio, and 32.2% nonparalytic polio; the death rate was 3.8%. In Iowa and Nebraska, the total number of reported cases

TABLE 23-1. *Distribution of infectious virus in infected individuals as measured by the induction of poliomyelitis in monkeys**

Material inoculated	Number of individuals	Number positive	Percentage positive
AUTOPSY			
Spinal cord and medulla	72	36	50
Cerebral cortex	21	0	0
Olfactory bulb	11	1	10
Hypophysis	5	0	0
Mesenteric lymph node	14	0	0
Thymus	1	0	0
Peyer's patch	1	0	0
Liver or spleen	3	0	0
Bile	6	0	0
Colon contents	19	5	26
Urine	9	0	0
Tonsil and adenoid	6	3	50
LIVING PATIENTS			
Cerebrospinal fluid	134	0	0
Nasal washings	139	0	0
Stool	53	11	20
Urine	9	0	0
CONTACT			
Stool	19	1	5

*Virus was isolated if the samples were taken within 3 weeks of onset of disease.
Data from Kessel JF, Moore FJ, Stimpert FD, Fisk RT. Occurrence of poliomyelitis virus in autopsies, patients and contacts. J Exp Med 1941;74:601–609.

was 417 (427 per 100,000), of which 30% were bulbar polio, 5.1% encephalitic polio, 56.4% nonbulbar paralytic polio, and 8.5% nonparalytic polio; the death rate was 6.8%.

Approximately 55,000 children were involved in the study, of whom half received gammaglobulin and half received gelatin. The severity of the 104 cases of paralysis in the study group was assessed, and the results are summarized graphically in Figure 23-4. Considering all paralytic cases (top panel of Fig. 23-4), there is no evidence of protection in the first week, but there is highly significant protection from week 2, which declines gradually to undetectable levels after week 8. If cases of mild residual paralysis are excluded (center panel), significant protection is also seen within 1 week of administration. Protection from the most severe residual paralysis (bottom panel) is complete. There is no effect on the severity of cases developing more than 1 week after administration of gammaglobulin.

This study demonstrated that low levels of antibody alone were sufficient to protect against poliomyelitis and thereby provided the theoretic basis for the development of active immunization methods. In terms of pathogenesis, it demonstrated that there was a stage more than 1 week before the development of paralysis in which the CNS disease could be completely blocked by antibody. The ameliorating effect of antibody given within 1 week of paralysis suggested that there was a period of 1 week or less during which virus spread could be inhibited but not totally prevented.

Vaccines Against Poliomyelitis

Two highly effective vaccines were developed against poliomyelitis in the 1950s. The formalin-inactivated virus prepa-

TABLE 23-2. *Distribution of infectious virus in autopsy material measured by infection of rhesus monkeys**

Tissue tested	Number positive/ Number examined
Olfactory bulb	0/7
Anterior perforated substance and adjacent corpus striatum	0/7
Anterior frontal and occipital portions of neopallial cortex	0/7
Motor cortex	4/7
Diencephalon	4/7
Mesencephalon	4/7
Medulla and pons	4/7
Spinal cord	6/7
Superior cervical sympathetic ganglia	0/7
Abdominal sympathetic ganglia	0/7
Suprarenals	0/7
Salivary glands	0/7
Cervical lymph nodes	0/7
Mesenteric lymph nodes	0/7
Axillary and inguinal lymph nodes	1/7
Lungs, liver, spleen, kidneys	1/7
Nasal mucosa	0/7
Pharyngeal mucosa with or without tonsils	4/7
Ileum (washed wall)	3/7
Ileum (contents)	4/7
Descending colon washed wall	1/7
Descending colon contents	6/6

*All samples were taken less than 1 week after the onset of symptoms.
Data from Sabin AB, Ward R. The natural history of human poliomyelitis. I. Distribution of virus in nervous and non-nervous tissues. J Exp Med 1941;73:771–793.

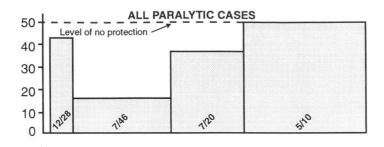

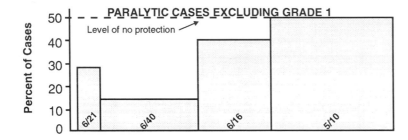

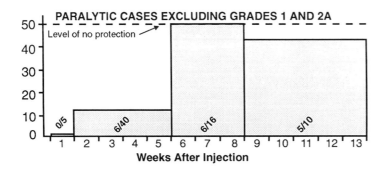

FIG. 23-4. Effect of passive immunoglobulin in protecting against paralytic poliomyelitis. The abscissa shows number of weeks after injection, and the ordinate shows the percentage of cases observed in children given immunoglobulin compared with those given gelatin placebo. A figure of 50% (bold dotted line) indicates equal numbers of cases in both groups (i.e., no protection). Top panel, all cases; center panel, mild cases (grade 1) excluded; bottom panel, severe cases only (grade 1 and grade 2A excluded). (Data from Hammon WD, Coriell LL, Wehrle PF, Stokes J. Evaluation of Red Cross gammaglobulin as a prophylactic agent for poliomyelitis. 4. Final report of results based on clinical diagnosis. JAMA 1953;151:1272–1285.)

rations devised by Salk, currently manufactured in a highly potent form,[94] have been used in Scandinavian countries, in the Netherlands, and increasingly in France with great success. The early, less potent preparations had a major impact on the incidence of poliomyelitis in the United States (see Fig. 23-2) before the introduction of the live attenuated strains developed by Sabin. The live attenuated strains establish a gut infection without causing disease and currently form the basis of the World Health Organization program to eliminate poliomyelitis. Both vaccines have been shown to interrupt virus transmission under the appropriate circumstances.

Inactivated poliovaccine was used exclusively in Finland for many years. An outbreak of poliomyelitis occurred in 1984 in which eight individuals presented with paralytic or nonparalytic poliomyelitis[28]; there is evidence that in the course of this outbreak much of the population was asymptomatically infected. The outbreak and virus circulation were attributed to a very low level of immunity in the population before the epidemic, partly because of reduced vaccination as a result of the decline of poliomyelitis as a public health issue, partly because of the use of old-style, low-potency inactivated vaccine, and possibly also because of the specific virus, which was an antigenically atypical type 3 strain. However, during the preceding 25 years, no poliovirus had been isolated from any

source in Finland,[28] presumably because virus circulation had been prevented by earlier, effective immunization strategies also involving inactivated vaccines.

In the Netherlands, two outbreaks of poliomyelitis occurred in a religious community that refuses vaccination; the first, in 1978, was caused by a type 1 strain, and the second, in 1992, was caused by a type 3 strain. In both outbreaks, the disease was essentially confined to the susceptible community and did not occur in potentially susceptible individuals in the population at large.[84] This implies that the virus did not circulate freely in the general population, where a high level of immunity had been generated by the use of potent IPV.

In studies of excretion of virus on challenge with OPV after immunization with either OPV or IPV, it has repeatedly been reported that IPV greatly reduces or abolishes shedding from the pharynx and respiratory tract but has only a slight effect on fecal shedding, whereas OPV effectively blocks both, although the intestinal immunity may not persist.[79,88] The success of IPV in breaking transmission is usually attributed to its effect on oropharyngeal spread, which is likely to be the major route in developed countries with high standards of sanitation, as opposed to fecal-oral spread. It is believed that IPV induces poor levels of immunoglobulin A in the gut and therefore has its primary effect through antibodies in the blood; its preferential inhibitory effect on shedding of virus from the pharynx rather than the gut therefore supports the role of antibodies in preventing dissemination of the infection from the gut to the CNS and suggests that the pharynx is a secondary site of infection. Alternatively, if circulating antibody crosses into the tonsils or oral secretions, it may prevent primary pharyngeal infection in immune but not in naive individuals. It implies that whatever the site of replication in the gut, it is relatively inaccessible to blood-borne antibodies. This is consistent with the finding that virus may be isolated from the feces of patients for weeks or even months after the development of antibodies, when it is no longer isolable from pharynx.[27]

Viremia in Poliomyelitis

A possible antibody-sensitive stage in viral pathogenesis is a viremia. Attempts to isolate poliovirus from the blood were unsuccessful until 1946, when an isolation was made.[95] A second isolation was made in 1949,[35] and the rarity with which virus was detected suggested that viremia was of no significance in pathogenesis. However, an alternative possibility was that the attempts at isolation were made late in the course of the disease, when antibody was already present in levels sufficient to clear the virus from the blood. This view was supported by experimental studies of oral infection of both monkeys and chimpanzees with either a type 2 or type 1 strain of poliovirus.[24] Of 39 cynomolgous monkeys given the type 2 strain, four were viremic on days 4 and 5. Of these, two became paralyzed on days 11 and 12 and two remained healthy. Of four chimpanzees, three were viremic on days 4 and 5. Viremia was detected in several cynomolgous monkeys fed the type 1 strain, on days 4, 5, and 6. Bodian reported similar findings.[3]

Viremia could be detected in human contacts of a paralytic patient and in children with signs of the minor illness.[25] Virus was isolated from the blood of 6 of 33 individuals infected with a type 1 strain; 18 of the 27 nonviremic samples had antibodies to the virus. Virus was also isolated from the throat and fecal samples of the viremic patients and could be found in the blood during the minor illness, during asymptomatic infection, and several days before a mild nonparalytic attack. Viremia in both animal models and human infections is therefore detectable. It is also detectable in recipients of the Sabin vaccine strains, especially type 2.[26] The relative rarity with which it is demonstrated may be explained by technical difficulties of timing and antibody response.

PENETRATION OF THE CENTRAL NERVOUS SYSTEM

Provocation Poliomyelitis

The viremic phase is now usually considered to be a major step in the process by which the virus gains access to the CNS, and this is consistent with the occurrence of "provocation" poliomyelitis. An analysis of paralytic poliomyelitis cases in 1949 in Australia indicated that recent vaccination against diphtheria and pertussis could be a factor in the site of paralysis.[49] In the Australian study, patients with known vaccination histories were scored for paralysis in the inoculated and uninoculated limbs after an injection of diphtheria toxoid or whole cell pertussis vaccine. The inoculated limb was more likely to be paralyzed than the others, especially in individuals receiving pertussis, in whom 22 of 24 limbs receiving the last inoculation were paralyzed, compared with 16 of 60 limbs that were either not inoculated or inoculated previously. The interval between the last inoculation and the onset of symptoms ranged from 5 to 32 days, except for two patients in whom the interval was approximately 62 days.

The studies of Bradford-Hill and Knowelden[7] in the United Kingdom concerned cases of poliomyelitis occurring from July to November of 1949. The sites of paralysis and the interval between the last injection and the onset of poliomyelitis are summarized for children younger than 2 years of age in Table 23-3. In those patients with no previous inoculations, 23% of arms and 57% of legs were paralyzed, giving a ratio of 1:2.5 for upper to lower limb paralysis, which is typical of poliomyelitis. In contrast, in those injected within 1 month of the onset of paralysis, the figures were 46% of arms and 39% of legs affected. Because it is known that 85% of the children had been injected in the arm, the data strongly indicate a bias toward paralysis in the injected limb. For patients injected 3 or more months before the onset of paralysis, 23% of arms and 55% of legs were involved, suggesting that the effect is of short duration.

A comparison was made between the inoculation histories of paralyzed patients and those of matched control subjects with no evidence of poliomyelitis, who were selected either by birth date or because they had a notified case of measles. The intervals between injection and the date of onset of paralytic poliomyelitis are shown in Table 23-4. More poliomyelitis patients than controls had been inoculated in the previous month (16 versus 1), but in all longer time intervals there was no difference between the groups. The duration of the provoking effect was therefore less than 1 month. In 26 of 33 cases, the onset of paralysis was 8 to 17 days after the injection.

The data from these studies strongly imply that a transient localized response to inoculation enables the virus to gain access to the CNS. The particularly marked effect observed with pertussis (which gives a strong local reaction) suggests that it is caused by inflammation. The data including the timing are consistent with the view that the virus, at least in these cases, enters from the blood during the antibody-sensitive phase, although other explanations are conceivable.

The Cutter Incident

In what became known as the Cutter incident, human subjects developed paralytic poliomyelitis after inadvertently being inoculated by the intramuscular route with live virulent virus present in inadequately inactivated vaccine. The incident involved batches of vaccine that were among the first released for use and is attributed to defects in the production process, which were rapidly corrected. The vaccine in current use has never been associated with poliomyelitis.

The outbreak attributable to the vaccine, which involved most areas of the United States, took place between mid-April and the end of June, 1955. The cases of poliomyelitis that occurred as a direct result of vaccination were partly obscured

TABLE 23-3. *Site of paralysis and inoculation history for poliomyelitis patients younger than 2 years of age**

	Interval between last injection and onset of paralysis (%)			
	Less than 1 month	1 to 3 months	More than 3 months	No inoculations
Arm	46	30	23	23
Leg	39	61	55	57
Trunk	11	9	15	9
Cranial nerve	4	0	7	11
Total number of patients	35	16	49	64
Ratio of upper to lower limb nodule	1:0.84	1:2	1:2.4	1:2.5

*Inoculation was with pertussis or diphtheria vaccine. Inoculation is assumed to have been given in the deltoid muscle, in accordance with usual practice, although this was not documented at the time.

Data from Bradford-Hill A, Knowelden J. Inoculation and poliomyelitis: a statistical investigation in England and Wales in 1949. Br Med J 1950;2:1–6.

by cases caused by wild-type poliovirus, but epidemiologic analysis demonstrated that of 94 cases reported among vaccinees and 126 among family contacts, 60 and 89, respectively, could be related to the vaccine.[59] Cases involved a type 1 strain, where the strain could be identified, and live type 1 virus was isolated from implicated batches of vaccine. It is estimated that at least 10% of recipients were infected, and on this assumption the rate of illness was 1 case per 100 to 1000 infections. Eighty-five percent of the cases in recipients of the implicated batches were paralytic, which is higher than expected. However, a similar high incidence of paralytic versus nonparalytic poliomyelitis was also observed in cases arising among contacts of recipients of the implicated batches, and it is therefore probably a reflection of the strain of virus used rather than the route of administration. The Mahoney strain used in the vaccine is known to be highly destructive of neurons in animals.

Forty-one of the 60 patients with vaccine-related poliomyelitis were paralyzed in the inoculated limb, compared with 3 out of 34 in a control group. This is consistent with facilitated access to the nerves in the inoculated area or the region of the spine that enervates it. Such facilitation may be caused by a high local concentration of virus, by direct damage from the injection, or by alteration of the blood-brain barrier in the region of the spine encrvating an area of trauma, as is believed to occur in provocation poliomyelitis.

Access to the nerves would then be followed by centripetal spread to the CNS.

About 65% of stool samples from affected vaccine recipients contained detectable virus, whereas stool samples from 29% of their unvaccinated and 15% of their vaccinated contacts gave virus isolates overall. However, for the cases occurring as a result of contact with a healthy but infected vaccine recipient, the isolation rates were much higher (80% overall, 75% in the younger age group of contacts) and were closer to those seen in normal epidemic poliomyelitis.[59]

The occurrence of the minor illness and the isolation of infectious virus from stools observed in a sample of the recipients indicates that the normal sites involved in transmission of virus to contacts were colonized after intramuscular administration, even if disease did not occur. However, the lower than normal frequency of isolation from affected vaccine recipients and their contacts implies that colonization of the gut and transmission were more limited relative to neural invasion after intramuscular administration of the strain than after its acquisition by contact with a vaccinee.

For cases among vaccine recipients, the median incubation period between exposure and paralytic disease was 10.7 days; for contacts, the distribution was broader, with a median of 21 days and a range of 12 to 49 days.[59] The two figures are broadly consistent on the basis of a number of reasonable assumptions concerning the time from injection to onset of ex-

TABLE 23-4. *Comparison of interval from inoculation for patients with poliomyelitis and control subjects*

	Interval from last inoculation (months)						
	0–1	1–3	3–6	6–12	More than 12 months	Not inoculated	Totals
Number of poliomyelitis cases	16	8	9	22	41	50	146
Number of controls	1	10	10	27	35	67	150

Data from Bradford-Hill A, Knowelden J. Inoculation and poliomyelitis: a statistical investigation in England and Wales in 1949. Br Med J 1950;2:1–6.

cretion and from onset of excretion to transmission to the family contact.

The Cutter incident illustrates that even after intramuscular inoculation, paralysis is a rare consequence of infection. The features of the outbreak were also consistent with the view that the neurotropism of a virus strain in an animal model may be a reflection of its neurotropism in the human host, because the Mahoney strain used in the vaccine was neurodestructive in animals and produced a high rate of paralytic poliomyelitis in both recipients and their contacts.

Animal Models

There is evidence in human infections that transport of virus from the peripheral nervous system to the CNS can occur, namely the preferential location of paralysis in the inoculated limb in both provocation polio and the Cutter incident. In certain studies in animal models, inoculation of peripheral sites (including nerves) with laboratory strains of virus resulted in a similar localization of paralysis to the inoculated limb. It could be shown that section of the nerve prevents paralysis,[5,6,29] but the experiments employed the highly neuroadapted MV strain. Use of the less neuroadapted Mahoney strain in monkeys showed that sciatic nerve block did not prevent spread of the virus after intramuscular inoculation of large amounts of virus.[58] In more recent times, Samuel and colleagues[83] have shown that inoculation of the Mahoney strain directly into the ulnar nerve of bonnet monkeys leads to paralysis, preferentially located in the inoculated limb, although there was often also extensive damage to the lumbar cord and paralysis of the hind limb. If neuronal transport was disrupted by bathing the nerve in colchicine, paralysis did not occur, although viremia and colonization of the gut were demonstrated by antibody responses and fecal excretion of virus. Moreover, intramuscular or subcutaneous inoculation of virus did not result in paralysis.

Ren and Racaniello[72] have shown neuronal transport of poliovirus in transgenic mice expressing the human receptor for poliovirus, which are susceptible to infection by a number of routes. When these mice were inoculated with either the type 1 Mahoney or the type 2 Lansing strain by the intramuscular route, paralysis developed first in the inoculated limb. When transgenic mice were inoculated in the hind limb footpad, transection of the sciatic nerve prevented paralysis. In contrast, infection of normal mice with the mouse-adapted Lansing strain did not result in preferential paralysis of the inoculated limb. This is consistent with local replication at the site of inoculation in the transgenic mice, allowing access to the peripheral nerves and thus to the CNS.

It seems reasonable that once virus has gained access to the nervous system, it can infect the CNS by passage along neurons from the site of entry. It does not necessarily follow that the virus can enter the CNS only from a peripheral nerve (although this may be true), or that it must do so directly from the blood without local replication in the vicinity of a nerve. The Cutter incident demonstrated that the preferred sites of replication, such as the gut and oropharynx, can be colonized by unusual routes; similarly, if the virus enters the CNS by any route, it may find its way to the lumbar cord, as in the bonnet monkey model of Samuel.[83]

MODELS OF PATHOGENESIS

An acceptable model of the pathogenesis of poliomyelitis must explain the occurrence of a biphasic disease in natural infections (in which a mild, apparently systemic infection may lead to the major disease) and the observed distribution of the virus in clinical specimens (which includes the gut and its contents, specific areas of the CNS, to a lesser degree the local and systemic lymphatic system, and, transiently, the blood). In addition, it must explain the effect of serum antibodies in preventing or ameliorating infection and provide a mechanism for penetration of the CNS consistent with the human and animal data.

Olfactory Hypothesis for Transmission of Poliovirus

In 1909, Landsteiner and Popper[38] reported the transmission of poliomyelitis to monkeys by intracerebral inoculation with material derived from an extract of spinal cord in a fatal human case. Flexner and Lewis reported in 1910 that poliomyelitis could be induced in monkeys by intranasal inoculation of virus, and Flexner and Clark showed that the olfactory lobes were infective 48 hours after intranasal inoculation of animals.[14] Others demonstrated a probable route from the nasopharyngeal mucosa to the spinal cord[11,12] and that section of the olfactory lobes prevented infection of monkeys by the nasal route.[40] Virus infectivity is detectable in washings or tissues from the nasopharynx in humans. The view therefore developed that poliovirus infection in humans was essentially neural in nature and that it was initiated through the neural tissue in the nose, from which it spread to the affected areas of the CNS. This hypothesis dominated work on polio pathogenesis for more than 30 years. Although it seems likely that if a virulent poliovirus were to be inoculated into the nose of human subjects, poliomyelitis would result, as an account of the natural pathogenesis of the human disease the model is now considered entirely wrong. This is based on a number of observations, one of which is that although infection of the olfactory bulbs is the rule in monkeys infected intranasally, it is rarely if ever histologically[75] or virologically demonstrable in human patients (see Tables 23-1 and 23-2). The model also fails to account for the presence of virus in nonneural sites or the effect of antibody on disease. The situation was further complicated by the use of the MV strain of poliovirus in many of the studies; this virus was maintained by intracerebral passage in monkeys and had become so highly adapted to growth in neural tissue that its pathogenesis is now thought to be atypical.

Lymphatic Model of Bodian

Bodian[4] reported that soon after chimpanzees were fed poliovirus, virus was found in the feces and local lymphoid tissues, including tonsils, Peyer's patches, and mesenteric and deep cervical lymph nodes, but not in other tissues examined (Table 23-5). Two viruses, one with a long incubation period and one with a short incubation period, were examined with the same results: after the gut was washed, the wall itself was free of infectious virus, but the Peyer's patches were not. If animals were examined a few days later in the course of infec-

TABLE 23-5. *Titer of virus in different tissues of chimpanzees, early after feeding poliovirus but before viremia or antibody response**

Tissue	Chimpanzee 147[†]	Chimpanzee 149[‡]	Chimpanzee 939[‡]
Feces	10	5,000	2,500
Throat swab	nt	nt	40,000
LYMPHOID TISSUES			
Tonsils	10	3,000	2,000
Peyer's patches	nt	nt	1,600
Cervical lymph nodes	nt	2,000	250
Mesenteric lymph nodes	100	nt	nt
Axillary, inguinal nodes	0	0	0
Thymus, spleen, bone marrow	0	0	0
ALIMENTARY TRACT			
Tongue, salivary glands, lung	0	0	0
Duodenum, jejunum, ileum, appendix, ascending colon, pancreas, liver	0	0	0
NEUROMUSCULAR TISSUES			
Trigeminal and coeliac ganglia	0	0	0
Biceps, brachii, diaphragm	0	0	0
Heart muscle	0	0	0
OTHER			
Bladder, kidney, adrenals	0	0	0
Uterus, ovary, testis, brown fat	0	0	0

nt, not tested.
*Titers are expressed as tissue culture infective dose per gram.
[†]10 days after feeding type 2 strain
[‡]4 days after feeding type 1 strain
Data from Bodian D. Emerging concept of poliomyelitis infection. Science 1955;122:105–108.

tion than those in Table 23-5, virus could be demonstrated in secondary sites, including brown fat, CNS, and somatic lymph nodes. A chimpanzee inoculated intramuscularly with virus produced infectious virus in the feces, presumably by infection of gut-associated lymphoid tissue (GALT) by means of viremia, analogous to the observations in humans in the Cutter incident and consistent with the view of poliovirus as a gut virus.

Bodian considered that it was unlikely that virus spread directly to the CNS from neurons innervating the gut, because there was no detectable virus in the gut tissue itself even when it was present in the associated lymphoid tissue and before it was found in the CNS. He therefore proposed the picture of poliovirus pathogenesis most commonly quoted today, which is presented in Figure 23-5. The features of the model are as follows. The primary sites of replication are the lymphatic tissues, initially the tonsils and the Peyer's patches; virus from the tonsils may go on to infect the Peyer's patches, which are in turn the source of virus in the feces. The deep cervical and mesenteric lymph nodes then become infected by drainage from the alimentary lymphoid tissue before the viremic phase occurs, and it is suggested that the blood-borne virus originates from these local lymph nodes. Virus is then disseminated independently to brown fat, other lymphatic structures, and the CNS. The CNS may be invaded directly by the blood-borne virus in the viremic phase without further replication in extraneural sites.

This model is consistent with the finding that low levels of passive antibody are able to prevent the development of paralytic poliomyelitis. The model requires that GALT should be a source of infection so long as virus is found in the gut contents. However, virus can be isolated from the feces for weeks after it can no longer be detected in the oropharynx.[27] This is usually interpreted to mean that the immune response has cleared the virus from the oropharynx, so that for the model to be correct, virus replicating in oropharyngeal lymphoid tissue would have to be affected differently from that replicating in intestinal lymphoid tissue. Moreover, as has been pointed out, IPV is believed to prevent infection of the tonsils although it does not greatly affect virus replication in the gut, and this is consistent with the view that in humans the tonsils are usually a secondary rather than a primary site of infection, producing virus only after the step susceptible to neutralization by antibody.

Mucosal Model of Sabin

Sabin[77] expressed a different and more complex view, summarized in Figure 23-6, in which the main primary sites of virus replication are muscosal, not lymphatic. It is based in part on the observation that even if antibody or immunization with killed virus fails to prevent disease, it can have an ameliorative effect on disease severity (see Fig. 23-4). Assuming

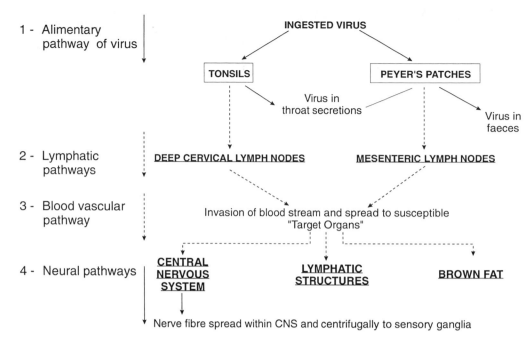

FIG. 23-5. Model of polio pathogenesis of Bodian, showing the progression from alimentary to lymphatic sites, viremia, and neuronal infection. Note the central importance of infection of lymphatic structures. (From Bodian D. Emerging concept of poliomyelitis infection. Science 1955;122:105–108.)

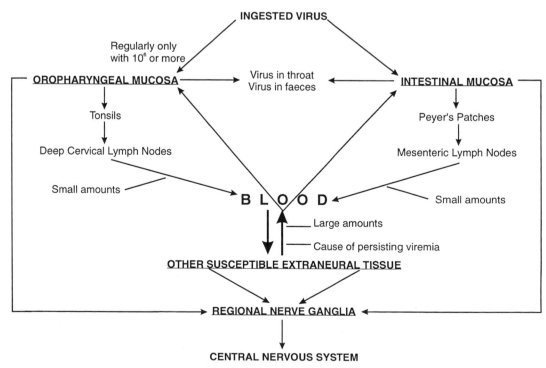

FIG. 23-6. Model of polio pathogenesis of Sabin, showing the interchange between oropharyngeal and intestinal mucosa, extraneural tissue, and regional nerve ganglia. Note the lesser importance of lymphatic structures. (From Sabin AB. Pathogenesis of poliomyelitis: reappraisal in the light of new data. Science 1956;123:1151–1157.)

that antibodies are unable to enter nerve cells, there appeared to be a stage before invasion of the CNS during which disease could be inhibited by antibody even if not prevented totally.

The model proposes that ingested virus replicates in the oropharyngeal or the intestinal mucosa, giving rise to virus in throat or feces, respectively. As a result, the local lymphoid tissue, namely the tonsils and the Peyer's patches, accumulate infectious virus without necessarily being replication sites, and then pass it on to the deep cervical or mesenteric lymph nodes. Small amounts of virus then leak from the lymphatic structures and are carried by the blood from the lymph nodes to other susceptible extraneural replication sites, which are the source of virus in the detectable viremic phase. The regional nerve ganglia may be infected by a number of routes, and the virus then migrates to the CNS; antibody would reduce the degree to which the regional ganglia became infected and thus reduce the severity of the disease.

A number of pieces of evidence were cited in support of this model. First, more virus could be found in the pharyngeal walls of infected chimpanzees than was reported in the tonsils by Bodian, implying that lymphoid tissues were quantitatively less significant in virus replication than other sites in the oropharynx, such as the mucosa. Second, in human volunteers virus multiplication in the throat was as extensive in those without tonsils and adenoids as in those with intact tonsils, suggesting that, at least in the pharynx, extensive replication must occur in nonlymphatic tissue. Third, in postmortem examination of patients who died from poliomyelitis, virus could not always be recovered from cervical and mesenteric lymph nodes even when it was still demonstrable in the pharyngeal mucosa and intestinal wall (see Table 23-2). Fourth, volunteers injected with the attenuated type 3 Leon virus failed to mount an immune response but did so if subsequently fed the virus. Assuming that the virus could reach the local lymphoid tissue after injection, it was not able to multiply sufficiently to generate an immune response; by extension, it was unlikely to multiply in the GALT. Collectively, these observations suggest that lymphoid tissue is a less important replication site than proposed by Bodian. Finally, the effect of antibody should be all or none if it acts to prevent neural infection as a direct result of viremia, because infection of an immunologically privileged site such as a nerve with a single virion should eventually be as disastrous as infection with several thousand.

The model accounts for the fact that the tonsils may be either a primary site of infection, as in the chimpanzees described by Bodian, or a secondary site, as implied by the effect of inactivated vaccine on pharyngeal infection. It conflicts with the data in Table 23-5 that the washed gut from infected chimpanzees was free of virus at a time when the Peyer's patches contained large amounts, unless this is supposed to be a problem of quantitative detection of virus on the mucosal surfaces. In addition, the observations in support of the model are not necessarily conclusive. For example, GALT could have different virologic properties from those of local nodes near the site of parenteral injection, and the ameliorative effect of antibody on the severity of paralytic poliomyelitis could be explained by the fact that antibody is now known to be able to affect viruses that are believed to be strictly neurotropic and may penetrate neurons.[56] The simplicity of the Bodian model makes it attractive, and it is the more commonly cited. Both models make predictions that are potentially testable in the light of current knowledge. As yet, although there have been studies of the sites of replication of virus in the spine of monkeys,[10] localization in extraneural sites has not been examined carefully.

ENTRY OF VIRUS INTO PEYER'S PATCHES IN THE GUT

Based on the location of virus in infected animals and the Bodian model of pathogenesis, it is widely held that the primary site of virus replication in the gut is the GALT or Peyer's patches. Histologically, these are accumulations of lymphoid cells under a layer of specialized epithelial cells on the internal wall of the intestines, termed membrane epithelial cells or M cells. M cells are found on mucosal surfaces in the oropharynx and respiratory system as well as at different levels of the gut, and there is good evidence that they function by sampling the luminal contents and passing material on to the lymphoid tissue.[97] It has been shown that both reovirus[98] and some pathogenic enteric bacteria[31,64] are readily taken up by M cells and transferred to the Peyer's patches, where they replicate. Similar evidence for the uptake of poliovirus has been presented, in which pieces from the small intestines of adults were incubated with type 1 poliovirus.[86] Virus could be detected adhering to the surface projections of the M cells, in coated pits, in vesicles, and in endosomes. The number of virus particles detected was small compared with that found in analogous studies of reovirus infection of mouse intestine, but no virus was detected in association with the absorptive epithelium. It is therefore likely that poliovirus gains access to the GALT through sampling of the gut contents by M cells.

Intestinal infection with polio is not associated with any detectable histopathology. The question of how the virus is returned to the gut contents from the lymphoid tissue in high titer (10^4 to 10^6 plaque forming units per gram of feces), as required by the Bodian model, is unanswered.

STRAINS OF VIRUS

It appears from the location of infectivity in cases of poliomyelitis in human and animal studies that poliovirus is able to multiply in vivo in a restricted number of locations, which include at least tissues associated with the gut and neuronal tissue of the CNS. In addition, the virus in the viremic phase may originate from other tissues, and replication in lymphoid tissues seems very likely. It may be assumed a priori that strains of virus differ in the degree to which they are able to replicate in the different loci. This expectation formed the basis for the selection by Sabin of the strains currently used as live attenuated vaccines throughout the world.

The MV strain of virus was propagated by intracerebral inoculation of monkeys for several years and was used in many studies of pathogenic routes in monkey model systems. For example, Lennette and Hudson[40] described the infection of rhesus monkeys by the intranasal route 5 months after sectioning of the olfactory tracts. No sectioned animal became affected, but nine normal control animals died of poliomyelitis. It is now recognized that, by virtue of its passage history, the MV strain had become highly neurotropic and was unable to cause paralysis if administered by nonneural routes or if direct neural transmission was blocked.

Naturally occurring variant strains can be isolated. Ramos-Alvirez and Sabin[70] obtained 1566 rectal swabs from healthy children in Ohio and isolated three type 2 and two type 3 polioviruses, as well as one coxsackie B virus and 25 echoviruses. The polioviruses were all avirulent when inoculated intracerebrally into cynomolgous monkeys, but they induced paralysis by the intraspinal route and by virtue of their origin were presumably well adapted to the human gut.

The use of mice in the passage of poliovirus is of interest in generating and identifying strains with novel pathogenic properties and is intriguing in itself in that only cells from Old World monkeys and higher primates can be infected in vitro. Armstrong[1] adapted the Lansing strain of type 2 poliovirus to mice, and Theiler[92] reported the isolation of a strain of Lansing after 50 rapid intracerebral passages in mice. This strain was unable to produce poliomyelitis in rhesus monkeys by the intracerebral route. Li and Schaeffer[42] reported adaptation of the type 1 Mahoney strain to mice; the strain, regarded as the archetypal poliovirus isolate, was originally isolated from a pool of three stool specimens from asymptomatic patients in Cleveland in 1941. The virus used had been passaged 14 times in monkeys and twice in vitro in monkey testes tissue culture and was then passaged either in vitro in testicular cultures or in mice alternating with in vitro culture. Four lines of virus were derived, and each could induce paralysis in mice or hamsters if injected intraspinally, although no other route of inoculation produced an effect. Monkeys inoculated intracerebrally remained asymptomatic, suggesting that the increase in mouse neurovirulence occurred at the expense of monkey neurovirulence. These strains eventually gave rise to the Sabin type 1 vaccine strain L Sc.[80] The type 3 strain Leon was also adaptable to mice,[41] but not to hamsters, and the type 2 strain MEF could infect mice by the intracerebral as well as the intraspinal route.

Sabin and colleagues[81] described the preparation of attenuated strains of type 1 (Mahoney), type 2 (Y-SK), and type 3 (Leon) virus. Passage at high multiplicities and short incubation times led to the preparation of virus of high titer in tissue culture but of low titer and neurovirulence in monkeys. For the type 1 virus, the product of the high-multiplicity passage grew significantly more rapidly than the original strain in monkey testicular cultures. Moreover, although inoculation by the intracerebral route produced neither paralysis nor lesions, cynomolgous monkeys could be infected by mouth without paralysis, implying effective replication in nonneural but not neural sites of replication. In addition, the material paralyzed mice when given intraspinally, in contrast to earlier passage material, which had no effect; this result is very similar to that reported by Li and Schaeffer. Passage of the Y-SK strain of stype 2 poliovirus in mice or monkeys also rapidly and reversibly altered its tropism (Table 23-6). The Leon strain was given 34 rapid passages in monkey kidney culture and produced neither paralysis nor lesions in monkeys when given by the intracerebral or intramuscular route. Although intramuscular injection gave rise to antibody, intracerebral inoculation did not, also implying extraneural replication. This strain, which gave rise to the Sabin type 3 vaccine strain,[80] could be shown to be immunogenic by the oral but not the parenteral route in human volunteers,[77] as described previously. Sabin also described the identification of strictly neurotropic viruses, which could be transmitted to other animals but not isolated in tissue culture.[76]

The use of different cell substrates or passage regimens therefore appears to be able to change the preferred replication sites of the virus.

VIRUS TROPISM

In both animal models and human infections, virus can be found in the gut and its contents, in certain areas of very specific nervous tissue, in brown fat, and in lymphoid tissue, but in very few other sites in significant quantities. There is evidence for replication and destruction of nervous tissue in the detection of viral nucleic acid by in situ hybridization in monkeys,[10] and it is reasonable to accept that high concentrations of virus are found in the loci in which the virus replicates. The same loci appear to be colonized when infection occurs by abnormal routes, implying that there are specific features of susceptible tissues that enable virus replication to occur, in addition to proximity to the normal portal of entry.

Holland and colleagues[23] demonstrated that rabbit kidney cells in vitro were not susceptible to infection with poliovirus, but that if the viral genome was introduced by transfection

TABLE 23-6. *Infectivity of the Y-SK strain of type 2 poliovirus after passage*

Virus history	Intracerebral titer ($\log_{10}$ PD50/g)		In vitro infectivity ($\log_{10}$ TCID50/g)	
	Mice	Cynomolgous monkey	Cynomolgous kidney	Cynomolgous testis
15 mouse passages	5.1	5.0	5.2	4.2
15 mouse passages + 2 cynomolgous brain passages	2.8	—	5.4	<1.0
15 mouse passages + 2 rhesus brain passages	<1.0	—	5.2	<1.0
30 mouse passages	4.2	—	6.2	5.2

PD50, median paralytic dose; TCID50, median tissue culture infectious dose.
Data from Sabin AB. Characteristics and generic potentialities of experimentally produced and naturally occurring variants of poliomyelitis virus. Ann NY Acad Sci 1995;61:924–938.

with naked nucleic acid, a single round of virus replication occurred. The block to infection must therefore reside at the level of attachment, penetration, or uncoating of the virus, and not at a subsequent replication stage. This implied the existence of specific cellular receptors for poliovirus, later confirmed by competition assays,[43] by the development of cell-specific monoclonal antibodies able to block infection by polioviruses but not other viruses,[55,62] and ultimately by the isolation of the gene encoding the receptor and the demonstration that nonsusceptible cells or mice in which the gene was artificially introduced became susceptible to infection.[34,50,68,71,72] The receptor is a previously unrecognized, three-domain protein of the immunoglobulin superfamily. One possible explanation of the pathogenesis was that the preferred sites of replication of the virus would express the receptor protein but others would not. However, the messenger RNA encoding the receptor is ubiquitous. An example of a Northern blot analysis of a range of human tissues is shown in Figure 23-7.[50] Antibodies raised against fusion proteins containing portions of the polio receptor were used in Western blot assays of tissues known to support poliovirus replication in vivo (motor cortex, cerebellar cortex, brain stem, spinal cord, and ileum) and of tissues such as kidney and liver, which do not.[17] All tissues reacted, implying that the receptor is expressed in all tissues examined, but there was a difference in the spectrum of proteins detected, which ranged from 30 to 150 kD in molecular weight. It is possible that the receptor occurs in different isoforms in different tissues, although there was no obvious correlation between the pattern of reactivity and virus susceptibility for a tissue.

Although kidney and testes do not appear to support the growth of poliovirus in vivo, cultures of fibroblasts from monkey kidney or epithelial cells from monkey testes evidently do (see previous discussion). Human amnion cells may be rapidly and totally infected with poliovirus when prepared as a dispersed cell culture but become chronically infected without destruction when grown in an intact organ culture

system.[8,22] It is therefore possible that the receptor is expressed but inaccessible to the virus in organs that are not susceptible, either for purely physical reasons or because the cells are coated with some matrix that the virus cannot penetrate. Alternatively, there may be a coreceptor.[85] The apparent tropism of the virus for particular sites obviously has yet to be explained.

The Sabin vaccine strains of poliovirus are of very low neurovirulence but retain the ability to grow in the gut. Sabin[78] reported a quantitative difference between the ability of virulent and of attenuated strains of type 1 poliovirus to bind to brain and spinal cord of cynomolgous monkeys, chimpanzees, and adult humans. Holland[22] found that the attenuated Sabin type 1 strain did not bind to human fetal brain or spinal cord under conditions in which the Mahoney strain did. In contrast, Kunin[37] found no difference in rhesus monkey brain tissue, and Harter and Choppin[20] found no difference in binding to either human or rhesus monkey brain or spinal cord for any of the three vaccine strains, compared with virulent strains. The view that neurotropism is reflected in the ability of the virus to bind to neural tissues is therefore unproven at best.

MOLECULAR BIOLOGY OF LIVE POLIOVIRUS VACCINES

The increased understanding of the molecular biology of the virus and the ability to manipulate it by recombinant DNA technology make it possible to address pathogenesis and the basis of neurovirulence and attenuation in a novel way. The genome of poliovirus is a single strand of RNA of about 7500 nucleotides that is covalently linked at the 5' end to a small virus-encoded protein, VPG, and ends in a polyadenylate tract of 40 to 100 residues. The genome is encased in a nonenveloped viral capsid made up of 60 copies of each of the four structural proteins, VP1, VP2, VP3, and VP4. The X-ray crystallographic structures of several virus strains have been solved.[13,21]

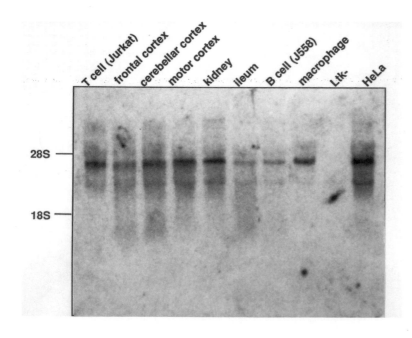

FIG. 23-7. Northern blot assay, showing tissue distribution of mRNA of the human polio receptor site in various human tissues. (From Mendelsohn CL, Wimmer E, Racaniello VR. Cellular receptor for poliovirus: molecular cloning, nucleotide sequence, and expression of a new member of the immunoglobulin superfamily. Cell 1989;56:855–865.)

The genome is of positive sense, and therefore infectious, being translated directly into virus-encoded proteins by the host cell machinery. Plasmid DNA copies of the genome are infectious or can be used as templates to produce infectious RNA[69]; in principle, the genome can therefore be manipulated at will to identify the genetic and molecular bases of particular phenotypes. The organization of the genome is shown in Figure 23-8. A single, large open reading frame of about 6500 nucleotides is preceded by a 5' noncoding region of about 750 nucleotides and followed by a 3' noncoding region of about 70 nucleotides and then the polyadenylate tract. The 5' noncoding region, which is abnormally long for a eukaryotic messenger RNA, acts as an internal ribosome binding site to which ribosomes may attach in the absence of a free capped 5' end.[67] The virus-encoded protease-2A acts in a way that has not been fully elucidated to shut off cap-dependent host protein synthesis, thereby enabling the virus to take over the translational machinery of the infected cell.

The ribosome is believed to translate the virus-encoded proteins as a single polypeptide or polyprotein, which is processed into the functional proteins by virus-encoded proteases. Protease-2A cleaves the structural proteins encoded by the 5' half of the genome as a unit from the remainder of the polyprotein by cleaving between VP1 and P2A while the polyprotein is in a nascent form, and the remainder of the cleavages required to produce the functional polypeptides are carried out by protease-3C or some precursor containing 3C. Apart from its effect in abolishing cap-dependent translation and the cleavage of P1 from the nascent polyprotein, protease-2A also cleaves 3CD in an alternative pathway, generating 3C' and 3D', and it almost certainly has additional functions.[48]

Replication of the genomic RNA is not fully understood, but nascent strands of RNA have a molecule of VPG covalently attached to the 5' end, and the process involves most of the nonstructural proteins in some way.

Assembly of the capsids involves the generation of pentamers, formed from five copies each of VP0, VP1, and VP3, where VP0 is the precursor of VP2 and VP4. Twelve pentamers may then assemble reversibly to give a dissociable empty capsid, or, with a single molecule of genomic RNA, to give a full mature virion in which VP0 is cleaved to VP2 and VP4 in a process thought to be autocatalytic. The mature virion is not readily reversibly dissociable. Numerous genomic sequences of polioviruses have been determined in whole or in part,[73,89] and there is extensive understanding of the molecular biology of the virus, including the molecular basis of its attenuation and reversion to virulence. By manipulation of cDNA copies of the genomes of the attenuated Sabin vaccine strains and of closely related strains isolated from patients with rare vaccine-associated poliomyelitis, or of the precursor strains from which the vaccine strains were derived, it has been possible to identify mutations that affect the virulence of the virus when it is given intraspinally into monkeys.[51] The mutations identified have a similar attenuating effect in the transgenic mouse model.[47,71]

For the type 3 strain, attenuating mutations have been identified in the 5' noncoding region at residue 472 and in the position of the genome-encoding amino acid 91 of the capsid protein VP3. An additional attenuating mutation in capsid protein VP1 at amino acid 6 has also been identified.[91] For type 2, a mutation in the 5' noncoding region at residue 481 and a change in capsid protein VP1 at amino acid 143 strongly affect virulence, and a mutation in VP4 may also have a weak effect.[47,71] For type 1, the situation is more complex, although it appears that there is also an effect of mutations in the 5' noncoding region, including one at residue 480, as well as mutations in the capsid region and in nonstructural proteins.[63]

The mutations in the 5' noncoding region all have been shown to reduce the efficiency of translation of the genomic RNA in cell-free systems to some extent[90] and to render virus growth sensitive to elevated temperatures in certain cell lines.[46] They are believed to act by weakening the complex secondary structure needed for internal binding of ribosomes, shown in Figures 23-9 and 23-10, by reducing the strength of base pairing. The mutation in VP3 in the type 3 strain has been shown to make virus growth sensitive to elevated temperatures in all cells examined, by preventing the assembly of protomeric capsid units of VP1, VP0, and VP3 into pentamers.[45]

FATE OF LIVE POLIOVIRUS VACCINES IN THE HUMAN GUT

The Sabin vaccine strains are believed to cause poliomyelitis an estimated 1 of every 530,000 first-time vaccine recipients and, because a full course of vaccination involves three doses, in 1 of every 2,000,000 vaccinees overall.[61] The nature of virus replicating in the gut and other sites has therefore been investigated to identify alterations as the virus adapts to its host. In 50% of primary vaccinees, virus excre-

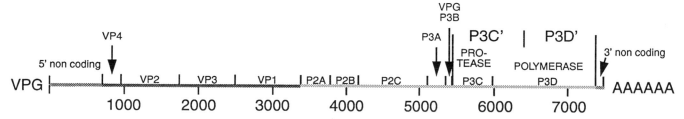

FIG. 23-8. Organization of the poliovirus genome, showing 5' noncoding region, structural proteins (VP4, VP2, VP3, VP1), nonstructural proteins (P2A, P2B, P2C; P3A, P3B, P3C, P3D, P3C', P3D'), and 3' noncoding region. VPG (P3B) is covalently linked to the 5' noncoding region, and the 3' terminus is polyadenylated. (From Minor PD. The molecular biology of poliovaccines. J Gen Virol 1992;73:3065–3077.)

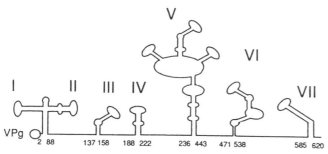

FIG. 23-9. Proposed secondary structure of poliovirus 5' noncoding region showing domains I to VII. (From Minor PD. The molecular biology of poliovaccines. J Gen Virol 1992;73:3065–3077.).

tion in the feces continues for 5 to 6 weeks, and in 1% for 10 weeks.[16] If, as is usually the case, the vaccine is given as a trivalent mixture of all three types, the type 2 strain is the most effective and the type 3 strain the least effective in infecting the gut. Because several doses are given, immunity to all three types is induced.

The nature of the virus excreted in the feces has now been examined at the molecular level in a considerable number of children. A summary of the results for the type 3 strain in one intensively studied child (Fig. 23-11) is shown in Figure 23-12.[54] Type 3 virus was excreted for a total of 73 days. The attenuating mutation in the vaccine strain at position 472 reverted to the virulent base at 48 hours after immunization, and by day 11 the virus isolated was drastically different from the vaccine. It not only lacked the temperature-sensitive phenotype associated with the attenuating mutation in VP3 and differed in antigenic sites defined by monoclonal antibodies, but also it was a recombinant virus in which the 3' portion of the genome from 2C onward was derived from type 2 and the re-

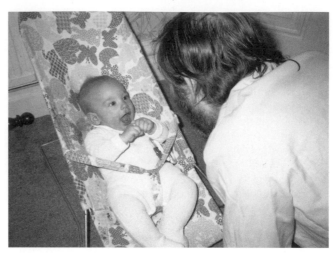

FIG. 23-11. The examiner and child study each other intensively.

mainder from type 3 virus. From day 42 until the end of the virus excretion period, the virus isolated was again different in antigenic sites and in being a more complex recombinant; it had 5' and 3' portions from type 3 virus and a central portion from type 2. The extent and rapidity of the variation in the virus is striking and has now been observed in a large number of children.[51]

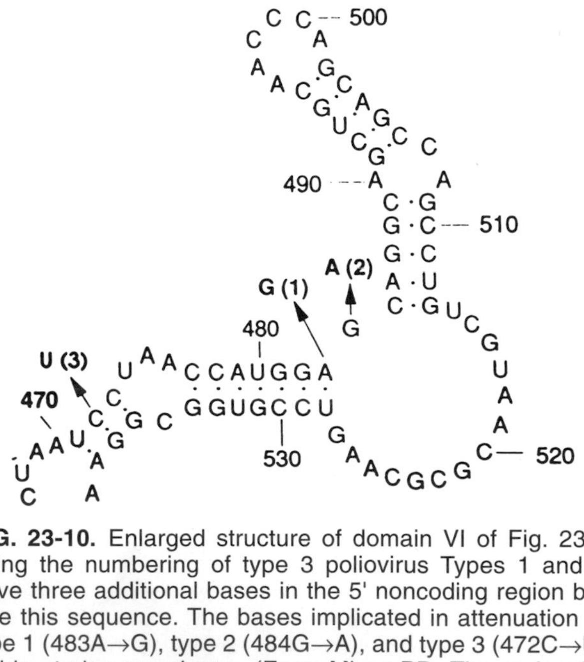

The changes associated with the attenuated phenotype are possibly to be expected in that attenuation is associated with poorer virus growth. However, it has been shown that suppression of the temperature-sensitive phenotype is virtually always effected by second-site suppression rather than by backmutation of the amino acid at residue 91 of VP3. The effect is to adjust the optimum growth temperature of the virus to 37°C, as found in the gut, rather than to either 34°C, as for the Sabin vaccine strain, or to 39°C, as for Leon, the precursor strain having the wild-type residue at VP3 91. Although many mutations act at the level of formation of the pentamers and therefore suppress the VP3 91 mutation directly, some act on capsid assembly or at other stages of virus assembly. The adaptation of the virus to its environment is therefore extremely subtle and precise, even in regard to optimum growth temperature. No difference in suppressor mutations has been found between isolates from healthy vaccinees and those from patients with paralytic poliomyelitis, and it is likely that paralysis caused by vaccination is essentially a chance phenomenon that cannot be explained by the occurrence of specific strains absent from healthy recipients.

The reason for the occurrence of recombinant type 3 viruses is not known, but virtually all type 3 isolates produced more than 11 days after vaccination have been recombinants with either type 2 or type 1. If the partner is type 2, a later recombination event occurs, almost certainly with a type 2 recombinant having the 3' portion of type 3 or type 1. Again, essentially similar viruses have been isolated from healthy vaccinees and from patients with vaccine-associated disease. In the limited number of cases tested, the intraspinal neurovirulence of the recombinant type 3 viruses is less than that of nonrecombinant viruses having the same mutations suppressing attenuation.[44] This supports the view that adaptation to the

C C -- 500
C A
A G
A A C G C A G C
G U C G C C
C G C
490 -- A A
C · G
G · C -- 510
G · C
A (2) A · U
G (1) C · G U C
480 G G
U (3) U A A C C A U G G A U
470 C · G C G G U G C C U A A
A A U · G G A C -- 520
U A G 530 A A C G C G
C A

FIG. 23-10. Enlarged structure of domain VI of Fig. 23-9 using the numbering of type 3 poliovirus Types 1 and 2 have three additional bases in the 5' noncoding region before this sequence. The bases implicated in attenuation of type 1 (483A→G), type 2 (484G→A), and type 3 (472C→U) Sabin strains are shown. (From Minor PD. The molecular biology of poliovaccines. J Gen Virol 1992;73:3065–3077.)

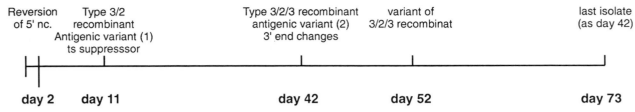

FIG. 23-12. Summary of evolution of type 3 poliovirus in baby DM. (From Minor PD, John A, Ferguson M, Icenogle JP. Antigenic and molecular evolution of the vaccine strain of type 3 poliovirus during the period of excretion by a primary vaccinee. J Gen Virol 1986;67:693–706.)

gut is not necessarily identical to adaptation to growth in neurons, although the pressure driving selection of the recombinants is not known.

The subtlety of the relation between the virus and its host may involve its antigenic properties. The sites recognized by neutralizing monoclonal antibodies of murine origin have been mapped by the isolation of antigenic mutants, and, in the mouse at least, the immunodominant antigenic feature of type 2 and type 3 virus, but not of type 1, corresponds to the most prominent structural feature at the fivefold pentameric apex of the virus particle. This site is extremely well conserved, although other sites vary slightly by point mutations acquired during the period of virus excretion. The dominant site is selectively cleaved by trypsin, which destroys both its immunogenicity and its antigenicity, so that the treated virus induces antibodies preferentially to other sites and does not react with antibodies to the dominant site.[30] Virus excreted by vaccinees is in the trypsin-treated form, as may be expected in view of its origin in the contents of the small intestine, which are rich in proteases.[53] Other than the Sabin strain, most strains of type 1 poliovirus do not have a proteolytically cleavable sequence in the corresponding region of the virus.

There are several views concerning the significance of this observation, including the possibility that it has none. First, the infectivity of many viruses is affected by proteolytic cleavage. Paramyxoviruses, orthomyxoviruses, and reoviruses all require proteolytic activation to infect cells, whereas foot-and-mouth disease virus is inactivated by trypsin cleavage. The specific cleavage of the poliovirus site may therefore affect its infectivity,[74] although not for the commonly used continuous cell line Hep2C.[54] A second possibility is that the phenomenon has a role in pathogenesis. According to this view, virus growing in the gut lacks an antigenic site compared with virus growing in the absence of proteases. Should virus invade and go through a single cycle outside the gut, the site is regenerated, and because it is the most immunogenic on the virus, the immune system is stimulated to recognize it overwhelmingly, thus terminating viremia with only limited consequence for the virus growing in the gut, which will continue to replicate. Studies of recipients of live attenuated vaccine have indicated some of the subtlety of the interactions between the virus and the host but have particularly concerned virus in feces, which is clearly only part of the story.

In addition, there are features of poliovirus molecular biology that are found in all isolates examined but whose function is unknown. The region of about 100 bases located before the initiation codon is the most poorly conserved sequence in the genome and can be deleted entirely by recombinant DNA techniques without affecting the phenotype of the virus in vitro.[36] Nonetheless, all isolates of polioviruses have a region corresponding to this sequence, in contrast to closely related rhinoviruses, in which it is absent. It is therefore essential in some way. The last stem loop in the predicted structure of the 5' noncoding region (see Fig. 23-9) is the most obvious and thermodynamically stable feature in the sequence, but it can be totally disrupted by deletions of the RNA sequence without affecting the in vitro phenotype.[36] The cleavage of 3CD by 2A (see Fig. 23-8) occurs in all poliovirus isolates examined except the Sabin type 3 strain and strains related to it. The basis for the lack of cleavage in the Sabin type 3 and related strains has been identified at the molecular level as a single amino acid change one residue from the cleavage site, but abolishing the cleavage has no known effect on the phenotype of the virus in culture.[39] It may be of interest that the recombinant type 3 strains generated in vaccinees gain and retain the 3CD cleavage site from the recombinant partners, consistent with the view that 3CD cleavage is selected for in vivo. These features of wild-type polioviruses have no identified function in virus growth in vitro, but their almost ubiquitous occurrence in isolates strongly suggests that they have some essential role in vivo and that the interactions of virus and host remain imperfectly understood.

SUMMARY AND CONCLUSIONS

Poliovirus infects the intestinal tract, where it may continue to replicate for several weeks. A systemic infection involving a short-lived viremia follows within a week of infection, and a number of lines of evidence show that the viremic phase is essential to the dissemination of the virus to the CNS in a normal infection. Access to the CNS may be by means of peripheral nerves, and damage is restricted to the motor neurons.

A large number of questions remain. The GALT is usually considered to be the primary site of replication in the intestine, but the evidence is conflicting, particularly regarding virus replication late in infection, when antibodies are found in the blood. The source of the virus in the viremic phase is not known, and although there is good evidence that viremia is in some form necessary to the development of the major disease, it is not clear whether virus gains access to the CNS directly from the blood or from local replication sites infected during the viremia. Similarly, transport of virus along peripheral nerves to the CNS is clearly possible, but it is not established whether this is the usual route of entry in a normal infection or whether there could also be more direct access by other routes. The highly specific location of virus in infected individuals remains unexplained.

Studies of the molecular biology of poliovirus infections demonstrate a number of extremely precise and subtle adaptations of virus to the host and suggest the existence of others. For obvious technical reasons, most of this work has involved gut-adapted virus or virus grown in vitro, so the adaptation of poliovirus to other tissues has not been closely examined even though it underlies the success of the live vaccine strains developed by Sabin. It is quite possible that poliomyelitis will be eradicated before the details of the interactions between the virus and its host are fully understood.

ABBREVIATIONS

CNS: central nervous system
GALT: gut-associated lymphoid tissue
IPV: inactivated polio vaccine
OPV: oral polio vaccine
VP1, VP2, VP3, VP4: structural capsid proteins of the poliovirus
VP0: precursor of VP2 and VP4

REFERENCES

1. Armstrong C. Successful transfer of the Lansing strain of poliomyelitis virus from the cotton rat to the white mouse. Pubic Health Rep 1939;54:2302–2305.
2. Bodian D. Poliomyelitis: pathological aspects. First International Polio Conference. Philadelphia: Lippincott, 1949.
3. Bodian D. Viraemia in experimental poliomyelitis. II. Viraemia and the mechanism of the "provoking" effect of injections or trauma. Am J Hyg 1954;60:358–370.
4. Bodian D. Emerging concept of poliomyelitis infection. Science 1955; 122:105–108.
5. Bodian D, Howe HA. Experimental studies of intraneural spread of poliomyelitis virus. Bull Johns Hopkins Hosp 1941;68:248–267.
6. Bodian D, Howe HA. The rate of progression of poliomyelitis virus in nerves. Bull Johns Hopkins Hosp 1941;69:79–85.
7. Bradford-Hill A, Knowelden J. Inoculation and poliomyelitis: a statistical investigation in England and Wales in 1949. Br Med J 1950;2:1–6.
8. Chany C, Gresser I, Vendrely C, Robbe-Fossat F. Persistent polioviral infection of the intact amniotic membrane. II. Existence of mechanical barrier to viral infection. Proc Soc Exp Biol Med 1966;123:960–968.
9. Christie AB. Infectious diseases: epidemiology and clinical practice. 3rd ed. New York: Churchill Livingstone, 1980.
10. Couderc T, Christodoulou C, Kopecka H, et al. Molecular pathogenesis of neural lesions induced by poliovirus type 1. J Gen Virol 1989; 70:2907–2918.
11. Faber HK, Gebhardt LP. Localisation of the virus of poliomyelitis in the central nervous system during the preparalytic period after intranasal instillation. J Exp Med 1933;57:993–954.
12. Fairbrother RW, Hurst EW. The pathogenesis of, and propagation of virus in, experimental poliomyelitis. J Pathol Bacteriol 1930;33:17–45.
13. Filman DJ, Syed R, Chow M, Minor PD, Macadam AJ, Hogle J. Structural factors that control conformational transitions and serotype specificity in type 3 poliovirus. EMBO J 1989;8:1567–1579.
14. Flexner S, Clark PF. A note on the mode of infection in epidemic poliomyelitis. Proc Soc Exp Biol Med 1912;10:1–2.
15. Fox JP. Epidemiology of poliomyelitis in populations before and after vaccination with inactivated viruses. In: Poliomyelitis: papers and discussions presented at the Fourth International Poliomyelitis Conference, 1958. Philadelphia: JB Lippincott, 1958;136–149.
16. Fox JP, Gelfand HM, Leblanc DR, Potash L, Clemmer DI, Laperta D. The spread of vaccine strains of poliovirus in the household and in the community in Southern Louisiana. In: International Poliomyelitis Conference, Copenhagen, 1960. Philadelphia: Lippincott, 1960:368–383.
17. Freistadt MS, Kaplan G, Racaniello VR. Heterogeneous expression of poliovirus receptor related proteins in human cells and tissues. Mol Cell Biol 1990;10:5700–5706.
18. Gear JHS. Non polio causes of polio like paralytic symptoms. Rev Infect Dis 1984;6(Suppl 2):S379–S384.
19. Hammon WD, Coriell LL, Wehrle PF, Stokes J. Evaluation of Red Cross gammaglobulin as a prophylactic agent for poliomyelitis. 4. Final report of results based on clinical diagnosis. JAMA 1953;151:1272–1285.
20. Harter DH, Choppin PW. Adsorption of attenuated and neurovirulent poliovirus strains to central nervous system tissues of primates. J Immunol 1965;95:730–736.
21. Hogle JM, Chow M, Filman DJ. The three dimensional structure of poliovirus at 2.9(arA) resolution. Science 1985;229:1358–1365.
22. Holland JJ. Receptor affinities as major determinants of enterovirus tissue tropism in humans. Virology 1961;15:312–326.
23. Holland JJ, MacLaren LC, Sylverton JT. The mammalian cell-virus relationship. IV. Infection of naturally insusceptible cells with enterovirus nucleic acid. J Exp Med 1959;110:65–80.
24. Horstmann DM. Poliomyelitis virus in blood of orally infected monkeys and chimpanzees. Proc Soc Exp Biol Med 1952;79:417–419.
25. Horstmann DM, McCallum RW, Masiola AD. Viremia in human poliomyelitis. J Exp Med 1954;99:355–369.
26. Horstmann DM, Opton EM, Klemperer R, Llado B, Vigneee AJ. Viraemia in infants vaccinated with oral poliovirus vaccine (Sabin). Am J Hyg 1964;79:47–63.
27. Horstmann DM, Ward R, Melnick JL. The isolation of poliomyelitis virus from human extraneural sources. III. Persistence of virus in stools after acute infection. J Clin Invest 1946;25:278–283.
28. Hovi T, Cantell K, Huovilainen A, et al. Outbreak of paralytic poliomyelitis in Finland: widespread circulation of antigenically altered poliovirus type 3 in a vaccinated population. Lancet 1986;1:1427–1432.
29. Hurst EW. A further contribution to the pathogenesis of experimental poliomyelitis: inoculation into the sciatic nerve. J Pathol Bacteriol 1930;33:1133–1143.
30. Icenogle JP, Minor PD, Ferguson M, Hogle JM. Modulation of the humoral response to a 12 amino acid site on the poliovirus virion. J Virol 1986;60:267–280.
31. Inman LR, Cantey JR. Specific adherence of Escherichia coli (strain RDEC-1) to membranous (M) cells of the Peyers patch in Escherichia coli diarrhoea in the rabbit. J Clin Invest 1983;71:1–8.
32. Kessel JF, Moore FJ, Stimpert FD, Fisk RT. Occurrence of poliomyelitis virus in autopsies, patients and contacts. J Exp Med 1941;74:601–609.
33. Kling C, Wernstedt W, Pettersen A. Recherches sur le mode de propagation de la paralysie infantile epidemique. z Immunitätsforsch 1912;12:316–323,657–670.
34. Koike S, Horie H, Ise I, et al. The poliovirus receptor protein is produced both as membrane-bound and secreted forms. EMBO J 1990;9:3217–3224.
35. Koprowski H, Norton TW, McDermott W. Isolation of poliomyelitis virus from human serum by direct inoculation into a laboratory mouse. Pubic Health Rep 1949;62:1467–1476.
36. Kuge S, Nomoto A. Construction of viable deletion and insertion mutants of the Sabin strain of type 1 poliovirus: function of the 5' non coding sequence in viral replication. J Virol 1987;61:1478–1487.
37. Kunin CM. Virus-tissue union and the pathogenesis of enterovirus infections. J Immunol 1962;88:556–569.
38. Landsteiner K, Popper E. Übertragung der Poliomyelitis acuta auf Affen. Ztschr f Immunitätsforsch u exper Therap Orig 1909;2:377–390.
39. Lee CK, Wimmer E. Proteolytic processing of poliovirus polyprotein: elimination of 2Apro-mediated alternative cleavage of polypeptide 3CD by in vitro mutagenesis. Virology 1988;166:405–414.
40. Lennette EH, Hudson NP. Relation of olfactory tracts to intravenous route of infection in experimental poliomyelitis. Proc Soc Exp Biol Med 1934;32:1444–1446.
41. Li CP, Habel K. Adaptation of Leon strain of poliomyelitis to mice. Proc Soc Exp Biol Med 1951;78:283–288.
42. Li CP, Schaeffer M. Adaptation of type 1 poliomyelitis virus to mice. Proc Soc Exp Biol Med 1953;82:477–481.

43. Lonberg-Holm KR, Crowell RL, Philipson L. Unrelated animal viruses share receptors. Nature 1976;259:679–681.

44. Macadam AJ, Arnold C, Howlett J, et al. Reversion of attenuated and temperature sensitive phenotypes of the Sabin type 3 strain of poliovirus in vaccinees. Virology 1989;174:408–414.

45. Macadam AJ, Ferguson G, Arnold C, Minor PD. An assembly defect as a result of an attenuating mutation in the capsid protein of the poliovirus type 3 vaccine strain. J Virol 1991;72:2475–2481.

46. Macadam AJ, Pollard SR, Ferguson G, et al. The 5' non-coding region of the type 2 poliovirus vaccine strain contains determinants of attenuation and temperature sensitivity. Virology 1991;181:451–458.

47. Macadam AJ, Pollard SR, Ferguson G, et al. Genetic basis of attenuation of the Sabin type 2 vaccine strain of poliovirus in primates. Virology 1993;192:18–26.

48. Macadam AJ, Ferguson G, Fleming T, Stone DM, Almond JW, Minor PD. Role for poliovirus protease 2A in cap independent translation. EMBO J 1994;13:924–927.

49. McCloskey BP. The relation of prophylactic inoculations to the onset of poliomyelitis. Lancet 1950;ii:659–663.

50. Mendelsohn CL, Wimmer E, Racaniello VR. Cellular receptor for poliovirus: molecular cloning, nucleotide sequence, and expression of a new member of the immunoglobulin superfamily. Cell 1989;56:855–865.

51. Minor PD. The molecular biology of poliovaccines. J Gen Virol 1992;73:3065–3077.

52. Minor PD, Brown F, King A, et al. Fifth report of the picornavirus study group of the International Committee on Taxonomy of viruses. In: Francki RIB, Fauquet CM, Knudson DL, Brown F, eds. Classification and nomenclature of viruses: fifth report of the International Committee on Taxonomy of Viruses. Arch Virology 1991;(Suppl 2):320–326.

53. Minor PD, Ferguson M, Phillips A, Magrath DI, Huovilainen A, Hovi T. Conservation in vivo of protease cleavage sites in antigenic sites of poliovirus. J Gen Virol 1987;68:1857–1865.

54. Minor PD, John A, Ferguson M, Icenogle JP. Antigenic and molecular evolution of the vaccine strain of type 3 poliovirus during the period of excretion by a primary vaccinee. J Gen Virol 1986;67:693–706.

55. Minor PD, Pipkin PA, Hockley D, Schild GC, Almond JW. Monoclonal antibodies which block cellular receptors of poliovirus. Virus Research 1984;1:203–212.

56. Morrison LA, Fields BN. Parallel mechanisms in neuropathogenesis of enteric virus infections. J Virol 1991;65:2767–2772.

57. Munsat TL. Poliomyelitis: new problems with an old disease. N Engl J Med 1991;324:1206–1207.

58. Nathanson N, Bodian D. Experimental poliomyelitis following intramuscular virus injection. 1. The effect of neural block on a neurotropic and a pantropic strain. Bull Johns Hopkins Hosp 1961;108:308–319.

59. Nathanson N, Langmuir AD. The Cutter incident: poliomyelitis following formaldehyde inactivated poliovirus vaccination in the United States during the spring of 1955. Am J Hyg 1963;78:16–81.

60. Nathanson N, Martin JR. The epidemiology of poliomyelitis: enigmas surrounding its appearance, epidemicity and disappearance. Am J Epidemiol 1979;110:672–692.

61. Nkowane BU, Wassilak SG, Oversteen WA, et al. Vaccine associated paralytic poliomyelitis in the United States: 1973 through 1984. JAMA 1987;257 1385–1340.

62. Nobis P, Zibirre R, Meyer G, Kuhne J, Warnecke G, Kock G. Production of a monoclonal antibody against an epitope on HeLa cells that is the functional poliovirus binding site. J Gen Virol 1985;6:2563–2569.

63. Omata T, Kohara M, Kuge S, et al. Genetic analysis of the attenuation phenotype of poliovirus type 1. J Virol 1986;58:348–358.

64. Owen RL, Pierce NF, Apple RT, Cray WC Jr. M Cell transport of *Vibrio* cholera from the intestinal lumen into Peyer's patches: a mechanism for antigen sampling and for microbial transepithelial migration. J Infect Dis 1986;153:1108–1118.

65. Patel V, Ferguson M, Minor PD. Antigenic sites on type 2 poliovirus. Virology 1993;192:361–364.

66. Paul JR. A history of poliomyelitis. New Haven: Yale University Press, 1971.

67. Pelletier J, Sonnenberg N. Internal initiation of translation of eukaryotic mRNA directed by a sequence derived from poliovirus RNA. Nature 1988;334:320–325.

68. Pipkin PA, Wood DJ, Racaniello VR, Minor PD. Characterisation of L cells expressing the human poliovirus receptor for the specific detection of polioviruses in vitro. J Virol Methods 1993;41:333–340.

69. Racaniello VR, Baltimore D. Cloned poliovirus complementary DNA is infectious in mammalian cells. Science 1981;214:916–919.

70. Ramos-Alvarez M, Sabin AB. Characteristics of poliomyelitis and other enteric viruses recovered in tissue culture from healthy American children. Proc Soc Exp Biol Med 1954;87:655–661.

71. Ren R, Moss EG, Racaniello VR. Identification of two determinants that attenuate vaccine-related type 2 poliovirus. J Virol 1991;65:1377–1382.

72. Ren R, Racaniello VR. Poliovirus spreads from muscle to the central nervous system by neural pathways. J Infect Dis 1992;166:747–752.

73. Rico-Hesse R, Pallansch MA, Nottay BK, Kew OM. Geographical distribution of wild type poliovirus type 1 genotypes. Virology 1987;160:311–322.

74. Roivainen M, Huovilainen A, Hovi T. Antigenic modification of polioviruses by host proteolytic enzymes. Arch Virol 1990;111:115–125.

75. Sabin AB. The olfactory bulbs in human poliomyelitis. Am J Dis Child 1940;60:1313–1318.

76. Sabin AB. Characteristics and genetic potentialities of experimentally produced and naturally occurring variants of poliomyelitis virus. Ann N Y Acad Sci 1955;61:924–938.

77. Sabin AB. Pathogenesis of poliomyelitis: reappraisal in the light of new data. Science 1956;123:1151–1157.

78. Sabin AB. Properties of attenuated polioviruses and their behaviour in human beings. In: St Whitlock OV, ed. Cellular biology, nucleic acids and viruses. New York Academy, New York 1957;5:113–127.

79. Sabin AB. Present position of immunization against poliomyelitis with live virus vaccine. Br Med J 1959;1:663–680.

80. Sabin AB, Boulger L. History of Sabin attenuated poliovirus oral live vaccine strains. J Biol Stand 1973;1:115–118.

81. Sabin AB, Henessen WA, Winsser J. Studies on variants of poliomyelitis virus. I. Experimental segregation and properties of avirulent variants of three immunologic types. J Exp Med 1954;99:551–576.

82. Sabin AB, Ward R. The natural history of human poliomyelitis. I. Distribution of virus in nervous and non-nervous tissues. J Exp Med 1941;73:771–793.

83. Samuel BU, Ponnuraj E, Rajasingh J, John TJ. Experimental poliomyelitis in bonnet monkey: clinical features, virology and pathology. In: Brown F, Lewis BP, eds. Poliovirus attenuation: molecular mechanisms and practical aspects. Dev Biol Stand 1993;78:71–78.

84. Schaap GJP, Bijker KH, Coutinto RA, Kapsenberg JG, van Wezel AL. The spread of wild poliovirus in the well vaccinated Netherlands in connection with the 1978 epidemic. Prog Med Virol 1984;29:124–140.

85. Shepley MP, Racaniello VR. A monoclonal antibody that blocks poliovirus attachment recognises the lymphocyte homing receptor CD44. J Virol 1994;68:1301–1308.

86. Sicinski P, Rowinski J, Warchol JB, et al. Poliovirus type 1 enters the human host through intestinal M cells. Gastroenterology 1990;98:56–58.

87. Simon J, Magrath D, Boulger L. The role of the defensive mechanism in experimental poliomyelitis. Prog Immunobiol Stand 1970;4:643–649.

88. Soloviev VD. Problems connected with live polio vaccine. Fifth International Poliomyelitis Conference, 1960. Philadelphia: Lippincott, 403–410.

89. Stanway G. Structure, function and evolution of picornaviruses. J Gen Virol 1990;71:2483–2501.

90. Svitkin Y, Cammack N, Minor PD, Almond JW. Translation deficiency of the Sabin type 3 poliovirus genome: association with an attenuating mutation C472-U. Virology 1990;175:103–109.

91. Tatem JM, Weeks-Levy C, Georgiu A, et al. A mutation present in the amino terminus of Sabin 3 poliovirus VP1 protein is attenuating. J Virol 1992;66:3194–3197.

92. Theiler M. Studies on poliomyelitis. Medicine (Baltimore) 1941;20:443–462.

93. Uhlig J, Wiegers K, Dernick R. A new antigenic site of poliovirus recognised by an intertypic, cross neutralizing monoclonal antibody. Virology 1990;178:606–610.

94. van Wezel AL, van Steenis G, van der Marel P, Osterhaus ADME. Inactivated poliovirus vaccine: current production methods and new developments. Rev Infect Dis 1984;6(Suppl 2):S335–S340.

95. Ward R, Horstmann DM, Melnick JL. The isolation of poliomyelitis virus from human extraneural sources. IV. Search for virus in the blood of patients. J Clin Invest 1946;25:284–286.

96. Wenner HA, Rabe EF. The recovery of virus from regional lymph nodes of fatal human cases of poliomyelitis. Am J Med Sci 1951; 222:292–299.

97. Wolf JL, Bye WA. The membranous epithelial (M) cell and the mucosal immune system. Ann Rev Med 1984;35:95–112.

98. Wolf JL, Rubin DH, Finberg R, et al. Intestinal M cells: a pathway for entry of reovirus into the host. Science 1981;212:471–472.

99. Yousef GE, Bell EJ, Mann GF, et al. Chronic enterovirus infection in patients with post viral fatigue syndrome. Lancet 1988;1:146–15

Viral Pathogenesis,
edited by Neal Nathanson, et al.
Lippincott–Raven Publishers, Philadelphia © 1997

CHAPTER 24

Rabies

Alan C. Jackson

INTRODUCTION

Rabies has been recognized since antiquity. The Latin word "rabies" is derived from the Sanskrit word *rabhas*, which means "to do violence."[146] The earliest known reference to rabies was in the pre-Mosaic Eshnunna Code of Mesopotamia in about 2300 BC[135] (Table 24-1). Ancient Chinese writings also indicate that rabid dogs were recognized centuries before the birth of Christ.[173] The writings of Democritus, Aristotle, Hippocrates, and Celsus describe the clinical features of rabies.[146,172] In 100 AD, Celsus recognized that the saliva of the biting animal contained the poisonous agent, and he recommended the practice of using caustics, burning, cupping, and sucking of the wounds of those bitten by rabid dogs.[62] In 1769, the pathologist John Morgagni speculated that rabies virus "does not seem to be carried through the veins, but by the nerves, up to their origins."[114]

In 1804, Zinke published a volume (in German) designed to prove that the infective agent of rabies was transmitted in infected saliva; this work contained the first recorded rational transmission experiments of a viral disease.[172] He took saliva from a rabid dog and painted it into incisions he had made in healthy animals, and the animals subsequently developed rabies.

In the 1880s, Pasteur (Fig. 24-1) experimentally transmitted rabies by inoculating central nervous system (CNS) material of rabid animals into the brains of other animals.[146] He also observed that sequential passage in the CNS led to attenuation for peripheral inoculation.[123] In 1885, Pasteur immunized a 9-year-old boy, Joseph Meister, who had been severely bitten by a rabid dog, with 13 inoculations of infected rabbit spinal cord material. Meister survived and it was assumed (but not proven) that he had been protected by the procedure. This material had previously been passaged and partially inactivated with progressively shorter periods of desiccation (from 15 days to 1 day).[122]

In 1889, DiVestea and Zagari[49] showed that inoculation of rabies virus into the sciatic nerve of a rabbit and a dog caused rabies, and that death could be prevented by sectioning and cauterizing the nerve after injection. They also noted that the clinical signs depended on the location of the inoculated nerve and the site at which it entered the CNS.

Definitive pathologic diagnosis of rabies became possible in 1903, when Negri[121] described the pathognomonic eosinophilic cytoplasmic inclusions in infected neurons. These inclusions were initially thought to represent protozoan organisms. They are now known as Negri bodies (Fig. 24-2), and they are associated with an accumulation of rabies virus particles and proteins. In 1958, Goldwasser and Kissling[67] used in-

A. C. Jackson: Departments of Medicine and Microbiology & Immunology, Queen's University, Kingston, Ontario, Canada.

TABLE 24-1. *Historic landmarks in clinical and experimental rabies*

Date	Event	Reference
2300 BC	Earliest known reference to rabies in Mesopotamia	Rosner, 1974[135]
400 BC	Description of animal rabies by Democritus	Wilkinson, 1977[172]
100 AD	Celsus recommends local prophylactic measures	Fleming, 1872[62]
1546	Description of human rabies by Fracastoro	Fracastoro, 1930[63]
1769	Morgagni speculates that the virus spreads in nerves	Morgagni, 1960[114]
1804	Experimental transmission of infection with saliva	Zinke, 1804[181]
1885	Pasteur immunizes Joseph Meister	Pasteur, 1885[122]
1889	Prevention of experimental rabies demonstrated by sectioning of the sciatic nerve	DiVestea and Zagari, 1889[49]
1892	Babes describes microglial nodules	Babes, 1892[4]
1903	Negri bodies are described	Negri, 1903[121]
1958	Fluorescent antibody staining of antigen in tissues	Goldwasser and Kissling, 1958[67]
1965	Experimental studies in mice using antigen detection	Johnson, 1965[91]

direct fluorescent antibody staining to demonstrate rabies virus antigens (RVAs) in tissues, and this technique has become important in rabies diagnosis. It also played an important role in the modern experimental pathogenesis studies of rabies in mice by Johnson[91] and in suckling hamsters by Murphy and coworkers.[116,117]

INFECTIOUS AGENT

Rabies virus is a member of the family *Rhabdoviridae,* which includes viruses that infect mammals, fish, insects, and plants.[21] Two genera infect mammals: lyssavirus and vesiculo-virus. Vesicular stomatitis virus is a vesiculovirus that causes a self-limiting vesicular disease with oral lesions in cattle. The lyssavirus genus is composed of rabies virus and the rabies-related viruses, including Lagos bat virus, Mokola virus, Duvenhage virus, and European bat lyssavirus types 1 and 2. A large number of rabies virus isolates (genotype 1 and serotype 1) from around the world have been characterized with monoclonal antibodies[142] and by limited nucleotide sequence analysis.[145] Lagos bat virus (genotype 2 and serotype 2) has been isolated from fruit-eating bats in Africa, where it has caused rabies in cats and a dog.[139] The reservoir of Mokola virus (genotype 3 and serotype 3) is believed to be in shrews; it has caused rabies in dogs and cats in Africa,[139] and a fatal human case was reported from Nigeria.[54] Duvenhage virus (genotype 4 and serotype 4) and European bat lyssavirus types 1 and 2 (genotypes 5 and 6)[18] have a reservoir in insectivorous bats, and these viruses have caused fatal cases of human rabies in both Africa[110] and Europe.[133] Other viruses, including ko-tonkan and Obodhiang, have distant serologic relationships to members of the genus Lyssavirus.[139]

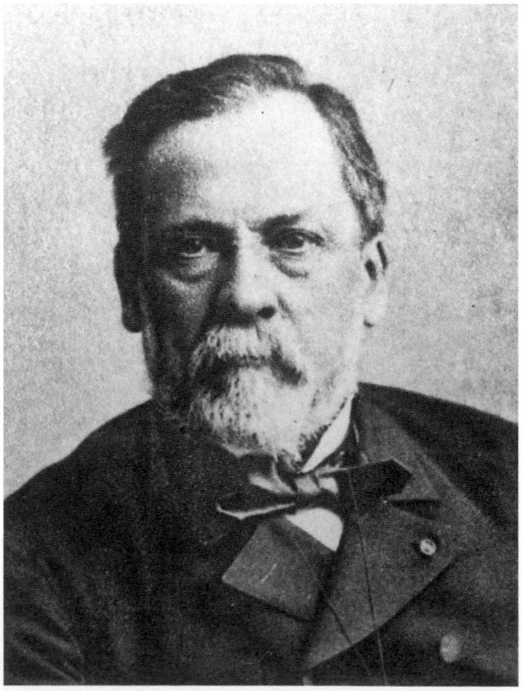

FIG. 24-1. Louis Pasteur. (From Vallery-Radot R. The life of Pasteur. Vol 2. London: Archibald Constable, 1902.)

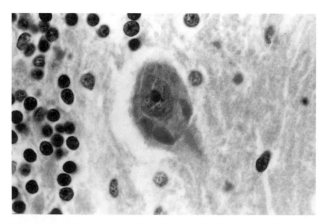

FIG. 24-2 A Purkinje cell in the cerebellum of an 8-year-old boy who died of rabies acquired from a dog. The eosinophilic inclusion bodies in the cytoplasm, called Negri bodies, contain viral particles. Hematoxylin and eosin stain; Magnification 750×.

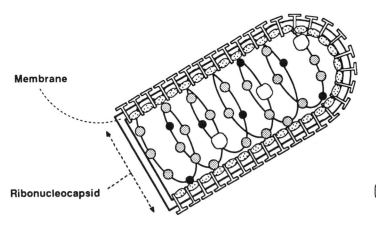

Membrane

Ribonucleocapsid

○ Nucleoprotein

● Phosphoprotein

○ Matrix protein

T Glycoprotein

☐ RNA-polymerase

FIG. 24-3. Schematic view of the rabies virus virion showing the genomic RNA, its five proteins, and the helical ribonucleocapsid core. (From Tordo N, Poch O. Structure of rabies virus. In: Campbell JB, Charlton KM, eds. Rabies. Boston: Kluwer Academic Publishers, 1988;25–45, with permission.)

Rabies virus is a single-stranded RNA virus of negative-sense polarity. Its structure and molecular biology have been reviewed.[151,175,176] The rabies virus genome consists of about 12,000 nucleotides, and it encodes five proteins, designated N, NS, M, G, and L. In the virion, there is a helical ribonucleocapsid core (Fig. 24-3) that consists of genomic RNA; N (nucleocapsid) protein, which protects the RNA from degradation and keeps it in a configuration for transcription; NS (phosphoprotein); and L (transcriptase) protein, which possesses enzymatic activities important for transcription and replication. The ribonucleocapsid core is surrounded by a lipid envelope derived from the host cell membrane. G (glycoprotein) spikes are embedded in the lipid membrane, and they are probably anchored by the M (matrix) protein in the interior.

SPREAD OF RABIES VIRUS IN THE HOST

There are a number of sequential steps in the pathogenesis of rabies after peripheral inoculation of rabies virus, including replication in peripheral tissues, spread along peripheral nerves and the spinal cord to the brain, dissemination within the CNS, and centrifugal spread along nerves to various organs, including the salivary glands (Fig. 24-4). Each of the pathogenetic steps is discussed individually in this chapter. Many of the pathogenesis studies have used strains of rabies virus, such as challenge virus standard (CVS), that have been sequentially passaged in animal brains. Genetic selection has resulted in attenuation of these strains for peripheral inoculation.

Events at the Site of Exposure

Under natural conditions, humans and animals have incubation periods that usually last for weeks after a bite exposure.[5,60] There is uncertainty about the events that occur during this relatively long incubation period. In a suckling hamster model, Murphy and coworkers[115,116] examined the site of viral entry after intramuscular inoculation in a hindlimb with a variety of rabies viruses. With CVS virus, a vampire bat isolate, and two rabies-related viruses (Lagos bat and Mokola), RVA was detected by immunofluorescence in stri-

ated muscle cells at 36 to 40 hours after inoculation, which was before there was evidence of any nervous system infection.[116] Similarly, with 10 of 12 street rabies virus isolates, antigen was observed in muscle on day 3 after inoculation. At that time, the only other evidence of infection was the presence of antigen in intramuscular nerves of the inoculated limb with two of the viruses.[115] Hence, muscle infection occurred before infection in the peripheral nervous system. The major shortcoming of this model is the very short incubation period and the possibility that the mechanism of viral penetration into the CNS is different from that occurring with natural rabies infection.

Charlton and Casey[29] found RVA in local extrafusal muscle fibers 7 days after intramuscular inoculation of skunks with street rabies virus; infection was first observed in the nervous system 10 days after inoculation. They also observed that RVA persisted in denervated skunk muscle fibers at the site of inoculation for 28 days.[30] Although early infection of muscle cells was shown in these models, muscle infection was not demonstrated to be a necessary pathogenetic step in the development of nervous system infection, and it did not explain the long incubation period.

Early infection of muscle or other extraneural tissues was not observed in the mouse models of either Johnson[91] or Coulon and colleagues.[37] Using a polymerase chain reaction (PCR) assay, Shankar and associates[138] did not detect virus-specific RNA in the masseter muscle of adult mice between 6 and 30 hours after inoculation of CVS virus in the muscle, although viral RNA was identified in trigeminal ganglia at 18 hours and in the brain stem at 24 hours after inoculation. These studies provide evidence that rabies virus is capable of direct entry into peripheral nerves without a replicative cycle in extraneural cells, but they do not provide an explanation for the long incubation period in natural rabies. The molecular and biologic events that take place at the site of viral entry during the incubation period remain an enigma. Further studies are needed in natural hosts with long incubation periods.

Lentz and colleagues[103] localized RVA with immunofluorescence in infected cultured chick myotubes and shortly after immersion of mouse diaphragms in a suspension of rabies virus. They found viral antigen at sites in neuromuscular junctions corresponding to the distribution of acetylcholine (ACH) receptors, which were stained with rhodamine-conjugated α-

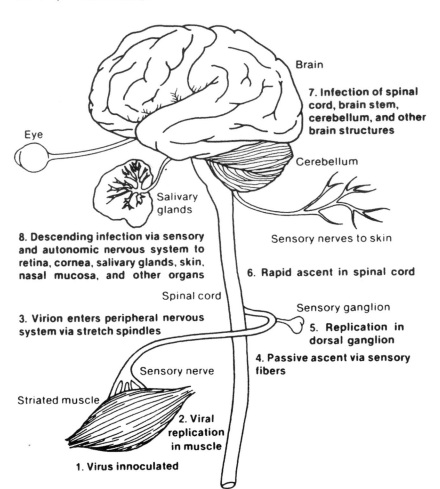

FIG. 24-4. Schematic representation of the pathogenesis of rabies virus after peripheral inoculation. (From Robinson PA. Rabies virus. In: Belshe RB, ed. Textbook of human virology. 2nd ed. St Louis: Mosby–Year Book, 1991;517–540, with permission.)

bungarotoxin. Pretreatment of myotubes with the nicotinic cholinergic antagonist α-bungarotoxin (irreversible) or treatment with *d*-tubocurarine (reversible) reduced the number of myotubes that became infected with rabies virus. Tsiang and associates[156] also showed that pretreatment of cultured rat myotubes with α-bungarotoxin had an inhibitory effect on infection. These studies have provided evidence that rabies virus binds to nicotinic ACH receptors in neuromuscular junctions.

Snake venom neurotoxins are polypeptides that bind to nicotinic ACH receptors, and Lentz and associates[104] compared the amino acid sequence of the rabies virus glycoprotein with that of snake venom neurotoxins. They found a significant sequence similarity between residues 151 to 238 of the rabies virus glycoprotein and the entire long neurotoxin sequence of 71 to 74 residues. The glycoprotein showed identity with residues in loop 2 of the neurotoxin (the "toxic loop"), which probably interacts with the binding site on the ACH receptor (Fig. 24-5). Lentz and coworkers suggested that binding of rabies virus to ACH receptors would localize and concentrate the virus on postsynaptic cells, which would facilitate subsequent uptake and transfer of virus to peripheral motor nerves.[103]

Reagan and Wunner[131] examined the in vitro susceptibility of L8 cells to rabies virus infection. L8 cells are rat skeletal muscle cells that differentiate from myoblasts without ACH

receptors to myotubes that elaborate high-density ACH receptors. They found that L8 myoblasts were fully susceptible to rabies virus infection, yet they failed to demonstrate significant binding of radiolabeled α-bungarotoxin. Four cell lines (BHK-21 cells, CER cells, mouse neuroblastoma cells, and *Aedes albopictus* clone C6/36) that are known to be susceptible to rabies virus infection in vitro also did not demonstrate significant binding of α-bungarotoxin. Therefore, the α-bungarotoxin binding sites of the nicotinic ACH receptor are not necessary for attachment and infection of cells in vitro. However, it is possible that different structures may serve as rabies virus receptors on different cell types.[102]

Spread to the Central Nervous System

Centripetal spread of rabies virus to the CNS occurs within motor and sensory axons of peripheral nerves. Sectioning of the sciatic nerve prevents the development of rabies after ipsilateral footpad inoculation of CVS,[10] indicating that the virus spreads to the spinal cord by means of the sciatic nerve. Tsiang[153] used colchicine, a microtubule-disrupting agent active for tubulin-containing cytoskeletal structures, to inhibit axonal transport in the sciatic nerve of rats. Colchicine was applied locally to the sciatic nerve with the use of elastomer

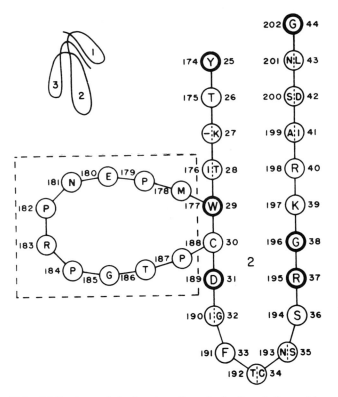

FIG. 24-5. A model showing the similarity of the rabies virus glycoprotein with the "toxic loop" of the neurotoxins. The segment of the glycoprotein (residues 174 to 202) corresponds to loop 2 of the long neurotoxins (Karlsson positions 25 to 44). Within circles, residues or gaps in the glycoprotein are shown on the left and those in the neurotoxin on the right. One letter is shown where the glycoprotein and toxin are identical. Bold circles are residues highly conserved or invariant among all the neurotoxins. A ten-residue insertion in the glycoprotein is enclosed in the box. The rabies virus sequence is that of the challenge virus standard (CVS) strain, and the neurotoxin sequence is that of *Ophiophagus hannah*, toxin b. The inset at upper left is a schematic representation of neurotoxin structure showing the positions of loops 1, 2, and 3. (From Lentz TL, Wilson PT, Hawrot E, Speicher DW. Amino acid sequence similarity between rabies virus glycoprotein and snake venom curaremimetic neurotoxins. Science 1984;226:847–848, with permission; copyright 1984 by the American Association for the Advancement of Science).

cuffs in order to obtain high local concentrations of the drug and avoid adverse systemic effects. Propagation of rabies virus was prevented in this study, and it provided strong evidence that rabies virus spreads from sites of peripheral inoculation to the CNS by retrograde fast axonal transport. Studies using human dorsal root ganglia neurons in a compartmentalized cell culture system showed that viral retrograde transport occurs at a rate of 50 to 100 mm/day.[155] Dorsal root ganglia and spinal cord neurons, including ventral horn cells, appear to be the earliest infected cells that are distant from the site of inoculation.[37,87,91]

Spread Within the Central Nervous System

In rodent models, after CNS neurons become infected there is rapid dissemination of rabies virus infection along neuroanatomic pathways. After peripheral inoculation, there is early involvement of the brain stem tegmentum and deep cerebellar nuclei.[87] Subsequently, the infection spreads to involve cerebellar Purkinje cells and neurons in the cerebral cortex. Rabies virus, like Borna disease virus,[24] spreads to the hippocampus relatively late. Rabies virus selectively infects pyramidal neurons of the hippocampus, and there is relative sparing of neurons in the dentate gyrus.[87] Rabies virus probably spreads within the CNS, as in the peripheral nervous system, by fast axonal transport. Gillet and colleagues[66] provided evidence for transport by this mechanism using stereotaxic brain inoculation in rats, and colchicine also inhibited transport within the CNS.[25,27] Studies on cultured rat dorsal root ganglia neurons showed that anterograde fast axonal transport of rabies virus occurs in the range of 100 to 400 mm/day.[157]

Spread From the Central Nervous System

Centrifugal spread, or viral spread from the CNS to peripheral sites along neuronal routes, is essential for transmission of rabies virus to its natural hosts. Salivary gland infection is necessary for the transfer of infectious oral fluids by rabid, biting animals. The salivary glands receive parasympathetic innervation from the facial nerve (via the submandibular ganglion or Langley's ganglion in some animals) and the glossopharyngeal nerve (via the otic ganglion), sympathetic innervation from the superior (or cranial) cervical ganglion, and afferent (sensory) innervation.[52] Dean and coworkers[41] found that unilateral excision of a portion of the lingual nerve and the cranial cervical ganglion of dogs and foxes resulted in very low viral titers in denervated salivary glands, compared with contralateral salivary glands, after street rabies virus infection. Murphy and colleagues[117] found RVA in mucous acinar cells of salivary glands, and Charlton and associates[31] provided evidence that widespread infection of salivary gland epithelial cells probably results from viral spread along multiple terminal axons rather than from spread between epithelial cells. Viral titers in salivary glands may be higher than in CNS tissues.[43]

In addition to salivary gland infection, Murphy and coworkers[117] found evidence of centrifugal spread involving the central, peripheral, and autonomic nervous systems in many peripheral sites. Infection was observed in the ganglion cell layer of the retina and in corneal epithelial cells, which are innervated by sensory afferents via the trigeminal nerve. Detection of RVA in corneal impression smears has been used as a diagnostic test for human rabies,[97] and rabies has been transmitted by corneal transplantation.[79] Infection is found in free sensory nerve endings of tactile hair.[117] Skin biopsies are probably the best method of confirming a diagnosis of rabies in humans.[23,163] Antigen may be demonstrated in small nerves of the skin taken from the nape of the neck, which is rich in hair follicles. Widespread infection is observed in sensory nerve end organs in the oral and nasal cavities, including the olfactory epithelium and taste buds in the tongue.

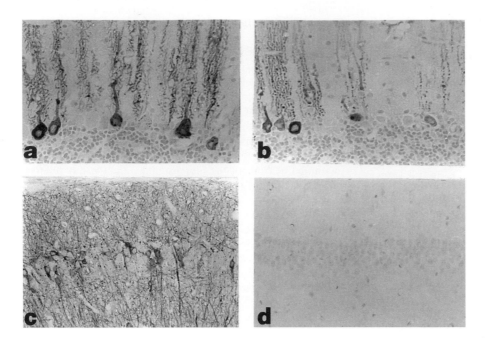

FIG. 24-6. Antigen was present in cerebellar Purkinje cells 5 days after inoculation with (**A**) challenge virus standard (CVS) and (**B**) RV194-2 rabies virus strains into the masseter muscle. Note the antigen in the dendritic processes of the Purkinje cells in the molecular layer. More antigen was present in the cerebellum with CVS than with the RV194-2 strain. Antigen was present in the CA1 region of the hippocampus 8 days after inoculation with CVS (**C**), but not after inoculation with RV194-2 (**D**). **A** and **B**, immunoperoxidase-hematoxylin staining, magnification 235×; **C** and **D**, immunoperoxidase-hematoxylin staining, magnification 140×. (Adapted from Jackson AC. Biological basis of rabies virus neurovirulence in mice: comparative pathogenesis study using the immunoperoxidase technique. J Virol 1991;65:537–540, with permission.)

Murphy and colleagues[117] also found infection of the autonomic nerves of the visceral organs, including the intestinal plexi, adrenal glands (sympathetic ganglion cells), and myocardium. Myocarditis has also been observed in human cases of rabies.[2,32,136] There is also evidence of infection in the lungs, pancreas, kidneys, and skeletal muscles.[42,117]

PATHOLOGY OF RABIES

In contrast to the dramatic clinical manifestations of rabies, which usually lead to a fatal outcome, its pathologic findings are relatively mild. There are inflammatory lesions of variable severity in the brain, spinal cord, and ganglia. Perivascular infiltrates, consisting primarily of mononuclear cells, and infiltration of inflammatory cells can be seen in the leptomeninges. Microglial nodules (Babes' nodules),[4] which are comprised mostly of activated microglia, are present in the CNS parenchyma, especially adjacent to neurons undergoing degeneration.[127]

Neuronal infection by rabies virus does not usually result in significant cytopathic changes, and neuronal degeneration is not prominent in rabies. However, chromatolytic changes in infected neurons may be prominent in infected cranial and spinal ganglia.[78,101,127] Neuronophagia (phagocytosis of infected neurons) is frequently observed in the brain and spinal cord, and Dupont and Earle[51] identified neuronophagia in 57% of 49 fatal human cases.

Eosinophilic inclusion bodies called Negri bodies can be identified in the cytoplasm of infected neurons,[121] and they are most prominent in large neurons such as cerebellar Purkinje cells (see Fig. 24-2). The morphology of Negri bodies varies in different species. They are very large in cattle but small and multiple in rabbits.[127] Negri bodies are present in about 70% of human patients with rabies.[51] Negri bodies contain RVA[67]; ultrastructural studies have shown viral particles embedded in an amorphous substance or matrix.[68] RVA can also be demonstrated in infected cells by immunofluorescent and immunohistochemical methods (Fig. 24-6A), and rabies virus genomic RNA and mRNAs encoding the rabies virus proteins can be detected with in situ hybridization[89] (Fig. 24-7).

Distinct pathologic features of paralytic rabies, as opposed to classic rabies, have not been defined. Chopra and associates[33] observed inflammatory infiltrates in the spinal cord and dorsal root ganglia and demyelinating lesions in the peripheral nerves of humans with paralytic rabies.

Electron microscopic studies have confirmed the viral nature of Negri bodies. Bullet-shaped mature viral particles (Fig.

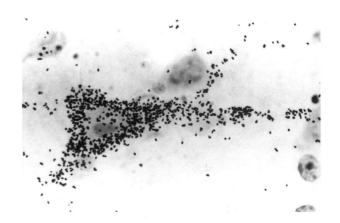

FIG. 24-7. In situ hybridization for rabies virus messenger RNA encoding the glycoprotein in a ventral horn cell of a mouse experimentally infected with the challenge virus standard (CVS) strain of fixed rabies virus. Grains are present in the perikaryon and in dendritic processes of the infected neuron. Hematoxylin stain; magnification 937×.

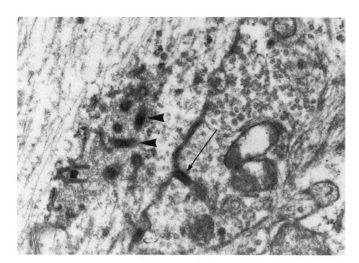

FIG. 24-8. Electron micrograph of the dorsal horn of the spinal cord of a skunk experimentally infected with street rabies virus. Note bullet-shaped virions (*arrowheads*) and viral matrix in a dendrite and a virion budding into an adjacent axon terminal at a synapse (*arrow*). Magnification 23,500×. (Courtesy of Dr. K.M. Charlton, Animal Diseases Research Institute, Nepean, Ontario, Canada.)

24-8) can be seen in infected neurons.[82] Budding of rabies virus from the neuronal plasma membrane has been observed in the brains of experimentally infected mice[80] and skunks.[29] Transneuronal transfer has been documented from dendrites to axons (see Fig. 24-8), indicating retrograde transsynaptic spread of the viral infection.[29]

ANIMAL MODELS OF RABIES VIRUS NEUROVIRULENCE

Viral neurovirulence can be defined as the capacity of a virus to cause disease of the nervous system, especially the CNS. It is usually analyzed in experimental models by comparing infections in a given host with those caused by closely related viruses, such as different strains, or a parent virus and a variant.[83] The ability of a virus to spread to the CNS from a peripheral site (neuroinvasiveness) is an important component of neurovirulence after inoculation through natural routes

of viral entry. The route of inoculation is important in evaluating neurovirulence experimentally. Intracerebral inoculation is commonly used for convenience, and many peripheral sites have also been used in different models, including footpad, intramuscular, intraperitoneal, and intraocular inoculation. Species, age, and immune status of the host are also important factors in neurovirulence.[61]

Variant viruses were selected in vitro from CVS with neutralizing antiglycoprotein monoclonal antibodies (MAR variants).[137] Mutations involving antigenic site III are located between positions 330 and 338 of the CVS glycoprotein. Variants with a single amino acid change at position 333, with loss of either arginine[48,137] or lysine,[158] have diminished virulence in mice after intracerebral inoculation, and variants with amino acid changes at other positions remain neurovirulent. Comparison of these "avirulent" variants with their parent viruses in mouse and rat models after inoculation by different routes has been a useful approach in understanding the biologic basis of rabies virus neurovirulence (Table 24-2). Both MAR variants RV194-2[48] and Av01[38] have substitution of a glutamine for the arginine of CVS at position 333 of the glycoprotein.

Events at the Site of Exposure

Avirulent rabies virus variants, but not the parent CVS strain, have been shown to cause infection in extraneural sites close to the site of inoculation in different models. Kucera and colleagues[99] observed that MAR variant Av01 infected the anterior epithelium of the lens after inoculation into the anterior chamber of the eye in rats (Fig. 24-9). After inoculation of MAR variant RV194-2 into the tongue of mice and rats, Torres-Anjel and associates[152] found local infection involving epithelial tissues, glandular cells, and muscles. In these models, the variant viruses demonstrated less restricted cellular tropism than CVS, which is highly neuronotropic.

Spread to the Central Nervous System

Coulon and coworkers[37] inoculated CVS and MAR variant Av01 into the forelimb muscles of mice and examined the spinal cord and dorsal root ganglia (sensory) neurons for the presence of RVA. Both viruses infected ventral horn (motor) cells and dorsal root ganglia at similar rates and efficiencies. After CVS and RV194-2 were inoculated into the masseter

TABLE 24-2. *Neurovirulence studies in animal models*

Species	Parent virus	Variant virus	Route of inoculation	Investigators
Mouse	CVS	RV194-2	Intracerebral	Dietzschold et al, 1985[47]
Mouse	CVS	Av01	Forelimb muscle	Coulon et al, 1989[37]
Mouse	CVS	RV194-2	Masseter muscle	Jackson, 1991[84]
Mouse, rat	CVS	RV194-2	Tongue	Torres-Anjel et al, 1984[152]
Mouse	CVS	Av01	Intranasal	Lafay et al, 1991[100]
Rat	CVS	Av01	Eye (anterior chamber)	Kucera et al, 1985[99]
Mouse	CVS	Av01	Neostriatum (stereotaxic)	Yang and Jackson, 1992[179]

CVS, challenge virus standard.
From Jackson AC. Animal models of rabies virus neurovirulence. In: Rupprecht CE, Dietzschold B, Koprowski H, eds. Curr Top Microbiol Immunol 1994;187:85–93, with permission.

muscles of mice, both viruses spread to the ipsilateral motor nucleus of the trigeminal nerve in the pons at similar rates.[84] RV194-2, but not CVS, spread to the ipsilateral trigeminal ganglion during the first 2 days after inoculation. There was no restriction in the pathways taken by the variants to the CNS in either of the models, and the variants were neuroinvasive.

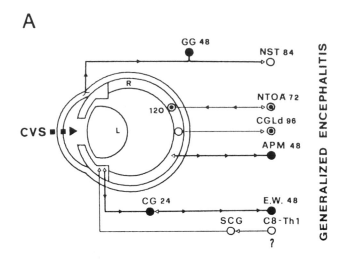

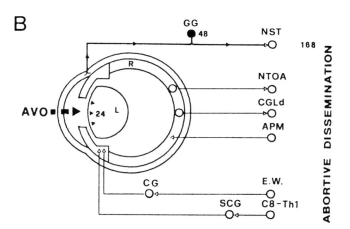

FIG. 24-9. Propagation of (**A**) the challenge virus standard (CVS) rabies virus strain and (**B**) the avirulent variant rabies virus strain AVO through the trigeminal (*top*), visual (*center*), and autonomic (*bottom*) interconnections between the eye and brain. Open arrows show direction of neurotransmission; closed arrows show direction of propagation of the virus. Peripheral and central neuronal somata are infected primarily (*closed circles*), secondarily (*dotted circles*), or not at all (*open circles*) at time intervals indicated in hours after inoculation. APM, area praetectalis medialis; C8-Th1, spinal preganglionic sympathetic neurons; CG, ciliary ganglion; CGLd, lateral geniculate body (dorsal part); E.W., Edinger-Westphal nucleus; GG, trigeminal (gasserian) ganglion; L, lens; NST, terminal trigeminal sensory nucleus; NTOA, terminal nuclei of the accessory optic system; R, retina; SCG, superior cervical sympathetic ganglion. (From Kucera P, Dolivo M, Coulon P, Flamand A. Pathways of the early propagation of virulent and avirulent rabies strains from the eye to the brain. J Virol 1985;55:158–162, with permission.)

Kucera and colleagues[99] developed an excellent model for studying the pathways of viral spread to the brain by inoculating rabies virus into the anterior chamber of the eye in rats. There are six potential neural pathways for viral spread to occur between the eye and brain (see Fig. 24-9). Rabies virus was localized in tissues with the use of immunofluorescent staining. After inoculation of CVS, antigen was initially detected at 24 hours in the ipsilateral ciliary ganglion, and later in the Edinger-Westphal nucleus of the oculomotor nerve (parasympathetic pathway). At 48 hours, spread had also occurred to the ipsilateral ganglion of the trigeminal nerve (an afferent sensory pathway) and to neurons of the contralateral area praetectalis medialis, which projects to the retina by means of preopticoretinal fibers. In contrast, Av01 propagated in the trigeminal pathway but not in either parasympathetic or preopticoretinal fibers. Neurons in the trigeminal ganglion were also infected at 48 hours, indicating a similar rate of spread. In this model, therefore, the avirulent MAR variant spreads to the brain by more restricted pathways than those used by its virulent parent virus.

Spread Within the Central Nervous System

Studies performed after masseter muscle[84] and intranasal[100] inoculation of mice indicate that the rate of spread of variants within the CNS is similar to that of the virulent parent viruses, indicating that there is probably not any difference in the axonal transport mechanism. The topographic distribution of CNS infections after inoculation of CVS and RV194-2 in the masseter muscle was quite similar.[84] The infections were widespread and involved major regions of the CNS, including the cerebral cortex, hippocampus, brain stem, cerebellum, and spinal cord. The same neuronal cell types were infected, although fewer neurons were infected by RV194-2, and viral spread was less efficient (see Fig. 24-6). After intranasal instillation of CVS and Av01, Lafay and coworkers[100] also observed that Av01 infected fewer olfactory neurons than CVS.

Intracerebral inoculation is a crude technique in which the inoculum spreads throughout the cerebrospinal fluid spaces, including the ventricular system and subarachnoid space.[113] A stereotaxic apparatus can deliver an inoculum into a precise location in the brain. Both Av01 and RV194-2 were found to be neurovirulent after stereotaxic inoculation into the neostriatum or cerebellum of adult mice,[179] although Av01 infected fewer neurons and deaths occurred later than after stereotaxic inoculation with CVS.[86] After inoculation of Av01 into the striatum, the infection was widespread in the brain, involving degenerative neuronal changes and marked infiltration with inflammatory cells. Serum neutralizing antibodies against rabies virus were produced later and in smaller quantities than after intracerebral inoculation. Av01 is probably neurovirulent after stereotaxic brain inoculation, because this route produces both a direct site of viral entry into the CNS and a low level of immune stimulation.

Spread From the Central Nervous System

In the model of Kucera and colleagues[99] using intraocular inoculation of rats, CVS spread from the nuclei of the accessory optic system to ganglionic cells of the retina in both eyes (see Fig. 24-9). Av01 did not show evidence of centrifugal spread in this model. In contrast, both CVS and RV194-2 spread to the trigeminal ganglia bilaterally after inoculation in a masseter muscle, indicating centrifugal spread.[84]

Summary of Neurovirulence in Animal Models

Analysis of avirulent (MAR) variants of CVS has given important insights into the mechanisms of rabies virus neurovirulence. Changes in cellular tropisms of variants have been observed close to the site of inoculation. Variants remain neuroinvasive, although there may be restrictions in their pathways to the CNS. After variants reach the CNS they spread widely, but interneuronal spread is inefficient, fewer neurons become infected than with CVS, and CNS cellular tropisms are unchanged. Variants are also capable of spreading centrifugally. The rate of viral spread centrally and peripherally is similar for variants and for CVS. A single amino acid change in the rabies virus glycoprotein clearly has dramatic effects on rabies virus neurovirulence. In the future, it will be challenging to determine the mode of action of specific viral gene products that affect neurovirulence in vivo.

BRAIN DYSFUNCTION IN RABIES

Despite the dramatic and severe clinical neurologic signs in rabies, the neuropathologic findings are usually quite mild[127]; the neuronal dysfunction therefore may result from alterations that are not detectable at the morphologic level. Studies performed in vitro have shown that rabies virus has little or no inhibitory effect on cellular RNA and protein synthesis.[53,109,159] The basis of the neuronal dysfunction in rabies at the cellular level is unknown. At the present time, the leading hypotheses to explain the neuronal dysfunction in rabies are defective neurotransmission and induction of nitric oxide.

Defective Neurotransmission

Tsiang[154] hypothesized that defective cholinergic neurotransmission may be the basis for neuronal dysfunction in rabies. He examined specific binding to muscarinic ACH receptors in CVS-infected rat brains with a ^{3}H-labeled antagonist, quinuclidinyl benzylate (QNB), and found that binding of ^{3}H-labeled QNB to infected brain homogenates was decreased by 96 hours after infection, compared with control animals, and it was markedly decreased at 120 hours (10 to 20 hours before death was expected to occur). The greatest reduction was found in the hippocampus, with smaller reductions in the cerebral cortex and in the caudate nucleus.

Jackson[85] examined cholinergic neurotransmission in CVS-infected and uninfected control mice. The enzymatic activities of choline acetyltransferase and acetylcholinesterase, which are required for the synthesis and degradation of ACH, were similar in the cerebral cortex and hippocampus of moribund CVS-infected mice and in control mice. In contrast to the findings in infected rats, binding to muscarinic ACH receptors, which was also assessed with ^{3}H-labeled QNB, was not significantly different in the cerebral cortex or hippocampus of CVS-infected and control mice. Scatchard plots were used to analyze the binding data in this study, and they provide a better analysis of the data than does expression of bound ^{3}H-labeled QNB as counts per minute.[134] It is possible that differences in the species (mouse versus rat) or in the route of inoculation (peripheral versus intracerebral) account for the different results in the two studies.

Binding of rabies virus to nicotinic ACH receptors in the brain could cause neuronal dysfunction, and there is evidence that rabies virus binds to nicotinic ACH receptors at the neuromuscular junction. Hanham and associates[71] used a monoclonal antirabies virus glycoprotein (G) antibody to generate (by immunization) an antiidiotypic antibody, B9, which binds to nicotinic ACH receptors. Furthermore, they found that B9 immunostaining of neuronal elements in the brains of rabies virus-infected mice was greatly reduced. This suggests that rabies virus may bind to nicotinic ACH receptors in the brain as well as the neuromuscular junction, but the pathogenetic significance of this binding in producing neuronal dysfunction in rabies has not yet been established.

Neurotransmitters other than ACH could be important in the pathogenesis of rabies, and serotonin (5-HT) has received the most attention. Serotonin has a wide distribution in the brain, and it is important in the control of sleep and wakefulness, pain perception, memory, and a variety of behaviors.[22,92] Alterations of sleep stages have been reported in experimental rabies in mice.[69,70] Ceccaldi and colleagues[26] examined binding to serotonin receptor subtypes in the brains of CVS-infected rats. Binding of 5-HT$_1$ sites using [^{3}H]5-HT was decreased in the cerebral cortex 5 days after inoculation of CVS into the masseter muscles. Binding of ligands specific for 5-HT$_{1A}$ and 5-HT$_{1B}$ sites was not affected. [^{3}H]5-HT binding assessed in the presence of drugs masking 5-HT$_{1A}$, 5-HT$_{1B}$, and 5-HT$_{1C}$ receptors was reduced by 50% in the cerebral cortex 3 days after inoculation, and binding remained at that level. These results suggest that rabies virus infection specifically affects 5-HT–like receptors in the cerebral cortex. Furthermore, the reduced binding was demonstrated before RVA was detected in the cerebral cortex. Hence, the effect on binding is unlikely to be caused by interaction between the virus and the receptor, or by either direct or indirect effects of viral replication in cortical neurons. There are important serotonergic projections from the dorsal raphe nuclei in the brain stem to the cerebral cortex, and Smart and Charlton[140] have reported early infection of the midbrain raphe nuclei in experimental rabies in skunks. It is possible that the reduced binding to 5-HT–like receptors is an indirect effect of infection at noncortical sites or that it is part of a physiologic response to the stress produced by infection. In support of impaired serotonergic neurotransmission in rabies, Bouzamondo and coworkers[19] have reported decreased potassium-evoked release of ^{3}H-serotonin in synaptosomes from the cerebral cortex of CVS-infected rats, indicating that there is also presynaptic involvement.

Induction of Nitric Oxide

Nitric oxide is a short-lived gaseous radical that acts as a biologic mediator for diverse cell types. It is produced by many different cells and mediates a variety of functions, including vasodilation, neurotransmission, immune cytotoxicity, production of synaptic plasticity in the brain, and neurotoxicity.[106,118] Nitric oxide is released by the enzyme nitric oxide synthase (NOS), which also produces other reactive oxides of nitrogen.[118] The constitutive NOS gene has been cloned from rat cerebellum,[20] and this system generates low levels of nitric oxide. In contrast, the NOS gene cloned from mouse macrophages is inducible (iNOS),[178] and the iNOS system can generate large quantities of nitric oxide over an extended time period.

Koprowski and associates[98] reported the induction of iNOS mRNA in mice experimentally infected with either street rabies virus or herpes simplex virus and rats infected with Borna disease virus. iNOS mRNA was detected by reverse transcription PCR in the brains of three of six paralyzed mice 9 to 14 days after inoculation of street rabies virus in the masseter muscle. iNOS expression was rapidly induced in the brains of rabid mice. Nitric oxide and other endogenous neurotoxins may mediate the neuronal dysfunction in rabies and other infectious diseases, including Borna disease.[98,180] The human immunodeficiency virus type 1 coat protein, gp120, is neurotoxic in primary cortical cultures, and nitric oxide probably contributes to the neurotoxicity.[40] Depletion of arginine from the incubation medium or the addition of either hemoglobin or nitroarginine to the medium reduces the neurotoxicity (iron in heme binds nitric oxide, and nitroarginine is a NOS inhibitor).

Nitric oxide mediates much of the antimicrobial activity of mouse macrophages against a variety of bacterial, fungal, protozoal, and helminthic pathogens.[119] There is recent evidence that nitric oxide also has antiviral activity. Croen[39] observed that replication of herpes simplex virus type 1 in the mouse RAW macrophage cell line, which is transformed with Abelson leukemia virus, was inhibited by interferon-γ and by bacterial lipopolysaccharide, both of which induce nitric oxide production. Competitive and noncompetitive inhibitors of NOS substantially reduced the antiviral effect of activated RAW macrophages. An exogenous donor of nitric oxide, S-nitroso-L-acetyl penicillamine (SNAP), reduced herpes simplex virus replication in a variety of cell lines, including RAW macrophages, and the antiviral effect of SNAP did not appear to result from a cytotoxic effect of nitric oxide. Karupiah and associates[95] showed that the ability of interferon-γ to inhibit replication of ectromelia, vaccinia, and herpes simplex virus type 1 in mouse RAW macrophages correlated with the cellular production of nitric oxide, and that viral replication was restored with exposure to NOS inhibitors. They also showed that a competitive inhibitor of iNOS, N-methyl-L-arginine, converted resolving ectromelia virus infection in mice into fulminant mousepox. It is uncertain at this time whether the dominant effects of iNOS expression in experimental rabies, which were reported by Koprowski and colleagues,[98] are antiviral or neurotoxic.

IMMUNE RESPONSE TO RABIES VIRUS

The rabies virus glycoprotein is the basic unit of the spikelike surface projections on the viral particle. It is the only RVA that induces the production of neutralizing antibodies, which confer protective immunity against a lethal challenge with rabies virus. Dietzschold and colleagues[46] reported that the rabies virus ribonucleoprotein (see Fig. 24-3), which consists of genomic RNA and the N, NS, and L proteins, can also confer protective immunity in a variety of species. It appears that rabies virus nucleoprotein induces T helper cells and the production of interferon-γ.[44] Xiang and associates[177] reported that mice immunized intramuscularly with a plasmid that expresses the rabies virus glycoprotein under the control of an SV40 early promoter produced a full spectrum of specific immune responses, including protection against viral challenge.

Humoral Immune Response

In natural infections, serum neutralizing antibody levels are usually low until the disease is advanced, and for this reason they are of limited value in the diagnosis of rabies. Rabies virus is sequestered from the immune system during the incubation period by unknown mechanisms. In contrast, serum neutralizing antibodies appear in about 4 to 6 days and reach a plateau level in about 2 weeks after immunization and in experimental infections.[166] In these situations, there is presumably much greater antigenic stimulation than in natural infections. If an animal survives a rabies virus infection, the serum antibody titer usually remains high for months to years. If recovery occurs in experimental infection after replication of rabies virus in the CNS, homogenates of brain tissue are capable of neutralizing infectious virus in a neutralization test.[14] This is presumably a result of intrathecal synthesis of antibody from immigrating B cells.[120]

Between 7 and 14 days after immunization of humans with rabies vaccine, there is a transition from an immunoglobulin M (IgM) to an IgG response.[160] Because rabies virus spreads neurally rather than by a viremia, IgM may be of limited value except in the neutralization of extracellular virus in bite wounds after postexposure immunization and, possibly, in antibody-dependent cellular cytotoxicity.[126,160] It is unclear whether "secretory" IgA plays any role in protection against the spread of rabies virus across mucosal surfaces.[160]

In addition to the neutralization of extracellular virus, neutralizing antibodies may bind to virus expressed on the cell surface and initiate complement-mediated lysis of infected cells.[171] Antibody-mediated cytolysis probably plays a role in vivo in immune protection and possibly also in immunopathology.[120]

Antibody may be important both in protection of the host from neuroinvasion of rabies virus and in clearance of the virus from the CNS. Dietzschold and colleagues[45] demonstrated that antiglycoprotein monoclonal antibodies inhibit rabies virus from spreading from cell to cell in monolayers of mouse neuroblastoma cells; one monoclonal antibody (1112-1) restricted rabies virus RNA transcription. Studies performed with immunofluorescence demonstrated endocytosis of the antibody, suggesting that antibodies may exert their inhibitory activity even after uptake by cells.

Cell-Mediated Immune Response

T lymphocytes act as helper cells for the induction of B-cell responses and the production of antibody, and they also act as effector cells for cellular immunity (cytotoxic T cells).[120] In both capacities, they play an important role in protection against rabies virus infection. The avirulent high-egg-passage strain of rabies virus causes lethal infection in T cell–deficient athymic nude mice, but it does not produce disease in normal littermates.[94] This occurs as a result of impaired T- and B-cell responses in the nude mice.

Wiktor and coworkers[167] observed that virus-specific cytotoxic T lymphocytes, which were assayed by ^{51}Cr release, appeared 4 days after rabies immunization, developed maximal activity at 6 days, and disappeared by 14 days. Furthermore, Wiktor and associates[168] observed that mice lethally infected with street rabies virus failed to develop cytotoxic T lymphocytes despite normal antibody production. This suggests that these animals have an impaired specific cellular immune response; if so, its mechanism is unknown.

In contrast to the short-lasting cytotoxic T cell response, there are brisk proliferative responses of spleen lymphocytes in vitro from rabies-immunized rabbits.[169] Maximum stimulation occurs 8 days after immunization with live or inactivated vaccines, and the responsiveness of sensitized lymphocytes is maintained for at least 175 days.

Macfarlan and coworkers[108] cleaved the rabies virus glycoprotein with cyanogen bromide into eight fragments in order to identify the domains of the glycoprotein that have the capacity to stimulate the proliferation of rabies virus–primed T lymphocytes. They found three peptide fragments with significant stimulatory activity under reducing (denaturing) conditions. Furthermore, two synthetic peptides (containing 13 and 27 residues), which included sequences from one of these fragments (residues 1 to 44), stimulated virus-primed T lymphocytes. The T lymphocytes that responded to either the intact viral glycoprotein or one of the synthetic peptides were Lyt-1–positive and Lyt-2–negative, indicating that they had the surface characteristics of helper T cells. The synthetic peptides also stimulated a minor population of Lyt-2–positive cells, which could be either cytotoxic or suppressor T cells. Analyses using cleavage by cyanogen bromide and limited tryptic digestion indicated that a nominal determinant of the rabies virus glycoprotein responsible for stimulating the cytotoxic T lymphocyte response is located between residues 130 and 178 of the glycoprotein.[107] Studies using T cell lines from human vaccine recipients showed cytotoxic T cell responses by a CD4+ T cell line against antigenic determinants of the rabies virus glycoprotein and ribonucleoprotein.[28]

Immunopathology

Immunosuppression results in increased severity of rabies and, in infection by attenuated strains, it can increase the mortality rate.[94,112,141] Studies using adoptive transfer of immune cells in immunosuppressed rabies virus–infected mice have shown that both T and B lymphocytes may reduce mortality and play a role in clearance of rabies virus from the CNS.[129]

In contrast, under certain conditions there is immune enhancement of rabies. Some humans who are immunized after a rabies exposure develop clinical rabies after a short incubation period; this has been called the early death phenomenon.[130] Experimental models have been useful in exploring immunopathologic mechanisms of the early death phenome-

non. Prabhakar and Nathanson[130] infected adult mice with the high-egg-passage Flury strain of rabies virus on the day that they received a lethal dose of total body irradiation. Four days later, the mice were reconstituted with normal or immune syngeneic spleen cells. Mice that received normal spleen cells or cells from donors immunized 30 days earlier died at a mean of 9 days after cell transfer. Spleen cells from donors immunized 7 days earlier conferred complete protection without signs of disease. In contrast, reconstitution with spleen cells obtained 3 days after secondary immunization of donors (secondary immune cells) resulted in 28% mortality, and these deaths occurred after a mean of only 3 days. These mice died with convulsions and tonic spasms, and histopathologic examination failed to demonstrate neuronal destruction or inflammation. The secondary immune spleen cells were separated into B- and T-cell–enriched populations. Immune B cells, but not immune T cells, and also anti–rabies virus antibody were capable of inducing early death. Smith and colleagues[144] also observed early death in street rabies virus–infected immunosuppressed mice that were given homologous immune serum.

The immune system can play a dual role during the course of rabies virus infection. The destruction of rabies virus–infected cells early in the course of infection results in immune clearance and prevention of clinical disease. If a large number of cells are infected, the immune response can enhance the disease and cause early death. The effects of antibody on infected cells play a critical role in the immunopathology of rabies.

CLINICAL RABIES

Human Rabies

Human rabies usually develops after rabies virus is transmitted through the saliva of a biting animal. Animal bites result in inoculation of rabies virus into subcutaneous tissues and muscle. Other types of exposure include contamination of an open wound, scratch, abrasion, or mucous membrane by saliva or CNS tissue, inhalation of aerosolized rabies virus (in bat caves[34] or laboratories[148,149,174]), and transplantation of rabies virus–infected tissues (i.e., cornea).[64,79,147]

Human rabies usually develops 1 to 3 months after an exposure, although rare cases have occurred after 1 year or longer.[143] Fishbein[60] stated that untreated persons develop rabies after 40% to 80% of head bites, 15% to 40% of hand or arm bites, and 0% to 10% of leg bites by a rabid animal. Nonspecific prodromal symptoms, including fever, chills, malaise, fatigue, insomnia, anorexia, headache, anxiety, and irritability, may last for a few days. About 50% of patients develop pain, paresthesias, or pruritus at or near the bite site, which may represent infection in local dorsal root ganglia.[73]

About 80% of patients develop the classic form of rabies (called furious or encephalitic rabies), and 20% have a paralytic form of disease. In classic rabies, patients have episodes of generalized arousal or hyperexcitability, which are separated by lucid periods.[161] Confusion, hallucinations, aggressive behavior, and seizures may occur. Fever is common, and there may be signs of autonomic dysfunction, including hypersalivation, sweating, and piloerection. Nuchal rigidity may be present, reflecting leptomeningeal inflammation. About half of the patients develop hydrophobia, which is a characteristic manifestation of rabies.[161] Patients may initially experience pain in the throat or difficulty swallowing. On attempts to swallow, they experience contractions of the diaphragm and other inspiratory muscles, which last for about 5 to 15 seconds (Fig. 24-10). Subsequently, the sight, sound, or even mention of water (or other liquids) may trigger these spasms, indicating that hydrophobia is reinforced by conditioning.[162] A draft of air on the skin may have the same effect (aerophobia). The hydrophobia of rabies is probably caused by selective infection of neurons that inhibit the inspiratory motor neurons in the region of the nucleus ambiguus in the brain stem.[161,162] There is often progression to paralysis, coma, and multiple organ failure. The disease is fatal, and death usually occurs within 14 days of the onset of clinical manifestations.

In paralytic rabies, flaccid muscle weakness develops early in the course of the disease. The weakness often begins in the bitten extremity and spreads to involve the other extremities and the facial muscles. Sphincter involvement, pain, and sensory disturbances may occur. Myoedema has been described at percussion sites.[76] Bulbar and respiratory muscles eventually become involved, resulting in death. Hydrophobia is unusual in this form of the disease, and survival in paralytic rabies is usually longer than in classic rabies.

The pathogenetic basis for the two different clinical forms of rabies has not been determined. In a small series, there were no marked differences in the regional distribution of RVA or in the inflammatory changes.[150] Patients with paralytic rabies may have defects in immune responsiveness, including lack of lymphocyte proliferative responses to RVA[77] and lower levels of serum cytokines than patients with classic rabies.[75]

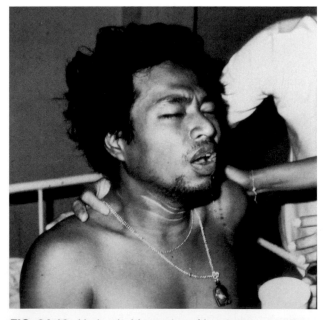

FIG. 24-10. Hydrophobic spasm of inspiratory muscles associated with terror in a patient with furious rabies encephalitis attempting to swallow water. (Copyright D.A. Warrell, Oxford University, UK.)

Analysis of the cerebrospinal fluid (CSF) is usually abnormal in patients with rabies. Anderson and associates[1] found a CSF pleocytosis (elevated number of white cells) in 59% of cases during the first week of illness and in 87% after the first week. The white cells are predominantly mononuclear cells, and the CSF protein concentration may be mildly elevated. Serum neutralizing antibodies against rabies virus are not usually present in unimmunized patients until after the tenth day of illness.[73] Rabies virus may occasionally be isolated from saliva, CSF, or urine sediment early in the illness.[1] RVA may be demonstrated during life in small nerves in skin biopsies or in corneal impression smears.[23,97,163] The diagnosis of rabies by brain biopsy has not been adequately assessed. Postmortem CNS tissues can be assessed for RVA and viral isolation.

Antiviral therapy and a variety of immunotherapies have been unsuccessful in the treatment of rabies.[72,111,164] Therapy is supportive, and survival may be prolonged with intensive care. Survival from rabies has been well documented in only three patients, all of whom had been immunized before the onset of clinical disease.[74,128,148,149]

Animal Rabies

Rabies virus can potentially infect all warm-blooded animals. There are virus, host, and environmental factors that influence the epidemiology of rabies, and the virus is maintained under natural conditions in a particular species in geographic areas of variable size. However, not all species are equally susceptible to infection by rabies virus.[6] Foxes have extremely high susceptibility, and opossums are one of the least susceptible species. Dogs have moderate susceptibility even though they are the most important vector worldwide.[6] Although the basis for species-related susceptibility is not understood, Baer and colleagues[9] have provided preliminary evidence that it may be related to the maximum number of binding sites (B_{max}) of nicotinic ACH receptors in skeletal muscle.

In animals, there are two clinical forms of rabies. In the furious form there is prominent aggressive behavior. In the dumb form, paralysis develops early and continues progressively until death[93]; the clinical course is quieter.[50] Although in individual animals either of the clinical forms may be more prominent in different phases of the disease, one form is often more characteristic of a specific species. For example, furious rabies is characteristic of cats, and dumb rabies is more common in dogs and cattle.[11]

Deviation from normal behavior is typical in animals with rabies. Nocturnal animals, such as skunks and bats, may become active during daylight hours. Animals often lose their normal fear of humans. Dogs may become more affectionate than usual (and lick their owners), become withdrawn, or become aggressive and bite humans, other animals, or inanimate objects[93,165] (Fig. 24-11). Hydrophobia does not occur in animals. Muscular weakness may cause difficulty swallowing, drooling of saliva, sagging of the lower jaw, and hoarseness in dogs and cattle.[11,93] Difficulty swallowing may lead the owner of a domestic animal to attempt to remove an object from its throat, resulting in an exposure. Tenesmus is common in cattle.[65] Aberrant sexual behavior and aggressiveness may also be observed in animals.

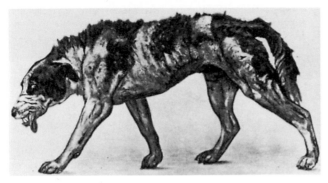

FIG. 24-11. A rabid dog. (From Bisseru B. Rabies. London: William Heinemann Medical Books, 1972, with permission.)

Recovery From Rabies

Although rabies is usually considered to be a uniformly fatal disease, animals may sometimes recover from rabies. Recovery from rabies has also been called abortive rabies, which can occur either with or without neurologic sequelae.[13] There have been a number of reports of survival after development of neurologic illness (Table 24-3), and most of these are in experimental animals. Because of limitations on laboratory diagnostic tests performed during life, a conclusive diagnosis of rabies may not be made in animals that recover. Animals clinically suspected of having rabies are usually killed before they have an opportunity to recover. For these reasons, reports may greatly underestimate the occurrence of recovery. The incidence of recovery in animals under natural conditions is unknown.

There are also rare reports of dogs with a carrier state. These clinically normal animals have excreted rabies virus in their saliva for prolonged periods of time (months or years).[55,56,58] It is unclear whether a carrier state in dogs has

TABLE 24-3. *Reports of recovery from rabies*

Species	Immunization status	Rabies strain	Route	Investigators
Human	Duck embryo	Bat	Natural exposure	Hattwick et al, 1972[74]
Human	Suckling mouse brain	Dog	Natural exposure	Porras et al, 1976[128]
Human	Immunized	Modified live rabies virus (parent was Street Alabama Dufferin)	Inhalation (laboratory accident)	Tillotson et al, 1977[149,150]
Dog	Unimmunized	Fixed rabies virus	Intravenous	Pasteur et al, 1882[124]
Dog	Unimmunized	Fixed rabies virus	Intravenous	Remlinger and Effendi, 1904[132]
Dog	Unimmunized	Vampire bat isolate	Intracerebral	Johnson, 1948[90]
Dog	Unimmunized	Low egg passage plus either low egg passage or bat isolate	Intracisternal, intraperitoneal	Bell et al, 1972[15]
Dog	Flury low egg passage	Street virus	Intramuscular	Arko et al, 1973[3]
Dog	Unimmunized	Dog isolate	Intramuscular	Fekadu and Baer, 1980[41]
Bat	Unimmunized	Bat isolate	Subcutaneous	Pawan, 1936[125]
Bat	Unimmunized	Bat isolate	Intracerebral	Constantine, 1967[36]
Pig	Unimmunized	Skunk	Natural exposure	Baer and Olson, 1972[8]
Guinea pig	Unimmunized	Dog isolate	Intramuscular	Bolin, 1959[17]
Donkey	Unimmunized	Donkey isolate	Intramuscular	Ferris et al, 1968[59]
Rat	Unimmunized	Skunk isolate	Intramuscular	Kitselman, 1964[96]
Mouse	Unimmunized	Fox, skunk, bat, and dog isolate	Intraperitoneal	Bell, 1964[12]
Mouse	Unimmunized	Bat isolate	Intraperitoneal	Lodmell et al, 1969[105]
Mouse	Flury high egg passage (intracerebral)	CVS and vampire bat isolate	Subcutaneous	Wiktor et al, 1972[170]
Mouse	Unimmunized	CVS ts 2	Subcutaneous	Iwasaki et al, 1977[81]
Mouse	Unimmunized	Fox, skunk, and bobcat isolates	Subcutaneous	Baer et al, 1977[7]
Mouse	Unimmunized	ERA/BHK	Subcutaneous	Smith, 1981[141]
Mouse	Unimmunized	Fox isolate	Subcutaneous	Jackson et al, 1989[88]

CVS, challenge virus standard.
Modified from Jackson AC, Reimer DL, Ludwin SK. Spontaneous recovery from the encephalitis in mice caused by street rabies virus. Neuropathol Appl Neurobiol 1989;15:459–475, with permission.

public health significance in countries where dog rabies is endemic.

SUMMARY

Rabies is a normally fatal viral infection of the nervous system in humans and animals with characteristic clinical manifestations. Considerable progress has been made in understanding the pathogenesis of rabies. Rabies virus is highly neurotropic. It binds to the nicotinic ACH receptor at the neuromuscular junction, and it spreads by an axonal transport mechanism in peripheral nerves and within the CNS, causing widespread infection of neurons. The combination of virus-induced behavioral changes in rabies vectors and centrifugal spread of the virus to salivary glands allows efficient transmission of the infection.

An understanding of the basis of rabies virus neurovirulence is emerging from studies on variants using a variety of animal models. A single amino acid change in the rabies virus glycoprotein has dramatic effects on the outcome of infection, including the efficiency and pathways of viral spread and cellular tropisms.

The events at the site of viral entry during the long incubation period of rabies remain poorly understood. The fundamental basis for neuronal dysfunction in rabies has not yet been determined, although defective neurotransmission and neurotoxicity caused by the induction of nitric oxide are current hypotheses. A better understanding of rabies pathogenesis may lead to advances in the treatment of rabies and other viral diseases.

ABBREVIATIONS

5-HT: serotonin
ACH: acetylcholine
CNS: central nervous system
CSF: cerebrospinal fluid
CVS: challenge virus standard (strain of rabies virus)
IgA, IgG, IgM: immunoglobulins
iNOS: inducible nitric oxide synthase
MAR: avirulent variant(s) of CVS rabies strain
NOS: nitric oxide synthase
PCR: polymerase chain reaction
QNB: quinuclidinyl benzylate
RVA: rabies virus antigen
SNAP: S-nitroso-L-acetyl penicillamine

REFERENCES

1. Anderson LJ, Nicholson KG, Tauxe RV, Winkler WG. Human rabies in the United States, 1960 to 1979: epidemiology, diagnosis, and prevention. Ann Intern Med 1984;100:728–735.
2. Araujo MDF, de Brito T, Machado CG. Myocarditis in human rabies. Rev Inst Med Trop Sao Paulo 1971;13:99–102.
3. Arko RJ, Schneider LG, Baer GM. Nonfatal canine rabies. Am J Vet Res 1973;34:937–938.
4. Babes V. Sur certains caracteres des lesions histologiques de la rage. Annales de L'Institut Pasteur 1892;6:209–223.
5. Baer GM. The natural history of rabies. 2nd ed. Boca Raton, Florida: CRC Press, 1991.
6. Baer GM, Bellini WJ, Fishbein DB. Rhabdoviruses. In: Fields BN, Knipe DM, eds. Virology. 2nd ed. Vol. 1. New York: Raven Press, 1990;883–930.
7. Baer GM, Cleary WF, Diaz AM, Perl DF. Characteristics of 11 rabies virus isolates in mice: titers and relative invasiveness of virus, incubation period of infection, and survival of mice with sequelae. J Infect Dis 1977;136:336–345.
8. Baer GM, Olson HR. Recovery of pigs from rabies. J Am Vet Med Assoc 1972;160:1127–1128.
9. Baer GM, Shaddock JH, Quirion R, Dam TV, Lentz TL. Rabies susceptibility and acetylcholine receptor. Lancet 1990;335:664–665. Letter.
10. Baer GM, Shanthaveerappa TR, Bourne GH. Studies on the pathogenesis of fixed rabies virus in rats. Bull World Health Org 1965;33:783–794.
11. Bedford PGC. Diagnosis of rabies in animals. Vet Rec 1976;99:160–162.
12. Bell JF. Abortive rabies infection. I. Experimental production in white mice and general discussion. J Infect Dis 1964;114:249–257.
13. Bell JF. Latency and abortive rabies. In: Baer GM, ed. The natural history of rabies. New York: Academic Press, 1975:331–354.
14. Bell JF, Lodmell DL, Moore GJ, Raymond GH. Brain neutralization of rabies virus to distinguish recovered animals from previously vaccinated animals. J Immunol 1966;97:747–753.
15. Bell JF, Sancho MI, Diaz AM, Moore GJ. Nonfatal rabies in an enzootic area: results of a survey and evaluation of techniques. Am J Epidemiol 1972;95:190–198.
16. Bisseru B. Rabies. London: William Heinemann Medical Books, 1972.
17. Bolin VS. Survival of a guinea pig following infection with street rabies virus: a case report. J Am Vet Med Assoc 1959;134:90–92.
18. Bourhy H, Kissi B, Lafon M, Sacramento D, Tordo N. Antigenic and molecular characterization of bat rabies virus in Europe. J Clin Microbiol 1992;30:2419–2426.
19. Bouzamondo E, Ladogana A, Tsiang H. Alteration of potassium-evoked 5-HT release from virus-infected rat cortical synaptosomes. Neuroreport 1993;4:555–558.
20. Bredt DS, Hwang PM, Glatt CE, Lowenstein C, Reed RR, Snyder SH. Cloned and expressed nitric oxide synthase structurally resembles cytochrome P-450 reductase. Nature 1991;351:714–718.
21. Brown F. The family Rhabdoviridae: general description and taxonomy. In: Wagner RR, ed. The rhabdoviruses. New York: Plenum Press, 1987:1–8.
22. Brownstein MJ. Serotonin, histamine, and the purines. In: Siegel GJ, Albers RW, Agranoff BW, Katzman R, eds. Basic neurochemistry. 3rd ed. Boston: Little, Brown and Company, 1981:219–231.
23. Bryceson ADM, Greenwood BM, Warrell DA, et al. Demonstration during life of rabies antigen in humans. J Infect Dis 1975;131:71–74.
24. Carbone KM, Duchala CS, Griffin JW, Kincaid AL, Narayan O. Pathogenesis of Borna disease in rats: evidence that intra-axonal spread is the major route for virus dissemination and the determinant for disease incubation. J Virol 1987;61:3431—3440.
25. Ceccaldi P, Ermine A, Tsiang H. Continuous delivery of colchicine in the rat brain with osmotic pumps for inhibition of rabies virus transport. J Virol Methods 1990;28:79–84.
26. Ceccaldi P, Fillion M, Ermine A, Tsiang H, Fillion G. Rabies virus selectively alters 5-HT$_1$ receptor subtypes in rat brain. Eur J Pharmacol 1993;245:129–138.
27. Ceccaldi PE, Gillet JP, Tsiang H. Inhibition of the transport of rabies virus in the central nervous system. J Neuropathol Exp Neurol 1989;48:620–630.
28. Celis E, Ou D, Dietzschold B, Koprowski H. Recognition of rabies and rabies-related viruses by T cells derived from human vaccine recipients. J Virol 1988;62:3128–3134.
29. Charlton KM, Casey GA. Experimental rabies in skunks: immunofluorescence light and electron microscopic studies. Lab Invest 1979;41:36–44.
30. Charlton KM, Casey GA. Experimental rabies in skunks: persistence of virus in denervated muscle at the inoculation site. Can J Comp Med 1981;45:357–362.
31. Charlton KM, Casey GA, Campbell JB. Experimental rabies in skunks: mechanisms of infection of the salivary glands. Can J Comp Med 1983;47:363–369.

32. Cheetham HD, Hart J, Coghill NF, Fox B. Rabies with myocarditis: two cases in England. Lancet 1970;1:921–922.

33. Chopra JS, Banerjee AK, Murthy JMK, Pal SR. Paralytic rabies: a clinico-pathological study. Brain 1980;103:789–802.

34. Constantine DG. Rabies transmission by nonbite route. Public Health Rep 1962;77:287–289.

35. Constantine DG. Transmission experiments with bat rabies isolates: responses of certain Carnivora to rabies virus isolated from animals infected by nonbite route. Am J Vet Res 1966;27:13–15.

36. Constantine DG. Bat rabies in the southwestern United States. Public Health Rep 1967;82:867–888.

37. Coulon P, Derbin C, Kucera P, Lafay F, Prehaud C, Flamand A. Invasion of the peripheral nervous systems of adult mice by the CVS strain of rabies virus and its avirulent derivative Av01. J Virol 1989;63:3550–3554.

38. Coulon P, Rollin P, Aubert M, Flamand A. Molecular basis of rabies virus virulence. I. Selection of avirulent mutants of the CVS strain with anti-G monoclonal antibodies. J Gen Virol 1982;61:97–100.

39. Croen KD. Evidence for an antiviral effect of nitric oxide: inhibition of herpes simplex virus type 1 replication. J Clin Invest 1993;91:2446–2452.

40. Dawson VL, Dawson TM, Uhl GR, Snyder SH. Human immunodeficiency virus type 1 coat protein neurotoxicity mediated by nitric oxide in primary cortical cultures. Proc Natl Acad Sci U S A 1993;90:3256–3259.

41. Dean DJ, Evans WM, McClure RC. Pathogenesis of rabies. Bull World Health Org 1963;29:803–811.

42. Debbie JG, Trimarchi CV. Pantropism of rabies virus in free-ranging rabid red fox Vulpes fulva. J Wildl Dis 1970;6:500–506.

43. Dierks RE. Electron microscopy of extraneural rabies infection. In: Baer GM, ed. The natural history of rabies. New York: Academic Press, 1975:303–318.

44. Dietzschold B, Gore M, Ertl H, Celis E, Otvos L, Koprowski H. Analysis of protective immune mechanisms induced by rabies nucleoprotein. In: Kolakofsky D, Mahy BWJ, eds. Genetics and pathogenicity of negative strand viruses. Amsterdam: Elsevier, 1989:295–305.

45. Dietzschold B, Kao M, Zheng YM, et al. Delineation of putative mechanisms involved in antibody-mediated clearance of rabies virus from the central nervous system. Proc Natl Acad Sci U S A 1992;89:7252–7256.

46. Dietzschold B, Wang H, Rupprecht CE, et al. Induction of protective immunity against rabies by immunization with rabies virus ribonucleoprotein. Proc Natl Acad Sci U S A 1987;84:9165–9169.

47. Dietzschold B, Wiktor TJ, Trojanowski JQ, et al. Differences in cell-to-cell spread of pathogenic and apathogenic rabies virus in vivo and in vitro. J Virol 1985;56:12–18.

48. Dietzschold B, Wunner WH, Wiktor TJ, et al. Characterization of an antigenic determinant of the glycoprotein that correlates with pathogenicity of rabies virus. Proc Natl Acad Sci U S A 1983;80:70–74.

49. DiVestea A, Zagari G. Sur la transmission de la rage par voie nerveuse. Ann Inst Pasteur (Paris) 1889;3:237–248.

50. Dumb rabies. Lancet 1978;2:1031–1032. Editorial.

51. Dupont JR, Earle KM. Human rabies encephalitis: a study of forty-nine fatal cases with a review of the literature. Neurology 1965;15:1023–1034.

52. Emmelin N. Nervous control of salivary glands. In: Code CF, ed. Handbook of physiology. Vol 2, Sec 6. Washington, DC: American Physiological Society, 1967:595–632.

53. Ermine A, Flamand A. RNA syntheses in BHK$_{21}$ cells infected by rabies virus. Ann Microbiol 1977;128:477–488.

54. Familusi JB, Osunkoya BO, Moore DL, Kemp GE, Fabiyi A. A fatal human infection with Mokola virus. Am J Trop Med Hyg 1972;21:959–963.

55. Fekadu M. Atypical rabies in dogs in Ethiopia. Ethiop Med J 1972;10:79–86.

56. Fekadu M. Latency and aborted rabies. In: Baer GM, ed. The natural history of rabies. 2nd ed. Boca Raton, Florida: CRC Press, 1991:191–198.

57. Fekadu M, Baer GM. Recovery from clinical rabies of 2 dogs inoculated with a rabies virus strain from Ethiopia. Am J Vet Res 1980;41:1632–1634.

58. Fekadu M, Shaddock JH, Baer GM. Intermittent excretion of rabies virus in the saliva of a dog two and six months after it had recovered from experimental rabies. Am J Trop Med Hyg 1981;30:1113–1115.

59. Ferris DH, Badiali L, Abou-Youssef M, Beamer PD. A note on experimental rabies in the donkey. Cornell Vet 1968;58:270–277.

60. Fishbein DB. Rabies in humans. In: Baer GM, ed. The natural history of rabies. 2nd ed. Boca Raton, Florida: CRC Press, 1991:519–549.

61. Flamand A, Coulon P, Pepin M, Blancou J, Rollin P, Portnoi D. Immunogenic and protective power of avirulent mutants of rabies virus selected with neutralizing monoclonal antibodies. In: Chanock RM, Lerner RA, eds. Modern approaches to vaccines: molecular and chemical basis of virus virulence and immunogenicity. Cold Spring Harbor, New York: Cold Spring Harbor Laboratory, 1984:289–294.

62. Fleming G. Rabies and hydrophobia: their history, nature, causes, symptoms, and prevention. London: Chapman & Hall, 1872:7–68.

63. Fracastoro G; Cave WC, trans. Rabies. In: Hieronymi Fracastorii. De contagione et contagiosis morbis et eorum curatione. Libri III. New York: Putnam, 1930:124–133.

64. Galian A, Guerin JM, Lamotte M, et al. Human-to-human transmission of rabies via a corneal transplant–France. MMWR Morb Mortal Wkly Rep 1980;29:25–26.

65. Gillespie JH, Timoney JF. The rhabdoviridae. In: Gillespie, Timoney, eds. Hagan and Bruner's infectious diseases of domestic animals. 7th ed. Ithaca: Cornell University Press, 1981:758–780.

66. Gillet JP, Derer P, Tsiang H. Axonal transport of rabies virus in the central nervous system of the rat. J Neuropathol Exp Neurol 1986;45:619–634.

67. Goldwasser RA, Kissling RE. Fluorescent antibody staining of street and fixed rabies virus antigens. Proc Soc Exp Biol Med 1958;98:219–223.

68. Gonzalez-Angulo A, Marquez-Monter H, Feria-Velasco A, Zavala BJ. The ultrastructure of Negri bodies in Purkinje neurons in human rabies. Neurology 1970;20:323–328.

69. Gourmelon P, Briet D, Clarencon D, Court L, Tsiang H. Sleep alterations in experimental street rabies virus infection occur in the absence of major EEG abnormalities. Brain Res 1991;554:159–165.

70. Gourmelon P, Briet D, Court L, Tsiang H. Electrophysiological and sleep alterations in experimental mouse rabies. Brain Res 1986;398:128–140.

71. Hanham CA, Zhao F, Tignor GH. Evidence from the anti-idiotypic network that the acetylcholine receptor is a rabies virus receptor. J Virol 1993;67:530–542.

72. Harmon MW, Janis B. Effects of cytosine arabinoside, adenine arabinoside, and G-azauridine on rabies virus in vitro and in vivo. J Infect Dis 1976;133:7–13.

73. Hattwick MAW. Human rabies. Public Health Rev 1974;3:229–274.

74. Hattwick MAW, Weis TT, Stechschulte CJ, Baer GM, Gregg MB. Recovery from rabies: a case report. Ann Intern Med 1972;76:931–942.

75. Hemachudha T, Panpanich T, Phanuphak P, Manatsathit S, Wilde H. Immune activation in human rabies. Trans R Soc Trop Med Hyg 1993;87:106–108.

76. Hemachudha T, Phanthumchinda K, Phanuphak P, Manutsathit S. Myoedema as a clinical sign in paralytic rabies. Lancet 1987;1:1210. Letter.

77. Hemachudha T, Phanuphak P, Sriwanthana B, et al. Immunologic study of human encephalitic and paralytic rabies: preliminary report of 16 patients. Am J Med 1988;84:673–677.

78. Herzog E. Histologic diagnosis of rabies. Arch Pathol 1965;39:279–280.

79. Houff SA, Burton RC, Wilson RW, et al. Human-to-human transmission of rabies virus by corneal transplant. N Engl J Med 1979;300:603–604.

80. Iwasaki Y, Clark HF. Cell to cell transmission of virus in the central nervous system. II. Experimental rabies in mouse. Lab Invest 1975;33:391–399.

81. Iwasaki Y, Gerhard W, Clark HF. Role of host immune response in the development of either encephalitic or paralytic disease after experimental rabies infection in mice. Infect Immun 1977;18:220–225.

82. Iwasaki Y, Liu DS, Yamamoto T, Konno H. On the replication and spread of rabies virus in the human central nervous system. J Neuropathol Exp Neurol 1985;44:185–195.

83. Jackson AC. Analysis of viral neurovirulence. In: Brosius J, Fremeau RT, eds. Molecular genetic approaches to neuropsychiatric diseases. San Diego: Academic Press, 1991:259–277.

84. Jackson AC. Biological basis of rabies virus neurovirulence in mice: comparative pathogenesis study using the immunoperoxidase technique. J Virol 1991;65:537–540.

85. Jackson AC. Cholinergic system in experimental rabies in mice. Acta Virol 1993;37:502–508.

86. Jackson AC. Animal models of rabies virus neurovirulence. In: Rupprecht CE, Dietzschold B, Koprowski H, eds. Curr Top Microbiol Immunol 1994;187:85–93.

87. Jackson AC, Reimer DL. Pathogenesis of experimental rabies in mice: an immunohistochemical study. Acta Neuropathol (Berl) 1989;78:159–165.

88. Jackson AC, Reimer DL, Ludwin SK. Spontaneous recovery from the encephalomyelitis in mice caused by street rabies virus. Neuropathol Appl Neurobiol 1989;15:459–475.

89. Jackson AC, Wunner WH. Detection of rabies virus genomic RNA and mRNA in mouse and human brains by using in situ hybridization. J Virol 1991;65:2839–2844.

90. Johnson HN. Derriengue: Vampire bat rabies in Mexico. Am J Hyg 1948;47:189–204.

91. Johnson RT. Experimental rabies: studies of cellular vulnerability and pathogenesis using fluorescent antibody staining. J Neuropathol Exp Neurol 1965;24:662–674.

92. Jouvet M. The role of monoaminergic neurons in the regulation and function of sleep. In: Petre-Quadens O, Schlag JD, eds. Basic sleep mechanisms. New York: Academic Press, 1974:207–236.

93. Kaplan, C, Turner GS, Warrell DA. Rabies: the facts. 2nd ed. Oxford: Oxford University Press, 1986.

94. Kaplan MM, Wiktor TJ, Koprowski H. Pathogenesis of rabies in immunodeficient mice. J Immunol 1975;114:1761–1765.

95. Karupiah G, Xie Q, Buller ML, Nathan C, Duarte C, MacMicking JD. Inhibition of viral replication by interferon-gamma–induced nitric oxide synthase. Science 1993;261:1445–1448.

96. Kitselman CH. Recovery of a rat from experimentally induced rabies. J Am Vet Med Assoc 1964;144:1113–1114.

97. Koch FJ, Sagartz JW, Davidson DE, Lawhaswasdi K. Diagnosis of human rabies by the cornea test. Am J Clin Pathol 1975;63:509–515.

98. Koprowski H, Zheng YM, Heber-Katz E, et al. In vivo expression of inducible nitric oxide synthase in experimentally induced neurologic diseases. Proc Natl Acad Sci U S A 1993;90:3024–3027.

99. Kucera P, Dolivo M, Coulon P, Flamand A. Pathways of the early propagation of virulent and avirulent rabies strains from the eye to the brain. J Virol 1985;55:158–162.

100. Lafay F, Coulon P, Astic L, et al. Spread of the CVS strain of rabies virus and of the avirulent mutant AvO1 along the olfactory pathways of the mouse after intranasal inoculation. Virology 1991;183:320–330.

101. Lapi A, Davis CL, Anderson WA. The gasserian ganglion in animals dead of rabies. J Am Vet Med Assoc 1952;120:379–384.

102. Lentz TL. Rabies virus receptors. Trends Neurosci 1985;8:360–364.

103. Lentz TL, Burrage TG, Smith AL, Crick J, Tignor GH. Is the acetylcholine receptor a rabies virus receptor? Science 1982;215:182–184.

104. Lentz TL, Wilson PT, Hawrot E, Speicher DW. Amino acid sequence similarity between rabies virus glycoprotein and snake venom curaremimetic neurotoxins. Science 1984;226:847–848.

105. Lodmell DL, Bell JF, Moore GJ, Raymond GH. Comparative study of abortive and nonabortive rabies in mice. J Infect Dis 1969;119:569–580.

106. Lowenstein CJ, Dinerman JL, Snyder SH. Nitric oxide: a physiologic messenger. Ann Intern Med 1994;120:227–237.

107. Macfarlan RI, Dietzschold B, Koprowski H. Stimulation of cytotoxic T-lymphocyte responses by rabies virus glycoprotein and identification of an immunodominant domain. Mol Immunol 1986;23:733–741.

108. Macfarlan RI, Dietzschold B, Wiktor TJ, et al. T cell responses to cleaved rabies virus glycoprotein and to synthetic peptides. J Immunol 1984;133:2748–2752.

109. Madore HP, England JM. Rabies virus protein synthesis in infected BHK-21 cells. J Virol 1977;22:102–112.

110. Meredith C, Rossouw AP, Van Praag Koch H. An unusual case of human rabies thought to be of chiropteran origin. S Afr Med J 1971;45:767–769.

111. Merigan TC, Baer GM, Winkler WG, et al. Human leukocyte interferon administration to patients with symptomatic and suspected rabies. Ann Neurol 1984;16:82–87.

112. Miller A, Morse HC, Winkelstein J, Nathanson N. The role of antibody in recovery from experimental rabies. I. Effect of depletion of B and T cells. J Immunol 1978;121:321–326.

113. Mims CA. Intracerebral injections and the growth of viruses in the mouse brain. Br J Exp Pathol 1960;41:52–59.

114. Morgagni JB, Alexander B. Wherein madness, melancholy, and hydrophobia, are treated of. In: The seats and causes of diseases investigated by anatomy. Vol. 1. New York: Hafner Publishing, 1960: 144–187.

115. Murphy FA, Bauer SP. Early street rabies virus infection in striated muscle and later progression to the central nervous system. Intervirology 1974;3:256–268.

116. Murphy FA, Bauer SP, Harrison AK, Winn WC. Comparative pathogenesis of rabies and rabies-like viruses: viral infection and transit from inoculation site to the central nervous system. Lab Invest 1973;28:361–376.

117. Murphy FA, Harrison AK, Winn WC, Bauer SP. Comparative pathogenesis of rabies and rabies-like viruses: infection of the central nervous system and centrifugal spread of virus to peripheral tissues. Lab Invest 1973;29:1–16.

118. Nathan C. Nitric oxide as a secretory product of mammalian cells. FASEB J 1992;6:3051–3064.

119. Nathan CF, Hibbs JB. Role of nitric oxide synthesis in macrophage antimicrobial activity. Curr Opin Immunol 1991;3:65–70.

120. Nathanson N, Gonzalez-Scarano F. Immune response to rabies virus. In: Baer GM, ed. The natural history of rabies. 2nd ed. Boca Raton, Florida: CRC Press, 1991:145–161.

121. Negri A. Beitrag zum Studium der Aetiologie der Tollwuth. Z Hyg Infektionskr 1903;43:507–528.

122. Pasteur L. Méthode pour prévenir la rage après morsure. C R Acad Sci III 1885;101:765–774.

123. Pasteur L, Chamberland M, Roux M. Physiologie experimentale: Nouvelle communication sur la rage. C R Acad Sci III 1884;98: 457–463.

124. Pasteur L, Chamberland M, Roux M, Thuillier M. Nouveaux faits pour servir à la connaissance de la rage. C R Acad Sci III 1882;95: 1187–1192.

125. Pawan JL. Rabies in the vampire bat of Trinidad, with special reference to the clinical course and the latency of infection. Ann Trop Med Parasitol 1936;30:401–422.

126. Pereira CA, Nozaki-Renard JN, Schwartz J, Eyquem A, Atanasiu P. Cytotoxicity reactions against target cells infected with rabies virus. J Virol Methods 1982;5:75–83.

127. Perl DP, Good PF. The pathology of rabies in the central nervous system. In: Baer GM, ed. The natural history of rabies. 2nd ed. Boca Raton, Florida: CRC Press, 1991:163–190.

128. Porras C, Barboza JJ, Fuenzalida E, Adaros HL, Oviedo de Diaz AM, Furst J. Recovery from rabies in man. Ann Intern Med 1976; 85:44–48.

129. Prabhakar BS, Fischman HR, Nathanson N. Recovery from experimental rabies by adoptive transfer of immune cells. J Gen Virol 1981;56:25–31.

130. Prabhakar BS, Nathanson N. Acute rabies death mediated by antibody. Nature 1981;290:590–591.

131. Reagan KJ, Wunner WH. Rabies virus interaction with various cell lines is independent of the acetylcholine receptor: brief report. Arch Virol 1985;84:277–282.

132. Remlinger P, Effendi M. Deux cas de guérison de la rage expérimentale chez le chien. Ann Inst Pasteur (Paris) 1904;18:241–245.

133. Roine RO, Hillbom M, Valle M, et al. Fatal encephalitis caused by a bat-borne rabies-related virus: clinical findings. Brain 1988;111: 1505–1516.

134. Rosenthal HE. A graphic method for the determination and presentation of binding parameters in a complex system. Anal Biochem 1967;20:525–532.

135. Rosner F. Rabies in the Talmud. Med Hist 1974;18:198–200.

136. Ross E, Armentrout SA. Myocarditis associated with rabies: report of a case. N Engl J Med 1962;266:1087–1089.

137. Seif I, Coulon P, Rollin PE, Flamand A. Rabies virulence: effect on pathogenicity and sequence characterization of rabies virus mutations affecting antigenic site III of the glycoprotein. J Virol 1985;53: 926–935.

138. Shankar V, Dietzschold B, Koprowski H. Direct entry of rabies virus into the central nervous system without prior local replication. J Virol 1991;65:2736–2738.

139. Shope RE. Rabies-like viruses. In: Webster RG, Granoff A, eds. Encyclopedia of virology. San Diego: Academic Press, 1994:1186–1190.

140. Smart NL, Charlton KM. The distribution of challenge virus standard rabies virus versus skunk street rabies virus in the brains of experimentally infected rabid skunks. Acta Neuropathol 1992;84:501–508.

141. Smith JS. Mouse model for abortive rabies infection of the central nervous system. Infect Immun 1981;31:297–308.

142. Smith JS. Rabies virus epitopic variation: use in ecologic studies. Adv Virus Res 1989;36:215–253.

143. Smith JS, Fishbein DB, Rupprecht CE, Clark K. Unexplained rabies in three immigrants in the United States: a virologic investigation. N Engl J Med 1991;324:205–211.

144. Smith JS, McClelland CL, Reid FL, Baer GM. Dual role of the immune response in street rabiesvirus infection of mice. Infect Immun 1982;35:213–221.

145. Smith JS, Orciari LA, Yager PA, Seidel HD, Warner CK. Epidemiologic and historical relationships among 87 rabies virus isolates as determined by limited sequence analysis. J Infect Dis 1992;166: 296–307.

146. Steele JH, Fernandez PJ. History of rabies and global aspects. In: Baer GM, ed. The natural history of rabies. 2nd ed. Boca Raton, Florida: CRC Press, 1991:1–24.

147. Thongcharoen P, Wasi C, Sirikavin S, et al. Human-to-human transmission of rabies via corneal transplant–Thailand. MMWR Morb Mortal Wkly Rep 1981;30:473–474.

148. Tillotson JR, Axelrod D, Lyman DO. Rabies in a laboratory worker–New York. MMWR Morb Mortal Wkly Rep 1977;26:183-184.

149. Tillotson JR, Axelrod D, Lyman DO. Follow-up on rabies–New York. MMWR Morb Mortal Wkly Rep 1977;26:249–250.

150. Tirawatnpong S, Hemachudha T, Manutsathit S, Shuangshoti S, Phanthumchinda K, Phanuphak P. Regional distribution of rabies viral antigen in central nervous system of human encephalitic and paralytic rabies. J Neurol Sci 1989;92:91–99.

151. Tordo N, Poch O. Structure of rabies virus. In: Campbell JB, Charlton KM, eds. Rabies. Boston: Kluwer Academic Publishers, 1988: 25–45.

152. Torres-Anjel MJ, Montano-Hirose J, Cazabon EPI, et al. A new approach to the pathobiology of rabies virus as aided by immunoperoxidase staining. Am J Assoc Vet Lab Diagn 1984;27:1–26.

153. Tsiang H. Evidence for an intraaxonal transport of fixed and street rabies virus. J Neuropathol Exp Neurol 1979;38:286–296.

154. Tsiang H. Neuronal function impairment in rabies-infected rat brain. J Gen Virol 1982;61:277–281.

155. Tsiang H, Ceccaldi PE, Lycke E. Rabies virus infection and transport in human sensory dorsal root ganglia neurons. J Gen Virol 1991;72:1191–1194.

156. Tsiang H, de la Porte S, Ambroise DJ, Derer M, Koenig J. Infection of cultured rat myotubes and neurons from the spinal cord by rabies virus. J Neuropathol Exp Neurol 1986;45:28–42.

157. Tsiang H, Lycke E, Ceccaldi P, Ermine A, Hirardot X. The anterograde transport of rabies virus in rat sensory dorsal root ganglia neurons. J Gen Virol 1989;70:2075–2085.

158. Tuffereau C, Leblois H, Benejean J, Coulon P, Lafay F, Flamand A. Arginine or lysine in position 333 of ERA and CVS glycoprotein is necessary for rabies virulence in adult mice. Virology 1989;172: 206–212.

159. Tuffereau C, Martinet-Edelist C. Shut-off of cellular RNA after infection with rabies virus. C R Acad Sci III 1985;300:597–600.

160. Turner GS. Immune response after rabies vaccination: basic aspects. Ann Inst Pasteur/Virol 1985;136E:453–460.

161. Warrell DA. The clinical picture of rabies in man. Trans R Soc Trop Med Hyg 1976;70:188–195.

162. Warrell DA, Davidson NM, Pope HM, et al. Pathophysiologic studies in human rabies. Am J Med 1976;60:180–190.

163. Warrell MJ, Looareesuwan S, Manatsathit S, et al. Rapid diagnosis of rabies and post-vaccinal encephalitides. Clin Exp Immunol 1988; 71:229–234.

164. Warrell MJ, White NJ, Looareesuwan S, et al. Failure of interferon alfa and tribavirin in rabies encephalitis. Br Med J 1989;299:830–833.

165. Webster LT. Rabies. New York: Macmillan, 1942:3–8.

166. Wiktor TJ. Cell-mediated immunity and postexposure protection from rabies by inactivated vaccines of tissue culture origin. Dev Biol Stand 1978;40:255–264.

167. Wiktor TJ, Doherty PC, Koprowski H. In vitro evidence of cell-mediated immunity after exposure of mice to both live and inactivated rabies virus. Proc Natl Acad Sci U S A 1977;74:334–338.

168. Wiktor TJ, Doherty PC, Koprowski H. Suppression of cell-mediated immunity by street rabies virus. J Exp Med 1977;145:1617–1622.

169. Wiktor TJ, Kamo I, Koprowski H. In vitro stimulation of rabbit lymphocytes after immunization with live and inactivated rabies vaccines. J Immunol 1974;112:2013–2019.

170. Wiktor TJ, Koprowski H, Rorke LB. Localized rabies infection in mice. Proc Soc Exp Biol Med 1972;140:759–764.

171. Wiktor TJ, Kuwert E, Koprowski H. Immune lysis of rabies virus-infected cells. J Immunol 1968;101:1271–1282.

172. Wilkinson L. The development of the virus concept as reflected in corpora of studies on individual pathogens: rabies–two millennia of ideas and conjecture on the aetiology of a virus disease. Med Hist 1977;21:15–31.

173. Wilkinson L. Understanding the nature of rabies: an historical perspective. In: Campbell JB, Charlton KM, eds. Rabies. Boston: Kluwer Academic Publishers, 1988:1–23.

174. Winkler WG, Fashinell TR, Leffingwell L, Howard P, Conomy JP. Airborne rabies transmission in a laboratory worker. JAMA 1973;226:1219–1221.

175. Wunner WH. The chemical composition and molecular structure of rabies viruses. In: Baer GM, ed. The natural history of rabies. 2nd ed. Boca Raton, Florida: CRC Press, 1991:31–67.

176. Wunner WH, Larson JK, Dietzschold B, Smith CL. The molecular biology of rabies viruses. Rev Infect Dis 1988;10(Suppl 4):S771–S784.

177. Xiang ZQ, Spitalnik S, Tran M, Wunner WH, Cheng J, Ertl HCJ. Vaccination with a plasmid vector carrying the rabies virus glycoprotein gene induces protective immunity against rabies virus. Virology 1994;199:132–140.

178. Xie Q, Cho HJ, Calaycay J, et al. Cloning and characterization of inducible nitric oxide synthase from mouse macrophages. Science 1992;256:225–228.

179. Yang C, Jackson AC. Basis of neurovirulence of avirulent rabies virus variant Av01 with stereotaxic brain inoculation in mice. J Gen Virol 1992;73:895–900.

180. Zheng YM, Schafer MK, Weihe E, et al. Severity of neurological signs and degree of inflammatory lesions in the brains of rats with Borna disease correlate with the induction of nitric oxide synthase. J Virol 1993;67:5786–5791.

181. Zinke GG. Neue Ansichten der Hundswuth; ihrer Ursachen und Folgen, nebst einer sichern Behandlungsart der von tollen Thieren gebissenen Menschen. Jena, Germany: Gabler, 1804.

Viral Pathogenesis,
edited by Neal Nathanson, et al.
Lippincott–Raven Publishers, Philadelphia © 1997

CHAPTER **25**

Lymphocytic Choriomeningitis Virus

Persephone Borrow and Michael B. A. Oldstone

INTRODUCTION

Lymphocytic choriomeningitis virus (LCMV) infection of
its natural host, the mouse, has proved to be one of the most
valuable model systems in the field of viral pathogenesis. A
remarkable number of key concepts in contemporary immunology and virology were first defined in studies using this
virus, including basic immunologic phenomena such as major
histocompatibility complex (MHC) restriction of T-cell recog-

nition[323–325]; the idea that, in addition to mediating viral clearance, antiviral immune responses may be instrumental in producing much of the tissue injury associated with acute and
persistent viral infections[65,100,101,193,203,204,247]; and the ability
of viruses to cause disease noncytopathically by interfering
with the differentiated functions of infected cells[213,214] (reviewed in Oldstone[195]).

One reason why LCMV immunobiology has been both so
interesting and so fruitful to study is that the outcome of infection of mice with this virus varies dramatically depending on
the age, immunocompetence, and genetic background of the
animals infected, the route of infection, and the strain and
dose of infecting virus (Fig. 25-1). For example, peripheral in-

P. Borrow and M. B. A. Oldstone: Department of Neuropharmacology, Division of Virology, The Scripps Research Institute,
La Jolla, California 92037.

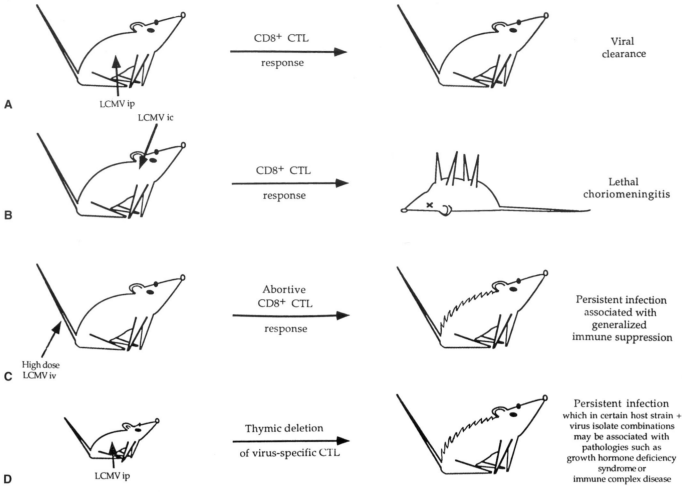

FIG. 25-1. **(A–D)** Examples of how the outcome of infection of mice with lymphocytic choriomeningitis virus (LCMV) may be different depending on the dose and strain of infecting virus, route of infection, and age and genetic background of the host. CTL, cytotoxic T lymphocyte.

oculation of adult immunocompetent mice with a moderate dose of most LCMV isolates (see Fig. 25-1A) results in induction of a protective immune response that mediates virus clearance in 10 to 14 days; clearance is predominantly mediated by virus-specific CD8+ cytotoxic T lymphocytes (CTL). Manipulation of this system has given valuable insight into the requirements for CTL induction, the specificity of CTL recognition, mechanisms involved in virus clearance, how immune memory is maintained after virus infection, and strategies by which viruses may evade clearance by the host response. However, if the route of infection and dose and strain of virus are appropriately adjusted, the antiviral immune response instead has predominantly immunopathologic consequences, resulting in lethal choriomeningitis (see Fig. 25-1B), hepatitis, or persistent infection associated with generalized immune suppression (see Fig. 25-1C). Further, if mice are infected with LCMV as neonates, thymic deletion of virus-specific CTL renders them unable to clear the infection, and a lifelong persistent infection develops (see Fig. 25-1D). Depending on the virus strain and genetic background of the animal involved, this may be associated with a variety of pathologies, including some which are directly mediated by

virus persistence in particular cell types (e.g., a growth hormone deficiency syndrome, alterations in thyroid function or behavioral abnormalities), and others that are immunopathologically mediated (e.g., immune complex disease).

This chapter attempts to provide a representative overview of the immunology and pathogenesis of this complex spectrum of virus-host interactions. It focuses on the more recent advances in the understanding of LCMV-immune system interactions, and the pathologic processes that are best understood. Further, LCMV infection of species other than its natural murine host is not discussed in any depth. The reader is referred to previous reviews[47,116,143,149,223,270] and information on LCMV infection of other species, including humans.[60,93,221,302]

OVERVIEW OF THE LYMPHOCYTIC CHORIOMENINGITIS VIRUS LIFE CYCLE

A complete understanding of the pathogenesis of any virus infection requires an amalgamation of information about the virus itself, its interaction with the host, and the host response to the virus. Unlike many other much-studied viruses, the basic virology (genetics, replication, and life cycle) of LCMV is less well understood than its in vivo interaction with its murine host. Here we will give just a brief overview of LCMV virology, highlighting those aspects of greatest importance to the discussion of LCMV-host interactions in the remainder of this chapter. For more detailed accounts, the reader is referred to reviews.[196,250,268]

Lymphocytic choriomeningitis virus is the prototypic member of the family *Arenaviridae*, which also includes human pathogens such as Lassa and Junin viruses.[221] It has lipid-enveloped virions that are somewhat pleomorphic but are typically spherical, with an average diameter of 90 to 110 nm,[52] and are covered with surface glycoprotein spikes. The virions enclose the viral nucleoprotein complexes, and frequently include host cell-derived ribosomes, which give the virus particles the "sandy" appearance from which the family name is derived. The viral genome consists of two single-stranded RNA segments of unequal length: a short (3.4 kilobase [kb]) S RNA, and a long (7.2 kb) L RNA. Each RNA segment has an ambisense coding strategy, encoding two proteins in opposite orientations, separated by an intergenic hairpin (Fig. 25-2). The S RNA encodes the approximately 75-kilodalton (kD) viral glycoprotein precursor (GP-C) at the 5′ end and the 63-kD viral nucleoprotein (NP) at the 3′ end,[240,244,245,254,271] whereas the L RNA encodes a 200-kD protein (L) that likely represents all or part of the virus-specific RNA polymerase at the 3′ end, and at the 5′ end an 11-kD protein (Z or p11) with sequence homology to zinc-binding proteins that have been implicated in transcriptional regulation in other systems.[252,253,266]

The viral glycoprotein precursor is posttranslationally processed to yield the two virion glycoproteins, GP-1 (44 kD) and GP-2 (35 kD).[319] Tetrameters of each of these proteins make up the spikes on the virion envelope. A model proposed by Burns and Buchmeier[51,52] suggests that the club-shaped head of the glycoprotein spike is made up of a homotetramer of disulfide-linked GP-1 molecules, and that this is associated by ionic interactions with a tetramer of transmembrane GP-2 molecules that form the stalk of the spike. GP-1 is the virion attachment protein that mediates interaction of LCMV with host cell surface receptors. Little is known about the latter, although the receptor for LCMV on rodent fibroblast cell lines has putatively been characterized as a 120- to 140-kD cell surface glycoprotein.[33] Whether this is the receptor used by LCMV on all cell types infected in vivo is not known. However, this protein is expressed in many tissues in the mouse (P. Borrow and M. B. A. Oldstone, 1996), and correspondingly LCMV can produce a widespread infection in vivo, as is strikingly illustrated by in situ hybridization with viral nucleic acid-specific probes on whole-body sections of mice persis-

tently infected with LCMV[31,269] (examples are shown in Fig. 25-8, later in the chapter). Within individual tissues, LCMV infects particular cell types (e.g., see Fazakerley and colleagues[91]). Receptor binding is one stage in the life cycle of viruses at which tropism for different cell types may be determined. Evidence indicates that differences in receptor binding properties between closely related isolates of LCMV are characteristics that play an important role in determining their in vivo pathogenicity, by dictating the efficiency with which they infect particular cell types in vivo. Two examples of this are discussed later in the chapter: 1) a difference in the ability of LCMV WE clones to infect growth hormone-producing cells in the anterior pituitary, which determines their ability to cause a growth hormone deficiency in neonatally infected C3H/St mice[276]; and 2) a difference in the ability of LCMV Armstrong variants to infect key antigen-presenting cell types in lymphoid tissues, which is one of the factors that determines their ability to induce a generalized immune suppression in adult mice (P. Borrow and colleagues, unpublished data).

After receptor binding, LCMV entry into host cells occurs by viropexis in large, smooth-walled vesicles[34]; an acid pH-dependent fusion event then takes place[34,73,74,102] to mediate transfer of the viral nucleoprotein complex into the cytoplasm, where viral replication takes place. The nature of the molecular events involved in viral transcription and replication is not completely understood (for a detailed discussion, the reader is referred to reviews[112,137,250,268]). It has been suggested that the ambisense coding strategy of LCMV (Fig. 25-3) allows for differential expression of the viral mRNAs. During a productive infection, NP mRNA, which can be directly transcribed from the viral genome, has been observed as early as 2 hours after infection, whereas the synthesis of GP-C mRNA cannot occur until viral RNA replication has commenced and full-length replicative intermediate viral-complementary RNA is available as a template for GP-C mRNA transcription. After processing in the Golgi (using host cell enzymes),[46,52,319] the viral envelope glycoproteins are transported to the cell surface, where virion assembly takes place. Virions bud from the cell surface, deriving their lipid envelope from the host cell plasma membrane. Virus release thus does not require cell lysis; indeed, LCMV-infected cells usually exhibit few cytopathic effects, although this is not always the case (e.g., infectious virus can be quantitated by plaque assay on Vero cells[88]).

That LCMV infection is usually noncytopathic is of great importance for virus-host interactions because it enables the virus to produce a persistent infection in vivo with high viral loads in many tissues without causing the rapid death of the host animal. How virus-host cell interactions differ during persistent versus acute infections with LCMV, and how per-

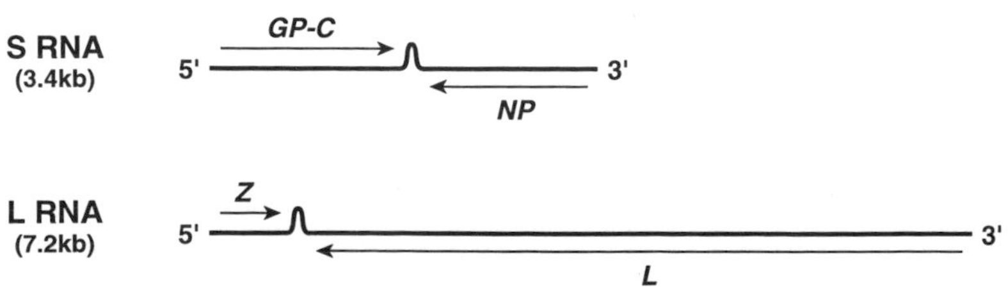

S RNA (3.4kb) 5′ —— GP-C → ⌐ ← NP —— 3′

L RNA (7.2kb) 5′ —— Z → ⌐ ← L —— 3′

FIG. 25-2. The genomic organization of lymphocytic choriomeningitis virus. GP-C, glycoprotein precursor; NP, nucleoprotein; L, putative viral polymerase; Z, zinc-binding protein.

Genome

5' ──── GP-C (+ve) ────⌒──── NP (-ve) ──── 3'

↓ transcription

NP mRNA ────

↓ translation

NP protein

↓ replication

Genome-complementary

3' ──── GP-C (-ve) ────⌒──── NP (+ve) ──── 5'

↓ transcription

──── **GP-C mRNA**

↓ translation

GP-C protein

↓ cleavage

GP-1 + GP-2 proteins   ↓ replication

Genome

5' ──── GP-C (+ve) ────⌒──── NP (-ve) ──── 3'

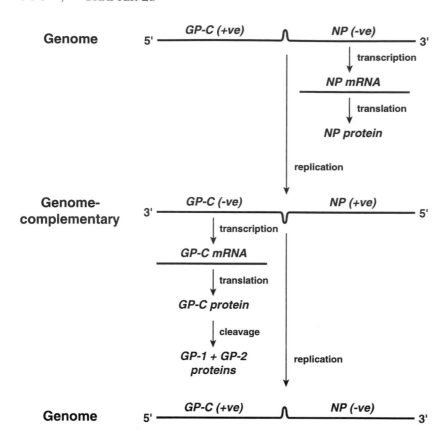

FIG. 25-3. How transcription, translation, and replication are thought to take place from the ambisense S RNA segment of lymphocytic choriomeningitis virus. A similar strategy is likely adopted for replication of the ambisense L RNA segment and production of the L and Z proteins. GP-C, glycoprotein precursor; NP, nucleoprotein.

sistent infections are established and maintained both in vitro and in vivo, are other poorly understood aspects of LCMV biology. A complex pattern of LCMV gene expression has been observed during persistent infection in vivo,[94,95] and it has been suggested that defective RNAs may be present, especially because interfering or defective interfering viruses have been described in persistent LCMV infections[121,142,231] (reviewed in Buchmeier and associates[47]). It has also been proposed that the ability of LCMV to regulate the expression of the different viral genes independently may play a part in the establishment and maintenance of persistent infection, perhaps contributing to the selective decrease in expression of the viral glycoprotein that has been observed during persistent LCMV infection[201] (reviewed in Francis and colleagues[96] and Lipkin and coworkers[161]). The latter not only may contribute to persistence at the cellular level, but may be a mechanism that enables LCMV to avoid immunologic surveillance, promoting viral persistence within the host.

A final virologic concept of key importance to the understanding of LCMV biology is that, like other RNA viruses, LCMV has a high mutation frequency, and viral variants are continually generated at high frequency during in vivo or in vitro viral replication. The virus thus exists not as a homogeneous population, but as a heterogeneous population or quasispecies (the reader is referred to a number of reviews[84,86,89,114,272]). Particular virus variants may have a growth advantage under certain conditions (e.g., within a specific host tissue), and will then be selected. For example, if mice are inoculated as neonates with the Armstrong strain of LCMV so that a widespread, lifelong, persistent infection is established, there is rapid selection within lymphoid tissues and the liver, and a slower selection in other tissues, such as

the heart, lung, and kidney, for viral variants that have a phenylalanine-to-leucine mutation at amino acid 260 in the viral glycoprotein GP-1.[90,296] LCMV Armstrong variants with this mutation have an enhanced ability to infect macrophages and related cells, such as Kupffer cells in the liver.[129,167,169] Even as long as 1 year postinfection, however, parental-type phenylalanine-possessing virus still predominates in the central nervous system (CNS), where neurons are the principal cell type infected[91,242]; phenylalanine-containing virus also predominates in the CNS of mice inoculated as neonates with a 1:10 ratio of phenylalanine:leucine-containing viruses.[77] This correlates with the ability of the parental virus to replicate more efficiently and outcompete leucine 260 variants in neuronal cell lines in vitro.[90,296] The differences in in vivo tropism and pathogenicity between LCMV Armstrong and one of its in vivo-selected variants, Armstrong-clone 13, when used to infect adult immunocompetent mice, are discussed in more detail later in the chapter.

THE IMMUNE RESPONSE TO LYMPHOCYTIC CHORIOMENINGITIS VIRUS

The Key Role Played by the Antiviral Immune Response in Lymphocytic Choriomeningitis Virus-Host Interactions

A large section of this chapter is devoted to the immune response to LCMV because the antiviral immune response plays a central part in determining the outcome of infection of mice with this virus. The immune response plays a protective role in mediating virus clearance, thus preventing the establishment of a persistent infection and its possible associated pathologic consequences; conversely, it may also mediate potentially lethal damage to the infected host. As mentioned in the introduction to this chapter, a large number of diverse host and viral factors can influence the outcome of LCMV infection of mice, making experiments carried out with different isolates of this virus often appear confusing. Most of these factors act by influencing the balance between virus replication and the host immune response, which, as diagrammed in Figure 25-4, is a pivotal determinant of the outcome of any LCMV infection.

As described in more detail later, the immune effector mechanism that plays the most dominant role in controlling LCMV replication and clearing the infection is the virus-specific CD8+ CTL response. Animals that are unable to mount a virus-specific CTL response (e.g., mice infected neonatally with LCMV) become persistently infected with the virus for life. This key host response is optimally induced when a low to moderate load of viral antigen is present in lymphoid tissues of adult immunocompetent mice, and it will then rapidly clear the infection. Immune effector mechanisms other than the CD8+ CTL response (e.g., interferons [IFNs] or antibody), even though they may not themselves be capable of mediating viral clearance, can nonetheless contribute to the outcome of infection by helping to keep the viral antigen load in lymphoid tissues within the optimal range for CTL induction. Any conditions under which virus replication is sufficiently favored to exceed the critical load of viral antigen in lymphoid tissues early after infection as the virus-specific CTL response is being induced result in "exhaustion" of antiviral CTL, and tip the balance in favor of virus persistence. Thus the dose of LCMV with which mice are initially infected and the route of inoculation are of importance, with intravenous (IV) inoculation and high virus doses favoring the rapid achievement of a high viral load in lymphoid tissues. Further, LCMV isolates that have a tropism for lymphoid tissues, a particularly rapid rate of replication, or are relatively resistant to host innate defense mechanisms such as IFN, more readily establish persistent infections in adult mice. Table 25-1 lists some of the more commonly used LCMV isolates, and compares them on the basis of these characteristics.

Although the factors shown in Figure 25-4 that tip the balance in favor of the virus promote the establishment of persistent infection, they may also protect the animal from immunopathologically mediated disease. For example, the CTL response induced in mice infected with a moderate dose of LCMV Armstrong causes a lethal choriomeningitis if the infection is initiated intracranially (IC); but mice infected IC

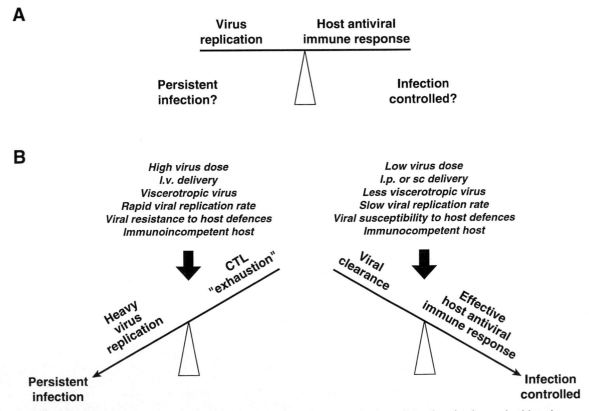

FIG. 25-4. The concept of virus-immune system balance in lymphocytic choriomeningitis virus (LCMV)-infected mice. **(A)** The balance between virus replication and the host immune response is a pivotal determinant of the outcome of any LCMV infection of mice. **(B)** Different factors may operate during acute infection of adult mice with LCMV to tip the balance in either direction. CTL, cytotoxic T lymphocyte.

TABLE 25-1. *Properties of some commonly used lymphocytic choriomeningitis virus (LCMV) isolates*

LCMV strain	Tropism for lymphohemopoietic tissues*	Interferon resistance or susceptibility†	Tendency to establish persistent infection in adult mice‡
WE docile	High	R	Greatest
Armstrong-clone 13	High	R	
Traub	High	R	
WE	Moderate	S	
WE aggressive	Moderate	S	
Armstrong	Low (neurotropic)	S	Least

*The in vivo tropism of the different LCMV isolates for visceral organs, in particular lymphatic tissues, versus the central nervous system, is indicated.[4,7,8,90,167,225,297]

†The replication of the different LCMV isolates is classified as relatively susceptible (S) or more resistant (R) to inhibition by interferon-α or -β or interferon-γ *in vivo* and *in vitro*.[176]

‡The relative ability of the different LCMV isolates to exhaust the virus-specific cytotoxic T-lymphocyte response and establish a persistent infection on intravenous inoculation into adult immunocompetent mice is shown.[8,121,177,179,180,224,225]

with an equal dose of LCMV Docile do not die of choriomeningitis.

Immune Response to Acute Lymphocytic Choriomeningitis Virus Infection

Intraperitoneal (IP) infection of adult immunocompetent mice with moderate doses of LCMV results in activation of a number of immune effector mechanisms, as a consequence of which infectious virus is cleared in 7 to 14 days (Fig. 25-5).

Interferon

Both type I (α and β) IFNs and IFN-γ are induced early after infection of mice with LCMV.[152,176] Experiments in which C57BL/6 mice were treated with antibodies that neutralize the activity of IFN-α/β or IFN-γ have shown that the role endogenous IFN production plays in controlling virus replication in vivo is LCMV strain dependent,[176] the replication of certain LCMV strains (e.g., Armstrong, Aggressive, and WE) being much more susceptible to inhibition by IFNs than that of others (e.g., Armstrong-clone 13, Docile, and Traub). Thus, treat-

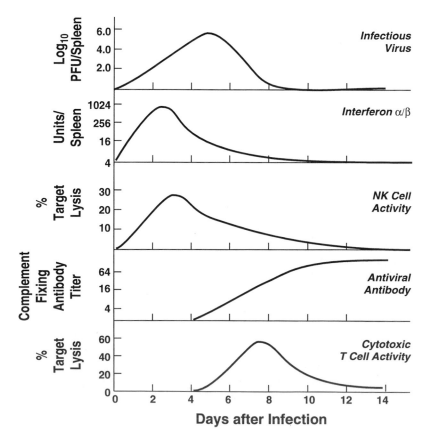

FIG. 25-5. The kinetics of several host responses elicited after intraperitoneal infection of adult mice with lymphocytic choriomeningitis virus, and the concomitant control of infectious virus. PFU, plaque-forming units; NK, natural killer. (Adapted with permission from Buchmeier MJ, Welsh RM, Dutko FJ, Oldstone MB. The virology and immunobiology of lymphocytic choriomeningitis virus infection. Adv Immunol 1980; 30:275–331.)

ment of mice with anti-IFN-γ antibody significantly enhanced the replication of the former but not the latter LCMV strains over the first 4 days postinoculation, and neutralization of IFN-α/β enhanced the replication of only the more susceptible LCMV strains early after infection, although an effect was seen with all LCMV strains by days 3 to 5 postinfection.

Although IFNs alone are unable completely to control the replication of even the most IFN-sensitive LCMV strains either in vivo or in vitro, IFN-mediated reduction of virus replication early early after infection nonetheless does make a critical contribution to the virus-immune system balance in vivo. This is demonstrated by the fact that the more IFN-resistant LCMV isolates that are able to replicate more rapidly in mice are more readily able to establish persistent infections in adult mice[176]; similarly, infection of mice treated with neutralizing antibody to IFN-α/β or IFN-γ, or of IFN-α/β- or IFN-γ-receptor knockout mice with even IFN-susceptible LCMV isolates can result in the establishment of persistent infection.[155,184,222,293,315] It appears that the enhanced virus replication that occurs in the absence of IFN-mediated control leads to "exhaustion" of LCMV-specific CD8+ CTL and thus failure to clear the infection.

Natural Killer Cells

Natural killer (NK) cells are a subpopulation of lymphocytes, activated by IFN-α/β production early after virus infection, that infiltrate infected tissues and may combat virus infections by their ability to recognize and lyse infected target cells in a nonvirus-specific, non–MHC-restricted fashion, or their ability to secrete cytokines such as IFN-γ and tumor necrosis factor-α.[304] Although NK cell activation occurs in close correlation with the generation of IFN-α/β in LCMV-infected mice,[29,30,308,309] several lines of evidence indicate that NK cells do not control LCMV replication in vivo (reviewed in Welsh[305]). For example, C57BL/6 mutant beige mice, which have markedly reduced NK cell activity, do not exhibit higher LCMV titers in the spleen than normal beige/+ littermates[306]; and depletion of NK cell activity with antibody to asialo-GM1 (a ganglioside expressed on NU cells and some other cell types) has little effect on the replication of either the Armstrong or WE strain of LCMV even during the early stages of infection.[49]

Antiviral Antibody

Antiviral antibody production occurs rapidly after infection of mice with LCMV: as reviewed in Buchmeier and coworkers,[47] antibody in the form of infectious virus-antibody complexes can be detected as early as 4 days after infection, whereas free antibody to LCMV is demonstrable by enzyme-linked immunosorbent assay or complement fixation by day 6 postinfection, and reaches peak titers in 2 to 3 weeks, which are then sustained for the life of the animal. Whereas most of the plasma cells producing virus-specific antibody are found in the spleen early (days 8 to 15) postinfection, bone marrow is the major site of long-term antibody production.[267] The rapid kinetics of antibody production after LCMV infection of mice likely results, at least in part, from the ability of virions to act as type II thymus-independent antigens and stimulate some an-

tibody production in a CD4+ T-cell–independent fashion,[36,47] although the production of high titers of antiviral IgG depends on T-cell–B-cell interaction.[3] Most of the virus-specific IgG produced after acute LCMV infection of mice is of the IgG2a isotype; this contrasts with the situation during persistent infection (discussed later), in which predominantly low-affinity IgG1 antibodies are produced.[282,287] This difference is likely the result of the cytokines present in lymphoid tissues during induction of the antiviral antibody response: the high levels of IFN-γ generated at early times after acute LCMV infection (discussed earlier) promote class switching to IgG2a.[92]

Although virus-specific antibody is produced early after acute infection of mice with LCMV, neutralizing antibodies are frequently generated only late, after 20 to 60 days.[117,143,144] The reason for this is unclear. It has been suggested that the delay before neutralizing antibodies reach detectable levels may be caused by immunopathologic destruction of the subset of B cells that produce LCMV-neutralizing antibodies by virus-specific CD8+ CTL.[26] This specific population of B cells may be targets for CTL-mediated destruction because they may be preferentially infected by LCMV. Although most B cells are not readily infected by LCMV, the surface immunoglobulin on B cells producing neutralizing antiviral antibodies may facilitate virus uptake by these cells, and hence their infection. That neutralizing antibodies are frequently not produced until after virus has already been eliminated suggests that antiviral antibodies are not of primary importance in virus clearance in mice acutely infected with LCMV. This is supported by experiments in which mice were depleted of B cells by treatment with anti-IgM antibody from birth and infected as adults with LCMV: although viral clearance was somewhat delayed, these mice were still able to eliminate the infection.[58,59,145] Further, as discussed in the following section, there is a wealth of evidence demonstrating that virus-specific CD8+ CTL are the primary mediators of protection in LCMV-infected mice.

However, although CTL are clearly sufficient to control LCMV infection of mice, antibodies do have a less well appreciated protective role, which is likely of greatest importance in resistance to reinfection. Treatment of mice with hyperimmune serum before IP infection with LCMV significantly reduced viral replication in the spleen and liver[278]; similarly, 10- and 14-day-old mice that received maternally derived anti-LCMV antibodies through nursing were protected from an otherwise lethal challenge with the Armstrong strain of LCMV.[23] Battegay and colleagues[24] showed that the way in which passively transferred neutralizing antibodies prevented lethal choriomeningitis in mice challenged IC with LCMV Armstrong was not by controlling local virus replication, but by reducing hematogenous spread and thus antigen load in lymphoid tissues. Antibodies thereby influenced induction of the primary CTL response and thus indirectly modulated the extent of T-cell–mediated immunopathology in the CNS. The same antibodies exhibited little or no protective effect on choriomeningitis induced by LCMV WE, a virus strain able to replicate faster in lymphoid tissues than LCMV Armstrong so that replication of the low dose of virus reaching lymphoid tissues was able to create a sufficient antigen load there to induce an immunopathologic CTL response.

Antibodies that have neutralizing activity against LCMV are all directed against the viral glycoprotein GP-1.[44,220,318] Investigating the mechanism by which passively transferred antibodies provide protection against LCMV in vivo, Baldridge and Buchmeier[23] found that not all monoclonal antibodies that neutralized LCMV infectivity in vitro mediated protection in vivo, but only those of the IgG2a (not those of the IgG1) isotype. Protection was independent of complement activation, but occurred by a Fc (fragment crystallizable)-dependent mechanism, possibly involving antibody-dependent cellular cytotoxicity.[23]

T-Lymphocyte Response

The key role played by T lymphocytes in mediating virus clearance (and also lethal immunopathology) in LCMV-infected mice has long been known (the reader is referred to reviews[47,143,150,197]). Since Rowe and associates[248] first demonstrated that neonatally thymectomized mice infected 3 to 4 weeks later with LCMV survived, but became persistently infected with the virus, a plethora of other depletion-reconstitution experiments have confirmed and reconfirmed the pivotal role of the cell-mediated immune response in LCMV-infected mice, and have refined our understanding of how viral clearance is mediated.

First, it has been demonstrated that T cells of the CD8+ subset, rather than CD4+ T cells, are the effector cell subpopulation that plays the principal role in virus clearance. Thus, in adoptive transfer experiments, transfer of CD8+ but not CD4+ cells from the spleen of LCMV-immune mice into infected animals reduced virus replication in the recipients.[21,329] Further, cloned, LCMV-specific MHC class I-restricted CD8+ CTL could also mediate virus clearance on transfer into syngeneic infected mice.[17,54,55,63,134] Similarly, mice depleted of CD4+ but not CD8+ T cells by in vivo treatment with subset-specific monoclonal antibodies,[128,154,178] CD4-deficient mice,[234] and MHC class II-deficient mice[62] generate strong virus-specific CTL responses and rapidly control acute LCMV infection, unlike CD8+ T-cell–depleted mice[154,178] and CD8-deficient[97] or β2-microglobulin-deficient mice.[62,148,183] LCMV clearance did occur from some CD8-deficient and β2-microglobulin-deficient animals, although with delayed kinetics,[97,183] which the latter authors attributed to the action of MHC class II-restricted CD4+ CTL produced in these mutant mice to compensate for the lack of CD8+ CTL. A further point demonstrated by this series of depleted or deficient mouse experiments is that CD4+ T cells are not required to provide help for generation of the virus-specific CD8+ CTL response.

Although CD4+ T cells are not required for clearance of acute LCMV infection, like IFNs and antiviral antibodies they nonetheless do make a contribution to the virus-immune system balance in vivo. For example, it was found that although CD4+ T-cell–depleted mice were perfectly capable of controlling an acute infection with LCMV Armstrong or low doses of viscerotropic LCMV isolates, they contracted a lifelong persistent infection when inoculated with slightly higher doses of viscerotropic LCMV variants that could be cleared (although slowly) by mice with intact CD4+ T cells.[25,166] In the absence of the contribution of CD4+ T cells to virus control in this more "borderline" infection situation, the viral load in lymphoid tissues likely reached sufficient levels to exhaust the CD8+ CTL response, resulting in a lifelong persistent infection.

The fact that the virus-specific CD8+ CTL response plays such an important role in determining the outcome of acute infection of mice with LCMV has stimulated an in-depth analysis of different aspects of this response, revealing many basic immunologic concepts and principles likely common to the control of other noncytopathic virus infections. These are discussed in the following subsections.

Antigen Recognition by Lymphocytic Choriomeningitis Virus-Specific CD8+ Cytotoxic T Lymphocytes

In 1974, Zinkernagel and Doherty made the seminal observation that recognition of antigen by LCMV-specific CTL occurs in an MHC-restricted fashion.[323,324] The molecular basis for this is now understood: CD8+ CTL bear antigen-specific T-cell receptors (TcR) that recognize specific eight- to nine-amino-acid–long peptides derived from viral proteins bound within a cleft in the α/β domains of host cell MHC class I molecules. Each MHC molecule binds only peptides with a particular secondary structure, and thus the viral epitopes presented to the immune system in mouse strains of different MHC haplotypes differ. Figure 25-6 illustrates the sequences of the principal CTL epitopes of LCMV Armstrong recognized in mice of the H-2^b (C57BL/6) and H-2^d (BALB/c) backgrounds, and their relative immundominance during the primary CTL response in naive animals. LCMV CTL epitopes were mapped using recombinant vaccinia viruses expressing individual LCMV proteins and truncated versions thereof to identify their approximate location, then synthetic peptides to pinpoint them more precisely[111,218,257,258,311–314] (reviewed in Klavinskis and associates[135] and Whitton[310]). The optimal length of each epitope and the relative binding affinities of the different peptides for MHC were determined by comparing the concentrations of peptides of different lengths required to sensitize target cells for CTL lysis, and to bind to MHC.[99]

After virus infection, the specificity of the primary CTL response generated is determined not only by the efficiency of presentation of different viral epitopes, but by the preexisting repertoire of T cells. Thus, although CTL clones from previously uninfected mice acutely infected with Pichinde or vaccinia virus do not recognize LCMV-infected target cells, many T-cell clones generated from LCMV-immune mice infected with Pichinde or vaccinia virus do cross-react with LCMV.[263] The infection history of an animal thus affects the immune response it mounts to subsequent infections (reviewed in Welsh and colleagues[307]).

Kinetics of the Virus-Specific Cytotoxic T-Lymphocyte Response During Acute Lymphocytic Choriomeningitis Virus Infection

The kinetics of the virus-specific CTL response during acute infection of adult immunocompetent mice with a moderate dose of most LCMV isolates correlates well with virus clearance[141,146,165] (see Fig. 25-5). Virus-specific CTL precursors (CTLp) are present at only a low frequency in an adult mouse that has not previously encountered LCMV. These cells are activated and start to proliferate after virus infection,

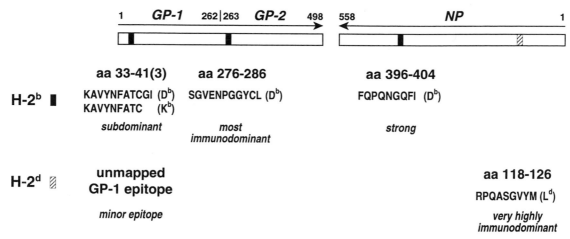

FIG. 25-6. The epitopes in the glycoproteins and nucleoprotein of lymphocytic choriomeningitis virus Armstrong recognized by cytotoxic T lymphocytes (CTL) in mice of the H-2b (e.g., C57BL/6) and H-2d (e.g., BALB/c) haplotypes. For each epitope, where known, the amino acid (aa) numbers and sequence of the optimal-length epitope, and the major histocompatibility complex molecule to which its recognition is restricted, are shown. The relative immunodominance of the different epitopes is also indicated; for example, on the H-2d background, more than 95% of the primary CTL response in naive animals is directed against the epitope at nucleoprotein (NP) aa 118–126. GP, glycoprotein. (Compiled from results in references 99, 218, 312, 314, and 315, and from unpublished observations of J.E. Gairin, CNRS, Toulouse, France, and M.B.A. Oldstone, The Scripps Research Institute, La Jolla, CA.)

and reach sufficient frequencies that their activity can readily be detected in in vitro ^{51}Cr release assays using primary splenocytes as the effector cells by about 5 days postinfection. The LCMV-specific CTL response reaches its peak at days 7 to 9 postinfection, by which time virus clearance is almost complete.[21,141,175]

In addition to the activation of LCMV-specific CD8+ T cells that occurs after LCMV infection, there appears to be substantial nonantigen-specific (bystander) T-cell proliferation[321] because total T-cell numbers may increase severalfold.[237] In fact, administration of the DNA precursor bromodeoxyuridine to mice for 7 days after LCMV infection has shown that more than 60% of lymph node and spleen CD8+ T cells are the progeny of dividing cells (compared with 10% in uninfected mice); division of CD4+ cells is much less marked.[290] The extent of cell division is particularly striking among memory-phenotype (CD44hi) CD8+ T cells, greater than 90% of which are bromodeoxyuridine positive 7 days postinfection. These data suggest that most of the CD8+ T cells that divide after LCMV infection are not virus specific. This intense, non–TcR-mediated bystander proliferation of CD8+ T cells is also observed after infection with other viruses, and appears to be stimulated by the production of cytokines, especially IFNs, that accompanies acute LCMV infection,[290] although some memory cells that cross-react with LCMV may also be stimulated in an antigen-specific fashion.[185,263]

This period of intense T-cell activation and proliferation is followed by a massive wave of apoptotic cell death that peaks about 11 days postinfection.[235] The mechanism by which this occurs is unclear. It may result simply from growth factor deprivation; alternatively, it may be associated with the susceptibility of activated T cells to apoptotic death. As discussed later in the chapter, the latter has been suggested to account for the temporary generalized suppression of T-cell responses to

other infectious agents and to mitogens that accompanies the LCMV-specific immune response.[53,236] There appears to be no selective sparing of LCMV-specific CTLp during the phase of cell death after the acute response to LCMV. However, the huge antigen-driven expansion of virus-specific cells that occurred earlier in the response results in the final postresponse frequency of LCMV-specific CTLp being considerably higher than in a nonimmune animal. This increased frequency of virus-specific CTLp is stably maintained for the life of the animal even in the absence of persisting viral antigen.[123,141]

At the cellular level, the mechanism by which virus-specific memory CD8+ T cells persist at high frequency is poorly understood. Antiviral CTLp in LCMV-immune mice exist in several different cell populations, as defined by phenotypic markers and activation state, including a subset of large blast-like cells expressing adhesion molecules and receptors for interleukin-2 (IL-2).[238] Thus, the population of virus-specific CD8+ T cells may be maintained in part through periodic cell division. Because memory is maintained even after LCMV has been completely cleared, the stimulus for this cell division is unclear. One possibility is that memory CD8+ T cells are stimulated through low-affinity interactions with cross-reactive antigens.[28] However, an alternate hypothesis is that because of the high sensitivity of memory-phenotype CD8+ T cells to cytokine-driven bystander proliferation, IFN produced in response to infection with completely unrelated viruses (or even bacteria) may periodically boost the memory cell population and maintain the frequency of virus-specific cells.[290] This hypothesis deserves serious consideration because CD8+ T cells that divide in response to IFN production differentiate into long-lived cells that maintain a memory phenotype.[290] Although CD4+ T cells are not required for induction of the acute CTL response to LCMV (discussed earlier), experiments using MHC class II-deficient and CD4+ T-cell–deficient mice have shown that this cell subpopulation does appear to be of importance for the generation and maintenance of CTL memory in LCMV-infected mice.[62,284,301] Just how CD4+ T cells function to support CD8+ CTL memory is unknown, but it is possible that they play a part in generating the correct cytokine milieu required for memory CTL turnover and maintenance.

Mechanism by Which CD8+ Cytotoxic T Lymphocytes Mediate Lymphocytic Choriomeningitis Virus Clearance During Acute Infection

Although it is well established that CD8+ CTL are the principal mediators of virus clearance from LCMV-infected mice, the mechanisms by which they bring about viral clearance are a subject of more debate. CD8+ CTL can combat virus infections in at least two ways: by cell contact-dependent lysis of virus-infected cells, and by production of antiviral cytokines such as IFN-γ. Unlike the former mechanism, cytokine-mediated viral clearance does not necessitate the destruction of virus-infected host cells.

An indication that the former rather than the latter type of mechanism is likely of greater importance in clearance of acute LCMV infection came from the observation[170] that adoptive transfer of either LCMV-specific CTL, or CTL specific for another arenavirus, Pichinde, that did not recognize LCMV-infected cells into mice infected with both viruses, resulted in a reduction in the splenic level of only the virus against which the transferred CTL were directed. For such a result to be obtained if a cytokine-mediated clearance mechanism were operating would require that the cytokines involved have an extremely localized effect. Further support for the importance of a direct lytic mechanism in clearance of acute LCMV infection comes from experiments with mice deficient in perforin. Although CD8+ T cells became activated when these animals were infected with LCMV, they failed to eliminate the virus.[126,303] By contrast, mice carrying the spontaneous mutations gld (nonfunctional Fas ligand) or lpr (inactive Fas) controlled acute LCMV infection with normal kinetics,[127] indicating that although perforin-dependent cytotoxicity is crucially involved in clearance of acute LCMV infection, there is no measurable involvement of Fas-dependent pathways.

That perforin-deficient mice were unable to eliminate LCMV indicates that cytokine production alone by CD8+ CTL is insufficient to mediate viral clearance of an acute infection. However, this does not mean that antiviral cytokines do not play any role in control of acute LCMV infection— they clearly can modulate the virus-immune response balance, as was discussed earlier in this chapter for IFNs. IFN-γ and tumor necrosis factor-α are two antiviral cytokines whose role in combating LCMV infection has been addressed in some detail. Although they are not essential for resolution of an acute infection of mice with LCMV Armstrong, because mice treated with antibodies to IFN-γ or tumor necrosis factor-α and IFN-γ–deficient mice are able to clear an acute infection with this virus,[131,157,284] IFN-γ does play an essential role in control of persistent LCMV infection, because T cells from IFN-γ–deficient mice, unlike T cells from intact animals, are unable to clear virus on adoptive transfer into persistently infected mice.[284] This is discussed in more detail later.

Establishment of Persistent Infection by Lymphocytic Choriomeningitis Virus

For a persistent infection with any virus to become established in vivo, two criteria must be met: the virus must adopt a sufficiently noncytopathic mode of replication that it does not kill the host, and the host immune system must fail to clear the virus infection. Because LCMV infection is generally noncytopathic, and the immune clearance of this virus is predominantly mediated by the virus-specific CD8+ CTL response, mice become persistently infected with LCMV whenever the antiviral CTL response fails. Three examples of situations in which this occurs, which illustrate different mechanisms for failure of CTL-mediated viral clearance, are shown in Figure 25-7.

Infection of Mice In Utero or Neonatally With Lymphocytic Choriomeningitis Virus

Naturally occurring persistent LCMV infection was first described by Traub,[291] who noted that infectious virus could be retained in the tissues of mice throughout the animals' lives without causing apparent harm. Such natural persistent infection results from in utero transmission of LCMV from persistently infected mothers to their offspring, but, as described by Hotchin and Cinits,[118] it can be modeled experimentally by inoculating newborn mice with LCMV within the first 24 to 48 hours of life. Seeking to explain the mechanism by which LCMV can persist in mice infected in utero, as described by Traub,[291] and not be eliminated by the immune system, and also Owen's[219] observations of chimeric cattle, Burnet and Fenner[50] postulated that clonal elimination of immunocompetent cells was the basis for immunologic tolerance to viruses and self antigens.

Mice persistently infected from birth with LCMV are not in fact tolerant to the virus at the B-cell level. Although many early attempts to detect antibody in the serum of carrier mice were negative (reviewed in Lehmann-Grube[143]), it was later shown[27,203–206] that antibody was in fact present, in the form of virus-antibody immune complexes. By contrast to the antibody produced in mice acutely infected with LCMV, the antiviral IgG in the serum of the LCMV carrier mice is predominantly low-affinity antibody of the IgG1 isotype.[282] Although serum from LCMV carrier mice may have a low level of neutralizing activity (reviewed in Buchmeier and colleagues[47]), antibody of the IgG1 subclass is not thought to mediate protection in vivo.[23] However, as discussed in more detail later in this chapter, the antiviral antibody made by LCMV carrier mice can result in the production of immune complex disease in susceptible mouse strains.[1,204,205,287]

Although antiviral antibodies are made by mice persistently infected from birth with LCMV, these mice usually do not exhibit LCMV-specific CD8+ CTL activity.[64,66] The defect in CTL activity is LCMV specific, because mice persistently infected from birth with LCMV mount normal immune responses on superinfection as adults with other viruses.[283] It

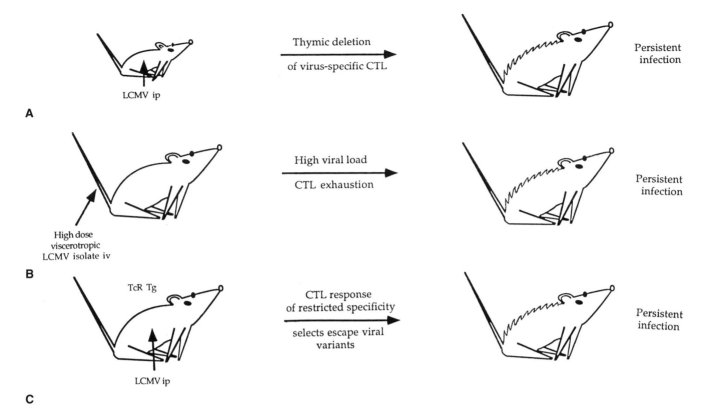

FIG. 25-7. Three examples of situations in which, for different reasons, lymphocytic choriomeningitis virus (LCMV) clearance by virus-specific CD8+ cytotoxic T lymphocytes (CTL) fails to occur, and a persistent infection is established. **(A)** Infection of mice neonatally (or in utero) with LCMV, which results in thymic deletion of virus-specific CTL. **(B)** LCMV infections in which virus rapidly replicates to high titers in lymphoid tissues (e.g., intravenous infection of mice with high doses of viscerotropic LCMV isolates, which are associated with exhaustion of the antiviral CTL response). **(C)** LCMV infection of virus-specific T-cell receptor transgenic (TcR Tg) mice, where the virtually monospecific CTL response selects for CTL escape viral variants. Further details are given in the text.

was postulated by early investigators[64,66,281] that if LCMV was present in mice soon after birth, T cells destined to become LCMV-specific CTL would be clonally eliminated by virtue of their ability to recognize the virus. It is now a well established concept that as T cells mature in the thymus they undergo a negative selection process, during which clones that bind with high affinity to antigens presented in the thymus are eliminated: this is an important mechanism contributing to the establishment and maintenance of self-tolerance. The generation of transgenic mice expressing a TcR specific for the major GP-1 epitope of LCMV recognized in association with H-2D[b226,228] has allowed direct investigation of the fate of CMV-specific T cells in mice neonatally infected with LCMV. TcR transgenic mice infected at birth with LCMV had drastically reduced numbers of CD4+ and CD8+ thymocytes and of peripheral T cells carrying the CD8 antigen, directly demonstrating that virus-specific cells were clonally deleted,[227] likely in the thymic cortex, where LCMV has been shown to be present in stromal cells in carrier mice.[130,173] Further work with this system has helped to cast some light on the mechanisms involved in T-cell selection and deletion (e.g., providing evidence for a differential avidity model of T-cell selection in the thymus).[20,230]

To summarize, if mice are infected with LCMV in utero or as neonates, viral antigens will be present in the thymus to cause deletion of specific T cells as they begin to mature, and thus the peripheral CD8+ T-cell repertoire that develops will lack sufficient LCMV-reactive CTL to clear the infection, resulting in persistence of virus for the life of the animal. That the lack of virus-specific CTL activity is the primary reason why LCMV carrier mice are unable to eliminate the virus is demonstrated by the fact that persisting virus can be cleared by adoptive transfer of splenocytes from syngeneic LCMV-immune mice[5,297] (reviewed in Oldstone[197]).

Jamieson and Ahmed[122] demonstrated that after clearance of LCMV from neonatal carrier mice by adoptive immunotherapy, the cured carrier mice were able to generate a host-derived virus-specific CTL response and resist a second LCMV challenge. The adoptively transferred CTL were able to infiltrate the thymus and clear all viral products from both medullary and cortical regions.[104,130] New LCMV-specific CTL differentiating from the bone marrow after elimination of virus from the thymus were then not tolerized, but matured and moved into the periphery to provide protection against reinfection.[124] LCMV-specific CTL could be developed even at a time when infectious virus and intracellular viral antigens, although cleared from the thymus, were still present in other tissues such as the kidney, testes, and brain (see later), suggesting that antigen in these sites did not tolerize newly developing T cells. In situ hybridization on whole-mouse sections with a LCMV S RNA segment-specific probe[269] illustrated that the kinetics of clearance of viral materials differs in different organs (Fig. 25-8); for example, whereas clearance of viral materials from most organs (e.g., liver, lungs, and spleen) occurs rapidly (by day 15), clearance from the kidney and central nervous system takes much longer (>60 days).[200] The delayed kinetics of viral nucleic acid clearance from the CNS may reflect the fact that the mechanism by which virus is cleared from this site differs from that by which virus is cleared from the periphery (e.g., neurons lack MHC class I expression in vivo and are thus not susceptible to lysis by LCMV-specific CTL).[125] Alternatively, because LCMV replication is known to be restricted in terminally differentiated neurons in vitro,[72] it could be envisioned that virus persistence in the CNS requires continuous reseeding from the periphery and that it takes several months for virus persisting in the CNS to decay when virus is cleared from the periphery and reseeding ceases.

Studies have demonstrated that there are differences in the requirements for clearance of persistent as contrasted to acute LCMV infections. First, although IFN-γ is not absolutely required for clearance of an acute infection with LCMV (although it does contribute to control of virus replication, as discussed previously), this cytokine does play an essential role in clearance of persisting virus, as demonstrated by the observation that splenocytes from LCMV-immune, IFN-γ–deficient mice are unable to clear LCMV from syngeneic normal carrier mice.[284] Given the widespread extent of infection in a mouse persistently infected with LCMV, it is understandable that a cytokine-mediated curative effector mechanism is of more importance that a direct cell contact-mediated lytic mecha-

nism in effecting viral clearance. This is also the case with other persistent viral infections.[108] Further, whereas CD8+ CTL alone can control an acute LCMV infection, CD4+ T-cell help is required if long-term control of persisting virus is to be achieved.[284] Whether CD4+ T cells are needed solely to sustain the CD8+ CTL response,[25,166,301] or also act directly to bring about viral clearance (e.g., by cytokine production) is not clear.

Lymphocytic Choriomeningitis Virus Infection in Which Virus Rapidly Replicates to High Titers in Lymphoid Tissues

Although acute infection of adult immunocompetent mice with LCMV normally induces a CTL response that rapidly clears the infection or causes lethal immunopathologic disease, it was realized in the 1960s (reviewed in Hotchin[116] and Lehmann-Grube[143]) that infection of mice with high doses of LCMV or with particular LCMV isolates tends to lead to persistent infection without lethal immunopathologic disease. Advances in the understanding of this phenomenon of "high-dose immune paralysis" were facilitated in the 1980s by isolation of LCMV variants from chronic carrier mice expressing distinct in vivo phenotypes that could more readily be dissected. The variants studied in most detail have been two non-clonal isolates from a mouse in which persistent infection had been initiated with WE (UBC), the Aggressive virus, which was lethal, and the Docile virus, which was not, after IC inoculation into normal mice[121,224,225]; and a plaque-purified isolate from a mouse in which persistent infection had been initiated with Armstrong, named Armstrong-clone 13, which, unlike the parental virus, established a persistent infection on

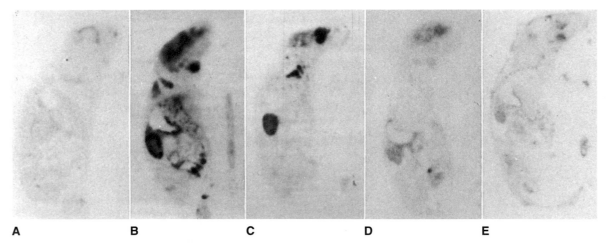

FIG. 25-8. Clearance of lymphocytic choriomeningitis virus (LCMV) nucleic acids from mice persistently infected with LCMV Armstrong after adoptive transfer of splenocytes from syngeneic LCMV-immune mice, illustrated by in situ hybridization to whole mouse sections using a ^{32}P-labeled cDNA probe specific for the S RNA segment of LCMV. The panels depict sections from **(A)** an uninfected control mouse, **(B)** a mouse persistently infected from birth with LCMV Armstrong, and mice persistently infected in a similar way sacrificed **(C)** 15, **(D)** 30, and **(E)** 120 days after receiving an adoptive transfer of 5 × 10[7] splenocytes from syngeneic LCMV-immune mice. (Data from Oldstone MBA, Blount P, Southern PJ, Lampert PW. Cytoimmunotherapy for persistent virus infection reveals a unique clearance pattern from the central nervous system. Nature 1986;321:239–243, with permission.)

IV inoculation into normal adult mice at a fairly high dose.[8] Although high levels of virus-specific CTL activity are mediated by splenocytes taken from mice infected 1 week previously with LCMV Aggressive or Armstrong, LCMV-specific CTL activity is low or undetectable at this time in mice becoming persistently infected with LCMV Docile or Armstrong-clone 13.

This phenomenon has been analyzed from both an immunologic and a virologic perspective. Immunologically, it has been found that a rapid-onset, transient CTL response can be detected in mice infected with LCMV Docile or Armstrong-clone 13,[32,177,180] but that in vitro restimulatable CTLp rapidly disappear, completely in the case of LCMV Docile,[180] or partially in the case of Armstrong-clone 13.[177] Because newly maturing virus-specific CTLp will subsequently be negatively selected in the infected thymus in LCMV Docile-infected mice, CTL tolerance becomes established and virus persists for the life of the animal. To determine whether the disappearance of LCMV-specific CTL activity after overwhelming LCMV Docile infection reflected anergy or peripheral clonal deletion of LCMV-specific CTL, Moskophidis and associates[180] adoptively transferred T cells from mice expressing a transgenic LCMV-specific TcR into syngeneic nontransgenic mice at different times after infection, and followed the fate of these indicator CTL in the recipient animals. They found that whether transferred at the same time as LCMV infection or 15 days later, the transgenic TcR-expressing T cells expanded rapidly for 6 days, then declined to undetectable levels by day 15. This result was not because of TcR downregulation, but because of peripheral deletion of virus-specific CTL, a phenomenon the authors termed "immune exhaustion." The mechanism underlying this phenomenon is unknown. The fact that CTL adoptively transferred on day 15, after the endogenous response had already disappeared, expanded vigorously makes it unlikely that limiting availability of cytokines or antigen presentation is responsible. Further, Moskophidis and associates[180] state that attempts to prevent exhaustion by repeated infusions of IL-1, IL-2, IFN-γ, or concentrated IL-rich supernatants were unsuccessful. Based on experiments analyzing high antigen dose-induced anergy or deletion of T or B cells in other systems (e.g., Guerder and Matzinger[107] and Schwartz[259]), the former authors hypothesize that prolonged engagement of clonotypic TcRs with viral peptide-MHC complexes may, above a critical threshold of antigenic stimulation, lead to anergy and disappearance of virus-specific CTLp before or soon after they become effector cells.[179].

Certainly the viral load reached early after infection in lymphoid tissues is a critical determinant of the production of CTL exhaustion in LCMV-infected mice. Any conditions that increase it favor CTL exhaustion and the establishment of persistent infection. These include: 1) high initial inoculum dose of virus[87,116,143,177,180]; 2) IV route of infection (as compared with IP or subcutaneous infection, after which the virus takes some time to spread to lymphoid tissues[8,177]); 3) genetic inability of the host to mount an optimal antiviral immune response, which depends on both MHC and non-MHC genes[13,179,208,279,327,328]; 4) virus tropism for lymphoid tissues, and more specifically for antigen-presenting cells within lymphoid tissues[4,7,9,32,129,167]; 5) rapid viral replication rate in vivo[167,224,225]; and 6) virus ability to resist control by host defense mechanisms (e.g., IFN resistance[176]) the amino acid mutation at GP residue 280 of LCMV Docile, which results in a lack of recognition by Db-restricted CTL directed against the epitope comprising GP amino acids 275 to 286.)[177]

Virologically, determination of the complete RNA sequence of the Armstrong and Armstrong-clone 13 LCMV isolates has revealed that these viruses differ at only five nucleotide positions, just two of which give rise to amino acid changes,[169,251,254] a phenylaline (F) (Armstrong) to leucine (L) charge at position 260 of the viral glycoprotein GP-1, and a lysine (K) (Armstrong) to glutanine (Q) charge at position 1079 of the viral polymerase. Studies with viral reassortants, revertants, and independently derived Armstrong variants have cast some light on how each of these amino acid differences affects the biologic properties of the two viruses and contributes to the observed difference[8] in their ability to establish persistent infections in adult mice. The amino acid change in GP-1, which is found in almost all virus isolates derived from the lymphoid tissues of mice persistently infected with Armstrong or its variants,[4,251] determines Armstrong-clone 13's preferential tropism for macrophages and dendritic cells,[32,167] acting by increasing the affinity of virus binding to the cellular receptor for LCMV, which is present at limitingly low levels on antigen-presenting cells (P. Borrow and colleagues, unpublished data). This change is necessary but not sufficient to produce the persistence phenotype.[169,251] Virus persistence in vivo also requires the change in the viral polymerase, which is responsible for the enhanced virus yield of Armstrong-clone 13 compared with Armstrong during replication in macrophages,[167] and likely also the IFN-resistance of the replication of Armstrong-clone 13,[176] although this has not yet been mapped. These studies indicate how just two amino acid mutations can cooperatively result in dramatic differences in the in vivo properties of a virus, the glycoprotein mutation enabling Armstrong-clone 13 to infect a large number of antigen-presenting cells in lymphoid tissues and the polymerase mutation enabling the virus to replicate to high titers in these cells and spread rapidly so that the developing virus-specific CTL response is aborted, and a persistent viral infection can be established.

Lymphocytic Choriomeningitis Virus Infection of Virus-Specific T-Cell Receptor Transgenic Mice

Although clearly an artificial system, LCMV infection of transgenic mice expressing an LCMV-specific TcR on a high percentage of peripheral T cells[227] models a situation in which the host antiviral CTL response is of limited specificity. Study of this model has revealed a third mechanism that can contribute to the failure of the antiviral CD8+ CTL response to control LCMV infection and hence the establishment of persistent infection, namely, selection of viral variants that can escape CTL recognition.[229]

Transgenic mice expressing the TcR Vα2 and Vβ8.1 chains derived from a CTL clone specific for LCMV GP-1 amino acids 32 to 42 plus Db on 75% to 90% of peripheral T cells mounted strong virus-specific CTL responses after infection with 10^6 plaque-forming units (PFU) of LCMV WE, as indicated by the ability of splenocytes taken 4 and 8 days postinfection to mediate lysis of LCMV-infected syngeneic target cells in vitro; however, virus was not eliminated from these mice. Bulk and most of the cloned LCMV isolates derived from TcR transgenic mice 8 or 15 days postinfection were found not to be recognized by day 8 spleen CTL from the TcR transgenic mice or CTL clones specific for the GP-1 32-42 epitope, although they were recognized by day 8 spleen CTL from nontransgenic mice and CTL clones specific for the other D^b-restricted GP epitope at amino acids 275 to 288. Sequence analysis indicated that the lack of recognition of viral clones by CTL specific for GP-1 32-42 was caused by amino acid changes within this sequence that interfered with TcR recognition.[229]

Because LCMV is an RNA virus, variants are generated at high frequency during its replication. The selective pressure exerted by a strong CTL response directed against a single epitope leads to emergence of viral variants containing mutations in the epitopic sequence that confer escape from CTL recognition, a phenomenon that can be reproduced in vitro by growing LCMV in tissue culture cell lines in the presence of virus-specific CTL clones.[2,158] Analysis of CTL escape variant viruses selected in vivo and in vitro has shown that mutations may confer CTL escape by affecting peptide binding to MHC class I or TcR recognition of mutant peptide-MHC complexes.[2,158,229]

The biologic importance that selection of CTL escape viral variants has in virus-immune system interactions in vivo is a subject of debate. Because infected hosts usually mount a CTL response directed against multiple viral epitopes (see, e.g., Fig. 25-6), the likelihood of selection of CTL-resistant variants is extremely low (discussed in Lewicki and coworkers[158]). Further, the plasticity of the immune system is such that immune responses to previously silent epitopes can emerge to combat viruses with mutations in the immunodominant epitopes, as illustrated by the finding that C57BL/6 mice infected with an in vitro-generated variant of LCMV Armstrong bearing mutations in all three of the CTL epitopes normally recognized in H-2^b mice were able to clear the infection by mounting a CTL response to a novel epitope in the L protein.[159,210] However, as modeled in the LCMV TcR-specific mice,[229] under circumstances in which the immune response is predominantly directed against a single viral epitope, CTL-resistant virus variants can, even if the immune system is able to evolve to recognize them, be selected in vivo. Their presence may tip the virus-immune system balance sufficiently in favor of the virus that a persistent infection becomes established. An in vivo illustration of this type of modulatory effect is that LCMV-specific TcR-transgenic mice in which CTL escape viral variants are selected become persistently infected if inoculated with 10^6 PFU of LCMV WE, but are able to clear infections initiated with 10^2 PFU of this virus. Similarly, LCMV WE variants with mutations conferring CTL escape in just the two glycoprotein epitopes, but not the nucleoprotein epitope recognized in H-2^b mice, were cleared with delayed kinetics from C57BL/6 mice.[182] Yet, variants of the slower-replicating, less viscerotropic LCMV Armstrong with mutations conferring CTL escape in all three immunodominant H-2^b-restricted epitopes could still be controlled in this mouse strain.[210]

IMMUNOPATHOLOGICALLY MEDIATED DISEASES IN LYMPHOCYTIC CHORIOMENINGITIS VIRUS-INFECTED MICE

That the immune response generated after virus infection not only has beneficial effects but may mediate much of the tissue damage associated with acute or persistent virus infec-

tions was first demonstrated by Rowe[247] using LCMV in a series of pioneering studies. He showed that death associated with acute LCMV infection in the mouse could be prevented by various immunosuppressive regimes. As reviewed by Buchmeier and colleagues,[47] this observation was subsequently confirmed and extended by many other investigators, including Cole and associates[65] and Gilden and coworkers,[100,101] who in adoptive transfer experiments demonstrated that acute lymphocytic choriomeningitis disease is T-cell–mediated. The concept of infection-associated immunopathology is now well established, and it is clear that damage may be mediated by cellular or humoral components of either the virus-specific immune response, or autoimmune responses that may be induced as a consequence of virus infection by a variety of different mechanisms (reviewed in Borrow and Oldstone[35]). Because LCMV is a noncytopathic virus that is well adapted to its natural murine host, many of the diseases associated with LCMV infection of mice are in fact immune mediated. Here we discuss four examples of diseases that occur in LCMV-infected mice as a result of damage to host tissues by the LCMV-specific immune response (Fig. 25-9), three of which are mediated by the CD8+ CTL response induced in mice acutely infected with LCMV (lethal choriomeningitis, hepatitis, and immunosuppression) and the fourth of which (immune complex disease) is a consequence of the chronic antiviral antibody production in mice persistently carrying virus after neonatal infection with LCMV. In addition, we describe two examples of diseases mediated by autoimmune responses induced as a consequence of LCMV infection in certain mouse strains (autoimmune lupus erythematosus-like disease, and autoimmune anemia). Further, we briefly discuss transgenic mouse models in which LCMV proteins have been expressed as "self" in different tissues, so that the consequences of a cell-mediated immune response that cross-reacts with an autoantigen being induced after virus infection can be simply investigated by infecting the mice with LCMV.

Diseases Mediated by the Lymphocytic Choriomeningitis Virus-Specific Immune Response

Lethal Choriomeningitis

Adult immunocompetent mice infected IC with moderate doses of most LCMV isolates usually contract an acute, fatal lymphocytic choriomeningitis, the disease from which LCMV derives its name. LCMV can also produce a similar meningitis in humans[262] (reviewed in Peters and colleagues[221]). The pathology of the murine disease was first described more than 40 years ago (reviewed in Buchmeier and colleagues[47] and Lehmann-Grube[143]). Mice begin to show signs of disease 4 to 5 days postinfection, including ruffled fur, a hunched posture, and blepharitis. This is followed by weight loss, lethargy, irritability, and increasing generalized motor seizures; death usually occurs 6 to 8 days postinfection. Histopathologic examination of the brain reveals massive accumulation of mononuclear cells in the meninges, choroid plexus, and ependyma (Fig. 25-10); the brain parenchyma is not greatly involved.[83,143] These sites of inflammation reflect the distribution of infected cells.[172,186,260]

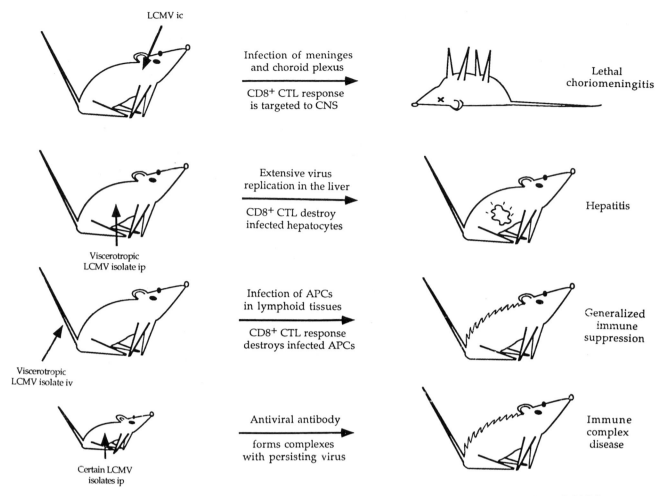

FIG. 25-9. Examples of diseases that may occur in lymphocytic choriomeningitis virus (LCMV)-infected mice as a result of damage to host tissues by the LCMV-specific immune response. CTL, cytotoxic T lymphocyte; APC, antigen-presenting cell.

The induction of inflammation and the development of clinical signs of disease can be prevented by immunosuppression, more specifically by the inhibition of T-cell responses (reviewed in Buchmeier and colleagues[47] and Lehmann-Grube[143]). Further, results from experiments involving adoptive transfers of lymphocyte subsets,[76,80] in vivo depletion of lymphocyte subsets from mice with CD4- or CD8-specific monoclonal antibodies,[154,178] or direct IC inoculation of virus-specific T-cell clones into mice,[22,134] have implicated LCMV-specific CD8+ CTL as the key effector T-cell population in this disease. Although CD4+ T cells are not essential for the development of lethal choriomeningitis, experiments with CD8-deficient or β_2-microglobulin–deficient mice have shown that CD4+ T cells can cause disease and weight loss in mice infected IC with LCMV that is sometimes lethal.[82,97,148,183,233]

The steps leading to the development of severe meningitis in mice infected IC with LCMV have been analyzed in some detail (reviewed in Allan and colleagues[12] and Doherty and coworkers[81]). Induction of an LCMV-specific immune response can be detected in the cervical lymph nodes after IC inoculation of the virus. There is an initial phase of massive, nonspecific recruitment of all classes of lymphocyte, followed by a wave of lymphocyte activation and proliferation that coincides with the development of CTL activity.[163] It is thought that LCMV-specific CD8+ effectors activated in the cervical lymph nodes enter the circulation and traffic to the CNS. Adoptive transfer experiments have demonstrated that the induction of severe meningitis requires class I histocompatibility between effector CD8+ T cells and a radiation-resistant CNS cell type, likely endothelial cells.[78,79] These experiments have been interpreted to suggest that CD8+ cells leave the circulation when they recognize endothelial cells presenting viral antigens in association with MHC class I at the blood-brain barrier. Persistent infection of cultured mouse brain endothelial cells with LCMV has been shown to enhance MHC class I expression on these cells.[98] The expression of adhesion molecules such as very late antigen-4 (VLA-4 or CD49b) and intercellular adhesion molecule-1 (ICAM-1 or CD54), and of macrophage-associated antigen-1 (mac-1 or CD11b/CD18) on activated CD8+ T cells is thought to facilitate their extravasation.[18,19,61,187] Relatively few virus-specific CD8+ CTL may be sufficient to mediate breakdown of the blood-brain barrier, an event that can be measured by protein leakage into the cerebrospinal fluid (CSF) and other techniques.[16,83,164] It is not

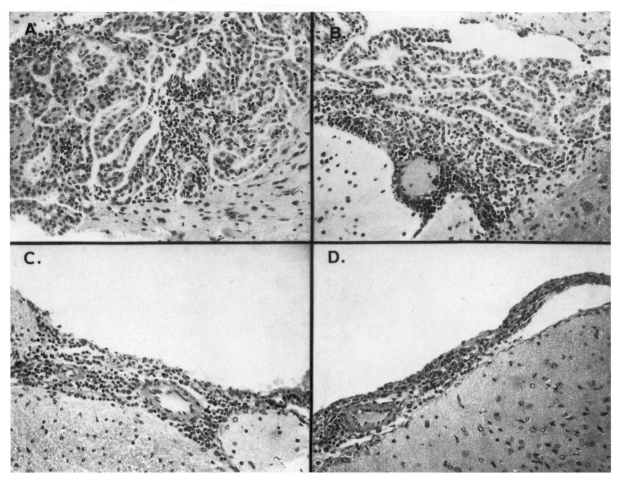

FIG. 25-10. Mononuclear cell infiltrates in the choroid plexus (**A, B**) and meninges (**C, D**) of a BALB/w mouse infected intracranially with 10³ plaque-forming units of lymphocytic choriomeningitis virus 6 days earlier. Hematoxylin and eosin-stain. (Reprinted with permission from Buchmeier MJ, Welsh RM, Dutko FJ, Oldstone MB. The virology and immunobiology of lymphocytic choriomeningitis virus infection. Adv Immunol 1980;30:275–331.)

clear whether impairment of blood-brain barrier integrity results from CTL lysis of infected endothelial cells or the production of cytokines such as IFN-γ by activated CD8+ T cells; however, this appears to be a critical event, which is followed by a massive extravasation of monocytes and antigen-nonspecific CD8+ T cells into the CSF. The CSF of C57BL/6 mice 6 days after IC infection with LCMV contains more than 10⁴ mononuclear cells/μL, and this increases to as high as 10⁵/μL over the following 24 hours,[13] probably in part because of cell concentration as the volume of CSF in the cisterna magna decreases with the acute swelling that accompanies the development of meningitis.[83] Approximately 30% of these cells are CD8+ T cells, at least one third of which express activation markers such as IL-2R (CD25) and phagocyteglycoprotein (PgP, CD44). These CD8+ cells include LCMV-specific CTL,[322] although at what frequency is unclear; the frequency of virus-specific CTLp as measured by limiting dilution assays is low,[57] but such assays do not reflect the level of activated effector cells present in a population. Surprisingly, few if any CD4+ T cells are present in the exudates. The reason for this is unclear: it may be that the local cytokine

milieu is inappropriate for their recruitment or retention. Functional assays indicate that some NK cells are present, but they do not seem to be essential for the disease process because beige mice and mice depleted of NK cells by treatment with antibody to asialo-GM1 4 or 5 days after IC infection with LCMV do not show a reduced susceptibility to the development of lethal choriomeningitis.[14] The remainder of the mononuclear cells in the CSF are predominantly monocyte-macrophages.

Although the events involved in the development of the CNS infiltrates characteristic of lymphocytic choriomeningitis are understood at least in outline, what actually causes the death of mice exhibiting lymphocytic choriomeningitis is unknown. Possibilities include:

1. The presence of inflammation and infiltrating cells may have physically deleterious effects, such as occlusion or the creation of pressure within the confines of the skull.
2. Cytokines and other mediators produced by the infiltrating CD8+ T cells or monocyte-macrophages may have pathogenic effects on the CNS: one candidate toxic mediator

would be nitric oxide, because mRNA for the inducible enzyme that produces it, nitric oxide synthase, has been found to be upregulated in cells (likely monocyte-macrophages) within the inflammatory infiltrates and in proximity to areas of LCMV infection in the brain.[56]

3. Lysis of infected cells or blood-brain barrier disruption may be critical.

Clarification awaits further investigation.

Hepatitis

Although the best known clinical consequence of acute LCMV infection of adult immunocompetent mice is the immunopathologically mediated lethal choriomeningitis that occurs in animals inoculated IC with the virus, it has long been known that immunocompetent mice inoculated IV or IP with LCMV can also show varying clinical signs of disease during the course of the infection, including a hepatitis that may occasionally be fatal.[113,116,143,316] The induction of hepatitis, which is also immunopathologically mediated, depends on both viral and host parameters.[153,326] Viral parameters influencing hepatitis include the LCMV strain, dose, and route of infection. Hepatitis is most severe under conditions in which extensive infection of the liver takes place, namely, in mice infected with hepatotropic LCMV isolates such as LCMV WE rather than LCMV Armstrong, which is more neurotropic; at higher rather than lower doses; and by the IV or IP rather than the subcutaneous route.[326] Host parameters influencing hepatitis include the genetic background of the mouse: A, ICR, and NMRI mice are very susceptible, C57BL and CBA mice are of intermediate susceptibility, and BALB/c and DBA/2 mice are least susceptible to LCMV WE-induced hepatitis. The genetic difference in their disease susceptibility does not appear to be MHC linked.[326] Also, as would be expected for an im-

munopathologically mediated disease, the immunocompetence of the host, more specifically the ability to mount a virus-specific T-cell response, is important: thus, nude mice and T-cell–depleted mice do not contract hepatitis[105,326] (Fig. 25-11).

Early after IV or IP inoculation of adult immunocompetent mice with LCMV WE, virus infection within the liver is predominantly confined to Kupffer cells, from where it spreads to involve other cell types, including hepatocytes.[109,162] Liver virus titers peak approximately 6 to 9 days postinfection, then decline thereafter. Histologic examination of the liver reveals disseminated spotty necroses, steatosis, a marked sinusoidal reaction, and lobular and (later) periportal mononuclear cell infiltrates[162] (see Fig. 25-11). Hepatocyte damage can be monitored by determination of serum levels of enzymes such as alanine aminotransferase, aspartate aminotransferase, and glutamate dehydrogenase; they may show a minor increase at 3 days postinfection, but do not exhibit marked increases until approximately 6 days postinfection; they reach their peak on days 9 to 12 postinfection, declining thereafter.[162,326] The kinetics of hepatocyte damage reflect the presence and lytic activity of lymphocytes within the liver. The mild, early increase in serum alanine aminotransferase levels coincides with the appearance of granulocytes and NK cells in the liver on day 3 postinfection, and the more significant later increase with larger infiltrates composed predominantly of CD8+ T lymphocytes and monocyte-macrophages, with some NK cells and smaller number of CD4+ T lymphocytes and B cells.[162,171] These infiltrates start to appear on days 5 to 6, peak on days 8 to 10, and begin to resolve on days 12 to 14 postinfection.

Depletion and adoptive transfer experiments have demonstrated that virus-specific CD8+ CTL are the critical effector cells that are both necessary and sufficient for the production of LCMV-associated hepatitis. Thus NK cell or B-cell depletion in fact enhances the severity of LCMV-induced hepatitis by allowing increased viral replication to occur in the

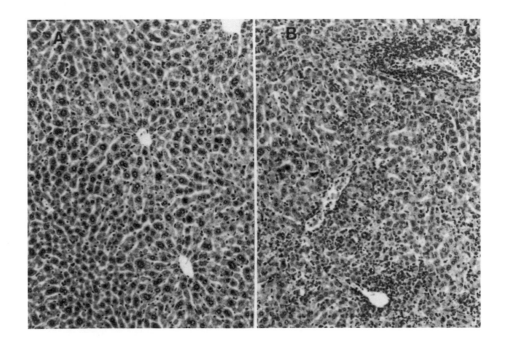

FIG. 25-11. Histologic appearance of livers from a *nu/nu* ICR mouse (**A**) and a *nu/+* animal (**B**) infected intravenously with 2 × 10⁵ plaque-forming units of lymphocytic choriomeningitis virus WE 6 days previously. Periportal mononuclear cell infiltrates associated with signs of focal liver cell destruction are evident in the section from the *nu/+* mouse, whereas no signs of inflammation are seen in the liver of its *nu/nu* counterpart. Hemotoxylin and eosin-stain. (From The Journal of Experimental Medicine1986; 164: 1075–1092, by permission of The Rockefeller University Press.)

liver,[49,162] whereas nude mice and irradiated mice fail to contract hepatitis altogether unless reconstituted with syngeneic LCMV-immune CD8+ T cells.[105,326] Interestingly, although CD4+ T cells are not essential for the development of hepatitis in normal mice infected with LCMV, in β$_2$-microglobulin–deficient mice that lack CD8+ T cells, a different type of LCMV hepatitis is developed that depends on CD4+ T cells,[105] confirming that in these mice, in which CD4+ T cells develop in the absence of CD8+ T cells, the CD4+ cell subset appears to adapt to take over some functions normally mediated by CD8+ T cells.

How do CD8+ T cells mediate hepatitis in LCMV-infected mice? In experiments in which CD8+ T cells were adoptively transferred into irradiated mice preinfected with LCMV WE, a rapid time- and dose-dependent linear increase in serum liver enzyme levels was observed, indicative of single-hit kinetics of liver cell death, which suggests that effector CD8+ T cells destroy infected hepatocytes by direct contact (as opposed to production of soluble toxic mediators).[326] Such a direct lytic mechanism seems possible given that the observed rise in serum alanine aminotransferase levels in mice infected IV with 2×10^6 PFU of LCMV WE2.2 is consistent with the destruction of only a small proportion (<5%) of hepatocytes.[109] Thus, unlike the example of CD8+ T-cell–dependent lethal choriomeningitis discussed previously, in which the pathogenetic mechanism is unclear, it appears that LCMV-associated hepatitis is a direct consequence of CD8+ CTL-mediated lysis of infected hepatocytes. This would account for the fact that this disease usually is not fatal: death does not occur except under conditions in which a particularly high proportion of hepatocytes are infected and rendered targets for CTL-mediated destruction.

Induction of a State of Generalized Immune Suppression

It has long been known that infection of adult immunocompetent mice with LCMV may be associated with a transient or more long-lasting suppression of both humoral and cell-mediated immune responses to a wide variety of antigens.[40,42,110,151,174] Many different groups have attempted to address the mechanisms underlying this phenomenon, and have reported apparently conflicting observations, with some mapping the immune defect to lymphocytes and others to antigen-presenting cells. Although LCMV infection-associated immune suppression is still not fully understood, it now appears that several different mechanisms may contribute to the generalized immune suppression observed in LCMV-infected mice. As is the case with many other aspects of LCMV-host interactions, their relative importance depends on the particular LCMV infection system being studied. The subject of LCMV infection-associated immune suppression is covered in this section of the chapter because the most clearly documented mechanism by which generalized immune suppression may be brought about after LCMV infection of mice is an immunopathologic one; however, other types of mechanism that can contribute to LCMV infection-associated immune suppression are also discussed here.

Acute infections of adult immunocompetent mice with LCMV that are rapidly cleared by the antiviral CTL response are associated with a transient suppression of in vivo immunologic responses,[42,110,151,174] which is also reflected in low in vitro lymphocyte proliferative responses to mitogens.[120,256] This first becomes apparent by days 2 to 3 postinfection, and reaches its peak by day 7; immune responses then gradually return to normal over a period of several weeks.[53,256] Although there is one report that ascribes this immune suppression to a defect in antigen-presenting cell function,[120] there is a strong body of evidence from both in vivo adoptive transfer experiments[38,277] and in vitro mixing experiments[53,256] suggesting that this immune defect predominantly resides at the level of lymphocyte responsiveness.

Many hypotheses have been suggested to account for this transient suppression of lymphocyte responsiveness. First, it has been proposed that LCMV infection of lymphocytes results in their lysis by viral or immune-mediated mechanisms, or alternatively causes a defect in their ability to respond to stimulation. This seems unlikely to play a major role because only a small proportion (<2%) of T cells and even fewer B cells are found to be infected during either acute or persistent LCMV infection in vivo.[6,37,85,129,212,232,288] LCMV efficiently binds to and infects lymphocytes from BB diabetic-prone rats, but not their diabetic-resistant counterparts, and a direct viral effect on lymphocytes may well be involved in the generalized immune suppression seen when BB diabetic-prone but not BB diabetic-resistant rats are infected IV with high doses of LCMV.[261,264] Second, uninfected lymphocytes could be lysed by LCMV-specific CTL if they picked up viral peptides.[37,139] However, if this mechanism were the cause of the in vivo immune suppression associated with LCMV infection, a huge decrease in total lymphocyte numbers would be observed. Although the ratio of CD4+ to CD8+ cells in the spleen is radically altered during acute LCMV infection, total T-cell numbers in fact increase, and B-lymphocyte numbers remain relatively constant.[53,256] Third, LCMV infection-associated hematopoietic defects[39,40,41,265] or viral interference with T-cell maturation[277] might be responsible for the transient decrease in immune responsiveness associated with acute LCMV infection in vivo. However, the immune suppression observed in vivo is not associated with a proportional decrease in peripheral T-cell numbers, making this hypothesis unlikely. A further hypothesis proposes that one of the LCMV-encoded proteins may be immunosuppressive (analogous to the p15E protein of feline leukemia virus). However, the fact that mice in which a persistent LCMV infection is established by neonatal inoculation with the virus do not exhibit a generalized immune suppression[110,151,174,216] despite having a high viral load in lymphoid tissues suggests that this is not the case.

The greatest insight into the basis of the transient lymphocyte unresponsiveness accompanying acute LCMV infection has come from in vitro studies.[53,236,255,256,275] These have shown that the defect in lymphocyte proliferative responses to antigens and mitogens is not caused by the presence of suppressive factors (e.g., prostaglandins[256] or transforming growth factor-β[275]) or a lack of necessary cytokines (e.g., IL-2). Although T cells from acutely infected mice secrete little or no IL-2 when stimulated with polyclonal activators, added IL-2 does not restore mitogen responsiveness.[255,256] IL-2 receptor expression is normal or elevated on T cells from mice acutely infected with LCMV, however, and is upregulated after in vitro stimulation of the cells with mitogens.[255,256] Further addition of IL-2 alone (without TcR ligation) stimulates activation and proliferation of T cells from mice infected 7 days previously with LCMV.[53,236] Although cell cycling in IL-2 alone does not induce apoptosis, it predisposes the cells to undergo a rapid apoptotic death on subsequent TcR-CD3 crosslinking.[236] This indicates that LCMV infection-induced lymphocyte unresponsiveness to mitogens in vivo is caused by apoptosis of activated lymphocytes, and suggests that sensitization by IL-2 of lymphocytes undergoing bystander proliferation during in vivo infection causes them to die on antigen recognition, which is likely the explanation for the generalized impairment of specific responses to nonviral antigens observed after LCMV infection of mice. Lymphocytes recover from this sensitized state as the antiviral immune response subsides, because T-cell responsiveness returns after LCMV infections of adult thymectomized mice.[53]

In summary, it appears that the main basis for the immune suppression that accompanies acute LCMV infection of adult mice is that, as the virus-specific CTL response is induced, antigen-nonspecific T lymphocytes are stimulated by the concomitant cytokine production to proliferate, and are sensitized to undergo an apoptotic death on antigen recognition. This suppression is transient because the general T-cell population recovers normal responsiveness after LCMV clearance and subsidence of the antiviral immune response.

This type of transient immune suppression accompanies the acute immune response to infection with many different viruses. However, LCMV infections may also (under conditions detailed later) be associated with a more long-lasting generalized suppression of immune responses, including those to other viruses,[246,249,283] diverse pathogens,[320] tumors,[136] and even the antibody response to LCMV itself.[181] This type of longer-lasting immune suppression is mediated by a very different mechanism from the transient suppression associated with the acute antiviral immune response. Unlike the latter, in which the immune defect resides at the level of responding lymphocytes, long-lasting immune suppression is associated with competent effector T and B cells, but severely impaired antigen presentation. This has been shown both by adoptive transfer experiments in vivo[15] and by in vitro mixing experiments.[32] Histologic and immunocytochemical analysis of lymphoid tissues from mice exhibiting this type of immune suppression has shown that the functional defect in antigen presentation results from a loss of essential antigen-presenting cells from lymphoid tissues: although red pulp macrophages are still present, marginal zone macrophages, follicular dendritic cells, and interdigitating dendritic cells are depleted.[32,188] As illustrated in Figure 25-12, the loss of these cells is associ-

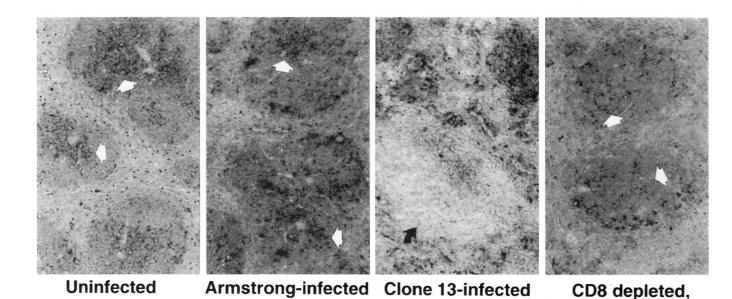

Uninfected   Armstrong-infected   Clone 13-infected   CD8 depleted, Clone 13-infected

FIG. 25-12. Loss of interdigitating periarterial dendritic cells associated with extensive destruction of the splenic architecture in mice infected intravenously (IV) with lymphocytic choriomeningitis virus (LCMV) Armstrong-clone 13. The four panels show immunocytochemical staining with the antibody NLDC 145, which recognizes a subpopulation of murine dendritic cells (hematoxylin counterstain, original magnification 40×) on spleen sections from (*left to right*) an uninfected BALB/c mouse; a BALB/c mouse infected IV 7 days previously with 2 × 10⁶ plaque-forming units (PFU) of LCMV Armstrong (a neurotropic LCMV isolate); a BALB/c mouse infected IV 7 days previously with 2 × 10⁶ PFU of LCMV Armstrong-clone 13 (a more viscerotropic variant); and a mouse depleted of CD8+ T cells before similar infection with LCMV Armstrong-clone 13. The white arrows indicate interdigitating periarterial dendritic cells, and the black arrow illustrates the loss of these important antigen-presenting cells from large areas of the spleen in the mouse infected with LCMV Armstrong-clone 13, associated with extensive destruction of the splenic architecture. That this damage is immunopathologically mediated is demonstrated by the fact that it is not observed in the animal from which CD8+ T cells were depleted before infection with LCMV Armstrong-clone 13. (Reprinted with permission from Borrow P, Evans CF, Oldstone MB. Virus-induced immunosuppression: immune system-mediated destruction of virus-infected dendritic cells results in generalized immune suppression. J Virol 1995;69:1059–1070.)

ated with extensive destruction of lymphoid tissue architecture.[15,147,188]

In the first few days after infections of mice that are associated with antigen-presenting cell loss, the cell types that are later lost are seen to be infected with LCMV.[32] The subsequent destruction of these infected cells is not a result of direct viral damage, but is mediated by virus-specific CD8+ CTL,[32,156] which, as the antiviral CTL response is induced, recognize the virus-infected antigen-presenting cells as targets and immunopathologically destroy them in their attempt to clear virus from the lymphoid tissues. The kinetics of induction of the generalized immune suppression mediated by this mechanism thus parallel those of the virus-specific CTL response,[246,249] and the loss of antigen-presenting cells and the induction of generalized immune suppression can be prevented by depleting mice of CD8+ T cells before LCMV infection.[32,156]

Whether generalized immune suppression mediated by this mechanism occurs when mice are infected with LCMV, and the severity and duration of the suppression produced, depend on a number of variables, including the LCMV isolate used, the dose and route of infection, and the host genetic background.[15,32,188,246] These variables affect the number of antigen-presenting cells that are infected and thus rendered targets for destruction by the antiviral CTL response. For example, LCMV Armstrong-clone 13 much more readily induces a generalized immune suppression than LCMV Armstrong, and this virus has a preferential tropism for critical antigen-presenting cell types in lymphoid organs. Three days after IV inoculation of mice with 2×10^6 PFU of Armstrong-clone 13, dendritic cells in the white pulp of the spleen are seen to be heavily infected with virus, whereas by contrast 3 days after IV inoculation of mice with the same dose of Armstrong, infection is predominantly confined to macrophages in the red pulp.[32,167]

The LCMV isolate used to infect mice and the dose administered affect not only the ease of induction and severity of immune suppression, but its duration, which may vary from weeks to months.[249] Recovery of immune responsiveness occurs in parallel with the histologic recovery of lymphoid tissues,[188] which is likely the result of repopulation of lymphoid tissues with antigen-presenting cells that have newly matured from bone marrow precursors. That this repopulation may take some time to occur is probably a reflection of the fact that LCMV infects not only antigen-presenting cells in lymphoid tissues but cells in the bone marrow, a site that is also infiltrated by activated NK cells and CD8+ T cells when the LCMV-specific immune response is mounted, and is thus also susceptible to immunopathologic damage, manifest as defects in hematopoiesis.[168,280] Although infection of bone marrow cells by different LCMV isolates has not been characterized in great depth, it seems likely that those LCMV isolates that cause the highest level of infection of antigen-presenting cells in lymphoid tissues and thus the most severe immune suppression may similarly infect cells in the bone marrow efficiently, thus explaining the duration of the in vivo immune suppression they produce.

Although immunopathologically mediated destruction of infected antigen-presenting cells is the key mechanism responsible for the generalized immune suppression seen in mice infected with LCMV isolates that infect antigen-presenting cells very efficiently in vivo, other mechanisms have also been de-

scribed that may make some contribution to the immune defects exhibited by these animals. For example, macrophages infected with Armstrong-clone 13 do not respond fully to stimulation with IFN-γ and are thus unable to control the growth of intracellular pathogens such as the fungus *Histoplasma capsulatum*.[295] Antibodies that neutralize IFN-α or -β restore responsiveness of LCMV-infected macrophages to IFN-γ, indicating that production of IFN-α or -β by the virus-infected macrophages antagonizes their responsiveness to IFN-γ.

Immune Complex Disease

The virus-specific CD8+ CTL response is not the only component of the antiviral immune response mounted by LCMV-infected mice that can mediate immunopathologic disease. Antiviral antibody production may also have immunopathologic consequences, leading under certain circumstances to immune complex-mediated disease (reviewed in Oldstone[193,194]). Immune complexes are formed during infections with a wide variety of RNA or DNA viruses when antiviral antibodies combine with the viral antigens against which they are directed, and, often after binding complement components, are cleared by the reticular endothelial system and mesangial cells. They are a hallmark of most, if not all, persistent virus infections in which the constant viral antigenic stimulation results in an ongoing antiviral antibody response and continuous formation of immune complexes (reviewed in Oldstone[193]). Persistent LCMV infection of mice initiated by neonatal infection is a classic example of this. As described earlier, mice neonatally infected with LCMV are not completely tolerant to the virus, but produce antiviral antibodies.[27,203–206] These are predominantly of the IgG1 isotype and are nonneutralizing.[23,282] Thus, they form complexes with viral antigens and virions, but do not control the infection, and infectious virus can be found in the circulation bound to antiviral IgG and complement.[204] Although many different strains of inbred mice can be persistently infected at birth with LCMV, produce antiviral antibodies, and form immune complexes, immune complex disease does not always result. Disease occurs only when the level of immune complex formation exceeds the rate of clearance sufficiently that high levels of immune complexes are deposited in tissues.

The tissue sites in which immune complexes predominantly tend to be deposited are the renal glomeruli, arteries, and choroid plexus (Fig. 25-13). Vessels with fenestrated endothelial cell linings entrap immune complexes very efficiently. Immunofluorescence microscopy of glomerular tissue from mice undergoing LCMV-induced immune complex disease shows an accumulation of host immunoglobulin, viral antigens, and various complement components in irregular granular deposits throughout capillary walls and mesangium (see Fig. 25-13). The specificity of the antibody in deposited complexes can be identified by eluting tissue-bound immunoglobulin and testing it for binding to viral antigens.[206] Whereas less than 1% of circulating antibody in mice persistently infected with LCMV is virus specific, immunoglobulin trapped in tissues is 10- to 50-fold enriched for antibodies that bind to the glycoproteins or nucleoprotein of LCMV.[45,202]

Deposition of antibody-antigen-complement complexes in mice persistently infected with LCMV leads to progres-

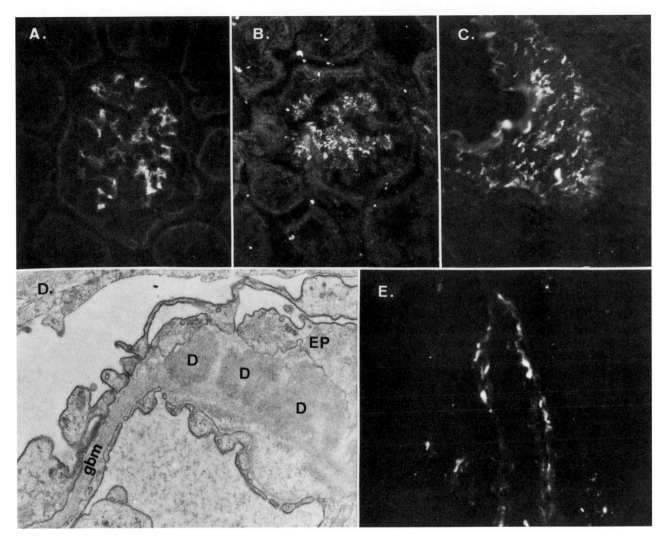

FIG. 25-13. Immune complex disease induced by lymphocytic choriomeningitis virus. (**A–C**) Immunofluorescent staining illustrates deposits of IgG (**A**) and viral antigen (**B**) in a glomerulus, and deposits of IgG in the renal arterial wall (**C**), of a persistently infected SWR/J mouse. (**D**) Electron micrograph of an affected glomerulus shows electron-dense deposits (D, D, D) in a subepithelial location. EP, epithelial cell; gbm, glomerular basement membrane. (**E**) Immunofluorescent staining for mouse IgG reveals immune complexes deposited along the choroid plexus of the lateral ventricle of a persistently infected SWR/J mouse. (Reprinted with permission from Buchmeier MJ, Welsh RM, Dutko FJ, Oldstone MB. The virology and immunobiology of lymphocytic choriomeningitis virus infection. Adv Immunol 1980;30:275–331.)

sive development of glomerulonephritis and arteritis.[204,205] A chronic inflammatory response is stimulated, during which foci of infiltrating cells, including polymorphonuclear leukocytes, plasma cells, and lymphocytes, are observed,[1,204,205] and tissue damage occurs. Local IFN production has been suggested to play an important role in the development of glomerulonephritis because IFN can have a toxic effect on rapidly dividing renal glomerular cells.[106,241,317] In support of this hypothesis, anti-IFN antibodies have been shown to inhibit the development of glomerulonephritis in mice infected at birth with LCMV.[106]

That this LCMV infection-associated immune complex disease is an immunopathologic consequence of the antiviral an-

tibody response is demonstrated by a number of lines of evidence. First, if mice infected at birth with LCMV are foster nursed on LCMV-immune mothers, they have a more rapid and severe onset of immune complex glomerulonephritis and arteritis than conventionally reared carrier mice, and a shorter life span.[207] Maternal antibody is found complexed to LCMV antigens in the glomeruli. Second, adoptive transfer of antiviral antibody into persistently infected mice or the parabiosis of an immune syngeneic mouse to a persistently infected mouse results in enhancement and severe manifestation of chronic LCMV disease.[205] Third, induction of LCMV infection-associated immune complex disease depends on both the mouse strain and infecting LCMV isolate (reviewed in

Oldstone[194]), and disease severity correlates with the level of antiviral antibody produced.

Thus, disease-susceptible inbred mouse strains are those that make high levels of antiviral antibody after neonatal infection with LCMV. For example, SWR/J mice persistently infected with LCMV Armstrong make 50-fold more LCMV nucleoprotein- and glycoprotein-specific antibody and have 7-fold higher levels of circulating complement-binding immune complexes than persistently infected BALB/WEHI mice, and show heavier deposits of virus-antibody complexes in their tissues, although both mouse strains carry the same load of infectious virus.[215] C3H/St and C57BL/6 mice are also low responders, although they respond slightly more strongly than BALB/WEHI mice. Disease susceptibility is determined by both MHC class II haplotype and background genes.[215,287] Although SWR/J mice persistently infected with LCMV Armstrong or E350 contain very high levels of circulating and trapped immune complexes, and mice infected with LCMV WE or Pasteur contain high levels, LCMV Traub elicits a much lower antiviral antibody response. Thus, SWR/J mice persistently infected with this virus isolate have low to negligible levels of circulating immune complexes, with minimal immune complex deposition in tissues, even though their viral load is similar to that in animals infected with LCMV Armstrong.[287] Both host and viral determinants thus influence susceptibility to the development of immune complex disease, acting by modulating the level of antiviral antibody production and the immunopathologic sequelae to this.

Diseases Mediated by Autoimmune Responses Induced in Lymphocytic Choriomeningitis Virus-Infected Mice

Autoimmune Lupus Erythematosus-Like Disease

New Zealand black (NZB) $\times$ New Zealand white (NZW) F1 hybrid mice spontaneously produce autoantibodies to DNA and RNA, and contract an immune complex disease that closely mimics systemic lupus erythematosus in humans.[140] As in humans, the (NZB $\times$ NZW) F1 systemic lupus erythematosus-like disease has a high incidence in females. In (NZB $\times$ NZW) F1 mice, complexes of anti-DNA antibodies with DNA and anti-RNA antibodies with RNA are deposited in the renal glomeruli, and a glomerulonephritis results that usually leads to death of the animals by 6 to 7 months of age. In NZB mice, the main manifestation of autoimmune disease is an autoimmune hemolytic anemia, although many animals also manifest antinuclear antibodies and a resultant glomerulonephritis that leads to death after 12 months of age or more. NZW mice, in contrast, do not spontaneously contract fatal autoimmune disease. When (NZB $\times$ NZW) F1 or NZB mice are persistently infected with LCMV, the kinetics of the autoimmune responses are dramatically speeded up, and the enhanced production of complexes of anti-DNA antibodies with DNA and anti-RNA antibodies with RNA results in death from glomerulonephritis by 2 to 3 months of age.[75,289] LCMV infection thus affects the course of the autoimmune disease in these animals.

When NZW mice are persistently infected with LCMV, however, they contract as severe a systemic lupus erythe-matosus-like disease as (NZB $\times$ NZW) F1 animals, and die at 3 to 4 months of age.[75,192,289] NZW mice thus have the potential for development of autoimmune disease, but do not do so unless infected with LCMV. These studies were the first to demonstrate that virus infection can play a direct role in the induction and course of an autoimmune disease. The mechanism by which LCMV infection induces autoimmune responses and enhances disease in these mice, and the origin of the nucleic acids found in the immune complexes, are unclear.

Autoimmune Anemia

As described earlier in this chapter, the Docile strain of LCMV is able to establish a lifelong persistent infection in adult mice. When C3HeB/FeJ mice are persistently infected as adults with this LCMV isolate, a severe anemia develops that ultimately resolves.[43] Although mice infected with LCMV Docile do exhibit hematopoietic abnormalities soon after infection, the anemia persists well beyond a strong erythroid compensatory response, indicating that peripheral loss or destruction of erythrocytes is the cause of the anemia, rather than defects in erythropoiesis.[43] There is no evidence of direct viral infection of erythrocytes. That erythrocyte destruction is in fact immune mediated has been demonstrated by the fact that cyclophosphamide treatment or CD4+ T-cell depletion abrogates or ameliorates it, whereas transfer of immune splenocytes into immunocompromised mice reestablishes it.[43,67,274] High quantities of antibody, predominantly of the IgG2a isotype, can be eluted from the erythrocytes of LCMV Docile-infected mice, and opsonization of erythrocytes can be demonstrated by macrophage phagocytosis. The level of opsonization corresponds with the course of anemia, suggesting that red blood cells are lost by erythrophagocytosis.[274,294]

Thus, it appears that the anemia induced after infection of C3HeB/FeJ mice with LCMV Docile results from the T-cell–dependent production of IgG2a autoantibodies to erythrocytes, which opsonize these cells for destruction by macrophages. The mechanism by which autoantibody production is triggered after LCMV infection of these mice is unclear. It seems unlikely that the pathogenic antibodies are LCMV-specific antibodies that cross-react with erythrocyte membrane epitopes (molecular mimicry), because antibody eluted from the erythrocytes of infected mice did not react with LCMV antigens in an enzyme-linked immunosorbent assay.[294] Stellrecht and Vella[273] showed that anemia-susceptible C3HeB mice, but not resistant B10.BR mice, showed gross elevations in serum IgG2a levels, and increased IgG1 and IgG2b levels, with a time course that correlated with the development of anemia, and suggested that autoantibody production occurred as a consequence of polyclonal B-cell activation. However, Coutelier and associates[67] were unable to confirm the difference in degree of polyclonal B-cell activation between the two mouse strains of differing disease susceptibility, and found that lactate dehydrogenase elevating virus, which is known to cause polyclonal B-cell activation, had no apparent effect on erythrocytes even though it also induced a sharp increase in plasma IgG levels.

Autoimmune Diseases Induced After Lymphocytic Choriomeningitis Virus Infection of Transgenic Mice Expressing Viral Antigens Under Tissue-Specific Promoters

The systemic lupus erythematosus-like disease and the transient anemia described earlier are examples of autoimmune diseases that are naturally triggered after LCMV infection of its murine host. It has been suggested that virus infections similarly play a role in the initiation of a number of autoimmune diseases of humans whose etiology is poorly understood, including insulin-dependent diabetes mellitus (IDDM) or multiple sclerosis (reviewed in Oldstone and colleagues[217]). One hypothesis as to how infectious agents such as viruses may contribute to the initiation and progression of these diseases suggests that during the immune response to infection, there may be concomitant activation of lymphocytes that recognize antigens in the target tissue (e.g., beta cells in the pancreatic islets of Langerhans for IDDM; CNS oligodendrocytes for multiple sclerosis). These may be self antigens that fortuitously cross-react with viral determinants, or, alternatively, may be viral antigens expressed at low levels in the cells of the target tissue after a previous exposure to the same or a closely related virus earlier in life. After activation, these lymphocytes would then home to the target tissue and mediate autoimmune damage to it.

As an experimental approach to testing this type of hypothesis, transgenic mice have been created that express the LCMV nucleoprotein or glycoproteins under control of tissue-specific promoters, such as the rat insulin promoter (RIP), which leads to expression of the transgene in the beta cells in the pancreatic islets of Langerhans,[191,211] or the myelin basic protein promoter, which leads to expression of the transgene in oligodendrocytes in the CNS.[115] In such transgenic mice, autoimmune disease does not develop spontaneously. However, when infected with LCMV, they generate cytotoxic T-lymphocyte responses to viral antigens, including those in the viral protein expressed in the pancreatic beta cells or CNS oligodendrocytes, thus demonstrating that the initial lack of response to the "transgenic self" antigen is not caused by clonal deletion of the T cells specific for this antigen, but rather just by lack of appropriate T-cell activation[191,211] (reviewed in Oldstone and colleagues[217]). After induction of the LCMV-specific immune response, activated lymphocytes infiltrate the transgene-expressing tissue (pancreas or CNS). In the RIP-LCMV mice, the immune response in the pancreas results in beta cell damage and development of IDDM.[191,211] The lag time before onset of diabetes was observed to differ in different lines of RIP-LCMV mice. It was found that the length of the lag period between infection of RIP-LCMV mice with LCMV and the development of clinical IDDM correlated with aberrant expression of the transgenic viral antigen at a low level in the thymus. Mice without thymic expression contracted a very rapid-onset diabetes mediated solely by CD8+ T cells, whereas in mice that expressed the transgenic viral protein in the thymus, the LCMV-specific CD8+ T cells of highest affinity were clonally deleted, and the LCMV-specific CD8+ T cells of lower affinity that matured into the periphery produced a delayed-onset diabetes dependent on CD4+ T-cell help.[298]

These transgenic models demonstrate that autoimmune disease can be triggered after virus infection as a consequence of activation of normally "silent" peripheral T cells with potential to recognize antigens expressed in host tissue during the antiviral immune response. Studies using the RIP-LCMV transgenic mouse lines have investigated how different cofactors may augment the development of autoimmune disease. Expression of B7-1 on pancreatic beta cells[300] and local production of tumor necrosis factor-α in the pancreas[190] were both found to enhance the induction of IDDM in RIP-LCMV mice infected with LCMV. Other studies have explored possible ways of preventing the development of autoimmune disease. It has been shown that inoculation of mice with soluble peptides encompassing the CTL epitopes of LCMV can, depending on the mode of immunization, induce tolerance by causing peripheral deletion of epitope-specific T cells,[10,138] and that such peptide-induced T-cell tolerance could prevent autoimmune diabetes induced by LCMV infection in RIP-GP transgenic mice.[11,189]

The autoimmune diseases induced after LCMV infection of transgenic mice expressing viral proteins under tissue-specific promoters are not discussed in any greater depth here because transgenic models for different diseases are discussed in Chapter 21. In addition, the reader is referred to reviews on these transgenic models for dissection of virus-induced autoimmune disease.[217,299]

VIRUS-MEDIATED DISEASES IN LYMPHOCYTIC CHORIOMENINGITIS VIRUS-INFECTED MICE

It is well known that viruses can directly produce disease in their hosts by destroying the cells in which they are replicating. A classic example of this is the paralytic disease poliomyelitis, which results from lytic infection of motor neurons in the anterior horn of the spinal cord by poliovirus. Relatively noncytopathic viruses, however, can produce disease in the absence of tissue destruction and inflammation by interfering with the differentiated functions (e.g., hormone production) of the cells they infect, leading to disturbances in homeostasis and disease at the whole-animal level (the reader is referred to reviews[68,71,195,199]). The concept that viruses can alter the differentiated or "luxury" functions of cells without disturbing their vital functions was first described in studies of murine neuroblastoma cells persistently infected with LCMV.[209] Although the cells survived and had normal levels of DNA, RNA, and total protein synthesis, the levels of acetylcholinesterase and choline acetyltransferase they produced were significantly decreased. Since this initial observation, a series of elegant studies have suggested that this mechanism of viral interference with the differentiated functions of host cells, in the absence of overt tissue damage, may underlie a number of disorders seen in mice persistently infected with LCMV, including growth hormone deficiency[70,133,213,243,292]; thyroid dysfunction[132]; alterations in behavior and learning[69,103,119]; and possibly also diabetes.[214,285] Further, studies in other infection systems have shown that this is a general mechanism that may contribute to a wide variety of diseases, possibly including some human disorders of unknown etiology (reviewed in de la Torre and associates[68], de la Torre and Oldstone[71], and Oldstone[195]).

Here we describe three different disorders that may be exhibited by mice persistently infected with LCMV in which this mechanism of viral interference with the differentiated functions of infected cells is thought to play a key role.

Growth Hormone Deficiency Syndrome

C3H/St mice infected neonatally with the Armstrong strain of LCMV exhibit a growth hormone deficiency syndrome (Fig. 25-14) manifest as growth retardation and severe hypoglycemia. Decreases in body weight and length become apparent when the mice are 5 to 7 days old, and by 15 days of age the weight of infected animals is approximately 50% of that of uninfected control animals.[213] These mice also exhibit severe hypoglycemia, which is thought to be the reason most of them die between 2 and 4 weeks of age.[214] The mechanisms

underlying the growth retardation have been analyzed in great detail, and this is probably the best understood example of a disease resulting from direct viral interference with the differentiated function of cells in the absence of cytolysis or inflammation.

The production of both the growth retardation and the severe hypoglycemia are mouse strain and virus isolate dependent. Whereas C3H/St and certain other mouse strains, including CBA/N mice, are susceptible to both phenomena when infected neonatally with LCMV Armstrong, other mouse strains (e.g., BALB/WEHI and SWR/J) are disease resistant.[198] Disease susceptibility is not MHC linked, and involves multiple genes.[286] Similarly, whereas the Armstrong and E350 strains of LCMV produce both growth retardation and hypoglycemia in C3H/St mice, and LCMV Pasteur does so to a lesser extent, LCMV WE and Traub have only a minimal effect on growth and do not cause hypoglycemia and death in most animals

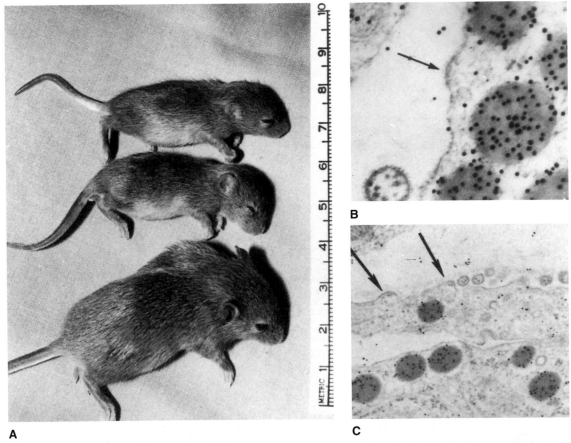

FIG. 25-14. Growth hormone deficiency syndrome induced by lymphocytic choriomeningitis virus (LCMV). **(A)** Two 15-day-old C3H/St mice that were persistently infected at birth with LCMV Armstrong, and a 15-day-old uninfected control animal. The almost 50% difference in size between the uninfected and infected animals is apparent. The disorder in growth is caused by diminished synthesis of growth hormone, which results from LCMV infection of growth hormone-producing cells in the anterior pituitary. **(B, C)** Electron micrographs taken by the late Peter Lampert that show LCMV budding (*arrows*) from growth hormone-producing cells in the anterior pituitary. Growth hormone-containing cells are identified by immunogold labeling using a growth hormone-specific antibody. (Reprinted with permission from Oldstone MBA, Ahmed R, Byrne J, Buchmeier MJ, Riviere Y, Southern P. Virus and immune responses: lymphocytic choriomeningitis virus as a prototype model of viral pathogenesis. Br Med Bull 1985;41:70–74.)

on the C3H/St background.[198] The clone 13 variant of LCMV Armstrong causes significant growth retardation, but does not cause hypoglycemia and death in C3H/St mice, indicating that the two disease phenomena may not have a common cause (J. C. de la Torre and colleagues, unpublished observation).

Whether growth retardation occurs in different murine host-virus isolate combinations correlates with the level of infection of growth hormone-producing cells in the anterior pituitary gland. Most (>90%) growth hormone-producing cells in the anterior pituitary of C3H/St mice infected with LCMV Armstrong contain viral antigen,[213] and mature virus particles can be detected budding from the surface of these cells by electron microscopy[243] (see Fig. 25-14), whereas LCMV Traub and WE infect far fewer growth hormone-producing cells (<15%) in the same mouse strain.[198] Studies with reassortant viruses generated between LCMV Armstrong and WE initially mapped the ability to infect growth hormone-producing cells and cause growth retardation in C3H/St mice to the viral S RNA segment.[239] More recently, LCMV clones have been isolated by plaque purification from the LCMV WE population that, unlike sister clones or the parental population, are able to cause growth retardation in C3H/St mice.[48] Sequence comparison of the S RNA segment of WE clones that do and do not cause disease in C3H/St mice has revealed that a single amino acid change in the viral glycoprotein correlates with disease-causing potential.[276] This amino acid difference affects the in vitro binding of the different LCMV WE clones to the putative cellular receptor for LCMV.[276] It is thus hypothesized that the virion attachment glycoprotein GP-1 plays a key role in dictating the ability of different LCMV isolates to produce growth retardation in vivo by determining the efficiency of infection of growth hormone-producing cells in the anterior pituitary.

How does LCMV replication in growth hormone-producing cells bring about growth retardation? It was initially reported by Oldstone and coworkers[213] that LCMV Armstrong infection of C3H/St mice resulted in a significant reduction (approximately 50% on day 16) in the level of growth hormone in the pituitary, and Valsamakis and colleagues[292] showed that this correlated with a fivefold reduction in the steady-state level of growth hormone mRNA. Further analysis revealed that this in turn was related to a reduction in initiation of transcription of this gene, which appeared to be selective. Transcriptional initiation of another pituitary gene, the precursor of thyroid-stimulating hormone (TSH-β) or of the housekeeping genes actin and proα2(1) collagen, were only minimally affected.[133]

A more in-depth characterization of the molecular mechanisms involved in LCMV-induced downregulation of growth hormone mRNA synthesis has been carried out in a tissue culture model system using a rat pituitary cell line (PC cells) that expresses both growth hormone and prolactin. Persistent infection of these cells by LCMV results in marked downregulation of growth hormone mRNA transcription but comparatively minimal interference with prolactin transcription.[70] Transfection experiments indicated that expression of the reporter gene chloramphenicol acetyltransferase in PC cells was significantly decreased by LCMV infection when the reporter gene was expressed under control of the growth hormone promoter.[70] By contrast, similar levels of chloramphenicol acetyltransferase activity were obtained in uninfected and LCMV-infected cells when chloramphenicol acetyltransferase expression was under control of either a cytomegalovirus immediate early promoter or a simian virus (SV40) promoter.[70] Further, the use of growth hormone promoter deletion mutants together with in vitro transcription assays using nuclear fractions from uninfected or LCMV-infected PC cells suggested that the viral effect on growth hormone promoter activity is caused by interference with the growth hormone transactivator GHF1 (Pit1).[70] Unpublished results by de la Torre and colleagues indicate that Pit1 mRNA levels are not reduced in LCMV-infected PC cells, but it is still not known whether Pit1 mRNA translation is affected, or alternatively whether Pit1's stability, intracellular location, interaction with another transcription factor, or interaction with the growth hormone promoter are altered.

Other studies of the molecular basis of LCMV's ability to downregulate growth hormone mRNA synthesis in PC cells have addressed which viral component(s) mediate the phenomenon. Infection of PC cells with a recombinant vaccinia virus expressing LCMV nucleoprotein, but not with a control vaccinia virus recombinant or one expressing LCMV glycoprotein, produced a significant decrease in the level of growth hormone mRNA, indicating that the viral nucleoprotein or its mRNA are sufficient to mediate this phenomenon.[48] In conjunction with the observation that during persistent infection of mice with LCMV, viral nucleoprotein levels remain high whereas expression of the viral glycoproteins is downregulated,[201] this result suggests that interaction of LCMV nucleoprotein or its mRNA with the Pit1 protein or its mRNA likely forms the molecular basis of the selective downregulation of growth hormone mRNA transcription and, in turn, growth hormone production, leading to growth retardation.

Although the basis of the growth retardation seen in C3H/St mice persistently infected with LCMV has been mapped in some detail, the cause of the hypoglycemia and death also exhibited by these mice is less clearly understood. Growth hormone is involved in regulation of glucose metabolism in addition to growth. However, it is not likely that the hypoglycemia seen in mice persistently infected with LCMV is solely a consequence of the decreased growth hormone production because, as explained earlier, the former can occur independently of the latter. Further, dwarfism in other systems is not routinely associated with severe hypoglycemia. The basis of the hypoglycemia thus requires further investigation.

Thyroid Dysfunction

Mice of many strains (including BALB/WEHI, C3H/St, and SWR/J) persistently infected congenitally or by neonatal inoculation with different LCMV isolates (including Armstrong, Pasteur, Traub, and WE) exhibit abnormalities in thyroid function manifest as a decrease in the level of circulating thyroid hormones triiodothyronine and thyroxine, which correlate with a reduction in the steady-state level of thyroglobulin mRNA in the thyroid.[132] This thyroid dysfunction is associated with LCMV persistence in the thyroid gland, particularly in the follicular epithelial cells, which secrete thyroglobulin, in the absence of necrosis and inflammation.[132] Although it has not been demonstrated whether the decrease in thyroid hormone production is in fact a direct effect of LCMV infection of the thyroid epithelial cells or a secondary consequence of viral perturbation of the hypothalamic-pituitary axis, it is likely that this may be a second example, analogous to the reduction in growth hormone production described earlier, of an endocrine disorder resulting from persisting virus selectively interfering with the regulation of production of a specific protein within a differentiated cell type.

Alterations in Behavior and Learning

Persistent LCMV infection is frequently not associated with clinical signs of severe disease. However, when tested as adults, apparently "normal" mice persistently infected with LCMV are found to exhibit neurobehavioral abnormalities.[103,119] These include an impaired spatial learning ability, as indicated by a deficit in the acquisition of discriminated avoidance performance[103] (Fig. 25-15), and a reduced tendency to explore a novel environment (although their baseline levels of locomotor activity are not affected).[103,119] During persistent infection of mice with LCMV, viral antigens and

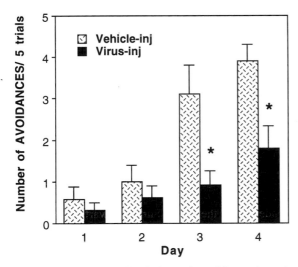

FIG. 25-15. Defects in discriminated avoidance learning in DBA/2J mice persistently infected at birth with lymphocytic choriomeningitis virus (LCMV) WE. Groups of 13 LCMV-infected and 7 vehicle-injected mice were tested five times per day over a 4-day period for ability to choose the safe arm of a Y-shaped maze and hence avoid receiving a mild electric shock: the mean + SEM number of avoidance responses is shown. The LCMV-infected animals exhibit deficits in learning to make a safe choice in this test compared with the uninfected controls. inj, injected; *$P < 0.05$. (Reprinted with permission from Gold LH, Brot MD, Polis I, et al. Behavioral effects of persistent lymphocytic choriomeningitis virus infection in mice. Behav Neural Biol 1994;62:100–109.)

nucleic acids in the CNS are localized almost exclusively within neurons. The highest levels of persisting virus are found in the hippocampus, neocortex, limbic system, and certain regions of the hypothalamus, with lower levels in the brain stem, thalamus, and basal ganglia.[91,242] Virus persistence occurs in the absence of necrosis and inflammation in the CNS. It thus seems likely that the neurobehavioral alterations seen in mice persistently infected with LCMV are a consequence of direct viral effects on the neuronal populations within which virus persists.

The details of all the effects LCMV persistence has on neuronal functioning, and the contributions each of these virus-induced deficits in neuronal functions may make to the neurobehavioral phenotype exhibited by mice persistently infected with LCMV, are incompletely understood. However, several pieces in the puzzle are emerging. One series of studies has linked neurochemical abnormalities affecting neurotransmitters to the LCMV-mediated neurologic deficits.[160,209] Thus, pharmacologic analysis has shown that mice persistently infected with LCMV have a hypersensitivity to the muscarinic cholinergic antagonist scopolamine, as revealed during their performance in tasks involving learning and motor activity.[103,119] Moreover, in vitro studies[209] have demonstrated that persistent infection of murine neuroblastoma cells with LCMV significantly lowered the intracellular levels of choline acetyltransferase. A cholinergic dysfunction occurring as a consequence of viral interference with neuronal production of key enzymes involved in neurotransmitter metabolism therefore may be one contributor to the learning deficits exhibited by mice persistently infected with LCMV.

One study[69] examined whether structural correlates of the CNS alterations described in mice persistently infected with LCMV could be found. Specifically, a search was made for alterations in synaptic density and neuronal plasticity, both of which can have profound effects on behavior. It was found that although the overall synaptic density in the neocortex and limbic structures of LCMV-infected mice was preserved, the expression of growth-associated protein-43 (GAP-43), a protein proposed to play an important role in the neuronal plasticity processes accompanying learning and memory, was significantly decreased in the molecular layer of the hippocampus.[69] In vitro analysis revealed that persistent infection with LCMV of PC12 cells, a cell line that undergoes differentiation from a chromaffin- to a neuron-like phenotype when grown in the presence of neurotrophic growth factor (NGF), prevented NGF induction of GAP-43 upregulation in these cells.[69] NGF-mediated upregulation of amyloid precursor protein in these cells was not affected. Just how LCMV infection affects NGF-mediated upregulation of GAP-43 expression in PC12 cells is not completely clear, but it may interfere with specific pathways of the NGF signal transduction mechanisms, including the protein kinase C-dependent pathway involved in stabilization of GAP-43 mRNA.[69] Similarly, LCMV persistence in neurons in vivo may interfere with the regulation of expression of GAP-43 in response to extracellular signals in the presynaptic terminals of the hippocampal circuitry, resulting in deficits in neuronal plasticity that contribute to the learning defects observed in mice persistently infected with this virus.

SUMMARY AND CONCLUSIONS

The overview presented in this chapter demonstrates just how valuable study of infection with LCMV has been in advancing the understanding of many aspects of virus-immune system interactions and viral pathogenesis. As discussed, a remarkable number of key concepts in immunology and virology that are applicable to many DNA and RNA virus infections were first defined in studies using LCMV. The complex spectrum of different outcomes of LCMV infection of mice also serves to illustrate the delicate balance in which virus-host interactions hang, and how seemingly small differences in either host or viral genetics can have a profound influence on the resolution of infection or the end-stage clinical picture.

Although a wealth of information is presented in this chapter, this review also demonstrates just how cursory our understanding of LCMV-host interactions remains. Of the wide spectrum of immunovirologic phenomena described here, few are understood in any detail. For example, although it is clear that the CTL response is exhausted after infection of mice with high doses of certain LCMV isolates, that mice that contract lymphocytic choriomeningitis die, and that adult mice persistently infected as neonates with LCMV exhibit behavioral abnormalities, the mechanisms behind each of these phenomena remain to be elucidated. The cornucopia of knowledge already gathered about many aspects of LCMV-host interactions makes this infection an ideal system in which to carry out a more in-depth analysis of these and other phenomena. Thus, future studies of LCMV infection of mice are likely to continue to yield many more conceptual advances in the understanding of viral pathogenesis.

ABBREVIATIONS

CNS: central nervous system
CSF: cerebrospinal fluid
CTL: cytotoxic T lymphocytes
CTLp: cytotoxic T-lymphocyte precursors
GAP: growth-associated protein-43
GP: glycoprotein
IC: intracranial
IDDM: insulin-dependent diabetes mellitus
IFN: interferon
IL: interleukin
IP: intraperitoneal
IV: intravenous
LCMV: lymphocytic choriomeningitis virus
MHC: major histocompatibility complex
NGF: neurotrophic growth factor
NK: natural killer
NP: nucleoprotein
NZB: New Zealand black (mice)
NZW: New Zealand white (mice)
PC: rat pituitary cell line
PFU: plaque-forming units
RIP: rat insulin promoter
TcR: T-cell receptor

ACKNOWLEDGMENTS

The authors thank Dr. Juan Carlos de la Torre and Dr. David Tough for stimulating discussions, their comments on parts of the manuscript, and their permission to refer to unpublished data; Dr. Michael Buchmeier and Dr. Lisa Gold for supplying material for figures; and Ms. Diana Frye for invaluable assistance with manuscript preparation. The authors are supported by NIH grants AI37430-01 (to Dr. Borrow) and AI09484-27, AG04342, and JDFDK49836-01 (to Dr. Oldstone). This is publication 9947-NP from the Viral-Immunobiology Laboratory, Department of Neuropharmacology, The Scripps Research Institute.

REFERENCES

1. Accinni L, Archetti I, Branca K, Hsu C, Andres G. Tubulo-interstitial (TI) renal disease associated with chronic lymphocytic choriomeningitis viral infection in mice. Clin Immunol Immunopathol 1978;11:395–405.
2. Aebischer T, Moskophidis D, Rohrer UH, Zinkernagel RM, Hengartner H. In vitro selection of lymphocytic choriomeningitis virus escape mutants by cytotoxic T lymphocytes. Proc Natl Acad Sci U S A 1991;88:11047–11051.
3. Ahmed R, Butler LD, Bhatti L. T4+ T helper cell function in vivo: differential requirement for induction of antiviral cytotoxic T-cell and antibody responses. J Virol 1988;62:2102–2106.
4. Ahmed R, Hahn CS, Somasundaram T, Villarete L, Matloubian M, Strauss JH. Molecular basis of organ-specific selection of viral variants during chronic infection. J Virol 1991;65:4242–4247.
5. Ahmed R, Jamieson BD, Porter DD. Immune therapy of a persistent and disseminated viral infection. J Virol 1987;61:3920–3929.
6. Ahmed R, King CC, Oldstone MB. Virus-lymphocyte interaction: T cells of the helper subset are infected with lymphocytic choriomeningitis virus during persistent infection in vivo. J Virol 1987;61:1571–1576.
7. Ahmed R, Oldstone MB. Organ-specific selection of viral variants during chronic infection. J Exp Med 1988;167:1719–1724.
8. Ahmed R, Salmi A, Butler LD, Chiller JM, Oldstone MB. Selection of genetic variants of lymphocytic choriomeningitis virus in spleens of persistently infected mice: role in suppression of cytotoxic T lymphocyte response and viral persistence. J Exp Med 1984;160:521–540.
9. Ahmed R, Simon RS, Matloubian M, Kolhekar SR, Southern PJ, Freedman DM. Genetic analysis of in vivo-selected viral variants causing chronic infection: importance of mutation in the L RNA segment of lymphocytic choriomeningitis virus. J Virol 1988;62:3301–3308.
10. Aichele P, Brduscha-Riem K, Zinkernagel RM, Hengartner H, Pircher H. T cell priming versus T cell tolerance induced by synthetic peptides. J Exp Med 1995;182:261–266.
11. Aichele P, Kyburz D, Ohashi PS, et al. Peptide-induced T-cell tolerance to prevent autoimmune diabetes in a transgenic mouse model. Proc Natl Acad Sci U S A 1994;91:444–448.
12. Allan JE, Dixon JE, Doherty PC. Nature of the inflammatory process in the central nervous system of mice infected with lymphocytic choriomeningitis virus. Curr Top Microbiol Immunol 1987;134:131–143.
13. Allan JE, Doherty PC. Consequences of a single Ir-gene defect for the pathogenesis of lymphocytic choriomeningitis. Immunogenetics 1985;21:581–589.
14. Allan JE, Doherty PC. Natural killer cells contribute to inflammation but do not appear to be essential for the induction of clinical lymphocytic choriomeningitis. Scand J Immunol 1986;24:153–162.
15. Althage A, Odermatt B, Moskophidis D, et al. Immunosuppression by lymphocytic choriomeningitis virus infection: competent effector T and B cells but impaired antigen presentation. Eur J Immunol 1992;22:1803–1812.

16. Andersen IH, Marker O, Thomsen AR. Breakdown of blood-brain barrier function in the murine lymphocytic choriomeningitis virus infection mediated by virus-specific CD8+ T cells. J Neuroimmunol 1991;31:155–163.

17. Anderson J, Byrne JA, Schreiber R, Patterson S, Oldstone MB. Biology of cloned cytotoxic T lymphocytes specific for lymphocytic choriomeningitis virus: clearance of virus and in vitro properties. J Virol 1985;53:552–560.

18. Andersson EC, Christensen JP, Marker O, Thomsen AR. Changes in cell adhesion molecule expression on T cells associated with systemic virus infection. J Immunol 1994;152:1237–1245.

19. Andersson EC, Christensen JP, Scheynius A, Marker O, Thomsen AR. Lymphocytic choriomeningitis virus infection is associated with long-standing perturbation of LFA-1 expression on CD8+ T cells. Scand J Immunol 1995;42:110–118.

20. Ashton-Rickardt PG, Bandeira A, Delaney JR, et al. Evidence for a differential avidity model of T cell selection in the thymus. Cell 1994;76:651–663.

21. Assmann-Wischer U, Simon MM, Lehmann-Grube F. Mechanism of recovery from acute virus infection. III. Subclass of T lymphocytes mediating clearance of lymphocytic choriomeningitis virus from the spleens of mice. Med Microbiol Immunol 1985;174: 249–256.

22. Baenziger J, Hengartner H, Zinkernagel RM, Cole GA. Induction or prevention of immunopathological disease by cloned cytotoxic T cell lines specific for lymphocytic choriomeningitis virus. Eur J Immunol 1986;16:387–393.

23. Baldridge JR, Buchmeier MJ. Mechanisms of antibody-mediated protection against lymphocytic choriomeningitis virus infection: mother-to-baby transfer of humoral protection. J Virol 1992;66: 4252–4257.

24. Battegay M, Kyburz D, Hengartner H, Zinkernagel RM. Enhancement of disease by neutralizing antiviral antibodies in the absence of primed antiviral cytotoxic T cells. Eur J Immunol 1993;23: 3236–3241.

25. Battegay M, Moskophidis D, Rahemtulla A, Hengartner H, Mak TW, Zinkernagel RM. Enhanced establishment of a virus carrier state in adult CD4+ T-cell-deficient mice. J Virol 1994;68:4700–4704.

26. Battegay M, Moskophidis D, Waldner H, et al. Impairment and delay of neutralizing antiviral antibody responses by virus-specific cytotoxic T cells. J Immunol 1993;151:5408–5415.

27. Benson L, Hotchin J. Antibody formation in persistent tolerant infection with lymphocytic choriomeningitis virus. Nature 1969;222: 1045–1047.

28. Beverly PCL. Is T-cell memory maintained by crossreactive stimulation? Immunol Today 1990;11:203–205.

29. Biron CA, Sonnenfeld G, Welsh RM. Interferon induces natural killer cell blastogenesis in vivo. J Leukoc Biol 1984;35:31–37.

30. Biron CA, Turgiss LR, Welsh RM. Increase in NK cell number and turnover rate during acute viral infection. J Immunol 1983;131: 1539–1545.

31. Blount P, Elder J, Lipkin WI, Southern PJ, Buchmeier MJ, Oldstone MBA. Dissecting the molecular anatomy of the nervous system: analysis of RNA and protein expression in whole body sections of laboratory animals. Brain Res 1986;382:257–265.

32. Borrow P, Evans CF, Oldstone MB. Virus-induced immunosuppression: immune system-mediated destruction of virus-infected dendritic cells results in generalized immune suppression. J Virol 1995;69:1059–1070.

33. Borrow P, Oldstone MB. Characterization of lymphocytic choriomeningitis virus-binding protein(s): a candidate cellular receptor for the virus. J Virol 1992;66:7270–7281.

34. Borrow P, Oldstone MB. Mechanism of lymphocytic choriomeningitis virus entry into cells. Virology 1994;198:1–9.

35. Borrow P, Oldstone MBA. Viruses. In: Frank MM, Austen KF, Claman HN, Unanue ER, eds. Samter's immunological diseases. Boston: Little, Brown, 1994:1379–1392.

36. Borrow P, Tishon A, Lee S, et al. CD40L-deficient mice show deficits in antiviral immunity and have an impaired memory CD8+ CTL response. J Exp Med 1996;183:2129–2142.

37. Borrow P, Tishon A, Oldstone MB. Infection of lymphocytes by a virus that aborts cytotoxic T lymphocyte activity and establishes persistent infection. J Exp Med 1991;174:203–212.

38. Bro-Jorgensen K, Guttler F, Jorgensen PN, Volkert M. T lymphocyte function as the principal target of lymphocytic choriomeningitis virus-induced immunosuppression. Infect Immun 1975;11:622–629.

39. Bro-Jorgensen K, Knudtzon S. Changes in hemopoiesis during the course of acute LCM virus infection in mice. Blood 1977;49:47–57.

40. Bro-Jorgensen K, Volkert M. Haemopoietic defects in mice infected with lymphocytic choriomeningitis virus. 1. The enhanced x-ray sensitivity of virus infected mice. Acta Pathologica et Microbiologica Scandinavica—Section B, Microbiology and Immunology 1972;80:845–852.

41. Bro-Jorgensen K, Volkert M. Haemopoietic defects in mice infected with lymphocytic choriomeningitis virus. 2. The viral effect upon the function of colony-forming stem cells. Acta Pathologica et Microbiologica Scandinavica—Section B, Microbiology and Immunology 1972;80:853–862.

42. Bro-Jorgensen K, Volkert M. Defects in the immune system of mice infected with lymphocytic choriomeningitis virus. Infect Immun 1974;9:605–614.

43. Broomhall KS, Morin M, Pevear DC, Pfau CJ. Severe and transient pancytopenia associated with a chronic arenavirus infection. J Exp Pathol 1987;3:259–269.

44. Bruns M, Cihak J, Muller G, Lehmann-Grube F. Lymphocytic choriomeningitis virus. VI. Isolation of a glycoprotein mediating neutralization. Virology 1983;130:247–251.

45. Buchmeier MJ, Oldstone MB. Virus-induced immune complex disease: identification of specific viral antigens and antibodies deposited in complexes during chronic lymphocytic choriomeningitis virus infection. J Immunol 1978;120:1297–1304.

46. Buchmeier MJ, Oldstone MB. Protein structure of lymphocytic choriomeningitis virus: evidence for a cell-associated precursor of the virion glycopeptides. Virology 1979;99:111–120.

47. Buchmeier MJ, Welsh RM, Dutko FJ, Oldstone MB. The virology and immunobiology of lymphocytic choriomeningitis virus infection. Adv Immunol 1980;30:275–331.

48. Buesa-Gomez J, Teng MN, Oldstone MBA, de la Torre JC. Variants able to cause growth hormone deficiency syndrome are present within the disease-nil WE strain of lymphocytic choriomeningitis virus. 1996 (submitted for publication).

49. Bukowski JF, Woda BA, Habu S, Okumura K, Welsh RM. Natural killer cell depletion enhances virus synthesis and virus-induced hepatitis in vivo. J Immunol 1983;131:1531–1538.

50. Burnet FM, Fenner F. The production of antibodies. Monograph of the Walter & Eliza Hall Institute 1949;142.

51. Burns JW, Buchmeier MJ. Protein-protein interactions in lymphocytic choriomeningitis virus. Virology 1991;183:620–629.

52. Burns JW, Buchmeier MJ. Glycoproteins of the arenaviruses. In: Salvato MS, ed. The arenaviridae. New York: Plenum Press, 1993: 17–35.

53. Butz EA, Southern PJ. Lymphocytic choriomeningitis virus-induced immune dysfunction: induction of and recovery from T-cell anergy in acutely infected mice. J Virol 1994;68:8477–8480.

54. Byrne JA, Oldstone MB. Biology of cloned cytotoxic T lymphocytes specific for lymphocytic choriomeningitis virus: clearance of virus in vivo. J Virol 1984;51:682–686.

55. Byrne JA, Oldstone MB. Biology of cloned cytotoxic T lymphocytes specific for lymphocytic choriomeningitis virus. VI. Migration and activity in vivo in acute and persistent infection. J Immunol 1986;136:698–704.

56. Campbell IL, Samimi A, Chiang CS. Expression of the inducible nitric oxide synthase: correlation with neuropathology and clinical features in mice with lymphocytic choriomeningitis. J Immunol 1994;153:3622–3629.

57. Ceredig R, Allan JE, Tabi Z, Lynch F, Doherty PC. Phenotypic analysis of the inflammatory exudate in murine lymphocytic choriomeningitis. J Exp Med 1987;165:1539–1551.

58. Cerny A, Huegin AW, Sutter S, Bazin H, Hengartner HH, Zinkernagel RM. Immunity to lymphocytic choriomeningitis virus in B cell-depleted mice: evidence for B cell and antibody-independent protection by memory T cells. Eur J Immunol 1986;16:913–917.

59. Cerny A, Sutter S, Bazin H, Hengartner H, Zinkernagel RM. Clearance of lymphocytic choriomeningitis virus in antibody- and B-cell-deprived mice. J Virol 1988;62:1803–1807.

60. Childs JE, Peters CJ. Ecology and epidemiology of arenaviruses and their hosts. In: Salvato MS, ed. The arenaviridae. New York: Plenum Press, 1993:331–384.

61. Christensen JP, Andersson EC, Scheynius A, Marker O, Thomsen AR. Alpha 4 integrin directs virus-activated CD8+ T cells to sites of infection. J Immunol 1995;154:5293–5301.

62. Christensen JP, Marker O, Thomsen AR. The role of CD4+ T cells in cell-mediated immunity to LCMV: studies in MHC class I and class II deficient mice. Scand J Immunol 1994;40:373–382.

63. Cihak J. In vivo antiviral effect of cytotoxic T lymphocyte clones specific for lymphocytic choriomeningitis virus. Microbiologica 1986;9:333–342.

64. Cihak J, Lehmann-Grube F. Immunological tolerance to lymphocytic choriomeningitis virus in neonatally infected virus carrier mice: evidence supporting a clonal inactivation mechanism. Immunology 1978;34:265–275.

65. Cole GA, Nathanson N, Prendergast RA. Requirement for theta-bearing cells in lymphocytic choriomeningitis virus-induced central nervous system disease. Nature 1972;238:335–337.

66. Cole GA, Prendergast RA, Henney CS. In vitro correlates of LCM virus-induced immune response. In: Lehmann-Grube F, ed. Lymphocytic choriomeningitis virus and other arenaviruses. Berlin, Heidelberg: Springer-Verlag, 1973:61–71.

67. Coutelier JP, Johnston SJ, El Idrissi M, el-A, Pfau CJ. Involvement of CD4+ cells in lymphocytic choriomeningitis virus-induced autoimmune anaemia and hypergammaglobulinaemia. J Autoimmun 1994;7:589–599.

68. de la Torre JC, Borrow P, Oldstone MBA. Viral persistence and disease: cytopathology in the absence of cytolysis. Br Med Bull 1991;47:838–851.

69. de la Torre JC, Mallory M, Brot M, et al. Viral persistence in neurons alters synaptic plasticity and cognitive functions without destruction of brain cells. Virology, 1996;220:508–515.

70. de la Torre JC, Oldstone MB. Selective disruption of growth hormone transcription machinery by viral infection. Proc Natl Acad Sci U S A 1992;89:9939–9943.

71. de la Torre JC, Oldstone MBA. The anatomy of viral persistence: mechanisms of persistence and associated disease. Adv Virus Res 1996;46:311–343.

72. de la Torre JC, Rall G, Oldstone C, Sanna PP, Borrow P, Oldstone MB. Replication of lymphocytic choriomeningitis virus is restricted in terminally differentiated neurons. J Virol 1993;67:7350–7359.

73. Di Simone C, Buchmeier MJ. Kinetics and pH dependence of acid-induced structural changes in the lymphocytic choriomeningitis virus glycoprotein complex. Virology 1995;209:3–9.

74. Di Simone C, Zandonatti MA, Buchmeier MJ. Acidic pH triggers LCMV membrane fusion activity and conformational change in the glycoprotein spike. Virology 1994;198:455–465.

75. Dixon FJ, Oldstone MBA, Tonietti G. Pathogenesis of immune complex glomerulonephritis of New Zealand mice. J Exp Med 1971;134:65s–71s.

76. Dixon JE, Allan JE, Doherty PC. The acute inflammatory process in murine lymphocytic choriomeningitis is dependent on Lyt-2+ immune T cells. Cell Immunol 1987;107:8–14.

77. Dockter J, Evans CF, Tishon A, Oldstone MBA. Competitive selection in vivo by a cell for one variant over another: implications for RNA virus quasispecies in vivo. J Virol 1996;70:1799–1803.

78. Doherty PC, Allan JE. Role of the major histocompatibility complex in targeting effector T cells into a site of virus infection. Eur J Immunol 1986;16:1237–1242.

79. Doherty PC, Allan JE. Differential effect of hybrid resistance on the localization of virus-immune effector T cells to spleen and brain. Immunogenetics 1986;24:409–415.

80. Doherty PC, Allan JE, Ceredig R. Contributions of host and donor T cells to the inflammatory process in murine lymphocytic choriomeningitis. Cell Immunol 1988;116:475–481.

81. Doherty PC, Allan JE, Lynch F, Ceredig R. Dissection of an inflammatory process induced by CD8+ T cells. Immunol Today 1990; 11:55–59.

82. Doherty PC, Hou S, Southern PJ. Lymphocytic choriomeningitis virus induces a chronic wasting disease in mice lacking class I major histocompatibility complex glycoproteins. J Neuroimmunol 1993; 46:11–17.

83. Doherty PC, Zinkernagel RM. T-cell mediated immunopathology in viral infections. Transplant Rev 1974;19:89–120.

84. Domingo E, Holland JJ. High error rates, population equilibrium and evolution of RNA replication systems. In: Domingo E, Holland JJ, Ahlquist P, eds. RNA genetics. Boca Raton, FL: CRC Press, 1988:3–36.

85. Doyle MV. Oldstone MB. Interactions between viruses and lymphocytes. I. In vivo replication of lymphocytic choriomeningitis virus in mononuclear cells during both chronic and acute viral infections. J Immunol 1978;121:1262–1269.

86. Duarte EA, Novella IS, Weaver SC, et al. RNA virus quasispecies: significance for viral disease and epidemiology. Infect Agents Dis 1994;3:201–214.

87. Dunlop MB, Blanden RV. Mechanisms of suppression of cytotoxic T-cell responses in murine lymphocytic choriomeningitis virus infection. J Exp Med 1977;145:1131–1143.

88. Dutko FJ, Oldstone MB. Genomic and biological variation among commonly used lymphocytic choriomeningitis virus strains. J Gen Virol 1983;64:1689–1698.

89. Eigen M. Viral quasispecies. Sci Am 1993;269:42–49.

90. Evans CF, Borrow P, de la Torre JC, Oldstone MB. Virus-induced immunosuppression: kinetic analysis of the selection of a mutation associated with viral persistence. J Virol 1994;68:7367–7373.

91. Fazakerley JK, Southern P, Bloom F, Buchmeier MJ. High resolution in situ hybridization to determine the cellular distribution of lymphocytic choriomeningitis virus RNA in the tissues of persistently infected mice: relevance to arenavirus disease and mechanisms of viral persistence. J Gen Virol 1991;72:1611–1625.

92. Finkelman FD, Katona IM, Mosmann TR, Coffman RL. IFN-gamma regulates the isotypes of Ig secreted during in vivo humoral immune responses. J Immunol 1988;140:1022–1027.

93. Fisher-Hoch SP. Arenavirus pathophysiology. In: Salvato MS, ed. The arenaviridae. New York: Plenum Press, 1993:299–323.

94. Francis SJ, Singh MK, Oldstone MB, Southern PJ. Analysis of lymphocytic choriomeningitis virus gene expression in acutely and persistently infected mice. Med Microbiol Immunol 1986;175:105–108.

95. Francis SJ, Southern PJ. Molecular analysis of viral RNAs in mice persistently infected with lymphocytic choriomeningitis virus. J Virol 1988;62:1251–1257.

96. Francis SJ, Southern PJ, Valsamakis A, Oldstone MB. State of viral genome and proteins during persistent lymphocytic choriomeningitis virus infection. Curr Top Microbiol Immunol 1987;133:67–88.

97. Fung-Leung WP, Kundig TM, Zinkernagel RM, Mak TW. Immune response against lymphocytic choriomeningitis virus infection in mice without CD8 expression. J Exp Med 1991;174:1425–1429.

98. Gairin JE, Joly E, Oldstone MB. Persistent infection with lymphocytic choriomeningitis virus enhances expression of MHC class I glycoprotein on cultured mouse brain endothelial cells. J Immunol 1991;146:3953–3957.

99. Gairin JE, Mazarguil H, Hudrisier D, Oldstone MB. Optimal lymphocytic choriomeningitis virus sequences restricted by H-2Db major histocompatibility complex class I molecules and presented to cytotoxic T lymphocytes. J Virol 1995;69:2297–2305.

100. Gilden DH, Cole GA, Monjan AA, Nathanson N. Immunopathogenesis of acute central nervous system disease produced by lymphocytic choriomeningitis virus. I. Cyclophosphamide-mediated induction by the virus-carrier state in adult mice. J Exp Med 1972;135:860–873.

101. Gilden DH, Cole GA, Nathanson N. Immunopathogenesis of acute central nervous system disease produced by lymphocytic choriomeningitis virus. II. Adoptive immunization of virus carriers. J Exp Med 1972;135:874–889.

102. Glushakova SE, Lukashevich IS. Early events in arenavirus replication are sensitive to lysosomotropic compounds. Arch Virol 1989; 104:157–161.

103. Gold LH, Brot MD, Polis I, et al. Behavioral effects of persistent lymphocytic choriomeningitis virus infection in mice. Behav Neural Biol 1994;62:100–109.

104. Gossmann J, Lohler J, Lehmann-Grube F. Entry of antivirally active T lymphocytes into the thymus of virus-infected mice. J Immunol 1991;146:293–297.

105. Gossmann J, Lohler J, Utermohlen O, Lehmann-Grube F. Murine

hepatitis caused by lymphocytic choriomeningitis virus. II. Cells involved in pathogenesis. Lab Invest 1995;72:559–570.

106. Gresser J, Morel-Maroger L, Verroust P, Riviere Y, Guillon JC. Anti-interferon globulin inhibits the development of glomerulonephritis in mice infected at birth with lymphocytic choriomeningitis virus. Proc Natl Acad Sci U S A 1978;75:3413–3416.

107. Guerder S, Matzinger P. A fail-safe mechanism for maintaining self-tolerance. J Exp Med 1992;176:553–564.

108. Guidotti LG, Ando K, Hobbs MV, et al. Cytotoxic T lymphocytes inhibit hepatitis B virus gene expression by a noncytolytic mechanism in transgenic mice. Proc Natl Acad Sci U S A 1994;91:3764–3768.

109. Guidotti LG, Borrow P, Hobbs MV, et al. Viral cross talk: intracellular inactivation of the hepatitis B virus during an unrelated viral infection of the liver. Proc Natl Acad Sci U S A 1996;93:4589–4594.

110. Guttler F, Bro-Jorgensen K, Jorgensen PN. Transient impaired cell-mediated tumor immunity after acute infection with lymphocytic choriomeningitis virus. Scand J Immunol 1975;4:327–336.

111. Hany M, Oehen S, Schulz M, et al. Anti-viral protection and prevention of lymphocytic choriomeningitis or of the local footpad swelling reaction in mice by immunization with vaccinia-recombinant virus expressing LCMV-WE nucleoprotein or glycoprotein. Eur J Immunol 1989;19:417–424.

112. Harnish DG, Polyak J, Rawls WE. Arenavirus replication: molecular dissection of the role of viral protein and RNA. In: Salvato MS, ed. The arenaviridae. New York: Plenum Press, 1993:157–174.

113. Hoffsten PE, Oldstone MB, Dixon FJ. Immunopathology of adoptive immunization in mice chronically infected with lymphocytic choriomeningitis virus. Clin Immunol Immunopathol 1977;7:44–52.

114. Holland JJ, de la Torre JC, Steinhauer DA. RNA virus populations as quasispecies. Curr Top Microbiol Immunol 1992;176:1–20.

115. Horwitz MS, Evans CF, Lazzarini RA, Oldstone MBA. A transgenic model for viral induced autoimmune-mediated demyelination. J Cell Biochem 1995;21A:144.

116. Hotchin JE. Persistent and slow virus infections. Monographs in Virology 1971;3:1–211.

117. Hotchin JE, Benson L, Sikora E. The detection of neutralizing antibody to lymphocytic choriomeningitis virus in mice. J Immunol 1969;102:1128–1135.

118. Hotchin JE, Cinits M. Lymphocytic choriomeningitis infection of mice as a model for the study of latent virus infection. Can J Microbiol 1958;4:149–163.

119. Hotchin JE, Seegal R. Virus-induced behavioral alteration of mice. Science 1977;196:671–674.

120. Jacobs RP, Cole GA. Lymphocytic choriomeningitis virus-induced immunosuppression: a virus-induced macrophage defect. J Immunol 1976;117:1004–1009.

121. Jacobson S, Pfau CJ. Viral pathogenesis and resistance to defective interfering particles. Nature 1980;283:311–313.

122. Jamieson BD, Ahmed R. T-cell tolerance: exposure to virus in utero does not cause a permanent deletion of specific T cells. Proc Natl Acad Sci U S A 1988;85:2265–2268.

123. Jamieson BD, Ahmed R. T cell memory: long-term persistence of virus-specific cytotoxic T cells. J Exp Med 1989;169:1993–2005.

124. Jamieson BD, Somasundaram T, Ahmed R. Abrogation of tolerance to a chronic viral infection. J Immunol 1991;147:3521–3529.

125. Joly E, Mucke L, Oldstone MB. Viral persistence in neurons explained by lack of major histocompatibility class I expression. Science 1991;253:1283–1285.

126. Kagi D, Ledermann B, Burki K, et al. Cytotoxicity mediated by T cells and natural killer cells is greatly impaired in perforin-deficient mice. Nature 1994;369:31–37.

127. Kagi D, Seiler P, Pavlovic J, Ledermann B, Burki K, Zinkernagel RM. The roles of perforin- and Fas-dependent cytotoxicity in protection against cytopathic and noncytopathic viruses. Eur J Immunol 1995;25:3256–3262.

128. Kasaian MT, Leite-Morris KA, Biron CA. The role of CD4+ cells in sustaining lymphocyte proliferation during lymphocytic choriomeningitis virus infection. J Immunol 1991;146:1955–1963.

129. King CC, de Fries R, Kolhekar SR, Ahmed R. In vivo selection of lymphocyte-tropic and macrophage-tropic variants of lymphocytic choriomeningitis virus during persistent infection. J Virol 1990;64:5611–5616.

130. King CC, Jamieson BD, Reddy K, Bali N, Concepcion RJ, Ahmed R. Viral infection of the thymus. J Virol 1992;66:3155–3160.

131. Klavinskis LS, Geckeler R, Oldstone MB. Cytotoxic T lymphocyte control of acute lymphocytic choriomeningitis virus infection: interferon gamma, but not tumour necrosis factor alpha, displays antiviral activity in vivo. J Gen Virol 1989;70:3317–3325.

132. Klavinskis LS, Notkins AL, Oldstone MB. Persistent viral infection of the thyroid gland: alteration of thyroid function in the absence of tissue injury. Endocrinology 1988;122:567–575.

133. Klavinskis LS, Oldstone MB. Lymphocytic choriomeningitis virus selectively alters differentiated but not housekeeping functions: block in expression of growth hormone gene is at the level of transcriptional initiation. Virology 1989;168:232–235.

134. Klavinskis LS, Tishon A, Oldstone MB. Efficiency and effectiveness of cloned virus-specific cytotoxic T lymphocytes in vivo. J Immunol 1989;143:2013–2016.

135. Klavinskis LS, Whitton JL, Oldstone MBA. Molecular anatomy of the cytotoxic T-lymphocyte responses to lymphocytic choriomeningitis. In: Salvato MS, ed. The arenaviridae. New York: Plenum Press, 1990:225–257.

136. Kohler M, Ruttner B, Cooper S, Hengartner H, Zinkernagel RM. Enhanced tumor susceptibility of immunocompetent mice infected with lymphocytic choriomeningitis virus. Cancer Immunol Immunother 1990;32:117–124.

137. Kolakofsky D, Garcin D. The unusual mechanism of arenavirus RNA synthesis. In: Salvato MS, ed. The arenaviridae. New York: Plenum Press, 1993:103–112.

138. Kyburz D, Aichele P, Speiser DE, Hengartner H, Zinkernagel RM, Pircher H. T cell immunity after a viral infection versus T cell tolerance induced by soluble viral peptides. Eur J Immunol 1993;23:1956–1962.

139. Kyburz D, Speiser DE, Aebischer T, Hengartner H, Zinkernagel RM. Virus-specific cytotoxic T cell-mediated lysis of lymphocytes in vitro and in vivo. J Immunol 1993;150:5051–5058.

140. Lambert PH, Dixon FJ. Pathogenesis of glomerulonephritis of NZB/W mice. J Exp Med 1968;127:507–522.

141. Lau LL, Jamieson BD, Somasundaram T, Ahmed R. Cytotoxic T-cell memory without antigen. Nature 1994;369:648–652.

142. Lehmann-Grube F. A carrier state of lymphocytic choriomeningitis virus in L cell cultures. Nature 1967;213:770–773.

143. Lehmann-Grube F. Lymphocytic choriomeningitis virus. Virol Monogr 1971;10:1–173.

144. Lehmann-Grube F. Lymphocytic choriomeningitis virus. In: Foster HL, Small JD, Fox JG, eds. The mouse in biomedical research. San Diego: Academic Press, 1972:231–266.

145. Lehmann-Grube F. Mechanism of recovery from acute virus infection. In: Bauer H, Klenk HD, Scholtissek C, eds. Modern trends in virology. Berlin, Heidelberg: Springer-Verlag, 1987:49–64.

146. Lehmann-Grube F, Assmann U, Loliger C, Moskophidis D, Lohler J. Mechanism of recovery from acute virus infection. I. Role of T lymphocytes in the clearance of lymphocytic choriomeningitis virus from spleens of mice. J Immunol 1985;134:608–615.

147. Lehmann-Grube F, Lohler J. Immunopathologic alterations of lymphatic tissues of mice infected with lymphocytic choriomeningitis virus. II. Pathogenetic mechanism. Lab Invest 1981;44:205–213.

148. Lehmann-Grube F, Lohler J, Utermohlen O, Gegin C. Antiviral immune responses of lymphocytic choriomeningitis virus-infected mice lacking CD8+ T lymphocytes because of disruption of the beta 2-microglobulin gene. J Virol 1993;67:332–339.

149. Lehmann-Grube F, Martinez-Peralta L, Bruns M, Lohler J. Persistent infection of mice with the lymphocytic choriomeningitis virus. In: Fraenkel-Conrat H, Wagner RR, eds. Comprehensive virology. New York: Plenum Press, 1983:43–103.

150. Lehmann-Grube F, Moskophidis D, Lohler J. Recovery from acute virus infection: role of cytotoxic T lymphocytes in the elimination of lymphocytic choriomeningitis virus from spleens of mice. Ann N Y Acad Sci 1988;532:238–256.

151. Lehmann-Grube F, Niemeyer IP, Lohler J. Lymphocytic choriomeningitis of the mouse. IV. Depression of the allograft reaction. Med Microbiol Immunol 1972;158:16–25.

152. Leist TP, Aguet M, Hassig M, Pevear DC, Pfau CJ, Zinkernagel RM. Lack of correlation between serum titres of interferon alpha, beta, natural killer cell activity and clinical susceptibility in mice infected

with two isolates of lymphocytic choriomeningitis virus. J Gen Virol 1987;68:2213–2218.

153. Leist TP, Althage A, Haenseler E, Hengartner H, Zinkernagel RM. Major histocompatibility complex-linked susceptibility or resistance to disease caused by a noncytopathic virus varies with the disease parameter evaluated. J Exp Med 1989;170:269–277.

154. Leist TP, Cobbold SP, Waldmann H, Aguet M, Zinkernagel RM. Functional analysis of T lymphocyte subsets in antiviral host defense. J Immunol 1987;138:2278–2281.

155. Leist TP, Eppler M, Zinkernagel RM. Enhanced virus replication and inhibition of lymphocytic choriomeningitis virus disease in anti-gamma interferon-treated mice. J Virol 1989;63:2813–2819.

156. Leist TP, Ruedi E, Zinkernagel RM. Virus-triggered immune suppression in mice caused by virus-specific cytotoxic T cells. J Exp Med 1988;167:1749–1754.

157. Leist TP, Zinkernagel RM. Treatment with anti-tumor necrosis factor alpha does not influence the immune pathological response against lymphocytic choriomeningitis virus. Cytokine 1990;2:29–34.

158. Lewicki H, Tishon A, Borrow P, et al. CTL escape viral variants. I. Generation and molecular characterization. Virology 1995;210:29–40.

159. Lewicki HA, Von Herrath MG, Evans CF, Whitton JL, Oldstone MB. CTL escape viral variants. II. Biologic activity in vivo. Virology 1995;211:443–450.

160. Lipkin WI, Battenberg EL, Bloom FE, Oldstone MB. Viral infection of neurons can depress neurotransmitter mRNA levels without histologic injury. Brain Res 1988;451:333–339.

161. Lipkin WI, Villarreal LP, Oldstone MBA. Whole animal section in situ hybridization and protein blotting: new tools in molecular analysis of animal models for human disease. Curr Top Microbiol Immunol 1989;143:33–54.

162. Lohler J, Gossmann J, Kratzberg T, Lehmann-Grube F. Murine hepatitis caused by lymphocytic choriomeningitis virus. I. The hepatic lesions. Lab Invest 1994;70:263–278.

163. Lynch F, Doherty PC, Ceredig R. Phenotypic and functional analysis of the cellular response in regional lymphoid tissue during an acute virus infection. J Immunol 1989;142:3592–3598.

164. Marker O, Nielsen MH, Diemer NH. The permeability of the blood-brain barrier in mice suffering from fatal lymphocytic choriomeningitis virus infection. Acta Neuropathol 1984;63:229–239.

165. Marker O, Volkert M. Studies on cell-mediated immunity to lymphocytic choriomeningitis virus in mice. J Exp Med 1973;137:1511–1525.

166. Matloubian M, Concepcion RJ, Ahmed R. CD4+ T cells are required to sustain CD8+ cytotoxic T-cell responses during chronic viral infection. J Virol 1994;68:8056–8063.

167. Matloubian M, Kolhekar SR, Somasundaram T, Ahmed R. Molecular determinants of macrophage tropism and viral persistence: importance of single amino acid changes in the polymerase and glycoprotein of lymphocytic choriomeningitis virus. J Virol 1993;67:7340–7349.

168. Matloubian M, Lau L, King CC, Wu-Hsieh B, Ahmed R. CD8+ T cell mediated hematopoietic dysfunction in chronic viral infection. In: IXth International Congress of Virology Abstracts, 1993;294.

169. Matloubian M, Somasundaram T, Kolhekar SR, Selvakumar R, Ahmed R. Genetic basis of viral persistence: single amino acid change in the viral glycoprotein affects ability of lymphocytic choriomeningitis virus to persist in adult mice. J Exp Med 1990;172:1043–1048.

170. McIntyre KW, Bukowski JF, Welsh RM. Exquisite specificity of adoptive immunization in arenavirus-infected mice. Antiviral Res 1985;5:299–305.

171. McIntyre KW, Welsh RM. Accumulation of natural killer and cytotoxic T large granular lymphocytes in the liver during virus infection. J Exp Med 1986;164:1667–1681.

172. Mims CA. Intracerebral injections and the growth of viruses in the mouse brain. British Journal of Experimental Pathology 1960;41:52–59.

173. Mims CA. Immunofluorescence study of the carrier state and mechanism of vertical transmission in lymphocytic choriomeningitis virus infection in mice. Journal of Pathology and Bacteriology 1966;91:395–402.

174. Mims CA, Wainwright S. The immunodepressive action of lymphocytic choriomeningitis virus in mice. J Immunol 1968;101:717–724.

175. Moskophidis D, Assmann-Wischer U, Simon MM, Lehmann-Grube F. The immune response of the mouse to lymphocytic choriomeningitis virus. V. High numbers of cytolytic T lymphocytes are generated in the spleen during acute infection. Eur J Immunol 1987;17:937–942.

176. Moskophidis D, Battegay M, Bruendler MA, Laine E, Gresser I, Zinkernagel RM. Resistance of lymphocytic choriomeningitis virus to alpha/beta interferon and to gamma interferon. J Virol 1994;68:1951–1955.

177. Moskophidis D, Battegay M, van den Broek M, Laine E, Hoffmann-Rohrer U, Zinkernagel RM. Role of virus and host variables in virus persistence or immunopathological disease caused by a non-cytolytic virus. J Gen Virol 1995;76:381–391.

178. Moskophidis D, Cobbold SP, Waldmann H, Lehmann-Grube F. Mechanism of recovery from acute virus infection: treatment of lymphocytic choriomeningitis virus-infected mice with monoclonal antibodies reveals that Lyt-2+ T lymphocytes mediate clearance of virus and regulate the antiviral antibody response. J Virol 1987;61:1867–1874.

179. Moskophidis D, Lechner F, Hengartner H, Zinkernagel RM. MHC class I and non-MHC-linked capacity for generating an anti-viral CTL response determines susceptibility to CTL exhaustion and establishment of virus persistence in mice. J Immunol 1994;152:4976–4983.

180. Moskophidis D, Lechner F, Pircher H, Zinkernagel RM. Virus persistence in acutely infected immunocompetent mice by exhaustion of antiviral cytotoxic effector T. Nature 1993;362:758–761.

181. Moskophidis D, Pircher H, Ciernik I, Odermatt B, Hengartner H, Zinkernagel RM. Suppression of virus-specific antibody production by CD8+ class I-restricted antiviral cytotoxic T cells in vivo. J Virol 1992;66:3661–3668.

182. Moskophidis D, Zinkernagel RM. Immunobiology of cytotoxic T-cell escape mutants of lymphocytic choriomeningitis virus. J Virol 1995;69:2187–2193.

183. Muller D, Koller BH, Whitton JL, LaPan KE, Brigman KK, Frelinger JA. LCMV-specific, class II-restricted cytotoxic T cells in beta 2-microglobulin-deficient mice. Science 1992;255:1576–1578.

184. Muller U, Steinhoff U, Reis LFL, et al. Functional role of type I and type II interferons in antiviral defense. Science 1994;264:1918–1921.

185. Nahill SR, Welsh RM. High frequency of cross-reactive cytotoxic T lymphocytes elicited during the virus-induced polyclonal cytotoxic T lymphocyte response. J Exp Med 1993;177:317–327.

186. Nathanson N, Monjan AA, Panitch HJ, Johnson ED, Petursson G, Cole GA. Viral immunology and immunopathology. San Diego: Academic Press, 1975.

187. Nielsen HV, Christensen JP, Andersson EC, Marker O, Thomsen AR. Expression of type 3 complement receptor on activated CD8+ T cells facilitates homing to inflammatory sites. J Immunol 1994;153:2021–2028.

188. Odermatt B, Eppler M, Leist TP, Hengartner H, Zinkernagel RM. Virus-triggered acquired immunodeficiency by cytotoxic T-cell-dependent destruction of antigen-presenting cells and lymph follicle structure. Proc Natl Acad Sci U S A 1991;88:8252–8256.

189. Oehen S, Ohashi PS, Aichele P, Burki K, Hengartner H, Zinkernagel RM. Vaccination or tolerance to prevent diabetes. Eur J Immunol 1992;22:3149–3153.

190. Ohashi PS, Oehen S, Aichele P, et al. Induction of diabetes is influenced by the infectious virus and local expression of MHC class I and tumor necrosis factor-alpha. J Immunol 1993;150:5185–5194.

191. Ohashi PS, Oehen S, Buerki K, et al. Ablation of "tolerance" and induction of diabetes by virus infection in viral antigen transgenic mice. Cell 1991;65:305–317.

192. Oldstone MBA. Autoimmunity and viruses fact or fiction: persistent LCM viral infection, anti-LCM viral immune response and tissue injury. Am J Clin Pathol 1971;56:299–302.

193. Oldstone MBA. Virus neutralization and virus-induced immune complex disease: virus-antibody union resulting in immunoprotection or immunologic injury—two sides of the same coin. Prog Med Virol 1975;19:84–119.

194. Oldstone MBA. Virus-induced immune complex formation and disease: definition, regulation and importance. In: Notkins AL, Oldstone MBA, eds. Concepts in viral pathogenesis. New York: Springer-Verlag, 1984:201–209.

195. Oldstone MBA. Virus can alter cell function without causing cell pathology: disordered function leads to imbalance of homeostasis and disease. In: Notkins AL, Oldstone MBA, eds. Concepts in viral pathogenesis. New York: Springer-Verlag, 1984:269–276.

196. Oldstone MBA. Arenaviruses: genes, proteins and expression. Curr Top Microbiol Immunol 1987;133.

197. Oldstone MBA. Immunotherapy for virus infection. Curr Top Microbiol Immunol 1987;134:211–229.

198. Oldstone MBA, Ahmed R, Buchmeier MJ, Blount P, Tishon A. Perturbation of differentiated functions during viral infection in vivo. I. Relationship of lymphocytic choriomeningitis virus and host strains to growth hormone deficiency. Virology 1985;142:158–174.

199. Oldstone MBA, Ahmed R, Byrne J, Buchmeier MJ, Riviere Y, Southern P. Virus and immune responses: lymphocytic choriomeningitis virus as a prototype model of viral pathogenesis. Br Med Bull 1985;41:70–74.

200. Oldstone MBA, Blount P, Southern PJ, Lampert PW. Cytoimmunotherapy for persistent virus infection reveals a unique clearance pattern from the central nervous system. Nature 1986;321: 239–243.

201. Oldstone MBA, Buchmeier MJ. Restricted expression of viral glycoprotein in cells of persistently infected mice. Nature 1982;300: 360–362.

202. Oldstone MBA, Buchmeier MJ, Doyle MV, Tishon A. Virus-induced immune complex disease: specific anti-viral antibody and C1q binding material in the circulation during persistent lymphocytic choriomeningitis virus infection. J Immunol 1980;124: 831–838.

203. Oldstone MBA, Dixon FJ. Lymphocytic choriomeningitis: production of antibody by "tolerant" infected mice. Science 1967;158: 1193–1195.

204. Oldstone MBA, Dixon FJ. Pathogenesis of chronic disease associated with persistent lymphocytic choriomeningitis viral infection. I. Relationship of antibody production to disease in neonatally-infected mice. J Exp Med 1969;129:483–505.

205. Oldstone MBA, Dixon FJ. Pathogenesis of chronic disease associated with persistent lymphocytic choriomeningitis viral infection. II. Relationship of anti-LCM viral response to tissue injury in chronic disease. J Exp Med 1970;131:1–20.

206. Oldstone MBA, Dixon FJ. Immune complex disease in chronic viral infection. J Exp Med 1971;134:32s–40s.

207. Oldstone MBA, Dixon FJ. Disease accompanying in utero viral infection: the role of maternal antibody in tissue injury after transplacental infection with lymphocytic choriomeningitis virus. J Exp Med 1972;135:827–838.

208. Oldstone MBA, Dixon FJ, Mitchell GF, McDevitt HO. Histocompatibility-linked genetic control of disease susceptibility: murine lymphocytic choriomeningitis virus infection. J Exp Med 1973; 137:1201–1212.

209. Oldstone MBA, Holmstoen J, Welsh RM. Alterations of acetylcholine enzymes in neuroblastoma cells persistently infected with lymphocytic choriomeningitis virus. J Cell Physiol 1977;91:459–472.

210. Oldstone MBA, Lewicki H, Borrow P, Hudrisier D, Gairin JE. Discriminated selection among viral peptides with the appropriate anchor residues: implications for the size of the cytotoxic T-lymphocyte repertoire and control of viral infection. J Virol 1995;69: 7423–7429.

211. Oldstone MBA, Nerenberg M, Southern PJ, Price J, Lewicki H. Virus infection triggers insulin-dependent diabetes mellitus in a transgenic model: role of anti-self (virus) immune response. Cell 1991;65:319–331.

212. Oldstone MBA, Salvato M, Tishon A, Lewicki H. Virus-lymphocyte interactions. III. Biologic parameters of a virus variant that fails to generate CTL and establishes persistent infection in immunocompetent hosts. Virology 1988;164:507–516.

213. Oldstone MBA, Sinha YN, Blount P, et al. Virus-induced alterations in homeostasis: alteration in differentiated functions of infected cells in vivo. Science 1982;218:1125–1127.

214. Oldstone MBA, Southern P, Rodriguez M, Lampert P. Virus persists in beta cells of islets of Langerhans and is associated with chemical manifestations of diabetes. Science 1984;224:1440–1443.

215. Oldstone MBA, Tishon A, Buchmeier MJ. Virus-induced immune complex disease: genetic control of C1q binding complexes in the circulation of mice persistently infected with lymphocytic choriomeningitis virus. J Immunol 1983;130:912–918.

216. Oldstone MBA, Tishon A, Chiller JM, Weigle WO, Dixon FJ. Effect of chronic viral infection on the immune system. I. Comparison of the immune responsiveness of mice chronically infected with LCM virus with that of noninfected mice. J Immunol 1973;110: 1268–1278.

217. Oldstone MBA, Von Herrath MG, Evans CF, Horwitz MS. Virus-induced autoimmune disease: transgenic approach to mimic insulin-dependent diabetes mellitus and multiple sclerosis. Curr Top Microbiol Immunol 1996;206:67–83.

218. Oldstone MBA, Whitton JL, Lewicki H, Tishon A. Fine dissection of a nine amino acid glycoprotein epitope, a major determinant recognized by lymphocytic choriomeningitis virus-specific class I-restricted H-2Db cytotoxic T lymphocytes. J Exp Med 1988;168: 559–570.

219. Owen RD. Immunogenetic consequences of vascular anastomoses between bovine twins. Science 1945;102:400–401.

220. Parekh BS, Buchmeier MJ. Proteins of lymphocytic choriomeningitis virus: antigenic topography of the viral glycoproteins. Virology 1986;153:168–178.

221. Peters CJ, Buchmeier MJ, Rollin PE, Ksiazek TG. Arenaviruses. In: Fields BN, Knipe DM, Howley PM, eds. Fields virology. 3rd ed. Philadelphia: Lippincott-Raven, 1996:1521–1551.

222. Pfau CJ, Gresser I, Hunt KD. Lethal role of interferon in lymphocytic choriomeningitis virus-induced encephalitis. J Gen Virol 1983; 64:1827–1830.

223. Pfau CJ, Thomsen AR. Lymphocytic choriomeningitis virus: history of the gold standard for viral immunobiology. In: Salvato MS, ed. The arenaviridae. New York: Plenum Press, 1993:191–198.

224. Pfau CJ, Valenti JK, Jacobson S, Pevear DC. Cytotoxic T cells are induced in mice infected with lymphocytic choriomeningitis virus strains of markedly different pathogenicities. Infect Immun 1982; 36:598–602.

225. Pfau CJ, Valenti JK, Pevear DC, Hunt KD. Lymphocytic choriomeningitis virus killer T cells are lethal only in weakly disseminated murine infections. J Exp Med 1982;156:79–89.

226. Pircher HP, Baenziger J, Schilham M, et al. Characterization of virus-specific cytotoxic T cell clones from allogeneic bone marrow chimeras. Eur J Immunol 1987;17:159–166.

227. Pircher HP, Burki K, Lang R, Hengartner H, Zinkernagel RM. Tolerance induction in double specific T-cell receptor transgenic mice varies with antigen. Nature 1989;342:559–561.

228. Pircher HP, Michalopoulos EE, Iwamoto A, et al. Molecular analysis of the antigen receptor of virus-specific cytotoxic T cells and identification of a new V alpha family. Eur J Immunol 1987;17: 1843–1846.

229. Pircher HP, Moskophidis D, Rohrer U, Burki K, Hengartner H, Zinkernagel RM. Viral escape by selection of cytotoxic T cell-resistant virus variants in vivo. Nature 1990;346:629–633.

230. Pircher HP, Rohrer UH, Moskophidis D, Zinkernagel RM, Hengartner H. Lower receptor avidity required for thymic clonal deletion than for effector T-cell function. Nature 1991;351:482–485.

231. Popescu M, Lehmann-Grube F. Defective interfering particles in mice infected with lymphocytic choriomeningitis virus. Virology 1977;77:78–83.

232. Popescu M, Lohler J, Lehmann-Grube F. Infectious lymphocytes in lymphocytic choriomeningitis virus carrier mice. J Gen Virol 1979; 42:481–492.

233. Quinn DG, Zajac AJ, Frelinger JA, Muller D. Transfer of lymphocytic choriomeningitis disease in beta 2-microglobulin-deficient mice by CD4+ T cells. Int Immunol 1993;5:1193–1198.

234. Rahemtulla A, Fung-Leung WP, Schilham MW, et al. Normal development and function of CD8+ cells but markedly decreased helper cell activity in mice lacking CD4. Nature 1991;353:180–184.

235. Razvi ES, Jiang Z, Woda BA, Welsh RM. Lymphocyte apoptosis during the silencing of the immune response to acute viral infections in normal, lpr, and Bcl-2-transgenic mice. Am J Pathol 1995;147: 79–91.

236. Razvi ES, Welsh RM. Programmed cell death of T lymphocytes during acute viral infection: a mechanism for virus-induced immune deficiency. J Virol 1993;67:5754–5765.

237. Razvi ES, Welsh RM. Apoptosis in viral infections. Adv Virus Res 1995;45:1–60.

238. Razvi ES, Welsh RM, McFarland HI. In vivo state of antiviral CTL precursors: characterization of a cycling cell population containing CTL precursors in immune mice. J Immunol 1995;154:620–632.

239. Riviere Y, Ahmed R, Southern P, Oldstone MB. Perturbation of differentiated functions during viral infection in vivo. II. Viral reassortants map growth hormone defect to the S RNA of the lymphocytic choriomeningitis virus genome. Virology 1985;142:175–182.

240. Riviere Y, Ahmed R, Southern PJ, Buchmeier MJ, Dutko FJ, Oldstone MB. The S RNA segment of lymphocytic choriomeningitis virus codes for the nucleoprotein and glycoproteins 1 and 2. J Virol 1985;53:966–968.

241. Riviere Y, Gresser I, Guillon JC, et al. Severity of lymphocytic choriomeningitis virus disease in different strains of suckling mice correlates with increasing amounts of endogenous interferon. J Exp Med 1980;152:633–640.

242. Rodriguez M, Buchmeier MJ, Oldstone MB, Lampert PW. Ultrastructural localization of viral antigens in the CNS of mice persistently infected with lymphocytic choriomeningitis virus (LCMV). Am J Pathol 1983;110:95–100.

243. Rodriguez M, von Wedel RJ, Garrett RS, Lampert PW, Oldstone MB. Pituitary dwarfism in mice persistently infected with lymphocytic choriomeningitis virus. Lab Invest 1983;49:48–53.

244. Romanowski V, Bishop DH. Conserved sequences and coding of two strains of lymphocytic choriomeningitis virus (WE and ARM) and Pichinde arenavirus. Virus Res 1985;2:35–51.

245. Romanowski V, Matsuura Y, Bishop DH. Complete sequence of the S RNA of lymphocytic choriomeningitis virus (WE strain) compared to that of Pichinde arenavirus. Virus Res 1985;3:101–114.

246. Roost H, Charan S, Gobet R, et al. An acquired immune suppression in mice caused by infection with lymphocytic choriomeningitis virus. Eur J Immunol 1988;18:511–518.

247. Rowe WP. Research report. NM 005048.14.01. Bethesda, MD: Naval Medical Research Institute, 1954.

248. Rowe WP, Black PH, Levey RH. Protective effect of neonatal thymectomy on mouse LCM infection. Proc Soc Exp Biol Med 1963;114:248–251.

249. Ruedi E, Hengartner H, Zinkernagel RM. Immunosuppression in mice by lymphocytic choriomeningitis virus infection: time dependence during primary and absence of effects on secondary antibody responses. Cell Immunol 1990;130:501–512.

250. Salvato MS. Molecular biology of the prototype arenavirus, lymphocytic choriomeningitis virus. In: Salvato MS, ed. The arenaviridae. New York: Plenum Press, 1993:133–156.

251. Salvato MS, Borrow P, Shimomaye E, Oldstone MB. Molecular basis of viral persistence: a single amino acid change in the glycoprotein of lymphocytic choriomeningitis virus is associated with suppression of the antiviral cytotoxic T-lymphocyte response and establishment of persistence. J Virol 1991;65:1863–1869.

252. Salvato MS, Shimomaye EM. The completed sequence of lymphocytic choriomeningitis virus reveals a unique RNA structure and a gene for a zinc finger protein. Virology 1989;173:1–10.

253. Salvato MS, Shimomaye E, Oldstone MB. The primary structure of the lymphocytic choriomeningitis virus L gene encodes a putative RNA polymerase. Virology 1989;169:377–384.

254. Salvato MS, Shimomaye EM, Southern PJ, Oldstone MBA. Virus-lymphocyte interactions. IV. Molecular characteristics of LCMV Armstrong (CTL$^+$) small genomic segment and that of its variant, clone 13 (CTL$^-$). Virology 1988;164:517–522.

255. Saron MF, Colle JH, Dautry-Varsat A, Truffa-Bachi P. Activated T lymphocytes from mice infected by lymphocytic choriomeningitis virus display high affinity IL-2 receptors but do not proliferate in response to IL-2. J Immunol 1991;147:4333–4337.

256. Saron MF, Shidani B, Nahori MA, Guillon JC, Truffa-Bachi P. Lymphocytic choriomeningitis virus-induced immunodepression: inherent defect of B and T lymphocytes. J Virol 1990;64:4076–4083.

257. Schulz M, Aichele P, Schneider R, Hansen TH, Zinkernagel RM, Hengartner H. Major histocompatibility complex binding and T cell recognition of a viral nonapeptide containing a minimal tetrapeptide. Eur J Immunol 1991;21:1181–1185.

258. Schulz M, Aichele P, Vollenweider M, et al. Major histocompatibility complex-dependent T cell epitopes of lymphocytic choriomeningitis virus nucleoprotein and their protective capacity against viral disease. Eur J Immunol 1989;19:1657–1667.

259. Schwartz RH. A cell culture model for T lymphocyte clonal anergy. Science 1990;248:1349–1356.

260. Schwendemann G, Lohler J, Lehmann-Grube F. Evidence for cytotoxic T-lymphocyte-target cell interaction in brains of mice infected intracerebrally with lymphocytic choriomeningitis virus. Acta Neuropathol 1983;61:183–195.

261. Schwimmbeck PL, Dyrberg T, Oldstone MB. Abrogation of diabetes in BB rats by acute virus infection: association of viral-lymphocyte interactions. J Immunol 1988;140:3394–3400.

262. Scott TFM, Rivers TM. Meningitis in man caused by filterable virus: 2 cases and method of obtaining virus from their spinal fluids. J Exp Med 1936;63:397–414.

263. Selin LK, Nahill SR, Welsh RM. Cross-reactivities in memory cytotoxic T lymphocyte recognition of heterologous viruses. J Exp Med 1994;179:1933–1943.

264. Shyp S, Tishon A, Oldstone MB. Inhibition of diabetes in BB rats by virus infection. II. Effect of virus infection on the immune response to non-viral and viral antigens. Immunology 1990;69:501–507.

265. Silberman SL, Jacobs RP, Cole GA. Mechanisms of hemopoietic and immunological dysfunction induced by lymphocytic choriomeningitis virus. Infect Immun 1978;19:533–539.

266. Singh MK, Fuller-Pace FV, Buchmeier MJ, Southern PJ. Analysis of the genomic L RNA segment from lymphocytic choriomeningitis virus. Virology 1987;161:448–456.

267. Slifka MK, Matloubian M, Ahmed R. Bone marrow is a major site of long-term antibody production after acute viral infection. J Virol 1995;69:1895–1902.

268. Southern PJ. Arenaviruses: the viruses and their replication. In: Fields BN, Knipe DM, Howley PM, eds. Fields virology. 3rd ed. Philadelphia: Lippincott-Raven, 1996:1505–1519.

269. Southern PJ, Blount P, Oldstone MBA. Analysis of persistent virus infections by in situ hybridization to whole-mouse sections. Nature 1984;312:555–558.

270. Southern PJ, Buchmeier MJ, Ahmed R, et al. Molecular pathogenesis of arenavirus infections. In: Brown F, Chanock RM, Lerner RA, eds. New approaches to immunization. New York: Cold Spring Harbor Laboratory Press, 1986:239–245.

271. Southern PJ, Singh MK, Riviere Y, Jacoby DR, Buchmeier MJ, Oldstone MB. Molecular characterization of the genomic S RNA segment from lymphocytic choriomeningitis virus. Virology 1987;157:145–155.

272. Steinhauer DA, Holland JJ. Rapid evolution of RNA viruses. Annu Rev Microbiol 1987;41:409–433.

273. Stellrecht KA, Vella AT. Evidence for polyclonal B cell activation as the mechanism for LCMV-induced autoimmune hemolytic anemia. Immunol Lett 1992;31:273–277.

274. Stellrecht-Broomhall KA. Evidence for immune-mediated destruction as mechanism for LCMV-induced anemia in persistently infected mice. Viral Immunol 1991;4:269–280.

275. Su HC, Leite-Morris KA, Braun L, Biron CA. A role for transforming growth factor-beta 1 in regulating natural killer cell and T lymphocyte proliferative responses during acute infection with lymphocytic choriomeningitis virus. J Immunol 1991;147:2717–2727.

276. Teng MN, Borrow P, Oldstone MBA, de la Torre JC. A single amino acid change in the glycoprotein of lymphocytic choriomeningitis virus is associated with the ability to cause growth hormone deficiency syndrome. 1996 (submitted for publication).

277. Thomsen AR, Bro-Jorgensen K, Jensen BL. Lymphocytic choriomeningitis virus-induced immunosuppression: evidence for viral interference with T-cell maturation. Infect Immun 1982;37:981–986.

278. Thomsen AR, Marker O. The complementary roles of cellular and humoral immunity in resistance to re-infection with LCM virus. Immunology 1988;65:9–15.

279. Thomsen AR, Marker O. MHC and non-MHC genes regulate elimination of lymphocytic choriomeningitis virus and antiviral cytotoxic T lymphocyte and delayed-type hypersensitivity mediating T lymphocyte activity in parallel. J Immunol 1989;142:1333–1341.

280. Thomsen AR, Pisa P, Bro-Jorgensen K, Kiessling R. Mechanisms of lymphocytic choriomeningitis virus-induced hemopoietic dysfunction. J Virol 1986;59:428–433.

281. Thomsen AR, Volkert M, Marker O. The timing of the immune response in relation to virus growth determines the outcome of the LCM infection. Acta Pathologica et Microbiologica Scandinavica 1979;87:47–54.

282. Thomsen AR, Volkert M, Marker O. Different isotype profiles of virus-specific antibodies in acute and persistent lymphocytic choriomeningitis virus infection in mice. Immunology 1985;55:213–223.

283. Tishon A, Borrow P, Evans C, Oldstone MB. Virus-induced immunosuppression. 1. Age at infection relates to a selective or generalized defect. Virology 1993;195:397–405.

284. Tishon A, Lewicki H, Rall G, Von Herrath M, Oldstone MB. An essential role for type 1 interferon-gamma in terminating persistent viral infection. Virology 1995;212:244–250.

285. Tishon A, Oldstone MB. Persistent virus infection associated with chemical manifestations of diabetes. II. Role of viral strain, environmental insult, and host genetics. Am J Pathol 1987;126:61–72.

286. Tishon A, Oldstone MB. Perturbation of differentiated functions during viral infection in vivo: in vivo relationship of host genes and lymphocytic choriomeningitis virus to growth hormone deficiency. Am J Pathol 1990;137:965–969.

287. Tishon A, Salmi A, Ahmed R, Oldstone MB. Role of viral strains and host genes in determining levels of immune complexes in a model system: implications for HIV infection. AIDS Res Hum Retroviruses 1991;7:963–969.

288. Tishon A, Southern PJ, Oldstone MB. Virus-lymphocyte interactions. II. Expression of viral sequences during the course of persistent lymphocytic choriomeningitis virus infection and their localization to the L3T4 lymphocyte subset. J Immunol 1988;140:1280–1284.

289. Tonietti G, Oldstone MBA, Dixon FJ. The effect of induced chronic viral infections on the immunologic diseases of New Zealand mice. J Exp Med 1970;132:89–109.

290. Tough DF, Borrow P, Sprent J. Intense bystander proliferation of T cells in vivo induced by viruses and type I interferon. Science 1996 (in press).

291. Traub E. Persistence of lymphocytic choriomeningitis virus in immune animals and its relation to immunity. J Exp Med 1936;63:847–861.

292. Valsamakis A, Riviere Y, Oldstone MB. Perturbation of differentiated functions in vivo during persistent viral infection. III. Decreased growth hormone mRNA. Virology 1987;156:214–220.

293. van den Broek MF, Muller U, Huang S, Aguet M, Zinkernagel RM. Antiviral defense in mice lacking both alpha/beta and gamma interferon receptors. J Virol 1995;69:4792–4796.

294. Vella AT, Pfau CJ. The presence of an anti-erythrocyte autoantibody in C3HeB/FeJ mice after lymphocytic choriomeningitis virus infection. Autoimmunity 1991;9:319–329.

295. Villarete L, de Fries R, Kolhekar S, Howard D, Ahmed R, Wu-Hsieh B. Impaired responsiveness to gamma interferon of macrophages infected with lymphocytic choriomeningitis virus clone 13: susceptibility to histoplasmosis. Infect Immun 1995;63:1468–1472.

296. Villarete L, Somasundaram T, Ahmed R. Tissue-mediated selection of viral variants: correlation between glycoprotein mutation and growth in neuronal cells. J Virol 1994;68:7490–7496.

297. Volkert M, Larsen JH. Studies on immunological tolerance to LCM virus. 3. Duration and maximal effect of adoptive immunization of virus carriers. Acta Pathologica et Microbiologica Scandinavica 1964;60:577–587.

298. Von Herrath MG, Dockter J, Oldstone MBA. How virus induces a rapid or slow onset insulin-dependent diabetes mellitus in a transgenic model. Immunity 1994;1:231–242.

299. Von Herrath MG, Evans CF, Horwitz MS, Oldstone MBA. Novel transgenic mouse models to dissect the pathogenesis of virus-induced autoimmune disorders of the islets of Langerhans and central nervous system. Immunol Rev 1996. In Press.

300. Von Herrath MG, Guerder S, Lewicki H, Flavell RA, Oldstone MBA. Coexpression of B7-1 and viral ("self") transgenes in pancreatic b cells can break peripheral ignorance and lead to spontaneous autoimmune diabetes. Immunity 1995;3:727–738.

301. Von Herrath MG, Yokoyama M, Dockter J, Oldstone MBA, Whitton JL. CD4-deficient mice have reduced levels of memory cytotoxic T lymphocytes after immunization and show diminished resistance to subsequent virus challenge. J Virol 1996;70:1072–1079.

302. Walker DH, Murphy FA. Pathology and pathogenesis of arenavirus infections. Curr Top Microbiol Immunol 1987;133:89–113.

303. Walsh CM, Matloubian M, Liu CC, et al. Immune function in mice lacking the perforin gene. Proc Natl Acad Sci U S A 1994;91:10854–10858.

304. Welsh RM. Natural killer cells and interferon. Crit Rev Immunol 1984;5:55–93.

305. Welsh RM. Regulation and role of large granular lymphocytes in arenavirus infections. Curr Top Microbiol Immunol 1996;134:185–209.

306. Welsh RM, Kiessling RW. Natural killer cell response to lymphocytic choriomeningitis virus in beige mice. Scand J Immunol 1980;11:363–367.

307. Welsh RM, Tay CH, Varga SM, O'Donnell CL, Vergilis KL, Selin LK. Lymphocyte-dependent "natural" immunity to virus infections mediated by both natural killer cells and memory T cells. Semin Virol 1996;7:95–102.

308. Welsh RM, Zinkernagel RM. Heterospecific cytotoxic cell activity induced during the first three days of acute lymphocytic choriomeningitis virus infection in mice. Nature 1977;268:646–648.

309. Welsh RM Jr. Cytotoxic cells induced during lymphocytic choriomeningitis virus infection of mice. I. Characterization of natural killer cell induction. J Exp Med 1978;148:163–181.

310. Whitton JL. Lymphocytic choriomeningitis virus CTL. Semin Virol 1990;1:257–262.

311. Whitton JL, Gebhard JR, Lewicki H, Tishon A, Oldstone MB. Molecular definition of a major cytotoxic T-lymphocyte epitope in the glycoprotein of lymphocytic choriomeningitis virus. J Virol 1988;62:687–695.

312. Whitton JL, Oldstone MBA. Class I MHC can present an endogenous peptide to cytotoxic T lymphocytes. J Exp Med 1989;170:1033–1038.

313. Whitton JL, Southern PJ, Oldstone MB. Analyses of the cytotoxic T lymphocyte responses to glycoprotein and nucleoprotein components of lymphocytic choriomeningitis virus. Virology 1988;162:321–327.

314. Whitton JL, Tishon A, Lewicki H, et al. Molecular analyses of a five-amino-acid cytotoxic T-lymphocyte (CTL) epitope: an immunodominant region which induces nonreciprocal CTL cross-reactivity. J Virol 1989;63:4303–4310.

315. Wille A, Gessner A, Lohler H, Lehmann-Grube F. Mechanism of recovery from acute virus infection. VIII. Treatment of lymphocytic choriomeningitis virus-infected mice with anti-interferon-gamma monoclonal antibody blocks generation of virus-specific cytotoxic T lymphocytes and virus elimination. Eur J Immunol 1989;19:1283–1288.

316. Wilsnack RE, Rowe WP. Immunofluorescent studies of the histopathogenesis of lymphocytic choriomeningitis virus infection. J Exp Med 1964;120:829–840.

317. Woodrow D, Ronco P, Riviere Y, et al. Severity of glomerulonephritis induced in different strains of suckling mice by infection with lymphocytic choriomeningitis virus: correlation with amounts of endogenous interferon and circulating immune complexes. J Pathol 1982;138:325–336.

318. Wright KE, Buchmeier MJ. Antiviral antibodies attenuate T-cell-mediated immunopathology following acute lymphocytic choriomeningitis virus infection. J Virol 1991;65:3001–3006.

319. Wright KE, Spiro RC, Burns JW, Buchmeier MJ. Post-translational processing of the glycoproteins of lymphocytic choriomeningitis virus. Virology 1990;177:175–183.

320. Wu-Hsieh B, Howard DH, Ahmed R. Virus-induced immunosuppression: a murine model of susceptibility to opportunistic infection. J Infect Dis 1988;158:232–235.

321. Yang H, Dundon PL, Nahill SR, Welsh RM. Virus-induced polyclonal cytotoxic T lymphocyte stimulation. J Immunol 1989;142:1710–1718.

322. Zinkernagel RM, Doherty PC. Cytotoxic thymus derived lymphocytes in cerebrospinal fluid of mice with lymphocytic choriomeningitis. J Exp Med 1973;138:1266–1269.

323. Zinkernagel RM, Doherty PC. Restriction of in vitro T cell-mediated cytotoxicity in lymphocytic choriomeningitis within a syngeneic or semiallogeneic system. Nature 1974;248:701–702.

324. Zinkernagel RM, Doherty PC. Immunologic surveillance against altered self components by sensitized T lymphocytes in lymphocytic choriomeningitis. Nature 1974;251:547–548.

325. Zinkernagel RM, Doherty PC. MHC-restricted cytotoxic T cells: studies on the biological role of polymorphic major transplantation antigens determining T-cell restriction specificity, function, and responsiveness. Adv Immunol 1979;27:51–177.

326. Zinkernagel RM, Haenseler E, Leist T, Cerny A, Hengartner H, Althage A. T cell-mediated hepatitis in mice infected with lymphocytic choriomeningitis virus: liver cell destruction by H-2 class I-restricted virus-specific cytotoxic T cells as a physiological correlate of the 51Cr-release assay? J Exp Med 1986;164:1075–1092.

327. Zinkernagel RM, Leist T, Hengartner H, Althage A. Susceptibility to lymphocytic choriomeningitis virus isolates correlates directly with early and high cytotoxic T cell activity, as well as with footpad swelling reaction, and all three are regulated by H-2D. J Exp Med 1985;162:2125–2141.

328. Zinkernagel RM, Pfau CJ, Hengartner H, Althage A. Susceptibility to murine lymphocytic choriomeningitis maps to class I MHC genes: a model for MHC/disease associations. Nature 1985;316: 814–817.

329. Zinkernagel RM, Welsh RM. H-2 compatibility requirement for virus-specific T cell-mediated effector functions in vivo. I. Specificity of T cells conferring antiviral protection against lymphocytic choriomeningitis virus is associated with H-2K and H-2D. J Immunol 1976;117:1495–502.

Viral Pathogenesis,
edited by Neal Nathanson, et al.
Lippincott–Raven Publishers, Philadelphia © 1997

CHAPTER 26

Avian and Murine Retroviruses

Harriet L. Robinson, Alan Rein, and Nancy A. Speck

N. A. Speck: Department of Biochemistry, Dartmouth Medical School, Hanover, New Hampshire 21701.

H. L. Robinson: Department of Pathology, University of Massachusetts Medical Center, Worcester, Massachusetts 01655.

A. Rein: Frederick Cancer Research Center, Frederick, Maryland 21701.

HISTORICAL PERSPECTIVE

The foundations for contemporary retrovirology arose from experimental observations in avian and murine models. The ease and accessibility of these models provided researchers with the experimental materials that led to the discovery of tumor-causing viruses, reverse transcriptase, and oncogenes. Each of these advances was realized by visionary individuals, nourished by the environments of "cutting-edge" institutions and empowered by pioneering technologies. In 1911, Peyton Rous, working at the Rockefeller University, used the filter to demonstrate that solid tumors could be caused by a filtrable agent.[128] Reverse transcriptase was discovered in 1970 when Howard Temin (at the University of Wisconsin, Madison) and David Baltimore (at the Massachusetts Institute of Technol-

ogy) demonstrated that virions of Rous sarcoma virus and murine leukemia viruses contained RNA-dependent DNA polymerases.[5,146] This novel enzymatic activity, now known as reverse transcription, revolutionized ideas about the flow of genetic information and the potential interactions of "RNA tumor viruses" with the genomes of their host cells. In 1976, Michael Bishop and Harold Varmus, working together at the University of California at San Francisco, used reverse transcriptase to prepare a complementary DNA representing the transforming region of Rous sarcoma virus. This complementary DNA hybridized with normal cellular DNAs, demonstrating that the transforming region of Rous sarcoma virus was related to a host cell gene.[140] This conceptually elegant, yet technically simple, experiment revealed a host cell "proto-oncogene" being converted into an "oncogene" by incorporation into a virus. Each of these accomplishments was recognized with a Nobel prize, with Peyton Rous receiving the 1966[129]; Howard Temin and David Baltimore, the 1975[6,145]; and Michael Bishop and Harold Varmus, the 1989 laureate.[13,156]

ESSENTIAL BACKGROUND

An RNA Virus With a DNA Intermediate

Retroviruses are RNA viruses that reverse transcribe their RNA into viral DNA when they infect a cell. The viral DNA moves to the nucleus, where it undergoes integration into the chromosomal DNA of the host cell. The integrated viral DNA is called a *provirus*. Host cell RNA polymerase II transcribes a single RNA species from the proviral DNA. This RNA can become virion RNA or serve as a messenger RNA (mRNA) for the synthesis of viral proteins. For most retroviruses, assembly of progeny virions takes place at the plasma membrane during viral budding. In many cases, infected cells do not die, but continuously produce virus while undergoing normal growth and differentiation.

The Long Terminal Repeat, U5, and U3

The genomic RNA and proviral DNA of retroviruses have similar gene orders but dissimilar ends (Fig. 26-1). Genomic RNAs have unique sequences at their 5' and 3' ends called *U5* and *U3*. Proviral DNAs have long terminal repeats (LTRs) at their ends. The LTRs provide essential cis-acting sequences for the synthesis and integration of proviral DNA. They also provide essential transcriptional control elements for the expression of viral RNA from proviral DNA. The LTRs are synthesized from viral U5 and U3 sequences during reverse transcription (see Fig. 26-1). The synthesis of the LTR from the ends of viral RNA represents an elegant mechanism by which retroviruses provide the DNA form of their genetic information with the transcriptional control elements for RNA expression.

gag, *pol*, and *env*

The three main genes of retroviruses, *gag*, *pol*, and *env*, encode precursor polyproteins. These polyproteins are designated by the same three letters as the genes, with the first letter of the polyprotein being uppercase. *Gag* (group-specific antigens) encodes the internal structural proteins. *Env* (envelope) encodes the transmembrane protein that mediates the adsorption and penetration of virus into cells. *Pol* (polymerase) encodes two enzymes that mediate reverse transcription (reverse transcriptase) and proviral integration (integrase). Codons for a third enzyme, an aspartyl protease, lie between Gag and Pol and may be part of the Gag or Pol polyprotein. After virus release, the protease mediates maturational cleavages of the Gag, Pol, and, in certain instances, Env polyproteins.

BASIC STRUCTURE OF RETROVIRUSES

Retroviruses are enveloped viruses with electron-dense cores[30,54] (Fig. 26-2). Mature virions are 80 to 120 nm in diameter. The envelope is formed from the host cell plasma membrane during budding. Oligomeric envelope glycoproteins are present as knobbed spikes that protrude from the envelope. The ribonucleoprotein core contains two identical copies of genomic RNA. These range from 7.2 to 11 kilobases (kb) in size, depending on the genus of the virus. The viral particle carries the three essential viral enzymes: reverse transcriptase, integrase, and protease.

ORIGIN OF RETROVIRUSES

The phylogeny of reverse transcriptase–containing elements suggests that retroviruses evolved from ancient retrotransposons[41,98] (Fig. 26-3). Retrotransposons are elements capable of moving from one chromosomal location to another by reverse transcribing RNA to DNA. Descendants of ancient retrotransposons include contemporary retrotransposons (e.g., the copia elements of *Drosophila*), retroviruses (see later and Chaps. 27 and 35), hepadnaviruses (see Chap. 31), and the cauliflower mosaic family of DNA plant viruses.

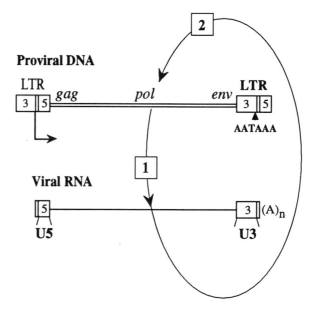

FIG. 26-1. Viral RNA and proviral DNA. Enzymatic steps in the production of viral RNA and proviral DNA are designated by numbers in boxes. (1) Host cell RNA polymerase II transcribes viral RNA from proviral DNA. This RNA is encapsidated into virus. The arrow with a right angle designates the transcription start site and AATAAA indicates the polyadenylation signal. (2) During the next round of infection, proviral DNA is produced from the viral RNA by reverse transcription and integration. During reverse transcription, unique sequences that form the 5´ and 3´ ends of viral RNA (U5 and U3, designated *5* and *3*) are duplicated to form the long terminal repeats (LTRs) that flank the integrated provirus (for details, see Fig. 26-10). The LTRs provide the transcriptional control elements necessary for the next cycle of viral RNA production by host cell RNA polymerase II. The narrow vertical rectangle between U3 and U5 in the LTR in proviral DNA, and flanking U5 and U3 in viral RNA, represents the R (repeat) sequence of viral RNA. The three basic genes of all retroviruses are *gag*, *pol*, and *env*.

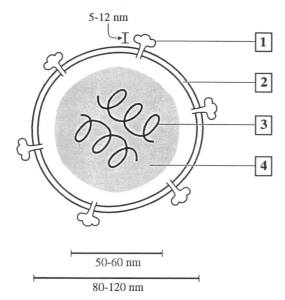

FIG. 26-2. A prototypic retroviral particle. The core structure is that of a type-C virus (see Fig. 26-4 for structures of other retroviruses). Important features are numbered in boxes. (1) Oligomeric forms of the envelope glycoprotein form knobbed spikes. These protrude 5 to 12 nm from the envelope of the virus. (2) The envelope, a lipid bilayer, is formed from the host cell plasma membrane during virus budding. (3) The electron-dense ribonucleoprotein core contains two identical copies of genomic RNA. These range from 7 to 11 kilobases in size. (4) The particles contain the three essential viral enzymes: reverse transcriptase, integrase, and protease.

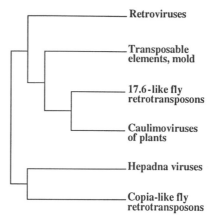

FIG. 26-3. Phylogeny of the reverse transcriptases of various eukaryotic elements. Retroviruses are one of several descendants of ancient retrotransposons that reverse transcribe their RNA to DNA. The 17.6 and copia elements are found in fruit flies. (Diagrammatic scale adapted from Mc-Clure MA. Evolutionary history of reverse transcriptase. In: Skalka AM, Goff SP, eds. Reverse transcriptase. Cold Spring Harbor, NY: Cold Spring Harbor Laboratory Press. 1993: 425–444; see also for a tree including more distantly related reverse transcriptase–containing elements [retroposons] and reverse transcriptase–encoding elements of bacteria [retrons]).

Genus	Representative Virus	Accessory Proteins	Virus Structure	Site of Assembly
Type-B	MMTV	Superantigen	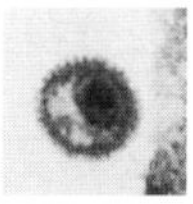	Cytoplasm
Type-C-MLV	MuLV	None	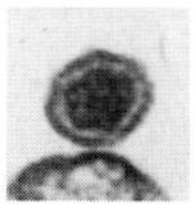	Plasma Membrane
Type-C-ALV	ALSV	None		Plasma Membrane
Type-D	MPMV	None	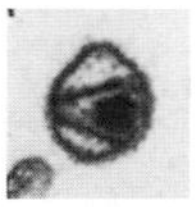	Cytoplasm
T-cell leukemia	HTLV-1	Tax, Rex	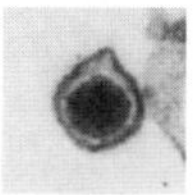	Plasma Membrane
Lentivirus	HIV-1	Vif, Vpr, Vpu, Tat, Rev, Nef	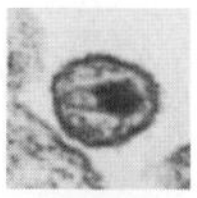	Plasma Membrane
Spumavirus	Human foamy virus	Bel-1, Bel-2, Bel-3	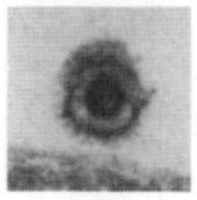	Cytoplasm

FIG. 26-4. Genera of retroviruses, characteristic accessory genes, and morphology. See text for background on classification. The micrographs present representative viral particles. The structures along the edges of the micrographs are plasma membrane surfaces of infected cells. "Site of assembly" refers to the site of core assembly. Notice the eccentric localization of the viral core in type B viruses, but not in other types of viruses. Also notice that the envelope glycoprotein spikes are seen most easily on the type B and spumaviruses. Type A particles are not included in the figure because these agents are replication-defective. Type A particles occur inside cells and do not bud from cells. MLV, murine leukemia virus; ALV, avian leukosis virus; MMTV, mouse mammary tumor virus; MuLV, the murine leukemia viruses discussed in this chapter; ALSV, the avian leukosis-sarcoma viruses discussed in this chapter; MPMV, Mason-Pfizer monkey virus; HTLV-1, human T-cell leukemia virus type 1; HIV-1, human immunodeficiency virus type 1. (Adapted from Coffin JM. Structure and classification of retroviruses. In: Levy JA, ed. The retroviridae. Vol 1. New York: Plenum Press, 1992:19–49.)

GENERA, SUBGENERA, AND GROUPS (SPECIES) OF RETROVIRUSES

Genera

Retroviruses are classified into seven genera on the basis of their genetic structures and sequence relationships[30] (Fig. 26-4). The retroviruses featured in this chapter belong to two genera: the type C murine leukemia viruses (MLVs) and the type C avian leukosis viruses (ALVs). The genomes of both these genera are limited to *gag*, *pol*, and *env* genes. Most other genera of retroviruses encode additional "accessory" proteins (see Fig. 26-4). The type C MLV and ALV viruses are placed in different genera based on sequence differences.[30]

Subgenera

The type C MLV genus includes three subgenera: mammalian type C viruses, reptilian type C viruses, and avian reticuloendotheliosis viruses. The use of *MLV* to designate a genus that includes mammalian, reptilian, and avian viruses reflects the historical importance of research with MLVs. This chapter addresses the mammalian type C virus subgenus of the type C MLV genus. Particular emphasis is placed on the murine leukemia virus (MuLV) group (or species) of the mammalian type C virus subgenus. Other groups of the mammalian type C virus subgenus include feline leukemia viruses (an endemic virus of household cats) and gibbon ape leukemia viruses.[30] The type C ALV genus includes only the avian leukosis sarcoma viruses (ALSVs) discussed in this chapter.

Historical Use of Structure for Classification

Before recombinant DNA technology allowed the classification of viruses by their sequence and genome structures, electron micrographs were used to classify retroviruses.[11,30] Type C viruses have centrally placed spherical (potentially icosahedral) cores. Type C viruses are first visualized in infected cells as they assemble during virus budding through the plasma membrane. Types A, B, and D, and more recently described morphologies associated with T-cell leukemia viruses and lentiviruses have other core structures, sites of particle assembly, or both[30,54] (see Fig. 26-4).

SUBGROUPS AND SUBTYPES OF RETROVIRUSES, THE IMPORTANCE OF RECEPTOR USAGE, AND THE PHENOMENON OF INTERFERENCE TO SUBGROUP CLASSIFICATION

Receptor-Based Subgroups: Use of Interference To Establish Receptor Usage

Each species (or group) of retroviruses is classified into subgroups on the basis of receptor usage. All members of a subgroup have envelope glycoproteins that use the same host cell receptor (see later). Receptor specificity is defined in tissue culture by a phenomenon called *viral interference*.[159,164]

Interference assays score whether a virus can superinfect cells previously infected with a virus of a known subgroup. Mechanistically, interference is mediated by the envelope glycoproteins of the preinfecting virus blocking the availability of receptors for the superinfecting virus. This block is receptor-specific. MuLVs belong to five different subgroups based on their patterns of receptor specificities. The ALSVs are classified into more than five different interference groups.

Subtypes

Each subgroup of retroviruses is classified further into subtypes. These subtypes represent envelope glycoproteins that use the same receptor but are blocked by different neutralizing antibodies. Subtypes of viruses can have substantial variation in the sequence of their envelope glycoproteins.

THE RETROVIRUS LIFE CYCLE: TIMING OF DNA, RNA, AND PROTEIN SYNTHESIS; ESTABLISHMENT OF CHRONIC VIRUS PRODUCERS; THE PRODUCED VIRUS

Establishing the Infection

Important steps in the retrovirus life cycle are entry, reverse transcription, integration of proviral DNA, and expression of proviral DNA (Fig. 26-5). These steps are accomplished within the time frame of a cell cycle. The first step, entry, reflects envelope-mediated binding and fusion of the virus with its target cell. Binding and post-binding fusion usually are rapid events. The next well-defined step of the virus life cycle is reverse transcription. The synthesis of the linear form of a complete provirus requires about 2 hours.[155] After reverse transcription, there is a several-hour lag (8 to 16 hours) before substantial proviral function is realized. This lag reflects the time required for the DNA-containing "preintegration complex" to gain access to and integrate into chromosomal DNA.[21] For MuLV and ALSV, mitosis, with its attendant breakdown of the nuclear membrane, is required for this access. Once the provirus is formed, viral protein synthesis occurs according to time frames associated with the transcription and translation of normal cell proteins. Gag proteins rapidly move to the plasma membrane, where they are incorporated into mature virions within 15 minutes from the time of synthesis.[3,160] Env proteins, which are routed through the rough endoplasmic reticulum and Golgi for glycosylation, require 1 to 2 hours to appear in virions.[45,75]

Chronic Virus Production

Once viral proteins are expressed by the integrated provirus, the infected cell enters a phase of chronic virus production. As chronic virus production is established, newly synthesized envelope glycoproteins establish interference. This limits superinfection and prevents potentially lethal mutations of the infected cell by continuing proviral insertions. The establishment of interference also limits the number of proviruses with which a cell has to share its synthetic machinery.

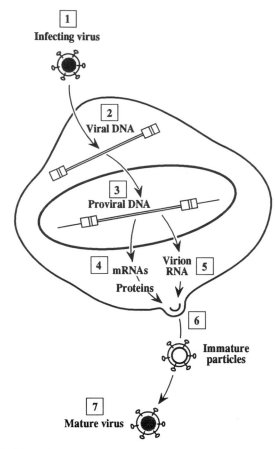

FIG. 26-5. Retroviral life cycle. Steps in the life cycle are represented by the numbers in boxes. (1) The virus envelope spikes interact with host cell receptors to mediate entry and release of the core structure into the cytoplasm. (2) The reverse transcriptase enzyme of the virus copies viral RNA into viral DNA, destroying the RNA in the process. (3) The viral DNA moves to the nucleus, where the viral integrase mediates integration to form proviral DNA. (4) The provirus is transcribed by host cell RNA polymerase II, producing mRNAs. A Gag-Pol mRNA is translated into Gag and Gag-Pol precursor polyproteins. An Env mRNA produces envelope glycoproteins. (5) The provirus also is transcribed to produce virion RNA. (6) The Gag precursor polyprotein localizes to the plasma membrane, where it mediates virion assembly and budding. (7) Maturation of the core structure occurs as the viral protease cleaves the Gag and Gag-Pol precursor polyproteins to their mature products. Once step 3 is accomplished, the infected cell enters a state of chronic virus production.

This is not a trivial consideration, because retroviruses have highly active transcriptional control elements.

Produced Virus

During the phase of chronic virus production, infected cells continuously produce from 1000 to 10,000 virus particles per day. Most of this virus never initiates an infection, with stocks containing many more physical particles (frequently 1000

times more) than infectious particles. The retroviruses present in a stock are a "quasispecies" (mixture) of closely related but nonidentical genomes. The average base substitution rate during reverse transcription is about 1×10^{-4} nucleotides (nt) per reverse transcription cycle.[8] This means that essentially every provirus carries one or more bases that are distinct from those of the infecting virion. The high error rate of reverse transcriptase is accentuated by frequent recombinational events between copackaged RNAs[72,158] (see Fig. 26-2 and later in this text). The high mutation and recombination rates provide a broad base of genetic variants that can undergo selection in infected hosts.

STRUCTURE AND FUNCTION OF ENVELOPE GLYCOPROTEINS

Conserved Features of Env Structure

The glycoproteins of retroviruses are comprised of a globular surface subunit (SU) that mediates receptor binding and a transmembrane anchor subunit (TM) that mediates fusion.[50,51,75] The glycoproteins of retroviruses have several conserved features[50,51] (Fig. 26-6A and B). All SU subunits have an N-terminal signal sequence and a C-terminal protease cleavage site. The signal sequence routes the Env polyprotein through the endoplasmic reticulum. The protease cleavage site (several basic amino acids) supports maturational cleavage of the Env to SU and TM by host cell proteases (see later). Internal to the SU subunit are two conserved turns ("hinge" regions). These are likely to support the formation of loops that contribute to SU function. All retroviral TM subunits contain two conserved hydrophobic regions. The first of these, at or near the N-terminus, is the fusion peptide. The second, an internal region, serves as a membrane anchor. Adjacent to the fusion domain is an ~60-amino acid (aa) region with the potential for forming extended helices. This conserved helical region is likely to play a role in structural transitions of the envelope spike.

Env Synthesis

Oligomers of Env precursor polyproteins assemble in the rough endoplasmic reticulum.[75] Host cell proteases (e.g., furan) cleave the polyproteins to SU and TM within the oligomer. The fusion domain is sequestered within the oligomer. The oligomers are transported to the plasma membrane for incorporation into particles. For mammalian type C viruses, the viral protease mediates a final maturational cleavage of TM in the particle.[33,81,116,120]

Two Functional Forms of Env Spikes

Different forms of the envelope spike mediate binding and post-binding fusion.[97] The binding form of the spike is the knobbed form of the spike seen on mature virions (see Figs. 26-4 and 26-6C). Post-binding entry is dependent on the transition of the binding form of the spike to a fusion form. Formation of the fusion form requires both unmasking of TM and structural changes in TM. Such a scenario can be envisioned as

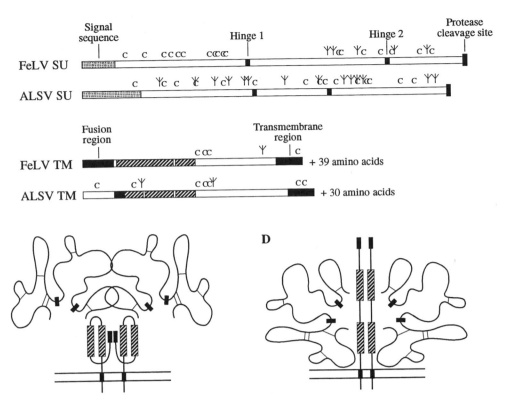

FIG. 26-6. Retroviral envelope glycoproteins. (**A** and **B**) Schematics highlighting conserved features in the SU and TM subunits of Env. The feline leukemia virus (FeLV) Env is used to represent its related murine leukemia virus Env. Conserved domains in SU include a leader sequence, two strong turns (hinge regions), and a recognition site for cellular proteases to cleave the Env precursor into SU and TM. Conserved regions in TM include two hydrophobic regions (*filled bars*): the fusion peptide and a transmembrane region. Sequences with the potential to form extended helices (*hatched bars*) are found adjacent to the fusion domain. The *forks* indicate glycosylation sites. C, cysteine residue; ALSV, avian leukosis-sarcoma virus. (**A, B** adapted from Gallaher WR, Ball JM, Garry RF, et al. A general model for the _surface glycoproteins of HIV and other retroviruses. AIDS Res and Human Retro 1995;11:191–202, and Gallaher WR, Ball JM, Garry RF, et al. A general model for the transmembrane proteins of HIV and other retroviruses. AIDS Res and Human Retro 1989;5:431–440.) (**C**) A schematic representing a hypothetical receptor-binding form of an Env spike. Notice the apical position of the SU binding domain and sequestration of the fusion region of TM. (**D**) A schematic representing a hypothetical fusion form of an Env spike. Notice the unmasking and erection of the fusion domain. The erection is stabilized by interactions between the conserved helices. The conserved regions in **C** and **D** have the same highlights as in **A** and **B**. Cross-lines within an SU loop represent disulfide bonds. For simplicity, two rather than three or four subunits of Env are included in the spike schematic. (**C, D** adapted from one of the possible forms of spikes in Mathews TJ, Wild C, Chen C-H, et al. Structural rearrangements in the transmembrane glycoprotein after receptor binding. Immun Rev 1994;140:93–104.)

displacement of SU accompanied by an erection of the fusion domain (see Fig. 26-6*D*). At this point, it is not known whether fusion requires additional cellular accessory molecules.

HOST CELL RECEPTORS AND HOST RANGE

Receptors and Host Range

Retroviruses use many different host cell molecules as receptors (Fig. 26-7). These define the host range and the tissue

tropism of the virus. Each group of viruses consists of subgroups that use different receptors. Each subgroup has a characteristic host range and tissue tropism that is defined by the presence and tissue distribution of its receptors.

Murine Leukemia Virus Subgroups and Receptors

Interference assays have identified five subgroups of MuLVs[165] (Table 26-1). Three of these subgroups use receptors with multiple membrane-spanning domains that normally

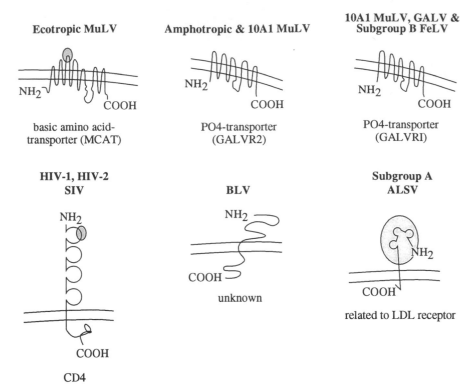

FIG. 26-7. Cellular receptors for retroviruses. Schematics indicate hypothetical structures. For some receptors, the binding regions for Env have been mapped (*shaded circles*). Two different members of the family of phosphate transporters are used by murine leukemia viruses (MuLVs). The 10A1 MuLV uses a receptor related to the receptors used by the gibbon ape leukemia virus (GALV) and subgroup B feline leukemia viruses (FeLVs). This receptor is termed GALVR1. The 10A1 virus also uses a second phosphate transporter, designated GALVR2 (see Table 26-1). Amphotropic MuLVs also use GALVR2 as their receptor. See Tables 26-1 and 26-2 and the text for more information and discussion of the evolutionary relation of receptors and subgroups of avian leukosis-sarcoma viruses (ALSVs) and MuLVs. MCAT, murine cationic amino acid transporter; BLV, bovine leukemia virus; HIV-1 and HIV-2, human immunodeficiency viruses; SIV, simian immunodeficiency virus. (Adapted from Weiss RA. Cellular receptors and viral glycoproteins involved in retrovirus entry. In: Levy JA, ed. The retroviridae. Vol 2. New York: Plenum Press 1993:1–108, and Coffin JM. Retroviridae: the viruses and their replication. In: Fields BN, Knipe DM, Howley PM, eds. Virology. 3rd ed. Philadelphia: Lippincott-Raven 1996:1767–1847.)

TABLE 26-1. *Subgroups and receptors for murine leukemia viruses*

Subgroup*	Origin†	Receptor locus	Receptor±	Host range
Ecotropic	Exogenous, endogenous	*Rec-1*	Basic amino acid transporter (MCAT-1)	Only rodents
MCF	Recombinant between ecotroic and endogenous	*Rmc-1‡*	Not known	Relative infectivities for rodents and non-rodents vary
Amphotropic	Exogenous, found in wild mice	*Ram-1*	PO4 transporter (GALVR2)	Rodents and non-rodents
10A1	Recombinant between amphotropic and endogenous	(1) *Ram-1* (2) Not mapped	(1) PO4 transporter (GALVR2) (2) PO4 transporter (GALVR1)	Rodents and non-rodents
Xenotropic	Endogenous	*Rmc-1‡*	Not known	Non-murine rodents, some wild mice

*The designations ecotropic, amphotropic, and xenotropic are derived from Greek. Ecotropic refers to infection of cells from one's own species; xenotropic, to infection of cells from other species; and amphotropic, to the ability to infect cells from one's own and other species.[91] MCF stands for mink cell focus-forming virus. This reflects the cells on which MCFs originally were detected.[65]

†For exogenous and endogenous origin, see text.

‡MCF and xenotropic subgroups use different alleles of *Rmc-1*.

±Acronyms in parentheses give designations for receptors. MCAT indicates the murine cationic amino acid transporter. GALVR denotes the gibbon ape leukemia virus receptor.

transport small molecules into cells[36] (see Fig. 26-7, *top row*). The receptor for ecotropic MuLVs transports basic amino acids into cells.[36] The receptors used by amphotropic and 10A1 MuLVs transport phosphate.[36,103,154] One of these phosphate transporters is the murine homolog of receptors used by two other mammalian type C viruses: gibbon ape leukemia virus and subgroup B feline leukemia viruses.[110,144,165] Receptors for the mink cell focus-forming virus (MCF) and xenotropic subgroups have not been identified. However, these receptors are allelic, because both map to the same genetic locus.[84]

Avian Leukosis Sarcoma Virus Subgroups and Receptors

Receptors for the five best-studied subgroups of ALSV map to three different loci. These are designated tumor virus (*tv*) *tva*, *tvb*, and *tvc*[165] (Table 26-2). Subgroup A viruses use receptors encoded at the *tva* locus. Subgroups B, D, and E viruses use different alleles or combinations of alleles of the *tvb* locus. Subgroup C viruses use receptors encoded at *tvc*. Only the product of the *tva* locus is known. This transmembrane protein has some homology to the low-density lipoprotein receptor[7,169] (see Fig. 26-7).

Diversity of Retroviral Receptors

Several generalizations can be made from a consideration of known retroviral receptors (see Fig. 26-7). First, receptors for different groups of viruses can have different structures. Only one feature is common to all the receptors: display on the surface of host cells. This diversity of receptor structure contrasts with the relatively conserved structures of retrovirus envelope glycoproteins (see Fig. 26-6*A* and *B*). This suggests that retroviral receptors may serve only to bind virus to cells, with post-binding fusion being mediated by the more conserved viral envelope glycoproteins.

Use of "Similar" Receptors by "Related" Viruses

A second interesting phenomenon is the use of similar receptors by related viruses. For example, subgroups of each of the three groups of mammalian type C viruses use the "GALVRI" host cell phosphate transporter as a receptor (Fig. 26-7). Three subgroups of ALSV (B, D, and E) use receptors that are encoded by different alleles of a single chicken locus (see Table 26-2). The MCF and xenotropic MuLVs use receptors that are alleles of the same murine locus (see Table 26-1).

The use of similar receptors by related viruses is likely to reflect Env-mediated interference selecting for variant viruses with envelope glycoproteins that can use different, yet related, receptors. An example of an Env that has evolved toward the use of a new receptor is found in the 10A1 recombinant (see Table 26-1). The 10A1 virus is a recombinant between amphotropic and endogenous MuLVs. 10A1 is able to use two different host cell PO4 transporters as receptors (see Fig. 26-7). Only one of these also is used by the amphotropic parent of 10A1. 10A1 exemplifies an amphotropic Env that has adapted to use a new phosphate transporter as a receptor.

Viral Selection of Hosts for "Resistant" Receptors

A third phenomenon is the apparent selection by retroviruses of their hosts for alternate forms of receptors. These "new" forms frequently are alleles of the original receptor. The new alleles presumably perform their essential host function, but no longer serve as a receptor for the "selecting" infection. Examples of this are found for the receptors for two relatively ancient infections of mice and chickens: the xenotropic MuLVs and the subgroup E ALVs (see Tables 26-1 and 26-2). Xenotropic virus receptors are present in essentially all rodents except mice (see Table 26-1). Similarly, subgroup E virus receptors are present in turkeys and quail, but are rare in chickens (see Table 26-2). The loci harboring both these receptors have multiple alleles. For fowl, the new alleles are limited to chickens (the host under selection). Discouragingly, for both mice and chickens, these "recent" alleles have

TABLE 26-2. *Subgroups and receptors for avian leukosis sarcoma viruses*

Subgroup*	Origin†	Receptor locus	Receptor	Host range±
A	Exogenous	*tva*	Transmembrane protein with LDL-like domain	Chickens, quail, turkeys
B	Exogenous	*tvb*‡	Unknown	Chickens
C	Exogenous	*tvc*	Unknown	Chickens, turkeys, ducks
D	Exogenous	*tvb*‡	Unknown	Chickens
E	Endogenous	*tvb*‡	Unknown	Quail, turkeys occasional chicken

*Five additional subgroups of avian leukosis viruses have been found in exogenous avian leukosis sarcoma viruses (ALSVs) (subgroup J) or recombinants between exogenous ALSVs and endogenous viruses of game birds (subgroups F, G, H, and I).[165]
†For exogenous and endogenous origins, see text.
‡Subgroups B, D, and E use different alleles or combinations of alleles at the *tvb* locus.[20,165]
±Only species with strong susceptibility are listed. For a more detailed consideration, see reference 165.
LDL, low-density lipoprotein.

A

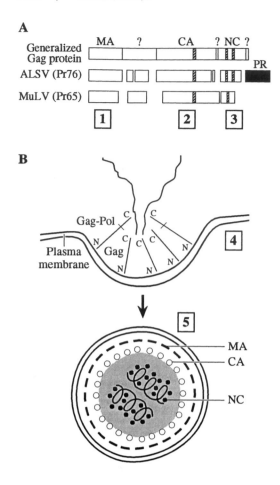

FIG. 26-8. Gag polyprotein structure and function in assembly. **(A)** Schematic designating subunits and functional domains in Gag precursor polyproteins. **(B)** Schematic depicting the function of the Gag and Gag-Pol polyproteins in assembly. (1) The N-terminal matrix (MA) region of Gag. For the murine leukemia virus (MuLV), modification of this region by myristylation provides part of the signal for localization at the plasma membrane. Sequences near the N-terminus of the avian leukosis-sarcoma (ALSV) Gag polyprotein also are important for localization at the plasma membrane. These sequences are acetylated. (2) The capsid (CA) region of the Gag polyprotein. A highly conserved region critical to assembly is highlighted by hatching. This region is called the MHR, or major homology region. (3) The nucleocapsid (NC) region of Gag. Zinc finger motifs embedded in basic residues are highlighted by hatching. These motifs play essential roles in encapsidation and infectivity. For ALSV, but not MuLV, protease (PR) is encoded in the Gag polyprotein. The question mark denotes nonconserved regions in Gag that have not been named. (4) Alignment of Gag and Gag-Pol precursor proteins in a nascent bud. Two copies of virion RNA are being encapsidated. This is being mediated by interactions of the encapsidation domains in the NC region of Gag with encapsidation sequences in the RNAs (see later). N, the N-terminal of the assembling polyproteins; C, the C-terminal of the assembling polyproteins. (5) Maturation of the viral particle occurs after proteolytic cleavage of the precursor polyproteins by the viral protease. The positions of MA, CA, and NC in the mature particle reflect their relative positions in the precursor. The Gag-Pol precursor polyproteins (and the Gag precursor in ALSV) also bring the essential viral enzymes into the particle. Envelope glycoprotein spikes are not included in the assembly diagram because their "recruitment" into particles is poorly understood. (Adapted from Wills JW, Craven RC. Form, function and use of retroviral Gag proteins. AIDS 1991;5:639–654, and Bolognesi DP, Montelaro RC, Frank H, Schafer W. Assembly of type C oncornaviruses: a model. Science 1978;199:183–186.)

become used by "more recent" subgroups of viruses (see Tables 26-1 and 26-2).

in CA termed the *major homology region*.[168] The most conserved region of Gag, nucleocapsid (NC), supports the encapsidation of viral RNA and additional functions that affect infectivity.[57,99] An encapsidation domain within NC contains zinc fingers embedded in a region of basic amino acids. Other prod-

STRUCTURE AND FUNCTION OF GAG-DERIVED PROTEINS AND PARTICLE FORMATION

In all retroviruses, the internal structural proteins are synthesized in the form of a precursor polyprotein, termed the *Gag polyprotein*[40,160,168] (Fig. 26-8). The Gag polyprotein has the capability of self-assembly into virus-like particles that bud from the plasma membrane (see Fig. 26-8*B*). The Gag polyprotein also contains signals for the incorporation of viral RNA into particles.

Functional Domains of Gag

The Gag precursor polyprotein encompasses several functional domains for virus assembly and structure (see Fig. 26-8*A*). The N-terminal matrix (MA) portion localizes the Gag precursor in cells. For most retroviruses, membrane association depends on modification of the N-terminus of the Gag polyprotein by a 14-carbon fatty acid, myristic acid.[88,119,122] A middle capsid (CA) portion is essential for virus assembly. Assembly is mediated in part by a highly conserved sequence

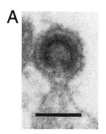 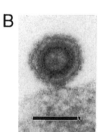 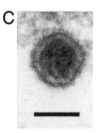

FIG. 26-9. Immature and mature virus particles. Electron micrographs of budding, immature, and mature murine leukemia virus particles. **(A)** Formation of the bud. Notice the crescent of the assembling virion and the presence of envelope glycoprotein spikes in the host cell plasma membrane. **(B)** An immature virus particle with an electron-lucent core. **(C)** A mature virus particle with a condensed electron-dense nucleoprotein core. Condensation of the core involves maturation of the dimer linkage between co-packaged RNAs and interactions of the nucleocapsid cleavage product of the Gag polyprotein with virion RNA. The bars represent 100 nm.

ucts derived from the Gag precursor are not conserved among the retroviruses and have not been named (see Fig. 26-8*A*).

Gag in Assembly

Each virus particle incorporates about 2000 monomers of the Gag polyprotein (see Fig. 26-8*B*). During virus maturation, the viral protease (PR) cleaves these monomers into the structural proteins of mature virus.[40,168] MA, CA, and NC are aligned in Gag in the same order (outside to inside) that they are found in mature virions.[17] The proteolytic cleavages allow "virus maturation," a morphologic change that forms the electron-dense cores of mature virus[33,81] (Fig. 26-9).

STRUCTURE AND FUNCTION OF THE PROTEASE

PR, an Aspartyl Protease

The sequence and structure of PR are related to those of the aspartyl or acid protease family, such as pepsin, cathepsin D, and renin.[82] The last two enzymes consist of two nearly identical domains, each of which contributes a highly conserved triplet (Asp-Thr/Ser-Gly) to the active site. The retroviral PR is synthesized as a single domain, similar in size and sequence to only one of the domains of the cellular proteases. The active form of the retroviral PR is a dimer formed by the noncovalent association of two monomers. PR is synthesized as part of the Gag or Gag-Pol polyprotein.

PR Function and Maturational Cleavages

Maturational cleavages of the Gag and Gag-Pol polyproteins are catalyzed by PR (see Fig. 26-8*B*).[33,81] The target sites for PR cleavage are diverse amino acid sequences.[82] In general, the target site is hydrophobic. This suggests that PR cleavage is controlled, in part, by the accessibility of sites within the native polyprotein.

STRUCTURE AND FUNCTION OF REVERSE TRANSCRIPTASE AND INTEGRASE, FORMATION OF THE LONG TERMINAL REPEAT, INTEGRATION, AND HOST CELL TARGETS FOR INTEGRATION

Multiple Functions of Reverse Transcriptase and Integrase

Reverse transcription and integration are catalyzed by the reverse transcriptase and integrase enzymes encoded in the Pol polyprotein.[82,167] Each of these enzymes accomplishes several functions. Reverse transcriptase copies RNA to DNA (a reverse transcriptase function),[5,46] digests the RNA strand of the RNA/DNA hybrid product (a ribonuclease H function),[104] and then copies the DNA strand of the hybrid product into DNA (a DNA polymerase function). Integrase cleaves the 3' termini of viral DNA to produce recessed ends (an endonucle-

ase function)[22,49] and catalyzes a nucleophilic attack of the recessed ends on chromosomal DNA (a polynucleotidyl transferase function).[22,49]

Structure and Function of Reverse Transcriptase

X-ray crystallographic analysis of the human immunodeficiency virus type 1 reverse transcriptase suggests that reverse transcriptase functions as a dimer in which one molecule provides catalytic functions and a second molecule provides structure.[18,82,167] The dimers of the human immunodeficiency virus type 1 reverse transcriptase are described as a hand with finger and thumb domains "holding" an incoming strand of template RNA and an outgoing strand of product DNA. Catalytic sites for polymerization and ribonuclease H activity lie along the palm, at an 18– to 20–base pair distance from each other. As viral RNA threads through the hand, it is copied and degraded.

Reverse Transcription and Formation of the Long Terminal Repeat

The LTRs of proviral DNA are produced during reverse transcription[74,82,155,167] (Fig. 26-10). Both strands of viral DNA are initiated using RNA primers (see Fig. 26-10, *step 1*). The binding sites for the primers define the boundaries of the terminal U5 and U3 regions of viral RNA. The 5' minus-strand primer is a host transfer RNA with homology to sequences adjacent to U5. This binding site is termed the *primer binding site* (designated pbs). The 3' plus-strand primer is a purine-rich fragment of viral RNA derived from sequences adjacent to U3. This primer (designated ppt for polypurine tract) is generated by ribonuclease H digestion of plus-strand viral RNA (see Fig. 26-10, *step 3*). Both primers initiate outward bound transcripts that rapidly reach the ends of their templates (see Fig. 26-10, *steps 1 and 3*). Complete copies of the viral genome are produced by reverse transcriptase undergoing strand transfers with these short initial products. The first strand transfer is to sequences at the other end of the template RNA, or of the copackaged second RNA molecule (see Fig. 26-10, *step 2*). This strand transfer is facilitated by the short repeated sequence (designated R) at both ends of viral RNA[155] (see Fig. 26-10, *step 2, region in ellipse*). The second strand transfer is between emerging plus- and minus-strand DNAs (see Fig. 26-10, *step 4*). This transfer may be facilitated by hybridization of the primer binding site region of the short outward bound plus-strand DNA to the primer binding site region of the elongating minus-strand DNA (see Fig. 26-10, *step 4, region in ellipse*). The two flanking LTRs are generated by reverse transcriptase duplicating the short outward-facing regions that underwent strand transfers (see Fig. 26-10, *step 4 leading to step 5*).

Recombination

The genomes of retroviruses undergo frequent recombinational events. These events occur during reverse transcription. The substrates for the recombination are copackaged RNA

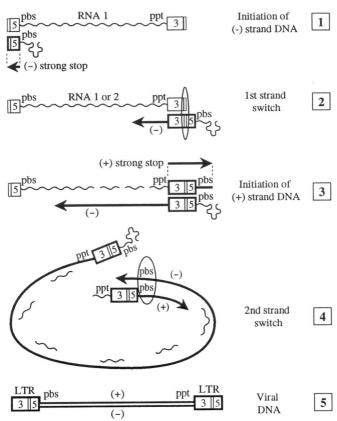

FIG. 26-10. The reverse transcription process: creation of the long terminal repeat (LTR) from U5 and U3. The U5, U3, and R regions are designated by boxes. Thin-lined boxes and wavy lines indicate viral RNA. Bold-lined boxes and bold lines designate the DNA products. Two copies of the RNA genome are present in the starting viral particle. These are designated RNA 1 and RNA 2. Both RNAs can provide template sequences for the synthesis of one proviral DNA. DNA synthesis starts near the ends of viral RNA and proceeds outward. These initial outward products, labeled (−) and (+) strong stop, are highlighted by bold arrows. Additional template (to achieve copying of internal viral sequences) is accomplished by "strand switches." (1) Minus-strand DNA synthesis starts near the 5′ end of viral RNA using tRNA^try (avian leukosis-sarcoma virus) or tRNA^pro (murine leukemia virus) as primers. These tRNAs are annealed by at least 18 nt at their 3′ ends to a region adjacent to U5 called the primer binding site (pbs). DNA synthesis proceeds to the 5′ end of the RNA genome through the U5 region and the terminally redundant R region. This product is known as minus-strand strong stop DNA. (2) The RNA portion of the RNA-DNA hybrid is digested by the RNase H activity of RT, exposing the single-stranded DNA strong stop product. This exposure facilitates hybridization of newly synthesized R DNA with the R region at the 3′ end of the same RNA, or the copackaged RNA (*ellipse*). This reaction represents the first strand switch. (3) After the first strand switch, minus-strand DNA synthesis proceeds through U3 and into *env.* When minus-strand DNA passes a polypurine-rich region adjacent to U3 (called ppt), RNAse H digestion generates the ppt plus-strand primer. Plus-strand DNA synthesis is initiated by the ppt primer using the 5′ strong stop DNA and the pbs region of its attached tRNA primer as templates. This produces plus-strand strong stop DNA. Meanwhile, minus-strand DNA synthesis continues through the genome using viral RNA as a template and removing the RNA template in its wake by RNase H activity. RNase H digestion products (*short, wavy lines*) provide additional primers for plus-strand DNA synthesis. (4) Complementarity for the second strand switch is provided by the pbs in plus-strand strong stop DNA annealing to its pbs complement in elongating minus-strand DNA (*ellipse*). (5) DNA synthesis then continues to produce a linear duplex of viral DNA. RNase H activity removes the primers. (Adapted from Whitcomb JM, Hughes SH. Retroviral reverse transcription and integration: progress and problems. Annu Rev Cell Biol 1992;8:275–306, and Katz RA, Skalka AM. The retroviral enzymes. Annu Rev Biochem 1994;63: 133–173.)

genomes. The genetic information in the copackaged genomes can undergo recombination during the strand switches (see Fig. 26-10, *steps 2 and 4*). The genomes also can undergo recombination by other phenomena, such as strand displacement.[82]

Integration

Integration is accomplished by the viral integrase.[82,167] Integrase endonucleolytically processes the ends of the linear duplex produced by reverse transcription (Fig. 26-11, *step 2*).

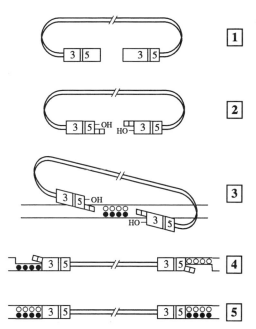

FIG. 26-11. Integration of retroviral DNA. (1) The blunt-ended, double-stranded, linear product of reverse transcription is the substrate for integration. The U5 and U3 regions that undergo endonucleolytic cleavage have been expanded to facilitate demonstration of their recession. (2) Integrase processes the double-stranded, blunt-ended product by cleaving two bases from the 3′ ends of both viral DNA strands. This exposes 3′ OH groups of a recessed C-A–dinucleotide sequence (shown as −OH in 2 and 3) that is characteristic of the ends of retrotransposons. Processing occurs in a preintegration complex in the cytoplasm. (3 and 4) The preintegration complex migrates to the nucleus, where IN catalyzes a nucleophilic attack of the 3′ OH groups on host DNA. The attack is made on PO4 groups at a fixed distance (4 to 6 base pairs, depending on the IN) on opposite strands of host DNA. This reaction joins viral and host strands together by a phosphodiester bond. (4 and 5) DNA repair converts the mismatched gaps at the ends of the provirus to double-stranded DNA. These form the short repeats of host sequences that flank integrated proviral DNA. The positions of the nucleophilic attack define the size of these repeats. (Adapted from Whitcomb JM, Hughes SH. Retroviral reverse transcription and integration: progress and problems. Annu Rev Cell Biol 1992;8:275–306.)

In all retroviruses, the processed ends are bounded by a 2–base pair sequence (CA) characteristic of the ends of transposable elements. A multimeric form of integrase inserts viral DNA into chromosomal DNA by a nucleophilic attack of the recessed ends on phosphates in the chromosomal DNA backbone[43] (see Fig. 26-11, *steps 3 and 4*). The attack on the two strands of target DNA is at a fixed distance (4 to 6 bases, depending on the retroviral group), with the repair of the ensuing gap creating the short repeats of chromosomal DNA that flank integrated proviruses (see Fig. 26-11, *steps 4 and 5*).

Host Cell Targets for Integration

Most integrations occur in regions of open or transcriptionally active chromatin.[127,157] Many of these open regions are tissue-specific in their expression. Data suggest that interaction of integrase with host cell transcription factors or "activator" proteins facilitates integration into transcriptionally active regions of chromatin.[80] Integrations show no significant preference for specific sequences.

Logistics

Virions typically contain 50 to 100 molecules of reverse transcriptase and integrase. These are produced by PR-mediated cleavages of Gag-Pol precursor polyproteins at the time of budding. Reverse transcription of viral RNA to DNA and endonucleolytic processing of the ends of the viral DNA occur in the cytoplasm in a capsid-containing preintegration complex.[21] For MuLVs and ALSVs, access of this complex to chromatin occurs during mitosis when nuclear membranes are not present. Newly synthesized viral DNA is not expressed until it has become integrated. This may reflect limited access of transcription factors to viral DNA in the preintegration complex.

TRANSCRIPTIONAL ACTIVITY OF THE LONG TERMINAL REPEAT

Basic Pattern of Transcription

Transcription of the integrated provirus depends on interaction of the transcriptional machinery of the host cell with LTR sequences[29,96] (Fig. 26-12A). Transcription is accomplished by RNA polymerase II. Transcription complexes initiate in the 5′ LTR, at the boundary between U3 and R. The complexes transcribe through the provirus, terminating transcription at host signals downstream of the 3′ LTR. Most of the transcripts are cleaved and polyadenylated at the R-U5 boundary in the 3′ LTR.[69] The remainder of the transcripts are cleaved and polyadenylated somewhere within the portion of the transcript derived from downstream cellular sequences. This last phenomenon sets the stage for disease induction by promoter insertions and the incorporation of host sequences into viral genomes (see later).

Functional Selectivity of 5′ and 3′ Long Terminal Repeats

Internal viral sequences in the vicinity of the 5′ and 3′ LTRs contribute to the functional selectivity of the two LTRs. A region near the 5′ LTR enhances transcriptional activity, contributing to the transcriptional dominance of this LTR.[16,52] The dominance of the 5′ LTR also reflects polymerase complexes initiated in the 5′ LTR passing over and masking transcription assembly sites in the 3′ LTR (a phenomenon referred to as *promoter occlusion*).[1,35] Processing of transcripts in the 3′ LTR is in response to the presence of polyadenylation signals in the U3 sequences transcribed from the 3' LTR[141] (see Fig. 26-12A).

Transcriptional Control Elements

Viral regulatory sequences for the binding of transcription factors reside in U3 (see Fig. 26-12B). These include a TATA box, upstream promoter sequences (CCAAT box), and an enhancer. The TATA box nucleates the assembly of RNA polymerase II complexes at the promoter to form the preinitiation complex. Proteins bound to the upstream CCAAT box and enhancer sequences then facilitate transcript initiation. Transcription can be efficient, with as much as 10% to 20% of the total mRNA of an in\fected cell being viral.[67,155]

Enhancer Elements

Retroviral enhancers have tightly packed binding sites for nuclear transcription factors (see Fig. 26-12B). Seven binding sites are found in the ~75–base pair enhancer of the Moloney MuLV.[138] Four of these are found in almost all MuLV enhancers.[56] These sites, termed LVb, core, NF1, and GRE, bind proteins from five distinct protein families. The LVb sites bind proteins in the *ets* family of transcription factors,[62] the core site binds proteins in the polyomavirus enhancer-binding protein 2/core-binding factor family,[133,162] the NF1 site binds a group of proteins referred to as nuclear factor-1,[121] and the GRE site binds both the helix-loop-helix E-box proteins and the glucocorticoid hormone receptor.[32,38,109] The conservation of these four sites in MuLV enhancers suggests that these pro-

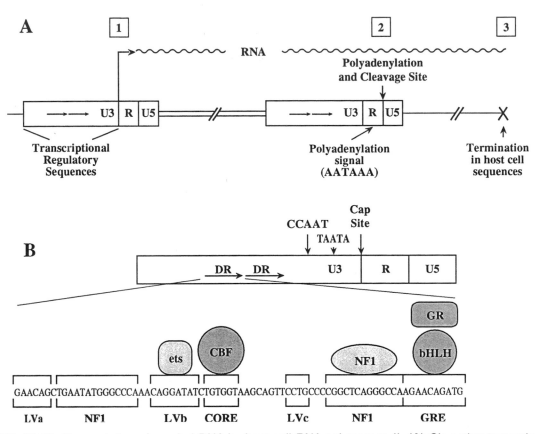

FIG. 26-12. Transcription of proviral DNA by host cell RNA polymerase II. (**A**) Cis-acting transcriptional control elements of a prototypic murine leukemia virus (MuLV). A provirus and its transcript are indicated. Notice that the two long terminal repeats (LTRs; whose sequences are identical) are playing different roles in transcription, with the 5′ LTR initiating transcripts and the 3′ LTR providing polyadenylation signals. Notice also that transcripts are terminating in downstream host sequences. This phenomenon is important to the incorporation of host cell sequences into retroviral genomes (see Figure 26-16). The double arrows in U3 represent two copies of enhancer sequences. The arrow with a right angle designates the transcription start site. (1) Initiation of transcripts in the 5′ LTR at the boundary between U3 and R. (2) Polyadenylation of transcripts in the 3′ LTR at the junction of R and U5. (3) Termination of transcripts in downstream host sequences. (**B**) Moloney MuLV enhancer sequence with binding sites for host cell transcription factors. Boxes represent binding sites for transcription factors. The designations for the binding sites are indicated below the boxes. Four of the sites are highly conserved in all mammalian C-type retroviral enhancers. The transcription factors for these sites are shown above their binding sites. (Adapted from Luciw PA, Leung NJ. Mechanisms of retrovirus replication. In: Levy JA, ed, The retroviridae. Vol 1. New York: Plenum Press 1992;159–298.)

teins cooperate to activate transcription in hematopoietic cells, the common target cells for MuLV replication. In contrast to the conservation of sequences in MuLV enhancer regions, other sequences in MuLV U3 regions are divergent. ALSV enhancers have little homology with MuLV enhancers.

High levels of transcriptional activity frequently are achieved by duplications of enhancer sequences (see Fig. 26-12B). Highly pathogenic viruses almost always contain at least two, and sometimes three or more, copies of a repeated enhancer sequence (see later).[39,89,93]

RNA AND PROTEIN SYNTHESIS

Overview of Virion and Messenger RNAs

Transcripts of viral RNA have two potential destinies. Some transcripts are incorporated into virions, where they serve as genomic RNA. Others become mRNAs. Both the genomic RNA and the viral mRNAs are capped and polyadenylated.[29] Full-length RNAs that are destined for virions transit through cells and into virus in a relatively short period (~1.5 hours).[90] RNAs that are destined for mRNA include full-length transcripts (indistinguishable from those found in virions) and spliced transcripts. Viral mRNAs are stable, functioning in protein synthesis for many hours.[90]

Viral Messenger RNAs and Protein Synthesis

MuLVs and ALVs have only two mRNAs: a full-length Gag-Pol mRNA and a subgenomic Env mRNA.[29,67] The full-length mRNA produces both Gag and Gag-Pol precursor polyproteins by initiating translation at the Gag start codon and translating, at a low frequency, across the Gag stop codon. For most retroviruses, translation across the Gag stop codon is accomplished by ribosomal frame-shifting.[77] Ribosomal frame-shifting occurs when ribosomes shift reading frames near the end of the Gag coding sequence, bypassing the Gag termination codon and continuing in the Pol reading frame. For mammalian type C viruses, Gag and Pol are encoded in the same reading frame. For these viruses, translation across the Gag stop codon is accomplished by the occasional translation of the Gag termination codon as an amino acid. This phenomenon is termed *read-through suppression*.[66] About 20 times more Gag polyprotein is produced than Gag-Pol polyprotein. The Env mRNA is used exclusively to translate Env.

PACKAGING SEQUENCES, DIMER LINKAGE OF COPACKAGED RNAS, AND MATURATION OF VIRAL RNA

The encapsidation of viral RNA into particles occurs during virus assembly. The genomic RNA in the virion is a dimer, composed of two identical molecules of full-length viral RNA. The structure of this dimeric RNA undergoes "maturation" after virus release.[48] This maturation appears to result from the interaction of NC with the viral RNA after NC is proteolytically cleaved from the Gag polyprotein.

Encapsidation Signals in Nucleocapsid and Viral RNA

The encapsidation process is accomplished by sequences in the Gag polyprotein recognizing sequences in viral RNA.[94,118] Important Gag sequences include zinc fingers and flanking basic residues in the NC region (see earlier). Important RNA sequences include "RNA packaging" sequences (termed ψ or *E sequences*). RNA packaging sequences are found in a several hundred–base pair region near U5. Deletion of ψ or E from a viral RNA reduces encapsidation. Conversely, insertion of ψ or E sequences into nonviral mRNAs renders these RNAs "packageable."

Dimer Linkage of Copackaged RNAs

The genomes of retroviruses consist of dimers of two identical copies of viral RNA.[9,12,155] The linkage between the monomers is believed to be near the 5' ends of the viral RNA in the same region encoding encapsidation signals. The thermostability of the dimers is consistent with the monomers being joined by hydrogen bonds or other weak, noncovalent bonds. Evidence suggests that the dimeric linkage may be initiated by a switch of some bases from intramolecular base-pairing in stem-loop structures to intermolecular base-pairing ("kissing loops").[135] This dimeric structure may be an element of the encapsidation signal.[48,115]

ENDOGENOUS AND EXOGENOUS VIRUSES

Germ Line Transmission of Endogenous But Not Exogenous Viruses

The transmission of retroviruses in nature is entwined with the replication of virion RNA through a proviral DNA intermediate. This proviral intermediate confers on the virus the potential to be transmitted as a normal host cell gene by chromosomal DNA.[4,28,79,85,95,113] Viral genomes that are transmitted by proviral DNA in eggs and sperm are termed *endogenous* viruses to distinguish them from the *exogenous* viruses that are transmitted by infection. Establishment of proviral DNA in the germ line is a rare event. Most infected animals do not sustain infections in germ cells. However, once a germ line infection is introduced, it tends, over a great many generations, to found a multicopy family of proviruses by further infections within the germ compartment. Most type C viruses have endogenous representatives.[30] In contrast, the T-cell leukemia viruses, the lentiviruses, and the spumaviruses do not have endogenous members.

Evolutionary Dominance of Endogenous Viruses

Once a virus has become endogenous to a species, its exogenous relatives tend to become extinct or evolve to use a different receptor. This reflects the expression of envelope glycoproteins by germ line proviruses interfering with superinfection by viruses that use the same receptor.[123] It also reflects the selection of host receptors for resistance to infection (see earlier). Key to early work with endogenous ALV was the realization that to grow an endogenous virus as an infectious agent (e.g., a chicken endogenous virus), it frequently was necessary to use an unrelated species (e.g., a quail or a turkey) that did not have interfering proviruses or "resistant" receptors.[163]

Characteristics of "Ancient" and "Recent" Groups of Endogenous Viruses

The germ lines of both mice and chickens contain several groups of endogenous proviruses[34,85] (for endogenous viruses of mice, see Table 26-3). The relative ages of these groups are reflected at least partially in the number of germ line proviruses, the defectiveness of the proviruses, and whether the group has exogenous members. The more ancient groups have large numbers of replication-defective proviruses (100 to 1000 per haploid genome; see IAP and VL30 groups in Table 26-3). The more recent groups have both exogenous and endogenous representatives (see MuLV and MMTV groups in Table 26-3). For these groups, the endogenous representatives typically are represented by less than 100 proviruses. These more recent proviruses encode both replication-competent and replication-defective viruses.

Coevolution of Endogenous Viruses With Their Hosts

With time, the genomes of vertebrates have acquired fairly large numbers of endogenous proviruses (more than 1000 per haploid mouse genome; see Table 26-3). Most of these are carried as unexpressed, replication-defective elements (see Table 26-3). Presumably, replication of endogenous viruses is detrimental to the survival of the host.

A subset of endogenous proviruses have introduced insertional mutations that alter the phenotype of their host. These confer phenotypes, such as coat color,[78] failure to develop hair,[142] or patterns of feathering[136] (see Table 26-3).

Malignancies Caused by Endogenous Viruses

Endogenous proviruses also are associated with the development of malignancies[25,85,107] (see later). This can happen when an endogenous provirus encodes a replication-competent cancer-inducing virus. Such is true for the endogenous mouse mammary tumor proviruses in GR mice and the AKV endogenous MuLV proviruses of AKR mice. Endogenous proviruses also can contribute to cancer induction by recombining with spreading replication-competent viruses to produce viruses with increased oncogenic potentials. An example of this is found in the MCF recombinants that contribute to the disease potential of ecotropic MuLV infections (see later).

Host Control of Endogenous Virus Expression

An important host mechanism for controlling the expression of endogenous proviruses is methylation.[61] Methylation can establish inactive chromatin structures that do not express the resident provirus. Inactive chromatin structures can undergo programmed activation (with concomitant activation of

TABLE 26-3. *Endogenous retroviruses of mice*

Group*	Approximate copy number†	Distribution‡	Comment±
IAP	1000	Mice, rats, hamsters, gerbils	Seen only as intracisternal A type particles; no known replication-competent members; expressed in many tumors where they cause insertional mutations[153]
VL30	150	Mice, rats	Only replication-defective representatives; RNA is efficiently encapsidated by MuLVs; sequences from VL30s contribute to the oncogenic potential of Harvey and Kirsten sarcoma viruses[14]
MuLVs	50	Mice, rats, hamsters	Proviruses belong to xenotropic and ecotropic subgroups; xenotropic proviruses are more ancient than ecotropic proviruses; most xenotroic proviruses are replication-defective; many ecotropic proviruses are replication-competent; the spread of ecotropic viruses (encoded by endogenous proviruses) as infectious agents causes cancer[25]; some MuLV germ line insertions affect phenotypes such as coat color[78,142]
MMTVs	30	Mice	Type B replication-defective and replication-competent proviruses; replication-competent proviruses cause mammary tumors[107]

*IAP, intracisternal type A particles; VL30, virus-like 30 sequences; MuLVs, murine leukemia viruses; MMTVs, mouse mammary tumor viruses. Two other groups of endogenous retroviruses are present in mice: B-26 and GLN-3.[85] Both are widespread in rodents, representing families of endogenous viruses that were established early in the evolution of rodents. GLN-3 and B-26 are limited to replication-defective elements.

†Number of endogenous proviruses per haploid mouse genome. Data are from reference 85.

‡Listed rodents include only those that have been analyzed and found to be positive for the indicated endogenous virus.

±The ecotropic subgroups of MuLVs and the MMTVs also have exogenous members. This table is limited to the endogenous members of these groups.

the resident provirus) during normal cell differentiation.[105] Activation of normally inactive chromatin structures also can occur in malignant cells that no longer are regulating their DNA synthesis (see Chap. 12). The presence of intracisternal A type particles and their associated insertional mutations in many mouse tumors may in part reflect this latter phenomenon[153] (see Table 26-3).

VERTICAL AND HORIZONTAL TRANSMISSION

Retrovirologists use the term *horizontal spread* to indicate the spread of virus within a group of animals. The term *vertical transmission* is used to designate the spread of virus from parent to child. This can occur by inheritance of germ line proviruses, by congenital infection (infection by shed virus up to or during the time of birth), or by shedding of virus in milk. Both exogenous and endogenous viruses can undergo horizontal and vertical transmission.

Spread of Exogenous Viruses

Avian and murine retroviruses of exogenous origin are shed in the reproductive tract, saliva, feces, and milk.[15,112,130] These patterns of shedding are supported by highly active replication of the virus in glandular tissues such as the salivary glands and pancreas, and in reproductive tissues such as the oviduct and testes.[42]

Spread of Endogenous Viruses

By definition, endogenous proviruses undergo vertical transmission in germ cells. However, replication-competent viruses of endogenous origin also can undergo shedding and infect other animals by congenital or horizontal infections. Replication-defective endogenous proviruses can "participate" in spreading infections by recombination with a replication-competent virus.[63] In certain instances, two replication-defective endogenous proviruses in the same cell can recombine to form spreading replication-competent infections.[124]

TWO MAJOR OUTCOMES OF INFECTION: TOLERIZATION AND A PERSISTENT VIREMIA, SEROCONVERSION AND A SMOLDERING INFECTION

Immunoincompetent Hosts

The long-term outcome of an infection depends on the immunocompetence of the host at the time of infection.[130] Hosts infected as newborns become largely tolerant to the infection. In such animals, the infection establishes a persistent viremia. The susceptible tissues of the host become fully infected.[126] Such animals carry highly active lifelong infections. These persistently viremic animals are the major source of virus within an endemic infection. Their oral, fecal, and reproductive secretions spread virus to social contacts. Congenital in-

fection of their progeny ensures a pool of persistently viremic carriers in the next generation.

Immunocompetent Hosts

In contrast to congenital transmission, which typically establishes a persistent viremia, horizontal spread of retroviruses to immunocompetent hosts usually results in seroconversion.[130] Seropositive mothers provide their offspring with maternal antibody that helps protect the infants from contact spread of virus while their immune systems mature. Offspring that were protected from infection early in life become seropositive if they subsequently are infected.

As a whole, seropositive hosts appear to contain rather than eliminate infections. Virus can be cultivated from the blood cells of seropositive hosts. Seropositive hosts also can undergo occasional virus shedding.[130]

USE OF VIRAL AND PROVIRAL DNA AS MARKERS FOR CLONAL AND POLYCLONAL DISEASES

Clonal and Polyclonal Diseases

The status of viral and proviral DNA in a diseased tissue can be used to determine whether a retrovirus-induced disease is clonal or polyclonal. If the disease results from the outgrowth of a single infected cell (a clonal outgrowth), the diseased tissue will carry the proviral insertions of the founding cell. These proviruses can be visualized on DNA blots of restriction endonuclease–digested DNAs, with discrete bands representing specific junctions of viral and proviral DNA. However, if the disease is caused by the abnormal growth of an infected tissue (a polyclonal disease), then DNA blots of the diseased tissue reveal a background smear of many different proviral-host junction fragments. This smear reflects the polyclonal disease originating from cells with many different sites of proviral insertion.

Other Uses of Junction Fragments

The discrete bands representing junction fragments of proviral and host sequences provide a means of identifying host sequences that are candidate targets for oncogenic insertions (see later). Junction fragments in tumors also can be used to determine the relation of tumor masses within an individual because metastases of a tumor have junction fragments that also are present in the primary tumor.

MOLECULAR MECHANISMS OF DISEASE INDUCTION

Insertional Mutagenesis

The establishment of a provirus requires the insertion of viral DNA into host chromosomal DNA. This process is called *insertional mutagenesis*, with the integration of each provirus representing an insertional mutation. A small subset of these insertions contribute to cancer induction by affecting host sequences involved in the control of cell growth[68,86,153] (see Chap. 11). In general, cancer-inducing insertions activate the expression of host proto-oncogenes. Activation can result from the stimulating effect of viral enhancer elements acting on host promoters. These are called *enhancer insertions*. Activation also can occur by synthesis of fused viral-host RNAs from promoter elements in a viral LTR. These are called *promoter insertions*. Finally, activation can occur by viral polyadenylation signals prematurely terminating host transcripts. This last group is called *terminator insertions*.

Enhancer Insertions

Enhancer insertions increase the expression of a normal host transcript by virtue of transcription factors that bind to the viral enhancer, acting on the host and the viral promoter (Fig. 26-13A). Tumor-inducing enhancer insertions cluster in specific regions of host DNA referred to as *common insertion sites* (see Chap. 11 for lists of common insertion sites and their associated tumors). Most enhancer insertions have transcriptional orientations that face outward with respect to their target proto-oncogene. This outward orientation may prevent the "collision" of transcription complexes initiated by the viral and cellular promoters (see Fig. 26-13A).

Extended Targets for Enhancer Insertions.

Enhancer insertions can act over long distances, with insertions that activate a common target occurring in several regions of an extended host sequence.[87,152,153] The proto-oncogene c-myc is a target for enhancer insertions in MuLV-induced T-cell lymphomas (see Fig. 26-13B). Enhancer insertions that upregulate c-myc expression are found in three regions of ~270 kb of chromosomal DNA. The first region is a ~2-kb region immediately upstream of c-myc. The second (Moloney leukemia virus integration region 4, Mlvi-4), is a ~1-kb region about 30 kb downstream of c-myc. The third region (Mlvi-1) is a ~16-kb region about 270 kb downstream from c-myc. Insertions in each of these regions activate c-myc transcription.

Promoter Insertions

In contrast to enhancer insertions that increase the activity of a cellular promoter, promoter insertions use a viral promoter to produce fused viral-host transcripts[68,153] (see Chap. 11; Fig. 26-14). Promoter insertions can initiate fused transcripts using viral promoters in the 5' LTR or the 3' LTR (see Fig. 26-14A and B, respectively).

5' Long Terminal Repeat Promoter Insertions.

5' LTR initiations occur in all promoter insertions that express a truncated host proto-oncogene or a fused viral-host protein (see Chap. 11). Transcripts initiated in the 5' LTR in-

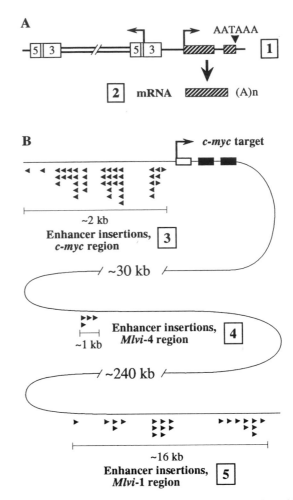

FIG. 26-13. Cancer induction by enhancer insertion. (**A**) A prototypic enhancer insertion. (**B**) Positions and orientations of thymoma-inducing enhancer insertions of *c-myc*. (1) The prototypic enhancer insertion is in the opposite transcriptional orientation as its target host gene (exons designated by *hatched rectangles*). This results in transcription complexes initiated by the viral and host promoters (*bent arrows*) moving in opposite directions. (2) A normal host mRNA is produced in response to the enhancer insertion. Tumor induction is caused by the viral enhancers deregulating the expression of the target mRNA. In **B**, arrowheads mark the orientation and approximate location of a series of thymoma-associated enhancer insertions for *c-myc*. Each arrowhead represents an insertion that occurred in an independent thymoma. The insertions cluster in three regions of an extended length (about 275 kilobases [kb]) of chromosomal DNA. The target gene for the insertions, *c-myc*, is represented by rectangles. Open rectangles represent noncoding exons of *c-myc*, and closed rectangles represent coding exons. (3 through 5) The three clusters of enhancer insertions for *c-myc*. (3) Forty-four examples of enhancer insertions that occurred immediately upstream of *c-myc*. Notice that all but two are in the opposite transcriptional orientation as *c-myc*. (4) Four examples of enhancer insertions in a region of about 1 kb of *Mlvi-4*. *Mlvi-4* lies about 30 kb downstream of *c-myc*. (5) Twenty-two examples of enhancer insertions in a region of about 16 kb of *Mlvi-1*. *Mlvi-1* lies about 270 kb downstream of *c-myc*. Notice that all the insertions in *Mlvi-4* and *Mlvi-1* face outward from *c-myc*. Data are for MuLV-induced thymomas in mice and rats.

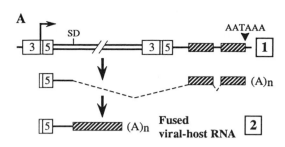

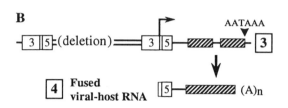

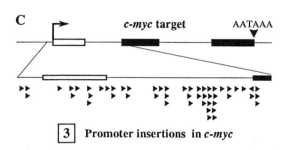

3 Promoter insertions in *c-myc*

FIG. 26-14. Cancer induction by promoter insertion. **(A)** A prototypic 5′ long terminal repeat (LTR) promoter insertion. **(B)** A prototypic 3′ LTR promoter insertion. **(C)** The positions of 3′ LTR promoter insertions in the chicken *c-myc* gene. Designations are the same as in Figure 26-13. (1) An inserted provirus mediating a 5′ LTR promoter insertion. A fused viral-host transcript is initiated in the 5′ LTR of the provirus and polyadenylated in downstream host sequences (the downstream host AATAAA polyadenylation signal is indicated). The fused transcript is spliced using viral and cellular splicing sequences. SD indicates the position of the dominant splice donor of the virus. 5′ LTR promotion also can be achieved by proviruses in which the 3′ LTR has undergone deletion. (2) A processed 5′ LTR–fused viral-host transcript. The line between the LTR and the hatched host sequences represents internal viral sequences. For insertions that truncate a host proto-oncogene, these internal viral sequences provide a translational start codon for the truncated host gene (see Chap. 11). (3) An inserted provirus that is mediating a 3′ LTR promoter insertion. Notice the deletion of sequences near the 5′ LTR in the inserted provirus. This deletion (and less frequent deletions of the complete 5′ LTR) allow the promoter elements in the 3′ LTR to be transcriptionally active (see text). (4) A fully processed viral-host RNA produced by the 3′ LTR promoter insertion. This RNA contains only LTR and host sequences. In most instances, the proteins produced by these insertions are normal host proteins. These proteins cause tumors because of the deregulation of their expression by the promoter insertion. (5) Approximate positions and orientations of 51 3′ LTR promoter insertions in the avian *c-myc* gene. These avian leukosis virus insertions caused B-cell lymphomas by upregulating the expression of *c-myc* RNA. In contrast to the enhancer insertions in Figure 26-13, which are upstream of the *c-myc* target, most of the promoter insertions are in the first noncoding exon and the first intron of *c-myc*. This places the insertions between the normal cellular promoter for *c-myc* and the *c-myc* start codon. (Adapted from Kung H-J, Boerkoel C, Carter TH. Retroviral mutagenesis of cellular oncogenes: a review with insights into the mechanisms of insertional activation. Curr Topics Micro Immunol 1991;171:1–18.)

clude internal viral sequences and downstream host sequences (see Fig. 26-14A). These internal viral sequences can provide an essential initiation codon for a truncated host protein. The internal viral sequences also can support the creation of fusion proteins in which the viral sequences increase the oncogenic potential of the target host sequence.[14]

3′ Long Terminal Repeat Promoter Insertions.

3′ LTR initiations are found in cancers that result from overexpression of an otherwise normal proto-oncogene product (see Fig. 26-14B). Proviruses that cause 3′ LTR initiations have characteristic patterns of deletion (see Chap. 11). These deletions allow the 3′ LTR (whose promoter activity is suppressed in a complete provirus) to become active (see earlier).

Figure 26-14C maps the approximate positions of 51 independent lymphoma-inducing insertions in the chicken *c-myc* gene. Each of these is a 3′ LTR promoter insertion. In contrast to enhancer insertions in the *c-myc* region, which are upstream of the first exon of *c-myc* (see Fig. 26-13B), all but 3 of the promoter insertions are within the first noncoding exon or the first intron of *c-myc*. Also in contrast to the enhancer insertions, which are predominantly in the opposite transcriptional orientation to *c-myc*, all the promoter insertions are in the same transcriptional orientation as *c-myc*.

Terminator Insertions

Terminator insertions activate proto-oncogene expression by providing termination signals for a host transcript[153] (see Chap. 11; Fig. 26-15A). Terminator insertions can truncate a gene product or stabilize a host transcript by removing sequences that confer instability on mRNAs.[134,153] Terminator insertions are in the same transcriptional orientation as their target gene, with shortening of the normal host transcript being accomplished by polyadenylation signals in the proviral 5′ LTR (see Fig. 26-15A).

Examples of lymphoma-inducing terminator insertions are given in Figure 26-15B. The insertions are clustered tightly immediately after the stop codon of their target gene, *pim-1* (see Fig. 26-15B). These insertions increase the levels of *pim-1* RNA in cells by stabilizing the transcript.[153]

Summary

Insertional mutations in 77 different regions of host cell sequences have been associated with retrovirus-induced cancers[153] (see Table 11-1 in Chap. 11). Twenty-eight of these have been associated with enhancer insertions, 10 with 5′ LTR promoter insertions, 11 with 3′ LTR promoter insertions, and 2 with terminator insertions. The target genes and activation

A

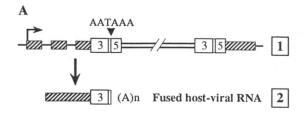

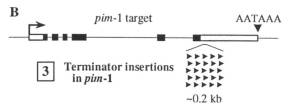

FIG. 26-15. Cancer induction by terminator insertion. (**A**) A prototypic terminator insertion. (**B**) The positions of terminator insertions in the *pim-1* host gene. Designations are as in Figure 26-13. (1) A provirus that is functioning as a terminator insertion. Notice that the provirus has integrated within a host exon. Transcripts initiated from the host promoter read into the provirus, where they are cleaved and polyadenylated by signals in the 5′ long terminal repeat. (2) The processed mRNA produced by the terminator insertion. This RNA has host sequences at its 5′ end and viral sequences at its 3′ end. (3) The approximate positions of 25 lymphoma-inducing terminator insertions in the murine *pim-1* gene. These murine leukemia virus insertions are located immediately after the stop codon for the *pim-1* protein (the *filled areas* in the exons represent protein-coding regions). All are in the same orientation as *pim-1*. These terminations increased the levels of the *pim-1* mRNA by removing 3′ nontranslated destabilizing elements (see text). (Adapted from Selten G, Cuypers HT, Boelens W, Robanus-Maandag E, Verbeek J, Domen J, van Beveren C, Berns A. The primary structure of the putative oncogene *pim-1* shows extensive homology with protein kinases. Cell 1986;46:603–611.)

mechanisms of the remaining insertions remain to be determined. Many of these are likely to be enhancer insertions that lie at some distance from their target proto-oncogene.

Viral Transduction of Host Sequences, Transforming Viruses and Helper Viruses, Acute Viruses and Nonacute Viruses

Creation of Transforming Viruses by Transduction of Host Sequences

The transmission of host information from one cell to another by a virus is termed *transduction*. Retroviral transductions are initiated by 5′ LTR promoter insertions that produce fused viral-host transcripts (see Fig. 26-14, *steps 1 and 2*, and Chap. 11; Fig. 26-16, *steps 1 and 2*). If packaging sequences for viral RNA are retained in the transcript, the fused transcript can be copackaged into a virion with normal viral RNA (see Fig. 26-16, *step 3*). During the next round of infection, reverse

transcriptase–mediated recombination can recombine viral sequences from the normal viral RNA with the fused transcript to generate a DNA that can integrate to become a provirus (see Fig. 26-16, *step 4*). This recombinant provirus expresses a "transducing" RNA that can undergo a normal retrovirus life cycle (see Fig. 26-16, *step 5*). The prefixes, "v" (viral) and "c" (cellular) are used to designate whether a gene is the transduced or the chromosomal form of a proto-oncogene.

Once a proto-oncogene sequence has been incorporated into a viral genome, it undergoes selection for mutations that increase its oncogenic potential.[117,149] In some instances, these mutations alter the types of tumors caused by the transduced sequence.[53,117]

Helper Viruses

In most instances, incorporation of host sequences into a viral genome is accompanied by the loss of sequences in *gag*, *pol*, or *env*. The loss of genes encoding essential viral proteins makes the transducing virus replication-defective. However, the transducing RNA can be transmitted if a co-infecting "helper" virus provides the transducing RNA with the proteins to form an infectious virus particle. The relation of the genome of a helper virus to the genomes of two transducing viruses is illustrated in Figure 26-17. The second transducing virus has incorporated sequences from two host proto-oncogenes (*c-erbA* and *c-erbB*).

Transducing viruses were among the first retroviruses to be isolated. These viruses were recognized by their ability to cause tumors in animals.[128] These viruses also could be detected in tissue culture by virtue of their ability to cause "foci" of transformed cells. Analyses of stocks of transducing viruses in tissue culture revealed that these stocks were mixtures of "transforming" viruses (the transducing viruses) and "nontransforming" viruses (the helper viruses).[64,131,147] Comparison of the genomes of transforming viruses and helper viruses provided the foundation for the identification of oncogenes in the transforming viruses and for the subsequent realization that these viral oncogenes had been created by transduction of sequences from host proto-oncogenes.[14,140,161]

Acute and Nonacute Viruses

Transforming viruses and helper viruses also are termed *acute* and *nonacute* viruses. This terminology reflects the different tempos of disease caused by transducing and nontransducing viruses. Inoculation of a transducing virus into a 1-day-old animal causes the rapid onset of a specific disease in virtually all infected animals. For example, viruses carrying the *src* gene cause a rapid onset of sarcomas, and viruses carrying the *erbB* gene cause a rapid onset of erythroblastosis. Most of these tumors are polyclonal, reflecting their growth from multiple cells, each transformed into a cancer cell by infection. By contrast, helper viruses (that do not carry oncogenes) are slow to cause disease. In this instance, disease induction requires several rare events, with the diseased tissue being a clonal outgrowth.

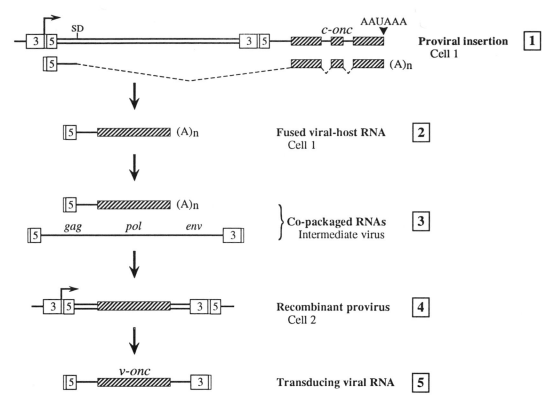

FIG. 26-16. Viral transduction of host sequences. (1) A 5′ long terminal repeat (LTR) promoter insertion initiates a transduction by producing a fused viral-host RNA. (2) This RNA is spliced. A fused viral-host RNA also can be produced by proviruses that have undergone deletion of the 3′ LTR. (3) If the spliced RNA includes encapsidation sequences (these are located near the 5′ LTR), it can be copackaged in a virion with a normal viral RNA. (4) During the next round of infection, the copackaged RNAs can recombine to give a recombinant provirus. (5) The recombinant provirus produces the transducing viral RNA. The transducing viral RNA can undergo transmission as an infectious agent in the presence of a helper virus (see text). Steps similar to those outlined earlier mediate recombination between two copackaged retroviral RNAs.

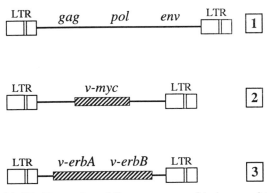

FIG. 26-17. Examples of the genomes of helper and transducing viruses. (1) An example of the genome of a helper virus. (2) An example of a virus that is transducing the *c-myc* gene. In the virus, *c-myc* is designated *v-myc* to distinguish it from its chromosomal counterpart. The transducing virus has lost part of *gag,* all of *pol,* and part of *env.* (3) An example of a virus that has transduced sequences from two host proto-oncogenes, *c-erbA* and *c-erbB.* This transducing virus also retains only a portion of its *gag* and *env* genes. LTR, long terminal repeat.

Use of Transforming Viruses to Identify Proto-oncogenes

The transduction of host sequences by avian and murine retroviruses has served to identify 27 different oncogenes (see Table 11-2 in Chap. 11). The characterization of these viruses and their associated host cell sequences has been of fundamental importance to our current view of the origins of cancer.

Two Cases in Which Defective Viral Genes Directly Cause Disease: Spleen Focus-Forming Virus and Murine Acquired Immunodeficiency Virus

There are two acute retroviruses in which modified viral genes (not transduced cellular genes) cause disease. One of these, spleen focus-forming virus (SFFV), has a defective envelope glycoprotein that induces hyperplasia of erythroid cells. The other, murine acquired immunodeficiency virus (MAIDS), has a defective Gag polyprotein that causes a gradual loss of immune function. Both the SFFV Env glycoprotein and the MAIDS Gag protein can directly cause the abnormal growth of their target cell.

Spleen Focus-Forming Virus env

The SFFV *env* gene causes hyperplasia by virtue of its interaction with the erythropoietin receptor.[10,92] This interaction makes erythroid cells hyperresponsive to, or completely independent of, erythropoietin. The SFFV *env* gene is derived from an MCF *env* (see Table 26-1). It differs from the MCF parent by a large deletion spanning the SU-TM junction and a frame shift near the C-terminus of TM.[132] These changes render the SFFV Env protein nonfunctional with respect to normal Env functions, requiring SFFV to be grown in the presence of a helper virus.[150] SFFV together with its helper virus are known as the *Friend complex* because of their discovery by Charlotte Friend.[47]

Murine Acquired Immunodeficiency Virus Gag

The MAIDS Gag protein causes the rapid proliferation and differentiation of B cells and CD4+ T cells, and the gradual loss of immune function.[106] Injection of mice with a replication-defective virus encoding only the N-terminal MA and p12 domains of the MAIDS Gag is sufficient to induce MAIDS in susceptible mice.[114] The myristylation site at the N-terminus of MA is necessary for disease induction, suggesting that pathogenesis may require localization of the "disease-inducing" Gag protein to the plasma membrane.[73]

Association of Disease With the Persistent Synthesis of Viral DNA

Occasional retrovirus-induced diseases are associated with the persistent synthesis of viral DNA in a diseased tissue.[108,125] In ALV-induced osteopetrosis, the persistent synthesis of viral DNA is associated with the abnormal growth and differentiation of osteoblasts.[137] Both the time of onset and the severity of osteopetrosis correlate with the level of viral DNA synthesis, which in turn correlates with the level of viral protein synthesis.[46,125]

In tissue culture, high levels of viral DNA synthesis are associated with cytopathic infections.[83,166] These high levels of viral DNA synthesis occur in infections that are slow to establish interference. The cytopathic effects can be prevented by the addition of neutralizing antibody to the infected culture. In ALV-induced osteopetrosis, the absence of disease in chickens that seroconvert is consistent with a role for multiple superinfection events in disease induction.[125]

MULTIPLE STEPS IN CANCER INDUCTION BY NONACUTE VIRUSES

In most instances, conversion of a normal cell to a malignant cell requires several mutations. For murine and avian retroviruses, the activation of more than one proto-oncogene is required for lymphoma induction[27,153] (see Chap. 11). The

hyperplasia induced by the defective SFFV Env also represents only one step toward a true leukemia.[10] Mice that survive the early polyclonal disease induced by the SFFV Env develop clonal outgrowths of leukemic cells. At least two steps are required for a hyperplastic SFFV-infected cell to become a leukemic cell. One of these is an enhancer insertion in the *spi-1* or *fli-1* host proto-oncogene (both members of the *ets* family of transcription factors). The second is inactivation of the p53 host cell tumor suppressor protein. This inactivation can be accomplished by a proviral insertion or other mutational events.

MANY PRIMARY AND SECONDARY TARGETS FOR DISEASE

Many Different Diseases

Nonacute avian and murine retroviruses have the potential for causing many different diseases. The specific diseases that occur depend on the virus strain, the genetic background of the host, and the timing of the infection.[58,85,112] MuLVs and ALVs induce B-cell and T-cell lymphomas, erythroleukemias, and myeloid leukemias.[19,60,85] MuLVs also induce neurologic diseases. These frequently are associated with hind limb paralysis.[85] ALVs also induce kidney tumors (nephroblastoma and adenocarcinoma), fibrosarcomas, and osteopetrosis.[19,112,125]

Primary and Secondary Diseases

For most virus-host combinations, the primary disease is a single clinicopathologic entity. Much lower incidences of other (secondary) diseases occur in the infected populations. In general, removal of the tissue that is the primary target for disease increases the incidence of secondary diseases. For example, if mice infected with the Gross passage A virus, a virus that induces primarily T-cell lymphoma, are thymectomized, they develop a high incidence of myeloid cancers.[59] Similarly, if chickens are bursectomized, removing the target tissue for B-cell lymphomas, higher incidences of osteopetrosis and kidney tumors are induced.[112]

LONG TERMINAL REPEAT AND *ENV* SEQUENCES AFFECT THE DISEASE POTENTIAL OF NONACUTE VIRUSES

The LTR and *env* regions of the genomes of nonacute viruses have the most influence on the disease potential of the virus.[19,44,85] This reflects the important roles that the LTR and *env* play in the timing and activity of infections in target tissues.

Long Terminal Repeat and *env* in the Timing of an Infection

An example of LTR and *env* playing important roles in the timing of an infection is found in ALV-induced B-cell lymphoma.[19] Developing B cells are susceptible to cancer induction by overexpression of *c-myc* only during the first few weeks of life.[148] If an infection fails to reach the bursa of Fabricius (the site of developing B cells) before 1 to 2 months of age, a lymphoma does not develop in the chicken. Two regions of the ALV genome affect lymphomogenic potential: *env* and LTR.[19] These two regions also determine how rapidly an infection spreads within a chicken and the ability of viruses to reach the bursa within the first weeks of life.[19]

Tissue-Specific Roles for the Long Terminal Repeat

An example of LTR sequences playing important "tissue-specific" activities in disease induction is found in MuLV-induced erythroleukemia. In studies using recombinants of Friend MuLV (the helper for SFFV; see earlier) and Moloney MuLV (a T-cell lymphoma–inducing virus), sequences within the Friend MuLV LTR were found to confer the ability to induce erythroleukemia.[24] These erythroleukemia-inducing sequences mapped to the enhancer region of the LTR[55,93] (see Fig. 26-12). The T-cell disease specificity of the Moloney MuLV also mapped to the enhancer region,[93] with small mutations within the enhancer converting the disease specificity to erythroleukemia.[55,139]

RECOMBINATION BETWEEN ENDOGENOUS AND EXOGENOUS VIRUSES PLAYS AN IMPORTANT ROLE IN THE DISEASE POTENTIAL OF MURINE LEUKEMIA VIRUSES

Generation of Mink Cell Focus-Forming Virus Recombinants in Ectropic Virus–Infected Mice

The study of the leukemogenic potential of MuLVs is closely connected with the study of recombinant MuLVs. Mice that are viremic for ecotropic MuLVs (as a result of exogenous infection or spontaneous activation of a replication-competent endogenous provirus) frequently become viremic for MCF recombinants[65] (see Table 26-1). MCFs arise by recombination between the replicating ecotropic virus and endogenous viruses. During these recombinational events, a large portion of the 5' end of the *env* gene (which plays a determining role in the receptor specificity of SU) and portions of the LTR are replaced with endogenous sequences.[143] After these recombinational events, both the original, ecotropic parent and the new MCF virus replicate in the mouse. Because these viruses use different receptors, there is no interference between them, and cells frequently are infected by both viruses.

Mink Cell Focus-Forming Virus Recombinants Confer Shorter Latency Periods

Mink cell focus-forming virus recombinants that are selected in tumors frequently have higher oncogenic potentials relative to the original ecotropic virus. These higher potentials are reflected in the ability to induce disease after a shorter period of latency.[26,76,85] Part of this increased oncogenic potential results from the presence of the recombinant Envs of MCFs. However, part also results from recombinational events in the LTR and other coding regions of MCF viruses.[71,111]

Recombinant Mink Cell Focus-Forming Virus Envs in Disease

It is not clear whether recombinant MCF envelope glycoproteins contribute to pathogenicity by giving the virus additional access to target cells, or by stimulating the growth of target cells by interacting with a signal transduction pathway. The similarity between the MCF Env and that of SFFV, which clearly exerts its effect by interacting with a growth factor receptor (see earlier), suggests that MCF glycoproteins may serve as mitogenic signals for T cells.[151]

Recombinant Mink Cell Focus-Forming Virus Long Terminal Repeats in Disease

The recombinant enhancers in MCF LTRs are likely to contribute to pathogenicity by increasing the ability of insertional mutations to activate host proto-oncogenes. The ultimate induction of disease always is associated with clonal outgrowths of cells that have undergone proviral insertions in one or more proto-oncogenes[153] (see Chap. 11).

RETROVIRAL VECTORS AND PACKAGING CELLS

Vectors

Retroviral vectors are used to transduce (permanently insert) transcriptionally active foreign genes into eukaryotic cells[23,102] (Fig. 26-18). The vectors consist of replication-defective genomes that carry the gene or genes to be introduced (much like a transducing virus; see Fig. 26-18A). Several regions of the retroviral genome are required in the vector for it to be able to undergo a retroviral life cycle. These include both 5' and 3' LTRs, primer binding sites for the initiation of reverse transcription, and ψ or E sequences for the incorporation of transcripts into virions. Many vectors also include a "selectable" marker that can be used to enrich cell populations for vector-expressing cells. Vectors are constructed in bacterial plasmids using recombinant DNA technology.

Packaging Cells

Because replication-competent retroviruses are potential pathogens, the medical application of retroviral vectors requires that they be produced in an infectious form in the absence of a replication-competent helper virus. Cells designed for the production of infectious vectors are termed *packaging cell lines* (see Fig. 26-18B). Such lines express Gag, Pol, and Env proteins from mRNAs that lack packaging signals. When a vector is expressed in a packaging cell line, the cells should produce infectious particles of the vector, but no replication-competent helper virus.

A

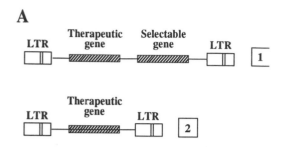

B

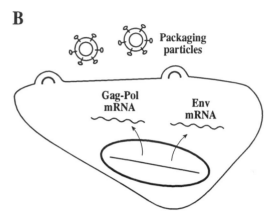

FIG. 26-18. (**A**) Examples of retroviral vectors. (1) Proviral form of the genome of a vector containing a therapeutically useful gene and a "selectable" gene. The presence of the selectable gene simplifies the isolation of cells infected with the vector. In practice, the selectable gene can be 5′ or 3′ of the therapeutic gene. The 3′ gene can be expressed from a separate promoter, or by splicing of a full-length mRNA. (2) Genome of a vector containing only a therapeutically useful gene. Both 1 and 2 include all the *cis*-acting sequences required for packaging, reverse transcription, integration, and expression. (**B**) Packaging cell used for production of infectious particles of a retroviral vector. Packaging cells synthesize viral proteins from Gag-Pol and Env mRNAs that lack sequences required for packaging. The proteins continually assemble into virus particles, but the particles contain no genomic RNA unless a "packageable" viral RNA is being produced in the cells. The production of packaged vector RNA is achieved by transfecting vector-encoding plasmid DNAs into the packaging cells.

The first packaging cell lines contained helper virus genomes from which packaging sequences had been deleted. However, recombination with packaging sequences in the vector or endogenous proviruses in the packaging cell frequently led to the appearance of fully replication-competent helper virus. More recently, packaging cell lines in which Env is expressed from a different mRNA from Gag and Gag-Pol have decreased the probability of such recombinational events.[37,101]

Medical Relevance

Retroviral vectors are useful both as reagents for research and as therapeutic agents, capable of introducing medically useful genes into diseased patients.[2,70,100] Although there remain technical problems in the successful therapeutic use of retroviral vectors, they are of potentially enormous significance because of their exquisite ability to stably transduce genes.

ABBREVIATIONS

ALSVs: avian leukosis sarcoma viruses; avian leukosis viruses are nontransducing viruses, avian sarcoma viruses are transducing viruses

ALV: avian leukosis virus, used in this chapter to denote the type C genus of retroviruses to which ALSV belong; also used to designate nontransducing members of the ALSV group of retroviruses

BLV: bovine leukemia virus

CA: the capsid protein, a subunit of Gag

c-erbA: a host cell proto-oncogene that can be converted to an oncogene by viral transduction

c-erbB: a host cell proto-oncogene that can be converted to an oncogene by insertional mutagenesis or viral transduction

c-myc: a host cell proto-oncogene that can be converted to an oncogene by insertional mutagenesis or viral transduction

E: encapsidation sequences for reticuloendotheliosis viruses; these are called ψ for MuLVs

env: a viral gene encoding the Env polyprotein

Env: a polyprotein that includes the SU and TM subunits of envelope glycoproteins

FeLVs: feline leukemia viruses

gag: a viral gene encoding the Gag polyprotein

Gag: group-specific antigen; a polyprotein that includes the internal structural proteins of retroviruses

GALVR1: gibbon ape leukemia virus receptor-1, a phosphate transporter that serves as a receptor for the 10A1 subgroup of MuLVs, the B subgroup of feline leukemia viruses, and gibbon ape leukemia viruses

GALVR2: gibbon ape leukemia virus receptor-2, a phosphate transporter that serves as a receptor for the 10A1 subgroup of MuLVs

LTR: long terminal repeat sequences at the ends of proviral DNA; contains cis-acting sequences for reverse transcription, integration, and transcription of viral RNA

MA: the matrix protein, a subunit of Gag

MAIDS: murine acquired immunodeficiency viruses

MCAT: murine cationic amino acid transporter, a basic amino acid transporter that serves as a receptor for ecotropic MuLVs

MCF: mink cell focus-forming virus

MLV: murine leukemia virus, used in this chapter to denote a type C genus of retroviruses that includes mammalian, avian, and reptilian subgenera

Mlvi-1: Moloney murine leukemia virus integration region-1, a region of host cell DNA that is associated with enhancer insertions that activate *c-myc* expression

Mlvi-4: Moloney murine leukemia virus integration region-4, a region of host cell DNA that is associated with enhancer insertions that activate *c-myc* expression

MuLV: murine leukemia virus, a subgroup of the mammalian type C subgenera of MLVs

NC: the nucleocapsid protein, a subunit of Gag

pol: a viral gene encoding reverse transcriptase and integrase

Pol: a polyprotein that includes reverse transcriptase and integrase

PR: the retroviral protease; PR can be encoded in the Pol polyprotein (MuLVs) or the Gag polyprotein (ALSV)

R: a short, direct repeat at the ends of viral RNA, the R sequence also is part of the LTR, where it resides between U3 and U5

Ram-1: receptor amphotropic, a locus in mice that encodes the GALVR2 receptor for the amphotropic subgroup of MuLVs

Rec-1: receptor ecotropic, a locus in mice that encodes the MCAT receptor for the ecotropic subgroup of MuLVs

Rmc-1: receptor MCF, a locus in mice that contains alleles encoding receptors for the MCF and xenotropic subgroups of MuLVs

SFFV: spleen focus-forming virus, an MuLV that causes erythroleukemias

SU: the receptor-binding subunit of Env

TM: the transmembrane subunit of Env

tva: a locus in chickens that encodes the receptor for subgroup A ALSV

tvb: a locus in chickens that encodes receptors for subgroups B, D, and E ALSV; different alleles at *tvb* encode receptors with different susceptibilities for subgroups B, D, and E viruses

tvc: a locus in chickens that encodes receptors for subgroup C ALSV

U3: unique sequences at the 3' end of viral RNA that become part of the LTR

U5: unique sequences at the 5' end of viral RNA that become part of the LTR

VL30: a group of endogenous viruses of mice that includes only replication-defective members

ψ: packaging sequences for MuLVs

ACKNOWLEDGMENTS

We are indebted to A.M. Skalka and S. Ruscetti for critical comments on portions of the chapter, to W. Gallaher for discussion of Figure 26-6, to P.N. Tsichlis for discussion of Figure 26-13, and to J.M. Coffin for provision of a preprint of reference. We thank M. Gonda and K. Nagashima for the electron micrographs used in Figure 26-9. We are indebted to the Biomedical Media Department of the University of Massachusetts Medical Center for help with the artwork, and to R. Reeves for invaluable bibliographic assistance.

REFERENCES

1. Adhya S, Gottesman M. Promoter occlusion: transcription through a promoter may inhibit its activity. Cell 1982;29:939–944.
2. Anderson WF. Human gene therapy. Science 1992;256:808–813.
3. Arcement LJ, Karshin WL, Naso RB, Arlinghaus RB. "gag" Polyprotein precursors of Rauscher murine leukemia virus. Virology 1977;81:284–297.
4. Astrin SM, Robinson HL, Crittenden LB, Buss EG, Wyban J, Hayward WS. Ten genetic loci in the chicken that contain structural genes for endogenous avian leukosis viruses. Cold Spring Harbor Symp Quant Biol 1980;44:1105–1109.
5. Baltimore D. RNA-dependent DNA polymerase in virions of RNA tumor viruses. Nature 1970;226:1209–1211.
6. Baltimore D. Nobel speech. Viruses, polymerases, and cancer. Science 1976;192:632–636.
7. Bates P, Young JAT, Varmus HE. A receptor for subgroup A Rous sarcoma virus is related to the low density lipoprotein receptor. Cell 1993;74:1043–1051.
8. Bebenek K, Kunkel T. The fidelity of retroviral reverse transcriptases. In: Skalka AM, Goff SP, eds. Reverse transcriptase. Cold Spring Harbor, NY: Cold Spring Harbor Laboratory Press, 1993:85–102.
9. Beemon K, Duesberg P, Vogt P. Evidence for crossing-over between avian tumor viruses based on analysis of viral RNAs. Proc Natl Acad Sci USA 1974;71:4254–4258.
10. Ben-David Y, Bernstein A. Friend virus-induced erythroleukemia and the multistage nature of cancer. Cell 1991;66:831–834.
11. Bernhard W. Electron microscopy of tumor cells and tumor viruses: a review. Cancer Res 1958;18:491–509.
12. Billeter MA, Parsons JT, Coffin JM. The nucleotide sequence complexity of avian tumor virus RNA. Proc Natl Acad Sci USA 1974; 71:3560–3564.
13. Bishop JM. Nobel lecture. Retroviruses and oncogenes II. Biosci Rep 1990;10:473–491.
14. Bishop JM, Varmus H. Functions and origins of retroviral transforming genes. In: Weiss R, Teich N, Varmus H, Coffin J, eds. RNA tumor viruses. Cold Spring Harbor, NY: Cold Spring Harbor Laboratory Press, 1982:999–1108.
15. Bittner JJ. Some possible effects of nursing on the mammary gland tumor incidence in mice. Science 1936;84:162.
16. Boerkoel CF, Kung H-J. Transcriptional interaction between retroviral long terminal repeats (LTRs): mechanism of 5' LTR suppression and 3' LTR promoter activation of *c-myc* in avian B-cell lymphomas. J Virol 1992;66:4814–4823.
17. Bolognesi DP, Montelaro RC, Frank H, Schafer W. Assembly of type C oncornaviruses: a model. Science 1978;199:183–186.
18. Boyer PL, Ferris AL, Clark P, et al. Mutational analysis of the fingers and palm subdomains of human immunodeficiency virus type-1 (HIV-1) reverse transcriptase. J Mol Biol 1994;243:472–483.
19. Brown DW, Blais BP, Robinson HL. Long terminal repeat (LTR) sequences, *env*, and a region near the 5' LTR influence the pathogenic potential of recombinants between Rous-associated virus types 0 and 1. J Virol 1988;62:3431–3437.
20. Brown DW, Robinson HL. Role of RAV-0 genes in the permissive replication of subgroup E avian leukosis viruses on line 15$_\beta$*ev*1 CEF. Virology 1988;162:239–242.
21. Brown PO. Integration of retroviral DNA. Curr Top Microbiol Immunol 1990;157:19–48.
22. Brown PO, Bowerman B, Varmus HE, Bishop JM. Retroviral integration: structure of the initial covalent product and its precursor, and a role for the viral IN protein. Proc Natl Acad Sci USA 1989;86: 2525–2529.
23. Cepko CL, Roberts BE, Mulligan RC. Construction and applications of a highly transmissible murine retrovirus shuttle vector. Cell 1984;37:1053–1062.
24. Chatis PA, Holland CA, Silver JE, Frederickson TN, Hopkins N, Hartley JW. A 3' end fragment encompassing the transcriptional enhancers of nondefective Friend virus confers erythroleukemogenicity on Moloney leukemia virus. J Virol 1984;52:248–254.
25. Chattopadhyay SK, Rowe WP, Teich NM, Lowy DR. Definitive evidence that the murine C-type virus inducing locus *Akv-1* is viral genetic material. Proc Natl Acad Sci USA 1975;72:906–910.
26. Cloyd MW, Hartley JW, Rowe WP. Lymphomogenicity of recombinant mink cell focus-inducing murine leukemia viruses. J Exp Med 1980;151:542–552.
27. Clurman BE, Hayward WS. Multiple proto-oncogene activations in avian leukosis virus-induced lymphomas: evidence for stage-specific events. Mol Cell Biol 1989;9:2657–2664.
28. Coffin J. Endogenous viruses. In: Weiss R, Teich N, Varmus H, Coffin J, eds. RNA tumor viruses. Cold Spring Harbor, NY: Cold Spring Harbor Laboratory Press, 1982:1109–1203.
29. Coffin JM. Retroviridae and their replication. In: Fields BN, Knipe DM, eds. Virology. 2nd ed. New York: Raven Press, 1990:1437–1500.
30. Coffin JM. Structure and classification of retroviruses. In: Levy JA, ed. The retroviridae. Vol 1. New York: Plenum Press, 1992:19–49.
31. Coffin JM. Retroviridae: the viruses and their replication. In: Fields

BN, Knipe DM, Howley PM, eds. Fields virology. 3rd ed. Philadelphia: Lippincott-Raven 1996:1767–1847.

32. Corneliussen B, Thornell A, Hallberg B, Grundstrom T. Helix-loop-helix transcriptional activators bind to a sequence in glucocorticoid response elements of retrovirus enhancers. J Virol 1991;65:6084–6093.

33. Crawford S, Goff SP. A deletion mutation in the 5' part of the *pol* gene of Moloney murine leukemia virus blocks proteolytic processing of the *gag* and *pol* polyproteins. J Virol 1985;53:899–907.

34. Crittenden LB. Retroviral elements in the genome of the chicken: implications for poultry genetics and breeding. Crit Rev of Poultry Biol 1991;3:73–109.

35. Cullen BR, Lomedico PT, Ju G. Transcriptional interference in avian retroviruses: implication for the promoter insertion model of leukaemogenesis. Nature 1984;307:241.

36. Cunningham JV, Kim JW. Cellular receptors for type C retroviruses. In: Wimmer E, ed. Cellular receptors for animal viruses. Cold Spring Harbor, NY: Cold Spring Harbor Laboratory Press, 1994:49–59.

37. Danos O, Mulligan RC. Safe and efficient generation of recombinant retroviruses with amphotropic and ecotropic host ranges. Proc Natl Acad Sci USA 1988;85:6460–6464.

38. DeFranco D, Yamamoto KR. Two different factors act separately or together to specify functionally distinct activities at a single transcriptional enhancer. Mol Cell Biol 1986;6:993–1001.

39. DesGroseillers L, Rassart E, Jolicoeur P. Thymotropism of murine leukemia virus is conferred by its long terminal repeat. Proc Natl Acad Sci USA 1983;80:4203–4207.

40. Dickson C, Eisenman R, Fan H, Hunter E, Teich N. Protein biosynthesis and assembly. In: Weiss R, Teich N, Varmus H, Coffin J, eds. RNA tumor viruses. Cold Spring Harbor, NY: Cold Spring Harbor Laboratory Press, 1982:513–648.

41. Doolittle RF, Feng DF, McClure MA, Johnson MS. Retrovirus phylogeny and evolution. Curr Top Microbiol Immunol 1990;157:1–18.

42. Dougherty RM, Di Stefano HS. Cytotropism of leukemia viruses. Prog Med Virol 1969;11:154–184.

43. Dyda F, Hickman AB, Jenkins TM, Engelman A, Craigie R, Davies DR. Crystal structure of the catalytic domain of HIV-1 integrase: similarity to other polynucleotidyl transferases. Science 1994;266:1981–1986.

44. Fan H. Influences of the long terminal repeats on retrovirus pathogenicity. Seminars in Virology 1990;1:165–174.

45. Fitting T, Kabat D. Evidence for a glycoprotein "signal" involved in transport between subcellular organelles. J Biol Chem 1982;257:14011–14017.

46. Foster RG, Lian JB, Stein G, Robinson HL. Replication of an osteopetrosis-inducing avian leukosis virus in fibroblasts, osteoblasts, and osteopetrotic bone. Virology 1994;205:179–187.

47. Friend C. Cell free transmission in adult Swiss mice of a disease having the character of a leukemia. J Exp Med 1957;105:307–318.

48. Fu W, Rein A. Maturation of dimeric viral RNA of Moloney murine leukemia virus. J Virol 1993;67:5443–5449.

49. Fujiwara T, Mizuuchi K. Retroviral DNA integration: structure of an integration intermediate. Cell 1988;54:497–504.

50. Gallaher WR, Ball JM, Garry RF, Griffin MC, Montelaro RC. A general model for the transmembrane proteins of HIV and other retroviruses. AIDS Res Hum Retroviruses 1989;5:431–440.

51. Gallaher WR, Ball JM, Garry RF, Martin-Amadee AM, Montelaro RC. A general model for the surface glycoproteins of HIV and other retroviruses. AIDS Res Hum Retroviruses 1995;11:191–202.

52. Gama Sosa MA, Rosas DH, DeGasperi R, Morita E, Hutchinson MR, Ruprecht RM. Negative regulation of the 5' long terminal repeat (LTR) by the 3' LTR in the murine proviral genome. J Virol 1994;68:2662–2670.

53. Gamett DC, Tracy SE, Robinson HL. Differences in sequences encoding the carboxyl-terminal domain of the epidermal growth factor receptor correlate with differences in the disease potential of viral *erbB* genes. Proc Natl Acad Sci USA 1986;83:6053–6057.

54. Gelderblom HR. Assembly and morphology of HIV: potential effect of structure on viral function. AIDS 1991;5:617–638.

55. Golemis E, Li Y, Frederickson TN, Hartley JW, Hopkins N. Distinct segments within the enhancer region collaborate to specify the type of leukemia induced by non defective Friend and Moloney viruses. J Virol 1989;63:328–337.

56. Golemis EA, Speck NA, Hopkins N. Alignment of U3 region sequences of mammalian type C viruses: identification of highly conserved motifs and implications for enhancer design. J Virol 1990;64:534–542.

57. Gorelick RJ, Henderson LE, Hanser JP, Rein A. Point mutants of Moloney murine leukemia virus that fail to package viral RNA: evidence for specific RNA recognition by a "zinc finger-like" protein sequence. Proc Natl Acad Sci USA 1988;85:8420–8424.

58. Gross L. "Spontaneous" leukemia developing in C3H mice following inoculation, in infancy, with AK-leukemic extracts, or AK-embryos. Proc Soc Exp Biol Med 1951;76:27–32.

59. Gross L. Development of myeloid (chloro-) leukemia in thymectomized C3H mice following inoculation of lymphatic leukemia virus. Proc Soc Exp Biol Med 1960;103:509–514.

60. Gross L. Mouse leukemia. In: Gross L, ed. Oncogenic viruses. 2nd ed. London: Pergamon Press, 1970:286–489.

61. Groudine M, Eisenman R, Weintraub H. Chromatin structure of endogenous retroviral genes and activation by an inhibitor of DNA methylation. Nature 1981;292:311–317.

62. Gunther CV, Graves BJ. Identification of ETS domain proteins in murine T lymphocytes that interact with the Moloney murine leukemia virus enhancer. Mol Cell Biol 1994;14:7569–7580.

63. Hanafusa T, Hanafusa H, Miyamoto T. Recovery of a new virus from apparently normal chick cells by infection with avian tumor viruses. Proc Natl Acad Sci USA 1970;67:1797–1803.

64. Hanafusa H, Hanafusa T, Rubin H. The defectiveness of Rous sarcoma virus. Proc Natl Acad Sci USA 1963;49:572–580.

65. Hartley JW, Wolford NK, Old LJ, Rowe WP. A new class of murine leukemia virus associated with development of spontaneous lymphomas. Proc Natl Acad Sci USA 1977;74:789–792.

66. Hatfield DL, Levin JG, Rein A, Oroszlan S. Translational suppression in retroviral gene expression. Adv Virus Res 1992;41:193–239.

67. Hayward WS. Size and genetic content of viral RNAs in avian oncovirus-infected cells. J Virol 1977;24:47–63.

68. Hayward WS, Neel BG, Astrin SM. Activation of a cellular *onc* gene by promoter insertion in ALV-induced lymphoid leukosis. Nature 1981;290:475–480.

69. Herman SA, Coffin JM. Differential transcription from the long terminal repeats of integrated avian leukosis virus DNA. J Virol 1986;60:497–505.

70. Hock RA, Miller AD. Retrovirus-mediated transfer and expression of drug resistance genes in human haematopoietic progenitor cells. Nature 1986;320:275–277.

71. Holland CA, Hartley JW, Rowe WP, Hopkins N. At least four viral genes contribute to the leukemogenicity of murine retrovirus MCF 247 in AKR mice. J Virol 1985;53:158–165.

72. Hu W-S, Pathak VK, Temin HM. Role of reverse transcriptase in retroviral recombination. In: Skalka AM, Goff SP, eds. Reverse transcriptase. Cold Spring Harbor, NY: Cold Spring Harbor Laboratory Press, 1993:251–274.

73. Huang M, Jolicoeur P. Myristylation of Pr60*gag* of the murine AIDS-defective virus is required to induce disease and notably for the expansion of its target cells. J Virol 1994;68:5648–5655.

74. Hughes SH, Shank PR, Spector DH, et al. Proviruses of avian sarcoma virus are terminally redundant, co-extensive with unintegrated linear DNA and integrated at many sites. Cell 1978;15:1397–1410.

75. Hunter E, Swanstrom R. Retrovirus envelope glycoproteins. Curr Top Microbiol Immunol 1990;157:187–253.

76. Ihle JN, Rein A, Mural R. Immunologic and virologic mechanisms in retrovirus-induced murine leukemogenesis. In: Klein G, ed. Advances in viral oncology. Vol 2. New York: Raven Press, 1984:95–137.

77. Jacks T, Varmus HE. Expression of the Rous sarcoma virus *pol* gene by ribosomal frameshifting. Science 1985;230:1237–1242.

78. Jenkins NA, Copeland NG, Taylor BA, Lee BK. Dilute (d) coat colour mutation of DBA-2J mice is associated with the site of integration of an ecotropic MuLV genome. Nature 1981;293:370–374.

79. Jenkins NA, Copeland NG, Taylor BA, Lee BK. Organization, distribution, and stability of endogenous ecotropic murine leukemia virus DNA sequences in chromosomes of *Mus musculus*. J Virol 1982;43:26–36.

80. Kalpana GV, Marmon S, Wang W, Crabtree GR, Goff SP. Binding and stimulation of HIV-1 integrase by a human homolog of yeast transcription factor SNF5. Science 1994;266:2002–2006.

81. Katoh I, Yoshinaka, Rein A, Shibuya M, Odaka T, Oroszlan S.

Murine leukemia virus maturation: protease region required for conversion from "immature" to "mature" core form and for virus infectivity. Virology 1985;145:280–292.

82. Katz RA, Skalka AM. The retroviral enzymes. Annu Rev Biochem 1994;63:133–173.

83. Keshet E, Temin HM. Cell killing by spleen necrosis virus is correlated with a transient accumulation of spleen necrosis virus DNA. J Virol 1979;31:376–388.

84. Kozak CA. Susceptibility of wild mouse cells to exogenous infection with xenotropic leukemia viruses: control by a single dominant locus on chromosome 1. J Virol 1985;55:690–695.

85. Kozak CA, Ruscetti S. Retroviruses in rodents. In: Levy JA, ed. The retroviridae. Vol 1. New York: Plenum Press, 1992:405–481.

86. Kung H-J, Boerkoel C, Carter TH. Retroviral mutagenesis of cellular oncogenes: a review with insights into the mechanisms of insertional activation. Curr Top Microbiol Immunol 1991;171:1–18.

87. Lazo PA, Lee JS, Tsichlis PN. Long-distance activation of the *myc* protooncogene by provirus insertion in *Mlvi-1* or *Mlvi-4* in rat T-cell lymphomas. Proc Natl Acad Sci USA 1990;87:170–173.

88. Lee PP, Linial ML. Efficient particle formation can occur if the matrix domain of human immunodeficiency virus type 1 Gag is substituted by a myristylation signal. J Virol 1994;68:6644–6654.

89. Lenz J, Haseltine WA. Localization of the leukemogenic determinants of SL3-3, an ecotropic, XC-positive murine leukemia virus of AKR mouse origin. J Virol 1983;47:317–328.

90. Levin JG, Rosenak MJ. Synthesis of murine leukemia virus proteins associated with virions assembled in actinomycin D-treated cells: evidence for persistence of viral messenger RNA. Proc Natl Acad Sci USA 1976;73:1154–1158.

91. Levy JA. Xenotropic viruses: murine leukemia viruses associated with NIH Swiss, NZB, and other mouse strains. Science 1973;182:1151–1153.

92. Li J-P, D'Andrea AD, Lodish HF, Baltimore D. Activation of cell growth by binding of Friend spleen focus-forming virus gp55 glycoprotein to the erythropoietin receptor. Nature 1990;343:762–764.

93. Li Y, Golemis E, Hartley JW, Hopkins N. Disease specificity of nondefective Friend and Moloney murine leukemia viruses is controlled by a small number of nucleotides. J Virol 1987;61:693–700.

94. Linial ML, Miller AD. Retroviral RNA packaging: sequence requirements and implications. In: Swanstrom R, Vogt P, eds. Retroviruses: strategies of replication. Berlin: Springer-Verlag, 1990:125–152.

95. Lowy DR, Rowe WP, Teich N, Hartley JW. Murine leukemia virus: high-frequency activation in vitro by 5-iododeoxyuridine and 5-bromodeoxyuridine. Science 1971;174:155–156.

96. Luciw PA, Leung NJ. Mechanisms of retrovirus replication. In: Levy JA, ed. The retroviridae. Vol 1. New York: Plenum Press, 1992:159–298.

97. Mathews TJ, Wild C, Chen C-H, Bolognesi DP, Greenberg ML. Structural rearrangements in the transmembrane glycoprotein after receptor binding. Immunol Rev 1994;140:93–104.

98. McClure MA. Evolutionary history of reverse transcriptase. In: Skalka AM, Goff SP, eds. Reverse transcriptase. Cold Spring Harbor, NY: Cold Spring Harbor Laboratory Press, 1993:425–444.

99. Meric C, Spahr PF. Rous sarcoma virus nucleic acid-binding protein p12 is necessary for viral 70S RNA dimer formation and packaging. J Virol 1986;60:450–459.

100. Miller AD. Human gene therapy comes of age. Nature 1992;357:455–460.

101. Miller AD, Buttimore C. Redesign of retrovirus packaging cell lines to avoid recombination to helper virus production. Mol Cell Biol 1986;6:2895–2902.

102. Miller AD, Rosman GJ. Improved retroviral vectors for gene transfer and expression. Biotechniques 1989;7:980–990.

103. Miller DG, Miller AD. A family of retroviruses that utilize related phosphate transporters for cell entry. J Virol 1994;68:8270–8276.

104. Mölling K, Bolognesi DP, Bauer H, Büsen W, Plassmann HW, Hausen P. Association of viral reverse transcriptase with an enzyme degrading the RNA moiety of RNA-DNA hybrids. Nat New Biol 1971;234:240–243.

105. Moroni C, Stoye JP, DeLamarter JF, et al. Normal B-cell activation involves endogenous retroviral antigen expression. Cold Spring Harbor Symp Quant Biol 1980;44:1205–1210.

106. Morse III HC, Chattopadhyay SK, Makino M, Fredrickson TN, Hügin AW, Hartley JW. Retrovirus-induced immunodeficiency in the mouse: MAIDS as a model for AIDS. AIDS 1992;6:607–621.

107. Muhlbock O, Bentvelzen P. The transmission of the mammary tumor viruses. Perspect Virol 1968;6:75–87.

108. Mullins JI, Chen CS, Hoover EA. Disease-specific and tissue-specific production of unintegrated feline leukaemia virus variant DNA in feline AIDS. Nature 1986;319:333–336.

109. Nielsen AL, Pallisgaard N, Pedersen FS, Jorgensen P. Murine helix-loop-helix transcriptional activator proteins binding to the E-box motif of the Akv murine leukemia virus enhancer identified by cDNA cloning. Mol Cell Biol 1992;12:3449–3459.

110. O'Hara B, Johann SV, Klinger HP, et al. Characterization of a human gene conferring sensitivity to infection by gibbon ape leukemia virus. Cell Growth Differ 1990;1:119–127.

111. Oliff A, Signorelli K, Collins L. The envelope gene and long terminal repeat sequences contribute to the pathogenic phenotype of helper-independent Friend viruses. J Virol 1984;51:788–794.

112. Payne LN. Biology of avian retroviruses. In: Levy JA, ed. The retroviridae. Vol 1. New York: Plenum Press, 1992:299–404.

113. Payne LN, Chubb RC. Studies on the nature and genetic control of an antigen in normal chick embryos which reacts in the COFAL test. J Gen Virol 1968;3:379–391.

114. Pozsgay JM, Beilharz MW, Wines BD, Hess AD, Pitha PM. The MA (p15) and p12 regions of the *gag* gene are sufficient for the pathogenicity of the murine AIDS virus. J Virol 1993;67:5989–5999.

115. Prats A-C, Roy C, Wang P, et al. *cis* Elements and *trans*-acting factors involved in dimer formation of murine leukemia virus RNA. J Virol 1990;64:774–783.

116. Ragheb JA, Anderson WF. pH-independent murine leukemia virus ecotropic envelope-mediated cell fusion: implications for the role of the R peptide and p12E TM in viral entry. J Virol 1994;68:3220–3231.

117. Raines MA, Maihle NJ, Moscovici C, Crittenden L, Kung H-J. Mechanism of c-*erbB* transduction: newly released transducing viruses retain poly(A) tracts of *erbB* transcripts and encode C-terminally intact *erbB* proteins. J Virol 1988;62:2437–2443.

118. Rein A. Retroviral RNA packaging: a review. Arch Virol 1994;S9:513–522.

119. Rein A, McClure MR, Rice NR, Luftig RB, Schultz AM. Myristylation site in Pr65^{gag} is essential for virus particle formation by Moloney murine leukemia virus. Proc Natl Acad Sci USA 1986;83:7246–7250.

120. Rein A, Mirro J, Haynes JG, Ernst SM, Nagashima K. Function of the cytoplasmic domain of a retroviral transmembrane protein: p15E-p2E cleavage activates the membrane fusion capability of the murine leukemia virus env protein. J Virol 1994;68:1773–1781.

121. Reisman D. Nuclear factor-1 (NF-1) binds to multiple sites within the transcriptional enhancer of Moloney murine leukemia virus. FEBS Lett 1990;277:209–211.

122. Rhee SS, Hunter E. Myristylation is required for intracellular transport but not for assembly of D-type retrovirus capsids. J Virol 1987;61:1045–1053.

123. Robinson HL, Astrin SM, Senior AM, Salazar FH. Host susceptibility to endogenous viruses: defective, glycoprotein-expressing proviruses interfere with infections. J Virol 1981;40:745–751.

124. Robinson HL, Eisenman R, Senior A, Ripley S. Low frequency production of recombinant subgroup E avian leukosis viruses by uninfected *V-15_B* chicken cells. Virology 1979;99:21–30.

125. Robinson HL, Miles BD. Avian leukosis virus-induced osteopetrosis is associated with the persistent synthesis of viral DNA. Virology 1985;141:130–143.

126. Robinson HL, Ramamoorthy L, Collart K, Brown DW. Tissue tropism of avian leukosis viruses: analyses for viral DNA and proteins. Virology 1993;193:443–445.

127. Rohdewohld H, Weiher H, Reik W, Jaenisch R, Breindl M. Retrovirus integration and chromatin structure: Moloney murine leukemia proviral integration sites map near DNase I-hypersensitive sites. J Virol 1987;61:336–343.

128. Rous P. Transmission of a malignant new growth by means of a cell-free filtrate. JAMA 1911;56:198.

129. Rous P. The challenge to man of the neoplastic cell. Nobel speech. Science 1967;157:24–28.

130. Rubin H, Cornelius A, Fanshier L. The pattern of congenital trans-

mission of an avian leukosis virus. Proc Natl Acad Sci USA 1961; 47:1058–1069.

131. Rubin H, Vogt PK. An avian leukosis virus associated with stocks of Rous sarcoma virus. Virology 1962;17:184–192.

132. Ruscetti S, Wolff L. Spleen focus-forming virus: relationship of an altered envelope gene to the development of a rapid erythroleukemia. Curr Top Microbiol Immunol 1984;112:21–39.

133. Satake M, Inuzuka M, Shigesada K, Oikawa T, Ito Y. Differential expression of subspecies of polyoma virus and murine leukemia virus enhancer core binding protein, PEBP2, in various hematopoietic cells. Jpn J Cancer Res 1992;83:714–722.

134. Selten G, Cuypers HT, Boelens W, et al. The primary structure of the putative oncogene *pim-1* shows extensive homology with protein kinases. Cell 1986;46:603–611.

135. Skripkin E, Paillart J-C, Marquet R, Ehresmann B, Ehresmann C. Identification of the primary site of the human immunodeficiency virus type 1 RNA dimerization in vitro. Proc Natl Acad Sci USA 1994;91:4945–4949.

136. Smith EJ, Fadly AM, Crittenden LB. Interactions between endogenous virus loci *ev6* and *ev21*. 2. Congenital transmission of EV21 viral product to female progeny from slow-feathering dams. Poult Sci 1990;69:1251–1256.

137. Smith RE. Avian osteopetrosis. Curr Top Microbiol Immunol 1982; 101:75–94.

138. Speck NA, Baltimore D. Six distinct nuclear factors interact with the 75-base-pair repeat of the Moloney murine leukemia virus enhancer. Mol Cell Biol 1987;7:1101–1110.

139. Speck NA, Renjifo B, Golemis E, Fredrickson N, Hartley JW, Hopkins N. Mutation of the core or adjacent LVb elements of the Moloney murine leukemia virus enhancer alters disease specificity. Genes Dev 1990;4:233–242.

140. Stehelin D, Varmus HE, Bishop JM, Vogt PK. DNA related to the transforming gene(s) of avian sarcoma viruses is present in normal avian DNA. Nature 1976;260:170–173.

141. Stoltzfus CM. Synthesis and processing of avian sarcoma retrovirus RNA. Adv Virus Res 1988;35:1–38.

142. Stoye JP, Fenner S, Greenoak GE, Moran C, Coffin JM. Role of endogenous retroviruses as mutagens: the hairless mutation of mice. Cell 1988;54:383–391.

143. Stoye JP, Moroni C, Coffin JM. Virological events leading to spontaneous AKR thymomas. J Virol 1991;65:1273–1285.

144. Takeuchi Y, Vile RG, Simpson G, O'Hara B, Collins MKL, Weiss RA. Feline leukemia virus subgroup B uses the same cell surface receptor as gibbon ape leukemia virus. J Virol 1992;66:1219–1222.

145. Temin HM. Nobel speech. The DNA provirus hypothesis. Science 1976;192:1075–1080.

146. Temin HM, Mizutani S. RNA-dependent DNA polymerase in virions of Rous sarcoma virus. Nature 1970;226:1211–1213.

147. Temin HM, Rubin H. Characteristics of an assay for Rous sarcoma virus and Rous sarcoma cells in tissue culture. Virology 1958;6: 669–688.

148. Thompson CB, Humphries EH, Carlson LM, Chen C-L H, Neiman PE. The effect of alterations in *myc* gene expression on B cell development in the bursa of Fabricius. Cell 1987;51:371–381.

149. Tracy SE, Woda BA, Robinson HL. Induction of angiosarcoma by a c-*erb*B transducing virus. J Virol 1985;54:304–310.

150. Troxler DH, Parks WP, Vass WC, Skolnick EM. Isolation of a fi-

broblast nonproducer cell line containing the Friend strain of the spleen focus-forming virus. Virology 1977;76:602–615.

151. Tsichlis PN, Bear SE. Infection by mink cell focus-forming viruses confers interleukin 2 (IL-2) independence to an IL-2-dependent rat T-cell lymphoma line. Proc Natl Acad Sci USA 1991;88:4611–4615.

152. Tsichlis PN, Sheperd BM, Bear SE. Activation of the *Mlvi-1/mis1/pvt-1* locus in Moloney murine leukemia virus-induced T-cell lymphomas. Proc Natl Acad Sci USA 1989;86:5487–5491.

153. van Lohuizen M, Berns A. Tumorigenesis by slow-transforming retroviruses: an update. Biochim Biophys Acta 1990;1032:213–235.

154. van Zeijl M, Johann SV, Closs E, et al. A human amphotropic retrovirus receptor is a second member of the gibbon ape leukemia virus receptor family. Proc Natl Acad Sci USA 1994;91:1168–1172.

155. Varmus H, Swanstrom R. Replication of retroviruses. In: Weiss R, Teich N, Varmus H, Coffin J, eds. RNA tumor viruses. Cold Spring Harbor, NY: Cold Spring Harbor Laboratory Press, 1982:369–512.

156. Varmus HE. Nobel speech. Retroviruses and oncogenes I. Biosci Rep 1990;10:413–430.

157. Vijaya S, Steffen DL, Robinson HL. Acceptor sites for retroviral integrations map near DNase I-hypersensitive sites in chromatin. J Virol 1986;60:683–692.

158. Vogt PK. Genetically stable reassortment of markers during mixed infection with avian tumor viruses. Virology 1971;46:947–952.

159. Vogt PK, Ishizaki R. Reciprocal patterns of genetic resistance to avian tumor viruses in two lines of chickens. Virology 1965;26:664–672.

160. Vogt VM, Eisenman R. Identification of a large polypeptide precursor of avian oncornavirus proteins. Proc Natl Acad Sci USA 1973; 70:1734–1738.

161. Wang LH, Duesberg PH, Kawai S, Hanafusa H. Location of envelope-specific and sarcoma-specific oligonucleotides on RNA of Schmidt-Ruppin Rous sarcoma virus. Proc Natl Acad Sci USA 1976;73:447–451.

162. Wang SW, Speck NA. Purification of core-binding factor, a protein that binds the conserved core site in murine leukemia virus enhancer. Mol Cell Biol 1992;12:89–102.

163. Weiss R. Interference and neutralization studies with Bryan strain Rous sarcoma virus synthesized in the absence of helper virus. J Gen Virol 1969;5:529–539.

164. Weiss R. Experimental biology and assay of RNA tumor viruses. In: Weiss R, Teich N, Varmus H, Coffin J, eds. RNA tumor viruses. Cold Spring Harbor, NY: Cold Spring Harbor Laboratory Press, 1982:209–260.

165. Weiss RA. Cellular receptors and viral glycoproteins involved in retrovirus entry. In: Levy JA, ed. The retroviridae. Vol 2. New York: Plenum Press, 1993:1–108.

166. Weller SK, Joy AE, Temin HM. Correlation between cell killing and massive second-round superinfection by members of some subgroups of avian leukosis virus. J Virol 1980;33:494–506.

167. Whitcomb JM, Hughes SH. Retroviral reverse transcription and integration: progress and problems. Annu Rev Cell Biol 1992;8:275–306.

168. Wills JW, Craven RC. Form, function and use of retroviral Gag proteins. AIDS 1991;5:639–654.

169. Young JA, Bates P, Varmus HE. Isolation of a chicken gene that confers susceptibility to infection by subgroup A avian leukosis and sarcoma viruses. J Virol 1993;67:1811 1816.

Viral Pathogenesis,
edited by Neal Nathanson, et al.
Lippincott–Raven Publishers, Philadelphia © 1997

CHAPTER 27

Visna-Maedi: The Prototype Lentiviral Disease

Opendra Narayan, Sanjay V. Joag, Yahia Chebloune, M.C. Zink, and
Janice E. Clements

INTRODUCTION

The pandemic caused by the human immunodeficiency virus (HIV) emphasizes the differences between its pathogenic mechanisms and those of other major human pathogens. The unchecked global toll that HIV has taken results from the convergence of several unique factors that favor the virus. Specifically, 1) the ability of HIV to exist as a swarm, resulting from a high rate of mutation of the virus and survival of pathogenic mutant genotypes that escape host immunity and cause infection in different organ systems; 2) its ability to integrate its DNA into host DNA and thus guarantee its survival; 3) its latent phase that involves replication in and dysregulation of host immune system cells, resulting in failure to induce curative immunity during infection; 4) its strategy in causing disease processes slow enough to ensure transmission; and 5) its apparent ability to cross host species barriers, are a combination that confers on HIV a most-formidable-virus status. All of these offensive strategies are pitted against a single weakness, its inefficient mode of transmission that requires the exchange of body fluids instead of excretions and aerosols.

O. Narayan and S. V. Joag: Department of Microbiology, Marion Merrell Dow Laboratory of Viral Pathogenesis, Kansas University Medical Center, Kansas City, Kansas 66160-7424.

Y. Chebloune: Institut National de la Recherche Agronomique (INRA), Ecole Nationale Veterinaire de Lyon, Lyon, France.

M. C. Zink and J. E. Clements: Division of Comparative Medicine, Johns Hopkins University School of Medicine, Baltimore, Maryland 21205.

The pathogenesis of the visna-maedi lentiviruses is examined from the perspective of the immunopathologic nature of the disease and the cell tropism of these viruses. The unique pathobiology of the lentiviruses in general results in part from their complex genetic structure and the activation of the virus from the quiescent proviral state by cellular and viral factors. An overview of the molecular biology and control of virus replication and gene expression is included.

PATHOGENESIS OF VISNA-MAEDI VIRUS INFECTION

Many of the concepts of pathogenesis mentioned previously, and discovered in HIV since the early 1980s, had begun to unfold in the 1950s in the course of studies by Bjorn Sigurdsson of an epizootic of slowly progressive pneumoencephalopathy, termed "maedi-visna," in Icelandic sheep.[108] *Visna* is Icelandic for wasting paralytic disease, and *maedi* for respiratory distress.[91] In addition to recording the clinical and histopathologic characteristics of the disease in the field, Sigurdsson isolated the etiologic virus (visna-maedi virus) in ovine cell cultures and showed that it caused multinucleated giant cell formation and lysis of the cells.[110]

Transmission experiments with visna-maedi virus established that the infection was persistent with a prolonged subclinical phase that lasted several months. The onset of disease was insidious, with gradual loss of flesh leading to cachexia in the animals (Fig. 27-1) and development of incoordination or respiratory distress. Disease progressed slowly over a period of months until death of the animals, with affected organs show-

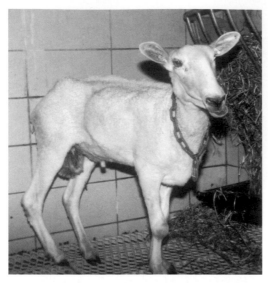

FIG. 27-1. Emaciated, 3-year-old Border Leicester ram, naturally infected with ovine progressive pneumonia virus and showing synovitis-arthritis and respiratory distress.

ing all of the typical histopathologic changes, as described earlier. Sigurdsson termed the syndrome "a slow infection" or "acute disease in slow motion," thereby establishing the concept of a type of viral pathogenesis that was distinctly different from that of classic acute diseases, such as influenza, poliomyelitis, and measles. Other investigators extended Sigurdsson's observations. Thormar's extensive studies on the biologic properties of visna virus in Iceland, and later in the United States, culminated with the demonstration that the agent was a species-specific retrovirus[67] that was cytopathic but not oncogenic, unlike all previously known pathogenic retroviruses. The fact that this retrovirus was exogenously transmitted also differentiated it from the then better-known endogenous retroviruses, such as strains of murine leukemia and avian leukosis viruses. Haase and Varmus confirmed the retroviral nature of visna virus with the demonstration of proviral DNA in infected cells.[42] These studies also established the major biologic properties of what would be a new taxonomic group of viruses, the lentiviruses, of which HIV would subsequently be identified as a member.[39] In addition to visna-maedi virus and HIV, the lentiviruses include the caprine arthritis-encephalitis virus (CAEV), the simian (SIV), the feline, and the bovine immunodeficiency viruses, and the equine infectious anemia virus (EIAV).

Visna is characterized histologically by chronic-active meningoencephalomyelitis and choroiditis with massive infiltrations of mononuclear cells around blood vessels in the neuropil (Fig. 27-2), development of microglial nodules in which the macrophages are activated and express major histocompatibility complex (MHC) class II antigens, and generalized astrogliosis. Focal malacia with dense infiltration of gitter cells frequently accompanies the inflammatory lesions. Pathologic changes also include areas of diffuse demyelination. Lesions in the spinal cord usually occur in the lateral and dorsal columns and are accompanied by a diffuse loss of myelin.[35,36,109,124]

Maedi is a classic interstitial pneumonia. Lesions consist of widespread infiltration of mononuclear cells into the interstitial spaces of the lung and around bronchi, and occur frequently in follicular arrangements (Fig. 27-3). Alveoli are obliterated by these infiltrations, and by thickening of the interalveolar septa. Macrophages are activated and express MHC II antigens. Diffuse proliferation of mesenchymal cells, including smooth muscle fibers, accompanies the inflammatory process.[21,37,54] Lymph nodes draining the lung undergo massive hyperplasia. In the Icelandic epizootic, affected sheep had either visna or maedi or both types of disease, although maedi was more prevalent.

Pathogenesis studies of visna by Petursson and colleagues confirmed and extended Sigurdsson's findings, with the newer studies showing that visna virus was cell associated and present in mononuclear cells in the peripheral blood, lymphoid tissues, and the brain of inoculated animals.[93] Further, comparative study of visna and experimental allergic encephalomyelitis in sheep established the close histologic parallels of the two syndromes and first suggested that the viral encephalopathy may have, in part, a cellular autoimmune pathogenesis.[92] Borrowing from their elegant studies showing that the pathogenesis of lymphocytic choriomeningitis virus infection in mice was mediated by cellular rather than humoral immune responses, Nathanson and coworkers inoculated sheep with visna-maedi virus, treated the animals with cyclophosphamide, and showed that this immunosuppressive therapy prevented development of early lesions of visna.[87] Although not definitive, this was the first illustration that the pathologic effects of the lentiviral infection were mediated by the cellular immune response to the virus, a finding shown also in HIV and SIV infections. In these latter infections, the early phase of infection is not only associated with a burst of virus replication, but the replication and histopathologic changes are associated with invasion of activated mononuclear cells into the central nervous system (CNS).[48,62,104]

Attempts to induce visna in American sheep by intracerebral inoculation of visna-maedi virus resulted in persistent in-

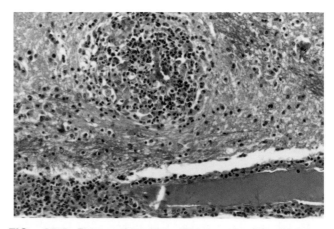

FIG. 27-2. Rare, visna-like disease in an American sheep,[106] showing encephalitis with intense perivascular accumulation of mononuclear cells in the neuropil. (Hematoxylin and eosin stain, magnification ×200.)

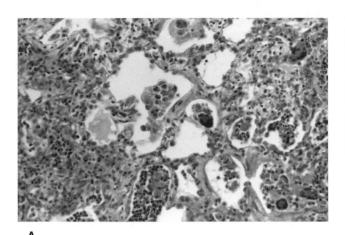
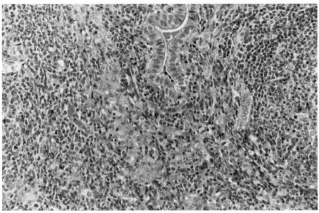

A   B

FIG. 27-3. Interstitial pneumonia typically caused by ovine lentivirus. (**A**) Alveolitis with sloughed macrophages into the alveoli; mononuclear cell infiltration in the interalveolar septa and collapse of alveoli by proliferating mononuclear cells. (**B**) Intense peribronchial accumulation of mononuclear cells, which become organized into follicular structures, shown in part on the right. (**A**, **B**, Hematoxylin and eosin stain, magnification ×200.)

fection and antigenic drift of the virus, but not progressive encephalopathy. Transient lesions of encephalitis developed in the animals at the site of inoculation in the brain, but these reactions led to scarification.[84] Inoculation of the same visna-maedi virus stock into Icelandic sheep caused encephalitis.[55] This established that genetic factors in the host played a role in regulating pathogenesis of the infection.

PATHOGENESIS OF CAPRINE ARTHRITIS-ENCEPHALITIS VIRUS INFECTION

In 1974, a new disease, caprine arthritis-encephalitis, was discovered in goats.[15] The etiologic virus (CAEV) is closely related to but distinct from Icelandic visna-maedi virus.[95] The predominant disease in goats is synovitis-arthritis, a syndrome that develops in adults with a pathogenesis following the same slow tempo as the ovine disease complex first described in Iceland.[18] The arthritic syndrome develops only in adults. The mammary gland is also a major target organ of the virus,[56] and studies in goats established that milk and colostrum were major sources of virus for transmission of the agent.[20,46] Further studies on goats showed that feeding of kid goats with milk pooled from several lactating animals, a practice that used to be prevalent in dairies, accounted for the massive infection of goats in industrialized countries, as opposed to the low incidence of infection in countries lacking facilities for mass production of milk.[1]

An intriguing new aspect of pathogenesis in the ovine-caprine disease complex was the finding of encephalopathy in neonatally infected goats.[15,16] This syndrome occurred sporadically in small herds in different parts of the world, and was associated with subclinical infection in the mothers. A rapidly progressive paralysis that was usually fatal within 2 months of birth developed in the kids. This disease is analogous to a rapid version of Icelandic visna. Histologically, lesions in both diseases are identical. The rapid course of the disease in newborn goats presaged the similar type of rapid onset of encephalopathy seen in newborn infants infected with HIV.[29] Inoculation of newborn goats intracerebrally with this virus resulted in severe inflammation at the site of inoculation and, in some animals, radiating inflammatory and demyelinating lesions from this site months later. Thus, unlike visna in U.S. sheep, the encephalitic syndrome was easily reproducible in goats.[17]

OTHER OVINE-CAPRINE LENTIVIRUS DISEASE SYNDROMES

Reexamination of maedi-visna disease complex in sheep in other parts of the world, after Sigurdsson's classic reports on the syndrome, showed that whereas maedi was a frequent occurrence, visna occurred only sporadically.[89,106] The dominant lentiviral disease in sheep in most parts of the world is the maedi-like disease called Montana lung disease[20] or ovine progressive pneumonia in the United States,[21] zwoergerziekte in Holland,[23] and Graaf-Reinet disease in South Africa,[80] among others. The disease in the United States was an indolent, sporadic syndrome that developed in adult animals, and was of only moderate importance to the sheep industry. In contrast, the disease outbreak in Iceland in the 1950s was prominent because it occurred in epizootic proportions after European rams had been introduced to diversify the gene pool of Icelandic sheep, which had become inbred after centuries of isolation from sheep in other parts of the world.[91] Ovine progressive pneumonia could be reproduced experimentally, with its typically long incubation period, protracted clinical course, and characteristic histopathologic changes. Both virus strain and breed of sheep affect outcome of infection with ovine progressive pneumonia virus (OPPV). Studies by Lairmore and colleagues had shown clearly that virus strains differ in virulence after intratracheal inoculation of virus into animals.[24,64] Border Leicester sheep in the United States and the Texel sheep in Holland seem particularly susceptible to disease.[80] Milking sheep in Europe also seem more prone to disease than sheep breeds that are reared for wool and meat. Lactating animals are more susceptible to mastitis, and the demonstration that the mammary gland is also a target organ for disease added a new dimension to the pathogenesis of infection.[56]

Comparison of the natural history of CAEV and visna-maedi virus in U.S. sheep, using polymerase chain reaction and DNA probes specific for each type of virus, showed that large numbers of sheep are infected with a virus more closely related to CAEV than to visna-maedi virus.[10,97] Moreover, the biologic properties of OPPV are more similar to those of CAEV than to those of visna-maedi virus, with respect to replication of the viruses in caprine cell cultures (CAEV and OPPV cause fusion; visna-maedi virus causes lysis) and failure to induce neutralizing antibodies (visna-maedi virus is a good inducer, CAEV and OPPV are poor inducers). Furthermore, arthritis occurs more frequently than CNS disease in naturally infected sheep. CAEV-like viruses may therefore be important in causing disease in sheep in this country. Goat milk is used on many sheep farms to feed orphan lambs, and this practice may have introduced virus across the species barrier.

CELL BIOLOGY OF OVINE-CAPRINE LENTIVIRUS INFECTIONS

Studies of the cell biology of the ovine-caprine viruses also provided another classic dimension of the *Lentivirus* genus—the ability to replicate in cells of the monocyte-macrophage lineage. Preliminary studies had shown that inoculation of visna-maedi virus or CAEV into phytohemagglutinin antigen (PHA)-treated peripheral blood mononuclear cells did not result in virus production.[40] Similarly, cultivation of PHA-treated mononuclear cells from blood or lymphoid tissues from infected animals also failed to yield infectious virus.[40] In contrast, cultivation of similar types of cell suspensions in medium that fostered differentiation of monocytes from the blood into macrophages led to productive virus replication in the cultivated macrophages.[40,85]

Comparison between primary sheep macrophages and sheep choroid plexus fibroblasts, the same type of cell culture used originally by Sigurdson and associates,[110] as host cells for virus replication, showed that in the macrophages, the virus budded into cytoplasmic vesicles where the particles accumulated until lysis of the cells, whereas in sheep choroid plexus fibroblasts, the virus matured at and budded from the plasma membrane of the cells. The morphogenesis of HIV follows a similar dual pathway, with virus accumulating intracellularly in macrophages and budding from the plasma membrane of infected T lymphocytes.

Studies on the molecular mechanism of this phenomenon showed that the enhancer region of visna-maedi viral long terminal repeats (LTR) contains AP-1 and AP-4 sites that bind inducible transcription factors Fos and Jun.[30,107] These nuclear-binding proteins participate in the differentiation of monocytes to macrophages, and during this process could activate transcription of viral RNA. The molecular aspects of infection by visna virus are detailed in Figure 27-5, later in the chapter. However, regulation of virus replication by transcription factors is probably only one of several mechanisms restricting virus replication in infected animals. In some animals studied longitudinally in the field, only unexpressed viral DNA could be found in peripheral blood mononuclear cells (by polymerase chain reaction),[97] and in such animals, this DNA could not always be expressed by cultivation and activation of macrophages from the animals.[10] In other animals, viral RNA but not virus production was found,[29] whereas in still others, viral proteins were identified in cultured macrophages, but no assembly of infectious virus particles occurred.[10] The onset of clinical disease correlated with virus production in macrophages in the affected tissues. This gave rise to production of cell-free virus in these local tissues. The enigma was that only the macrophages in the pathologically affected tissues were in a virus-productive phase. Macrophages from other tissues expressed variable levels of virus RNA, but these showed minimal evidence of virus production. Although bone marrow cells were high producers, Kupffer macrophages in liver were relatively poor producers of viral RNA.[34]

In addition to maturational factors in macrophages that induced virus production, T lymphocytes interacting with infected macrophages produced virus-specific cytokines, including an interferon-γ-like substance that caused activation of macrophages and enhanced expression of MHC II antigen.[54,83] This substance, found in cell cultures, was found in synovial fluid of arthritic joints in CAEV-infected goats[57] and in supernatant fluids of lymphocytes cultivated from lungs with progressive pneumonia lesions.[63] Whether production of this cytokine was an epiphenomenon or had a role in pathogenesis of the lesion is not known. However, production of this cytokine may explain activation of macrophages in the lesions, as well as the occurrence of free virus in the inflamed tissues. Cultivation of lymphocytes from these lesions failed to produce virus, whereas macrophages cultivated from the infected tissues produced cell-free virus for several days in culture. Thus, lesions in vivo were associated exclusively with productive virus replication in local tissue macrophages, the encephalitic lesions being associated with virus production in microglia, pneumonia with virus production in alveolar macrophages, and arthritis with virus production in synovial macrophages.

Another characteristic of the lentiviral lesion was the presence of high levels of antibodies against the viral glycoproteins at the site. Such antibodies were present in synovial fluid of arthritic joints of CAEV-infected goats.[51,52] Large numbers of plasma cells were also found in lesions of visna[35] and progressive pneumonia,[54] suggesting that immunoglobulins were produced locally at these sites also. A suggestion that these antibodies may be important in pathogenesis of the lesions came from two studies showing that immunization of infected sheep and goats with viral antigens led to increased severity of lesions.[73,86] Thus, the local tissue lesions were characterized by productive virus replication in the macrophages, activated macrophages, production of novel cytokines including an interferon-γ-like substance, and larger amounts of anti-viral antibodies. All of these factors are also present in HIV-induced encephalopathy and maedi-like pneumonia, and may therefore be generic to lesions caused by lentiviruses.

ROLE OF NEUTRALIZING ANTIBODIES IN LENTIVIRUS INFECTIONS

Studies of the persistent infection in sheep with visna-maedi virus showed that the animals expressed neutralizing antibodies to the virus, but new neutralization-resistant variants appeared subsequently in these animals. Gudnadottir first reported on this phenomenon,[41] which was confirmed later by Lutley and associates.[68] Further studies on the phenomenon were performed in our laboratory using plaque-purified visna-maedi virus to infect American sheep.[81,82] These experiments showed that antibody-escape variants developed subsequent to appearance of neutralizing antibodies. An unusual feature was that parental virus did not disappear, thus distinguishing antigenic drift in visna-maedi virus from the same phenomenon in chronic trypanosomiasis and malaria, with which it had been compared. Studies on antigenic drift of visna-maedi virus were extended to ovine cell cultures using plaque-purified virus for inoculation, followed by addition of "early" and "late" sera from infected sheep to select variants. Infected cultures treated with early neutralizing antibodies selected non-neutralizable variants of the virus within days of initiation of the treatment. "Late" sera with broadly neutralizing antibodies did not select variants, however, suggesting that antigenic variation did not continue indefinitely in individual animals.[79] The genetic basis of the antigenic variation phenomenon was illustrated by Clements and coworkers, who showed, using RNA fingerprint analyses of viral RNA, that the biologic effects of antigenic variation were associated with mutations and single-base deletions and substitutions, and that these changes accumulated in the viral RNA as the agent became more resistant to neutralization.[11,12] Antigenic drift of HIV was also demonstrated in cell culture[119] and in a macaque infected with $SIV_{mac}239$,[49] but the phenomenon was best illustrated in horses infected with another lentivirus, EIAV. Kono and associates' studies on this animal infection illustrated that the sequential episodes of fever and hemolytic crisis characteristic of horses infected with EIAV were associated with new antigenic variants of the virus.[61] Montelaro and colleagues' analysis of antigenic variation of EIAV confirmed the genetic basis of the phenomenon and provided new data, showing that mutations of the virus had occurred at random before neutralizing antibodies had developed in the animals. Variants of EIAV were then selected from a preexisting swarm by the neutralizing antibodies that appeared early after infection.[99] This phenomenon is relevant to HIV, which, like EIAV, replicates explosively during the first few weeks of infection, leading to viremia. Because viral mutation is a function of the rate of virus replication, the viral swarm effect, illustrated first in EIAV infection, could easily have allowed development of a few antigenic variants that would escape neutralizing antibodies induced by the dominant virus in the swarm. In animals infected with OPPV, however, neutralizing antibodies to the virus developed only rarely, unlike in sheep infected with Icelandic visna-maedi virus.

INSIGHTS FROM SIMIAN IMMUNODEFICIENCY VIRUS$_{MAC}$ INFECTION IN MACAQUES

The initial reports on the cell biology of HIV replication in cell culture and in people with acquired immunodeficiency syndrome (AIDS) had illustrated the unusually strong tropism of the virus for activated CD4+ T lymphocytes[6,94] and appeared to suggest that cells of the macrophage lineage were not as important in pathogenesis. Yet, this conflicted with data that people with HIV-associated neurologic disease had mainly macrophage-tropic virus in brain tissue, similar to sheep with visna.[29,60,105] This eventually led to the realization that the neurotropic stains of HIV were actually dual tropic viruses,[44] whereas viruses associated with AIDS were T-cell tropic.[115] The visna model seemed irrelevant to this question because in sheep and goats only a tissue-specific disease developed, and not AIDS, in keeping with the biologic property of the virus, which is macrophage but not T-cell tropic.

The pathogenesis of SIV_{mac} infection in rhesus macaques resembles that of HIV more than any other animal model.[66,76] The simian agents include viruses that are tropic for CD4+ T cells and others that are dual tropic for T cells and macrophages. Moreover, macaques infected with SIV_{mac} may manifest AIDS, immunosuppression, and neurologic disease. The following summary shows that despite the link between T-cell–tropic virus and AIDS, the experimental studies on the neurologic disease are reminiscent of visna. $SIV_{mac}239$ proved to be an ideal virus to begin these studies because this virus was derived from an infectious molecular clone that also was pathogenic.[58,78] Inoculation of this virus into PHA-treated blast cells and monocyte-derived macrophages derived from rhesus macaque peripheral blood showed that the virus replicated productively with fusion cytopathic effect in the T cells, but inefficiently in macrophages.[75] This virus infected macrophages, but the precursor proteins gp160 and core protein p55 did not undergo complete cleavage.[113] Inoculation of this virus into macaques duplicated the T-cell tropism seen in vitro.[103] Activated infected T cells appeared in lymphoid tissues and blood, accompanied by plasma viremia. The activated infected cells appeared in the cerebrospinal fluid, and this was associated with low-grade meningitis without productive virus replication in the neuropil.[48,62,103] The virus failed to replicate in neuropil even after intracerebral inoculation into animals. Infectious virus was not recovered from macrophages cultivated from any tissues (bone marrow, blood, spleen, lung, and brain), although homogenates of the lymphoid tissues had cell-free infectious virus. Many of the animals infected with $SIV_{mac}239$ became immunosuppressed during the following 2 years, and opportunistic infections or lymphoma developed.[25,26,103] None of our animals (about 20) had neurologic disease, although this syndrome had been reported from the Desrosiers laboratory.[26]

Simian immunodeficiency virus$_{mac}$239 was "neuroadapted" by two sequential passages of infectious bone marrow cells intracerebrally into uninfected macaques.[104] In two of two animals in the second passage, severe neurologic disease and interstitial pneumonia developed. Further studies on these and other animals in which encephalitis developed showed that the only animals that had CNS disease were those that had become severely immunosuppressed.[50] Thus, SIV that was mainly T-cell–tropic caused AIDS and transient meningitis, but no encephalitis. CNS disease was associated with selection of macrophage-tropic virus from bone marrow, but expression of this virus in brain occurred only in animals that had become severely immunosuppressed.[7] Animals infected with dual-tropic virus but that did not become severely immunosuppressed did not have CNS disease. One interpretation of the findings is that among viruses with dual tropism, expression of the macrophage tropic potential in the brain may be predicated on previous expression of the T-cell–tropic potential of the virus in lymphocytes, causing immunosuppression. Alternatively, two viruses may be involved in the pathogenesis, one with tropism for T cells, causing immunosuppression, and the other with tropism for macrophages, causing CNS disease.

The mechanisms of CNS disease in macaques required reevaluation of the pathogenesis of visna, whose etiologic virus replicates only in macrophages. In light of the SIV experience, does development of visna require immunosuppression in the animal? If so, are Icelandic sheep more susceptible to immunosuppression than non-Icelandic sheep (which are resistant to visna)? Reports on the pathologic process of visna by Georgsson and colleagues in Iceland[35] and Zink and associates in the United States[125] have suggested that cells morphologically similar to lymphocytes had viral RNA when evaluated by immunocytochemical and in situ hybridization procedures. It is possible that T cells may be defectively infected with visna-maedi virus and, in this setting, this could lead to clonal deletion of this subset of T cells specific to visna-maedi virus. This would bring the pathogenesis of visna more in line with that seen in macaques and humans. However, only future studies will elucidate these questions.

GENETIC STRUCTURE OF VISNA-MAEDI, CAPRINE ARTHRITIS-ENCEPHALITIS, AND SIMIAN IMMUNODEFICIENCY VIRUSES

The unique pathologic process, cell tropism, and regulated levels of viral gene expression characteristic of lentivirus infections of sheep are caused in part by the viruses' genetic structure. The virus genomes are more complex than those of other retroviruses, and encode regulatory genes that are important in replication and gene expression. In addition, productive virus replication in target cells in vivo requires cellular activation and the interaction of cellular and viral proteins.

The genomes of lentiviruses, like other retroviruses, are positive-stranded RNA molecules that range in size from 8.5 to 9.4 kilobases. Two copies of the viral genome are present in the virion. The high rate of recombination in retroviruses and lentiviruses occurs during reverse transcription of the genomic RNA from virions that contain two RNA molecules that have slightly different genetic compositions.

The genome of lentiviruses contains the structural (*gag* and *env*) genes and enzymatic (*pol*) genes typical of the retrovirus family (Fig. 27-4). However, in addition to these genes, lentivirus genomes encode regulatory genes that mediate the level of viral expression (*tat* and *rev*) as well as "auxiliary" genes that have functions that are being elucidated (*vif*,

vpr/vpx, *vpu*, and *nef*). These genes are referred to as "auxiliary" because they are not strictly required for virus replication in vitro in cell lines. In addition, different subsets of these genes are found in the genomes of lentiviruses. However, in more recent studies these auxiliary genes are emerging as important in vivo in the development of disease and thus in the pathogenesis of these virus infections. Lentiviruses can be separated roughly into two groups based on their cellular tropism. The lentiviruses of sheep, goats, and horses (visna-maedi virus, CAEV, and EIAV) replicate strictly in monocytes and macrophages, whereas the primate lentiviruses (HIV-1, HIV-2, and the SIVs) have dual tropisms for CD4+ lymphocytes as well as monocytes and macrophages. The genomic complexity of the dual-tropic lentiviruses is greater and this is reflected in the number of auxiliary genes present in the genome (see Fig. 27-4).

The RNA genomes of the lentiviruses contain repeated regions (R) at the 5' and 3' ends and unique 5' and 3' (U5 and U3) that are important in the process of reverse transcription of the genomic RNA into DNA. These regions comprise the LTR found in all retroviruses (see Fig. 27-4). The U3 region of the LTR of lentiviruses contains the enhancer and promoter elements that control transcription of viral RNA. The enhancer elements are recognized by cellular transcription factors that activate basal transcription of the viral genome (Fig. 27-5). All viral mRNA transcripts initiate transcription at the cap site (+1) in the 5' LTR and terminate in the 3' LTR at the polyadenylation signal (see Fig. 27-5). Transcription of lentiviral genomes initially depends on the presence in the cell of the appropriate cellular transcription factors. The specific cellular transcription factors used by a particular lentivirus are in part determined by the virus's cellular tropism. Thus, one of the cellular factors that activate transcription of SIV (see Fig. 27-2) is NF-κB, a transcription factor present in activated T lymphocytes and monocytes.[32] In contrast, visna-maedi virus and CAEV use the transcription factors c-Jun and c-Fos (that bind to AP-1 sequences) found in activated or differentiated macrophages.[30,107] In addition to these well characterized transcription factors, there are sites for additional cellular factors in the U3 region of all lentiviruses. These factors may provide lentiviruses with the capacity to be activated at the transcriptional level in many different cellular environments. The U3 region of the lentivirus genome has a high degree of heterogeneity. This may allow for the selection of viruses that can replicate in particular cells and organs.

The lentiviral *gag*, *pol*, and *env* genes encode the proteins that comprise the infectious viral particle. The capsid protein and the other Gag proteins provide the structural framework for the virus and interact at the cell membrane with the viral glycoproteins. The precise events leading to encapsidation of the viral RNA genome (two copies of viral RNA), along with the tRNA primer and reverse transcriptase, are not fully understood. Lentiviruses bud from the cell membrane in a fashion similar to the oncogenic retroviruses. However, in some biologically important cell types such as macrophages and endothelial cells, the lentiviruses also bud internally into intracellular vacuoles, providing a reservoir of infectious virus particles that are not exposed on the cell surface and cannot be recognized by the immune system.

In addition to the structural and enzymatic proteins, a number of the auxiliary proteins are also present in lentivirus parti-

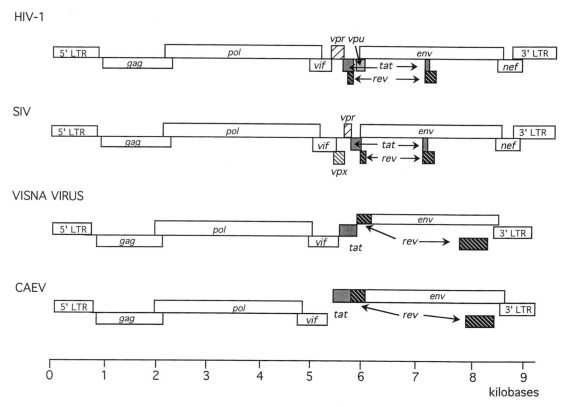

FIG. 27-4. The structure of lentivirus DNA. The genetic organization of visna-maedi virus, caprine arthritis-encephalitis virus (CAEV), human immunodeficiency virus-1 (HIV-1), and simian immunodeficiency virus (SIV) are presented as examples of the difference in the genomic complexity of these lentiviruses. LTR, long terminal repeat.

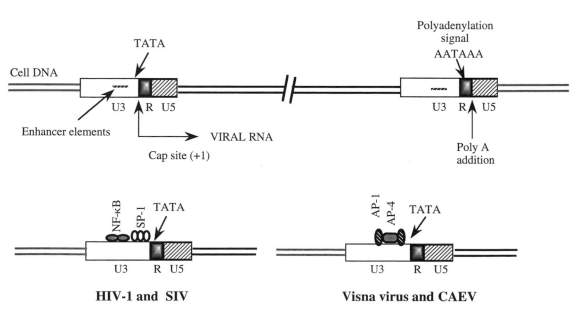

FIG. 27-5. Transcriptional control elements of lentiviruses. The long terminal repeat contains the U3, R, and U5 regions. The U3 region contains the transcriptional regulatory sequences called enhancers and promoters. The R region contains the cap site, which is the start of viral RNA synthesis and the signal for polyadenylation of the RNA. The core enhancer element is shown in the lower portion for human immunodeficiency virus-1 (HIV-1), simian immunodeficiency virus (SIV), visna-maedi virus, and caprine arthritis-encephalitis virus (CAEV). Nf–κB, nuclear factor κB.

cles. The Vif (viral infectivity factor) protein is present in the virus and appears to facilitate the infectivity and spread of virus, particularly in primary lymphocytes and macrophages.[53,65,88,112,118] Mutations in the *vif* gene prevent virus spread by cell-free virus, as well as by cell to cell spread. The *vpu* gene is also found in the virion.[114] The function of this protein in the virus life cycle is not clear, but it has been suggested that Vpu forms an ion channel and is important in the formation and release of viral particles.[123] Another function of the Vpu protein is the degradation of CD4, the cellular receptor for HIV-1 and HIV-2.[38,121] The Vpu protein has been shown to be a type 1 integral membrane protein, and forms oligomers in the infected cell.[69] A number of the lentiviruses package the Rev protein in the virion. This protein binds to a structured element in the genomic RNA and may be present in the viral particles because of this interaction (*rev* gene function is described later in this chapter).

SPECIFIC CHARACTERISTICS OF LENTIVIRUS REPLICATION

The lentiviruses are able to replicate in nondividing terminally differentiated cells. This implies that cellular DNA replication is not required for integration of the viral DNA into the cellular genome, unlike in oncogenic retroviruses. It is still an open question whether the auxiliary genes of the lentiviruses play a role in altering the nondividing cell to provide the necessary enzymes and metabolites for viral DNA replication and integration.

Replication of the lentivirus RNA genome into the double-stranded DNA proceeds by mechanisms similar to those elucidated for the other retroviruses. Lentiviral DNA then integrates randomly into the host cell chromosome. Early studies on replication of visna-maedi virus had suggested that viral DNA had an episomal relation to cellular DNA,[43] but subsequent molecular cloning of the integrated genomes of CAEV, EIAV, visna-maedi virus, SIV, and HIV-1 provided definitive evidence that lentiviruses do indeed integrate into the cellular DNA.[4,9,31,96,120,122] A study in our laboratory extended these observations, showing that SIV$_{mac}$ DNA integrated into the DNA of primary macaque macrophages inoculated with the virus.[3]

A new gene segment located between RNase H and IN, in the *pol* gene of nonprimate lentiviruses, has been identified.[72] The genomes of EIAV, visna-maedi virus, and CAEV contain this genetic element, but it is lacking in the *pol* genes of the primate lentiviruses. This region encodes a functional deoxyuridine triphosphatase (dUTPase) activity in feline immunodeficiency virus,[28] EIAV,[116] and visna-maedi virus (S.L. Payne, Case Western Reserve University School of Medicine, Cleveland, Ohio, unpublished observations) that has been found in gradient-purified virions. Thus, these viruses bring this protein into the cell on infection. Genetic analysis of this gene in EIAV has provided evidence that deletion of the dUTPase domain in an infectious clone results in functional reverse transcriptase and a virus that replicates to wild-type levels in cell lines. However, this dUTPase-deficient EIAV replicated poorly in cultures of primary equine macrophages. These data suggest that the virus-encoded dUTPase is required for efficient replication in macrophages. The function of the dUTPase in the genomes of nonprimate lentiviruses is unclear. However, the monocyte–macrophage is the primary target cell for these viruses in vivo, and this viral-encoded enzyme activity may reflect the adaptation to replication in these nondividing cells. Cellular dUTPases are cell cycle regulated, and one of their roles in cellular DNA replication is thought to be the prevention of uracil incorporation into DNA.[27,74] Thus, it is attractive to speculate that lentiviral dUTPase may serve a similar function during replication in nondividing cells, where cellular dUTPase levels might be low.

The ability of lentiviruses to replicate in nondividing cells distinguishes them from other groups of retroviruses. The presence of a group of auxiliary genes that are dispensable for replication of lentiviruses in some cell types, but not in others, suggests that these gene products may play critical roles in lentivirus replication in certain cell types in vivo. It is possible that the presence of different subsets of auxiliary genes confers species specificity and a unique pathobiologic process to each member of the lentivirus group.

REGULATION OF LENTIVIRUS GENE EXPRESSION BY VIRAL PROTEINS

Lentivirus replication can be separated into early and late phases. The regulatory proteins Tat, Rev, and Nef are expressed in the early phase and are the only viral proteins made during this period.[19] These proteins are translated from fully spliced viral mRNAs, in contrast to the other structural, enzymatic, and auxiliary proteins that are translated from unspliced or partially spliced viral RNAs. The Tat protein functions to increase transcription from the viral LTR and is similar to other viral transactivators in its interactions with basal transcription factors in the cell to activate transcription. This leads to the production of increased levels of viral RNA that is spliced in the cell and the synthesis of increasing levels of the Rev protein. A critical level of the Rev protein is required in the cell to shift to the late stage of viral replication. This is characterized by the transport of unspliced and partially spliced viral RNAs from the nucleus. This regulation of viral gene expression is observed only in the lentiviruses and retroviruses that encode Tat and Rev proteins (human T-lymphotropic virus [HTLV]-I, HTLV-II, and the spumaviruses have analogous gene products).

The *tat* gene of lentiviruses functions to increase viral gene expression at both the transcriptional and posttranscriptional levels.[13,19] In the SIV RNAs (as in HIV-1, HIV-2, and EIAV), a stem-loop structure called TAR (tat-activating region) located at the 3' end of the viral mRNA serves as a binding site for the tat protein and cellular proteins that function to increase gene expression from the viral promoter as well as to increase elongation of RNA. In contrast, visna-maedi virus and CAEV lack a TAR element and have tat proteins that act in a more indirect fashion.[33] Data obtained for the visna-maedi virus tat protein have shown that it is a transcriptional activator that contains a typical acidic-hydrophobic domain that does not bind directly to DNA or RNA.[8] The mechanism of action of this protein is more analogous to the transactivator proteins of adenovirus (E1a), HTLV-1 (Tax), and herpes simplex (VP16), which interact with cellular proteins to activate transcription.[45,47,98,111] The visna-maedi virus Tat protein activates transcription by means of the AP-1 site most proximal to the TATA box.[33] It also activates transcription of heterologous promoters (viral and cellular) that contain AP-1 sites. To dissect the functional domains of the visna-maedi virus Tat protein, the yeast gal 4 DNA binding domain was fused to the entire Tat protein or segments of the protein. An acidic-hydrophobic region at the amino terminus of the protein was found to contain the activation domain of the visna-maedi virus Tat protein.[8]

The Rev protein facilitates the export of unspliced viral mRNAs from the nucleus and the association of these viral RNAs with polyribosomes.[2,5] Rev proteins of lentiviruses share little amino acid homology, but have common functions that can be attributed to two separate functional domains.[77] One is a basic domain that acts as a nucleolar localization signal. Transiently expressed Rev proteins of HIV-1 and visna-maedi virus localize in the nucleolus of transfected cells.[71,100,117] It has been shown that the Rev proteins of visna-maedi virus and CAEV localize in the nucleolus of infected primary cells in culture.[101,102] The functional significance of Rev localization in the nucleolus is still under investigation. This cellular localization may be related to the association of Rev with cellular RNAs and proteins and the normal trafficking pattern of those cellular components.

Rev functions by binding through a basic domain in the protein to a highly structured RNA element (the Rev-responsive element, or RRE) present in the *env* gene of lentiviruses.[14,70,90] Rev protein binds to RNA through the RRE and facilitates the transport of unspliced and partially spliced viral mRNAs into the cytoplasm. The Rev protein may cause the utilization of an alternative RNA-processing pathway that bypasses the splicing machinery and promotes the transport of the viral RNAs through the nucleolus. Cellular RNAs that are not processed by the cellular splicing machinery are found in the nucleolus. The Rev proteins of visna-maedi virus and CAEV localize in the nucleolus regardless of whether viral RNAs are present in the cell.[101,102] Thus, nucleolar localization is independent of binding to the RRE in the viral RNA.

The Rev protein facilitates the expression of the unspliced viral RNA that encodes the structured proteins in the viral core (Gag proteins) and the enzymatic proteins in the *pol* gene. The singly spliced *env* gene also depends on the Rev protein for expression. Thus, late viral gene expression is initiated when these structural and enzymatic proteins are expressed in the infected cell. Further stages of lentivirus maturation are being studied and the roles of the other auxiliary genes (such as *vpu*) in these processes are beginning to be understood.[69]

The Nef protein, the third early gene product, is not required for virus replication in cell culture. However, the SIV$_{mac}$ *nef* gene is required in vivo for efficient virus replication and disease progression.[22,59] SIV$_{mac}$ mutants that have deletions in the *nef* gene cause infection in rhesus macaques but do not cause disease, and after a year in the animal protect against infection with wild-type virus.[22] The mechanism of action of the Nef protein is not completely understood; however, the expression in cells of either the HIV-1 or SIV$_{mac}$ Nef proteins results in the downregulation of CD4 (the cellular receptor for both viruses) on the surface of cells. Thus, the *nef* gene may function to reduce the amount of CD4 on the surface of infected cells, facilitating the expression of the Env proteins on the cell surface without interactions with CD4. The Nef protein is clearly important in the pathogenesis of SIV and may also be important in HIV-1. It is curious that the strictly monocyte-macrophage–tropic lentiviruses do not contain a *nef* gene. This may be related to the use of receptors other than CD4 that may have lower affinities and thus not require downregulation on the surface of the infected cell. Alternatively, these other lentiviruses may have gene products that function in an analogous fashion to the Nef protein, and once the receptors for these viruses are identified, a virus protein may be identified. In bovine immunodeficiency virus a truncated form of the transmembrane protein is expressed, and it has been postulated by Garvey and coworkers that this protein may be the Nef equivalent in the nonprimate lentiviruses.[31]

SUMMARY AND CONCLUSIONS

In summary, despite the apparently vast difference between the HIV disease complex and maedi-visna in sheep, numerous parallels in the mechanisms of virus replication, the intimate interactions between virus and infected cell, the host response to the agent, and the tempo of clinical disease confirm the common ground between the two systems. Whereas in many cases animal models of human disease are developed after characterization of the human syndrome, the maedi-visna syndrome preceded HIV and, in many ways, its pathogenesis predicted many aspects of the biology of HIV. The syndrome therefore fully merits its designation as one of the classic models of human disease.

ABBREVIATIONS

AIDS: acquired immunodeficiency syndrome
CAEV: caprine arthritis-encephalitis virus
CNS: central nervous system
dUTPase: deoxyuridine triphosphatase
EIAV: equine infectious anemia virus
HIV: human immunodeficiency virus
HTLV: human T-cell leukemia virus
LTR: long terminal repeat
MHC: major histocompatibility complex
OPPV: ovine progressive pneumonia virus
PHA: phytohemagglutinin
RRE: Rev-responsive element
SIV: simian immunodeficiency virus
TAR: tat-activating region

ACKNOWLEDGMENTS

Supported by grants NS-23039, AI-32369, NS-32208, NS-28357, NS-12127, AI-29382, NS-32203, and RR-06753 from the National Institutes of Health, Bethesda, Maryland. The authors thank Jean Pemberton and Maryann Brooks for typing the manuscript.

REFERENCES

1. Adams DS, Oliver RE, Ameghino E, et al. Global survey of serologic evidence of caprine arthritis-encephalitis virus infections. Vet Rec 1984;115:493–495.
2. Ahmed YF, Hanly SM, Malim MH, Cullen BR, Greene WC. Structure function analysis of the HTLV-1 rex and HIV-1 rev RNA response elements: insights into the mechanisms of rex and rev functions. Genes Dev 1991;4:1014–1022.
3. Anderson MG, McEntee MF, Narayan O, Clements JE. Integration of SIV DNA in primary macrophages. 1994.
4. Andresson OS, Elser JE, Tobin GJ, et al. Nucleotide sequence and biological properties of a pathogenic proviral molecular clone of neurovirulent visna virus. Virology 1993;193:89–105.
5. Arrigo SJ, Chen ISY. Rev is necessary for translation but not cytoplasmic accumulation of HIV-1, vif, vpr, and env/vpu 2 RNAs. Genes Dev 1991;5:808–819.
6. Barre-Sinoussi F, Chermann JC, Rey F, et al. Isolation of a T-lymphotropic retrovirus from a patient at risk for acquired immune deficiency syndrome. Science 1983;220:868–871.
7. Baskin GB, Murphey-Corb M, Roberts ED, Didier PJ, Martin LN. Correlates of SIV encephalitis in rhesus monkeys. J Med Primatol 1992;21:59–63.
8. Carruth LM, Hardwick JM, Morse BA, Clements JE. Visna virus Tat protein: a potent transcription factor with both activator and repressor domains. J Virol 1994;68:6137–6146.
9. Chakrabarti L, Guyader M, Alizon M, et al. Sequence of simian immunodeficiency virus from macaque and its relationship to other human and simian retroviruses. Nature 1987;328:543–547.
10. Chebloune Y, Karr B, Sheffer D, et al. Variations in lentiviral gene expression in monocyte-derived macrophages from naturally infected sheep. J Gen Virol 1996 (in press).
11. Clements JE, D'Antonio N, Narayan O. Genomic changes associated with antigenic variation of visna virus. II. Common nucleotide sequence changes detected in variants from independent isolations. J Mol Biol 1982;158:415–434.
12. Clements JE, Pedersen FS, Narayan O, Haseltine WA. Genomic changes associated with antigenic variation of visna virus during persistent infection. Proc Natl Acad Sci U S A 1980;77:4454–4458.
13. Clements JE, Wong-Staal F. Molecular biology of lentiviruses. Semin Virol 1992;3:137–146.
14. Cochrane AW, Chen CH, Rosen CA. Specific interaction of the human immunodeficiency virus rev protein with a structured region in the env mRNA. Proc Natl Acad Sci U S A 1990;87:1198–1202.
15. Cork LC, Hadlow WJ, Crawford TB, Gorham JR, Pyper RC. Infectious leukoencephalomyelitis of goats (CAEV). J Infect Dis 1974;129:134–141.
16. Cork LC, Hadlow WJ, Gorham JR, Piper RC, Crawford TB. Pathology of viral leukoencephalomyelitis of goats. Acta Neuropathol (Berl) 1974;29:281–292.
17. Cork LC, Narayan O. The pathogenesis of viral leukoencephalomyelitis-arthritis of goats. I. Persistent viral infection with progressive pathologic changes. Lab Invest 1980;42:596–602.
18. Crawford TB, Adams DS, Cheevers WP, Cork LC. Chronic arthritis in goats caused by a retrovirus. Science 1980;207:997–999.
19. Cullen BR. Mechanism of action of regulatory proteins encoded by complex retroviruses. Microbiol Rev 1992;56:375–394.
20. Cutlip RC, Lehmkuhl HD, Brogden KA, Bolin SR. Mastitis associated with ovine progressive pneumonia virus infection in sheep. American Journal of Veterinary Pathology 1985;46:326–328.
21. Cutlip RC, Lehmkuhl HD, Schmerr MJ, Brogden KA. Ovine progressive pneumonia (maedi-visna) in sheep. Vet Microbiol 1988;17:237–250.
22. Daniel MD, Kirchhoff F, Czajak SC, Sehgal PK, Desrosiers RC. Protective effects of a live attenuated SIV vaccine with a deletion in the nef gene. Science 1992;258:1938–1941.
23. DeBoer GF. Virus, the causative agent for both progressive interstitial pneumonia (maedi) and meningo encephalitis (visna) in sheep. Res Vet Sci 1975;18:15–25.
24. DeMartini JC, Brodie SJ, de la Concha Bermejillo A, Ellis JA, Lairmore MD. Pathogenesis of lymphoid interstitial pneumonia in natural and experimental ovine lentivirus infection. Clin Infect Dis 1993;17(Suppl 1):S236–S242.
25. Desrosiers RC. Simian immunodeficiency viruses. Annu Rev Microbiol 1988;42:607–625.
26. Desrosiers RC, Hansen Moosa A, Mori K, et al. Macrophage-tropic variants of SIV are associated with specific AIDS-related lesions but are not essential for the development of AIDS. Am J Pathol 1991;139:29–35.
27. Duker NJ, Grant CL. Alterations in the levels of deoxyuridine triphosphatase, uracil DNA glycosylase and AP endonuclease during the cell cycle. Exp Cell Res 1980;125:493–497.
28. Elder JH, Lerner DL, Hasselkus Light CS, et al. Distinct subsets of retroviruses encode dUTPase. J Virol 1992;66:1791–1794.
29. Epstein LG, Sharer LR, Joshi VV, Fojas MM, Koenigsberger MR, Oleske JM. Progressive encephalopathy in children with acquired immune deficiency syndrome. Ann Neurol 1985;17:488–496.
30. Gabuzda DH, Hess JL, Small JA, Clements JE. Regulation of the visna virus long terminal repeat in macrophages involves cellular factors that bind sequences containing AP-1 sites. Mol Cell Biol 1989;9:2728–2733.
31. Garvey KJ, Oberste MS, Elser JE, Braun MJ, Gonda MA. Nucleotide sequence and genome organization of biologically active proviruses of the bovine immunodeficiency like virus. Virology 1990;175:391–409.
32. Gaynor R. Cellular transcription factors involved in the regulation of HIV-1 gene expression. AIDS 1992;6:347–363.
33. Gdovin SL, Clements JE. Molecular mechanisms of visna virus tat: identification of the targets for transcriptional activation and evidence for a post-transcriptional effect. Virology 1992;188:438–450.
34. Gendelman HE, Narayan O, Molineaux S, Clements JE, Ghotbi Z. Slow, persistent replication of lentiviruses: role of tissue macrophages and macrophage precursors in bone marrow. Proc Natl Acad Sci U S A 1985;82:7086–7090.
35. Georgsson G, Houwers DJ, Palsson P, Petursson G. Expression of viral antigens in the central nervous system of visna-infected sheep: an immunohistochemical study on experimental visna induced by virus strains of increased neurovirulence. Acta Neuropathol 1989;77:299–306.
36. Georgsson G, Martin JR, Klein J, Palsson PA, Nathanson N, Petursson G. Primary demyelination in visna: an ultrastructural study of Icelandic sheep with clinical signs following experimental infection. Acta Neuropathol 1982;57:171–178.
37. Georgsson G, Palsson PA. The histopathology of maedi, a slow viral pneumonia of sheep. Vet Pathol 1971;8:63–80.
38. Geraghty RJ, Panganiban AT. Human immunodeficiency virus type 1 Vpu has a CD4- and an envelope glycoprotein-independent function. J Virol 1993;67:4190–4194.
39. Gonda MA, Wong-Staal F, Gallo RC, Clements JE, Narayan O, Gilden RV. Sequence homology and morphologic similarity of HTLV-III and visna virus, a pathogenic lentivirus. Science 1985;227:173–177.
40. Gorrell MD, Brandon MR, Sheffer D, Adams RJ, Narayan O. Ovine lentivirus is macrophagetropic and does not replicate productively in T lymphocytes. J Virol 1992;66:2679–2688.
41. Gudnadottir M. Visna-maedi in sheep. Prog Med Virol 1974;18:336–349.
42. Haase AT, Varmus HE. Demonstration of DNA provirus in the lytic growth of visna virus. Nature 1973;245:237–239.
43. Harris JD, Blum H, Scott J, Traynor B, Venture P, Haase A. Slow virus visna: reproduction in vitro of virus from extrachromosomal DNA. Proc Natl Acad Sci U S A 1984;81:7212–7215.
44. Ho DD, Rota TR, Hirsch MS. Infection of monocyte/macrophages by human T-lymphotropic virus type III. J Clin Invest 1986;77:1712–1715.
45. Horikoshi N, Maguire K, Kralli A, Maldonado E, Reinberg D, Weinmann R. Direct interaction between adenovirus E1A protein and the TATA box binding transcription factor IID. Proc Natl Acad Sci U S A 1991;88:5124–5128.
46. Houwers DJ, Pekelder JJ, Akkermans JW, van der Molen EJ, Schreuder BE. Incidence of indurative lymphocytic mastitis in a flock of sheep infected with maedi-visna virus. Vet Rec 1988;122:435–437.
47. Ingles CJ, Shales M, Cress WD, Triezenberg SJ, Greenblatt J. Reduced binding of TFIID to transcriptionally compromised mutants of VP16. Nature 1991;88:588–590.

48. Joag SV, Adams RJ, Foresman L, et al. Early activation of PBMC and appearance of antiviral CD8[+] cells influence the prognosis of SIV-induced disease in rhesus macaques. J Med Primatol 1994;23:108–116.

49. Joag SV, Anderson MG, Clements JE, et al. Antigenic variation of molecularly cloned SIV$_{mac}$239 during persistent infection in a rhesus macaque. Virology 1993;195:406–412.

50. Joag SV, Stephens EB, Galbreath D, et al. SIV$_{mac}$ chimeric virus whose env gene was derived from SIV-encephalitic brain is macrophage-tropic but not neurovirulent. J Virol 1995;69:1367–1369.

51. Johnson GC, Adams DS, McGuire TC. Pronounced production of polyclonal immunoglobulin G1 in the synovial fluid of goats with caprine arthritis encephalitis virus infection. Infect Immun 1983;41:805–815.

52. Johnson GC, Barbet AF, Klevjer-Anderson P, McGuire TC. Preferential immune response to virion surface glycoproteins by caprine arthritis encephalitis virus infected goats. Infect Immun 1983; 41:657–665.

53. Kan NC, Franchini G, Wong-Staal F, et al. Identification of HTLV-III/LAV or gene product and detection of antibodies in human sera. Science 1986;231:1553–1555.

54. Kennedy PGE, Narayan O, Ghotbi Z, Hopkins J, Gendelman HE, Clements JE. Persistent expression of Ia antigen and viral genome in visna-maedi virus-induced inflammatory cells: possible role of lentivirus-induced interferon. J Exp Med 1985;162:1970–1982.

55. Kennedy PGE, Narayan O, Zink MC, Hess J, Clements JE, Adams RJ. The pathogenesis of visna, or lentivirus induced immunopathologic disease of the central nervous system. In: Gilden DH, Lipton, H, eds. Clinical and molecular aspects of viral illness of the nervous system. Boston: Martinus Nijhoff, 1988;394–421.

56. Kennedy-Stoskopf S, Narayan O, Strandberg JD. The mammary gland as a target organ for infection with caprine arthritis-encephalitis virus. J Comp Pathol 1985;95:609–617.

57. Kennedy-Stoskopf S, Zink C, Narayan O. Pathogenesis of ovine lentivirus-induced arthritis: phenotypic evaluation of T lymphocytes in synovial fluid, synovium, and peripheral circulation. Clin Immunol Immunopathol 1989;52:323–330.

58. Kestler HW, Naidu YN, Kodama T, et al. Use of infectious molecular clones of simian immunodeficiency virus for pathogenesis studies. J Med Primatol 1989;18:305–309.

59. Kestler HW, Ringler DJ, Mori K, et al. Importance of the nef gene for maintenance of high virus loads and for development of AIDS. Cell 1991;65:651–662.

60. Koenig S, Gendelman HE, Orenstein JM, et al. Detection of AIDS virus in macrophages in brain tissue from AIDS patients with encephalopathy. Science 1986;233:1089–1093.

61. Kono Y, Kobayashi K, Fukunaga Y. Antigenic drift of equine infectious anemia virus in chronically infected horses. Archiv fur die Gesamte Virusforschung 1973;41:1–10.

62. Lackner AA, Vogel P, Ramos RA, Kluge JD, Marthas M. Early events in tissues during infection with pathogenic (SIVmac239) and nonpathogenic (SIVmac1A11) molecular clones of SIV. Am J Pathol 1994;145:428–439.

63. Lairmore MD, Butera ST, Callahan GN, DeMartini JC. Spontaneous interferon production by pulmonary leukocytes is associated with lentivirus-induced lymphoid interstitial pneumonia. J Immunol 1988;140:779–785.

64. Lairmore MD, Poulson JM, Adduci TA, DeMartini JC. Lentivirus-induced lymphoproliferative disease: comparative pathogenicity of phenotypically distinct ovine lentivirus strains. Am J Pathol 1988;130:80–90.

65. Lee TH, Coligan JE, Allan JS, McLane MF, Groopman JE, Essex M. A new HTLV-III/LAV protein encoded by a gene found in cytopathic retroviruses. Science 1986;231:1546–1549.

66. Letvin NL, Daniel MD, Sehgal PK, et al. Induction of AIDS-like disease in macaque monkeys with T-cell tropic retrovirus STLV-III. Science 1985;230:71–73.

67. Lin FH, Thormar H. Characterization of ribonucleic acid from visna virus. J Virol 1971;7:582–587.

68. Lutley R, Petursson G, Georgsson G, Palsson PA, Nathanson N. Antigens drift in visna: virus variation during long term infection of Icelandic sheep. J Gen Virol 1983;64:1433–1440.

69. Maldarelli F, Chen MY, Willey RL, Strebel K. Human immunodeficiency virus type 1 Vpu protein is an oligomeric type I integral membrane protein. J Virol 1993;67:5056–5061.

70. Malim M, Hauber J, Le SY, Maizel J, Cullen B. The HIV-1 rev trans-activator acts through a structured target sequence to activate nuclear export of unspliced viral mRNA. Nature 1989;338:254–257.

71. Malim M, Tiley L, McCarn D, Rusche J, Hauber J, Cullen BR. HIV-1 structural gene expression requires binding of the rev trans-activator to its RNA target sequence. Cell 1990;60:675–683.

72. McGeoch DJ. Protein sequence comparisons show that the pseudoproteases encoded by poxviruses and certain retroviruses belong to the deoxyuridine triphosphatase family. Nucleic Acids Res 1990;18:4105–4110.

73. McGuire TC, Adams DS, Johnson GC, Klevjer-Anderson P, Barbee DE, Gorham JR. Retrovirus challenge of vaccinated on persistently infected goats causes acute arthritis. Am J Vet Res 1986;47:537–540.

74. McIntosh EM, Ager DD, Gadsden MH, Haynes RH. Human dUTP prophosphatase: cDNA sequence and potential biological importance of the enzyme. Proc Natl Acad Sci U S A 1992;89:7020–8024.

75. Mori K, Ringler DJ, Desrosiers RC. Restricted replication of simian immunodeficiency virus strain 239 in macrophages is determined by env but is not due to restricted entry. J Virol 1993;67:2807–2814.

76. Murphey-Corb M, Martin LN, Rangan SRS, et al. Isolation of an HTLV-III related retrovirus from macaques with simian AIDS and its possible origin in asymptomatic mangabeys. Nature 1986;321:435–437.

77. Myers G, Pavlakis G. Evolutionary potential of complex retroviruses. The Retroviridae 1991;1:1–37.

78. Naidu YM, Kestler HW, Li Y, et al. Characterization of infectious molecular clones of simian immunodeficiency virus (SIV$_{mac}$) and human immunodeficiency virus type 2: persistent infection of rhesus monkeys with molecularly cloned SIV$_{mac}$. J Virol 1988;62:4691–4696.

79. Narayan O, Clements JE, Griffin DE, Wolinsky JS. Neutralizing antibody spectrum determines the antigenic profiles of emerging mutants of visna virus. Infect Immun 1981;32:1045–1050.

80. Narayan O, Cork LC. Lentiviral diseases of sheep and goats: chronic pneumonia leukoencephalomyelitis and arthritis. Rev Infect Dis 1985;7:89–98.

81. Narayan O, Griffin DE, Chase J. Antigenic drift of visna virus in persistently infected sheep. Science 1977;197:376–378.

82. Narayan O, Griffin DE, Clements JE. Virus mutation during "slow infection": temporal development and characterization of mutants of visna virus recovered from sheep. J Gen Virol 1978;41:343–352.

83. Narayan O, Sheffer D, Clements JE, Tennekoon G. Restricted replication of lentiviruses: visna viruses induce a unique interferon during interaction between lymphocytes and infected macrophages. J Exp Med 1985;162:1954–1969.

84. Narayan O, Strandberg JD, Griffin DE, Clements JE, Adams RJ. Aspects of the pathogenesis of visna in sheep. In: Mimms CA, Cuzner ML, Kelly RE, eds. Symposium on viruses and demyelinating diseases. New York: Academic Press, 1984:125–140.

85. Narayan O, Wolinsky JS, Clements JE, Strandberg JD, Griffin DE, Cork LC. Slow virus replication: the role of macrophages in the persistence and expression of visna viruses of sheep and goats. J Gen Virol 1982;59:345–356.

86. Nathanson N, Martin JR, Georgsson G, Palsson PA, Lutley RE, Petursson G. The effect of post-infection immunization on the severity of experimental visna. J Comp Pathol 1981;91:185–191.

87. Nathanson N, Panitch H, Palsson PA, Peturrson G, Georgsson G. Pathogenesis of visna. II. Effect of immunosuppression upon the central nervous system lesions. Lab Invest 1976;35:444–451.

88. Oberste MS, Gonda MA. Conservation of amino-acid sequence motifs in lentivirus Vif proteins. Virus Genes 1992;6:95–102.

89. Oliver RE, Gorham JR, Parish SF, Hadlow WJ, Narayan O. Ovine progressive pneumonia: pathologic and virologic studies on the naturally occurring disease. Am J Vet Res 1981;42:1554–1559.

90. Olsen CW, Cochrane AW, Dillon PJ, Nalin CM, Rosen CA. Interaction of the HIV type 1 rev protein with a structured region in env mRNA is dependent on multimeric formation mediated through a basic stretch of amino acids. Genes Dev 1990;4:1357–1364.

91. Palsson PA. Maedi and visna in sheep. In: Kimberlin RH, ed. Slow

viral disease of animals and man. Amsterdam: North-Holland, 1976: 17–43.

92. Panitch H, Petursson G, Georgsson G, Palsson PA, Nathanson N. Pathogenesis of visna. III. Immune responses to central nervous system antigens in experimental allergic encephalomyelitis and visna. Lab Invest 1976;35:452–460.

93. Petursson G, Nathanson N, Geysson G, Parritch H, Palsson PA. Pathogenesis of visna. I. Sequential virologic, serologic and pathologic studies. Lab Invest 1976;35:402–412.

94. Popovic M, Sarngadharan MG, Read E, Gallo RC. Detection, isolation and continuous production of cytopathic retroviruses HTLV-III from patients with AIDS and pre-AIDS. Science 1984;224:497–500.

95. Pyper JM, Clements JE, Molineaux SM, Narayan O. Genetic variation among lentiviruses: homology between visna virus and caprine arthritis-encephalitis virus is confined to the 5' gag-pol region and a small portion of the env gene. J Virol 1984;51:713–721.

96. Ratner L, Fisher A, Jagodzinski LL, et al. Complete nucleotide sequences of functional clones of the AIDS virus. AIDS Res Hum Retroviruses 1987;3:57–69.

97. Rimstad E, East NE, Torten M, Higgins J, DeRock E, Pedersen NC. Delayed seroconversion following naturally acquired caprine arthritis-encephalitis virus infection in goats. Am J Vet Res 1993;54:1858–1862.

98. Roberts SGE, Ha I, Maldonado E, Reinberg D, Green MR. Interaction between an acidic activator and transcription factor TFIIB is required for transcriptional activation. Nature 1993;363:741.

99. Salinovich O, Payne SL, Montelaro RC, Hussain KA, Issel CJ, Schnorr KL. Rapid emergence of novel antigenic and genetic variants of EIAV during persistent infection. J Virol 1986;57:71–80.

100. Saltarelli MJ, Schoborg RV, Pavlakis GN, Clements JE. Identification of the caprine arthritis encephalitis virus Rev protein and its cis-acting Rev-responsive element. Virology 1994;199:47–55.

101. Schoborg RV, Clements JE. The Rev protein of visna virus is localized to the nucleus of infected cells. Virology 1994;202:485–490.

102. Schoborg RV, Saltarelli MJ, Clements JE. A REV protein is expressed in caprine arthritis-encephalitis virus (CAEV) infected cells and is required for efficient viral replication. Virology 1994;202:1–15.

103. Sharma DP, Anderson M, Zink MC, et al. Pathogenesis of acute infection in rhesus macaques with a lymphocyte-tropic strain of simian immunodeficiency virus. J Infect Dis 1992;166:738–746.

104. Sharma DP, Zink MC, Anderson M, et al. Derivation of neurotropic simian immunodeficiency virus from exclusively lymphocytetropic parental virus: pathogenesis of infection in macaques. J Virol 1992;66:3550–3556.

105. Shaw GM, Harper ME, Hahn BH, Gallo RC. HTLVIII infection in brains of children and adults with AIDS. Science 1984;227:177–181.

106. Sheffield WD, Narayan O, Strandberg JD, Adams RJ. Visna-maedi-like disease associated with an ovine retrovirus infection in a Corriedale sheep. Vet Pathol 1980;17:544–552.

107. Shih DS, Carruth LM, Anderson M, Clements JE. Involvement of FOS and JUN in the activation of visna virus gene expression in macrophages through an AP-1 site in the viral LTR. Virology 1992;190:84–91.

108. Sigurdsson B. Observations on three slow infections of sheep: maedi, paratuberculosis, rida, a slow encephalitis of sheep with general remarks on infections which develop slowly, and some of their special characteristics. Br Vet J 1954;110:255–270.

109. Sigurdsson B, Palsson PA, Grissom H. Visna, a demyelinating transmissable disease of sheep. J Neuropathol Exp Neurol 1957;16:389–403.

110. Sigurdsson B, Thormar H, Palsson PA. Cultivation of visna virus in tissue culture. Archiv fur die Gesamte Virusforschung 1960;10:368–381.

111. Smith MR, Greene WC. Identification of HTLV-1 tax trans-activator mutants exhibiting novel transcriptional phenotypes. Genes Dev 1990;4:1875–1885.

112. Sodroski J, Goh WC, Rosen C, et al. Replicative and cytopathic potential of HTLV-III/LAV with or gene deletions. Science 1986;231:1549–1553.

113. Stephens EB, McClure HM, Narayan O. The proteins of lymphocyte and macrophage tropic strains of SIV are processed differently in macrophages. Virology 1995;206:535–544.

114. Strebel K, Klimkait T, Maldarelli F, Martin MA. Molecular and biochemical analysis of human immunodeficiency virus type 1 vpu protein. J Virol 1989;63:3784–3791.

115. Tersmette M, Gruters RA, de Wolf F, et al. Evidence for a role of virulent human immunodeficiency virus (HIV) variants in the pathogenesis of acquired immunodeficiency syndrome: studies on sequential HIV isolates. J Virol 1989;63:2118–2125.

116. Threadgill DS, Steagall WK, Flaherty MT, et al. characterization of equine infectious anemia virus dUTPase: growth properties of a dUTPase-deficient mutant. J Virol 1993;67:2592–2600.

117. Tiley LS, Brown PH, Le SY, Maizel JV, Clements JE, Cullen BR. Visna virus encodes a post-transcriptional regulator of viral structural gene expression. Proc Natl Acad Sci U S A 1990;87:7497–7501.

118. von Schwedler U, Song J, Aiken C, Trono D. Vif is crucial for HIV type 1 proviral DNA synthesis in infected cells. J Virol 1993;67:4945–4955.

119. Watkins BA, Reitz MSJ, Wilson CA, Aldrich K, Davis AE, Robert Guroff M. Immune escape by human immunodeficiency virus type 1 from neutralizing antibodies: evidence for multiple pathways. J Virol 1993;67:7493–7500.

120. Whetter L, Archambault D, Perry S, et al. Equine infectious anemia virus derived from a molecular clone persistently infects horses. J Virol 1990;64:5750–5756.

121. Willey RL, Maldarelli F, Martin MA, Strebel K. Human immunodeficiency virus type 1 vpu protein regulates the formation of intracellular gp120-CD4 complexes. J Virol 1992;66:226–234.

122. Yaniv A, Dahlberg JE, Tronick SR, Chiu IM, Aaronson SA. Molecular cloning of integrated caprine arthritis-encephalitis virus. Virology 1985;145:340–345.

123. Yao X, Goettlinger H, Haseltine WA, Cohen E. Envelope glycoprotein and CD4 independence of Vpu-facilitated human immunodeficiency virus type 1 capsid export. J Virol 1992;66:5119–5126.

124. Zink MC, Gorrell MD, Narayan O. The neuropathogenesis of visna virus infection in sheep. Neurosciences 1991;3:125–130.

125. Zink MC, Yager JA, Myers JD. Pathogenesis of caprine arthritis encephalitis virus: cellular localization of viral transcripts in tissues of infected goats. Am J Pathol 1990;136:843–854.

Viral Pathogenesis,
edited by Neal Nathanson, et al.
Lippincott–Raven Publishers, Philadelphia © 1997

CHAPTER 28

Reovirus

Herbert W. Virgin IV, Kenneth L. Tyler, and Terence S. Dermody

H. W. Virgin: Center for Immunology, Departments of Pathology and Molecular Microbiology, Washington University School of Medicine, St. Louis, Missouri 63110.
K. L. Tyler: Departments of Neurology, Microbiology, Immunology, and Medicine, University of Colorado Health Science Center and Neurology Service, Denver VA Medical Center, Denver, Colorado 80262.

T. S. Dermody: Departments of Pediatrics and Microbiology and Immunology, and Elizabeth B. Lamb Center for Pediatric Research, Vanderbilt University School of Medicine, Nashville, Tennessee 37232.

HISTORY AND PRINCIPLES

Mammalian reoviruses are nonenveloped, double-stranded RNA (dsRNA) viruses of the genus *Orthoreovirus*, family *Reoviridae*. The biology of reoviruses has been reviewed in detail.[139,205] In this chapter, we focus on mammalian reoviruses as models for analysis of viral pathogenesis at the level of the cell and the host.

Reoviruses infect humans, but are not associated with significant morbidity or mortality (reviewed in Tyler and Fields[205]). Despite the lack of a specific human disease association, experimental infection of animals with reovirus has been extremely valuable for analyzing how viruses cause disease (pathogenesis), the mechanisms underlying the severity of disease (virulence), and the basis for associations between infection and damage to specific cells or tissues (tropism). Indeed, principles that govern our understanding of viral pathogenesis frequently have been derived from studies of reovirus pathogenesis (reviewed in Morrison and Fields[129] and Nibert and colleagues[138]). The primary experimental model for analysis of reovirus pathogenesis has been infection of newborn or, more recently, adult severe combined immunodeficient (SCID) mice.[71,75,76,180]

Reoviruses are respiratory and enteric viruses that spread systemically in mice after primary replication in the lungs or intestine. The prominence of neurologic illness (either encephalitis or hydrocephalus) in infected neonatal mice has focused research on how these viruses enter and damage the nervous system. More recently, other reovirus-induced diseases such as hepatitis, pneumonitis, and myocarditis have been investigated. Using these systems in parallel with experiments in cell culture and in vitro, sequential stages in infection of the cell and the host have been delineated and analyzed.

The application of genetic techniques to analysis of viral pathogenesis has been a particularly important aspect of studies in the reovirus model system. Because of the segmented nature of the reovirus genome, genetic approaches allow identification of genome segments, and therefore proteins, involved in a particular stage of pathogenesis or step in infection of the cell. Structural information about the virion and structural intermediates in the virus replication cycle has clarified interpretation of both pathogenetic and genetic studies. The extensive background knowledge of stages of reovirus pathogenesis in animals and steps in reovirus infection of cells has facilitated analysis of how the immune system, especially humoral immunity, protects the host. In this chapter, we review relationships between viral proteins and structures, sequential steps in virus infection of cells and animals, and mechanisms of immunity, to provide a picture of how reoviruses interact with the host.

Original Isolation, Nomenclature, and Serotypes

The prototypic reoviruses were isolated from the gastrointestinal tract of humans or animals as part of a search for viral causes of human and veterinary disease (Table 28-1; reviewed in Tyler and Fields[205]). Albert Sabin subsequently proposed that these viruses be grouped as **r**espiratory **e**nteric **o**rphan

viruses on the basis of their structure and lack of associated human disease.[165] Leon Rosen collected a large number of reoviruses from around the world, and, using serologic techniques (hemagglutination inhibition), classified reoviruses into serotypes 1, 2, and 3.[156] "Strain" and "clone" have been used interchangeably to designate reovirus strains, and these designations are maintained in this chapter to be consistent with the literature. Prototype reoviruses serotype 1 strain Lang (T1L), serotype 2 strain Jones (T2J), and serotype 3 strains Abney (T3A) and Dearing (T3D) were each isolated from humans.[157,165] Reovirus serotype 3 clone 9 (T3C9) was isolated from a mouse,[83] whereas serotype 3 strain 8B (8B) is a myocarditic reassortant virus isolated from a mouse coinfected with T1L and T3D.[181]

The division of reoviruses into groups based on serotype has been useful because these groupings have consistently predicted important differences in pathogenesis and biochemistry. Thus, the reovirus serotypes are related in a number of ways, and yet are distinct in aspects of structure and pathogenesis. Serotypes 1 and 3 have been most extensively studied both structurally and pathogenetically, and thus, T1L and T3D are the best characterized viruses. Many of the field isolates collected by Rosen have become useful tools for addressing issues and mechanisms first defined by the prototypic reoviruses T1L and T3D.[43,84,94,234] T3D has been used extensively as a model for analysis of neurologic disease caused by reovirus, but this strain grows poorly in intestinal tissue and is much more virulent after intramuscular, intraperitoneal, or intracerebral inoculation than after peroral inoculation (see section on Stages in Infection of the Host). Therefore, T3C9, which is highly infectious after peroral inoculation and causes neurologic disease similar to that caused by T3D, has been used to produce serotype 3 disease after peroral inoculation.

Although prototype reoviruses have been extensively passaged in cell culture, sequences of the same genome segments determined by different groups have been remarkably consistent (reviewed in Nibert and associates[139]). This may be a result of the double-stranded nature of the reovirus genome and tight constraints on mutations tolerated in proteins that must retain the capacity to assemble stably and infect cells. The relative lack of mutations in viruses with different passage histories is an important property of reovirus, and has no doubt contributed to the success of reassortant genetic analysis, which would be confounded if mutations accumulated rapidly during tissue culture passage.

TABLE 28-1. *Prototype reoviruses used for pathogenesis studies*

Virus and serotype	Designation
Serotype 1 strain Lang	T1L
Serotype 2 strain Jones	T2J
Serotype 3 strain Abney	T3A
Serotype 3 strain Dearing	T3D
Serotype 3 clone 9	T3C9
Serotype 3 strain 8B	8B

THE INFECTIOUS AGENT

Reovirus Structure: Forms for Specific Purposes

Reoviruses have a dsRNA genome consisting of 10 discrete genome segments encoding 11 known proteins (Table 28-2). The reovirus structural proteins are arranged as two intercalated concentric shells (Fig. 28-1). There are eight structural proteins and three nonvirion-associated proteins. The functions of the nonvirion-associated proteins are not well understood. The ten genome segments fall into three size classes, large (L), medium (M), and small (S).[139] Genome segments are numbered within their size classes (see Table 28-2). Sequences have been determined for each of the segments of T3D, and many of the segments of T1L. The protein products of each genome segment have been identified (reviewed in Nibert and associates[139]). Protein products of different sized genome segments are referred to by size (σ proteins from the S segments, μ proteins from the M segments, and λ proteins from the L segments). Because the genome segments and proteins of the virus were identified independently, the number designations of the proteins are not always the same as the number designations of the corresponding genome segment (see Table 28-2). For example, both structural protein $\sigma1$ and nonvirion-associated protein $\sigma1s$ are encoded by the S1 segment, but $\mu1$ is encoded by segment M2. Nine of the ten segments encode single proteins, whereas the S1 segment is bicistronic, encoding the larger $\sigma1$ protein and the smaller $\sigma1s$ protein[58,89,168] (see Table 28-2; Fig. 28-2). In one other case (the M1 segment encoding core protein $\mu2$), alternate translation initiation sites may generate two forms of the same protein from a single segment,[154] although the larger of the two potential products has not been detected biochemically[154] (M. Roner, personal communication, October, 1995).

For reoviruses, the proteins of the icosahedral virion are arranged as two concentric shells, the outer capsid and core[51,139] (see Fig. 28-1). The outer capsid provides stability in the environment and serves as the first interface between the virus and its host. The core contains the dsRNA genome segments and mediates viral transcription. As the virus interacts with the host or cultured cells, the outer capsid of the virus is sequentially uncoated by proteolysis, giving rise to at least one distinct structural form that is intermediate between the intact virion and the core (see Fig. 28-1). This particle, termed the infectious subvirion particle (ISVP), has a number of important functions, including binding to intestinal microfold cells (M cells) and penetration of cell membranes. Virions, ISVPs, and cores have been studied extensively, both structurally and biochemically, and each plays an important role in virus-host interactions and viral replication.

Protein Constituents of Virions, Infectious Subvirion Particles, and Cores

Four reovirus proteins constitute the outer capsid. Six hundred copies each of proteins $\sigma3$ (encoded by segment S4) and $\mu1/\mu1C$ (encoded by segment M2), constitute most of the virion surface. The outer capsid has 60 copies of $\lambda2$ (encoded by segment L2), which are arranged as pentamers at each of the 12 vertices, and either 36 or 48 copies of $\sigma1$ (encoded by segment S1), which are arranged as oligomers at each of the 12 vertices. Each outer capsid protein has specific functions in interactions with cells and animal hosts. The $\sigma1$ protein mediates attachment of the virus to cells. Protein $\sigma3$ is the outermost reovirus capsid protein, and proteolysis of $\sigma3$ plays an important role in the transition from virion to ISVP, a process important for viral infectivity and entry into the host. Protein $\mu1/\mu1C$ plays a role in virus interactions with membranes.[116,136,202]

Uncoating of virions to ISVPs involves removal of outer capsid protein $\sigma3$, cleavage of the $\mu1/\mu1C$ protein to δ and ϕ,

---

TABLE 28-2. *Reovirus genome segments, encoded proteins, and their locations in viral particles*

Genome segment	Particles containing encoded protein	Encoded protein	Mass (kd) of protein	Copies in Virion
S1	Virion, ISVP	$\sigma1$	51	36–48
S1	Nonvirion associated	$\sigma1s$	14	—
S2	Virion, ISVP, core	$\sigma2$	47	120–180
S3	Nonvirion associated	σNS	41	—
S4	Virion	$\sigma3$	41	600
M1	Virion, ISVP, core	$\mu2$	83	12
M2	Virion, ISVP	$\mu1$	76	600
M3	Nonvirion associated	μNS	80	—
L1	Virion, ISVP, core	$\lambda3$	142	12
L2	Virion, ISVP, core	$\lambda2$	144	60
L3	Virion, ISVP, core	$\lambda1$	137–143	120

ISVP, infectious subvirion particle. Adapted from Dryden KA, Wang G, Yeager M, et al. Early steps in reovirus infection are associated with dramatic changes in supramolecular structure and protein conformation: analysis of virions and subviral particles by cryoelectron microscopy and image reconstruction. J Cell Biol 1993;122:1023–1041; and Nibert ML, Schiff LA, Fields BN. Reoviruses and their replication. In: Fields BN, Knipe DM, Howley PM, eds. Fields virology. 3rd ed. Philadelphia: Lippincott–Raven, 1996:1557–1596. Uncertainties in the numbers in the table are discussed in these references.

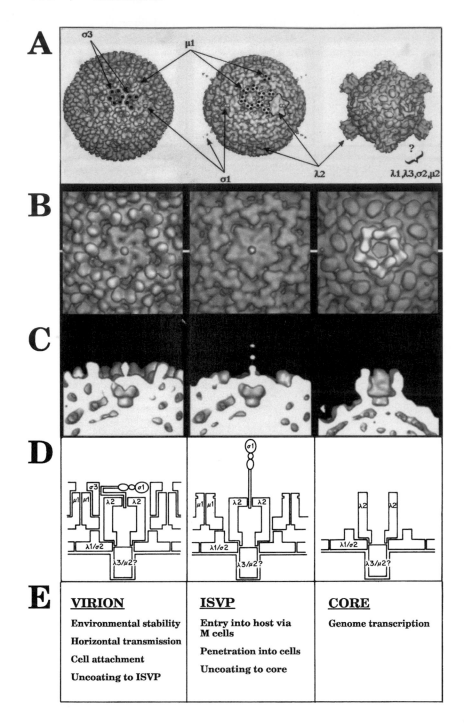

FIG. 28-1. Reovirus forms with specific biologic roles. Each panel of the figure shows (*left to right*) virions, infectious subvirion particles (ISVPs), and cores. (**A–C**) Image reconstructions from multiple cryoelectron micrographs. (Reconstructions made with the help of Kelly Dryden (Harvard Medical School, Boston, MA), based on images in Yeager M, Dryden KA, Olson NH, Greenberg HB, Baker TS. Three-dimensional structure of rhesus rotavirus by cryoelectron microscopy and image reconstruction. J Cell Biol 1990;110:2133–2144.) (**A**) External views of the reovirus virion, the ISVP, and the core. Specific proteins are identified with arrows directed to structures on the surface of the reconstructed images. (**B**) Enlarged view of the core spike and its surrounding structures. Note that the core spike changes conformation significantly when ISVPs are converted to cores with consequent opening of a channel in the core spike. (**C**) Cross-sectional reconstruction of the core spike. The cross-section is taken at the level shown by the white lines outside of the images in (**B**). (**D**) Schematic of the likely arrangement of viral proteins at and surrounding the core spike. The indentations in the µ1 protein in ISVPs denote that the protein is proteolytically cleaved as part of the conversion of virions to ISVPs. Note the changes in conformation in both the σ1 and λ2 proteins between virions, ISVPs, and cores. (**E**) Functions of different reovirus particles. M cell, microfold cell. (Adapted from Nibert ML, Fields BN. Early steps in reovirus infection of cells. In: Wimmer E, ed. Cellular receptors for animal viruses. Cold Spring Harbor, NY: Cold Spring Harbor Laboratory Press, 1994: 341–364.)

and extension of the σ1 protein outward from the surface of the virion (see Fig. 28-1; reviewed in Nibert and associates[139]). Further processing of ISVPs results in loss of σ1 and removal of µ1 cleavage fragments. The resulting particles, referred to as cores, catalyze transcription of viral dsRNA genome segments.[21,185] The core contains 120 copies of λ1, 120 to 180 copies of σ2, and 60 copies of λ2.[51] The specific arrangement of λ1 and σ2 in the core is not defined. The λ2 pentamer extends from the outer capsid of the virion into the core and is therefore available for interactions with outer capsid proteins σ1, σ3, and µ1/µ1C as well as core proteins pres-

ent at the base of the viral vertex (reviewed in Dryden and colleagues[51]). In addition to forming the core spike, λ2 participates in RNA synthesis as a guanylyl transferase.[34,118] The M1 and L1 segments encode minor core proteins (µ2 and λ3, respectively) present in approximately 12 copies per virion (reviewed in Dryden and colleagues[51]), consistent with an association between µ2 and λ3 at each of the 12 vertices. In addition, cryoelectron microscopy studies suggest that λ3 and possibly µ2 are associated with λ2 at the base of the viral vertex[51] (K. Dryden, M. Nibert, and B. N. Fields, personal communication). Protein λ3 can physically associate with com-

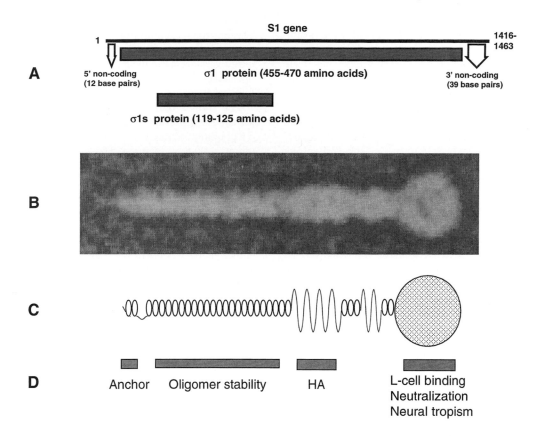

FIG. 28-2. Structure of the reovirus S1 genome segment and its protein products σ1 and σ1s. **(A)** Schematic of the S1 genome segment. The lengths of the segment differ between prototype reoviruses, with the T1L S1 segment containing 1463 nucleotides and the T3D S1 segment containing 1416 nucleotides. Beneath the genome segment schematic, filled boxes show the S1 segment protein products, σ1 and σ1s, and the relation between the open reading frames for σ1 and σ1s. **(B)** Reconstruction of the structure of the σ1 oligomer from multiple electron microscopic views. Prominent features include the globular head and two nodular densities in the tail adjacent to the head. **(C)** Line drawing of a σ1 monomer. Regions of α-helix (coils) and β-sheet (curved lines) in the σ1 tail, and the globular head (filled circle) are predicted by patterns of conserved apolar residues in an alignment of deduced σ1 amino acid sequences. **(D)** The relation between portions of the σ1 monomer and known biologic properties of the σ1 protein. HA, hemagglutination; L cell, L929 fibroblasts. (Figure prepared with the assistance of Mehmet Goral, MD, Vanderbilt University School of Medicine, Nashville, TN.)

plexes of λ2 and core protein λ1, and has RNA-dependent RNA polymerase activity.[192] Protein λ3 likely requires other core proteins to generate template specificity. The function of μ2 is not known,[154,226,241] although temperature-sensitive mutants that map to the M1 segment are compromised in RNA synthesis at nonpermissive temperatures (reviewed in Nibert and associates[139]).

The Reovirus Attachment Protein σ1

Many important properties, including viral attachment to cells, tropism in the central nervous system (CNS), and pathways of spread in the host, have been linked (using reassortant genetics) to the reovirus S1 segment, which encodes the σ1 and σ1s proteins. By virtue of its function as the viral attachment protein[101,225] and its importance in multiple aspects of reovirus biology, the σ1 protein has been the subject of intense study. The nonvirion-associated σ1s protein has received less attention than σ1; however, it is possible that some biologic properties mapped to the S1 segment are attributable to σ1s and not σ1.

Domains of the serotype 3 σ1 protein responsible for the binding of σ1 to cells have been partially characterized. Much less is known about cell-attachment domains of the serotype 1 σ1 protein, although the T1L and T3D σ1 proteins share some common structural features and some antibody epitopes.[78,135] The nature of the cellular receptors to which reoviruses bind is controversial. Carbohydrates are a part of the receptor for all three reovirus serotypes,[10,70,145–147] and sialic acid is the carbohydrate bound by serotype 3 reovirus.[70,146,147] Carbohydrates bound by serotype 1 and serotype 2 strains have not been identified. Cellular receptors important for reovirus infection are discussed in more detail in the section on Stages in Infection of the Cell.

The σ1 protein consists of an elongated fibrous tail topped with a globular head[64,65] (see Fig. 28-2). In intact virions, σ1 forms an oligomer,[15,103,193] which is located at the 12 fivefold vertices of the virion icosahedron where it associates with core spike protein, λ2.[51,64,65,193] Data suggest that the oligomeric species of σ1 is either a trimer[103,106,193] or a tetramer.[15,64] Predictions of secondary structure and hydrophobicity of σ1 proteins of prototype[135] and field isolate[43] reovirus strains have been used to correlate σ1 sequence features with morphologic characteristics digitally imaged by electron microscopy.[64] A model of σ1 structure (see Fig. 28-2) suggests that amino acid sequences in the σ1 tail form a tandem arrangement of α-helix and β-sheet structural motifs. Sequences in the σ1 head likely assume a more complex arrangement of secondary structures.[64,135] Amino acid sequences predicted to form α-helix in the σ1 tail are important for stabilizing σ1 oligomers,[104] and a short, amino-terminal domain of σ1 anchors the protein to the virion.[105,117]

Reoviruses bind to erythrocytes and numerous types of cultured cells. Binding to erythrocytes is detected as hemagglutination (HA). The importance of HA capacity in reovirus pathogenesis has not been defined. Nonetheless, studies of reovirus HA have contributed important information about interactions of σ1 with cellular receptors. For serotype 3 reoviruses, σ1 binding to sialic acid is important for HA, and the capacity to produce HA is determined by sequences in the σ1 tail.[42] Large deletions in the tail of expressed T3D σ1 lead to loss of HA capacity, whereas binding to murine L929 fibroblasts is retained.[133] Serotype 3 strains that do not produce HA contain single amino acid substitutions at positions 198, 202, and 204, which are located in the larger of two predicted β-sheet structures in the σ1 tail[42] (see Fig. 28-2). These sequences are also important for serotype 3 reovirus infection of murine erythroleukemia (MEL) cells, an erythroid precursor cell line.[164]

In contrast to the importance of the σ1 tail in HA and infection of MEL cells, several lines of evidence suggest that the σ1 head is important for binding to other types of cells, including L cells,[53,106,133,203] ependymal cells,[199] thymoma cells,[35,167,231] rat neuroblastoma cells,[35] explanted mouse and rat cortical neurons,[46] and cells in various regions of the mouse CNS.[93,190,209] Mutagenesis studies suggest that the receptor-binding domain in the σ1 head includes a series of noncontiguous amino acids.[203] Point mutations[203] and nested deletions[53] in the σ1 head abrogate binding of expressed σ1 to L cells. It has been suggested that a monoclonal anti-idiotype antibody (87.92.6), which is directed against a σ1-specific monoclonal antibody (9BG5) whose target epitope lies within the globular head of σ1, contains an internal image of the σ1 receptor-binding domain. The antigen-binding region of this anti-idiotype antibody contains an amino acid sequence that is similar to amino acids 317 to 332 within the σ1 head,[231] and synthetic peptides derived from this sequence inhibit binding of T3D to cultured cells.[232] Amino acid substitutions in the σ1 proteins of neutralization-resistant variants of T3D selected by anti-σ1 mono-

clonal antibodies occur in the head at positions 340 and 419.[16,93] These variants demonstrate dramatic alterations in their tropism within the mouse CNS.[93,190] Mutations in these antibody-selected variants are in the σ1 open reading frame, but not the σ1s open reading frame,[16] a distinction important for attributing differences in neurotropism to σ1 rather than σ1s.

The studies outlined previously suggest that, at least for serotype 3 reoviruses, sequences in either the head or tail of σ1 play important roles in receptor-binding depending on the target cell. For example, HA-negative serotype 3 reovirus strains grow in L cells to titers comparable to those of HA-positive strains, but fail to bind to MEL cells.[164] This pattern of growth indicates that sequences in the σ1 tail, which are important for binding to sialic acid, are more important for binding to MEL cells than L cells. When the σ1 head is removed from virions by proteolysis, binding to L cells becomes more dependent on sialic acid, demonstrating that the head and tail of σ1 contain independent receptor-binding domains.[134] These findings are consistent with a model of serotype 3 reovirus cell attachment in which σ1 mediates two binding events, one involving an interaction between the σ1 tail and sialic acid and another involving an interaction between the σ1 head and an as yet unidentified moiety on the same or discrete cell surface molecule.[42] In the case of L cells and other types of cells, interactions between the σ1 tail and the abundant ligand sialic acid may constitute the initial binding event, which is followed by interactions between the σ1 head and a second target. For attachment of serotype 3 reovirus to MEL cells, a receptor for the σ1 head may not exist, or may be of such low affinity that binding of sialic acid by the σ1 tail constitutes the critical binding step.

The Segmented Reovirus Genome and Principles of Reassortant Genetics

The most important advantage of reovirus as a model system is the availability of genetic tools for pathogenetic studies. Although mutant viruses have been evaluated in detail, the strength of the system has been the availability of reassortant genetics as a means to identify genome segments associated with various aspects of the virus-host interaction. Soon after the initial isolation of reoviruses, it became clear that the genome consists of dsRNA. Subsequent studies showed that the genome consists of ten individual genome segments encoding one or two proteins (reviewed in Nibert and associates[139]). Thus, genetic studies linking a genome segment to a particular phenotype link one or at most two proteins to that phenotype. Although the segmented nature of the genome created the potential for use of reassortants as genetic tools, it was the discovery that genome segments from different viruses exhibit polymorphic migration patterns in polyacrylamide gels that made reassortant genetic analysis practical (reviewed in Sharpe and Fields[175,176]).

Coinfection of a cell with two reovirus strains gives rise to progeny (reassortant viruses) that contain different combinations of parental genome segments (Fig. 28-3). This phenomenon is different from recombination, in which distinct portions of the same genome segment are derived from separate parental viruses. Recombination has not been demonstrated for reoviruses. Reoviruses containing different combinations

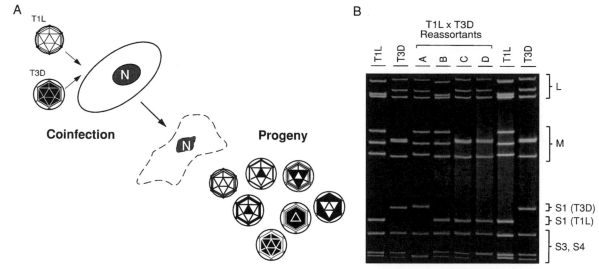

FIG. 28-3. Reassortment of genome segments during infection of a cell with different reoviruses. **(A)** Cell being infected with two reovirus strains, T1L and T3D. As virus replicates, genome segments of T1L and T3D are assorted in different combinations into progeny virions, as schematically indicated here. N, nucleus. **(B)** After plaque purification, reassortant progeny can be analyzed by sodium dodecyl sulfate-polyacrylamide gel electrophoresis. Genomic double-stranded RNA prepared from parental T1L and T3D, as well as the T1L × T3D reassortants, is electrophoresed and the mobilities of genome segments compared. The parental origin of genome segments in a reassortant virus is established by comparing the mobilities of reassortant and parental genome segment. For example, reassortant A in **(B)** has the S1 genome segment derived from T3D, whereas reassortants B through D have the S1 genome segment derived from T1L. (Figure prepared with the assistance of Mehmet Goral and Steven Rodgers, Vanderbilt University School of Medicine, Nashville, TN.)

of parental genome segments are properly termed "reassortants" rather than "recombinants" because each genome segment is derived exclusively from one or the other parental virus. Although most reassortants have been generated using coinfection, novel methods such as microinjection of reovirus cores into cells have been useful for generating monoreassortants.[126] Monoreassortants are viruses containing nine genome segments from one virus and a single genome segment from another virus. Monoreassortants can be particularly useful when analyzing reassortant genetic data, but have the potential drawback that a single mutation could result in false mapping of a viral phenotype (discussed in Sharpe and Fields[175]). However, monoreassortants can provide important information when the mapping is corroborated by other reassortants.

Reassortant genetic analysis has been particularly valuable in studies of reovirus pathogenesis. For example, T1L spreads hematogenously and T3D spreads neurally[207] (Fig. 28-4). This phenotypic difference was defined using sciatic nerve section in neonatal mice. Thus, section of the sciatic nerve in the leg into which reovirus is inoculated by the intramuscular route eliminates spread of T3D, but not T1L, to the nervous system (see Fig. 28-4). Section of the contralateral sciatic nerve does not alter spread of T3D to the CNS. In addition, T1L appears in all parts of the nervous system simultaneously, whereas T3D first appears in the portion of the nervous system innervating the site of inoculation. Thus, despite the fact that T3D can be found in blood and T1L can be found in neurons innervating the site of inoculation,[63] the primary route of spread of T3D is neural and T1L is hematogenous.

To determine the genome segments important for neural versus hematogenous spread, reassortants between T1L and T3D were generated by coinfecting cells with the two viruses, and then picking plaques to isolate progeny virus (see Fig. 28-3). Polyacrylamide gel analysis shows that the T1L and T3D dsRNA genome segment mobilities are sufficiently distinct to allow unambiguous definition of whether a genome segment comes from one or the other parent (see Fig. 28-3). T1L × T3D reassortants were evaluated for their capacity to spread to the CNS by neural or hematogenous routes (see Fig. 28-4). Reassortant viruses using primarily a neural route appeared in higher titers in the portion of the spinal cord innervating the site of inoculation, whereas hematogenously spreading reassortants are found in all regions of the spinal cord simultaneously (see Fig. 28-4). Results from reassortant studies are analyzed by comparing the phenotype measured with the parental origin of genome segments in the panel of reassortants. In the example provided, the S1 segment is responsible for the capacity to spread by the neural or hematogenous route because viruses containing the T3D S1 segment spread neurally, whereas viruses carrying the T1L S1 segment spread hematogenously.

Applicability and Interpretation of Reassortant Genetic Data

Reassortant genetics has been a powerful tool for identification of viral genes important for various stages in reovirus pathogenesis. However, the approach has several important

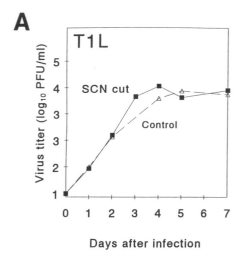
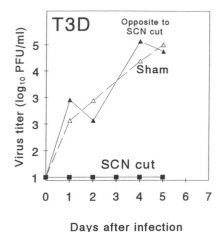

A

T1L — Virus titer (log₁₀ PFU/ml) vs Days after infection. SCN cut, Control.

T3D — Virus titer (log₁₀ PFU/ml) vs Days after infection. Opposite to SCN cut, Sham, SCN cut.

B

Virus	Outer Capsid		CS*	Core					NV@			Pattern of Spread#
	M2	S1 (σ1)	S4	L2	L1	L3	M1	S2	M3	S1 (σ1s)	S3	
T1L	L	L	L	L	L	L	L	L	L	L	L	Hematogenous
EB144	D	L	L	L	L	L	L	L	D	L	D	Hematogenous
EB126	L	L	L	D	D	D	D	D	L	L	D	Hematogenous
H24	L	L	D	L	L	L	L	L	L	L	L	Hematogenous
3HA1	D	L	D	D	D	D	D	D	D	L	D	Hematogenous
H17	D	L	L	D	D	D	L	D	D	L	D	Hematogenous
EB145	D	L	D	D	D	D	D	D	L	L	D	Hematogenous
T3D	D	D	D	D	D	D	D	D	D	D	D	Neural
H30	D	D	D	D	D	D	D	D	D	D	L	Neural
EB143	L	D	L	L	D	L	L	L	L	D	L	Neural
1HA3	L	D	L	L	L	L	L	L	L	D	L	Neural
G2	L	D	L	D	L	L	L	L	L	D	L	Neural

*Reassortant reoviruses were generated from cells infected with T1L and T3D. "L" indicates that the reassortant genome segment was derived from T1L while "D" indicates that the genome segment was derived from T3D.

% CS= Core spike

@ NV= Non-virion associated proteins are encoded by these genome segments.

Neural versus hematogenous spread was determined by inoculating viruses into either the hindlimb or forelimb and then determining the viral titer in the superior and inferior spinal cords 2-3 days later. Viruses present in higher titers in the portion of the spinal cord enervating the site of inoculation than in other regions of the spinal cord were judged to have spread neurally. Viruses that reached both superior and inferior spinal cord equally well regardless of site of inoculation were judged to have spread hematogenously

FIG. 28-4. Use of reassortant genetics to identify genome segments important for a defined stage in pathogenesis. (**A**) Results of experiments demonstrating that reoviruses T1L and T3D differ in the primary route used to spread to the central nervous system (CNS). In the experiment presented on the left side of (**A**), T1L was injected into one hindlimb footpad, and the titer of virus in the inferior spinal cord determined at different times after inoculation. When the sciatic nerve (SCN) was cut in the same limb inoculated with T1L, spread to the inferior spinal cord was unaffected. "Control" in this panel refers to mice that had not been operated on. Thus, T1L does not require an intact SCN for spread to the nervous system. In the experiment presented on the right side of (**A**), T3D was inoculated into the hindlimb. When the SCN was cut in the same limb inoculated with T3D, spread to the inferior spinal cord was blocked. Section of the contralateral SCN did not alter spread to the inferior spinal cord. This shows that T3D spreads by the SCN to the inferior spinal cord. PFU, plaque-forming units. (**B**) Table comparing the routes of spread used by a series of T1L × T3D reassortant viruses. This analysis was performed using the fact that the neurally spreading T3D strain appears in the inferior spinal cord before appearing in the superior spinal cord, whereas the hematogenously spreading T1L strain appears in all regions of the CNS simultaneously. Thus, significant differences in viral titer between inferior and superior spinal cord are seen when a neurally spreading virus is inoculated. In contrast, differences in titer between inferior and superior spinal cord are minimal when a hematogenously spreading virus is inoculated. When the parental gene segments in reassortants that spread neurally or hematogenously are compared, the S1 genome segment was found to determine the route of spread of reassortant viruses. (Adapted from Tyler KL, McPhee DA, Fields BN. Distinct pathways of viral spread in the host determined by reovirus S1 gene segment. Science 1986;233:770–774.)

limitations (reviewed in Ramig and Ward[151] and Sharpe and Fields[175]). One potential concern is the reported high rate of mutations in many RNA viruses. As isolation of reassortants involves several passages in tissue culture, a high spontaneous mutation rate could give rise to reassortant progeny that differ from parental viruses on the basis of accumulated mutations rather than the presence of different combinations of parental genome segments. However, it has been shown that, at least for the S1 genome segment, isolation of a reassortant did not result in accumulation of new mutations.[93] In addition, sequences obtained by different research groups from prototype strains passaged extensively in different laboratories diverge minimally.[139]

The most important limitation of reassortant genetic analysis is that it permits evaluation only of viral properties that differ between two viruses. Thus, a property shared by all viruses in equal measure cannot be analyzed genetically using reassortants, whereas a viral property that limits a phenotype in a particular genetic context will be prominent in a reassortant genetic analysis. A consequence of this is the fact that genetic mapping of a single phenotype using reassortants derived from crosses of different parental strains may not consistently identify a single genome segment as important for a phenotype. Although this important concept was first clearly defined with rotaviruses,[29] data from reovirus confirms this point. For example, three different reassortant crosses have been used to identify genome segments important for the efficient induction of myocarditis.[178,179] When T1L × T3D reassortants are used to evaluate myocarditic potential, the M1 and L2 segments are important for determining the difference between T1L and T3D. In contrast, when reassortants between T3A and G16 (a nonmyocarditic T1L × T3D reassortant) are evaluated, the M1, L1, and S1 segments are important. Thus, genome segments associated with myocarditis induction differ between the two crosses used. The L1 and S1 segments are important when T3A and G16 reassortants are analyzed, but not when T1L × T3D reassortants are evaluated. A possible explanation for this apparent discrepancy is that the T3D and T1L L1 and S1 segments function similarly in myocarditis induction, with the result that T1L × T3D reassortant analysis does not identify L1 and S1 as determinants of the difference between T1L and T3D. Similarly, the T3A and G16 L2 segments are likely similar as regards myocarditis induction, resulting in the lack of an impact of L2 on the myocarditic potential of T3A × G16 reassortants. This type of strain dependence of genetic mapping data does not invalidate the importance of a given genome segment in a specific cross. For example, the same genome segments important for myocarditis in neonatal mice are important for virulence in adult SCID mice,[76] validating the in vivo importance of these genome segments and the proteins they encode.

Another issue that affects the use and interpretation of reassortant genetics is the fact that the panel of reassortants used for a given experiment is a small subset of the 1024 reassortants (2^{10}) that could in theory be generated if reassortment is completely random and all reassortant progeny could be isolated. Analysis of available reassortant pools shows that genome segment reassortment is nonrandom.[139] That is, certain combinations of genome segments are rarely found in reassortant progeny, or are found only when mutations in other segments are present (M. Nibert and K. Coombs, personal communication). Lack of random reassortment could occur at the level of the genome segments (certain combinations of segments might not assort into progeny virions), or at the level of selection of progeny during reassortant isolation (certain combinations of genome segments are lethal or result in progeny that do not grow well). Studies with temperature-sensitive reovirus mutants, and their revertants,[124,150] suggest that there are tight constraints on protein-protein interactions in the viral capsid. Thus, genome segments could be incompatible if the proteins they encode do not function well together as a unit. If a phenotype being evaluated by reassortant genetic techniques involves combinations of genome segments that do not randomly reassort, it may be difficult to determine independent contributions of individual genome segments.[76]

Although genome segments involved in a phenotype can be identified using reassortant analysis, specific domains of a particular protein important for the phenotype can be identified only when minimal sequence variation exists between genome segments. Domains of the protein can be evaluated by mutagenizing expressed protein when in vitro assays are available (see section on The Reovirus Attachment Protein σ1). A current limitation of the reovirus system is that it has not yet been possible to reinsert genome segments containing targeted mutations to test hypotheses directly using mutant viruses. Progress in addressing this issue is crucial to the future expansion of reovirus as an experimental model. Encouraging results from both reovirus[155] and rotavirus[30] suggest that this limitation can be overcome.

Methods of Reassortant Genetic Analysis

Analysis of reassortant data has evolved over the years. Initially, important properties of the virus were defined using monoreassortants. For example, a virus containing nine genome segments from T3D and the S1 segment from T1L can be compared with a virus containing nine genome segments from T1L and the S1 segment of T3D. If a property differing between T1L and T3D depends on the S1 segment, these two monoreassortants should differ in that property. Even when monoreassortants are not available, other mapping results are clear by direct inspection of the data (see Fig. 28-4). In these cases there is a one-to-one correspondence between the experimental variable analyzed and the parental origin of a single genome segment. However, as the biologic window used to evaluate a panel of reassortants expands, the likelihood increases that multiple genome segments are involved. For example, although one genome segment determines differences between neurotropism of T1L and T3D,[204,221,224] four genome segments are important determinants of differences in virulence of T1L and T3D in adult SCID mice.[76] This increasing complexity has necessitated the application of statistical methods to reassortant genetic mapping.[76,122,178,179]

Proper application of statistical methods to reassortant analysis requires that a large number of reassortants be used.[76,178] In addition, attention must be paid to whether the data generated in a particular experiment are normally distributed. Normally distributed data can properly be analyzed by either rank sum or regression analysis, whereas rank sum methods should be used for data that are not normally distrib-

TABLE 28-3. *Sequence relatedness of different T1L and T3D proteins*

Genome segment	Encoded Protein	Number of amino acids	Number of amino acid differences between T1L and T3D
S1	σ1	470 (T1L) 455 (T3D)	122
S2	σ2	418	5
S3	σNS	366	10
S4	σ3	365	12
M1	μ2	736	10
M2	μ1	708	20
L2	λ2	1267	22

uted.[76,178] All reassortant analysis rests on the assumption that the primary determinant of experimental outcome is the genetic constitution of the viruses used. This was quantitated in one study,[76] in which genetic constitution of viruses was found to be responsible for between 66% and 94% of the variance in experimental data. Regression analysis allows assessment of factors other than genetic constitution of reassortants that can contribute to variance in experimental data, including possible contributions of mutant viruses and nonrandom combinations of genome segments in a reassortant panel.[76]

Reassortment of Reovirus Genome Segments in Nature

The study of reovirus evolution has provided insight into strategies by which reoviruses survive in nature. Reovirus

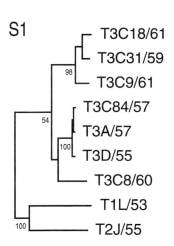

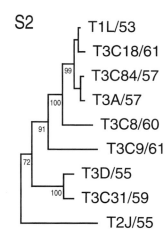

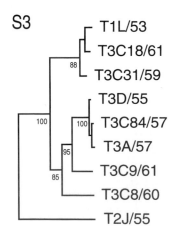

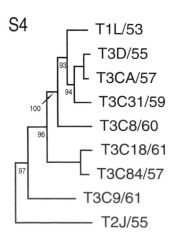

FIG. 28-5. Minimum-length phylogenetic trees based on S1, S2, S3, and S4 segment nucleotide sequences of T1L, T2J, T3D, and six serotype 3 reovirus field-isolate strains. S1, S2, S3, and S4 phylogenetic trees were constructed from σ1-encoding, σ2-encoding, σNS-encoding, and σ3-encoding sequences, respectively, using the branch-and-bound algorithm of the parsimony program, PAUP. Each tree is rooted at the midpoint of its longest branch. Values indicated at selected branchings of the trees represent the percentage of bootstrap analyses (of 1000) that support the groupings shown at each node. Trees prepared by Mehmet Goral and Terrence Dermody, Vanderbilt University School of Medicine, Nashville, TN, based on data in references 28, 43, 74, 94.

evolution appears to occur by accumulation of point mutations and genome segment reassortment. Influences on these processes include immune selection,[73] tissue adaptation,[75,76] and other as yet unidentified factors. With the exception of S1 segment products σ1 and σ1s, amino acid sequences of reovirus proteins of prototype strains are highly conserved (Table 28-3; reviewed in Nibert and associates[139]). The extensive variation seen in the σ1 protein is consistent with its role in many serotype-associated properties of reoviruses (e.g., hematogenous vs. neural spread).

Two lines of evidence suggest that reassortment of reovirus genome segments occurs in nature. First, reassortment occurs in animals coinfected with different reovirus strains.[227] Second, analysis of protein-coding sequences of the S1,[43] S2,[28] S3,[74] and S4[94] segments shows that topologies of phylogenetic trees for these genome segments are distinct (Fig. 28-5). That is, the evolutionary relationships between different genome segments do not correlate with the viral strains from which the sequences are derived. This provides direct evidence that, at least for reovirus S-class genome segments, reassortment occurs in nature. Similarly, analysis of these sequences shows that sequence variability does not correlate with host species, geographic site, or date of isolation. This observation suggests that reovirus strains containing genome segments with divergent sequences cocirculate among different host species in a given geographic site.

STAGES IN INFECTION OF THE CELL

Overview of Reovirus Infection of the Cell

The reovirus replication cycle has been extensively reviewed[137,139] (Fig. 28-6). After attachment to cellular recep-

tors, virions are delivered by receptor-mediated endocytosis to an endocytic compartment, where the viral outer capsid is uncoated by pH-dependent proteases. Uncoating of the outer capsid leads to generation of ISVPs (see Figs. 28-1 and 28-6), which likely penetrate endosomes, leading to delivery of viral cores or viral RNA into the cytoplasm. ISVPs also can be generated extracellularly by proteases. Extracellular generation of ISVPs occurs naturally in the intestinal lumen and experimentally when proteases such as chymotrypsin are used to digest virions. Entry of extracellularly generated ISVPs into cells is pH independent and probably results from direct penetration of the plasma membrane rather than receptor-mediated endocytosis. Cores are transcriptionally active and release ten capped, nonpolyadenylated mRNAs. These RNAs also serve as template for synthesis of genomic dsRNA. After synthesis of viral structural proteins and dsRNA genome segments, progeny virions are assembled and released concomitant with lysis of the infected cell. The replication cycle is entirely cytoplasmic, although the nucleus is necessary for efficient viral replication because enucleation of target cells decreases the yield of viral progeny (reviewed in Nibert and associates[139]). A summary of the relationships between individual genome segments and proteins and stages in reovirus infection of the cell is shown in Table 28-4.

Reovirus Attachment to Cells

Although reovirus attachment protein σ1 has been studied in detail, cellular receptors to which σ1 binds are not well understood. Reovirus infects most human and mouse cell types in culture, suggesting that the virus can use either multiple cell surface molecules for entry or that a structure important for viral attachment is common to most or all mouse and hu-

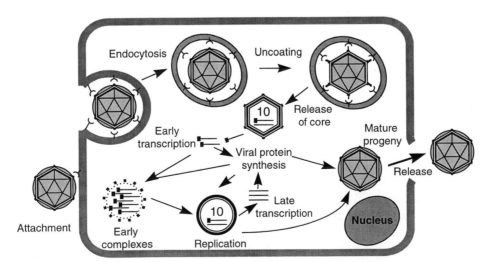

FIG. 28-6. The reovirus replication cycle. Reoviruses attach to cellular receptors, which have not been identified with certainty, and virions enter cells by receptor-mediated endocytosis. Within an endocytic compartment, the viral outer capsid is uncoated by pH-dependent proteases to generate infectious subvirion particles (ISVPs). ISVPs penetrate membranes of endocytic vesicles, resulting in delivery of the viral core or mRNA into the cytoplasm. Transcription of the viral genome occurs within the core. After synthesis of viral proteins and replication of viral genomic double-stranded RNA, progeny virions are assembled and exit the cell in conjunction with cell lysis. (Figure prepared by Mehmet Goral, MD, Vanderbilt University School of Medicine, Nashville, TN.)

TABLE 28-4. *Reovirus protein involvement in interactions with the cell, host, and immune system*

Genome segment	Protein	Protein interactions with:		
		Cell	Host	Immune system
S1	σ1	Hemagglutinin Cell attachment Extended in ISVP Inhibition DNA synthesis Apoptosis Interaction with microtubules	Neurotropism Oily fur syndrome	Defines serotype Antibodies protect, neutralize, inhibit hemagglutination, block binding to cells, inhibit neural spread, block ^{51}Cr release, aggregate virions Determines hemagglutination inhibition capacity of anti-σ3 antibodies
	σ1s	See Nibert et al, 1996[139]	None known	None known
	σ1 or σ1s	Maintenance of persistent infection of L cells	Neural versus hematogenous spread Growth in neonatal* and SCID† intestine Growth in SCID brain SCID virulence Neonatal myocarditis Oily fur syndrome (biliary atresia)	Target for cytotoxic T lymphocytes (in addition to other reovirus proteins)
S2	σ2	Binds single-stranded RNA, see Nibert et al, 1996[139]	None known	None known
S3	σNS	Binds dsRNA, role in assortment, see Nibert et al, 1996[139]	None known	None known
S4	σ3	Inhibition of protein and RNA synthesis Cleavage in endosome leads to ISVP Establishment of persistent infection of L cells Zinc metalloprotein Binds dsRNA	Heat sensitivity Cleavage in intestinal lumen leads to ISVP	Antibodies protect, neutralize, inhibit hemagglutination, block internalization, block cleavage and generation of ISVP by chymotrypsin, inhibit intracellular uncoating, aggregate virions
M1	μ2	Yield in cardiac myocytes RNA synthesis	Neonatal myocarditis SCID hepatitis SCID virulence Growth in SCID liver	None known
M2	μ1	Membrane interaction, release of ^{51}Cr Protease sensitivity Cleavage in endosome leads to ISVP Apoptosis Myristoylated Transcriptase activation	Neonatal neurovirulence Ethanol sensitivity Cleavage in intestinal lumen leads to ISVP	Antibodies protect, inhibit neutralization, block hemagglutination, inhibit ^{51}Cr release, aggregate virions, block membrane penetration by ISVPs
M3	μNS	See Nibert et al, 1996[139]	None known	None known
L1	λ3	RNA-dependent RNA polymerase pH optimum for transcription Yield in cardiac myocytes	Neonatal myocarditis SCID hepatitis SCID virulence Growth in SCID liver, brain, intestine	None known
L2	λ2	Guanyl transferase Nucleotide binding Generation of mutants during high multiplicity of infection passage in L cells	Growth in neonatal and SCID intestine Efficiency of horizontal spread Neonatal myocarditis SCID hepatitis SCID virulence Growth in SCID liver and brain	Antibodies neutralize, inhibit hemagglutination
L3	λ1	Yield in cardiac myocytes and L cells Binds dsRNA Zinc metalloprotein	None known	None known

*Refers to neonatal NIH(s) mice.
†Refers to adult CB17 SCID mice.
ISVP, infectious subvirion particles; dsRNA, double-stranded RNA; SCID, severe combined immunodeficient.

man cells. The fact that a variety of cell types from different species can support reovirus replication has led to considerable controversy about the identity of cellular receptors for reovirus. Identification of reovirus receptors is further complicated by the capacity of these viruses to bind many cell surface proteins,[32,33] not all of which may result in productive viral infection. Receptors for reovirus, defined as those cellular components that bind virus specifically resulting in initiation of the virus replication cycle, have not been identified. Studies using a variety of cell types indicate that most cells contain between 40,000 to 500,000 viral receptors. Viral binding is usually of high affinity with reported K_d values between 3×10^{-9} and 1×10^{-10} M.[7,10,57]

Serotype-specific cell and tissue tropism,[144,204,220,221] as well as serotype-dependent capability to bind certain types of brain[45,199] and erythroid[42,164] cells in culture, suggest that reoviruses use more than one receptor. L cells may have a unique receptor for serotype 3 reovirus, as well as a receptor to which both serotypes 1 and 3 can bind.[7] Carbohydrate molecules serve as a component of the receptor for all three reovirus serotypes, and binding to carbohydrate results in HA.[10,145,147] There is general agreement that sialic acid residues participate in the attachment of serotype 3 reoviruses to a variety of cultured cells and erythrocytes.[70,146,147] The principal sialylated glycoprotein of human erythrocytes, glycophorin A, is bound by serotype 3 reoviruses,[42,147] but not serotype 1 reoviruses.[42] Serotype 3 reovirus binding to L cells can be competitively inhibited by free sialic acid and sialylated oligosaccharide.[69,146] In addition, monoclonal antibodies to several outer capsid proteins block both HA and viral binding to glycophorin containing sialic acid.[215] Enzymatic removal of sialic acid reduces serotype 3 reovirus binding to target cells.[10,69,134,145] In addition to HA, binding of serotype 3 reovirus to sialylated glycoprotein is required for productive infection of some types of cells, such as MEL cells,[164] and interactions with sialylated receptors contribute to binding other types of cells, including L cells.[69,145,146] The erythrocyte molecule bound by serotype 1 reoviruses is unknown. However, sialic acid is not involved in binding of serotype 1 reovirus to erythrocytes.[145]

Anti-idiotypic monoclonal antibody 87.92.6, which blocks serotype 3 reovirus binding to murine thymoma and rat neuroblastoma cells,[141] was used to recover a potential reovirus receptor protein from a thymoma cell line.[35] This protein shares several biochemical properties with the β-adrenergic receptor, including apparent molecular weight, tryptic digestion pattern, and isoelectric point.[36] It was proposed that this binding may involve a $β_2$-receptor subtype or a binding site near the antagonist domain of the β receptor.[47,109] However, the suggestion that the β-adrenergic receptor serves as a functional receptor for serotype 3 reovirus is controversial. It is clear that reovirus binding to target cells is not associated with activation of the β-adrenergic receptor. Cell attachment by reovirus neither blocks activation of β-adrenergic receptors nor induces their downregulation.[31,169] Similarly, downregulation of cell surface β-adrenergic receptors by agonist binding does not interfere with the subsequent capacity of reovirus to bind these cells. Reovirus infects cells lacking β-adrenergic receptors, such as L cells,[31] and receptors for reovirus and β-adrenergic agonists and antagonists are differentiable on A431 cells, an epidermoid carcinoma line rich in β-adrenergic receptors.[31] Therefore, it is unlikely that the β-adrenergic receptor is the sole receptor for serotype 3 reoviruses.

The epidermal growth factor (EGF) receptor has been reported to play a role in determining the efficiency of reovirus growth in fibroblasts.[194,197] T3D replicates poorly and causes minimal cytopathic effect in fibroblasts lacking the EGF receptor. Transfection of these cells with the EGF receptor results in marked enhancement of T3D growth and cytopathicity. A functional EGF receptor appears to be required for these effects because mutant receptors do not result in enhanced efficiency of viral infection. The mechanism by which the EGF receptor enhances reovirus infectivity remains to be established.

Entry Into Cells and Proteolytic Uncoating of the Virion

After viral attachment to cells, electron microscopy shows virions in clathrin-coated pits, suggesting that virion uptake occurs by receptor-mediated endocytosis[20,195] (see Fig. 28-6). Within late endosomes or lysosomes, viral outer capsid proteins σ3 and μ1 are subject to proteolysis by cellular proteases, yielding ISVPs[21,27,182,195] (see Figs. 28-1 and 28-6). In this uncoating process, σ3 is degraded and released from the virion. The μ1 protein is present on the surface of the virion as cleaved μ1N and μ1C fragments (reviewed in Nibert and associates[139]). On conversion to ISVPs, μ1C is cleaved and changes in conformation.[51] Cleavage of μ1C generates a large amino-terminal subfragment (δ) and a smaller carboxy-terminal subfragment (φ), which remain associated with the ISVP.[136] The fact that fragments of μ1C remain on the ISVP surface provides a rationale for the association of the M2 segment, which encodes μ1, with the capacity of ISVPs to interact with membranes,[116] the capacity of a μ1-specific monoclonal antibody to block HA by ISVPs,[215] and the capacity of μ1-specific antibodies to inhibit membrane penetration by ISVPs.[81]

Infectious subvirion particles generated in the endocytic compartment are probably identical to those generated either in the intestinal lumen of perorally infected mice[13,19] or by in vitro digestion of virions with chymotrypsin or trypsin.[21,182,195] The uncoating of virions to ISVPs is critical to virus infectivity. This was shown using ammonium chloride, a weak base that increases pH of intracellular vesicles. Ammonium chloride reversibly inhibits reovirus growth and intracellular uncoating.[119,195] However, if virus is treated in vitro with chymotrypsin, the resulting ISVPs grow well in ammonium chloride-treated cells. This shows that ammonium chloride blocks viral growth by inhibiting intracellular uncoating, and proves that proteolytic uncoating to ISVPs is a critical step in virus infection.[195] Monoclonal antibodies specific for σ3 that protect against lethal infection also block this intracellular step in the viral replication cycle[216] (see section on Immunity and Stages in Infection of the Cell and Host). The susceptibility of virions to proteolysis in vitro maps to the μ1-encoding M2 segment.[48,50]

Penetration of Processed Virions Into the Cytoplasm

Significant evidence supports a direct role for ISVPs in the penetration of reovirus particles across cell membranes. ISVPs generated in vitro mediate release of ^{51}Cr from preloaded L cells.[20,82,116] This result suggests that ISVPs are capable of direct penetration of cell membranes, resulting in leakage of ^{51}Cr from the cell because of formation of pores or disruption of membrane integrity. Further evidence supporting direct penetration of membranes by ISVPs comes from the demonstration that ISVPs induce conductance through artificial planar bilayers, presumably by generating pores through which ions pass.[202]

Reassortant analysis shows that strain-specific differences in ^{51}Cr release by ISVPs map to the μ1-encoding M2 segment, indicating the importance of μ1 in membrane interaction.[116] This conclusion is further supported by the finding that monoclonal antibodies specific for μ1 inhibit virus-mediated release of ^{51}Cr from cells.[81] In addition, ethanol-resistant mutants consistently show diminished release of ^{51}Cr from cells, a property mapped to specific mutations in the μ1 protein.[82,228] Protein μ1 interactions with membranes may be important in vivo because the M2 segment determines strain-specific differences in virulence of serotype 3 reovirus in the mouse CNS.[84]

Transcription and Assortment of Genome Segments and Release of Virions

Transcription of reovirus genome segments occurs in two distinct stages (reviewed in Nibert and associates[139]). Uncoating of ISVPs to cores results in activation of viral transcription, which results in release of ten capped, nonpolyadenylated mRNA transcripts.[21,27,182,183] These transcripts act as template for both translation and minus-strand synthesis, leading to formation of progeny dsRNA. Whole virion cores are required for transcription because disruption of the core abolishes transcriptional activity.[87,90,229] Several genome segments that are important determinants of reovirus pathogenesis (L1, L2, and M1[76,178]; see section on Stages in Infection of the Host) encode proteins that in part form the core and likely play critical roles in viral transcription or replication. The L1 segment product, λ3, is an important component of the viral polymerase,[192] and determines strain-specific differences in the pH optimum of transcription.[48] The L2 segment-encoded λ2 protein is the viral guanylyl transferase[34,118] and likely mediates capping of viral transcripts. The μ2 protein encoded by segment M1 also likely plays a role in transcription because temperature-sensitive mutants that map to M1 fail to synthesize dsRNA efficiently at the nonpermissive temperature (reviewed in Nibert and associates[139]).

The mechanism by which the ten reovirus genome segments are assorted into progeny virions is not known. The assortment process is highly efficient because particle–to–plaque-forming units (PFU) ratios approaching one have been reported,[189] although particle-to-PFU ratios of 100 are more typically encountered. Signals involved in assortment are not known, but common 5' tetranucleotide and 3' pentanucleotide sequences on viral genome segments[9] and predicted secondary structures of message-sense RNAs[28,94,108,240] could play a role in virus assembly.

Assembly of reovirus particles is a dynamic process that is tightly linked with genome replication and late transcription. After completion of minus-strand synthesis, particles are generated that are capable of late transcription.[127,186,239,242] Mature virions are formed by addition of a full component of viral structural proteins and released from infected cells by lysis. The mechanism of cell lysis and virion release is not understood, but is presumably critical for spread within and between hosts.

Interferons and Reovirus

Reoviruses and their dsRNA genomes are potent inducers of interferon,[79,100,115,186] but the role that interferon plays in host defenses against reovirus infections in vivo is not known. Interferon induction varies between viral strains, with T3D being a better inducer than T1L.[175] Reovirus strains may also differ in their sensitivity to exogenous interferon-β.[88] Interferon inhibits reovirus growth through inhibition of translation of viral proteins.[230]

Although reoviruses are potent inducers of interferon, they are relatively resistant to its effects. Specific viral proteins have been implicated in reovirus resistance to the antiviral effects of interferon. By virtue of its capacity to bind dsRNA,[85,170] outer capsid protein σ3 serves to block activation of the interferon-induced kinase, protein kinase RNA (PKR).[86,110] After activation by dsRNA, PKR phosphorylates eIF-2α, resulting in inhibition of translational initiation.[140,166] Thus, by sequestering dsRNA, σ3 prevents PKR activation, which allows viral protein synthesis to proceed. This mechanism likely explains how σ3 affects the expression of reporter genes, and determines differences in the capacity of reovirus strains to influence cellular protein synthesis.[171,174,201]

Effects of Reovirus Infection on the Cell

Cells infected with reovirus produce large, perinuclear cytoplasmic inclusions that contain viral dsRNA[72,184] and proteins,[60,188] as well as complete and incomplete viral particles.[40,72] Microtubules and intermediate filaments are associated with these inclusions,[39,152,172,188] and vimentin filament organization is progressively disrupted during the course of reovirus infection.[172] Although an intact microtubular network is not required for productive reovirus infection of cultured cells,[11,39,187] microtubules are important for fast axonal transport of reovirus within nerves in infected mice.[207] Reovirus infection is associated with inhibition of host cell DNA synthesis[67,153,173] as well as RNA[99,174] and protein synthesis.[41,56,132,174] In addition, cells infected with reovirus also exhibit changes in growth factor receptor number and signaling capacity.[125,194,212] The importance to viral pathogenesis of these reovirus-induced effects on infected cells has not been extensively analyzed.

Reoviruses induce apoptosis as part of their cytopathic effect in cultured cells.[208] L cells infected with reovirus show ultrastructural features of apoptosis, and DNA extracted from these cells forms oligonucleosome-length ladders characteristic of cells undergoing apoptosis (Fig. 28-7). T3D induces apoptosis to a greater extent than T1L, and these differences are determined by the S1 segment.[208] Apoptosis is induced by replication-incompetent ultraviolet light-inactivated reovirus and inhibited by anti-σ1 monoclonal antibodies, suggesting that the σ1 product of the S1 segment is responsible for induc-

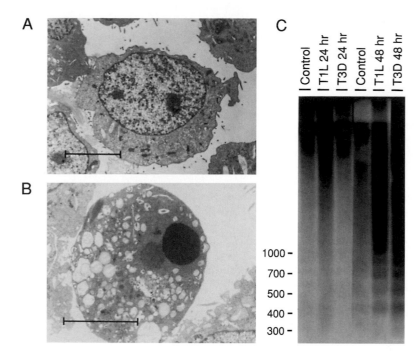

FIG. 28-7. Induction of apoptosis by reovirus. **(A)** Uninfected L929 fibroblasts and **(B)** L929 fibroblasts cells infected with T3D for 18 hours were prepared for electron microscopy.[208] Infection with T3D causes cytoplasmic and nuclear membrane blebbing, cytoplasmic vacuolization, and compaction and condensation of nuclear chromatin. **(C)** Agarose gel electrophoresis of low–molecular-weight cellular DNA extracted from mock-infected L929 fibroblasts (Control), or L929 fibroblasts infected with either T1L and T3D for 24 or 48 hours. Cellular DNA was purified and resolved with agarose gel electrophoresis, transferred to a nitrocellulose filter, and hybridized with ^{32}P-labeled L929 fibroblast genomic DNA. Size markers are indicated to the left in base pairs. (Modified from Tyler KL, Squier MKT, Rogers SE, et al. Differences in the capacity of reoviruses to induce apoptosis are determined by viral attachment protein sigma-1. J Virol 1995;69:6972– 6979.)

ing apoptosis and that viral replication is not essential for this process.[208] The mechanism by which reovirus induces apoptosis remains to be defined, although it may be related to the capacity of reovirus to induce DNA synthesis inhibition. Like strain-specific differences in apoptosis induction exhibited by reovirus, differences in DNA synthesis inhibition are determined by the S1 segment.[173] It remains to be established whether reovirus-induced apoptosis functions principally as a host defense mechanism, a virus-induced process that facilitates viral replication, or an inadvertent by-product of virus-cell interaction.

Persistent Reovirus Infections of Cultured Cells

Reoviruses have served as useful models for defining mechanisms of virus-cell coevolution during persistent viral infections of tissue culture cells. Although usually cytolytic, reoviruses establish persistent infections of many types of cells in culture.[5,107,123,125,196,212] Reoviruses do not establish persistent infections of immunocompetent animals; however, prolonged infections of SCID mice (>100 days) have been reported[75,76] (see section on Stages in Infection of the Host). Cell cultures persistently infected with reovirus produce high titers of virus for long periods of time, and most cells show evidence of viral infection.[2,5,44,196,212] Studies using L cells have identified two phases of persistent infection: establishment and maintenance. Specific viral proteins play distinct roles in these phases of reovirus persistence.

Establishment of persistently infected L-cell cultures occurs when infection is initiated with viral stocks passaged serially at high multiplicity of infection.[4,5,22,44] Such stocks contain a variety of viral mutants,[3,6] and some of these mutants appear to facilitate establishment of persistent infection. Mu-

tations in the S4 segment are especially important for the establishment of persistent infection.[4] The L2 segment product λ2 is important for generation of mutations that allow persistent infection to be established.[22] The type of host cell also can determine whether persistent infection is established. Persistent infections of 3T3,[212] CHO,[196] MDCK,[125] and SC1[41] cells can be established using wild-type reovirus stocks, which lack the capacity to establish persistent infections of L cells.[4] In some cases, the capacity of cells to support establishment of persistent infection is linked to resistance to reovirus-induced inhibition of cellular protein synthesis.[41,52]

Viral and Cellular Mutants Selected During Persistent Infection of Cultured Cells

During maintenance of L-cell cultures persistently infected with reovirus, mutations are selected in both viruses and cells.[2,44] The fact that viruses adapt to growth in mutant cells during these persistent infections suggests a model for selection of viral variants analogous in some respects to organ-specific selection of viral variants in vivo (see section on Stages in Infection of the Host).[75] Cytolytic reoviruses used to establish a persistently infected culture lead to selection of mutant cells that are less permissive for viral replication. These cellular mutants in turn lead to selection of mutant viruses capable of infecting the mutant cells. Prolonged maintenance of the persistent infection requires a balance between cellular resistance to viral infection and viral cytopathic effect. Viral mutants selected during maintenance of persistent infections of L-cell cultures have delayed clearance in the neonatal mouse CNS,[130] suggesting that the mutations carried by these viruses are contained in proteins important for viral pathogenesis. However, viral mutants selected during persistent infection of

L-cells contain different types of mutations than those selected during chronic infections of SCID mice.[75] These findings suggest that different selection pressures lead to selection of viral variants during chronic reovirus infections in cultured cells and in vivo.

Early steps in the reovirus replication cycle are altered by the mutations in both cells and viruses selected during maintenance of reovirus persistence. When persistently infected cultures are cured of infection by passage in medium containing anti-reovirus antibody, the resulting cells support the growth of viruses isolated from persistently infected cultures (termed PI viruses) significantly better than that of parental viruses.[2,44] Although these cured cells do not support efficient growth of parental virus, they do support the growth of ISVPs derived from parental virus.[44] This suggests that a mutation in cured cells affects a step or steps in reovirus replication before formation of ISVPs. Similarly, PI viruses have mutations that affect early steps in their replication. PI viruses exhibit normal infection and growth in L cells treated with ammonium chloride,[44] which blocks infection by parental virus through inhibition of virion uncoating.[195] The relationship of these findings to the observation that ammonium chloride can facilitate the establishment of persistent infection[26] is not known. However, it appears likely that early pH-sensitive steps in the reovirus growth cycle are important in determining cellular injury and survival, and that viral and cellular factors affecting these processes favor the establishment and maintenance of persistent infections.[44]

The genome segments responsible for the capacity of PI viruses to grow efficiently in cells cured of persistent infection have been mapped in one study.[91] Reassortant viruses containing an S1 segment derived from a PI virus parent grew to high titer in cured cells, suggesting that mutations in S1 (in addition to cellular mutations) are important for maintenance of persistent reovirus infection. It is not known which of the S1 segment products (σ1 or σ1s) determines the observed differences in the capacity of PI viruses to grow better than wild-type virus in cured cells.

STAGES IN INFECTION OF THE HOST

Overview of Reovirus Infection of the Host

The stages in reovirus pathogenesis have been reviewed.[129,138,175,176,205] Genome segments important for determining the efficiency and nature of reovirus infection at many of these stages have been identified using reovirus mutants and reassortant viruses. The roles of individual genome segments and proteins in reovirus pathogenesis are summarized in Table 28-4. Several important concepts have been derived from these studies. The linkage of specific viral genome segments and proteins to carefully delineated stages in viral pathogenesis has provided a model for understanding how virus-induced disease occurs. The role of viral attachment protein σ1 in multiple aspects of pathogenesis has received particular attention, giving rise to the concept that attachment to specific cells in vivo plays a major role in determining viral tropism and disease expression. More recent studies have identified proteins that form the virion vertex as important determinants of virulence, damage to organs such as liver and heart, and growth in different organs. Finally, data show that the viral gene segments important for organ tropism differ for each organ, giving rise to the concept of organ-specific virulence genes. Why one genome segment is more important in one set of organs than another has not been defined.

Stability in the Environment

The first stage of reovirus infection is transmission to a susceptible host, a process that is enhanced by environmental stability. Perhaps the two most important environmental variables determining stability of viruses are temperature and humidity (reviewed in Tyler and Fields[205]). Reoviruses are quite stable under ambient environmental conditions and can be isolated from such environmental sources as river water, stagnant water, and sewage (reviewed in Tyler and Fields[205]).

Genetic studies indicate that the viral outer capsid plays a key role in viral stability in the environment. Analysis of the genetic basis for environmental stability has been possible because strain-specific variations exist. T2J is the most thermolabile, T1L is the most thermostable, and T3D shows an intermediate phenotype.[50] Temperature-related loss in viral infectivity appears to result from loss of σ1 from virions.[50] The S4 segment, encoding outer capsid protein σ3, determines the sensitivity of reovirus strains to temperature inactivation.[50] Reoviruses are relatively resistant to desiccation and survive for long periods in the presence of high (>90%) relative humidity.[1] The efficiency of reovirus growth is influenced by pH. Viral yield drops sharply at pH less than 6.5 and is optimal between pH 6.8 to 7.5.[59] At extremely alkaline pH (e.g., pH 11), σ1 is lost from virions with an associated decline in infectivity.[50] Sensitivity to alkaline pH parallels temperature sensitivity, with T1L being more resistant than T3D, and T2J being most sensitive.[50] Studies of the effects of a variety of additional physical and chemical inactivating agents indicate that the S1, S4, and M2 segments encoding reovirus outer capsid proteins are the key determinants of reovirus stability.[49,50,228] For example, mutations in the μ1 protein are associated with resistance to ethanol.[228]

Entry of Virus Into the Host

As implied by their name, reoviruses enter into animal hosts by both respiratory and enteric routes (reviewed in Tyler and Fields[205]). Little is known about mechanisms of reovirus entry by these routes in humans. However, viral entry has been extensively investigated in mice, and these studies have provided principles (such as the importance of M cells in viral entry) that have proved applicable to pathogens that include bacteria and other viruses.

After inoculation into the upper gastrointestinal tract of mice, reoviruses adhere selectively to surface projections and stunted microvilli on the luminal surface of M cells.[14,235–237] These specialized epithelial cells overlie focal aggregates of lymphoid tissue (Peyer's patches) in the intestine. Electron microscopic studies of the fate of virus in the intestinal tract indicate that virions are endocytosed by M cells and then transported across these cells within cytoplasmic vesicles.[235,237] Virus that reaches the submucosal zone by traveling across M cells can either spread to adjacent intestinal tissue by infecting the basal surface of intestinal epithelial cells,[158,162,219] or disseminate within the host by using neural, lymphoid, or hematogenous pathways.[92,131]

The respiratory tract contains focal aggregates of lymphoid tissue that are analogous to Peyer's patches found in the gastrointestinal tract, and M cells are found within the epithelial cell layer overlying this bronchus-associated lymphoid tissue. Immediately after intratracheal inoculation of T1L into adult rats, virus preferentially adheres to the apical surface of bronchial M cells.[128] Within 30 to 60 minutes after inoculation, virus is present within membrane-bound cytoplasmic vesicles, and then subsequently in the intercellular space on the basal side of M cells. These findings, combined with earlier studies on virus spread in the gastrointestinal tract, indicate that transepithelial transport of reovirus across M cells provides a general mechanism by which pathogens cross mucosal surfaces and subsequently gain access to visceral organs.

Studies indicate that proteolytic enzymes present in the intestinal lumen are required for efficient infection of the host by the peroral route. Reovirus virions undergo proteolytic uncoating to ISVPs in the intestinal lumen similar to that seen during viral entry into cells[8,13,19] (see Figs. 28-1 and 28-6). This proteolytic uncoating results in removal of outer capsid protein σ3, cleavage of μ1/μ1C, and extension of the viral attachment protein σ1.[65,134] Intraluminal conversion of virions to ISVPs is a prerequisite for viral adherence to M cells.[8] Inhibition of the intraluminal conversion of native virions to ISVPs results in marked loss of the capacity of reoviruses to initiate intestinal infection and grow in intestinal tissue.[8,13] This shows the dual functional import of the ISVP form of reoviruses, which plays a critical role in infection of cells and entry into the host (see Figs. 28-1 and 28-6).

In addition to being transported across M cells, T1L infects intestinal epithelial cells.[162,235] Infection appears to begin in the crypts of Lieberkuhn at sites adjacent to Peyer's patches. Virus may spread from M cells to the underlying lymphoid follicles and then to basal crypt epithelial cells by lymphatics or cell-to-cell spread.[14,162] Studies in cell culture show that reoviruses can selectively infect polarized epithelial cells at either their apical or basolateral surface and, after assembly and maturation, can also show a selective pattern of release from the apical or basolateral surface (reviewed in Tyler and Fields[205]). The potential importance of polarized infection for viral entry and dissemination in vivo has not been clearly established.[7,14,158,162,219] Apical release allows viral reentry into the lumen of the intestinal tract and thereby facilitates local infection and cell-to-cell spread along the intestinal epithelium, and may provide shed virus for transmission between hosts. Conversely, basolateral release of virus allows access to subepithelial tissues and facilitates dissemination of virus within the host. It is also possible that transport of reovirus into bile may contribute to infection of intestinal tissues and horizontal transmission.[159,161]

Studies using T1L × T3D reassortant viruses show that the viral S1 and L2 segments, encoding the σ1, σ1s, and λ2 proteins, are the major determinants of the capacity of reovirus to grow and survive in intestinal tissue of neonatal mice.[18] The efficiency of viral replication in the intestine correlates directly with the amount of virus shed in the stool, with T1L being shed in 1000- to 10,000-fold greater amounts than T3D.[95] Virus shed in the stool appears to be an important source for transmission of reovirus infection.[95] The efficiency with which different reovirus strains spread from orally infected mice to uninfected mice in the same litter parallels the degree of viral growth in intestine and shedding in stool, and is determined by the viral L2 segment.[95] These data are consistent with a model in which the L2 segment, encoding the core spike protein λ2, determines the efficiency of horizontal spread through effects on total viral replication in the intestine, and thus shedding of infectious virus in stool. Studies of reovirus growth in SCID mice confirm the importance of the S1 and L2 segments in determining reovirus growth in the intestine, and also suggest a role for the L1 segment in influencing intestinal reovirus titers.[76]

Spread of Virus Within the Host

After peroral inoculation and subsequent replication in intestinal tissue, reoviruses are capable of disseminating within the host to produce systemic infection.[92,131,205] There are two major pathways for viral dissemination within the infected host (reviewed in Tyler and Fields[205]). Viruses may spread through nerves from the site of entry to distant target organs, or through lymphatics and the bloodstream. Reoviruses are capable of using both of these routes of spread. In general, one route or the other predominates for the well characterized prototype viruses (see Fig. 28-4). For example, T3C9 can be sequentially traced as it spreads from the intestinal tract to submucosal lymphoid tissue to neurons of the myenteric plexus.[129,131] Virus then spreads through the vagus nerve to reach neurons within the dorsal motor nucleus of the vagus within the brain stem.[129,131] In contrast, T1L spreads by lymphatics from Peyer's patches to mesenteric lymph nodes and finally to blood and spleen.[92] After inoculation into the respiratory tract, T1L spreads by lymphatics from bronchus-associated lymphoid tissue to bronchial lymph nodes and then enters the blood stream.[128] After intramuscular inoculation, reovirus T1L and T3D show similar differences in the principal pathway of spread to spinal cord and brain, with T3D spreading primarily through nerves and T1L through the bloodstream[63,207] (see Fig. 28-4). Studies using T1L × T3D reassortant viruses show that the viral S1 segment is the major determinant of the pattern of viral spread in the infected host[92,207] (see Fig. 28-4).

Neural spread of T3D appears to be mediated by fast axonal transport.[207] Pharmacologic agents such as colchicine, which cause disruption of microtubules and inhibit fast but not slow axonal transport, block neural transport of T3D. Selective inhibitors of slow axonal transport do not inhibit neural spread of reovirus. Ultrastructural studies of reovirus-infected cells consistently demonstrate an association of reovirus particles with cellular microtubules,[40,172,188] and binding of virions to isolated microtubules can be demonstrated in vitro.[11] Transport of serotype 3 reoviruses can be demonstrated within motor, sensory, and autonomic fibers and can occur in both anterograde and retrograde directions.[63,131,207] The pattern of spread indicates that transneuronal transport of reovirus occurs, but it remains to be established whether this is restricted to spread across synapses or occurs at other locations such as axons.

T1L spreads from the respiratory tract, gastrointestinal tract, and muscle primarily through the bloodstream. The mechanisms by which reoviruses are carried in the blood (plasma vs. cell associated) have not been defined. Viral antigen can be detected within capillary endothelium[63] and viral particles can be seen by electron microscopy within endothelial cells. In addition, both T1L and T3D bind to cultured rat endothelial cells in vitro.[210] In vitro studies also show that reoviruses can bind to erythrocytes, lymphocytes, and macrophage-like cells (see section on Reovirus Attachment to Cells, and Burstin and coworkers[23]). In addition, reovirus can infect undifferentiated hematopoietic precursor cells, including MEL,[164] K562 erythroleukemia cells,[33] and HL60 human promyelocytic leukemia cells.[55] However, it remains to be established whether hematopoietic cells play a role in viral transport in vivo.

Cell and Tissue Tropism and Receptor Recognition

Studies with reovirus reassortants were among the first to show that a genome segment (S1) encoding a viral attachment protein is a primary determinant of tissue tropism.[204,221,224] The importance of the σ1 protein in determining viral tropism also has been established by a variety of in vivo studies. T1L and T3D differ in their tropism within the CNS after intracerebral inoculation into newborn mice. T3D infects neurons and produces a necrotizing meningoencephalitis. In contrast, T1L primarily infects the ependymal cells lining cerebral ventricles, resulting in hydrocephalus. Studies with T1L × T3D reassortants indicate that the viral S1 segment, encoding σ1 and σ1s, is the major determinant of these patterns.[221,224] Because σ1 is the viral attachment protein, an attractive hypothesis is that the interaction between σ1 and cellular receptors explains differences in tropism between T1L and T3D. However, the bicistronic nature of the S1 segment leaves open the possibility that σ1s plays a role in tropism. The fact that T1L can be detected in neurons of the spinal cord after intramuscular inoculation[63] suggests that differences in tropism between T1L and T3D may be influenced by factors other than interactions of σ1 protein with cell surface receptors. However, correlations between cell attachment and tropism have been found in studies of viral binding to isolated ependymal cells and neurons.[45,199] Additional evidence for the importance of the σ1 protein, rather than the σ1s protein, in neurotropism comes from T3D variants that contain single amino acid substitutions within the globular head of σ1. These variants show an altered pattern of CNS tropism compared with wild-type T3D.[93,190,191] Mutations in the S1 segments of these viruses are contained within the coding sequences for σ1 but not σ1s, arguing strongly that σ1 is the principal determinant of reovirus neurotropism[16,93] (see Table 28-4).

Host Factors Contributing to Viral Tropism

In addition to S1 and other viral determinants of tropism (see section on Organ-Specific Virulence Genes), host factors play an important role in determining disease outcome. For example, preexisting hepatic injury alters the localization and extent of reovirus-induced hepatic disease.[149,163] Neonatal mice are much more susceptible to lethal infection than adult mice.[198] Although the basis for this age-dependent loss of permissiveness is not known, it appears that different parts of the CNS acquire resistance to reovirus-mediated damage at different ages.[198] The immunocompetence of the mouse also affects the expression of reovirus-induced disease. Adult immunocompetent mice are resistant to lethal infection, but adult SCID mice are killed by reovirus.[71,75,76,198] Specific types of immune responses can alter viral tropism and disease phenotype. For example, protection against lethal T3D-induced encephalitis by adoptive transfer of σ1-specific monoclonal antibody 9BG5 is associated with prevention of cortical destruction, but late development of striking hippocampal inflammation.[209] Intramuscular or intracranial inoculation of neonatal mice with T3D regularly generates viral titers of 10^8 to 10^9 PFU per brain. In contrast, titers in the brain of adult SCID mice, despite their lack of functional immunity, range from 10^3 to 10^4 PFU per brain.[71,76] Although neonatal mice infected with serotype 3 reoviruses die of severe meningoencephalitis, adult SCID mice contract hepatitis or myocarditis.[71,76,180] These data strongly argue that factors such as innate immunity and tissue maturation are important determinants of reovirus tropism.

Pathology and Disease

Central Nervous System

Studies of reovirus infection of the CNS have provided key evidence for the role of the S1 segment and σ1 protein in determining tropism. Serotype 3 reoviruses produce meningoencephalitis in newborn mice with necrosis and a variable inflammatory response that is concentrated in the cortex, limbic system, thalamus, basal ganglia, cerebellum, brain stem, and spinal cord.[121,205,221] In contrast, serotype 1 viruses produce minimal neuronal injury and predominantly infect ependymal cells lining the cerebral ventricles.[96,120,148,205,221] Hydrocephalus develops in animals as a consequence of ependymal cell sloughing and obstruction of the aqueduct of Sylvius as well as blockage of cerebrospinal fluid outflow from the fourth ventricle. Differences between T1L and T3D in CNS tropism have been mapped to the S1 segment using reassortant viruses.[221,224] The S1 segment also determines the capacity of reoviruses to infect discrete populations of cells in the pituitary[144] and retina,[204] and is a major determinant of reovirus growth in brain tissue of adult SCID mice.[76] T3D variant viruses containing mutations in the globular head of the σ1 protein have attenuated neurovirulence and a restricted pattern of CNS tropism.[16,93,190,191] These variants continue to infect and injure limbic structures, but fail to produce significant injury to the cortex. Whether this change in tropism relates to the cell attachment property of σ1, or another property linked to the S1 segment such as inhibition of DNA synthesis or induction of apoptosis, is not clear.

Although all serotype 3 reovirus strains exhibit tropism for neurons, they vary in their capacity to grow in the CNS and produce lethal meningoencephalitis after intracerebral inoculation.[84] Genetic studies with reassortants derived from virulent and avirulent serotype 3 strains indicate that the viral M2 segment, encoding outer capsid protein μ1, is a major determinant of neurovirulence for serotype 3 strains. The specific property of μ1 responsible for influencing neurovirulence is not known, but a number of intriguing possibilities are apparent when structural and biologic properties of μ1 are considered (see Table 28-4). For example, a role for μ1 in neurovirulence could involve μ1 function in either membrane penetration or protease sensitivity.

Cardiorespiratory System

Reoviruses produce myocarditis in neonatal mice and SCID mice.[178–181] Variations in efficiency with which reovirus isolates produce myocarditis occur between viruses of different serotypes and between different strains within one serotype. Reovirus-induced myocardial necrosis often occurs in the absence of a significant inflammatory response, suggesting that direct viral injury accounts for most of the observed disease. This view is supported by studies in SCID mice. Reovirus-induced myocarditis develops in SCID mice, demonstrating that neither anti-viral immunity nor autoimmunity are required for myocardial damage caused by reovirus infection. Indeed, in distinction to hypotheses in some other viral models of myocarditis, both antibody and immune cells protect against, rather than potentiate, reovirus-induced myocardial injury.[180]

Variations in the efficiency of myocarditis induction correlate with the cytopathicity of reovirus isolates in cultured myocardial cells.[17,181] One of the most efficiently myocarditic reovirus isolates is 8B (see Table 28-1). 8B was derived through in vivo selection and reassortment in a mouse coinfected with T1L and T3D.[181] T3D is nonmyocarditic, and T1L causes myocarditis less efficiently than 8B.[178,179,181] The enhanced myocarditic capacity of strain 8B thus demonstrates that the biologic properties of reassortant viruses are not invariably constrained by the properties of parental viruses from which they are derived.

Studies of reovirus myocarditis provided the first example of the importance of viral core proteins in pathogenesis. Studies of reassortant viruses that were generated by crossing efficiently myocarditic reoviruses, such as 8B or T3A (see Table 28-1), and poorly myocarditic or nonmyocarditic viral strains show that the viral M1 segment, encoding viral core protein μ2, is strongly associated with myocarditis induction.[178,179] More recent studies have extended this original observation by showing that the L1 segment (encoding the λ3 core protein), the L2 segment (encoding the λ2 core spike protein), and the S1 segment (encoding σ1 and σ1s) are also determinants of the myocarditic phenotype of certain reovirus strains.[178] These same four genome segments play important roles in virulence and tissue tropism in adult SCID mice.[76] In sum, the L1, L2, S1, and M1 segments encode structural proteins constituting the reovirus vertex (see Fig. 28-1, Table 28-2). Thus, these studies demonstrate the importance of the vertex in pathogenesis. It has been suggested that vertex-associated proteins influence myocarditis and virulence in SCID mice through their actions on cellular macromolecular synthesis, by affecting the stability of reovirus core particles, or by altering the rate of viral RNA synthesis.[76,178]

Reoviruses produce pneumonia after inoculation into adult rats.[128] As discussed earlier, studies of the early stages of reovirus infection in rat lung have indicated that viral entry occurs through M cells overlying bronchus-associated lymphoid tissue.[128] The lung may also play a role in clearance of T1L from the bloodstream in infected animals.[211,213]

Hepatobiliary System

Reovirus can produce hepatobiliary infection in mice.* Reoviruses infect bile duct epithelial cells, producing chronic obstructive jaundice and biliary atresia,[234] and hepatocytes, producing cell death and diffuse hepatitis.[71,76] The liver also serves as an important site for the clearance of reovirus from the bloodstream[211,213] and for the entry of infectious virus into the biliary system.[161] The fact that hepatitis occurs in SCID mice suggests that viral injury to the liver, like that to the heart, is the result of direct viral replication rather than immune mediated.[71,76,180] Other experiments suggest that both CD4 and CD8 T cells play a role in controlling hepatobiliary disease in neonatal mice.[217] The similarity of the pathologic picture seen in neonatal mice after inoculation with certain reovirus strains to human biliary atresia (see, e.g., Virgin and Tyler[217] and Wilson and colleagues[234]) led to a number of studies designed to address the potential role of reoviruses in the induction of human hepatobiliary disease (reviewed in Tyler and Fields[205]). The role of reoviruses in inducing human disease remains speculative.

The capacity of T1L to infect hepatocytes is enhanced by antecedent hepatic injury caused by surgical trauma or hepatotoxins such as carbon tetrachloride.[149,163] Injury to the liver may induce hepatocyte activation and replication, which in turn facilitates reovirus infection.[149,163] This view is supported by in vitro studies using murine hepatocarcinoma cells.[200] In these cells, the capacity to support T1L replication correlates with ongoing cell division because T1L antigen is found in dividing but not quiescent hepatocytes. Earlier in vitro studies with other cell types also suggest that transformed cells are more susceptible to reovirus infection than their nontransformed counterparts.[52]

Several studies have addressed the role of specific genome segments in hepatobiliary disease induced by reoviruses. Studies using T1L × T3D reassortants in SCID mice indicate that three viral genome segments, M1, L2, and L1, encoding structural components of the reovirus vertex, are determinants of viral growth in liver and the severity of hepatitis[76] (Fig. 28-8). Of these segments, the association between M1 and severity of hepatitis is most significant. Thus, for the liver as well as the heart, the M1 segment plays a major role in determining the extent of tissue injury. No role was found for the S1 segment in reovirus-induced hepatitis in SCID mice.[76]

In another model system, inoculation of neonatal outbred mice, the S1 segment plays a role in determining the outcome of hepatic disease.[234] Neonatal outbred mice inoculated perorally with T3A contract the "oily fur syndrome," a disease in which mice show stunted growth and oily-appearing fur. Mice with the oily fur syndrome have striking biliary disease and, thus, the clinical syndrome was attributed to biliary atresia.[234] The efficiency of viral replication is not an important determinant of which viral strains induce the oily fur syndrome. This distinguishes this model from the adult SCID mouse model, in which replication and hepatitis induction are tightly linked.[76] Reassortant analysis shows that the T3A S1 segment is an important determinant of the capacity to induce the oily fur syndrome. A direct assessment of the relationship between the S1 segment and biliary disease has not been conducted, but it was

---

* References 71, 76, 149, 159, 161, 163, 217, 218, 234.

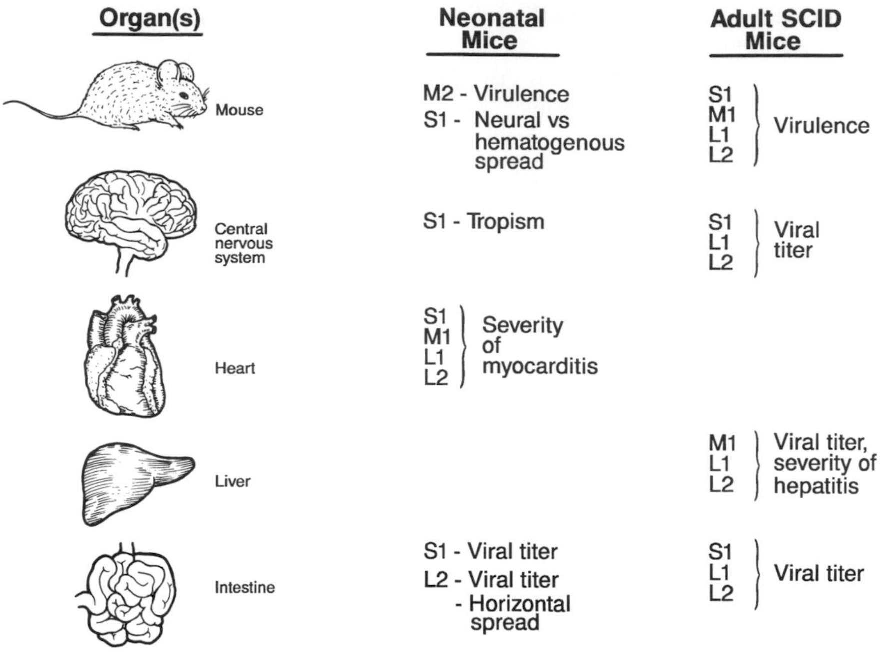

Organ(s)	Neonatal Mice	Adult SCID Mice
Mouse	M2 - Virulence S1 - Neural vs hematogenous spread	S1 M1 L1 L2 } Virulence
Central nervous system	S1 - Tropism	S1 L1 L2 } Viral titer
Heart	S1 M1 L1 L2 } Severity of myocarditis	
Liver		M1 L1 L2 } Viral titer, severity of hepatitis
Intestine	S1 - Viral titer L2 - Viral titer - Horizontal spread	S1 L1 L2 } Viral titer

FIG. 28-8. Organ-specific virulence genes. Genome segments demonstrated to be important for either growth or tropism in the organ schematically depicted are shown. SCID, severe combined immunodeficient.

suggested that proteins encoded by the S1 segment could be involved in generation of biliary atresia.[234] Regions of the S1 segment associated with the capacity of reovirus strains to induce the oily fur syndrome were evaluated by comparing sequences of viruses that vary in their capacity to induce this disease. Sequence polymorphisms that correlate with oily fur syndrome induction are found in regions encoding both head and tail domains of σ1 (see Fig. 28-2). Because these changes are outside of the σ1s reading frame, these findings argue that σ1 is an important determinant of the outcome of hepatic disease in newborn immunocompetent mice.

Gastrointestinal Tract

In addition to identifying a critical role for M cells and ISVPs in entry into the host, studies of reovirus infection of the intestine show that both the viral S1 and L2 segments play an important role in determining the capacity of reoviruses to grow in the intestine of neonatal mice.[18,76,95] Perhaps related to this capacity to grow efficiently in intestinal tissue, the S1 segment is a determinant of the capacity to spread to visceral organs after peroral inoculation,[92] and the L2 segment is a determinant of efficient horizontal transmission of reovirus infection to littermates.[95] In SCID mice, the S1, L1, and L2 segments are important determinants of intestinal growth.[76] Other studies have found that sites of T1L- and T3D-induced gastrointestinal disease differ after intravenous challenge, and that the S1 segment plays an important part in determining these differences.[160] The contribution of the S1 segment to strain-specific differences in reovirus growth and tropism in intestine has been hypothesized to reside in differences in the susceptibility of σ1 protein to cleavage by intestinal proteases.[18,54,134,238] However, S1 is a determinant of intestinal replication after intraperitoneal inoculation, a situation in which exposure of virions to lumenal proteases may not be important.[76] The role of the σ1s protein in intestinal growth and tropism has not been evaluated.

Endocrine System

Both T1L and T3D can injure tissues of the endocrine system. Autoantibodies against target cell antigens[77] and decreases in levels of circulating hormones are observed during reovirus infection, although their pathogenetic roles have not been defined. Because both T1L and T3D injure the endocrine pancreas, they have been used as animal models of virus-induced islet cell injury (reviewed in Tyler and Fields[205]). In mice infected with T1L, autoantibodies to insulin, reduced serum insulin levels, and transient abnormalities in glucose tolerance develop.[144] In addition to the pancreas, reovirus infection can also result in thyroiditis. Thyroid infection results in the production of thyroid autoantibodies and the induction of major histocompatibility complex (MHC) proteins.[142] Reovirus infection is associated with upregulation of MHC proteins in other situations as well.[25,143,144] Reoviruses also infect the pituitary.[144] T1L infects the growth hormone-producing cells of the anterior pituitary and is associated with decreased circulating growth hormone, which may contribute to impaired growth in infected animals.

Organ-Specific Virulence Genes

One of the important findings from analysis of the roles of reovirus gene segments in multiple models of disease is the fact that different genome segments are important in different organs, a finding that supports the concept of organ-specific virulence genes. For example, in the adult SCID mouse model, genome segments L1, L2, and S1 are important determinants of virulence and growth in brain and intestine. No role for the M1 segment is detected in brain or intestine, despite the use of sensitive statistical techniques.[76] In contrast, viral yield as well as the number of hepatic inflammatory lesions in the liver of SCID mice are determined by segments L1, L2, and M1, whereas no role for the S1 segment is observed. Similarly, in neonatal mice, the M1, L1, L2, and S1 segments play an important role in induction of myocarditis,[178,179] whereas M2 and S1 are important in the CNS (see section on Pathology and Disease in the Central Nervous System). Similar to results from studies using adult SCID mice, L2 and S1 are important for controlling viral growth in the neonatal mouse intestine.[18,95]

One model to explain the finding that different genome segments are important in specific organs is sequential involvement of different proteins in reovirus replication. In this model, viral proteins vary in their importance in specific tissues because the rate-limiting step in viral growth or clearance differs from organ to organ. For example, if the S1 segment-encoded σ1 attachment protein is important for growth in CNS or intestine, then steps in viral replication related to attachment or entry might be rate limiting in CNS or intestine. In the liver, the M1 segment-encoded μ2 protein would provide a rate-limiting function in viral replication or clearance, whereas S1 segment-encoded proteins would not be rate limiting. Alternatively, the host response controlling viral replication might be distinct in different organs. In this model, viral genome segments important in determining viral growth or tissue injury would be involved in steps in viral replication that are targeted by tissue-specific host factors (e.g., cytokines).

Biology of Mutants Selected During Chronic Infection In Vivo

Reoviruses usually cause either lethal infection or are cleared from the host. Thus, although reoviruses produce persistent infections in cell culture, there is no in vivo model of persistent reovirus infection. PI viruses isolated from persistently infected L cells show delayed clearance from the CNS, but are ultimately cleared by immunocompetent animals.[130] The fact that these viruses are cleared more slowly than wild-type T3D suggests that mutations affecting the process of viral entry regulate clearance of virus in vivo. Another model for evaluation of reovirus mutation during prolonged infection is chronic T3D infection of adult SCID mice. T3D grows poorly in adult SCID mouse intestine and brain, and kills mice 80 to 100 days after inoculation.[75,76] When viruses are plaque-purified from adult SCID mice 87 days after inoculation, mutant viruses with altered pathogenetic phenotypes are found.[75] One such variant grows better than T3D in both SCID and neonatal mouse intestine and is more infectious than T3D after oral inoculation. Another grows better in SCID mouse brain and is more virulent in SCID mice than T3D, but retains poor (T3D-like) oral infectivity. Thus, variants arise that appear suited to specific stages in reovirus pathogenesis. Variants selected in vivo lack the phenotypes (efficient growth in cured cells or

cells treated with ammonium chloride) found in PI viruses isolated from persistently infected L cells.[75]

IMMUNITY AND STAGES OF INFECTION OF THE CELL AND HOST

Overview of Immunity to Reoviruses

Although the pathogenesis of reovirus in multiple organs has been studied for many years, interest in reovirus immunity has intensified in more recent years. This area has attracted attention because of the potential for integrating an understanding of functions of specific proteins at different stages in pathogenesis with information about protein-specific immunity (see Table 28-4). Although a number of studies have evaluated activities of anti-reovirus antibodies, less is known about T-cell recognition of reovirus antigens and the potential influence of T cells on reovirus pathogenesis.

The reovirus system illustrates several important concepts about mechanisms of antibody action in vivo and in vitro. For example, studies using monoclonal antibodies clearly demonstrate that antibody can block neural spread of virus without affecting replication at the primary site of infection. Viral susceptibility to the action of antibody can be determined by viral proteins other than the antibody's target antigen. The lack of clear correlation between in vivo protective capacity of antibodies and their in vitro properties led to the discovery that some protective antibodies act by inhibiting steps in viral replication subsequent to cell attachment. Finally, studies show that circulating IgG (independent of IgA) can play an important role in clearance of virus infection from the intestine.

Many studies have defined the in vitro activities of antibodies specific for various reovirus proteins, but initially these studies contributed more information about the structure and function of reovirus proteins than the nature of protective immunity. In addition, because so much of reovirus biology is related to reovirus serotype, study of serotype-specific immune responses has overshadowed investigation of immune responses that are not serotype specific. Because serotype specificity is primarily determined by epitopes on the σ1 protein, this focus has tended to emphasize immunity to σ1. More recently, the presence of cross-reactivity between serotypes has attracted more attention, with consequent demonstration of protective responses to non-σ1 epitopes.

All recognized anti-reovirus immune responses are specific for protein antigens. There is no evidence for reovirus-specific anti-carbohydrate, anti-lipid, or anti-dsRNA immune responses. It is important to recognize that there is tremendous conservation of amino acid sequences in proteins from prototypic and field isolate reovirus strains (see Table 28-3). For example, the σ3 protein contains 365 amino acids, and T1L and T3D are different at only 11 amino acid positions. Thus, it is not surprising that a significant component of both T- and B-cell immunity is not serotype specific. For example, polyclonal antibodies raised against prototypic strain T1L precipitates T3D proteins,[66] and even the serotype-defining σ1 protein has some serotype–cross-reactive epitopes.[66,78,215]

Serotype-Specific and Cross-Reactive Recognition of Reovirus Antigens by Antibody

There are both serotype-specific and serotype-independent antigens on reoviruses.[156] The availability of reassortant genetic techniques allowed rapid identification of targets of certain serotype-specific responses. Reassortant analysis shows that the S1 segment-encoded σ1 protein is the primary determinant of serotype-specific neutralization.[222] This conclusion is in agreement with the fact that the σ1 protein is more polymorphic than any other structural reovirus protein (see Table 28-3). Several studies show that most of the neutralizing monoclonal antibodies specific for σ1 exhibit serotype-specific binding or neutralization of prototype reovirus strains.[24,78,214,215] In addition, monoclonal antibodies specific for T1L and T3D σ1 proteins show serotype-specific binding to a panel of nonprototype serotype 1 and serotype 3 reoviruses.[215] These observations support the use of σ1-specific monoclonal antibodies, such as 9BG5 and 5C6, for determining the serotype of reovirus isolates.[74]

In contrast to σ1-specific monoclonal antibodies, monoclonal antibodies specific for other outer capsid proteins typically cross-react with proteins from prototype reoviruses of different serotypes.[78,215] Although these antibodies are cross-reactive, certain antibodies specific for the σ3, μ1, and λ2 capsid proteins consistently bound better to a panel of serotype 3 viruses than a panel of serotype 1 viruses.[215] This is similar to results of earlier experiments demonstrating that some monoclonal antibodies specific for proteins other than σ1 selectively precipitated proteins of one serotype more efficiently than other serotypes.[102] Even polyclonal antibody raised against prototype reoviruses shows some level of serotype specificity in immunoprecipitating σ3, λ2, and μ1.[66] The apparent higher avidity of certain monoclonal antibodies to σ3, λ2, and μ1 from serotype 3 than serotype 1 viruses may reflect subtle differences in the conformation of outer capsid proteins in serotype 1 and serotype 3 viruses. Alternatively, the σ1 proteins of serotype 1 and serotype 3 reoviruses might differ in their interactions with outer capsid proteins σ3, μ1, and λ2, causing changes in the conformation of these proteins and consequent serotype-dependent epitope recognition by monoclonal antibodies.

T-Cell Responses to Reoviruses

T-cell responses are induced during reovirus infection. This has been best demonstrated by evaluating changes in T-cell populations in intestinal tissue after peroral inoculation. After peroral challenge with T1L, both Peyer's patches and intraepithelial lymphocyte preparations have cytotoxic T-lymphocyte (CTL) precursors that generate reovirus-specific CTL after in vitro stimulation.[111,114] These cells are MHC restricted.[113,114] Reovirus infection is also followed by development of IgA memory cells and both CD4 T cells and virus-specific helper cell responses.[111,114] Although CTL responses, and likely CD4 responses, to reovirus clearly occur, the physiologic importance of these responses is less clear. A number of studies show that immune cells protect against reovirus infec-

tion.[37,180,217] However, in mice with an interrupted β₂-microglobulin gene, which have a significant deficiency in CD8 T cells, reovirus is cleared from the intestine with normal kinetics.[12] This finding suggests that normal levels of CTLs are not required for clearance of reovirus from the intestine, but does not rule out that these cells, or perhaps CD4 T cells, have some role in the normal response to reovirus.[217]

Few studies have been conducted to identify the protein antigens recognized by reovirus-specific T cells. In particular, newer methods to map peptides responsible for T-cell recognition by MHC class I or class II restricted T cells have not been performed. However, reassortant genetic analysis has defined certain proteins as targets. Initial studies of CTL killing of reovirus-infected cells suggested that a prominent part of the CTL response to reovirus is serotype specific[61,62] and directed to products of the S1 segment (σ1 or σ1s). Although serotype-specific killing was observed, significant cross-reaction between targets infected with viruses of different serotypes was seen. Similar data, demonstrating that serotype-specific T-cell responses can be directed to S1 segment products, was obtained during evaluation of the delayed-type hypersensitivity response of BALB/c mice to rechallenge with reovirus.[223] Further analysis clearly showed that although serotype-specific CTL exist, many reovirus-specific CTLs cross-react with viruses of different serotypes.[80,111,112] Thus, there must be CTL epitopes on multiple reovirus proteins in addition to either σ1 or σ1s.

An anti-idiotypic monoclonal antibody raised against the T3D σ1-specific neutralizing monoclonal antibody 9BG5 can be used to immunize mice.[177] The subsequent delayed-type hypersensitivity response is directed against σ1.[177] This same anti-idiotypic antibody elicited serotype-specific anti-reovirus antibody in several strains of mice, and mothers immunized with the anti-idiotype monoclonal antibody give birth to pups resistant to viral infection.[68] The molecular basis of this cross-reactive recognition of viral epitopes by T cells and antibody specific for the anti-idiotypic antibody is likely related to the presence of sequences in the variable domain of the anti-idiotype with homology to sequences in the σ1 protein.[231,233]

Neutralization of Reovirus Infectivity

Neutralization of reovirus by antibody is usually measured as plaque reduction,[78,215] but the mechanism of neutralization has not been fully delineated for reovirus. Certain monoclonal antibodies (e.g., monoclonal antibody 9BG5, which is specific for T3D σ1) are efficient at plaque reduction neutralization and also efficiently block binding of virus to L cells.[24,214,216] A number of very efficient neutralizing anti-σ1 monoclonal antibodies also aggregate virions,[78] but the role of virion aggregation in plaque reduction neutralization has not been completely defined. Although serotype-specific neutralization can be observed using polyclonal sera, polyclonal anti-T1L serum efficiently neutralizes T3D, and vice versa.[78,214] Monoclonal antibodies specific for σ1 often have plaque reduction activity,[24,78,215] as do some monoclonal and monospecific antibodies to λ2 and σ3.[78] Mechanisms responsible for plaque-reduction neutralization by anti-σ3 and anti-λ2 monoclonal antibodies have not been defined.

Hemagglutination Inhibition and the Genetics of Viral Susceptibility to Antibody Action

Polyclonal anti-reovirus antibodies can inhibit virion-mediated HA.[156] This is likely the result, at least for antibodies specific for the viral hemagglutinin σ1, of antibody blocking the interaction between the virion and the erythrocyte surface. Monoclonal antibodies specific for σ3 and μ1 also efficiently inhibit HA,[78,215] which shows that antibody specific for one outer capsid protein (σ3) can inhibit the function of another outer capsid protein (σ1). The HA-inhibiting capacity of monoclonal anti-σ3 antibodies depends on the target virus. For example, monoclonal antibody 8F12 (specific for both T3D and T1L σ3) inhibits HA by T1L more efficiently than T3D, whereas monoclonal antibody 4F2 (specific for both T1L and T3D σ3) inhibits HA by T3D more efficiently than T1L. These differences are not explained by the avidity of anti-σ3 monoclonal antibodies for T1L versus T3D,[215] but instead may be the result of strain-dependent interactions between σ1 and σ3. Reassortant genetic analysis showed that strain-specific differences in HA inhibition capacity of anti-σ3 monoclonal antibodies is determined by the S1 segment. Thus, monoclonal antibody 4F2, which is specific for σ3, inhibits HA by reassortant viruses containing the T3D but not the T1L S1 segment.[215] This shows that the primary determinant of susceptibility to antibody action can be a protein other than the antibody's target antigen. This is an important concept because the efficacy of subunit vaccines may depend on viral proteins other than the vaccine antigen.

Adoptive Transfer of Protection Against Reovirus-Induced Disease

Antibody (both monoclonal and polyclonal, both serotype-specific and serotype cross-reactive) can protect against lethal infection with serotype 3 reoviruses (T3D and T3C9).[38,206,209,214] In addition, antibody can protect against T1L-induced hydrocephalus[206] and 8B-induced myocarditis.[180] Antibody has been used prophylactically to prevent lethal disease and as treatment for established CNS infection.[214] Pups born of immune dams are resistant to lethal challenge with reovirus,[38] and this protection appears to be related to both transplacental transfer of antibody and antibody in breast milk.[38] Immunization of dams with monoclonal anti-idiotype also protects pups from reovirus infection.[68]

Adoptive transfer of immune spleen cells protects neonatal mice from lethal infection with either perorally administered T3C9 or intramuscularly administered T3D.[217] Protection against hydrocephalus caused by T1L and myocarditis caused by 8B also has been observed.[180,217] In this adoptive transfer model, both CD4 and CD8 T cells are required for maximal protection against T3D, T3C9, or 8B.[180,217] Further evidence for a role of both CD4 and CD8 T cells in protection against reovirus-induced disease comes from experiments using monoclonal antibodies to deplete CD4 and CD8 T cells in vivo.[217] In these experiments, depletion of CD4 and CD8 T cells increased the severity and changed the nature of T3C9-induced liver disease. Adoptive transfer of Peyer's patch cells protects

adult SCID mice against lethal infection[71] and neonatal mice against peroral challenge with T3C9.[37] This shows that protective immune cells are present in the intestine, which is the primary portal of viral entry into the host.

Role of Antibody at Defined Pathogenetic Stages

Spread Within the Host

The effect of antibody at different stages in reovirus pathogenesis has been evaluated in detail (Fig. 28-9), based on extensive studies defining the stages in reovirus pathogenesis (see section on Stages in Infection of the Host). Monoclonal antibodies specific for outer capsid proteins σ1,[206,209,214] σ3,[206] and μ1[206] can be protective in vivo. One prominent in vivo mechanism of antibody action is inhibition of neural spread of virus from primary sites in muscle and intestine to the nervous system. T3D spreads from hind-limb muscle to the CNS by the sciatic nerve, whereas T3C9 spreads from the intestine to the CNS by the vagus nerve. Monoclonal antibody-mediated protection against T3D-induced disease after intramuscular inoculation is associated with inhibition of spread to the inferior spinal cord, in some cases without effects on primary replication.[206,209] In addition, viral spread within the CNS, for example from the brain to the retina or from the inferior to the superior spinal cord, is inhibited by adoptively transferred antibody.[209] Consistent with these findings, monoclonal antibodies inhibit spread of T3C9 from the intestine by the vagus nerve to the brain, in many cases without altering T3C9 titer in intestine.[206,209] Thus, in two distinct disease models, antibody inhibits neural spread from primary sites of infection when effects on primary replication are minimal or absent. Mechanisms by which antibody inhibits neural spread independent of replication at the primary site of inoculation have not been defined.

Effects on Primary Replication in the Intestine

Although the capacity of antibody to protect against systemic disease with reovirus and the capacity of adoptively transferred immune cells to control intestinal virus replication are clear, less is known about mechanisms responsible for controlling viral replication, and finally clearing virus, from primary sites of infection. Certain monoclonal antibodies inhibit viral replication after intramuscular inoculation with T3D, establishing that antibodies can act at primary sites.[206] The importance of B cells and antibody at a natural portal of entry, the intestine, has been addressed in a study comparing the clearance of reovirus T3C9 from the intestine after peroral inoculation of adult immunocompetent and immunocompromised mice. SCID mice and mice with targeted interruptions of either the transmembrane exon of IgM (B-cell and antibody deficient[97]) or the β_2-microglobulin component of MHC class I molecules (CD8 T-cell deficient[98]) were compared.[12] SCID mice failed to clear intestinal infection after peroral inoculation, whereas immunocompetent mice cleared virus within 7 days. This confirms that functional lymphocytes are important

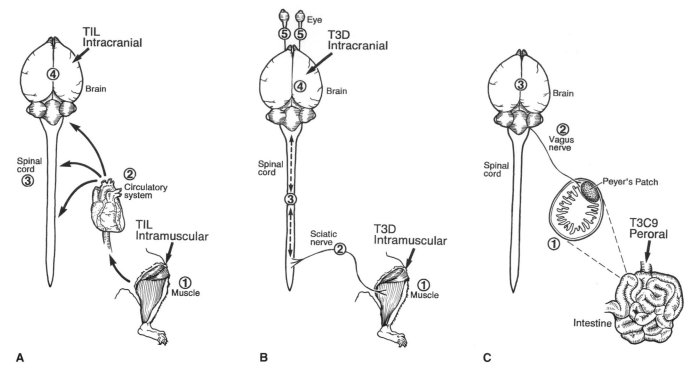

FIG. 28-9. Role of antibody at specific stages in pathogenesis of reovirus infection. The numbers in each panel denote sites at which antibody has specific functions. (**A**) For hematogenous spread after intramuscular or intracranial inoculation of T1L, antibody can 1) inhibit replication in muscle, 2) decrease viremia independent of effects on replication in muscle, 3) inhibit spread to or growth in the spinal cord, 4) inhibit spread to or growth in the brain, and prevent development of hydrocephalus. (**B**) For neural spread after intramuscular or intracranial inoculation of T3D, antibody can 1) inhibit replication in muscle, 2) inhibit neural spread to or growth in the spinal cord independent of effects on replication in muscle, 3) inhibit spread to or growth in and spread by the spinal cord, 4) inhibit growth in the brain and prevent lethal encephalitis, and 5) inhibit neural spread to or growth in the eye from the brain. (**C**) For neural spread after peroral inoculation of T3C9, antibody can 1) enhance intestinal clearance of virus after peroral inoculation of adult B-cell–deficient mice (however, circulating IgG does not affect primary replication early [days 3 to 5] after peroral inoculation of neonatal mice); 2) inhibit neural spread to or growth in the brain by the vagus nerve; and 3) inhibit growth in the brain and prevent lethal encephalitis.

for clearance of virus from the intestine.[71,76] Despite the prominent CD8 CTL response documented in intestine after peroral inoculation of reovirus, mice with an interrupted β_2-microglobulin gene cleared T3C9 from the intestine with normal kinetics. In contrast, mice deficient in B cells and antibody failed to control T3C9 replication in intestine between 7 and 11 days after inoculation, demonstrating an important role for B cells in intestinal clearance. This was confirmed in studies showing that adoptive transfer of immune B cells into SCID mice allowed control of intestinal infection. In addition, systemic administration of IgG specific for reovirus reconstituted the ability of B-cell–deficient mice to clear primary infection from the intestine,[12] showing that circulating IgG can play a protective role at mucosal surfaces independent of IgA.

Effect of Antibody on Virus-Cell Interactions

Although a number of activities of antibody in vitro have been examined, more recent studies have focused on the role of antibodies after virus-antibody complexes bind to the cell. These studies were undertaken because, in the reovirus system, antibody-mediated protection does not consistently correlate with in vitro properties of antibodies including antibody isotype, antibody avidity, plaque-reduction neutralization, HA inhibition, or inhibition of viral binding to target cells.[206,209,214] For example, several monoclonal antibodies specific for the $\sigma 3$ outer capsid protein are nonneutralizing but are protective in vivo.[206] Monoclonal antibody-mediated protection against T3D-induced CNS disease is seen in mice depleted of serum complement,[214] arguing against a critical role for complement in protection by antibody. Thus, the available data in the reovirus system strongly argue against reliance on in vitro properties of antibody (such as neutralization) as predictors of in vivo efficacy of antibody responses.

These findings led to a search for other actions of antibodies that might explain their protective capacity (Fig. 28-10). It was observed that antibodies specific for $\sigma 3$ and $\mu 1$ inhibited replication of virus already bound to the cell surface.[216] This effect on postbinding events is a consistent predictor of in

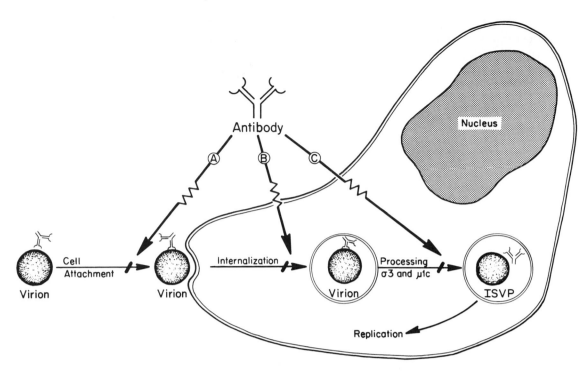

FIG. 28-10. Effects of antibody on virus-cell interactions. Antibodies specific for virion outer capsid proteins inhibit multiple stages in the interaction between reoviruses and the cell. Antibody effect A: some antibodies specific for the σ1 protein block cell attachment of virus to the cell. Antibody effect B: an antibody specific for the σ3 protein, when bound to the virus before virus binding to the cell, inhibits internalization of the virus. antibody effect C: antibodies specific for the σ3 protein, when bound to the virus before the virus binds to the cell, block the intracellular proteolytic uncoating of the virion to the infectious subviral particle (ISVP) form. (From Virgin HW, Mann MA, Tyler KL. Protective antibodies inhibit reovirus internalization and uncoating by intracellular proteases. J Virol 1994;68:6719–6729, with permission.)

vivo protective capacity.[206,216] Multiple mechanisms contribute to antibody-mediated inhibition of viral growth (see Fig. 28-10). First, some monoclonal antibodies inhibit reovirus internalization. In addition, monoclonal anti-σ3 antibodies inhibit intracellular proteolytic uncoating of the reovirus outer capsid, and augment the action of ammonium chloride (which also inhibits virion uncoating).[216] This is an effect of antibody on proteolysis of σ3 because antibodies also blocked uncoating of virions by chymotrypsin in vitro. Antibodies specific for the μ1 outer capsid protein inhibit membrane penetration by ISVPs, suggesting an additional intracellular site of antibody action.[81] These studies suggest that subunit vaccine design might be effectively directed to epitopes critical for postbinding steps in viral replication, and that antiviral drugs might be combined with antibodies targeted to the same steps in viral replication.

FUTURE DIRECTIONS

The value of the reovirus system as a model for studies of viral pathogenesis has been the availability of structural, biochemical, genetic, pathogenetic, and immunologic tools that can be applied to an analysis of viral disease in an integrated fashion. Thus, it is the merging of these different approaches focused by genetic analysis that has been the key to success in this system. In the future, these aspects of the reovirus model will continue to be useful. However, significant challenges exist. In particular, the ability to make targeted mutations in reovirus genes would add significantly to reassortant genetic analysis. This approach would allow definition of important motifs, regions, and individual amino acids in genome segments already shown to be critical for one or more aspects of reovirus interactions with cells, hosts, and the immune system. Analysis of variant viruses also promises to delineate better regions of proteins important for specific properties of the virus.

Although genetic approaches hold much promise, basic questions about reovirus pathogenesis remain. How does a virus enter a neuron? How do viruses spread in nerves? Why are some genes more important than others in one or another organ? What cellular and viral factors are important for reovirus transcription and replication? How are genome segments assorted into progeny virions? What can be learned from the structure of the different forms of reovirus virions about the biologic roles of these structures? What is pathogenetically important about the reovirus vertex? What is the structural basis for interactions between reovirus proteins that share a role at a given step in infection of the cell or host? What mechanisms underlie the role of single proteins and single amino acid changes in determining tissue tropism? These and other questions will require integration of old and new methodologies to approach important problems central to an understanding of the relationship between viruses and their hosts.

ABBREVIATIONS

8B: reovirus serotype 3 strain 8B
CNS: central nervous system
CTL: cytotoxic T lymphocyte
dsRNA: double-stranded RNA
EGF: epidermal growth factor
HA: hemagglutination
ISVP: infectious subvirion particle
L929 fibroblast: L929 fibroblast cell line
M cell: microfold cell
MEL: murine erythroleukemia
MHC: major histocompatibility complex
PFU: plaque-forming units
PI virus: persistent infection virus
SCID: severe combined immunodeficient
T1L: reovirus serotype 1 strain Lang
T2J: reovirus serotype 2 strain Jones
T3A: reovirus serotype 3 strain Abney
T3C9: reovirus serotype 3 clone 9
T3D: reovirus serotype 3 strain Dearing

DEDICATION

We dedicate this chapter to the memory of Dr. Bernard N. Fields, whose pioneering work in the field of reovirus pathogenesis, genetics, and structure provides much of the framework on which reovirus research now stands. The chapter was started during the latter stages of the illness that led to his premature passing, but still he provided suggestions about principles he wished to impart, as well as a strong and abiding enthusiasm for the future of research in reovirus pathogenesis and viral pathogenesis in general, and it is fair to say that his spirit permeates much of the work summarized in the chapter. As investigators, we derived much of our current appreciation for science and approach to research from Dr. Fields. We hope that we have done him, and the field he loved, justice in this chapter.

REFERENCES

1. Adams DJ, Spendlove JC, Spendlove RS, Barnett BB. Aerosol stability of infectious and potentially infectious reovirus particles. Appl Environ Microbiol 1982;44:903–908.
2. Ahmed R, Canning WM, Kauffman RS, Sharpe AH, Hallum JV, Fields BN. Role of the host cell in persistent viral infection: coevolution of L cells and reovirus during persistent infection. Cell 1981; 25:325–332.
3. Ahmed R, Chakraborty PR, Graham AF, Ramig RF, Fields BN. Genetic variation during persistent reovirus infection: presence of ex-
tragenically suppressed temperature-sensitive lesions in wild-type virus isolated from persistently infected L cells. J Virol 1980; 34:383–389.
4. Ahmed R, Fields BN. Role of the S4 gene in the establishment of persistent reovirus infection in L cells. Cell 1982;28:605–612.
5. Ahmed R, Graham AF. Persistent infections in L cells with temperature-sensitive mutants of reovirus. J Virol 1977;23:250–262.
6. Ahmed R, Kauffman RS, Fields BN. Genetic variation during persistent reovirus infection: isolation of cold-sensitive and temperature-sensitive mutants from persistently infected L cells. Virology 1983;131:71–78.
7. Ambler L, Mackay M. Reovirus 1 and 3 bind and internalize at the apical surface of intestinal epithelial cells. Virology 1991;184: 162–169.
8. Amerongen HM, Wilson GR, Fields BN, Neutra MR. Proteolytic processing of reovirus is required for adherence to intestinal M cells. J Virol 1994;68:8428–8432.
9. Antczak JB, Chmelo R, Pickup DJ, Joklik WK. Sequences at both termini of the ten genes of reovirus serotype 3 (strain Dearing). Virology 1982;121:307–319.
10. Armstrong GD, Paul RW, Lee PWK. Studies on reovirus receptors of L cells: virus binding characteristics and comparison with reovirus receptors of erythrocytes. Virology 1984;138:37–48.
11. Babiss LE, Luftig RB, Weatherbee JA, Weihing RR, Ray UR, Fields BN. Reovirus serotypes 1 and 3 differ in their in vitro association with microtubules. J Virol 1979;30:863–874.
12. Barkon ML, Haller BL, Virgin HW. Circulating IgG can play a critical role in clearance of intestinal reovirus infection. J Virol 1996; 70:1109–1116.
13. Bass DM, Bodkin D, Dambrauskas R, Trier JS, Fields BN, Wolf JL. Intraluminal proteolytic activation plays an important role in replication of type 1 reovirus in the intestines of neonatal mice. J Virol 1990;64:1830–1833.
14. Bass DM, Trier JS, Dambrauskas R, Wolf JL. Reovirus type 1 infection of small intestinal epithelium in suckling mice and its effect on M cells. Lab Invest 1988;55:226–235.
15. Bassel-Duby R, Nibert ML, Homcy CJ, Fields BN, Sawutz DG. Evidence that the sigma 1 protein of reovirus serotype 3 is a multimer. J Virol 1987;61:1834–1841.
16. Bassel-Duby R, Spriggs DR, Tyler KL, Fields BN. Identification of attenuating mutations on the reovirus type 3 S1 double-stranded RNA segment with a rapid sequencing technique. J Virol 1986;60: 64–67.
17. Baty CJ, Sherry B. Cytopathogenic effect in cardiac myocytes but not in cardiac fibroblasts is correlated with reovirus-induced acute myocarditis. J Virol 1993;67:6295–6298.
18. Bodkin DK, Fields BN. Growth and survival of reovirus in intestinal tissue: role of the L2 and S1 genes. J Virol 1989;63:1188–1193.
19. Bodkin DK, Nibert ML, Fields BN. Proteolytic digestion of reovirus in the intestinal lumens of neonatal mice. J Virol 1989;63:4676–4681.
20. Borsa J, Morash BD, Sargent MD, Copps TP, Lievaart PA, Szekely JG. Two modes of entry of reovirus particles into L cells. J Gen Virol 1979;45:161–170.
21. Borsa J, Sargent MD, Lievaart PA, Copps TP. Reovirus: evidence for a second step in the intracellular uncoating and transcriptase activation process. Virology 1981;111:191–200.
22. Brown EG, Nibert ML, Fields BN. The L2 gene of reovirus serotype 3 controls the capacity to interfere, accumulate deletions and establish persistent infection. In: Compans RW, Bishop DHL, eds. Double-stranded RNA viruses. New York: Elsevier, 1983:275–287.
23. Burstin SJ, Brandriss MW, Schlesinger JJ. Infection of a macrophage-like cell line, P388D1 with reovirus: effects of immune ascitic fluids and monoclonal antibodies on neutralization and on enhancement of viral growth. J Immunol 1983;130:2915–2919.
24. Burstin SJ, Spriggs DR, Fields BN. Evidence for functional domains on the reovirus type 3 hemagglutinin. Virology 1982;117: 146–155.
25. Campbell IL, Harrison LC, Ashcroft RG, Jack I. Reovirus infection enhances expression of class I MHC proteins on human beta-cell and rat RINm5F cell. Diabetes 1988;37:362–365.
26. Canning WM, Fields BN. Ammonium chloride prevents lytic growth of reovirus and helps to establish persistent infection in mouse L cells. Science 1983;219:987–988.

27. Chang CT, Zweerink HJ. Fate of parental reovirus in infected cells. Virology 1971;46:544–555.

28. Chappell JD, Goral MI, Rodgers SE, dePamphilis CW, Dermody TS. Sequence diversity within the reovirus S2 gene: reovirus genes reassort in nature and their termini are predicted to form a panhandle motif. J Virol 1994;68:750–756.

29. Chen D, Burns JW, Estes MK, Ramig RF. Phenotypes of rotavirus reassortants depend on the recipient genetic background. Proc Natl Acad Sci U S A 1989;86:3743–3747.

30. Chen D, Zeng Q-Y, Wentz MJ, Gorziglia M, Estes MK, Ramig RF. Template-dependent, in vitro replication of rotavirus RNA. J Virol 1994;68:7030–7039.

31. Choi AH, Lee PW. Does the beta-adrenergic receptor function as a reovirus receptor? Virology 1988;163:191–197.

32. Choi AH, Paul RW, Lee PW. Reovirus binds to multiple plasma membrane proteins of mouse L fibroblasts. Virology 1990;178:316–320.

33. Choi AHC. Internalization of virus binding proteins during entry of reovirus into K562 erythroleukemia cells. Virology 1994;200:301–306.

34. Cleveland DR, Zarbl H, Millward S. Reovirus guanylyltransferase is L2 gene product lambda 2. J Virol 1986;60:307–311.

35. Co MS, Gaulton GN, Fields BN, Greene MI. Isolation and biochemical characterization of the mammalian reovirus type 3 cell-surface receptor. Proc Natl Acad Sci U S A 1985;82:1494–1498.

36. Co MS, Gaulton GN, Tominaga A, Homcy CJ, Fields BN, Greene MI. Structural similarities between the mammalian beta-adrenergic and reovirus type 3 receptors. Proc Natl Acad Sci U S A 1985;82:5315–5318.

37. Cuff CF, Cebra CK, Lavi E, Molowitz EH, Rubin DH, Cebra JJ. Protection of neonatal mice from fatal reovirus infection by immune serum and gut derived lymphocytes. Adv Exp Med Biol 1991;310:307–315.

38. Cuff CF, Lavi E, Cebra CK, Cebra JJ, Rubin DH. Passive immunity to fatal reovirus serotype 3-induced meningoencephalitis mediated by both secretory and transplacental factors in neonatal mice. J Virol 1990;64:1256–1263.

39. Dales S. Association between the spindle apparatus and reovirus. Proc Natl Acad Sci U S A 1962;50:268–275.

40. Dales S, Gomatos P, Hsu KC. The uptake and development of reovirus in strain L cells followed with labelled viral nucleic acid and ferritin-antibody conjugates. Virology 1965;25:193–211.

41. Danis C, Mabrouk T, Garzon S, Lemay G. Establishment of persistent reovirus infection in SC1 cells: absence of protein synthesis and increased levels of double-stranded RNA-activated protein kinase. Virus Res 1993;27:253–265.

42. Dermody TS, Nibert ML, Bassel Duby R, Fields BN. A sigma 1 region important for hemagglutination by serotype 3 reovirus strains. J Virol 1990;64:5173–5176.

43. Dermody TS, Nibert ML, Bassel Duby R, Fields BN. Sequence diversity in S1 genes and S1 translation products of 11 serotype 3 reovirus strains. J Virol 1990;64:4842–4850.

44. Dermody TS, Nibert ML, Wetzel D, Tong X, Fields BN. Cells and viruses with mutations affecting viral entry are selected during persistent infections of L cells with mammalian reoviruses. J Virol 1993;67:2055–2063.

45. Dichter MA, Weiner HL. Infection of neuronal cell cultures with reovirus mimics in vitro patterns of neurotropism. Ann Neurol 1984;16:603–610.

46. Dichter MA, Weiner HL, Fields BN, et al. Antiidiotypic antibody to reovirus binds to neurons and protects from viral infection. Ann Neurol 1986;19:555–558.

47. Donta ST, Shanley JD. Reovirus type 3 binds to antagonist domains of the beta-adrenergic receptor. J Virol 1990;64:639–641.

48. Drayna D, Fields BN. Activation and characterization for the reovirus transcriptase: genetic analysis. J Virol 1982;41:110–118.

49. Drayna D, Fields BN. Biochemical studies on the mechanism of chemical and physical inactivation of reovirus. J Gen Virol 1982;63:161–170.

50. Drayna D, Fields BN. Genetic studies on the mechanism of chemical and physical inactivation of reovirus. J Gen Virol 1982;63:149–160.

51. Dryden KA, Wang G, Yeager M, et al. Early steps in reovirus infection are associated with dramatic changes in supramolecular structure and protein conformation: analysis of virions and subviral particles by cryoelectron microscopy and image reconstruction. J Cell Biol 1993;122:1023–1041.

52. Duncan, MR, Stanish SM, Cox DC. Differential sensitivity of normal and transformed human cells to reovirus infection. J Virol 1978;28:444–449.

53. Duncan R, Horne D, Strong JE, et al. Conformational and functional analysis of the C-terminal globular head of the reovirus cell attachment protein. Virology 1991;182:810–819.

54. Duncan R, Lee PWK. Localization of two protease-sensitive regions separating distinct domains in the reovirus cell-attachment protein sigma 1. Virology 1994;203:149–152.

55. el-Ghorr AA, Gordon DA, George K, Maratos-Flier E. Regulation of expression of the reovirus receptor on differentiated HL60 cells. J Gen Virol 1992;73:1961–1968.

56. Ensminger WD, Tamm I. Cellular DNA and protein synthesis in reovirus-infected L cells. Virology 1969;39:357–359.

57. Epstein RL, Powers ML, Rogart RB, Weiner HL. Binding of iodine-125 labelled reovirus to cell surface receptors. Virology 1984;133:46–55.

58. Ernst H, Shatkin AJ. Reovirus hemagglutinin mRNA codes for two polypeptides in overlapping reading frames. Proc Natl Acad Sci U S A 1985;82:48–52.

59. Fields BN, Eagle H. The pH-dependence of reovirus synthesis. Virology 1973;52:581–583.

60. Fields BN, Raine CS, Baum SG. Temperature-sensitive mutants of reovirus type 3: defects in viral maturation as studied by immunofluorescence and electron microscopy. Virology 1971;43:569–578.

61. Finberg R, Spriggs DR, Fields BN. Host immune response to reovirus: CTL recognize the major neutralization domain of the viral hemagglutinin. J Immunol 1982;129:2235–2238.

62. Finberg R, Weiner HL, Fields BN, Benacerraf B, Burakoff SJ. Generation of cytolytic T lymphocytes after reovirus infection: Role of S1 gene. Proc Natl Acad Sci U S A 1979;76:442–446.

63. Flammand A, Gagner J-P, Morrison LA, Fields BN. Penetration of the nervous systems of suckling mice by mammalian reoviruses. J Virol 1991;65:123–131.

64. Fraser RD, Furlong DB, Trus BL, Nibert ML, Fields BN, Steven AC. Molecular structure of the cell˜2Dattachment protein of reovirus: correlation of computer-processed electron micrographs with sequence-based predictions. J Virol 1990;64:2990–3000.

65. Furlong DB, Nibert ML, Fields BN. Sigma 1 protein of mammalian reoviruses extends from the surfaces of viral particles. J Virol 1988;62:246–256.

66. Gaillard RK, Joklik WK. The antigenic determinants of most of the proteins coded by the three serotypes of reovirus are highly conserved during evolution. Virology 1980;107:533–536.

67. Gaulton GN, Greene MI. Inhibition of cellular DNA synthesis by reovirus occurs through a receptor-linked signaling pathway that is mimicked by antiidiotypic, antireceptor antibody. J Exp Med 1989;169:197–211.

68. Gaulton GN, Sharpe AH, Chang DW, Fields BN, Greene MI. Syngeneic monoclonal internal image anti-idiotopes as prophylactic vaccines. J Immunol 1986;137:2930–2936.

69. Gentsch JR, Pacitti AF. Effect of neuraminidase treatment of cells and effect of soluble glycoproteins on type 3 reovirus attachment to murine L cells. J Virol 1985;56:356–364.

70. Gentsch JR, Pacitti AF. Differential interaction of reovirus type 3 with sialylated receptor components on animal cells. Virology 1987;161:245–248.

71. George A, Kost SI, Witzleben CL, Cebra JJ, Rubin DH. Reovirus-induced liver disease in severe combined immunodeficient (SCID) mice: a model for the study of viral infection, pathogenesis, and clearance. J Exp Med 1990;171:929–934.

72. Gomatos PJ, Tamm I, Dales S, Franklin RM. Reovirus type 3: physical characteristics and interactions with L cells. Virology 1962;17:441–454.

73. Gombold JL, Ramig RF. Passive immunity modulates genetic reassortment between rotaviruses in mixedly infected mice. J Virol 1989;63:4525–4532.

74. Goral MI, Grundy MM, Dermody TS. Sequence diversity within the reovirus S3 gene: reoviruses evolve independently of host species, geographic locale, and date of isolation. Virology 1996;216:265–271.

75. Haller BL, Barkon ML, Li X, et al. Brain and intestine-specific variants of reovirus serotype 3 strain Dearing are selected during chronic infection of severe combined immunodeficient mice. J Virol 1995;69:3933–3937.

76. Haller BL, Barkon ML, Vogler G, Virgin HW. Genetic mapping of reovirus virulence and organ tropism in severe combined immunodeficient mice: organ specific virulence genes. J Virol 1995;69:357–364.

77. Haspel MV, Onodera T, Prabhakar BS, Horita M, Suzuki H, Notkins AL. Virus-induced autoimmunity: monoclonal antibodies that react with endocrine tissues. Science 1983;220:304–306.

78. Hayes EC, Lee PW, Miller SE, Joklik WK. The interaction of a series of hybridoma IgGs with reovirus particles: demonstration that the core protein lambda 2 is exposed on the particle surface. Virology 1981;108:147–155.

79. Henderson DR, Joklik WK. The mechanism of interferon induction by UV-irradiated reovirus. Virology 1978;91:389–406.

80. Hogan KT, Cashdollar LW. Clonal analysis of the cytotoxic T-lymphocyte response to reovirus. Viral Immunol 1991;4:167–175.

81. Hooper JW, Fields BN. Monoclonal antibodies to reovirus sigma-1 and mu-1 proteins inhibit chromium release from mouse L cells. J Virol 1996;70:672–677.

82. Hooper JW, Fields BN. Role of the reovirus mu-1 protein in virion stability and chromium release from host cells. J Virol 1996;70:459–467.

83. Hrdy DB, Rosen L, Fields BN. Polymorphism of the migration of double-stranded RNA segments of reovirus isolates from humans, cattle, and mice. J Virol 1979;31:104–111.

84. Hrdy DB, Rubin DH, Fields BN. Molecular basis of reovirus virulence: role of the M2 gene in avirulence. Proc Natl Acad Sci U S A 1982;79:1298–1302.

85. Huismans H, Joklik WK. Reovirus-coded polypeptides in infected cells: isolation of two native monomeric polypeptides with high affinity for single-stranded and double-stranded RNA, respectively. Virology 1976;70:411–424.

86. Imani F, Jacobs BL. Inhibitory activity for the interferon-induced protein kinase is associated with the reovirus serotype 1 sigma 3 protein. Proc Natl Acad Sci U S A 1988;85:7887–7891.

87. Ito Y, Joklik WK. Temperature-sensitive mutants of reovirus. I. Patterns of gene expression by mutants of groups C, D, and E. Virology 1972;50:189–201.

88. Jacobs BL, Ferguson RE. The Lang strain of reovirus serotype 1 and the Dearing strain of reovirus serotype 3 differ in their sensitivities to beta interferon. J Virol 1991;65:5102–5104.

89. Jacobs BL, Samuel CE. Biosynthesis of reovirus-specified polypeptides: the reovirus s1 mRNA encodes two primary translation products. Virology 1985;143:63–74.

90. Joklik WK. The reovirus particle. In: Joklik WK, ed. The reoviridae. New York: Plenum Press, 1983:9–78.

91. Kauffman RS, Ahmed R, Fields BN. Selection of a mutant S1 gene during reovirus persistent infection of L cells: role in maintenance of the persistent state. Virology 1983;131:79–87.

92. Kauffman RS, Wolf JL, Finberg R, Trier JS, Fields BN. The sigma 1 protein determines the extent of spread of reovirus from the gastrointestinal tract of mice. Virology 1991;124:403–410.

93. Kaye KM, Spriggs DR, Bassel Duby R, Fields BN, Tyler KL. Genetic basis for altered pathogenesis of an immune selected antigenic variant of reovirus type 3 (Dearing). J Virol 1986;59:90–97.

94. Kedl R, Schmechel S, Schiff L. Comparative sequence analysis of the reovirus S4 genes from 13 serotype 1 and serotype 3 field isolates. J Virol 1995;69:552–559.

95. Keroack M, Fields BN. Viral shedding and transmission between hosts determined by reovirus L2 gene. Science 1986;232:1635–1638.

96. Kilham L, Margolis G. Hydrocephalus in hamsters, ferrets, rats and mice following inoculations with reovirus type 1. Lab Invest 1969; 21:183–188.

97. Kitamura D, Roes J, Kuhn R, Rajewsky K. A B cell-deficient mouse by targeted disruption of the membrane exon of the immunoglobulin mu chain gene. Nature 1991;350:423–426.

98. Koller BH, Marrack P, Kappler JW, Smithies O. Normal development of mice deficient in beta 2M, MHC class I proteins, and CD8+ T cells. Science 1990;248:1227–1230.

99. Kudo H, Graham AF. Selective inhibition of reovirus induced RNA in L cells. Biochim Biophys Acta 1966;24:150–155.

100. Lai M-HT, Joklik WK. The induction of interferon by temperature-sensitive mutants of reovirus, UV-irradiated reovirus, and subviral reovirus particles. Virology 1973;51:191–204.

101. Lee PW, Hayes EC, Joklik WK. Protein sigma 1 is the reovirus cell attachment protein. Virology 1981;108:156–163.

102. Lee PW, Hayes EC, Joklik WK. Characterization of anti˜2Dreovirus immunoglobulins secreted by cloned hybridoma cell lines. Virology 1981;108:134–146.

103. Leone G, Duncan R, Lee PW. Trimerization of the reovirus cell attachment protein (sigma 1) induces conformational changes in sigma 1 necessary for its cell-binding function. Virology 1991;184: 758–761.

104. Leone G, Duncan R, Mah DC, Price A, Cashdollar LW, Lee PW. The N-terminal heptad repeat region of reovirus cell attachment protein sigma 1 is responsible for sigma 1 oligomer stability and possesses intrinsic oligomerization function. Virology 1991;182:336–345.

105. Leone G, Mah DC, Lee PW. The incorporation of reovirus cell attachment protein sigma 1 into virions requires the N-terminal hydrophobic tail and the adjacent heptad repeat region. Virology 1991; 182:346–350.

106. Leone G, Maybaum L, Lee PWK. The reovirus cell attachment protein possesses two independently active trimerization domains: basis of dominant negative effects. Cell 1992;71:479–488.

107. Levy JA, Henle G, Henle W, Zajac BA. Effect of reovirus type 3 on cultured Burkitt's tumour cells. Nature 1968;220:607–608.

108. Li JK-K, Keene JD, Scheible PP, Joklik WK. Nature of the 3'-terminal sequence of the plus and minus strands of the S1 gene of reovirus serotypes 1, 2, and 3. Virology 1980;105:41–51.

109. Liu J, Co MS, Greene MI. Reovirus type 3 and [125I]-iodocyanopindolol bind to distinct domains on the beta-adrenergic like receptor. Immunol Res 1988;7:232–238.

110. Lloyd RM, Shatkin AJ. Translational stimulation by reovirus polypeptide sigma 3: substitution for VAI-RNA and inhibition of phosphorylation of the alpha-subunit of eukaryotic initiation factor-II. J Virol 1992;66:6878–6884.

111. London SD, Cebra JJ, Rubin DH. Intraepithelial lymphocytes contain virus-specific, MHC-restricted cytotoxic cell precursors after gut mucosal immunization with reovirus serotype 1/Lang. Reg Immunol 1989;2:98–102.

112. London SD, Cebra JJ, Rubin DH. The reovirus-specific cytotoxic T cell response is not restricted to serotypically unique epitopes associated with the virus hemagglutinin. Microb Pathog 1989;6:43–50.

113. London SD, Cebra-Thomas JA, Rubin DH, Cebra JJ. CD8 lymphocyte subpopulations in Peyer's patches induced by reovirus serotype 1 infection. J Immunol 1990;144:3187–3194.

114. London SD, Rubin DH, Cebra JJ. Gut mucosal immunization with reovirus serotype 1/L stimulates virus-specific cytotoxic T cell precursors as well as IgA memory cells in Peyer's patches. J Exp Med 1987;165:830–847.

115. Long WF, Burke DC. Interferon production by double-stranded RNA: a comparison of interferon induction by reovirus RNA to that by a synthetic double-stranded polynucleotide. J Gen Virol 1971; 12:1–11.

116. Lucia-Jandris P, Hooper JW, Fields BN. Reovirus M2 gene is associated with chromium release from mouse L cells. J Virol 1993;67: 5339–5345.

117. Mah DC, Leone G, Jankowski JM, Lee PW. The N-terminal quarter of reovirus cell attachment protein sigma 1 possesses intrinsic virion-anchoring function. Virology 1990;179:95–103.

118. Mao ZX, Joklik WK. Isolation and enzymatic characterization of protein lambda 2, the reovirus guanylyltransferase. Virology 1991; 185:377–386.

119. Maratos Flier E, Goodman MJ, Murray AH, Kahn CR. Ammonium inhibits processing and cytotoxicity of reovirus, a nonenveloped virus. J Clin Invest 1986;78:1003–1007.

120. Margolis G, Kilham L. Hydrocephalus in hamsters, ferrets, rats and mice following inoculations with reovirus type 1. Lab Invest 1969; 21:189–198.

121. Margolis G, Kilham L, Gonatas NK. Reovirus type III encephalitis: observations of virus-cell interactions in neural tissues. I. Light microscopy studies. Lab Invest 1971;24:91–109.

122. Matoba Y, Sherry B, Fields BN, Smith TW. Identification of the viral genes responsible for growth of strains of reovirus in cultured mouse heart cells. J Clin Invest 1991;87:1628–1633.

123. Matsuzaki N, Hinshaw VS, Fields BN, Greene MI. Cell receptors for the mammalian reovirus: reovirus specific T-cell hybridomas

can become persistently infected and undergo autoimmune stimulation. J Virol 1986;60:259–266.

124. McPhillips TH, Ramig RF. Extragenic suppression of temperature-sensitive phenotype in reovirus: mapping suppressor mutations. Virology 1984;135:428–439.

125. Montgomery LB, Kao CY, Verdin E, Cahill C, Maratos Flier E. Infection of a polarized epithelial cell line with wild-type reovirus leads to virus persistence and altered cellular function. J Gen Virol 1991;72:2939–2946.

126. Moody MD, Joklik WK. The function of reovirus proteins during the reovirus multiplication cycle: analysis using monoreassortants. Virology 1989;173:437–446.

127. Morgan EM, Zweerink HJ. Characterization of transcriptase and replicase particles isolated from reovirus infected cells. Virology 1975;68:455–466.

128. Morin MJ, Warner A, Fields BN. A pathway of entry of reoviruses into the host through M cells of the respiratory tract. J Exp Med 1994;180:1523–1527.

129. Morrison LA, Fields BN. Parallel mechanisms in neuropathogenesis of enteric virus infections. J Virol 1991;65:2767–2772.

130. Morrison LA, Fields BN, Dermody TS. Prolonged replication in the mouse central nervous system of reoviruses isolated from persistently infected cell cultures. J Virol 1993;67:3019–3026.

131. Morrison LA, Sidman RL, Fields BN. Direct spread of reovirus from the intestinal lumen to the central nervous system through vagal autonomic nerve fibers. Proc Natl Acad Sci U S A 1991;88:3852–3856.

132. Munemitsu SM, Samuel CE. Biosynthesis of reovirus-specified polypeptides: multiplication rate but not yield of reoviruses serotype 1 and serotype 3 correlates with the level of virus mediated inhibition of cellular protein synthesis. Virology 1984;136:133–143.

133. Nagata L, Masri SA, Pon RT, Lee PW. Analysis of functional domains on reovirus cell attachment protein sigma 1 using cloned S1 gene deletion mutants. Virology 1987;160:162–168.

134. Nibert ML, Chappell JD, Dermody TS. Infectious subvirion particles of reovirus type 3 Dearing exhibit a loss in infectivity and contain a cleaved sigma-1 protein. J Virol 1995;69:5057–5067.

135. Nibert ML, Dermody TS, Fields BN. Structure of the reovirus cell-attachment protein: a model for the domain organization of sigma 1. J Virol 1990;64:2976–2989.

136. Nibert ML, Fields BN. A carboxy-terminal fragment of protein mu1/mu1C is present in infectious subvirion particles of mammalian reoviruses and is proposed to have a role in penetration. J Virol 1992;66:6408–6418.

137. Nibert ML, Fields BN. Early steps in reovirus infection of cells. In: Wimmer E, ed. Cellular receptors for animal viruses. Cold Spring Harbor, NY: Cold Spring Harbor Laboratory Press, 1994:341–364.

138. Nibert ML, Furlong DB, Fields BN. Mechanisms of viral pathogenesis: distinct forms of reoviruses and their roles during replication in cells and host. J Clin Invest 1991;88:727–734.

139. Nibert ML, Schiff LA, Fields BN. Reoviruses and their replication. In: Fields BN, Knipe DM, Howley PM, eds. Fields virology. 3rd ed. Philadelphia: Lippincott-Raven, 1996:1557–1596.

140. Nilsen TW, Maroney PA, Baglioni C. Inhibition of protein synthesis in reovirus-infected HeLa cells with elevated levels of interferon-induced protein kinase activity. J Biol Chem 1982;257:14593–14596.

141. Noseworthy JH, Fields BN, Dichter MA, et al. Cell receptors for the mammalian reovirus. I. Syngeneic monoclonal anti-idiotype antibody identifies a cell surface receptor for reovirus. J Immunol 1983;131:2533–2538.

142. Onodera T, Awaya A. Anti-thyroglobulin antibodies induced with recombinant reovirus infection in BALB/c mice. Immunology 1990;71:581–585.

143. Onodera T, Jenson AB, Yoon J-Y, Notkins AL. Virus-induced diabetes mellitus: reovirus infection of pancreatic beta cells in mice. Science 1978;201:529–531.

144. Onodera T, Toniolo A, Ray UR, Jenson AB, Knazek RA, Notkins AL. Virus-induced diabetes mellitus. XX. Polyendocrinopathy and autoimmunity. J Exp Med 1981;153:1457–1473.

145. Pacitti AF, Gentsch JR. Inhibition of reovirus type 3 binding to host cells by sialylated glycoproteins is mediated through the viral attachment protein. J Virol 1987;61:1407–1415.

146. Paul RW, Choi AH, Lee PW. The alpha-anomeric form of sialic acid is the minimal receptor determinant recognized by reovirus. Virology 1989;172:382–385.

147. Paul RW, Lee PW. Glycophorin is the reovirus receptor on human erythrocytes. Virology 1987;159:94–101.

148. Phillips PA, Alpers MP, Stanley NF. Hydrocephalus in mice inoculated neonatally by the oronasal route with reovirus type 1. Science 1970;168:858–859.

149. Piccoli DA, Witzleben CL, Guico CJ, Morrison A, Rubin DH. Synergism between hepatic injuries and a nonhepatotropic reovirus in mice: enhanced hepatic infection and death. J Clin Invest 1990;86:1038–1045.

150. Ramig RF, Fields BN. Revertants of temperature-sensitive mutants of reovirus: evidence for frequent extragenic suppression. Virology 1979;92:155–167.

151. Ramig RF, Ward RL. Genomic segment reassortment in rotaviruses and other reoviridae. Adv Virus Res 1991;39:163–207.

152. Rhim JS, Jordan LE, Mayor HD. Cytochemical, fluorescent-antibody, and electron microscopic studies in the growth of reovirus (ECHO 10) in tissue culture. Virology 1962;17:342–355.

153. Roner MR, Cox DC. Cellular integrity is required for inhibition of initiation of cellular DNA synthesis by reovirus type 3. J Virol 1985;53:350–359.

154. Roner MR, Roner LA, Joklik WK. Translation of reovirus RNA species m1 can initiate at either of the first two in frame codons. Proc Natl Acad Sci U S A 1993;90:8947–8951.

155. Roner MR, Sutphin LA, Joklik WK. Reovirus RNA is infectious. Virology 1990;179:845–852.

156. Rosen L. Serologic groupings of reovirus by hemagglutination inhibition. American Journal of Hygiene 1960;71:242–249.

157. Rosen L, Hovis JF, Mastrota FM, Bell JA, Huebner RJ. Observations on a newly recognized virus (Abney) of the reovirus family. American Journal of Hygiene 1960;71:258–265.

158. Rubin DH. Reovirus serotype 1 binds to the basolateral membrane of intestinal epithelial cells. Microb Pathog 1987;3:215–219.

159. Rubin DH, Costello T, Witzleben CL, Greene MI. Transport of infectious reovirus into bile: class II major histocompatibility antigen-bearing cells determine reovirus transport. J Virol 1987;61:3222–3226.

160. Rubin DH, Eaton MA, Anderson AO. Reovirus infection in adult mice: the virus hemagglutinin determines the site of intestinal disease. Microb Pathog 1986;1:79–87.

161. Rubin DH, Eaton MA, Costello T. Reovirus type 1 is secreted into the bile. J Virol 1986;60:726–728.

162. Rubin DH, Kornstein MJ, Anderson AO. Reovirus serotype 1 intestinal infection: a novel replicative cycle with ileal disease. J Virol 1985;53:391–398.

163. Rubin DH, Morrison AH, Witzleben CL, Guico CJ, Piccoli DA. Site of reovirus replication in liver is determined by the type of hepatocellular insult. J Virol 1990;64:4593–4597.

164. Rubin DH, Wetzel JD, Williams WV, Cohen JA, Dworkin C, Dermody TS. Binding of type 3 reovirus by a domain of the sigma 1 protein important for hemagglutination leads to infection of murine erythroleukemia cells. J Clin Invest 1992;90:2536–2542.

165. Sabin AB. Reoviruses. Science 1959;130:1387–1389.

166. Samuel CE, Duncan R, Knutson GS, Hershey JWB. Mechanism of interferon action: increased phosphorylation of protein synthesis initiation factor eIF-2 alpha in interferon-treated reovirus-infected mouse L-929 fibroblasts in vivo and in vitro. J Biol Chem 1984;259:13451–13457.

167. Saragovi HU, Fitzpatrick D, Raktabutr A, Nakanishi H, Kahn M, Greene MI. Design and synthesis of a mimetic from an antibody complementarity-determining region. Science 1991;253:792–795.

168. Sarkar G, Pelletier J, Bassel Duby R, Jayasuriya A, Fields BN, Sonenberg N. Identification of a new polypeptide coded by reovirus gene S1. J Virol 1985;54:720–725.

169. Sawutz DG, Bassel Duby R, Homcy CJ. High affinity binding of reovirus type 3 to cells that lack beta adrenergic receptor activity. Life Sci 1987;40:399–406.

170. Schiff LA, Nibert ML, Co MS, Brown EG, Fields BN. Distinct binding sites for zinc and double-stranded RNA in the reovirus outer capsid protein sigma 3. Mol Cell Biol 1988;8:273–283.

171. Seliger LS, Giantini M, Shatkin AJ. Translational effects and sequence comparisons of the three serotypes of the reovirus S4 gene. Virology 1992;187:202–210.

172. Sharpe AH, Chen LB, Fields BN. The interaction of mammalian reoviruses with the cytoskeleton of monkey kidney CV-1 cells. Virology 1982;120:399–411.

173. Sharpe AH, Fields BN. Reovirus inhibition of cellular DNA synthesis: role of the S1 gene. J Virol 1981;38:389–392.

174. Sharpe AH, Fields BN. Reovirus inhibition of cellular RNA and protein synthesis: role of the S4 gene. Virology 1982;122:381–391.

175. Sharpe AH, Fields BN. Pathogenesis of reovirus infection. In: Joklik WK, ed. The reoviridae. New York: Plenum Press, 1983:229–285.

176. Sharpe AH, Fields BN. Pathogenesis of viral infections: basic concepts derived from the reovirus model. N Engl J Med 1985; 312:486–497.

177. Sharpe AH, Gaulton GN, McDade KK, Fields BN, Greene MI. Syngeneic monoclonal antiidiotype can induce cellular immunity to reovirus. J Exp Med 1984;160:1195–1205.

178. Sherry B, Bloom MA. Multiple viral core proteins are determinants of reovirus-induced acute myocarditis. J Virol 1994;68:8461–8465.

179. Sherry B, Fields BN. The reovirus M1 gene, encoding a viral core protein, is associated with the myocarditic phenotype of a reovirus variant. J Virol 1989;63:4850–4856.

180. Sherry B, Li X-Y, Tyler KL, Cullen JM, Virgin HW. Lymphocytes protect against and are not required for reovirus induced myocarditis. J Virol 1993;67:6119–6124.

181. Sherry B, Schoen FJ, Wenske E, Fields BN. Derivation and characterization of an efficiently myocarditic reovirus variant. J Virol 1989;63:4840–4849.

182. Silverstein SC, Astell C, Levin DH, Schonberg M, Acs G. The mechanism of reovirus uncoating and gene activation in vivo. Virology 1972;47:797–806.

183. Silverstein SC, Dales S. The penetration of reovirus RNA and initiation of its genetic function in L-strain fibroblasts. J Cell Biol 1968;36:197–230.

184. Silverstein SC, Schur PH. Immunofluorescent localization of double-stranded RNA in reovirus-infected cells. Virology 1970;41:564–566.

185. Skehel JJ, Joklik WK. Studies on the in vitro transcription of reovirus RNA catalyzed by reovirus cores. Virology 1969;39:822–831.

186. Skup D, Millward S. mRNA capping enzymes are masked in reovirus progeny subviral particles. J Virol 1980;34:490–496.

187. Spendlove RS, Lennette EH, Chin JN, Knight CO. Effect of anti-mitotic agents on intracellular reovirus antigen. Cancer Res 1964;24:1826–1833.

188. Spendlove RS, Lennette EH, Knight CO, Chin JH. Development of viral antigens and infectious virus on HELA cells infected with reovirus. J Immunol 1963;90:548–553.

189. Spendlove RS, McClain ME, Lennette EH. Enhancement of reovirus infectivity by extracellular removal or alteration of the virus capsid by proteolytic enzymes. J Gen Virol 1970;8:83–93.

190. Spriggs DR, Bronson RT, Fields BN. Hemagglutinin variants of reovirus type 3 have altered central nervous system tropism. Science 1983;220:505–507.

191. Spriggs DR, Fields BN. Attenuated reovirus type 3 strains generated by selection of hemagglutinin antigenic variants. Nature 1982; 297:68–70.

192. Starncs MC, Joklik WK. Reovirus protein lambda 3 is a poly(C)-dependent poly(G) polymerase. Virology 1993;193:356–366.

193. Strong JE, Leone G, Duncan R, Sharma RK, Lee PW. Biochemical and biophysical characterization of the reovirus cell attachment protein sigma 1: evidence that it is a homotrimer. Virology 1991;184:23–32.

194. Strong JE, Tang D, Lee PW. Evidence that the epidermal growth factor receptor on host cells confers reovirus infection efficiency. Virology 1993;197:405–411.

195. Sturzenbecker LJ, Nibert M, Furlong D, Fields BN. Intracellular digestion of reovirus particles requires a low pH and is an essential step in the viral infectious cycle. J Virol 1987;61:2351–2361.

196. Taber R, Alexander V, Whitford W. Persistent reovirus infection of CHO cells resulting in virus resistance. Virology 1976;17:513–524.

197. Tang D, Strong JE, Lee PW. Recognition of the epidermal growth factor receptor by reovirus. Virology 1993;197:412–414.

198. Tardieu M, Powers ML, Weiner HL. Age dependent susceptibility to reovirus type 3 encephalitis: role of host and viral factors. Ann Neurol 1983;13:602–607.

199. Tardieu M, Weiner HL. Viral receptors on isolated murine and human ependymal cells. Science 1982;215:419–421.

200. Taterka J, Sutcliffe M, Rubin DH. Selective reovirus infection of murine hepatocarcinoma cells during cell division: a model of viral liver infection. J Clin Invest 1994;94:353–360.

201. Tillotson L, Shatkin AJ. Reovirus polypeptide sigma 3 and N-terminal myristoylation of polypeptide mu 1 are required for site-specific cleavage to mu 1C in transfected cells. J Virol 1992;66:2180–2186.

202. Tosteson MT, Nibert ML, Fields BN. Ion channels induced in lipid bilayers by subvirion particles of the nonenveloped mammalian reoviruses. Proc Natl Acad Sci U S A 1993;90:10549–10552.

203. Turner DL, Duncan R, Lee PW. Site-directed mutagenesis of the C-terminal portion of reovirus protein sigma 1: evidence for a conformation-dependent receptor binding domain. Virology 1992;186:219–227.

204. Tyler KL, Bronson RT, Byers KB, Fields BN. Molecular basis of viral neurotropism: experimental reovirus infection. Neurol. 1985;35:88–92.

205. Tyler KL, Fields BN. Reoviruses. In: Fields BN, Knipe DM, Howley PM, eds. Fields virology. 3rd ed. Philadelphia: Lippincott-Raven, 1996:1597–1623.

206. Tyler KL, Mann MA, Fields BN, Virgin HW. Protective anti-reovirus monoclonal antibodies and their effects on viral pathogenesis. J Virol 1993;67:3446–3453.

207. Tyler KL, McPhee DA, Fields BN. Distinct pathways of viral spread in the host determined by reovirus S1 gene segment. Science 1986;233:770–774.

208. Tyler KL, Squier MKT, Rogers SE, et al. Differences in the capacity of reoviruses to induce apoptosis are determined by viral attachment protein sigma-1. J Virol 1995;69:6972–6979.

209. Tyler KL, Virgin HW, Bassel Duby R, Fields BN. Antibody inhibits defined stages in the pathogenesis of reovirus serotype 3 infection of the central nervous system. J Exp Med 1989;170:887–900.

210. Verdin EM, King GL, Maratos-Flier E. Characterization of a common high-affinity receptor for reovirus serotypes 1 and 3 on endothelial cells. J Virol 1989;63:1318–1325.

211. Verdin EM, Lynn SP, Fields BN, Maratos Flier E. Uptake of reovirus serotype 1 by the lungs from the bloodstream is mediated by the viral hemagglutinin. J Virol 1988;62:545–551.

212. Verdin EM, Maratos Flier E, Carpentier JL, Kahn CR. Persistent infection with a nontransforming RNA virus leads to impaired growth factor receptors and response. J Cell Physiol 1986;128:457–465.

213. Verdin EM, Maratos Flier E, Kahn CR, et al. Visualization of viral clearance in the living animal. Science 1987;236:439–442.

214. Virgin HW, Bassel Duby R, Fields BN, Tyler KL. Antibody protects against lethal infection with the neurally spreading reovirus type 3 (Dearing). J Virol 1988;62:4594–4604.

215. Virgin HW, Mann MA, Fields BN, Tyler KL. Monoclonal antibodies to reovirus reveal structure/function relationships between capsid proteins and genetics of susceptibility to antibody action. J Virol 1991;65:6772–6781.

216. Virgin HW, Mann MA, Tyler KL. Protective antibodies inhibit reovirus internalization and uncoating by intracellular proteases. J Virol 1994;68:6719–6729.

217. Virgin HW, Tyler KL. The role of immune cells in protection against and control of reovirus infection in neonatal mice. J Virol 1991; 65:5157–5164.

218. Walters MN, Leak PJ, Joske R, Stanley NF, Perret D. Murine infection with reovirus. III. Pathology of infection with types I and II. Br J Exp Pathol 1965;46:200–212.

219. Weiner DB, Girard K, Williams WV, McPhillips T, Rubin DH. Reovirus type 1 and type 3 differ in their binding to isolated intestinal epithelial cells. Microb Pathog 1988;5:29–40.

220. Weiner HL, Ault KA, Fields BN. Interaction of reovirus with cell surface receptors. I. Murine and human lymphocytes have a receptor for the hemagglutinin of reovirus type 3. J Immunol 1980;124:2143–2148.

221. Weiner HL, Drayna D, Averill DR, Fields BN. Molecular basis of reovirus virulence: role of the S1 gene. Proc Natl Acad Sci U S A 1977;74:5744–5748.

222. Weiner HL, Fields BN. Neutralization of reovirus: the gene responsible for the neutralization antigen. J Exp Med 1977;146:1305–1310.

223. Weiner HL, Greene MI, Fields BN. Delayed hypersensitivity in mice infected with reovirus. I. Identification of host and viral gene products responsible for the immune response. J Immunol 1980; 125:278–282.

224. Weiner HL, Powers ML, Fields BN. Absolute linkage of virulence and central nervous system cell tropism of reoviruses to viral hemagglutinin. J Infect Dis 1980;141:609–616.

225. Weiner HL, Ramig RF, Mustoe TA, Fields BN. Identification of the gene coding for the hemagglutinin of reovirus. Virology 1978; 86:581–584.

226. Weiner JR, Bartlett JA, Joklik WK. The sequences of reovirus serotype 3 genome segments M1 and M3 encoding the minor protein mu 2 and the major non-structural protein muNS, respectively. Virology 1989;169:293–304.

227. Wenske EA, Chanock SJ, Krata L, Fields BN. Genetic reassortment of mammalian reoviruses in mice. J Virol 1985;56:613–616.

228. Wessner DR, Fields BN. Isolation and characterization of ethanol-resistant reovirus mutants. J Virol 1993;67:2442–2447.

229. White CK, Zweerink HJ. Studies on the structure of reovirus cores: selective removal of polypeptide lambda-2. Virology 1976;70: 171–180.

230. Wiebe ME, Joklik WK. The mechanism of inhibition of reovirus replication by interferon. Virology 1975;66:229–240.

231. Williams WV, Guy HR, Rubin DH, et al. Sequences of the cell-attachment sites of reovirus type 3 and its anti-idiotypic/antireceptor antibody: modeling of their three-dimensional structures. Proc Natl Acad Sci U S A 1988;85:6488–6492.

232. Williams WV, Kieber Emmons T, Weiner DB, Rubin DH, Greene MI. Contact residues and predicted structure of the reovirus type 3-receptor interaction. J Biol. Chem. 1991;266:9241–9250.

233. Williams WV, London SD, Weiner DB, et al. Immune response to a molecularly defined internal image idiotype. J Immunol 1989; 142:4392–4400.

234. Wilson GAR, Morrison LA, Fields BN. Association of the reovirus S1 gene with serotype 3-induced biliary atresia in mice. J Virol 1994;68:6458–6465.

235. Wolf JL, Dambrauskas R, Sharpe AH, Trier JS. Adherence to and penetration of the intestinal epithelium by reovirus type 1 in neonatal mice. Gastroenterology 1987;92:82–91.

236. Wolf JL, Kaufmann RS, Finberg R, Dambrauskas R, Fields BN, Trier J. Determinants of reovirus interaction with intestinal M cells and absorptive cells of murine intestine. Gastroenterology 1983; 85:291–300.

237. Wolf JL, Rubin DH, Finberg R, et al. Intestinal M cells: A pathway for entry of reovirus into the host. Science 1981;212:471–472.

238. Yeung MC, Lim D, Duncan R, Shahrabadi MS, Cashdollar LW, Lee PW. The cell attachment proteins of type 1 and type 3 reovirus are differentially susceptible to trypsin and chymotrypsin. Virology 1989;170:62–70.

239. Zarbl H, Skup D, Millward S. Reovirus progeny subviral particles synthesize uncapped mRNA. J Virol 1980;34:497–505.

240. Zou S, Brown EG. Identification of sequence elements containing signals for replication and encapsidation of the reovirus M1 genome segment. Virology 1992;186:377–388.

241. Zou S, Brown EG. Nucleotide sequence comparison of the M1 genome segment of reovirus type 1 Lang and type 3 Dearing. Virus Res 1992;22:159–164.

242. Zweerink HJ, Ito Y, Matsuhisa T. Synthesis of reovirus double-stranded RNA within virion-like particles. Virology 1972;50:349–358.

PART IV

Systems Pathogenesis

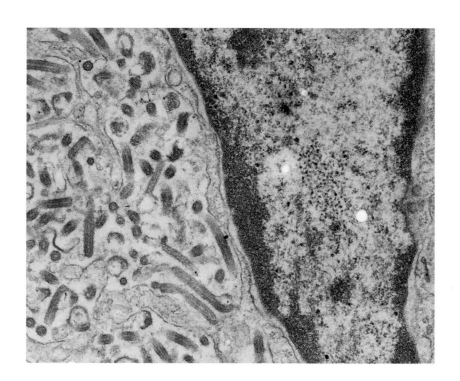

Viral Pathogenesis,
edited by Neal Nathanson, et al.
Lippincott–Raven Publishers, Philadelphia © 1997

CHAPTER **29**

Respiratory Diseases

Peter F. Wright

INTRODUCTION

The respiratory tract shares with the gastrointestinal tract a substantial burden of exposure to viruses and resultant viral disease. There are a unique set of virus-cell interactions that initiate and sustain viral infection and that impose on these mucosal surfaces the need to create unique sets of host defense mechanisms. In the respiratory tract, the defense mechanisms can be classified as anatomic, nonspecific inhibitory, and viral-specific inhibitory or protective.[38,39] Likewise, in an evolutionary dance in which the virus is the more nimble partner, there are a series of adaptations that viruses have made to the respiratory tract. This chapter addresses respiratory tract structure and nonspecific defense mechanisms, patterns of viral replication, and the specific immune responses at this primary site of viral-host interaction.

IMPLICATIONS OF RESPIRATORY TRACT ANATOMY FOR VIRAL INFECTIONS

The nose has a convoluted set of bony turbinates which create air turbulence during the inspiratory-expiratory exchange of more than 12,000 L of air per day. The role of the nasophar-

ynx is to remove large particulate matter and to begin the warming and humidifying of inspired air.

The designation of the lower respiratory tract as the tracheobronchial tree is apt, because there are 8 to 24 successive branchings before the alveoli are reached. The arborization is largely completed by birth, but afterward the alveoli mature and the diameters of airways increase. The initial small size and increased resistance of the bronchioles may contribute to the unusual severity of respiratory disease in the first 6 months of life. The relative size of the airways also influences the initial distribution of viruses in their aerosolized form in the airway. After initial replication in the upper respiratory tract, a virus may spread from cell to cell or by inhalation to the lower tract.

A temperature differential exists from the nose (33°C) to the alveoli, which approach core body temperature. Rhinoviruses that replicate preferentially in the upper respiratory tract exhibit optimal growth at the cooler temperatures of the nasal epithelium. The temperature differential has been used as a rationale for the development of temperature-sensitive viruses as live attenuated respiratory viral vaccines for respiratory syncytial virus (RSV), parainfluenza type 3, and influenza. Such vaccines would have a safety factor conferred by limitation of growth in the warmer lower respiratory tract.

Mucosal Surface of the Respiratory Tract

The primary interaction of respiratory viruses and the host occurs at the epithelial surface. The vestibule of the nose is

　P. Wright: Departments of Pediatrics and Microbiology/Immunology, Vanderbilt University Medical Center, Nashville, Tennessee 37232.

lined by squamous epithelial cells, and the nasopharynx is lined by an epithelium that is composed of several cell types. Posteriorly, there is a narrow zone of transitional epithelium followed by a ciliated epithelium with numerous mucous goblet cells. Within the superior aspect of the nose is a specialized olfactory epithelium, which provides a direct connection between the central nervous system and the respiratory tract. The olfactory epithelium is a potential pathway for viral entry into the central nervous system.[52]

In response to viral infection, inflammation, or allergy, the nasal epithelium becomes swollen and edematous, with resultant obstruction. The pathophysiology of this event, particularly during viral infection, is not well understood. Nonetheless, the swelling is responsible for many of the symptoms of upper respiratory tract infection that contribute to bacterial superinfection in the contiguous sinuses and middle ear space.[15,22,25]

The other primary ostium for entry into the respiratory tract is the mouth. The oral mucosa is composed of a nonciliated stratified squamous epithelium that is less permissive than the nasopharyngeal mucosa for the replication of many of the classic respiratory viruses (e.g., rhinovirus).[8] However, primary herpes simplex type 1 is often localized to the gingiva, buccal cavity, and oropharynx. In addition, a number of viruses, including mumps and cytomegalovirus, replicate in the acinar tissue of the salivary glands. The primary secretion of the salivary glands, amylase, has not been implicated in viral pathogenesis.

The trachea and bronchi are lined by a pseudostratified epithelium with representation of six types of cells: ciliated, serous, goblet, brush, basal, and Clara cells. The last is a nonciliated secretory cell that, in the rat, has been implicated in the production of a protease that effectively cleaves the influenza hemagglutinin, a step in virus replication that is critical for productive viral infection.[29]

In the alveoli, there are two cells—alveolar type 1 cells with an attenuated cytoplasm, though which oxygen exchange occurs, and alveolar type II cells, granular cells with many mitochondria that are responsible for surfactant production and are the source of regenerating cells in the alveolus. Underlying all of the respiratory epithelium is a continuous basement membrane, which maintains a relatively tight lining to the respiratory tract.

Small numbers of circulating cells are also normally found within the airway. When bronchoalveolar lavage is performed in nonsmoking adults, approximately 15×10^6 cells can be recovered from the airway. They are 85% macrophages, 7% to 12% lymphocytes, 1% to 2% neutrophils, and 1% to 5% ciliated cells. The lymphocytes are 50% CD4+ helper-inducer phenotype, 30% CD8+ suppressor-cytotoxic phenotype, 7% natural killer cells, 5% to 10% B cells, and approximately 5% nontypeable.[47]

Interactions Between Virus and Epithelial Cells

The epithelial cell types discussed represent the relatively limited number of cell types in which initial virus replication in the respiratory tract presumably must occur. Very little is known about the initiation of virus replication in the epithelial cell and whether viruses are selective in their growth among these different cell types. Limited studies in human embryonic tracheal organ cultures suggest that RSV may grow exclusively in ciliated cells.[24] Growth of influenza, adenovirus, coronavirus 229E, and rhinovirus has been shown to occur in epithelial cells surrounding bits of epithelial tissue,[65] and influenza A in a human adenoid organ culture,[11] but these systems have not allowed definition of the specific cell types infected. Many viruses enter and are released from cells from either the apical or basolateral surface. As may be predicted, the mucosal viruses that have been examined exhibit apical preference.[61]

The mechanisms of virus destruction of individual epithelial cells probably vary by virus. The destruction of epithelium and loss of ciliary function contribute to secondary bacterial invasion, manifested as sinusitis, otitis, and pneumonia. It has been shown that vitamin A has a critical role in recovery of the integrity of the respiratory epithelium from injury.[7] The administration of exogenous vitamin A has a beneficial effect in children with severe measles.[27] Serum vitamin A levels drop acutely during RSV infection, and the lowest values are asso-

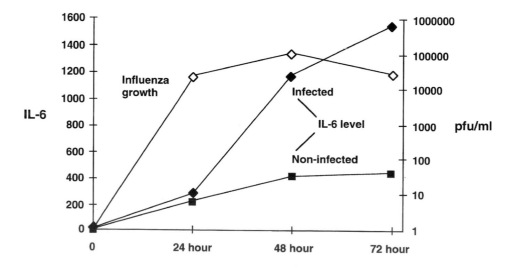

FIG. 29-1. Production of interleukin-6 (IL-6) by epithelial cells in tissue culture during influenza infection. PFU, plaque forming units. (Experiment of Yasuhiro Endo; unpublished results, 1994.)

ciated with the most severe disease.[37] Clinical trials of the possible benefit of vitamin A in RSV and other respiratory viral infections are underway.

In the process of infection of epithelial cells, viruses may induce cytokine production. These cytokines may be responsible for clinical symptoms and may play a role in the induction of the immune response.[46] Among the cytokines produced by epithelial cells interleukin-6 (IL-6) may be of particular significance, because its production is enhanced during influenza virus infection of epithelial cells in culture (Fig. 29-1) and it has been shown to have an important role in converting immunoglobulin A (IgA)–committed B cells to plasma cells.[32] Also, production of cytokines by virally infected epithelial cells may be the signal to initiate immune induction (see later discussion).

The cellular receptors for the respiratory viruses that are limited in their growth to the respiratory mucosa are either not known or appear to be ubiquitous; examples include sialic acid for influenza virus and the cell adhesion molecule, ICAM-1, as the major rhinovirus receptor. Virus receptor specificity does not account, by itself, for localization to the mucosal surface. As mentioned with respect to viral entry, there is good evidence that viruses can be polarized in their release from epithelial cells. Two respiratory viruses that have been studied, influenza and Sendai, bud only at the apical surface.[61] This facilitates cell-to-cell spread of virus and release into the luminal cavity of the respiratory tract. However, it poses the question of how antigen presentation occurs to the secretory and systemic immune systems with these superficially replicating viruses. Possible mechanisms include entry through specialized cells such as M cells, uptake by macrophages in the respiratory lumen, and sampling by dendritic cell populations in the epithelium.

PATTERNS OF VIRUS REPLICATION IN THE RESPIRATORY TRACT

Virtually all viral classes have adapted to growth in the respiratory tract (Table 29-1). The respiratory tract is a primary site of viral replication for a large number of viruses which then diverge into three pathogenetic pathways: (1) acute infection with replication confined to the respiratory mucosal surface, (2) persistent viral infection on the respiratory mucosa, and (3) initial replication on the respiratory mucosa followed by systemic spread.

Virus may reach the respiratory tract by several different routes, including nose-hand-nose transmission[21] and aerosol transmission. The average sneeze generates an aerosol consisting of particles from 100 to 2000 μm in diameter, which exits the nose with a velocity of 100 feet/second and travels an average of 2 to 5 feet. The average cough disperses material from the oropharynx and lower respiratory tract at a velocity of up to 850 feet/second. Routes of transmission vary for different viruses. For example, RSV is most efficiently spread by direct contact,[23] measles is effectively spread through aerosols,[28] and smallpox and varicella can spread via fomites through ventilation systems.[20] Presumably, relative temperature and humidity, as well as crowding and exposure, influence the poorly understood seasonality of many of the respiratory viruses.

TABLE 29-1. *Patterns of respiratory viral replication*

Pattern of infection	Viruses

Acute infection with replication confined to the respiratory mucosal surface	Paramyxoviruses
	  Parainfluenza 1, 2, 3
	  Respiratory syncytial virus
	Orthomyxoviruses
	  Influenza A, B, C
	Coronaviruses
	Picornaviruses
	  Rhinoviruses
	Herpesvirus
	  Herpes simplex

Persistent replication on the respiratory mucosal surface	Herpesviruses Epstein-Barr virus Adenoviruses Papillomavirus

Systemic replication after primary replication on the respiratory mucosal surface	Paramyxoviruses
	  Mumps
	  Measles
	Herpesviruses
	  Varicella
	  Human herpesvirus 6
	  Cytomegalovirus
	Togaviruses
	  Rubella
	Bunyaviruses
	Arenaviruses
	Parvovirus
	Picornavirus
	  Poliovirus
	Poxviruses
	Reovirus

Acute Infections With Replication Confined to the Respiratory Surface

Viruses with replication confined to the respiratory tract (see Table 29-1) typically replicate for 10 to 14 days during primary infection. Live, attenuated, intranasally administered viral vaccines can serve as a surrogate for understanding patterns of replication in the seronegative child. The timing of administration of virus and prior serologic status is known, and the vaccinees are monitored with daily sampling of their respiratory secretions for height of virus replication. A typical pattern of replication for parainfluenza type 3 virus is shown in Figure 29-2. This pattern is very stereotypic for the orthomyxoviruses and paramyxoviruses that have been studied. A better understanding of the events that terminate these viral infections is needed. In adults and seropositive children, both the duration and height of virus shedding are much more limited.

The onset of illness may be as early as 48 to 72 hours after the initiation of infection, as in the case with influenza. With other viruses such as RSV, there appears to be a biphasic illness, with early upper respiratory tract illness followed 4 to 7 days later by the onset of lower respiratory tract illness. This second phase of illness may be immune mediated, or it may represent the sequential spread of the viral infection to lower respiratory tract sites.

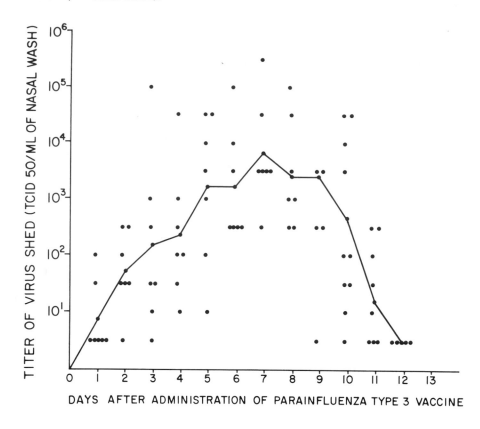

FIG. 29-2. Replication of a live attenuated parainfluenza type 3 virus in the upper respiratory tract. Volunteer human subjects were infected by administration of aerosolized virus. Nasal washes were collected at daily intervals. TCID50, median tissue culture infectious dose. (From Wright PF. Parainfluenza viruses. In: Belshe RB, ed. Textbook of human virology. St Louis: Mosby–Year Book, 1991:345.)

Persistent Infections

Some viruses have a more permanent symbiotic relation with the respiratory epithelium (see Table 29-1). The first virus recognized to behave in this manner was adenovirus.[50] The common childhood types of adenovirus (types 1, 2, and 5) can be recovered from adenoidal tissue in at least 50% of adenoids removed at surgery. Although acute adenovirus infection is associated with illness,[10] the persistent infection is asymptomatic. If adenoid epithelial cells are grown in tissue culture, the persistent adenovirus is expressed after 1 to 3 weeks, with a cytopathic effect that engulfs the cells in 24 to 48 hours. The consensus is that the virus is persisting in the lymphoid elements of the adenoids.[26] The appearance of adenovirus cytopathology in these cultures can be limited by exposure of the cells to immune globulin, suggesting that horizontal, extracellular transmission of virus maintains the persistent infection. Adenovirus has the capability to downregulate the expression of major histocompatibility complex (MHC) class I antigens on the cell surface, which may be a mechanism for allowing evasion of the immune system.[4] There is also a suggestion that the expression of the putative adenovirus receptor on lymphoid cells may vary and that, under some circumstances, adenovirus infection of lymphocytes may be blocked at the level of internalization, with capping of viruses on the lymphocyte surface.[55] The tropism of particular adenovirus strains for the respiratory tract, eye, urinary tract, or gastrointestinal tract is unexplained, as is the predominance of types 1, 2 and 5 in childhood respiratory disease and of types 4, 7, and 21 in acute respiratory disease among military personnel.

Epstein-Barr virus (EBV) also has the ability to establish a chronic infection in the respiratory tract. Using in situ hybridization, EBV DNA was detected in the oropharyngeal epithelial cell population during acute infection, consistent with its etiologic role in nasopharyngeal carcinoma.[56] A marker for these infections is the virus-specific IgA response. In one epithelial cell line, HT-29, polymeric IgA promotes entry of EBV into the otherwise refractory epithelial cells,[56] perhaps because of the ability of polymeric IgA to be transcytosed into epithelial cells by secretory component (see later discussion). These observations may explain why a virus, generally thought to be tropic for B lymphocytes, causes infection of epithelial cells.

Initial Infection Followed by Systemic Spread

A wide range of viruses normally considered in the context of systemic infection have the respiratory tract as their portal of entry and site of initial replication (see Table 29-1). Measles can serve as a model for such infections. After initial replication in the respiratory epithelium, measles virus is thought to spread to regional lymph nodes, after which a sustained viremia is produced.

NONSPECIFIC VIRAL DEFENSE MECHANISMS IN THE RESPIRATORY TRACT

Within the respiratory tract, there are a series of anatomic and nonspecific barriers through which a virus must pass to gain access to the epithelial cell. Filtration in the nose removes particles smaller than 0.5 μm and greater than 10 μm. An important clearance mechanism is provided by the mucociliary transport system, which carries secretions to the back of the throat, where they may be swallowed or expectorated. Mucus is released into the larger airways from discrete mucous-producing glands populated by goblet cells, which produce a mucus blanket that overlies the respiratory epithelium. Mucus itself is made up of complex mucopolysaccharides and forms a physical barrier to virus attachment and entry as well as a carpet on which the virus rides to the back of the nasopharynx and out of the lung, propelled by cilia beating 1000 to 1500 times per minute. In the course of an established viral infection, mucociliary transport and epithelial cell integrity are disrupted.[5] The mechanism of increase in mucus production, which is such a prominent part of respiratory viral infection, is not well explained, nor is its role as a potential host defense understood. However, coughing and sneezing, in addition to being means of transmission of viruses, are in themselves defense mechanisms for clearing secretions.[58]

A number of nonspecific soluble factors may influence viral attachment and growth in the respiratory tract. Proteases play a role in facilitating the growth of respiratory viruses, such as influenza, that depend on cleavage of their surface glycoproteins for replication. Deficiency in the protease inhibitor α_1-antitrypsin causes a chronic obstructive pulmonary disease, which may be a result of failure to inactivate a number of proteases intrinsic to the lung or secreted from the peripheral circulation. Sources of proteases in the respiratory tract include mast cells, neutrophils, and bacteria. *Staphylococcus aureus* strains produce a protease that cleaves the influenza hemagglutinin, enhancing the pathogenicity of influenza in mixed infection.[60]

Lysozyme and lactoferrin are soluble proteins that have antibacterial action but are not known to have antiviral effects. The soluble proteins recovered from the lung on bronchoalveolar lavage include very low levels of complement (which could potentially enhance viral neutralization by antibody and contribute to cytotoxic killing of cells), secretory IgA, IgG, free secretory component, α_1-antitrypsin, transferrin, and albumin—the last of which is a transudate from plasma.[48]

ANATOMY AND BIOLOGY OF THE MUCOSAL IMMUNE SYSTEM

The accepted model of the mucosal immune system is that immune induction is initiated by antigen, which is presented after uptake by microfold cells within local lymphoid tissue aggregates such as Peyer's patches or tonsils. Antigen-committed cells, primarily of the IgA isotype, enter the systemic circulation and home to mucosal sites, leaving the systemic circulation preferentially in high endothelial cells of postcapillary venules. A specialized transport system delivers immunoglobulin by transcytosis across epithelial cells to the mucosal surface. In aggregate, the cell populations involved in respiratory tract immunity are referred to as bronchus-associated lymphoid tissue (BALT). However, the structure and function of BALT in antigen presentation and the resulting mucosal immune response are less well defined than that of the enteric-associated lymphoid system, GALT.

The ring of lymphoid organs in the posterior nasopharynx that includes the tonsils and adenoids (Waldeyer's ring) appears to play an important role in stimulating the specific immune response,[30] as witnessed by the lower total IgA and impaired response to live oral poliovirus vaccine children who have had these structures surgically removed.[42] Forty percent of the lymphoid cells in the adenoid are CD3+ T cells, of which three quarters are CD4+ and the remainder are CD8+. The majority of the B cells are either IgM- or IgG-committed, with 10% of the cells IgA+, most of which are of the IgA_1 subtype[1] (H. Kiyono, personal communication, 1994).

In the upper respiratory tract, IgA is predominantly polymeric and largely of the IgA_1 subclass. IgM can also be transported across the epithelial cell and may become the predominant isotype in the face of IgA deficiency. IgA deficiency is estimated to occur in 1 of every 400 persons, and it is associated with an increase in frequency and severity of upper respiratory tract infections; however, the increase in infections in IgA deficiency is not as great as may be expected, perhaps because of a compensatory increase in IgM transport.

In the lower respiratory tract, collections of lymphoid tissue surround the bronchioles. In a study of comparative anatomy of the lung, BALT was seen in all rats and mice but not in higher mammals including cats and humans.[43] The lower respiratory tract is a normally sterile environment, and its associated immune system may not be as extensive as that in the enteric system. The T cells of the lower respiratory tract are approximately 60% CD4+ cells and 40% CD8+ cells, a proportion similar to that of the adenoids. Antigen-processing cells, including macrophages and dendritic cells, are also found in the lymphoid aggregates of the respiratory tract. The antibody produced is mainly of the IgA class, the IgA subclass depending on the site in the mucosal system at which antigen presentation occurs. In the respiratory tract, it is predominantly IgA_1.

In the lower respiratory tract, there appears to be a more prominent defensive role for IgG antibody. In animal models of RSV infection, administration of a passive antibody protects against infection in the lung.[45] Serum levels of viral antibodies probably correlate with protection because of the ability of IgG to diffuse into the airway. A prophylactic effect of hyperimmune RSV immunoglobulin has been reported in infants with bronchopulmonary dysplasia.[18]

The role of IgE as a mediator of acute and sustained allergic reactions in the lung has been studied extensively in patients with asthma. It appears to act through basophils and mast cells with the release of histamine, proteases and cytokines, particularly tumor necrosis factor-α. Mast cells are a prominent component of the respiratory layer, and, through their histamine-releasing function, they play a role in the bronchoconstriction of asthma. A direct link between mast cell function and viral pathogenesis has not been established. Mast cell degranulation serves to recruit other inflammatory cells into the airway, including monocytes, lymphocytes, platelets, and neutrophils, which in turn release a cascade of other cytokines.[14] The IgE response may play an important role in directing the clinical response to RSV infection toward bronchiolitis and contribute to the triggering of asthma by viral infections.[62]

Localized cell-mediated immune function is poorly defined. Intraepithelial lymphocytes are scattered though the epithelial layer,[44] but it is not clear that they are as common in the respiratory tract as they are in the gastrointestinal tract, where they have been shown to mediate cytotoxic cellular responses to rotavirus.[41]

Neutrophils appear to have little direct antiviral function, although their chemotactic function may be inhibited by viruses such as influenza.[64] Scattered macrophages may be seen within the alveolar walls and free in the bronchial cavities. These cells remove foreign and infectious particles from the airways and probably participate in the presentation of viral antigen to the local bronchial and systemic immune systems.

Commonality of the Mucosal System

It was originally thought that the components of the mucosal immune system were biologically linked, based on the demonstration that animals reconstituted with cells from Peyer's patches repopulated both gut and bronchial lamina propria.[51] The protection afforded against adenoviral respiratory illness by an enteric vaccine[9] and the demonstration of virus-specific IgA antibodies in breast milk after respiratory and enteric infection[13] were further evidence of a shared system. However, it is becoming evident that the mucosal system is more fragmented than previously thought. The distribution of immunoglobulin isotypes varies in different areas of the mucosal system, and the optimal induction of protection from natural infection or vaccine may be site specific.[31] A study of live polio virus vaccine administered into the distal arm of a colostomy demonstrated a much higher antibody response in the site of replication, a limited response elsewhere in the gut, and no measurable nasopharyngeal antibody.[42a] Even within the respiratory tract there may be differences in inductive capabilities between the upper respiratory tract, where there is clearly lymphoid tissue proximate to the airway, and the lung, where lymphoid tissue is less prominent.

Antigen Presentation

Current concepts of the mucosal immune response involve induction through specialized lymphoreticular tissues. In the intestinal tract, these have been well described and involve a unique epithelium with specialized antigen-transporting cells, the microfold (M) cells. The M cells in the gastrointestinal tract overlie lymphoid aggregates, Peyer's patches, and have been shown to have specialized ability to trap and present virus to the immune system. There is debate about the existence of M cells in the respiratory tract, although they have been shown to be prevalent in the nasopharyngeal lymphoid tissue in some species.[2]

Mucosal Immune Induction

Because antigen presentation is a key determinant of the type of immune response generated—that is, toward cytotoxic T cell dominance (Th1) or toward immunoglobulin production (Th2)—it becomes critical to know whether mucosally replicating viruses replicate in antigen-presenting cells or only in epithelial cells.[3] Viruses replicating in epithelial cells produce proteins that are degraded in endosomes to peptides and presented on the cell surface in the context of MHC II,

which is expressed only on a limited set of cells, particularly macrophages. Through the appropriate cytokines, primarily IL-4, a Th2 response would be predicted; this is characterized by IL-4, IL-5, IL-6, and IL-10, which drive the helper T cell population toward stimulation and differentiation of B cells, with resultant antibody production. The major viral proteins recognized in this paradigm would be surface proteins.

If respiratory viruses replicate in specialized antigen-presenting cells, antigen should be presented primarily in the context of MHC I. After assembly with MHC I in the endoplasmic reticulum, viral peptides, mainly representing internal viral proteins such as the influenza nucleoprotein, are carried to the plasma membrane. If presentation in the context of MHC I is an important component of antigen presentation, a Th1 response would be predicted, with IL-12 being an important cytokine in induction[53] and the major response being mediated by IL-2 and interferon-γ. The immune response should be manifested by a cell-mediated immune response with delayed-type hypersensitivity and cytotoxicity. However, the evidence for replication of influenza, RSV, or rhinovirus in mononuclear cells is limited.

Expression of Immunoglobulin A

After induction of the immune response, there is circulation of dimeric IgA, joined by a J chain produced in the plasma cell, which selectively exits the circulatory system in high endoplasmic venules. Secretory component acts as a receptor for polymeric immunoglobulins on the basolateral cell surface of epithelial cells. IgA is then transported across the epithelial cell to the apical surface in conjunction with secretory component in a process called transcytosis.[33] At the apical surface, a cleavage event occurs, and IgA is released, with retention of a tail of the secretory component.

The recognition of the intracellular transport of IgA has opened up a new area of interest—that is, that IgA may neutralize virus intracellularly. Antibody would not have to be directed at the proteins classically associated with virus neutralization, because steps in virus assembly would also be blocked by antibody directed against any of the structural viral proteins during binding of protein and by antibody within the cell during transcytosis.

It has been shown that IgA has a memory, and on reexposure to viral antigen after natural infection there is a rapid increase in influenza-specific IgA in the upper respiratory tract.[66] This may to some extent compensate for the relatively short duration of the primary IgA response.

Role of Immunity in Respiratory Viral Infection

The immune system has two very different roles: termination of primary viral infection and prevention of reinfection. In experimental murine RSV infection, the depletion of antibody by treatment with anti-μ antiserum has no effect on termination of primary RSV infection.[16] If either CD4+ or CD8+ cells are depleted, primary infection is more prolonged. The termination of respiratory virus replication (10 to 14 days; see Fig. 29-2) usually occurs before a primary mucosal or humoral immune response can be measured, suggesting that cellular host defenses may play a role in clearing a primary infection.

It is assumed, but actually proven in only a few cases, that the mucosal immune system is the primary defense against reinfection of viruses in the respiratory tract. The clearest demonstration of the preeminent role of the mucosal immune system occurs with the parainfluenza viruses, for which a very strong correlation between the level of virus-specific IgA antibody in nasal secretions and protection against experimental infection is seen.[57] With RSV and influenza, that correlation is harder to demonstrate.[34] The problem is in part a result of the difficulty of quantitating specific IgA activity in secretions that are diluted during collections of varying efficiency. The contribution of serum antibody to protection makes it difficult to isolate the effect of mucosal antibody. For example, infants with high transplacental maternal antibody values do not get as severe RSV infections in infancy, and high levels of serum antibody induced by inactivated influenza vaccine protect against influenza.

Recurrent infection is commonly seen with respiratory viruses. One difficulty in mounting an effective host response against the acute respiratory viruses is their capacity for antigenic variation. For example, there are multiple relatively stable serotypes of adenovirus, and influenza virus has the ability to undergo antigenic drift through mutation on a yearly basis and periodically to produce an entirely novel human pathogen through emergence of reassortant virus from animal reservoirs. Rhinoviruses also have multiple serotypes with little evidence for heterotypic immunity. These examples suggest that cell-mediated immunity directed against common internal proteins has little role in prevention of reinfection with respiratory viruses. Again, live attenuated vaccines have provided an insight, in that response to a H3N2 vaccine infection is identical regardless of prior infection with the heterotypic H1N1 virus. This is contrast to murine models of influenza, in which heterotypic immunity is mediated by cytotoxic T cells that recognize shared epitopes on the more constant internal proteins, notably the nucleoprotein. The possibility that parainfluenza type 3 may be immunosuppressive through infec-

tion of lymphocytes and that this contributes to reinfection has recently been raised.[59]

Reinfection has also been studied in animal models. The mode of antigen presentation on primary RSV immunization in the mouse determines the subsequent cytokine response on challenge. A killed or subunit vaccine as the primary immunogen induces a Th2 response on challenge with live virus and is accompanied by illness in the mouse.[17] In contrast, prior live virus infection of the respiratory tract induces a protective response that is characterized by a Th1 cytokine pattern.

Age influences the respiratory immune response. Elderly persons respond much less well to influenza vaccine than do younger adults. The immunocompetence of children younger than 6 months of age is just being explored. With live influenza vaccine, the response is influenced by the age of the child and the level of maternal antibody.[19] Similar complex influences on the primary immune response have been seen in natural RSV infection.[36] The duration of serum antibody after primary infection is also limited. With RSV a sawtooth pattern of antibody titers is seen, with a sustained antibody response manifested only after 3 to 4 infections.

PREVENTION OF RESPIRATORY VIRUS ILLNESS

The impact of respiratory illness at the extremes of life is hard to overestimate. Influenza causes excess mortality among elderly persons, and viruses such as RSV account for a large number of hospitalizations for pneumonia and bronchiolitis in infancy. In young children, otitis media and its sequelae account for almost a quarter of visits to pediatricians.[67] In healthy adults, respiratory viruses contribute to loss of productivity and account for a major market for symptomatic relief of respiratory ailments. It has proved difficult to immunize against acute viral respiratory infections for reasons that are enumerated in Table 29-2.

There are two examples of successful immunization against acute respiratory viral infections. The first is immunization against influenza with an inactivated vaccine consisting of

TABLE 29-2. *Difficulties in prevention of acute respiratory viral infection*

Category	Examples
Viral factors	Antigenic variation (influenza)
	Multiple serotypes (rhinoviruses, adenoviruses)
Immunologic factors	Short incubation period allowing little time for induction or even immune memory recall
	Apparent short duration of IgA mucosal response
	Systemic administration of antigen that does not induce optimal mucosal immunity
	Mucosal administration of antigen subject to rapid clearance
	Systemic administration of inactivated vaccine has been associated with enhanced illness (RSV)
Epidemiologic factors	Efficient rapid spread with frequent exposure
	Symptom complex (Many viruses can cause a similar illness, such as "influenza," lowering perception of vaccine efficacy against a single agent)
	Differing definition of efficacy–prevention versus amelioration of disease

intact or disrupted virions.[6] The efficacy of inactivated influenza vaccine has been demonstrated in a healthy adult population to be comparable to that of live attenuated vaccines,[12] and in elderly persons, despite reduced immunogenicity, it prevents influenza and its complications, leading to reductions in respiratory mortality.[40] It presumably works through boosting of serum and perhaps local antibody, and efficacy has been correlated with the level of serum hemagglutinating antibody.[63] Live attenuated influenza vaccines may find their role in immunization of pediatric populations or in mass immunization in the face of a new pandemic strain.[12]

The second example is the use of an enteric-coated live adenovirus vaccine in military personnel to prevent epidemics of acute respiratory illness that previously occurred with regularity among new recruits.[9] This vaccine stimulates serum antibody but may also provide protection through the commonality of the mucosal immune system by stimulation of respiratory mucosal immunity generated during replication in the gastrointestinal tract.[35]

The great bulk of pediatric respiratory illness is viral and remains a major challenge for future immunization research. Each virus has established an independent pathogenetic niche within the human host, and an understanding of pathogenesis underlies the success of future efforts at respiratory disease prevention.

ABBREVIATIONS

BALT: bronchus-associated lymphoid tissue
EBV: Epstein-Barr virus
GALT: gut-associated lymphoid tissue
ICAM-1: intercellular adhesion molecule-1
IgA, IgA$_1$, IgE, IgG, IgM: immunoglobulins
IL-2, IL-4, IL-5, IL-6, IL-10, IL-12: interleukins
MHC: major histocompatibility complex
RSV: respiratory syncytial virus
Th1: CD8 cytokine immune response pattern
Th2: B cell immune response pattern

ACKNOWLEDGMENTS

The author would like to acknowledge the contributions of Patrick Sniezek and Micki Estes in the preparation of this manuscript.

REFERENCES

1. Bernstein JM, Yamanaka N, Nadal D. Immunobiology of the tonsils and adenoids. In: Ogra PL, Stober W, Mestecky J, et al, eds. Handbook of mucosal immunology. San Diego: Academic Press, 625–640.
2. Bienenstock J, Clancy R. Bronchial mucosal lymphoid tissue. In: Ogra PL, et al. Handbook of mucosal immunology. San Diego: Academic Press, 529–550.
3. Braciale TJ, Braciale VL. Antigen presentation: structural themes and functional variations. Immunol Today 1991;12:124–129.
4. Burgert HG, Krist S. An adenovirus type 2 glycoprotein blocks cell surface expression of human histocompatibility class 1 antigens. Cell 1985;41:987–997.
5. Carson J, Collier AM, Hu SS. Acquired ciliary defects in nasal epithelium of children with acute viral upper respiratory infections. N Engl J Med 1985;312:463–468.
6. Centers for Disease Control. Recommendations of the ACIP: prevention and control of influenza. Part I, Vaccines. MMWR Morb Mortal Wkly Rep 1994;43–45(RR-9).
7. Chytil F. The lungs and vitamin A. Am J Physiol 1992;6:L517–L527.
8. Douglas RG Jr. The common cold: relief at last. N Engl J Med 1986;314:114–115.
9. Edmondson WP, Purcell RH, Gundelfinger BF, Love JWP, Ludwig W, Chanock RM. Immunization by selective infection with type 4 adenovirus grown in human diploid tissue culture. JAMA 1966;195:453–459.
10. Edwards KM, Thompson J, Paolini J, Wright PF. Adenovirus infections in young children. Pediatrics 1985;76:420–424.
11. Edwards KM, Snyder PN, Stephens DS, Wright PF. Human adenoid organ culture: a model to study the interaction of influenza A with human nasopharyngeal mucosa. J Infect Dis 1986;153:41–47.
12. Edwards KM, Dupont WD, Westrich MK, Plummer WD Jr, Palmer PS, Wright PF. A randomized controlled trial of cold-adapted and inactivated vaccines for the prevention of influenza A disease. J Infect Dis 1994;169:68–76.
13. Fishaut M, Murphy D, Neifert M, McIntosh K, Ogra PL. Bronchomammary axis in the immune response to respiratory syncytial virus. J Pediatr 1981;99:186–191.
14. Galli SJ. New concepts about the mast cell. Seminars in Medicine at the Beth Israel Hospital, Boston. N Engl J Med 1993;328:257–265.
15. Giebink GS. Studies of *Streptococcus pneumoniae* and influenza virus vaccines in the chinchilla otitis media model. Pediatr Infect Dis J 1989;8:S42-4.
16. Graham BS, Bunton LA, Rowland J, Wright PF, Karzon DT. Respiratory syncytial virus infection in anti-µ treated mice. J Virol 1991;65:4936–4942.
17. Graham BS, Henderson GS, Tang W, Lu X, Neuzil KM, Colley DG. Priming immunization determines T helper cytokine mRNA expression patterns in lungs of mice challenged with respiratory syncytial virus. J Immunol 1993;151:2032–2040.
18. Groothuis JR, Simoes EA, Levin MJ, et al. Prophylactic administration of respiratory syncytial virus immune globulin to high-risk infants and young children. N Engl J Med 1993;329:1524–1530.
19. Gruber WC, Darden P, Still JG, Lohr J, Wright PF, and the NIH/Wyeth-Ayerst ca influenza vaccine investigators group. Pediatr Res 1994;35:181A.
20. Gustafson TL, Lavely GB, Brawner ER, Hutcheson RH, Wright PF, Schaffner W. An outbreak of airborne nosocomial varicella. Pediatrics 1982;70:550–556.
21. Gwaltney JM Jr, Hendley JO. Rhinovirus transmission: one if by air, two if by hand. Am J Epidemiol 1978;107:357–361.
22. Gwaltney JM Jr, Phillips CD, Miller RD, Riker DK. Computed tomographic study of the common cold. N Engl J Med 1994;330:25–30.
23. Hall CB, Douglas RG. Modes of transmission of respiratory syncytial virus. J Pediatr 1981;99:1000–1003.
24. Henderson FW, Hu SC, Collier AM. Pathogenesis of respiratory syncytial virus infection in ferret and fetal human tracheas in organ culture. Am Rev Respir Dis 1978;118:29–37.
25. Henderson FW, Collier AM, Sanyal MA, et al. A longitudinal study of respiratory viruses and bacteria in the etiology of acute otitis media with effusion. N Engl J Med 1982;306:1377–1383.
26. Horvath J, Palkonyay L, Weber J. Group C adenovirus DNA sequences in human lymphoid cells. J Virol 1986;59:189–192.
27. Hussey GD, Klein M. A randomized, controlled trial of vitamin A in children with severe measles. N Engl J Med 1990;323:160–164.
28. Istre GR, McKee PA, West GR, et al. Measles spread in medical settings: an important focus of disease transmission. Pediatrics 1987;79:356–358.
29. Kido H, Yokogoshi Y, Sakai K, et al. Isolation and characterization of a novel trypsin-like protease found in rat bronchiolar epithelial Clara cells. J Biol Chem 1992;267:13573–13579.
30. Kuper CF, Koornstra PJ, Hameleers DMH, et al. The role of nasopharyngeal lymphoid tissue. Immunol Today 1992;13:2192–2194.
31. McGhee JR, Kiyono H. New perspectives in vaccine development: mucosal immunity to infections. Infect Agents Dis 1993;2:55–73.
32. McGhee JR, Fujihashi K, Lue C, Beagley KW, Mestecky J, Kiyono H. Role of IL-6 in human antigen-specific and polyclonal IgA responses. In: Mestecky J, Blair C, Ogra PL, eds. Symposium on im-

munology of milk and the neonate (1990 Miami, Fla.). New York: Plenum Press, 113–121.

33. Mestecky J, Cummins L, Russell MW. Selective transport of IgA. Gastrol Clin North Am 1989;20:441–471.

34. Mills JV, Van Kirk JE, Wright PF, Chanock RM. Experimental respiratory syncytial virus infection of adults. J Immunol 1971;107:123–130.

35. Mueller RE, Muldoon RC, Jackson GG. Communicability of enteric live adenovirus type 4 vaccine in families. J Infect Dis 1969;119:60–66.

36. Murphy BR, Graham BS, Prince GA, et al. The serum and nasal wash IgG and IgA antibody response of infants and children to respiratory syncytial virus F and G glycoproteins following primary infection. J Clin Microbiol 1986;23:1009–1014.

37. Neuzil KM, Gruber WC, Chytil F, Stahlman MT, Engelhardt B, Graham B. Serum vitamin A levels in respiratory syncytial virus infection. J Pediatr 1994;124:433–436.

38. Newhouse M, Sanchis J, Bienenstock J. Lung defense mechanisms. N Engl J Med 1976;295:990–998.

39. Newhouse M, Sanchis J, Bienenstock J. Lung defense mechanisms. N Engl J Med 1976;295:1045–1052.

40. Nichol KL, Margolis KL, Wuorenma J, Von Sternberg T. The efficacy and cost effectiveness of vaccination against influenza among elderly persons living in the community. N Engl J Med 1994;331:778–784.

41. Offit PA, Cunningham SL, Dudzik KI. Memory and distribution of virus-specific cytotoxic T lymphocytes (CTLs) and CTL precursors after rotavirus infection. J Virol 1991;65:1318–1324.

42. Ogra PL, Karzon DT. Distribution of poliovirus antibody in serum, nasopharynx and alimentary tract following segmental immunization of lower alimentary tract with poliovaccine. J Immunol 1969;102:1423–1430.

42a. Ogra PL, Karzon DT. Formation and function of poliovirus antibody in different tissues. In Progress in medical virology. Basel: S Karger, 1971:156–93.

43. Pabst R, Gehrke I. Is the bronchus-associated lymphoid tissue (BALT) an integral structure of the lung in normal mammals, including humans? Am J Respir Cell Mol Biol 1990 3:131–135.

44. Pawankar R, Okuda M. A comparative study of the characteristics of intraepithelial and lamina propria lymphocytes of the human nasal mucosa. Allergy 1993;48:99–105.

45. Prince GA, Hemming VG, Horswood RL, Chanock RM. Immunoprophylaxis and immunotherapy of respiratory syncytial virus infection in the cotton rat. Virus Res 1985;3:193–206.

46. Proud D, Gwaltney JM Jr, Hendley JO, Dinarello C, Gillis S, Schleimer RP. Increased levels of interleukin-1 are detected in nasal secretions of volunteers during experimental rhinovirus colds. J Infect Dis 1994;169:1007–1013.

47. Reynolds HY. Bronchoalveolar lavage. Am Rev Respir Dis 1987;135:250–263.

48. Reynolds HY, Newball HH. Analysis of proteins and respiratory cells obtained from human lungs by bronchial lavage. J Lab Clin Med 1974;84:559–573.

49. Ross BB, Gramiak R, Rahn H. Physical dynamics of the cough mechanism. J Appl Physiol 1955;8:264–268.

50. Rowe WP, Huebner RJ, Gillmore LK, Parrott RH, Ward TG. Isolation of a cytopathogenic agent from human adenoids undergoing spontaneous degeneration in tissue culture. Proc Soc Exp Biol Med 1953;84:570–573.

51. Rudzik R, Clancy RL, Perey DYE, Day RP, Bienenstock J. Repopulation with IgA containing cells of bronchial and intestinal lamina propria after transfer of homologous Peyer's patch and bronchial lymphocytes. J Immunol 1975;114:1599–1604.

52. Schlitt M, Lakeman A, Wilson ER, et al. A rabbit model of focal herpes simplex encephalitis. J Infect Dis 1986;153:732–735.

53. Scott P. IL-12: initiation cytokine for cell-mediated immunity. Science 1993;260:496–497.

54. Sieg S, Muro-Cachco C, Robertson S, Huang Y, Kaplan D. Infection and immunoregulation of T lymphocytes by parainfluenza virus type 3. Proc Natl Acad Sci U S A 1994;91:6293–6297.

55. Silver L, Anderson CW. Interaction of human adenovirus serotype 2 with human lymphoid cells. Virology 1988;165:377–387.

56. Sixbey JW, Yao Q. Immunoglobulin A–induced shift of Epstein-Barr virus tissue tropism. Science 1992;255:1578–1580.

57. Smith CB, Purcell RH, Bellanti JA, Chanock RM. Protective effect of antibody to parainfluenza type 1 virus. N Engl J Med 1966;275:1145–1452.

58. Stromberg BV. Sneezing: its physiology and management. The Eye, Ear, Nose and Throat Monthly 1975;54:12–6.

59. Townsend AR, Rothbard J, Goch FM, Bahadur G, Wraith D, McMichael AJ. The epitopes of influenza nucleoprotein recognized by cytotoxic T lymphocytes can be defined with short synthetic peptides. Cell 1986;44:959–468.

60. Tashiro M, Ciborowski P, Klenk H-D, Pulverer G, Rott R. Role of *Staphylococcus aureus* in the development of influenza pneumonia. Nature 1987;325:536–537.

61. Tucker SP, Compans RW. Virus infection of polarized epithelial cells. Adv Virus Res 1993;42:187–247.

62. Welliver RC, Wong DT, Middleton E Jr, Sun M, McCarthy N, Ogra PL. Role of parainfluenza virus specific IgE in pathogenesis of croup and wheezing subsequent to infection. J Pediatr 1982;101:889–896.

63. Wenzel RP, Hendley JO, Sande MA, Gwaltney Jr JM. Serum and nasal antibody responses to parenteral vaccination. JAMA 1973;226:435–438.

64. Wheeler JG, Winkler LS, Seeds M, Bass D, Abramson JS. Influenza A virus alters structural and biochemical functions of the neutrophil cytoskeleton. J Leukocyte Biol 1990;47:332–343.

65. Winther B, Gwaltney JM, Hendley JO. Respiratory virus infection of monolayer cultures of human nasal epithelial cells. Am Rev Respir Dis 1990;141:839–845.

66. Wright PF, Murphy BR, Kervina M, Lawrence EM, Phelan MA, Karson DT. Secretory immunological response after intranasal inactivated influenza A virus vaccinations: evidence for immunoglobulin A memory. Infect Immun 1983;4:1092–1095.

67. Wright PF, Sell SH, McConnell KB, et al. Impact of recurrent otitis media on middle ear function, hearing, and language. J Pediatr 1988;113:581–587.

Viral Pathogenesis,
edited by Neal Nathanson, et al.
Lippincott–Raven Publishers, Philadelphia © 1997

CHAPTER 30

Viral Enteric Diseases

Margaret E. Conner and Robert F. Ramig

INTRODUCTION

The gastrointestinal (GI) tract is a highly developed organ with numerous functions. Consistent with its function in the digestion and adsorption of foodstuffs and the resorbtion of water, it has an extremely large surface area relative to its contents. This surface area also presents a large target to infec-

tious agents, including viruses, and contains many specialized cell types that can serve as targets for specific viruses. However, the gut is also a hostile environment for infectious agents. To infect the epithelial surfaces lining the gut, a virus must survive the acidic environment of the stomach and then the bile salts of the upper small intestine. If these barriers are surmounted, the virus must then penetrate the mucus coating the gut to find the proper receptors and cell type to initiate infection. If the host has experienced a previous infection, the virus may encounter a vigorous local immune response that can neutralize the virus before infection or clear infected cells

M. E. Conner and R. F. Ramig: Division of Molecular Virology, Baylor College of Medicine, Houston, Texas 77030.

by specific lysis. However, many infectious agents have adapted to survive in this environment, because GI infections rank second only to respiratory infections as a cause of infectious morbidity.[95,171]

In this chapter, we survey viruses associated with infections of the GI tract, with particular emphasis on current knowledge of pathogenesis. Among these viruses are 1) nonenteropathogenic viruses that are found in feces in the absence of GI disease, 2) opportunistic gut viruses that are particularly important in immunocompromised individuals, and 3) viruses associated with gastroenteritis whose primary site of replication is the GI system. Among the many enteric viruses, relatively less is known about the pathogenesis of the large group of viruses associated with gastroenteritis, because they have in general been refractory to growth in tissue or organ culture. As a result, relatively few diagnostic reagents have been developed, which, in turn, has limited our understanding of the natural history of most of these viral infections. Predominant among the viruses associated with gastroenteritis that have been adapted to tissue culture are the group A rotaviruses. The ability to grow rotaviruses has allowed the development of diagnostic methods, as well as studies of replication, molecular biology, and experimental infection, with the result that rotavirus pathogenesis is probably the best understood among the gastroenteritis viruses. Therefore, the bulk of this chapter is devoted to the rotaviruses.

VIRUSES ASSOCIATED WITH THE GASTROINTESTINAL TRACT

Given the inability to cultivate many of the viruses associated with GI tract infection, the most fruitful early approach to identification of viral agents in individuals with GI disease was electron microscopic examination of feces. However, many specimens from control subjects contained viruses, and many specimens from diseased individuals contained more than a single morphologic type of virus. This indicated that simple presence of a virus was not indicative of GI infection, and that in cases of GI infection viruses could be present that were not the etiologic agent of the GI disease. Indeed, some viruses found in the GI tract have been shown to be nonenteropathogenic, and others have been shown to be opportunistic infections that did not contribute to GI disease.

Nonenteropathogenic Viruses Found in the Gut

Numerous viruses found in feces are not associated with primary infection or disease of the GI tract (Table 30-1). These viruses belong to three major taxonomic groups, the enteroviruses, reoviruses, and adenoviruses, and are typified by a fecal-oral or respiratory mode of spread. Viruses in this group are relatively easy to culture, and often are grown in tissue culture in attempts to isolate the agents of GI disease.

The viruses of this group, of which poliovirus is probably the paradigm, share a common natural history. The virus enters the GI tract orally and undergoes primary replication in the lymphoid tissues associated with the pharynx and gut. Viremia may occur, leading to secondary systemic spread and disease

TABLE 30-1. *Nonenteropathogenic human viruses found in feces*

Virus group	Specific viruses
Enteroviruses	Poliovirus (types 1–3)
	Coxsackievirus A (types 1–24)
	Coxsackievirus B (types 1–6)
	Echovirus (types 1–34)
	Enterovirus (types 68–71)
	Hepatitis A virus (type 72)
Reoviruses	Reovirus (types 1–3)
Adenoviruses	Adenovirus (types 1–39)

Modified from Farthing MJG. Gut viruses: a role in gastrointestinal disease? In: Farthing MJG, ed. Viruses and the gut. London: Smith Kline & French Laboratories, 1989:1–4.

unrelated to the GI portal of entry and site of primary replication. Virus is shed into the gut from the site of primary infection and appears in the feces for several days or weeks. These viruses have little or no ability to disrupt structure or function within the GI tract and are not established agents of any GI disease. However, they may appear in the feces as agents commensal with the agent responsible for GI disease.[109,222]

Opportunistic Gastrointestinal Viruses

A number of viruses that are not classically associated with infection of the gut can infect the GI tract under certain conditions (Table 30-2), often in a sexually transmitted mode in immunocompromised individuals. These opportunistic infections can be life threatening. In addition to these opportunistic viruses, viruses normally associated with nonpathogenic GI infection can cause particularly severe and prolonged disease in the immunocompromised.

Human immunodeficiency virus (HIV) is thought to have its primary affect on GI infection through immunosuppression, so that infections with other agents, including viruses that are normally self-limiting, become prolonged or lifelong. However, there is some evidence that HIV may be a direct enteric pathogen, because some HIV-infected patients have severe diarrheal disease in the absence of other enteropathogens.[183] In these cases, villus atrophy and fat maladsorption were noted,[225] and the HIV genome has been demonstrated in cells of the deep

TABLE 30-2. *Opportunistic gastrointestinal viruses of humans*

Virus	Disease
Human immunodeficiency virus	Chronic diarrhea and malabsorption
Herpes simplex virus	Esophagitis, proctitis
Cytomegalovirus	Esophagitis, gastritis, duodenitis, proctocolitis
Human papillomavirus	Anal warts, anal cancer

Modified from Farthing MJG. Gut viruses: a role in gastrointestinal disease? In: Farthing MJG, ed. Viruses and the gut. London: Smith Kline & French Laboratories, 1989:1–4.

crypts of the duodenum and rectal mucosa.[232] In some parts of the world, a predominant clinical symptom of HIV infection is "slim disease," accompanied by diarrhea and weight loss suggesting significant GI involvement.[297] Severe GI involvement has also been noted in HIV-infected children.[211]

Viruses of the herpes family can involve the GI tract, particularly in immunocompromised people.[367] Herpes simplex virus has long been recognized as a cause of proctitis in male homosexuals.[127] Disseminated cytomegalovirus infection is common in patients with acquired immunodeficiency syndrome, including cytomegalovirus infections of the GI tract,[182] and GI involvement is found in about 30% of patients with disseminated cytomegalovirus infection.[179]

Anogenital warts caused by papillomaviruses are a common sexually transmitted infection, and may be particularly severe in the immunocompromised. These infections may progress to neoplasia, although progression at the anus is less frequent than is carcinoma of the cervix.[298]

Viruses Associated With Gastroenteritis

The viruses associated with gastroenteritis represent a large number of taxonomic groups and a wide array of viral morphologies. Because these viruses have in general been difficult to cultivate, most members of this group were first associated with GI disease by electron microscopic examination of feces or biopsy specimens. The need to impose some sort of classification scheme on this array of viruses led to a scheme based solely on morphology. Here we attempt to group the viruses based on taxonomic groups established by the International Committee on Taxonomy of Viruses (Table 30-3). These viruses target specific cell types in the GI tract. Figure 30-1 provides a schematic summary of GI histology and localization of infection with the various viruses.

Parvoviruses

Human parvoviruses have not been directly linked to GI disease. However, animal viruses, such as feline parvovirus, feline panleukopenia virus, mink enteritis virus, and canine parvovirus form a group of closely related viruses that cause enteritis in animal hosts.[258] These viruses replicate in rapidly dividing cells. In utero and in the preweanling young, the primary focus for parvovirus infections is the central nervous system. However, after weaning, the GI tract becomes a site of rapid cell turnover and a target of parvovirus infection. Infection of the rapidly dividing crypt cells results in a shortening and blunting of the villi with a strong inflammatory response. Destruction of the maturing enterocytes causes hemorrhagic enteritis and dehydration, with a high mortality. Thus, infection of the animal GI tract with parvoviruses is an age-dependent phenomenon, with GI disease occurring after weaning.[258]

Adenoviruses

Although adenoviruses are often found in fecal specimens, they have not usually been associated with GI disease. In the mid-1980s, two previously uncultivatable fecal adenoviruses were adapted to culture and found to represent serotypes 40 and 41, forming a new subgenus (F) among the human adenoviruses.[44,153,177] Numerous studies have shown that types 40 and 41 are causative agents of diarrheal disease[354] and that adenovirus gastroenteritis accounts for about 7% to 8% of childhood diarrhea.[33] Enteric adenoviruses typically are associated with a mild disease compared with rotavirus infection, but with a more prolonged diarrhea (10.8 days, vs. 5.9 days for rotavirus) and less severe vomiting and fever.[343]

TABLE 30-3. *Viruses associated with gastroenteritis*

Virus	GI cell type infected	GI distribution of virus-induced injury
Animal parvoviruses	Dividing cells of the crypt	Small intestine
Adenovirus	Mature enterocytes	Apices of villi, small intestine
Calicivirus	Mature enterocytes	Sides of villi, proximal small intestine
Astrovirus	Mature enterocytes	Apices of villi, small intestine (ovine)
	M cells covering domes	Peyer's patches, proximal small intestine (bovine)
Rotavirus	Mature enterocytes	Apices of villi in proximal or distal small intestine, depending on host
Coronavirus	Mature enterocytes	Small intestine
	Surface and crypt cells	Large intestine
Toroviruses	Villus enterocytes crypt → apex	Distal small intestine
	M cells covering domes	Peyer's patches
	Surface and crypt cells	Large intestine
Mini-reoviruses	?	?
Picobirnaviruses	?	?

GI, gastrointestinal; M cells, microfold cells.

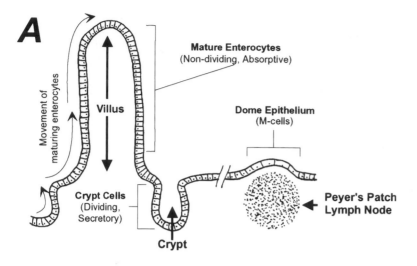

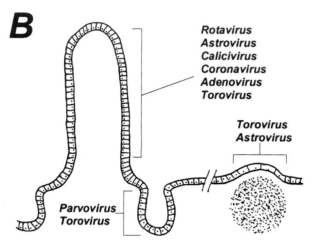

FIG. 30-1. Structure of small intestinal epithelium and locations targeted by gastrointestinal viruses. (A) Cross-section through a villus and crypt showing the location of the crypt cells, which are dividing and secretory, and the mature enterocytes, which are nondividing and absorptive. At the right is illustrated the specialized epithelium of the dome epithelium (M cells) that covers Peyer's patch lymph nodes. (B) The cell types infected by the various groups of viruses associated with gastroenteritis are indicated.

Caliciviruses

Numerous animal caliciviruses associated with gastroenteritis have been described, beginning with vesicular exanthema viruses of swine in 1932, although the first human calicivirus was not isolated until 1976.[81] Many caliciviruses have a characteristic morphology with 32 cups (calices) on their surface, but others have an indistinct, fuzzy appearance. This morphologic variation by electron microscopy led to placement of viruses now known to be caliciviruses in groups thought to be distinct. Most prominent of the viruses that had been classified only on the basis of morphology were those of the Norwalk virus group, which are now understood to be members of the calicivirus group based on a virion composed of a single capsid protein[138] and organization of the viral genome.[165] Norwalk group viruses cause an epidemic form of gastroenteritis in humans that is usually mild, and a provisional diagnosis of calicivirus infection can be made if there are no bacterial or parasitic pathogens, vomiting and diarrhea are of sudden onset and occur in more than 50% of cases, the incubation period is 24 to 48 hours, and the duration of disease is 12 to 60 hours.[173] Limited studies of Norwalk infection in volunteers have shown blunting of villi and crypt hyperplasia, but the mucosa remained intact[368]; however, this picture is

likely incomplete because only the proximal GI tract could be examined. In contrast, some animal caliciviruses cause severe gastroenteritis with high mortality.[80] In bovine infections with Newbury agent, where detailed anatomic studies have been done, the lesions were restricted to the proximal small intestine, with involvement apparently limited to the enterocytes on the sides of the villi.[143]

Astroviruses

Astroviruses were first associated with outbreaks of gastroenteritis in humans in 1975,[7] and have been associated with diarrheal disease in a number of animal species.[186] However, bovine astroviruses do not cause diarrheal disease but have been shown to infect the microfold cells overlying the Peyer's patches of the proximal small intestine.[373] In sheep, which have a disease similar to that in humans, virus is found replicating in the mature enterocytes at the apices of the villi of the small intestine. Disease associated with astroviruses is usually mild, with little vomiting and diarrhea of relatively short duration, and astroviruses are not considered a major cause of diarrheal disease in humans.[186]

Rotaviruses

Seven serogroups (A to G) of rotavirus have been recognized that share a common morphology, but have distinctive common antigens.[285] Group A rotaviruses are the major cause of endemic gastroenteritis in children and the young of mammalian species. The group A rotaviruses have been studied extensively and their pathogenesis is probably the best understood of the gastroenteric viruses. They are covered extensively later in this chapter.

In general, the significance of the non-group A rotaviruses as enteric pathogens is not readily evaluated, because most of them have not been adapted to cell culture and have been isolated relatively rarely. However, the group B rotaviruses have been associated with major epidemics of adult diarrhea in China[160] and group C rotaviruses with outbreaks affecting children and adults in Japan.[347] In pigs, in which infections with group A, B, and C viruses have been compared, the group B and C viruses caused less severe diarrhea than did group A virus.[285]

Coronaviruses

Human enteric coronaviruses were first described in 1975,[56] whereas in animals a viral enteric disease caused by what is now known to be a coronavirus was described as early as 1945 as transmissible gastroenteritis virus of swine.[96] The role of human enteric coronaviruses in enteric disease is unclear because a large proportion of normal control subjects excrete the virus.[55] However, a relatively strong link has been made between human enteric coronaviruses and necrotizing enterocolitis in neonates.[57,274] In contrast, animal coronaviruses have been demonstrated as the causative agent of severe diarrheal disease in a number of domestic animal species. Transmissible gastroenteritis virus is perhaps the best studied example, and produces outbreaks of diarrhea that affect swine of all ages and is often fatal in neonatal pigs. The primary site of replication for transmissible gastroenteritis virus is the mature enterocytes covering the intestinal villi, but other animal enteric coronaviruses also infect the epithelial cells of the large intestine.[263]

Toroviruses

A group of highly pleomorphic, membrane-bound viruses were isolated from calves (Breda virus) and horses (Berne virus) with diarrheal disease, and subsequently from cases of gastroenteritis in children and adults.[17,366,374] These viruses have been placed into the genus *Torovirus* of the *Coronaviridae* family.

In cattle, torovirus infects the distal small intestine and the large intestine with involvement of the epithelium from the crypt to the apex of the villus. Toroviruses appear to infect preferentially the microfold cells covering Peyer's patches.[373] Diarrheal disease associated with torovirus infection varies in severity, with severe disease usually occurring in the young.

Other Agents

In the past few years, a number of new agents have been identified in fecal specimens from individuals with diarrheal disease. Whether these agents cause diarrhea is unknown, but the large proportion of diarrheal disease for which no pathogen has been identified (30% to 70%[21]) suggests that other enteropathogenic agents will be identified. For example, *minireoviruses* were detected in electron microscopic surveys and were described as second to rotavirus in causing diarrhea in the study population.[319] However, one of these agents has been demonstrated to be a calicivirus,[190] which brings into question the distinctness of this group based on morphologic characteristics alone. Viruses with two segments of double-stranded RNA, termed *picobirnaviruses*, were found in surveys of fecal samples from individuals with gastroenteritis using electrophoresis of extracted RNA.[264] The virions of picobirnaviruses appeared to be quite labile because they could not be visualized until purified preparations were fixed with glutaraldehyde. A causative role for picobirnaviruses in diarrheal disease is not established.[111]

Overview of Pathophysiology of Viruses Associated With the Gastrointestinal Tract

Infection of the GI tract with the viruses described previously probably causes diarrhea by a variety of mechanisms. Most of these viruses infect the enterocytes or crypt cells lining the mucosa of various regions of the GI tract (see Table 30-3), with several possible consequences.[142,226,267,323] The enterocytes lining the villus surfaces in normal intestine are nonproliferating cells differentiated to have digestive and adsorptive functions (see Fig. 30-1). Adsorption across the enterocytic epithelium usually occurs by diffusion of solutes along electrochemical or osmotic gradients or by active transport. The transport of water is passive along osmotic gradients. In contrast, the cells of the crypt are the undifferentiated progenitors of the enterocytes, which differentiate to absorptive function as they migrate from the crypt and up the sides of the villus. Crypt cells actively secrete Cl^- ions. Thus, the transport of solutes and water across the intestinal epithelium results from a balance between adsorption in the villi and secretion in the crypts, with villus adsorption normally exceeding crypt secretion for a net absorption.

Viruses that infect and destroy the nondividing, absorptive enterocytes on the villus result in a generalized reduction of the net digestive and absorptive capacity of the small intestine, a functional deficit known as *malabsorption*. As a result of reduced digestion and absorption, undigested or partially digested material remains in the lumen of the small intestine, where it holds water by osmotic effect. As the undigested material enters the large intestine, fermentation results in lower–molecular-weight molecules that increase the osmotic gradient holding water in the lumen. The result is diarrhea when the absorptive capacity of the large intestine is exceeded. The absorptive capacity of the large intestine can also be reduced by viruses that infect the epithelium of the large intestine, increasing the water load and leading to diarrhea. The situation is somewhat different for viruses that infect the dividing, secretory cells of the crypts. In this case, depletion of crypt cells results in a reduced ability to replace the absorptive cells of the villi as they migrate toward the tips and are sloughed away. Thus, as the infection progresses, the digestive and absorptive capacity of the small intestine is impaired because the absorptive cells are not replaced. Depletion of the absorptive cells secondary to infection of the crypt cells leads to a functional deficit known as *secondary malabsorption*. Many of the viruses discussed previously cause a more severe diarrhea in neonates and the young than in older animals and adults. This is thought to result from the relatively slow rate of proliferation of cells in the crypts and migration of enterocytes along the villus in neonates. With age and the development of the intestinal flora, the rate of crypt cell proliferation and the rate of migration of enterocytes along the villus surface increases, so that older animals repair the absorptive surface of the intestine more rapidly after viral infection. Thus, *age affects* are seen in GI virus infections, with viruses targeting enterocytes tending to cause more severe diarrhea in the young and, conversely, viruses targeting the crypt cells tending to cause more severe diarrhea in older individuals.

EPIDEMIOLOGY AND CLINICAL IMPACT OF GUT VIRUSES

Among enteric infectious diseases, those causing diarrheal disease have the greatest impact. Diarrheal diseases affect all ages, but are most severe among the young. The Institute of Medicine estimated that 60% of all diarrheal illnesses and 90% of associated deaths occurred in children younger than 5 years of age.[164] The average child contracts diarrheal disease several times during each of the first 5 years of life,[21] and diarrheal disease is responsible for 25% to 30% of all deaths in this age group in developing countries.[318] The relative roles of the various etiologic agents vary, with bacteria playing an important role in children in developing countries, whereas in developed areas of the world viruses play predominant roles. In both settings, rotaviruses are responsible for the greatest proportion of childhood diarrhea. However, in 30% to 70% of episodes of diarrhea, no pathogen is identified.[21] Among people older than 5 years of age, diarrheal disease appears to be less prominent, although this may result from reduced clinical severity in this age group. However, the elderly and immunodeficient are at particularly high risk for diarrheal disease. In the older age group, viruses account for the largest proportion of diagnosed diarrhea, but most disease episodes still have no identified etiologic agent.[21]

Epidemiology

Among the viral agents causing diarrhea, two patterns of disease are noted. *Endemic diarrhea* is seen in children and has been associated predominantly with infection by rotaviruses, caliciviruses, and astroviruses. Nearly every child is infected with these agents in the first few years of life. *Epidemic diarrhea* occurs in outbreaks and is associated primarily with Norwalk-like viruses, and group B and C rotaviruses. The outbreaks often have an identifiable source such as contaminated water, food, or shellfish. The division between endemic and epidemic disease patterns is not absolute, but this broad characterization provides a framework for understanding the disease patterns associated with viral agents of diarrheal disease.[21]

Because the viruses associated with GI disease have in general been refractory to cultivation, relatively few well characterized reagents have been available for diagnosis and epidemiologic studies. Although the use of patient sera has allowed some progress to be made with the noncultivatable viruses, and the generation of reagents through the application of recombinant DNA technology holds promise for future progress with these viruses, the greatest progress has been made with the cultivatable group A rotaviruses.

It has become clear that group A rotaviruses are the major etiologic agents of serious diarrheal disease in infants and young children throughout the world. The acquisition of rotavirus antibody at an early age is indicative of widespread distribution of the virus worldwide, with greater than 90% of children having antibody by age 3 years.[170] In developed countries the incidence of rotavirus in children hospitalized with gastroenteritis has been variously estimated at 35% to 52%.[32,86,181] Furthermore, in the United States rotavirus diarrhea in the 1- to 4-year age group is estimated to include over one million cases per year with approximately 150 deaths,[152] a high morbidity with a low mortality. The low mortality rate most likely reflects the use of fluid replacement therapy in developed countries.[170] Prospective community-based studies revealed significant rotavirus infection, although at rates lower than those in hospitalized children. Of particular interest was the 88% symptomatic infection rate in the 36-month and younger age group. In developing areas of the world, studies of children receiving treatment for diarrheal disease revealed that 34% to 46% had rotavirus as the identified pathogen.[31,307] The burden of rotavirus diarrheal disease in children in the developing world was estimated to be over 125 million cases annually. Over 18 million of the cases were relatively severe, and it was estimated that they resulted in 873,000 deaths per year.[164] A prospective study in Bangladesh revealed that enterotoxigenic *Escherichia coli* and *Shigella* species were the most common pathogens associated with community disease in children, but rotavirus was the third most common pathogen. However, dehydration occurred significantly more often with rotavirus infection than with enterotoxigenic *E coli* or shigellae, suggesting that rotavirus disease was more life threatening.[29,30] Rotavirus infections are also documented in older children and adults but are usually asymptomatic except in the elderly, in whom immunity may wane, and in the immunocompromised.[170]

Rotavirus disease has a seasonal pattern of occurrence in the United States and other developed countries, with peaks in the winter.[32] However, this seasonal pattern is not seen in other settings.[170]

Age Distribution of Gastrointestinal Disease

As noted earlier, most of the viruses causing diarrheal disease produce the most severe disease in relatively young children. This may be partially based on the physiology of the developing GI tract and the differential response to infection with age.[226] However, the high rate of acquisition of antibodies to many of these viruses suggests that protective antibody may play a role in preventing infection in older people or that immunity results in subclinical infections.[199]

Nutritional Effects and Coinfections With Other Enteropathogens

Infectious diseases are known to be a factor in the development of malnutrition in infants and children.[175] It has been suggested that repeated diarrheal infections may promote the development of malnutrition by damaging the intestinal mucosa so that absorption is deficient over an extended period of time.[201] Diarrheal diseases may also be more clinically severe in malnourished individuals, as has been demonstrated for rotaviruses in humans and in animal models.[254,278]

Gastrointestinal viruses are frequently isolated in combination with other potential viral, bacterial, or parasitic pathogens, from individuals with diarrheal disease. The question is whether one of the infectious agents caused disease, or if the agents acted synergistically to produce more severe disease. Inoculation of mice with rotavirus induced mild diarrhea with no deaths, and *E coli* B44 induced severe diarrhea, with 45% of mice dying. Inoculation of mice with the combination of rotavirus and *E coli* B44 resulted in severe diarrhea and death in 84% of the animals, suggesting a synergism between the agents of diarrhea.[233]

It seems likely that the combination of malnutrition and coinfections with other enteropathogenic agents contributes to the severity of viral diarrhea in the developing world.

Transmission

The viruses associated with GI infection and diarrheal disease appear to be transmitted primarily by the fecal-oral route.[27,81,153,167,186,258,263] Most, although not all of these agents (e.g., Norwalk virus[105]) are shed in vast quantities in the feces so that the slightest contamination with feces would provide a relatively large inoculum. There is speculation that some of these viruses can be spread by a respiratory route, but definitive proof is lacking.

VACCINATION POTENTIAL

The impact of diarrheal disease on a worldwide basis is staggering. The unfortunate fact is that this burden of disease and death falls disproportionately on preschool-age children, with over 10,000 estimated to die of diarrheal disease each day.[167,169]

Antigenic Complexity

Characterization of the antigens and definition of serotypes of the enteric viruses have been difficult because many of the viruses are not cultivable. This has prevented production of high-quality, specific antisera and has made classic neutralization assays unavailable. Therefore, provisional typing of many of the enteric viruses has been performed using immunoelectron microscopy, crossprotection studies, or comparisons of nucleotide and amino acid homologies.

It has become clear, however, that there is a high degree of antigenic diversity among the enteric viruses. Rotaviruses, for example, are antigenically diverse with numerous serotypes (see section on Genes, Gene Products, and Virus Structure). Multiple serotypes or genogroups have been identified for each of the enteric virus groups: adenovirus (two serotypes), astrovirus (eight serotypes), calicivirus (at least four serotypes, three genogroups), coronavirus (four antigenic groups with multiple serotypes), and torovirus (at least two serotypes). The antigenic diversity observed among these viruses indicates that multiple infections with different serotypes of each virus are possible, and that development of vaccines is likely to require inclusion of antigens to stimulate immunity to multiple serotypes.[21,167]

Immune Correlates of Protection

Immune correlates of protection have not been identified for most of the enteric viruses. With most of these agents, diarrheal disease is primarily observed in the young, implying that immune protection restricts disease in older animals. However, caliciviruses are associated with epidemic outbreaks of diarrheal disease in all age groups, suggesting that the epidemiology or immune response differs somewhat from other enteric viruses.[105,168] As a result, there is conflict as to whether caliciviruses induce immune protection. For example, in a study in children, serum antibody to Sapporo calicivirus clearly correlated with protection from disease, but not infection.[105] In contrast, short-term protection from disease has been observed in some adult volunteers, but in other volunteers it appeared that antibody was associated with more severe disease.[105] This example illustrates our poor understanding of immunity to the disease produced by enteric viruses.

Vaccination Strategies

The disproportionate burden of diarrheal disease falls on the young and mandates that vaccination strategies be aimed at this population. However, there is a series of obstacles to effective vaccination of the young. Among these are the prevalence of the viral agents of diarrheal disease, so that potential vaccinees have a relatively high level of maternally derived antibody. This passively acquired antibody can decrease immune response to protein antigens and restrict replication of live attenuated-virus vaccines so that immunogenicity is decreased. This group of potential vaccinees is also immunologically naive, so that vaccines must be extremely safe and nonreactogenic. Thus, a fine balance between attenuation and immunogenicity must be achieved if live attenuated-virus vaccines are to be used.[229]

Vaccines against enteric infections must stimulate immune responses at the local site of infection, the GI tract. Immunization of mucosal surfaces is a field in its infancy, but several general comments are relevant. First, in general, more efficacious mucosal immunity is stimulated by presentation of immunogens at mucosal sites than by systemic presentation, but it has been relatively difficult to induce effective mucosal immunity.[210,355] Second, oral infection or immunization typically stimulates production of IgA, which is the predominant isotype in the intestine. Third, stimulation of high levels of mucosal immunity would be expected with the use of live replicating vaccines, but issues of safety may limit this approach. Fourth, development of new delivery systems and mucosal adjuvants is underway and is likely to facilitate formulation of both live virus and recombinant antigen strategies for mucosal immunization. Finally, creation of effective vaccines against viruses that cause GI illness will require a better understanding of the correlates of protection and how best to induce protective mucosal immune responses.

THE ROTAVIRUS MODEL OF ENTERIC DISEASE

The group A rotaviruses cause the largest proportion of serious diarrheal disease of the young. As a result of this predominant position, these agents are the most studied of the viral enteropathogens. The remainder of this chapter describes our understanding of the pathogenesis of the group A rotaviruses.

General Features of the Rotaviruses

A number of features of the genome structure, proteins, capsid structure, and replication of rotaviruses must be understood for the discussion to follow.

Rotavirus Genes, Gene Products, and Virus Structure

The rotavirus genome consists of 11 discrete molecules, or segments, of double-stranded RNA (Fig. 30-2). In cells infected with two viruses, the segments can segregate independently, leading to formation of progeny that contain 11 segments that are of mixed parental origin. This ability to reassort segments provides the basis for segregation analysis, which has been used to identify genetic determinants of important viral phenotypes.[272]

Each of the genome segments encodes a single primary gene product (see Fig. 30-2), although certain segments encode smaller gene products of undefined function.[102] Six of the protein species are found in the virion structure (VP1, VP2, VP3, VP4, VP6, and VP7). The remaining five proteins are nonstructural (NSP1, NSP2, NSP3, NSP4, and NSP5), being found only in infected cells. Among the structural proteins, three (VP4, VP6, and VP7) are of particular interest. VP6 is the most prevalent (780 copies) protein in the virion. VP6 is highly antigenic and contains epitopes that allow the identification of rotavirus subgroups. VP4 is present in 120 copies in the virion and is a minor constituent. Cleavage of VP4 is required for infectivity. VP4 contains neutralization epitopes that define the P (protease-sensitive) serotype. Ten P serotypes have been defined by neutralization, but studies of amino acid homology have identified 20 P genotypes, 10 of which correspond to the P serotypes defined by neutralization. VP7 is a prevalent (780 copies) glycoprotein that contains epitopes that define the G (glycoprotein) serotype. Fourteen G serotypes have been defined that correspond to 14 amino acid homology groups. Thus, the neutralization serology of rotaviruses is determined by two proteins, VP4 and VP7.

Structurally, rotaviruses consist of three concentric protein capsids (see Fig. 30-2). The innermost capsid layer has VP2 on its surface, and contains VP1, VP3, and the genome within.[268] This single-layered particle is surrounded by VP6, which comprises the intermediate capsid layer. The double-layered particles with VP6 on the surface express a virion-associated, RNA-dependent RNA polymerase activity that is required for transcription and initiation of infection. However, double-layered particles cannot bind to cells and initiate infection directly. The outermost capsid layer is composed of VP4 and VP7. VP7 comprises the smooth surface of the triple-layered particle, and dimers of VP4 comprise the spikes that emanate from the surface. Triple-layered particles can bind to cells to initiate infection and are the only particle type that can be neutralized by anti-VP4 and anti-VP7 antibodies.

Rotavirus Replication

The replication cycle of rotavirus is schematically illustrated in Figure 30-3. The details of this life cycle were determined in cultured cells,[102] but the essentials appear to be similar in vivo. The salient steps of the life cycle, in order, can be summarized as follows.

1. Triple-layered particles bind to a rotavirus-specific cellular receptor. The viral attachment protein appears to be VP4, but the cellular receptor has not been identified.
2. The virus penetrates into the cell by either direct penetration of the plasma membrane, or by receptor-mediated endocytosis. The productive mode of entry appears to be direct membrane penetration, and entry by receptor-mediated endocytosis appears to be nonproductive. Penetration requires protease cleavage of VP4 into VP5* and VP8*, both of which remain associated with the virion.
3. The virus is uncoated by the removal of VP4 and VP7. Ca^{2+} is required for the integrity of the outer capsid, and it is thought to be removed when the triple-layered particle encounters the cytoplasm, where the $[Ca^{2+}]$ is too low to maintain outer capsid structure.
4. Removal of the outer capsid activates the virion-associated, RNA-dependent RNA polymerase, and mRNAs are transcribed and extruded from the double-layered particle.
5. The mRNAs are translated by the cellular translation apparatus.
6. When sufficient proteins have been made, mRNAs complex with viral structural and nonstructural proteins to form nascent subviral particles that resemble single-layered particles, but also contain nonstructural proteins. This process occurs at cytoplasmic sites called viroplasms, which are concentrations of viral protein and RNA.
7. In the nascent single-layered particles, the mRNA is replicated ([-]-strands are synthesized), leading to the ultimate formation of particles containing double-stranded RNA. At the end of the replication process, nonstructural proteins are lost and VP6 is added, forming double-layered particles.
8. The nascent double-layered particles formed at the periphery of viroplasms bud through the membrane of adjacent endoplasmic reticulum (ER). In this budding pro-

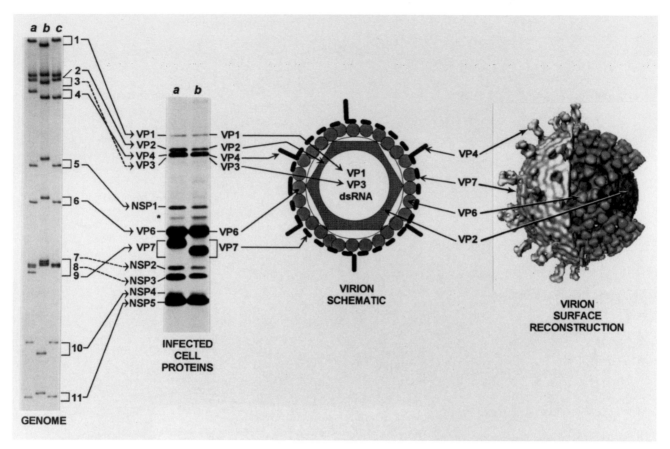

FIG. 30-2. The rotavirus genome, protein species, coding assignments, and location of proteins within the virion structure. (**A**) Genome. The electrophoretic profiles of three virus strains are shown. Lane a, bovine rotavirus strain B223; lane b, simian rotavirus variant SA11-4F; lane c, a reassortant derived from a cross of B223 with SA11-4F. In the reassortant segments, 4 and 9 are derived from the SA11-4F parent and the remaining segments from the B223 parent. Note different rates of mobility for genome segments of different viruses, and the ability of segments to be derived from both parents in reassortants. (**B**) Infected cell proteins. The electrophoretic profiles of the intracellular proteins of two rotavirus strains are shown. Lane a, strain B223; lane b, strain SA11-4F. Note that the mobility of the protein species differs between strains only for some of the protein species. The asterisk indicates a host cell protein. The segment in which each of the viral proteins is encoded is indicated by an arrow. (**C**) Virion schematic. The locations of the viral structural proteins within the three capsid layers of the virus particle are indicated. dsRNA, double-stranded RNA. (**D**) Virion surface reconstruction. A cryo-electron microscopic reconstruction of a rotavirus particle with various capsid layers removed. Arrows indicate the protein species found on the surface of each of the three capsid layers. (Reconstruction courtesy of Dr. B.V.V., Prasad, Baylor College of Medicine, Houston, TX.)

cess, VP7, which is synthesized as an integral ER protein, and VP4 are added to the particles, which possesses a transient envelope derived from the ER membrane.

9. In the lumen of the ER, triple-layered particles mature through final assembly of VP4 and VP7 into the outer capsid layer and loss of the membrane.

10. Mature, infectious, triple-layered particles are released by cell lysis.

Animal Models of Rotavirus Pathogenesis

Rotaviruses have a broad host range and generally similar pathogenesis in all infected species. Thus, development of an-

imal models did not require adaptation of heterologous strains to model host species. The use of animal models of rotavirus infection has provided key insights in our understanding of the pathogenesis of both human and animal rotaviruses. However, studies of rotavirus pathogenesis are complicated by the ubiquitous distribution and early age of rotavirus infection in human and animal populations. This has required generation and rigorous maintenance of rotavirus-naive animals for the model systems. Five animal models, two small laboratory animal (rabbit and mouse) and three large (cow, pig, and sheep), have been used to define parameters of rotavirus infection, pathologic process, disease, immune response, and vaccine efficacy. The salient features of each model are summarized and compared with features of human infection in Table 30-4.

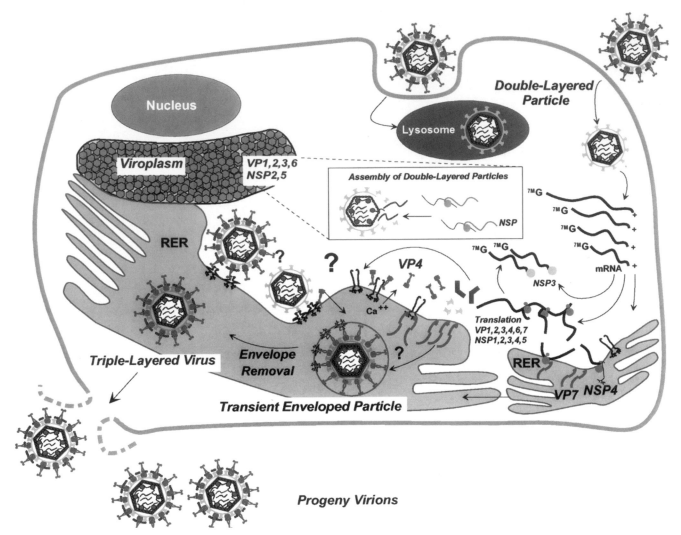

FIG. 30-3. The rotavirus replication cycle. A schematic representation of the rotavirus replication cycle based on information gathered from infection of cells in tissue culture. RER, rough endoplasmic reticulum. (From Estes MK. Rotaviruses and their replication. In: Fields BN, Knipe DM, Howley PM, eds. Fields Virology. 3rd ed. Philadelphia: Lippincott–Raven, 1996:1625–1654, with permission.)

This section is limited to presentation of group A rotavirus infections because they are the most common worldwide and are used in most studies of pathogenesis.

Large Animal Models

Much of the early work on rotavirus pathogenesis used large animals, usually either colostrum-deprived or gnotobiotic models. Because transfer of maternal antibodies across the placenta does not occur in cows, pigs, or sheep, neonates removed from their dams before ingestion of colostrum (colostrum-deprived) receive no rotavirus-specific humoral or cell-mediated immunity from the dam. Colostrum-deprived animals are housed in isolation immediately after birth to prevent contamination with exogenous rotaviruses from the environment. Colostrum-deprived animals have some of the nat-

ural microflora in the intestine and near-normal immune systems. Gnotobiotic animals are delivered by cesarean section to preclude exposure to rotavirus during or after birth. Gnotobiotes are housed under germ-free conditions, have no microflora in the intestine, and are free of rotavirus-specific humoral and cell-mediated immune responses. The immune system in gnotobiotic animals is underdeveloped because they lack normal microflora in the intestine. Large animal models have been of limited use because of size, costs, and the limited availability of isolation or germ-free facilities, factors that preclude their use in large-scale studies.

Bovine Model

Many studies have examined infection of calves with rotaviruses of bovine origin (homologous infection). Natural ro-

TABLE 30-4. Comparative features of rotavirus infections of humans and experimental animals

Species	Transplacental transfer of antibody	Age of infection		Age of clinical disease		Infection with multiple glycoprotein (G) serotypes		Virus inducing experimental clinical disease	
		Natural	Experimental	Natural	Experimental	Natural	Experimental	Homologous	Heterologous
Human	Yes	All	—	0.5–2 y	—	Yes	—	Yes	—
Bovine	No	1–10 wk	≤10 wk	1–10 wk	Birth to 6 mo	Yes	Yes	Yes	Yes
Porcine	No	>1 wk	Birth to ≥8 wk	1–8 wk	Birth to ≥8 wk	Yes	Yes	Yes	Yes
Ovine	No	≥2 wk	1–12 d	≥2 wk	≤12 d	?	?	Yes	No
Lapine	Yes	1–2 mo	Birth to ≥9 mo	≤3 mo	No	No?	Yes	Yes	No
Murine									
Neonate	Yes	?	Birth to 2 wk	≤2 wk	≤2 wk	No?	Yes	Yes	Yes
Adult	Yes	?	2 wk to ≥1 y	No	No	No?	Yes	No	No

tavirus infections in calves younger than 1 week of age usually result in subclinical infections, although subclinical infections also occur in older calves[34,88,215] (see Table 30-4). Symptomatic infection in calves usually begins at about 1 to 2 weeks of age, but infections and disease are reported in both naturally and experimentally infected calves up to 8 to 10 weeks of age.[40,34,219,370] Diarrhea is more severe and mortality higher in younger calves, followed by a decrease in mortality with age, possibly as a result of age-related changes in the intestine (see section on Age-Related Host Factors) or acquisition of active immunity to rotavirus. Several G and P serotypes commonly circulate in the bovine population worldwide.[287] Calves also can be infected with some heterologous rotaviruses of several serotypes. Diarrhea is observed with some but not all heterologous strains, and often is less severe.[54,220,221,378,379]

Ovine Model

Compared with infections in piglets and calves, rotavirus infection in lambs results in less severe histopathologic changes and mild clinical disease[214,310,311,313] (see Table 30-4).

Some of the earliest studies on rotavirus immunity were performed in sheep. The protective effect of antibody in the intestine at the time of virus challenge was established in the ovine model.[313,315-317] In these studies, lambs were allowed colostrum and then divided in two groups that either nursed on antibody-positive ewes or were reared on antibody-negative milk before challenge with rotavirus. Lambs nursing on antibody-positive ewes were protected from rotavirus challenge, whereas most of the lambs that did not have antibody in the intestine at the time of challenge were not protected. Limited protection was noted in lambs with high levels of serum antibody but no detectable intestinal antibody, indicating that in some instances, serum antibody obtained from colostrum afforded partial protection.

Porcine Model

The piglet is a monogastric animal with intestinal physiology resembling that of humans.[289] Piglets have been used extensively because large litters can be derived from one sow, and the size of the young allows housing in germ-free isolators up to approximately 8 weeks of age. A significant limitation of the gnotobiotic piglet model is underdevelopment of the immune system. Therefore, infection and immune response may not be completely analogous to infections in children. Although challenge studies are readily performed, the time between primary and challenge inoculation is somewhat limited (3 to 4 weeks) because of the need to remove the piglets from the germ-free isolators at approximately 8 weeks of age. Both natural and experimental rotavirus infections in piglets can be severe, causing pronounced histologic changes in the intestine.[136,216,287,328]

The piglet is unique among the animal models because piglets are susceptible to infection by rotavirus isolates from other species,[35,42,87,144,224,321,334,336,377] and diarrhea has been observed after inoculation with some heterologous rotaviruses (see Table 30-4). The ability to infect gnotobiotic piglets and produce diarrheal disease with human rotavirus strains[42,87,289,336,377] provides a model system to study active immunity and protection from clinical disease with human virus isolates. Studies indicate that piglets can be infected with piglet-adapted human virus up to at least 6 weeks of age.[289] As observed in other models, culture adaptation of challenge strains leads to attenuation of virulence in piglets.[36,50,289,342]

Small Animal Models

Small animal models have several advantages over large animal models, including cost effectiveness, the ability to incorporate large numbers of animals in studies, the feasibility of isolation of large numbers of infected animals, short gestations and multiparous births, and the availability of rotavirus-naive animals.

Lapine Model

The rabbit was originally proposed as a model of rotavirus infection because the epidemiology of natural rotavirus infections indicated that rabbits were susceptible to infection to at least 2 to 3 months of age, several easily cultivable strains of rabbit rotavirus had been reported, and a small animal model was needed for active immunity studies. Unlike large animals, rabbit kits receive anti-rotavirus antibody from the dam both transplacentally and lactogenically. Rotavirus is endemic in commercial rabbit populations and natural infections occur by 1 to 3 months of age.[93,94,265] Several investigators have established rotavirus-free rabbit colonies.

Several rabbit rotavirus strains (serotype G3, P?) have been isolated and adapted to cell culture.[53,265,293,327,331] Rabbits have been experimentally infected with homologous rabbit strains and heterologous simian virus. Most homologous viruses replicate well in rabbits, whereas limited replication has been observed with one rabbit virus and the heterologous virus.[71,72,330] Homologous strains are readily transmitted to uninoculated control animals, whereas the heterologous virus is not.[71]

Rabbits from 1 week to 9 months of age are susceptible to homologous virus infection, allowing conduct of long-term studies of immunity or vaccine protective efficacy.[68,71,72,330] Therefore, the rabbit is an infection model in which protection from challenge can be assessed by reduction of virus or antigen shedding. Although rotavirus infections are associated with diarrhea in naturally infected rabbits, little or no diarrhea is seen when rabbits are experimentally infected with homologous or heterologous viruses.[71,147,265,330] Increased fluidity of small intestinal contents of experimentally infected rabbits is noted, and it was hypothesized that the failure to induce diarrhea resulted from the large absorptive capacity of the rabbit cecum,[71,72,330] or the natural avirulence or cell culture attenuation of the viruses tested. Although diarrhea is not observed, experimental infection of rabbits produces histopathologic lesions in the small intestine (Fig. 30-4) that are consistent with those observed in other animal species (see section on Pathologic Lesions in Rotavirus Infection).[103,124,330]

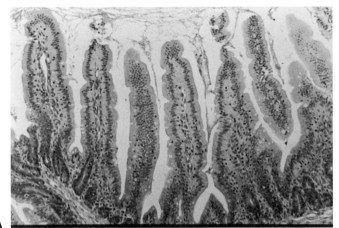

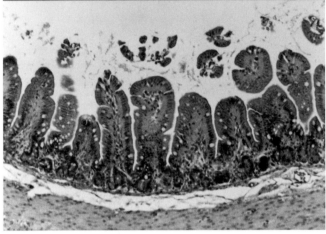

FIG. 30-4. Histopathology of rabbit ileum after oral infection with rabbit rotavirus strain Ala. **(A)** Section of ileum from a 45-day-old, uninfected, control rabbit showing normal villus height and appearance of the villus epithelium. **(B)** Section of ileum from a 34-day-old rabbit, 18 hours after infection with rabbit rotavirus strain Ala. Note the shortening of the villi and increased vacuolation of the villus epithelium. **(A, B,** Hematoxylin and eosin stain, original magnification × 200.)

Murine Model

Two mouse models of rotavirus infection have been developed (see Table 30-4). In the neonatal mouse model, both infection and disease (diarrhea) occur, whereas in the adult mouse model infection occurs without disease. The neonatal model has been used primarily to examine passive immunity based on transfer of antibody from mother to neonate, and challenge during the first or second week of life. The adult model was developed primarily to provide a small animal model of active immunity. The mouse model has several advantages over other animal models: rotavirus-naive outbred, inbred, and gene-knockout mice are available, and a large array of immunologic reagents are commercially available that allow conduct of immunologic studies not readily performed in the other outbred animal model systems. The neonatal and adult mouse models have somewhat different characteristics and are discussed separately.

The nomenclature and identity of murine rotavirus strains is confusing because many independent isolates have been referred to as epidemic diarrhea of infant mice virus. A new nomenclature has been proposed that should clarify the identity of murine rotavirus strains.[50] At least six strains of murine rotavirus have been isolated, but only since the mid-1980s has the virus been adapted to cell culture.[50,139,326] Adaptation to culture has usually resulted in loss of virulence.[50] Five murine strains have been tentatively identified as G3 type viruses, based on amino acid sequence homology of VP7, and all are cross-protective in the adult mouse model.[50,99] The amino acid sequences of VP4 molecules indicate that the murine strains fall into two P types.[99,296]

Neonatal Mouse Model. Early studies demonstrated that inoculation of murine rotavirus strains in mice results in infection and disease only in mice younger than 15 days of age.[1,107,185,277,304,369] The basis of age restriction was postulated to be the result of maturation of enterocytes in the small intestine leading to "closure" of the intestine, with decreased nonspecific macromolecular transport, at 15 to 17 days of age,[369] or of a decrease in rotavirus receptors on epithelial cells with increasing age.[277] The neonatal mouse model was used for a number of studies examining the rotavirus pathologic process, protection from infection and disease mediated by passive immunity, definition of genes involved in virulence, and identification of proteins important in producing protective antibodies. Active immunity and protection were examined in only a single study[375] because a strong active immune response could not be demonstrated at an age when animals remained susceptible to disease.

Infection of neonatal mice with murine rotavirus strains results in productive replication with excretion of antigen, diarrhea, and development of mild intestinal histopathologic lesions. Shedding of viral antigen is initially detected within 1 to 2 days postinoculation, often is biphasic with peaks at approximately 2 and 6 days postinoculation, and usually terminates by 7 to 10 days postinoculation.[50,107,191,192,270,304,320]

Neonatal mice are also susceptible to infection and manifest diarrhea after oral inoculation with many heterologous rotavirus strains.[19,107,131,178,244,270,277,304] Limited or abortive virus replication occurs in mice infected with heterologous rotaviruses, as evidenced by the high dose of virus required to induce disease, failure of virus excretion titers to exceed input titers, mild or absent pathologic changes in the intestine, failure routinely to observe viral particles in small intestinal epithelial cells, and failure of transmission of infection from inoculated to contact animals.[139,191,192,244,270]

Adult Mouse Model. The adult mouse model was developed specifically to examine active immunity to, and protection from, rotavirus infection and to evaluate vaccine strategies.[213,362,363] Mice of different ages were inoculated and examined for evidence of infection, either virus excretion or seroconversion. All mice orally inoculated with tissue culture-adapted murine virus (epidemic diarrhea of infant mice virus) from 4 to 180 days of age were infected as determined by virus shedding and seroconversion and were protected from homologous challenge up to 4 months after primary infection.[362,363]

Characterization of rotavirus infection of adult mice with four animal-passaged murine rotavirus strains has been reported.[50] All four strains replicate in adult mice. Differences in the median shedding dose (SD_{50}) are observed among the strains. After an incubation period of 1 to 2 days, mice shed virus for 4 to 6 days with a monophasic shedding profile. Excretion of rotavirus antigen in adults is at levels similar to those seen in neonatal mice, but no disease or histopathologic changes are observed in any adults. However, there is an increase in fecal fluidity and a change in color of small intestinal contents. In adults inoculated with animal-passaged virus, detectable levels of intestinal anti-rotavirus IgA are first observed at 5 days postinoculation, which coincides with the decline in viral antigen shedding.[50] Mice challenged with the same strain, or a different strain of murine virus 6 weeks after primary infection, are totally protected from reinfection. Anamnestic intestinal IgA responses are not observed after challenge, but some increase in serum IgG is seen. Long-term serologic and mucosal immune responses persist for up to 1 year after oral infection of neonatal mice with 10^5 plaque-forming units of simian Rhesus rotavirus (RRV).[302]

Common Features of Infection and Disease in Humans and Animal Models

Many of the features of rotavirus infection and disease are similar in the various animal models, varying only in degree or detail.

Rotavirus Infection

The most consistent clinical signs of rotavirus infection include a watery diarrhea, anorexia, depression, dehydration, and sometimes vomiting.[27,170,287] Deaths attributed to rotavirus infections result from severe dehydration secondary to loss of fluids from diarrhea or vomiting. Diarrhea is observed in natural infections of most species, but is variable in animal models after infections with heterologous virus strains. Other signs of infection include low-grade fever and abdominal distention or discomfort. Failure to thrive has been reported in children in developing countries where rotavirus infections may exacerbate malnutrition or be synergistic with other enteropathogens,[176,200,202,203] and has also been reported in domestic animals.[144,371]

The incubation period of rotavirus infection varies from 11 hours to 4 to 6 days.[27,170,287] Virus particles are observed in stools or intestinal contents as early as 12 hours postinfection and persist for variable lengths of time from 1 to 14 days. Virus is usually shed in large quantities (10^9 to 10^{10} particles/g) and shedding can precede diarrhea or can persist beyond cessation of diarrhea. Long-term persistence of virus excretion and diarrhea has been reported in immunocompromised children and mice.[276,294]

Rotavirus is stable, and large quantities may contaminate the environment. Infection appears to be transmitted by direct fecal-oral contact or through fomites.[51,189,349,370] Because high concentrations of virus are shed, and the minimal infectious dose is low ($<$1 to 100 tissue culture infectious units),[50,73,132,259,342,357] minimal environmental contamination is required to transmit infection.

Pathologic Lesions in Rotavirus Infection

The severity and localization of rotavirus infection varies in different animal species and between studies (reviewed in Greenberg and colleagues[136]). These variations result from many factors, including inoculum used (virus strain and titer), immune status of host, age at infection, method of assessing infection, and host intestinal physiology.

Pathologic changes induced by rotavirus infection are almost exclusively limited to enterocytes in the small intestine.[25,85,144,218,260,262,310,335] Microscopically, cytolytic changes occur in infected villus enterocytes and, in severe disease, sloughing of enterocytes may expose the basement membrane at villus tips. Blunting and atrophy of villi is common, and villus fusion may occur in some species. In severe infections villi virtually disappear.[329] Decreased villus height and crypt hyperplasia result in significantly reduced mucosal-to-serosal surface ratios.[79,124,217,218,311] This change in ratio indicates a relative loss of absorptive cells and an increase in secretory cells, producing changes in gut homeostasis.[79,124,217,218,226,311] Rotavirus infections do not produce a significant inflammatory response, and only mild mononuclear infiltration of the lamina propria usually is observed. Similar pathologic changes occur during subclinical infections, although the extent and severity of the lesions usually are much less than in animals with diarrhea.[34,124,145,275] Macroscopic changes in the intestine usually are not observed, although in piglets there is thinning of the intestinal wall and disappearance of chyle in the mesenteric lymphatics.[136] Histopathologic changes usually appear within 24 hours of infection, and are maximal between 24 and 68 hours postinfection.[66,79,124,145,218,257,260,310,320,329]

The anatomic segment (duodenum $\rightarrow$ jejunum $\rightarrow$ ileum) of the small intestine that is affected varies between species and between homologous and heterologous infections, but the significance of these variations is not understood.[87,224,262,371] In piglets and lambs, the most pronounced histopathologic changes usually are observed in the distal intestine (jejunum, ileum).[214,216,310] In calves, the most pronounced changes occur in the proximal intestine (duodenum, jejunum), but there are changes throughout the length of the small intestine.[145,218,262,275] In mice, the most pronounced changes are observed in the proximal to middle small intestine (duodenum, jejunum).[66,257,320] Pathologic lesions in rabbits are observed throughout the small intestine.[103,124,330] In calves and mice, infection appears to begin proximally and proceed distally.[136,218,220]

Rotavirus-induced lesions in the small intestine of large animal models (piglets, calves, lambs) appear to be the direct result of damage to epithelial cells caused by virus replication, because sites of replication usually correlate with the sites of pathologic changes.[79,260,310,328] The correlation of replication sites and lesions is less clear in mice because the pathologic process and virus replication is limited.[66,257,270,320] In rabbits, pathologic changes were observed throughout the small intestine, suggesting that replication is also generalized and not localized.[103,124,330]

Ultrastructural changes in infected epithelial cells are similar to those reported in cultured cells.[4,144,231,261,288] Changes vary from cell to cell, with normal enterocytes adjacent to damaged cells. Infected epithelial cells appear swollen, often show a disruption or loss of microvilli, and can be separated from the basement membrane of the villus. The ER appears distended and double-layered virus particles often are seen budding into the cisternae of the ER. Tubular viral structures are occasionally observed in the cytoplasm. Electron-dense viroplasms are observed in the cytoplasm of cells adjacent to regions of morphogenesis at the ER. Cells often contain many vacuoles that appear filled with lipid-like materials. Margination of nuclear chromatin and irregular or convoluted nuclear membranes have been reported.

Both murine and heterologous rotaviruses induce diarrhea in neonatal mice, but unlike other species examined, infection results in only mild histopathologic changes.[66,107,191,192,244,257,270,304,320] Villus atrophy and blunting, swelling and loss of enterocytes from villi, and mononuclear infiltration of the lamina propria are all quite limited. Crypt hyperplasia is not observed. In the mouse, vacuolation of enterocytes is more extensive and is often the most prominent finding. Infection of neonatal mice with murine viruses causes slightly more severe changes in the small intestine than infection by heterologous viruses. No histopathologic changes are observed in adult mice infected with murine rotavirus.[50]

Detection of infection by immunocytochemical staining or electron microscopy shows that scattered enterocytes rather than foci are infected by murine rotaviruses, and few cells are infected by this criterion in heterologous infections.[66,91,191,192,270,320] When infected cells are detected, they appear at the tips of the villus and appear to be limited to the proximal and middle small intestine.[66,257] Induction of diarrhea in neonatal mice with heterologous strains requires inoculation of very high doses, and studies indicate that both the virulence (DD_{50}) and SD_{50} of the murine strains are 10^4- to 10^5-fold lower than for heterologous strains.[50,110,270] The virtual absence of changes in the small intestine of mice that are readily infected and manifest diarrhea is a challenge to explain (see section on Mechanisms of Rotavirus Diarrhea Induction).

Pathophysiology of Rotavirus Infection

Tropism in the Infected Individual

Rotaviruses replicate in the nondividing mature enterocytes of the villus epithelium of the small intestine (see Fig. 30-1). This tropism suggests that differentiated enterocytes express factors required for efficient infection and replication. Whether differentiation of villus enterocytes results in expression of a viral receptor or some other cell product that allows permissive replication is not known. In vitro, rotavirus infection is promoted by proteolytic cleavage of the spike protein VP4,[3,11,104,133,208,328] and similar cleavage may be required for infectivity in vivo. The cleavage of VP4 does not affect binding to receptors, but is important for penetration of virus into the cell.[64,120,121,166] The low protease concentration in the immature GI tract has been suggested as an explanation for asymptomatic infections of very young neonates.

Studies using the heterologous simian virus RRV and crude enterocyte extracts showed that an enterocyte brush border glycoprotein of apparent molecular weight 300 to 330 kD bound the virus and VP4.[15] However, the protein's identity and direct proof that it functions as the rotavirus receptor are lacking. Similar studies using porcine virus in piglets identified a cell surface monoganglioside that would specifically compete with cells for virus binding.[280] Other studies have suggested that binding of rotavirus to cells in vitro occurs by two mechanisms, one sialic acid dependent and the other sialic acid independent. Animal strains of rotavirus appear to bind to receptors in both sialic acid-dependent and independent modes, whereas human virus strains appear to use only the sialic acid-independent mode.[119,223,384] The ability of animal viruses to use a sialic acid-independent mode of binding was demonstrated by the isolation of mutants that could efficiently infect cells from which sialic acid had been removed.[88] The identity of the rotavirus receptor or receptors is unclear.

The rotavirus viral attachment protein has been variously reported to be either of the outer capsid proteins VP4[78] or VP7[283] or the nonstructural protein NSP2.[16] The best evidence indicates that VP4 is the viral attachment protein because VP4 is required for binding of virus particles, or baculovirus-expressed virus-like particles (VLP), to cells,[41,78,195,266] and antibodies to the VP8* cleavage product of VP4 specifically block binding of virus to cells.[281]

Penetration of rotaviruses into host cells depends on proteolytic cleavage of VP4.[64,120,121,166] Several studies have shown that rotaviruses can enter cells by two mechanisms: direct penetration of the plasma membrane, which appears to be the permissive route,[166,324,325] and receptor-mediated endocytosis, which does not result in productive infection.[196,266,269] The route and kinetics of virus penetration is influenced by the cleavage state of VP4. Virus with cleaved VP4 enters the cell by direct penetration ($t_{1/2}$ = 3 to 5 minutes), whereas virus with uncleaved VP4 enters by endocytosis ($t_{1/2}$ = 30 to 50 minutes).[166,324] Additional support for productive virus entry by direct penetration related to VP4 cleavage includes 1) virus particles with cleaved VP4 are lipophilic for both liposomes and isolated cellular membrane vesicles[230,282]; 2) VP4 contains a highly conserved domain that shares homology with the fusion domains of alphaviruses[197]; 3) rotaviruses can mediate fusion of cells from without[108]; and 4) treatment of cells with inhibitors of endocytosis has minimal effect on infection with virus containing cleaved VP4.[166] Although these data support the hypothesis that virus entry occurs by a VP4 cleavage-dependent, direct penetration mechanism, all the evidence is indirect.

After penetration, uncoating must occur to allow transcription so that replication can proceed. A number of studies support the hypothesis that uncoating occurs when the entering virus particle encounters the low $[Ca^{2+}]$ environment of the cytoplasm, where the $[Ca^{2+}]$ falls below that required to maintain the integrity of the outer capsid.[67,196] Comparison of rotavirus infections in permissive and semipermissive cells, or of permissive and nonpermissive viruses in a single cell line, indicates that virus binding and internalization occurred but that there is a block in uncoating (S. Jafar and R. F. Ramig, unpublished data, 1995).[14]

Thus, it is possible that rotavirus tropism is determined both by binding of virus to receptor, and by a subsequent event such as penetration or uncoating, or both. In any event, it is clear that the spike protein VP4 must be proteolytically cleaved for productive infection to occur.

Infection at Extraintestinal Sites

Although rotaviruses primarily target the villus epithelium of the small intestine, this tissue tropism is not absolute and rotaviruses can initiate infections at extraintestinal sites. Pathologic lesions, isolation of infectious rotavirus, or detection of rotavirus antigen have been occasionally reported at extraintestinal sites in infected animals or humans. These sites include the lamina propria, mesenteric lymph nodes, lungs, liver, kidney, and bile ducts.[91,125,144,218,260,279,310,329,344] Extraintestinal infections are thought to play an insignificant role in disease because they are rarely observed and often are transitory.

Infection of mice with the heterologous simian RRV strain resulted in extraintestinal infection with spread of virus to the liver and resulting biliary atresia.[279,344] Hepatitis and death occurred in immunocompromised mice, and transient hepatitis was observed in malnourished and normal mice.[344] Subsequent in vitro studies with various animal and human virus strains indicated that some strains are capable of replicating in liver-derived HepG2 cells, whereas other strains are not.[178,271,295] Genetic experiments implicated VP4 as the determinant of growth phenotype in HepG2 cells,[271] and the restriction to growth of some strains was determined to be at the level of uncoating (S. Jafar and R. F. Ramig, unpublished data). The apparent tropism of rotaviruses to liver cells may explain findings of abnormal liver function associated with rotavirus diarrhea in children.[52,140,172,180,184] Additional evidence for liver infections in humans was obtained when the presence of rotavirus antigen was demonstrated in liver and kidney from immunocompromised children.[125] The use of RRV as a live-virus oral vaccine in children has raised concerns about safety, especially with regard to its use in developing countries where there is a higher prevalence of malnourishment and immune depression.[125,344] However, there have been no reports of long-lasting liver abnormalities or hepatitis after vaccination with RRV.

Neurologic symptoms, including encephalopathy and convulsions, have been reported in children with rotavirus diarrhea or rotavirus in their stool.[148,174,234,292,346] Whether the neurologic symptoms are the result of rotavirus replication in neurologic tissue is unknown. Rotaviruses can undergo at least limited replication in neuronal cells in vitro,[346,364,365] and direct inoculation of rotavirus into the brain and spinal cords of monkeys results in pathologic lesions.[89] Rotavirus RNA has been detected by reverse transcription and polymerase chain reaction in the blood and cerebrospinal fluid of children with concomitant convulsions and rotavirus diarrhea.[234,348] Electrolyte levels were normal in the cerebrospinal fluid of these patients, suggesting that the symptoms were not secondary to electrolyte imbalances associated with dehydration.[174,346]

Mechanisms of Rotavirus Diarrhea Induction

The pathophysiologic mechanisms by which rotaviruses induce diarrhea are unclear. Proposed mechanisms for induction of diarrhea by rotavirus include malabsorption secondary to enterocyte death, villus ischemia, and toxin-like effects of the nonstructural protein NSP4, or toxin-like effects of a viral structural protein. One or all of these proposed mechanisms may be important in the disruption of fluid homeostasis in the intestine that leads to diarrhea. The relative importance of each of these mechanisms may depend on a variety of viral and host factors.

Malabsorptive Diarrhea

Malabsorption secondary to enterocyte death is the most generally accepted mechanism of rotavirus diarrhea induction (see section on Viruses Associated With Gastroenteritis).

Diarrhea Resulting From Villus Ischemia

In mice, pathologic lesions are mild after infection with either homologous or heterologous rotaviruses, although severe diarrhea is observed in neonates.[66,257,270,320] Therefore, diarrhea is unlikely to result from malabsorption secondary to enterocyte destruction. Villus ischemia has been observed in mice with rotavirus-induced diarrhea.[257,320] In the absence of significant enterocyte damage, it has been proposed that diarrhea could result from virus-induced release of an unknown vasoactive agent from infected epithelial cells, causing a local villus ischemia and subsequent functional damage to, but not loss of, enterocytes.[257] Villus ischemia has not been described in rotavirus infections of other species, so the general significance of this observation is unknown.

Toxin-Induced Diarrhea

Although enterotoxins are important mediators of bacterial diarrheas, they have not been reported in viral diarrheas. However, studies have demonstrated that the nonstructural protein NSP4 (or a peptide representing amino acids 114 to 135 of NSP4) induced diarrhea in mice when administered by intraperitoneal or intraileal routes.[12] The induction of diarrhea by NSP4 protein or peptide showed the same age dependence as oral infection with native virus. Diarrhea was observed more quickly after administration of NSP4, but was of shorter duration, than after virus infection. Enterotoxin-like activity of the peptide was specifically blocked by anti-NSP4 or anti-peptide serum. Studies in vitro indicated that NSP4 induced intracellular $[Ca^{2+}]_i$ increases, and electrophysiologic studies of the small intestinal epithelium showed that NSP4 increased cyclic adenosine monophosphate-dependent Cl^- secretion.[12,332,333] A new model of rotavirus-induced diarrhea has been proposed in which there are two receptors for rotavirus, one for binding and entry of rotavirus and a second age-dependent receptor specific for NSP4. Virus entry through the first receptor would result in rotavirus gene expression but not necessarily productive infection or disease. Released NSP4 from the initial virally infected cell binds to its receptor and triggers a receptor-mediated signal transduction pathway, resulting in increased intracellular $[Ca^{2+}]_i$ and increased Cl^- secretion by the intestinal epithelium.[12,332,333] The diarrhea caused by the enterotoxin-like action of NSP4 would be of a secretory type, with water following the osmotic gradient established by the secretion of Cl^- ions. Older animals lacking the NSP4 receptor would be susceptible to rotavirus infection through the virus receptor, but would not be susceptible to diarrhea induced through the NSP4 receptor.

A toxin-like effect has been reported when high concentrations of psoralin-inactivated RRV were administered orally to mice and diarrhea was induced.[301] The diarrhea did not appear to result from incomplete inactivation of the virus because no detectable viral antigen was shed, and stool from the initially inoculated mice was not infectious for other mice. The mechanism and significance of this toxin-like effect remains to be determined, but the result suggests that a structural protein or proteins can have toxin-like activity.

Viral Factors Associated With Disease Severity

Virulent and avirulent rotavirus strains have been described in animals and humans, but the factors that control rotavirus virulence are not yet fully understood. It appears that virulence is multigenic and that a dynamic interplay of viral and host factors determines the clinical outcome of infection. In rotaviruses it is not yet possible to introduce changes into a gene and rescue the altered gene into infectious virus for use in infection studies. Therefore, investigations of virulence are limited to studies using genetic reassortants and strains that naturally vary in virulence, or to comparisons of the nucleotide and amino acid sequences of viruses.

Symptomatic Versus Asymptomatic Infections

Subclinical infections are common in humans and animals in both natural and experimental infections. Comparisons have been made between symptomatic (virulent) and asymptomatic (avirulent) infections to establish the determinants of clinical disease.[34,39,54,145,163,342]

Several studies in calves with homologous viruses have compared infection with virulent and avirulent strains.[34,37–39,145] There were no significant differences in the peak titers and duration of virus shedding, but the onset of diarrhea was earlier and small intestinal enterocyte involvement was significantly more extensive with virulent strains.[34,145] These results suggest that the virulent virus replicates more extensively than avirulent virus, resulting in sufficient lesions to induce diarrhea.[145] The age at which animals became refractory to disease differed among the rotavirus isolates, indicating that induction of clinical disease depends on both host and virus factors.[34]

Endemic infections are common in hospital newborn nurseries, and approximately 90% of these infections are asymptomatic.[27,62,228,356] The neonatal nursery strains were genetically stable and were found to share a VP4 that differs from VP4 of viruses causing symptomatic illness.[2,27,112,115,128,129] These results led to the hypothesis that nursery strains are naturally attenuated, and that the unusual VP4 might be related to virulence.[27,112,128,129,158] However, electropherotypically and serotypically identical rotaviruses have been isolated from both asymptomatic neonates and symptomatic older children in the same hospital ward, suggesting that asymptomatic neonatal infection may also result directly from host factors.[322,353]

Adaptation of rotaviruses to cell culture often results in attenuation of virulence.[34,39,50,289] Reversion of an avirulent virus to a virulent phenotype has been documented after sequential passage of the virus in the homologous large animal host.[36] Passage of avirulent virus in the mouse and rabbit models has not resulted in reversion to virulent phenotype (M. E. Connor, unpublished data).[43] The genetic changes responsible for the phenotypic changes in virulence are under investigation.[47,48]

Viral Virulence Determinants

The studies outlined previously demonstrated that, host variables being constant, there are viral factors that determine the virulence of rotavirus infection. Numerous attempts have been made to identify the viral virulence determinants using the reassortment strategy so elegantly applied in studies of reovirus virulence and pathogenesis.[338]

An initial study examined the genetic basis of virulence by comparing the virulence (DD_{50}) in neonatal mice infected with reassortants derived from two parental heterologous (bovine and simian) strains of differing DD_{50}.[239] Virulence was found to segregate with genome segment 4 (encodes VP4) from the more virulent parent. In another experiment using the neonatal mouse model, virulence could not be mapped to any single gene or gene constellation in reassortants derived from the heterologous virus strains SA11-4F and B223 (R. F. Ramig and D. Chen, unpublished data). However, these experiments must be interpreted with caution because both parental viruses were heterologous and replicated poorly in mice (see following discussion).

Subsequent studies attempted to overcome possible problems with heterologous viruses by using a highly virulent homologous virus as one of the parents for generation of reassortants. These studies suggest that virulence is multigenic and that the choice of viral strains and hosts may affect the constellation of genes determining virulence. In neonatal mice infected with reassortants derived from murine rotavirus (highly virulent) and heterologous simian RRV (low virulence), VP4 was not a determinant of virulence.[43] No single murine rotavirus gene was found to segregate absolutely with virulence. Genome segment 5, encoding NSP1, was significantly associated with virulence ($P < 0.008$) and segment 7, encoding NSP3, was weakly associated with virulence ($P < 0.027$). In the pig model, reassortants derived from the highly virulent SB-1A porcine strain and the avirulent human DS-1 strain were analyzed for virulence.[155] Transfer of any one of DS-1 genome segments 3 (VP3), 4 (VP4), 9 (VP7), and 10 (NSP4) onto the virulent SB-1A genetic background rendered the reassortant avirulent. Transfer of the combination of SB-1A genome segments 3 (VP3), 4 (VP4), 9 (VP7), and 10 (NSP4) onto the avirulent DS-1 genetic background converted the reassortant to the virulent phenotype. Transfer of any of the porcine genes singly, or in combinations of two or three, failed to generate virulent reassortants. Thus, virulence required the simultaneous presence of four genes from the virulent parent.

These studies have implicated genes encoding both structural and nonstructural proteins in virulence, and imply that virulence may be regulated at many levels, including binding, entry, and uncoating of virus, as well as at later stages in the replication cycle. Although the use of genetic reassortants is a powerful tool, results of segregation analysis must be interpreted cautiously because the recipient genetic background has been shown to affect the expression of particular phenotypes.[59,60,187] This suggests that any identification of virulence determinants made using a particular pair of parental viruses should be confirmed using a different pair of parental viruses.

Host Range

Rotaviruses have a broad host range in cultured cells, but natural transmission of virus between species has been difficult to document. The first clear indication that host range might be genetically determined came from extensive analysis of sequence data. NSP1 (genome segment 5) was found to be the most divergent of all the rotavirus gene products, varying from 36% to 92% amino acid homology. However, phylogenetic analysis revealed a clustering of NSP1 sequences according to species of origin.[100,159,380] This finding led to the hypothesis that NSP1 and segment 5 might be the host range determinant.

The ability to transmit infection to contact animals, a property usually observed only in homologous infections, has been used as a proxy to examine host range in reassortment experiments to identify the host range determinant. In the neonatal mouse model, genome segment 5 (NSP1) was found to segregate with transmission to a significant level,[43,194] although the association was not absolute. In contrast, in the rabbit model, a reassortant containing genome segment 5 from homologous ALA rotavirus and the other ten genes from the heterologous SA11 rotavirus replicated poorly in rabbits and was not able to spread to contact animals (M. E. Conner and R. F. Ramig, unpublished data). It is clear that additional studies will be required to identify further the host range determinants of rotavirus.

Host Factors Associated With Rotavirus Disease Severity

Enteric diseases often show variations that are related to host factors such as nutritional status, parasite load, immune function, level of exposure to enteric agent, age, and so forth.[306] Rotavirus infection and induction of diarrhea in both children and animals may be affected by a number of these host factors.

Malnutrition and Parasite Load in the Host

It is well documented that malnutrition can have profound effects on nonimmune and immune defense functions and the ability to rapidly repair intestinal epithelial cell damage.[306] Impairment of any of these functions may result in more severe rotavirus infections in malnourished children or animals.[146,321] Rotavirus infections in malnourished mice result in more severe diarrhea, a significant decrease in the incubation period and the minimal infectious dose, more extensive infection of enterocytes, and loss of mucosal barrier function with increased permeability and higher risk of spread of rotavirus to the liver and subsequent hepatitis.[227,235,254,278,345] Malnutrition also may be an important risk factor in children. In a prospective study of rotavirus diarrhea, malnourished children were more likely to be hospitalized with rotavirus-induced diarrhea.[82] Malnourished children had lower serum antibody titers to rotavirus and other enteric and respiratory pathogens than did well nourished children, suggesting that malnutrition may adversely affect the immune response and render children more susceptible to subsequent rotavirus infections.[47] Undernourished children have reduced levels of gastric acid and pepsin synthesis, which may reduce the gastric acid barrier to rotavirus infection.[306] Studies in neonatal and adult mice show that higher levels of gastric acid and pepsin in the adult mice reduce the infectivity of RRV.[13]

Concurrent infections of the intestine with rotavirus and other enteric pathogens can increase the severity of diarrhea. Synergistic infection and disease has been noted in mice, rabbits, foals, calves, and pigs infected with both a rotavirus and one of the following enteropathogens: coronavirus, E coli, Cryptosporidium species, or Salmonella species.[20,106,188,233,309,339-341] Similar synergy has been noted in concurrent infections in children.[303]

Age-Related Host Factors

Symptomatic rotavirus infection with dehydrating diarrhea is primarily observed in children between 6 to 24 months of age,[27] and in animals within the first 1 to 2 months of life.[287] A number of host-related factors that may contribute to the observed age distribution of rotavirus diarrhea are discussed in the following.

Age-Dependent Receptor Expression. Expression of a receptor functional for rotavirus must persist throughout life as evidenced by infection in all age groups (see Table 30-4).[27,34,72,122,287,302,362] The model proposed for the enterotoxin-like action of NSP4 may explain this conundrum. The proposed NSP4-specific receptor that leads to induction of diarrheal disease may be expressed in an age-dependent manner.[12] Thus, although the primary receptor used by rotaviruses to initiate infection may not be differentially expressed with age, a secondary receptor involved in disease induction may be age dependent and account for the severity of disease in the young.

Age-Dependent Protease Expression. Efficient entry of rotavirus into cells, followed by multiple rounds of replication, depends on the cleavage of VP4 by proteolytic enzymes. The production of proteolytic enzymes in the intestine is developmentally regulated, and concentrations increase with age. Rotavirus infections in newborns may therefore be less virulent because of decreased entry of rotavirus into enterocytes secondary to low levels of protease in the intestinal tract.[136]

Age-Dependent Mucin Expression. Mucus in the intestine serves as a barrier to prevent access of pathogens to the epithelium. The functional properties of mucins may vary with age because developmental changes in the terminal glycosylation of mucins have been documented.[306] Mucins in the intestine and in milk have been shown to inhibit rotavirus replication in vitro and to inhibit replication and reduce duration of diarrhea in mice.[58,382–384] Therefore, the composition of mucins in the intestine at the time of infection may play a role in determining the severity of rotavirus infection.

Age-Dependent Epithelial Cell Replacement and Fluid Absorption. The rate of replacement of intestinal epithelial cells can vary with age and between species, and be decreased in malnourished individuals.[226,306] The ability more quickly to repair or replace epithelium damaged by rotavirus infection may reduce the severity of diarrhea in older animals. Loss of fluids in the small intestine may be compensated by the ability of the large intestine to absorb the excess fluid. Fluid absorption in the large intestine increases with age, so that older animals may be able to resorb excess fluid and experience less severe diarrhea than younger animals.[226]

Host Immune Status

The neonate acquires passive immunity from its mother, either transplacentally or by ingestion of colostrum and milk (see Table 30-4). Because virtually all mothers have antibody to rotaviruses as a result of previous infections, rotavirus antibody is passively transferred to the neonate. The presence of sufficient levels of rotavirus antibody in the intestine from ingestion of milk can protect neonatal animals from rotavirus disease.[69,241,242,286,315–317] The role that passively transferred antibody plays in protection and prevention of rotavirus infection or disease in children is controversial. Comparisons of rotavirus infection and diarrhea rates in breast-fed versus non-breast-fed infants have not shown a clear and consistent protective role of maternal antibody, although less severe disease was associated with breast-feeding in some studies.[27,97,98,126,145,236,237] In contrast, two more recent studies indicate that breast-feeding reduces the severity and postpones rotavirus infection by several months.[65,206] Rotavirus infection of human neonates often is asymptomatic, but it is unclear if the lack of clinical symptoms is the result of the presence of maternal antibody or of the relative virulence of the rotavirus strains infecting neonates.[27]

Immune Response to Rotavirus Infection

Studies of the immune response to rotavirus infections in humans and animals are complicated by several factors. First, rotaviruses are ubiquitous and result in virtually 100% morbidity in young children and animals. This makes it difficult to study the primary immune response. Second, repeated infections are common, with secondary infections often involving different viral serotypes and leading to asymptomatic infection. The absence of information on previous serotypic exposure history, severity of previous infections, and interval since the most recent infection complicates interpretation of data.

Third, the primary site of rotavirus replication and immune response is the intestine, a relatively inaccessible site. Results from studies of rotavirus immune responses in natural infections of children and animals must be interpreted with these issues in mind. Experimental studies in animal models pose fewer problems, primarily because prior exposure can be controlled. However, the fact that the results may be influenced by factors such as the host species and age, virus strain and dose, and study design must be kept in mind.

Humoral Immune Responses to Rotavirus Infection

Studies in animal models indicate that rotavirus infection induces a rapid humoral immune response in both the intestine and serum, with production of IgM followed by IgG and IgA. Intestinal antibody has been detected as early as 3 days postinoculation, and by 1 to 2 weeks rotavirus-specific neutralizing and nonneutralizing antibodies and antibody-secreting cells are detected in the intestine and blood.[68,72,91,110,284,290,300,302,350] IgA appears to be the predominant intestinal isotype response in animals and humans, although IgG also has been detected in some studies.[68,72,75,76,141,150,193,236,237,289,300,302,350] The effect of immunizing dose on the magnitude of the immune response has been studied in rabbits and mice. Dose had little effect on the magnitude of the immune response after infection with homologous strains, presumably because efficient viral replication allowed an optimal antigenic load to be achieved.[73,110,139,212] In contrast, the magnitude of the immune response to heterologous virus strains is dose dependent.[110] The duration of the immune response after oral rotavirus infection exceeds 1 year in animal models.[73,302] The situation is somewhat different in children, in whom multiple infections usually occur during the first few years of life until the immune response exceeds a protective level.[27,61,75,76,141,206] Possibly this reflects the fact that primary infections in children occur in the presence of rotavirus antibody, whereas studies in animal models have pursued an understanding of immunity in naive animals.

Rotavirus Antigens

Oral or parenteral inoculation of animals with rotavirus elicits antibodies to both structural and nonstructural proteins. The most vigorous response is usually directed to the surface protein of double-layered particles, VP6. Anti-VP6 antibodies are, however, not neutralizing. The two proteins of the outer capsid layer, VP4 and VP7, both elicit neutralizing antibodies.[239] The relative roles of VP4 and VP7 in the immune response and protection are not understood, although sufficient levels of passively or actively acquired intestinal antibody to either protein confers protection from challenge.[6,99,156,198,207,243] The relative importance of VP4 and VP7 in induction of active immune responses has been difficult to measure and has not been clearly defined.[300,359,360,361]

A possible role for anti-VP6 antibody has been suggested after demonstration that administration of anti-rotavirus IgA monoclonal antibody, by a backpack tumor model in mice, protected from infection and cleared chronic rotavirus infection.[137,308] The same antibodies administered orally were not protective, and not all anti-VP6 monoclonal antibodies and none of the anti-VP4 monoclonal antibodies were protective in the model, so the significance of the observation remains to be determined.

Humoral Anti-Rotavirus Immunity and Protection From Disease

It is thought that immune protection from rotavirus disease is mediated by mechanisms that prevent invasion of susceptible enterocytes, that limit the spread of infection, or both. Passive immunization studies in animals demonstrated that serum neutralizing antibody alone was insufficient for protection, and that neutralizing antibody in the intestine was required.[241,242,315–317] Intestinal antibody, especially IgA, has been shown to be of primary importance in or a predictor of protection.[50,75,110] Epitope-specific responses to VP7 and VP4 also appear to correlate with protection from infection.[134,135,205,299]

Immunizations in animal models have shown that the primary neutralizing immune response is in general homotypic, and that the immune response does not broaden to include other serotypes to which the animal has not yet been exposed.[18,72,241,242,312,314] It appears that a homotypic response also develops in children after their first rotavirus infection.[27,61] Heterotypic immune responses are induced by some virus strains, suggesting these strains present a broader range of cross-reactive epitopes.[26,70,77]

No single immune correlate of protection has been identified. Because rotaviruses infect and replicate at a mucosal site, it is expected that induction of a local mucosal immune response will be most effective in protection. Indeed, both intestinal IgA and IgG have been shown to provide protection from rotavirus challenge in passive and active immunity models. However, in some studies heterotypic protection was observed in the absence of detectable neutralizing antibodies to the challenge strain in the intestine,[38,358,376] whereas in other studies heterotypic protection was not observed.[156,372] These conflicting results remain unexplained, although they may relate to the particular virus strains and doses used in primary inoculation and challenge. Heterologous simian RRV (G3, P3) and bovine neonatal calf diarrhea virus (NCDV) (G6, P1) rotaviruses were able to induce active protection in mice inoculated orally at 5 to 7 days of age, and challenged 6 weeks later with murine EHP (G3, P17).[110] Protection was virus strain and dose related, and the intestinal anti-rotavirus IgA titer correlated with protection. Thus, heterologous viruses that were able to induce intestinal anti-rotavirus IgA responses after primary infection protected from challenge. Doses of heterologous virus that induced disease, but failed to induce intestinal IgA, did not protect from challenge, indicating that there is little correlation between clinical disease per se and subsequent protection.[110,362] In contrast, both virulent and attenuated homologous murine viruses were highly effective inducers of intestinal IgA and serum IgG antibody and protection, regardless of immunizing dose.[50]

Oral inoculation with live, replicating virus is expected to induce the highest levels of antibody in the intestine and protection from rotavirus infection and disease. However, parenteral immunization with rotavirus or VLP can also induce intestinal antibody and protection. Parenteral immunization

with live or inactivated rotavirus, empty rotavirus capsids, or VLPs has been shown to induce active and passive protection from rotavirus challenge in mice and rabbits.[68,213,241,246,305] In rabbits, protection from rotavirus challenge was associated with the presence of IgG, but not IgA, in the intestine.[68–70] These results may correlate with data from sheep and calves, in which very high levels of circulating antibody can afford protection from rotavirus challenge.[23,315] The suggestion has been made that, in the young, protection may be mediated by IgG that "leaks" from the circulation into the gut, if the levels of circulatory IgG are sufficiently high.[68,151]

Cellular Immune Responses to Rotavirus Infection

Cell-mediated immunity is an important component of the immune response to rotavirus infections.[237,238] Most of the information on cell-mediated immunity comes from studies in mice, although studies in cattle substantially support the findings in mice. Most evidence indicates that cell-mediated immunity is important for clearance of viral infection, but plays an insignificant role in protection against disease.

Viral Antigens Eliciting Cell-Mediated Immunity

Rotavirus-specific cytotoxic T lymphocytes broadly cross-react with target cells infected with different rotavirus serotypes,[248] indicating heterotypic recognition of targets. Studies to identify the target antigen indicated that VP7 elicited splenic cytotoxic T lymphocytes at high frequency.[118,240] Other studies indicated that rotavirus-induced cytotoxic T lymphocytes recognized targets expressing VP4 or VP6 to levels slightly above background levels.[117,240] Thus, VP7 appears to be the primary target of anti-rotavirus cell-mediated immunity. However, the induction of cytotoxic T lymphocytes after immunization with baculovirus-expressed VP1, VP3, VP4, VP6, or VP7 has been reported,[90,117] indicating that the cytotoxic T-cell repertoire generated after rotavirus has the potential to be broader than suggested by the studies cited previously. An immunodominant cytotoxic T-lymphocyte epitope on VP7 has been identified that overlaps the H2 signal peptide of VP7.[118] The cross-reactivity of the cytotoxic T lymphocytes suggests that any other epitopes will lie in conserved regions of the protein.

The route of inoculation determined the site where cytotoxic T lymphocytes were first detected. Oral inoculation induced cytotoxic T lymphocytes at higher frequency in Peyer's patches than did parenteral inoculation.[238,245,247]

T-helper cells are also elicited after inoculation, either orally or parenterally, with live or inactivated rotaviruses.[45,238] T-helper cell responses have also been detected in humans.[250,251,337,381]

Cell-Mediated Anti-Rotavirus Immunity and Protection From Disease

Cytotoxic T lymphocytes have been implicated in protection from rotavirus disease in a limited number of studies involving passive transfer of T cells to naive mice.[249,253] However, studies using gene knockout (J_HD-deficient or β_2-

microglobulin–deficient) or immune-deficient (severe combined immunodeficient [SCID] or RAG-2) mice indicate that antibody, and not cell-mediated immunity, provides protection from infection and disease.[116] In addition, depletion of CD8+ lymphocytes or suppression of mitogenic responses in calves previously infected with rotavirus did not adversely affect protection from challenge, suggesting that cell-mediated immunity is not required for protection.[255,256] Thus, data support only a minor role in protection for cell-mediated immunity.

Cell-Mediated Anti-Rotavirus Immunity and Clearance of Infection

Severe combined immunodeficient and RAG-2 knockout mice lack both functional T and B cells. Infection of SCID or RAG-2 mice with rotavirus results in persistent infection with continued shedding of virus.[116,276] Adoptive transfer of rotavirus-specific major histocompatibility complex class I-restricted CD8+ T cells to persistently infected SCID mice results in clearance of the infection as assayed by cessation of virus shedding.[92] However, permanent clearance is mediated only by transfer of CD8+ cells from donors previously immunized by the intraperitoneal but not oral route.[92] More recent studies in J_HD-deficient or β_2-microglobulin–deficient mice indicate that CD8+ T cells play a role in virus clearance but are not required for this function.[116] β_2-Microglobulin–deficient mice that lack CD8+ T cells exhibit only slightly delayed clearance of virus infection. Antibody-deficient J_HD mice usually resolved virus infection normally, but when depleted of CD8+ T cells they shed rotavirus chronically. Therefore, resolution of primary rotavirus infection can be mediated by both antibody and CD8+ T cells. CD8+ T-cell–mediated clearance is heterotypic and not serotype restricted.[90] Finally, transfer of CD8+ T cells generated in animals immunized with baculovirus-expressed VP1, VP4, VP6, and VP7 can mediate clearance of persistent infection, whereas cells from animals immunized with VP2, NSP1, NSP3, or NSP4 do not mediate clearance. The mechanism by which CD8+ T cells mediate clearance has not been reported.

Vaccination Against Rotavirus Infection and Disease

The position of the group A rotaviruses as the cause of the most severe diarrheal disease in children has led to a focus on developing vaccination strategies and vaccines for rotavirus, and the following discussion concentrates on the vaccination problem for rotaviruses.

Complexity of Antigenic Structure

Rotaviruses are characterized by many different serologic types as determined by neutralization tests. Neutralization of rotavirus can be mediated by either of the two proteins (VP4 and VP7) that comprise the outermost capsid of the virion.[158,243] Reciprocal neutralization studies between various viruses have revealed that there are at least 14 distinct serologic types (serotypes or G-types) of VP7 and 10 distinct

serotypes (P-types) of VP4 (reviewed in Hoshino and Kapikian[154]). Furthermore, new G- and P-types continue to be identified. The situation is further complicated by the ability of the G and P antigens, encoded on separate segments of the segmented genome of rotavirus, to reassort into progeny viruses with new nonparental combinations of the G and P antigens.[158,243,272] Thus, the potential for diversity of neutralization types in the rotaviruses is high. The problem of antigenic diversity may be lessened by the fact that human G serotypes 1 through 4 are by far the most frequently isolated (>95%[204]).

Immune Correlates of Protection

Children previously infected with rotavirus are protected against severe disease after reinfection, suggesting immune protection.[24] The immunologic mechanisms responsible for the protection remain poorly understood. The current understanding of immune correlates of protection have been reviewed by Offit[236] and are summarized in the following. 1) Protective anti-viral neutralizing antibodies are directed at epitopes on both of the outer capsid proteins, VP4 and VP7.[158,243] 2) The presence of adequate levels of neutralizing antibody at the mucosal surface protects from disease. These antibodies can be present passively or actively induced at the mucosal surface by oral or parenteral immunization.[242,252,315–317] 3) Rotavirus-specific cytotoxic T lymphocytes are induced after infection or immunization,[247] and may play a role in heterotypic protection.[248] Cytotoxic T lymphocytes can also decrease the time of virus shedding and can clear persistent infections.[92] Thus, protection is associated with the humoral and cellular arms of the host immune system. The relative importance of each of these determinants is yet to be determined.

Vaccination Strategies

The disproportionate burden of diarrheal disease that falls on the young mandates that vaccination strategies be aimed at this population. However, there is a series of obstacles to effective vaccination of the young. Among these are the prevalence of the viral agents of diarrheal disease, so that potential vaccinees have a relatively high level of maternally derived antibody because of maternal boosting. This passively acquired antibody can decrease immune response to protein antigens and restrict replication of live attenuated-virus vaccines so that immunogenicity is decreased. Because infants are immunologically naive, vaccines must be extremely safe and nonreactogenic. A fine balance between attenuation and immunogenicity must be achieved if live attenuated-virus vaccines are to be used.[229]

The goal of rotavirus vaccination strategies is not the eradication of the disease, but the prevention of the severe, dehydrating diarrheas that lead to hospitalization or death.[167] Most efforts have concentrated on live attenuated-virus vaccines because it is postulated that a replicating antigen will provide a more effective stimulus to the host immune system, and will effectively stimulate production of local IgA in particular. These efforts and their results have been reviewed.[74,167,169,351] Here, we concentrate on strategies, and discuss results with specific vaccine candidates for which a clear picture has emerged.

Attenuated Human Rotaviruses as Vaccines

The earliest strategy for vaccination against rotavirus disease involved attenuation by tissue culture and animal passage, followed by safety and antigenicity testing of human rotavirus strain Wa. This approach was based on the observation that children convalescing from rotavirus infection often had neutralizing antibodies to additional serotypes besides the serotype that caused the infection.[379] More recently, in a different approach to attenuation of a human vaccine candidate virus, the human rotavirus strain M37 has been tested,[113,114] because it was isolated from the asymptomatic infection of a neonate and appeared to be naturally attenuated. The rationale for use of virus from asymptomatic infection as a vaccine strain was the observation that neonates in whom subclinical infections develop in the first 2 weeks of life are protected against clinically significant rotavirus diarrhea through 3 years of age.[24] However, in vaccine trials M37 had only limited efficacy and was withdrawn.[351,352]

The Jennerian Approach to Rotavirus Vaccination

The observation that calves infected with bovine rotavirus produced antibodies capable of neutralizing serotypically heterologous human strains[379] led to the approach of using animal rotavirus strains as surrogates for human viruses in vaccination strategies. This approach is called "Jennerian" in reference to Jenner's use of cowpox as a surrogate antigen to induce immunity to smallpox. This approach has the advantage that animal virus strains are often naturally attenuated in humans, or can be attenuated by relatively few tissue culture passages.[169] The Jennerian approach has been applied using several animal virus strains as vaccine candidates, including bovine virus strains RIT4237 and WC3 and the simian virus strain MMU18006.[74] These candidate vaccines have progressed through phase I and II and into field trials. None of these vaccine candidates has been found to protect from infection, and the protection from clinically significant disease has been variable. Although results of initial trials in developed countries appeared encouraging, none of candidate strains had acceptable efficacy in developing countries.[74] The RIT4237 and WC3 strains have been withdrawn,[351] and the MMU18006 and WC3 strains are being developed further using the modified strategy outlined next.

The Modified Jennerian Approach to Rotavirus Vaccination

The MMU18006 candidate strain showed reasonable efficacy in trials in which the challenge virus was human G serotype 3 strain, suggesting that this vaccine candidate was inducing serotypically homologous protection. This observation led to formulation of a multivalent approach in which the VP7 gene of MMU18006 was replaced by natural reassortment with the VP7 gene of human G serotypes 1, 2, and 4 (human G serotypes 1 through 4 are the most common serotypes associated with human disease, accounting for >95% of diagnoses). A mixture of MMU18006 (G serotype 3) together with reassortants carrying human VP7 genes representing G serotypes 1, 2, and 4 would constitute a tetravalent vaccine with the potential to induce immune response to G serotypes 1 through 4.[169] A major dilemma encountered in these trials was the failure to induce responses to all four components of the vaccine, but adjusting the doses of the individual components appears to have overcome this problem. Trials with both MMU18006 and WC3 tetravalent vaccines are underway and have shown promise against severe disease.[22,63,351] Although this approach is promising, the emergence of new serotypes of rotavirus in humans[83,84,123] suggests that incorporation of additional G serotypes into the multivalent vaccine may be necessary.

Antigen Expression From Replicating Nonrotaviral Vaccine Vectors

Replicating viral vectors or vaccines for other nonenteric diseases have the potential to express and induce antibodies to foreign antigens. Vaccinia virus[5] and adenovirus[130] have both been engineered to express rotavirus-neutralizing antigens. The vaccinia virus-based expression system has been used to immunize mice, and expressed wild-type VP7, or a construct with the VP7 gene modified so that VP7 was expressed on the cell surface, was able to induce protection in the passive protection model in mice.[6] An attenuated bacterial vector (*Salmonella typhimurium* SL32612) has been tested for expression of a VP7-β-galactosidase fusion protein, but anti-rotaviral antibodies were not detected after inoculation of mice with this vector.[291]

Nonreplicating Antigens for Rotavirus Vaccination

Nonreplicating antigen approaches to vaccination against rotavirus disease have the advantage of using noninfectious antigen, but it is difficult to present the immune system with sufficient amounts of antigen to induce a protective immune response. Several approaches are under evaluation:

1. Inactivated whole virus injected parenterally has induced protection in a rabbit model of active immunization.[68]
2. Expression of rotaviral VP7 or VP4 in bacterial expression systems, either alone or as fusion protein, and vaccination of animals with the product has resulted in the induction of low levels of neutralizing antibody,[8,10,209] but protection studies have not been reported.
3. Rotavirus VP7 has been expressed in the eukaryote *Dictyostelium discoideum*.[101] The expressed protein is antigenic, but immunogenicity has not been reported.
4. Rotavirus antigens have been expressed in the baculovirus expression system in eukaryotic (insect) cells.[198,273] The expressed proteins are made in high yield and have in general been immunogenic when semipurified protein was used to inoculate model animals. Baculovirus-expressed VP4 has been shown to induce passive protection from challenge in a mouse model system.[198]

5. Coexpression of combinations of rotavirus structural genes in the baculovirus expression system results in the assembly of the viral proteins into empty VLP.[78] VP2, VP4, VP6, and VP7 VLP have been shown to provide partial protection after vaccination of rabbits in an active protection model.[69,70]

6. Synthetic peptides representing rotavirus epitopes have been investigated as a potential approach to vaccination. Most peptides examined have been poorly immunogenic, suggesting that neutralizing epitopes of rotavirus are often conformational.[9] In one case, coupling VP4- or VP7-specific peptides to a carrier antigen before inoculation into mice resulted in passive protection against challenge in that model.[161,162]

7. DNA vaccination of mice with plasmids encoding either VP4, VP6, or VP7 has been reported to induce protection against murine virus challenge.[149]

SUMMARY AND CONCLUSIONS

Viral enteric infectious diseases cause a tremendous disease burden, especially on the young. The propensity of these viruses to cause more severe disease in the young makes the development of safe and effective vaccines a high-priority goal. Relatively little is known about most of the viruses in this group because many of them cannot be grown in culture. The application of new technologies to these viruses, particularly the noncultivatable viruses, is yielding useful information at an ever-increasing rate. The new data promise to reveal basic information on the pathogenesis of viral infections, as well as assisting in identifying correlates of protection that will be useful in rational vaccine formulation. Of particular importance are the identification of molecular mechanisms involved in the pathogenic process, identification of the humoral and cellular immune correlates of protection, and development of methods of effectively inducing local immune responses. These will be difficult problems, given the antigenic diversity that is characteristic of these viruses. However, the future is bright and it seems likely that results leading to rational vaccines or antivirals will emerge in the near future.

ABBREVIATIONS

ER: endoplasmic reticulum
G serotype: glycoprotein serotype
GI: gastrointestinal
HIV: human immunodeficiency virus
P serotype: protease-sensitive serotype
RRV: Rhesus rotavirus
SCID: severe combined immunodeficient
VLP: virus-like particles

ACKNOWLEDGMENTS

The authors thank the editors of this volume for their help and encouragement during the preparation of this chapter.

The work of the authors was supported by research grants AI16887, AI36385, and AI24998 from the National Institutes of Health, grant MIMV2718130 from the World Health Organization, and grant 004949-029 from the Texas Higher Education Coordinating Board Advanced Technology Program.

REFERENCES

1. Adams WR, Kraft LM. Epizootic diarrhea of infant mice: identification of the etiologic agent. Science 1963;141:359–360.
2. Albert MJ, Unicomb LE, Barnes GL, Bishop RF. Cultivation and characterization of rotavirus strains infecting newborn babies in Melbourne, Australia, from 1975 to 1979. J Clin Microbiol 1987;25:1635–1640.
3. Almeida JD, Hall T, Banatvala JE, Totterdell BM, Chrystie IL. The effect of trypsin on the growth of rotavirus. J Gen Virol 1978;40:213–218.
4. Altenburg BC, Graham DY, Estes MK. Ultrastructural study of rotavirus replication in cultured cells. J Gen Virol 1980;46:75–85.
5. Andrew ME, Boyle DB, Coupar BE, Whitfeld PL, Both GW, Bellamy AR. Vaccinia virus recombinants expressing the SA11 rotavirus VP7 glycoprotein gene induce serotype-specific neutralizing antibodies. J Virol 1987;61:1054–1060.
6. Andrew ME, Boyle DB, Coupar BEH, Reddy D, Bellamy AR, Both GW. Vaccinia-rotavirus VP7 recombinants protect mice against rotavirus-induced diarrhoea. Vaccine 1992;10:185–191.
7. Appleton H, Higgins PG. Viruses and gastroenteritis in infants. Lancet 1975;1:1297.
8. Arias CF, Ballado T, Plebanski M. Synthesis of the outer-capsid glycoprotein of the simian rotavirus SA11 in *Escherichia coli*. Gene 1986;47:211–219.
9. Arias CF, Garcia G, Lopez S. Priming for rotavirus neutralizing antibodies by a VP4 protein-derived synthetic peptide. J Virol 1989;63:5393–5398.
10. Arias CF, Lizano M, Lopez S. Synthesis in *Escherichia coli* and immunological characterization of a polypeptide containing the cleavage sites associated with trypsin enhancement of rotavirus SA11 infectivity. J Gen Virol 1987;68:633–642.
11. Babiuk LA, Mohammed K, Spence L, Fauvel M, Petro R. Rotavirus isolation and cultivation in the presence of trypsin. J Clin Microbiol 1977;6:610–617.
12. Ball JM, Tian P, Zeng CQ, Morris A, Estes MK. Age-dependent diarrhea is induced by a viral nonstructural glycoprotein. Science 1996;272:101–104.
13. Bass DM, Baylor M, Broome R, Greenberg HB. Molecular basis of age-dependent gastric inactivation of rhesus rotavirus in the mouse. J Clin Invest 1992;89:1741–1745.
14. Bass DM, Baylor MR, Chen C, Mackow EM, Bremont M, Greenberg HB. Liposome-mediated transfection of intact viral particles reveals that plasma membrane penetration determines permissivity of tissue culture cells to rotavirus. J Clin Invest 1992;90:2313–2320.
15. Bass DM, Mackow ER, Greenberg HB. Identification and partial characterization of a rhesus rotavirus binding glycoprotein on murine enterocytes. Virology 1991;183:602–610.
16. Bass DM, Mackow ER, Greenberg HB. NS35 and not VP7 is the soluble rotavirus protein which binds to target cells. J Virol 1990;64:322–330.
17. Beards GM, Hall C, Green J, Flewett TH, Lamouliatte F, Du Pasquier P. An enveloped virus in stools of children and adults with gastroenteritis that resembles the Breda virus of calves. Lancet 1984;1:1050–1052.
18. Beards GM, King JA, Mazhar S, Landon J, Desselberger U. Homotypic and heterotypic immune responses to group A rotaviruses in parenterally immunized sheep. Vaccine 1993;11:262–266.
19. Bell LM, Clark HF, O'Brien EA, Kornstein MJ, Plotkin SA, Offit PA. Gastroenteritis caused by human rotaviruses (serotype three) in a suckling mouse model. Proc Soc Exp Biol Med 1987;184:127–132.
20. Benfield DA, Francis DH, McAdaragh JP, et al. Combined rotavirus and K99 *Escherichia coli* infection in gnotobiotic pigs. Am J Vet Res 1988;49:330–337.

21. Bern C, Glass RI. Impact of diarrheal diseases worldwide. In: Kapikian AZ, ed. Viral infections of the gastrointestinal tract. 2nd ed. New York: Marcel Dekker, 1994:1–26.

22. Bernstein DI, Glass RI, Rodgers G, Davidson BL, Sack DA. Evaluation of rhesus rotavirus monovalent and tetravalent reassortant vaccines in US children. US Rotavirus Vaccine Efficacy Group. JAMA 1995;273:1191–1196.

23. Besser TE, Gay CC, McGuire TC, Evermann JF. Passive immunity to bovine rotavirus infection associated with transfer of serum antibody into the intestinal lumen. J Virol 1988;62:2238–2242.

24. Bishop RF, Barnes GL, Cipriani E, Lund JS. Clinical immunity after neonatal rotavirus infection: a prospective longitudinal study in young children. N Engl J Med 1983;309:72–76.

25. Bishop RF, Davidson GP, Holmes IH, Ruck BJ. Virus particles in epithelial cells of duodenal mucosa from children with acute non-bacterial gastroenteritis. Lancet 1973;2:1281–1283.

26. Bishop RF, Tzipori SR, Coulson BS, Unicomb LE, Albert MJ, Barnes GL. Heterologous protection against rotavirus-induced disease in gnotobiotic piglets. J Clin Microbiol 1986;24:1023–1028.

27. Bishop RF. Natural history of rotavirus infections. In: Kapikian AZ, ed. Viral infections of the gastrointestinal tract. 2nd ed. New York: Marcel Dekker, 1994:131–167.

28. Black RE, Brown KH, Becker S. Malnutrition is a determining factor in diarrheal duration, but not incidence, among young children in a longitudinal study in Bangladesh. Am J Clin Nutr 1984;39:87–94.

29. Black RE, Brown KH, Becker S, Alim ARMA, Huq I. Longitudinal studies of infectious diseases and physical growth of children in rural Bangladesh. II. Incidence of diarrhea and association with known pathogens. Am J Epidemiol 1982;115:315–324.

30. Black RE, Brown KH, Becker S, Yunus M. Longitudinal studies of infectious diseases and physical growth of children in rural Bangladesh. I. Patterns of morbidity. Am J Epidemiol 1982;115:305–314.

31. Black RE, Merson MH, Rahman MH, et al. A 2 year study of bacterial, viral and parasitic agents associated with diarrhea in rural Bangladesh. J Infect Dis 1980;142:660–664.

32. Brandt CD, Kim HW, Rodriguez WJ, et al. Pediatric viral gastroenteritis during eight years of study. J Clin Microbiol 1983;18:71–78.

33. Brandt CD, Kim HW, Rodriguez WJ, et al. Adenoviruses and pediatric gastroenteritis. J Infect Dis 1985;151:437–443.

34. Bridger JC. A definition of bovine rotavirus virulence. J Gen Virol 1994;75:2807–2812.

35. Bridger JC, Brown JF. Antigenic and pathogenic relationships of three bovine rotaviruses and a porcine rotavirus. J Gen Virol 1984;65:1151–1158.

36. Bridger JC, Burke B, Beards GM, Desselberger U. The pathogenicity of two porcine rotaviruses differing in their in vitro growth characteristics and genes 4. J Gen Virol 1992;73:3011–3015.

37. Bridger JC, Hall GA, Parsons KR. A study of the basis of virulence variation of bovine rotaviruses. Vet Microbiol 1992;33:169–174.

38. Bridger JC, Oldham G. Avirulent rotavirus infections protect calves from disease with and without inducing high levels of neutralizing antibody. J Gen Virol 1987;68:2311–2317.

39. Bridger JC, Pocock DH. Variation in virulence of bovine rotaviruses. J Hyg (London) 1986;96:257–264.

40. Bridger JC, Woode GN. Neonatal calf diarrhoea: identification of a reovirus-like (rotavirus) agent in faeces by immunofluorescence and immune electron microscopy. Br Vet J 1975;131:528–535.

41. Bridger JC, Woode GN. Characterization of two particle types of calf rotavirus. J Gen Virol 1976;31:245–250.

42. Bridger JC, Woode GN, Jones JM, Flewett TH, Bryden AS, Davies H. Transmission of human rotaviruses to gnotobiotic piglets. J Med Microbiol 1975;8:565–569.

43. Broome RL, Vo PT, Ward RL, Clark HF, Greenberg HB. Murine rotavirus genes encoding outer capsid proteins VP4 and VP7 are not major determinants of host range restriction and virulence. J Virol 1993;67:2448–2455.

44. Brown M. Selection of nonfastidious adenovirus species in 293 cells inoculated with stool specimens containing adenovirus 40. J Clin Microbiol 1985;22:205–209.

45. Bruce MG, Campbell I, Xiong Y, Redmond M, Snodgrass DR. Recognition of rotavirus agents by mouse L3T4-positive T helper cells. J Gen Virol 1994;75:1859–1866.

46. Brüssow H, Benitez O, Uribe F, Sidoti J, Rosa K, Cravioto A. Rotavirus-inhibitory activity in serial milk samples from Mexican women and rotavirus infections in their children during their first year of life. J Clin Microbiol 1993;31:593–597.

47. Brüssow H, Sidoti J, Dirren H, Freire WB. Effect of malnutrition in Ecuadorian children on titers of serum antibodies to various microbial agents. Clinics in Diagnostic and Laboratory Immunology 1995;2:62–68.

48. Burke B, Bridger JC, Desselberger U. Temporal correlation between a single amino acid change in the VP4 of a porcine rotavirus and a marked change in pathogenicity. Virology 1994;202:754–759.

49. Burke B, McCrae MA, Desselberger U. Sequence analysis of two porcine rotaviruses differing in growth in vitro and in pathogenicity: distinct VP4 sequences and conservation of NS53, VP6 and VP7 genes. J Gen Virol 1994;76:2205–2212.

50. Burns JW, Krishnaney AA, Vo PT, Rouse RV, Anderson LJ, Greenberg HB. Analyses of homologous rotavirus infection in the mouse model. Virology 1995;207:143–153.

51. Butz AM, Fosarelli P, Dick J, Cusack T, Yolken R. Prevalence of rotavirus on high-risk fomites in day-care facilities. Pediatrics 1993;92:202–205.

52. Carlson JA, Middleton PJ, Szymanski MT, Huber J, Petric M. Fatal rotavirus gastroenteritis: an analysis of 21 cases. Am J Dis Child 1978;132:477–479.

53. Castrucci G, Ferrari M, Frigeri F, Cilli V, Perucca L, Donelli G. Isolation and characterization of cytopathic strains of rotavirus from rabbits: brief report. Arch Virol 1985;83:99–104.

54. Castrucci G, Ferrari M, Frigeri F, Traldi V, Angelillo V. A study on neonatal calf diarrhea induced by rotavirus. Comp Immunol Microbiol Infect Dis 1994;17:321–331.

55. Caul EO. Human coronaviruses. In: Kapikian AZ, ed. Viral infections of the gastrointestinal tract. 2nd ed. New York: Marcel Dekker, 1994:603–625.

56. Caul EO, Clarke SKR. Coronavirus propagated from patient with non-bacterial gastroenteritis. Lancet 1975;2:853–854.

57. Chany C, Moscovici O, Lebon P, Rousset S. Association of coronavirus infection with neonatal necrotizing enterocolitis. Pediatrics 1982;69:209–214.

58. Chen CC, Baylor M, Bass DM. Murine intestinal mucins inhibit rotavirus infection. Gastroenterology 1993;105:84–92.

59. Chen D, Burns JW, Estes MK, Ramig RF. Phenotypes of rotavirus reassortants depend upon the recipient genetic background. Proc Natl Acad Sci U S A 1989;86:3743–3747.

60. Chen D, Estes MK, Ramig RF. Specific interactions between rotavirus outer capsid proteins VP4 and VP7 determine expression of a cross-reactive, neutralizing VP4-specific epitope. J Virol 1992;66:432–439.

61. Chiba S, Nakata S, Ukae S, Adachi N. Virological and serological aspects of immune resistance to rotavirus gastroenteritis. Clin Infect Dis 1993;16(Suppl 2):S117–S121.

62. Chrystie IL, Totterdell BM, Banatvala JE. Asymptomatic endemic rotavirus infections in the newborn. Lancet 1978;1:1176–1178.

63. Clark HF, Offit PA, Ellis RW, et al. WC3 reassortant vaccines in children. Proceedings of the Sapporo International Symposium on Viral Gastroenteritis, June 28–July 10, Tomakomai, Hokkaido, Japan, 1995. Arch Virol 1996 (in press).

64. Clark SM, Roth JR, Clark ML, Barnett BB, Spendlove RS. Trypsin enhancement of rotavirus infectivity: mechanism of enhancement. J Virol 1981;39:816–822.

65. Clemens J, Rao M, Ahmed F, et al. Breast-feeding and the risk of life-threatening rotavirus diarrhea: prevention or postponement? Pediatrics 1993;92:680–685.

66. Coelho KIR, Bryden AS, Hall C, Flewett TH. Animal model: pathology of rotavirus infection in suckling mice: a study by conventional histology, immunofluorescence, ultrathin sections, and scanning electron microscopy. Ultrastruct Pathol 1981;2:59–80.

67. Cohen J, Laporte J, Charpilienne A, Scherrer R. Activation of rotavirus RNA polymerase by calcium chelation. Arch Virol 1979;60:177–186.

68. Conner ME, Crawford SE, Barone C, Estes MK. Rotavirus vaccine administered parenterally induces protective immunity. J Virol 1993;67:6633–6641.

69. Conner ME, Crawford SE, Barone C, Estes MK. Rotavirus or virus-like particles administered parenterally induce active immunity. In: Proceedings of the Modern Approaches to New Vaccines, 11th Annual Meeting, Cold Spring Harbor, New York, September, 1994.

70. Conner ME, Crawford SE, Barone C, et al. Rotavirus subunit vac-

cines. Proceedings of the Sapporo International Symposium on Viral Gastroenteritis, June 28–July 10, Tomakomai, Hokkaido, Japan, 1995. Arch Virol 1996 (in press).

71. Conner ME, Estes MK, Graham DY. Rabbit model of rotavirus infection. J Virol 1988;62:1625–1633.

72. Conner ME, Gilger MA, Estes MK, Graham DY. Serologic and mucosal immune response to rotavirus infection in the rabbit model. J Virol 1991;65:2562–2571.

73. Conner ME, Graham DY, Estes MK. Determination of the duration of a primary immune response and the ID_{50} of ALA rabbit rotavirus in rabbits. 1996 (submitted for publication).

74. Conner ME, Matson DO, Estes MK. Rotavirus vaccines and vaccination potential. Curr Top Microbiol Immunol 1994;185:286–337.

75. Coulson BS, Grimwood K, Hudson IL, Barnes GL, Bishop RF. Role of coproantibody in clinical protection of children during reinfection with rotavirus. J Clin Microbiol 1992;30:1678–1684.

76. Coulson BS, Grimwood K, Masendycz PJ, et al. Comparison of rotavirus immunoglobulin A coproconversion with other indices of rotavirus infection in a longitudinal study in childhood. J Clin Microbiol 1990;28:1367–1374.

77. Coulson BS, Tursi JM, McAdam WJ, Bishop RF. Derivation of neutralizing monoclonal antibodies to human rotaviruses and evidence that an immunodominant neutralization site is shared between serotypes 1 and 3. Virology 1986;154:302–312.

78. Crawford SE, Labbe M, Cohen J, Burroughs MH, Zhou Y-J, Estes MK. Characterization of virus-like particles produced by the expression of rotavirus capsid proteins in insect cells. J Virol 1994; 68:5945–5952.

79. Crouch CF, Woode GN. Serial studies of virus multiplication and intestinal damage in gnotobiotic piglets infected with rotavirus. J Med Microbiol 1978;11:325–334.

80. Cubitt DW. Caliciviruses. In: Farthing MJG, ed. Viruses and the gut. London: Smith Kline & French Laboratories, 1989:182–84.

81. Cubitt DW. Caliciviruses. In: Kapikian AZ, ed. Viral infections of the gastrointestinal tract. 2nd ed. New York: Marcel Dekker, 1994: 549–568.

82. Dagan R, Bar-David Y, Sarov B, et al. Rotavirus diarrhea in Jewish and Bedouin children in the Negev region of Israel: epidemiology, clinical aspects and possible role of malnutrition in severity of illness. Pediatr Infect Dis J 1990;9:314–321.

83. Das BK, Gentsch JR, Hoshino Y, et al. Characterization of the G serotype and genogroup of New Delhi newborn rotavirus strain 116E. Virology 1993;197:99–107.

84. Das M, Dunn SJ, Woode GN, Greenberg HB, Durga Rao C. Both surface proteins (VP4 and VP7) of an asymptomatic neonatal rotavirus strain (I321) have high levels of sequence identity with the homologous proteins of a serotype 10 bovine rotavirus. Virology 1993;194:374–379.

85. Davidson GP, Barnes GL. Structural and functional abnormalities of the small intestine in infants and young children with rotavirus enteritis. Acta Paediatr Scand 1979;68:181–186.

86. Davidson GP, Bishop RF, Townlee RR, Holmes IH, Ruck BJ. Importance of a new virus in acute sporadic enteritis in children. Lancet 1975;1:242–245.

87. Davidson GP, Gall DG, Petric M, Butler DG, Hamilton JR. Human rotavirus enteritis induced in conventional piglets: intestinal structure and transport. J Clin Invest 1977;60:1402–1409.

88. de Leeuw PW, Ellens DJ, Straver PJ, van Balken JA, Moerman A, Baanvinger T. Rotavirus infections in calves in dairy herds. Res Vet Sci 1980;29:135–141.

89. Delem A, Berge E, Brucher JM, Lobmann M, Zygraich N. The neurovirulence of human and animal rotaviruses in cercopithecus monkeys. J Biol Standard 1985;13:107–114.

90. Dharakul T, Labbe M, Cohen J, et al. Immunization with baculovirus-expressed recombinant rotavirus proteins VP1, VP4, VP6, and VP7 induces CD8+ T lymphocytes that mediate clearance of chronic rotavirus infection in SCID mice. J Virol 1991;65: 5928– 5932.

91. Dharakul T, Riepenhoff-Talty M, Albini B, Ogra PL. Distribution of rotavirus antigen in intestinal lymphoid tissues: potential role in development of the mucosal immune response to rotavirus. Clin Exp Immunol 1988;74:14–19.

92. Dharakul T, Rott L, Greenberg HB. Recovery from chronic rotavirus infection in mice with severe combined immunodeficiency: virus clearance mediated by adoptive transfer of immune CD8+ T lymphocytes. J Virol 1990;64:4375–4382.

93. DiGiacomo RF, Thouless ME. Age-related antibodies to rotavirus in New Zealand rabbits. J Clin Microbiol 1984;19:710–711.

94. DiGiacomo RF, Thouless ME. Epidemiology of naturally occurring rotavirus infection in rabbits. Lab Anim Sci 1986;36:153–156.

95. Dingle JH, Badger GF, Jordan WS. Illness in the home: a study of 25,000 illnesses in a group of Cleveland families. Cleveland: Western Reserve University Press, 1964:19.

96. Doyle LP, Hutchings LM. A transmissible gastroenteritis in pigs. J Am Vet Med Assoc 1946;108:257–259.

97. Duffy LC, Byers TE, Riepenhoff-Talty M, La Scolea LJ, Zielezny M, Ogra PL. The effects of infant feeding on rotavirus-induced gastroenteritis: a prospective study. Am J Public Health 1986;76: 259–263.

98. Duffy LC, Riepenhoff-Talty M, Byers TE, et al. Modulation of rotavirus enteritis during breast-feeding: implications on alterations in the intestinal bacterial flora. Am J Dis Child 1986;140:1164–1168.

99. Dunn JD, Burns JW, Cross TI, et al. Comparisons of VP4 and VP7 of five murine rotavirus strains. Virology 1994;203:250–259.

100. Dunn SJ, Cross TL, Greenberg HB. Comparison of the rotavirus nonstructural protein NSP1 (NS53) from different species by sequence analysis and Northern blot hybridization. Virology 1994;203:178–183.

101. Emslie KR, Miller JM, Slade MB, Dormitzer PR, Greenberg HB, Williams KL. Expression of the rotavirus SA11 protein VP7 in the simple eukaryote Dictyostelium discoideum. J Virol 1995;69: 1747–1754.

102. Estes MK. Rotaviruses and their replication. In: Fields BN, Knipe DM, Howley PM, eds. Fields virology. 3rd ed. Philadelphia: Lippincott–Raven, 1996:1625–1654.

103. Estes MK, Conner ME, Gilger MA, Graham DY. Molecular biology and immunology of rotavirus infections. Immunol Invest 1989; 18:571–581.

104. Estes MK, Graham DY, Mason BB. Proteolytic enhancement of rotavirus infectivity: molecular mechanisms. J Virol 1981;39:879–888.

105. Estes MK, Hardy ME. Norwalk virus and other enteric calicivirus. In: Blaser MJ, Smith PD, Ravdin JI, Greenberg HG, Guerrant RL, eds. Infections of the gastrointestinal tract. New York: Raven Press, 1995:1009–1034.

106. Eugster AK, Whitford HW, Mehr LE. Concurrent rotavirus and Salmonella infections in foals. J Am Vet Med Assoc 1978;173: 857–858.

107. Eydelloth RS, Vonderfecht SL, Sheridan JF, Enders LD, Yolken RH. Kinetics of viral replication and local and systemic immune responses in experimental rotavirus infection. J Virol 1984; 50:947–950.

108. Falconer MM, Gilbert JM, Roper AM, Greenberg HB, Gavora JS. Rotavirus-induced fusion from without in tissue culture cells. J Virol 1995;69:5582–5591.

109. Farthing MJG. Gut viruses: a role in gastrointestinal disease? In: Farthing MJG, ed. Viruses and the gut. London: Smith Kline & French Laboratories, 1989:1–4.

110. Feng N, Burns JW, Bracy L, Greenberg HB. Comparison of mucosal and systemic humoral immune responses and subsequent protection in mice orally inoculated with a homologous or heterologous rotavirus. J Virol 1994;68:7766–7773.

111. Flewett TH. Search for new viruses. In: Farthing MJG, ed. Viruses and the gut. London: Smith Kline & French Laboratories, 1989: 96–100.

112. Flores J, Midthun K, Hoshino Y, et al. Conservation of the fourth gene among rotaviruses recovered from asymptomatic newborn infants and its possible role in attenuation. J Virol 1986;60:972–979.

113. Flores J, Perez-Schael I, Blanco M, et al. Comparison of reactogenicity and antigenicity of M37 rotavirus vaccine and rhesus-rotavirus-based quadrivalent vaccine. Lancet 1990;336:330–334.

114. Flores J, Preez-Schael BM, White L, et al. Comparison of reactogenicity and antigenicity of M37 rotavirus vaccine and rhesus-rotavirus-based quadrivalent vaccine. Lancet 1990;2:330–334.

115. Flores J, Sears J, Green KY, et al. Genetic stability of rotaviruses recovered from asymptomatic neonatal infections. J Virol 1988;62: 4778–4781.

116. Franco MA, Greenberg HB. Role of B cells and cytotoxic T lymphocytes in clearance of and immunity to rotavirus infection in mice. J Virol 1995;69:7800–7806.

117. Franco MA, Lefevre P, Willems P, Tosser G, Lintermanns P, Cohen

J. Identification of cytotoxic T cell epitopes on the VP3 and VP6 rotavirus proteins. J Gen Virol 1994;75:589–596.

118. Franco MA, Prieto I, Labbe M, Poncet D, Borras-Cuesta F, Cohen J. An immunodominant cytotoxic T cell epitope on the VP7 rotavirus protein overlaps the H2 signal peptide. J Gen Virol 1993;74:2579–2586.

119. Fukudome K, Yoshie O, Konno T. Comparison of human, simian, and bovine rotaviruses for requirement of sialic acid in hemagglutination and cell adsorption. Virology 1989;172:196–205.

120. Fukuhara N, Yoshie O, Kitaoka S, Konno T. Role of VP3 in human rotavirus internalization after target cell attachment via VP7. J Virol 1988;62:2209–2218.

121. Fukuhara N, Yoshie O, Kitaoka S, Konno T, Ishida N. Evidence for endocytosis-independent infection by human rotavirus. Arch Virol 1987;97:93–99.

122. Gelberg HB. Studies on the age resistance of swine to group A rotavirus infection. Vet Pathol 1992;29:161–168.

123. Gerna G, Sarasini A, Parea M, et al. Isolation and characterization of two distinct human rotavirus strains with G6 specificity. J Clin Microbiol 1992;30:9–16.

124. Gilger MA, Conner ME, Estes MK, Graham DY. Effect of rotavirus infection on rabbit small intestinal structure. Gastroenterology 1988;94:A-146

125. Gilger MA, Matson DO, Conner ME, Rosenblatt HM, Finegold MJ, Estes MK. Extraintestinal rotavirus infections in children with immunodeficiency. J Pediatr 1992;120:912–917.

126. Glass RI, Stoll BJ, Wyatt RG, Hoshino Y, Banu H, Kapikian AZ. Observations questioning a protective role for breast-feeding in severe rotavirus diarrhea. Acta Paediatr Scand 1986;75:713–718.

127. Goodell SE, Quinn TC, Mkrtichian PA-C, Schuffler MD, Holmes KK, Corey L. Herpes simplex proctitis in homosexual men: clinical, sigmoidoscopic and histopathological features. N Engl J Med 1983;308:868–871.

128. Gorziglia M, Green K, Nishikawa K, et al. Sequence of the fourth gene of human rotaviruses recovered from asymptomatic or symptomatic infections. J Virol 1988;62:2978–2984.

129. Gorziglia M, Hoshino Y, Buckler-White A, et al. Conservation of amino acid sequence of VP8 and cleavage region of 84-kDa outer capsid protein among rotaviruses recovered from asymptomatic neonatal infection. [Published erratum appears in Proc Natl Acad Sci U S A 1987;84:2062] Proc Natl Acad Sci U S A 1986;83:7039–7043.

130. Gorziglia M, Kapikian AZ. Expression of the OSU rotavirus outer capsid protein VP4 by an adenovirus recombinant. J Virol 1992;66:4407–4412.

131. Gouvea VS, Alencar AA, Barth OM, et al. Diarrhoea in mice infected with a human rotavirus. J Gen Virol 1986;67:577–581.

132. Graham DY, Dufour GR, Estes MK. Minimal infective dose of rotavirus. Arch Virol 1987;92:261–271.

133. Graham DY, Estes MK. Proteolytic enhancement of rotavirus infectivity: biology mechanism. Virology 1980;101:432–439.

134. Green KY, Kapikian AZ. Identification of VP7 epitopes associated with protection against human rotavirus illness or shedding in volunteers. J Virol 1992;66:548–553.

135. Green KY, Taniguchi K, Mackow ER, Kapikian AZ. Homotypic and heterotypic epitope-specific antibody responses in adult and infant rotavirus vaccinees: implications for vaccine development. J Infect Dis 1990;161:642–679.

136. Greenberg HB, Clark HF, Offit PA. Rotavirus pathology and pathophysiology. Curr Top Microbiol Immunol 1994;185:255–283.

137. Greenberg HB, Franco M, Feng N, Siadat-Pajouh M. Determinants of immunity to rotavirus in the mouse model. Proceedings of the Sapporo International Symposium on Viral Gastroenteritis, June 28–July 10, Tomakomai, Hokkaido, Japan, 1995. Arch Virol 1996 (in press).

138. Greenberg HB, Valdesuso JE, Kalica AR, et al. Proteins of Norwalk virus. J Virol 1981;37:994–999.

139. Greenberg HB, Vo PT, Jones R. Cultivation and characterization of three strains of murine rotavirus. J Virol 1986;57:585–590.

140. Grimwood K, Coakley JC, Hudson IL, Bishop RF, Barnes GL. Serum aspartate aminotransferase levels after rotavirus gastroenteritis. J Pediatr 1988;112:597–600.

141. Grimwood K, Lund JC, Coulson BS, Hudson IL, Bishop RF, Barnes

GL. Comparison of serum and mucosal antibody responses following severe acute rotavirus gastroenteritis in young children. J Clin Microbiol 1988;26:732–738.

142. Hall GA. Mechanisms of mucosal injury: animal studies. In: Farthing MJG, ed. Viruses and the gut. London: Smith Kline & French Laboratories, 1989:27–29.

143. Hall GA, Bridger JC, Brooker BE, Parsons, KR, Ormerod E. Lesions of gnotobiotic calves experimentally infected with a calicivirus-like (Newbury) agent. Vet Pathol 1984;21:208–215.

144. Hall GA, Bridger JC, Chandler RL, Woode GN. Gnotobiotic piglets experimentally infected with neonatal calf diarrhoea reovirus-like agent (rotavirus). Vet Pathol 1976;13:197–210.

145. Hall GA, Bridger JC, Parsons KR, Cook R. Variation in rotavirus virulence: a comparison of pathogenesis in calves between two rotaviruses of different virulence. Vet Pathol 1993;30:223–233.

146. Hall GA, Parsons KR, Waxler GL, Bunch KJ, Batt RM. Effects of dietary change and rotavirus infection on small intestinal structure and function in gnotobiotic piglets. Res Vet Sci 1989;47:219–224.

147. Hambraeus BAM, Hambraeus LEJ, Wadell G. Animal model of rotavirus infection in rabbits: protection obtained without shedding of viral antigen. Arch Virol 1989;107:237–251.

148. Herrmann B, Lawrenz-Wolf B, Seewald C, Wehinger H. 5th day convulsion of the newborn infant in rotavirus infections. Monatsschrift Kinderheilkunde 1993;141:120–123.

149. Herrmann JE, Chen SC, Fynan EF, Santoro JC, Greenberg HB, Robinson HL. DNA vaccines against rotavirus infections. Proceedings of the Sapporo International Symposium on Viral Gastroenteritis, June 28–July 10, Tomakomai, Hokkaido, Japan, 1995. Arch Virol 1996 (in press).

150. Hjelt K, Grauballe PC, Andersen L, Schitz PO, Howitz P, Krasilnikoff PA. Antibody response in serum and intestine in children up to six months after a naturally acquired rotavirus gastroenteritis. J Pediatr Gastroenterol Nutr 1986;5:74–80.

151. Hjelt K, Sorensen CH, Nielsen OH, Krasilnikoff PA. Concentrations of IgA, secretory IgA, IgM, secretory IgM, IgD, and IgG in the upper jejunum of children without gastrointestinal disorders. J Pediatr Gastroenterol Nutr 1988;7:867–871.

152. Ho M-S, Glass RI, Pinsky PF, Anderson LL. Rotavirus as a cause of diarrheal morbidity and mortality in the United States. J Infect Dis 1988;158:1112–1116.

153. Horowitz MS. Adenoviruses. In: Fields BN, Knipe DM, eds. Virology. 2nd ed. New York: Raven Press, 1990:1723–1740.

154. Hoshino Y, Kapikian AZ. Rotavirus antigens. Curr Top Microbiol Immunol 1994;185:179–227.

155. Hoshino Y, Saif LJ, Kang S-Y, Sereno MM, Chen W-K, Kapikian AZ. Identification of group A rotavirus genes associated with virulence of a porcine rotavirus and host range restriction of a human rotavirus in the gnotobiotic piglet model. Virology 1995;209:274–280.

156. Hoshino Y, Saif LJ, Sereno MM, Chanock RM, Kapikian AZ. Infection immunity of piglets to either VP3 or VP7 outer capsid protein confers resistance to challenge with a virulent rotavirus bearing the corresponding antigen. J Virol 1988;62:744–748.

157. Hoshino Y, Sereno MM, Midthun K, Flores J, Kapikian AZ, Chanock RM. Independent segregation of two antigenic specificities (VP3 and VP7) involved in neutralization of rotavirus infectivity. Proc Natl Acad Sci U S A 1985;82:8701–8704.

158. Hoshino Y, Wyatt RG, Flores J, Midthun K, Kapikian AZ. Serotypic characterization of rotaviruses derived from asymptomatic human neonatal infections. J Clin Microbiol 1985;21:425–430.

159. Hua J, Mansell EA, Patton JT. Comparative analysis of the rotavirus NS53 gene: conservation of basic and cysteine-rich regions in the protein and possible stem-loop structures in the RNA. Virology 1993;196:372–378.

160. Hung T, Chen G, Wang C, et al. Waterborne outbreak of rotavirus diarrhoea in adults in China caused by a novel rotavirus. Lancet 1984;2:1139–1142.

161. Ijaz MK, Alkarmi TO, el-Mekki AW, Galadari SH, Dar FK, Babiuk LA. Priming and induction of anti-rotavirus antibody response by synthetic peptides derived from VP7 and VP4. Vaccine 1995;13:331–338.

162. Ijaz MK, Attah-Poku SK, Redmond MJ, Parker MD, Sabara MI, Babiuk LA. Heterotypic passive protection induced by synthetic peptides corresponding to VP7 and VP4 of bovine rotavirus. [Pub-

lished errata appear in J Virol 1991;65:5130 and 1992;66:614] J Virol 1991;65:3106–3113.

163. Ijaz MK, Dent D, Haines D, Babiuk LA. Development of a murine model to study the pathogenesis of rotavirus infection. Exp Mol Pathol 1989;51:186–204.

164. Institute of Medicine. New vaccine development: establishing priorities. Washington, DC: National Academy Press, 1986.

165. Jiang X, Wang K, Graham DY, Estes MK. Norwalk virus genome cloning and characterization. Science 1990;250:1580–1583.

166. Kaljot KT, Shaw RD, Rubin DH, Greenberg HB. Infectious rotavirus enters cells by direct cell membrane penetration, not by endocytosis. J Virol 1988;62:1136–1144.

167. Kapikian AZ. Jennerian and modified jennerian approach to vaccination against rotavirus diarrhea in infants and young children. In: Kapikian AZ, ed. Viral infections of the gastrointestinal tract. 2nd ed. New York: Marcel Dekker, 1994:409–417.

168. Kapikian AZ. Norwalk and norwalk-like viruses. In: Kapikian AZ, ed. Viral infections of the gastrointestinal tract. 2nd ed. New York: Marcel Dekker, 1994:471–518.

169. Kapikian AZ. Rhesus rotavirus-based human rotavirus vaccines and observations on selected non-Jennerian approaches to rotavirus vaccination. In: Kapikian AZ, ed. Viral infections of the gastrointestinal tract. 2nd ed. New York: Marcel Dekker, 1994: 443–470.

170. Kapikian AZ, Chanock RM. Rotaviruses. In: Fields BN, Knipe DM, eds. Virology. 2nd ed. New York: Raven Press, 1990;1353–1404.

171. Kapikian AZ, Wyatt RG, Greenberg HB, et al. Approaches to immunization of infants and young children against gastroenteritis due to rotaviruses. Rev Infect Dis 1980;2:459–469.

172. Kapikian AZ, Wyatt RG, Levine MM, Black RE, Greenberg HB, Flores J, Kalica AR, Hoshino Y, Chanock RM. Studies in volunteers with human rotaviruses. Dev Biol Stand 1983;53:209–218.

173. Kaplan JE, Feldman R, Campbell DS, Lookabaugh C, Gary GW. The frequency of a Norwalk-like pattern of illness in outbreaks of acute gastroenteritis. Am J Pubic Health 1982;72:1329–1332.

174. Keidan I, Shif I, Keren G, Passwell JH. Rotavirus encephalopathy: evidence of central nervous system involvement during rotavirus infection. Pediatr Infect Dis J 1992;11:773–775.

175. Keusch GT, Scrimshaw NS. Selective primary health care: strategies for control of disease in the developing world. XXII. The control of infection to reduce the prevalence of infantile and childhood malnutrition. Rev Infect Dis 1986;8:273–287.

176. Khoshoo V, Bhan MK, Jayashree S, Kumar R, Glass RI. Rotavirus infection and persistent diarrhoea in young children. Lancet 1990;336:1314–1315.

177. Kidd AH, Madeley CR. In vitro growth of some fastidious adenoviruses from stool specimens. J Clin Pathol 1981;34:213–216.

178. Kitamoto N, Ramig RF, Matson DO, Estes MK. Comparative growth of different rotavirus strains in differentiated cells (MA104, HepG2, and CaCo-2). Virology 1991;184:729–737.

179. Klatt EC, Shibata D. Cytomegalovirus infection in the acquired immunodeficiency syndrome: clinical and autopsy findings. Arch Pathol Lab Med 1988;112:540–544.

180. Konno T, Suzuki H, Imai A, Ishida N. Reovirus-like agent in acute epidemic gastroenteritis in Japanese infants: fecal shedding and serologic response. J Infect Dis 1977;135:259–266.

181. Konno T, Suzuki H, Katsushima N, et al. Influence of temperature and relative humidity on human rotavirus infection in Japan. J Infect Dis 1983;147:125–128

182. Kotler DP, Culpepper-Morgan JA, Tierny AR, Klein EB. Treatment of disseminated cytomegalovirus infection with 9-(1,3-dihydroxy-2-propoxymethyl) guanine: evidence of prolonged survival in patients with the acquired immunodeficiency syndrome. AIDS Res 1986;2:299–308.

183. Kotler DP, Gaetz HP, Lange M, Klein EB, Holt PR. Enteropathy associated the the acquired immunodeficiency syndrome. Ann Intern Med 1984;101:421–428.

184. Kovacs A, Chan L, Hotrakitya C, Overturf G, Portnoy B. Serum transaminase elevations in infants with rotavirus gastroenteritis. J Pediatr Gastroenterol Nutr 1986;5:873–877.

185. Kraft LM. Studies on the etiology and transmission of epidemic diarrhea of infant mice. J Exp Med 1957;106:743–755.

186. Kurtz JB. Astroviruses. In: Kapikian AZ, ed. Viral infections of the gastrointestinal tract. 2nd ed. New York: Marcel Dekker, 1994:569–580.

187. Lazdins I, Coulson BS, Kirkwood C, et al. Rotavirus antigenicity is affected by the genetic context and glycosylation of VP7. Virology 1995;209:80–89.

188. Lecce JG, Balsbaugh RK, Clare DA, King MW. Rotavirus and hemolytic enteropathogenic Escherichia coli in weanling diarrhea of pigs. J Clin Microbiol 1982;16:715–723.

189. Lecce JG, King MW, Dorsey WE. Rearing regimen producing piglet diarrhea (rotavirus) and its relevance to acute infantile diarrhea. Science 1978;199:776–778.

190. Lew JF, Kapikian AZ, Jiang X, Estes MK, Green KY. Identification of "minireovirus" as a Norwalk-like virus in pediatric patients with gastroenteritis. J Virol 1994;68:3391–3396.

191. Little LM, Shadduck JA. Pathogenesis of rotavirus infection in mice. Infect Immun 1982;38:755–763.

192. Little LM, Shadduck JA. Pathogenesis of rotavirus infections. Prog Food Nutr Sci 1983;7:179–187.

193. Losonsky GA, Reymann M. The immune response in primary asymptomatic and symptomatic rotavirus infection in newborn infants. J Infect Dis 1990;161:330–332.

194. Ludert JE, Broome RL, Feng N, Greenberg HB. Comparison of homologous and heterologous rotavirus infection in mouse intestinal loops. In: Proceedings of the American Society for Virology, 14th Annual Meeting, Austin, TX, July 8–12, 1995. Abstract.

195. Ludert JE, Feng N, Yu JH, Broome RL, Hoshino Y, Greenberg HB. Genetic mapping indicates that VP4 is the rotavirus cell attachment protein in vitro and in vivo. J Virol 1995 (in press).

196. Ludert JE, Michelangeli F, Gil F, Liprandi F, Esparza J. Penetration and uncoating of rotaviruses in cultured cells. Intervirology 1987;27:95–101.

197. Mackow ER, Shaw RD, Matsui SM, Vo PT, Dang MN, Greenberg HB. The rhesus rotavirus gene encoding protein VP3: location of amino acids involved in homologous and heterologous rotavirus neutralization and identification of a putative fusion region. Proc Natl Acad Sci U S A 1988;85:645–649.

198. Mackow ER, Vo PT, Broome R, Bass D, Greenberg HB. Immunization with baculovirus-expressed VP4 protein passively protects against simian and murine rotavirus challenge. J Virol 1990; 64:1698–1703.

199. Madeley CR. Epidemiology and clinical impact of gut viruses. In: Farthing MJG, ed. Viruses and the gut. London: Smith Kline & French Laboratories, 1989:5–15.

200. Mata L. Diarrheal disease as a cause of malnutrition. Am J Trop Med Hyg 1992;47(Suppl):16–27.

201. Mata L, Jimenez P, Allen MA. Diarrhea and malnutrition: breast feeding intervention in a transitional population. In: Holme T, Holmgren J, Merson, MH, Mollby R., eds. Acute Enteric Infections in Children: New Prospects for Treatment and Prevention, New York, Elsevier, 1981; 233–251.

202. Mata L, Simhon A, Urrutia JJ, Kronmal RA. Natural history of rotavirus infection in the children of Santa Maria Cauque. Prog Food Nutr Sci 1983;7:167–177.

203. Mata L, Simhon A, Urrutia JJ, Kronmal RA, Fernandez R, Garcia B. Epidemiology of rotaviruses in a cohort of 45 Guatemalan Mayan Indian children observed from birth to the age of three years. J Infect Dis 1983;148:452–461.

204. Matson DO, Estes MK, Burns JW, Greenberg HB, Taniguchi K, Urasawa S. Serotype variation of human group A rotaviruses in two regions of the USA. J Infect Dis 1990;162:605–614.

205. Matson DO, O'Ryan ML, Pickering LK, et al. Characterization of serum antibody responses to natural rotavirus infections in children by VP7-specific epitope-blocking assays. J Clin Microbiol 1992;30:1056–1061.

206. Matson DO, Velazquez FR, Calva JJ, et al. Protective immunity against group A rotavirus infection and illness in infants. Proceedings of the Sapporo International Symposium on Viral Gastroenteritis, June 28–July 10, Tomakomai, Hokkaido, Japan, 1995. Arch Virol 1996 (in press).

207. Matsui SM, Offit PA, Vo PT, et al. Passive protection against rotavirus-induced diarrhea by monoclonal antibodies to the heterotypic neutralization domain of VP7 and the VP8 fragment of VP4. J Clin Microbiol 1989;27:780–782.

208. Matsuno S, Inouye S, Kono R. Plaque assay of neonatal calf diar-

rhea virus and the neutralizing antibody in human sera. J Clin Microbiol 1977;5:1–4.

209. McCrae MA, McCorquodale JG. Expression of a major bovine rotavirus neutralisation antigen (VP7c) in *Escherichia coli*. Gene 1987;55:9–18.

210. McGhee JR, Kiyono H. Mucosal immunity to vaccines: current concepts for vaccine development and immune response analysis. In: Ciardi JE, ed. Genetically engineered vaccines. New York: Plenum Press, 1992:3–12.

211. McLoughlin LC, Nord KS, Joshi VV, Oleske JM, Conner EM. Severe gastrointestinal involvement in children with acquired immunodeficiency syndrome. J Pediatr Gastroenterol Nutr 1987;6:517–524.

212. McNeal MM, Broome RL, Ward RL. Active immunity against rotavirus infection in mice is correlated with viral replication and titers of serum rotavirus IgA following vaccination. Virology 1994;204:642–650.

213. McNeal MM, Sheridan JF, Ward RL. Active protection against rotavirus infection of mice following intraperitoneal immunization. Virology 1992;191:150–157.

214. McNulty MS, Allan GM, Pearson GR, McFerran JB, Curran WL, McCracken RM. Reovirus-like agent (rotavirus) from lambs. Infect Immun 1976;14:1332–1338.

215. McNulty MS, Logan EF. Longitudinal survey of rotavirus infection in calves. Vet Rec 1983;113:333–335.

216. McNulty MS, Pearson GR, McFerran JB, Collins DS, Allan GM. A reovirus-like agent (rotavirus) associated with diarrhoea in neonatal pigs. Vet Microbiol 1976;1:55–63.

217. Mebus CA, Rhodes MB, Underdahl NR. Neonatal calf diarrhea caused by a virus that induces villous epithelial cell syncytia. Am J Vet Res 1978;39:1223–1228.

218. Mebus CA, Stair EL, Underdahl NR, Twiehaus MJ. Pathology of neonatal calf diarrhea induced by a reo-like virus. Vet Pathol 1971;8:490–505.

219. Mebus CA, Underdahl NR, Rhodes MB, Twiehaus MJ. Calf diarrhea (scours): reproduced with a virus from a field outbreak. Nebraska Agricultural Experimental Station Research Bulletin 1969;223:2–16.

220. Mebus CA, Wyatt RG, Kapikian AZ. Intestinal lesions induced in gnotobiotic calves by the virus of human infantile gastroenteritis. Vet Pathol 1977;14:273–282.

221. Mebus CA, Wyatt RG, Sharpee RL, et al. Diarrhea in gnotobiotic calves caused by the reovirus-like agent of human infantile gastroenteritis. Infect Immun 1976;14:471–474.

222. Melnick JL. Enteroviruses: polioviruses, coxsackieviruses, echoviruses, and newer enteroviruses. In: Fields BN, Knipe DM, eds. Virology. 2nd ed. New York: Raven Press, 1990:549–605.

223. Mendez E, Arias CF, Lopez S. Binding of sialic acids is not an essential step for the entry of animal rotaviruses to epithelial cells in culture. J Virol 1994;67:5253–5259.

224. Middleton PJ, Petric M, Szymanski MT. Propagation of infantile gastroenteritis virus (orbi-group) in conventional and germfree piglets. Infect Immun 1975;12:1276–1280.

225. Miller ARO, Griffin GE, Batman PA, et al. Jejunal mucosal architecture and fat absorption in male homosexuals infected with human immunodeficiency virus. QJM 1988;69:1009–1019.

226. Moon HW. Pathophysiology of viral diarrhea. In: Kapikian AZ, ed. Viral infections of the gastrointestinal tract. 2nd ed. New York: Marcel Dekker, 1994:27–52.

227. Morrey JD, Sidwell RW, Noble RL, Barnett BB, Mahoney AW. Effects of folic acid malnutrition on rotaviral infection in mice. Proc Soc Exp Biol Med 1984;176:77–83.

228. Murphy AM, Albrey MB, Hay PJ. Rotavirus infections in neonates. Lancet 1975;2:452–453. Letter.

229. Murphy BR, Chanock RM. Immunization against viruses. In: Fields BN, Knipe DM, eds. Virology. 2nd ed. New York: Raven Press, 1990:469–502.

230. Nandi P, Charpilienne A, Cohen J. Interaction of rotavirus particles with liposomes. J Virol 1992;66:3363–3367.

231. Narita M, Fukusho A, Shimizu Y. Electron microscopy of the intestine of gnotobiotic piglets infected with porcine rotavirus. J Comp Pathol 1982;92:589–597.

232. Nelson JA, Clayton AW. Human immunodeficiency virus detected in bowel epithelium from patients with gastrointestinal symptoms. Lancet 1988;1;259–262.

233. Newsome PM, Coney KA. Synergistic rotavirus and *Escherichia coli* diarrheal infection of mice. Infect Immun 1985;47:573–574.

234. Nishimura S, Ushijima H, Shiraishi H, et al. Detection of rotavirus in cerebrospinal fluid and blood of patients with convulsions and gastroenteritis by means of the reverse transcription polymerase chain reaction. Brain Dev 1993;15:457–459.

235. Noble RL, Sidwell RW, Mahoney AW, Barnett BB, Spendlove RS. Influence of malnutrition and alterations in dietary protein on murine rotaviral disease. Proc Soc Exp Biol Med 1983;173:417–426.

236. Offit PA. Immunologic determinants of protection against rotavirus disease. Curr Top Microbiol Immunol 1994;185:229–254.

237. Offit PA. Rotaviruses: immunological determinants of protection against infection and disease. Adv Virus Res 1994;44:161–202.

238. Offit PA. Virus-specific cellular immune response to intestinal infection. In: Kapikian AZ, ed. Viral infections of the gastrointestinal tract. 2nd ed. New York: Marcel Dekker, 1994:89–100.

239. Offit PA, Blavat G, Greenberg HB, Clark HF. Molecular basis of rotavirus virulence: role of gene segment 4. J Virol 1986;57:46–49.

240. Offit PA, Boyle DB, Both GW, et al. Outer capsid glycoprotein VP7 is recognized by cross-reactive, rotavirus-specific, cytotoxic T lymphocytes. Virology 1991;184:563–568.

241. Offit PA, Clark HF. Maternal antibody-mediated protection against gastroenteritis due to rotavirus in newborn mice is dependent on both serotype and titer of antibody. J Infect Dis 1985;152:1152–1158.

242. Offit PA, Clark HF. Protection against rotavirus-induced gastroenteritis in a murine model by passively acquired gastrointestinal but not circulating antibodies. J Virol 1985;54:58–64.

243. Offit PA, Clark HF, Blavat G, Greenberg HB. Reassortant rotaviruses containing structural proteins VP3 and VP7 from different parents induce antibodies protective against each parental serotype. J Virol 1986;60:491–496.

244. Offit PA, Clark HF, Kornstein MJ, Plotkin SA. A murine model for oral infection with a primate rotavirus (simian SA11). J Virol 1984;51:233–236.

245. Offit PA, Cunningham SL, Dudzik KI. Memory and distribution of virus-specific cytotoxic T lymphocytes (CTLs) and CTL precursors after rotavirus infection. J Virol 1991;65:1318–1324.

246. Offit PA, Dudzik KI. Noninfectious rotavirus (strain RRV) induces an immune response in mice which protects against rotavirus challenge. J Clin Microbiol 1989;27:885–888.

247. Offit PA, Dudzik KI. Rotavirus-specific cytotoxic T lymphocytes appear at the intestinal mucosal surface after rotavirus infection. J Virol 1989;63:3507–3512.

248. Offit PA, Dudzik KI. Rotavirus-specific cytotoxic T lymphocytes cross-react with target cells infected with different rotavirus serotypes. J Virol 1988;62:127–131.

249. Offit PA, Dudzik KI. Rotavirus-specific cytotoxic T lymphocytes passively protect against gastroenteritis in suckling mice. J Virol 1990;64:6325–6328.

250. Offit PA, Hoffenberg EJ, Pia ES, Panackal PA, Hill NL. Rotavirus-specific helper T cell responses in newborns, infants, children, and adults. J Infect Dis 1992;165:1107–1111.

251. Offit PA, Hoffenberg EJ, Santos N, Gouvea V. Rotavirus-specific humoral and cellular immune response after primary, symptomatic infection. J Infect Dis 1993;167:1436–1440.

252. Offit PA, Shaw RD, Greenberg HB. Passive protection against rotavirus-induced diarrhea by monoclonal antibodies to surface proteins vp3 and vp7. J Virol 1986;58:700–703.

253. Offit PA, Svoboda YM. Rotavirus-specific cytotoxic T lymphocyte response of mice after oral inoculation with candidate rotavirus vaccine strains RRV or WC3. J Infect Dis 1989;160:783–788.

254. Offor E, Riepenhoff-Talty M, Ogra PL. Effect of malnutrition on rotavirus infection in suckling mice: kinetics of early infection. Proc Soc Exp Biol Med 1985;178:85–90.

255. Oldham G, Bridger JC. The effect of dexamethasone-induced immunosuppression on the development of faecal antibody and recovery from and resistance to rotavirus infection. Vet Immunol Immunopathol 1992;32:77–92.

256. Oldham G, Bridger JC, Howard CJ, Parsons KR. In vivo role of

lymphocyte subpopulations in the control of virus excretion and mucosal antibody responses of cattle infected with rotavirus. J Virol 1993;67:5012–5019.

257. Osborne MP, Haddon SJ, Spencer AJ, et al. An electron microscopic investigation of time-related changes in the intestine of neonatal mice infected with murine rotavirus. J Pediatr Gastroenterol Nutr 1988;7:236–248.

258. Pattison JR. Parvoviruses. In: Fields BN, Knipe DM, eds. Virology. 2nd ed. New York: Raven Press, 1990:1765–1784

259. Payment P, Morin É. Minimal infective dose of the OSU strain of porcine rotavirus. Arch Virol 1990;112:277–282.

260. Pearson GR, McNulty MS. Pathological changes in the small intestine of neonatal pigs infected with a pig reovirus-like agent (rotavirus). J Comp Pathol 1977;87:363–375.

261. Pearson GR, McNulty MS. Ultrastructural changes in small intestinal epithelium of neonatal pigs infected with pig rotavirus. Arch Virol 1979;59:127–136.

262. Pearson GR, McNulty MS, Logan EF. Pathological changes in the small intestine of neonatal calves naturally infected with reo-like virus (rotavirus). Vet Rec 1978;102:454–458.

263. Pensaert M, Callebaut P, Cox E. Enteric coronaviruses of animals. In: Kapikian AZ, ed. Viral infections of the gastrointestinal tract. 2nd ed. New York: Marcel Dekker, 1994:627–696.

264. Pereira HG, Fialho AM, Flewett TH, Telxeira JM, Andrade ZP. Novel viruses in human feces. Lancet 1988;2:103–104.

265. Petric M, Middleton PJ, Grant C, Tam JS, Hewitt CM. Lapine rotavirus: preliminary studies on epizoology and transmission. Canadian Journal of Comparative Medicine 1978;42:143–147.

266. Petrie BL, Graham DY, Estes MK. Identification of rotavirus particle types. Intervirology 1981;16:20–28.

267. Phillips AD. Mechanisms of mucosal injury: human studies. In: Farthing MJG, ed. Viruses and the gut. London: Smith Kline & French Laboratories, 1989:30–40.

268. Prasad BVV, Chiu W. Structure of rotaviruses. In: Ramig R, ed. Rotaviruses. Berlin: Springer-Verlag, 1994:9–29.

269. Quan CM, Doane FW. Ultrastructural evidence for the cellular uptake of rotavirus by endocytosis. Intervirology 1983;20:223–231.

270. Ramig RF. The effects of host age, virus dose, and virus strain on heterologous rotavirus infection of suckling mice. Microb Pathog 1988;4:189–202.

271. Ramig RF, Galle KL. Rotavirus genome segment 4 determines viral replication phenotype in cultured liver cells (HepG2). J Virol 1990; 64:1044–1049.

272. Ramig RF, Ward RL. Genomic segment reassortment in rotaviruses and other reoviridae. Adv Virus Res 1991;39:163–208.

273. Redmond MJ, Ijaz MK, Parker MD, et al. Assembly of recombinant rotavirus proteins into virus-like particles and assessment of vaccine potential. Vaccine 1993;11:273–281.

274. Resta S, Luby JP, Rosenfeld CR, Seigel JD. Isolation and propagation of a human enteric coronavirus. Science 1985;229:978–981.

275. Reynolds DJ, Hall GA, Debney TG, Parsons KR. Pathology of natural rotavirus infection in clinically normal calves. Res Vet Sci 1985;38:264–269.

276. Riepenhoff-Talty M, Dharakul T, Kowalski E, Michalak S, Ogra PL. Persistent rotavirus infection in mice with severe combined immunodeficiency. J Virol 1987;61:3345–3348.

277. Riepenhoff-Talty M, Lee PC, Carmody PJ, Barrett HJ, Ogra PL. Age-dependent rotavirus-enterocyte interactions. Proc Soc Exp Biol Med 1982;170:146–154.

278. Riepenhoff-Talty M, Offor E, Klossner K, Kowalski E, Carmody PJ, Ogra PL. Effect of age and malnutrition on rotavirus infection in mice. Pediatr Res 1985;19:1250–1253.

279. Riepenhoff-Talty M, Schaekel K, Clark HF, et al. Group A rotaviruses produce extrahepatic biliary obstruction in orally inoculated newborn mice. Pediatr Res 1993;33:394–399.

280. Rolsma MD, Gelberg HB, Kuhlenschmidt MS. Assay for evaluation of rotavirus-cell interactions: identification of an enterocyte ganglioside fraction that mediates group A porcine rotavirus recognition. J Virol 1994;68:258–268.

281. Ruggeri FM, Greenberg HB. Antibodies to the trypsin cleavage peptide VP8* neutralize rotavirus by inhibiting binding of virions to target cells in culture. J Virol 1991;65:2211–2219.

282. Ruiz M-C, Alonso-Torre SR, Charpilienne A, et al. Rotavirus interaction with isolated membrane vesicles. J Virol 1994;68: 4009–4016.

283. Sabara M, Gilchrist JE, Hudson GR, Babiuk LA. Preliminary characterization of an epitope involved in neutralization and cell attachment that is located on the major bovine rotavirus glycoprotein. J Virol 1985;53:58–66.

284. Saif LJ. Development of nasal, fecal and serum isotype-specific antibodies in calves challenged with bovine coronavirus or rotavirus. Vet Immunol Immunopathol 1987;17:425–439.

285. Saif LJ, Jiang B. Nongroup A rotaviruses of humans and animals. Curr Top Microbiol Immunol 1994;185:339–371.

286. Saif LJ, Redman DR, Smith KL, Theil KW. Passive immunity to bovine rotavirus in newborn calves fed colostrum supplements from immunized or nonimmunized cows. Infect Immun 1983;41: 1118–1131.

287. Saif LJ, Rosen BI, Parwani AV. Animal rotaviruses. In: Kapikian AZ, ed. Viral infections of the gastrointestinal tract. 2nd ed. New York: Marcel Dekker, 1994:279–367.

288. Saif LJ, Theil KW, Bohl EH. Morphogenesis of porcine rotavirus in porcine kidney cell cultures and intestinal epithelial cells. J Gen Virol 1978;39:205–217.

289. Saif LJ, Ward LA, Yuan L, Rosen BI, To TL. The gnotobiotic piglet as a model for studies of disease pathogenesis and immunity to human rotaviruses. Proceedings of the Sapporo International Symposium on Viral Gastroenteritis, June 28–July 10, Tomakomai, Hokkaido, Japan, 1996. Arch Virol 1996 (in press).

290. Saif LJ, Weilnau P, Miller K, Stitzlein L. Isotypes of intestinal and systemic antibodies in colostrum- fed and colostrum-deprived calves challenged with rotavirus. Adv Exp Med Biol 1987;216: 1815–1823.

291. Salas-Vidal E, Plebañski M, Castro S, et al. Synthesis of the surface glycoprotein of rotavirus SA11 in the aroA strain of *Salmonella typhimurium* SL3261. Res Microbiol 1990;141:883–886.

292. Salmi TT, Arstila P, Koivikko A. Central nervous system involvement in patients with rotavirus gastroenteritis. Scand J Infect Dis 1978;10:29–31.

293. Sato K, Inaba Y, Miura Y, Tokuhisa S, Matumoto M. Isolation of lapine rotavirus in cell cultures: brief report. Arch Virol 1982; 71:267–271.

294. Saulsbury FT, Winkelstein JA, Yolken RH. Chronic rotavirus infection in immunodeficiency. J Pediatr 1980;97:61–65.

295. Schwarz KB, Moore TJ, Willoughby RE Jr, Wee S-B, Vonderfecht SL, Yolken RH. Growth of group A rotaviruses in a human liver cell line. Hepatology 1990;12:638–643.

296. Sereno MM, Gorziglia MI. The outer capsid protein VP4 of murine rotavirus strain Eb represents a tentative new P type. Virology 1994;199:500–504.

297. Serwadda D, Mugerwa RD, Sewankambo NK, et al. Slim disease: a new disease in Uganda and its association with HTLVIII infection. Lancet 1985;2:849–852.

298. Shah KV, Howley PM. Papillomaviruses. In: Fields BN, Knipe DM, eds. Virology. 2nd ed. New York: Raven Press, 1990:1651–1676.

299. Shaw RD, Fong KJ, Losonsky GA, et al. Epitope-specific immune responses to rotavirus vaccination. Gastroenterology 1987;93:941–950.

300. Shaw RD, Groene WS, Mackow ER, Merchant AA, Cheng EH. VP4-specific intestinal antibody response to rotavirus in a murine model of heterotypic infection. J Virol 1991;65:3052–3059.

301. Shaw RD, Hempson SJ, Mackow ER. Rotavirus diarrhea is caused by nonreplicating viral particles. J Virol 1995;69:5946–5950.

302. Shaw RD, Merchant AA, Groene WS, Cheng EH. Persistence of intestinal antibody response to heterologous rotavirus infection in a murine model beyond 1 year. J Clin Microbiol 1993;31:188–191.

303. Shepherd RW, Truslow S, Walker-Smith JA, et al. Infantile gastroenteritis: a clinical study of reovirus-like agent infection. Lancet 1975;2:1082–1084.

304. Sheridan JF, Eydelloth RS, Vonderfecht SL, Aurelian L. Virus-specific immunity in neonatal and adult mouse rotavirus infection. Infect Immun 1983;39:917–927.

305. Sheridan JF, Smith CC, Manak MM, Aurelian L. Prevention of rotavirus-induced diarrhea in neonatal mice born to dams immunized with empty capsids of simian rotavirus SA-11. J Infect Dis 1984; 149:434–438.

306. Sherman PM, Lichtman SN. Pediatric considerations relevant to en-

teric infections. In: Blaser MJ, Smith PD, Ravdin JI, Greenberg HB, Guerrant RL, eds. Infections of the gastrointestinal tract. New York: Raven Press, 1995:143–162.

307. Shukry S, Zaki AM, DuPont HL, Shoukry I, el Tagi M, Hamed Z. Detection of enteropathogens in fatal and potentially fatal diarrhea in Cairo, Egypt. J Clin Microbiol 1986;24:959–962.

308. Siadatpajouh M, Burns JW, Ruggeri F, Greenberg HB. Novel protection of rotavirus murine model by an anti-VP6 IgA monoclonal antibody. In: Proceedings of the American Society for Virology, 14th Annual Meeting, Austin, TX, July 8–12 1995. Abstract.

309. Snodgrass DR. Mixed infections in the intestinal tract. In: Saif LJ, Theil KW, eds. Viral diarrheas of man and animals. Boca Raton, FL: CRC Press, 1990:279–286.

310. Snodgrass DR, Angus KW, Gray EW. Rotavirus infection in lambs: pathogenesis and pathology. Arch Virol 1977;55:263–274.

311. Snodgrass DR, Ferguson A, Allan F, Angus KW, Mitchell B. Small intestinal morphology and epithelial cell kinetics in lamb rotavirus infections. Gastroenterology 1979;76:477–481.

312. Snodgrass DR, Fitzgerald TA, Campbell I, et al. Homotypic and heterotypic serological responses to rotavirus neutralization epitopes in immunologically naive and experienced animals. J Clin Microbiol 1991;29:2668–2672.

313. Snodgrass DR, Herring JA, Gray EW. Experimental rotavirus infection in lambs. J Comp Pathol 1976;86:637–642.

314. Snodgrass DR, Ojeh CK, Campbell I, Herring AJ. Bovine rotavirus serotypes and their significance for immunization. J Clin Microbiol 1984;20:342–346.

315. Snodgrass DR, Wells PW. Passive immunity in rotaviral infections. J Am Vet Med Assoc 1978;173:565–568.

316. Snodgrass DR, Wells PW. Rotavirus infection in lambs: studies on passive protection. Arch Virol 1976;52:201–205.

317. Snodgrass DR, Wells PW. The immunoprophylaxis of of rotavirus infections in lambs. Vet Rec 1978;102:146–148.

318. Snyder JD, Merson MH. The magnitude of the global problem of acute diarrhoeal disease: a review of the active surveillance data. Bull World Health Organ 1982;60:605–613.

319. Spratt HC, Marks MI, Gomersall M, Gill P, Pai CH. Nosocomial infantile gastroenteritis associated with minirotavirus and calicivirus. J Pediatr 1978;93:922–926.

320. Starkey WG, Collins J, Wallis TS, et al. Kinetics, tissue specificity and pathological changes in murine rotavirus infection of mice. J Gen Virol 1986;67:2625–2634.

321. Steel RB, Torres-Medina A. Effects of environmental and dietary factors on human rotavirus infection in gnotobiotic piglets. Infect Immun 1984;43:906–911.

322. Steele AD, Garcia D, Sears J, Gerna G, Nakagomi O, Flores J. Distribution of VP4 gene alleles in human rotaviruses by using probes to the hyperdivergent region of the VP4 gene. J Clin Microbiol 1993;31:1735–1740.

323. Stephen J. Functional abnormalities in the intestine. In: Farthing MJG, ed. Viruses and the gut. London: Smith Kline & French Laboratories, 1989:41–44.

324. Suzuki H, Kitaoka S, Konno T, Sato T, Ishida N. Two modes of human rotavirus entry into MA 104 cells. Arch Virol 1985;85:25–34.

325. Suzuki H, Kitaoka S, Sato T, et al. Further investigation on the mode of entry of human rotavirus into cells. Arch Virol 1986;91:135 144.

326. Tajima T, Suzuki E, Ushijima H, et al. Isolation of murine rotavirus in cell cultures: brief report. Arch Virol 1984;82:119–123.

327. Tanaka TN, Conner ME, Graham DY, Estes MK. Molecular characterization of three rabbit rotavirus strains. Arch Virol 1988;98:253–265.

328. Theil KW, Bohl EH, Agnes AG. Cell culture propagation of porcine rotavirus (reovirus-like agent). Am J Vet Res 1977;38:1765–1768.

329. Theil KW, Bohl EH, Cross RF, Kohler EM, Agnes AG. Pathogenesis of porcine rotaviral infection in experimentally inoculated gnotobiotic pigs. Am J Vet Res 1978;39:213–220.

330. Thouless ME, DiGiacomo RF, Deeb BJ, Howard H. Pathogenicity of rotavirus in rabbits. J Clin Microbiol 1988;26:943–947.

331. Thouless ME, DiGiacomo RF, Neuman DS. Isolation of two lapine rotaviruses: characterization of their subgroup, serotype and RNA electropherotypes. Arch Virol 1986;89:161–170.

332. Tian P, Estes MK, Hu Y, Ball JM, Zeng CQ-Y, Schilling WP. The rotavirus nonstructural glycoprotein NSP4 mobilizes Ca^{2+} from the endoplasmic reticulum. J Virol 1995;69:5763–5772.

333. Tian P, Hu Y, Schilling WP, Lindsay DA, Eiden J, Estes MK. The nonstructural glycoprotein of rotavirus affects intracellular calcium levels. J Virol 1994;68:251–257.

334. Torres A, Ji-Huang L. Diarrheal response of gnotobiotic pigs after fetal infection and neonatal challenge with homologous and heterologous human rotavirus strains. J Virol 1986;60:1107–1112.

335. Torres-Medina A, Underdahl NR. Scanning electron microscopy of intestine of gnotobiotic piglets infected with porcine rotavirus. Canadian Journal of Comparative Medicine 1980;44:403–411.

336. Torres-Medina A, Wyatt RG, Mebus CA, Underdahl NR, Kapikian AZ. Diarrhea caused in gnotobiotic piglets by the reovirus-like agent of human infantile gastroenteritis. J Infect Dis 1976;133:22–27.

337. Totterdell BM, Banatvala JE, Chrystie IL, Ball G, Cubitt WD. Systemic lymphoproliferative responses to rotavirus. J Med Virol 1988;25:37–44.

338. Tyler KL, Fields BN. Reoviruses. In: Fields BN, Knipe DM, Howley PM, eds. Fields virology. 3rd ed. Philadelphia: Lippincott-Raven, 1996:1597–1623.

339. Tzipori SR, Makin TJ, Smith ML, Krautil FL. Clinical manifestations of diarrhea in calves infected with rotavirus and enterotoxigenic Escherichia coli. J Clin Microbiol 1981;13:1011–1016.

340. Tzipori S, Makin T, Smith M, Krautil F. Enteritis in foals induced by rotavirus and enterotoxigenic Escherichia coli. Aust Vet J 1982;58:20–23.

341. Tzipori S, Smith M, Halpin C, Makin T, Krautil F. Intestinal changes associated with rotavirus and enterotoxigenic Escherichia coli infection in calves. Vet Microbiol 1983;8:35–43.

342. Tzipori S, Unicomb L, Bishop R, Montenaro J, Vaelioja LM. Studies on attenuation of rotavirus: a comparison in piglets between virulent virus and its attenuated derivative. Arch Virol 1989;109:197–205.

343. Uhnoo I, Olding-Stenkvist E, Kreuger A. Clinical features of acute gastroenteritis associated with rotavirus, enteric adenoviruses and enteropathogenic bacteria. Arch Dis Child 1986;61:732–738.

344. Uhnoo I, Riepenhoff-Talty M, Dharakul T, et al. Extramucosal spread and development of hepatitis in immunodeficient and normal mice infected with rhesus rotavirus. J Virol 1990;64:361–368.

345. Uhnoo IS, Freihorst J, Riepenhoff-Talty M, Fisher JE, Ogra PL. Effect of rotavirus infection and malnutrition on uptake of a dietary antigen in the intestine. Pediatr Res 1990;27:153–160.

346. Ushijima H, Bosu K, Abe T, Shinozaki T. Suspected rotavirus encephalitis. Arch Dis Child 1986;61:692–694.

347. Ushijima H, Honma H, Mukoyama A, et al. Detection of group C rotaviruses in Tokyo. J Med Virol 1989; 27: 299–303.

348. Ushijimi H, Xin K-Q, Nishimura S, Morikawa S, Abe T. Detection and sequencing of rotavirus VP7 gene from human materials (stools, sera, cerebrospinal fluids, and throat swabs) by reverse transcription and PCR. J Clin Microbiol 1994;32:2893–2897.

349. Van R, Morrow AL, Reves RR, Pickering LK. Environmental contamination in child day care centers. Am J Epidemiol 1991;133:460–470.

350. van Zaane D, Ijzerman J, de Leeuw PW. Intestinal antibody response after vaccination and infection with rotavirus of calves fed colostrum with or without rotavirus antibody. Vet Immunol Immunopathol 1986;11:45–63.

351. Vesikari T. Bovine rotavirus-based rotavirus vaccines in humans. In: Kapikian AZ, ed. Viral infections of the gastrointestinal tract. 2nd ed. New York: Marcel Dekker, 1994:419–442.

352. Vesikari T, Ruuska T, Koivu H-P, Green KY, Flores J, Kapikian AZ. Evaluation of the M37 human rotavirus vaccine in 2- to 6-month-old infants. Pediatr Infect Dis J 1991;10:912–917.

353. Vial PA, Kotloff KL, Losonsky GA. Molecular epidemiology of rotavirus infection in a room for convalescing newborns. J Infect Dis 1988;157:668–73.

354. Wadell G, Allard, A, Johansson M, Svensson L, Uhnoo I. Enteric adenoviruses. In: Kapikian AZ, ed. Viral infections of the gastrointestinal tract. 2nd ed. New York: Marcel Dekker, 1994:519–547.

355. Walker RI. New strategies for using mucosal vaccination to achieve more effective immunization. Vaccine 1994;12:387–400.

356. Walther FJ, Bruggeman C, Daniels-Bosman MS, et al. Symptomatic and asymptomatic rotavirus infections in hospitalized children. Acta Paediatr Scand 1983;72:659–663.

357. Ward RL, Bernstein DI, Young EC, Sherwood JR, Knowlton DR,

Schiff GM. Human rotavirus studies in volunteers: determination of infectious dose and serological response to infection. J Infect Dis 1986;154:871–880.

358. Ward RL, Clemens JD, Knowlton DR, et al. Evidence that protection against rotavirus diarrhea after natural infection is not dependent on serotype-specific neutralizing antibody. J Infect Dis 1992;166:1251–1257.

359. Ward RL, Knowlton DR, Greenberg HB, Schiff GM, Bernstein DI. Serum-neutralizing antibody to VP4 and VP7 proteins in infants following vaccination with WC3 bovine rotavirus. J Virol 1990;64: 2687–2691.

360. Ward RL, Knowlton DR, Schiff GM, Hoshino Y, Greenberg HB. Relative concentrations of serum neutralizing antibody to VP3 and VP7 proteins in adults infected with a human rotavirus. J Virol 1988;62:1543–1549.

361. Ward RL, McNeal MM, Sander DS, Greenberg HB, Bernstein DI. Immunodominance of the VP4 neutralization protein of rotavirus in protective natural infections of young children. J Virol 1993;67: 464–468.

362. Ward RL, McNeal MM, Sheridan JF. Development of an adult mouse model for studies on protection against rotavirus. J Virol 1990;64:5070–5075.

363. Ward RL, McNeal MM, Sheridan JF. Evidence that active protection following oral immunization of mice with live rotavirus is not dependent on neutralizing antibody. Virology 1992;188:57–66.

364. Weclewicz K, Kristensson K, Greenberg HB, Svensson L. The endoplasmic reticulum-associated VP7 of rotavirus is targeted to axons and dendrites in polarized neurons. J Neurocytol 1993;22: 616–626.

365. Weclewicz K, Svensson L, Billger M, Holmberg K, Wallin M, Kristensson K. Microtubule-associated protein 2 appears in axons of cultured dorsal root ganglia and spinal cord neurons after rotavirus infection. J Neurosci Res 1994;36:173–182.

366. Weiss M, Stect F, Horzinek MC. Purification and partial characterization of a new enveloped RNA virus (Berne virus). J Gen Virol 1983;64:1849–1858.

367. Whitley RJ. Herpes simplex viruses. In: Fields BN, Knipe DM, eds. Virology. 2nd ed. New York: Raven Press, 1990:1843–1887.

368. Widerlite L, Trier JS, Blacklow NR, Schreiber DS. Structure of the gastric mucosa in acute infectious nonbacterial gastroenteritis. Gastroenterology 1975;68:425–430.

369. Wolf JL, Cukor G, Blacklow NR, Dambrauskas R, Trier JS. Susceptibility of mice to rotavirus infection: effects of age and administration of corticosteroids. Infect Immun 1981;33:565–574.

370. Woode GN. Epizootiology of bovine rotavirus infection. Vet Rec 1978;103:44–46.

371. Woode GN, Bridger J, Hall GA, Jones JM, Jackson G. The isolation of reovirus-like agents (rota-viruses) from acute gastroenteritis of piglets. J Med Microbiol 1976;9:203–209.

372. Woode GN, Kelso NE, Simpson TF, Gaul SK, Evans LE, Babiuk L. Antigenic relationships among some bovine rotaviruses: serum neutralization and cross-protection in gnotobiotic calves. J Clin Microbiol 1983;18:358–364.

373. Woode GN, Pohlenz JF, Kelso-Gourley NE, Fagerland JA. Astrovirus and bredavirus infections of dome cell epithelium of bovine ileum. J Clin Microbiol 1984;19:623–630.

374. Woode GN, Reed DE, Runnels MA, Herrig MA, Hill HT. Studies with an unclassified virus isolated from diarrheic calves. Vet Microbiol 1982; 7:221–240.

375. Woode GN, Zheng S, Melendy DR, Ramig RF. Studies on rotavirus homologous and heterologous active immunity in infant mice. Viral Immunol 1989;2:127–132.

376. Woode GN, Zheng SL, Rosen BI, Knight N, Gourley NE, Ramig RF. Protection between different serotypes of bovine rotavirus in gnotobiotic calves: specificity of serum antibody and coproantibody responses. J Clin Microbiol 1987;25:1052–1058.

377. Wyatt RG, James WD, Bohl EH, et al. Human rotavirus type 2: cultivation in vitro. Science 1980;207:189–191.

378. Wyatt RG, Kapikian AZ, Mebus CA. Induction of cross-reactive serum neutralizing antibody to human rotavirus in calves after in utero administration of bovine rotavirus. J Clin Microbiol 1983; 18:505–508.

379. Wyatt RG, Mebus CA, Yolken RH, et al. Rotaviral immunity in gnotobiotic calves: heterologous resistance to human virus induced by bovine virus. Science 1979;203:548–550.

380. Xu L, Tian Y, Tarlow O, Harbour D, McCrae MA. Molecular biology of rotaviruses. IX. Conservation and divergence in genome segment 5. J Gen Virol 1994;75:3413–3421.

381. Yasukawa M, Nakagomi O, Kobayashi Y. Rotavirus induces proliferative response and augments non-specific cytotoxic activity of lymphocytes in humans. Clin Exp Immunol 1990;80:49–55.

382. Yolken RH, Ojeh C, Khatri IA, Sajjan U, Forstner JF. Intestinal mucins inhibit rotavirus replication in an oligosaccharide-dependent manner. J Infect Dis 1994;169:1002–1006.

383. Yolken RH, Peterson JA, Vonderfecht SL, Fouts ET, Midthun K, Newburg DS. Human milk mucin inhibits rotavirus replication and prevents experimental gastroenteritis. J Clin Invest 1992;90: 1984–1991.

384. Yolken RH, Willoughby R, Wee SB, Miskuff R, Vonderfecht S. Sialic acid glycoproteins inhibit in vitro and in vivo replication of rotaviruses. J Clin Invest 1987;79:148–154.

Viral Pathogenesis,
edited by Neal Nathanson, et al.
Lippincott–Raven Publishers, Philadelphia © 1997

CHAPTER 31

Viral Hepatitis

Francis V. Chisari and Carlo Ferrari

  F.V. Chisari: Department of Molecular and Experimental Medicine, The Scripps Research Institute, La Jolla, California 92037.
  C. Ferrari: Department of Infectious Diseases, The University of Parma, 43100 Parma, Italy.

INTRODUCTION

Viral hepatitis is a common inflammatory liver disease of variable severity. It is caused by several different types of virus that can produce either transient or persistent infection. Although hepatitis sometimes occurs as a relatively mild systemic manifestation of many different infections, it is most commonly caused by one of five primarily hepatotropic agents that have been designated the hepatitis viruses A, B, C, D, and E.[4] Persistent infection by three of these viruses (B, C, and D) is often associated with chronic liver disease that can lead to the development of cirrhosis and hepatocellular carcinoma (HCC). Several hundred million people throughout the world are persistently infected by these viruses, with the concomitant cirrhosis and HCC being major health issues in areas where these infections are endemic. In this chapter, we focus on the host-virus interactions that determine the outcome of infection by these viruses, with particular emphasis on the role of the host immune response in viral clearance and in the pathogenesis of the associated liver disease.

The Hepatitis Viruses

Although they all infect the human hepatocyte, the five hepatitis viruses differ from each other at several very important levels (Table 31-1). For example, the hepatitis B virus (HBV, a member of the hepadnavirus family) possesses a dou-ble-stranded circular DNA genome, whereas the others are single-stranded RNA viruses, and their genomes are sufficiently distinct to classify them in separate virus families. Specifically, the hepatitis A virus (HAV, a picornavirus), hepatitis C virus (HCV, a flavivirus), and hepatitis E virus (HEV, unclassified) display linear RNA genomes with positive polarity. In contrast, the hepatitis delta virus (HDV, classified with plant viroids and satellite RNAs) exhibits negative polarity, and, because of extensive base pairing within its circular RNA, its single-stranded genome probably exists as a double-stranded, unbranched, rod-like structure. HDV is also unique because it cannot spread from cell to cell on its own, and it uses the envelope proteins encoded by HBV for this purpose. Thus, HBV coinfection is an absolute requirement for maintenance of the HDV life cycle.

These important genomic differences are reflected in the biologic and pathogenetic properties of each of these viruses, and in the diseases that they induce. For example, HAV and HEV are transmitted only enterically, by the fecal-oral route, whereas the other viruses are transmitted parenterally, by the percutaneous and transmucosal exchange of infected blood and body fluids. In addition to the epidemiologic implications

TABLE 31-1. *Properties of the hepatitis viruses*

Classification	A	B	C	D	E
	Picornavirus	Hepadnavirus	Flavivirus	Plant virus satellites	Unclassified
Virus					
Diameter (nm)	27–32	42	30–60	36	27–34
Enveloped	No	Yes	Yes	Yes	Unknown
Genome					
Size (kb)	7.5	3.2	9.4	1.6	7.5
Structure	Linear	Circular	Linear	Circular	Linear
Strandedness	Single	Double	Single	Single	Single
Polarity	Plus	NR	Plus	Minus	Plus
Poly (A)	Yes	NR	Variable	No	Yes
Integration	No	Yes	No	No	No
Cell culture					
Infectious	Yes	No	Yes	No	No
Cytopathic	No	No	No	±	?
Host range	Human	Human	Human	Human	Human
	Chimpanzee	Chimpanzee	Chimpanzee	Chimpanzee	Chimpanzee
	Monkey	Woodchuck		Woodchuck	Monkey
		Pekin duck			
		Ground squirrel			
Transmission	Enteric	Parenteral	Parenteral	Parenteral	Enteric
Hepatitis	Acute	Acute	Acute	Acute	Acute
		Chronic	Chronic	Chronic	
Pathogenesis	Immune	Immune	Immune	Immune(?)	Unknown
Hepatocellular Carcinoma	No	Yes	Yes	Yes	No
New cases per year in U.S.	130,000	200,000	150,000	7500	0
Deaths per year in U.S.					
Fulminant hepatitis	90	125	?	35	0
Chronic hepatitis	0	5–6000	8–10,000	1000	0
Chronic hepatitis incidence (millions)					
U.S.	0	1	3	0.07	0
Worldwide	0	300–400	50–100	?	0

NR, not reported.

of these differences, it is possible that the route of entry of each virus may influence its tissue distribution as well as the character of the antiviral host response, both of which may influence the tendency of each virus to become persistent. For example, although all of these viruses can cause severe (and sometimes fatal) acute hepatitis, the enterically transmitted viruses are never associated with persistent infection or chronic liver disease, which do occur after infection by the parenterally transmitted viruses. In addition, because the parenterally transmitted viruses can be passed neonatally from mother to infant (and perhaps transplacentally to the fetus), they have the additional opportunity to become persistent because of the immunologic immaturity of the infected host. Whether this interesting relation between route of infection and disease outcome is causal or incidental is an important question with many ramifications, and it deserves serious further examination.

Another important feature of these viruses is their high mutation rate, a result of the lack of proofreading function of the RNA polymerase and reverse transcriptase enzymes that replicate their genomes (HBV, a DNA virus, replicates by reverse transcription of a pregenomic RNA). This creates the opportunity for selection to occur if a mutation confers even a small positive growth advantage to a mutant viral genome or deletes a recognition site for the host immune response. The existence of substantial nucleotide and amino acid sequence heterogeneity in different isolates of HBV and HCV, and the emergence of specific mutations in the HBV genome in individual patients are well established events that may contribute to the pathogenesis and natural history of the associated diseases.

The Disease Spectrum

When the incidence of infection due to all five of the hepatitis viruses is combined, it is estimated that between 400,000 to 500,000 new cases of acute viral hepatitis occur each year in the United States (see Table 31-1). Most of these diseases are self-limited nonfatal infections, but 15,000 to 20,000 people in the United States will die each year from the complications of chronic viral hepatitis, which affects as many as 4 million people in this country. In addition to causing liver disease, most of these viruses also cause assorted extrahepatic manifestations that are generally explainable on the basis of immune complex formation, including skin rashes, arthralgias, glomerulonephritis, polyarteritis nodosa, and cryoglobulinemia.

In the case of HBV, as much as 10% of acutely infected adults and 90% of acutely infected neonates fail to clear the virus and contract chronic hepatitis. For HCV, it has been conservatively estimated that up to 90% of acutely infected adults become persistently infected. Reflecting these figures, it is thought that approximately 300 to 400 million people are chronically infected by HBV throughout the world, and that at least 50 million people are persistently infected by HCV. These chronically infected people suffer from liver diseases of varying severity, ranging from the clinically inapparent "healthy" carrier state at one end of the spectrum to the most severe cases of chronic active hepatitis at the other, and people can move from one disease category to another at varying times during the course of their infection. The most seriously affected patients are at risk for development of the life-threatening complications of cirrhosis and HCC. Indeed, for HBV it has been estimated that the lifetime risk of HCC in men infected at birth is approximately 40%,[18] and for chronic HCV infection the risk may be quite similar.

The Available Experimental Systems

The pathogenetic mechanisms that cause viral hepatitis and HCC in patients with chronic hepatitis are not very well defined because the experimental systems that are traditionally used to examine these questions are not available for these viruses.

For example, except for HAV and the Pekin duck counterpart of HBV, none of these viruses is infectious for its natural target cell in vitro. In addition, except for humans, the chimpanzee, and certain monkeys, the human hepatitis viruses are not infectious in vivo, and the natural hosts for the duck, woodchuck (woodchuck hepatitis virus [WHV]), and ground squirrel (ground squirrel hepatitis virus [GSHV]) hepadnaviral homologues of HBV are outbred species whose immune systems are not well defined. Although these in vivo models, and a wealth of clinical correlative studies in humans, have contributed enormously to our understanding of the natural history and pathogenetic potential of these viruses, they do not permit definitive analysis of the role played by the immune response in viral clearance, disease pathogenesis, and hepatocarcinogenesis.

Accordingly, investigators have been forced to develop nontraditional (e.g., transgenic) animal models to study the direct and indirect consequences of viral gene expression, and to use alternative methods for the detection and characterization of the virus-specific immune response in infected patients. Although none of these models is an entirely satisfactory substitute for the infection of genetically defined cell lines in vitro or the infection of inbred animals in vivo, they have nonetheless yielded a great deal of pathogenetically relevant information that, together with the aforementioned clinical and animal studies, have led to a fairly good concept of the pathogenesis of viral hepatitis that is developed in the remainder of this chapter.

The Central Hypothesis

Most studies suggest that the hepatitis viruses are not directly cytopathic, or at least not highly cytopathic, for the infected hepatocyte.[55,59,223] Because the disease spectrum associated with these viruses is extraordinarily variable, as illustrated for HBV in Figure 31-1, it has been a long-standing prediction that the host response to these viruses must play a critical role in the pathogenesis of the associated diseases. Indeed, based on fairly extensive studies of HBV pathogenesis in humans and animal models, there is considerable evidence that viral hepatitis is initiated by an antigen-specific antiviral intrahepatic cellular immune response that sets in motion a cascade of antigen-nonspecific cellular and molecular effector systems that actually cause most of the damage to the liver.

With respect to HBV, there is a great deal of evidence that both the cellular and humoral limbs of the immune response

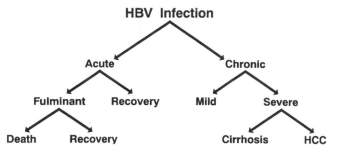

FIG. 31-1. Spectrum of liver disease after hepatitis B virus (HBV) infection. HBV infection is transient in approximately 90% of adults and 10% of neonates, and persistent in the rest. Most cases of acute hepatitis are asymptomatic (subclinical), and less than 1% of clinically apparent acute infections are fulminant. Approximately one third of chronic hepatitis infections are severe enough to be associated with the sequelae of cirrhosis and hepatocellular carcinoma. Worldwide, more than 300 million people are chronically infected by HBV. *Acute hepatitis B* is characterized by the presence of IgM anti-core serum antibodies (which convert to IgG with clinical recovery and convalescence), and the transient (<6 months) presence of hepatitis B surface antigen (HBsAg), hepatitis B precore antigen (HBeAg), and viral DNA, with clearance of these markers followed by seroconversion to anti-HBsAg and anti-HBeAg. More than 90% of cases of adult-onset infection fall into this category. The remaining 5% to 10% of cases of adult-onset infection, and over 90% of cases of neonatal infection become chronic, and may continue for the life span of the patient. *Chronic hepatitis B* is a prolonged (>6 months) infection with persistent serum levels of HBsAg and IgG anti-core antibodies and the absence of an anti-HBsAg antibody response by commercial immunoassays. HBV DNA and HBeAg are often detectable at high concentrations, but may disappear if viral replication ceases or if mutations occur that prevent the synthesis of the viral precore protein precursor of HBeAg. The associated inflammatory liver disease is variable in severity. It is always much milder than the usual case of acute hepatitis, but it can last for decades, and when it is severe (chronic active hepatitis), it often proceeds to regenerative nodule formation and fibrous scarring (cirrhosis), and after many decades it is associated with more than a 100-fold increase in the risk for the development of hepatocellular carcinoma (HCC).

are required for viral clearance to occur. Data also suggest that noncytolytic intracellular viral inactivation by certain inflammatory cytokines released by virus-activated lymphomononuclear cells may play an important role in the clearance of at least some of these viruses from the infected cell (Fig. 31-2). It is the purpose of this chapter to review and interpret the evidence that pertains to the foregoing hypothesis. Most of the data that we discuss have been derived from studies dealing with HBV pathogenesis because this virus has been most extensively studied at this level. Although we believe that the principles we present are likely to be pertinent to all of the hepatitis viruses, we emphasize that they are neither universal nor all-inclusive, so that generalization beyond HBV must take this into account.

THE HEPATITIS B VIRUS GENOME AND LIFE CYCLE

As previously reviewed,[54] the HBV virion contains a circular, partially double-stranded DNA genome approximately 3200 base pairs (3.2 kb) in length (Fig. 31-3). The long (minus) strand of the viral DNA encodes a greater-than-genome-length, 3.5-kb pregenomic RNA that is reverse transcribed as an early step in viral replication. The minus strand also encodes 3.5-, 2.4-, 2.1-, and 0.7-kb mRNA species that are translated into the structural (envelope, nucleocapsid) and nonstructural (polymerase, transactivating protein) proteins of the virus. Because the experimental systems and concepts that have led to an understanding of HBV pathogenesis touch on many aspects of the structure and function of each of these gene products, we provide a brief review of their characteristics and of the regulatory elements that control their expression.

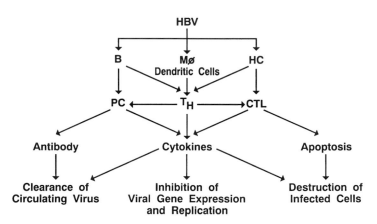

FIG. 31-2. Hypothetic course of hepatitis B virus (HBV) immunopathogenesis. Eradication of HBV infection depends on the coordinate and efficient development of humoral and cell-mediated immune responses against HBV proteins. Antibodies secreted by plasma cells (PC) derived from antigen-specific B cells (which usually recognize viral antigens in their native conformation) are mostly responsible for the neutralization of free circulating viral particles. Cytotoxic T cells (CTL) that recognize endogenous viral antigens in the form of short peptides associated with human leukocyte antigen (HLA) class I molecules on the surface of the infected hepatocytes (HC) are the main effectors for the elimination of intracellular virus. They can do this by at least two different mechanisms: direct attachment to the cell membrane, causing the infected cell to undergo apoptosis; and the release of soluble cytokines that can downregulate viral gene expression, leading to the elimination of intracellular virus without destruction of the infected cell. Both humoral and cytotoxic functions are more or less stringently regulated by the helper effect of the CD4+ T cells (T$_H$) that recognize exogenous viral antigens, released or secreted by liver cells, in the form of short peptides that associate with HLA class II molecules in the endosomal compartment of professional antigen-presenting cells such as B cells, macrophages (Mø), and dendritic cells.

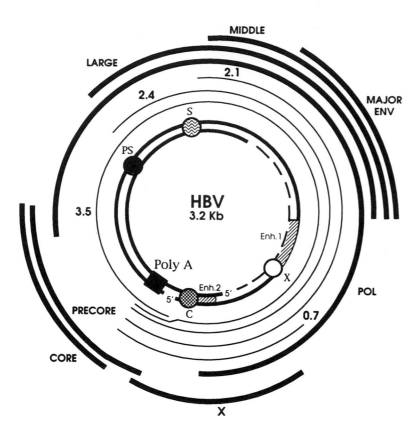

FIG. 31-3. Genetic organization of the hepatitis B virus (HBV) genome, with its transcripts and proteins. The HBV genome is a 3.2-kilobase pair (kb), circular, double-stranded DNA molecule (innermost concentric lines) containing four promoters (PS, S, C, and X; shown as circles) that drive the synthesis of four viral transcripts (shown as thin lines) that are 3.5, 2.4, 2.1, and 0.7 kb in length. These transcripts encode the viral nucleocapsid (core, precore), polymerase (POL), envelope (ENV; large, middle, and small [major]), and transcriptional transactivating (X) proteins (shown as bold lines), and the 3.5-kb mRNA also serves at the pregenomic RNA template for reverse transcription for first-strand DNA synthesis during viral replication. Two viral enhancers (Enh) are present that facilitate liver-specific expression. A single polyadenylation (Poly A) site ensures that all viral transcripts have common 3′ termini.

Hepatitis B Virus Regulatory Elements

Four promoter elements regulate expression of the various HBV genes. The *core promoter* is located just upstream of the first translational start codon in the nucleocapsid open reading frame. It contains several binding sites for transcriptional transactivators such as CCAAT/enhancer binding protein (C/EBP) and Sp1 that may contribute to its transcriptional activity in vivo.[190,363] It encodes a greater-than-genome-length (3.5 kb) transcript that serves as the RNA pregenome template for reverse transcription and production of DNA minus strands during viral replication.[35,265,316,351] It also encodes the viral precore, core, and polymerase proteins.[80,81] In view of the importance of these transcripts and polypeptides in viral replication, this promoter is transcriptionally quite active in most HBV infected tissue. Evidence suggests that elements within this promoter region (Enh 2) exert a major influence on the tissue specificity of HBV gene expression[356] by virtue of their interaction with liver-specific transcription factors.[140,166]

Two independent promoters control envelope gene expression. The *preS promoter* is relatively silent transcriptionally compared with the core and S promoters.[269] It is located just upstream of the first translational start codon in the envelope[35,250,299,351] region, and it encodes a 2.4-kb transcript from which the large envelope polypeptide is produced. Transcription initiation from this promoter occurs preferentially in differentiated hepatoma cells[46] by virtue of interaction of promoter sequences with a liver-specific nuclear factor similar to rat hepatocyte nuclear factor (HNF-1).[269] The *S promoter* is located within the envelope coding region just upstream of the

translation start site of the middle envelope polypeptide.[80,81,265,270] It is transcriptionally very active and is regulated by positive and negative elements,[72] including several Sp1 binding sites that probably contribute to the level of expression from this promoter during viral infection.[268] It encodes a 2.1-kb transcript that controls production of the middle and major envelope polypeptides. The usual balance between the S and preS promoters normally leads to the relative underproduction of the large envelope polypeptide with respect to the others, perhaps because elements within the S promoter exert a strong negative influence on the activity of the preS promoter.[33] It now appears that dysregulated overproduction of the large envelope polypeptide carries significant structural and pathologic consequences (see discussion later).

Like the preS promoter, the *X gene promoter* is transcriptionally quite silent in vivo and its RNA is characteristically a low-abundance species, being usually undetectable by Northern blot analysis of infected tissue.[164] Nonetheless, the X promoter is very active in vitro in several hepatoma cell lines, raising the possibility that the *X* mRNA may have a very short half-life.[269] In view of the transcriptional transactivating properties of the X gene product,[292,308,329] it has been postulated that dysregulated *X* expression may have important pathophysiologic consequences, including hepatocarcinogenesis (see discussion later).

Another *enhancer* element (Enh 1), which increases the level of HBV promoter activity and viral replication in liver cells,[8,166,274,293,326] is present between the envelope and *X* open reading frames. This enhancer is also active in many other cell types[340] such that the liver specificity of HBV expression is thought to be determined primarily by the Enh 2 element in the nucleocapsid promoter region.[356] Enhancer 1 has been shown to bind or to contain binding sites for several general and liver-specific transcription factors such as nuclear factor-1 (NF-1), HNF-1, C/EBP, EBP-1, and enhancer factor-C (EF-C).[166,248,253,274] This enhancer element also displays glucocorticoid inducibility together with a glucocorticoid response element located elsewhere in the genome.[326]

Hepatitis B Virus Proteins

The *nucleocapsid* open reading frame contains two in-phase start codons that define two overlapping (core and precore) polypeptides the shorter of which (core, hepatitis B core antigen [HBcAg]) is a cytoplasmic and nuclear protein that self-assembles to form the viral nucleocapsid. The carboxy-terminal region of the core protein includes an arginine-rich domain that contains nuclear localization sequences[78,357] and an overlapping sequence required for encapsidation of the 3.5-kb viral RNA pregenome.[229] Core particles are assembled from core protein dimer precursors in a spontaneous, concentration-dependent process that can occur in the absence of other viral components.[290,367–369] It is thought that core particles transport the viral replication complex to the nucleus for amplification and that they also associate with viral envelope at the endoplasmic reticulum (ER) membrane for virion assembly and export (see discussion later).

A longer counterpart (precore) of the core protein is translocated, by a signal peptide at its extreme amino-terminus,[310] into the ER, from which it is secreted as hepatitis B precore antigen (HBeAg) after truncation of amino- and carboxy-terminal residues.[249,287] The precore protein is clearly not required for viral replication,[49] and its role in the viral life cycle is undefined. Nonetheless, the presence of HBeAg in the serum of infected patients is a good serologic marker of viral replication.

It has been suggested that the cellular immune response to the nucleocapsid antigens is an important factor in viral clearance in HBV infection because they elicit a strong human leukocyte antigen (HLA) class I- and class II-restricted T-cell response in infected patients.* In this context, it is interesting that HBV has been reported to suppress interferon (IFN)-β transcription by a transacting mechanism that has been traced to the core protein.[331,333] The extent to which this process may contribute to HBV pathogenesis remains to be determined.

The *envelope* open reading frame contains three in-phase translation start codons that define the amino termini of three overlapping polypeptides, the expression of which is transcriptionally regulated. The relative abundance of these three proteins plays an important role in viral particle morphogenesis. The major and middle envelope polypeptides assemble into small, 22-nm spherical particles by budding into the lumen of the ER, and they are rapidly secreted after passage and glycosylation in the Golgi apparatus.[76,77,254,255] The large envelope polypeptide appears to be an essential component of the infectious virion (Dane particle), and may play an important structural role in complete virus particle assembly. The large envelope polypeptide also exerts an important structural influence on the formation of the abundant, noninfectious

subviral particles that are characteristic of HBV infection.[61,207,218,251,309] Depending on the relative molar ratio of the large envelope polypeptide to the major and middle envelope polypeptides within a given cell, either short, secretable filaments are formed or long, nonsecretable, branching filaments are produced that accumulate within the ER and lead to the development of "ground glass" hepatocytes and may ultimately contribute to the death of the cell.[60,112,113]

Considerable evidence indicates that available recombinant HBV envelope vaccines induce vigorous immune responses to the preS antigen and hepatitis B surface antigen (HBsAg).[12,41,42,93,95,99,157] In addition, it has been shown that in patients with acute viral hepatitis B who ultimately clear the virus, a strong polyclonal and multispecific cytotoxic T-lymphocyte (CTL) response develops to several envelope antigens,[230] and that class I- and class II-restricted, envelope-specific T cells are present in the intrahepatic infiltrate in patients with chronic hepatitis.[11–13] Furthermore, in transgenic mice, HBsAg-specific, class I-restricted CTL cause hepatitis[6,7,224] and inhibit HBV gene expression[121] and viral replication,[123] demonstrating the potential importance of these antigens in the pathogenesis of HBV infection in man.

The *X* open reading frame encodes a *transcriptional transactivating protein* that positively regulates transcription from HBV and other viral, and cellular, promoters[67,292,308,330,332] in vitro. It has been shown that the X protein is important for the establishment of WHV infection.[51,370] Despite the fact that the X protein is present in trace quantities in infected tissue, presumably because of the low abundance of its RNA and its short half-life as a protein,[279] it is immunogenic at the B- and T-cell levels,[159,312] possibly because it transactivates such immunologically important cellular genes as HLA-DR,[146] major histocompatibility complex (MHC) class I,[366] and intercellular adhesion molecule-1.[147] The role of the anti-X-protein–specific immune response in viral clearance and disease pathogenesis, however, is undefined at this time. Data suggest that the X gene product is not a DNA-binding protein; instead, it complexes with cellular transcription factors and modifies their ability to bind to regulatory elements, thereby influencing the transcription process in a general fashion rather than by directly binding DNA target sequences itself.[67,194,298,334] Furthermore, it has been shown that the X protein complexes with the p53 tumor suppressor protein and inhibits its sequence-specific DNA-binding capacity, transcriptional activation function, and, perhaps, its indirect DNA repair function in vitro.[346] Because of these properties, it has been proposed that dysregulated expression of the X gene product may be involved in hepatocarcinogenesis in chronic HBV infection.[353] It has also been shown that high-level expression of the X gene product is associated with the development of HCC in the absence of any associated liver disease in some lineages of transgenic mice.[173]

The *polymerase* open reading frame encodes the viral polymerase protein, which is translated by internal ribosomal initiation of the 3.5-kb core mRNA.[155,169] The polymerase protein contains DNA-dependent DNA polymerase, reverse transcriptase, and RNAse H domains as well as a 5' DNA-binding protein that serves as a primer for reverse transcription of the viral pregenome.[15,16,24,192,286,342] The polymerase gene products also play essential roles in encapsidation and replication of the viral genome[14,138,184] by binding to a hairpin structure at the 5' end of the 3.5-kb pregenomic RNA that serves both as a packaging signal[138,160] and as the template for initiation of reverse

---

*References 19, 21, 92, 96, 97, 125, 217, 221, 257, 258, 325.

HBV Life Cycle

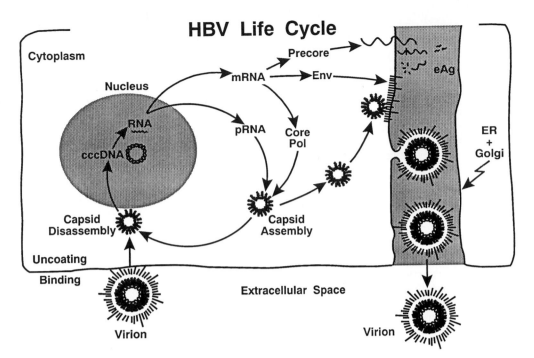

FIG. 31-4. Schematic representation of the hepatitis B virus (HBV) life cycle. The HBV virion presumably binds to an unidentified receptor at the hepatocyte surface; viral nucleocapsids enter the cell and migrate to the nucleus, where capsid disassembly is thought to occur, thereby allowing the immature viral genome to be transported into the nucleus. In the nucleus, second-strand DNA synthesis is completed and the gaps in both strands are repaired to yield a covalently closed circular (ccc; supercoiled) DNA molecule that serves as the template for transcription of viral RNAs. These transcripts are polyadenylated and the mRNA are transported into the cytoplasm, where they are translated into the various viral proteins. The envelope (Env) proteins insert themselves as integral membrane proteins into the lipid membrane of the endoplasmic reticulum (ER). The viral core (Core) and polymerase (Pol) proteins encapsidate the pregenomic viral RNA (pRNA) and form new viral nucleocapsids (capsids) that can follow two different intracellular pathways, one of which leads to the formation and secretion of new virions, whereas the other leads to amplification of the viral genome inside the cell nucleus. In the virion assembly pathway, the capsids migrate to the ER, where they associate with the envelope proteins and bud into the lumen of the ER, from which they are rapidly secreted by the Golgi apparatus out of the cell. In the genome amplification pathway, the capsids migrate to the nuclear membrane, disassemble, and deliver their nascent viral genome to amplify the intranuclear pool of supercoiled viral DNA. The precore protein contains a signal sequence that transports it into the ER lumen, where its amino- and carboxy-termini are trimmed and the resultant polypeptide is secreted as precore antigen (eAg). The X protein contributes to the efficiency of HBV gene expression and replication by a series of complex pathways, including interaction with cellular transcription factors. These pathways are not precisely defined, so they are not shown.

transcription of the viral pregenome.[343] The polymerase protein is quite immunogenic during acute and chronic infection,[271,347,362] and the terminal protein has been shown to inhibit the cellular response to IFN.[103] It is likely that the immune response to this protein may play an important role in the pathogenesis of chronic hepatitis.

The Viral Life Cycle

As previously reviewed,[62] the mechanism of viral entry into the hepatocyte is not known, although there is evidence that attachment may be mediated by the interaction of a domain in the preS[1] region of the large envelope polypeptide[232] with one

or more structures on the hepatocyte membrane. Several candidate receptors for HBV have been suggested, including the polyalbumin receptor,[191] the transferrin receptor,[105] the interleukin (IL)-6 receptor,[234] endonexin II,[132] and apolipoprotein H,[208] among others. At present, however, the molecular basis for viral attachment and entry is not known for HBV or for any of the other hepatitis viruses.

The replication of HBV is unique among DNA viruses in that it involves reverse transcription of an RNA pregenome.[316] Based on this seminal observation and subsequent studies from several laboratories,* a model of the HBV life cycle

---

*References 187, 202, 213, 215, 219, 275, 289, 316, 327, 351.

within the hepatocyte has emerged,[273] and it appears that similar mechanisms may be operative within lymphoid cells.[176]

As illustrated in Figure 31-4, after entry and presumptive uncoating, viral plus strand DNA synthesis is completed within the nucleocapsid particle, which delivers the viral genome to the nucleus by nuclear localization signals located at the carboxy-terminus of HBcAg (see previous discussion). Data from a transgenic mouse model suggest that nucleocapsid particles do not enter the nucleus (see discussion later). This suggests that capsid disassembly probably occurs on the cytoplasmic face of the nuclear membrane and that the viral genome is released into the nucleus, where DNA repair enzymes process and join the viral minus and plus strands, yielding the covalently closed circular DNA molecule that serves as the template for transcription of the viral pregenomic and messenger RNAs.[316]

After its transport into the cytoplasm, the RNA pregenome becomes incorporated into a nascent core particle by interacting with core and polymerase proteins that have been translated from their respective mRNAs. Within these nucleocapsid particles, new DNA minus strands are synthesized by reverse transcription of the pregenomic RNA. Newly formed DNA minus strands serve as the template for DNA plus strand synthesis, and plus strand elongation converts the linear DNA intermediates into a relaxed, circular, double-stranded molecule.

Some of these core particles are transported back to the nucleus in a process that effectively amplifies the pool of HBV genomes within the cell.[327] Other core particles associate with viral envelope proteins that exist as integral membrane proteins in the ER, into which they bud, and are ultimately secreted as infectious virion to initiate new rounds of infection in susceptible cells. With each cycle of viral and host cell replication there is a chance that the viral DNA may integrate into the host genome. The chances that this will occur are greatly increased during chronic infection. Integration is often associated with extensive rearrangement of viral and host flanking sequences that can modulate the expression of viral and host genes (see discussion later).

STUDIES IN ANIMAL MODELS

Experimental approaches to HBV pathogenesis have been severely hampered because the host range of HBV is limited to humans, chimpanzees, and the great apes, and because in vitro culture systems for the propagation of HBV do not exist. Thanks to the discovery and characterization of several related viruses in woodchucks, ground squirrels, and Pekin ducks that, collectively, comprise the hepadnavirus family, many of these obstacles have been circumvented.

Woodchuck Hepatitis Virus

The discovery of a naturally occurring hepadnavirus in woodchucks,[307] and its association with acute and chronic liver disease and HCC,[262,307] laid the groundwork for much of our current understanding of hepadnavirus biology and pathogenesis. For example, similar to HBV, neonatal infection by WHV invariably leads to persistent infection and HCC,

whereas adult-onset infection leads to acute, self-limited hepatitis and viral clearance.[175] Discovery of the extrahepatic replication of WHV,[174] especially its ability to replicate efficiently in lymphomononuclear cells,[48,175–177,263] reinforced the concept that HBV is not strictly hepatotropic, and that extrahepatic reservoirs of virus may exist that can contribute to viral persistence and serve as a continuing source of virus and viral antigens to maintain the immune response long after seroconversion and recovery from acute viral hepatitis (see discussion later). These virus depots may also seed hepatic allografts after liver transplantation.

The WHV model has also greatly strengthened the concept that the antiviral T-cell response plays a critical role in viral clearance and disease pathogenesis, because cyclosporin A-treated woodchucks with suppressed T-cell function fail to terminate WHV infection when infected as adults.[70] This model also documented the dependence of HDV on coincident or preceding HBV infection.[231] Because of the ability to infect the woodchuck liver by direct intrahepatic injection of cloned WHV genomes, it has been shown that the precore protein is dispensable for viral replication,[52] but that the X protein is not.[50,370]

Perhaps the greatest contribution of the woodchuck model lies in the area of hepatocarcinogenesis (see section on Mechanisms of Hepatocarcinogenesis). More recently, the woodchuck model has been used to examine the physiologic basis for viral clearance during acute WHV infection. The results of these studies are compatible with a hypothesis that has been forthcoming from a transgenic mouse model of viral hepatitis[121] (see discussion later) that, in addition to destroying infected hepatocytes, the immune response can also deliver a noncytolytic signal that eliminates the virus from the hepatocyte without causing the death of the infected cell.[161]

Other Hepadnaviruses

The discovery of a related hepadnavirus in Beechey ground squirrels (GSHV)[195] and the demonstration that chronic infection by this virus also led to HCC[196] firmly established the oncogenic potential of HBV. These studies further corroborated that hepadnaviruses do not carry an acutely transforming oncogene, but, rather, that HCC develops after many years of antecedent infection and liver disease. Extension of the hepadnavirus family to Pekin ducks[204] created the opportunity to define the molecular aspects of the viral life cycle (see previous discussion; reviewed in Summers[315]) because it is possible to transmit the virus readily to adult and unborn animals[203] and to infect cultured primary hepatocytes[328] and a transformed avian hepatoma cell line.[68] The duck model has been particularly useful to study antiviral drug activity in vivo and in vitro[68,108,130,238,259,361] and to examine the role of certain physiologic events, especially hepatocellular turnover, in viral clearance.[156]

The Transgenic Mouse Model

Despite the enormous strides that were made possible by the availability of the foregoing animal models, the outbred nature of these species and the lack of reagents to define their immune responses to these viral antigens have severely hampered the analysis of hepadnaviral immunobiology and immunopathogenesis. The same is true for the other hepatitis viruses. With the advent of embryo microinjection technology, it became evident that many questions relating to HBV biology and pathogenesis might be directly examined by introduction of partial or complete copies of the HBV genome into transgenic mice.

Complete Hepatitis B Virus Genome Transgenic Mice

As previously reviewed,[56] using constructs containing only HBV-derived regulatory sequences, several laboratories[9,10,34,63,89,115,124,170] have produced transgenic mice that preferentially express all of the viral gene products, and even replicate the virus, in the liver (hepatocyte). These mice also express the viral gene products in kidney tubular epithelial cells, sometimes preferentially, and they also display sporadic and unpredictable expression in miscellaneous other tissues that are unique to each transgenic lineage, presumably reflecting integration site influences.

These studies demonstrated that HBV has the potential to be expressed and to replicate in many cells besides the hepatocyte, that viral gene expression is developmentally regulated,[73] and that it is positively regulated by androgens[90] and glucocorticoids,[90] providing insight into the male predominance of HBV infection and the increased viral burden associated with steroid therapy of chronic hepatitis B in humans. Together with evidence of extrahepatic viral DNA and virus expression in infected patients and the various hepadnavirus models (reviewed in Korba and colleagues[177]), these data strongly suggest that the relative liver specificity of HBV must reflect multiple constraints at the levels of viral entry, replication, and gene expression, and that none of these constraints is absolutely specific for the human hepatocyte.

An important by-product of these studies was the demonstration that most of the HBV gene products, and the process of viral replication itself, are not directly cytopathic for the hepatocyte, at least at the levels attained in these animals.[9,89] This feature has made it possible to examine the pathogenetic consequences of the immune response to these viral antigens in vivo in these animals, providing an exceptional opportunity to examine the molecular and cellular basis for viral clearance and liver disease during HBV infection in humans (see discussion later).

Function and Effects of the Large Envelope Polypeptide

In separate studies, it was shown that the HBV large envelope protein assembles into long, branching, filamentous HBsAg particles that become trapped in the ER and are not secreted.[60,61] It was subsequently shown that the progressive accumulation of these subviral filamentous particles leads to a dramatic expansion of the ER in the hepatocyte,[60] eventually causing ultrastructural and histologic changes that are characteristic of the ground glass hepatocytes found in the liver of chronically infected patients with integrated HBV DNA.[112,113] Prolonged storage of high concentrations of these long subviral filaments in the ER was shown to be directly cytotoxic to the hepatocyte, initiating a storage disease characterized by chronic hepatocellular necrosis and a secondary inflammatory and regenerative response in the transgenic mice[60,102] that in-

exorably leads to HCC.[62,74,291] A more detailed consideration of this subject is presented in the section on Mechanisms of Hepatocarcinogenesis.

Hepatocytotoxic Effects of Bacterial Lipopolysaccharide and Interferon-γ in Ground Glass Hepatocytes

Although the pathophysiologic basis for the death of the HBsAg-loaded hepatocyte in this model is not well understood, it has been shown that the ground glass cell is hypersensitive to certain endogenous stimuli that normally are not toxic to the HBsAg-negative hepatocyte. Specifically, it has been shown that these animals are exquisitely sensitive to the hepatocytotoxic effects of bacterial lipopolysaccharide and IFN-γ, but not to other inflammatory cytokines, and that the degree of hepatocellular injury observed after lipopolysaccharide administration is a direct function of the amount of HBsAg retained in the ER.[116] The pathophysiologic basis for this effect is not known.

Development of a Model of Immune-Mediated Acute Hepatitis in Hepatitis B Surface Antigen Transgenic Mice

Based on observations in infected patients (discussed in the section on Studies in Infected Patients: Hepatitis B Virus), it is generally assumed that an MHC-restricted cytolytic immune response to virally encoded antigens expressed at the surface of the hepatocyte plays an important role in viral clearance and in the pathogenesis of HBV-induced liver disease. Because of the narrow host range of HBV and its nontransmissibility in routine cell culture systems, it was necessary to develop an HBV transgenic mouse model system to test this hypothesis (Fig. 31-5). In these studies, it was shown that transgenic mice that express HBV envelope antigens in their hepatocytes[352] contract acute viral hepatitis after adoptive transfer of CD8+, MHC class I (Ld)-restricted, HBsAg 28-39 (IPQSLDSWWTSL)-specific CTL lines and clones that produce IFN-γ when they recognize HBsAg.[6,224]

In the course of those studies, it was demonstrated that the earliest detectable pathologic event that occurs after the entry of these CTL into the liver is their attachment to HBsAg-positive hepatocytes, which they trigger to undergo apoptosis (Fig. 31-6). This was the first direct demonstration that antigen-specific immune effector mechanisms can destroy HBV-positive hepatocytes in vivo. As such, it provided the first direct proof of the hypothesis that HBV-induced liver disease has an immunologic basis.

Cytotoxic T-Lymphocyte–Induced Acute Viral Hepatitis Is a Multistep Process

In an extension of these studies, it was demonstrated that the severity of the CTL-induced necroinflammatory liver disease in these animals depended on the route of CTL administration, the production of IFN-γ by the CTL, the number of HBsAg-positive hepatocytes present within the liver, the amount of HBsAg within each hepatocyte, and the sex of the recipient. Furthermore, by quantitative morphometric histopathologic

Adoptive Transfer of HBsAg Specific CTL to HBsAg Transgenic Mice

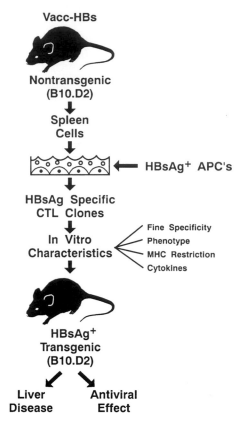

FIG. 31-5. Experimental strategy used to examine the pathogenetic and antiviral effects of hepatitis B virus (HBV)-specific, major histocompatibility complex (MHC) class I-restricted, cytotoxic T lymphocytes (CTL) in transgenic mice that express the corresponding viral antigen in their hepatocytes. Nontransgenic mice are immunized with a vaccinia virus (Vacc-HBs) that expresses the HBV envelope proteins. Spleen cells from these animals are cultured to produce CTL lines that are cloned and characterized in vitro. MHC class I-restricted CD8+ CTL that recognize hepatitis B surface antigen (HBsAg)-positive target cells and secrete interferon-γ and tumor necrosis factor-‡ are injected intravenously into syngeneic transgenic mice whose hepatocytes express HBsAg. The pathogenetic and antiviral consequences of CTL activation in the liver are monitored at the biochemical, histopathologic, and molecular levels. APCs, antigen-presenting cells.

analysis of the liver at different time points after the injection of CTL, it was shown that the disease progresses through a series of clearly definable steps in an orderly fashion.

Step 1 begins, within 1 hour of CTL administration, with antigen recognition by the CTL and delivery of a signal that results in the death of the hepatocyte by apoptosis, as described earlier. This event appears to be limited to very few cells, however, possibly because free-ranging CTL movement is severely limited by the architectural constraints of solid tissue. The direct CTL-target cell interaction results in widely scattered, acidophilic Councilman bodies (apoptotic hepato-

cytes) that are characteristic of acute viral hepatitis in humans.[318] To our knowledge, this is the first definitive demonstration that class I-restricted CTL can directly destroy their target cells in vivo.

Step 2 begins between 4 to 12 hours later, when the CTL recruit many host-derived inflammatory cells into their immediate vicinity, resulting in the formation of necroinflammatory foci, and by the extension of hepatocellular necrosis to the periphery of necroinflammatory foci, well beyond the CTL, indicating that the hepatocytes were being killed by cells other than the CTL themselves. The histopathologic features of step 2 were abrogated by lethal irradiation, which also caused a 24-hour delay in the disease process, indicating that radiation-sensitive lymphocytes and neutrophils probably contribute importantly to this aspect of the disease. It is likely that step 2 is mediated by secretion of one or more cytokines by the antigen-activated CTL, but the identity of the responsible factors has not been established at this point.

Like most cases of human acute hepatitis, the disease is always transient in these mice, is relatively mild (destroying no more than 5% of the hepatocytes), and is never fatal, unless the hepatocytes retain HBsAg because they express the large envelope polypeptide (see previous discussion). In that case, the disease extends to step 3, which kills nearly half of the mice within 3 days of CTL injection.

Step 3 is characterized by massive hepatocellular necrosis, a lymphomononuclear inflammatory cell infiltrate, and Kupffer cell hyperplasia, and it resembles the histopathologic features of HBV-induced fulminant hepatitis in humans.[318] The inflammatory cells, especially the macrophages, outnumber the injected CTL by at least 100-fold at this point in the disease process. Step 3 can be completely prevented by the prior administration of neutralizing antibodies to IFN-γ or by the inactivation of macrophages by multiple injections of carrageenan.[7]

Collectively, these observations suggest that most of the histopathologic manifestations of the liver disease in this model, except hepatocellular apoptosis, are mediated by antigen-nonspecific cytokines and effector cells that have been activated by the virus-specific T cells, and not by the CTL themselves. The striking similarities between the immunopathologic and histopathologic features of the current model and acute viral hepatitis in humans suggest that similar events probably contribute importantly to the pathogenesis of the human disease as well (Fig. 31-7).

Cytotoxic T Lymphocytes Can Inhibit Hepatitis B Virus Gene Expression and Viral Replication Without Killing the Hepatocyte

It is interesting that the CTL-induced liver disease in these transgenic mice is always transient, resolving within 7 days of CTL administration. While studying the basis for this observation it was learned that, in addition to initiating the foregoing immunopathologic response, the CTL also downregulate the expression and replication of HBV by all of the hepatocytes in the liver *without killing them.*[121]

Indeed, using transgenic mice containing the complete viral genome that sustain relatively little liver disease after CTL administration, hepatocellular HBV gene expression was found to be profoundly suppressed by noncytolytic regulatory sig-

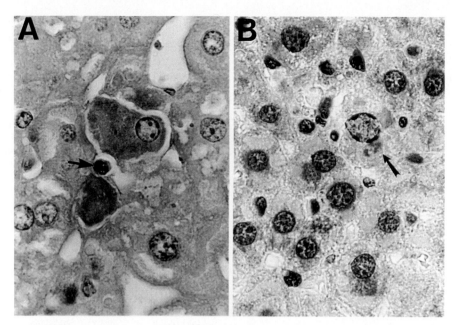

FIG. 31-6. Hepatitis B surface antigen (HBsAg)-specific cytotoxic T lymphocytes (CTL) are directly cytopathic for HBsAg-positive hepatocytes and trigger them to undergo apoptosis. Within 1 hour after HBsAg-specific CTL labeled in vitro with bromodeoxyuridine (*arrow*) are injected into HBsAg transgenic mice, they are seen to enter the liver, bind to selected hepatocytes, and induce nuclear chromatin margination, nuclear and cytoplasmic condensation and fragmentation, cytoplasmic blebbing, and cell shrinkage, the characteristic cytologic features of apoptosis (**A**), and DNA fragmentation (**B**, *arrow*) revealed by in situ end labeling using the terminal transferase reaction (**B**). (Immunohistochemical stain for bromodeoxyuridine; original magnification ×600. Modified and reproduced, with permission, from Ando K, Guidotti LG, Wirth S, et al. Class I restricted cytotoxic T lymphocytes are directly cytopathic for their target cells in vivo. J Immunol 1994;152: 3245–3253.)

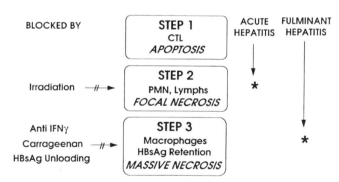

FIG. 31-7. Class I-restricted immunopathogenesis is a multistep process in hepatitis B surface antigen (HBsAg) transgenic mice. The ability of hepatitis B virus (HBV)-specific cytotoxic T lymphocytes (CTL) to induce the HBV hepatocyte to undergo apoptosis (step 1) represents a critical initiating event, but most of the liver cell injury is caused by the antigen-nonspecific inflammatory cells that the CTL recruit. The CTL induce a stereotypic response in which polymorphonuclear cells (PMN) and nonspecific lymphomononuclear cells (Lymphs) amplify the effects of the CTL locally, forming discrete necroinflammatory foci (step 2) surrounding each CTL. The CTL also release inflammatory cytokines such as interferon-γ (IFNγ; step 3) that activate intrahepatic macrophages and destroy a subset of HBsAg-positive hepatocytes that retain the large HBsAg polypeptide in their endoplasmic reticulum ("ground glass" hepatocytes). The striking histopathologic similarities between this model and human viral hepatitis suggest that similar immunopathogenetic mechanisms may be operative in the natural disease.

nals delivered by the HBsAg-specific CTL (Fig. 31-8). In further studies,[123] it has been shown that all of the viral gene products, including the 3.5- and 2.1-kb viral RNAs, their translation products (HBcAg, HBeAg, and HBsAg), and episomal replicative DNA intermediates, are susceptible to this remarkable effect, suggesting that a strong intrahepatic immune response to HBV could suppress viral replication and, if the supercoiled viral genome is eliminated by this process, perhaps even "cure" infected hepatocytes of the virus without killing them. In addition, the data suggest that a weak immune response could actively contribute to viral persistence and chronic liver disease by reducing the expression of viral antigens sufficiently for most but not all of the infected cells to escape immune recognition.

The regulatory effect of the CTL does not merely represent the destruction of HBsAg-positive hepatocytes, for several reasons. First, HBV steady-state mRNA was reduced more than 95% in transgenic mice despite the fact that no more than 5% of the hepatocytes were destroyed by the CTL, whereas virtually 100% of the hepatocytes express HBV RNA by in situ hybridization. Hence, the magnitude of the reduction in HBV gene expression greatly exceeds the amount of cell death in these animals. Second, it is possible to dissociate the cytopathic and regulatory effects of the CTL by the prior administration of antibodies to IFN-γ or tumor necrosis factor (TNF)-α, which completely abrogate the regulatory effect without affecting disease severity. Finally, the kinetics of the pathogenetic and regulatory effects of the CTL are quite different: namely, the peak of disease activity occurs on day 2,

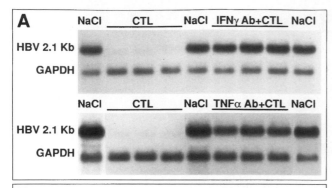

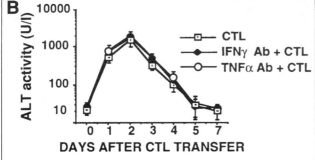

FIG. 31-8. Hepatitis B virus (HBV)-specific cytotoxic T lymphocytes (CTL) inhibit hepatocellular HBV gene expression by a noncytolytic process in vivo. Five days after hepatitis B surface antigen (HBsAg)-specific CTL are injected into HBsAg transgenic mice, the viral RNA is no longer detectable (**A**). This is completely prevented by pretreatment with antibodies to interferon-γ (IFNγ) and tumor necrosis factor-$\ddagger$ (TNF$\ddagger$), indicating that these cytokines mediate this property of the CTL. The CTL also cause a moderately severe hepatitis in these animals (**B**) that is not affected by the anti-lymphokine antibodies, demonstrating that the regulatory (antiviral?) and cytopathic effects of the CTL are independent of each other. GAPDH, cellular housekeeping gene used to normalize each lane for total RNA content; ALT, alanine aminotransferase, a liver enzyme that is released into the blood by injured hepatocytes and serves as a marker of liver disease; Ab, antibody. (Adapted, with permission, from Guidotti LG, Ando K, Hobbs MV, et al. Cytotoxic T lymphocytes inhibit hepatitis B virus gene expression by a noncytolytic mechanism in transgenic mice. Proc Natl Acad Sci U S A 1994;91:3764–3768.)

whereas reduction of HBV mRNA does not begin until day 3 and is maximal on day 5 after CTL administration in both lineages.

It is likely that IFN-γ and TNF-α act interdependently to inhibit HBV gene expression, because the CTL effect is blocked completely by monoclonal antibodies specific for each cytokine. Because IFN-γ is a powerful macrophage activator, it is quite possible that its effect is mediated by TNF-α produced by activated macrophages. This hypothesis is strengthened by the observation that recombinant TNF-α also inhibits HBV gene expression in these mice,[115] as does IL2, and that the regulatory effect of IL2 is mediated by TNF-α[122] through a posttranscriptional mechanism that selectively accelerates the degradation of cytoplasmic HBV mRNA.[126]

The foregoing observations provide a glimpse into previously unsuspected, noncytolytic immunologic events that could contribute to viral clearance or persistence during HBV infection. Because of the obvious pathogenetic and therapeutic potential of this system, the extracellular and intracellular pathways that transmit the regulatory message from the CTL to the viral genome and the target sequences within HBV that respond to the regulatory signals are important areas for future investigation. Together with the compelling evidence that the immune system can also destroy antigen-positive hepatocytes and cause an acute necroinflammatory liver disease in these animals, the stage is set for a consideration of the evidence that similar events might be responsible for viral clearance and persistence during HBV infection in humans.

STUDIES IN INFECTED PATIENTS: HEPATITIS B VIRUS

Antibody Response to Hepatitis B Virus

The antibody response to HBV envelope antigens is a T-cell–dependent process[211] that plays a critical role in viral clearance by complexing with free viral particles and removing them from the circulation and by preventing their attachment and uptake by susceptible cells.

As generally observed in most viral infections, the HBV proteins critical for induction of neutralizing antibodies are glycoproteins expressed on the surface of the viral particles,* specifically, HBsAg, preS1, and preS2. Accordingly, anti-HBV surface protein antibodies appear soon after clearance of HBsAg, whereas they usually are not detectable in persistently infected patients with chronic hepatitis. These antibodies also contribute to the pathogenesis of several extrahepatic syndromes associated with HBV infection, including glomerulonephritis, cryoglobulinemia, polyarteritis nodosa, and the prodromal syndromes of urticaria and arthralgia, by forming antigen-antibody complexes.

These anti-envelope antibodies are not thought to cause liver disease. Because they are produced by patients who clear the virus and recover from acute hepatitis, and are usually undetectable in the serum of patients with chronic HBV infection, they are thought to play an important role in viral clearance. This concept must be reexamined, however, in view of the serologic profiles emerging from more recent studies using reagents that can detect these antibodies in the presence of excess antigen. These studies reveal that anti-envelope antibodies are indeed produced by most patients with chronic hepatitis B, but they are complexed with surface antigens secreted by the infected liver and present at high concentrations in the serum.[201] Accordingly, the HBV-specific B-cell response may be entirely intact in chronic hepatitis.

The role of the antibody response to the nucleocapsid antigens (HBcAg and HBeAg) and to the nonstructural HBV proteins in HBV pathogenesis is still a debated issue.[47,91,311,312,347,362] It is generally accepted that these antibodies do not express neutralizing activity because they are present in high titers in pa-

*References 2, 17, 31, 79, 152, 172, 233, 245.

tients with chronic HBV infection. This may be caused in part by chronic B-cell stimulation by HBcAg, which has been shown to function as a T-cell–independent as well as a T-cell–dependent antigen.[211] Passively administered anti-HBeAg antibodies, however, have protected chimpanzees against HBV infection,[313] suggesting that they play some currently obscure role in HBV pathogenesis.

Antigen-Specific T-Cell Response to Hepatitis B Virus

As we have reviewed,[57,58] the peripheral blood and intrahepatic T-cell response to HBV-encoded antigens has been studied extensively in vaccine recipients and infected patients. In general, the T-cell response to HBV is vigorous, polyclonal, and multispecific in patients with acute hepatitis who ultimately clear the virus, and it is relatively weak and more restricted in patients with chronic hepatitis who do not (Table 31-2). Many class I- and class II-restricted T-cell epitopes

have been defined in the various HBV proteins. The class II-restricted, CD4+ helper T-cell response is focused principally on the nucleocapsid antigens of HBV in acutely infected patients, whereas the envelope and polymerase antigens are more often targeted by the class I-restricted CD8+ CTL response in these patients.

CD4+ T-Cell Response in Acute Hepatitis B

In general, HLA class II-restricted CD4+ T cells recognize peptide fragments derived from extracellular antigens that are proteolytically processed in acidified endosomes or lysosomes after endocytosis by specialized antigen-presenting cells (macrophages, dendritic cells, B cells).[114] Viral peptides are seen by the T-cell receptor in association with HLA class II molecules.

Virtually all patients with self-limited acute hepatitis produce a vigorous HLA class II-restricted peripheral blood T-

TABLE 31-2. *Immune responses to hepatitis B virus (HBV) and hepatitis C virus (HCV) proteins in patients with acute and chronic HBV and HCV infections*

Virus	Antigen	B-cell response Antibody		T-cell response CD4		CD8	
		Acute	Chronic	Acute	Chronic	Acute	Chronic
HBV	PreS1	++*†	+	+	ND	ND	ND
	PreS2	++	+	+	±§	ND	±
	HBsAg	++	+‡	+	±	+++‖	ND
	HBcAg	+++	+++	+++	±¶	+++	±
	HBeAg	++	+	+++	±	+++	±
	Polymerase	+	+	ND	ND	+++	±
	HBxAg	+	+	ND	±	ND	ND
HCV	Core	+++	+++	ND	++	ND	++
	E1	+#	++	ND	+	ND	++
	E2/NS1	+	++	ND	+	ND	++
	NS2	ND	ND	ND	ND	ND	++
	NS3	+++	+++	ND	+	ND	++
	NS4	++	++	ND	++	ND	++
	NS5	++	++	ND	±	ND	++

*Because extensive and sequential studies of the antibody response to preS1, preS2, polymerase, and HBxAg in HBV-infected patients are missing, the relevance of these responses could be underestimated.

†Anti-preS1 antibodies to the putative attachment site of HBV to the hepatocyte membrane are detectable in self-limited acute hepatitis but not in chronic HBV infection.

‡Anti-envelope and anti-e antibodies are produced by most patients with chronic HBV infection but they are frequently undetectable by commercial immunoassays because of the presence of an excess of circulating antigens.

§HBV envelope- and HBcAg-specific CD4+ T cells are detectable within the liver of patients with chronic infection, but their frequency appears to be low.

¶The CD4-mediated responses to HBcAg and HBeAg, which are generally weak or undetectable in the peripheral blood of patients with chronic HBV infection, can increase during exacerbations of chronic liver disease.

Available information on the CD8 response against the different HBV proteins is so far limited to the HLA-A2–restricted responses that have been analyzed with synthetic peptides containing the HLA-A2 binding motifs.

#Little information is available about the kinetics of the anti-envelope antibodies in acute hepatitis C.

±, very weak response; +, weak response; ++, moderate response; +++, strong response; ND, not determined; CD4, helper T cells; CD8, cytotoxic T cells; PreS, promoter controlling envelope gene expression; HBsAg, hepatitis B surface antigen; HBcAg, hepatitis B core antigen; HBeAg, hepatitis B precore antigen; HBxAg, hepatitis B X protein antigen; E, envelope; NS, nonstructural; HLA, human leukocyte antigen.

cell response directed against several epitopes within HBcAg and HBeAg (Fig. 31-9), a few of which appear to be strongly immunodominant and widely recognized by patients with different HLA backgrounds.[92,96] Surprisingly, the CD4+ T-cell response to the HBV envelope antigens is relatively weak in these patients, despite the fact that it is frequently strong in vaccine recipients who have been immunized with plasma-derived or recombinant HBsAg.[41,42,95,157]

The nucleocapsid specific response is temporally associated with the clearance of HBV envelope antigens and infectious virus from the serum in acutely infected patients, suggesting that it may be required for efficient virus elimination. This notion is reinforced by the fact that the CD4+ T-cell response to the nucleocapsid is weak in patients with chronic HBV infection who do not spontaneously clear the virus.[96,98,158] Because the kinetics and vigor of the CD4+ nucleocapsid-specific T-cell response during acute hepatitis parallel those of the HLA class I-restricted CTL response to all of the viral antigens[217,230,257] (see discussion later), it is possible that these T cells facilitate the induction of virus-specific CTL.

In addition, viral clearance is probably facilitated by the direct cooperation between HBcAg-specific helper T cells and HBV envelope-specific B cells, through a mechanism of "intermolecular" help, leading to amplification of the virus-neutralizing anti-envelope antibody response. It is well known that B cells can be helped to produce antibodies by T cells of different antigen specificity, provided that different viral antigens are coexpressed in the same protein or present in the same viral particle, thereby creating a physical link between helper T cells and antibody-producing B cells. For instance, HBV envelope-specific B cells, which bind virions by receptors for native HBV surface protein and preS determinants, can process viral particles (that contain HBcAg) and present specific epitopes derived from HBcAg degradation to HBcAg-specific T cells, which, in turn, can provide T-cell help to envelope-specific B cells, resulting in the production of anti-envelope antibodies.[212] This mechanism may be critical for anti-HBsAg production in view of the weak HLA class II-restricted T-cell response to the envelope antigens in these patients, despite their ability to produce a strong anti-envelope antibody response.

It has been suggested that an anti-envelope T-cell response may occur during the preclinical incubation period of disease.[341] If this is correct, it can be speculated that HBV envelope-specific T cells could become either exhausted as a result of infection with high doses of virus, or paralyzed by the high concentrations of envelope antigens that may occur when early immune responses fail completely and rapidly to eradicate infection. Under these conditions, the nucleocapsid-specific helper T-cell population could indeed provide the crucial immunoregulatory T cells for the development of protective antiviral immunity. It is also possible, however, that class II-restricted T cells of all HBV antigen specificities could be anergized rather than activated if they can recognize antigen on the surface of infected hepatocytes that are induced to express class II by the inflammatory response, because such cells would not express the costimulatory molecules (e.g., B7) that are needed to activate CD4+ T cells after antigen recognition.

CD4+ T-Cell Response in Chronic Hepatitis B

During chronic HBV infection, the peripheral blood HLA class II-restricted T-cell response to all viral antigens, including HBcAg and HBeAg, is much less vigorous than in patients with acute hepatitis[96,158] (see Fig. 31-9). In neonatal infection, this is probably explainable on the basis of neonatal tolerance. During adult-onset infection, however, the basis for this important difference is not clear, but it probably plays a critical role in the development of viral persistence (see sections on Neonatal Tolerance and Tolerance During Adult-Onset Infection). These T cells are present in the liver at low frequency.[94,97] The response appears to be accentuated during acute exacerbations of disease, which are often preceded by increased serum HBV DNA and HBeAg concentrations that can drop dramatically as the flare in disease activity subsides.[325] In contrast, during these reactivation episodes, serum HBsAg concentrations usually remain unchanged and the proliferative response to HBV envelope antigens remains weak or undetectable.

The scenario emerging from these data is that the class II-restricted, nucleocapsid-specific T-cell response, and perhaps

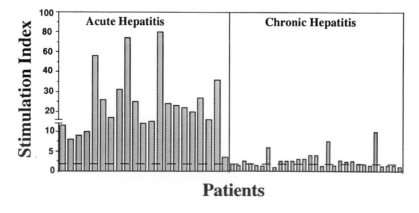

FIG. 31-9. The class II-restricted T-cell response to the hepatitis B virus nucleocapsid protein during acute and chronic hepatitis. The CD4+ proliferative T-cell response to hepatitis B core antigen and hepatitis B precore antigen is vigorous in patients with acute hepatitis who clear the virus, and it is weak or not detectable in chronically infected patients who do not clear the virus. (Adapted, with permission, from Ferrari C, Penna A, Bertoletti A, et al. Cellular immune response to hepatitis B virus-encoded antigens in acute and chronic hepatitis B virus infection. J Immunol 1990;145:3442–3449.)

the temporally associated flare of liver disease, may depend on the attainment of a critical level of viral replication indicated by the expression of HBV nucleocapsid antigens.[200,201] According to this hypothesis, nucleocapsid-specific T cells could play a key immunoregulatory role, whereas envelope-specific T-cell activity may be suppressed by the persistently elevated levels of circulating HBsAg.

It has been shown that the evolution of certain infections may be profoundly influenced by the specific pattern of lymphokines stimulated by the infectious agent. Results from a murine model of leishmaniasis and from human leprosy suggest that T helper 1-like (Th1-like) responses, dominated by the production of IL2, IFN-γ, and TNF-β, are particularly effective against intracellular pathogens; T helper 2-like (Th2-like) responses, such as those induced by helminths and associated with preferential secretion of IL4, IL5, IL6, and IL10, are instead critical for antibody responses and therefore important for protection against extracellular pathogens.[256] Preliminary data indicate that in chronic HBV infection, a Th1-like response is strongly represented in the intrahepatic lymphomononuclear infiltrate.[13,94]

CD8+ T-Cell Response in Acute Hepatitis B

Antiviral CTL are believed to play a major role in eradication of infection by virtue of their capacity to identify and kill virus-infected cells through recognition of viral peptides presented by HLA class I molecules.[358] In addition, the ability of CTL to clear certain viruses, including HBV, from infected cells by noncytolytic pathways is becoming increasingly appreciated (see section on Cytotoxic T Lymphocytes Can Inhibit Hepatitis B Virus Gene Expression), and may ultimately prove to be the most important antiviral function of the CTL.

Because of the restricted host range of HBV and its lack of infectivity in vitro, the CTL response to this virus has been difficult to study. Thanks to the emerging understanding of the molecular basis for antigen recognition, an experimental strategy to study the CTL response to HBV has been developed. HLA class I-restricted CD8+ T cells recognize peptides that are usually 8 to 11 residues long derived from the intracellular cytosolic processing of endogenously synthesized viral antigens that are transported into the ER, where those peptides that display specific amino acid motifs attach to the antigen-binding groove of the resident HLA class I molecules.*Therefore, by combining the use of HBV-derived synthetic peptides containing these motifs to stimulate the expansion of HBV-specific CTL, and eukaryotic expression vectors that direct the synthesis of the corresponding native viral proteins in human cells so that they may be processed and presented to the peptide-stimulated CTL in the context of the corresponding HLA class I molecules,[21,125,257] it is possible to detect HBV-specific CTL in peripheral blood mononuclear cell cultures from patients with acute viral hepatitis. Most of the CTL epitopes identified thus far using this approach (Fig. 31-10) are 9-mers or 10-mers that contain the HLA-A2 binding motif with leucine in position 2 and valine at the carboxy-terminus.[19,230]

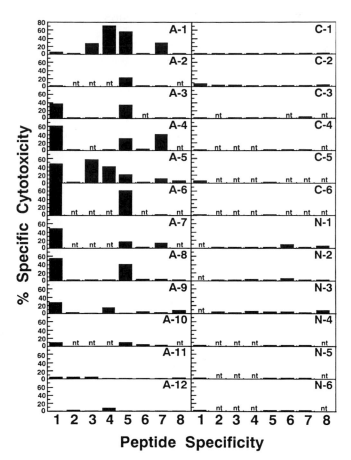

FIG. 31-10. The human leukocyte antigen (HLA) class I-restricted T-cell response to multiple hepatitis B virus (HBV) envelope and nucleocapsid epitopes during acute and chronic hepatitis. The CD8+, HLA-A2–restricted cytotoxic T-cell response to one nucleocapsid epitope and seven different HBV envelope epitopes is vigorous, polyclonal, and multispecific in patients with acute hepatitis, and weak or nonexistent in patients with chronic hepatitis. (Adapted, with permission, from Nayersina R, Folwer P, Guilhot S, et al. HLA A2 restricted cytotoxic T lymphocyte responses to multiple hepatitis B surface antigen epitopes during hepatitis B virus infection. J Immunol 1993;150:4659–4671.)

Several novel and pathogenetically relevant aspects of the HLA class I-restricted response to HBV antigens have emerged as a result of these studies in acutely infected patients. First, patients with acute self-limited infection manifest a vigorous, polyclonal, HLA class I-restricted CTL response against multiple epitopes in the HBV envelope, nucleocapsid, and polymerase proteins[230,257,271] (see Fig. 31-10). Second, several of the epitopes, especially core 18 to 27, envelope 183 to 191, envelope 250 to 258, envelope 335 to 343, and polymerase 455 to 463, are recognized by most of the infected patients, whereas the rest are seen by a minority of subjects, suggesting that a CTL response hierarchy exists for this virus. Third, this hierarchy is influenced by the HLA-A2 binding affinity of the peptides and the degree to which they are conserved among HBV isolates, but other, undefined factors must

---

*References 85, 106, 128, 149, 154, 206, 220, 267, 276, 301, 339, 358, 364.

play a role because many of the highest-affinity and well conserved peptides do not elicit a CTL response in acutely infected patients. Finally, a number of CTL epitopes have been identified within viral sequences that are critical for specific viral functions. For example, the nuclear localization and genome encapsidation signals of HBcAg span nucleocapsid residues 141 to 151, which contain an important CTL epitope that is dually recognized by HLA A31- and HLA Aw68-restricted CTL.[217] Similarly, an important topogenic sequence in the transmembrane domain of HBsAg overlaps an HLA-A2–restricted CTL epitope located between HBV envelope residues 250 to 269.[230] These factors, plus the polyclonality and multispecificity of the CTL response, mitigate against the emergence of viral escape mutants during acute viral hepatitis.

Although these observations indicate a strong relationship between the vigor and polyclonality of the CTL response and viral clearance, they do not prove that this is a causal relationship. The clearest and most direct evidence that this is true is provided by the transgenic mouse experiments described earlier in the final three sections under The Transgenic Mouse Model. Those studies suggest that the clearance of HBV from all infected hepatocytes may be mediated principally by the antiviral cytokines released by HBV-specific CTL rather than the destructive effect of the CTL. Indeed, as discussed later in the sections on Neonatal Tolerance and Tolerance During Adult-Onset Infection, the number of infected hepatocytes in the liver can exceed the number of HBV-specific CTL in the body so greatly that antigen-specific destruction of all the infected cells by the CTL would appear to be physically impossible.

CD8+ T-Cell Response in Chronic Hepatitis B

In contrast to the vigorous CTL response that is detectable in the peripheral blood of most patients who successfully clear the virus, HBV persistence is typically associated with a weak or undetectable, virus-specific CTL response (see Fig. 31-10). As was discussed previously for the class II-restricted T-cell response to HBV, whereas neonatal tolerance is probably responsible for the lack of an antiviral immune response and viral persistence after mother-infant transmission, the immunologic basis for CTL nonresponsiveness to HBV during adult-onset infection is not understood. Nonetheless, the evidence suggests that the vigor of the CTL response to HBV plays a principal role in determining whether an infected person clears the virus.[217,230,257,271] It also suggests that the weak CTL response may actually cause the indolent necroinflammatory liver disease that is characteristic of chronic HBV infection. Experiments indicate that although the HBV-specific CTL precursor frequency is greatly diminished in the peripheral blood of chronically infected patients, such CTL are nonetheless present in the periphery,[20] and they are also present in the infected liver.[11] Thus, it appears that HBV-specific T cells have not been clonally deleted in these patients. Instead, the data suggest that they have not undergone clonal expansion to the same extent as they do in patients who clear the virus. Once again, the reason for this difference is not understood, and this question represents one of the most important areas remaining to be elucidated in HBV immunobiology and pathogenesis.

Mechanisms of Viral Persistence

The dramatic difference between the strength of the antiviral T-cell response in acute and chronic HBV infection suggests that it is an important determinant of viral clearance and persistence. For a noncytopathic virus to persist, it must either not induce an effective antiviral immune response or it must be able to evade or overwhelm it. Several different mechanisms exist whereby a virus can elude recognition by the immune system.

Neonatal Tolerance

Clonal deletion of HBV-specific T cells could play an important role in the chronic infection that develops in infants born to infected mothers. The cellular basis for this observation has been investigated in a transgenic mouse model of neonatal tolerance to HBeAg.[210] In these studies, nontransgenic progeny of transgenic mothers were tolerant to both HBeAg and HBcAg at the T-cell level, presumably because of the transplacental passage of low–molecular-weight HBeAg resulting in the clonal deletion of MHC class II-restricted HBeAg-helper T cells in the developing thymus. This mechanism should not be operative, however, for the immune response to large particulate antigens (such as HBsAg) or to antigens contained within viral particles (such as polymerase) that are known to be immunogenic at the T-cell level but cannot cross the normal placental barrier. In the presence of placental disease, however, intrauterine infection can occur, and then the foregoing process of central tolerance to all of the viral antigens can occur.

Intrapartum or postpartum infection can also lead to viral persistence by delaying the onset of the antiviral immune response, because of the immaturity of the immune system, until the virus has spread throughout the liver. The number of potentially infected hepatocytes is vast (approximately 10^{11} per liver), and the number of HBV-specific T cells that can be produced is relatively small (consider that the total number of lymphocytes in the body is also approximately 10^{11} cells, and that antigen-specific T-cell frequencies during acute HBV infection are at best between 1 in 1000 and 1 in 10,000 total T cells). In view of these facts, once an infection is established in even a significant minority of the hepatocytes, it may never be possible for the immune response to eradicate it, at least not by the traditional mechanisms of direct, T-cell–mediated destruction of infected cells, because it is probably physically impossible for these T cells to reach all of the infected hepatocytes. Furthermore, these late-developing T cells may be inactivated if their T-cell receptors bind specific antigen on nonprofessional antigen-presenting cells (e.g., hepatocytes) that lack the necessary costimulatory molecules (e.g., B7) that must simultaneously engage receptors on the T cells (e.g., CD28) to activate them instead of triggering them to become anergic or undergo apoptosis.

Perinatal tolerance is probably responsible for most of the persistent HBV infections in the world because perinatal infection is the most common mode of transmission of HBV in Asia and Africa, where most of the chronic HBV infections occur.

Tolerance During Adult-Onset Infection

In adult-onset infection, immunologic tolerance may also be caused by an imbalance between the timing and vigor of the immune response and the kinetics and extent of the infection, coupled with the inactivation of HBV-specific T cells by the incomplete signals delivered by infected nonprofessional antigen-presenting epithelial cells (i.e., hepatocytes). Once again, in our opinion, the sheer mass of potentially infectible cells in the liver greatly exceeds the direct sterilizing capacity of the immune response by several orders of magnitude. In this scenario, viral clearance would occur when the immune response develops before the virus spreads to a critical mass of hepatocytes, beyond which it may be ineradicable simply because there are not enough antigen-specific T cells to reach and destroy all of the infected hepatocytes, as discussed previously. Therefore, the viral and host factors that determine the kinetics of the immune response and the rate of viral spread are probably the primary determinants of viral clearance or persistence in these and other viral infections. Even in the context of an early and vigorous immune response, however, it is likely that the noncytolytic antiviral activities of virus-specific T cells, mediated by diffusible products, such as IFN-γ and TNF-α, which they release on antigen recognition, may actually be primarily responsible for viral clearance during HBV infection. According to this hypothesis, the attendant liver disease could be viewed as an undesirable consequence of antigen-specific T-cell recognition that plays a minor role in viral clearance, and that clearance is principally mediated by the antiviral cytokines that the same T cells release when they recognize infected cells. Future efforts should be directed toward the identification of these host and viral factors, to the development of assays to predict their occurrence early during viral infection, and to the establishment of immunostimulatory and antiviral strategies to tip this balance in favor of the host.

In addition to the foregoing, several other events may also contribute to viral persistence. These events are discussed in the paragraphs that follow. These processes, however, are not likely to be the primary cause of viral persistence. Instead, they can probably occur only after the infection is already persistent, under which circumstances they can tip the balance further in favor of the virus, and thereby consolidate the persistence of the virus in the previously chronically infected host.

Evasion of Immune Recognition

Infection of Immunologically Privileged Sites

Infection of peripheral tissues that cannot be easily reached by lymphocytes, or exposure of antigen on cell types that do not express MHC molecules, is ignored by the immune system. By this mechanism, viruses could persist and replicate, eluding lymphocyte recognition at the site of replication. Consistent with this mechanism of persistence, it has been demonstrated[5] that HBV-specific, class I-restricted CTL injected intravascularly into HBV transgenic mice can recognize and destroy HBV antigen-positive hepatocytes but ignore the same antigens expressed in other tissues (e.g., brain, kidney, testis, pancreas, gastrointestinal tract) in the same animals because their access to antigen at these sites is precluded by microvascular anatomic barriers in these tissues that do not exist in the sinusoidal structure of the liver. The same process may occur during natural HBV or HCV infection because replicative forms of these viruses have been detected in mesenteric lymph nodes, spleen, kidney, pancreas, brain, and in some endocrine tissues, including testis, ovary, and adrenal and thyroid glands.[247,359] Virions released from such immunologically protected sites could infect liver cells, where they would maintain the antiviral specific CTL response as well as the associated chronic liver disease.

Alteration of Recognition Molecules on the Surface of Infected Cells

Studies with adenoviruses, cytomegalovirus, and Epstein-Barr virus reveal that expression of HLA and other accessory molecules can be influenced by the viruses themselves, leading to inefficient recognition of infected cells by CTL and virus escape from immune clearance.[29,109,236,246] Although there is no evidence that HBV exerts a direct negative influence on the expression of HLA or accessory molecules, the findings that HBV can suppress transcription of the IFN-β[350] and can inhibit the cellular response to IFN-α and IFN-γ[103] suggest that HBV may have the capacity to downregulate these accessory molecules indirectly. Another mechanism through which viruses can evade lymphocyte recognition is by downregulating the expression of their own proteins.[246] It is well known that HBV can integrate into the host genome, which interrupts at least one of the coding regions of the virus, thereby reducing its accessibility to the immune system.

Selective Immune Suppression

Viruses such as HBV and HCV that infect lymphocytes and monocytes have the potential to cause either selective or generalized immunosuppression of the host.[246] Global immunosuppression does not occur during infection by any of the hepatitis viruses. In contrast, virus-specific defects in T-cell responsiveness are characteristic of chronic hepatitis, especially during HBV infection. Because HBV virions and defective HBV envelope particles have been shown to enter the class II processing pathway in T cells after uptake by the transferrin receptor, HBV peptide-HLA class II complexes could in theory target T cells for elimination by HLA class II-restricted CTL,[99,105] similar to the mechanism responsible for elimination of gp120-specific T cells in human immunodeficiency virus infection.[183,300] It also has been shown that exogenous HBsAg can enter the class I processing pathway in a variety of cell types, including B and T cells, that can subsequently be killed by class I-restricted CTL.[281,282] Thus, it is conceivable that HBV-specific T cells drawn to the site of antigen synthesis could also take up viral envelope antigens, process and present them to neighboring envelope-specific CTL, and be eliminated. Similarly, HBsAg-specific B cells could be killed by class I-restricted, envelope antigen-specific CTL after antigen uptake by the immunoglobulin receptor.[12]

Finally, HBcAg-specific CD8+ T cells have been detected in the liver of patients with chronic hepatitis B that can specifically suppress the CD4+ proliferative T-cell response to HBV.[97] Although it is reasonable to speculate that these pathways might contribute to viral persistence during chronic HBV infection, this is strictly an untested hypothesis.

Virus Mutations

Escape from T-cell recognition by antigenic variation represents an effective strategy that viruses with high mutation rates, such as HBV and HCV, can in theory adopt to persist within their host. Nonetheless, several conditions must be fulfilled for a mutant virus to be selected by the immune pressure exerted by the CTL response, which may limit the likelihood of this type of event. First, the CTL response in the infected person must be selectively focused on the epitope where mutations arise; the CTL response against the variant epitope must be crucial for virus elimination; and no vital biologic functions of the virus must be affected by the mutational event.

During acute HBV infection, most patients manifest a strong, polyclonal CTL response against multiple epitopes in the viral envelope, nucleocapsid, and polymerase proteins that is vigorous enough to be detected in the peripheral blood.[217,230,257] In this condition, the likelihood of mutant selection by the CTL response is probably low because abrogation of the response against the variant epitope will not make the infected cell invisible to CTL if other epitopes are simultaneously expressed on the same cell. Thus, the enormous diversity of the T-cell repertoire, which allows T cells to "see" at the same time different details of viral structure, provides the immune system with a powerful tool to counteract the continuous attempts of the virus to escape recognition by antigenic variation. The possibility of mutant virus selection seems to be more likely in patients with chronic HBV infection in which the CTL response is weak and narrowly focused, as suggested by the identification of epitope-inactivating mutations in the context of a narrow repertoire of CTL specificities.[230,257]

Besides altering the amino acid sequence of an immunodominant epitope, a single base substitution can also influence the antiviral immune response by giving rise to new translational stop codons within an open reading frame, with abrogation of synthesis of an entire viral protein, as reported for the preC variants of HBV.[23,40] If the affected protein is critical for the development of a protective immune response, it is conceivable that viral variants that cannot produce that protein might have a survival advantage. Finally, mutant viruses could display a positive growth advantage entirely independent of any immunologic advantage, if they could replicate more efficiently than the parental wild-type virus, as suggested by reports that certain mutations in the preC region can increase the conformational stability and, perhaps, the efficiency of the viral encapsidation signal, which plays a critical role in viral replication.[131,189]

Besides rendering CTL epitopes invisible to T-cell recognition, substitutions of T-cell receptor contact sites can also influence the CTL response by creating analog peptides that can still interact with the T-cell receptor but are unable to deliver a full stimulatory signal, thus acting as antagonists. Natural variants of the HBV core 18 to 27 CTL epitope that interfere with recognition of the wild-type epitope, acting as T-cell receptor antagonists, have been identified in two patients with chronic hepatitis.[22] This property could give the variant virus a selective survival advantage over the wild-type virus if the CTL response in these patients is focused solely or predominantly on this epitope.

Suppression of Viral Gene Expression by the Immune Response

Finally, certain soluble products of the immune response, especially IFN-γ, TNF-α, and IL2, have been shown to suppress HBV gene expression and replication by the hepatocyte in vivo in a transgenic mouse model (see Studies in Animal Models). As previously discussed, this process could lead to viral clearance if it is strong enough to eliminate the virus from all of the infected hepatocytes in patients as efficiently as it does in transgenic mice. Alternatively, a less-than-vigorous immune response could actively contribute to viral persistence and chronic liver disease by downregulating viral gene expression only partially, such that most but not all of the cells can escape immune recognition.

THE HEPATITIS C VIRUS

Hepatitis C virus is an RNA virus that causes acute and chronic liver disease.[64,66,143,181] A high proportion of infected patients fail to clear the virus and contract chronic infection, which is associated with an increased incidence of HCC.[66,237,277] The mechanisms responsible for these lesions are not understood. HCV contains a positive-stranded RNA genome of about 9401 nucleotides, consisting of a single, uninterrupted long open reading frame that encodes a polyprotein of 3010 to 3011 amino acids.[65,143,167,320] Its genetic organization and some regions of amino acid homology indicate that HCV is distantly related to the *Flaviviridae* family, which includes the human flaviviruses (yellow fever viruses, dengue viruses, Japanese encephalitis viruses) and the animal pestiviruses (bovine viral diarrhea virus, hog cholera virus, and border disease virus of sheep).[65,214] Like other flaviviruses, HCV contains a small 5' untranslated region followed by an uninterrupted open reading frame coding for several structural and nonstructural proteins, derived from a single polyprotein precursor. This precursor molecule is processed posttranslationally or cotranslationally by proteases encoded by the viral genome and by the host.* The gene order in the HCV genome is 5'-C-E1-E2/NS1-NS2-NS3-NS4A-NS4B-NS5A-NS5B-3'.[120]

The far amino-terminal region contains a highly basic domain, which is thought to encode a 19- to 22-kD RNA-binding nucleocapsid protein, and is followed by two glycoproteins of about 33 kD (E1) and 72 kD (E2/NS1).[143] By analogy to pestiviral structure, E1 and E2/NS1 are believed to be components of the viral envelope.[142] In flaviviruses, the counterpart to HCV E2 is nonstructural protein 1, which is a major

---

*References 65, 84, 118, 119, 134, 135, 167, 260, 278, 320, 324.

antigenic determinant.[305] It is known that active immunization with purified E2/NS1 or transfer of anti-E2/NS1 antibodies confers protection against rechallenges of the same flavivirus.[283–285] HCV structural proteins are generated from the polyprotein precursor by cleavages that occur after hydrophobic stretches and appear to be catalyzed in the ER lumen by host signal peptidases.[134]

Processing of the nonstructural proteins is mediated by viral proteases contained within the NS2 and NS3 proteins. A serine proteinase that mediates cleavages between NS3/4A, NS4A/4B, NS4B/5A, and NS5A/5B is located in the amino-terminal one-third of the NS3 protein.[118,324] A second proteinase, which is located in the carboxy-terminal portion of the NS2 protein and extends into the NS3 region overlapping with the serine-proteinase domain, is responsible for cleavage between NS2 and NS3.[119,135] The NS3 protein also contains motifs characteristic of NTPases and helicases.[65,117,214,317] NS4 is a hydrophobic nonstructural protein of unknown function. NS5 appears to be the RNA polymerase: it is highly conserved and contains a GDD motif characteristic of a large number of viral RNA polymerases.[162,261] HCV does not replicate through DNA intermediate forms, and integrated molecules of the virus have not been detected thus far in the host genome.[143]

Several partial and complete nucleotide sequences have been derived from geographically widespread HCV isolates (Japan, Europe, the United States, and so forth).[*] The data indicate substantial sequence diversity within, and especially between, each geographic area.[302] Multiple HCV variants also have been isolated from the same patient.[198,199,227,241] The degree of similarity between isolates at the amino acid level varies from region to region. The nucleocapsid protein has the highest sequence homology (97% to 100%) between all isolates sequenced to date.[150,320,321] In contrast, the E1 and E2/NS1 regions present the highest degree of sequence variability among different isolates[143]; in particular, the amino-terminal portion of E2/NS1 contains a hypervariable region of 30 amino acids, which shows extensive variation between virtually all known isolates.[133,143,348]

Hepatitis C virus is transmitted parenterally and it is the most common cause of posttransfusion hepatitis.[338] The most striking feature of hepatitis C is its tendency toward chronicity, with reported frequencies usually exceeding 50% of the cases. The clinical course of HCV infection is similar to that of HBV-induced hepatitis. The onset is usually insidious and about 75% of the cases tend to be anicteric. Serum alanine aminotransferase elevation can be monophasic, with a rapid increase and a subsequent rapid decrease, or multiphasic. It seems that the monophasic type of infection is usually self-limiting, whereas the multiphasic form is more likely to progress to chronic liver disease.[69]

STUDIES IN INFECTED PATIENTS: HEPATITIS C VIRUS

The mechanisms whereby HCV causes acute hepatocellular injury and initiates the sequence of events leading to chronic liver disease and ultimately to HCC are not well understood. Analysis of the direct cytopathic effects of HCV for host liver

*References 53, 65, 133, 134, 150, 167, 180, 239, 242, 243, 320, 323.

cells has been hampered by the lack of suitable tissue culture systems. It is possible that both direct, virus-related or indirect (i.e., immunologically mediated) mechanisms may play an important role. Several clinical observations underline the contribution of the host immune response to liver cell injury: 1) chronic infection without evidence of liver cell injury is common; and 2) immunosuppression reduces the severity of liver cell injury in chronic hepatitis C.[139]

Although the immune response almost certainly plays an important, perhaps a central, role in HCV pathogenesis, one reproducible fact confounds our understanding of the process. Specifically, chimpanzees can be repetitively infected when they are exposed to the same infectious inoculum of HCV after recovery from a previous infection and the development of what would otherwise appear to be a perfectly competent immune response.[86,264] Although this may be the result of the well known propensity of the virus to mutate, and the presence of diverse viral quasispecies in any given inoculum, the apparent absence of a protective neutralizing humoral or cellular response to common conserved determinants in the various viral proteins is puzzling.

There is no known reason to suspect that the immune response to this virus is extremely narrow or focused only on subtype-specific determinants. Consequently, it is reasonable to wonder if HCV is relatively unresponsive to the antigen-nonspecific antiviral signals delivered by antigen-activated T cells that can noncytolytically control the replication of other viruses, including HBV. This would allow HCV to persist indefinitely in the face of an otherwise vigorous immune response, as appears to be the case in most patients infected by HCV. Much remains to be done in this area, and the discussion that follows should be interpreted with the caveat that the antiviral and pathogenetic consequences of the immune responses to be described have not been established.

Antibody Response to Hepatitis C Virus

In the absence of efficient in vitro systems to support and measure virus replication,[295,296] the neutralizing capacity of the different anti-HCV antibodies remains largely undefined. Nonetheless, HCV-specific neutralizing antibodies have been demonstrated in the plasma of chronically infected patients by in vitro neutralization of the capacity of HCV-positive inocula to infect continuous T-cell lines[294] and chimpanzees.[87] Although these antibodies can protect against infection by HCV strains previously present in the patients from which they are derived, they fail to neutralize viral strains prevalent in the patient at the time the antibodies are detected. Because the neutralizing antibody response appears to be directed against epitopes[168,266,349] located within the highly variable HCV envelope proteins,[133,322,348] it is likely that the humoral immune response contributes to viral heterogeneity by selecting for mutant viruses that lack the corresponding epitopes. In this way, the "neutralizing" antibody response to HCV may contribute more to viral persistence than to viral clearance.

Using various antigen-binding immunoassays, the kinetics of the antibody response to HCV structural and nonstructural antigens has been sequentially studied in large populations of patients from the early stages of acute infection through the development of chronic hepatitis. Immunodominant epitopes within envelope, core, NS3, and NS4 antigens have been identified,* but no clear antibody patterns associated either with virus replication or with different disease outcomes have been defined thus far.[88] It is not possible, therefore, to assign or deny the anti-HCV antibody response any role in HCV pathogenesis.

CD4+ T-Cell Response to Hepatitis C Virus

Using recombinant HCV proteins to stimulate HCV-specific T cells in the peripheral blood and intrahepatic T-cell infiltrate, the HLA class II-restricted T-cell response to HCV has been studied in patients with chronic HCV infection and in subjects apparently recovered from acute hepatitis.[25,100,288] In contrast to the relatively weak antiviral T-cell response in patients with chronic hepatitis B, the T-cell response to HCV proteins is quite vigorous in patients with chronic hepatitis C, and the response is even more vigorous after recovery from acute HCV infections.

CD4+ T cells from chronically infected patients are characteristically polyclonal and multispecific for more than one viral antigen. A clear hierarchy of T-cell responsiveness to HCV proteins has been defined in these patients. Specifically, core and NS4 are recognized by most patients, whereas the putative envelope proteins (E1 and E2/NS1) and NS5 are immunogenic for a small proportion of patients. The high immunogenicity of NS4 at the T-cell level has been confirmed by the isolation of NS4-specific T cells from the liver of patients with chronic hepatitis C.[216] Remarkably, CD4 T cells sequestered within the inflamed liver are functionally and clonotypically different from NS4-specific T cells present in the peripheral blood, suggesting a specific compartmentalization of some T cells at the site of infection. The presence of a vigorous HLA class II-restricted T-cell response in patients with chronic HCV infection despite persistence of the virus, represents an important difference in the pathobiology of chronic HBV and HCV infections and probably reflects different pathogenetic mechanisms operative during infection by these hepatotropic viruses.

CD8+ T-Cell Response to Hepatitis C Virus

Similar to the foregoing, HLA class I-restricted HCV-specific CD8+ CTL are detectable in the peripheral blood and the lymphocytic infiltrate in patients with chronic hepatitis C.[45,178,179] A similar CTL response has been demonstrated in the liver of acutely infected chimpanzees, and the response has been shown to persist indefinitely after infection, indicating that the virus can persist in the presence of these CTL.[82]

The CTL identified thus far in infected patients are able to recognize both conserved and variable regions of the HCV core, E1, E2/NS1, NS2, NS4, and NS5 antigens in the context of several different HLA molecules.[45,171,178,179,297] Moreover, the response is often polyclonal and multispecific in individual chronically infected patients. CTL clones have been isolated from the intrahepatic compartment using only antigen-nonspecific stimuli, implying that these cells must be present at high

frequency within the intrahepatic infiltrate.[178,179] In contrast, it is necessary to expand the peripheral blood CTL precursor population with HCV-derived peptides to demonstrate a CTL response to HCV. Nonetheless, the HCV-specific CTL response is probably stronger than the response to HBV because it can be relatively easily detected in the periphery during chronic infection, whereas the response to HBV cannot, and because virus-specific lesional T cells seem to be more highly represented in HCV-infected than in HBV-infected livers.

This difference suggests that distinct mechanisms are likely to be involved in the immunopathogenesis of viral hepatitis due to HCV and HBV infection. A critical factor that probably influences the pathogenetic mechanisms operative in these two infections is the relative antigen load, which is very high in HBV infection and very low for HCV. Although high antigen load may be responsible for T-cell exhaustion during chronic HBV infection, this pathway probably does not contribute to HCV persistence, where more active viral escape mechanisms may play a more important role in view of the extremely high mutation rate of this virus. Once again, however, selection of mutant viruses is most likely to occur in the context of a weak and narrowly focused immune response, which is probably the primary determinant of viral persistence in these patients.

OTHER HEPATITIS VIRUSES

Little is known about the pathogenetic role of the immune response in HDV and HEV infection. Indeed, it is not clear whether these viruses are directly cytopathic, although HEV carries a high mortality rate in pregnant women,[163] suggesting the possibility of hormonal regulation of HEV replication perhaps leading to the production of very high (cytopathic?) levels of virus in the hepatocyte. For HDV, a cytopathic effect has been reported in certain cell lines transfected with HDV genomic constructs.[193] However, transgenic mice that express the HDV large and small antigens show no evidence of liver disease.[127]

Hepatitis A virus-induced hepatitis, however, appears to be a T-cell–mediated disease. HAV-specific CTL seem to play a central role in the pathogenesis of hepatitis A because HLA class I-restricted, HAV-specific CTL have been detected in the intrahepatic infiltrate of patients with acute hepatitis A.[336] This contrasts with the previous notion that liver cell injury was principally caused by a direct cytopathic effect of the virus, but it is in accordance with the histopathologic picture in acute HAV infection, characterized by diffuse inflammatory infiltrate typical of an immune-mediated pathologic process. Cytotoxic cells seem to be preferentially concentrated at the site of tissue damage, because antiviral CTL are either absent or present at very low frequency in the peripheral blood of HAV-infected patients.

ALTERNATIVE DISEASE PATHWAYS

Even though the HLA class I-restricted cytotoxic T-cell response is probably responsible for most of the liver damage in HAV, HBV, and HCV infections, other immune mechanisms may also contribute to the pathogenesis of hepatocellular injury in these diseases. For example, the finding that some HBV-

---

*References 1, 43, 44, 101, 141, 151, 222, 228, 244, 303.

infected cells display HBeAg on the surface membrane in a conformation that is recognizable by anti-HBeAg antibodies suggests that this antigen might serve as a target for an antibody-mediated elimination of HBV-infected cells.[287] This is in keeping with the observation that seroconversion from HBeAg to anti-HBeAg frequently correlates with virus clearance, and that HBV infection can be delayed or prevented in chimpanzees by passive immunization with anti-HBeAg antibodies.[313]

The demonstration that HBV envelope-specific, cytotoxic CD4+ HLA class II-restricted T-cells isolated from hepatitis B vaccine recipients can recognize not only exogenous[42] but endogenously synthesized viral antigens[258] illustrates that these lymphocytes may also participate in the clearance of virus infected liver cells. CD4+ cytotoxic T-cell clones have been described in influenza[26] and vesicular stomatitis[30] virus-infected mice, and in influenza-,[165] measles-,[153] and herpes simplex-infected humans.[355] Moreover, experiments in β_2-microglobulin–deficient mice demonstrate that HLA class II-restricted CD4+ cells can be cytotoxic for lymphocytic choriomeningitis virus-infected cells, causing death of infected mice even in the absence of CD8+ CTL.[225] These results show that the cytolytic activity of CD4+ cells can be expressed in vivo, therefore suggesting that it might be relevant for viral pathogenesis.

The observation that hepatocytes express HLA class II molecules after HBV infection provides additional support to a possible role of CD4+ CTL in liver immunopathogenesis.[337] Thus, infected and uninfected hepatocytes that endocytose viral antigens might be susceptible to destruction by CD4+ HLA class II-restricted CTL.

Finally, lymphokines released by activated T cells can recruit and activate antigen-nonspecific effector cells (e.g., macrophages, neutrophils, and natural killer cells), and they can also be directly cytopathic for virus-infected and -uninfected hepatocytes. All these processes take place in proximity to antigen-activated T cells that are needed to initiate this cascade of events. In this way, antigen-nonspecific effector mechanisms can be focused at the site of virus replication and antigen presentation and amplify the consequences of the antigen-specific immune response (see section on Studies on Animal Models).

MECHANISMS OF HEPATOCARCINOGENESIS

Perhaps the most devastating consequence of chronic HBV and HCV infection is the development of HCC. This represents an enormous, global public health problem, because between 300 to 400 million people are chronically infected by each of these viruses throughout the world. Although the precise incidence of HCC in chronic HCV infection has not yet been established, there is extensive epidemiologic evidence that long-term chronic HBV infection carries more than a 100-fold increased risk of HCC, and it has been estimated that men chronically infected by HBV from birth carry a 40% lifetime risk for development of HCC.[18] The lifetime risk of HCC is even higher in woodchucks (100%) and ground squirrels (67%) chronically infected with their respective hepadnaviruses.[272] No other known virus or environmental factor approaches the carcinogenic potential of HBV except, perhaps, heavy cigarette smoking, which has been estimated to increase the risk of lung cancer between 10- to 60-fold in men who smoke two packs a day for 20 years.[335]

The mechanisms responsible for malignant transformation in chronic HBV and HCV infection are incompletely defined. Because the interval between infection and hepatoma is usually several decades, it appears that these viruses are neither directly nor acutely oncogenic. Several alternative mechanisms that have been proposed are summarized in the following sections. For HBV at least, the carcinogenic stimulus is so strong that many, if not all of these alternatives are likely to be valid, and it is reasonable to suspect that they can coexist in the same infected liver, where they synergize to transform the infected hepatocyte.

Chromosomal Integration and Insertional Activation of Cellular Protooncogenes by Hepatitis B Virus

During chronic HBV infection, viral integration occurs and integrated viral DNA is detected in virtually all cases of HBV-associated chronic hepatitis and HCC. The integrated viral DNA is clonal in HCC, suggesting that integration might play a direct role in the transformation process. Viral DNA integration is random, however, with respect to the host genome, suggesting that if it does play a role, different cellular genes must be disrupted in individual tumors. All HBV integrations are associated with microdeletions in the flanking cellular DNA.[205] In addition, larger deletions, inversions, duplications, amplifications, and translocations of cellular genomic sequences have been described in HBV-associated HCC.[272] Thus, it appears that HBV integration can cause genomic integration site instability that could contribute to the oncogenic potential of this virus. No common cellular gene should be affected by this process, however.

The role of HBV integrants as insertional activators of oncogene expression has been intensively studied. Thus far, integration in the vicinity of genes associated with growth control and differentiation has been observed in only two of the many cases of HBV-associated HCC that have been examined (retinoic acid receptor, cyclin A).[71,345] Thus, insertional activation of cellular protooncogenes does not seem to be a common pathway for HBV-induced hepatocarcinogenesis in infected humans. In the WHV-infected woodchuck model, however, insertional activation of c-myc and N-myc genes is a common event[104,145] that clearly plays a critical role in hepatocarcinogenesis in these animals. Amplification of c-myc occurs quite commonly in GSHV-infected ground squirrel HCC, but it is independent of the GSHV integration site. Thus, although enhanced c-myc expression occurs in both woodchuck and ground squirrel HCC, two different mechanisms are operative. It appears, therefore, that insertional myc activation is a woodchuck-specific event and that the mechanisms responsible for hepatocarcinogenesis in HBV-infected humans, GSHV- and WHV-infected ground squirrels, and HBsAg transgenic mice (see discussion later) are quite different from those at work in the WHV-infected woodchuck. Because HCV does not integrate into the host genome during chronic infection, and because the associated HCC do not contain integrated viral sequences, it is clear that other events must deregulate growth control in the liver during HCV infection.

Integration Site-Independent Changes in Cellular Protooncogenes and Tumor Suppressor Genes During Hepatocarcinogenesis

Noninsertional activation of the known cellular growth control genes is also uncommon in human HCC,[110,111] although increased expression of c-myc,[136] N-ras,[319] c-Ha-ras, c-fos, and c-fms has been reported in sporadic human hepatomas[365] with and without associated HBV or HCV infection. The only growth control gene that is known to be frequently activated in HBV- and WHV-induced HCC is the gene for insulin-like growth factor-II (IGF2), which is transcriptionally reactivated in a high percentage of human and woodchuck hepatomas.[36,37,38,107] Transgenic mouse studies, however, suggest that IGF2 reactivation appears to occur at a relatively late stage of disease (see discussion later), suggesting that it could contribute to the promotion or progression but not to the initiation of hepatocarcinogenesis in these systems. Because all of these genes are activated in the regenerating liver, they may simply reflect increased hepatocellular turnover rather than causative events in hepatocyte transformation. To the extent that hepatocellular proliferation plays a role in transformation, however (see discussion later), these genes could be viewed as contributing factors in the individual tumors in which they have been found. The diversity of activated protooncogenes associated with HBV-induced HCC suggests that the hepatocyte may be unusually susceptible to transforming events, perhaps because of its high intrinsic proliferative potential, which implies the existence of growth control pathways that may not be shared with most parenchymal cells.

Furthermore, there is a growing body of evidence that tumor suppressor gene inactivation may play an important role in the development of HCC. Indeed, loss of heterozygosity has been identified in human tumors at chromosomes 1p, 4q, 5q, 8q, 10q, 11p, 13q, 16q, and 17p.[32,304,306,344] Loss of heterozygosity at these and related loci is often indicative of loss of tumor suppressor alleles,[197] and the nondeleted allele is often inactivated by point mutations in many human tumors.[197] The structure and expression of the p53 antioncogene is abnormal in some HCC cell lines.[27] Strikingly, loss of one allele of the p53 gene has been reported in up to 60% of HBV-associated HCC, principally by unknown mechanisms, although in two cases loss of 17p13, and therefore p53, was associated with HBV integrations at that site.[272]

Point mutations in the p53 locus (located on human chromosome 17p13), especially in the 249th codon, have been reported to be common in human HCC.[28,144] Although the apparent targeting of a single codon suggests the involvement of chemical carcinogens (probably aflatoxins) in these tumors, and decreases the likelihood that the point mutations are related to the underlying HBV infection, nonetheless they illustrate the important role this antioncogene can play in hepatocarcinogenesis. In addition, p53 point mutations (not affecting codon 249) have been reported in 8 of 22 cases of advanced HCC in Japan.[226] These eight cases of HCC also presented either loss of the Rb gene, or loss of heterozygosity at chromosome 13q, suggesting the involvement of two tumor suppressor genes in late stages of hepatocarcinogenesis, as already reported in small cell lung cancers[360] and soft tissue sarcomas.[314]

The Hepatitis B Virus X Gene and Hepatocellular Carcinoma

Because the HBV X gene product displays transcriptional transactivating properties and can transactivate cellular genes (e.g., c-myc and c-jun) associated with cellular growth control, it has been suggested that unregulated expression of this gene may contribute to the malignant transformation of the infected hepatocyte. It has also been reported that the HBV X protein inhibits p53 gene function in vitro,[346] strengthening the evidence for a role of this viral transactivator in hepatocarcinogenesis. In support of this hypothesis, it has been shown that high-level expression of the HBV X gene can lead to HCC in transgenic mice,[173] although others have not observed the induction of HCC in independently derived X gene transgenic mouse strains.[185] Although this discrepancy might be related to differences in the strength and duration of X protein expression and different mouse genetic background influences in the various transgenic models, the long interval before tumor development in the HCC-susceptible lineages indicates that X gene expression alone is not sufficient for carcinogenesis, and that other events, presumably genetic mutations or chromosomal abnormalities, are necessary for HCC to develop. In addition, X protein expression has been observed in only a minority of human HCC, suggesting that if deregulated X gene expression plays a role in hepatocarcinogenesis, it does so only in a small percentage of tumors.[272]

Chronic Hepatitis Itself Is Sufficient to Cause Hepatocellular Carcinoma

Almost all cases of HCC occur in the setting of many years of antecedent chronic hepatitis due to a wide array of viral and nonviral etiologies. Chronic active hepatitis is characterized by indolent and progressive liver cell injury with associated hepatocellular regeneration (i.e., cellular DNA synthesis) and inflammation (i.e., the production of mutagens), which can precipitate widespread random genetic and chromosomal damage and lead to the development of HCC. Indeed, similar events are thought to contribute to the development of gastric carcinoma in patients with chronic gastritis and to colon cancer in patients with ulcerative colitis.[240]

As described previously in the section on Studies on Animal Models, transgenic mice that overexpress the HBV large envelope polypeptide have a storage disease that leads to the development of HCC.[62] In this model, severe, prolonged hepatocellular injury initiates a programmed response within the liver, characterized by inflammation, Kupffer cell hyperplasia, hepatocellular regenerative hyperplasia, transcriptional deregulation, and aneuploidy, that inexorably progresses to HCC.[62,74] Thus, the inappropriate expression of a single structural viral gene is sufficient to set in motion a complex series of events that ultimately leads to malignant transformation. The incidence of HCC in this model corresponds to the frequency, severity, and age of onset of liver cell injury, which itself corresponds to the intrahepatic concentration of HBsAg and is influenced by genetic background and sex.

Hepatocellular turnover in these mice, relative to nontransgenic controls, is increased nearly 100-fold for at least a year before the onset of HCC.[148] Also, oxygen radical production

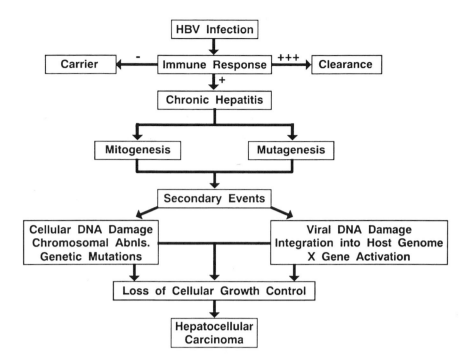

FIG. 31-11. The chronic injury leading to hepatocellular carcinoma hypothesis. According to this hypothesis, a vigorous (+++) immune response to hepatitis B virus (HBV) leads to viral clearance, whereas an absent (−) immune response leads to the "healthy" carrier state, and an intermediate (+) immune response produces chronic hepatitis. This indolent necroinflammatory liver disease is characterized by chronic liver cell necrosis that stimulates a sustained regenerative response. The inflammatory component includes activated macrophages that are a rich source of free radicals. The collaboration of these mitogenic and mutagenic stimuli has the potential to cause cellular and viral DNA damage, chromosomal abnormalities, genetic mutations, and the like that deregulate cellular growth control in a multistep process that eventually leads to hepatocellular carcinoma.

is greatly increased and the antioxidant (glutathione and catalase) content is greatly decreased in the liver of these mice. These changes are associated with a dramatic increase in oxidative DNA damage to hepatocellular genomic DNA.[129] It is reasonable to assume that these events could lead to the development of random mutations throughout the liver cell genome that eventually contribute to the development of HCC.

In view of the prolonged antecedent hepatocellular injury, regeneration, and oxidative DNA damage, it is likely that transformation occurs by a multistep process in this transgenic model. Because transformation was observed in two independent lineages, without evidence of transgene rearrangement or instability, direct insertional activation of a cellular oncogene is improbable. Rather, it likely involves activating or inactivating mutations in multiple cellular genes that are spatially and functionally independent of the integrated HBV sequences.

IGF2 and *mdr-3* gene expression is transcriptionally activated in most of the transgenic mouse hepatomas.[182,280] These genes are not overexpressed during the preneoplastic phase of the disease, however, suggesting that they represent late changes associated with tumor progression but not with tumor initiation in this model. The importance of these findings is underscored by the contrasting fact that no changes in *p53*, *Rb-1*, *Ha-ras*, *Ki-ras*, *N-ras*, *c-myc*, *N-myc*, *erb-A*, *erb-B*, *src*, *mos*, *abl*, *sis*, *fms*, *fes*, *fos*, *jun*, the genes for transforming growth factor-α, transforming growth factor-β, platelet-derived growth factor-α, platelet-derived growth factor-β, epidermal growth factor receptor, retinoic acid receptor-β, HNF-1, C/EBP, or cyclic AMP response element B (CREB) DNA copy number, gene structure, steady-state RNA levels, or protein content were detected in any of the tumors.[252] Obviously, the cellular genome is vast, as are the opportunities for growth-promoting mutations and chromosomal abnormalities outside of these loci.

The link between injury and transformation is strengthened by the fact that HCC has not been observed in any HBV transgenic lineage that does not display liver cell injury* except for the mice that express the transactivating *X* gene, as discussed earlier. The pathogenetic importance of injury in this regard is further strengthened by the development of nodular regenerative activity and HCC in livers of transgenic mice sustaining neonatal hepatitis as a consequence of the hepatocellular retention of α₁-antitrypsin.[75] Additional support for this hypothesis is the fact that human HCC occurs in the context of necrosis, inflammation, and regeneration (cirrhosis) in several diseases other than hepatitis B, such as chronic hepatitis C (reviewed in Alter[3]), alcoholism,[186] hemochromatosis,[235] glycogen storage disease,[188] α₁-antitrypsin deficiency,[39,83] and primary biliary cirrhosis.[209]

These results suggest that severe, prolonged hepatocellular injury induces a preneoplastic proliferative and inflammatory response that places the dividing hepatocyte at risk for development of multiple random mutations or other chromosomal changes, including viral integration, some of which program the cell for unrestrained growth (Fig. 31-11). In the transgenic mouse model, injury is secondary to the overproduction of a viral gene product. Although this process may occur during viral infection, it is more likely that immunologic mechanisms play a dominant role in humans (see section on Studies in Infected Patients: Hepatitis B Virus). Regardless of etiology or pathogenesis, however, it appears that chronic liver cell injury is a premalignant condition initiating a cascade of events characterized by increased rates of cellular DNA synthesis and pro-

---

*References 9, 10, 34, 63, 73, 89, 90, 137, 354.

duction of endogenous mutagens coupled with compromised cellular detoxification and repair functions, which eventually cooperate to increase the mutation rate to a level compatible with the acquisition of the multiple genetic and chromosomal changes necessary to transform one or a few of the hepatocytes that clonally expand into HCC that eventually kills the host.

SUMMARY AND CONCLUSIONS

The diversity of clinical syndromes and disease manifestations associated with each of the hepatitis viruses strongly suggests that the outcome of these infections is determined by the quality and vigor of the antiviral immune response produced by each infected individual. As illustrated for HBV in Figure 31-12, all limbs of the immune response must cooperate productively to terminate this viral infection. Individual differences in the efficiency of viral antigen processing by hepatocytes and professional antigen-presenting cells, or at the level of antigen recognition and responsiveness by B and T lymphocytes, affect the strength of the antiviral immune response and the extent to which it contributes to viral clearance and liver disease.

As summarized in Table 31-2 and Figures 31-9 and 31-10, patients who successfully clear the virus during an episode of acute viral hepatitis acquire strong, polyclonal class I- and class II-restricted T-cell responses to HBV, whereas these responses are weak and perhaps more oligoclonal in patients who fail to clear the virus and contract chronic liver disease of varying severity. Although a great deal is now known about

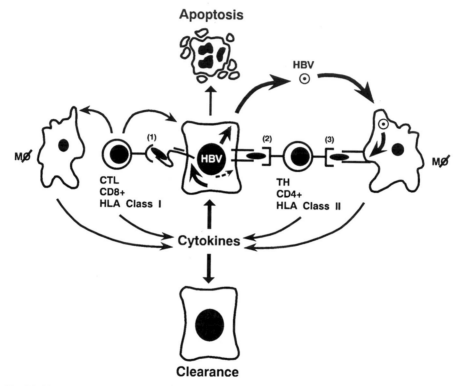

FIG. 31-12. Multiple pathways of hepatitis B virus (HBV) pathogenesis. The HBV-infected hepatocyte (central figure) synthesizes viral proteins that are degraded and enter the human leukocyte antigen (HLA) class I processing pathway (*bold arrow* between 6 and 9 o'clock inside the cell) or assemble into viral particles and are secreted from the cell (*bold arrow* pointing toward 1 o'clock and exiting the cell). Small quantities of newly synthesized and degraded viral antigen may also enter the class II processing pathway, but this is an inefficient process (*dashed arrow* between 4 and 6 o'clock inside the cell). Peptide antigen bound by class I is presented to the T-cell receptor (1) of CD8+ cytotoxic T lymphocytes (CTL), which become activated and perform at least three different functions. First, they trigger the antigen-presenting hepatocyte to undergo programmed cell death (apoptosis). Second, they release factors that recruit inflammatory cells and activate macrophages in their immediate vicinity. Third, the CTL and the recruited-activated antigen-nonspecific inflammatory cells secrete inflammatory cytokines, such as interferon-γ and tumor necrosis factor-‡, that can amplify their local cytopathic effects, thereby worsening the disease, but by diffusion they can also bind to infected hepatocytes at a distance from the CTL and activate them to produce antiviral molecules that destroy the virus while leaving the cell alive and healthy (clearance). In addition, these cytokines can induce the hepatocyte to synthesize HLA class II molecules. If any viral antigen enters the class II antigen-presenting pathway under these conditions, it could be recognized by the T-cell receptor (2) of CD4+ helper T cells (TH) that can perform the same functions as the CTL. Secreted viral particles can be phagocytosed by intrahepatic macrophages (Mø) and dendritic cells (not shown) that process the antigens and efficiently present them in the context of HLA class II to the T-cell receptor (3) of CD4+ TH cells with the same downstream effects.

the effector limb of these responses, the factors that determine whether a given individual will mount an effective immune response to this virus are poorly understood, and represent the greatest challenge for investigation in the future.

At the effector level, it appears that several pathways can be activated to eliminate the virus, either by killing the infected cells or by eliminating the virus from within the cell without killing it. As illustrated in Figure 31-12, the first, and dominant, pathway (1) is by means of the CD8+ cytotoxic T cell that recognizes endogenously synthesized HBV antigens presented by HLA class I molecules at the hepatocyte membrane. On antigen recognition, these cells perform several antiviral functions. First, they are directly cytopathic for the antigen-presenting hepatocyte by triggering it to undergo apoptosis (see also Fig. 31-6). Second, they secrete lymphokines that recruit antigen-nonspecific inflammatory cells that amplify their cytopathic effect and worsen the severity of disease by at least an order of magnitude (see also Fig. 31-7). Third, they secrete other cytokines that noncytolytically inhibit HBV gene expression and viral replication by destabilizing the viral RNA (see also Fig. 31-8), thereby interrupting the viral life cycle (see Fig. 31-4) and possibly contributing to viral clearance without destroying the infected liver and killing the host.

The second (2) and third (3) pathways shown in Figure 31-12 involve antigen recognition by CD4+, HLA class II-restricted T cells. Although the second pathway is not likely to be very important because endogenously synthesized viral antigen does not associate efficiently with HLA class II molecules inside of the cell, intrahepatic macrophages express high levels of HLA class II and they can efficiently process and present phagocytosed antigen to the class II-restricted T cells, which could then release their own set of cytokines, as discussed earlier. According to this notion, the third pathway, reminiscent of a classic delayed-type hypersensitivity reaction, is probably quite active in the infected liver. This suggests that the class II-restricted T cells may contribute to viral clearance and immunopathogenesis much in the same way as the class I-restricted CTL, except for their direct cytopathic effect, which actually appears to contribute very little to the overall severity of liver disease.

According to this scenario, viral clearance depends on the development of a vigorous intrahepatic immune response, with the severity of the associated liver disease being determined by the number of infected hepatocytes and the balance between the cytopathic and antiviral regulatory effects of the intrahepatic inflammatory cells. If the overall response is weak, or if the cytopathic component of the response is stronger than its antiviral regulatory component, the virus might be expected to persist with an associated liver disease of varying severity, setting up the mitogenic and mutagenic environment that favors the development of chromosomal and genetic damage leading to malignant transformation and HCC (see also Fig. 31-11).

If the foregoing hypothesis is correct, strategies designed to boost the HBV-specific immune response (e.g., CTL immunotherapy) or to alter the balance between the cytopathic and the regulatory components of the response (e.g., specific cytokine immunotherapy) may be able to terminate persistent infection and ameliorate the severity and consequences of the chronic liver disease that accompanies persistent HBV infection. In the meanwhile, much remains to be done before our understanding of the immunobiology and pathogenesis of HBV and the other hepatitis viruses is complete.

ABBREVIATIONS

C/EBP: CCAT/enhancer binding protein
CTL: cytotoxic T lymphocyte
E: envelope
ER: endoplasmic reticulum
GSHV: ground squirrel hepatitis virus
HAV: hepatitis A virus
HBcAg: hepatitis B core antigen
HBeAg: hepatitis B precore antigen
HBsAg: hepatitis B surface antigen
HBV: hepatitis B virus
HCC: hepatocellular carcinoma
HCV: hepatitis C virus
HDV: hepatitis delta virus
HEV: hepatitis E virus
HLA: human leukocyte antigen
IFN: interferon
HNF: hepatocyte nuclear factor
IL: interleukin
MHC: major histocompatibility complex
NS: nonstructural
TNF: tumor necrosis factor
WHV: woodchuck hepatitis virus

ACKNOWLEDGMENTS

We are indebted to our colleagues, whose work is summarized in this review, for permitting us to include some of their data before publication and for sharing their thoughts and ideas with us as we wrote the manuscript. We are particularly grateful to Drs. Luca Guidotti, Claudio Pasquinelli, Stephane Guilhot, Patrick Gilles, Takashi Moriyama, Kazuki Ando, Tetsuya Ishikawa, Andreas Cerny, Barbara Rehermann, Antonio Bertoletti, Gabriele Missale, Antonietta Valli, Albertina Cavalli, and Amalia Penna for their important contributions to our laboratories during the past several years, and to Ms. Patricia Fowler for outstanding technical contributions to all aspects of our research. We also thank Dr. Miriam Alter for expert consultation in the area of viral epidemiology, Drs. Allan Redeker, John Person, John McHutchison, Paul Pockros, Tiziana Giuberti, and Franco Fiaccadori for their important clinical collaboration, and Ms. Bonnie Weier for invaluable assistance with manuscript preparation. Sections of this chapter have been previously published in Hepatology 1995;22:1316–1325, Springer Seminars in Immunopathology 1995;17:261–281, and Annual Review of Immunology 1995;13:29–60, and have been modified and reproduced with permission from the publishers. These studies were supported by grants AI20001, AI26626, CA40489, CA54560 and RR00833 from the National Institutes of Health. This is manuscript number 8679-MEM from The Scripps Research Institute, La Jolla, California.

REFERENCES

1. Akatsuka T, Donets M, Scaglione L, et al. B cell epitopes on the hepatitis C virus nucleocapsid protein determined by human monospecific antibodies. Hepatology 1993;18:503–510.
2. Alberti A, Cavalletto D, Pontisso P, Chemello L, Tagariello G, Belussi F. Antibody response to pre-S2 and hepatitis B virus induced liver damage. Lancet 1988;1:1421–1424.

3. Alter HJ. Transfusion-associated non-A, non-B hepatitis: the first decade. In: Zuckerman AJ, ed. Viral hepatitis and liver disease. New York: Alan R. Liss, 1988:534–542.

4. Alter MJ, Mast EE. The epidemiology of viral hepatitis in the United States. Gastroenterol Clin North Am 1994;23:437–455.

5. Ando K, Guidotti LG, Cerny A, Ishikawa T, Chisari FV. CTL access to tissue antigen is restricted in vivo. J Immunol 1994;153: 482–488.

6. Ando K, Guidotti LG, Wirth S, et al. Class I restricted cytotoxic T lymphocytes are directly cytopathic for their target cells in vivo. J Immunol 1994;152:3245–3253.

7. Ando K, Moriyama T, Guidotti LG, et al. Mechanisms of class I restricted immunopathology: a transgenic mouse model of fulminant hepatitis. J Exp Med 1993;178:1541–1554.

8. Antonucci TK, Rutter WJ. Hepatitis B virus (HBV) promoters are regulated by the HBV enhancer in a tissue-specific manner. J Virol 1989;63:579–583.

9. Araki K, Miyazaki J-I, Hino O, et al. Expression and replication of hepatitis B virus genome in transgenic mice. Proc Natl Acad Sci U S A 1989;86:207–211.

10. Babinet C, Farza H, Morello D, Hadchouel M, Pourcel C. Specific expression of hepatitis B surface antigen (HBsAg) in transgenic mice. Science 1985;230:1160–1163.

11. Barnaba V, Franco A, Alberti A, Balsano C, Benvenuto R, Balsano F. Recognition of hepatitis B envelope proteins by liver-infiltrating T lymphocytes in chronic HBV infection. J Immunol 1989;143: 2650–2655.

12. Barnaba V, Franco A, Alberti A, Benvenuto R, Balsano F. Selective killing of hepatitis B envelope antigen-specific B cells by class I restricted, exogenous antigen specific T lymphocytes. Nature 1990; 345:258–260.

13. Barnaba V, Franco A, Paroli M, et al. Selective expansion of cytotoxic T lymphocytes with a CD4+CD56+ surface phenotype and a T helper type 1 profile of cytokine secretion in the liver of patients chronically infected with hepatitis B virus. J Immunol 1994;152: 3074–3087.

14. Bartenschlager R, Junker-Niepmann M, Schaller H. The P gene product of hepatitis B virus is required as a structural component for genomic RNA encapsidation. J Virol 1990;64:5324–5332.

15. Bavand M, Feitelson M, Laub O. The hepatitis B virus-associated reverse transcriptase is encoded by the viral pol gene. J Virol 1989; 63:1019–1021.

16. Bavand MR, Laub O. Two proteins with reverse transcriptase activities associated with hepatitis B virus-like particles. J Virol 1988;62:626–628.

17. Beasley RP, Hwang LY, Stevens CE, et al. Efficacy of hepatitis B immune globulin for prevention of perinatal transmission of the hepatitis B virus carrier state: final report of a randomized double-blind, placebo-controlled trial. Hepatology 1983;3:135–141.

18. Beasley RP, Lin C-C, Hwang LY, Chen C-S. Hepatocellular carcinoma and hepatitis B virus: a prospective study of 22,707 men in Taiwan. Lancet 1981;2:1129–1133.

19. Bertoletti A, Chisari FV, Penna A, et al. Definition of a minimal optimal cytotoxic T cell epitope within the hepatitis B virus nucleocapsid protein. J Virol 1993;67:2376–2380.

20. Bertoletti A, Costanzo A, Chisari FV, et al. Cytotoxic T lymphocyte response to a wild type hepatitis B virus epitope in patients chronically infected by variant viruses carrying substitutions within the epitope. J Exp Med 1994;180:933–943.

21. Bertoletti A, Ferrari C, Fiaccadori F, et al. HLA class I-restricted human cytotoxic T cells recognize endogenously synthesized hepatitis B virus nucleocapsid antigen. Proc Natl Acad Sci U S A 1991;88: 10445–10449.

22. Bertoletti A, Sette A, Chisari FV, et al. Natural variants of cytotoxic epitopes are T cell receptor antagonists for antiviral cytotoxic T cells. Nature 1994;369:407–410.

23. Bonino F, Brunetto MR, Rizzetto M, Will H. Hepatitis B virus unable to secrete e antigen. Gastroenterology 1991;100:1138–1141.

24. Bosch V, Bartenschlager R, Radziwill G, Schaller H. The duck hepatitis B virus P-gene codes for protein strongly associated with the 5'-end of the viral DNA minus strand. Virology 1988;166:475–485.

25. Botarelli P, Brunetto MR, Minutello MA, et al. T-lymphocyte response to hepatitis C virus in different clinical courses of infection. Gastroenterology 1993;104:580–587.

26. Braciale TJ, Morrison LA, Sweetser MT, Sambrook J, Gething MJ, Braciale VL. Antigen presentation pathways to class I and class II MHC-restricted T lymphocytes. Immunol Rev 1987;98:95–114.

27. Bressac B, Galvin KM, Liang TJ, Isselbacher KJ, Wands JR, Ozturk M. Abnormal structure and expression of p53 gene in human hepatocellular carcinoma. Proc Natl Acad Sci U S A 1990;87: 1973– 1977.

28. Bressac B, Kew M, Wands J, Ozturk M. Selective G to T mutations of p53 in hepatocellular carcinoma from southern Africa. Nature 1991;350:429–431.

29. Browne H, Smith G, Beck S, Minson T. A complex between the MHC class I homologue encoded by human cytomegalovirus and β2 microglobulin. Nature 1990;347:770–772.

30. Browning M, Reiss CS, Huang A. The soluble viral glycoprotein of vesicular stomatitis virus efficiently sensitized target cells for lysis by CD4+ T lymphocytes. J Virol 1990;64:3810–3816.

31. Budkowska A, Dubreuil P, Capel F, Pillot J. Hepatitis B virus pre-S gene-encoded antigenic specificity and anti-pre-S antibody: relationship between anti-pre-S response and recovery. Hepatology 1986;6:360–368.

32. Buetow KH, Murray JC, Israel JL, et al. Loss of heterozygosity suggests tumor suppressor gene responsible for primary hepatocellular carcinoma. Proc Natl Acad Sci U S A 1989;86:8852–8856.

33. Bulla G, Siddiqui A. Negative regulation of the hepatitis B virus pre-S1 promotor by internal DNA sequences. In: Abstracts of papers presented at the 1988 meeting on molecular biology of hepatitis B virus. La Jolla, CA: University of California San Diego, 1988:64.

34. Burk RD, DeLoia JA, ElAwady MK, Gearhart JD. Tissue preferential expression of the hepatitis B virus (HBV) surface antigen gene in two lines of HBV transgenic mice. J Virol 1988;62:649–654.

35. Buscher M, Reiser W, Will H, Schaller H. Transcripts and the putative RNA pregenome of duck hepatitis B virus: implications for reverse transcription. Cell 1985;40:717–724.

36. Cariani E, Lasserre C, Kemeny F, Franco D, Brechot C. Expression of insulin-like growth factor II, α-fetoprotein and hepatitis B virus transcripts in human primary liver cancer. Hepatology 1991;13: 644–649.

37. Cariani E, Lasserre C, Seurin D, et al. Differential expression of insulin-like growth factor II mRNA in human primary liver cancers, benign liver tumors, and liver cirrhosis. Cancer Res 1988;48:6844– 6849.

38. Cariani E, Seurin D, Lasserre C, Franco D, Binoux M, Brechot C. Expression of insulin-like growth factor II (IGF-II) in human primary liver cancer: mRNA and protein analysis. J Hepatol 1990; 11:226–231.

39. Carlson J, Eriksson S. Chronic "cryptogenic" liver disease and malignant hepatoma in intermediate alpha-1-antitrypsin deficiency identified by a pi 2-specific monoclonal antibody. Scand J Gastroenterol 1985;20:835–841.

40. Carman WF, Thomas HC. Genetic variation in hepatitis B virus. Gastroenterology 1992;102:711–719.

41. Celis E, Kung PC, Chang TW. Hepatitis B virus-reactive human T lymphocyte clones: antigen specificity and helper function for antibody synthesis. J Immunol 1984;132:1511–1516.

42. Celis E, Ou D, Otvos L. Recognition of hepatitis B surface antigen by human T lymphocytes: proliferative and cytotoxic responses to a major antigenic determinant defined by synthetic peptides. J Immunol 1988;140:1808–1815.

43. Cerino A, Boender P, LaMonica N, Rosa C, Habets W, Mondelli MU. A human monoclonal antibody specific for the N terminus of the hepatitis C virus nucleocapsid protein. J Immunol 1993;151: 7005–7015.

44. Cerino A, Mondelli MU. Identification of an immunodominant B cell epitope on the hepatitis C virus nonstructural region defined by human monoclonal antibodies. J Immunol 1991;147:2692–2696.

45. Cerny A, McHutchison JG, Pasquinelli C, et al. Cytotoxic T lymphocyte response to hepatitis C virus-derived peptides containing the HLA A2.1 binding motif. J Clin Invest 1995;95:521–530.

46. Chang H-K, Ting LP. The surface gene promoter and the human hepatitis B virus displays a preference for differentiated hepatocytes. Virology 1989;170:176–183.

47. Chang LJ, Dienstag J, Ganem D, Varmus H. Detection of antibodies against hepatitis B polymerase antigen in hepatitis ZB virus-infected patients. Hepatology 1989;10:332–337.

48. Chemin I, Baginski I, Vermot-Desroches C, et al. Demonstration of woodchuck hepatitis virus infection of peripheral blood mononu-

clear cells by flow cytometry and polymerase chain reaction. J Gen Virol 1992;73:123–129.

49. Chen H-S, Kew MC, Hornbuckle WE, et al. The precore gene of the woodchuck hepatitis virus genome is not essential for viral replication in the natural host. J Virol 1992;66:5682–5684.

50. Chen HS, Kaneko S, Girones R, et al. The woodchuck hepatitis virus X gene is important for establishment of virus infection in woodchucks. J Virol 1993;67:1218–1226.

51. Chen HS, Kaneko S, Girones R, et al. The woodchuck hepatitis virus X gene is important for establishment of virus infection in woodchucks. J Virol 1994;67:1218–1226.

52. Chen HS, Kew MC, Hornbuckle WE, et al. The precore gene of the woodchuck hepatitis virus genome is not essential for viral replication in the natural host. J Virol 1992;66:5682–5684.

53. Chen P-J, Lin M-H, Tai K-F, Liu P-C, Lin C-J, Chen D-S. The Taiwanese hepatitis C virus genome: sequence determination and mapping at the 5' termini of viral genomic and antigenomic RNA. Virology 1992;188:102–113.

54. Chisari FV. Analysis of hepadnavirus gene expression, biology and pathogenesis in the transgenic mouse. Curr Top Microbiol Immunol 1991;168:85–101.

55. Chisari FV. Hepatitis B virus biology and pathogenesis. In: Friedmann T, ed. Molecular genetic medicine. San Diego: Academic Press, 1992:67–104.

56. Chisari FV. Hepatitis B virus transgenic mice: insights into the virus and the disease. Hepatology 1995;22:1316–1325.

57. Chisari FV, Ferrari C. Hepatitis B virus immunopathogenesis. Annu Rev Immunol 1995;13:29–60.

58. Chisari FV, Ferrari C. Hepatitis B virus immunopathology. Springer Semin Immunopathol 1995;17:261–281.

59. Chisari FV, Ferrari C, Mondelli MU. Hepatitis B virus structure and biology. Microb Pathog 1989;6:311–325.

60. Chisari FV, Filippi P, Buras J, et al. Structural and pathological effects of synthesis of hepatitis B virus large envelope polypeptide in transgenic mice. Proc Natl Acad Sci U S A 1987;84: 6909–6913.

61. Chisari FV, Filippi P, McLachlan A, et al. Expression of hepatitis B virus large envelope polypeptide inhibits hepatitis B surface antigen secretion in transgenic mice. J Virol 1986;60:880–887.

62. Chisari FV, Klopchin K, Moriyama T, et al. Molecular pathogenesis of hepatocellular carcinoma in hepatitis B virus transgenic mice. Cell 1989;59:1145–1156.

63. Chisari FV, Pinkert CA, Milich DR, et al. A transgenic mouse model of the chronic hepatitis B surface antigen carrier state. Science 1985;230:1157–1160.

64. Choo Q-L, Kuo G, Weiner AJ, Overby LR, Bradley DW, Houghton M. Isolation of a cDNA clone derived from a blood-borne non-A, non-B viral hepatitis genome. Science 1989;244:359–362.

65. Choo Q-L, Richman KH, Han JH, et al. Genetic organization and diversity of the hepatitis C virus. Proc Natl Acad Sci U S A 1991; 88:2451–2455.

66. Choo Q-L, Weiner AJ, Overby LR, Kuo G, Houghton M, Bradley DW. Hepatitis C virus: the major causative agent of viral non-A, non-B hepatitis. Br Med Bull 1990;46:423–441.

67. Colgrove R, Simon G, Ganem D. Transcriptional activation of homologous and heterologous genes by the hepatitis B virus X gene product in cells permissive for viral replication. J Virol 1989;63: 4019–4026.

68. Condreay LD, Aldrich CE, Coates L, Mason WS, Wu T-T. Efficient duck hepatitis B virus production by an avian liver tumor cell line. J Virol 1990;64:3249–3258.

69. Cordoba J, Camps J, Esteban JI. The clinical picture of acute and chronic hepatitis C. In: Reesink HW, ed. Hepatitis C virus. Basel: Karger, 1994:69–88.

70. Cote PJ, Korba BE, Steinberg H, et al. Cyclosporin A modulates the course of woodchuck hepatitis virus infection and induces chronicity. J Immunol 1991;146:3138–3144.

71. de The H, Marchio A, Tiollais P, Dejean A. A novel steroid thyroid hormone receptor-related gene inappropriately expressed in human hepatocellular carcinoma. Nature 1987;330:667–670.

72. De-Medina T, Faktor O, Shaul Y. The S promoter of hepatitis B virus is regulated by positive and negative elements. Mol Cell Biol 1988;8:2449–2455.

73. DeLoia JA, Burk RD, Gearhart JD. Developmental regulation of hepatitis B surface antigen expression in two lines of hepatitis B virus transgenic mice. J Virol 1989;63:4069–4073.

74. Dunsford HA, Sell S, Chisari FV. Hepatocarcinogenesis due to chronic liver cell injury in hepatitis B virus transgenic mice. Cancer Res 1990;50:3400–3407.

75. Dycaico MJ, Grant SG, Felts K, et al. Neonatal hepatitis induced by alpha 1-antitrypsin: a transgenic mouse model. Science 1988;242: 1409–1412.

76. Eble BE, Lingappa VR, Ganem D. Hepatitis B surface antigen: an unusual secreted protein initially synthesized as a transmembrane polypeptide. Mol Cell Biol 1986;6:1454–1463.

77. Eble BE, MacRae DR, Lingappa VR, Ganem D. Multiple topogenic sequences determine the transmembrane orientation of hepatitis B surface antigen. Mol Cell Biol 1987;7:3591–3601.

78. Eckhardt SG, Milich DR, McLachlan A. Hepatitis B virus core antigen has two nuclear localization sequences in the arginine-rich carboxyl terminus. J Virol 1991;65:575–582.

79. Emini EA, Larson V, Eichberg J, et al. Protective effect of a synthetic peptide comprising the complete preS2 region of the hepatitis B virus surface protein. J Med Virol 1989;28:7–12.

80. Enders GH, Ganem D, Varmus H. Mapping the major transcripts of ground squirrel hepatitis virus: the presumptive template for reverse transcriptase is terminally redundant. Cell 1985;42:297–308.

81. Enders GH, Ganem D, Varmus HE. 5'-terminal sequences influence the segregation of ground squirrel hepatitis virus RNAs into polyribosomes and viral core particles. J Virol 1987;61:35–41.

82. Erickson AL, Houghton M, Choo QL, et al. Hepatitis C virus-specific CTL responses in the liver of chimpanzees with acute and chronic hepatitis C. J Immunol 1993;151:4189–4199.

83. Eriksson S, Carlson J, Velez RN. Risk of cirrhosis and primary liver cancer in alpha-1-antitrypsin deficiency. N Engl J Med 1986; 314: 736–740.

84. Failla C, Tomei L, De Francesco R. Both NS3 and NS4A are required for proteolytic processing of hepatitis C virus nonstructural proteins. J Virol 1994;68:3753–3760.

85. Falk K, Roetzschke O, Stevanovic S, Jung G, Rammensee H-G. Allele-specific motifs revealed by sequencing of self-peptides eluted from MHC molecules. Nature 1991;351:290–296.

86. Farci P, Alter HJ, Govindarajan S, et al. Lack of protective immunity against reinfection with hepatitis C virus. Science 1992;258: 135–140.

87. Farci P, Alter HJ, Wong DC, et al. Prevention of hepatitis C virus infection in chimpanzees after antibody-mediated in vitro neutralization. Proc Natl Acad Sci U S A 1994;91:7792–7796.

88. Farci P, London W, Wong DC, et al. The natural history of infection with hepatitis C virus (HCV) in chimpanzee: comparison of serologic responses measured by first and second generation assays and relationship to HCV viremia. J Infect Dis 1992;165: 1006–1011.

89. Farza H, Hadchouel M, Scotto J, Tiollais P, Babinet C, Pourcel C. Replication and gene expression of hepatitis B virus in a transgenic mouse that contains the complete viral genome. J Virol 1988;62: 4144–4152.

90. Farza H, Salmon AM, Hadchouel M, et al. Hepatitis B surface antigen gene expression is regulated by sex steroids and glucocorticoids in transgenic mice. Proc Natl Acad Sci U S A 1987;84:1187–1191.

91. Feitelson MA, Millman I, Duncan GD, Blumberg BS. Presence of antibodies to the polymerase gene product(s) of hepatitis B and woodchuck hepatitis virus in natural and experimental infections. J Med Virol 1988;24:121–126.

92. Ferrari C, Bertoletti A, Penna A, et al. Identification of immunodominant T cell epitopes of the hepatitis B virus nucleocapsid antigen. J Clin Invest 1991;88:214–222.

93. Ferrari C, Cavalli A, Penna A, et al. Fine specificity of the human T cell response to the hepatitis B virus preS1 antigen. Gastroenterology 1992;103:255–263.

94. Ferrari C, Mondelli MU, Penna A, Fiaccadori F, Chisari FV. Functional characterization of cloned intrahepatic, hepatitis B virus nucleoprotein-specific helper T cell lines. J Immunol 1987;139: 539–544.

95. Ferrari C, Penna A, Bertoletti A, et al. The preS1 antigen of hepatitis B virus is highly immunogenic at the T cell level in man. J Clin Invest 1989;84:1314–1319.

96. Ferrari C, Penna A, Bertoletti A, et al. Cellular immune response to hepatitis B virus-encoded antigens in acute and chronic hepatitis B virus infection. J Immunol 1990;145:3442–3449.

97. Ferrari C, Penna A, Giuberti T, et al. Intrahepatic, nucleocapsid antigen-specific T cells in chronic active hepatitis B. J Immunol 1987; 139:2050–2058.

98. Ferrari C, Penna A, Sansoni P, et al. Selective sensitization of peripheral blood T lymphocytes to hepatitis B core antigen in patients with chronic active hepatitis type B. Clin Exp Immunol 1986;66: 497–506.

99. Ferrari C, Pilli M, Penna A, et al. Autopresentation of hepatitis B virus envelope antigens by T cells. J Virol 1992;66:2536–2540.

100. Ferrari C, Valli A, Galati L, et al. T-cell response to structural and nonstructural hepatitis C virus antigens in persistent and self-limited hepatitis C virus infections. Hepatology 1994;19:286–295.

101. Ferrone P, Mascolo G, Zaninetti M, et al. Identification of four epitopes in hepatitis C virus core protein. J Clin Microbiol 1993;31: 1586–1591.

102. Filippi P, Buras J, McLachlan A, et al. Overproduction of hepatitis B virus large envelope polypeptide causes filament storage, ground glass cell formation, hepatocellular injury and nodular hyperplasia in transgenic mice. In: Zuckerman AJ, ed. Viral hepatitis and liver disease. New York: Alan R. Liss, 1988:632–640.

103. Foster GR, Ackrill AM, Goldin RD, Kerr IM, Thomas HC, Stark GR. Expression of the terminal protein region of hepatitis B virus inhibits cellular responses to interferons a and gamma and double-stranded RNA. Proc Natl Acad Sci U S A 1991;88:2888–2892.

104. Fourel G, Trepo C, Bougueleret L, et al. Frequent activation of N-myc genes by hepadnavirus insertion in woodchuck liver tumours. Nature 1990;347:294–298.

105. Franco A, Paroli M, Testa U, et al. Transferrin receptor mediates uptake and presentation of hepatitis B envelope antigen by T lymphocytes. J Exp Med 1992;175:1195–1205.

106. Fremont DH, Matsumara M, Stura EA, Peterson PA, Wilson IA. Crystal structures of two viral peptides in complex with murine MHC class I H-2Kb. Science 1992;257:919–927.

107. Fu XX, Cu CY, Lee Y, et al. Insulinlike growth factor II expression and oval cell proliferation associated with hepatocarcinogenesis in woodchuck hepatitis virus carriers. J Virol 1988;62:3422–3430.

108. Fukuda R, Okinaga S, Akagi S, et al. Alteration of infection pattern of duck hepatitis B virus by immunomodulatory drugs. J Med Virol 1988;26:387–396.

109. Gabathuler R, Levy F, Kvist S. Requirements for the association of adenovirus type 2 E3/19K wild type and mutant proteins with HLA antigens. J Virol 1990;64:3679–3685.

110. Ganem D. Of marmots and men. Nature 1990;347:230–232.

111. Ganem D, Varmus HE. The molecular biology of the hepatitis B virus. Annu Rev Biochem 1987;56:651–693.

112. Gerber MA, Hadziyannis S, Vissoulis C, Schaffner F, Paronetto F, Popper H. Hepatitis B antigen: nature and distribution of cytoplasmic antigen in hepatocytes of carriers (37912). Proc Soc Exp Biol Med 1974;145:863–867.

113. Gerber MA, Hadziyannis S, Vissoulis C, Schaffner F, Paronetto F, Popper H. Electron microscopy and immunoelectronmicroscopy of cytoplasmic hepatitis B antigen in hepatocytes. Am J Pathol 1974; 75:489–502.

114. Germain RN. MHC-dependent antigen processing and peptide presentation: providing ligands for T lymphocyte activation. Cell 1994; 76:287–299.

115. Gilles PN, Fey G, Chisari FV. Tumor necrosis factor-alpha negatively regulates hepatitis B virus gene expression in transgenic mice. J Virol 1992;66:3955–3960.

116. Gilles PN, Guerrette DL, Ulevitch RJ, Schreiber RD, Chisari FV. Hepatitis B surface antigen retention sensitizes the hepatocyte to injury by physiologic concentrations of gamma interferon. Hepatology 1992;16:655–663.

117. Gorbalenya AE, Donchenko AP, Koonin EV, Blinov VM. N-terminal domains of putative helicases of flavi- and pestiviruses may be serine proteases. Nucleic Acids Res 1989;17:3889–3897.

118. Grakoui A, McCourt DW, Wychowski C, Feinstone SM, Rice CM. Characterization of the hepatitis C virus-encoded serine proteinase: determination of proteinase-dependent polyprotein cleavage sites. J Virol 1993;67:2832–2843.

119. Grakoui A, McCourt DW, Wychowski C, Feinstone SM, Rice CM. A second hepatitis C virus-encoded proteinase. Proc Natl Acad Sci U S A 1993;90:10583–10587.

120. Grakoui A, Wychowski C, Lin C, Feinstone SM, Rice CM. Expression and identification of hepatitis C virus polyprotein cleavage products. J Virol 1993;67:1385–1395.

121. Guidotti LG, Ando K, Hobbs MV, et al. Cytotoxic T lymphocytes inhibit hepatitis B virus gene expression by a noncytolytic mechanism in transgenic mice. Proc Natl Acad Sci U S A 1994;91: 3764–3768.

122. Guidotti LG, Guilhot S, Chisari FV. Interleukin 2 and interferon alpha/beta downregulate hepatitis B virus gene expression in vivo by tumor necrosis factor dependent and independent pathways. J Virol 1994;68:1265–1270.

123. Guidotti LG, Ishikawa T, Hobbs MV, Matzke B, Schreiber R, Chisari FV. Intracellular inactivation of the hepatitis B virus by cytotoxic T lymphocytes. Immunity 1996;4:25–36.

124. Guidotti LG, Matzke B, Schaller H, Chisari FV. High level hepatitis B virus replication in transgenic mice. J Virol 1995;69:6158–6169.

125. Guilhot S, Fowler P, Portillo G, et al. Hepatitis B virus (HBV) specific cytolytic T cell response in humans: production of target cells by stable expression of HBV-encoded proteins in immortalized human B cell lines. J Virol 1992;66:2670–2678.

126. Guilhot S, Guidotti LG, Chisari FV. Interleukin-2 downregulates hepatitis B virus gene expression in transgenic mice by a post-transcriptional mechanism. J Virol 1993;67:7444–7449.

127. Guilhot S, Huang S, Xia YP, LaMonica N, Lai MMC, Chisari FV. Expression of the hepatitis delta virus large and small antigens in transgenic mice. J Virol 1994;68:1052–1058.

128. Guo H-C, Jardetzky TS, Garrett TPJ, Lane WS, Strominger JL, Wiley DC. Different length peptides bind to HLA-Aw68 similarly at their ends but bulge out in the middle. Nature 1992;360:364–366.

129. Hagen TM, Wehr C, Huang S-N, et al. Extensive oxidative DNA damage in hepatocytes of transgenic mice with chronic active hepatitis destined to develop hepatocellular carcinoma. Proc Natl Acad Sci U S A 1994;91:12808–12812.

130. Haritani H, Uchida T, Okuda Y, Shikata T. Effect of 3'-azido-3'-deoxythymidine on replication of duck hepatitis B virus in vivo and in vitro. J Med Virol 1989;29:244–248.

131. Hasegawa K, Huang J, Rogers SA, Blum HE, Liang TJ. Enhanced viral replication of a hepatitis B virus mutant associated with an epidemic of fulminant hepatitis. J Virol 1994;68:1651–1659.

132. Hertogs K, Leenders WPJ, Depla E, et al. Endonexin II, present on human liver plasma membranes, is a specific binding protein of small hepatitis B virus envelope protein. Virology 1993;197: 549–557.

133. Hijikata M, Kato N, Ootsuyama Y, Nakagawa M, Ohkoshi S, Shimotohno K. Hypervariable regions in the putative glycoprotein of hepatitis C virus. Biochem Biophys Res Commun 1991;175:220–228.

134. Hijikata M, Kato N, Ootsuyama Y, Nakagawa M, Shimotohno K. Gene mapping of the putative structural region of the hepatitis C virus genome by in vitro processing analysis. Proc Natl Acad Sci U S A 1991;88:5547–5551.

135. Hijikata M, Mizushima H, Akagi T, et al. Two distinct proteinase activities required for the processing of putative nonstructural precursor protein of hepatitis C virus. J Virol 1993;67:4665–4675.

136. Himeno Y, Fukuda Y, Hatanaka M, Imura H. Expression of oncogenes in human liver disease. Liver 1988;8:208–212.

137. Hino O, Nomura K, Ohtake K, Kawaguchi T, Sugano H, Kitagawa T. Instability of integrated hepatitis B virus DNA with inverted repeat structure in a transgenic mouse. Cancer Genet Cytogenet 1989;37:273–278.

138. Hirsch RC, Lavine JE, Chang L, Varmus HE, Ganem D. Polymerase gene products of hepatitis B viruses are required for genomic RNA packaging as well as for reverse transcription. Nature 1990;344: 552–555.

139. Hollinger FB. Hepatitis B virus. In: Fields BN, Knipe DM, eds. Virology. New York: Raven Press, 1990:2171–2236.

140. Honigwachs J, Faktor O, Dikstein R, Shaul Y, Laub O. Liver-specific expression of hepatitis B virus is determined by the com-

bined action of the core gene promoter and the enhancer. J Virol 1989;63:919–924.

141. Hosein B, Fang CT, Popovsky MA, Ye J, Zhang M, Wang CY. Improved serodiagnosis of hepatitis C virus infection with synthetic peptide antigen from capsid protein. Proc Natl Acad Sci U S A 1991;88:3647–3651.

142. Houghton M, Selby M, Weiner A, Choo Q-L. Hepatitis C virus: structure, protein products and processing of the polyprotein precursor. In: Reesink HW, ed. Hepatitis C virus. Basel: Karger, 1994: 1–11.

143. Houghton MA, Weiner A, Han J, Kuo G, Choo Q-L. Molecular biology of the hepatitis C virus: implications for diagnosis, development and control of viral disease. Hepatology 1990;14:381–388.

144. Hsu IC, Metcalf RA, Sun T, Welsh JA, Wang NJ, Harris CC. Mutational hotspot in the p53 gene in human hepatocellular carcinoma. Nature 1991;350:427–428.

145. Hsu T-Y, Moroy T, Etiemble J, et al. Activation of c-myc by woodchuck hepatitis virus insertion in hepatocellular carcinoma. Cell 1988;55:627–635.

146. Hu K-Q, Vierling JM, Siddiqui A. Trans-activation of HLA-DR gene by hepatitis B virus X gene product. Proc Natl Acad Sci U S A 1990;87:7140–7144.

147. Hu K-Q, Yu CH, Vierling JM. Up-regulation of intracellulare adhesion molecule-1 transcription by hepatitis B virus X protein. Proc Natl Acad Sci U S A 1992;89:11441–11445.

148. Huang S-N, Chisari FV. Strong, sustained hepatocellular proliferation precedes hepatocarcinogenesis in hepatitis B surface antigen transgenic mice. Hepatology 1995;21:620–626.

149. Hunt DF, Henderson RA, Shabanowitz J, et al. Characterization of peptides bound to the class I MHC molecule HLA-A2.1 by mass spectrometry. Science 1992;255:1261–1263.

150. Inchauspe G, Zebedee S, Lee D-H, Sugitani M, Nasoff M, Prince AM. Genomic structure of the human prototype strain H of hepatitis C virus: comparison with the American and Japanese isolates. Proc Natl Acad Sci U S A 1991;88:10292–10296.

151. Ishida C, Matsumoto K, Fukada K, Matsushita K, Shiraki H, Maeda Y. Detection of antibodies to hepatitis C virus (HCV) structural proteins in anti-HCV-positive sera by an enzyme-linked immunosorbent assay using synthetic peptides as antigens. J Clin Microbiol 1993;31:936–940.

152. Itho Y, Takai E, Ohnuma H, et al. A synthetic peptide vaccine involving the product of the pre-S(2) region of hepatitis B virus DNA: protective efficacy in chimpanzees. Proc Natl Acad Sci U S A 1986; 83:9174–9178.

153. Jacobson S, Sekaly RP, Jacobson CL, McFarland HF, Long EO. HLA class II-restricted presentation of cytoplasmic measles virus antigens to cytotoxic T cells. J Virol 1989;63:1756–1762.

154. Jardetzky TS, Lane WS, Robinson RA, Madden DR, Wiley DC. Identification of self peptides bound to purified HLA-B27. Nature 1991;353:326–329.

155. Jean-Jean O, Weimer T, De Recondo AM, Will H, Rossignol JM. Internal entry of ribosomes and ribosomal scanning involved in hepatitis B virus P gene expression. J Virol 1989;63:5451–5454.

156. Jilbert AR, Wu T-T, England JM, et al. Rapid resolution of duck hepatitis B virus infections occurs after massive hepatocellular involvement. J Virol 1992;66:1377–1388.

157. Jin Y, Shih W-K, Berkower I. Human T cell response to the surface antigen of hepatitis B virus (HBsAg): endosomal and nonendosomal processing pathways are accessible to both endogenous and exogenous antigen. J Exp Med 1988;168:293–306.

158. Jung MC, Spengler U, Schraut W, et al. Hepatitis B virus antigen-specific T-cell activation in patients with acute and chronic hepatitis B. J Hepatol 1991;13:310–317.

159. Jung MC, Stemler M, Weimer T, et al. Immune response of peripheral blood mononuclear cells to HBx antigen of hepatitis B virus. Hepatology 1990;13:637–643.

160. Junker-Niepmann M, Bartenschlager R, Schaller H. A short cis-acting sequence is required for hepatitis B virus pregenome encapsidation and sufficient for packaging of foreign RNA. EMBO J 1990; 9:3389–3396.

161. Kajino K, Jilbert AR, Saputelli J, Aldrich CE, Cullen J, Mason WS. Woodchuck hepatitis virus infections: very rapid recovery after a prolonged viremia and infection of virtually every hepatocyte. J Virol 1994;68:5792–5803.

162. Kamer G, Argos P. Primary structural comparison of RNA-dependent polymerases from plant, animal and bacterial viruses. Nucleic Acids Res 1984;12:7269–7282.

163. Kane MA, Bradley DW, Shrestha SM, et al. Epidemic non-A, non-B hepatitis in Nepal: recovery of a possible etiologic agent and transmission studies in marmosets. JAMA 1984;252:3140–3145.

164. Kaneko S, Miller RH. X-region-specific transcript in mammalian hepatitis B virus-infected liver. J Virol 1988;62:3979–3984.

165. Kaplan DR, Griffith R, Braciale VL, Braciale TJ. Influenza virus-specific human cytotoxic T cell clones: heterogeneity in antigenic specificity and restriction by class II MHC products. Cell Immunol 1984;88:193–206.

166. Karpen S, Banerjee R, Zelent A, Price P, Acs G. Identification of protein-binding sites in the hepatitis B virus enhancer and core promoter domains. Mol Cell Biol 1988;8:5159–5165.

167. Kato N, Hijikata M, Ootsuyama Y, et al. Molecular cloning of the human hepatitis C virus genome from Japanese patients with non-A, non-B hepatitis. Proc Natl Acad Sci U S A 1990;87:9524–9528.

168. Kato N, Sekiya H, Ootsuyama Y, et al. Humoral immune response to hypervariable region 1 of the putative envelope glycoprotein (GP70) of hepatitis C virus. J Virol 1993;67:3923–3930.

169. Kawamoto S, Yamamoto S, Ueda K, Nagahata T, Chisaka O, Matsubara K. Translation of hepatitis B virus DNA polymerase from the internal AUG codon, not from the upstream AUG codon for the core protein. Biochem Biophys Res Commun 1990;171:1130–1136.

170. Kim C-M, Koike K, Saito I, Miyamura T, Jay G. HBx gene of hepatitis B virus induces liver cancer in transgenic mice. Nature 1991; 351:317–320.

171. Kita H, Moriyama T, Kaneko T, et al. HLA-B44-restricted cytotoxic T lymphocytes recognizing an epitope on hepatitis C virus nucleocapsid protein. Hepatology 1993;18:1039–1044.

172. Klinkert MQ, Theilmann L, Pfaff E, Schaller H. Pre-S1 antigens and antibodies early in the course of acute hepatitis B virus infection. J Virol 1986;58:522–525.

173. Koike K, Moriya K, Iino S, et al. High level expression of hepatitis B virus HBx gene and hepatocarcinogenesis in transgenic mice. Hepatology 1994;19:810–819.

174. Korba BE, Brown TL, Wells FV, et al. Natural history of experimental woodchuck hepatitis virus infection: molecular virologic features of the pancreas, kidney, ovary, and testis. J Virol 1990;64:4499–4506.

175. Korba BE, Cote PJ, Wells FV, et al. Natural history of woodchuck hepatitis virus infections during the course of experimental viral infection: molecular virologic features of the liver and lymphoid tissues. J Virol 1989;63:1360–1370.

176. Korba BE, Wells F, Tennant BC, Cote PJ, Gerin JL. Lymphoid cells in the spleens of woodchuck hepatitis virus-infected woodchucks are a site of active viral replication. J Virol 1987;61:1318–1324.

177. Korba BE, Wells F, Tennant BC, Yoakum GH, Purcell RH, Gerin JL. Hepadnavirus infection of peripheral blood lymphocytes in vivo: woodchuck and chimpanzee models of viral hepatitis. J Virol 1986; 58:1–8.

178. Koziel MJ, Dudley D, Afdhal N, et al. Hepatitis C virus (HCV)-specific cytotoxic T lymphocytes recognize epitopes in the core and envelope proteins of HCV. J Virol 1993;67:7522–7532.

179. Koziel MJ, Dudley D, Wong JT, et al. Intrahepatic cytotoxic T lymphocyte specific for hepatitis C virus in persons with chronic hepatitis. J Immunol 1992;149:3339–3344.

180. Kremsdorf D, Porchon C, Kim JP, Reyes GR, Brechot C. Partial nucleotide sequence analysis of a French hepatitis C virus: implications for HCV genetic variability in the E2/NS1 protein. J Gen Virol 1991;72:2557–2561.

181. Kuo G, Choo Q-L, Alter HJ, et al. An assay for circulating antibodies to a major etiologic virus of human non-A, non-B hepatitis. Science 1989;244:362–364.

182. Kuo MT, Zou J-Y, Teeter LD, Ikeguchi M, Chisari FV. Activation of multidrug resistance (P-glycoprotein) mdr3/mdr1a gene during the development of hepatocellular carcinoma in hepatitis B virus transgenic mice. Cell Growth Differ 1992;3:531–540.

183. Lanzavecchia A, Roosnek E, Gregory T, Berman P, Abrignani S. T cells can present antigens such as HIV gp120 targeted to their own surface molecules. Nature 1988;334:530–532.

184. Lavine J, Hirsch R. A system for studying the selective encapsidation of hepadnavirus FNA. J Virol 1989;63:4257–4263.

185. Lee T-H, Finegold MJ, Shen R-F, DeMayo JL, Woo SL, Butel JS. Hepatitis B virus transactivator X protein is not tumorigenic in transgenic mice. J Virol 1990;64:5939–5947.

186. Lieber CS, Garro A, Leo MA, Mak KM, Worner T. Alcohol and cancer. Hepatology 1986;6:1005–1019.

187. Lien J-M, Aldrich CE, Mason WS. Evidence that a capped oligoribonucleotide is the primer for duck hepatitis B virus plus-strand DNA synthesis. J Virol 1986;57:229–236.

188. Limmer J, Fleig WE, Leupold D, Bittner R, Ditschunest H, Berger H-G. Hepatocellular carcinoma in type 1 glycogen storage disease. Hepatology 1988;8:531–537.

189. Lok ASF, Akarca U, Greene S. Mutations in the precore region of hepatitis B virus serve to enhance the stability of the secondary structure of the pregenome encapsidation signal. Proc Natl Acad Sci U S A 1994;91:4077–4081.

190. Lopez-Cabrera M, Letovskyk J, Hu KQ, Siddiqui A. Multiple liver specific factors bind to the hepatitis B virus core/pregenomic promoter: trans-activation and repression by CCAAT/enhancer binding protein. Proc Natl Acad Sci U S A 1990;87:5069–5073.

191. Machida A, Kishimoto S, Ohnuma H, et al. A hepatitis B surface antigen polypeptide (P31) with the receptor for polymerized human as well as chimpanzee albumins. Gastroenterology 1983;85:268–274.

192. Mack DH, Bloch W, Nath N, Sninsky JJ. Hepatitis B virus particles contain a polypeptide encoded by the largest open reading frame: a putative reverse transcriptase. J Virol 1988;62:4786–4790.

193. Macnaughton TB, Gowans EJ, Jilbert AR, Burrell CJ. Hepatitis delta virus RNA, protein synthesis and associated cytotoxicity in a stably transfected cell line. Virology 1990;177:692–698.

194. Maguire HF, Hoeffler JP, Siddiqui A. HBV X protein alters the DNA binding specificity of CREB and ATF-2 by protein-protein interactions. Science 1991;252:842–844.

195. Marion PL, Oshiro LS, Regnery DC, Scullard GH, Robinson WS. A virus in Beechey ground squirrels which is related to hepatitis B virus of man. Proc Natl Acad Sci U S A 1980;77:2941–2945.

196. Marion PL, Van Davelaar MJ, Knight SS, et al. Hepatocellular carcinoma in ground squirrels persistently infected with ground squirrel hepatitis virus. Proc Natl Acad Sci U S A 1986;83:4543–4546.

197. Marshall CJ. Tumor suppressor genes. Cell 1991;64:313–326.

198. Martell M, Esteban JI, Quer J, et al. Hepatitis C virus (HCV) circulates as a population of different but closely related genomes: quasispecies nature of HCV genome distribution. J Virol 1992;66:3225–3229.

199. Martell M, Esteban JI, Quer J, et al. Dynamic behavior of hepatitis C virus quasispecies in patients undergoing orthotopic liver transplantation. J Virol 1994;68:3425–3436.

200. Maruyama T, Iino S, Koike K, Yasuda K, Milich DR. Serology of acute exacerbation in chronic hepatitis B. Gastroenterology 1993;105:1141–1151.

201. Maruyama T, McLachlan A, Iino S, Koike K, Kurokawa K, Milich DR. The serology of chronic hepatitis B infection revisited. J Clin Invest 1993;91:2586–2595.

202. Mason WS, Aldrich C, Summers J, et al. Asymmetric replication of duck hepatitis B virus DNA in liver cells (free minus-strand DNA). Proc Natl Acad Sci U S A 1982;79:3997–4001.

203. Mason WS, Halpern MS, England JM, et al. Experimental transmission of duck hepatitis B virus. Virology 1983;131:375–384.

204. Mason WS, Seal S, Summers J. Virus of Pekin ducks with structural and biological relatedness to human hepatitis B virus. J Virol 1980;36:829–836.

205. Matsubara K, Tokina T. Integration of hepatitis B virus DNA and its implications for hepatocarcinogenesis. Mol Biol Med 1990;7: 243–260.

206. Matsumara M, Fremont DH, Peterson PA, Wilson IA. Emerging principles for the recognition of peptide antigens by MHC class I molecules. Science 1992;257:927–934.

207. McLachlan A, Milich DR, Raney AK, et al. Expression of hepatitis B virus surface and core antigens: Influences of pre-S and precore sequences. J Virol 1987;61:683–780.

208. Mehdi H, Kaplan MJ, Anlar FY, et al. Hepatitis B virus surface antigen binds to apolipoprotein H. J Virol 1994;68:2415–2424.

209. Melia WM, Wilkinson ML, Portmann BC, Johnson PJ, Williams R. Hepatocellular carcinoma in the non-cirrhotic liver: a comparison with that complicating cirrhosis. QJM 1984;53:391–400.

210. Milich DR, Jones JE, Hughes JL, Price J, Raney AK, McLachlan A. Is a function of the secreted hepatitis B e antigen to induce immunologic tolerance in utero? Proc Natl Acad Sci U S A 1990;87: 6599–6603.

211. Milich DR, McLachlan A. The nucleocapsid of hepatitis B virus is both a T-cell-independent and a T-cell-dependent antigen. Science 1986;234:1398–1401.

212. Milich DR, McLachlan A, Thornton GB, Hughes JL. Antibody production to the nucleocapsid and envelope of the hepatitis B virus primed by a single synthetic T cell site. Nature 1987;329: 547–549.

213. Miller RH, Marion PL, Robinson WS. Hepatitis B viral DNA-RNA hybrid molecules in particles from infected liver are converted to viral DNA molecules during an endogenous DNA polymerase reaction. Virology 1984;139:64–72.

214. Miller RH, Purcell RH. Hepatitis C virus shares amino acid sequence similarity with pestiviruses and flaviviruses as well as members of two plant virus supergroups. Proc Natl Acad Sci U S A 1990;87:2057–2061.

215. Miller RH, Tran C-T, Robinson WS. Hepatitis B virus particles of plasma and liver contain viral DNA-RNA hybrid molecules. Virology 1984;139:53–63.

216. Minutello MA, Pileri P, Unutmaz D, et al. Compartmentalization of T-lymphocyte to the site of disease: intrahepatic CD4+ T-cells specific for the protein NS4 of hepatitis C virus in patient with chronic hepatitis. J Exp Med 1993;178:17–26.

217. Missale G, Redeker A, Person J, et al. HLA-A31 and HLA-Aw68 restricted cytotoxic T cell responses to a single hepatitis B virus nucleocapsid epitope during acute viral hepatitis. J Exp Med 1993; 177:751–762.

218. Molnar-Kimber KL, Jarocki-Witek V, Dheer SK, et al. Distinctive properties of the hepatitis B virus envelope proteins. J Virol 1988; 62:407–416.

219. Molnar-Kimber KL, Summers JW, Mason WS. Mapping of the cohesive overlap of duck hepatitis B virus DAN and of the site of initiation of reverse transcription. J Virol 1984;51:181–191.

220. Monaco JJ. A molecular model of MHC class-I-restricted antigen processing. Immunol Today 1992;13:173–179.

221. Mondelli M, Vergani GM, Alberti A, et al. Specificity of T lymphocyte cytotoxicity to autologous hepatocytes in chronic hepatitis B virus infection: evidence that T cells are directed against HBV core antigen expressed on hepatocytes. J Immunol 1982;129:2773–2778.

222. Mondelli MU, Cerino A, Boender P, et al. Significance of the immune response to a major, conformational B cell epitope on the hepatitis C virus NS3 region defined by a human monoclonal antibody. J Virol 1994;68:4829–4836.

223. Mondelli MU, Chisari FV, Ferrari C. The cellular immune response to nucleocapsid antigens in hepatitis B virus infection. Springer Seminars in Immunopathology, Springer-Verlag 1990;12:25–31.

224. Moriyama T, Guilhot S, Klopchin K, et al. Immunobiology and pathogenesis of hepatocellular injury in hepatitis B virus transgenic micc. Science 1990;248:361–364.

225. Muller D, Koller BH, Whitton JL, LaPan KE, Brigman KK, Frelinger JA. LCMV-specific, class II-restricted cytotoxic T cells in β2-microglobulin-deficient mice. Science 1992;255:1576–1578.

226. Murakami Y, Hayashi S, Sekiya T. Aberrations of the tumor suppressor p53 and retinoblastoma genes in human hepatocellular carcinomas. Cancer Res 1991;51:5520–5525.

227. Murakawa K, Esumi M, Kato T, Kambara H, Shikata J. Heterogeneity within the nonstructural protein 5-encoding region of hepatitis C viruses from a single patient. Gene 1992;117:229–232.

228. Nasoff MS, Zebedee SL, Inchauspé G, Prince AM. Identification of an immunodominant epitope within the capsid protein of hepatitis C virus. Proc Natl Acad Sci U S A 1991;88:5462–5466.

229. Nassal M. The arginine-rich domain of the hepatitis B virus core protein is required for pregenome encapsidation and productive viral positive-strand DNA synthesis but not for virus assembly. J Virol 1992;66:4107–4116.

230. Nayersina R, Folwer P, Guilhot S, et al. HLA A2 restricted cytotoxic T lymphocyte responses to multiple hepatitis B surface antigen epitopes during hepatitis B virus infection. J Immunol 1993;150:4659–4671.

231. Negro F, Korba BE, Forzani B, et al. Hepatitis delta virus (HDV) and woodchuck hepatitis virus (WHV) nucleic acids in tissues of HDV-infected chronic WHV carrier woodchucks. J Virol 1989;63:1612–1618.

232. Neurath AR, Kent SB, Strick N, Parker K. Identification and chemical synthesis of a host cell receptor binding site on hepatitis B virus. Cell 1986;46:429–436.

233. Neurath AR, Kent SBH. The pre-S region of hepadnavirus envelope proteins. Adv Virus Res 1988;34:65–142.

234. Neurath AR, Strick N, Sproul P. Search for hepatitis B virus cell receptors reveals binding sites for interleukin 6 on the virus envelope protein. J Exp Med 1992;175:461–469.

235. Niederau C, Fischer R, Sonnenberg A, Stremmel W, Trampisch HJ, Strohmeyer G. Survival and causes of death in cirrhotic and in noncirrhotic patients with primary hemochromatosis. N Engl J Med 1985;313:1256–1262.

236. Nilsson T, Jackson M, Peterson PA. Short cytoplasmic sequences serve as retention signals for transmembrane proteins in the endoplasmic reticulum. Cell 1989;58:707–718.

237. Nishioka K, Watanabe J, Furuta S, et al. A high prevalence of antibody to the hepatitis C virus in patients with hepatocellular carcinoma in Japan. Cancer 1991;67:429–433.

238. Niu J, Wang Y, Qiao M, et al. Effect of *Phyllanthus amarus* on duck hepatitis B virus replication in vivo. J Med Virol 1990;32:212–218.

239. Ogata N, Alter HJ, Miller RH, Purcell RH. Nucleotide sequence and mutation rate of the H strain of hepatitis C virus. Proc Natl Acad Sci U S A 1991;88:3392–3396.

240. Ohshima H, Bartsch H. Chronic infections and inflammatory processes as cancer risk factors: possible role of nitric oxide in carcinogenesis. Mutat Res 1994;305:253–264.

241. Okamoto H, Kojima M, Okada SI, et al. Genetic drift of hepatitis C virus during an 8.2 year infection in a chimpanzee: variability and stability. Virology 1992;190:894–899.

242. Okamoto H, Kurai K, Okada S-I, et al. Full-length sequence of a hepatitis C virus genome having poor homology to reported isolates: comparative study of four distinct genotypes. Virology 1992;188:331–341.

243. Okamoto H, Okada S, Sugiyama Y, et al. Nucleotide sequence of genomic RNA of hepatitis C virus isolated from a human carrier: comparison with reported isolates for conserved and divergent regions. J Gen Virol 1991;72:2697–2704.

244. Okamoto H, Tsuda F, Machida A, et al. Antibodies against synthetic oligopeptides deduced from the putative core gene for the diagnosis of hepatitis C virus infection. Hepatology 1992;15:180–186.

245. Okamoto H, Usuda S, Imai M, et al. Antibody to the receptor for polymerized human serum albumin in acute and persistent infection with hepatitis B virus. Hepatology 1986;6:354–359.

246. Oldstone MBA. Viral persistence. Cell 1989;56:517–520.

247. Omata M. Significance of extrahepatic replication of hepatitis B virus. Hepatology 1990;12:364–366.

248. Ostapchuk P, Scheirle G, Hearing P. Binding of nuclear factor EF-C to a functional domain of the hepatitis B virus enhancer region. Mol Cell Biol 1989;9:2787–2797.

249. Ou J-H, Yeh CT, Yen TSB. Transport of hepatitis B virus precore protein into the nucleus after cleavage of its signal peptide. J Virol 1989;63:5238–5243.

250. Ou J, Rutter WJ. Hybrid hepatitis B virus-host transcripts in a human hepatoma cell. Proc Natl Acad Sci U S A 1985;82:83–87.

251. Ou JH, Rutter WJ. Regulation of secretion of the hepatitis B virus major surface antigen by the preS-1 protein. J Virol 1987;61: 782–786.

252. Pasquinelli C, Bhavani K, Chisari FV. Multiple oncogenes and tumor suppressor genes are structurally and functionally intact during hepatocarcinogenesis in hepatitis B virus transgenic mice. Cancer Res 1992;52:2823–2829.

253. Patel NU, Jameel S, Isom H, Siddiqui A. Interactions between nuclear factors and the hepatitis B virus enhancer. J Virol 1989;63:5293–5301.

254. Patzer EJ, Nakamura GR, Simonsen CC, Levinson AD, Brands R. Intracellular assembly and packaging of hepatitis B surface antigen particles occur in the endoplasmic reticulum. J Virol 1986;58:884–892.

255. Patzer EJ, Nakamura GR, Yaffe A. Intracellular transport and secretion of hepatitis B surface antigen in mammalian cells. J Virol 1984;51:346–353.

256. Paul WE, Seder RA. Lymphocyte responses and cytokines. Cell 1994;76:241–251.

257. Penna A, Chisari FV, Bertoletti A, et al. Cytotoxic T lymphocytes recognize an HLA-A2-restricted epitope within the hepatitis B virus nucleocapsid antigen. J Exp Med 1991;174:1565–1570.

258. Penna A, Fowler P, Bertoletti A, et al. Hepatitis B virus (HBV)-specific cytotoxic T-cell (CTL) response in humans: characterization of HLA class II-restricted CTLs that recognize endogenously synthesized HBV envelope antigens. J Virol 1992;66:1193–1198.

259. Petcu DJ, Aldrich CE, Coates L, Taylor JM, Mason WS. Suramin inhibits in vitro infection by duck hepatitis B virus, Rous sarcoma virus, and hepatitis delta virus. Virology 1988;167:385–392.

260. Pizzi E, Tramontano A, Tomei L, et al. Molecular model of the specificity pocket of the hepatitis C virus proteinase: implications for substrate recognition. Proc Natl Acad Sci U S A 1994;91:888–892.

261. Poch O, Sauvaget I, Delarue M, Tordo N. Identification of four conserved motifs among RNA-dependent polymerase encoding elements. EMBO J 1989;8:3867–3874.

262. Popper H, Roth L, Purcell RH, Tennant BC, Gerin JL. Hepatocarcinogenicity of the woodchuck hepatitis virus. Proc Natl Acad Sci U S A 1987;84:866–870.

263. Potts RC, Sherif MM, Robertson AJ, Gibbs JH, Brown RA, Beck JS. Serum inhibitory factor in lepromatous leprosy: its effect on the pre-S-phase cell-cycle kinetics of mitogen-stimulated normal human lymphocytes. Scand J Immunol 1981;14:269–280.

264. Prince AM, Brotman B, Huima T, Pascual D, Jaffery M, Inchauspe G. Immunity in hepatitis C infection. J Infect Dis 1992;165: 438–443.

265. Rall LB, Standring DN, Laub O, Rutter WJ. Transcription of hepatitis B virus by RNA polymerase II. Mol Cell Biol 1983;3:1766–1773.

266. Ralston R, Thudium K, Berger K, et al. Characterization of hepatitis C virus envelope glycoprotein complexes expressed by recombinant vaccinia viruses. J Virol 1993;67:6753–6761.

267. Rammensee H-G, Falk K, Rotzschke O. Peptides naturally presented by MHC class I molecules. Annu Rev Immunol 1993;11:213–244.

268. Raney AK, Le HB, McLachlan A. Regulation of transcription from the hepatitis B virus major surface antigen promoter by the Sp1 transcription factor. J Virol 1992;66:6912–6921.

269. Raney AK, Milich DR, Easton AJ, McLachlan A. Differentiation-specific transcriptional regulation of the hepatitis B virus large surface antigen gene in human hepatoma cell lines. J Virol 1990;64:2360–2368.

270. Raney AK, Milich DR, McLachlan A. Characterization of hepatitis B virus major surface antigen gene transcriptional regulatory elements in differentiated hepatoma cell lines. J Virol 1989;63:3919–3925.

271. Rehermann B, Person J, Redeker A, et al. The cytotoxic T lymphocyte response to multiple hepatitis B virus polymerase epitopes during and after acute viral hepatitis. J Exp Med 1995;181:1047–1058.

272. Robinson WS. Molecular events in the pathogenesis of hepadnavirus-associated hepatocellular carcinoma. Annu Rev Med 1994;45:297–323.

273. Robinson WS, Miller RH, Marion PL. Hepadnaviruses and retroviruses share genome homology and features of replication. Hepatology 1987;7:64S-73S.

274. Roossinck MJ, Jameel S, Loukin SH, Siddiqui A. Expression of hepatitis B viral core region in mammalian cells. Mol Cell Biol 1986;6:1393–1400.

275. Rosenthal N, Kress M, Gruss P, et al. BK viral enhancer element and a human cellular homolog. Science 1983;222:749–755.

276. Rotzschke O, Falk K, Deres K, et al. Isolation and analysis of naturally processed viral peptides as recognized by cytotoxic T cells. Nature 1990;348:252–254.

277. Saito I, Miyamura T, Ohbayashi A, et al. Hepatitis C virus infection is associated with the development of hepatocellular carcinoma. Proc Natl Acad Sci U S A 1990;87:6547–6549.

278. Santolini E, Migliaccio G, La Monica N. Biosynthesis and biochemical properties of the hepatitis C virus core protein. J Virol 1994;68: 3631–3641.

279. Schek N, Bartenschlager R, Kuhn C, Schaller H. Phosphorylation and rapid turnover of hepatitis B virus X-protein expressed in HepG2 cells from a recombinant vaccinia virus. Oncogene 1991;6: 1735–1744.

280. Schirmacher P, Held WA, Chisari FV, Yang D, Rogler CE. Reactivation of insulin-like growth factor II during hepatocarcinogenesis in transgenic mice suggests a role in malignant growth. Cancer Res 1992;52:2549–2556.

281. Schirmbeck R, Melber K, Kuhröber A, Janowicz ZA, Reimann J. Immunization with soluble hepatitis B virus surface protein elicits murine H-2 class I-restricted CD8+ cytotoxic T lymphocyte responses in vivo. J Immunol 1994;152:1110–1119.

282. Schirmbeck R, Melber K, Mertens T, Reimann J. Antibody and cytotoxic T-cell responses to soluble hepatitis B virus (HBV) S antigen in mice: implication for the pathogenesis of HBV-induced hepatitis. J Virol 1994;68:1418–1425.

283. Schlesinger JJ, Brandriss MW, Cropp CB, Monath TP. Protection against yellow fever in monkeys by immunization with yellow fever virus nonstructural protein NS1. J Virol 1986;60:1153–1155.

284. Schlesinger JJ, Brandriss MW, Walsh EE. Protection against 17D yellow fever encephalitis in mice by passive transfer of monoclonal antibodies to the nonstructural glycoprotein gp48 and by active immunization with gp48. J Immunol 1985;135:2805–2809.

285. Schlesinger JJ, Brandriss MW, Walsh EE. Protection of mice against dengue 2 virus encephalitis by immunization with the dengue 2 virus nonstructural glycoprotein NS1. J Gen Virol 1987;68: 853–857.

286. Schlicht H-J, Radziwill G, Schaller H. Synthesis and encapsidation of duck hepatitis B virus reverse transcriptase do not require formation of core-polymerase fusion proteins. Cell 1989;56:85–92.

287. Schlicht HJ, Schaller H. The secretory core protein of human hepatitis B virus is expressed on the cell surface. J Virol 1989;63:5399–5404.

288. Schupper H, Hayashi P, Scheffel J, et al. Peripheral blood mononuclear cell responses to recombinant hepatitis C virus antigens in patients with chronic hepatitis C. Hepatology 1993;18:1055–1060.

289. Seeger C, Ganem D, Varmus HE. Biochemical and genetic evidence for the hepatitis B virus replication strategy. Science 1986;232:477–484.

290. Seifer M, Zhou S, Standring DN. A micromolar pool of antigenically distinct precursors is required to initiate cooperative assembly of hepatitis B virus capsids in Xenopus oocytes. J Virol 1993;67: 249–257.

291. Sell S, Hunt JM, Dunsford HA, Chisari FV. Synergy between hepatitis B virus expression and chemical hepatocarcinogens in transgenic mice. Cancer Res 1991;51:1278–1285.

292. Seto E, Yen TSB, Peterlin BM, Ou J-H. Trans-activation of the human immunodeficiency virus long terminal repeat by the hepatitis B virus X protein. Proc Natl Acad Sci U S A 1988;85:8286–8290.

293. Shaul Y, Rutter WJ, Laub O. A human hepatitis B viral enhancer element. EMBO J 1985;4:427–430.

294. Shimizu YK, Hijikata M, Iwamoto A, Alter HJ, Purcell RH, Yoshikura H. Neutralizing antibodies against hepatitis C virus and the emergence of neutralization escape mutant viruses. J Virol 1994; 68:1494–1500.

295. Shimizu YK, Iwamoto A, Hijikata M, Purcell RH, Yoshikura H. Evidence for in vitro replication of hepatitis C virus genome in a human T cell line. Proc Natl Acad Sci U S A 1992;89:5477–5481.

296. Shimizu YK, Purcell RH, Yoshikura H. Correlation between the infectivity of hepatitis C virus in vivo and its infectivity in vitro. Proc Natl Acad Sci U S A 1993;90:6037–6041.

297. Shirai M, Akatsuka T, Pendleton CD, et al. Induction of cytotoxic T cells to a cross-reactive epitope in the hepatitis C virus nonstructural RNA polymerase-like protein. J Virol 1992;66:4098–4106.

298. Siddiqui A, Gaynor R, Srinivasan A, Mapoles J, Farr RW. Transactivation of viral enhancers including long terminal repeat of the human immunodeficiency virus by the hepatitis B virus X protein. Virology 1989;173:764–766.

299. Siddiqui A, Jameel S, Mapoles J. Transcriptional control elements of hepatitis B surface antigen gene. Proc Natl Acad Sci U S A 1986;83:566–570.

300. Siliciano RF, Lawton T, Knall C, et al. Analysis of host-virus interactions in AIDS with anti-gp120 T cell clones: effect of HIV sequence variation and a mechanism for CD4+ cell depletion. Cell 1988;54:561–575.

301. Silver ML, Guo H-C, Strominger JL, Wiley DC. Atomic structure of a human MHC molecule presenting an influenza virus peptide. Nature 1992;360:367–369.

302. Simmonds P. Variability of hepatitis C virus genome. In: Reesink HW, ed. Hepatitis C virus. Basel: Karger, 1994:12–35.

303. Simmonds P, Rose KA, Graham S, et al. Mapping of serotype-specific, immunodominant epitopes in the NS4 region of hepatitis C virus (HCV): use of type-specific peptides to serologically differentiate infections with HCV type 1, 2 and 3. J Clin Microbiol 1993; 31:1493–1503.

304. Slagle BL, Zhou Y-Z, Butel JS. Hepatitis B virus integration event in human chromosome 17p near the p53 gene identifies the region of the chromosome commonly deleted in virus-positive hepatocellular carcinomas. Cancer Res 1991;51:49–54.

305. Smith GW, Wright PW. Synthesis of proteins and glycoproteins in dengue type 2 virus-infected Vero and Aedes albopticus cells. J Gen Virol 1985;66:559–571.

306. Smith M, Hiroshige S, Murray J. Evidence in human hepatomas for structural chromosome changes and alteration in the expression of genes in the region 4q21-4q27. Am J Hum Genet 1986;39:A220. Abstract.

307. Snyder RL, Summers J. Woodchuck hepatitis virus and hepatocellular carcinoma. In: Essex M, Todaro G, zur Hausen H, eds. Viruses in naturally occurring cancers: Cold Spring Harbor conferences on cell proliferation. Vol 7. Cold Spring Harbor, NY: Cold Spring Harbor Laboratories, 1980:447–458.

308. Spandau DF, Lee CH. Transactivation of viral enhancers by the hepatitis B virus X protein. J Virol 1988;62:427–434.

309. Standring DN, Ou J-H, Rutter WJ. Assembly of viral particles in Xenopus oocytes: pre-surface-antigens regulate secretion of the hepatitis B viral surface envelope particle. Proc Natl Acad Sci U S A 1986;83:9338–9342.

310. Standring DN, Ou JH, Masiarz FR, Rutter WJ. A signal peptide encoded within the precore region of hepatitis B virus directs the secretion of a heterogeneous population of e antigens in Xenopus oocytes. Proc Natl Acad Sci U S A 1988;85:8405–8409.

311. Stemler M, Hess J, Braun R, Will H, Schroder CH. Serological evidence for expression of the polymerase gene of human hepatitis B virus in vivo. J Gen Virol 1988;69:689–693.

312. Stemler M, Weimer T, Tu Z-X, et al. Mapping of B-cell epitopes of the human hepatitis B virus X protein. J Virol 1990;64:2802–2809.

313. Stephan W, Prince AM, Brotman B. Modulation of hepatitis B infection by intravenous application of an immunoglobulin preparation that contains antibodies to hepatitis B e and core antigens but not to hepatitis B surface antigen. J Virol 1984;51:420–424.

314. Stratton MR, Moss S, Warren W, et al. Mutation of the p53 gene in human soft tissue sarcomas: association with abnormalities of the RB1 gene. Oncogene 1990;5:1297–1301.

315. Summers J. The replication cycle of hepatitis B viruses. Cancer 1988;61:1957–1962.

316. Summers J, Mason WS. Replication of the genome of a hepatitis B-like virus by reverse transcription of an RNA intermediate. Cell 1982;29:403–415.

317. Suzich JA, Tamura JK, Palmer-Hill F, et al. Hepatitis C virus NS3 protein polynucleotide-stimulated nucleoside triphosphatase and comparison with the related pestivirus and flavivirus enzymes. J Virol 1993;67:6152–6158.

318. Suzuki Y, Remington JS. The effect of anti-IFN-g antibody on the protective effect of Lyt-2+ immune T cells against toxoplasmosis in mice. J Immunol 1990;144:1954–1956.

319. Takada S, Koike K. Activated N-*ras* gene was found in human hepatoma tissue but only in a small fraction of the tumor cells. Oncogene 1989;4:189–193.

320. Takamizawa A, Mori C, Fuke I, et al. Structure and organization of the hepatitis C virus genome isolated from human carriers. J Virol 1991;65:1105–1113.

321. Takeuchi K, Kubo Y, Boonmar S, et al. The putative nucleocapsid and envelope protein genes of hepatitis C virus determined by comparison of the nucleotide sequences of two isolates derived from an experimentally infected chimpanzee and healthy human carriers. J Gen Virol 1990;71:3027–3033.

322. Taniguchi S, Okamoto H, Sakamoto M, et al. A structurally flexible and antigenically variable N-terminal domain of the hepatitis C virus E2/NS1 protein: implication for an escape from antibody. Virology 1993;195:297–301.

323. Thiel H-J, Stark R, Weiland E, Rümenapf T, Meyers G. Hog cholera virus: molecular composition of virions from a pestivirus. J Virol 1991;65:4705–4712.

324. Tomei L, Failla C, Santolini E, De Francesco R, La Monica N. NS3 is a serine protease required for processing of hepatitis C virus polyprotein. J Virol 1994;67:4017–4026.

325. Tsai SL, Chen PJ, Lai MY, et al. Acute exacerbations of chronic type B hepatitis are accompanied by increased T cell responses to hepatitis B core and e antigens: implications for hepatitis e antigen seroconversion. J Clin Invest 1992;89:87–96.

326. Tur-Kaspa R, Burk RD, Shaul Y, Shafritz DA. Hepatitis B virus contains a glucocorticoid-responsive element. Proc Natl Acad Sci U S A 1986;83:1627–1631.

327. Tuttleman J, Pourcel C, Summers J. Formation of the pool of covalently closed circular viral DNA in hepadnavirus infected cells. Cell 1986;47:451–460.

328. Tuttlemen J, Pugh J, Summers J. In vitro experimental infection of primary duck hepatocyte cultures with duck hepatitis B virus. J Virol 1986;58:17–25.

329. Twu J-S, Schloemer RH. Transcriptional trans-activating function of hepatitis B virus. J Virol 1987;61:3448–3453.

330. Twu JS, Chu K, Robinson WS. Hepatitis B virus X gene activated kB-like enhancer sequences in the long terminal repeat of human immunodeficiency virus 1. Proc Natl Acad Sci U S A 1989;86:5168–5172.

331. Twu JS, Lee CH, Lin PM, Schloemer RH. Hepatitis B virus suppresses expression of human beta-interferon. Proc Natl Acad Sci U S A 1988;85:252–256.

332. Twu JS, Schloemer RH. Transcriptional trans-activating function of hepatitis B virus. J Virol 1987;61:3448–3453.

333. Twu JS, Schloemer RH. Transcription of the human beta interferon gene is inhibited by hepatitis B virus. J Virol 1989;63:3065–3071.

334. Unger T, Shaul Y. The X protein of the hepatitis B virus acts as a transcription factor when targeted to its responsive element. EMBO J 1990;9:1889–1895.

335. United States Department of Health and Human Services. The health consequences of smoking: nicotine addiction. A report of the Surgeon General. DHHS (Centers for Disease Control) Publication no. 88-8406. Washington, DC: US Government Printing Office, 1988.

336. Vallbracht A, Maier K, Stierhof Y-D, Wiedmann KH, Flehming B, Fleicher B. Liver-derived cytotoxic T cells in hepatitis A virus infection. J Infect Dis 1989;160:209–217.

337. van den Oord JJ, de Vos R, Desmet VJ. In situ distribution of major histocompatibility complex products and viral antigens in chronic hepatitis B virus infection: evidence that HBc-containing hepatocytes may express HLA-DR antigens. Hepatology 1986;6:981–989.

338. Van der Poel CL. Hepatitis C virus: epidemiology, transmission and prevention. In: Reesink HW, ed. Hepatitis C virus. Basel: Karger, 1994:137–163.

339. VanBleek GM, Nathenson SG. Isolation of an endogenously processed immunodominant viral peptide from the class I H-2K^b molecule. Nature 1990;348:213–216.

340. Vannice JL, Levinson AD. Properties of the human hepatitis B virus enhancer: position effects and cell-type nonspecificity. J Virol 1988;62:1305–1313.

341. Vento S, Rondanelli EG, Ranieri S, O'Brien CJ, Williams R, Eddleston AL. Prospective study of cellular immunity to hepatitis-B-virus antigens from the early incubation phase of acute hepatitis B. Lancet 1987;2:119–122.

342. Wang GH, Seeger C. The reverse transcriptase of hepatitis B virus acts as a protein primer for viral DNA synthesis. Cell 1992;71:663–670.

343. Wang GH, Seeger C. Novel mechanism for reverse transcription in hepatitis B viruses. J Virol 1993;67:6506–6512.

344. Wang HP, Rogler CE. Deletions in human chromosome arms 11p and 13q in primary hepatocellular carcinomas. Cytogenet Cell Genet 1988;48:72–78.

345. Wang J, Chenivesse X, Henglein B, Brechot C. Hepatitis B virus integration in a cyclin A gene in a hepatocellular carcinoma. Nature 1990;343:555–557.

346. Wang XW, Forrester K, Yeh H, Feitelson MA, Gu J-R, Harris CC. Hepatitis B virus X protein inhibits p53 sequence-specific DNA binding, transcriptional activity and associated with transcription factor ERCC3. Proc Natl Acad Sci U S A 1994;91:2230–2234.

347. Weimer T, Weimer K, Tu ZX, Jung C, Pape GR, Will H. Immunogenicity of human hepatitis B virus P-gene derived proteins. J Immunol 1989;143:3750–3759.

348. Weiner AJ, Brauer MJ, Rosenblatt J, et al. Variable and hypervariable domains are found in the regions of HCV corresponding to the flavivirus envelope and NS1 proteins and the pestivirus envelope glycoproteins. Virology 1991;180:842–848.

349. Weiner AJ, Geysen HM, Christopherson C, et al. Evidence for immune selection of hepatitis C virus (HCV) putative envelope glycoprotein variants: potential role in chronic HCV infection. Proc Natl Acad Sci U S A 1992;89:3468–3472.

350. Whitten TM, Quets AT, Schloemer RH. Identification of the hepatitis B virus factor that inhibits expression of the beta interferon gene. J Virol 1991;65:4699–4704.

351. Will H, Reiser W, Weimer T, et al. Replication strategy of human hepatitis B virus. J Virol 1987;61:904–911.

352. Wirth S, Guidotti LG, Ando K, Schlicht HJ, Chisari FV. Breaking tolerance leads to autoantibody production but not autoimmune liver disease in HBV envelope transgenic mice. J Immunol 1995;154:2504–2515.

353. Wollersheim M, Debelka U, Hofschneider PH. A transactivating function encoded in the hepatitis B virus X gene is conserved in the integrated state. Oncogene 1988;3:545–552.

354. Yamamura K, Tsurimoto T, Ebihara T, et al. Methylation of hepatitis B virus DNA and liver-specific suppression of RNA production in transgenic mouse. Jpn J Cancer Res 1987;78:681–688.

355. Yasukawa M, Zarling JM. Human cytotoxic T cell clones directed against herpes simplex virus-infected cells. I. Lysis restricted by HLA class II MB and DR antigens. J Immunol 1984;133:422–427.

356. Yee JK. A liver-specific enhancer in the core promoter region of human hepatitis B virus. Science 1989;246:658–661.

357. Yeh C-T, Liaw Y-F, Ou J-H. The arginine-rich domain of hepatitis B virus precore and core proteins contains a signal for nuclear transport. J Virol 1990;64:6141–6147.

358. Yewdell JW, Bennink JR. Cell biology of antigen processing and presentation to major histocompatibility complex class I molecule-restricted T lymphocytes. Adv Immunol 1992;52:1–123.

359. Yoffe B, Burns DK, Bhatt HS, Combes B. Extrahepatic hepatitis B virus DNA sequences in patients with acute hepatitis B infection. Hepatology 1990;12:187–192.

360. Yokota J, Wada M, Shimosato Y, Terada M, Sugimura T. Loss of heterozygosity on chromosomes 3, 13 and 17 in small-cell carcinoma and chromosome 3 in adenocarcinoma of the lung. Proc Natl Acad Sci U S A 1987;84:9252–9256.

361. Yokota T, Konno K, Chonan E, et al. Comparative activities of several nucleoside analogs against duck hepatitis B virus in vitro. Antimicrob Agents Chemother 1990;34:1326–1330.

362. Yuki N, Hayashi N, Kasahara A, et al. Detection of antibodies against the polymerase gene product in hepatitis B virus infection. Hepatology 1990;12:193–198.

363. Zhang P, Raney AK, McLachlan A. Characterization of functional Sp1 transcription factor binding sites in the hepatitis B virus nucleocapsid promoter. J Virol 1993;67:1472–1481.

364. Zhang W, Young ACM, Imarai M, Nathenson SG, Sacchettini JC. Crystal structure of the major histocompatibility complex class I H-2K^b molecule containing a single viral peptide: implications for peptide binding and T cell receptor recognition. Proc Natl Acad Sci U S A 1992;89:8403–8408.

365. Zhang XK, Huang DP, Chiu DK, Chiu JF. The expression of oncogenes in human developing liver and hepatomas. Biochem Biophys Res Commun 1987;142:932–938.

366. Zhou DX, Taraboulos A, Ou JH, Yen TSB. Activation of class I major histocompatibility complex gene expression by hepatitis B virus. J Virol 1990;64:4025–4028.

367. Zhou S, Standring DN. Production of hepatitis B virus nucleocapsidlike core particles in *Xenopus* oocytes: assembly occurs mainly in the cytoplasm and does not require the nucleus. J Virol 1991;65: 5457–5464.

368. Zhou S, Standring DN. Hepatitis B virus capsid particles are assembled from core-protein dimer precursors. Proc Natl Acad Sci U S A 1992;89:10046–10050.

369. Zhou S, Yang SQ, Standring DN. Characterization of hepatitis B virus capsid particle assembly in *Xenopus* oocytes. J Virol 1992;66: 3086–3092.

370. Zoulim F, Saputelli J, Seeger C. Woodchuck hepatitis virus X protein is required for viral infection in vivo. J Virol 1994;68: 2026–2030.

Viral Pathogenesis,
edited by Neal Nathanson, et al.
Lippincott–Raven Publishers, Philadelphia © 1997

CHAPTER 32

Viral Hemorrhagic Fevers

Clarence J. Peters

INTRODUCTION

A number of viral infections of humans are regularly associated with a syndrome that is described as viral hemorrhagic fever (HF). These viruses are all zoonotic and generally circulate in nature without involving humans. Usually, they are maintained as chronic rodent infections or in arthropod-vertebrate-arthropod cycles (Table 32-1). The rodent infections induced by arenaviruses are often associated with prolonged or lifelong viremia and vertical transmission.[26] In contrast, Hantaviruses are thought to produce chronic rodent infections involving only brief viremia but long-term shedding of virus from mucosal surfaces into respiratory secretions, urine, saliva, and feces.[104] Arthropod-borne viruses usually induce chronic infections in the arthropod host. In some cases, such as Rift Valley fever virus, there is thought to be an important element of vertical transmission in the arthropod vector, but in others there is a low level of vertical transmission that cannot perpetuate the virus but may serve as a fail-safe mechanism. The persistence of HF viruses in the natural environment is

therefore usually a consequence of a persistent infection in one of the reservoir hosts and may also involve a special mechanism for intergenerational transmission, operative in each generation or perhaps only as a backup.[151] There are interesting contrasts between the pathogenesis in reservoir hosts and that in the human disease target; pathogenesis in arthropods is discussed in Chapter 14 and in one representative rodent arenavirus infection in Chapter 25.

The pathogenesis of most of these infections is poorly understood for several reasons. The diseases share one or more epidemiologic characteristics that compromise our ability to study them: occurrence in areas with little modern infrastructure, sporadic and unpredictable timing, and poor surveillance. Animal models, particularly nonhuman primates and guinea pigs, have proved useful in several of the diseases. For these viruses, the mouse is a poor surrogate, and the many immunologic and genetic approaches available in the murine system cannot be brought to bear on realistic models of the human disease. Finally, most of the viruses require special containment for safe research, and the funding for research on diseases such as these, with their major impact outside North America and Europe, is low.

The data presented here point to an additional complication in the study of these diseases. The actual pathophysiology is complex, and the mechanisms of disease fall within the realm

C. J. Peters: Special Pathogens Branch, Division of Viral and Rickettsial Diseases, Centers for Disease Control and Prevention, Atlanta, Georgia 30333.

TABLE 32-1. *Viruses associated with the hemorrhagic fever (HF) syndrome and their diseases*

Virus	Disease name	Geographic range	Maintenance	Perpetuation in reservoir(s)
ARENAVIRIDAE				
Junin	Argentine HF	Argentine pampas	Horizontal and vertical transmission in a field rodent, *Calomys musculinus*	Chronic virus shedding, sometimes with chronic viremia
Machupo	Bolivian HF	Bolivia, Beni Province	Horizontal and vertical transmission in a field rodent, *Calomys callosus*	Chronic virus shedding, sometimes with chronic viremia
Guanarito	Venezuelan HF	Venezuela, Portuguesa State	Chronic infection of field rodent *Zygodontomys brevicauda*	Chronic virus shedding, sometimes with prolonged or chronic viremia
Sabia	?	? rural area near Sao Paulo, Brazil	Presumably chronic infection of unidentified rodents	?
Lassa	Lassa fever	West Africa	Chronic infection of rodents of the genus *Mastomys*; vertical transmission	Chronic virus shedding and chronic viremia
BUNYAVIRIDAE				
Rift Valley fever	Rift Valley fever	Sub-Saharan Africa	Vertical infection of flood-water *Aedes* mosquitoes; unknown amount of amplification by infected vertebrates. Other mosquito species become infected by viremic vertebrates, particularly during epidemics.	Chronic infection of mosquito, including transovarial transmission in specific *Aedes* reservoir species. Transient viremic infection of vertebrate amplifier.
Crimean-Congo HF	Crimean-Congo HF	Africa, Middle East, Balkans, southern countries of the former Soviet Union, western China	Tick-mammal-tick infection; vertical infection occurs in ticks.	Ticks chronically infected; infection survives stages of maturation of tick. Transient viremic infection of vertebrate amplifier.
Hantaan, Seoul, Puumala, and others	Hemorrhagic fever with renal syndrome (HFRS)	Worldwide, depending on rodent reservoir	Horizontal infection in a single rodent genus or species	Rodents are chronically infected and shed virus on mucosal surfaces but are not thought to be chronically viremic
Sin Nombre, Black Creek Canal, and others	Hantavirus pulmonary syndrome (HPS)	Americas	As for viruses causing HFRS	Unknown; possibly as for viruses causing HFRS
FILOVIRIDAE				
Marburg, Ebola	Filovirus HF	Africa, ?Philippines	Unknown	Unknown
FLAVIVIRIDAE				
Yellow fever	Yellow fever	Africa, South America	Mosquito-primate-mosquito	Chronic infection of mosquito. Transient viremia in vertebrate.
Dengue	Dengue hemorrhagic fever, dengue shock syndrome (DHF/DSS)	Tropics and subtropics worldwide	Mosquito-primate-mosquito	Chronic infection of mosquito. Transient viremia in vertebrate. Human is overwhelmingly the most important primate involved.
Kyasanur forest disease (KFD)	KFD	Limited area of Mysore State, India	Tick-vertebrate-tick	Chronic infection of tick surviving maturation through stages. Transient viremia in vertebrate.
Omsk hemorrhagic fever (OHF)	OHF	Western Siberia	Poorly understood cycle involving ticks, voles, muskrats, and possibly waterborne transmission	Needs further study

of cytokine and lipid mediator research. These are areas of rapid progress and considerable controversy, so that causal inferences increasingly require interactions among the disciplines of virology, cell biology, immunology, and pathophysiology.

THE DISEASES AND THE VIRUSES

Clinical Characteristics

The HFs are acute febrile diseases that begin with a prodromal phase which is usually characterized by combinations of myalgia, prostration, dizziness, and mild vascular abnormalities seen as flushing or conjunctival injection. As the disease progresses, evidence of increased vascular permeability becomes more marked, with proteinuria and nondependent edema such as periorbital edema; in some diseases, prominent lumbar pain occurs and is correlated with the appearance of retroperitoneal edema. Manifestations of vascular damage are also present in the form of petechiae, and, in severe cases, there is progression to ecchymoses and frank hemorrhage from mucous membranes. Lowering of blood pressure also is seen commonly; in severe cases, hypotension culminates in shock. Shock is the most common cause identified for fatal outcome, although hemorrhage and central nervous system involvement are often prominent in fatal cases. The hemodynamic alterations are in excess of what can be accounted for by fluid shifts or blood loss and are poorly understood.

There are also a number of accompanying signs and symptoms suggesting multisystem involvement. Participation of the lung in the disease process is commonly manifested through a tendency toward development of pulmonary edema after administration of intravenous fluid and the appearance of occasional infiltrates that could represent direct viral involvement, localized pulmonary edema, or secondary infection; Hantavirus pulmonary syndrome (HPS) is the exception in this case (see later discussion). Abdominal pain, nausea and vomiting, diarrhea, and, at times, constipation are common indications of gastrointestinal tract involvement. Proteinuria, mild azotemia, and urinary sediment abnormalities are found, but significant renal failure out of proportion to the degree of cardiovascular compromise is not usual, except in hemorrhagic fever with renal syndrome (HFRS) or the terminal stages of yellow fever. Abnormalities of serum enzymes are present, although they vary by disease, and the level of aspartate aminotransferase (AST) is usually high in proportion to that of alanine aminotransferase (ALT), suggesting nonhepatic origin in many cases.

Severe cases usually have a prominent neurologic component, often with confusion, stupor, coma, and convulsions. It is unknown whether these findings are a direct viral effect, because confounding metabolic problems occur.[29] However, some patients with Argentine HF have a purely neurologic picture. This and the presence of glial nodules and perivascular cuffing in Marburg disease autopsies leaves little doubt that there is direct involvement in these two diseases, and clinical judgment favors it in other HFs as well.[91,177,178] Three of the HF viruses (those causing Rift Valley fever, Omsk HF, and Kyasanur Forest disease) are clearly associated with viral encephalitis, which occurs independently of or after the HF syndrome.

Some of the clinical characteristics have been summarized in Table 32-2. In spite of the similarities among the disease syndromes, there are significant differences in the pace of the disease (incubation and time course), in the case-infection ratio, and in some of the typical clinical findings. It would be difficult or impossible to distinguish a given patient's disease, but when groups of patients and their epidemiologic characteristics are taken into account, the different HFs are distinctive.

Pathologic Features

Pathologic features vary by disease syndrome, but one frequent characteristic is the lack of anatomic lesions sufficiently severe to explain the demise of the human or animal host. This is particularly true for the arenaviruses.[190] In several of the diseases, particularly those caused by arenaviruses and filoviruses, inflammatory cells are not seen in lesions. In most HFs, the pathologic and clinical findings suggest that the microvasculature is the focus of the problem; large-vessel lesions are not usually seen, and massive hemorrhage is not usually the root cause of serious clinical difficulties. In many respects, the viral HFs resemble the rickettsial diseases such as Rocky Mountain spotted fever, which have extensive endothelial involvement.

Characteristics of the Viruses

The viruses as well as the diseases share several characteristics. They are all single-stranded RNA viruses with a relatively small genome (less than 5×10^6 D) and a lipid envelope. All except dengue have been associated with airborne infections by small-particle aerosols, particularly in the laboratory setting. This is not unexpected in the case of rodent-borne viruses, which are thought to spread to humans largely by the airborne route and which may even be transmitted among their natural reservoir hosts by aerosols at times, but it is somewhat surprising for viruses such as yellow fever or Rift Valley fever, which are strongly associated with arthropod transmission in their natural cycle and in their spread to humans. Of the zoonotic RNA viruses not associated with HF, a smaller proportion are also clearly aerosol-infectious (e.g., Venezuelan equine encephalitis virus).

There are also differences among the viruses. The differences in replicative strategies of the four families represented are well known, and some of their other properties particularly relevant to this discussion are summarized in Table 32-3. Their abilities to induce a cytopathic effect, respond to interferon (IFN), or interact with the immune system are clearly different and greatly influence the pathogenesis of the diseases` they cause.

PATTERNS OF PATHOGENESIS

Endothelial Infection and Damage

The endothelium of the capillary bed is the largest surface area exposed to blood and plays a critical role in maintaining

TABLE 32-2. *Clinical characteristics of the hemorragic fevers (HF)**

Disease	Typical incubation (days)	Typical time to death or improvement (days)	Case:infection ratio	Case mortality (%)	Characteristic features
ARENAVIRIDAE					
South American HF (Junin, Machupo, Guanarito, and Sabia viruses)	10–14	10–14	Most infections (>50%) probably result in disease	15% to 30%	Patients typically have hypotension, shock, obvious bleeding, and neurologic symptoms such as dysarthria and intention tremor. Some have virtually pure neurologic syndrome.
Lassa fever	10–14	10–14	Unknown. Some studies suggest most infections result in mild febrile illness	15%	Severe prostration and shock; not associated with such florid hemorrhagic or neurologic manifestations as the South American HF except in severe cases. Less thrombocytopenia. Deafness a sequela in 20%.
BUNYAVIRIDAE					
Rift Valley Fever HF	2–4	3–7	Only small proportion of infections result in HF (1%)	High (50%)	Severe disease associated with bleeding, shock, anuria, icterus. Encephalitis and retinal vasculitis also occur, but there is no particular overlap with HF syndrome.
Crimean-Congo	3–6	7–10	Estimates vary, 20% to 100% virus strain differences?	15% to 30%	Most severe bleeding and ecchymoses of all the HF.
HF with renal syndrome	14–21	5–14	High (>3/4) for Hantaan and low for Puumala (5%)	5% to 15% for Hantaan, <1% for Puumala	Bleeding during febrile prodrome and subsequent shock and renal failure. Puumala infections similar course but much milder
Hantavirus pulmonary syndrome	14–21	5–10	Very high	40–50 for Sin Nombre virus	Febrile prodrome followed by acute pulmonary edema and shock
FILOVIRIDAE					
Filovirus HF	5–7	7–9	Probably high	25% for Marburg. 50% to 90% for Sudan and Zaire subtypes of Ebola. 0/4 for Reston subtype of Ebola	Most severe of the HF. Marked weight loss and prostration. Maculopapular rash common. Patients have had late sequelae (hepatitis, uveitis, orchitis) often with virus isolation from biopsy or aspiration.
FLAVIVIRIDAE					
Yellow fever	3–6	7–10	Estimates vary with epidemic	20%	Acute febrile period. Defervesence accompanied in severe cases by jaundice, renal failure
Dengue HF with dengue shock syndrome (DHF/DSS)	Unknown (dengue fever commonly 5–6)	4–7	Varies with virus and host immune status. One estimate: .007% of nonimmune and 1% of heterologous immune.	Varies with surveillance and epidemic; probably <1%.	High fever for 3–5 days, then shock lasting 1–2 days. DHF is not equated to DSS. DSS is the most dangerous manifestation and is caused by an acute vascular leak.
Kyasanur forest disease and Omsk HF	3–7	10–12	Variable	0.5–9%	Typical biphasic disease with a febrile or hemorrhagic period often followed by central nervous system involvement. Similar to tickborne encephalitis except hemorrhagic manifestations are not characteristic of first phase of tickborne encephalitis.

*These data are the best available estimates and are intended to provide an overall impression and not a detailed examination of the diseases.

TABLE 32-3. *Some properties of the viruses and the primate immune response*

Virus	Cytopathic effect*	Antiviral effects†	Neutralization by convalescent serum in vitro‡	Timing of antibody response§	Speculative role of cell-mediated immunity
ARENAVIRIDAE					
Junin, Machupo	+/-	Low	++	Recovery	Important adjunct
Lassa	+/-	Low	+	Positive fluorescent antibody and ELISA results often appear early in disease without evident clinical or virologic improvement; neutralization only found weeks after recovery	Determining
BUNYAVIRIDAE					
Rift Valley fever	+++	High	+++	Recovery	Minor; neutralizing antibody dominates
Crimean-Congo hemorrhagic fever	+	High	++	Recovery	?
Hantaan	+/-	High	+++	Onset of disease	Probably important; immunopathology suspected for cellular and humoral responses
Sin Nombre	+/-	?	+++	Onset of disease	Probably important; immunopathology suspected
FILOVIRIDAE					
Marburg, Ebola	+/-, ++	Low	+/-	Recovery	Determining? Early convalescent, antibody nonneutralizing in vitro, nonprotective in passive transfer to animals
FLAVIVIRIDAE					
Yellow fever	++	High	+++	After fever, onset of "intoxication"	Minor
Dengue	+	High	+++	Homologous: recovery; preexisting heterologous implicated in dengue shock syndrome	Deleterious in disease induction; important adjunct in recovery.

*An arbitrary scale in which +/- indicates that most strains produce inconstant and only modest visible cytopathic effect in most mammalian cells, although viruses may interfere with luxury functions and produce plaques under agar overlay with neutral red; +++ indicates that most strains result in complete cell sheet destruction in most mammalian cells tested.

†Sensitivity to the antiviral effects of interferon-α or -α/β mixtures in typical in vitro assays. Low indicates less than 50% inhibition by 100's of units and high indicates inhibition by 10's or fewer units. Junin virus is sensitive to the antiviral effects of gamma interferon-γ in vitro.

‡An arbitrary scale in which +/- indicates that it is difficult to demonstrate neutralization in vitro under any circumstances. + indicates that fresh serum, adequate complement, and low dilutions of serum are needed to show neutralization best expressed as a log neutralization index. +++ indicates that serum dilution neutralization titers of >500 are readily shown with heated serum in the absence of complement.

§Recovery refers to onset of improvement in the patients' signs and symptoms of disease.

the integrity of the vascular compartment as well as the liquid, noncoagulated state of the blood. The endothelial monolayer is anticoagulant through its electrically charged, nonwetting surface. The tendency to thrombosis is regulated through several mechanisms, including the opposing physiologic activities of thrombomodulin and prostacyclin. Endothelial coverage of the basement membrane prevents contact and activation of platelets or the coagulation cascade by collagen or the basement membrane substrate, and healthy endothelial cells assure that the procoagulant "tissue factor" they contain does not come in contact with blood. Endothelial cells are highly reactive to cytokines and other soluble mediators and in turn can be actively secretory.[117,118]

If normal endothelium is damaged or retracts, platelets plug the opening, and the clotting cascade may also result in polymerization of fibrinogen to form a coagulum. Lesions of the endothelium may readily be restored by this means, or they may progress to hemorrhage that is worsened if thrombocytopenia limits the normal reparative reaction of the platelets. Another consequence of endothelial dysfunction or excessive procoagulant activity in blood is clotting in situ, with downstream damage to the tissues irrigated by the capillary and triggering of the cascade of disseminated intravascular coagulation (DIC).

Endothelial cells are readily infected in vitro by HF viruses and numerous other agents.[5,170,200] In vivo, Hantaviruses are unique in their marked predilection for endothelial cell infection; most infected cells are endothelial cells, and a relatively high proportion of endothelial cells are infected.[102,202,203] The potential functional significance of endothelial infection with other HF viruses is not as clear. The authors of the first published study of viral antigen distribution in HF patients remarked on the extensive infection of macrophages and the minor involvement of endothelial cells.[81] However, human and animal model studies of most HFs have identified patchy involvement of cells thought to be endothelial in nature.[4,12,31,53] The significance of the small number of infected areas is unclear, because even the scattered lesions seen in immunostained planar microscopic sections could presumably result in considerable compromise in linear tubular structures such as capillaries. There has been no three-dimensional quantitative assessment of such lesions and their possible impact.

Infection of endothelial cells could lead directly to altered properties with respect to coagulation and platelets, but this has not been studied sufficiently to permit any conclusions. These infected sites are also candidate causes for the increase in vascular permeability and for the petechial hemorrhages seen so often in skin and internal organs. However, many of these viruses are relatively noncytopathic in most cultured cells and may be so in vivo (Table 32-4). Indirect effects of viral infection on endothelium through induction of soluble mediators of inflammation may be more important than direct effects in some situations.[45,47]

The morphology of endothelial cells is not notably altered by conventional histopathologic examination, although swelling and other difficult-to-interpret changes are sometimes reported. Only in the case of the filoviruses has localized coagulation been observed in association with endothelial lesions, but there are insufficient studies in several of the HFs to dismiss this possibility.

Hemorrhage

One of the hallmarks of these diseases is the presence of a hemorrhagic diathesis, although the degree of hemorrhage is not usually marked in Lassa fever and even less so in HPS. The pathogenesis of hemorrhage differs in the different diseases. One of the most important considerations is the presence or absence of DIC as a mechanism. This process leads to multiple microscopic areas of hypoxemic tissue damage as a result of occlusion of small vessels; however, these fibrin clots are often taken up by fibrinolysis, leaving no histologic trace of their presence. The consumption of clotting factors, generation of fibrin split products, and activation of fibrinolysis in turn lead to a systemic hypocoagulable state. Activation of factor XII also has the potential to activate complement and kinin pathways. In this situation, there are falling levels of factor XII, decreases of other intrinsic pathway factors, and appearance of vasoactive kinins and complement components.[107] Platelets are trapped and destroyed in the fibrin webs in capillaries, and the multiple microscopic clots are lysed by the usual mechanisms, leading to the circulation of their degradation products, which are a source of diagnostic information and also have anticoagulant properties.

Well-founded criteria have evolved for the diagnosis of DIC in general medical conditions by means of clinical findings and commonly available laboratory test results. The usual requirements for implicating DIC are prolonged prothrombin time, thrombocytopenia, hypofibrinogenemia, and evidence of fibrinolysis (e.g., demonstration of circulating fibrin split products).[30,163] Even with these guidelines, however, it is difficult to assess the presence of DIC in the HFs. The diseases are often accompanied by variable degrees of hepatic damage and liver hypoxia from shock, resulting in decreased synthesis of some clotting factors and retarded clearance of fibrin split products. Cytokines can induce either increases or decreases in synthesis of clotting factors, pentraxins, and other proteins by hepatocytes, macrophages, and endothelial cells.[51,117] Finally, the increase in vascular permeability can result in extravasation of proteins such as coagulation factors without any change in their synthetic or catabolic rates.[195] The level of thrombocytes is also potentially affected by multiple factors during the course of the disease, including direct viral infection of megakaryocytes, induction of mediator molecules affecting platelet production, virus-platelet interactions, and even the effects of the antiviral drug ribavirin in increasing platelet production.

As an example of the type of predisposing vascular lesion that may occur, endothelial monolayers may contract under the influence of thrombin, tumor necrosis factor-alpha (TNF-α),[22] complement component C5b67,[164] infected macrophage supernatants,[47] or other stimuli to leave gaps in the cell sheet; a gap could serve as a nidus for hemorrhage or microvascular coagulation. Some of these stimuli also result in other potentially deleterious changes in endothelial cells, including induction of procoagulant activity, secretion of cytokines, and recruitment of leukocytes through expression of adhesion molecules.[118]

One of the most dramatic experimental models of viral-induced hemorrhage has been described only in murine hepatitis virus infection and has not been adequately explored in the HFs. In genetically susceptible mouse strains, infection

TABLE 32-4. *Pathogenetic features of the hemorrhagic fevers (HFs)*

Disease	Genesis of hemorrhage	Pathogenetic findings	Virologic findings	Speculative pathogenesis
ARENAVIRIDAE				
South American HFs	Thrombocytopenia, vascular damage	Very high interferon-α Elevated TNF-α. No activation C, no significant immune compexes. CD8 and to greater extent CD4 lymphocytes decreased	Viremic during acute illness. Disappearance of viremia and appearance of N and indirect fluorescent antibody antibodies coincide with improvement	Induction of mediators of inflammation and shock has important role in pathophysiology, perhaps coupled with direct viral effects. Recovery by humoral and cellular immunity
Lassa fever	Platelet dysfunction, vascular damage	Lymphopenia	Viremic during acute illness. Indirect fluorescent antibodies appear early with no effect on disease course. Disappearance of viremia coincides with clinical improvement. N antibodies late and inefficient	Probably similar to South American HFs, but virus less neuroinvasive and there is less thrombocytopenia. Recovery is virtually exclusively a result of cellular immunity.
BUNYAVIRIDAE				
Rift Valley fever	Viral damage and DIC in model primate model	Early interferon response important in determining outcome in primate model	Viremic during acute illness. Disappearance of viremia coincides with improvement and appearance of N antibodies	Cytopathic virus attacks endothelium with induction of DIC unless early interferon response protects endothelium. Recovery largely by N antibody response.
Crimean-Congo HF	DIC		Viremic during acute illness	
HFRS	DIC	Kinin and C activation well documented. Extensive endothelial involvement by virus in experimental rodent models. Immune complexes found by nonspecific tests but not characterized.	Virus difficult to isolate from acute patient sera. Disease occurs at a time when indirect fluorescent antibody, N, and ELISA responses are rising and there are numerous circulating DR + CD8 + cells in blood	DIC, complement activation, bradykinin, and perhaps other mediators cause vascular damage and instability with shock and local hemodynamic factors leading to renal failure. Endothelium extensively infected. Probably an important immunopathologic component
HPS	Usually no hemorrhage. DIC in severe cases	Pulmonary endothelium extensively involved by viral antigen and both T cells and activated macrophages present in lung interstitum. Less antigen and virtually no lymphoid infiltrates at other sites in body.	Virus difficult to isolate from patient sera, although viral genetic sequences present for several days after onset. Disease occurs at a time when Indirect fluorescent antibody and ELISA responses are rising and there are numerous circulating DR + CD8 + cells in blood.	Immune T cells infiltrate the lung where capillary infection is extensive; T-cell products result in acute pulmonary edema directly or through the secretions of activated macrophages, lymphocytes, or endothelial cells. Cause of shock unknown.
FILOVIRIDAE				
Filovirus HF	Viral damage, ?DIC	Extensive involvement of macrophages and endothelial cells (depending on virus strain)	Virus readily isolated from blood and usually no sign of effective immune response in fatal infections.	Direct and indirect viral damage to endothelium and extensive liberation of macrophage products. Direct viral cytopathology.
FLAVIVIRIDAE				
Yellow fever	Hepatic failure, DIC doubtful	Initial infection of Kupfer cells and later extensive hepatic involvement with accompanying B-cell necrosis in speen. Acute tubular necrosis also common.	Viremic during first 4 days illness or "febrile period." Antibodies detectable subsequently, the "period of intoxication"	Acute viremic illness directly inflicts damage on liver and other organs. In severe cases subsequent hepatorenal syndrome and other physiologic derangements produce disease and death.
Dengue hemorrhagic fever, dengue shock syndrome	Vascular damage, thrombocyto-penia, local factors	Macrophage is overwhelmingly the most important target cell. The syndrome is largely caused by increased vascular permeability with albumin leak, hemoconcentration, shock.	Most cases are "secondary" in that prior infection with another serotype of dengue has occured previously. High-titered, broadly-reactive antibodies and crossreactive T lymphocytes present at onset of DSS. Virus difficult to isolate from acute sera or organs unless mosquito inoculation is used.	Antibody-induced enhancement of macrophage infection leads to more extensive viremia. Viremia and secondary antibody response activate C system. Cross-primed T cells secrete interferon-γ, enhancing Fc receptor expression, which further enhances infection. T cells (particularly CD8 +) responsible produce multiple mediators of shock through secretion and interactions with infected macrophages.

DIC, disseminated intravascular coagulation; ELISA, enzyme-linked immunosorbent assay.

with this coronavirus leads to T lymphocyte–dependent microcirculatory thrombosis and resultant hepatic necrosis. The key event is induction of procoagulant activity or tissue factor in mononuclear cells.[105]

Among the arenavirus infections, there is clear evidence that DIC is not an important component, based on detailed studies in human Argentine HF,[37,124] clinical data from Lassa fever patients, and data from most animal models.[120,149] Argentine HF shows only minor abnormalities in clotting factors that indicate limited activation of the coagulation pathway and also an increase in fibrinolysis.[69] Hemorrhage must be attributed to some form of vascular damage aggravated by thrombocytopenia.

Diminished platelet activity is a major correlate of bleeding in the arenavirus HFs, as evidenced by the very common presence of hemorrhage in the South American HFs, with their characteristic thrombocytopenia,[9] but the appearance of hemorrhage only in the most severely ill Lassa fever patients.[120]

Thrombocytopenia may not be the only important platelet-related defect. Platelets normally aggregate in response to stimuli such as collagen or epinephrine, but this function is diminished in Lassa fever,[34,48] Argentine HF,[36] HFRS,[142] and dengue hemorrhagic fever with dengue shock syndrome (DHF/DSS),[180] as well as in nonhuman primate models of Lassa fever, Bolivian HF, and yellow fever (P. B. Jahrling, T. M. Cosgriff, C. J. Peters, unpublished observations, 1988.

In human Lassa fever, marked loss of platelet aggregation is associated with severe disease and clinical evidence of bleeding.[34] However, even the most seriously affected Lassa fever patients usually have only modestly decreased platelet counts. Lassa patients with abnormal aggregation also have a plasma inhibitor that inhibits platelet aggregation if it is incubated with normal platelets in vitro.[34] One candidate to mediate the loss of platelet function in some of the HFs is nitric oxide. This compound is a common mediator of disease, can be synthesized in platelets and other cells, is inducible by cytokines in macrophages and vascular endothelium, and blocks platelet aggregation.[160]

In other HFs, DIC does appear to play an important role. In Marburg disease, for example, clinical laboratory data strongly suggest the presence of DIC early in the course and persisting throughout the clinical episode.[52,119] Pathology studies often demonstrate endothelial lesions, and direct viral infection of endothelium can be shown by both electron microscopy and immunohistochemistry, particularly in nonhuman primates infected with the Reston and Zaire subtypes of Ebola virus.[12,53,76,132,134] Intravascular clotting is seen as well, and it is particularly frequent in necropsy tissues from macaques infected with the Sudan subtype of Ebola virus.

There are no coagulation data from human Rift Valley fever, but in primate models of Rift Valley fever there is extensive DIC.[32,150] Satisfactory studies of viral antigens in monkey tissues to demonstrate endothelial infection have not been performed, but there is extensive involvement of endothelium in the rat model.[4] It has been speculated that the highly cytopathic nature of the Rift Valley fever virus-cell interaction leads to endothelial damage and DIC, amplifying the direct virus-induced necrotic damage present in infected parenchymal cells of the liver and other organs.[152]

Coagulation tests in human Crimean-Congo HF also suggest that DIC is a regular feature of the disease and appears early.[80,181] DIC has been suggested as the basis for vascular damage in yellow fever, but the presence of severe liver damage complicates the interpretation of the data (T. M. Cosgriff, personal communication), and this must be regarded as an open question.

Shock

Severe HF is always associated with circulatory shock, yet the pathophysiology is not well understood. In general, inadequate perfusion of the tissues of the body can be attributed to several mechanisms: failure of the heart as a pump, improper regulation of flow resistance and capacitance in the vascular tree, or inadequate circulating volume in the vascular system. Even in well-studied conditions, such as hemorrhagic or septic shock, the underlying mechanisms for the intractable progression are not well understood.[14,15,143]

No anatomic lesion of the heart has been found to explain shock in the HF syndrome. Many patients dying of HF have electrocardiographic abnormalities as well as the same nonspecific changes in the myocardium that are often found in terminal shock from many causes; nevertheless, there is usually no evidence for direct viral invasion of the heart muscle or viral myocarditis. In Junin and Machupo virus infections of nonhuman primates, lesions of the autonomic nervous system are present and could be relevant to the vascular collapse seen in these diseases; such lesions have not been described in humans.[149] Diminished circulating blood volume, secondary to leakage of plasma because of increased vascular permeability, may contribute to circulatory embarrassment but is not the sole cause.[14]

It has been asserted that "viral shock" is essentially the same as septic shock or the sepsis syndrome. For example, physiologic observations in immunosuppressed leukemic or posttransplantation patients with cytomegaloviremia showed a pattern of high cardiac output and low systemic vascular resistance,[38,139] resembling to some extent the pattern seen in bacterial sepsis.[15,143] However, measurements of cardiovascular variables of HFRS patients in Korea found low cardiac output and high systemic vascular resistance throughout the hypotensive phase of illness,[43] a pattern similar to that seen in HPS in North America.[39,63] DHF/DSS patients also have a similar pattern.[156] A single hypotensive patient with Crimean-Congo HF was studied and was found to have a high cardiac output and low systemic vascular resistance with a falling cardiac output as the disease progressed.[187] There is a considerable need for further exploration of this aspect of the pathogenesis of human HF, but the observed patterns suggest significant functional differences compared with patients with bacterial sepsis.

Because Pichinde virus, an arenavirus from Colombia that is not pathogenic for humans, can be adapted to infect inbred strain 13 guinea pigs with a virologic[77,77a] and pathologic picture[7,31,77a,149] that resembles human Lassa fever, potentially relevant physiologic observations have been made in that animal model. The guinea pig appears normal for approximately 7 days after infection, after which fever and weight loss begin. During this period, viremia becomes detectable and most of the infected cells are macrophages. As the viremia progresses, macrophage infection becomes more abundant, and epithelial cells of several organs begin to show viral antigen. However, only a few dramatic histologic lesions are seen: focal necrosis in liver and adrenal, mild interstitial pneumonitis in the lung, marginal zone necrosis in the splenic white pulp, and an unusual intestinal lesion with villus blunting. Immunohistochemistry shows that the degree of infection in the liver and adrenal is far more extensive than the mild areas of inflammation and focal necrosis visualized histologically. Exhaustive studies of the heart fail to detect viral antigen or viral titers suggesting myocardial infection.

In contrast to the relatively modest pathologic lesions at the light microscopic level in Pichinde-infected guinea pigs, there are extensive physiologic changes in the cardiovascular system which lead to the death of the animal. There is a progressive decrease in cardiac index (volume of blood pumped each minute normalized to the body surface area) by about 50%. This is compensated by a rise in the systemic vascular resistance, which maintains the blood pressure until the last stages of infection, at about day 14 to 18.[157] The fall in cardiac index is probably caused by the action of mediators such as leukotrienes,[114] platelet activating factor,[158,159] or β-endorphins[62] that are present in the guinea pig model and are known to decrease cardiac function in other systems. Both TNF-α and interleukin-6 (IL-6) are also produced by macrophages from these infected guinea pigs.[7,8] Furthermore, central and peripheral nervous system abnormalities are seen in the levels of vasoactive amines, such as catecholamines, dopamine, and serotonin,[62,62a] and in patterns of atrial natriuretic peptide.[61]

The mechanism by which these several potent physiologic regulators are increased in the Pichinde-infected guinea pig is not known, in part because of the many positive and negative signals interchanged among these molecules, both in their secretion and in their final activities.[15] The finding of increased concentrations of multiple molecular messengers known to have deleterious effects in sepsis cannot be fortuitous; of the nine mediators strongly associated with shock in human sepsis, five are known to be activated in the Pichinde-infected guinea pig.[134]

We can speculate how one particular pathway could function, using TNF-α and leukotrienes as an example. TNF-α is detected in the plasma early after infection of the strain 13 guinea pig,[8] and it, in turn, can induce IL-1.[188] These two cytokines can readily account for the fever, weight loss, and inappetence that are seen.[149] TNF-α itself has many effects potentially contributory to the HF syndrome; it can increase endothelial cell permeability, enhance tissue factor and other procoagulant functions, upregulate vascular adhesion molecules, activate macrophages, alter prostaglandin synthesis, and lead to many more direct and indirect effects.[22,46,117,118,188] TNF-α functions as a direct cardiodepressant by uncoupling the β-adrenergic receptor stimulation of myocardial contractility.[103] In addition, TNF-α induces the secretion of sulfidopeptide leukotrienes,[33,72] which produce potent coronary vasoconstriction and myocardial depression[49,155] with both decreased cardiac output and increased systemic vascular resistance after their acute infusion. Abnormal amounts of these leukotrienes are present in the blood of the Pichinde-infected guinea pig by both bioassay and radioimmunoassay.[114] Furthermore, treatment of guinea pigs with FPL-55712, a leukotriene antagonist, prolonged survival from 14 days to between 18 and 21 days, with an associated slowing of weight loss.[149] Intravenous infusion of the same drug in acute experiments improved the decreased cardiac output.[115] TNF-α also increases secretion of platelet activating factor, perhaps through

IL-1,[20,117] and this cardiodepressant lipid mediator is present in increased concentration in the Pichinde-infected guinea pig.[158,159] Although hemorrhage is not a prominent feature in this model, it is potentially important that TNF-α induces procoagulant activity in endothelial cell cultures.[13]

The mechanisms by which these various mediators are induced in Pichinde-infected guinea pigs are unknown. The fact that immunosuppression fails to ameliorate fatal guinea pig infection with the related arenavirus Junin, along with the lack of cellular infiltrates such as are found in the brain in the lymphocytic choriomeningitis virus (LCMV) immunopathologic meningitis model or in the lung of humans with fatal HPS, suggests that the immune system may not be a major participant.

Significant pulmonary functional compromise is present in the Pichinde-infected guinea pig, as well. There is increased airways resistance, particularly late in disease and in younger animals.[60,157,167,168] Although mild pulmonary edema is present, decreased ventilation is primarily attributable to accumulation of lymphocytes in association with infected macrophages or bronchial epithelium in or near small bronchi[168] and could be an important element in the final collapse of the animal.

Clinical observations of nondependent edema and serous effusions suggest that there are generalized increases in capillary permeability leading to extravasation of fluid and decrease in circulating blood volume in arenaviral and other HFs, but measurements of capillary permeability in the Pichinde-infected strain 13 guinea pig have not given clearcut results. The response to fluid infusion mirrors the expectations from observations of human disease. Administration of saline (crystalloid) results in some increase in cardiac output but rapidly brings on pulmonary edema and death; volume expansion with a higher-molecular-weight solute such as albumin (colloid) improves cardiac output and does not precipitate pulmonary edema so rapidly.[149] However, permeability (measured by the escape of albumin from the circulation) has repeatedly been found to be normal, except for measurements very late in experimental infections. Studies of local fluxes have shown that abnormalities in effective pore size are present in some vascular beds but are masked by other processes such as dehydration.[82,83] Individual organ measurements have shown only modest increases.[82,157,167,168]

The findings of florid activation of both cytokine and lipid mediators in the Pichinde-infected guinea pig in the absence of obvious morphologic causes for the physiologic findings strongly suggest that these mediators are the cause of the derangements, both in the model and probably in human arenavirus diseases. However, as in the septic shock syndrome,[15,134] it is not yet possible to trace the interrelations of the different interlocking sequences of induction and secretion or to use inhibitors to block the abnormalities. The most important single finding in the Pichinde-infected guinea pig is the presence of early myocardial dysfunction without direct viral invasion of the heart; this forces us to consider these indirect pathogenetic pathways.

To Live or Die

The substantial mortality rates in the HFs emphasize the question of why patients survive or succumb to the infection.

Although the mechanisms are not known, there are early indicators of mortality in almost all the HFs, suggesting the importance of events occurring soon after infection for survival. These prognostic factors have practical implications in evaluating treatment modalities as well as theoretic importance; they permit assurance of comparability among treatment and control groups and selective enrollment of high-risk patients, leading to smaller trials with increased power.[148]

Viremia measured at the time of clinical presentation predicts outcome in both Lassa fever[79] and Crimean-Congo HF.[172] Several clinical pathology measurements determined early in the course of disease also predict a fatal outcome in Crimean-Congo HF, yellow fever, and Lassa fever.[79,148,181]

Another common thread among infections by arenaviruses, Crimean-Congo HF virus, and filoviruses lies in the immune system. Patients who die usually have not developed a significant immune response at the time of death.[19,37,79,119,196] In the case of the arenavirus disease Argentine HF, there is a difference in the human leukocyte antigen haplotype, with an excess of the B7 haplotype when severe and mild cases are compared, but it is not clear whether this reflects a genetic difference in the immune response.[165] In all these diseases, there is prominent necrosis and fibrinoid deposition around germinal centers in the spleen and lymph nodes, a lesion that would be expected to be immunosuppressive. Indeed, in LCMV infection of the mouse, this same lesion may be important in blunting the immune response and may be a consequence of cytotoxic T lymphocyte destruction of infected antigen-presenting cells.[138]

INDIVIDUAL DISEASES

Arenaviridae

Arenaviruses cause relatively prolonged infections compared with other HF viruses such as the *Bunyaviridae,* infect macrophages extensively in humans and experimental animals, are often controlled by cellular immunity, and are relatively insensitive to the antiviral effects of IFN.[31,54,57,116,149,152] Pathologic changes at necropsy are usually slight, although there may be reticuloendothelial necrosis in some animal models.[149,190] Both in animal models and in human HF, death usually occurs in the setting of continuing viremia without an effective immune response. In contrast, arenavirus infections of the natural rodent hosts may produce lifelong infection, with macrophages being a prominent antigen-containing cell, but have minimal effect on the host.[26] Two passaged arenaviruses that became attenuated for primates also developed increased pathogenicity for their rodent reservoir host.

South American Hemorrhagic Fevers

All four of the South American arenaviruses known to cause the HF syndrome (see Table 32-1) have similar clinical pictures. Argentine HF, caused by Junin virus, has been studied in the most detail. Human infection with Junin virus induces a lymphopenia with a marked reduction in CD8+ lymphocytes, accompanied by a loss of responsiveness to mitogens and cutaneous anergy.[41,186] The very high serum IFN levels correlate with the severity of disease and contribute to

many of the clinical findings.[108] In addition, patients have high serum levels of TNF-α,[70] which is probably indicative of a more generalized increase in cytokine secretion, a leading candidate for the mechanism of disease and shock. DIC, inflammatory immune complexes, and complement activation have been excluded as important pathogenetic mechanisms.[37] Hemorrhage is very common and is thought to reflect vascular damage and thrombocytopenia with contributions from a mild coagulopathy and fibrinolysis.[69] Some viral strains cause typical hemorrhagic disease in guinea pigs or monkeys, but others produce a primarily a neurologic disease. In monkeys, the disease induced by virus innoculation correlated with type of human disease from E use?.[86,122,123]

The recovery stage usually begins at about day 10 to 12 and is accompanied by the detection of indirect fluorescent antibodies and neutralizing antibodies coincident with the disappearance of viremia.[37,41] Patients with Argentine HF rapidly develop neutralizing and cytolytic antibodies as they recover, and these antibodies are relatively complement independent, in contrast to those produced after Lassa fever.[89] These antibodies have been used therapeutically. Within 24 hours of infusion of convalescent plasma, viremia becomes undetectable, symptoms and signs of disease are markedly improved, and lymphocyte mitogen responsiveness is restored. The rapid clinical and virologic response to infusion of convalescent plasma with adequate neutralizing antibody content is convincing evidence that humoral immunity can play an important role in recovery.[42] The likelihood that cellular immunity is important as well is suggested by the fact that nonhuman primates are protected against Junin and Machupo viruses by administration of live attenuated Junin vaccine[11] even in the absence of neutralizing antibodies.

Although passive antibody treatment reduces the mortality of acute Argentine HF from between 15% and 30% to less than 1%, approximately one in ten treated survivors develops a late neurologic syndrome about 1 month later.[42,41] Abnormalities of cranial nerves, cerebellar function, and sensorium are accompanied by fever and headache. Virus has not been isolated from cerebrospinal fluid, and brain tissue has not been available for study. Nevertheless, antibody titers in cerebrospinal fluid are elevated, and the peak serum humoral response is delayed. The most likely pathogenesis is a failure to eradicate virus from the brain at the time of passive antibody administration, followed by a delayed active immune response in the central nervous system.

Observations in the guinea pig model also support the dual importance of antibodies and cellular immunity in recovery. Immunosuppression exacerbates the disease rather than sparing the animals, as is the case with the most commonly studied arenavirus model, the mouse infected intracranially with LCMV.[87] Passive antibody infusion protects the Junin virus–infected guinea pig, and there is a late neurologic syndrome in a proportion of survivors, as is observed after therapy in humans.[85]

An important in vitro correlate of survival in the guinea pig model is the development of spleen cell cytotoxicity against Junin-infected target cells. Studies with anti–T-cell monoclones, cell separation experiments, and inhibition with aggregated gammaglobulin all indicate that killing is accomplished by antibody-dependent cellular cytotoxicity and not by T-cell–mediated cytolysis.[88] In this system, cellular cytotoxicity requires both the activation of effector cells during the infection and the presence of virus-specific antibodies. Normal guinea pig spleen cells are poor effectors in the presence of exogenous antibody; spleen cells from guinea pigs infected with a lethal Junin strain can mediate cellular toxicity if antibodies are added, but they are ineffective by themselves. The role of antibody-dependent cellular cytotoxicity in recovery is similar to that of cytotoxic T lymphocytes in poorly cytopathic arenavirus infections—namely, the elimination of infected host cells. The importance of elimination of infected cells can be shown in a heterologous system in which human immunoglobulin G (IgG) but not its antigen-binding F(ab')$_2$ fragment is protective for guinea pigs in passive transfer experiments.[84] Both preparations are equally effective in neutralizing virus in vitro, but multiple infusions of the F(ab')$_2$ pool do not modify survival, mean time to death, or postmortem virus titer.

Lassa Fever

Lassa fever clinically resembles the South American HFs with a few exceptions: neurologic involvement is less common, leukopenia is not a regular feature, and thrombocytopenia is not usual.[120] The pathogenesis of neural deafness, which occurs in approximately 20% of patients with Lassa fever, is not understood.[35] Its frequent occurrence after Lassa fever supports the idea that idiopathic sudden-onset deafness, which is so common in the United States and has a similar audiologic profile, may also be viral in origin and that studies of Lassa fever patients could provide better information on therapy.[111]

The duration of viremia during Lassa fever is commonly 7 to 14 days or longer, and the level of viremia is closely correlated with the prognosis.[79] The level of AST similarly predicts the outcome; relatively low levels (e.g., 150 U/mL of serum) begin to indicate a poor prognosis, suggesting that death is not caused by extensive hepatitis.

The antibody response to Lassa virus and its significance in recovery are different from those of Junin virus and resemble what is seen with another Old World arenavirus, the phylogenetically related LCMV. During Lassa virus infection, binding antibodies detectable in fluorescent antibody and enzyme-linked immunosorbent assay (ELISA) tests may be detected within the first few days of disease but are not associated with clinical improvement.[79] Viremia disappears and clinical disease fades without the appearance of neutralizing, protective antibodies. Weeks later, antibodies that are capable of both in vitro neutralization and passive protection are detected.[74,75,78,149] Even when neutralizing antibodies do appear, they are of low titer and are highly complement dependent.[149] Formal tests in strain 13 guinea pigs show that spleen cells mediate protection in passive transfer and that protective antibodies appear only much later, in parallel with the development of in vitro neutralizing antibodies.[149]

Bunyaviridae

Rift Valley Fever

Rift Valley fever virus usually causes a 3- to 5-day undifferentiated febrile illness, but a small fraction of human infections (estimated at 1% to 2%) result in complicated illness. These more severe illnesses are characterized by one of three

different syndromes without any necessary overlap: viral HF, encephalitis, and retinal vasculitis.

Inbred rat strains also vary in their response to the virus. A benign, transient viremia develops in some rat strains; in others, encephalitis; and in still others, severe liver necrosis with vascular infection resembling viral HF.[1,3,4,154] Early determinants of the virus-host interaction are important in controlling the outcome, and IFN plays a major role. Susceptible rat strains have very high virus titers—10^7 to 10^8 plaque forming units per milliliter of serum or per gram of tissue in serum, liver, and other organs—within 24 hours of inoculation and are dead before 48 hours. Many tissues, including vascular endothelium, are infected, but death is attributable to extensive hepatic necrosis. Resistant rats carry a single mendelian dominant gene that results in a 10^6-fold higher median lethal dose and a 10^4-fold lower viremia. The independence of this genetic mechanism from the immune response can be demonstrated by cyclophosphamide immunosuppression of genetically resistant animals; their early viremia is identical to that of intact animals of the same rat strain but 10^5-fold lower than that of genetically susceptible rats. Serum virus titers of these immunosuppressed, genetically resistant rats continue to rise for about 5 days, but in intact genetically resistant rats viremia is undetectable by day 2. Immunosuppressed rats die late (day 4 to 11) with multiple organ involvement.

The primacy of antibody in recovery in the rat model can also be demonstrated by giving passive neutralizing antibody to the immunosuppressed rats in order to mimic the titers seen in active antibody synthesis. This produces a normal recovery. Both delayed-type hypersensitivity (G. A. Anderson, unpublished data) and cytolytic T lymphocytes (M. Balady, unpublished data) can be demonstrated by 7 to 10 days after infection in surviving rodents, but they appear several days after the control of virus infection. High-titered neutralizing antibodies may appear as early as 2 days after inoculation in resistant rodent species. The rapidity of the antibody response can also be seen in infected lambs, which can develop an effective neutralizing antibody response titer with rising from less than 1:10 on day 4 after infection to 1:320 24 hours later.[147]

Other studies have failed to determine the exact action of the rat resistance gene. It is not associated with rat major histocompatibility complex (MHC) haplotype, nor does it segregate with mixed lymphocyte culture (MLC) markers in F2 crossbreeding (C. J. Peters, unpublished observations, 1985). It does not affect the neutralizing antibody response to inactivated Rift Valley fever vaccine or the clearance of injected virus.[1] Pretreatment of resistant rat strains with anti-IFN globulin or administration of IFN to susceptible rat strains can mask the phenotype, but IFN responses cannot meaningfully be compared because of the widely differing stimuli to IFN production in the two strains.

If the resistance gene is isolated from the resistant Lewis rat strain on the susceptible Wistar-Furth background, the resulting congenic resistant rat strain is virtually identical to the parental Lewis strain in its response to Rift Valley fever virus.[3] Radiation bone marrow chimeras indicate that the locus of resistance or susceptibility is in the hepatocyte and not in the transplanted marrow-derived macrophages.[1] This was further supported by the differential susceptibility of isolated hepatocytes to the virus.

Only certain Rift Valley fever virus strains induce overwhelming infection in genetically susceptible rats. These strains grow to higher titers and form larger plaques in susceptible rat hepatocytes and are relatively resistant to the antiviral effects of rat IFN measured in rat cells.[2] All strains have a similar sensitivity to human IFN, and there are no correlations between IFN sensitivity and the source of the virus isolate.

The pathogenesis of Rift Valley fever in rhesus monkeys more closely resembles the situation in humans.[150] Infected animals may show only mild fever and anorexia, but many progress to more severe disease with cutaneous petechiae, hemorrhages, vomiting, and rash. About 20% of rhesus monkeys die with midzonal hepatitis and classic DIC, including microangiopathic hemolytic anemia and the presence of intravascular thrombi postmortem.[32,150] Viremia occurs within 24 hours after intravenous infection and tends to be higher and more prolonged in more severely ill animals. The best correlation with disease severity, however, is the early IFN response.[129] Seventeen macaques were infected with Rift Valley fever virus intravenously, and all became viremic. Animals with detectable serum IFN by 6 to 12 hours had an asymptomatic course; those with IFN first found at 24 hours usually had no disease or nonfatal disease, but both animals with IFN first detected in the sample taken at 30 hours died. Pretreatment of monkeys with 5×10^5 U/kg recombinant IFN-α or purified human leukocyte IFN prevents clinically apparent disease.[130] Delaying IFN treatment until 6 hours after infection or using doses as low as 5×10^3 U/kg still had marked protective effects. Human recombinant IFN-γ (104 to 106 U/kg intravenously begun the day before infection) also modulated viremia and disease, although less efficiently than IFN-α.[128] No synergism with IFN-α was detected after a suboptimal dose of 5×10^3 U/kg IFN-α was combined with 10^4 U/kg of IFN-γ.

Recovery of rhesus macaques,[131,150,152] as in other Rift Valley fever models,[40,136,146] appeared to be determined by the neutralizing antibody response. In most monkeys, there is a close correlation between the disappearance of viremia and antigenemia and the appearance of the humoral response, with antibodies usually detected by IgM capture ELISA shortly before neutralizing antibodies. A few monkeys circulate antigen (thought to be nucleocapsid) for 12 to 24 hours after development of antibodies and clearance of infectivity; an analogous phenomenon may produce the saddleback fever curve described in some humans recovering from Rift Valley fever.

Antibodies are also effective in prophylaxis; as little as 0.025 mL/kg of convalescent serum prevents viremia in subcutaneously-inoculated rhesus monkeys.[150] This amount produces no detectable passive titer in recipients, and its similarity to the quantities of IgG needed for hepatitis A protection suggests the feasibility of using Cohn fractionated immune serum globulin from endemic areas for protection of humans during epidemics.

Crimean-Congo Hemorrhagic Fever

Little is known about the pathogenesis of this disease, in part because of the lack of a realistic animal model for study. Observations on patients strongly support the presence of DIC as one of the mechanisms of disease and also establish that viremia continues throughout disease, with clinical recovery coinciding with appearance of antibodies in blood and disappearance of circulating virus.[19,80] The finding of early prognostic indicators, such as markedly abnormal serum AST or ALT and coagulation tests,[181] suggests that early limitation of virus replication before the potential onset of a virus-specific immune response is an important determinant of survival.

Hantaviruses

These viruses resemble arenaviruses in many respects; they are noncytopathic, are carried by apparently normal chronically infected rodents, and cause serious human disease with a longer than usual incubation period (2 to 3 weeks). However, in contrast to arenaviruses, in which a successful immune response and disappearance of viremia herald recovery, human Hantavirus disease appears coincident with the immune response.

Hemorrhagic Fever With Renal Syndrome

HFRS is severe and in parts of Asia is common; more than 100,000 cases occur annually in China. This disease is the most important HF in the world, challenged only by yellow fever, which is preventable by vaccination, and dengue, which can be attacked through mosquito control. The clinical picture is divided into sequential phases: fever, shock or hypotension, oliguria, and polyuria.[104] DIC, kinin activation, and complement activation all are well documented during the shock phase. Patients presenting early in their course have thrombocytopenia, evidence of platelet consumption, abnormal levels of serum fibrin degradation products, fibrinogen catabolism, and usually abnormal partial thromboplastin times, prothrombin times, bleeding times, and fibrinogen levels.[105] Increased fibrinolytic activity is also present. The overall picture is one of active DIC accompanied by modest evidence of hemorrhage. The hemorrhagic state continues after the DIC resolves, as the bleeding diathesis of uremia supervenes.

The pathogenesis of the DIC is not known. In rodent models, extensive infection of endothelium has been documented,[102] and these same cells are involved in the human disease.[102,202] The extent of infection of human endothelial cells, the functional changes of infected endothelial cells, and their relation to disease induction are still not known.

DIC in HFRS is also accompanied by other signs of activation of the factor XII–dependent intrinsic or contact pathway, particularly kinin generation.[68,163,173] It is not known whether factor XII is activated by the same process as is responsible for the DIC, particularly because these processes are dissociated in endotoxin-induced disease.[107] The resulting bradykinin is thought to contribute to the hypotension and increased vascular permeability seen during this phase of illness. Complement activation by classic pathways, and probably by alternative pathways as well, is documented.[105,197,198] One possible mechanism is the action of a factor XII fragment on C1, with subsequent activation of the classic pathway.[56] The presence of DIC is correlated with decreased C3 levels, perhaps suggesting a relation between coagulation abnormalities and complement activation.[105] Immune complexes have also been detected in serum by several tests, including C1q precipitation, platelet aggregation, and conglutinin binding.[105,145] The antigens present in the putative immune complexes measured by generic binding tests have never been determined, but in one series immune complex levels correlated with a decrease in immunochemical C3 levels.[105]

Viral antigen is found in endothelium and also in macrophages throughout the body in patients dying with acute disease,[102] and renal biopsies from recovering patients have shown antigen in tubule cells.[95] In contrast to HPS (see later discussion), there is no particular predilection for finding antigen in the target organ, the kidney,[202,203] nor are there prominent inflammatory infiltrates at sites of lesions.

The genesis of the renal failure is poorly understood, but it is probably caused by a combination of systemic shock, local renal circulatory conditions, and factors unique to HFRS. The kidney receives about one fourth of the cardiac output, but the intrarenal circulation is complicated and is regulated by mechanical, neural, and hormonal influences. In fatal HFRS, intrarenal edema is histologically visible and grossly evident as the kidney capsule is cut. The kidney, in addition to its tightly applied capsule, is constrained by the retroperitoneal fascia, which is bulging with extensive edema, further compromising renal circulation. At times, gross renal hemorrhage occurs.[112] Studies of renal function during the evolution of disease show a loss of renal plasma flow that is gradual and relatively independent of blood pressure, accompanied by a fall in glomerular filtration that is more dependent on the systemic circulation.[50,182] The renal medulla is congested and is the site of microscopic hemorrhages, particularly in the subcortical region.[177,202]

Close study of individually dissected nephrons from fatal cases of HFRS reveals tubulonecrotic lesions scattered throughout the nephron but most commonly near the corticomedullary junction.[140,141] It is precisely this region of the kidney that is most susceptible to hypoxic damage because of the low partial pressure of oxygen associated with the renal medullary circulation and the high metabolic demands of the cells in this zone of the kidney.[17] In addition, intracellular metabolites can be toxic in the presence of hypoxic insults.[174] The roles of the several recognized physiologically active circulating mediators that influence the intrarenal circulation[28] in Hantaan virus–induced renal failure, including atrial natriuretic peptide,[27] TNF-α,[199] renin,[94] complement fragments, kinins, and others,[23] have not been defined. There is very little evidence to suggest that the deposition of circulating immune complexes has an important role in the pathogenesis of the renal syndrome.[95]

In contrast to most of the HFs, the immune response in *Hantavirus* infections has its onset before the patient presents for medical care. Both antigen-binding (fluorescent and ELISA) and virus-neutralizing antibodies,[73,104] as well as circulating activated CD8+ T lymphocytes,[25,106] are readily detectable in Hantaan virus infections. Presumably as a consequence of the immune response, virus has been difficult to isolate from acute serum or blood, although viral RNA can be detected.[71] These immune responses represent mechanisms for inducing disease as well as for limiting virus replication. The relative lack of cytopathology by Hantaviruses replicating in endothelial[200] and other cells suggests that immune or other mechanisms may be required for disease induction.

The lack of adequate animal models for Hantavirus disease has been an obstacle to progress in the field. Suckling mice inoculated with the prototype Hantaan virus strain manifest encephalitis 10 to 14 days later, approximately at the time of de-

velopment of the humoral immune response.[121] Viremia is cleared, and animals die with high titers of serum neutralizing antibodies, histologic evidence of encephalitis, and mononuclear cell infiltrates in the brain. Lymphoid organs show evidence of an active response. Virus-specific T lymphocytes are also present and are capable of mediating virologic recovery in mice.[10] Neutralizing monoclones to viral glycoproteins can also mediate protection in the suckling mouse model, but high dilutions of these monoclones as well as nonneutralizing glycoprotein-specific monoclones have Fc-dependent in vitro enhancing properties.[6,201] Other rodent models have been used to show that immunogens such as baculovirus-expressed proteins or vaccinia virus recombinants with glycoproteins or nucleocapsid protein can protect against infection, as measured by viral antigen accumulation in lungs.[169]

Hantavirus Pulmonary Syndrome

Although HPS disease was first described in 1993, there are already important clues to its pathogenesis and clear parallels to HFRS.[135] It differs from typical cases of the adult respiratory distress syndrome clinically,[39,127] pathologically,[137,203] and in its pathogenesis.[98,203] Several viruses in the Americas, usually carried by sigmodontine rodents, have been implicated as causing the syndrome. The agent, most commonly Sin Nombre virus, is usually acquired by the airborne route.[21,179]

The typical incubation of about 2 to 3 weeks presumably provides a period for replication of the virus and viremic spread throughout the body. The earliest clinical manifestations are fever, myalgia, and malaise, which last a median of 4 days before the onset of dyspnea or other respiratory symptoms brings the patient to the hospital. At this point in the disease, the patient's blood provides important evidence of the underlying process: hemoconcentration reflects the extravasation of fluid into the lung, hypoxemia is present, tachycardia and mild hypotension are usual, antibody is detectable in blood, and there are large numbers of circulating activated CD8 lymphocytes.[30,63,92,98,137,203] Pulmonary involvement progresses rapidly, and about 40% of patients die, usually within 48 hours of hospitalization. The basic physiologic lesion is pulmonary edema, which is evident on the chest radiograph and by the protein-rich fluid aspirated from the endotracheal tubes of very sick patients and is confirmed at autopsy. An independent process appears to lead to circulatory shock as well.

The cause of the increased permeability responsible for the lung process is unknown. The features of HPS differ in several ways from the usual ones hypothesized for the many causes of adult respiratory distress syndrome[175] associated with sepsis, trauma, and the more common pulmonary insults: there is little epithelial cell damage, the hyaline membranes are acellular and scanty, multiorgan failure is not a usual concomitant, and, above all, there are usually few or no polymorphonuclear leukocytes found in the lung. Viral antigen is very extensive in the pulmonary capillaries.[203] There is usually little necrosis or hemorrhage, which suggests that the lesion may be one of cellular dysfunction and may be reversible. The virus causes no obvious morphologic changes in cell culture, but its direct effects on endothelial cell barrier function have never been examined. These effects may be examined by in vitro infection of endothelial cell monolayers with Sin Nombre virus, which can readily be achieved, particularly with primary human pulmonary endothelial cultures (T. Voss, unpublished results).

There are numerous infiltrating mononuclear cells in the lungs. These are identifiable by morphology and by antigenic markers as CD8 lymphocytes, CD4 lymphocytes, and activated macrophages.[137,203] It is plausible that the T lymphocytes present in the interstitial areas of the lung secrete molecules that act directly on the endothelial cells or that they activate macrophages to secrete effector messengers that increase permeability.

Several candidates exist for increasing pulmonary vascular permeability in HPS, particularly TNF-α. There are also examples of immune-mediated reactions that increase the plausibility of this hypothesis. For example, infusion of the T cell–specific monoclonal antibody OKT3 in humans results in marked release of cytokines, including TNF-α, IFN-γ, and IL-2; physiologic correlates of fever, hypertension, and tachycardia begin within 2 hours and are followed at 5 to 7 hours by hypoxemia, hypotension, and decreased vascular resistance.[33] Although these changes do not parallel those of HPS exactly, the abrupt onset of the condition after T-cell stimulation with resulting shock and pulmonary edema provides a useful parallel. Early data on cytokine expression, including plasma concentrations,[176] mRNA in tissues (A. Ansari et al, unpublished observations), and immunohistochemical detection in tissues (S. R. Zaki, unpublished observations) support their participation in the process.

There are remarkable similarities between HFRS and HPS, including the noncytopathic character of the viruses, the presumed immunopathologic mechanism for disease, the occurrence of shock, and the importance of changes in vascular permeability. There are also some significant pathogenetic differences. In HPS, the increase in vascular permeability is virtually confined to the thoracic cavity, presumably because the lung is the only site where abundant viral antigen and activated T lymphocytes are found in proximity.[203] The ingress of effector lymphocytes into the pulmonary parenchyma is undoubtedly directed by adhesion molecules, and there is preliminary evidence of intercellular adhesion molecule-1 expression on pulmonary endothelium in patients (S. R. Zaki, unpublished observations, 1995). Neither is the flushing and conjunctival injection of HFRS a feature of HPS. Although almost all HPS patients have some degree of thrombocytopenia and most have a prolonged partial thromboplastin time, only a minority develop severe thrombocytopenia, DIC, or frank bleeding, in contrast to the usual presence of DIC in HFRS. An interesting feature of HPS is the frequent occurrence of dizziness, which may be severe and may be associated with true vertigo[93,127] (C. J. Peters, unpublished observations). This may have a counterpart in the invasion by another Hantavirus, Seoul virus, of the labyrinth of experimentally inoculated rats and guinea pigs.[183]

There are few data that deal directly with the mechanisms of virus elimination in HPS patients, despite evidence of activation of both the humoral and cellular immune systems[98,137] (F. A. Ennis, unpublished observations). Although a large number of infected endothelial cells are found in the lungs and elsewhere, there is little evidence of vascular disruption in survivors[39] or in most patients dying of the disease.[137,203] If the disease process in survivors is similar to that mirrored in necropsy tissues, extensive pulmonary capillary infection

must be resolved, either because the infection itself is self-limiting or through the intercession of the immune system. The elimination or downregulation of virus infection presumably involves noncytolytic mechanisms such as those described for T cells in some poxvirus[161] or coronavirus[144] infections, or for antibody in alphavirus encephalitis.[58]

Filoviridae

The diseases caused by Marburg and the four distinct subtypes of Ebola virus share considerable similarity; they have a marked impact on the body economy, and patients are usually extremely ill. Viral particles or viral antigens are found in endothelial cells, macrophages, and parenchymal cells of organs throughout the body.[12,53,76,133,132] Examination of material from the 1995 Zaire Ebola outbreak has emphasized the extensive infection of the reticuloendothelial system but has also shown marked involvement of epithelial cells and fibroblasts, with accompanying collagen fragmentation (S. R. Zaki, unpublished observations, 1995). There is even involvement of fibroblasts, capillaries, and sweat glands in the skin. This rampant viral replication suggests the need for antiviral drugs or effective immunotherapy, in addition to adequate supportive care, if the host is to survive.

Mechanisms of disease production include direct viral cytopathology, particularly in the case of the Zaire subtype of Ebola virus. There is obvious necrosis in productively infected cells in numerous organs, including liver and spleen. Evidence for DIC is found in some virus-host combinations. In vitro data suggest the potential for cytokine participation,[45,170] and preliminary analysis of circulating blood cells from patients in the 1995 Zaire epidemic shows increased levels of cytokine mRNA, particularly TNF-α (F. Villenger, P. E. Rollin, et al, unpublished data).

Nonhuman primates dying with the Reston subtype of Ebola[75a,76] and humans with the Zaire subtype[76,196] (T. G. Ksiazek, unpublished observations) may develop an early humoral immune response, but death is thought to occur with uncontrolled viremia. The lack of an effective immune response is unexplained, although there are several speculative possibilities. The extensive lymphoid lesions present provide a plausible anatomic explanation.[12,132] Furthermore, a frame-shift transcriptional mechanism results in synthesis of a soluble glycoprotein that is secreted by cultured cells[156] (A. Sanchez, unpublished observations) and is found in the circulation in Ebola patients (A. Sanchez, unpublished observations, 1995). Other possibilities include the hypotheses that the extensively glycosylated glycoproteins[46,55] are masked from the immune system or that the conserved 17-amino-acid motif found in filovirus glycoproteins and in the p15E protein of murine leukemia viruses may be immunosuppressive.[153,189]

It has been difficult to detect neutralizing antibodies in human patients or experimental animals that survive filovirus infection, and the few attempts to demonstrate protection by passive transfer of antibodies have failed to show a positive effect on disease. Late, poorly active neutralizing antibodies, similar to those found after Lassa fever, may develop in Reston subtype survivors.[76] It has been possible to protect experimental animals from challenge with virulent virus with the use of hyperimmune serum, although preliminary data suggest antibody enhancement in some systems (P. B. Jahrling, A. L. Schmaljohn, unpublished observations).

Flaviviridae

Yellow Fever

The classic clinical picture of severe yellow fever is often divided into a febrile period and a so-called phase of intoxication.[91] The febrile phase actually corresponds to the period of viremia and viral cytopathogenic effect, which typically lasts about 4 days. During the afebrile, "toxic" period that follows, the patient suffers the consequences of viral damage to the liver and other organs. The clinical picture ranges from a mild hepatitis to a severe, virtually complete hepatic necrosis. Fatally infected patients enter the stage of intoxication with circulating serum antibody and no viremia; virus usually can be isolated from organs such as liver and spleen after death.

The viremia in yellow fever disappears approximately 4 days after disease onset, coincident with detection of serum antibody. Because of the brisk in vitro neutralization and the efficacy of neutralizing antibody transfer in the primate model and in limited human experiments, it is likely that antibody is critical in recovery. Although the immune response has controlled viremia before the onset of severe disease, it does not appear to have a deleterious or immunopathologic role, because humans may die with "hyperacute" disease,[91] and analysis of monkey infections shows no correlation between the presence of antibodies and onset of typical yellow fever pathology.[148]

Initial infection in nonhuman primates first involves the Kupffer cells and then extends to nearby hepatocytes.[184] Studies have failed to identify extensively infected endothelial cells or obvious morphologic causes for shock, increased vascular permeability, and death except for the extensive hepatic necrosis seen in many cases. Once again, the importance of soluble mediators in the pathophysiology of the disease is suggested. The final stages of illness often resemble those seen in other severe hepatic diseases, such as the hepatorenal syndrome.[44] Studies of rhesus monkeys dying from yellow fever have shown decreases in renal plasma flow and glomerular filtration rate and other changes suggesting hepatorenal syndrome and leading to anuria, with tubular necrosis occurring only as a late, shock-associated finding.[125] Furthermore, terminal yellow fever in rhesus macaques is associated with abnormalities of water and electrolyte regulation in critical areas of the brain such as the medulla oblongata.[113]

Dengue Hemorrhagic Fever With Dengue Shock Syndrome

There are four phylogenetically different dengue viruses, which share a similar febrile clinical syndrome, vector specificity, and several antigenic determinants.[110] Dengue fever can be caused by dengue-1, -2, -3, or -4 viruses and is a temporarily prostrating febrile disease that carries little or no risk of a fatal outcome.[65,166] Dengue fever is often associated with thrombocytopenia, and patients not infrequently experience minor hemorrhage, particularly epistaxis. Patients with gastrointestinal pathology may hemorrhage from that lesion during the course of dengue fever,[185] much as with the use of coumadin anticoagulants. There is no associated virus-related shock, and patients almost always recover promptly and completely.

In contrast to uncomplicated dengue infection, there are rare instances in which infection with these viruses causes a primary HF syndrome with shock,[59,162,171] which appears to be dependent on both host and virus strain. Relatively little is known about the pathogenesis of this disease.

In areas where multiple dengue viruses are transmitted, infections of an individual immune to one or more dengue viruses with a heterologous serotype may lead to DHF/DSS. Only a small proportion (possibly 1%) of secondary infections are associated with severe disease, and the case-fatality rate is low (<1%) if supportive treatment is available.[16,64] Nevertheless, the morbidity and the enormous number of dengue infections worldwide make this an important disease.

DSS typically begins as a febrile illness with fever and other manifestations of uncomplicated dengue, but about 4 days into the hospital course the patient abruptly manifests increased vascular permeability and hypotension progressing to shock. This occurs at about the time of termination of viremia, defervescence, and development of a maculopapular rash.[66,65] Although hemorrhage commonly occurs in these patients, there may be a dissociation between the presence of bleeding and the major life-threatening manifestation of shock; hence, the name DHF/DSS.

Epidemiologic observations coupled with careful laboratory correlations have yielded important clues to the pathogenesis of this disease. Infection with one dengue virus leads to lifelong immunity to the same dengue virus but only a few months' protection against heterologous viruses.[166] The homologous immunity is presumably a result of long-term synthesis of high-avidity neutralizing antibody and residual cellular immunity. The mechanism of heterologous immunity is less well understood but may be based primarily on mediation of cellular immunity by crossreacting CD8 lymphocytes.[18]

Second infections with a heterologous dengue virus occur mainly in geographic areas where large populations of the vector mosquito, Aedes aegypti, are present and multiple dengue viruses circulate. In this setting, heterologous antibodies do not protect but may enhance infection of the major target cell for dengue replication, the macrophage.[66,67] The relevance of antibody-dependent enhancement to DHF/DSS was demonstrated by prospective studies in Thai school children that showed a correlation between the occurrence of DHF/DSS and circulating in vitro enhancing antibodies.[97] Infants may also develop DHF/DSS, which is hypothesized to be caused by antibody-dependent enhancement from maternal antibody. The latter phenomenon has been shown to be important by the close temporal association of its occurrence with the loss of protective neutralizing maternal antibodies and the resulting presence of enhancing antibodies[96] and by its virtual absence in the 1981 Cuban epidemic, in which mothers uncommonly had heterologous dengue antibodies to transfer to the newborn.[16] Many examples of in vitro antibody-mediated enhancement have been reported, but dengue is the only example in which the in vivo relevance is fully supported by laboratory and epidemiologic evidence. Other flavivirus diseases (e.g., yellow fever) usually show no effect or modest cross-protection from previous flavivirus infection.[126]

The enhancing antibodies are thought to increase virus burden in macrophages, the major site of dengue replication. An important mechanism underlying DHF/DSS may also be a brisk immune response primed by crossreacting epitopes that results in formation of large quantities of immune complexes. Antigen-antibody complexes activate complement, resulting in a phlogistic response and increased vascular permeability. In support of this hypothesis, both decreases in complement components and presence of circulating immune complexes by the Raji cell assay correlate with the severity of DSS.[195]

In addition to potential antibody-mediated mechanisms of immunopathology, T-cell activation can be responsible for deleterious effects.[101] Crossreactive CD4+ T lymphocyte clones secrete IFN-γ when stimulated in vitro, leading to increased expression of Fc receptors in macrophages and increased infection by enhancing antibodies.[100] High levels of IFN-γ are found in sera from patients with dengue and DHF/DSS.

T cells are also candidate effectors in DHF/DSS. Analysis of serum levels of several molecules associated with T-cell activation has shown increases in soluble CD4, IL-2, soluble IL-2R, and IFN-γ in dengue and in DHF/DSS. Serum levels of soluble CD4 and soluble IL-2R are higher in DHF/DSS than in uncomplicated dengue, and soluble CD8 is elevated in comparison with either normal subjects or patients with dengue fever.[99] Primary dengue infection establishes memory CD4+ and CD8+ T-cell clones that can be stimulated in vitro by heterologous dengue serotypes to secrete proinflammatory cytokines and to display lytic activity for MHC-matched infected cells.[18,100] The presence of these T cells provides a potential in vivo mechanism for destruction of the extensively infected macrophages, with release of cytokines and other active mediator molecules.[18] The lytic activity may further be enhanced by upregulation of MHC restriction elements caused by the high levels of IFN-α and IFN-γ present in serum of patients with dengue or DHF/DSS.[99] The same mechanisms that induce DHF/DSS are also responsible for recovery from dengue and DHF/DSS. The onset of the DSS usually coincides with defervescence, which is associated with the appearance of the maculopapular rash in uncomplicated dengue.[65] The immune response eliminates virus but also induces the shock syndrome. Little virus but very high levels of neutralizing antibodies are found in patients presenting with DSS. In addition to the hypothesized participation of immune complexes in pathogenesis, there is also the possibility that CD8+ T lymphocytes may lyse infected macrophages, resulting in release of large quantities of mediators of shock.

In uncomplicated dengue fever, participation of T cells in recovery is inferred but has not been proved.

Kyasanur Forest Disease and Omsk Hemorrhagic Fever

Kyasanur Forest disease presents much like other HFs, with fever, headache, and severe myalgia giving way to hypotension and hemorrhage lasting 1 to 2 weeks. Many patients appear to recover but then develop a second bout of fever beginning about 3 weeks into their illness and accompanied by signs of encephalitis.[193,194] This pattern of diphasic illness resembles that of other tickborne flaviviruses such as louping ill and tickborne encephalitis, except that the first phase of illness is rarely associated with hemorrhagic or circulatory abnormalities in those diseases.

Viremia is detectable during the early phase of illness, both in humans[194] and in a realistic monkey model of infection in *Macaca radiata*.[90,191] The appearance of antibody corresponds to the termination of the hemorrhagic phase, but virus is readily isolated from brain tissue. Immunohistochemistry identifies a prominent component of lymphocyte and macrophage infection in the macaque model.[90]

The pathogenesis of Kayasanur Forest disease has not been well explained, but several interesting observations have been made. There is typically a striking bradycardia and maximum hypotension at the time of defervescence at about the end of the first week of disease; the reason for this was not found in careful studies of the model infection of *Macaca radiata*, including careful histopathologic examination of the heart and autonomic nervous system.[191] The bleeding diathesis is accompanied by, and in part caused by, thrombocytopenia of uncertain origin. The thrombocytopenia, anemia, and a marked leukopenia have been related to the common finding of erythrophagocytosis and agglutinins against hematologic elements.[24,192]

Omsk HF pursues a similar clinical course, and the pathogenetic issues are thought to be essentially the same.[177]

SUMMARY

HFs are acute, severe viral infections that are responsible for thousands of deaths annually and whose pathogenesis is poorly understood. Viral HF is a syndrome caused by members of four virus families. Several common features of the clinical disease, such as flushing, hypotension, and increased vascular permeability, are probably caused by systemic release of soluble mediators included in the spectrum of cytokines, lipid molecules, and other participants in the systemic bacterial sepsis syndrome and other inflammatory states.[15] The hemodynamic picture in the diseases that have been studied (HFRS, HPS, and DHF/DSS) is different from that of septic shock in that there is a low cardiac output and high systemic vascular resistance, suggesting the important participation of cardiodepressants. Studies of arenavirus-infected guinea pigs implicate leukotrienes, platelet activating factor, and TNF-α as candidate mediators.

Hemorrhagic manifestations may result from direct viral damage to endothelium, but soluble mediators can cause endothelial cell retraction in vitro and can shift the anticoagulant state toward thrombosis and inflammation, suggesting other possible mechanisms for either capillary damage and subsequent hemorrhage or initiation of local coagulation. Some of these viruses infect macrophages much more prominently than endothelial cells, providing an important potential source for cytokine or lipid mediators, through either direct viral stimulation or immune interactions. Clinically relevant DIC occurs in some diseases but not in others. Thrombocytopenia is common and is most severe in patients who have bleeding manifestations.

In arenavirus and filovirus diseases, IFN plays a relatively minor virus-regulatory role and cellular immunity is a major factor in recovery. Growth of *Bunyaviridae* and *Flaviviridae* is efficiently inhibited by IFN, and antibody is more important in terminating those infections. In most HFs, clinical recovery corresponds temporally to control of virus replication by the immune response. In contrast, Hantavirus diseases appear to be induced by the immune response. Patients presenting with HFRS or HPS usually have activated CD8 lymphocytes in their blood and rising antibody titers. DHF/DSS usually occurs in persons with a previous infection with a heterologous dengue virus, and the immune response appears to both increase the extent of infection and participate in disease induction. Virus replication is enhanced by crossreacting, nonneutralizing antibodies and T-cell mechanisms, such as IFN-γ upregulation of Fc receptors, which increase the efficiency of enhancing antibodies. Immune complexes and T-cell cytokine–mediated immunopathology are important for producing severe clinical disease.

ABBREVIATIONS

ALT: alanine aminotransferase
AST: aspartate aminotransferase
C1, C1q, C3, C5b67: components of complement
DHF/DSS: dengue hemorrhagic fever with dengue shock syndrome
DIC: disseminated intravascular coagulation
ELISA: enzyme-linked immunosorbent assay
F(ab')$_2$: antigen-binding fragment of IgG
HF: hemorrhagic fever
HFRS: hemorrhagic fever with renal syndrome
HPS: hantavirus pulmonary syndrome
IgG, IgM: immunoglobulins
IL-1, IL-2, IL-2R, IL-6: interleukins
IFN, IFN-α, IFN-γ: interferons
LCMV: lymphocytic choriomeningitis virus
MHC: major histocompatibility complex
TNF-α: tumor necrosis factor-alpha

ACKNOWLEDGMENTS

I would like to thank my colleagues who have shared their opinions and experiences with me. The documentation of this chapter relies strongly on reviews to keep the references within a manageable number so that many original contributions are only indirectly acknowledged, and I apologize to the authors whose publications are not directly referenced.

REFERENCES

1. Anderson GW. Viral and host determinants of resistance to Rift Valley fever in a rat model. Baltimore: Johns Hopkins University School of Hygiene and Public Health, 1988. Doctoral dissertation.
2. Anderson GW Jr, Peters CJ. Viral determinants of virulence for Rift Valley fever (RVF) in rats. Microb Pathog 1988;5:241–250.
3. Anderson GW Jr, Rosebrock JA, Johnson AJ, Jennings GB, Peters CJ. Infection of inbred rat strains with Rift Valley fever virus: development of a congenic resistant strain and observations on age-dependence of resistance. Am J Trop Med Hyg 1991;44:475–480.
4. Anderson GW Jr, Slone TW, Peters CJ. Pathogenesis of Rift Valley fever virus (RVFV) in inbred rats. Microb Pathog 1987;2:283–293.
5. Andrews BS, Theofilopoulos AN, Peters CJ, Loskutoff DJ, Brandt WE, Dixon FJ. Replication of dengue and Junin viruses in cultured rabbit and human endothelial cells. Infect Immun 1978;20:776–781.
6. Arikawa J, Yao JS, Yoshimatsu K, Takashima I, Hashimoto N. Protective role of antigenic sites on the envelope protein of Hantaan virus defined by monoclonal antibodies. Arch Virol 1992;126:271–281.
7. Aronson JF, Herzog NK, Jerrells TR. Pathological and virological features of arenavirus disease in guinea pigs: comparison of two Pichinde virus strains. Am J Pathol 1994;145:228–235.
8. Aronson JF, Herzog NK, Jerrells TR. Tumor necrosis factor and the pathogenesis of Pichinde virus infection in guinea pigs. Am J Trop Med Hyg 1995;52:262–269.
9. Arribalzaga RA. Una nueva enfermedad epidemica a germen desconocido: hipertermia, nefrotoxica, leucopenica y enantematica. Dia Medico (Buenos Aires) 1955;27:1204–1210.
10. Asada H, Tamura M, Kondo K, et al. Role of T lymphocyte subsets in protection and recovery from Hantaan virus infection in mice. J Gen Virol 1987;68:1961–1969.
11. Barrera Oro JG, Lupton HW, Jahrling PB, Meegan J, Kenyon RH, Peters CJ. Cross-protection against Machupo virus with Candid #1 live-attenuated Junin virus vaccine. I. The postvaccination prechallenge immune response. Second International Conference on the Impact of Viral Diseases on the Development of Latin American Countries and the Caribbean Region, Buenos Aires, Argentina, March 1988:20–26.
12. Baskerville A, Fisher-Hoch SP, Neild GH, Dowsett AB. Ultrastructural pathology of experimental Ebola hemorrhagic fever virus infection. J Pathol 1985;147:199–209.
13. Bevilacqua MP, Pober JS, Majeau GR, Fiers W, Cotran RS, Gimbrone MA. Recombinant tumor necrosis factor induces procoagulant activity in cultured human vascular endothelium. Proc Natl Acad Sci U S A 1986;83:4533–4537.
14. Blalock A. Acute circulatory failure as exemplified by shock and haemorrhage. Surg Gynecol Obstet 1934;58:551–566.
15. Bone RT. The pathogenesis of sepsis. Ann Intern Med 1991; 115:457—469.
16. Bravo JR, Guzman MG, Kouri GP. Why dengue haemorrhagic fever in Cuba? I. Individual risk factors for dengue haemorrhagic fever/dengue shock syndrome (DHF/DSS). Trans R Soc Trop Med Hyg 1987;81:816–820.
17. Brezis M, Rosen S. Hypoxemia of the renal medulla: its implications for disease. N Engl J Med 1995;332:647–655.
18. Bukowski JF, Kurane I, Lai CJ, Bray M, Falgout B, Ennis FA. Dengue virus–specific cross-reactive CD8+ human cytotoxic T lymphocytes. J Inf Dis 1989;63:5086–5091.
19. Burt FJ, Leman PA, Abbott JC, Swanepoel R. Serodiagnosis of Crimean-Congo haemorrhagic fever. Epidemiol Infect 1994;113: 551–562.
20. Bussolino F, Breviario F, Tetta C, Aglletta M, Mantovani A, Dejana E. Interleukin 1 stimulates platelet-activating factor production in cultured human endothelial cells. J Clin Invest 1986;77:2027–2033.
21. Butler JC, Peters CJ. 1994. Hantaviruses and Hantavirus pulmonary syndrome. Clin Infect Dis 1994;19:387–395.
22. Camussi G, Turello E, Bussolino F, Baglioni C. Tumor necrosis factor alters cytoskeletal organization and barrier function of endothelial cells. Int Arch Allergy Appl Immunol 1991;96:84–91.
23. Carmines PK, Fleming JT. Control of the renal microvasculature by vasoactive peptides. FASEB J 1990;4:3300–3309.
24. Chatterjea JB, Swarup S, Pain SK, Rao RL. Haematological and biochemical studies in Kyasanur Forest disease. Brit J Exp Pathol 1963;51:419–435.
25. Chen LB, Yang WS. Abnormalities of T cell immunoregulation in hemorrhagic fever with renal syndrome. J Infect Dis 1990;161: 1016–1019.
26. Childs JC, Peters CJ. Ecology and epidemiology of arenaviruses and their hosts. In: Salvato MS, ed. The Arenaviridae. New York: Plenum, 1993:331–373.
27. Cho KW, Kim SH, Koh GY, et al. Plasma concentration of atrial natriuretic peptide in different phases of Korean hemorrhagic fever. Nephron 1989;51:215–219.
28. Chou SY, Porush JG, Fauber PF. Renal medullary circulation: hormonal control. Kidney Int 1990;37:1–13.

29. Cohen MS, Kwei HE, Chin CC, Ge HC. CNS manifestations of epidemic hemorrhagic fever. Arch Intern Med 1983;143:2070–2072.

30. Colman RW, Robboy SJ, Minna JD. Disseminated intravascular coagulation (DIC): an approach. Am J Med 1972;52:679–689.

31. Connolly BM, Jensen AB, Peters CJ, Geyer SJ, Barth JF, McPherson RA. Pathogenesis of Pichinde virus infection in strain 13 guinea pigs: an immunocytochemical, virologic, and clinical chemistry study. Am J Trop Med Hyg 1993;49:10–24.

32. Cosgriff TM, Morrill JC, Jennings GB, et al. The hemostatic derangement produced by Rift Valley fever virus in rhesus monkeys. Rev Infect Dis 1989;11:S807–S814.

33. Costanzo-Nordin MR. Cardiopulmonary effects of OKT3: determinants of hypotension, pulmonary edema, and cardiac dysfunction. Transplant Proc 1993;25:21–24.

34. Cummins D, Fisher-Hoch SP, Walshe KJ, et al. A plasma inhibitor of platelet aggregation in patients with Lassa fever. Br J Haematol 1989;72:543–548.

35. Cummins D, McCormick JB, Bennett D, et al. Acute sensorineural deafness in Lassa fever. JAMA 1990;264:2093–2096.

36. Cummins D, Molinas FC, Lerer G, Maiztegui JI, Faint R, Machin SJ. A plasma inhibitor of platelet aggregation in patients with Argentine hemorrhagic fever. Am J Trop Med Hyg 1990;42:470–475.

37. De Bracco MME, Rimoldi MT, Cossio PM, et al. Argentine hemorrhagic fever: alterations of the complement system and anti—Juninvirus humoral response. N Engl J Med 1978;299:216—221.

38. Deutschman CS, Konstantinides KN, Tsai M, Simmons RL, Cerra FB. Physiology and metabolism in isolated viral septicemia. Arch Surg 1987;122:21–25.

39. Duchin JS, Koster F, Peters CJ, et al. Hantavirus pulmonary syndrome: a clinical description of 17 patients with a newly recognized disease. N Engl J Med 1994;330:949–955.

40. Easterday BC. Rift Valley fever. Adv Vet Sci 1965;10:65–127.

41. Enria D, Franco SG, Ambrosio A, Vallejos D, Levis S, Maiztegui J. Current status of the treatment of Argentine hemorrhagic fever. Med Microbiol Immunol (Berl) 1986;175:173–176.

42. Enria D, Maiztegui JI. Antiviral treatment of Argentine hemorrhagic fever. Antiviral Res 1994;23:23—31.

43. Entwisle G, Hale E. Hemodynamic alterations in hemorrhagic fever. Circulation 1957;15:414–425.

44. Epstein M. Hepatorenal syndrome: emerging perspectives of pathophysiology and therapy. J Am Soc Nephrol 1994;4:1735–1753.

45. Feldmann H, Bugany H, Mahner F, Klenk H-D, Drenckhahn D, Schnittler H-J. Virus-induced endothelial permeability triggered by affected macrophages. FASEB J 1994;8:A756.

46. Feldmann H, Nichol ST, Klenk H-D, Peters CJ, Sanchez A. Characterization of filoviruses based on differences in structure and antigenicity of the virion glycoprotein. Virology 1994;199:469–473.

47. Feldmann H, Zaki S, Rollin PE, Klenk H-D, Peters CJ, Schnittler H-J. Virus-activated macrophages induce endothelial leakage: a concept to investigate pathogenesis in an in vitro model. Ninth International Conference on Negative Strand Viruses, Estoril, Portugal, October 1994. Elsevier, 1995:2–7.

48. Fisher-Hoch S, McCormick JB, Sasso D, Craven RB. Hematologic dysfunction in Lassa fever. J Med Virol 1988;26:127–135.

49. Ford-Hutchinson A, Letts G. Biological actions of leukotrienes. Hypertension 1986;8(Suppl II):44–49.

50. Froeb HF, McDowell ME. Renal function in epidemic hemorrhagic fever. Am J Med 1954;16:671–676.

51. Gauldie J, Richards C, Harnish D, Lansdorp P, Baumann H. Proc Natl Acad Sci U S A 1987;84:7251–7255.

52. Gear JSS, Cassel GA, Gear AJ, et al. Outbreak of Marburg virus disease in Johannesburg. Br~20Med J 1975;4:489–493.

53. Geisbert TW, Jahrling PB, Hanes MA, Zack PM. Association of Ebola-related Reston virus particles and antigen with tissue lesions of monkeys imported to the United States. J Comp Pathol 1992;106:137–152.

54. Genovesi EV, Johnson AJ, Peters CJ. Susceptibility and resistance of inbred strains of Syrian golden hamsters (Mesocricetus auratus) to wasting disease caused by lymphocytic choriomeningitis virus: pathogenesis of lethal and non-lethal infections. J Gen Virol 1988;69:2209–2220.

55. Geyer H, Will C, Feldmann H, Klenk H-D, Geyer R. Carbohydrate structure of Marburg virus glycoprote. Glycobiology 1992;2: 299–312.

56. Ghebrehiwet B, Silverberg M, Kaplan AP. Activation of the classical pathway of complement by Hageman factor fragment. J Exp Med 1981;153:665–676.

57. Gonzalez PH, Cossio PM, Arana RM, Maiztegui JI, Laguens RP. Lymphatic tissue in Argentine hemorrhagic fever. Arch Pathol Lab Med 1980;104:250—254.

58. Griffin DE, Levine B, Ubol S, Harkwick JM. The effects of alphavirus infection on neurons. Ann Neurol 1994;35:S23–S27.

59. Gubler DJ, Reed D, Rosen L, Hitchcock JC. Epidemiologic, clinical, and virologic observations on dengue in the Kingdom of Tonga. Am J Trop Med Hyg 1978;27:581–589.

60. Guo ZM, Liu CT. Pulmonary responses of conscious strain 13 guinea pigs to Pichinde virus infection. Lab Anim Sci 1991;41:581–584.

61. Guo ZM, Liu CT. Role of atrial natriuretic peptide (ANP) in disturbed water and electrolyte metabolism of guinea pigs infected with Pichinde virus. Lab Anim Sci 1995 (in press).

62. Guo ZM, Liu CT, Peters CJ. Possible involvement of endogenous beta-endorphin in the pathophysiological mechanisms of Pichinde virus–infected guinea pigs. Proc Soc Exp Biol Med 1992;200:343–348.

62a. Guo ZM, Qian C, Peters CJ, Liu CT. Changes in platelet-activating factor, catecholamine, and serotonin concentrations in brain, cerebrospinal fluid, and plasma of Pichinde virus–infected guinea pigs. Lab Anim Sci 1993;43:569–574.

63. Hallin GW, Simpson SQ, Crowell RE, et al. Cardiopulmonary manifestations of hoatavirus pulmonary syndrome. Crit Care Med 1996; 24:252–258.

64. Halstead SB. The pathogenesis of dengue: molecular epidemiology in infectious disease. Am J Epidemiol 1981;114:632–648.

65. Halstead SB. Dengue and dengue hemorrhagic fever. In: Feigin Cherry JD, ed. Textbook of pediatric infectious disease. Philadelphia: WB Saunders, 1987:1510–1521.

66. Halstead SB. Antibody, macrophages, dengue virus infection, shock, and hemorrhage: a pathogenic cascade. Rev Infect Dis 1989; 11(Suppl 4):S830–S839.

67. Halstead SB, O'Rourke EJ. Dengue viruses and mononuclear phagocytes. I. Infection enhancement by non-neutralizing antibody. J Exp Med 1977;146:201–217.

68. Han JS, Lee JS, Lee SK, Kim S, Koh CS, Lee M. Activation of kallikrein-kinin in hemorrhagic fever with renal syndrome (Korean hemorrhagic fever with renal syndrome). Korean J Intern Med 1989;37:11–27.

69. Heller MV, Marta RF, Sturk A, et al. Early markers of blood coagulation and fibrinolysis activation in Argentine hemorrhagic fever. Thromb Haemost 1995;73:368–373.

70. Heller MV, Saavedra MC, Falcoff R, Maiztegui JI, Molinas FC. Increased tumor necrosis factor-alpha levels in Argentine hemorrhagic fever. J Infect Dis 1992;166:1203–1204.

71. Hjelle B, Spiropoulou CF, Torrez-Martinez N, Morzunov S, Peters CJ, Nichol ST. Detection of Muerto Canyon virus RNA in peripheral blood mononuclear cells from patients with Hantavirus pulmonary syndrome. J Infect Dis 1994;170:1013–1017.

72. Huber M, Beutler B, Keppler K. Tumor necrosis factor α stimulates leukotriene production in vivo. Eur J Immunol 1988;18:2085–2088.

73. Huggins JW, Hsiang CM, Cosgriff TM, et al. Prospective, double-blind, concurrent, placebo controlled clinical trial of intravenous ribavirin therapy of hemorrhagic fever with renal syndrome. J Infect Dis 1991;164:1119–1127.

74. Jahrling PB. Protection of Lassa virus—infected guinea pigs with Lassa-immune plasma of guinea pig, primate, and human origin. J Med Virol 1983;12:93—102.

75. Jahrling PB, Frame JD, Rhoderick JB, Monson MH. Endemic Lassa fever in Liberia. IV. Selection of optimally effective plasma for treatment by passive immunization. Trans R Soc Trop Med Hyg 1985;79:380–384.

75a. Jahrling PB, Geisbert TW, Dalgard DW, et al. Preliminary report: isolation of Ebola virus from monkeys imported to USA. Lancet 1990; 335:502–505.

76. Jahrling PB, Geisbert TW, Jaax NK, Hanes MA, Ksiazek TG, Peters CJ. Experimental infection of cynomolgus macaques with Ebola (Reston subtype) filoviruses from the 1989–1990 US epizootics. Arch Virol 1996 (in press).

77. Jahrling PB, Hesse RA, Eddy GA, et al. Lassa fever infection in rhesus monkeys: pathogenesis and treatment with ribavirin. J Infect Dis 1980;141:580–589.

77a. Jahrling PB, Hesse RA, Rhoderick JB, Elwell MA, Moe JB. Pathogenesis of a Pichinde virus strain adapted to produce lethal infections in guinea pigs. Infect Immun 1981;32:872–880.

78. Jahrling PB, Peters CJ. Passive antibody therapy of Lassa fever in cynomolgus monkeys: importance of neutralizing antibody and Lassa virus strain. Infect Immun 1984;44:528–533.

79. Johnson KM, McCormick JB, Webb PA, Smith ES, Elliott LH, King IJ. Clinical virology of Lassa fever in hospitalized patients. J Infect Dis 1987;155:456—464.

80. Joubert JR, King JB, Rossouw, Cooper R. A nosocomial outbreak of Crimean-Congo haemorrhagic fever at Tygerberg Hospital. III. Clinical pathology and pathogenesis. S Afr Med J 1985;68:722–728.

81. Karmyshev VYA, Leshchinskaya EV, Butenko AM, et al. Results of laboratory and clinical-morphological investigations of Crimean hemorrhagic fever. 1973;2:17–22.

82. Katz MA, Starr JF. Pichinde virus infection in strain 13 guinea pigs reduces intestinal protein reflection coefficient with compensation. J Infect Dis 1990;162:1304–1308.

83. Katz MA, Starr JF. Influence of volume expansion on capillary transport in the gut of Pichinde virus–infected strain 13 guinea pigs. J Med Virol 1991;35:60–64.

84. Kenyon RH, Condie RM, Jahrling PB, Peters CJ. Protection of guinea pigs against experimental Argentine hemorrhagic fever by purified human IgG: importance of elimination of infected cells. Microb Pathog 1990;9:219–226.

85. Kenyon RH, Green DE, Eddy DE, Peters CJ. Treatment of Junin virus–infected guinea pigs with immune serum: development of late neurological disease. J Med Virol 1986;20:207–218.

86. Kenyon RH, Green DE, Maiztegui JI, Peters CJ. Viral strain dependent differences in experimental Argentine hemorrhagic fever (Junin virus) infection in guinea pigs. Intervirology 1988;29:133– 143.

87. Kenyon RH, Green DE, Peters CJ. Effect of immuno-suppression on experimental Argentine hemorrhagic fever in guinea pigs. J Virol 1985;53:75–80.

88. Kenyon RH, Peters CJ. Cytolysis of Junin infected target cells by immune guinea pig spleen cells. Microb Pathog 1986;1:453–464.

89. Kenyon RH, Peters CJ. Actions of complement on Junin virus. Rev Infect Dis 1989;11:S771–S776.

90. Kenyon RH, Rippey MK, McKee KT, Zack PM, Peters CJ. Infection of *Macaca radiata* with viruses of the tick-borne encephalitis group. Microb Pathog 1992;13:398–409.

91. Kerr JA. The clinical aspects and diagnosis of yellow fever. In: Strode GR, ed. Yellow fever. New York: McGraw-Hill, 1951:385–425.

92. Ketai LH, Williamson MR, Telepak RJ, et al. Hantavirus pulmonary syndrome (HPS): radiographic findings in 16 patients. Radiology 1994;191:665–668.

93. Khan AS, Ksiazek TG, Zaki SR, et al. Fatal Hantavirus pulmonary syndrome in an adolescent. Pediatrics 1995;95:276–280.

94. Kim S, Cho BY, Lee JS, et al. A study on plasma renin activity in Korean hemorrhagic fever.

95. Kim S, Kang ET, Kim YG, et al. Localization of Hantaan viral envelope glycoproteins by monoclonal antibodies in renal tissues from patients with Korean hemorrhagic fever. Am J Clin Pathol 1993; 100:398–403.

96. Kliks SC, Nimmanitya S, Nisalak A, Burke DS. Evidence that maternal dengue antibodies are important in the development of dengue hemorrhagic fever in infants. Am J Trop Med Hyg 1988; 38:411–419.

97. Kliks SC, Nisalak A, Brandt WE, Wahl L, Burke DS. Antibody-dependent enhancement of dengue virus growth in human monocytes as a risk factor for dengue hemorrhagic fever. Am J Trop Med Hyg 1989;40:444–451.

98. Ksiazek TG, Peters CJ, Rollin PE, et al. Identification of a new North American Hantavirus that causes acute pulmonary insufficiency. Am J Trop Med Hyg 1995;52:117–123.

99. Kurane I, Innis BL, Nimmannitya S, et al. Activation of T lymphocytes in dengue virus infections. 1991;88:1473–1480.

100. Kurane I, Innis BL, Nisalak A, et al. Human T cell responses to dengue virus antigens. J Clin Invest 1989;83:506–513.

101. Kurane I, Rothman AL, Livingston PG, et al. Immunopathologic mechanisms of dengue hemorrhagic fever and dengue shock syndrome. Arch Virol 1994;(Suppl)9:59–64.

102. Kurata T, Sata T, Aoyama Y, et al. Systemic deposition of viral antigens in the vascular endothelia of hemorrhagic fever with renal syndrome. In: Kano K, Mori S, Sugisaki T, Torisu M, eds. Cellular, molecular, and genetic approaches to immunodiagnosis and immunotherapy. Tokyo: University of Tokyo Press, 1987:305–312.

103. Lange LG, Schreiner GF. Immune mechanisms of cardiac disease. N Engl J Med 1994;330:1129–1135.

104. Lee HW. Korean hemorrhagic fever. Prog Med Virol 1982;28:96–113.

105. Lee M, Kim BK, Kim S, et al. Coagulopathy in hemorrhagic fever with renal syndrome (Korean hemorrhagic fever). Rev Infect Dis 1989;11(Suppl 4):S877–S883.

106. Lee JH, Kim GH, Kim YG, Kang ET, Han JS, Lee JS. The changes of peripheral lymphocyte subsets in Korean hemorrhagic fever. Korean J Nephrol 1992;11:343–357.

107. Levi M, ten Cate H, van der Poll T, van Deventer JH. Pathogenesis of disseminated intravascular coagulation in sepsis. JAMA 1993; 270:975–979.

108. Levis SC, Saavedra MC, Ceccoli C, et al. Correlation between endogenous interferon and the clinical evolution of patients with Argentine hemorrhagic fever. J Interferon Res 1985;5:383—389.

109. Levy G, Abecassis M. Activation of the immune coagulation system by murine hepatitis virus strain 3. Rev Infect Dis 1989;11(Suppl 4): S712–S721.

110. Lewis JA, Chang GJ, Lanciotti RS, Kinney RM, Mayer LW, Trent DW. Phylogenetic relationships of dengue-2 viruses. Virology 1993; 197:216–224.

111. Liao BS, Byl FM, Adour KK. Audiometric comparison of Lassa fever hearing loss and idiopathic sudden hearing loss: evidence for a viral cause. Otolaryngol Head Neck Surg 1992;106:226–229.

112. Lim TH, Lee JS, Choi BI, et al. An explanation of renal hemodynamics in acute renal failure based on sequential CT in patients with Korean hemorrhagic fever. J Comput Assist Tomogr 1987;11: 474–479.

113. Liu CT, Griffin MJ. Changes in body fluid compartments, tissue water and electrolyte distribution, and lipid concentrations in rhesus macaques with yellow fever. Am J Vet Res 1982;43:2013–2018.

114. Liu CT, Jahrling PB, Peters CJ. Evidence for the involvement of sulfidopeptide leukotrienes in the pathogenesis of Pichinde virus infection in strain 13 guinea pigs. Prostaglandins Leukot Med 1986;24: 129–138.

115. Liu CT, Peters CJ. Improvement of cardiovascular functions with a sulfidopeptide leukotriene antagonist (FPL-55712) in a guinea pig model of viral hemorrhagic fever. Pharmacologist 1987;29:196.

116. Maiztegui JI, Laguens RP, Cossio PM, et al. Ultrastructural and immunohistochemical studies in five cases of Argentine hemorrhagic fever. J Infect Dis 1975;132:35–43.

117. Mantovani A, Bussolino F, Dejana E. Cytokine regulation of endothelial cell function. FASEB J 1992;6:2591–2599.

118. Mantovani A, Dejana E. Cytokines as communication signals between leukocytes and endothelial cells. Immunol Today 1989; 10:370–375.

119. Martini GA, Siegert R, eds. Marburg virus disease. Berlin: Springer-Verlag, 1971.

120. McCormick JB, King IJ, Webb PA, et al. A case-control study of the clinical diagnosis and course of Lassa fever. J Infect Dis 1987; 155:445–455.

121. McKee KT, Kim GR, Green DE, Peters CJ. Hantaan virus infection in suckling mice: virologic and pathologic correlates. J Med Virol 1985;17:107–117.

122. McKee KT, Mahlandt BG, Maiztegui JI, Eddy GA, Peters CJ. Experimental Argentine hemorrhagic fever in rhesus macaques: viral strain–dependent clinical response. J Infect Dis 1985;152:218– 221.

123. McKee KT Jr, Mahlandt BG, Maiztegui JG, Green DE, Peters CJ. Virus-specific factors in experimental Argentine hemorrhagic fever in rhesus macaques. J Med Virol 1987;22:99–111.

124. Molinas FC, de Bracco MME, Maiztegui JI. Hemostasis and the complement system in Argentine hemorrhagic fever. Rev Infect Dis 1989;11(Suppl 4):762–767.

125. Monath TP, Brinker KR, Chandler FW, Kemp GE, Cropp CB. Pathophysiologic correlations in a rhesus monkey model of yellow fever with special observations on the acute necrosis of B cell areas of lymphoid tissues. Am J Trop Med Hyg 1981;30:431–443.

126. Monath TP, Craven RB, Adjukiewicz A, et al. Yellow fever in the Gambia, 1978–1979: epidemiologic aspects with observations on

the occurrence of Orungo virus infections. Am J Trop Med Hyg 1980;29:912–928.

127. Moolenaar RL, Dalton C, Lipman HB, et al. Clinical features that differentiate Hantavirus pulmonary syndrome from three other acute respiratory illnesses. Clin Infect Dis 1995;21:643–649.

128. Morrill JC, Czarniecki CW, Peters CJ. Recombinant human interferon-gamma modulates Rift Valley fever virus infection in the rhesus monkey. J Interferon Res 1991;11:297–304.

129. Morrill JC, Jennings GB, Cosgriff TM, Gibbs PH, Peters CJ. Prevention of Rift Valley fever in rhesus monkeys with interferon-alpha. Rev Infect Dis 1989;11:S815–S825.

130. Morrill JC, Jennings GB, Johnson AJ, Cosgriff AM, Gibbs PH, Peters CJ. Pathogenesis of Rift Valley fever in rhesus monkeys: role of interferon response. Arch Virol 1990;110:195–212.

131. Morrill JC, Knauert FK, Ksiazek TG, Meegan JM, Peters CJ. Rift Valley fever infection of rhesus monkeys: implications for rapid diagnosis of human disease. Res Virol 1989;140:139–146.

132. Murphy FA. Pathology of Ebola virus infection. In: Pattyn, SR, ed. Ebola virus haemorrhagic fever. Amsterdam: Elsevier/North-Holland, 1978:43–59.

133. Murphy FA, Simpson DIH, Whitfield SG, Zlotnik I, Carter GB. Marburg virus infection in monkeys. Lab Invest 1971;24:279–291.

134. Neugebauer EA, Holaday JW. Handbook of mediators in septic shock. Boca Raton: CRC Press, 1993.

135. Nichol ST, Spiropoulou CF, Morzunov S, et al. Genetic identification of a Hantavirus associated with an outbreak of acute respiratory illness. Science 1993;262:914–917.

136. Niklasson BS, Meadors GF, Peters CF. Active and passive immunization against Rift Valley fever virus infection in Syrian hamsters. Acta Pathol Microbiol Immunol Scand 1984;92:197–200.

137. Nolte KB, Feddersen RM, Foucar K, et al. Hantavirus pulmonary syndrome in the United States: a pathological description of a disease caused by a new agent. Hum Pathol 1995;26:110–120.

138. Odermatt B, Eppler M, Leist TP, Hengartner H, Zinkernagel RM. Virus-triggered acquired immunodeficiency by cytotoxic T-cell–dependent destruction of antigen-presenting cells and lymph follicle structure. Proc Natl Acad Sci U S A 1991;88:8252—8256.

139. Okrent DG, Abraham E, Winston D. Cardiorespiratory patterns in viral septicemia. Am J Med 1987;83:681–686.

140. Oliver J. The spectrum of structural change in acute renal failure. Mil Med 1955;229–232.

141. Oliver J, MacDowell MC. The renal lesion in epidemic hemorrhagic fever. J Clin Invest 1957;36:99–133.

142. Park S, Lee M. Platelet functions in Korean hemorrhagic fever. Korean J Hematol 1982;17:115–120.

143. Parrillo JR. Pathogenetic mechanisms of septic shock. N Engl J Med 1993;328:1471–1477.

144. Pearce BD, Hobbs MV, McGraw TS, Buchmeier MJ. Cytokine induction during T-cell–mediated clearance of mouse hepatitis virus from neurons in vivo. J Virol 1994;68:5483–5495.

145. Penttinen K, Lahdevirta J, Kekomaki R, et al. Circulating immune complexes, immunoconglutinins, and rheumatoid factors in nephropathia epidemica. J Infect Dis 1981;143:15–21.

146. Peters CJ, Anderson GW. Pathogenesis of Rift Valley fever. In: Goldblum N, Swartz TA, Klingberg MA, eds. Contributions to epidemiology and statistics. Vol 3. Basel: S Karger, 1981:21–41.

147. Peters CJ, Ennis WH, Turell MJ, Niklasson B. Rapid detection of Rift Valley fever antigen in the serum of infected lambs. Res Virol 1989;140:43–46.

148. Peters CJ, Huggins JW, Jahrling PB. Antiviral therapy for yellow fever. Annals of the International Symposium on Yellow Fever and Dengue, Rio de Janeiro, Brazil, May 1988. 1991:134–152.

149. Peters CJ, Jahrling PB, Liu CT, Kenyon RH, McKee KT Jr, Barrera-Oro JG. Experimental studies of arenaviral hemorrhagic fevers. Current topics in microbiology and immunology. Vol 134. Heidelberg: Springer-Verlag, 1987:5–68.

150. Peters CJ, Jones D, Trotter R, et al. Experimental Rift Valley fever in rhesus macaques. Arch Virol 1988;99:31–34.

151. Peters CJ, LeDuc JW. Viral hemorrhagic fevers: persistent problems, persistence in reservoirs. In: Mahy BWJ, Compans RW, eds. Immunobiology and pathogenesis of persistent virus infections. Chur, Switzerland: Harwood Academic Publishers, 1995.

152. Peters CJ, Liu C-T, Anderson GW Jr, Morrill JC, Jahrling PB. Pathogenesis of viral hemorrhagic fever: Rift Valley fever and Lassa fever contrasted. Rev Infect Dis 1989;11:S743–S749.

153. Peters CJ, Sanchez A, Feldmann H, Rollin PE, Nichol S, Ksiazek TG. Filoviruses as emerging pathogens. Semin Virol 1994;5:147–154.

154. Peters CJ, Slone TW. Inbred rat strains mimic the disparate human response to Rift Valley fever. J Med Virol 1982;10:45–54.

155. Pfeffer MA, Pfeffer JM, Lewis RA, Braunwald E, Corey EJ, Austen DF. Systemic hemodynamic effects of leukotrienes C4 and D4 in the rat. Am J Physiol 1983;244:H628–H633.

156. Pongpanich B, Kumponpant S. Studies of dengue hemorrhagic fever. V. Hemodynamic studies of clinical shock associated with dengue hemorrhagic fever. J Pediatr 1973;83:1073–1077.

157. Qian C, Jahrling PB, Peters CJ, Liu CT. Cardiovascular and pulmonary responses to Pichinde virus infection in strain 13 guinea pigs. Lab Anim Sci 1994;44:600–607.

158. Qian C, Liu CT, Peters CJ. Increased platelet-activating factor (PAF) concentrations in hearts and lungs of Pichinde virus–infected guinea pigs. J Lipid Mediat 1992;5:261–270.

159. Qian C, Liu CT, Peters CJ. Metabolism of platelet-activating factor (PAF) in neutrophils isolated from Pichinde virus–infected guinea pigs. J Leukoc Biol 1992;51:210–213.

160. Radomski MW, Palmer RMJ, Moncada S. Modulation of platelet aggregation by an L-arginine–nitric oxide pathway. Trends Pharmacol Sci 1991;12:87–88.

161. Ramsay AJ, Ruby J, Ramshaw IA. A case for cytokines as effector molecules in the resolution of virus infection. Immunol Today 1993;14:155–157.

162. Rosen L. Disease exacerbation caused by sequential dengue infections: myth or reality? Rev Infect Dis 1989;11:S840–S842.

163. Rubin RN, Colman RW. Disseminated intravascular coagulation: approach to treatment. Drugs 1992;44:963–971.

164. Saadi S, Platt JL. Transient perturbation of endothelial integrity induced by natural antibodies and complement. J Exp Med 1995;181:21–31.

165. Saavedra MdC, Feuillade MR, Levis S, Maiztegui JI, Haas E. Antigenos de histocompatibilidad en la fiebre hemorrhagica Argentina. XXX Renunion Anual de la Sociedad Argentina de Investigation Clinica, Mar del Plata, November 1985.

166. Sabin AB. Research on dengue during World War II. Am J Trop Med Hyg 1952;1:30–50.

167. Schaeffer RC, Bitrick MS. Death after Pichinde virus infection in large and small strain 13 guinea pigs. J Infect Dis 1993;167:1059–1064.

168. Schaeffer RC, Bitrick MS, Connolly B, Jensen AB, Gong FC. Pichinde virus–induced respiratory failure due to obstruction of the small airways: structure and function. Exp Lung Res 1993;19:715–729.

169. Schmaljohn CS, Chu YK, Schmaljohn AL, Dalrymple JM. Antigenic subunits of Hantaan virus expressed by baculovirus and vaccinia virus recombinants. J Virol 1990;64:3162–3170.

170. Schnittler HJ, Mahner F, Drenckhahn D, Klenk HD, Feldmann H. Replication of Marburg virus in human endothelial cells: a possible mechanism for the development of viral hemorrhagic disease. J Clin Invest 1993;91:1301–1309.

171. Scott RM, Nimmannitya S, Bancroft WB, Mansuwan P. Shock syndrome in primary dengue infections. Am J Trop Med Hyg 1976;25:866–874.

172. Shepherd AJ, Swanepoel R, Leman PA, Shepherd SP. Comparison of methods for isolation and titration of Crimean-Congo hemorrhagic fever virus. J Clin Microbiol 1986;24:654–656.

173. Sidelnikov Y, Obukhova G. Components of kinin system, blood histamine and serotonin in patients with hemorrhagic fever with renal syndrome. Vopr Med Khim 1990;36:47–49.

174. Siegel NJ, Devarajan P, Why SV. Renal cell injury: metabolic and structural alterations. Pediatr Res 1994;36:129–136.

175. Simon RH, Ward PA. Adult respiratory distress syndrome. In: Gaillin JI, Goldstein IM, Snyderman R, eds. Inflammation: basic principles and clinical correlates. 2nd ed. New York: Raven Press, 1992.

176. Simpson SQ, Mapel V, Koster FT, Montoya J, Bice DE, Williams AJ. Evidence for lymphocyte activation in the Hantavirus pulmonary syndrome. Chest 1995;108:975.

177. Smorodintsev AA, Kazbintsev LI, Chudakov VG. Virus hemorrhagic fevers. Jerusalem: Israel Program for Scientific Translations, 1964.

178. Solbrig MV. Lassa virus and central nervous system diseases. In: Salvato MS, ed. The Arenaviridae. New York: Plenum Press, 1993: 325—330.

179. Spiropoulou CF, Morzunov S, Feldmann H, Sanchez A, Peters CJ, Nichol ST. Genome structure and variability of a virus causing Hantavirus pulmonary syndrome. Virology 1994;200:715–723.

180. Srichaikul T, Nimmannitya S, Sripaisarn T, Kamolsilpa M, Pulgate C. Platelet function during the acute phase of dengue hemorrhagic fever. Southeast Asian J Trop Med Public Health 1989;20:19–25.

181. Swanepoel R, Gill DE, Shepherd AJ, Leman PA, Mynhardt JH, Harvey S. The clinical pathology of Crimean-Congo hemorrhagic fever. Rev Infect Dis 1989;11(Suppl 4):S794–S800.

182. Syner JC, Markels RA. Continuous renal clearance studies in epidemic hemorrhagic fever. US Armed Forces Med J 1955;6:807–822.

183. Tamura M, Ogino S, Matsunaga T, et al. Experimental labyrinthitis in guinea pigs caused by a Hantavirus. ORL J Otorhinolaryngol Relat Spec 1991;53:1–5.

184. Tiggert WD, Berge TO, Gochenour L, et al. Experimental yellow fever. Trans N Y Acad Sci 1960;22:323–333.

185. Tsai CJ, Kuo CH, Chen PC, Changcheng CS. Upper gastrointestinal bleeding in dengue fever. Am J Gastroenterol 1991;86:33–35.

186. Vallejos DA, Ambrosio AM, Feuillade MR, Maiztegui JI. Lymphocyte subsets alteration in patients with Argentine hemorrhagic fever. J Med Virol 1989;27:160–163.

187. van Eeden PJ, van Eeden SF, Joubert JR, King JB, van de Wal BW, Michell WL. A nosocomial outbreak of Crimean-Congo haemorrhagic fever at Tygerberg Hospital Part II. Management of patients. S Afr Med J 1985;68:718–721.

188. Vassalli P. The pathophysiology of tumor necrosis factor. Annu Rev Immunol 1992;10:411–452.

189. Volchkov VE, Blinov VM, Netesov SV. The envelope glycoprotein of Ebola virus contains an immunosuppressive-like domain similar to oncogenic retroviruses. FEBS Lett 1992;305:181–184.

190. Walker DH, Murphy FA. Pathology and pathogenesis of arenavirus infections. Current topics in microbiology and immunology 1987; 133:89–113.

191. Webb HE, Burston J. Clinical and pathological observations with special reference to the nervous system in Macaca radiata infected with Kyasanur Forest disease virus. Trans R Soc Trop Med Hyg 1966;60:325–331.

192. Webb HE, Chatterjea JB. Clinico-pathological observations on monkeys infected with Kyasanur Forest disease virus, with special reference to the haemopoietic system. 1962;8:401–413.

193. Webb HE, Rao RL. Kyasanur Forest disease: a general clinical study in which some cases with neurological complications were observed. Trans R Soc Trop Med Hyg 1961;55:284–298.

194. Work TH, Trapido H, Murthy PN, Rao RL, Bhatt PN, Kulkarni KG. Kyasanur Forest disease. III. A preliminary report on the nature of the infection and clinical manifestations in human beings. Indian J Med Sci 1957;11:619–645.

195. World Health Organization. Pathogenetic mechanisms in dengue hemorrhagic fever: report of an international collaborative study. Bull World Health Organ 1973;48:117.

196. World Health Organization. Ebola haemorrhagic fever in Zaire, 1976: report of an international commission. Bull World Health Organ 1978;56:271–93.

197. Xian-shi G, Dao-qin W, Shi-he Y, Dong-you Y. Activation of the alternative complement pathway in patients with epidemic hemorrhagic fever. Chin Med J (Engl) 1984;97:283–290.

198. Yan D, Gu X, Dao-qin W, Yang S. Studies on immunopathogenesis in epidemic hemorrhagic fever: sequential observations on activation of the first complement component in sera from patients with epidemic hemorrhagic fever. J Immunol 1981;127:1064–1069.

199. Yang CW, Bang BK. Changes of serum levels of tumor necrosis factor-alpha in patients with hemorrhagic fever with renal syndrome. J Catholic Med Coll 1992;45:819–830.

200. Yanigahara R, Silverman DJ. Experimental infection of human vascular endothelial cells by pathogenic and nonpathogenic Hantaviruses. Arch Virol 1990;111:281–286.

201. Yao JS, Arikawa J, Kariwa H, Yoshimatsu K, Takashima I, Hashimoto N. Effect of neutralizing monoclonal antibodies on Hantaan virus infection of the macrophage P388D1 cell line. Jpn J Vet Res 1992;40:87–97.

202. Zaki SR. Hantavirus-associated diseases. In: Schwartz D, Connor D, Chandler F, eds. Diagnostic pathology of infectious diseases. Norwalk, Connecticut: Appleton & Lange, 1995.

203. Zaki SR, PW Greer, LM Coffield, et al. Hantavirus pulmonary syndrome: pathogenesis of an emerging infectious disease. Am J Pathol 1995;146:552–579.

Viral Pathogenesis,
edited by Neal Nathanson, et al.
Lippincott–Raven Publishers, Philadelphia © 1997

CHAPTER 33

Viral Infections of the Fetus and Neonate

Ann M. Arvin

INTRODUCTION

Several of the human herpesviruses have the potential to infect the fetus and the newborn infant, with consequences that range from completely asymptomatic, subclinical infection to life-threatening or fatal disease. Among this group of viruses, cytomegalovirus (HCMV) is most likely to produce fetal injury as a result of intrauterine infection and herpes simplex virus (HSV), especially HSV-2, is the most important cause of severe neonatal disease resulting from viral transmission at the time of delivery. Varicella-zoster virus (VZV) can also result in serious intrauterine and perinatal disease. In contrast, Epstein-Barr virus (EBV) is a very rare cause of symptomatic fetal or neonatal infections. Human herpesvirus 6 (HHV-6) seems to be acquired most often in infancy, but pathologic effects have not been observed in the fetus or newborn.

Differences in the propensity of the various human herpesviruses to infect the fetus or newborn, or to cause clinical disease if infection occurs, are an intriguing but poorly understood aspect of virus-host interactions. Nevertheless, certain

basic characteristics of the pathogenesis of herpesvirus infections in the fetus and newborn are common to other human viruses. Because all of the herpesviruses establish latency and reactivate periodically after initial infection, fetal and neonatal herpesvirus infections also illustrate unique features that depend on whether virus infection of the mother is primary or recurrent. Much of what is known about the functional capacities of the fetal and neonatal immune system to respond to specific viral pathogens has emerged from studies of herpesvirus immunity.

EPIDEMIOLOGY OF INTRAUTERINE AND NEONATAL HERPESVIRUS INFECTIONS

Extensive clinical evidence indicates that most fetal and neonatal herpesvirus infections are acquired from the mother. These observations are confirmed by the finding that HCMV, HSV, and HHV-6 isolates recovered from mothers and their infected infants have identical DNA restriction enzyme profiles.[1,69]

The capacity of a viral pathogen to cause infection and disease is usually defined by the attack rate and the incidence of symptomatic illness that it produces among susceptible individuals. In the unique circumstance of pregnancy, virulence

A. M. Arvin: Departments of Pediatrics and Microbiology/Immunology, Stanford University School of Medicine, Stanford, California 94305

for the fetus or newborn is determined in part by the inherent potential of the virus to infect and damage the developing host, but fetal and neonatal risks are also related to whether the maternal infection is primary. The higher risk associated with primary maternal infections means that the epidemiologic patterns of infection in women of childbearing age must be considered before concluding that a particular virus is more or less pathogenic for the fetus and newborn.

The percentage of women of childbearing age who remain susceptible to the viral pathogen, and therefore may acquire a new infection during pregnancy, has a direct impact on fetal and neonatal risk. This principle is illustrated very well by the epidemiology of herpesvirus transmission and disease (Table 33-1). The rate of intrauterine HCMV infection is about 1 in 100 infants born in the United States each year, but disease is unusual; 90% to 95% of infected infants have no signs of fetal damage. The sequelae observed among 5% to 10% of infants who are infected in utero are almost always caused by primary maternal HCMV infection complicating the pregnancy. Many women are infected with HCMV in childhood; most instances of asymptomatic intrauterine HCMV infection are caused by transmission of the virus to the fetus from about 0.2% of these persistently infected mothers.[59] A second peak of HCMV acquisition is observed in adolescents and young women, reflecting transmission by sexual contact. This route of transmission probably accounts for the primary maternal infections that occur during pregnancy.

Primary maternal infection acquired late in gestation has a direct impact on the risk of herpesvirus transmission and disease resulting from perinatal exposure. Because HSV-2 infection is a sexually transmitted disease, the majority of young adult women are susceptible. The rate of acquisition of HSV-2 among pregnant women is about 0.5%, which is comparable to the incidence among nonpregnant adults.[10] The attack rate for disease in the newborn period approaches 50% if the mother develops primary HSV-2 infection in late gestation.[12,54] Seroepidemiologic studies done using assays that detect antibodies to type-specific proteins of HSV-2, such as glycoprotein G (gG), indicate that 25% or more of pregnant women of all socioeconomic classes have had a prior infec-

tion with HSV-2.[54] These women may have HSV-2 reactivation at delivery, but the risk of perinatal transmission from recurrent maternal HSV-2 is less than 5%. Primary maternal infection acquired near term is rare compared with the high prevalence of HSV-2 infections acquired before pregnancy, but the difference in transmission rates means that these infections account for about half of the estimated 1200 cases of neonatal HSV infection that occur annually in the United States. A comparison of HSV-1 and HSV-2 also illustrates the significance of epidemiologic variables as opposed to virulence factors in determining the risk of perinatal infection. HSV-1 accounts for much less neonatal disease than HSV-2 in the United States because primary HSV-1 infection usually occurs in childhood. Nevertheless, HSV-1 is as likely to be life-threatening for newborns as HSV-2 if it is acquired from a mother with primary infection or from another contact by an infant born to a seronegative mother.[68]

In contrast to the other herpesviruses, VZV is transmitted efficiently by the respiratory route, causing annual epidemics of varicella with high rates of infection during childhood. VZV is an uncommon intrauterine pathogen, in part because of the low incidence of maternal varicella, which was identified as a complication of only 0.07% of pregnancies in one large series.[13] If primary maternal VZV infection occurs during pregnancy, the risk of congenital varicella syndrome is approximately 3%; perinatal transmission causes neonatal varicella, with an attack rate of about 30%, among infants born to women with varicella at term.[13,26,50]

Primary EBV infection during pregnancy is very unusual because only about 1% to 3% of pregnant women remain susceptible to this virus.[27,44] Its association with fetal infection is uncertain. As evidenced by antibodies to early antigen (EA) as a marker, 55% of pregnant women had evidence of EBV reactivation, compared with 22% to 32% of nonpregnant adults, but none of the infants born to these women had signs of intrauterine infection.[20] HHV-6 is acquired by most children within the first few years of life, leaving very few adult women at risk for primary infection. Only one case of possible intrauterine HHV-6 has been reported; if perinatal transmission occurs, it has not caused identifiable disease in newborn infants.[6]

TABLE 33-1. *Epidemiology of primary and recurrent maternal herpesvirus infections during pregnancy and risk of viral transmission to the fetus or newborn infant*

Virus	Prevalence of infection in adult women (%)		Proportion of susceptible women acquiring primary infection in a single pregnancy (%)	Risk of fetal damage from maternal infection during pregnancy		Risk of neonatal disease from maternal infection at delivery	
	Susceptible	Prior infection		Primary	Recurrent	Primary	Recurrent
HCMV	20	80	1–4	18%	Very rare	Very rare*	Very rare
HSV-2	75	25	0.5	Rare	Rare or none	50%	<5%
VZV	5	95	0.07	2–3%	Rare or none	30%	None
EBV	2	98	<0.01	Rare or none	None	None	None
HHV-6	1	99	<0.01	Rare or none	None	None	None

HCMV, human cytomegalovirus; HSV-2, herpes simplex virus type 2; VZV, varicella-zoster virus; EBV, Epstein-Barr virus; HHV-6, human herpesvirus type 6.
*Neonatal disease rates are distinguished from asymptomatic infection in the case of HCMV.

MECHANISMS OF ENHANCED FETAL AND NEONATAL RISK FROM PRIMARY MATERNAL INFECTION

The two major pathogenic mechanisms that account for the higher fetal and neonatal risks associated with primary maternal herpesvirus infections acquired during pregnancy or at term are (1) more extensive viral replication in the mother who lacks immunity and (2) delayed or limited transplacental transfer of virus-specific maternal immunoglobulin G (IgG) antibodies to the infant.

Viral Replication

Maternal viremia, which is probably critical for intrauterine infection, is characteristic of primary infection with HCMV and VZV. VZV is detectable in peripheral blood mononuclear cells (PBMCs) that have the morphologic appearance of lymphocytes, for several days before and after the appearance of the cutaneous varicella rash.[43] Viremia is probably a factor in VZV pathogenesis, because the congenital varicella syndrome is associated with primary infection acquired during pregnancy; maternal herpes zoster, in which viral replication is localized to cutaneous dermatomal sites, does not cause this unique syndrome. Case reports of disseminated HSV suggest that the pathogenesis of primary HSV infection includes a viremic phase in some pregnant women, which may explain the rare instances of transplacental HSV infection.[38]

HSV-2 illustrates the contribution of enhanced viral replication to the increased risk of perinatal transmission to the newborn infant as a result of primary maternal infection. The sites of replication include the cervix and the lower genital tract, increasing the opportunity for exposure of the infant to higher titers of infectious virus during primary infection.[12,68] Primary oral gingivostomatitis may be accompanied by asymptomatic HSV-1 replication in the genital tract, allowing exposure of the infant at delivery to the virus at a remote site even though HSV-1 recurrences are limited to the oral mucosa. In the case of HCMV, antibody titers to specific proteins are higher in mothers who transmit the virus to their infants, indicating greater antigenic stimulation from enhanced virus replication.[11] Higher titers of virus in the birth canal probably contribute to perinatal transmission of HCMV from mothers with recent primary infection.

Like HCMV, EBV can be detected in peripheral blood cells during and after primary infection, but EBV rarely causes fetal infection. Differences in the extent to which viral latency is maintained could explain the difference in rates of transmission to the fetus. EBV is perpetuated in an episomal, nonreplicating form within latently infected B lymphocytes, whereas HCMV detected in peripheral blood cells probably represents infectious virus taken up from other sites of active viral replication. Paralleling the lack of transplacental transmission, EBV is a very rare cause of transfusion-acquired infection, even among immunocompromised patients, whereas HCMV transmission by blood products is well documented.[70] Information is very limited, but initial studies indicate that HHV-6 is also rarely transmitted transplacentally, even though it persists in PBMCs. Better understanding of EBV and HHV-6 latency should help to explain why these viruses rarely infect the fetus despite their presence in peripheral blood cells of almost all pregnant women.

Maternal IgG Antibodies

Transplacentally acquired IgG antibodies to herpesvirus proteins have an important role in protecting the fetus and newborn from transplacental or perinatal transmission of infectious virus and from severe disease if infection occurs. Definite correlations of higher risk with low or absent virus-specific maternal antibodies at the time of fetal or neonatal exposure are established for HCMV, HSV-2, and VZV.

The risk of sequelae in infants with congenital HCMV infection is predictable from the maternal antibody status before conception.[23] In one large, prospective study, signs of congenital infection were present at birth in 18% of 189 infants born to seronegative women who acquired HCMV during pregnancy; 13% of these 189 infants had severe mental impairment (intelligence quotient [IQ] <70) in later childhood. In contrast, all infants with intrauterine HCMV infection whose mothers were seropositive before pregnancy were asymptomatic at birth, and none had an IQ of less than 70.[23] Neonatal HCMV infection is also modified by maternally derived IgG antibodies to the virus. Premature infants born to seropositive mothers are less likely to develop pneumonia and other complications of transfusion-acquired HCMV than those who have no passive antibodies to the virus.[66]

Transplacentally acquired neutralizing antibodies prevent infection by blocking virus attachment and entry into cells, whereas antibodies that mediate cellular cytotoxicity (ADCC) act with leukocytes to induce cell lysis before the release of new infectious virus. The protective role of passively acquired antibodies with these functions is illustrated by studies of perinatal HSV transmission.[51,54,63,64] Infants with maternally derived IgG antibodies to HSV-2 in cord blood are at very low risk of infection despite exposure to infectious virus. In our studies, neutralizing antibody titers to HSV were more than 1:20 in 79% of infants exposed to maternal HSV-2 reactivation, antibodies to HSV-2 gG were detected in 91%, ADCC antibody titers were high, and none of the infants became infected.[42,63,64] In contrast, all infants with symptomatic neonatal HSV disease lacked neutralizing antibodies to HSV or had titers less than 1:20, and their ADCC and type-specific antibodies to HSV-2 gG were also low or undetectable. HSV-1 and HSV-2 are closely related antigenically, and antibodies to the glycoproteins B and D mediate cross-neutralization of the two virus types. Nevertheless, the evidence correlating type-specific antibodies with better protection from HSV-2 disease indicates that transplacentally acquired antibodies require a high degree of specificity for the infecting agent in order to prevent maternal-infant transmission of viral pathogens.[5,64]

The pathogenesis of neonatal infection may be altered if transplacentally acquired antibodies interfere with viral replication after infection is established. In our experience, infants with the disseminated form of neonatal herpes infection were less likely to have neutralizing, ADCC, and HSV-2 gG antibodies than infants who had localized mucocutaneous or central nervous system disease.[42,64] These observations suggest that passively transferred antibodies sometimes protect the infant from progressive disease by limiting cell-to-cell spread after infection and by blocking attachment and cell entry at the initial site of virus inoculation.

Maternal varicella in late gestation provides a natural experiment that documents the impact of the maternal IgG response on disease.[13,26] Infants exposed to maternal varicella in cases in which the mother's rash began more than 4 days before delivery are born with varicella lesions or have rash within the first 5 days, but they do not develop disseminated VZV infection. The 4-day interval between the onset of maternal infection and delivery permits the transfer of maternal VZV antibodies of the IgG subclass to the fetus. This clinical circumstance proves that the transplacental transfer of antiviral antibodies is highly efficient in late gestation, because high titers of VZV IgG antibodies do not appear in serum until at least 2 to 4 days after the onset of varicella. Infants who are born less than 4 days after the onset of maternal varicella lack transplacentally acquired VZV antibodies and are at risk for life-threatening varicella in the newborn period. The attack rate is reduced significantly by giving varicella-zoster immune globulin to these infants at birth. However, some infants develop severe, progressive varicella despite passive antibody prophylaxis, indicating that the balance between the virus inoculum and virus-specific passive antibody titers is critical in determining the outcome of neonatal exposure to viral pathogens.

PATHOGENESIS OF FETAL INFECTION

Viral Transmission to the Fetus

The two pathways that permit infection of the fetus are virus transmission across the placenta and infection that ascends from the maternal genital tract. The consensus is that human herpesvirus infections acquired in utero most often represent transplacental rather than ascending infection.

Transplacental Transmission

Important progress has been made in understanding the anatomy and functions of the placenta, with implications concerning virus transmission to the fetus.[7] Figure 33-1 illustrates the relation between the maternal and fetal circulations within the placenta and possible mechanisms involved in the pathogenesis of intrauterine herpesvirus infections.[7] Maternal blood flows through the intervillous spaces of the placenta. In order

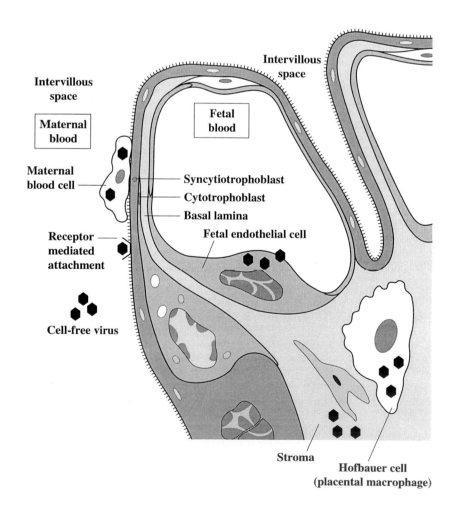

FIG. 33-1. The cytoarchitecture of the placenta and potential mechanisms of transplacental transmission of herpesviruses. (Modified from Benirschke K, Kaufman P. Pathology of the human placenta. 2nd ed. New York: Springer-Verlag, 1990.)

to gain access to the fetal circulation, infectious virus or infected maternal cells must move from the maternal blood or peripheral blood cells in these spaces and traverse the trophoblast and its basal lamina as well as the basement membrane and endothelial cells composing the fetal villous capillaries. An intervening phase of infection of the stromal cells may occur before virus moves across fetal capillary cells.[7,58]

As the first step in transmission to the fetus, the virus must cross the trophoblast, which consists of the syncytiotrophoblast and the cytotrophoblast. The syncytiotrophoblast is a multinucleated cell layer that provides an epithelial-like surface lining the whole extent of the intervillous spaces. This cell layer separates the fetal structures of the placenta from maternal blood flowing through these spaces. It is referred to as the trophoblast because it appears to form a continuous syncytium, rather than being made up of adjacent but distinct cells. The cytotrophoblast is just beneath the syncytiotrophoblast and is the probable source of new cellular components during gestation. The surface of the syncytiotrophoblast is covered with microvilli that are exposed constantly to maternal blood flow and have surface receptors involved in transplacental transfer of proteins. Specific receptors for insulin and various growth factors as well as Fc receptors involved in IgG transport have been identified in the microvilli. The fetal blood vessels form the villous tree, ending in the fetal capillaries located within the terminal villi; sections of the endothelial cell walls of the fetal capillaries lie next to the inner basal lamina of the trophoblast (see Fig. 33-1). The fetal capillaries are surrounded by the stromal cells that make up the mesenchymal core of the chorionic villi. The stromal cells are fixed connective tissue cells of probable fibroblast lineage, which are arranged in a loose network in which the characteristic placental Hofbauer cells are distributed. Hofbauer cells are considered to be fetal macrophages; they may be replaced by cell division or by recruitment of new cells from the fetal circulation.

The initial pathogenic event involved in transplacental transmission of viruses probably depends on whether the virus exists in a cell-free state in maternal plasma or is carried in maternal peripheral blood cells. Herpesviruses usually circulate within peripheral blood cells, but HCMV may be an exception, because recent studies using polymerase chain reaction methods demonstrated HCMV DNA in plasma as well as in leukocytes.[69] If the positive polymerase chain reaction signal indicates the presence of cell-free virus, HCMV could attach to virus receptor binding sites and infect the trophoblast directly. Alternatively, HCMV may not be detected in plasma by standard tissue culture methods because it is complexed with IgG antibodies; in this case, the Fc receptors on the trophoblast could mediate the transfer of virus-IgG complexes. Assuming that HCMV viremia is not exclusively intracellular, the higher rates of intrauterine transmission compared with other herpesviruses could be explained by this difference in the pathogenesis of maternal infection.

Some information about the next step, in which the virus enters the trophoblast layer of the placenta, is available for HCMV.[60] Immunohistochemical staining of placentas from pregnancies in which the fetus had symptomatic HCMV disease shows that only the immediate early proteins of HCMV are detectable in the trophoblast. Because early and late viral proteins are required to make new infectious virus, this obser-

vation suggests that transmission to the fetus does not require a complete cycle of replication in the trophoblast. Some in vitro studies indicate that trophoblast cells support HCMV and HSV replication, and others suggest that these cells are not permissive.[49] Interpreting these variable results is difficult because culture conditions cannot reproduce the complex environment of growth factors, cytokines, and native cells of the placenta. Conceptually, the trophoblast phase of virus transfer could be transient and not accompanied by the production of new virions, acting only to move the infectious virus particle or viral DNA into stromal cells in the chorionic villi or into endothelial cells of the fetal capillaries. There are transtrophoblastic channels or pores, from 17 to 25 nm diameter, in guinea pig trophoblast[7]; smaller viruses may cross the trophoblast through these channels, but the unenveloped HCMV virion is 105 nm in diameter.[1] Biologic mechanisms are probably more important than physical pathways in the transport of complex viral pathogens to the fetus.

If maternal viremia is cell-associated, infectious virus may enter the syncytiotrophoblast and cytotrophoblast by cell-to-cell spread, or intact, infected maternal blood cells may cross the trophoblast. Cell-to-cell spread is a likely mechanism if maternal macrophages harbor the pathogen, because these cells, especially activated macrophages expressing increased major histocompatibility class II antigen, are observed in close association with the trophoblast during all stages of gestation.[37] Virus that enters the trophoblast layer may or may not replicate at this site before spreading into stromal cells of the chorionic villi or into the endothelial cells of the fetal capillaries. Viral antigens have been detected in fetal capillary endothelium in cases of HCMV and HSV placentitis, and herpesviruses replicate in endothelial cells in vitro. Dissemination of infectious virus may occur by direct release from endothelial cells into the fetal circulation, or, as has been described with HCMV in other clinical circumstances, infected endothelial cells may detach and be carried to other sites by hematogenous routes.[31]

Intact maternal lymphocytes are detected in the fetal circulation, but migration of these cells across the trophoblast, including both the superficial and basal laminae, and through the fetal capillary endothelium into the fetal circulation, appears to be a rare event. Whether cell-associated viremia causes fetal infection by this mechanism could depend on the type of peripheral blood cell that is infected and on the number of virus-infected cells in the maternal circulation. There is no definitive evidence that transfer of intact, infected maternal cells is a pathogenic mechanism leading to fetal infection, but the transmission of VZV from mothers with varicella in late gestation supports the possibility. VZV viremia is entirely cell-associated, with about 1 in 30,000 to 100,000 mononuclear cells containing the virus, and viremia precedes the appearance of the mucocutaneous rash by 24 to 48 hours.[43] Infants who are delivered during this 2-day interval, before any possible exposure to the virus in maternal mucocutaneous lesions, develop infection. The direct transfer of VZV-infected maternal peripheral blood cells to the fetus seems to be the most likely explanation for these cases of neonatal varicella.

The hierarchy of fetal infection rates associated with different herpesviruses may be explained if the highest risk is associated with the presence of virus in plasma as well as in leukocytes or mononuclear cells, as illustrated by HCMV. An intermediate risk may result if viremia is completely cell-associated, as in VZV, and there may be little or no risk if virus is confined to mucocutaneous sites only, as usually occurs during primary HSV infection in the healthy host. Comparison of HCMV and VZV with HSV suggests that viremia, whether cell-associated or not, is a necessary condition for transplacental transmission of herpesviruses. The fact that intrauterine EBV infections are extremely rare indicates that viremia is not a sufficient condition, because primary EBV infection is associated with a very high frequency of infected circulating cells. Because VZV appears to infect T lymphocytes and EBV infects B lymphocytes, the cell type that carries the virus in peripheral blood may determine transmissibility. Failure to document fetal transmission results in part from the low frequency of primary EBV infection during pregnancy, but even this low rate should result in the birth of approximately 2500 exposed infants each year in the United States.[22]

Whether the transplacental transmission of herpesviruses requires a phase of active virus replication in stromal cells of the chorionic villi is not known. The capacity of HCMV to infect stromal cells of the chorionic villi has been demonstrated by detection of inclusion-containing cells, immunohistochemical staining for viral proteins, and in situ hybridization.[29,48,56,57] Chorionic villitis caused by HSV or VZV is rare but has also been reported.[2,24,38a,68] Foci of cells expressing HSV-2 antigens were observed within the chorionic villi, and the presence of complete virions was confirmed by electron microscopy in the placenta from an infant of 30 weeks gestation.[48] VZV infection of the placenta is characterized by focal necrosis with inclusion-containing cells.[7,21] Only one case of chorionic villitis associated with EBV has been reported.[50]

Chronic infection of the chorionic villi is not essential for herpesvirus transmission, because normal placental histology is described in some cases of in utero HCMV infection.[1] Nevertheless, chronic lymphoplasmacytic villitis, with diffuse stromal hyperplasia, is common when the fetus or infant has signs of intrauterine damage. Only a few percent of the antigen-positive cells are classic inclusion-bearing cells, but immediate early, early, and late HCMV proteins are detected in many placental cells by immunologic methods. Whether the cells involved in this process represent fetal macrophages (Hofbauer cells) or connective tissue fibroblasts is uncertain.[58,60]

Although it is not essential, multifocal infection of the chorionic villi probably facilitates virus transmission to the fetus. Virus-induced cell lysis and the associated inflammatory reaction disrupt the cellular and basal lamina barriers to the fetal circulation, and extensive stromal replication probably enhances cell-to-cell spread of virus into capillary endothelial cells. In HCMV placentitis, diffuse infection and focal necrosis of the stromal cells in the chorionic villi are accompanied by evidence of infection of adjacent macrophages and endothelial cells.[60] Viral pathogens that are capable of escaping destruction by the villous macrophages (Hofbauer cells) or that replicate actively in these cells may be more likely to reach the fetal circulation. Effective restriction of herpesvirus replication to placental cells is also possible, because extensive histopathologic changes have been observed in cases in which the fetus escaped HCMV infection.[35]

Herpesvirus transmission is not likely to occur during the earliest stage after conception, which is the interval required for implantation of the embryo and differentiation of the structures that constitute the interface between the maternal and fetal circulation. Implantation is considered to be complete and maternal erythrocytes are observed in the developing lacunae at about 11 days after fertilization, and formation of secondary villi begins at about 14 days.[7] Therefore, embryonic infection is unlikely if the maternal infection resolves within 10 to 14 days after conception.

Maternal virus infections may cause fetal morbidity indirectly by precipitating spontaneous abortion or premature delivery. Studies of women who acquire HCMV, HSV, or VZV during pregnancy do not show an increase above the background incidence of miscarriage, which is about 3%, and the few anecdotal reports of spontaneous abortion associated with primary HSV infections indicate that it is a rare event.[1,62,68] Induction of preterm labor is observed when maternal varicella complicates late pregnancy, and a disproportionate number of infants with neonatal herpes infection are born prematurely. One hypothesis is that maternal macrophages are activated by exposure to interferon-γ (IFN-γ) produced by antigen-stimulated lymphocytes and release high concentrations of prostaglandin E_2, triggering labor.[37] However, primary maternal HCMV infection is not associated with preterm labor, even if there is widespread chorionic villitis, indicating that herpesviruses often do not precipitate this reaction.[48,51]

Ascending Infection

The second possible route of intrauterine viral infection is ascending infection with transfer of virus from the maternal genital tract to the fetus across intact membranes. Fetal infection by the ascending route is a very rare mechanism of herpesvirus transmission, except in a few cases of intrauterine HSV disease. Intrauterine HSV infection has been associated with histopathologic changes of chorioamnionitis and inflammation along the umbilical cord, referred to as funisitis; in one case, cells expressing HSV antigens were detected in a region of the fetal membranes that was probably next to the cervix as well as in outer sections of the cord.[35] Cervical cells support HSV replication, and high titers of infectious virus can be recovered from this site for several weeks, especially during primary maternal infection. Cells of the chorioamnionic membranes may be infected by local extension from the cervix or by maternal viremia, followed by release of infectious virus into the amniotic fluid. In most circumstances, maternal IgG antibodies present in the amniotic fluid probably protect the fetus from effective inoculation of mucous membranes by neutralizing the virus.[54,68]

Cell Tropism and Pathologic Consequences of Fetal Infection

The risk of intrauterine transmission varies significantly among the human herpesviruses, but the pathologic effects of fetal infection exhibit many similarities. The spectrum ranges from asymptomatic infection to lethal damage. The herpesviruses injure the fetus as a direct result of cytopathic and in-flammatory damage within developing organs (embryopathy) rather than by virtue of teratogenic effects like those associated with intrauterine exposure to drugs or environmental toxins. The fetal inflammatory response probably magnifies virus-induced tissue destruction in some target organs. Along with virus-induced cytopathology, infants who are severely affected by congenital HCMV, VZV, or HSV infection have generalized intrauterine growth retardation resulting from placental insufficiency caused by chronic infection.

As is true of other viral pathogens, the risk of herpesvirus infection of the fetus must be differentiated from the risk of fetal damage. Virus transmission to the fetus early in gestation increases the incidence of symptomatic infection. For example, the rate of HCMV transmission is about 50% whether primary maternal infection occurs before or after the first 22 weeks of gestation, but about a third of infants exposed to neonatal HCMV infection during the first half of gestation have sequelae, whereas none of the infants with later maternal infection develop clinical signs of intrauterine HCMV.[62] High titers of maternal IgG antibodies to HCMV gB and higher HCMV IgM antibodies at the first prenatal visit (8 to 16 weeks) correlate with the risk of hearing loss in infants who are otherwise asymptomatic, confirming that maternal infection in early gestation is the definitive risk factor for fetal damage.[9] The incidence of virus transmission to the fetus is also comparable after early- and late-gestation exposures to VZV, but the congenital varicella syndrome is associated with fetal exposure during the first half of gestation.[13,26,51]

Infants with intrauterine HCMV, VZV, or HSV disease have infection of multiple organs, indicating that these viruses cause viremia in the fetus. Viral replication in fetal tissues may be potentiated by the high rate of cell division occurring in early development. The in vitro replication of HCMV, VZV, and HSV is most efficient in subconfluent human fetal cell monolayers. Virus tropism for the developing central nervous system produces severe morbidity. Severely affected infants who have intrauterine HCMV, VZV, or HSV infection are born with microcephaly caused by generalized or focal encephalitis and cerebral atrophy. At birth, these infants often have little or no intact cortical tissue, scattered calcifications, and, occasionally, large porencephalic cysts or hydrocephalus. Infants with HCMV infection of the central nervous system have multinucleated, inclusion-bearing cells within both white and gray matter. Neuronal cells with cyto-pathic changes characteristic of HCMV are prominent, but inclusions are also detected in glial cells and in the choroid plexus, ependyma, and meninges.[1] Areas of focal necrosis throughout the brain parenchyma evolve to gliosis and calci-fications. Similar pathologic changes occur with intrauterine VZV and HSV encephalitis.[26,38,68] Some destruction of brain tissue is probably secondary to virus-induced vasculitis, ischemia, and infarctions caused by direct herpesvirus infection of vascular endothelial cells or by the fetal inflammatory response.

Chorioretinitis and other ocular anomalies are common with symptomatic HCMV, VZV, or HSV intrauterine infection. Chorioretinitis is probably a consequence of the capacity of these viruses to produce acute vasculitis. Continued local viral replication has been demonstrated by the recovery of

HCMV from vitreous fluid, and VZV has been detected by polymerase chain reaction.[1] Other signs of herpesvirus tropism for ocular tissues of the fetus include microopthalmia, cataracts, and optic neuritis with atrophy of the optic discs.

The liver is the second major organ that is usually infected during intrauterine HCMV, HSV, or VZV infection. In HCMV, inclusions are present in hepatocytes and in Kupffer cells; cholangitis, with signs of viral infection of epithelial cells of the biliary ducts, and cholestasis are prominent histopathologic abnormalities.[1,62] Transient ascites followed by calcification in the liver is detected in utero and after birth. HCMV hepatitis may occur without associated encephalitis, demonstrating that infection of one major organ in utero does not always mean that other potential target organs will be damaged. Early reports suggested that hepatic infection caused cirrhosis or biliary atresia, but subsequent studies indicated that HCMV hepatitis usually resolves without irreversibly damaging the liver or biliary tract.[62] Although the pathologic mechanism is not known, infants with congenital HCMV infection often develop transient hepatomegaly and abnormal hepatocellular function with jaundice in the newborn period. This clinical observation suggests that a phase of increased viral replication in the liver is initiated after birth but subsides without producing chronic liver dysfunction. In contrast to disseminated VZV and HSV infections acquired at delivery, HCMV hepatitis is usually not fulminant and rarely progresses to hepatic failure.

Like hepatitis, the hematologic abnormalities associated with symptomatic congenital HCMV infection are usually not evident at birth, but most infants develop postnatal thrombocytopenia, anemia, and pancytopenia.[1] In exceptional cases, anemia associated with intrauterine HCMV is severe enough to cause nonimmune hydrops in utero; intrauterine HSV-1 infection resulting in hydrops fetalis has also been described.[30] Intradermal erythropoiesis, with the classic "blueberry muffin" rash, has been observed in a few infants with congenital HCMV infection, indicating persistent interference with bone marrow function. Some hematologic changes may be caused by splenomegaly and hypersplenism associated with chronic HCMV replication in utero. Thrombocytopenia may also be caused by direct viral lysis of megakaryocytes. Although low platelet counts, anemia, and neutropenia can persist for weeks or months after birth, these abnormalities usually resolve spontaneously.

Historically, intrauterine HCMV infection was first differentiated from congenital syphilis and referred to as congenital inclusion disease after the detection of desquamated cells with inclusions in urine. Very high titers of HCMV (approximately 10^{-4} to 10^{-5} times the median tissue culture infective dose in 0.2 mL) are excreted in the urine of infants with intrauterine HCMV infection, whether or not the infant has symptomatic disease.[1,62] Nevertheless, the kidneys show no pathologic changes, although cells of the distal convoluted tubules and collecting ducts contain viral inclusions, and virus-infected cells can be demonstrated by in situ hybridization and im-munohistochemical staining for viral protein expression.

Viral tropism for alveolar cells of the lung, with associated inflammatory reactions that produce life-threatening pneu-monitis, is characteristic of severe HCMV infection in other immunocompromised populations, including patients with human immunodeficiency virus (HIV) infection and bone marrow transplant recipients. HCMV pneumonitis is also the major pathologic disorder in infants who develop symptomatic HCMV infection after perinatal transmission from blood products.[70] In contrast, infants with intrauterine HCMV infection rarely have severe pulmonary disease, even though pathologic examination of lung tissue shows extensive viral infection. This clinical difference correlates with an absent or limited interstitial inflammatory process in the lungs and indicates that the host response, in addition to the cell tropism of the virus, is a critical determinant of organ damage. Infants with intrauterine VZV or HSV infection may have involvement of the lung, but they usually have no signs of pulmonary disease, in contrast to the life-threatening pneumonitis associated with perinatally acquired VZV or HSV infections. Identification of host factors that reduce inflammation in infants who have intrauterine infections that do not appear to be active postnatally, even if the same virus infects the newborn, warrants further investigation.

In addition to their similarities in cell tropism, HCMV, VZV, and HSV exhibit characteristic pathologic differences. For example, HCMV usually infects the salivary glands and the cells of the inner ear that constitute the organ of Corti and the cochlea.[1] The most striking anomalies of the congenital varicella syndrome are unusual cutaneous defects with cicatricial skin scarring and atrophy of an extremity.[32,51] Evidence of damage to the autonomic nervous system also indicates that VZV has tropism for cells of the developing peripheral nervous system as well as for brain parenchyma.

The failure to establish and maintain viral latency is an important characteristic of host-virus interactions in HCMV, VZV, or HSV infection of the fetus. The high titers of virus in urine of infants with congenital HCMV persist for months to years after birth, whereas adults with primary HCMV infection have transient virus excretion.[52,53] The occurrence of herpes zoster in infancy, without any preceding episode of varicella, is often the only evidence of VZV transmission in infants who were exposed to maternal varicella during pregnancy.[13] Herpes zoster results from VZV reactivation and is otherwise rare in childhood. Infants who have intrauterine HSV infection are often born with widely scattered, cutaneous lesions and have extensive, frequent recurrences of skin vesicles for months or years.[38]

PATHOGENESIS OF NEONATAL INFECTION

Viral Transmission to the Newborn

The usual route for perinatal herpesvirus transmission is by inoculation of mucous membranes with infectious virus present in the maternal genital tract. HSV and HCMV can be recovered from oropharyngeal secretions of the infant immediately after delivery.[4] The infant is usually protected from ascending infection across intact membranes, but some infants acquire HSV despite cesarean delivery from mothers whose membranes were apparently intact, indicating that this barrier may not be effective at preventing HSV spread after the onset of labor. The generalized immunosuppressive effects of pregnancy may influence whether herpesviruses are present in the genital tract at delivery. The incidence of HCMV reacti-

vation involving the cervix increases from 2.7% in the first trimester to 6.9% in the third trimester.[62] Active infection occurs at term in about 1% to 2% of women who are seropositive for HSV-2, but the stage of gestation has little effect on the frequency of asymptomatic or clinical HSV-2 reactivations.[49] If the mother has varicella in late gestation, the infant may be exposed to infectious virus in maternal lesions during or after delivery as well as by transplacental transfer of virus just before birth. Hematogenous transmission may result from placental leakage and maternal-fetal transfusion during the birth process, but it is probably a rare cause of perinatal herpesvirus transmission.

The incidence of perinatal transmission of herpesviruses varies depending on the pathogen and whether the maternal infection is a primary one. As described previously, the attack rate for neonatal HSV infection approaches 50% if the mother has a primary infection, compared with less than 5% if the infant is exposed to recurrent maternal infection.[54] In contrast, HCMV is often transmitted to the newborn infant from recurrent maternal infection; in one large, prospective study, the perinatal transmission rate was 57% if infants were exposed to cervical HCMV reactivation.[62] The risk of neonatal varicella after perinatal exposure to primary maternal VZV infection is about 30% unless the infant receives varicella-zoster immune globulin, but maternal herpes zoster at term is not associated with VZV transmission to the infant.[13,26] Documentation of EBV transmission at delivery is difficult for technical reasons, but it may occur, because EBV DNA is detected in cervical specimens and serologic studies suggest that EBV reactivation is more common during pregnancy.[20,21,61,66] Many children have serologic evidence of EBV infection by 12 to 24 months, but perinatally acquired infections cannot be differentiated from those caused by later exposures to EBV in oral secretions of the mother or other immune contacts.[3]

Breastfeeding is an important potential mechanism of perinatal transmission for many viruses, including HCMV. Exposure to HCMV in breast milk, without exposure to cervical reactivation, resulted in transmission to 63% of infants.[62] Nosocomial transmission is less common in herpesvirus infections than for other viral pathogens, but nursery outbreaks of varicella have been reported.[26] Newborn infants can be inoculated with HSV from individuals who have herpes labialis or by transmission on hands or fomites from another infected infant in the nursery.[68]

Cell Tropism and Pathologic Consequences of Neonatal Infection

Although HCMV transmission to the newborn is very common, it is almost always subclinical; perinatal HSV and VZV infections, on the other hand, are usually life-threatening. Many infants who are exposed to HSV at delivery do not develop clinical signs of neonatal herpes, but these infants are asymptomatic because they have escaped infection.[47,55]

The initial manifestations of neonatal HSV infection are localized mucocutaneous infection, disseminated disease, or meningoencephalitis.[47,68] Infants fail to restrict HSV replication to mucocutaneous sites, and life-threatening complications occur in about 70% of cases unless antiviral therapy is given. Infants with disseminated HSV-1 or HSV-2 disease usually have pneumonitis, hepatitis, and cardiovascular collapse, with or without meningoencephalitis. The involvement of multiple organs, the appearance of scattered vesicular skin lesions, and the recovery of infectious virus from blood demonstrate that viremia is the underlying pathogenic mechanism. The consequence of uncontrolled viral replication is fulminant disease that is fatal in 50% of cases even with antiviral therapy. Histopathologic evidence of necrosis is seen in the liver, lungs, spleen, and adrenal glands, and virus is recovered from most tissues. HSV-2 encephalitis in the newborn usually begins in the temporal or parietal lobes but progresses rapidly to extensive, bilateral disease. Transplacentally acquired antibodies do not always prevent this process, presumably because the virus is less accessible if it is spreading by neural pathways.

The cell tropism of VZV during the newborn period resembles progressive varicella in immunocompromised patients.[13,26] Deficient control of cell-associated viremia is evident from the dissemination of the virus to lungs, liver, central nervous system, bone marrow, and other organs. Varicella pneumonitis, fulminant hepatitis, and disseminated intravascular coagulopathy are the life-threatening pathologic consequences of perinatal VZV infection.

Symptomatic perinatal HCMV infection is limited to disease in premature or high-risk newborns, especially those born to seronegative mothers, who acquire the virus from blood products.[62,70] These infants have pneumonia, hepatitis, and thrombocytopenia, but HCMV is much less virulent even in high-risk, premature infants than is HSV or VZV acquired perinatally.

EBV is the only herpesvirus for which a possible association between perinatal or early neonatal infection and oncogenicity has been proposed, because of a serologic correlation between high titers of antibodies to EBV viral capsid antigen and the subsequent occurrence of Burkitt lymphoma in African children.[18] If this hypothesis is correct, EBV resembles the increased oncogenic potential of animal tumor viruses for infection occurring in the neonatal period.[3]

HOST FACTORS THAT INFLUENCE HERPESVIRUS PATHOGENESIS IN THE FETUS AND NEWBORN

Maternal Immunity

Altered maternal immunity may facilitate intrauterine or perinatal transmission of herpesviruses by reducing the capacity to localize viral replication to mucocutaneous sites, to terminate viremia, or to maintain latency (Table 33-2). Some mothers of infants with congenital HCMV infection have diminished T-cell recognition of HCMV antigens in vitro, but poor responses do not correlate definitively with virus transmission to the fetus.[1] The risk of dissemination during maternal VZV or HSV infection appears to increase in later gestation, suggesting a cumulative suppression of cellular immunity during pregnancy.[13,51] Maternal cellular immune responses are not likely to modify the course of infection in the fetus or newborn directly, and early studies suggesting that antigen-specific T cells are transferred in utero have not been confirmed.

The transplacental transfer of virus-specific maternal IgG antibodies has a definitive impact on herpesvirus pathogenesis in the fetus and newborn. IgG transport is a passive process in early gestation; IgG antibodies are detectable in fetal blood at 8 weeks, but titers remain low until about 20 weeks.[67] Therefore, the fetus may be at greater risk of infection and sequelae

TABLE 33-2. *Host factors that influence viral pathogenesis in the fetus and newborn*

MATERNAL IMMUNITY

Potential for increased viral replication during primary infection due to impaired maternal immune responses
Effect of gestational stage on transplacental transfer of virus-specific IgG antibodies
Potential for less effective maintenance of herpesvirus latency

PLACENTAL MECHANISMS

Macrophages
    Viral inhibitory functions
    Susceptibility to viral replication

DEVELOPING FETAL IMMUNE SYSTEM

B lymphocytes
    Diminished IgG production
    Delayed switching from IgM to IgG production
T lymphocytes
    Absent or diminished induction of antigen-specific T-cells
    Diminished IFN-γ production
Nonspecific responses
    Absent or diminished IFN-α production
    Diminished natural killer cell function
    Limited antibody dependent cellular cytotoxicity

early in gestation because of limited transfer of antiviral antibodies, even though primary infection elicits equivalent IgG titers among pregnant women who are infected early or late in gestation. Active transport, in which maternal IgG antibodies are transferred across the trophoblast by receptor-dependent mechanisms, results in a gradual increase in fetal IgG concentrations from 20 weeks' gestation to birth. Infant IgG titers at birth are usually about 10% higher than maternal titers to the same antigen, which is also true of IgG antibodies to herpesviruses. Sites in the Fc region of the IgG heavy chain determine placental transfer; the efficient transfer of herpesvirus antibodies indicates that they are processed, as expected, by the trophoblast transport mechanisms.[19] Virus-specific IgA antibodies, which are probably important in blocking mucosal inoculation, cannot be transferred across the placenta, but IgG antibodies with neutralizing and other antiviral activities are detected at mucosal sites in newborn infants.[40] The increase in transplacental IgG transfer during late gestation is likely to affect the outcome of perinatal exposure to viral pathogens. For example, lower antibody titers among exposed preterm infants may account for the disproportionate number of premature infants who develop neonatal herpes.[68]

Placental Immune Mechanisms

The analysis of immune cells in normal placentas demonstrates that approximately 75% are lymphocytes, 15% are monocytes, and 10% are granulocytes (8%); the lymphocytes are predominantly T cells (65%), as opposed to B cells (8%).[28] The lymphocyte populations in HCMV villitis consist of fetal-derived T cells with very few B cells, but plasma cells of fetal origin that produce both IgG and IgM antibodies are common.[58] The antigen specificity of placental lymphocytes in pregnancies complicated by intrauterine infection has not been investigated. The fetal trophoblast does not express class I or class II major histocompatibility complex (MAC) molecules, so virus-specific CD4+ or CD8+ T cells would not be expected to recognize and lyse virus-infected cells.[7] Fetal-derived placental macrophages (Hofbauer cells) comprise the predominant inflammatory cell population in the stromal regions of the chorionic villi of placentas from HCMV-infected fetuses.[29,57,60] Based on evidence from in situ hybridization and protein expression studies, these cells fail to control viral replication and become actively infected with HCMV.[57] Cytokines are produced by placental cells, but the role of these responses in the pathogenesis of intrauterine viral infections is not known.[37] Natural killer (NK) cells are abundant in the placenta, but their functional activity is low.

The Developing Immune System

The fetal immune system has the cellular components required to respond to infectious agents from as early as 12 weeks, but assessments of humoral and cell-mediated immunity to the herpesviruses among infants infected in utero or at the time of delivery indicate that antiviral immune responses are functionally limited. Both B-cell and T-cell responses appear to require a period of physiologic maturation postnatally in order to be effective in vivo against these and other pathogens.[8,67]

Humoral Immunity

Defining the functional capacity of fetal or neonatal B cells to produce virus-specific antibodies is difficult because maternal and infant IgG antibodies cannot be differentiated. Neonatal HSV infection caused by primary maternal HSV infection provides an opportunity to assess the humoral immune response of the newborn to a viral pathogen in the absence of transplacental antibodies.[39,63,64] In this circumstance, only 19% of infants produce HSV neutralizing antibodies within 4 weeks, compared with 100% of adults, and only 36% of infants have evidence of endogenous antibody production measured by the appearance of antibodies to a new HSV protein.[39,63] IgM- and IgG-secreting B lymphocytes are present as early as 12 weeks' gestation, but even at birth, 80% to 90% of B lymphocytes have surface IgM and IgD instead of the predominance of IgG or IgA that is characteristic of adult cells. These phenotypic differences may indicate altered B-cell function that affects virus-specific antibody production by the immature host. Instead of representing a protective response, high virus-specific antibody titers to some viral proteins may reflect the extent of viral replication and tissue damage, as suggested by the finding that antibodies to HSV ICP4 are increased in infants with neonatal herpes who have frequent cutaneous recurrences and a poor neurologic outcome.[39]

In contrast to IgG antibody production, 76% of infants with neonatal herpes infection develop IgM antibodies to HSV during the acute phase of infection.[63] In vitro studies show that B cells from newborns respond to T-dependent antigens but IgM antibodies predominate, suggesting that infant B cells do not make the switch to IgG production efficiently.[67] The analysis of humoral immunity in infants with HSV infection indicates that these in vitro observations reflect limitations of the host response that are relevant in vivo.

Cellular Immunity

Cellular immunity is critical in controlling the replication of herpesviruses in vivo.[45] An effective host response requires the induction of T cells that recognize viral antigens processed and presented in the context of major histocompatibility antigens. T cells that recognize epitopes of viral proteins produce Th1 and Th2 cytokines and function as helper cells for antibody production or as cytotoxic cells. Thymocytes are detected in the developing fetus by 8 weeks, and absolute numbers of CD4+ and CD8+ T cells are equivalent in infants and adults.[67] Nevertheless, infants with herpesvirus infections clearly have deficiencies in T-cell recognition of viral proteins. For example, infants with HCMV acquired in utero have poor in vitro T-cell proliferation in response to HCMV antigens, but this is not associated with a decreased response to mitogens.[1,52,53] The relevance of this response to the control of viral replication is suggested by the cessation of chronic virus excretion in the urine after HCMV-specific T cells appear. The eventual acquisition of cellular immunity in these infants demonstrates that diminished T-cell recognition of HCMV is not caused by induction of permanent tolerance with clonal deletion of HCMV-specific T cells in utero. Perinatal HCMV infection is also associated with prolonged failure to develop T-cell recognition of HCMV antigens, prolonged viruria, and termination of virus excretion in urine after T-cell responses develop.[52] The low proliferation response in infants reflects a lower number of responder T cells that recognize HCMV antigens compared with adults who are immune to HCMV.[36] The immunologic basis for the delayed acquisition of antigen-specific T cells is not known, but the defect is not caused by diminished antigen presentation by mononuclear cells and cannot be overcome by the use of concentrated glycoproteins to stimulate T cells.[25]

The deficiencies in cellular immunity observed with chronic intrauterine and perinatal HCMV infection are also observed in infants with acute HSV infection in the newborn period.[63] Premature infants and infants who have symptoms within the first week of life are significantly less likely to develop HSV-specific T-cell responses and are more likely to have progressive, disseminated infection.[63] The capacity to develop HSV-specific helper T cells may affect antibody responses, because 80% of infants with neutralizing antibody responses have positive T-cell proliferation to HSV antigen, compared with only 19% of those without such responses. Failure to develop T-cell immunity may be caused by direct thymic destruction by the virus, as was reported in four of six infants with fatal, disseminated HSV infection.[48] As in the case of HCMV, HSV-specific responder cell frequencies in infants are less than one third the frequencies measured in adults; decreased proliferation in response to HSV appears to be intrinsic to T cells, because antigen presentation by infant macrophages to HLA-matched B cells is intact.[36] The assessment of classic antiviral cytotoxic T-cell responses has not been accomplished in infants with herpesvirus infections for technical reasons.

The relation between deficient virus-specific T-cell responses and failure to maintain latency after intrauterine herpesvirus infection is suggested by the high frequency of reactivation in infants with mucocutaneous HSV infection and the occurrence of herpes zoster in infants exposed to VZV in utero.[33] T-cell proliferation in response to VZV antigens is diminished in infants with evidence of intrauterine VZV infection, with responses only about one third of those measured in older children and adults.[51]

NK cells, which can lyse virus-infected cells even if the individual has had no exposure to the foreign antigens, are probably an important initial immune mechanism against herpesviruses.[45] Fetal NK cells are limited in number until relatively late in gestation, being undetectable at 20 weeks' gestation but appearing at 27 weeks.[63] Although the experiments were not done with purified subpopulations, when probable NK activity of neonatal PBMCs was assessed against HSV or HCMV-infected target cells, lysis was diminished significantly in comparison with adult NK function.[41,40] Passive antibodies to herpesviruses can act with effector cells that mediate ADCC. Newborn monocytes appear to function effectively in ADCC responses and, although newborn PBMCs have low lymphocyte ADCC effector activity compared with those of adults, the differences are relative and not absolute.[40]

IFN-α production by leukocytes is a nonspecific host response to viral infection that has direct antiviral effects and also enhances NK activity. Cells from healthy, uninfected infants are able to respond to HSV stimulation in vitro with IFN-α concentrations equivalent to those of adults.[16] However, IFN-α production by PBMCs is diminished in infants with HSV infection.[63] IFN-γ is an important cytokine in the response to viral pathogens because it enhances the clonal expansion of B cells with cytotoxic function and amplifies the antigen-specific host response. Newborn PBMCs have diminished IFN-γ mRNA production in vitro.[14,67] This deficiency may be important in herpesvirus pathogenesis in vivo, because IFN-γ production in response to HSV antigen stimulation is delayed in infected infants compared with adults with acute HSV infection.[15,17]

COMPARISON OF HERPESVIRUS PATHOGENESIS WITH OTHER VIRAL DISEASES OF THE FETUS AND NEWBORN

Several other viral pathogens are well recognized for their potential to infect and damage the fetus and the newborn infant, including rubella, enteroviruses, parvovirus B19, hepatitis B, and HIV. Intrauterine and perinatal infections caused by these viruses exhibit many similarities, as well as some differences, from those caused by the human herpesviruses.

Before the introduction of the live attenuated vaccine, rubella was more important than HCMV as a cause of serious fetal infection.[17a] Maternal viremia is presumed to lead to transplacental transmission, with the timing of maternal infection during gestation being the most important variable in determining the risk of fetal damage. Rubella is more likely to cause maternal symptoms than HCMV, but it may also cause fetal injury when it is subclinical. Transmission in early pregnancy is even more common than in HCMV, with rates of approximately 75% during the first 14 weeks of gestation, and transmission continues at high rates during later pregnancy. However, as with HCMV, serious fetal sequelae are essentially limited to maternal infections complicating early gestation. Infection restricted to the placenta, without associated fetal infection, is documented in rubella and in HCMV. Infants with congenital rubella have prolonged excretion of the virus at multiple sites and poor humoral and cell-mediated immune responses to the virus, but rubella differs from HCMV in its capacity to cause nonspecific as well as virus-specific deficiencies in the host immune response. Infants with congenital rubella may have persistent hypogammaglobulinemia and altered CD4/CD8 T-cell ratios. The tissue pathology of intrauterine rubella infection is characterized by relatively few infected cells, a limited inflammatory response, and evidence that vasculitis is an important mechanism for inducing organ damage, as it may also be in HCMV. The implementation of immunization programs has established that prevention of primary maternal infection eliminates the risk of congenital rubella.

The enteroviruses, including polioviruses, coxsackieviruses, and echoviruses, cause frequent epidemics that affect women of childbearing age, and infection is associated with viremia.[16] Nevertheless, there is little evidence that these pathogens are transferred transplacentally in early gestation, and only rare cases of late-gestation transmission have been identified (e.g., coxsackie B virus causes myocarditis in utero after maternal infection acquired near term). Perinatal transmission is documented, often from mothers who have had recent acute febrile illnesses, and is probably caused by fecal carriage with inoculation of the infant during delivery. The enteroviruses resemble HSV in their capacity to cause acute, life-threatening disease in this circumstance. The pathologic mechanism is direct cytopathic damage; fulminant hepatitis with hepatic necrosis, with or without meningoencephalitis, is common, as it is in disseminated neonatal HSV infection.

Parvovirus B19 causes viremia during primary infection and can be transmitted transplacentally, although the incidence of transmission is not well defined.[65] This virus is unique as an intrauterine pathogen because of its tropism for human erythroid precursors. The fetus is vulnerable to severe intrauterine anemia and nonimmune hydrops, because fetal erythrocytes have a shorter survival time and fetal growth requires a rapid increase in the erythrocyte pool. Parvovirus B19 also causes unusual placental pathology, characterized by erythroblastosis and vasculitis of villous capillaries. Nonimmune hydrops occurs in other fetal infections, including HCMV, but the damage from intrauterine parvovirus infection is attributed only to this mechanism. The pathologic consequences result from hypoxic damage to multiple organs, including the brain, hemosiderin deposits in the liver, and congestive heart failure.

Hepatitis B infects women of childbearing age in many geographic areas, but it is rarely transmitted to the fetus in utero despite chronic maternal infection or acquisition by the mother during the first trimester.[71] How the placenta provides such an effective barrier to this virus is not known, but surface antigen is not detected in cord blood from infants of mothers with chronic infection. Prevention of almost all cases by active and passive immunization against hepatitis B in the newborn period proves that most transmission is caused by exposure at delivery.

Fetal or neonatal transmission of HIV is one of the most tragic consequences of the HIV epidemic.[46] Chronic maternal viremia allows transfer of the virus to the fetus or to the infant during delivery. Information about the pathogenesis is limited, but extensive placental infection has been demonstrated in some cases, and chorioamnionitis may occur. Viral genome sequences and expression of HIV proteins can be detected in Hofbauer and endothelial cells, but, as with the herpesviruses, infection of the placenta is not invariably associated with fetal or nonneonatal infection. Discordant transmission is observed among twins and in subsequent infants born to the same mother. Attempts to correlate transmission with maternal virus load in peripheral blood CD4+ T cells or with stage of disease have produced inconsistent results.[46] An important study demonstrated a decrease in the infant infection rate from 25% to 8% after HIV-infected mothers were treated with zidovudine during pregnancy and the infants were treated for 6 weeks after birth, suggesting that intrapartum transmission is a major risk factor. The cell tropism of HIV in the fetus and newborn resembles infection in older individuals; early reports of a congenital infection syndrome have not been substantiated. In contrast to the herpesviruses, fatal disease follows HIV transmission to the fetus or newborn even if maternal infection is acquired before pregnancy. In this infection, transplacentally acquired antibodies to the virus have limited potential to affect disease progression.

SUMMARY AND CONCLUSIONS

In addition to its scientific interest, understanding of the pathogenesis of herpesvirus infections in the fetus and newborn has direct relevance to clinical diagnosis and intervention. Diagnostic problems arise in evaluating pregnancies complicated by maternal herpesvirus infections, because the virus may infect the fetus in utero without causing damage. For example, HCMV can be isolated from amniotic fluid owing to urinary excretion by the infected fetus, but the infant is usually completely healthy. Because many infants with intrauterine HCMV, HSV, or VZV infections do not produce IgM antibodies, a negative serologic result does not exclude infection, and, as in the case of virologic methods, a positive result does not mean that the fetus will have sequelae. With respect to intervention, passive antibodies given to mothers who are experiencing primary herpesvirus infections in early gestation do not have predictable protective efficacy because of limitations in IgG transfer. Early antiviral therapy is essential to compensate for the limited capacity of the newborn immune system to restrict herpesviruses. Finally, the significant enhancement of risk when maternal herpesvirus infections are primary means that the development of effective vaccines is likely to have a major impact on the incidence of herpesvirus disease in fetuses and newborn infants.

ABBREVIATIONS

ADCC: antibody-dependent cell-mediated cytotoxicity
EA: early antigen
EBV: Epstein-Barr virus
gB, gG: type-specific glycoproteins
HCMV: human cytomegalovirus
HHV-6: human herpesvirus type 6
HIV: human immunodeficiency virus
HLA: human leukocyte antigen
HSV, HSV-1, HSV-2: herpes simplex virus
IFN-α, IFN-γ: interferons
IgA, IgD, IgG, IgM: immunoglobulins
IQ: intelligence quotient
NK: natural killer (cells)
PBMC: peripheral blood mononuclear cell
VZV: varicella-zoster virus

REFERENCES

1. Alford CA, Britt WJ. Cytomegalovirus. In: Fields BN, Knipe BN, et al, eds. Virology. 2nd ed. New York: Raven Press, 1990:2011–2054.
2. Altshuler G. Pathogenesis of congenital herpes virus infection: case report including a description of the placenta. Am J Dis Child 1974; 127:427–432.
3. Andiman WA. The Epstein-Barr virus and EB virus infections in childhood. J Pediatr 1979;95:171–182.
4. Arvin AM, Hensleigh PA, Au DS, et al. Failure of antepartum maternal cultures to predict the infant's risk of exposure to herpes simplex virus at delivery. N Engl J Med 1986;315:796–800.
5. Ashley RL, Militoni J, Burchett S, et al. HSV-2 type specific antibody correlates of protection in infants exposed to HSV-2 at birth. J Clin Invest 1992;90:511–514.
6. Aubin J-T. Intrauterine transmission of human herpes virus 6. Lancet 1992;340:2.
7. Benirschke K, Kaufman P. Pathology of the human placenta. 2nd ed. New York: Springer-Verlag, 1990.
8. Billington WB. The normal fetomaternal immune relationship. Baillieres Clin Obstet Gynaecol 1992;6:417–438.

9. Boppana SB, Pass RF, Britt WJ. Virus-specific antibody responses in mothers and their newborn infants with asymptomatic congenital cytomegalovirus infections. J Infect Dis 1993;167:72–77.

10. Boucher FD, Yasukawa LL, Bronzan RN, Hensleigh PA, Arvin AM, Prober CG. A prospective evaluation of primary genital herpes simplex virus type 2 infections acquired during pregnancy. Pediatr Infect Dis J 1990;9:499–504.

11. Britt WJ, Vugler LG. Antiviral antibody responses in mothers and their newborn infants with clinical and subclinical congenital cytomegalovirus infections. J Infect Dis 1990;161:214–219.

12. Brown ZA, Vontver LA, Denedetti J, et al. Effects on infants of a first episode of genital herpes during pregnancy. N Engl J Med 317; 1246–1251.

13. Brunell PA. Varicella in pregnancy, the fetus and the newborn: problems in management. J Infect Dis 1992;166(Suppl 1):S42–S47.

14. Bryson YJ, Winter HS, Gard SE, et al. Deficiency of immune interferon production by leukocytes of normal newborns. Cell Immunol 1980;55:191–200.

15. Burchett SK, Corey L, Mohan KM, et al. Diminished IFN-γ and lymphocyte proliferation in neonatal and postpartum primary herpes simplex virus infection. J Infect Dis 1992;167:813–818.

16. Cherry J. Enteroviruses. In: Remington J, Klein J, eds. Infectious diseases of the fetus and newborn. 4th ed Philadelphia: WB Saunders, 1994:404–446.

17. Chilmonczyk BA, Levin MJ, McDuffy R, et al. Characterization of the human newborn response to herpesvirus antigen. J Immunol 1985;134:4184–4188.

17a.Cooper LZ, Preblud S, Alford CA. Rubella. In: Remington J, Klein J, eds. Infectious diseases of the fetus and newborn. 4th ed. Philadelphia: WB Saunders, 1994:268–311.

18. de The G, Geser A, Day NE, et al. Epidemiological evidence for causal relationship between Epstein-Barr virus and Burkitt's lymphoma from Ugandan prospective study. Nature 1978;274:756–760.

19. Down JA, Kawakami M, Klein MH, Dorrington KJ. Proteins associated with activity of Fc receptors on isolated human placental syncytiotrophoblast microvillous plasma membranes. Placenta 1989;10: 227–246.

20. Fleisher G, Bologonese R. Persistent Epstein-Barr virus infection and pregnancy. J Infect Dis 1983;147:982–986.

21. Fleisher G, Bologonese R. Epstein-Barr virus infections in pregnancy: a prospective study. J Pediatr 1984;104:374–379.

22. Fleisher G, Bologonese R. Infectious mononucleosis during gestation: report of three women and their infants studies prospectively. Pediatr Infect Dis 1984;3:308–331.

23. Fowler KB, Stagno S, Pass RF, Britt WJ, Boll TJ, Alford CA. The outcome of congenital cytomegalovirus infection in relation to maternal antibody status. N Engl J 1992;326:663–667.

24. Garcia AGP. Fetal infection in chickenpox and alastrim with histopathologic study of the placenta. Pediatrics 1963;32:895–901.

25. Gehrz RC, Liu Y-NC, Peterson ES, Fuad SA. Role of antigen-presenting cells in congenital cytomegalovirus-specific immunodeficiency. J Infect Dis 1987;156:198–202.

26. Gershon A. Chickenpox, measles and mumps. In: Remington J, Klein J, eds. Infectious diseases of the fetus and newborn. Philadelphia: WB Saunders, 1990:395–419.

27. Gervais F, Joncas JH. Seroepidemiology in various population groups of the greater Montreal area. Comp Immunol Microbiol Infect Dis 1979;2:207–213.

28. Goldsobel A, Ank B, Spina C, Giorgi J, Stiehm ER. Phenotypic and cytotoxic characteristics of the immune cells of the human placenta. Cell Immunol 1986;97:335–343.

29. Greco MA, Wieczorek R, Sachdev R, et al. Phenotype of villous stromal cells in placentas with cytomegalovirus, syphilis, and nonspecific villitis. Am J Pathol 1992;141:835–842.

30. Greene D, Watson WJ, Wirtz PS. Non-immune hydrops associated with congenital herpes simplex infection. S D J Med 1993;46:219–220.

31. Grefte A, van der Giessen M, van Son W, The TH. Circulating cytomegalovirus (CMV)–infected endothelial cells in patients with an active CMV infection. J Infect Dis 1993;167:270–277.

32. Grose C. Varicella-zoster virus: pathogenesis of the human diseases, the virus and viral replication. In: Hyman R, ed. The natural history of varicella-zoster virus. New York: CRC Press, 1987:1–66.

33. Grose C. Congenital varicella-zoster virus infection and the failure to establish virus-specific cell-mediated immunity. Mol Biol 1989;6: 453–462.

34. Harrison CJ, Waner JL. Natural killer cell activity in infants and children excreting cytomegalovirus. J Infect Dis 1985;151:301–307.

35. Hayes K, Gibas H. Placental cytomegalovirus infection without fetal involvement following primary infection in pregnancy. J Pediatr 1971;79:401–405.

36. Hayward AR, Herberger MJ, Groothuis J, Levin MR. Specific immunity after congenital or neonatal infection with cytomegalovirus or herpes simplex virus. J Immunol 1984;133:2469–2473.

37. Hunt JS. Macrophages in human uteroplacental tissues: a review. Am J Reprod Immunol 1989;21:119–122.

38. Hutto C, Arvin AM, Jacobs R, et al. Intrauterine herpes simplex virus infections. J Pediatr 1987;110:97–101.

38a.Hyde SR, Giacoia GP. Congenital herpes infection: placental and umbilical cord findings. Obstet Gynecol 1993;81:852–855.

39. Kahlon J, Whitley RJ. Antibody response of the newborn after herpes simplex virus infection. J Infect Dis 1988;158:925–933.

40. Kohl S. The neonatal human's immune response to herpes simplex virus infection: a critical review. Pediatr Infect Dis J 1989;8:67–74.

41. Kohl S, Harmon MW. Human neonatal leukocyte interferon production and natural killer cytotoxicity in response to herpes simplex virus. J Interferon Res 1983;3:461–463.

42. Kohl S, West MS, Prober CG, Sullender WM, Loo LS, Arvin AM. Neonatal antibody-dependent cellular cytotoxic antibody levels are associated with the clinical presentation of neonatal herpes simplex virus infection. J Infect Dis 1989;160:770–776.

43. Koropchak CM, Solem SM, Diaz PS, Arvin AM. Investigation of varicella-zoster virus infection of lymphocytes by in situ hybridization. J Virol 1989;63:2392–2395.

44. Le CT, Chang S, Lipson MH. Epstein-Barr virus infections during pregnancy. Am J Dis Child 1983;137:466–468.

45. Lopez C, Arvin AM, Ashley R. Immunity to herpesvirus infections in humans. In: Roizman B, Whitley RJ, Lopez C. The human herpesviruses. New York: Raven Press, 1993;397–425.

46. Mueller BU, Pizzo PA. Acquired immunodeficiency syndrome in the infant. In: Remington J, Klein J, eds. Infectious diseases of the fetus and newborn. 4th ed. Philadelphia: WB Saunders, 1994:377–403.

47. Nahmias A, Norrild B. Herpes simplex viruses 1 and 2: basic and clinical aspects. Dis Mon 1979;25:5–42.

48. Nakamura Y, Yamamoto S, Tanaka S, et al. Herpes simplex viral infection in human neonates: an immunohistochemical and electron microscopic study. Hum Pathol 1985;16:1091–1097.

49. Norskov-Lauritsen N, Aboagye-Mathiesen G, Juhl CB, et al. Herpes simplex virus infection of cultured human term trophoblast. J Med Virol 1992;36:162–166.

50. Ornoy A, Dudai M, Sadovsky E. Placental and fetal pathology in infectious mononucleosis: a possible indicator for Epstein-Barr virus teratogenicity. Diagn Gynecol Obstet 1982;4:11–16.

51. Paryani SG, Arvin AM. Intrauterine infection with varicella-zoster virus after maternal varicella. N Engl J Med 1986;314:1542–1546.

52. Pass RF, Dworsky ME, Whitley RJ, et al. Specific lymphocyte blastogenic responses in children with cytomegalovirus and herpes simplex virus infections acquired early in infancy. Infect Immun 1981;34: 166–170.

53. Pass RF, Stagno S, Britt WJ, Britt WJ. Specific cell-mediated immunity and the natural history of congenital infection with cytomegalovirus. J Infect Dis 1983;148:953–961.

54. Prober CG, Arvin AM. Genital herpes and the pregnant woman. In: Remington J, Swartz M, eds. Current clinical topics in infectious diseases. Vol 10. London: Blackwell Scientific Publications 1989:1–26.

55. Prober CG, Sullender WM, Lew-Yasukawa L, Au DS, Yeager AS, Arvin AM. Low risk of herpes simplex virus infections in neonates exposed to virus at the time of vaginal delivery to mothers with recurrent genital herpes simplex virus infections. N Engl J Med 1987; 316:240–244.

56. Schwartz DA, Caldwell E. Herpes simplex virus infection of the placenta: the role of molecular pathology in the diagnosis of viral infection of placental-associated tissues. Arch Pathol Lab Med 1991;115: 1141–1144.

57. Schwartz DA, Khan R, Stoll B. Characterization of the fetal inflammatory response to cytomegalovirus placentitis. Arch Pathol Lab Med 1992;116:21–27.

58. Schwartz DA, Nahmias AJ. Human immunodeficiency virus and the placenta: current concepts of vertical transmission in relation to other viral agents. Ann Clin Lab Sci 1991;21:264–274.

59. Shrier RD, Nelson JA, Oldstone MBA. Detection of human cytomegalovirus in peripheral blood lymphocytes in a natural infection. Science 1985;230:1048–1051.

60. Sinzger C, Muenterfering H, Loening T, et al. Cell types infected in human cytomegalovirus placentitis identified by immunohistochemical double staining. Virchows Arch A Pathol Anat Histopathol 1993; 423:249–256.

61. Sixbey JW, Lemon SJ, Pagano JS. A second site of Epstein-Barr virus shedding: the uterine cervix. Lancet 1986;2:1122–1124.

62. Stagno S. Cytomegalovirus. In: Remington J, Klein J, eds. Infectious diseases of the fetus and newborn. 4th ed. Philadelphia: WB Saunders, 1994:331–353.

63. Sullender WM, Miller JL, Yasukawa LL, et al. Humoral and cellular immunity in neonates with herpes simplex virus infection. J Infect Dis 1987;155:28–37.

64. Sullender WM, Yasukawa LL, Schwartz M, et al. Type-specific antibodies to herpes simplex virus type 2 (HSV-2) glycoprotein G in pregnant women, infants exposed to maternal HSV-2 infection at delivery and infants with neonatal herpes. J Infect Dis 1988;157: 164–171.

65. Torok TJ. Human parvovirus B19. In: Remington J, Klein J, eds. Infectious diseases of the fetus and newborn. 4th ed. Philadelphia: WB Saunders, 1994:668–702.

66. Visintine A, Gerber P, Nahmias AJ. Leukocyte transforming agent (Epstein-Barr virus) in newborn infants and older individuals. J Pediatr 1976;89:571.

67. Wilson C. Developmental immunology and role of host defenses in neonatal susceptibility. In: Remington J, Klein J, eds. Infectious diseases of the fetus and newborn. Philadelphia: WB Saunders, 1990: 17–67.

68. Whitley RJ, Arvin AM. Herpes simplex virus infections. In: Remington J, Klein J, eds. Infectious diseases of the fetus and newborn. 4th ed. Philadelphia: WB Saunders, 1994:354–376.

69. Wolf DG, Spector SA. Early diagnosis of human cytomegalovirus disease in transplant recipients by DNA amplification in plasma. Transplantation 1993;56:330–334.

70. Yeager AS, Grumet FC, Hafleigh EB, Arvin AM, Bradley JS, Prober CG. Prevention of transfusion-acquired cytomegalovirus infections in newborn infants. J Pediatr 1980;98:281–287.

71. Zeldis JB, Crumpacker CS. Hepatitis. In: Remington J, Klein J, eds. Infectious diseases of the fetus and newborn. 4th ed. Philadelphia: WB Saunders, 1994:805–834.

Viral Pathogenesis,
edited by Neal Nathanson, et al.
Lippincott–Raven Publishers, Philadelphia © 1997

CHAPTER 34

HIV Infection and Associated Diseases

William A. O'Brien and Roger J. Pomerantz

INTRODUCTION

Human immunodeficiency virus types 1 and 2 (HIV-1 and HIV-2) are members of the subfamily *Lentivirinae* of the *Retroviridae* family. HIV-1 is more prevalent in the United States and Europe, whereas HIV-2 is seen primarily in West Africa, the Caribbean, and South America. Although animal lentiviruses were first identified more than 90 years ago, human lentiviruses have been recognized for little more than a decade[16,99] and have been found in association with the acquired immunodeficiency syndrome (AIDS) and with a variety of other diseases that occur in the early stages of HIV infection. Both HIV-1 and HIV-2 can cause immune deficiency, but HIV-1 infection appears to be more virulent.[175] Because HIV-1 has been more intensively studied, most of this review focuses on HIV-1 infection.

Despite rapid characterization of the structure and life cycle of HIV-1, the mechanisms whereby it produces disease are poorly understood. There are many barriers to our understand-

ing of HIV-1 pathogenesis, including the remarkable genetic diversity among HIV-1 strains, the diverse responses to infection among individuals, and the limitations of experimental models.

The truly problematic aspect of HIV-1 infection is how the principal target cell, the CD4+ lymphocyte, which is crucial for a variety of host immune responses, is depleted over a period of several years as a result of infection. Depletion of CD4+ lymphocytes leads to progressive immunoincompetence, which not only results in impairment of the host's ability to inhibit HIV-1 replication but also allows the emergence of numerous opportunistic pathogens associated with AIDS.

MOLECULAR BIOLOGY OF HIV

Structural Genes of HIV

Lentiviruses are characterized by a single-stranded RNA genome and RNA-dependent DNA polymerase (reverse transcriptase) carried in infectious virions.[279] The HIV genome is approximately 9.7 kb in size and exists within the virion as a dimer with two identical RNA strands.[195] Retroviral particles consist of an outer lipid envelope and associated glycoproteins surrounding a core that contains RNA genome associated with nucleoproteins (Fig. 34-1). Three structural genes, present in all retroviruses, encode proteins required for pro-

W. A. O'Brien: Division of Infectious Diseases, West Los Angeles Veterans Affairs Medical Center and UCLA, Los Angeles, California 90073.

R. J. Pomerantz: Division of Infectious Diseases, Dept. of Medicine, Thomas Jefferson University, Philadelphia, Pennsylvania 19107.

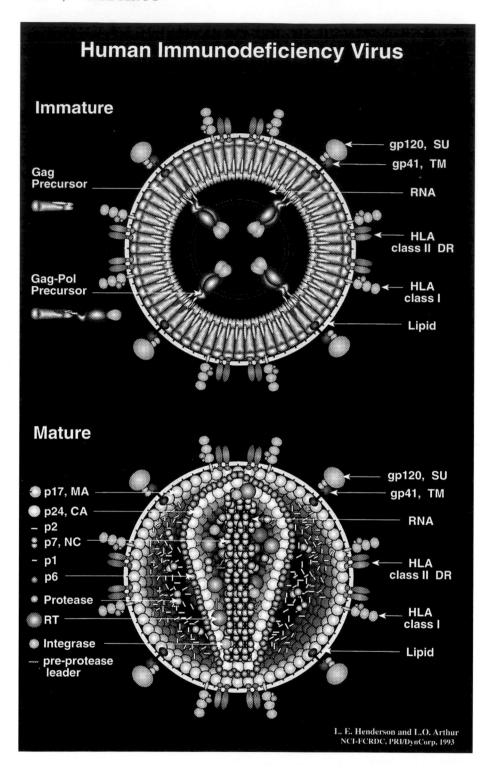

Human Immunodeficiency Virus

Immature

gp120, SU
gp41, TM
RNA

Gag
Precursor

HLA
class II DR

Gag-Pol
Precursor

HLA
class I

Lipid

Mature

p17, MA
p24, CA
p2
p7, NC
p1
p6

Protease
RT

Integrase
pre-protease
leader

gp120, SU
gp41, TM

RNA

HLA
class II DR

HLA
class I

Lipid

L. E. Henderson and L.O. Arthur
NCI-FCRDC, PRI/DynCorp, 1993

FIG. 34-1. Structure of the HIV-1 virion. HLA, human leukocyte antigen; RNA, ribonucleic acid; RT, reverse transcriptase; MA, matrix; CA, capsid; NC, nucleocapsid, SU, surface, TM, transmembrane.

duction of infectious progeny virions. The *gag* gene encodes a precursor protein which is cleaved after translation to form nucleocapsid products. The principal *gag* product in HIV-1 is a 24-kD protein (p24). The *pol* gene encodes the highly conserved enzymatic proteins protease, reverse transcriptase, integrase, and ribonuclease H. The *env* gene encodes a glycosylated precursor protein (gp160), which is cleaved to produce an external glycoprotein (gp120) involved in recognition and binding to target cell receptors and a smaller, hydrophobic transmembrane protein (gp41) involved in membrane fusion; gp120 is noncovalently bound to gp41 and can be shed from the surface of the virion.

Novel HIV-1 and HIV-2 Genes

In HIV and the primate lentivirus simian immunodeficiency virus (SIV), there are complex regulatory systems not found in other retroviruses. These auxiliary genes are encoded in six overlapping open reading frames, which are well conserved within each primate lentivirus group (Fig. 34-2), suggesting that these proteins play an important role in the viral life cycle. The precise roles of these novel genes in the virus life cycle, however, remain ill defined. Two of these auxiliary HIV genes (*tat* and *rev*) are required for replication in all host cells.[88,254] Mutations in the other four genes have variable effects, depending on the experimental system. The *tat* (*trans*-activator of transcription) gene encodes a 14-kD protein utilizing exons in three distinct regions of the HIV genome and is synthesized early after infection.[10,255] The Tat protein enhances HIV gene expression by interacting with cellular factors and binding to *trans*-activation–responsive (TAR) RNA sequences located in the 5' end of all HIV transcripts[17,230] (Fig. 34-3). Tat may increase HIV gene expression by stabilizing mRNA transcripts and facilitating elongation.[89,103] The *rev* (regulator of expression of virion proteins) gene also encodes a protein translated from multiply-spliced RNAs.[88,254] The Rev protein binds to HIV RNAs in the nucleus through sequences located within the *env* gene termed the Rev-responsive element (RRE).[72,171,305] Rev acts after transcription to facilitate the cytoplasmic accumulation and translation of RRE-containing RNAs.[8,172] Consequently, Rev is required for the expression of structural proteins and indirectly downregulates its own expression, as well as that of *tat* and *nef*.

The role of the gene products of the other four HIV accessory genes in viral replication are less well understood. The *nef* gene is present in all primate lentiviruses and is highly immunogenic. In early studies, a functional *nef* gene was associated with a modest decrease in efficiency of viral spread in cell culture, compared with *nef*-deficient viruses, and the gene product was therefore named negative factor (Nef).[46,168] A role as a specific repressor of HIV transcription was proposed,[3] although this result was not reproduced by others.[116,145] The Nef protein is associated with membrane structures and appears to downregulate surface expression of CD4 by inducing endocytosis and degradation of CD4 in lysosomes.[4,76,101,112] Therefore, Nef may be involved with either protein transport or transmembrane signaling. There appear to be differences in the effects of Nef on HIV replication in vivo and those seen in culture. The role of Nef has been analyzed using mutant strains derived from the SIV_{mac239} strain having premature stop codons or large deletions that result in a truncated Nef protein.[143] Although there was no difference in replicative ability between mutant and wild-type *nef* strains in culture, monkeys infected with SIV_{mac239} strains encoding a functional Nef protein had much higher levels of virus replication and exhibited dramatic clinical progression. Animals infected by SIV strains having point mutations in *nef* overcame the stop signal by spontaneous point mutations, which appeared rapidly and gave rise to high levels of virus replication. Therefore, at least in SIV, *nef* appears to be required for vigorous virus replication in vivo as well as for pathogenic effects. Similar results have been obtained for HIV-1: there was little difference in replication between wild-type and Nef-deficient strains in culture, yet there was attenuated replication and T-lymphocyte depletion in a murine model having a reconstituted human hematopoietic system[130] (see Models for

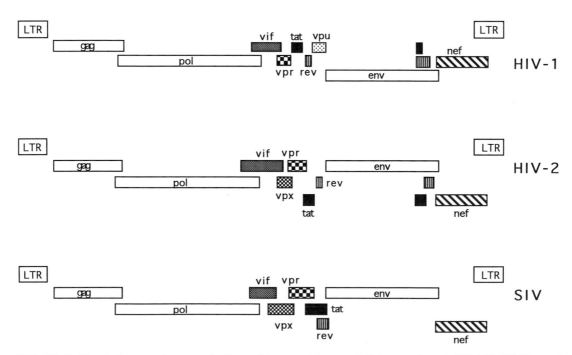

FIG. 34-2. Proviral genomic organization of human immunodeficiency virus-1 (HIV-1), HIV-2, and simian immunodeficiency virus (SIV). Location of regions encoding precursors for known virion proteins are shown. LTR, long terminal repeat.

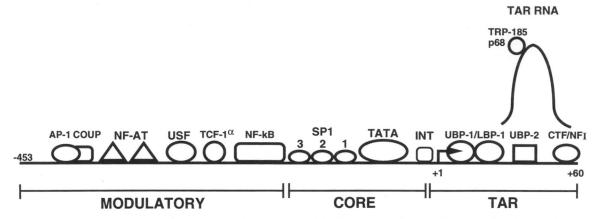

FIG. 34-3. Schematic diagram of cellular factors binding to the human immunodeficiency virus (HIV-1) long terminal repeat (LTR). HIV-1 replication is regulated by LTR DNA- and RNA-binding proteins. These include binding sites for activator protein (AP-1), chicken ovalbumin upstream promoter (COUP), nuclear factor of activated T cells (NF-AT), upstream stimulatory factor (USF), T-cell factor-1α (TCF-1α), nuclear factor kappa B (NF-kB), SP1, TATA, initiator (INT), untranslated binding protein-1 (UBP-1) or leader binding protein-1 (LBP-1), UBP-2, and cellular transcription factor/nuclear factor-1 (CTF/NF1). TAR, *trans*-activation-responsive sequence.

Studying HIV-1 Infection). Using low multiplicity of infection, diminished infectivity and replication was also shown for Nef− HIV-1 in primary cell cultures.[189,256] HIV-1 sequences having deletions in *nef* were found in multiple blood samples over a period of 10 years in a patient with nonprogressive HIV-1 infection, suggesting that *nef*-deficient strains are attenuated.[146] The mechanism for this function of *nef* has not been defined.

The *vif* (viral infectivity factor) gene encodes a late gene product found to be essential for the spread of HIV-1 in peripheral blood lymphocytes and in primary macrophages[281] as well as in some, but not all, established cell lines.[98,235] Early studies demonstrated that mutations in *vif* can decrease infectivity of HIV-1 particles by as much as 1000-fold,[93,263] but this was dependent on cell type. In addition to a role in viral particle formation, Vif appears to be important for both cell-to-cell and cell-free transmission. Thus, Vif may compensate for cell functions important for production of virus that are present in some cell lines but not in primary cells.

The *vpr* (virion protein R) gene encodes a 15-kD protein associated with the nucleocapsid protein p6,[216] which is present within HIV-1 virions in abundant quantities.[57,156,166] Although dispensable for replication in CD4+ lymphocytes,[14,74] Vpr appears to augment both HIV-1 and HIV-2 replication in macrophages[119,291] and has been implicated in nuclear localization of viral nucleic acids in nondividing cells.[120] Vpr has weak transactivation properties for the HIV long terminal repeat (LTR) and other promoters[57] and may act in *trans* to modestly increase HIV-2 expression in macrophages.[119]

The *vpu* (virion protein U) gene is present in HIV-1 but not in HIV-2 or SIV. Vpu is necessary for intracellular dissociation of gp160 and CD4 through degradation of CD4 in the endoplasmic reticulum.[293,294] Although not essential for replication, Vpu may play a role in proper and efficient virion assembly and release,[107,264,272] and it has been implicated in CD4 downregulation. Vpu may also facilitate export of virus

capsid proteins.[297] The *vpx* (virion protein X) gene is not present in HIV-1, but is present and produced in large amounts by HIV-2 and SIV.[299] The *vpx* gene is not essential for viral replication, but mutations can modestly impair virus production.[139,173,301] The Vpx protein is present in the virion outside the core structure, suggesting a role in virus penetration or uncoating.[300] As the precise functions of these accessory genes are better defined, insights will be gained into the HIV-1 replication process, particularly the interaction with cellular factors.

HIV-1 LIFE CYCLE

HIV replication is similar to that of other retroviruses[279] and involves reverse transcription of the RNA viral genome to form a double-stranded DNA provirus (Fig. 34-4). HIV genetic sequences are present for the lifetime of the cell. The early steps of replication lead to establishment of infection in target cells, but the virus may be dormant in some cell types, requiring activation for viral gene expression.

HIV infection is initiated by binding of the viral envelope to a cellular receptor. HIV is one of the few retroviruses for which the cellular receptor, the CD4 molecule, has been identified.[71,147,170] CD4 is expressed on the surface of the T-helper lymphocyte subset and, in lesser quantities, on mononuclear phagocytes; these are the principal target cells in vivo. There may be other cell surface molecules involved in virus binding and entry, however, because transfection of the CD4 gene into some nonpermissive cell types does not confer susceptibility to all HIV strains.[49] In addition, cells that do not detectably express CD4 antigen can be infected in vitro by some HIV-1 strains,[39,118,160,268] and HIV-1 infection has been detected in a variety of non–CD4-bearing cells in infected individuals.[201,223,221,292] Alternative routes of HIV entry besides CD4 have been identified, but their biologic significance is uncertain.[21,29,117,126,266] In contrast to other retroviruses, HIV does

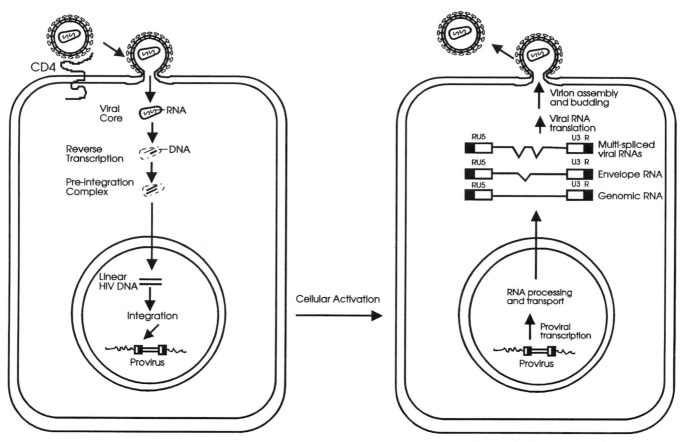

FIG. 34-4. Retrovirus life cycle. After binding to the surface of the host cell, the viral core enters by virus-cell membrane fusion. A double-stranded DNA copy is synthesized from genomic RNA by virion-associated reverse transcriptase. The viral core is transported to the nucleus, and the provirus is formed by integration into the host genome. Viral RNA can be expressed from the provirus, typically after cell activation, and viral proteins are synthesized on host ribosomes. Progeny virions are formed by budding through the membrane of infected cells.

not enter cells through receptor-mediated endocytosis.[260] Instead, after the binding events, a pH-independent fusion of viral and cell membranes occurs, and the viral core is taken up into the cytoplasm.[177]

Once inside the cell, virion-associated reverse transcriptase synthesizes a linear, double-stranded DNA copy of the viral genome. Although initially thought to occur only in the cytoplasm of newly infected cells,[302] reports indicate that viral DNA generated by partial reverse transcription is contained within HIV-1 virions, both in those purified from culture[164,274] and in those purified from peripheral blood plasma of HIV-infected individuals.[307] Enzymes and primers required for this process are contained within the virion. The kinetics of reverse transcription are more rapid in CD4+ lymphocytes than in macrophages, which suggests that cellular factors are also involved.[207] The viral preintegration complex is actively transported to the cell nucleus through interactions with the *gag* matrix protein (p17), possibly involving Vpr.[35,120] Integration of full-length viral DNA occurs by colinear insertion into chromosomal DNA to form the provirus. Viral genes are replicated along with host chromosomal DNA and therefore persist for the life of the cell. Lentiviruses differ from other classes of

retroviruses in their ability to replicate in nondividing as well as in dividing cells. This may require special functions, supplied by some of the accessory genes, to permit translocation of the preintegration complex and integration into nonreplicating genomic DNA.

Expression of HIV genes is directed by complex regulatory systems that involve both cellular and viral proteins. Whereas establishment of infection is mediated largely by viral factors, the later steps of the HIV life cycle require host factors to perform synthesis, processing of viral RNA, and translation of viral mRNA on host ribosomes. Signals for initiation of transcription are found in the 5' LTR region, which is formed by duplication of the terminal ends of the viral genome during reverse transcription (see Fig. 34-3). There are also enhancer regions of the LTR, which can increase the level of transcription after binding of host regulatory proteins[104]; these include the cellular transcription factors, Sp1,[132] and nuclear factor kappa B (NFκB),[198] as well as a negative regulatory element.[167] After translation of viral mRNAs on host ribosomes and proteolytic cleavage of precursor proteins, virions are assembled in the cytoplasm and are released from the cell by budding through the cell surface membrane. Cellular proteins have been found in association with virions and may have been acquired during budding.[9,18,241] These antigens may be important both for host immune response and for binding and entry into target cells.

GENETIC VARIATION

Variability of molecular sequence between isolates of HIV-1 arises as a result of nucleotide incorporation errors and abnormal strand transfers during reverse transcriptase.[23,269] Genetic variability is also driven by factors that select for new mutants, particularly in vivo, including the abilities to replicate rapidly, to escape neutralization or other immune clearance mechanisms, and to resist actions of antiretroviral drugs.

Genetic variation is not distributed evenly throughout the genome. Although some regions (e.g., *gag*, *tat*) are well conserved, other regions show marked differences, particularly the *env* region.[113,197] Genetic diversity within a single individual has been demonstrated,[109,114,152,185] but these strains are more closely related than are those between different patients, suggesting that virus populations found in a single individual arose from a common progenitor strain.

There appear to be geographic influences on HIV variation. Based on similarities in the *env* or *gag* genes, at least eight sequenced subtypes of HIV-1 and five of HIV-2 have been designated as distinct clades.[100,165,197] Divergent strains of HIV-1 have been reported from Cameroon, in West Central Africa, now characterized as subtype O.[75,111,278] Infection with these strains is not detected by many of the current serologic tests, mandating modification of these assays and increased vigilance for new variants.

The extent of HIV-1 genetic sequence heterogeneity differs at various stages of disease and appears to be related to level of HIV-1 accumulation (viral load), duration of infection, and evasion of host immune responses. For instance, the sequences are homogenous during acute infection, although there are high levels of viral replication.[180,213,308] This suggests that only one or a limited number of HIV-1 strains are transmitted in acute infection. Circulating virus levels fall after the acute phase, at 4 to 8 weeks, although there may be abundant virus replication at these early disease stages in lymph nodes.[82,214] Sequence diversity remains limited but gradually increases as the virus load grows.[180] During advanced stages of disease, the virus load is typically high, and marked sequence heterogeneity can be detected. The increased sequence heterogeneity is associated with emergence of new phenotypes, including strains that exhibit greater cytopathicity and more rapid replication kinetics in vitro.[48,90,243,271] Many of these strains can be characterized by the ability to induce multicell syncytia in MT2 cells. These syncytium-inducing (SI) strains are not detected during acute transmission,[308] for reasons that are not clear. It has been suggested that HIV-1 strains that are adapted to T-cell lines (TCLs), which tend to have the SI phenotype, have more exposed CD4 binding and antibody neutralization sites.[206,296] Therefore, SI strains could be more readily suppressed by the immune system early in infection. At later disease stages, coincident with decline of immune responsiveness, SI strains often appear and are associated with CD4+ lymphocyte decline and disease progression[68,243] (see Development of AIDS). The increased sequence diversity is also associated with increasing antigenic diversity, which enhances escape from immune surveillance.[202]

TROPISM

Genetic diversity can produce other viral phenotypes thought to be important for determining the course of clinical disease. One such trait is the differential ability of viruses to replicate in various cell types, termed cell tropism. Although CD4+ lymphocytes are the predominant target cell for HIV-1 infection in circulating blood, and almost all clinical virus strains replicate efficiently in this cell type, there is greater range of infection efficiency in mononuclear phagocytes (MPs).[64,275] The predominance of macrophage-tropic HIV-1 strains during the stable, asymptomatic period[243] and their presence through all stages of infection suggest a role for these strains in viral persistence. In addition, most HIV-1 viruses in extravascular and extralymphoid tissues are associated with MPs,[181] and a variety of HIV-related diseases may arise as a result of local virus production in MPs. In particular, the AIDS dementia complex is thought to be a consequence of HIV infection of MPs in the central nervous system (CNS), and it is likely that different HIV-1 strains vary in their potential for induction of clinical brain disease. In support of this concept, HIV-1 strains recovered from brain tissue of patients who died with AIDS dementia replicate efficiently in MPs.[47,152,163] Although macrophage-tropic strains are genetically distinct, they are more closely related to each other than to strains exhibiting different cell tropisms.[60,197]

HIV-1 strains also vary in their ability to replicate in transformed TCLs. Because of the uniformity of clonal populations of transformed T cells and their ability to grow indefinitely in culture, these cells were used for most studies of HIV-1 pathogenesis undertaken in the mid-1980s,[16,99] and the original virus isolates identified as the causative agent of AIDS were derived after prolonged passage in transformed T cells. However, virus strains that emerge from these continuous cultures are adapted for efficient growth in these cells and are phenotypically distinct from primary virus strains. Most of these TCL-adapted virus strains replicate in peripheral blood lymphocytes (PBLs), exhibit the SI phenotype, and replicate inefficiently in MPs. In general, virus strains appear to have reciprocal tropisms for either MPs or transformed TCLs,[61,128,203,252] but all replicate in primary lymphocyte cultures.

Phenotypic differences in cell tropism have been mapped, by recombinant virus studies using highly macrophage-tropic strains and TCL-adapted strains, to the gp120 portion of the HIV-1 envelope.[205,252,290] This region of *env* includes the major neutralization domain, variable region 3 (V3). This 30- to 40-amino-acid domain forms a loop, stabilized by a disulfide-linked cysteine bridge, which has been shown to independently confer the macrophage-tropic phenotype.[128] Cell tropism for transformed TCL maps to a similar region of gp120, and viral determinants of tropism for TCL and MP tend to be mutually exclusive.[50,128,203,252] Although the same CD4 receptor is involved in entry into both MP and T cells,[59,69,71] HIV-1 strains can exhibit different tropisms based on differences in Env, the virus attachment protein. Presumably, this is because the V3 loop, which is not involved in CD4 binding, is involved in a later step in entry during which there are interactions with other cellular accessory proteins.

Although the V3 domain is crucial for cell tropism, other regions of gp120 also appear to be involved in the viral entry process. Distinct envelope regions appear to interact to produce a complex structure, with generation of conformational epitopes of the highly glycosylated gp120/gp41 hetero-oligomer that are involved in the entry process.[138,257,258,295] Mutations at distant gp120 sites can modify phenotypic characteristics directed by V3.[28,190,242,246,291] In addition, gp41 is involved in fusion of the viral and target cell membranes.[97,151,260] It is likely that a second cellular receptor, in addition to CD4, is involved in postbinding interactions with the V3 region of gp120, as well as with gp41. The cell surface peptidase CD26 has been proposed to fulfill this function,[37] but this hypothesis appears unlikely.[6,32,38,157] Moreover, the putative second cellular receptor may differ in various cell types, and for different strains, because HIV-1 strains that replicate efficiently in PBLs vary in efficiency of entry into MPs. Finally, new conformation-dependent envelope epitopes apparently involved in HIV-1 entry appear after CD4 binding.[138,190,237,273] HIV-1 entry therefore appears to involve a multistep process with complex and sequential interactions between envelope and target cells.

Viral replication differences in macrophages have also been attributed to domains exclusive of envelope, notably *vpr*, which may be essential for replication in nondividing cells.[119,291] Although viral entry appears to be a critical step in determining cell tropism,[222,242] later steps may also be involved under some circumstances. Several reports indicate that TCL-adapted strains appear to enter macrophages and initiate reverse transcription but are blocked at a later stage in the replication cycle.[63,127,192,238] These putative postentry blocks are influenced by products of the *env* gene, which are believed to function during virus entry.

RESTRICTED REPLICATION

In addition to virus-defined restrictions on HIV replication, there are also cell-specific restrictions. Although PBLs and MPs are both susceptible to infection with most replication-competent primary virus strains, there are differences in the levels of virus production from these cells, depending on activation state. In normal adults, more than 99% of circulating CD4+ lymphocytes are quiescent, and virus production is limited in these cells compared with activated and proliferating CD4+ lymphocytes. HIV entry and initiation of reverse transcription is efficient in both quiescent and activated CD4+ lymphocytes; however, completion of reverse transcription and integration of full-length viral DNA is inefficient in quiescent cells.[262,302,303] Whereas reverse transcription and provirus formation occur within 6 hours in activated CD4+ lymphocytes, reverse transcription is arrested at an intermediate stage in resting cells, and there is very little accumulation of full-length viral DNA. In these cells, there appears to be low-level virus expression, predominantly of singly- and multiply-spliced mRNAs.[224] On cellular stimulation, there is first an increase in the regulatory mRNAs, and then an increase in the unspliced RNAs, which encode structural proteins.[224,247] Therefore, the ordered appearance of mRNA transcripts seen during acute in vitro infection may also be invoked in infected cells on release from the latently infected state.[144]

HIV replication in MPs represents a third scenario. In general, these cells do not divide but can be productively infected with apparent integration, even after cell proliferation is impaired by irradiation of cells.[288] Reverse transcription in MPs appears to proceed by slower kinetics than in activated T cells,[144,207,302] requiring 36 to 48 hours after virus entry for accumulation of full-length viral DNA. The kinetics of reverse transcription can be accelerated in MPs by addition of exogenous nucleotide precursors, but this is not the case for quiescent PBLs.[303] Although MP nucleoside concentrations are low, utilization of these precursors may also be inefficient, because the accelerated rate is still much slower than that seen in activated CD4+ lymphocytes. MPs also differ in susceptibility to HIV-1 infection based on activation state. Fresh monocytes, in culture less than 1 day, are much less susceptible to productive virus infection than are MPs recovered from the lungs of the same patient or blood monocytes activated by adherence to plastic in culture.[226] Virus production from MPs or TCLs can be increased further by activation with lectins or cytokines.[95,94,153] This activation appears to induce cell factors that interact with the HIV LTR to increase virus expression and levels of virus production.

THE DEVELOPMENT OF AIDS

AIDS is a clinical syndrome which has been defined by the appearance of diseases that result from impaired cellular immunity in the absence of explanation other than HIV infection.[42,43] Almost all HIV-infected individuals develop AIDS over a variable period of time as a result of a progressive, relentless virus infection that is associated with a gradual increase of virus load. This leads to an inexorable deterioration of immunity, particularly cell-mediated immunity (CMI), which is most closely associated with the decline in circulating CD4+ lymphocyte number. In 1992, decline of CD4+ lymphocyte count below 200 cells/µL was added to the Centers for Disease Control case definition,[43] because this level is strongly associated with disease and clinical outcome. The appearance of opportunistic infections and other manifestations of HIV-1 infection is closely linked to stages defined by circulating CD4+ lymphocyte count (Table 34-1). Minor opportunistic diseases, such as rash and diarrhea, occur at early stages (CD4+ lymphocytes >500/µL), and cachexia and neurologic dysfunction occur at late stages (CD4+ lymphocytes <100/µL).

Although the mechanisms for destruction of T lymphocytes and competent immunity are not known, they are certain to be complex and multifactorial. In the remainder of this section, we discuss possible mechanisms for the development of AIDS by reviewing virologic, immunologic, and cofactor determinants of disease.

Viral Factors

HIV Quantitation and AIDS

There is a clear association between increasing amounts of viral burden and clinical progression.[64,82,186,214,232,239] Until recently, quantitative viral measurements, such as the level of

TABLE 34-1. *Relation of CD4+ lymphocyte count and onset of particular HIV–related diseases*

CD4+ count (cells/µL)	Disease
>500	Asymptomatic Shingles Lymphadenopathy syndrome Rash Diarrhea
200–500	Vaginal candidiasis Thrush Oral hairy leukoplakia Kaposi's sarcoma Recurrent herpes simplex virus infection
<200	*Pneumocystis carinii* pneumonia *Candida* esophagitis Cervical dysplasia Cryptococcal meningitis

<100	Disseminated
	   cytomegalovirus infection
	Disseminated
	   Mycobacterium avium
	   complex infection
	HIV encephalopathy
	Wasting

HIV-1 p24 antigen in blood, were too insensitive to be useful for monitoring of viral load. Culture methods can be used to quantitate infectious virus in blood,[65,122,219] but they require propagation of virus in the laboratory and may not be sensitive. In contrast, amplification methods for detection of HIV-specific DNA or RNA can identify and quantify viral sequences at any stage of disease.[125,186,219,232,239] Viral DNA measurements assess the abundance of provirus, which is an indication of the viral reservoir, although not necessarily of productive infection. Moreover, viral DNA may also represent virus-specific nucleic acids from defective strains incapable of completing the viral life cycle. HIV-1 RNA measurements can be used to indicate active expression and replication.[78,196] In addition, there are marked decreases in plasma HIV-1 RNA after initiation of therapies known to provide clinical benefit.[7,58,123,140,149,287] When applied to plasma, this assay measures all virus particles and typically yields values two to four orders of magnitude greater than those detected by culture methods.[219]

The high levels of circulating virus seen after acute infection are suppressed by the host immune response within 1 or 2 months.[70,150] Despite the marked decline in circulating virus, there is ongoing virus replication in lymphoid tissue during the early, clinically latent stage of disease.[82,214] Measurements at different stages of disease show progressively higher levels of virus replication in later stages.[64,65,122,186,219,232,239,248] In some patients, marked increases in levels of virus replication are associated with an abrupt drop in CD4+ lymphocyte count,[64,68] although some researchers argue that the correlation between increasing virus load and the rate of CD4+ lym-

phocyte depletion is weak.[218] High levels of virus replication can occasionally be seen in patients at earlier stages of disease, but loss of ability to control virus replication is a hallmark of late-stage disease. Increases in HIV replication may accelerate loss of CD4+ lymphocytes (see later discussion), but the magnitude of these effects may be modulated by viral phenotype.

HIV-1 Replicative Ability

As the viral burden increases in later stages of disease, HIV-1 variants exhibiting increased replication kinetics and cytopathicity appear.[48,90,228,271] This enhanced replication capacity may accelerate the increase in viral load as well as CD4+ lymphocyte depletion through the cytopathic effect of syncytium induction. During the early phase of HIV infection, host immunity appears to control viral replication, particularly of SI strains, and emergence of these cytopathic strains coincides with failing host immunity. The dynamic relation between HIV-1 replication and CD4+ lymphocyte loss was recently demonstrated.[123,287] In these studies, the turnover rates of plasma virus and virus-producing cells were calculated after administration of potent antiretroviral drugs, and both were shown to have a halflife of only 2 days. Therefore, there is continuous and highly productive replication of HIV-1, and viral factors that lead to increased virus replication ability may hasten the decline of CD4+ lymphocytes.

Drug-resistant strains rapidly emerge in patients who have received antiretroviral treatment (see Treatment of HIV-1 Infection). Levels of active virus replication fall after initiation of effective antiretroviral therapy[123,219,287] but increase again after several months, at least in part because of emergence of resistant strains. Therefore, in late-stage disease, HIV-1 variants emerge that can elude both host immune suppressive mechanisms and pharmacologic inhibitions.

CD4+ Lymphocyte Depletion

The hallmark of clinical progression in HIV infection is the depletion of CD4+ lymphocytes. Among the potential mechanisms for this phenomenon are virus-induced cytopathicity, immune clearance, normal homeostatic mechanisms, and the actions of secondary mediators such as cytokines. The relative impacts on progression from each of these phenomena remain to be elucidated. One probable mechanism of cell killing of CD4+ lymphocytes is a direct result of HIV-1 infection. Scanning electron micrographs of T-cell infection in vitro have demonstrated an exuberant budding process, with hundreds to thousands of virions released from an infected cell.[105]

Cell death has been associated with direct toxicity from viral envelope proteins. Addition of gp120 to cultured brain cells was shown to cause cell killing in a dose-dependent manner.[31,79,135] This toxicity appears to be related to direct damage to the cell membrane. There is a rapid influx of calcium into cells exposed to gp120, possibly because of enhanced sensitivity of *N*-methyl-o-aspartate (NMDA) receptors, resulting in disturbances in membrane integrity and cell function.[79] This phenomenon has not been demonstrated for PBMCs, and it is possible that toxic effects in those cells are unrelated to inter-

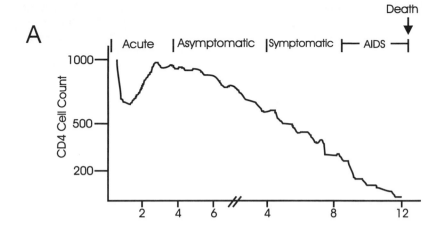

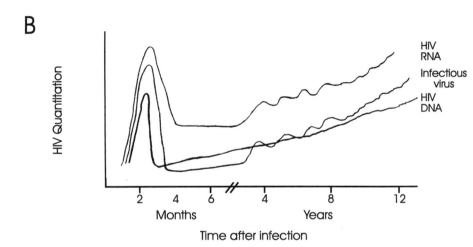

FIG. 34-5. Clinical and virologic correlates of human immunodeficiency virus (HIV) infection. (**A**) The pattern of CD4+ lymphocyte depletion and clinical disease over time after acute infection. Particular HIV-associated diseases or conditions tend to occur at intermediate and late stages (CD4+ lymphocyte counts 200 to 500/μL and <200/μL, respectively). (**B**) HIV quantitation at different stages of disease. HIV RNA levels range from 10^2 to more than 10^6 copies per milliliter, HIV DNA from 10 to 10^5 copies per 10^6 cells, and plasma infectious virus from 0 to 10^4 tissue culture infectious doses (TCID) per milliliter of plasma.

actions with the CD4 molecule. The transmembrane protein, gp41, can also be toxic to cells, and it shares structural similarities with well-described neurotoxins.[188] Tat also shares similarities with neurotoxins and can be toxic to PBMCs in culture.[102] Tat may also induce cytokine production and has been implicated in the genesis of Kaposi's sarcoma (KS), an AIDS-associated neoplasm.[83,84]

Alternatively, cytopathic effects may be related to syncytium induction after interaction of gp120 expressed on the surface of infected CD4+ lymphocytes with CD4 epitopes on uninfected cells. In this case, both infected and uninfected bystander CD4+ lymphocytes could be killed. However, CD4+ lymphocyte depletion occurs in patients without SI strains, and syncytia are rarely detected in vivo, so this latter mechanism may not be the principal cause of CD4+ lymphocyte depletion.

Another potential mechanism of CD4+ lymphocyte depletion is immune clearance of infected cells. Viral proteins expressed in infected cells may act as targets for immune clearance through antibody-dependent cell-mediated cytotoxicity or through direct lysis by cytotoxic T lymphocytes (CTLs). CMI responses play a critical role in the outcome of many acute viral infections.[179,225] In general, clearance of virus typically coincides with the development of virus-specific class I

major histocompatibility complex (MHC)–restricted CD8+ CTLs.[150] HIV-specific memory CTLs can be distinguished from other antiviral memory CTLs in HIV-infected individuals by their increased numbers during the asymptomatic phase of infection[124,234] and their marked depletion during end-stage disease.[41] The high frequencies of HIV-specific CTLs reported early in disease are attributed to persistent viral replication, which results in chronic activation and expansion of CTLs.[124] Moreover, these cells probably participate in the clearance of virus during acute infection.[150] On the other hand, the presence of elevated levels of CTLs at later time points may simply reflect increases in viral burden, because they do not appear to be capable of preventing disease progression. It has been suggested that CTLs play a protective role in HIV disease through direct lysis of infected CD4+ lymphocytes.[25] However, it can also be argued that lysis of infected cells indirectly contributes to clinical disease progression by removal of CD4+ lymphocytes from circulation.[306]

Third, it has been suggested that homeostatic mechanisms controlling the total CD4+ lymphocyte level may contribute to depletion of the CD4+ lymphocyte compartment.[1,174,259] In this model, CD4+ lymphocytes are replaced without regard to subset, thereby maintaining a balance of total CD4+ lymphocytes but a deficit in the CD4+ lymphocytes that are selectively depleted during HIV infection. This mechanism may be particularly important in light of recent evidence that CD4+ lymphocyte turnover is quite rapid, with an average circulating halflife of just 2 to 3 days.[123,287]

HIV infection results in a chronic activation of the immune system with spontaneous activation of B lymphocytes, demonstrated by increased levels of circulating antibody and increased cytokine production. Cytokines secreted from T lymphocytes and macrophages act as secondary mediators and may contribute to CD4+ lymphocyte depletion. For instance, tumor necrosis factor-alpha (TNF-α, or cachectin) has been demonstrated to enhance HIV-1 replication in latently infected cells.[94,220] Interleukin-1 (IL-1) is believed to have the capacity to stimulate HIV-1 expression in vitro, but the level of enhancement is significantly weaker than that observed with TNF-α, and apparent contradictions in the literature are evident.[95,148,209] Furthermore, a variety of hematopoietic growth factors, including granulocyte-monocyte colony-stimulating factor (GM-CSF), monocyte-CSF, and IL-3, have been demonstrated to upregulate latent HIV-1 expression in tissue culture.[136,153] In HIV-infected individuals, there is spontaneous production of TNF-α and IL-6 in PBMC cultures[229] as well as spontaneous release of GM-CSF by alveolar macrophages and production of IL-1 in monocyte cultures.[158] In this view, HIV-1 replication may be enhanced in vivo, through overexpression of cytokines.

Elevated levels of cytokines have also been demonstrated in the blood and body fluids of HIV-1–infected individuals. Elevated levels of TNF-α and IL-6 persist in the blood of these patients and tend to increase during disease progression.[282] IL-6 levels in plasma may be elevated as much as 16-fold in some HIV-1–infected individuals, compared with normal controls.[30] In vivo production of GM-CSF is also evident in HIV-1–infected donors. Agostini and colleagues[2] detected as much as 36 pg/mL of GM-CSF in unconcentrated bronchoalveolar lavage fluid from HIV-1–infected patients. In light of these data, it appears likely that a variety of cytokines, including TNF-α, GM-CSF, granulocyte-CSF, monocyte-CSF, IL-3, IL-6, and possibly IL-1, modulate HIV-1 expression in vivo and may serve to accelerate disease progression in the infected host.

Finally, in HIV-infected individuals, there may be a paradoxical CD4+ lymphocyte response to immune stimulation. Rather than stimulating lymphocyte proliferation, these cells may undergo a sequence of events known as programmed cell death, or apoptosis.[110,270] This active process requires protein synthesis and results in fragmentation of cellular DNA by endogenous endonuclease into small fragments. This has been demonstrated in vitro by exposing primed CD4+ lymphocytes from HIV-infected patients to influenza or tetanus antigen,[110] and it has been proposed as a mechanism of lymphocyte depletion in lymph nodes for cells previously exposed to HIV antigens.[87] It has not been shown whether this mechanism is involved in CD4+ lymphocyte depletion in vivo,[184] but recent data suggest that CD4+ lymphocyte destruction is directly related to the level of virus replication.[123,287]

T-Lymphocyte Dysfunction

Initially, there is a competent and broad immune response that brings HIV infection somewhat under control at the outset.[87] Patients with chronic HIV-1 infection, however, develop a profound deficiency in CMI, presumably in part because of the selective loss of the CD4+ T helper (Th)–lymphocyte response to antigen.[54] Before CD4+ lymphocyte depletion, however, there are functional defects in these cells, with failure to proliferate in response to T-cell receptor stimulation by recall antigens and mitogens.[55,183,187,249] In both symptomatic and asymptomatic HIV-1–infected individuals, there is also a progressive dysfunction in the Th-lymphocyte response to various T-lymphocyte stimulants. This deterioration occurs in a cascade; loss in reactivity is reported to occur first in response to recall antigens and is followed by loss of reactivity to alloantigens and, finally, to mitogens such as phytohemagglutinin.[245] Moreover, coexpression among T lymphocytes of CD28, an important receptor involved in signal transduction and IL-2 production in response to antigens,[161] is markedly decreased in HIV-infected individuals.[26,108] The mechanisms for these alterations in Th-lymphocyte function remain unresolved, but a number of hypotheses have been proposed, including (1) selective loss of Th memory lymphocytes,[233,240,276] (2) defects in antigen presentation to the memory cells,[169] (3) induction of suppressor factors or suppressor cells,[53,141,155] and (4) altered patterns of expression of immunoregulatory cytokines, resulting in a shift from a predominantly Th1-type response (characterized by cytokines that promote CMI responses) to a Th2-type response (characterized by cytokines that tend to influence humoral-mediated responses).[55,245] In addition, there are declines in cytolytic activity mediated by virus-specific class I MHC–restricted CD8+ CTLs as well as CD56 natural killer cells.[150,234] In chronic viral infections, CD4+ lymphocytes appear to be required for production of virus-specific CD8+ CTLs,[176] and loss of anti-HIV CD8+ CTLs at late stages of disease may be caused by decreased CD4+ lymphocyte number.

Macrophage Dysfunction

MPs are important in the host immune response for antigen presentation to T lymphocytes and for direct killing of intracellular pathogens. There is compelling clinical evidence of MP dysfunction in AIDS, but it is not clear whether this is caused by a direct effect of HIV infection or by a decrease in T-lymphocyte number and T-lymphocyte dysfunction.[12] Blood-derived macrophages from HIV-positive individuals exhibit impaired phagocytosis for *Histoplasma capsulatum*.[45] Defects in phagocytosis were also reported for *Staphylococcus aureus* in macrophages from symptomatic but not from asymptomatic HIV-positive patients,[265] suggesting that diminution of macrophage function is associated with loss of CD4+ T-lymphocyte number and function. Changes in macrophage phagocytosis with more advanced disease could also be a result of increasing viral load. Soluble gp120 can impair macrophage phagocytosis.[253,283] Moreover, HIV-induced impairment of macrophage function allows more rapid growth of *H capsulatum*,[45] *M avium*,[67] *Cryptococcus neoformans*,[86] *S aureus*,[286] and *Candida pseudotropicalis*.[12] Impairment of macrophage function may therefore contribute to the emergence of numerous opportunistic infections at more advanced stages of disease.

In addition to their function in antigen presentation and intracellular killing, MPs secrete a variety of cytokines. Aberrant secretion of cytokines and other soluble factors by these cells has been implicated in the pathogenesis of CNS disease, in loss of control of viral latency, and in T-lymphocyte killing.[19,22,106,182,289] Because macrophages are distributed widely in extravascular tissues and are involved in complex cytokine circuits, it is difficult to examine the true role of infected macrophages for HIV-1 pathogenesis with the use of in vitro systems.

Cofactors

One of the hallmarks of lentivirus infections is a relatively long time period between infection and the development of disease. The mechanisms responsible for progression remain to be elucidated. One potential mechanism relates to events that lead to HIV-1 induction from mononuclear cells by activation, as has been shown to occur in HIV-infected patients who received the influenza vaccine. Ten of 20 patients exhibited a fourfold or greater increase in HIV RNA in PBMCs at 1 or 2 weeks after vaccination; similar increases were not seen in 15 nonvaccinated controls.[204] The linkage between vaccine-induced increases in HIV-1 replication and clinical progression has not been proved, but progression is associated with increases in virus load. Increases in viral burden over time may be the result of many such inductions of HIV-1 replication, caused by vaccines, infections, or other immunologic stimuli. It is difficult to precisely define mechanisms of progression, because regulation of the rate of clinical progression is probably multifactorial in nature, involving virologic, genetic, and environmental stimuli.

Coinfection with heterologous viruses may also result in enhancement of HIV-1 replication and a more rapid degeneration of the immune system, with acceleration of clinical progression. Herpes simplex virus type 1 (HSV-1) DNA can activate expression of a latent murine retrovirus.[27] Other ubiquitous human herpesviruses, including human cytomegalovirus, Epstein-Barr virus, human herpesvirus type 6, HSV-1, and HSV-2, may also act as cofactors in HIV-1 disease[154] and can lead to synergy of HIV-1 and herpesvirus replication in coinfected cells.[121] In addition to the in vivo data, there are a multitude of in vitro studies demonstrating upregulation of HIV-1 by herpesvirus proteins through a region of the HIV-1 promoter that is distinct from the Tat-responsive element, TAR.[200] Another role for herpesvirus coinfection in AIDS is suggested by the presence of herpesvirus-like sequences in lesions of KS.[44] Although it has been suggested that there is a cofactor responsible for the KS seen in HIV infection, a causal link between these sequences and AIDS-KS remains to be established.

In support of the concept that herpesvirus coinfection may enhance disease progression, it has been reported that consistent use of the antiherpes drug acyclovir at a dose sufficient to suppress HSV recurrence significantly prolonged survival in a well-characterized patient cohort.[261] Symptomatic episodes of HSV infection were associated with a trend toward shortened survival time. This observation was supported by another report,[66] but in neither study was there an effect on clinically apparent cytomegalovirus infection.

Additional environmental factors may affect control of virus replication. Ingestion of alcohol may lead to increased HIV-1 replication through an effect on CD8+ lymphocytes.[11,13] In a case report, rapid clinical progression was seen in an individual with alcoholism.[96]

TREATMENT OF HIV-1 INFECTION

Antiretroviral Drugs

There are limited options for treatment of HIV-1 infection, and only four antiretroviral drugs (all nucleoside reverse transcriptase inhibitors) were approved for human use by the U.S. Food and Drug Administration prior to 1995.[304,33,56] In addition, only one clinical trial has demonstrated a survival benefit,[91] perhaps because reverse transcriptase inhibitors have only modest effect on HIV-1 replication, which is usually not sustained. Furthermore, there are significant toxicities associated with use of these drugs. Zidovudine (azidothymidine, or AZT) was initially tested in high doses in patients with advanced disease, and there was a clear demonstration of benefit.[91] Subsequent studies in HIV-infected individuals at earlier stages of disease demonstrated a modest effect in delay of clinical progression, but at no point in any of the studies was a survival benefit observed.[62,92,115,280] Potential mechanisms for the failure of long-term benefits from this agent include development of drug resistance induced by prolonged monotherapy, which may lead to increasing viral levels and allow emergence of more pathogenic HIV-1 strains.[227] The optimal time for initiation of zidovudine treatment is controversial, but no studies have reported a treatment benefit for HIV-infected patients with CD4+ lymphocyte counts greater than 500 cells/μL.

Three other reverse transcriptase inhibitors—didanosine (dideoxyinosine, or ddI), zalcitabine (dideoxycytidine, or ddC), and stavudine (didehydro-deoxythymidine, or d4T)—have been approved and have provided modest benefits in patients in whom zidovudine is not tolerated or who have clinically progressed on zidovudine therapy.[304,85,133,298] However, these agents are associated with peripheral neuropathy, and resistance can also develop rapidly. Improved control of this infection appears to be possible using combination therapy with both reverse transcriptase inhibitors and other agents such as protease inhibitors that affect different steps of the HIV life cycle.

Although other agents have been tested for efficacy in treatment of HIV infection, resistant HIV-1 strains emerge rapidly in patients treated with nonnucleoside reverse transcriptase inhibitors.[277] A promising class of antiretroviral agents are the protease inhibitors, which interfere with the retroviral enzymes required for processing of viral proteins. However, viral resistance can also develop to this class of agents.[210]

A variety of gene therapy approaches have been attempted to express recombinant constructs intracellularly. These include introduction of ribozymes to cleave viral RNA,[208,236,300] antisense molecules that bind to specific HIV-1 RNA species or yield triplex formation in specific areas of HIV-1 proviral DNA,[34,162] and intracellular antibody production and intracellular dominant negative inhibitors.[20,80,81,199,217] Although in vitro data are promising, improved delivery into primary cells from patients and sustained expression of recombinant constructs is required before these methods can be tested in vivo.

Vaccines

Initially, there was great optimism that an effective vaccine would soon be available once the virus that causes AIDS was identified. The recognition of the V3 region of gp120 as a neutralizing domain led to development of recombinant envelope vaccines designed to induce neutralizing antibody. Unfortunately, these prototypic vaccines tend to generate neutralizing antibody only for the virus strain from which the vaccine was derived.[187]

Development of an effective, prophylactic HIV vaccine will be extremely difficult for several reasons. Of greatest concern is the tremendous genetic variability of HIV and the propensity for rapid genetic drift in response to immunologic or pharmacologic pressures.

Second, it is not yet clear which immune responses are necessary to control HIV infection. Although humoral immunity has been found to provide protection from infection with many other viruses (see Chap. 7) and the V3 of Env region has been identified as an important neutralizing domain for HIV, the specific epitopes that should be targeted by a vaccine have not been identified. Moreover, because CMI appears to be important in controlling acute infection,[150] it may be a crucial protective response, perhaps invoking CTLs specific for more conserved viral epitopes.[131] HIV-1 exposed individuals who are not infected may have potent anti-HIV CMI responses, suggesting that this natural response may be effective in preventing acute infection.[51,52,231] This is an important new direction for HIV vaccine development. There is also good evidence for a soluble factor, elaborated by CD8+ lymphocytes, that inhibits HIV replication.[284] Characterization of this factor and strategies to stimulate its production may be part of a prophylactic HIV program.

Third, because sexual transmission is an important mode of HIV infection, it is necessary to prevent cell-to-cell transfer of HIV in addition to infection by cell-free virus, and protection must act at mucosal surfaces. Vaccine strategies that stimulate mucosal anti-HIV immunoglobulin A secretion would appear to be crucial for protective anti-HIV immunity.

Fourth, an effective immune response to this virus may not be achievable. Initial infection invokes a broadbased immune response, including both Th1 and Th2 components, that is typical for many virus infections. For HIV, this response dramatically suppresses but does not eliminate virus replication. Virus spreads through lymphoid tissue and gradually depletes CD4+ lymphocytes to the point at which immune surveillance is incompetent. It is possible that the same scenario could occur in individuals given preexposure immunization, regardless of its effectiveness.

Finally, no ideal animal model exists in which to test potential vaccines (see Models for Studying HIV-1 Infection). The only animal species that can be infected with low doses of HIV are the great apes. However, chimpanzees do not manifest an AIDS-like disease,[285] and they are expensive and not readily available. Infection of rhesus macaques with the SIV isolate SIV$_{mac239}$ results in an AIDS-like syndrome, including CD4+ lymphocyte depletion and opportunistic infections.[142] Nonetheless, there are substantial genetic and antigenic differences between HIV and SIV, and an SIV vaccine would not be applicable for protection against HIV infection in human beings.

The ability of a vaccine to provide sustained protection from viral infection may be enhanced by use of a live attenuated virus. Such an approach, in which low-level virus infection from a strain unable to cause disease continues to stimulate protective immunity over many years, has proven effective in the development of vaccines against polio and smallpox (see

Chap. 16). The potential for protection from an attenuated retroviral vaccine has been shown in the SIV system. Rhesus macaques infected with *nef*-deficient SIV strains remain disease free without CD4 depletion for several years and are also protected by infection from wild-type SIV strains, even with high inoculum challenge.[73] This strategy may also be effective for an HIV vaccine, but there are concerns about the possibility of recombination or backmutation in vivo, which could result in a pathogenic virus infection.

Even if an effective vaccine can be developed, there will probably be rapid selection for spread of HIV-1 subtypes not prevented by the vaccine. The potential need for different vaccine formulations in different geographic regions, and for frequent vaccine reformulation to respond to viral genetic drift, will probably increase the cost of vaccination, particularly in regions where multiple HIV clades coexist. This may impair the ability to apply vaccine strategies for prevention of transmission in developing regions, where the benefit would be greatest.

LONG-TERM NONPROGRESSORS

In contrast to the scenario of progressive immune deterioration in most HIV-infected individuals, a small fraction (<5%) of those infected for 10 to 12 years or more have not exhibited clinical signs of disease progression, maintain a healthy and functional immune system, and have high, stable CD4+ lymphocyte levels and a low viral burden.[64,250] Long-term nonprogressors may be defined as those individuals infected for at least 10 years who have stable CD4+ lymphocyte counts greater than 500 cells/μL and an absence of HIV-related symptoms.[40,215] Although these individuals form a heterogeneous group in terms of HLA determinants, age, and racial background, there are several common features. The viral load, both in lymphoid tissue and circulating in blood, remains low despite the long duration of the infection.[40,215] HIV-1 strains isolated from these patients may be relatively attenuated, with lower replicative capabilities and less cytopathicity than is seen with HIV-1 isolates from patients with AIDS. Inability to deplete CD4+ lymphocytes may be a result of a lower level of replication, as suggested by the identification of *nef*-deficient strains in a long-term nonprogressor.[146] This is consistent with observations in persons infected with HIV-2, in which in vitro cytopathicity is less and disease progression is slower.[175]

A more important explanation for long-term survival with HIV-1 infection in these patients may be their immune response. There are consistently higher titers of neutralizing antibody in these patients, perhaps explaining in part the difficulty of recovering virus from plasma.[40,215] In addition, strong virus-specific class I MHC–restricted (CD8+) CTLs are found. This response is usually associated with clearance of the virus after acute infection and may also be important for surveillance and stringent control of viral replication. Further evidence for the importance of the CD8+ CTL response is demonstrated in HIV-1–seronegative and uninfected individuals who have been exposed to HIV. In some of these persons, HIV-specific CTL responses can be demonstrated, suggesting that this response can also be protective.[51,52,231] Detailed characterization of immune response in long-term nonprogressors may suggest ways in which virus replication can be better contained in patients faced with progressive disease. It may also provide insights into which specific immune responses should be targeted for augmentation in immunotherapies. Finally, it is likely that individuals who are long-term nonprogressors may be heterogeneous, with many mechanisms leading to relatively low viral load and absence of disease.

MODELS FOR STUDYING HIV-1 INFECTION

The goal of model systems is to mimic the in vivo situation in order to investigate HIV pathogenesis and response to therapies without incurring risks or hazards to HIV-infected patients. A variety of model systems have been developed, including both in vitro and animal systems. We focus our discussion on the most promising models, all of which depend on primary target cells for infection, rather than TCLs.

Primary Cell Systems

Because HIV was first recovered in TCLs, it seemed logical to use these as in vitro model systems to study virus replication; most of the studies reported in the mid-1980s used the prototypic HIV strain IIIB in such cell lines. Although much useful information was obtained, there are fundamental differences in replication of TCL-adapted and primary virus strains. For example, TCL-adapted strains are restricted for replication in MPs, but almost all primary strains are able to replicate to some extent in these cells. Adaptation to growth in TCLs results in biochemical changes in the HIV envelope, which leads to quite different interactions with the virus receptor, CD4. TCL-adapted strains shed the noncovalently-linked gp120 much more readily than primary strains,[191,206,296] and gp120 density appears to be much higher for primary strains. These fundamental differences misled investigators as basic work was moved from the benchtop to clinical trials. This was particularly true for soluble CD4 therapy and, as discussed previously, for vaccines. Soluble CD4 was shown in laboratory studies to efficiently neutralize HIV infection (IIIB strain) using clinically achievable soluble CD4 concentrations.[134] This therapy proved not to be useful, however, mostly because of inherent resistance to soluble CD4 neutralization by primary HIV strains.[69]

It is clear that, to approximate clinical HIV infection as closely as possible, in vitro systems employing primary virus strains and primary human cells are needed. This is important not just to determine mechanisms of virus entry but also to study regulation of virus replication. A drawback to this model is variability in donor target cells, because the uniformity of target cells provided by transformed TCLs is not available in primary cell systems. In addition, it is difficult to examine the diversity of virus strains in this system, because only a limited number of primary strains can be examined at one time.

Primate Models

To fully understand the pathogenesis of AIDS, in vivo model systems that involve interaction of HIV replication and immune response are essential. Although a variety of animal systems have been used to study retrovirus pathogenesis, most standard animal model systems cannot be infected by HIV-1, and those that can be infected do not display pathology after infection. Investigators have relied on animal viruses, genetically distinct from HIV-1, that cause AIDS-like disease in their hosts. The best primate models involve SIV infection of rhesus macaques or HIV-1 infection of chimpanzees. The latter animals do not develop immunodeficiency, however, and they are a scarce and endangered species.[77] It is therefore desirable to develop other primate models.

Like HIV, SIV strains exhibit tremendous genetic diversity, particularly in the hypervariable *env* regions. The variants also differ in cell tropism and in replicative and cytopathic properties. In animals that develop immunodeficiency, there are several features shared with HIV infection and AIDS that make the SIV-macaque system a useful model for pathogenesis. SIV strains that evolve in the animal over time are less efficiently neutralized than the infecting virus.[36] This appears to be related to generation of new N-linked glycosylation site motifs.[211] In addition, viruses isolated from macaques that have progressed to simian AIDS are similar in phenotype to HIV strains frequently detected late in HIV infection in humans and likewise exhibit more rapid replication and greater cytopathicity. Macaques also develop CNS disease, and this may be a useful model for the study of the neuropathogenesis of HIV.[246] In contrast to HIV, however, the V3 region of SIV does not appear to be as important in determining viral phenotype as other variable regions.[15,212] Because the V3 region of HIV appears to be so important for the pathogenesis of AIDS, the SIV-macaque model is somewhat limited. One approach to address this limitation has been to use chimeric viruses comprising both SIV and HIV regions, which can mimic certain properties of HIV yet be suitable for in vivo testing in simian systems.[129,159,251] Chimeric viruses may also be useful for vaccine assessment, if it can be established that immune responses to these viruses resemble those found in natural HIV-1 infection in humans.

SCID Mouse Models

Novel models have been developed using mice with severe combined immune deficiency (SCID). These animals are unable to undergo immunoglobulin or T-cell rearrangement and therefore are unable to reject xenografts.[244] Injection of human PBLs into SCID mice resulted in long-term reconstitution of human T and B lymphocytes and macrophages, although in different proportions than found in peripheral blood.[193] These animals could be infected by HIV-1 after intraperitoneal injection, and T lymphocytes could be depleted by HIV infection.[194] Important limitations of this model relate primarily to the limited number of human cell types that can be inoculated and the marked phenotypic differences in human cells in this model compared with those circulating in blood.[267] Human adult lymphocytes in these reconstituted animals are generally activated (xenoreactive) and anergic to further stimulation, in contrast to human peripheral blood, in which more than 99% of cells are quiescent.

Another model using SCID mice involves implantation of human fetal thymus and liver into the renal capsule.[178] A better representation of the human hematopoietic system ensues after this implantation, and these animals also can be infected by HIV.[178] HIV-1 infection results in depletion of T lymphocytes and human thymus tissue in these animals, which allows assessment of mechanisms of immune destruction caused by HIV-1 infection.[5,24,137] Both of these murine models appear to be suitable for testing efficacy of antiretroviral compounds.

CONCLUSIONS

Substantial progress has been made toward our understanding of the molecular structure and mechanisms of replication of HIV-1 in the relatively short time since this virus was discovered. Delineation of the mechanisms of disease pathogenesis, however, has been much more difficult, particularly the mechanisms of loss of CD4 lymphocytes. This is probably a complex and multifactorial process involving viral factors, host factors, and exogenous cofactors. The key step in developing more effective therapies is to identify the components of an effective immune response and to develop an improved understanding of the regulation of HIV replication. Although cellular activation in general appears to augment HIV replication, the specific factors involved in viral induction, and particularly in viral downregulation, deserve further study. The increasing number of available antiretroviral agents and their use in combination hold great promise to markedly reduce HIV-1 replication, perhaps sustained over many years. Future strategies should also target control of replication by through enhancement of antiretroviral immunity or through modulation of factors important for virus control. Both of these strategies are amenable to gene therapy approaches.

ADDENDUM

Cellular Receptors

Recent studies have demonstrated that various chemokines, including MIP-1α, MIP-1β, and RANTES, appear to be involved with the inhibition of HIV-1 replication in T-lymphocytic and monocytic cells. These chemokines may be expressed from both CD8− and CD4+ T-lymphocytes.[6a,56a]

In addition, very recent data have demonstrated that chemokine receptors act as co-receptors for HIV-1 and are involved in tropism for various cell types. These transmembrane proteins, found on many immune system cells, appear to bind areas of the envelope glycoproteins of these lentiviruses. Different cytokine receptors function as co-receptors for HIV-1, in T-cell lines and primary monocyte/macrophages. The transmembrane G protein-coupled receptor for T-lymphocytotropic strains of HIV-1 has been name Fusin, and the receptor for non-syncitia-inducing macrophage-tropic viral isolates is the β-chemokine receptor CC-CKR-5. These studies may be critically important for understanding the basic tropism and pathogenesis of HIV-1. Preliminary data have shown that certain individuals who are multiply exposed to HIV-1 and do not seroconvert, and possibly some long-term non-progressor HIV-1-infected individuals, have high levels of chemokines, which may block these co-receptors for HIV-1. Further studies will be critical to determine whether novel compounds can be developed to block these co-receptors for HIV.[89a,78a,216a]

Antiretroviral Therapy

Several important reports in 1995 and 1996 advanced both the understanding of HIV-1 replication in vivo and concepts for inhibiting HIV-1 replication. Based on an analysis of the rate of decline of HIV particles in plasma following initiation of antiretroiral therapy, minimum estimates of HIV-1 production and clearance were derived which indicated that over one billion virions per day, with a t½ of two days.[123,287,217a] The relatively brief benefit seen with reverse transcriptase inhibitor monotherapy is explained by the dramatic levels of HIV-1 replication and the inability to reduce these levels substantially enough to prevent the rapid emergence of resistant HIV-1 strains.

The superiority of antiretroviral therapy combinations over monotherapy was demonstrated in two large multicenter clinical trials in Europe and the United States. Decreased clinical progression rates and mortality in subjects given combination therapy were observed as compared with zidovudine monotherapy. In the U.S. study, plasma HIV RNA levels were also decreased more with combination than with zidovudine monotherapy. These were clinical endpoint trials, which involved thousands of study subjects followed for several years, and which will be increasingly difficult to conduct as more therapeutic alternatives become available. It appears that the decrease in plasma HIV RNA seen with antiretroviral therapy explains most of the clinical benefit resulting from therapy.[204a] Combination therapy with lamivudine and zidovudine resulted in more improvement in plasma HIV-1 RNA and CD4 lymphocyte count than either drug alone.[84a]

Although clinical benefit was not demonstrated, the concept that drug efficacy can be assessed by the effect of HIV-1 replication levels has resulted in an acceleration of drug approvals. Seven new antiretroviral drugs were approved by the Food and Drug Administration from November 1995 to June 1996, bringing the total to 11. The protease inhibitors saquinavir, ritonavir, and indinavir are particularly important among the new approvals; they have the potential to reduce HIV-1 replication levels by over 2 logs (>99%) as compared with 0.5 logs (67%) for most of the reverse transcriptase inhibitors. Use of two- and three-drug combinations that include protease inhibitors can reduce plasma HIV-1 RNA to undetectable levels (<200 to 500 copies/mL), which may greatly delay or prevent emergence of resistance and allow for dramatic improvements in clinical outcome.

ABBREVIATIONS

AIDS: acquired immunodeficiency syndrome
AZT: azidothymidine (zidovudine)
CMI: cell-mediated immunity
CNS: central nervous system
CSF: colony-stimulating factor
CTL: cytotoxic T lymphocyte
ddI: dideoxyinosine (didanosine)
ddC: dideoxycytidine (zalcitabine)
d4T: didehydro-deoxythymidine (stavudine)
GM-CSF: granulocyte-monocyte colony-stimulating factor
HIV-1, HIV-2, HIV strain IIIB: human immunodeficiency virus
HSV: herpes simplex virus

IL-1, IL-2, IL-3, IL-6: interleukins
KS: Kaposi's sarcoma
LTR: long terminal repeat
MHC: major histocompatibility complex
MP: mononuclear phagocyte
NFκB: nuclear factor kappa B
NMDA: *N*-methyl-o-aspartate
PBL: peripheral blood lymphocyte
PBMC: peripheral blood mononuclear cell
RRE: Rev-responsive element
SCID: severe combined immune deficiency
SI: syncytium-inducing (strain of HIV)
SIV, SIV$_{mac239}$ strain: simian immunodeficiency virus
TAR: *trans*-activation–responsive element
TCL: T-cell line
Th: T helper (lymphocyte)
TNF-α: tumor necrosis factor-alpha
V3: variable region 3 (of gp120)

ACKNOWLEDGMENTS

We thank Drs. Kathie Grovit-Ferbas and John Ferbas for helpful comments, Saeed Sadeghi for artwork, and Mizue Aizeki for manuscript preparation. William O'Brien is supported by Department of Veterans Affairs medical research funds and by PHS grant AI29897, and Roger Pomerantz by PHS grants AI31836 and AI33810.

REFERENCES

1. Adleman LM, Wofsy D. T-cell homeostasis: implications in HIV infection. J Acquir Immune Defic Syndr 1993;6:144–152.
2. Agostini C, Trentin L, Zambello R, et al. Release of granulocyte-macrophage colony-stimulating factor by alveolar macrophages in the lung of HIV-1 infected patients. J Immunol 1992;149:3379–3385.
3. Ahmed N, Venkatesan S. Nef protein of HIV-1 is a transcriptional repressor of HIV-1 LTR. Science 1988;241:1481–1485.
4. Aiken C, Konner J, Landau NR, Lenburg ME, Trono D. Nef induces CD4 endocytosis: requirement for a critical dileucine motif in the membrane-proximal CD4 cytoplasmic domain. Cell 1994;76:853–864.
5. Aldrovandi GM, Feuer G, Gao L, et al. The SCID-hu mouse as a model for HIV-1 infection. Nature 1993;363:732–736.
6. Alizon M, Dragic T. CD26 antigen and HIV fusion? Science 1994;264:1161–1162.
6a. Alkhatib G, Combadiere C, Broder CC, et al. CC CKR5: A RANTES, MIP-1α, MIP-1β receptor as a fusion cofactor for macrophage-tropic HIV-1. Science 1996;1:1955–1958.
7. Aoki-Sei S, Yarchoan R, Kageyama S, et al. Plasma HIV-1 viremia in HIV-1 infected individuals assessed by polymerase chain reaction. AIDS Res Hum Retroviruses 1992;8:1263–1270.
8. Arrigo JS, Chen ISY. Rev is necessary for translation but not cytoplasmic accumulation of HIV-1 *vif, vpr,* and *env/vpu* 2 RNAs. Genes Dev 1991;5:808–819.
9. Arthur LO, Bess JW Jr, Sowder RC II, et al. Cellular proteins bound to immunodeficiency viruses: implications for pathogenesis and vaccines. Science 1992;258:1935–1938.
10. Arya SK, Guo C, Josephs SF, Wong-Staal F. Trans-activator gene of human T-lymphotropic virus type III (HTLV-III). Science 1985;229:69–73.
11. Bagasra O, Kajdacsy-Balla A, Lischner HW, Pomerantz RJ. Alcohol intake increases human immunodeficiency virus type 1 replication in human peripheral blood mononuclear cells. J Infect Dis 1993;167:789–797.
12. Baldwin GC, Fleischmann J, Chung Y, Koyanagi Y, Chen ISY, Golde DW. Human immunodeficiency virus causes mononuclear phagocyte dysfunction. Proc Natl Acad Sci U S A 1990;87:3933–3937.
13. Balla AK, Lischner HW, Pomerantz RJ, Barasra O. Human studies on alcohol and susceptibility to HIV infection. Alcohol 1994;11:99–103.
14. Balotta C, Lusso P, Crowley R, Gallo RC, Franchini G. Antisense phosphorothioate oligodeoxynucleotides targeted to the *vpr* gene inhibit human immunodeficiency virus type 1 replication in primary human macrophages. J Virol 1993;67:4409–4414.
15. Banapour B, Marthas ML, Ramos RA, et al. Identification of viral determinants of macrophage tropism for simian immunodeficiency virus SIV$_{mac}$. J Virol 1991;65:5798–5805.
16. Barre-Sinoussi F, Chermann JC, Rey F, et al. Isolation of a T-lymphotropic retrovirus from a patient at risk for acquired immunodeficiency virus (AIDS). Science 1983;220:868–870.
17. Barry PA, Pratt-Lowe E, Unger RE, Luciw PA. Cellular factors regulate transactivation of human immunodeficiency virus type 1. J Virol 1991;65:1392–1399.
18. Benkirane M, Blanc-Zouaoui D, Hirn M, Devaux C. Involvement of human leukocyte antigen class I molecules in human immunodeficiency virus infection of CD4-positive cells. J Virol 1994;68:6332–6339.
19. Benveniste EN. Cytokine circuits in brain: implications for AIDS dementia complex. Assoc Res Nervous Mental Dis 1994;72:71–88.
20. Bevec D, Dobrovnik M, Hauber J, Bohnlein E. Inhibition of human immunodeficiency virus type 1 replication in human T cells by retroviral-mediated gene transfer of a dominant-negative Rev transactivator. Proc Natl Acad Sci U S A 1992;89:9870–9874.
21. Bhat S, Spitalnik SL, Gonzalez-Scarano F, Silberberg DH. Galactosyl ceramide or a derivative is an essential component of the neural receptor for human immunodeficiency virus type 1 envelope glycoprotein gp120. Proc Natl Acad Sci U S A 1991;88:7131–7134.
22. Blumberg BM, Gelbard HA, Epstein LG. HIV-1 infection of the developing nervous system: central role of astrocytes in pathogenesis. Virus Res 1994;32:253–267.
23. Bobenek K, Kunkel TA. The fidelity of retroviral reverse transcriptases. In: Skalka A, Goff S, eds. Reverse transcriptase. Cold Spring Harbor, NY: Cold Spring Harbor Laboratory Press, 1993:85–102.
24. Bonyhadi ML, Rabin L, Salimi S, et al. HIV induces thymus depletion in vivo. Nature 1993;363:728–732.
25. Borrow P, Lewick H, Hahn BH, Shaw GM, Oldstom MBA. Virus-specific CD8+ cytotoxic T-lymphocyte activity associated with control of viremia in primary human immunodeficiency virus type. J Virol 1994;68:6103–6110.
26. Borthwick NJ, Bofill M, Gombert WM, et al. Lymphocyte activation in HIV-1 infection. II. Functional defects of CD28− T cells. AIDS 1994;8:431–441.
27. Boyd AL, Enquist L, Vande Woude GF, Hampar B. Activation of mouse retrovirus by herpes simplex virus type 1 cloned DNA fragments. Virology 1980;103:228–236.
28. Boyd MT, Simpson GR, Cann AJ, Johnson MA, Weiss R. A single amino acid substitution in the V1 loop of human immunodeficiency virus type 1 gp120 alters cellular tropism. J Virol 1993;67:3649–3652.
29. Boyer V, Desgranges C, Trabaud MA, Fischer E, Kazatchkine MD. Complement mediates human immunodeficiency virus type 1 infection of a human T cell line in CD4− and antibody-independent fashion. J Exp Med 1991;173:1151–1158.
30. Breen EC, Rezai AR, Nakajima K, et al. Infection with HIV is associated with elevated IL-6 levels. J Immunol 1990;144:480–484.
31. Brenneman DE, Westbrook GL, Fitzgerald SP, et al. Neuronal cell killing by the envelope protein of HIV and its prevention by vasoactive intestinal peptide. Nature 1988;335:639–642.
32. Broder CC, Nussbaum O, Gutheil WG, Bachovchin WW, Berger EA. CD26 antigen and HIV fusion? Science 1994;264:1156–1159. Letter.
33. Browne MJ, Mayer KH, Chafee SBD, et al. 2',3'-Didehydro-3'-deoxythymidine (d4T) in patients with AIDS or AIDS-related complex: a phase I trial. J Infect Dis 1993;167:21–29.
34. Buck HM, Koole LH, van Genderen MHP, et al. Phosphate-methylated DNA aimed at HIV-1 RNA loops and integrated DNA inhibits viral infectivity. Science 1990;248:208–212.

35. Bukrinsky MI, Haggerty S, Dempsey MP, et al. A nuclear localization signal within HIV-1 matrix protein that governs infection of non-dividing cells. Nature 1993;365:666–669.

36. Burns DPW, Collignon C, Desrosiers RC. Simian immunodeficiency virus mutants resistant to serum neutralization arise during persistent infection of rhesus monkeys. J Virol 1993;67:4104–4113.

37. Callebaut D, Krust B, Jacotot E, Hovanessian AG. T cell activation antigen CD26 as a cofactor for entry of HIV in CD4+ cells. Science 1993;262:2045–2050.

38. Camerini D, Planelles V, Chen ISY. CD26 antigen and HIV fusion? Science 1994;264:1160–1161.

39. Cao Y, Friedman-Kien AE, Huang Y, et al. CD4-independent, productive human immunodeficiency virus type 1 infection of hepatoma cell lines in vitro. J Virol 1990;64:2553–2559.

40. Cao Y, Qin L, Linqi Z, Safrit J, Ho DD. Virologic and immunologic characterization of long-term survivors of human immunodeficiency virus type 1 infection. N Engl J Med 1995;332:201–208.

41. Carmichael A, Jin X, Sissons P, Borysiewicz L. Quantitative analysis of the human immunodeficiency virus type 1 (HIV-1)–specific cytotoxic T lymphocyte (CTL) response at different stages of HIV-1 infection: differential CTL responses to HIV-1 and Epstein-Barr virus in late disease. J Exp Med 1993;177:249–256.

42. Centers for Disease Control. Revision of the CDC surveillance case definition for acquired immunodeficiency syndrome. MMWR Morb Mortal Wkly Rep 1987;36:1S–15S.

43. Centers for Disease Control. 1993 Revised classification system for HIV infection and expanded surveillance case definition for AIDS among adolescents and adults. MMWR Morb Mortal Wkly Rep 1992;41:RR-17.

44. Chang Y, Cesarman E, Pessin MS, et al. Identification of herpesvirus-like DNA sequences in AIDS-associated Kaposi's sarcoma. Science 1994;266:1865–1869.

45. Chaturvedi S, Frame P, Newman SL. Macrophages from human immunodeficiency virus–positive persons are defective in host defense against *Histoplasma capsulatum*. J Infect Dis 1995;171:320–327.

46. Cheng-Mayer C, Lannello P, Shaw K, Luciw PA, Levy JA. Differential effects of *nef* on HIV replication: implications for viral pathogenesis in the host. Science 1989;246:1629–1632.

47. Cheng-Mayer C, Quiroga M, Tung JW, Dina D, Levy JA. Viral determinants of human immunodeficiency virus type 1 T-cell or macrophage tropism, cytopathic, and CD4 antigen modulation. J Virol 1990;64:4390–4398.

48. Cheng-Mayer C, Seto D, Tateno M, Levy JA. Biologic features of HIV-1 that correlate with virulence in the host. Science 1988;240:80–82.

49. Chesebro B, Nishio J, Perryman S, et al. Identification of HIV envelope gene sequences influencing viral entry into CD4-positive HeLa cells, T-cell leukemia cells and macrophages. J Virol 1991;65:5782–5789.

50. Chesebro B, Wehrly K, Nishio J, Perryman S. Macrophage-tropic human immunodeficiency virus isolates from different patients exhibit unusual V3 envelope sequence homogeneity in comparison with T-cell-tropic isolates: definition of critical amino acids involved in cell tropism. J Virol 1992;66:6547–6554.

51. Clerici M, Giorgi JV, Chou CC, et al. Cell-mediated immune response to human immunodeficiency virus type 1 in seronegative homosexual men with recent sexual exposure. J Infect Dis 1992;165:1012–1019.

52. Clerici M, Levin J, Kessler H, et al. HIV-specific T-helper activity in seronegative health care workers exposed to contaminated blood. JAMA 1994;271:42–46.

53. Clerici M, Roilides E, Via CS, Pizzo PA, Shearer GM. A factor from CD8 cells of human immunodeficiency virus–infected patients suppresses HLA self-restricted T helper cell responses. Proc Natl Acad Sci U S A 1992;89:8424–8428.

54. Clerici M, Stocks NI, Zajac RA, Boswell RN, Via CS, Shearer GM. Circumvention of defective CD4 T helper cell function in HIV-infected individuals by stimulation with HLA alloantigens. J Immunol 1990;144:3266–3271.

55. Clerici M, Stocks NI, Zajac RA, et al. Detection of three distinct patterns of T helper cell dysfunction in asymptomatic, human immunodeficiency virus–seropositive patients: independence of CD4+ cell numbers and clinical staging. J Clin Invest 1989;84:1892–1899.

56. Clumeck N. Current use of anti-HIV drugs in AIDS. J Antimicrob Chemother 1993;32(Suppl A):133–138.

56a. Cocchi F, DeVico AL, Garzino-Demo A, et al. Identification of RANTES, MIP-1α, MIP-1β as the major HIV-suppressive factors produced by CD8+ T cells. Science 1995;270:1881–1815.

57. Cohen EA, Dehni G, Sodroski JG, Haseltine WA. Human immunodeficiency virus *vpr* product is a virion-associated regulatory protein. J Virol 1990;64:3097–3099.

58. Collier AC, Coombs RW, Fischl MA, et al. Combination therapy with zidovudine and didanosine compared with zidovudine alone in HIV-1 infection. Ann Intern Med 1993;119:786–793.

59. Collman R, Godfrey B, Cutilli J, et al. Macrophage-tropic strains of human immunodeficiency virus type 1 utilize the CD4 receptor. J Virol 1990;66:4468–4476.

60. Collman RB, Godfrey J, Cutilli A, et al. An infectious molecular clone of an unusual macrophage-tropic and highly cytopathic strain of human immunodeficiency virus type 1. J Virol 1992;66:7517–7521.

61. Collman R, Hassan NF, Walker R. Infection of monocyte-derived macrophages with human immunodeficiency virus type. J Exp Med 1989;170:1149–1163.

62. Concorde Coordinating Committee. MRC/ANRS randomised double-blind controlled trial of immediate and deferred zidovudine in symptom-free HIV infection. Lancet 1994;343:871–881.

63. Connor RI, Ho DD. Human immunodeficiency virus type 1 variants with increased replicative capacity develop during the asymptomatic stage before disease progression. J Virol 1994;68:4400–4408.

64. Connor RI, Mohri H, Cao Y, Ho DD. Increased viral burden and cytopathicity correlate temporally with CD4+ T-lymphocyte decline and clinical progression in human immunodeficiency virus type 1–infected individuals. J Virol 1993;67:1772–1777.

65. Coombs RW, Collier AC, Allain JP, et al. Plasma viremia in human immunodeficiency virus infection. N Engl J Med 1989;321:1626–1631.

66. Cooper DA, Perhson PO, Pedersen C, et al. The efficacy and safety of zidovudine alone or as cotherapy with acyclovir for the treatment of patients with AIDS and AIDS-related complex: a double-blind, randomized trial. AIDS 1993;7:197–207.

67. Crowle AJ, Ross ER, Cohn DL, Gilden J, May MH. Comparison of the abilities of *Mycobacterium avium* and *Mycobacterium intracellulare* to infect and multiply in cultured human macrophages from normal and human immunodeficiency virus–infected subjects. Infect Immun 1992;60:3697–3703.

68. Daar ES, Chernyavskiy T, Zhao J-Q, Krogstad P, Chen IYS, Zack JA. Sequential determination of viral load and phenotype in human immunodeficiency virus type 1 infection. AIDS Res Hum Retroviruses 1995;11:3–9.

69. Daar ES, Li XL, Moudgil T, Ho DD. High concentrations of recombinant soluble CD4 are required to neutralize primary HIV-1 isolates. Proc Natl Acad Sci U S A 1990;87:6574–6578.

70. Daar ES, Moudgil T, Meyer RD, Ho DD. Transient high levels of viremia in patients with primary human immunodeficiency virus type 1 infection. N Engl J Med 1991;324:961–964.

71. Dalgleish AG, Beverley PCL, Clapham PR, Crawford DH, Greaves MF, Weiss RA. The CD4 (T4) antigen is an essential component of the receptor for the AIDS retrovirus. Nature 1984;312:763–767.

72. Daly TJ, Cook KS, Gray GS, Malone TE, Rusche JR. Specific binding of HIV-1 recombinant Rev protein to the Rev-responsive element in vitro. Nature 1989;342:816–819.

73. Daniel MD, Kirchhoff F, Czajak SC, Sehgal PK, Desrosiers RC. Protective effects of a live attenuated SIV vaccine with a deletion in the nef gene. Science 1992;258:1938–1942.

74. Dedera D, Hu W, Vander Heyden N, Ratner L. Viral protein R of human immunodeficiency virus types 1 and 2 is dispensable for replication and cytopathogenicity in lymphoid cells. J Virol 1989;63:3205–3208.

75. De Leys R, Vanderborght B, vanden Haesevelde M, et al. Isolation and partial characterization of an unusual human immunodeficiency retrovirus from two persons of west-central American origin. J Virol 1990;64:1207–1216.

76. Desrosiers RC. HIV with multiple gene deletions as a live attenuated vaccine for AIDS. AIDS Res Hum Retroviruses 1992;8:411–421.

77. Desrosiers RC, Letvin NL. Animal models for acquired immunodeficiency syndrome. Rev Infect Dis 1987;9:438–446.

78. Dewar RL, Highbarger HC, Sarmiento MD, et al. Application of branched DNA signal amplification to monitor human immunodeficiency virus type 1 burden in human plasma. J Infect Dis 1994;170: 1172–1179.

78a. Dragic T, Litwin V, Allaway GP, et al. HIV-1 entry into CD4+ cells is mediated by the chemokine receptor CC-CKR-5. Nature 1996;5:667–648.

79. Dreyer EB, Kaiser PK, Offermann JT, Lipton SA. HIV-1 coat protein neurotoxicity prevented by calcium channel antagonists. Science 1990;248:364–367.

80. Duan L, Bagasra O, Laughlin MA, Oakes JW, Pomerantz RJ. Potent inhibition of human immunodeficiency virus type 1 replication by an intracellular anti-Rev single-chain antibody. Proc Natl Acad Sci U S A 1994;91:5075–5079.

81. Duan L, Zhang H, Oakes JW, Bagasra O, Pomerantz RJ. Molecular and virological effects of intracellular anti-Rev single-chain variable fragments on the expression of various human immunodeficiency virus type 1 strains. Hum Gene Ther 1994;5:1315–1324.

82. Embretson J, Zupancic M, Ribas JL, et al. Massive covert infection of helper T lymphocytes and macrophages by HIV during the incubation period of AIDS. Nature 1993;362:359–362.

83. Ensoli B, Barillari G, Salahuddin SZ, Gallo RC, Wong-Staal F. Tat protein of HIV-1 stimulates growth of cells derived from Kaposi's sarcoma lesions of AIDS patients. Nature 1990;345:84–86.

84. Ensoli B, Gendelman R, Markham P, et al. Synergy between basic fibroblast growth factor and HIV-1 Tat protein in induction of Kaposi's sarcoma. Nature 1994;371:674–680.

84a. Eron TJ, Benoit SL, Jemsek J, et al. N.A. HIV working party. N Engl J Med 1995;333:1662–1669.

85. Eron JJ, Johnson VA, Merrill DP, Chou TC, Hirsch MS. Synergistic inhibition of replication of human immunodeficiency virus type 1, including that of a zidovudine-resistant isolate, by zidovudine and 2',3'-dideoxycytidine in vitro. Antimicrob Agents Chemother 1992;36:1559–1562.

86. Estevez ME, Ballart IJ, Diez RA, Planes N, Scaglione C, Sen L. Early defect of phagocytic cell function in subjects at risk for acquired immunodeficiency syndrome. Scand J Immunol 1986;24: 215–221.

87. Fauci AS. Multifactorial nature of human immunodeficiency virus disease: implications for therapy. Science 1993;262:1011–1018.

88. Feinberg MB, Jarrett RF, Aldovini A, Gallo RC, Wong-Staal F. HTLV-III expression and production involve complex regulation at the levels of splicing and translation of viral RNA. Cell 1986;46:807–817.

89. Feng S, Holland EC. HIV-1 tat trans-activation requires the loop sequence within tar. Nature 1988;334:165–167.

89a. Feng Y, Broder CC, Kennedy PE, Berger EA. HIV-1 entry cofactor: functional cDNA cloning of a seven-transmembrane G protein-coupled receptor. Science 1996;272:872–877.

90. Fenyo EM, Morfeldt-Manson L, Chiodi F, et al. Distinct replicative and cytopathic characteristics of human immunodeficiency virus isolates. J Virol 1988;62:4414–4419.

91. Fischl MA, Richman DD, Grieco MH, et al. The efficacy of azidothymidine (AZT) in the treatment of patients with AIDS and AIDS-related complex. N Engl J Med 1987;317:185–191.

92. Fischl MA, Richman DD, Hansen N. The safety and efficacy of zidovudine (AZT) in the treatment of mildly symptomatic human immunodeficiency virus type 1 (HIV) infection: a double-blind, placebo-controlled trial. Ann Intern Med 1990;112:727–737.

93. Fisher AG, Ensoli B, Ivanoff L, et al. The sor gene of HIV-1 is required for efficient virus transmission in vitro. Science 1987;237: 888–893.

94. Folks TM, Clouse KA, Justement J, et al. Tumor necrosis factor induces expression of human immunodeficiency virus in a chronically infected T-cell clone. Proc Natl Acad Sci U S A 1989;86:2365–2368.

95. Folks TM, Justement J, Kinter A, Dinarello CA, Fauci AS. Cytokine-induced expression of HIV-1 in a chronically infected promonocytic cell line. Science 1987;238:800–802.

96. Fong IW, Read S, Wainberg MA, Chia WK, Major C. Alcoholism and rapid progression to AIDS after seroconversion. Clin Infect Dis 1994;19:337–338.

97. Freed EO, Delwart EL, Buchschacher JGL, Panganiban AT. A mutation in the human immunodeficiency virus type 1 transmembrane glycoprotein gp41 dominantly interferes with fusion and infectivity. Proc Natl Acad Sci U S A 1992;89:70–74.

98. Gabuzda DH, Lawrence K, Langhoff E, et al. Role of vif in replication of human immunodeficiency virus type 1 in CD4+ T lymphocytes. J Virol 1992;66:6489–6495.

99. Gallo RC, Sarin PS, Gelmann EP, et al. Isolation of human T cell leukemia virus in acquired immune deficiency syndrome (AIDS). Science 1983;220:865–867.

100. Gao F, Yue L, Robertson DL, et al. Genetic diversity of human immunodeficiency virus type 2: evidence for distinct sequence subtypes with differences in virus biology. J Virol 1994;68:7433–7447.

101. Garcia JV, Miller AD. Serine phosphorylation independent downregulation of cell-surface CD4 by nef. Nature 1991;350:508–511.

102. Garry RF and Koch G. Tat contains a sequence related to snake neurotoxins. AIDS 1992;6:1541–1542.

103. Gatignol A, Buckler-White A, Berkhout B, Jeang K-T. Characterization of a human TAR RNA-binding protein that activates the HIV-1 LTR. Science 1991;251:1597–1600.

104. Gaynor R. Cellular transcription factors involved in the regulation of HIV-1 gene expression. AIDS 1992;6:346–363.

105. Gelderblom H, Ozel M, Hausmann EHS, Winkel T, Pauli G, Koch MA. Fine structure of human immunodeficiency virus (HIV), immunolocalization of structural proteins and virus-cell relation. Micron Microsc 1988;19:41–60.

106. Genis P, Jett M, Bernton EW, et al. Cytokines and arachidonic metabolites produced during human immunodeficiency virus (HIV)-infected macrophage-astroglia interactions: implications for the neuropathogenesis of HIV disease. J Exp Med 1992;176:1703–1718.

107. Geraghty RJ, Panganiban AT. Human immunodeficiency virus type 1 Vpu has a CD4− and an envelope glycoprotein-independent function. J Virol 1993;67:4190–4194.

108. Giorgi JV, Boumsell L, Autran B. Reactivity of T cell section monoclonal antibodies with circulating CD4+ and CD8+ T cells in HIV disease and following in vitro activation. In: Schlossman S, Boumsell L, Gilks W, et al, ed. Leukocyte typing. V. White cell differentiation antigens. Oxford: Oxford University Press, 1995:446–461.

109. Goodenow M, Huet T, Saurin W, Kwok S, Sninsky J, Wain-Hobson S. HIV-1 isolates are rapidly evolving quasispecies: evidence for viral mixtures and preferred nucleotide substitutions. J Acquir Immune Defic Syndr 1989;2:344–352.

110. Groux H, Torpier G, Monte D, Mouton Y, Capron A, Ameisen JC. Activation-induced death by apoptosis in CD4+ T cells from human immunodeficiency virus-infected asymptomatic individuals. J Exp Med 1992;175:331–340.

111. Gurtler LG, Hauser PH, Eberle J, et al. A new subtype of human immunodeficiency virus type 1 (MVP-5180) from Cameroon. J Virol 1994;68:1581–1585.

112. Guy B, Kieny M, Riviere Y, et al. HIV F/3' orf encodes a phosphorylated GTP-binding protein resembling an oncogenic product. Nature 1987;330:266–269.

113. Hahn BH, Gonda MA, Shaw GM, et al. Genomic diversity of the acquired immune deficiency syndrome virus HTLV-III: different viruses exhibit greatest divergence in their envelope genes. Proc Natl Acad Sci U S A 1985;82:4813–4817.

114. Hahn BH, Shaw GM, Taylor ME, et al. Genetic variation in HTLV-III/LAV over time in patients with AIDS or at risk for AIDS. Science 1986;232:1548–1553.

115. Hamilton JD, Hartigan PM, Simberoff MS, et al. Early versus later zidovudine therapy for patients with symptomatic human immunodeficiency virus infection: results of a randomized, double-blind VA cooperative study. N Engl J Med 1992;326:437–443.

116. Hammes SR, Dixon EP, Malim MH, Cullen BR, Greene WC. Nef protein of human immunodeficiency virus type 1: evidence against its role as a transcriptional inhibitor. Proc Natl Acad Sci U S A 1989;86:9549–9553.

117. Harouse JM, Bhat S, Spitalnik SL, et al. Inhibition of entry of HIV-1 in neural cell lines by antibodies against galactosyl ceramide. Science 1991;253:320–323.

118. Harouse JM, Kunsch C, Hartle HT, et al. CD4-independent infection of human neural cells by human immunodeficiency virus type 1. J Virol 1989;63:2527–2533.

119. Hattori N, Michaels F, Fargnoli K, Marcon L, Gallo RC, Granchini G. The human immunodeficiency virus type 2 *vpr* gene is essential for productive infection of human macrophages. Proc Natl Acad Sci U S A 1990;87:8080–8084.

120. Heinzinger NK, Bukrinsky MI, Haggerty SA, et al. The Vpr protein of human immunodeficiency virus type 1 influences nuclear localization of viral nucleic acids in nondividing host cells. Proc Natl Acad Sci U S A 1994;91:7311–7315.

121. Heng MC, Heng SY, Allen SG. Co-infection and synergy of human immunodeficiency virus-1 and herpes simplex virus. Lancet 1994;343:255–258.

122. Ho DD, Moudgil T, Alam M. Quantitation of human immunodeficiency virus type 1 in the blood of infected persons. N Engl J Med 1989;321:1621–1625.

123. Ho DD, Neumann AU, Perelson AS, Chen W, Leonard JM, Markowitz M. Rapid turnover of plasma virions and CD4 lymphocytes in HIV-1 infection. Nature 1995;373:123–126.

124. Hoffenbach A, Langlade-Demoyen P, Dadaglio G, et al. Unusually high frequencies of HIV-specific cytotoxic T lymphocytes in humans. J Immunol 1989;142:452–462.

125. Holodniy M, Katzenstein DA, Sengupta S, et al. Detection and quantification of human immunodeficiency virus RNA in patient serum by use of the polymerase chain reaction. J Infect Dis 1991;163:862–866.

126. Homsy J, Meyer M, Tateno M, Clarkson S, Levy JA. The Fc and not CD4 receptor mediates antibody enhancement of HIV infection in human cells. Science 1989;244:1357–1360.

127. Huang Z-B, Potash MJ, Simm M, et al. Infection of macrophages with lymphotropic human immunodeficiency virus type 1 can be arrested after viral DNA synthesis. J Virol 1993;67:6893–6896.

128. Hwang SS, Boyle TJ, Lyerly HK, Cullen BR. Identification of envelope V3 loop as the primary determinant of cell tropism in HIV-1. Science 1991;253:71–74.

129. Igarashi T, Shibata R, Hasebe I, et al. Persistent infection with SIV$_{mac}$ chimeric virus having tat, rev, vpu, env, and nef of HIV type 1 in macaque monkeys. AIDS Res Hum Retroviruses 1994;10:1021–1029.

130. Jamieson BD, Aldrovandi GM, Planelles V, et al. Requirement of human immunodeficiency virus type 1 *nef* for in vivo replication and pathogenicity. J Virol 1994;68:3478–3485.

131. Johnson RP, Hammond SA, Trocha A, Siliciano RF, Walker BD. Induction of a major histocompatibility complex class I restricted cytotoxic T-lymphocyte response to a highly conserved region of human immunodeficiency virus type 1 (HIV 1) gp120 in seronegative humans immunized with a candidate HIV-1 vaccine. J Virol 1994;68:3145–3153.

132. Jones KA, Kadonaga JT, Luciw PA, Tjan R. Activation of the AIDS retrovirus promoter by the cellular transcription factor, Spl. Science 1986;232:755–759.

133. Kahn JA, Lagakos SW, Richman DD, et al. A controlled trial comparing continued zidovudine with didanosine in human immunodeficiency virus infection. N Engl J Med 1992;327:581–587.

134. Kahn JO, Allan JD, Hodge TL, et al. The safety and pharmacokinetics of recombinant soluble CD4 (rCD4) in subjects with the acquired immunodeficiency syndrome (AIDS) and AIDS-related complex. Ann Intern Med 1990;112:254–261.

135. Kaiser PK, Offermann JT, Lipton SA. Neuronal injury due to HIV-1 envelope protein is blocked by anti-gp120 antibodies but not by anti-CD4 antibodies. Neurology 1990;40:1757–1761.

136. Kalter DC, Nakamura M, Turpin JA, et al. Enhanced HIV-1 replication in macrophage colony-stimulating factor–treated monocytes. J Immunol 1991;146:3396–3404.

137. Kaneshima H, Su L, Bonyhadi ML, Connor RI, Ho DD, McCune JM. Rapid-high, syncytium-inducing isolates of human immunodeficiency virus type 1 induce cytopathicity in the human thymus of the SCID-hu mouse. J Virol 1994;68:8188–8192.

138. Kang C-Y, Hariharan K, Nara PL, Sodroski J, Moore JP. Immunization with a soluble CD4-gp120 complex preferentially induces neutralizing anti-human immunodeficiency virus type 1 antibodies directed to conformation-dependent epitopes of gp120. J Virol 1994;68:5854–5862.

139. Kappes JC, Conway JA, Lee S-W, Shaw GM, Hahn BH. Human immunodeficiency virus type 2 vpx protein augments viral infectivity. Virology 1991;184:197–209.

140. Katzenstein DA, Winters M, Bubp J, Israelski D, Winger E, Merigan TC. Quantitation of human immunodeficiency virus by culture and polymerase chain reaction in response to didanosine after long-term therapy with zidovudine. J Infect Dis 1994;169:416–419.

141. Kekow J, Wachsman W, McCutchan JA, Cronin M, Carson DA, Lotz M. Transforming growth factor beta and noncytopathic mechanisms of immunodeficiency in human immunodeficiency virus infection. Proc Natl Acad Sci U S A 1990;87:8321–8325.

142. Kestler HW, Kodama T, Ringler D, et al. Induction of AIDS in rhesus monkeys by molecularly cloned simian immunodeficiency virus. Science 1990;248:1109–1112.

143. Kestler HW, Ringler DJ, Mori K, et al. Importance of the *nef* gene for maintenance of high virus loads and for development of AIDS. Cell 1991;65:651–662.

144. Kim S, Byrn R, Groopman J, Baltimore D. Temporal aspects of DNA and RNA synthesis during human immunodeficiency virus infection: evidence for differential gene expression. J Virol 1989;63:3708–3713.

145. Kim S, Ikeuchi K, Byrn R, Groopman J, Baltimore D. Lack of a negative influence on viral growth by the *nef* gene of human immunodeficiency virus type 1. Proc Natl Acad Sci U S A 1989;86:9544–9548.

146. Kirchhoff F, Greenough TC, Brettler DB, Sullivan JL, Desrosiers RC. Brief report: absence of intact *nef* sequences in a long-term survivor with nonprogressive HIV-1 infection. N Engl J Med 1995;332:228–232.

147. Klatzmann K, Champagne E, Chamaret S, et al. T-lymphocyte T4 molecule behaves as the receptor for human retrovirus LAV. Nature 1984;312:767–768.

148. Kobayashi N, Hamaoto Y, Koyanagi Y, Chen IS, Yamamoto N. Effect of interleukin-1 in the augmentation of human immunodeficiency virus gene expression. Biochem Biophys Res Commun 1989;165:715–721.

149. Kojima E, Shirasaka T, Anderson B, et al. Monitoring the activity of antiviral therapy for HIV infection using a polymerase chain reaction method coupled with reverse transcription. AIDS 1993;(Suppl 2):S101–105.

150. Koup RA, Safrit JT, Cao Y, et al. Temporal association of cellular immune responses with the initial control of viremia in primary human immunodeficiency virus type 1 syndrome. J Virol 1994;68:4650–4655.

151. Kowalski M, Potz J, Basiripour L, et al. Functional regions of the human immunodeficiency virus envelope glycoprotein. Science 1987;237:1351–1355.

152. Koyanagi Y, Miles S, Mitsuyasu RT, Merryl JE, Vinters HV, Chen ISY. Dual infection of the central nervous system by AIDS viruses with distinct cellular tropisms. Science 1987;236:819–822.

153. Koyanagi Y, O'Brien WA, Zhao JQ, Golde DW, Gasson JC, Chen ISY. Cytokines alter production of HIV from primary mononuclear phagocytes. Science 1988;241:1673–1675.

154. Laurence J. Molecular interactions among herpesviruses and human immunodeficiency viruses. J Infect Dis 1990;162:338–346.

155. Laurence J, Gottlieb AB, Kunkel HG. Soluble suppressor factors in patients with acquired immune deficiency syndrome and its prodrome: elaboration in vitro by T lymphocyte–adherent cell interactions. J Clin Invest 1983;72:2072–2081.

156. Lavallee C, Yao XJ, Ladha A, Gottlinger H, Haseltine WA, Cohen EA. Requirement of the Pr55*gag* precursor for incorporation of the Vpr product into human immunodeficiency virus type 1 viral particles. J Virol 1994;68:1926–1934.

157. Lazaro I, Naniche D, Signoret N, et al. Factors involved in entry of the human immunodeficiency virus type 1 into permissive cells: lack of evidence of a role for CD26. J Virol 1994;68:6535–6546.

158. Lepe-Zuniga JL, Mansell PWA, Hersh EM. Idiopathic production of interleukin-1 in acquired immune deficiency syndrome. J Clin Microbiol 1987;25:1695–1700.

159. Li J, Lord CI, Haseltine W, Letvin NL, Sodroski J. Infection of cynomolgus monkeys with a chimeric HIV-1/SIV$_{mac}$ virus that expresses HIV-1 envelope glycoproteins. J Acquir Immun Defic Syndr 1992;5:639–646.

160. Li XL, Moudgil T, Vinters HV, Ho DD. CD4-independent, productive infection of a neuronal cell line by human immunodeficiency virus type 1. J Virol 1990;64:1383–1387.

161. Linsley PS, Ledbetter JA. The role of CD28 receptor during T cell responses to antigen. Ann Rev Immunol 1993;11:191–212.

162. Lisziewicz J, Sun D, Klotman M, Agrawal S, Zamecnik P, Gallo R. Specific inhibition of human immunodeficiency virus type 1 replication by antisense oligonucleotides: an in vitro model for treatment. Proc Natl Acad Sci U S A 1992;89:11209–11213.

163. Liu Z-Q, Wood C, Levy JA, Cheng-Mayer C. The viral envelope gene is involved in the macrophage tropism of an HIV-1 strain isolated from the brain. J Virol 1990;64:6143–6153.

164. Lori F, Veronese FM, DeVico AL, Lusso P, Reitz MS, Gallo RC. Viral DNA carried by human immunodeficiency virus type 1 virions. J Virol 1992;66:5067–5074.

165. Louwagie J, McCutchan F, Peeters M, et al. Phylogenetic analysis of gag genes from 70 international HIV-1 isolates provides evidence for multiple genotypes. AIDS 1993;7:769–780.

166. Lu Y-L, Spearman P, Ratner L. Human immunodeficiency virus type 1 viral protein R localization in infected cells and virions. J Virol 1993;67:6542–6550.

167. Lu Y, Touzjian N, Stenzel M, Dorfman T, Sodroski JG, Haseltine WA. Identification of cis-acting repressive sequences within the negative regulatory element of human immunodeficiency virus type 1. J Virol 1990;64:5226–5229.

168. Luciw PA, Cheng-Mayer C, Levy JA. Mutational analysis of the human immunodeficiency virus: the orf-B region down-regulates virus replication. Proc Natl Acad Sci U S A 1987;84:1434–1438.

169. Macatonia SE, Patterson S, Knight SC. Suppression of immune responses by dendritic cells infected with HIV. Immunology 1989;67: 285–289.

170. Maddon PJ, Dalgleish AG, McDougal JS, Clapham PR, Weiss RA, Axel R. The T4 gene encodes the AIDS virus receptor and is expressed in the immune system and the brain. Cell 1986;47:333–348.

171. Malim MH, Hauber J, Fenrick R, Cullen BR. Immunodeficiency virus rev trans-activator modulates the expression of the viral regulatory genes. Nature 1988;335:181–183.

172. Malim MH, Hauber J, Le S-Y, Maizel JV, Cullen BR. The HIV-1 rev trans-activator acts through a structured target sequence to activate nuclear export of unspliced viral mRNA. Nature 1989;338:254–257.

173. Marcon L, Michaels F, Hattori N, Fargnoli K, Gallo RC, Franchini G. Dispensable role of the human immunodeficiency virus type 2 Vpx protein in viral replication. J Virol 1991;65:3938–3942.

174. Margolick JB, Donnenberg AD, Munoz A, et al. Changes in T and non-T lymphocyte subsets following seroconversion to HIV-1: stable CD3+ and declining CD3- populations suggest regulatory responses linked to loss of CD4 lymphocytes. J Acquir Immune Defic Syndr 1993;6:153–161.

175. Marlink R, Kanki P, Thior I, et al. Reduced rate of disease development after HIV-2 infection as compared to HIV-1. Science 1994; 265:1587–1590.

176. Matloubian M, Concepcion RJ, Ahmed R. CD4+ cells are required to sustain CD8+ cytotoxic T-cell responses during chronic viral infection. J Virol 1994;68:8056–8063.

177. McClure MO, Marsh M, Weiss RA. Human immunodeficiency virus infection of CD4-bearing cells occurs by a pH-independent mechanism. EMBO J 1988;7:513–518.

178. McCune JM, Namikawa R, Kaneshima H, Shultz LD, Leiberman M, Weissman IL. The SCID-hu mouse: murine model for the analysis of human hematolymphoid differentiation and function. Science 1988;241:1632–1639.

179. McMichael AJ, Gotch FM, Noble GR, Beare PAS. Cytotoxic T-cell immunity to influenza. N Engl J Med 1983;309:13–17.

180. McNearney T, Hornickova Z, Markham R, et al. Relationship of human immunodeficiency virus type 1 sequence heterogeneity to stage of disease. Proc Natl Acad Sci U S A 1992;89:10247–10251.

181. Meltzer MS, Gendelman HE. Mononuclear phagocytes as targets, tissue reservoirs, immunoregulatory cells in human immunodeficiency virus disease. Curr Top Microbiol Immunol 1992;181:239–263.

182. Merrill JE, Koyanagi Y, Chen ISY. Interleukin-1 and tumor necrosis factors can be induced from mononuclear phagocytes by human immunodeficiency virus type 1 binding to the CD4 receptor. J Virol 1989;63:4404–4408.

183. Meyaard L, Otto SA, Hooibrink B, Miedema F. Quantitative analysis of CD4+ T cell function in the course of human immunodefi-

184. Meyaard L, Otto SA, Keet IP, Roos MT, Miedema F. Programmed death of T cells in human immunodeficiency virus infection: no correlation with progression to disease. J Clin Invest 1994;93:982–988.

185. Meyerhans A, Cheyneir R, Alber J, et al. Temporal fluctuations in HV quasispecies in vivo are not reflected by sequential HIV isolations. Cell 1989;58:901–910.

186. Michael NL, Vahey M, Burke DS, Redfield RR. Viral DNA and mRNA expression correlate with the stage of human immunodeficiency virus (HIV) type 1 infection in humans: evidence for viral replication in all stages of HIV disease. J Virol 1992;66:310–316.

187. Miedema F, Petit AJ, Terpstra FG, et al. Immunological abnormalities in human immunodeficiency virus (HIV)–infected asymptomatic homosexual men: HIV affects the immune system before CD4+ T helper cell depletion occurs. J Clin Invest 1988;82:1908–1914.

188. Miller MA, Garry RF, Jaynes JM, Montelaro RC. A structural correlation between lentivirus transmembrane proteins and natural cytolytic peptides. AIDS Res Hum Retroviruses 1991;7:511–519.

189. Miller MD, Warmerdam MT, Gaston I, Greene WC, Feinberg MB. The human immunodeficiency virus-1 nef gene product: a positive factor for viral infection and replication in primary lymphocytes and macrophages. J Exp Med 1994;179:101–113.

190. Moore JP, Ho DD. Antibodies to discontinuous or conformationally sensitive epitopes on the gp120 glycoprotein of human immunodeficiency virus type 1 are highly prevalent in sera of infected humans. J Virol 1993;67:863–875.

191. Moore JP, McKeating JA, Huang Y, Ashkenazi A, Ho DD. Virions of primary human immunodeficiency virus type 1 isolates resistant to soluble CD4 (sCD4) neutralization differ in sCD4 binding and glycoprotein gp120 retention from sCD4-sensitive isolates. J Virol 1991;66:235–243.

192. Mori K, Ringler DJ, Desrosiers RC. Restricted replication of simian immunodeficiency virus strain 239 in macrophages is determined by env but is not due to restricted entry. J Virol 1993;67:2807–2814.

193. Mosier DE, Gulizia RJ, Baird SM, Wilson DB. Transfer of a functional human immune system to mice with severe combined immunodeficiency. Nature 1988;335:256–259.

194. Mosier DE, Gulizia RJ, Baird SM, Wilson DB, Spector DH, Spector SA. Human immunodeficiency virus infection of human-PBL-SCID mice. Science 1991;851:791–794.

195. Muesling MA, Smith DH, Cabradilla CV, Benton CV, Lasky LA, Capon DJ. Nucleic acid structure and expression of the human AIDS/lymphadenopathy retrovirus. Nature 1985;313:450–453.

196. Mulder J, McKinney N, Christopherson C, et al: Rapid and simple PCR assay for quantitation of human immunodeficiency virus type 1 RNA in plasma: application to acute retroviral infection. J Clin Microbiol 1994;32:292–300.

197. Myers G, Korber B, Wain-Hobson S, Smith RF, Paulakis GN, eds. Human retroviruses and AIDS 1993: a compilation and analysis of nucleic acid and amino acid sequences. Los Alamos, NM: Los Alamos National Laboratory, 1993.

198. Nabel G, Baltimore D. An inducible transcription factor activates expression of human immunodeficiency virus in T cells. Nature 1987;326:711–713.

199. Nabel GJ, Fox BA, Post L, Thompson CB, Woffedin C. A molecular genetic intervention for AIDS: effects of a transdominant negative form of Rev. Hum Gene Ther 1994;5:79–92.

200. Nabel GJ, Rice SA, Knipe DM, Baltimore D. Alternative mechanisms for activation of human immunodeficiency virus enhancer in T cells. Science 1988;239:1299–1302.

201. Nelson JA, Wiley CA, Reynolds-Kohler C, Reese CE, Margaretten W, Levy JA. Human immunodeficiency virus detected in bowel epithelium from patients with gastrointestinal symptoms. Lancet 1988; 1:259–262.

202. Nowak MA, Anderson RM, McLean AR, Wolfs TFW, Goudsmit J, May RM. Antigenic diversity thresholds and the development of AIDS. Science 1991;254:963–969.

203. O'Brien WA, Chen ISY, Ho DD, Daar ES. HIV-1 resistance to soluble CD4 is conferred by domains of gp120 that determine cell tropism. J Virol 1992;66:3125–3130.

204. O'Brien WA, Grovit-Ferbas K, Namazi A, et al. HIV-1 replication can be increased in peripheral blood of seropositive patients following influenza vaccination. Blood 1995;86:1082–1089.

204a. O'Brien WA, Hartigan PM, Martin D, et al. Changes in plasma HIV-1 RNA and CD4+ lymphocyte counts and the risk of progression to AIDS. N Engl J Med 1996;334:496–502.

205. O'Brien WA, Koyanagi Y, Namazie A, et al. HIV-1 tropism for mononuclear phagocytes can be determined by regions of gp120 outside the CD4-binding domain. Nature 1990;348:69–73.

206. O'Brien WA, Mao S-H, Cao Y, Moore JP. Macrophage and T-cell tropic HIV-1 strains differ in their susceptibility to neutralization by soluble CD4 at different temperatures. J Virol 1994;68:5264–5269.

207. O'Brien WA, Namazi A, Mao S-H, Kalhor H, Zack JA, Chen ISY. Kinetics of HIV-1 reverse transcription in blood mononuclear phagocytes are slowed by limitations of nucleotide precursors. J Virol 1994;68:1258–1263.

208. Ojwang JO, Hampel A, Looney DJ, Wong-Staal F, Rappaport J. Inhibition of human immunodeficiency virus type 1 expression by a hairpin ribozyme. Proc Natl Acad Sci U S A 1992;89:10802–10806.

209. Osborn L, Kinkel S, Nabel GJ. Tumor necrosis factor α and interleukin-1 stimulate the human immunodeficiency virus enhancer by activation of the nuclear factor κB. Proc Natl Acad Sci U S A 1989;86:2336–2340.

210. Otto MJ, Garber S, Winslow DL, et al. In vitro isolation and identification of human immunodeficiency virus (HIV) variants with reduced sensitivity to C-2 symmetrical inhibitors of HIV type 1 protease. Proc Natl Acad Sci U S A 1993;90:7543–7547.

211. Overbaugh J, Rudensey LM. Alterations in potential sites for glycosylation predominate during evolution of the simian immunodeficiency virus envelope gene in macaques. J Virol 1992;66:5937–5948.

212. Overbaugh J, Rudensey LM, Papenhausen MD, Benveniste RE, Morton WR. Variation in simian immunodeficiency virus env is confined to V1 and V4 during progression to simian AIDS. J Virol 1991;65:7025–7031.

213. Pang S, Schlesinger Y, Daar ES, Moudgil T, Ho DD, Chen ISY. Rapid generation of sequence variation during primary HIV-1 infection. AIDS 1992;6:453–460.

214. Pantaleo G, Graziosi C, Demarest JF, et al. HIV infection is active and progressive in lymphoid tissue during the clinically latent stage of disease. Nature 1993;362:355–358.

215. Pantaleo G, Menzo S, Vaccarezza M, et al. Studies in subjects with long-term nonprogressive human immunodeficiency virus infection. N Engl J Med 1995;332:209–216.

216. Paxton W, Connor RI, Landau NR. Incorporation of Vpr into human immunodeficiency virus type 1 virions: requirement for the p6 region of gag and mutational analysis. J Virol 1993;67:7229–7237.

216a. Paxton WA, Martin SR, Tse D, et al. Relative resistance to HIV-1 infection of CD4 lymphocytes from persons who remain uninfected despite multiple high-risk sexual exposures. Nature Med 1996;2:412–417.

217. Pearson L, Garcia J, Wu F, Modesti N, Nelson J, Gaynor RA. Transdominant Tat mutant that inhibits Tat-induced gene expression from the human immunodeficiency virus long terminal repeat. Proc Natl Acad Sci U S A 1990;87:5079–5083.

217a. Perelson AS, Avidan UN, Markowitz M, et al. HIV-1 dynamics in vivo: virion clearance rate, infected cell life-span, and viral generation time. Science 1996;271:1582–1586.

218. Phillips AN, Sabin CA, Elford J, et al. Viral burden in HIV infection. Nature 1994;367:24.

219. Piatak M, Saag MS, Yang LC, et al. High levels of HIV-1 in plasma during all stages of infection determined by competitive PCR. Science 1993;259:1749–1754.

220. Poli G, Kintner A, Justement JS, et al. Tumor necrosis factor α functions in an autocrine manner in the induction of human immunodeficiency virus expression. Proc Natl Acad Sci U S A 1990;87:782–785.

221. Pomerantz RJ, de la Monte SM, Donegan SP, et al. Human immunodeficiency virus (HIV) infection of the uterine cervix. Ann Intern Med 1988;108:321–326.

222. Pomerantz RJ, Feinberg MB, Andino R, Baltimore D. The long terminal repeat is not a major determinant of the cellular tropism of human immunodeficiency virus type 1. J Virol 1991;65:1041–1045.

223. Pomerantz RJ, Kuritzkes DR, de la Monte SM, et al. Infection of the retina by human immunodeficiency virus type 1. N Engl J Med 1987;317:1643–1647.

224. Pomerantz RJ, Trono D, Feinberg MB, Baltimore D. Cells nonproductively infected with HIV-1 exhibit an aberrant pattern of viral RNA expression: a molecular model for latency. Cell 1990;61:1271–1276.

225. Quinnan GVJ, Kirmani N, Rook AH, et al. Cytotoxic T cells in cytomegalovirus infection. N Engl J Med 1982;307:7–13.

226. Rich EA, Chen ISY, Zack JA, Leonard ML, O'Brien WA. Increased susceptibility of differentiated mononuclear phagocytes to productive infection with human immunodeficiency virus expression. Proc Natl Acad Sci U S A 1992;87:176–183.

227. Richman DD. Resistance of clinical isolates of human immunodeficiency virus to antiretroviral agents. Antimicrob Agents Chemother 1993;37:1207–1213.

228. Richman DD, Bozzett SA. The impact of syncytium-inducing phenotype of human immunodeficiency virus on disease progression. J Infect Dis 1993;169:968–974.

229. Rieckmann P, Poli G, Kehrl JH, Fauci AS. Activated B lymphocytes from human immunodeficiency virus infected individuals induce virus expression in infected T cells and monocytes. J Exp Med 1991;173:1–5.

230. Rosen CA, Sodroski JG, Haseltine WA. The location of cis-acting regulatory sequences in the human T cell lymphotropic virus type III (HTLV-III/LAV) long terminal repeat. Cell 1985;41:813–823.

231. Rowland-Jones SL, Nixon DF, Aldhous MC, et al. HIV-specific cytotoxic T cell activity in an HIV-exposed but uninfected infant. Lancet 1993;341:860–861.

232. Saag MS, Crain MJ, Decker WD, et al. High-level viremia in adults and children infected with human immunodeficiency virus: relation to disease stage and CD4+ lymphocyte levels. J Infect Dis 1991;164:72–80.

233. Sabbaj S, Para MF, Fass RJ, Adams PW, Orosz CG, Whitacre CC. Quantitation of antigen-specific immune responses in human immunodeficiency virus (HIV)–infected individuals by limiting dilution analysis. J Clin Invest 1992;12:216–224.

234. Safrit JT, Andrews CA, Zhy T, Ho DD, Koup RA. Characterization of HIV-1-specific cytotoxic T lymphocyte clones isolated during acute seroconversion: recognition of autologous virus sequences within a conserved immunodominant epitope. J Exp Med 1994;179:463–472.

235. Sakai H, Shibata R, Sakuragi J-I, Sakuragi S, Kawamura M, Adachi A. Cell-dependent requirement of human immunodeficiency virus type 1 Vif protein for maturation of virus particles. J Virol 1993;67:1664–1666.

236. Sarver N, Cantin EM, Chang PS, et al. Ribozymes as potential anti-HIV-1 therapeutic agents. Science 1989;247:1222–1225.

237. Sattentau QJ, Moore JP. Conformational changes induced in the human immunodeficiency virus envelope glycoprotein by soluble CD4 binding. J Exp Med 1991;174:407–415.

238. Schmidtmayerova H, Bolmont C, Baghdiguian S, Hirsch I, Cherman J-C. Distinctive pattern of infection and replication of HIV-1 strains in blood-derived marophages. Virology 1992;190:124–133.

239. Schnittman SM, Greenhouse JJ, Psallidopoulos MC, et al. Increasing viral burden in CD4+ T cells from patients with human immunodeficiency virus (HIV) infection reflects rapidly progressive immunosuppression and clinical disease. Ann Intern Med 1990;113:438–443.

240. Schnittman SM, Lane HC, Greenhouse J, Justement JS, Baseler M, Fauci AS. Preferential infection of CD4+ memory T cells by human immunodeficiency virus type 1: evidence for a role in the selective T-cell functional defects observed in infected individuals. Proc Natl Acad Sci U S A 1990;87:6058–6062.

241. Schols D, Pauwels R, Desmyter J, De Clerco E. Presence of class II histocompatibility DR proteins on the envelope of human immunodeficiency virus demonstrated by FACS analysis. Virology 1992;189:374–376.

242. Schuitemaker H, Groenink M, Meyaard L, et al. Early replication steps but not cell type-specific signalling of the viral long terminal repeat determine HIV-1 monocytotropism. AIDS Res Hum Retroviruses 1993;9:669–675.

243. Schuitemaker H, Koot M, Kootstra NA, et al. Biological phenotype of human immunodeficiency virus type 1 clones at different stages of infection: progression of disease is associated with a shift from monocytotropic to T-cell-tropic virus populations. J Virol 1992;66:1354–1360.

244. Schuler W, Weiler IJ, Schuler A, et al. Rearrangement of antigen receptor genes is defective in mice with severe combined immunodeficiency. Cell 1986;46:963–972.

245. Schulick RD, Clerici M, Dolan MJ, Shearer GM. Limiting dilution analysis of interleukin-2–producing T cells responsive to recall and alloantigens in human immunodeficiency virus–infected and uninfected individuals. Eur J Immunol 1993;23:412–417.

246. Schultz TF, Reeves JD, Hoad JG, et al. Effect of mutations in the V3 loop of HIV-1 gp120 on infectivity and susceptibility to proteolytic cleavage. AIDS Res Hum Retroviruses 1993;9:159–166.

247. Seshamma T, Bagasra O, Trono D, Baltimore D, Pomerantz RJ. Blocked early-stage latency in the peripheral blood cells of certain individuals infected with human immunodeficiency virus type 1. Proc Natl Acad Sci U S A 1992;89:10663–10667.

248. Shaw GM, Harper ME, Hahn BH, et al. HTLV-III infection in brains of children and adults with AIDS encephalopathy. Science 1985;227:177–181.

249. Shearer GM, Bernstein DC, Tung KS, et al. A model for the selective loss of major histocompatibility complex self-restricted T cell immune responses during the development of acquired immune deficiency syndrome (AIDS). J Immunol 1986;137:2514–2521.

250. Sheppard HW, Lang W, Ascher MS, Vittinghoff E, Winkelstein W. The characterization of non-progressors: long-term HIV-1 infection with stable CD4+ T-cell levels. AIDS 1993;7:1159–1166.

251. Shibata R, Kawamura M, Sakai H, Hayami M, Ishimoto A, Adachi A. Generation of a chimeric human and simian immunodeficiency virus infectious to monkey peripheral blood mononuclear cells. J Virol 1991;65:3514–3520.

252. Shioda T, Levy JA, Cheng-Mayer C. Macrophage and T cell-line tropisms of HIV-1 are determined by specific regions of the envelope gp120 gene. Nature 1991;349:167–169.

253. Shiratsuchi H, Johnson JL, Toossi Z, Ellner JJ. Modulation of the effector function of human monocytes for *Mycobacterium avium* by human immunodeficiency virus-1 envelope glycoprotein gp120. J Clin Invest 1994;93:885–891.

254. Sodroski J, Goh WC, Rosen C, Dayton A, Terwillinger EF, Haseltine W. A second post-transcriptional *trans*-activator gene required for HTLV-III replication. Nature 1986;321:412–417.

255. Sodroski J, Patarca R, Rosen C, Wong-Staal F, Haseltine W. Location of the *trans*-activating region of the genome of human T-cell lymphotropic virus type III. Science 1985;229:74–77.

256. Spina CA, Kwoh TJ, Chowers MY, Guatelli JC, Richman DD. The importance of *nef* in the induction of human immunodeficiency virus type 1 replication from primary quiescent CD4 lymphocytes. J Exp Med 1994;179:115–123.

257. Stamatatos L, Cheng-Mayer C. Evidence that the structural conformation of envelope gp120 affects human immunodeficiency virus type 1 infectivity, host range, and syncytium-forming ability. J Virol 1993;67:5635–5639.

258. Stamatatos L, Werner A, Cheng-Meyer C. Differential regulation of cellular tropism and sensitivity to soluble CD4 neutralization by the envelope gp120 of human immunodeficiency virus type 1. J Virol 1994;68:4973–4979.

259. Stanley SK, Fauci AS. T cell homeostasis in HIV infection: Part of the solution, or part of the problem? J Acquir Immune Defic Syndr 1993;6:142–143. Editorial.

260. Stein BS, Gowda SD, Lifson JD, Penhallow RC, Bensch KG, Engleman EG. pH-Independent HIV entry into CD4+ T cells via virus envelope fusion to the plasma membrane. Cell 1987;49:659–668.

261. Stein DS, Graham NM, Park LP, et al. The effect of the interaction of acyclovir with zidovudine on progression to AIDS and survival. Ann Intern Med 1994;121:100–108.

262. Stevenson M, Stanwick TL, Dempsey MP, Lamonica CA. HIV-1 replication is controlled at the level of T cell activation and proviral integration. EMBO J 1990;9:1551–1560.

263. Strebel K, Daugherty D, Clouse K, Cohen D, Folks T, Martin MA. The HIV "A" (*sor*) gene product is essential for virus infectivity. Nature 1987;328:728–731.

264. Strebel K, Klimkait T, Matin MA. A novel gene of HIV-1, *vpu*, and its 16-kilodalton product. Science 1988;241:1221–1223.

265. Szkaradkiewicz A. Phagocytosis and microbicidal capacity of human monocytes in the course of HIV infection. Immunol Lett 1992;33:145–150.

266. Takeda A, Tuazon CU, Ennis FA. Antibody-enhanced infection taken by HIV-1 via Fc receptor-mediated entry. Science 1988;242:580–583.

267. Tary-Lehmann M, Saxon A. Human mature T cells that are anergic in vivo prevail in SCID mice reconstituted with human peripheral blood. J Exp Med 1991;175:503–516.

268. Tateno M, Gonzalez-Scarano F, Levy JA. Human immunodeficiency virus can infect CD4-negative human fibroblastoid cells. Proc Natl Acad Sci U S A 1989;86:4287–4290.

269. Temin HM. Retrovirus variation and reverse transcription: abnormal strand transfers result in retrovirus genetic variation. Proc Natl Acad Sci U S A 1993;90:6900–6903.

270. Terai C, Kornbluth RS, Pauza CD, Richman DD, Carson DA. Apoptosis as a mechanism of cell death in cultured T lymphoblasts acutely infected with HIV. J Clin Invest 1991;87:1710–1715.

271. Tersmette M, Gruters RA, de Wolf F, et al. Evidence for a role of virulent human immunodeficiency virus (HIV) variants in the pathogenesis of acquired immunodeficiency syndrome: studies on sequential HIV isolates. J Virol 1989;63:2118–2125.

272. Terwilliger EF, Cohen EA, Lu Y, Sodroski JG, Haseltine WA. Functional role of human immunodeficiency virus type 1 *vpu*. Proc Natl Acad Sci U S A 1989;86:5163–5167.

273. Thali M, Moore JP, Furman C, et al. Characterization of conserved human immunodeficiency virus type 1 gp120 neutralization epitopes exposed upon gp120-CD4 binding. J Virol 1993;67:3978–3988.

274. Trono D. Partial reverse transcripts in virions from human immunodeficiency and murine leukemia viruses. J Virol 1992;66:4893–4900.

275. Valentin A, Albert J, Fenyo EM, Asjo B. Dual tropism for macrophages and lymphocytes is a common feature of primary human immunodeficiency virus type 1 and 2 isolates. J Virol 1994;68:6684–6689.

276. van Noesel CJ, Gruters RA, Terpstra FG, Schellekens PT, van Lier RA, Miedema F. Functional and phenotypic evidence for a selective loss of memory T cells. J Clin Invest 1990;86:293–299.

277. Vandamme AM, Debyser Z, Pauwels R, et al. Characterization of HIV-1 strains isolated from patients treated with TIBO R82913. AIDS Res Hum Retroviruses 1994;10:39–46.

278. vanden Haesevelde M, Decourt J, De Leys RJ, et al. Genomic cloning and complete sequence analysis of a highly divergent African human immunodeficiency virus isolate. J Virol 1994;68:1586–1596.

279. Varmus H. Retroviruses. Science 1988;240:1427–1435.

280. Volberding PA, Lagakos SW, Koch MA. Zidovudine in asymptomatic human immunodeficiency virus infection: a controlled trial in persons with fewer than 500 CD4-positive cells per cubic millimeter. N Engl J Med 1990;322:941–949.

281. von Schwedler U, Song J, Aiken C, Trono D. *vif* is crucial for human immunodeficiency virus type 1 proviral DNA synthesis in infected cells. J Virol 1993;67:4945–4955.

282. von Sydow M, Sonnerborg A, Gaines H, Strannegard O. Interferon-alpha and tumor necrosis factor-alpha in serum of patients in various stages of HIV-1 infection. AIDS Res Hum Retroviruses 1991;7:375–380.

283. Wagner RP, Levitz SM, Tabuni A, Kornfeld H. HIV-1 envelope protein (gp120) inhibits the activity of human bronchoalveolar macrophages against *Cryptococcus neoformans*. Am Rev Respir Dis 1992;146:1434–1438.

284. Walker CM, Erickson A, Hsueh F, Levy J. Inhibition of human immunodeficiency virus replication in acutely infected CD4+ cells by CD8+ cells involves a noncytotoxic mechanism. J Virol 1991;65:5921–5927.

285. Wantanabe M, Ringler DJ, Fultz PV, et al. A chimpanzee-passaged human immunodeficiency virus isolate is cytopathic for chimpanzee cells but does not induce disease. J Virol 1991;65:3344–3348.

286. Washburn RG, Tuazon CU, Bennett JE. Phagocytic and fungicidal activity of monocytes from patients with acquired immunodeficiency syndrome. J Infect Dis 1985;151:565–566.

287. Wei X, Ghosh SK, Taylor ME, et al. Viral dynamics in human immunodeficiency virus type 1 infection. Nature 1995;373:117–122.

288. Weinberg JB, Matthew TJ, Cullen BR, Malim MH. Productive human immunodeficiency virus type 1 (HIV-1) infection of nonproliferating human monocytes. J Exp Med 1991;174:1477–1482.

289. Wesselingh SL, Power C, Glass JD, et al. Intracerebral cytokine messenger RNA expression in acquired immunodeficiency syndrome dementia. Ann Neurol 1993;33:576–582.

290. Westervelt P, Gendelman HE, Ratner L. Identification of a determinant within the HIV-1 surface envelope glycoprotein critical for productive infection of cultured primary monocytes. Proc Natl Acad Sci U S A 1991;88:3097–3101.

291. Westervelt P, Trowbridge DB, Epstein LG, et al. Macrophage tropism determinants of human immunodeficiency virus type 1 in vivo. J Virol 1992;66:2577–2582.

292. Wiley CA, Schrier RR, Nelson JA, Lampert PW, Oldstone MBA. Cellular localization of human immunodeficiency virus infection within the brains of acquired immune deficiency syndrome patients. Proc Natl Acad Sci U S A 1986;83:7089–7093.

293. Willey RL, Maldarelli F, Martin MA, Strebel K. Human immunodeficiency virus type 1 Vpu protein induces rapid degradation of CD4. J Virol 1992;66:7193–7200.

294. Willey RL, Maldarelli F, Martin MA, Strebel K. Human immunodeficiency virus type 1 Vpu protein regulates the formation of intracellular gp160-CD4 complexes. J Virol 1992;66:226–234.

295. Willey RL, Ross EK, Buckler-White AJ, Theodore TS, Marting MA. Functional interaction of constant and variable domains of human immunodeficiency virus type 1 gp120. J Virol 1989;63:3595–3600.

296. Willey RL, Theodore TS, Martin MA. Amino acid substitutions in the human immunodeficiency virus type 1 gp120 V3 loop that change viral tropism also alter physical and functional properties of the virion envelope. J Virol 1994;68:4409–4419.

297. Yao XJ, Garzon S, Boisvert F, Haseltine WA, Cohen EA. The effect of vpu on HIV-1 induced syncytia formation. J Acquir Immune Defic Syndr 1993;6:135–141.

298. Yarchoan R, Mitsuay H, Thomas RV, et al. In vivo activity against HIV and favorable toxicity profile of 2',3'-dideosyinosine. Science 1989;245:412–415.

299. Yu X-F, Ito S, Essex M, Lee T-H. A naturally immunogenic virion-associated protein specific for HIV-2 and SIV. Nature 1988;335:262–265.

300. Yu X-F, Matsuda Z, Yu Q-C, Lee T-H, Essex M. Vpx of simian immunodeficiency virus is localized primarily outside the virus core in mature virions. J Virol 1993;67:4386–4390.

301. Yu X-F, Yu Q-C, Essex M, Lee T-H. The vpx gene of simian immunodeficiency virus facilitates efficient viral replication in fresh lymphocytes and macrophages. J Virol 1991;65:5088–5091.

302. Zack JA, Arrigo SJ, Weitsman SR, Go AS, Haislip A, Chen ISY. HIV-1 entry into quiescent primary lymphocytes: molecular analysis reveals a labile, latent viral structure. Cell 1990;61:213–222.

303. Zack JA, Haislip AM, Krogstad P, Chen ISY. Incompletely reverse-transcribed human immunodeficiency virus type 1 genomes in quiescent cells can function as intermediates in the retroviral life cycles. J Virol 1992;66:1717–1725.

304. Zalcitabine approved under accelerated drug review policy. Clin Pharm 1992;11:747.

305. Zapp ML, Green MR. Sequence specific RNA binding by the HIV-1 Rev protein. Nature 1989;342:714–717.

306. Zarling JM, Ledbetter JA, Sias J, et al. HIV infected humans but not chimpanzees have circulating cytotoxic T lymphocytes that lyse uninfected CD4+ cells. J Immunol 1990;144:2992–2998.

307. Zhang H, Bagasra O, Niikura M, Poiesz BJ, Pomerantz RJ. Intravirion reverse transcripts in the peripheral blood plasma of human immunodeficiency virus type-1 infected individuals. J Virol 1994;68:7591–7597.

308. Zhu T, Mo H, Wang N, et al. Genotypic and phenotypic characterization of HIV-1 in patients with primary infection. Science 1993;261:1179–1181.

Viral Pathogenesis,
edited by Neal Nathanson, et al.
Lippincott–Raven Publishers, Philadelphia © 1997

CHAPTER **35**

Viral Diseases of the Central Nervous System

Acute Infections

Kenneth L. Tyler and Francisco Gonzalez-Scarano

INTRODUCTION

Acute viral infections of the central nervous system (CNS) are an important cause of human morbidity, particularly in children. Their significance is evidenced by the intensive efforts at vaccination that have led to a marked diminution in clinical cases of poliovirus and measles. Investigators have developed several excellent models with which to study viral entry, spread, and the mechanisms of disease production in the nervous system. In this chapter, we review the best-established factors, limiting the number of examples to those that illustrate key principles.

For purposes of dissecting the pathogenetic process in the CNS, we have divided viral replication into two large areas: replication that occurs in tissues outside the nervous system and leads to the process of penetration of the CNS (neuroinva-

siveness) and replication that occurs within the CNS, involves neural elements, and leads to either dysfunction or death of the cell (neurovirulence). Because they are an attempt at simplification, these terms may have slightly different meanings for different models, and for some viruses the properties of neuroinvasiveness and neurovirulence overlap. However, the concepts provide a useful framework to study viral diseases of the CNS, particularly those that cause acute infections.

Viruses that infect the CNS enter the host through a variety of routes, including the skin, respiratory tract, gastrointestinal tract, genitourinary tract, and conjunctiva.[83,128,213] General mechanisms of virus entry are described in Chapter 2. In this chapter, consideration is limited to mechanisms by which virus spreads to the nervous system.

DISSEMINATION OF VIRUS TO THE NERVOUS SYSTEM

Hematogenous Spread

To produce neurologic disease, viruses must spread from their original site of entry in the host to the nervous system. This spread may occur through the bloodstream or within

K. L. Tyler: Departments of Neurology, Medicine, Microbiology, and Immunology, University of Colorado Health Science Center, and Neurology Service (127) Denver VA Medical Center, Denver, Colorado 80262.
F. Gonzalez-Scarano: Departments of Neurology and Microbiology, University of Pennsylvania School of Medicine, Philadelphia, Pennsylvania 19104-6146.

nerves (see later discussion), and the two processes are not mutually exclusive. Varicella-zoster virus (VZV) spreads to the skin through the bloodstream to produce the classic rash of chickenpox; it is then thought to undergo retrograde transport in the axons of sensory neurons to reach the trigeminal and dorsal root ganglia, where it becomes latent. Reactivation from latency is associated with axoplasmic transport of virus from ganglion cells to skin, where local infection results in the appearance of shingles. It has been proposed that certain neurotropic flaviviruses may spread from the bloodstream to olfactory bulb neurons, and then through olfactory neurons to the CNS.[130] Different strains of a single virus can show striking differences in their capacity to spread through nerves or through the bloodstream. Variations in the predominant pattern of spread used by different viral strains have been demonstrated for poliovirus and reovirus.[144,201] Figure 35-1 demonstrates the key steps involved in the dissemination to the CNS of a neurotropic agent, St. Louis encephalitis virus, for which the level of viremia is a key determinant of CNS infection.

Entry into the bloodstream may result from direct inoculation of virus. This may occur after an insect or animal bite or iatrogenically as a result of the use of contaminated needles or transfusion of infected blood products. If this passive inocula-

tion–derived viremia is of sufficient magnitude, it may allow virus to reach the CNS and initiate infection. This has been demonstrated experimentally after bunyavirus infection and in certain instances of human immunodeficiency virus (HIV) infection in humans.[33,60,153]

The typical sequence of events in the viremic spread of viruses in the host was initially delineated by Fenner in his studies of ectromelia.[45,213] An initial, low-titer, primary viremia is generated by early replication of virus near its original site of entry into the host. For some viruses, this primary viremia may be partly induced by experimental subcutaneous or intramuscular injection or by direct intravenous injection of virus, as in the bite of a mosquito. Important sites of primary replication can include skeletal muscle, brown fat, and connective tissue.[57,140,143] Some viruses can productively infect endothelial cells, which allows progeny virus to directly enter the bloodstream and, if cerebral vascular endothelial cells are involved, may also provide a route of invasion into the CNS[7,30,49,105,120,151,159,222] (see later discussion). Primary viremia spreads virus to the reticuloendothelial system and other organs, where further replication leads to a more sustained, higher-titer, secondary viremia that facilitates further dissemination of virus. For some viruses, including certain togaviruses and bunyaviruses, there appears to be a direct

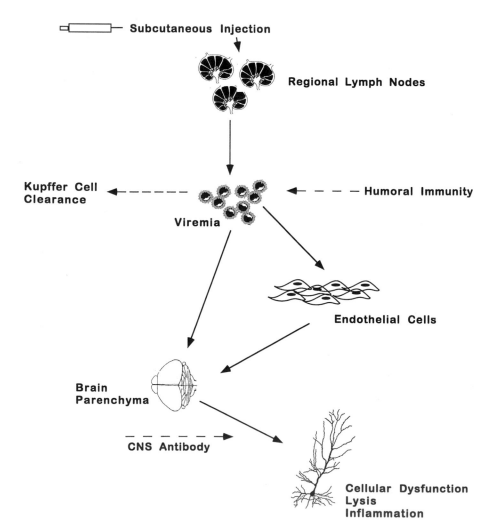

FIG. 35-1. Pathogenesis of viral infections of the central nervous system (CNS). The sequential steps involved in CNS entry are depicted using the pathogenesis of St. Louis Encephalitis virus as a model. (Adapted from Nathanson N. Pathogenesis. In: Monath TP, ed. St. Louis encephalitis. Washington, DC: American Public Health Association, 1980:201–236.)

correlation between the capacity to generate a high-titer viremia and the subsequent capacity to invade the CNS.[75,80,128,143,167]

Early spread of virus from the site of entry to regional lymphatic tissue, such as the gut-associated and bronchus-associated lymphoid tissues, provides access to efferent lymphatic vessels. Efferent lymphatics ultimately drain into the thoracic duct, allowing virus to enter the systemic circulation.[1] This sequence of events may be important in the pathogenesis of picornaviruses, such as poliovirus[15,16] and certain togaviruses.[118,143] Figure 35-2 illustrates the entry of reovirus into M cells overlying bronchus-associated lymphoid tissue.

The magnitude and duration of viremia represent a balance between virus entering the circulation and the host's capacity to clear circulating virus. Clearance of viremia is mediated primarily by phagocytic cells within the reticuloendothelial system. Their capacity to clear virus is in turn influenced by such factors as the presence of opsonizing antibodies and complement components, virion size, surface charge, and the nature of virion surface proteins.[128] Conversely, factors that inhibit the phagocytic capacity of macrophages and other cells may enhance viremia and potentiate infection.[133,221]

Certain neurotropic viruses are capable of replicating within phagocytic cells such as macrophages.[128,152] These cells may then actually transport virus or contribute to continuing viremia rather than terminating it. Replication in macrophages occurs with certain togaviruses (lactate dehydrogenase elevating virus), lentiviruses,[61,154] coronaviruses (mouse hepatitis virus),[8] arenaviruses (lymphocytic choriomeningitis virus, LCMV), cytomegalovirus (CMV),[76,116] herpes simplex virus (HSV),[71,132] and reoviruses.[18] Differences in the capacity of macrophages from newborn animals and from adults to handle viral infection efficiently may also play a role in determining age-related susceptibility to certain neurotropic viruses, including HSV.[71,81,132]

Viruses that travel in the bloodstream may do so either free in the plasma or in association with cells. Viruses that can be found in cell-free plasma include HIV, bunyaviruses, picornaviruses, and togaviruses[160] (see later discussion). Many neurotropic viruses are associated with infection of lymphoid cells and cells of monocyte-macrophage lineage, including HIV and other lentiviruses, Epstein-Barr virus, CMV, LCMV, JC virus, poliovirus, measles virus, and mumps virus.* Infection of polymorphonuclear neutrophils has been reported during influenza virus infection,[165] but its pathogenic significance remains unclear.

Neural Spread

Transport of virus within neurons provides a mechanism for viruses to spread from the periphery to and within the CNS.[53,83,86,96,198,199,200] The possibility that viruses could spread through nerves was first demonstrated by Pasteur for rabies virus and subsequently by others.[6,51,100,104,138,139,195] Neural spread has been demonstrated conclusively for a wide variety of neurotropic viruses, including HSV,[97,99,203,204,205] poliovirus,[74,144,170] certain togaviruses,[173,175] coronaviruses,[9,155,156]

---

*References 24, 29, 31, 37, 40, 42, 48, 116, 121, 154, 185, 191

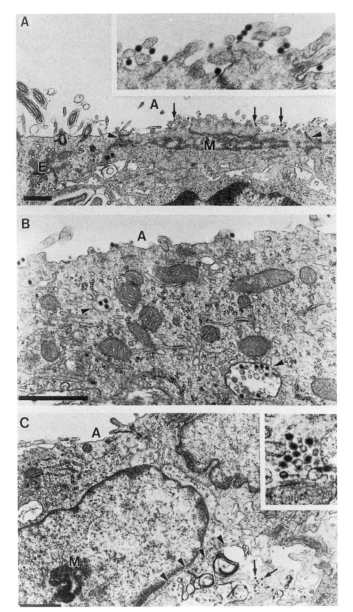

FIG. 35-2. Entry of reoviruses into M cells overlying bronchus-associated lymphoid tissue: $10^{11.8}$ particles of reovirus type 1 Lang were instilled into the tracheas of adult rats, and tissue was obtained and fixed for electron microscopy at 30 and 60 minutes after inoculation. In each of the three photomicrographs, the length of the bar represents 1.0 μm. **(A)** Virus particles (*arrows*) bound to M cells (*M*). Adjacent epithelial cell (*E*) does not demonstrate any viral particles. The inset shows virus particles bound to the surface of an M cell (original magnification ×40,000). **(B)** Reovirus particles within membrane-bound vesicles (*arrowheads*) inside M cells, 60 minutes after inoculation. **(C)** Virus particles (*arrows*) in the intercellular space beneath an M cell (*M*). The inset shows the particle pool at higher magnification (×49,000). (Reprinted from Morin MJ, Warner A, Fields BN. A pathway for entry of reoviruses into the host through M cells of the respiratory tract. J Exp Med 1994;180:1523–1527 with permission.)

reoviruses,[46,135,201] pseudorabies virus,[20,21] and Borna disease virus.[19,131] This list includes both enveloped and nonenveloped viruses, and those with both RNA and DNA genomes, indicating that neural spread is used by viruses with highly varied structural properties and replicative strategies.

Studies in a wide variety of experimental systems have led to the recognition that there are a number of common features to neural spread by viruses. First, prior replication in nonneural tissue is not essential for the subsequent initiation of neural spread, as shown by studies with rabies virus[177] and poliovirus[74] and with a number of viruses in in vitro systems. Second, although sequential infection of perineural cells (e.g., Schwann cells) may provide a potential pathway for neural spread,[82] the pathogenetically important pathway appears to be axoplasmic transport within neurons. This has been demonstrated repeatedly, both by ultrastructural studies showing virions within axons[27,70,163] and by studies in cultured neurons in vitro.[114,115,194,197,220] Third, depending on factors such as viral strain and site of inoculation, viruses may utilize motor, sensory, or autonomic nerve fibers for transport and may be transported either toward the cell body (retrograde) or toward the cell periphery (anterograde). HSV spreads through sensory neurons to reach sensory ganglia; certain reovirus strains spread through autonomic fibers from the gut to reach the brain stem;[135] and certain poliovirus strains spread from muscle through motor fibers to reach spinal cord motor neurons.[144,170] These should be considered as examples rather than as unique or mutually exclusive pathways, because each of these viruses can be shown to be transported in neuronal pathways of a variety of functional specificities.

Neurons transport macromolecules by means of structurally and molecularly distinct pathways of fast and slow axonal transport. Kinetic and pharmacologic studies indicate that viruses are almost exclusively dependent on the microtubule-associated system of fast axonal transport. To date, there is no evidence that viruses use slow axonal transport for dissemination. Fast axonal transport results in the movement of materials at rates of 100 to 400 mm/day, with retrograde being somewhat slower than anterograde transport. Calculated rates of viral transport within nerves in in vivo studies have consistently been slower than this rate (typically <20 mm/day),[74,77,99,201] perhaps reflecting the time required for additional events, including target cell binding, penetration, and, in some cases, processing of viral protein. Measured rates of transport in cell culture systems are typically[196,197,220] but not invariably[115] faster and approach the rate for fast axonal transport of macromolecules.

The molecular mechanisms by which viruses undergo axoplasmic transport have not been defined. It is presumed that viruses, like macromolecules, are transported within vesicles linked to microtubules. However, certain viruses that undergo axoplasmic transport, such as reoviruses, can also bind directly to isolated microtubules,[5] raising the possibility that extravesicular transport of viruses could also occur.

Pharmacologic studies add further support for the importance of microtubules in virus transport. Agents that disrupt the microtubular structure essential for fast axonal transport, including colchicine, taxol, nocodazole, and vinca alkaloids, can be shown to inhibit viral transport in vivo and in culture systems.[13,25,26,96,99,115,194,201] Agents that disrupt cellular intermediate filaments, which are involved in slow axonal trans-

port, do not inhibit viral transport.[201] Inhibition of viral transport has also been reported after administration of a selective inhibitor of retrograde transport[98] or of an inhibitor of axonal transport in sensory neurons (capsaicin).[183]

Studies in a number of different viral systems indicate that viruses are capable of moving from muscle to nerve and transneuronally at both synaptic and nonsynaptic sites.[21,96,125,184,201,203,204,205] Transneuronal transfer of virus may be facilitated by polarized release of virions from neurons, in a process analogous to polarized release of virions from epithelial cells.[38] After infection of muscle cells, rabies virus particles accumulate near the neuromuscular junction.[137,195] Although the observation remains controversial, it has been suggested that the nicotinic acetylcholine receptor, found on muscle cells at the neuromuscular junction, may function as a rabies receptor.[17,62,107] For some neurotropic viruses, including HSV and rabies virus, it has been suggested, based on studies of viral binding and entry into cultured neurons, that the synaptic terminals of neurons may contain a high density of receptor molecules that serve to promote entry into neurons at these points.[115,206,207,220] Similarly, there may be structural features of the synaptic region, perhaps related to the normal process of exocytosis of neurotransmitter vesicles, that also facilitate viral release.[39]

Advances have been made in identification of the roles played by specific viral genes and the proteins they encode in determining the capacity of viruses to utilize different pathways of spread in the infected host. Reovirus strains differ in their principal pathway of spread to the CNS after intramuscular or footpad inoculation in mice. Reovirus serotype 1 Lang (T1L) spreads primarily through the bloodstream, whereas reovirus serotype 3 Dearing (T3D) spreads through nerves. Studies using intertypic T1L × T3D reassortants show that the reovirus S1 gene, which encodes the outer capsid protein s1, is the principal determinant of the pattern of spread.[201] Spread of reoviruses from the gut to extraintestinal organs such as the spleen and liver is also determined by the S1 gene.[89]

Genes responsible for determining the capacity of HSV to spread to the CNS after peripheral inoculation have been extensively investigated. The capacity of HSV to spread from footpad to spinal cord and from cornea to brain has been mapped to regions of the genome that encode the HSV DNA polymerase, thymidine kinase, the p40 nucleoprotein, and the gB envelope protein.[148,192] Mutations within both the gB and gD envelope glycoproteins have also been found to be important in the neuroinvasiveness of certain HSV strains.[78,218] The mechanism by which nonstructural genes, such as the DNA polymerase,[35] influence the neuroinvasiveness of HSV strains remains to be established but may be related to effects on replication within either primary or neuronal cells. In the case of pseudorabies virus, patterns of neuronal uptake and transport may be influenced by changes in the gI and gp63 glycoproteins.[22,23,94,212]

PENETRATION OF VIRUS INTO THE CENTRAL NERVOUS SYSTEM

The capacity of viruses to invade the CNS (neuroinvasiveness) depends in part on their route of spread (Fig. 35-3).

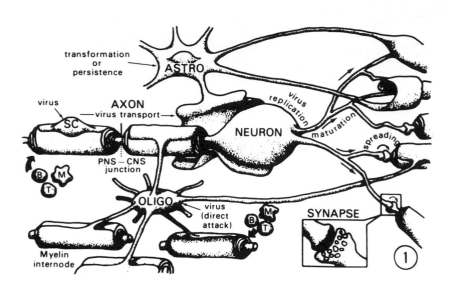

FIG. 35-3. Schematic representation of the interactions between viruses and cell types within the nervous system. Virus can be transported to the neuronal cell body by retrograde axonal transport, where replication takes place. Virus can then be spread along the dendrites and, in some cases, to and across synapses. Myelin-forming cells (oligodendrocytes [OLIGO] and Schwann cells [SC]) can be directly attacked by viruses or destroyed by direct or cytokine-mediated activity associated with macrophages (M) or lymphocytes (B and T). Astrocytes (ASTRO) and neurons may be sites for viral persistence. CNS, central nervous system; PNS, peripheral nervous system. (Reprinted from terMeulen V. Introduction: virus-cell interaction in the nervous system. Sem Neurosci 1991;3:81, with permission.)

Some neurons, such as the motor neurons of the spinal cord, have cell bodies within the CNS but send their axons outside the CNS. For some viruses, such as rabies virus, and in experimental models of infection with viruses such as poliovirus and reovirus T3D, spread of virus from the periphery to motor neurons may be all that is required for initiation of CNS invasion. Primary sensory neurons have their cell bodies in peripheral ganglia that reside outside the CNS. However, these bipolar neurons send axons directly into the CNS. Infection of cells such as dorsal root ganglion cells or trigeminal ganglion cells therefore provides direct access into the CNS. This pathway of CNS invasion has repeatedly been demonstrated in murine models of HSV infection.

A special circumstance also exists in the case of olfactory neurons.[83] Olfactory receptor cells are first-order sensory neurons, with rods that are exposed in the epithelium of the nasal mucosa. These cells synapse directly with second-order neurons within the olfactory bulb. Infection of olfactory rod cells with subsequent infection of mitral cell neurons in the olfactory bulb provides a direct pathway for invasion of the CNS. The importance of this pathway has never been demonstrated conclusively for human infections, but its potential has repeatedly been shown in experimental models of CNS viral infection, including those involving poliovirus,[43,74] coronaviruses,[10,106,155,156] vesicular stomatitis virus,[174] and HSV.[3]

Neural spread may also be an important pathway for CNS invasion by certain neurotropic enteroviruses.[134] For example, after oral inoculation, reovirus serotype 3 clone 9 (T3C9) infects the neurons in the intestinal myenteric plexuses adjacent to ileal Peyer's patches and then subsequently spreads to the neurons of the dorsal motor nucleus of the vagus in the brain stem.[135] A similar pattern of spread is seen after injection of pseudorabies virus into the stomach wall of rats.[21] Hemagglutinating encephalomyelitis virus of swine, an enteric coronavirus, also has the capacity to infect enteric neurons.

The pathways used by blood-borne viruses to leave the bloodstream and invade the CNS are complex.[83,86,128] The blood vessels of the CNS are separated from the brain parenchyma by a series of anatomic structures that jointly compose the blood-brain barrier. In most regions of the CNS, cerebral capillary endothelial cells are interconnected by tight junctions (zona occludens). These cells are in turn surrounded by a dense basement membrane. Perivascular astrocytes oppose their processes to this basement membrane, forming the outermost layer of the blood-brain barrier. Disruption of this barrier may facilitate viral invasion of the CNS.[176] In addition, there are a number of regions within the CNS where the blood-brain barrier is incomplete or not fully developed. These areas include the choroid plexus, posterior pituitary, and circumventricular organs (area postrema, median eminence, subfornical and subcommisural organs). In these regions, the capillary endothelium is fenestrated and the basement membrane is sparse and often not surrounded by astrocytic foot processes. Perhaps the most extensively studied of these regions in terms of its potential to facilitate CNS invasion by blood-borne viruses has been the choroid plexus.

Viruses can spread from the bloodstream through fenestrated choroid plexus microvascular endothelial cells to enter the stroma of the choroid plexus.[83] They can then infect the choroid plexus epithelial cells, which directly abut the ventricular spaces. Transport of virus across choroid plexus epithelial cells provides the virus direct access to the cerebrospinal fluid (CSF). Once in the CSF, viruses can spread to infect the ependymal cells lining the ventricles and, subsequently, the adjacent brain tissue. This pattern of sequential spread from bloodstream through choroid plexus to CSF to ependymal cells and brain parenchyma has been shown for a number of viruses, including mumps virus,[68] certain arboviruses,[113] and rat parvovirus.[110] It could account for the propensity of viruses, including mumps virus, reovirus T1L, and certain togaviruses, to produce striking degrees of hydrocephalus in infected animals,[32,85,92,127,158] and in some cases in humans.[83] Lentiviruses[65,142] can be grown in choroid plexus epithelial cells in culture, and reovirus T1L can infect cultured

TABLE 35-1. *Putative receptors for selected neurotropic viruses*

Virus	Family	Receptor	Investigators
Poliovirus	*Picornaviridae*	PVR	Mendelsohn et al, 1989[126]
Rhinovirus		ICAM-1	Greve et al, 1989[56]
Echovirus 1.8		Integrin VLA-2	Bergelson et al, 1992[11]
Reovirus T3 (Dearing)	*Reoviridae*	Sialic acid	—
Rotavirus SA11		Gangliosides	—
Measles virus	*Myxoviridae*	CD46	Naniche et al, 1993[141]
Sendai virus		Gangliosides	Haywood, 1974[66]
Influenza A, B		Sialic acid	—
Mouse hepatitis virus	*Coronaviridae*	Carcinoembrionic antigen	Williams et al, 1991[215]
Herpes simplex virus	*Herpesviridae*	Heparan sulfate	Spear, 1993[183]
Epstein-Barr virus		CD21 (CR2)	McClure, 1992[124]
Rabies virus	*Rhabdoviridae*	Acetylcholine receptor	Superti et al, 1986[187]
		Gangliosides	Wunner et al, 1984[216]
		Phospholipids	Regan and Wunner, 1985[166]
HIV-1	*Retroviridae*	CD4	Maddon et al, 1986[117]
		Galactosylceramide	Harouse et al, 1991[64]; Fantini et al, 1993[44]
MuLV		Amino acid transporter	Kim et al, 1991[93]
Sindbis virus	*Togaviridae*	Laminin receptor	Wang et al, 1992[210]
Semliki Forest virus		HLA, H2-K, H2-D	

HIV, human immunodeficiency virus; HLA, human leukocyte antigen; ICAM, intercellular adhesion molecule; MuLV, murine leukemia virus; PVR, poliovirus receptor.

Adapted from Haywood AM. Virus receptors: binding, adhesion strengthening, and changes in viral structure. J Virol 1994;68:1–5.

ependymal cells,[190] perhaps providing in vitro analogs to events that occur in vivo.

For viruses that do not invade the CNS in areas where the blood-brain barrier is incomplete, an alternative strategy is to either directly infect or be transported across brain capillary endothelial cells.[7,83] This may serve as a mechanism for CNS invasion by picornaviruses,[30,222] togaviruses,[151] bunyaviruses,[84] and certain retroviruses[120,159] (see later discussion). Other viruses, including CMV, reoviruses, and lentiviruses, are capable of infecting endothelial cells in vitro,[49,105,136,208,209] suggesting that endothelial cell infection may be a mechanism of CNS invasion for a large group of blood-borne viruses. Diapedesis of virally infected leukocytes may provide another mechanism by which viruses can cross the endothelial cell barrier.[47,154,186] This process may be facilitated by the induction of cell surface molecules such as leukocyte function antigen-1, intercellular adhesion molecules, and integrins.[4,69,171]

TROPISM

The term cell tropism is used to designate the differential ability of viruses to infect specific target cells. Susceptibility of individual cell types to the effects of a virus is a major component of its organotropism (the capacity to infect specific organs), and its host range is determined by which species are susceptible to viral infection. Because the CNS contains some of the most complex cells within any organism, there is an enormous potential variability in the infectability of cells by different viruses. For many neurotropic viruses, the specificity of the cellular targets is not well defined, but for others, particularly the more chronic infections, this specificity appears to be a key determinant of their pathogenesis in the CNS.

Viral tropism is frequently defined at the level of entry, and host cell receptors, which interact with the viral attachment proteins, are a key determinant of cellular susceptibility. However, the number of cellular receptors for neurotropic viruses that have been identified is relatively small (Table 35-1). Furthermore, in many instances cellular receptors do not define susceptibility to infection. In some situations, viral entry may proceed appropriately but replication is blocked at later steps. This has been demonstrated in HIV infection of quiescent cells, in which reverse transcription is arrested before completion.[219] In the next sections, we describe examples to illustrate the principles of tropism for CNS cells.

Neuroinvasiveness

Direct infection of endothelial cells appears to be a mechanism for the penetration of viruses from several families and for at least two retroviruses: simian immunodeficiency virus (SIV) and a neurotropic form of murine leukemia virus (MuLV).[149] Like its human counterpart, SIV can penetrate the nervous system and cause symptomatology indicative of degenerative disease. Many of the lesions associated with SIV encephalopathy are perivascular, suggesting that neuroinvasiveness is hematogenous,[103] and viral antigens and nucleic acids have been observed in endothelial cells of the CNS[103] as well as other cells, including microglia. Starting from a molecular clone of a nonneurotropic SIV strain (SIV$_{mac239}$), Sharma and colleagues[178] derived a neurovirulent strain (SIV$_{mac239}$/17E-BR) and demonstrated that there were distinct sequences associated with neurotropism. Most of these were in the *env* region, which encodes the glycoproteins, including the viral-attachment protein gp120, and therefore indirectly implicate the process of cellular entry. Using the same viral isolates, Mankowski and associates[119] demonstrated the presence of nucleic acid in the endothelia of animals infected with the neurovirulent strain. Furthermore, when primary endothelial cultures established from macaque brain were exposed to each SIV strain, SIV$_{mac239}$/17E-BR replicated to high titers, but the parent SIV$_{mac239}$ failed to replicate.

These experiments correlated the ability to infect brain capillary endothelial cells with neuroinvasiveness. An additional finding was that the productive endothelial infection by SIV$_{mac239}$/17E-BR was not inhibited by soluble CD4, in contrast to infection of several CD4+ cell lines tried in parallel.[119] This observation suggests that entry of this SIV strain into endothelial cells is not mediated by the principal SIV receptor and points toward the possibility that efficient utilization of a specific alternative receptor is responsible for the enhanced neuroinvasiveness of the SIV$_{mac239}$/17E-BR strain. Confirmation of this hypothesis awaits further delineation of the entry pathway for SIV, and perhaps other lentiviruses, into cerebral capillary endothelial cells.

Endothelial cells are also the target of another retroviral infection, that induced by TR1.3, a strain of Friend MuLV.[149] In neonatal mice, TR1.3 infects CNS endothelial cells, leading to apparent syncytia formation in vivo and to a syncytia-forming phenotype in vitro. Endothelial cell infection is associated with the development of seizures and tremors, and death is mediated in a high proportion of cases by brain hemorrhages. Using chimeras constructed between molecular clones of TR1.3 and FB29, a similar but nonneuroinvasive MuLV, Park and associates[150] demonstrated that tropism for endothelial cells was determined by a 600-bp region of the *env* gene that differed between the two strains by only three amino acids. Using the molecular clone of the nonneuroinvasive strain, these researchers substituted each of the three amino acids to resemble the TR1.3 sequence. A single substitution (of a glycine for a tryptophan at amino acid 102) resulted in the conversion of the FB29 clone to a neurovirulent phenotype, associating the infectivity of endothelial cells with a specific sequence in SU, the viral-attachment protein.

Because only mice inoculated on postpartum days 0 to 3 demonstrated endothelial infection, the relation between receptor expression and infection was then studied. Analysis of the distribution and expression of the ecotropic MuLV receptor demonstrated that this receptor is expressed in cerebral endothelial cells only during early development, paralleling the susceptibility to viral infection.[122] Therefore, in this system, the ability of the virus to penetrate a specific and critical cell type in the CNS is strictly correlated with the presence of its specific receptor.

Neurovirulence and Specific Cellular Receptors

HIV

The ability to infect the nervous system, and particularly neural cells, is termed neurovirulence, and infection of neural elements also depends on the presence of specific receptors at the cell surface. Specific receptor interactions appear to define the relation between nervous system cells and HIV. In the CNS, HIV can cause both acute and chronic problems, the former including meningitis, meningoencephalitis, and cranial neuropathies. Some of these acute syndromes have been fatal. More commonly, HIV causes a chronic infection of the CNS, and virus can be isolated from the CSF, which may contain a chronic inflammatory reaction. A severe encephalopathy with motor symptomatology and dementia (HIV dementia or AIDS dementia complex) develops in as many as 30% of HIV-infected individuals.[52,123] The pathogenesis of this syndrome is being investigated extensively, and its precise mechanism remains obscure. However, it is clearly related to HIV infection, because the virus can be recovered from the brain and investigators have correlated the presence of HIV genome with the development of dementia.

The cell membrane protein, CD4, is the principal HIV receptor (see Table 35-1), and it would be expected that those cells expressing CD4 would be the principal cell type involved in CNS infection. Indeed, productive infection of the CNS by HIV, as defined by the detection of either viral RNA or proteins with appropriate techniques, is observed primarily in microglia, the resident CNS macrophage.[157,214] That CD4 is present in human microglia has not been formally proved, because it is difficult to demonstrate it in cells with low levels of expression.[28] However, in vitro infection of microglia by HIV strains is abolished by pretreatment with anti-CD4 antibodies,[179,211] which indicates that receptor specificity is a principal determinant of neural-cell tropism. Nevertheless, HIV can also infect other, CD4-negative cell types within the CNS, both in vitro[63] and in vivo.[14,193] Sensitive methodologies such as in situ polymerase chain reaction amplification have shown that other cell types, including neurons, may harbor the provirus, but the level of infectivity is much lower[147]; there are also many examples of cultured and primary cells derived from the nervous system that can be infected with HIV. Although the initial studies demonstrating the importance of CD4 in HIV entry suggested that a related molecule was expressed in high amounts in brain,[117] subsequently it was shown that, except for microglia, CNS cells do not express CD4. Therefore, alternative receptors may mediate entry in astrocytes, oligodendrocytes, and neurons. Galactosylceramide has been proposed as a potential binding molecule in some tissue culture cells,[64,217] and it could act to mediate HIV infection of glia, but other molecules must perform the same function, because cerebral endothelial cells can be infected with HIV but do not express galactosylceramide.[136]

Poliovirus

The role of receptor specificity as a component of neurovirulence has been studied extensively for poliovirus. Poliovirus has a well-defined host range and can infect only primates or primate tissues, but early experiments with RNA transfections demonstrated that the species barrier could be overcome by directly delivering the genomic material into normally resistant cells.[72,73,164] This implicated the early steps of receptor binding and entry in the natural resistance to infection exhibited by nonprimate cells. Identification of the poliovirus receptor (PVR), a member of the immunoglobulin supergene family,[126] was the first step toward a definitive proof of this concept, the second being the development of transgenic mice expressing PVR.[168,169] Transgenic mice expressing PVR in many tissues are susceptible to peritoneal or intracranial injection of poliovirus and develop a paralytic disease that resembles human and primate poliovirus infection.[169] Therefore, expression of its receptor is the primary determinant of poliovirus infection in a nonprimate species.

Nevertheless, PVR expression does not explain the pathogenesis of poliovirus in mice completely. Some tissues that expressed the receptor in transgenic mice (e.g., spleen) did not support viral replication.[169] Furthermore, perhaps because of potential artefact resulting from more widespread expression of PVR in transgenic animals, replication in the mouse CNS did not follow precisely the pattern in natural infections. This correlates with the fact that, in humans, expression of the PVR is more widespread than the pattern of infection would suggest (see Chap. 23). The existence of a coreceptor (CD44) has been suggested as a possible explanation for these findings.[180]

Poliovirus strains vary significantly in their neurovirulence, and vaccines strains are, of course, attenuated in this property. This variability could also be explained theoretically by enhanced affinity for the PVR by neurovirulent strains and, conversely, by a less avid interaction between PVR and the viral attachment proteins of attenuated vaccine strains. However, a careful study of the attenuated type 3 Sabin strain[12] demonstrated that the dissociation constant binding of this strain to HeLa cells was almost identical to that of a more virulent serotype (type 1 Mahoney). This finding is consistent with the fact that the reversion of attenuation in vaccine strains is genetically associated with the noncoding regions of the poliovirus genome, and not with the regions that encode its capsid proteins[2] (see Chap. 23). Therefore, although the association between poliovirus and PVR is a critical determinant of neural infection, several other factors are important in determining the outcome and distribution of infectivity.

Measles Virus

Measles virus presents a situation similar to that of poliovirus, in which natural infection is limited to primates. Nevertheless, the measles virus can be adapted to growth in brains of rats and other species, and vaccine strains have been prepared in chick embryos. Measles virus is neurotropic and can cause a variety of neurologic syndromes, including an acute encephalopathy that may be immune mediated, a chronic disease (subacute sclerosing panencephalitis) that is associated with specific, perhaps defective strains, and an inclusion-body encephalitis.[146] A receptor for measles virus, CD46, has been identified (see Table 35-1), and hamster cell lines engineered to express this protein become susceptible to infection with wild-type measles virus.[36] CD46 is expressed ubiquitously in primate tissues, and measles virus infects a variety of tissues during the acute phase of the disease. Therefore, the presence of CD46 is a critical determinant of species susceptibility to measles virus and explains its global tropism among primate cells. The fact that the virus can be adapted to growth in the brains of some nonprimate species[109] indicates that it can use alternative receptors within some brain cells.

MOLECULAR AND GENETIC DETERMINANTS OF VIRULENCE

The properties of neuroinvasiveness and neurovirulence have been analyzed in a number of viruses with neurotropic potential that are responsible for acute infections. Among the wide number, we have selected a few that illustrate the principles of neuroinvasion and neurovirulence.

Neuroinvasiveness and Envelope Genes

Viruses of the California serogroup (genus bunyavirus, family *Bunyaviridae*) are human pathogens that are responsible for many cases of pediatric encephalitis in areas where their mosquito vectors are endemic (e.g., midwestern United States). A mouse model of encephalitis demonstrates many of the features of the human disease, with peripheral replication in muscle leading to an active plasma viremia and subsequent neuroinvasion. Age-dependent susceptibility, an important characteristic of the clinical disease, is also reproduced in the murine model.[58,60]

Different strains of the California serogroup vary in their ability to infect the murine nervous system. For example, La Crosse virus, the most studied American strain, causes a fatal disease in newborn mice after a subcutaneous inoculation of less than 1 plaque-forming unit (PFU); in contrast, the brain-passaged 181/57 strain of Tahyna virus is highly attenuated after peripheral inoculation, requiring 10,000 PFU per median lethal dose.[80] Furthermore, because bunyaviruses have a segmented, negative-stranded genome, genetic reassortment among antigenically related wild-type strains can readily be achieved by coinfection at high input multiplicity.[79] These features have allowed the dissection of the genetic underpinnings of neurologic infections in these viruses.

To study the property of neuroinvasiveness, reassortants between neuroinvasive La Crosse and noninvasive Tahyna 181/57 were prepared and tested by subcutaneous inoculation into suckling mice (Table 35-2).[79] The reassortants are designated according to the origin of their large (L) segment, which encodes the polymerase protein, their middle (M) segment, which encodes the two glycoproteins and a nonstructural protein, and the small (S) segment, which encodes the nucleocapsid protein and a nonstructural protein. A reassortant labelled TLT contains the L segment from Tahyna, the M segment from La Crosse, and the S segment from Tahyna. As demonstrated in Table 35-2, those reassortants containing the M segment from La Crosse virus (TLT, TLL, and LLT) were almost as virulent as the La Crosse parent (LLL), whereas the opposite was true for reassortants containing the Tahyna M segment. For all of

TABLE 35-2. *Bunyavirus neuroinvasiveness maps to the M segment*

Genotype*	Virus	PFU/LD50 suckling mice†	Comparative neuroinvasiveness
LLL (La Crosse)	Original	−0.3	++++
TLT	B1-11A	−0.3	++++
	B1-26A	0.2	++++
LLT	A1-3A	−0.3	++++
	B1-29A	0.1	++++
TLL	P1-2GG	0.1	++++
LTL	F1-18A	3.2	+
	F2-18A	3.2	+
TTL	F1-2A	3.3	+
	F2-2A	3.7	−
LTT	B1-1A	3.9	−
	V1-1A	3.2	+
TTT (Tahyna)	181-57	4.2	−

*The three-letter viral genotype designates the derivation of the L, M, and S segments, respectively. L, segment derived from La Crosse virus; T, segment derived from Tahyna virus.

†Plaque-forming units per median lethal dose, denoted as $\log_{10}$.

Adapted from Janssen R, Gonzalez-Scarano F, Nathanson N. Mechanisms of bunyavirus virulence: comparative pathogenesis of a virulent strain of La Crosse and an avirulent strain of Tahyna virus. Lab Invest 1984;50:447–455.

these experiments, an essential requirement is robust replication of all reassortants in a default cell line such as BHK-21.

Because neuroinvasiveness is associated with replication in muscle, a tissue culture model using differentiated mouse muscle cells (C2C12) was used to determine whether the reassortant viruses differed in their ability to infect this tissue.[59] As determined by immunofluorescence assay, reassortant viruses containing the La Crosse M segment RNA infected a greater proportion of myotubes (differentiated muscle pheno-

type) than either parent the Tahyna virus or those reassortants containing its M segment.[59] These findings are illustrated in Figure 35-4.

Because the M segment encodes the glycoproteins, these results implicate these surface proteins in neuroinvasiveness. A definitive mechanistic explanation for the importance of the glycoproteins, such as evidence that the initial interaction between the viruses and the cells is more efficient for one or the other strain, awaits the identification of the receptor for California serogroup viruses, which circumstantial evidence indicates is likely to be the same for all strains.[152a] However, experiments with a mutant La Crosse virus obtained by selection with a monoclonal antibody directed against the G1 glycoprotein[54] indicated that cell entry is a critical determinant of neuroinvasiveness: the monoclonal antibody resistant variant, V22, was much less neuroinvasive than the parent La Crosse. The mutant was less efficient than the parent virus at mediating cell-to-cell fusion, and maximal fusion occurred at pH 5 rather than pH 6.[55] These experiments implicated one of the two glycoproteins in neuroinvasiveness and associated the phenotype with alteration in a function that is involved in the entry process of enveloped viruses.

Most California serogroup viruses, and certainly both La Crosse and Tahyna, are able to infect brain cells if injected intracerebrally, indicating that both strains are equally neurovirulent. We were unable to relate this property to any specific segment by study of reassortants from wild-type viruses.

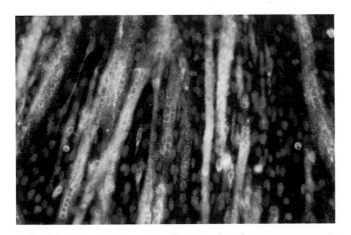

FIG. 35-4. Replication of La Crosse virus in mouse myocyte cultures. Differentiated C2C12 cells forming myotubes were infected with La Crosse virus and stained by indirect immunofluorescence with anti–La Crosse antibodies 24 hours later. Robust replication of virus is seen in the myotubes but lower levels in the undifferentiated myocytes. (Magnification ×170) (Griot C, Pekosz A, Davidson R, et al. Replication in cultured C2C12 muscle cells correlates with the neuroinvasiveness of California serogroup viruses. Virology 1994;201: 399–403.)

Polymerases, Core Proteins, and Nonstructural Proteins

To map the property of neurovirulence, a new strain of a California virus was selected by passage in tissue culture, using a paradigm previously shown to be effective in Sinbis virus, and tested by intracerebral inoculation of adult mice.[41]

A reassortant virus obtained by a coinfection of Tahyna and La Crosse viruses (see previous section) with genotype TLL was passaged in tissue culture 25 times, and neuroattenuated plaques were further screened. The neuroattenuated virus, RFC/25B.5, or B.5, was more than 100,000-fold less virulent than either parent or other reassortants with the same genotype. Even if tested by intracerebral inoculation of suckling mice—which are exquisitely sensitive to these agents—B.5 was at least tenfold less virulent than the parent viruses.

The B.5 reassortant was then backcrossed to viruses with the reciprocal genotype to generate a full panel of reassortants that isolated each of the B.5 genes. Furthermore, revertant viruses were obtained by virtue of the temperature sensitivity of the B.5 clone. In each instance, the avirulent phenotype was mapped to the L segment, which encodes the viral polymerase.[60] Therefore, in this group of viruses, the interaction between the viral polymerase and cellular factors can determine replication in the nervous system. Because the B.5 virus expresses the La Crosse glycoproteins, it is assumed that the interaction between the virus and cellular receptors, and indeed the entry process itself, proceeds as efficiently as in La Crosse virus.

Noncoding Regions of the Genome

Robust replication within the CNS has also been mapped to noncoding regions of viruses. The clearest examples occur in the picornaviruses, and more extensive discussions on the subject are presented in Chapters 23 (poliovirus) and 36 (Theiler's murine encephalomyelitis virus). A brief summary of the poliovirus example is appropriate to demonstrate that neurovirulence can be associated with unexpected regions of the genome.

The earliest information regarding the regions of the poliovirus genome that are associated with neurovirulence was obtained by comparing the sequences of the attenuated Sabin type 3 strain (P3/Leon/12a1b) with those of its parent type 3 strain and revertant neurovirulent strains.[90,129,145] An U-C reversion at position 472 in the 5' noncoding region (NTR) was found to be particularly common in the neurovirulent revertants. Its importance was later confirmed after introduction of this mutation into an infectious molecular clone resulted in attenuation of the mutated clone. Further work has confirmed the importance of this region for both type 1 and type 2 polioviruses. For type 1, a mutation at position 480 is associated with reduced virulence; for type 2, mutants in base 481 have a similar effect.

How does a mutation in an untranslated region affect neurovirulence? The most accepted hypothesis suggests that this region is involved in the interaction between the poliovirus RNA and ribosomes, which are thought to bind internally in several picornaviruses with roughly similar genomic organization.[2] Computer models indicate that the 5' NTR region has extensive secondary structure and that the region around these mutations forms a distinctive stem-loop structure[181] (see Chap. 23). Introduction of several mutations that potentially disrupt this theoretical structure has also resulted in attenuation of the virus. Using cell-free systems, Svitkin and colleagues[188,189] were able to demonstrate that in vitro translation of mutant RNA was less efficient than translation of wild-type RNA. Others have suggested that the binding of specific initiation factors to the mutant RNA may be decreased.[102] Some

mutations in the region are also known to lead to a temperature-sensitive (ts) phenotype, which is associated with the attenuation.

Mutations in the 5' NTR have also been found to attenuate Sindbis virus neurovirulence in a mouse model.[101] In that system, mutations in the 3' NTR were also capable of decreasing replication in mouse brain cells and, in fact, may have been more effective attenuators. Moreover, several double mutants containing mutations in both NTRs were even more attenuated. As with mutations in the poliovirus 5' NTR, several of the Sindbis mutants demonstrated a ts phenotype.

SELECTED MECHANISMS OF NEUROVIRULENCE

Cell Death

The most deleterious, and to some extent best described, effect of an acute neurotropic viral infection is the death of neuronal cells. This may eventually result in death of the organism, as is typical for many experimental models involving bunyaviruses, alphaviruses, rabies virus, and herpesviruses. Cell death induced by viral infection has traditionally been ascribed to a variety of mechanisms, including interference with host cell RNA transcription and transport, inhibition of host cell RNA translation and DNA replication, and disruption of the cytoskeleton. Most of these mechanisms are specific for virus families. Some viruses may even kill neural cells by promotion of cell-to-cell fusion and the formation of polykaryons. However, for the most part, there is inadequate understanding of the precise mechanisms involved in the mediation of neuronal death or dysfunction, other than to extrapolate information that has been obtained with tissue culture models. These models usually consist of simpler cell types and do not represent the full range of injury that may be sustained by a highly specialized cell like the neuron.

Much attention has been directed toward programmed cell death (apoptosis) as a potential mechanism for CNS tissue injury in viral infections. Programmed cell death is an important regulatory mechanism for the elimination of superfluous cells in the nervous system, particularly during development, and the machinery for induction of apoptosis is present in CNS cells. Starting from the observation that Sindbis virus establishes a persistent, productive infection of differentiated cultured neurons, Levine and colleagues[108] established that Sindbis virus kills a number of undifferentiated cell lines by a process involving programmed cell death. Further, they indirectly demonstrated an inverse relation between expression of the *bcl-2* gene, an antagonist of the apoptotic process, and the establishment of these chronic infections in primary dorsal root ganglia. A cell line engineered to overexpress bcl-2 was not susceptible to Sindbis virus-induced neuropathology, in contrast to its parent line. These observations indicate that Sindbis virus neuropathology may be mediated by the induction of apoptosis and suggest that the relative resistance of older animals to the deleterious effects of the virus[87] is caused by the fact that postmitotic neurons are less susceptible to apoptosis.

More recently, Ubol and associates[202] obtained a neurovirulent strain of Sindbis virus by serial passage in mouse brain and showed that, in contrast to the wild-type virus from which it was derived, it caused a fatal encephalitis in 3- to 4-week-old mice. In vitro, this neurovirulent strain was able to induce extensive cytopathology in a cell line that expresses high levels of bcl-2, suggesting that overcoming this effect was the mechanism for its enhanced virulence. The neurovirulence of this strain was mapped to a single amino acid in the E2 surface glycoprotein.[202] Definitive proof of the relation between bcl-2, neurovirulence, and age-dependent susceptibility awaits the use of transgenic mice expressing high levels of bcl-2 early in their development. Nevertheless, these seminal experiments have suggested an important mechanism of virus-induced cell death.

Specific tropisms for subpopulations of neuronal cells may influence the pattern of neurovirulence. For example, poliovirus preferentially infects and kills neuronal cells residing in the anterior horn of the spinal cord, resulting in its characteristic neurologic symptomatology, focal paralysis. VZV, in contrast, appears to infect neurons in sensory ganglia, leading to a rash in a dermatomal distribution and to herpetic and postherpetic pain.[50] Figure 35-5 demonstrates the tropism of La Crosse bunyavirus for Purkinje cells in the cerebellum of an adult mouse inoculated intracranially, another example of tropism for a specific neural cell population.

How such specific tropism arises is unclear. As discussed in previous sections, the presence of PVR does not fully explain the distribution of poliovirus in infected transgenic mice. It is likely that predilection for some subpopulations is multifactorial and relates to both cell membrane and intracellular proteins.

Dysfunction Without Cell Death

Most experimental models, whether in vivo or in vitro, concentrate on cell death as a manifestation of infection or virulence, but there is considerable although mostly circumstantial evidence that viruses can cause cellular dysfunction without death. This could account for the recovery that typically occurs

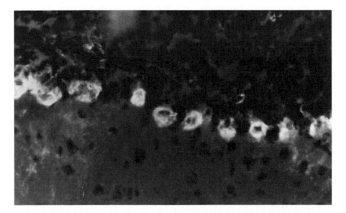

FIG. 35-5. Replication of La Crosse virus in Purkinje cells of the cerebellum. La Crosse viral antigen is shown in Purkinje cells of the cerebellar cortex in an adult mouse after intracerebral inoculation. This demonstrates the neuronotropism of some viral strains. (Immunofluorescent stain using hyperimmune rabbit anti-LaCrosse virus antiserum; magnification ×500.) (From Janssen R, Gonzalez-Scarano F, Nathanson N. Mechanisms of bunyavirus virulence: comparative pathogenesis of a virulent strain of La Crosse and an avirulent strain of Tahyna virus. Lab Invest 1984;50:447–455.)

after encephalitis. A classic example occurs in poliovirus, in which respiratory failure is a significant problem that, if managed well by artificial respiration, can eventually resolve. The postpolio syndrome, a neuromuscular deterioration that occurs many years after a clinical case of polio, is now accepted not to be the result of a persistent poliovirus infection. An interesting—and viable—hypothesis proposes that, after the acute infection, a proportion of motor neurons remain alive but damaged. With age, these eventually deteriorate or even die off, leading to additional symptoms in a limb previously affected.

VZV may also lead to dysfunctional sensory neurons. Postherpetic neuralgia, a painful condition in which severe burning pain occurs in the distribution of the previous bout of herpes zoster, may be the result of neuronal damage during an acute VZV infection. It has been suggested that VZV can decrease the expression of glial fibrillary acidic protein in explant cultures of astrocytes.[91]

One of the most enigmatic problems in neurovirology is the pathophysiology of HIV dementia, alluded to in earlier sections. In this syndrome, infection of microglial cells, perhaps coupled with a minimal infection of neurons, astrocytes, and oliogodendrocytes, results in deterioration of neurologic function with both motor and cognitive symptoms. In spite of the apparent neuronal origin of the problem, there is minimal neuronal pathology, and the presence of neuronal death is controversial. The most prevalent hypotheses suggest that neuronal dysfunction is mediated either by viral gene products secreted by infected microglia or by cytokines or other products of macrophage activation that are toxic to neurons.

A number of HIV gene products have been implicated in toxicity to neurons, mostly in systems using neurons from nonprimate species. The viral receptor-attachment protein, gp120, has been the subject of most of these studies, and several investigators have demonstrated toxicity to rat retinal ganglion and hippocampal neurons. This toxicity is associated with a rise in intracellular calcium and suggests that N-methyl-D-aspartate (NMDA) is involved in gp120-mediated toxicity.[88,111,112] One group of investigators has indicated that nitric oxide may be involved as well.[34] The viral transactivator, tat, has also been implicated in neuronal changes.[95,172]

Although most of these experiments have used neuronal death or gross morphologic changes as their end point, subtler changes may occur at lower concentrations of the toxins or in different neuronal subtypes. Alternatively, a number of cytokines have been suspected as having a role in development of neurons and astrocytes. The interactions between inflammatory cells and neural cells within the CNS may be deleterious without actual cell killing. Cell toxicity has been observed in cultured brain cells exposed to the supernatants of infected macrophages.[161,162] In one study, cytopathic changes in fetal neurons and glia resulted from cocultivation with an HIV-infected monocytoid cell line.[190]

SUMMARY

In this chapter, we have attempted to provide a framework for understanding the pathogenesis of acute infections of the nervous system, from the point of entry into the organism, through the site of primary replication, to the penetration of the target organ, the CNS. To develop these concepts, a few well-studied models were described, but there are many others that could not be covered in this relatively short chapter. The brain has a well-developed barrier to the systemic circulation, and understanding of the mechanism of viral penetration of this organ yields information that is generally applicable. Part of the attractiveness of CNS models—and the reason they are relatively abundant—is that the brain is an important target organ for many viruses.

Another attractive feature of many of these models is that they use a well-studied laboratory species, the mouse, which allows exploration of the host response as a component of pathogenesis. Even in instances (e.g., poliovirus) in which virus tropism is limited by species, the development of transgenic mice has extended the usefulness of this animal for studies of pathogenesis.

The brain is also the site of many infections whose pathogenesis involves chronic and latent infection. The principles underlying the study of these, an equally rich area, are the subject of Chapter 36.

ABBREVIATIONS

CMV: cytomegalovirus
CNS: central nervous system
CSF: cerebrospinal fluid
E2: a surface glycoprotein of Sindbis virus
G1: a surface glycoprotein of La Crosse virus
HIV: human immunodeficiency virus
HSV: herpes simplex virus
L: large segment (of bunyavirus genome)
LCMV: lymphocytic choriomeningitis virus
M: middle segment (of bunyavirus genome)
LCMV: lymphocytic choriomeningitis virus
MuLV: murine leukemia virus
NTR: noncoding [untranslated] region
PFU: plaque-forming unit
PVR: poliovirus receptor
S: small segment (of bunyavirus genome)
SIV, SIV$_{mac239}$: simian immunodeficiency virus
T1L, T3D, T3C9: reovirus serotypes
TR1.3, FB29: strains of MuLV
ts: temperature-sensitive
SIV: simian immunodeficiency virus
VZV: varicella-zoster virus

ACKNOWLEDGMENTS

Supported by PHS Grants NS-30606, NS-20904 (to F. G-S) and NS 32228 and a Merit Grant from the Department of Veterans Affairs (to KLT).

REFERENCES

1. Albrecht P. Pathogenesis of neurotropic arbovirus infection. Curr Top Microbiol Immunol 1968;43:44–91.
2. Almond JW. Poliovirus neurovirulence. Semin Neurosci 1991;3: 101–108.
3. Anderson J, Field H. The distribution of herpes simplex virus type 1 antigen in the mouse central nervous system after different routes of inoculation. J Neurol Sci 1983;60:181–195.
4. Attibele N, Wyde PR, Trial J, Smole SC, Smith CW, Rossen RD. Measles virus-induced changes in leukocyte function antigen 1 ex-
pression and leukocyte aggregation: possible role in measles virus pathogenesis. J Virol 1993:67:1075–1079.
5. Babiss L, Luftig R, Weatherbee J, Weihing R, Ray U, Fields BN. Reovirus serotypes 1 and 3 differ in their in vitro association with microtubules. J Virol 1979;30:863–874.
6. Bak I, Markham C, Cook M, Stevens J. Intra-axonal transport of herpes simplex virus in the rat central nervous system. Brain Res 197;136,415–429.
7. Bang F, Luttrell C. Factors in the pathogenesis of virus diseases. Adv Virus Res 1961;8:199–244.
8. Bang F, Warwick A. Mouse macrophages as host cells for the mouse hepatitis virus and the genetic basis of their susceptibility. Proc Natl Acad Sci U S A 1960;46:1065–1075.
9. Barnett EM, Perlman S. The olfactory nerve and not the trigeminal nerve is the major site of CNS entry for mouse hepatitis virus, strain JHM. Virology 1993;194:185–191.
10. Barthold SW. Olfactory neural pathways in mouse hepatitis virus nasoencephalitis. Acta Neuropathol (Berl) 1988;76:502–506.
11. Bergelson JM, Shepley MP, Chan BMC, Hemler ME, Finberg RW. Identification of the integrin VLA-2 as a receptor for echovirus 1. Science 1992;255:1718–1720.
12. Bibb JA, Witherell G, Bernhardt G, Wimmer E. Interaction of poliovirus with its cell surface binding site. Virology 1994;201:107–115.
13. Bijlenga G, Heaney T. Post-exposure local treatment of mice infected with rabies with two axonal flow inhibitors, colchicine and vinblastine. J Gen Virol 1978;39:381–385.
14. Saito Y, Sharer LR, Epstein LG, et al. Overexpression of nef as a marker for restricted HIV-1 infection of astrocytes in postmortem pediatric central nervous tissues. Neurology 1994;44:474–481.
15. Bodian D. Emerging concepts of poliomyelitis infection. Science 1955;122:105–108.
16. Bodian D. Poliomyelitis: pathogenesis and histopathology. In: Rivers TM, Horsfall FL Jr, eds. Viral and rickettsial infections of man. Philadelphia: JB Lippincott, 1959:479–498.
17. Burrage TG, Tignor GH, Smith AL. Rabies virus binding at neuromuscular junctions. Virus Res 1985;2:273–289.
18. Burstin SJ, Brandriss MW, Schlesinger JJ. Infection of a macrophage-like cell line P388D1 with reovirus: effects of immune ascitic fluids and monoclonal antibodies on neutralization and enhancement of viral growth. J Immunol 1983;130:2915–2919.
19. Carbone KM, Duchala CS, Griffin JW, Kincaid AL, Narayan O. Pathogenesis of Borna disease virus in rats: evidence that intra-axonal spread is the major route for dissemination and determinant for disease incubation. J Virol 1987;61:431–3440.
20. Card JP, Rinaman L, Lynn RB, et al. Pseudorabies virus infection of the rat central nervous system: ultrastructural characterization of viral replication, transport, and pathogenesis. J Neurosci 1993;13: 2515–2539.
21. Card JP, Rinaman L, Schwaber JS, et al. Neurotropic properties of pseudorabies virus: uptake and transneuronal passage in the rat central nervous system. J Neurosci 1990;10:1974–1994.
22. Card JP, Whealy ME, Robbins AK, Enquist LW. Pseudorabies virus envelope glycoprotein gI influences both neurotropism and virulence during infection of the rat visual system. J Virol 1992;66: 3032 3041.
23. Card JP, Whealy ME, Robbins AK, Moore RY, Enquist LW. Two alpha-herpesvirus strains are transported differentially in the rodent visual system. Neuron 1991;6:957–969.
24. Carillo C, Borca MV, Alfonso CL, Onisk DV, Rock DL. Long-term persistent infection of swine monocytes/macrophages with African swine fever virus. J Virol 1994;68:580–583.
25. Ceccaldi PE, Ermine A, Tsiang H. Continuous delivery of colchicine in the rat brain with osmotic pumps for inhibition of rabies virus transport. J Virol Methods 1990;28:79–84.
26. Ceccaldi PE, Gillet JP, Tsiang H. Inhibition of the transport of rabies virus in the central nervous system. J Neuropathol Exp Neurol 1989;48:620–630.
27. Charlton K, Casey G. Experimental rabies in skunks: immunofluorescent, light, and electron microscopic studies. Lab Invest 1979;41: 36–44.
28. Collman R, Godfrey B, Cutilli J, et al. Macrophage-tropic strains of human immunodeficiency virus type 1 utilize the CD4 receptor. J Virol 1990;64:4468–4476.

29. Coombs RW, Collier RC, Allain JP, et al. Plasma viremia in human immunodeficiency virus infection. N Engl J Med 1989;321:1626–1631.

30. Couderc T, Hogle J, Le Blay H, Horaud F, Blondel B. Molecular characterization of mouse-virulent poliovirus type 1 mahoney mutants: involvement of residues of polypeptides VP1 and VP2 located on the inner surface of the capsid protein shell. J Virol 1993;67:3808–3817.

31. Darr ES, Mondgil T, Meyer RD, et al. Transient high levels of viremia in patients with primary human immunodeficiency virus type 1 infection. N Engl J Med 1991;324:961–964.

32. Davis LE. Communicating hydrocephalus in newborn hamsters and cats following vaccinia virus infection. J Neurosurg 1981;54:767–772.

33. Davis LE, Hjelle BL, Miller VE, et al. Early viral brain invasion in iatrogenic human immunodeficiency virus infection. Neurology 1992;42:1736–1739.

34. Dawson VL, Dawson TM, Uhl GR, Snyder SH. Human immunodeficiency virus type 1 coat protein neurotoxicity mediated by nitric oxide in primary cortical cultures. Proc Natl Acad Sci U S A 1993;90:3256–3259.

35. Day S, Lausch R, Oakes J. Evidence that the gene for herpes simplex virus type 1 DNA polymerase accounts for the capacity of an intertypic recombinant to spread from eye to central nervous system. Virology 1988;163:166–173.

36. D(auo)rig RE, Marcil A, Chopra A, Richardson CD. The human CD46 molecule is a receptor for measles virus (Edmonston strain). Cell 1993;75:295–303.

37. Dorries K, Vogel E, Gunther S, Czub S. Infection of human polyomaviruses JC and BK in peripheral blood leukocytes from immunocompetent individuals. Virology 1994;198:59–70.

38. Dotti CG, Simons K. Polarized sorting of viral glycoproteins to the axon and dendrites of hippocampal neurons in culture. Cell 1990;62:63–72.

39. Dubois-Dalcq M, Hooghe-Peters E, Lazzarini R. Antibody induced modulation of rhabdovirus infection of neurons in vitro. J Neuropathol Exp Neurol 1980;39:507–522.

40. Embretson J, Zupancic M, Ribas JL, et al. Massive covert infection of helper T lymphocytes and macrophages by HIV during the incubation period of AIDS. Nature 1993;362:359–362.

41. Endres M, Valsamakis A, Gonzalez-Scarano F, Nathanson N. A neuroattenuated bunyavirus variant: derivation, characterization and revertant clones. J Virol 1990;64:1927–1933.

42. Esolen LM, Ward BJ, Moench TR, Griffin DE. Infection of monocytes during measles. J Infect Dis 1993;168:47–52.

43. Faber H. The pathogenesis of poliomyelitis. Springfield, Illinois: CC Thomas, 1955.

44. Fantini J, Cook DG, Nathanson N, Spitalnik SL, Gonzalez-Scarano F. Infection of colonic epithelial cells by type 1 human immunodeficiency virus is associated with cell surface expression of galactosylceramide. Proc Natl Acad Sci U S A 1993;90:2700–2704.

45. Fenner F. Mousepox (infectious ectromelia of mice): a review. J Immunol 1949;63:341–373.

46. Flamand A, Gagner JP, Morrison LA, Sidman R, Fields BN. Penetration of the nervous system of suckling mice by mammalian reoviruses. J Virol 1991;65:123–131.

47. Fournier J-G, Tardieu M, Lebon P, et al. Detection of measles virus RNA in lymphocytes from peripheral blood and brain perivascular infiltrates of patients with subacute sclerosing panencephalitis. N Engl J Med 1985;313:910–915.

48. Freistadt MS, Fleit HB, Wimmer E. Poliovirus receptor on human blood cells: a possible extraneural site of poliovirus replication. Virology 1993;195:798–803.

49. Friedman H, Macarek E, MacGregor RA, Wolfe J, Kefalides N. Virus infection of endothelial cells. J Infect Dis 1981;143:266–273.

50. Gilden DH, Mahalingam R, Dueland AN, Cohrs R. Herpes zoster: pathogenesis and latency. In: Melnick JL, ed. Progress in medical virology. Basel, Switzerland: S Karger, 1992:19–75

51. Gillet JP, Derer P, Tsiang H. Axonal transport of rabies virus in the central nervous system of the rat. J Neuropathol Exp Neurol 1986;45:619–634.

52. Glass JD, Wesselingh SL, Selnes OA, McArthur JC. Clinical-neuropathological correlation in HIV-associated dementia. Neurology 1993;43:2230–2237.

53. Gonzalez-Scarano F, Tyler KL. Molecular pathogenesis of neurotropic viral infections. Ann Neurol 1987;22:565–574.

54. Gonzalez-Scarano F, Janssen RS, Najjar JA, Pobjecky N, Nathanson N. An avirulent G1 glycoprotein variant of La Crosse bunyavirus with defective fusion function. J Virol 1985;54:757–763.

55. Gonzalez-Scarano F, Pobjecky N, Nathanson N. La Crosse bunyavirus can mediate pH-dependent fusion from without. Virology 1984;132:2212–2225.

56. Greve JM, Davis G, Meyer AM, et al. The major human rhinovirus receptor is ICAM-1. Cell 1989;56:839–847.

57. Grimley P, Friedman R. Arboviral infection of voluntary striated muscles. J Infect Dis 1970;122:45–52.

58. Griot C, Gonzalez-Scarano F, Nathanson N. Molecular determinants of the virulence and infectivity of California serogroup bunyaviruses. Ann Rev Microbiol 1994;47:117–138.

59. Griot C, Pekosz A, Davidson R, et al. Replication in cultured C2C12 muscle cells correlates with the neuroinvasiveness of California serogroup viruses. Virology 1994;201:399-403.

60. Griot C, Pekosz A, Lukac D, et al. Polygenic control of neuroinvasiveness in California serogroup bunyaviruses. J Virol 1993;67:3861–3867.

61. Haase AT. Pathogenesis of lentiviruses infections. Nature 1986;322:130–136.

62. Hanham CA, Zhao F, Tignor GH. Evidence from the anti-idiotype network that the acetylcholine receptor is a rabies virus receptor. J Virol 1993;67:530–542.

63. Harouse JM, Kunsch C, Hartle HT, et al. CD4-independent infection of human neural cells by human immunodeficiency virus type 1. J Virol 1989;63:2527–2533.

64. Harouse JM, Laughlin MA, Pletcher C, Friedman, HM, Gonzalez-Scarano F. Entry of HIV-1 into glial cells proceeds via an alternate, efficient pathway. J Leukoc Biol 1991;49:605–609.

65. Harouse JM, Wroblewska Z, Laughlin MA, Hickey WF, Schonwetter BS, Gonzalez-Scarano F. Human choroid plexus cells can be latently infected with human immunodeficiency virus. Ann Neurol 1989;25:406–411.

66. Haywood AM. Characteristics of Senday virus receptors in a model membrane. J Mol Biol 1974;83:427-436.

67. Haywood AM. Virus receptors: binding, adhesion strengthening, and changes in viral structure. J Virol 1994;68:1–5.

68. Herndon RM, Johnson RT, Davis LE, Descalzi LR. Ependymitis in mumps virus meningitis: electron microscopic studies of cerebrospinal fluid. Arch Neurol 1974;30:475–479.

69. Hildreth JEK, Orentas R. Involvement of a leukocyte adhesion receptor (LFA-1) in HIV induced syncytium formation. Science 1989;244:1075.

70. Hill T, Field H, Roome A. Intra-axonal location of herpes simplex virus particles. J Gen Virol 1972;15:253–255.

71. Hirsch MS, Zisman B, Allison AC. Macrophages and age-dependent resistance to herpes simplex virus in mice. J Immunol 1970;104:1160–1165.

72. Holland JJ. Receptor affinities as major determinants of enterovirus tissue tropisms in humans. Virology 1961;15:312–326.

73. Holland JJ, MacLaren LC, Sylverton JT. The mammalian cell-virus relationship. IV. Infection of naturally insusceptible cells with enterovirus nucleic acid. J Exp Med 1959;110:65–80.

74. Howe H, Bodian D. Neural mechanisms in poliomyelitis. New York: Commonwealth Fund, 1942.

75. Huang CH, Wong C. Relation of the peripheral multiplication of Japanese B encephalitis virus to the pathogenesis of infection in mice. Acta Virol 1963;7:322–330.

76. Ibanez CE, Schrier R, Ghazal P, Wiley C, Nelson JA. Human cytomegalovirus productively infects differentiated macrophages. J Virol 1991;65:6581–6588.

77. Iwasaki Y, Liu D, Yamamoto T, Konno H. On the replication and spread of rabies virus in the human central nervous system. J Neuropathol Exp Neurol 1985;44:185–195.

78. Izumi KM, Stevens JG. Molecular and biological characterization of a herpes simplex virus type 1 (HSV-1) neuroinvasiveness gene. J Exp Med 1990;172:487–496.

79. Janssen RS, Nathanson N, Endres MJ, Gonzalez-Scarano F. Virulence of La Crosse virus is under polygenic control. J Virol 1986;59:1–7.

80. Janssen R, Gonzalez-Scarano F, Nathanson N. Mechanisms of bunyavirus virulence: comparative pathogenesis of a virulent strain of La Crosse and an avirulent strain of Tahyna virus. Lab Invest 1984; 50:447–455.

81. Johnson RT. The pathogenesis of herpes virus encephalitis. II. A cellular basis for the development of resistance with age. J Exp Med 1964;120:359–374.

82. Johnson RT. The pathogenesis of herpes encephalitis. I. Virus pathway to the nervous system of suckling mice demonstrated by fluorescent antibody staining. J Exp Med 1964;119:343–356.

83. Johnson RT. Viral infections of the nervous system. New York: Raven Press, 1982.

84. Johnson RT. Pathogenesis of La Crosse virus in mice. In: Calisher C, Thompson W, eds. California serogroup viruses. New York: Alan R Liss, 1983:139–144.

85. Johnson RT, Johnson KP, Edmonds CJ. Virus-induced hydrocephalus: development of aqueductal stenosis in hamsters after mumps infection. Science 1967;157:1066–1067.

86. Johnson RT, Mims CA. Pathogenesis of viral infections of the nervous system. N Engl J Med 1968;278:23–30,84,92.

87. Johnson RT, McFarland HF, Levy SE. Age-dependent resistance to viral encephalitis: studies of infections due to Sinbis virus in mice. J Infect Dis 1972;125:257– 262.

88. Kaiser PK, Offermann JT, Lipton SA. Neuronal injury due to HIV-1 envelope protein is blocked by anti-gp120 antibodies but not by anti-CD4 antibodies. Neurology 1990;40:1757–1761.

89. Kauffman R, Wolf J, Finberg R, Trier J, Fields B. The sigma 1 protein determines the extent of spread of reovirus from the gastrointestinal tract of mice. Virology 1983;124:403–410.

90. Kawamura N, Kohara M, Abe S, et al. Determinants in the 5' noncoding region of poliovirus Sabin 1 RNA that influence the attenuation phenotype. J Virol 1989;63:1302–1309.

91. Kennedy PGE, Major EO, Williams RK, Straus SE. Down-regulation of glial fibrillary acidic protein expression during acute lytic varicella-zoster virus infection of cultured human astrocytes. Virology 1994;205:558–562.

92. Kilham-Margolis G. Hydrocephalus in hamsters, ferrets, rats and mice following infection with reovirus type 1. Lab Invest 1969; 21:183–188.

93. Kim JW, Closs EI, Albritton LM, et al. Transport of cationic amino acids by the mouse ecotropic retrovirus receptor. Nature 1991; 352:725–728.

94. Kinman TG, De Wind N, Oei-Lie N, Pol JMA, Berns AJM, Gielkens ALJ. Contribution of single genes within the unique short region of Aujesky's disease virus (suid herpesvirus type 1) to virulence, pathogenesis and immunogenicity. J Gen Virol 1992;73: 243–251.

95. Kolson DL, Buchhalter J, Collman R, et al. HIV-1 tat alters normal organization of neurons and astrocytes in primary rodent brain cell cultures: RGD sequence dependence. AIDS Res Hum Retrovir 1993;9:677–685.

96. Kristensson K. Implications of axoplasmic transport for the spread of viruses in the nervous system. In: Weiss DG, Gorio A, eds. Axoplasmic transport in physiology and pathology. New York: Springer-Verlag, 1982:153–158.

97. Kristensson K, Ghetti B, Wisniewski H. Study on the propagation of herpes simplex virus (type 2) into the brain after intraocular injection. Brain Res 1974;69:189–201.

98. Kristensson K, Lycke E, Roytta M, Svennerholm B, Vahlne A. Neuritic transport of herpes simples virus in rat sensory neurons in vitro: effects of substances interacting with microtubular function and axonal flow (nocodazde, taxol and erythro-9-3(2-hydroxynonyl)adenine). J Gen Virol 1986;67:2023–2028.

99. Kristensson K, Lycke E, Sjostand J. Spread of herpes simplex virus in peripheral nerves. Acta Neuropathol 1971;17:44–53.

100. Kucera P, Dolivo M, Coulon P, Flamand A. Pathways of the early propagation of virulent and avirulent rabies strains from the eye to the brain. J Virol 1985;55:158–162.

101. Kuhn RJ, Griffin DE, Zhang H, Niesters HGM, Strauss JH. Attenuation of Sindbis virus neurovirulence by using defined mutations in nontranslated regions of the genome RNA. J Virol 1992;66:7121–7127.

102. La Monica N, Racaniello VR. Differences in replication of attenuated and neurovirulent polioviruses in human neuroblastoma cell line SH-SY5Y. J Virol 1989;63:2357–2360.

103. Lackner AA, Smith MO, Munn RJ, et al. Localization of SIV in the CNS of rhesus monkeys. Am J Pathol 1991;139:609–621.

104. Lafay F, Coulon P, Astic L, et al. Spread of the CVS strain of rabies virus and of the avirulent mutant Av01 along the olfactory pathways of the mouse after intranasal inoculation. Virology 1991;183:320–330.

105. Lathey JL, Wiley CA, Verity MA, Nelson JA. Cultured human brain capillary endothelial cells are permissive for infection by human cytomegalovirus. Virology 1990;176:266–273.

106. Lavi E, Fishman PS, Highkin MK, et al. Limbic encephalitis after inhalation of murine coronavirus. Lab Invest 1988;58:31–36.

107. Lentz TL, Burrage TG, Smith AL, Crick J, Tignor GH. Is the acetylcholine receptor a rabies virus receptor? Science 1982;215:182–184.

108. Levine B, Huang Q, Isaacs JT, Reed JC, Griffin DE, Hardwick JM. Conversion of lytic to persistent alphavirus infection by *bcl-2* cellular oncogene. Nature 1993;361:739–742.

109. Liebert UG, ter Meulen V. Virological aspects of measles virus–induced encephalitis in Lewis and BN rats. J Gen Virol 1987;28: 1715–1722.

110. Lipton HL, Johnson RT. The pathogenesis of rat virus infections in the newborn hamster. Lab Invest 1972;27:508–513.

111. Lipton SA. Calcium channel antagonists and human immunodeficiency virus coat protein-mediated neuronal injury. Ann Neurol 1991;30:110–114.

112. Lipton SA, Sucher NJ, Kaiser PK, Dryer EB. Synergistic effects of the HIV coat protein and NMDA receptor-mediated neurotoxicity. Neuron 1991;7:111.

113. Liu C, Voth D, Rodina P, Shauf L, Gonzalez G. A comparative study of the pathogenesis of western equine and eastern equine encephalomyelitis virus infections in mice by intracerebral and subcutaneous inoculations. J Infect Dis 1970;122:53–63.

114. Lycke E, Kristensson K, Svennerholm B, Vahlne A, Ziegler R. Uptake and transport of herpes simplex virus in neurites of rat dorsal root ganglia cells in culture. J Gen Virol 1984;65:55–64.

115. Lycke E, Tsiang H. Rabies virus infection of cultured rat sensory neurons. J Virol 1987;61:2733–2741.

116. Maciejewski JP, Bruening EE, Donahue RE, et al. Infection of mononuclear phagocytes with human cytomegalovirus. Virology 1993;195:327–336.

117. Maddon PJ, Dalgleish AG, McDougal JS, Clapham PR, Weiss RA, Axel R. The T4 gene encodes the AIDS virus receptor and is expressed in the immune system and the brain. Cell 1986;47:333-348.

118. Malkova D. The role of the lymphatic system in experimental infection with tick-borne encephalitis. Acta Virol 1960;4:233–240.

119. Mankowski JL, Spelman JP, Ressetar HG, et al. Neurovirulent simian immunodeficiency virus replicates productively in endothelial cells of the central nervous system in vivo and in vitro. J Virol 1994;68:8202–8208.

120. Masuda M, Hoffman PM, Ruscetti SK. Viral determinants that control the neuropathogenicity of PVC-211 murine leukemia virus in vivo determine brain capillary endothelial cell tropism in vitro. J Virol 1993;67:4580–4587.

121. Matloubian M, Kolhekar SR, Somasundaram T, Ahmed R. Molecular determinants of macrophage tropism and viral persistence: importance of single amino acid changes in the polymerase and glycoprotein of lymphocytic choriomeningitis virus. J Virol 1993;67: 7340–7349.

122. Matuschke B, Park B, Gaulton G. Regulation of developmental susceptibility to TR1.3 murine leukemia virus neurologic disease by differential expression of the ecotropic receptor on cerebral vessel endothelium. Sixth Workshop on the Pathogenesis of Animal Retroviruses, November 1994.

123. McArthur JC, Hoover DR, Bacellar H, et al. Dementia in AIDS patients: incidence and risk factors. Neurology 1993;43:2245–2251.

124. McClure JE. Cellular receptor for Epstein-Barr virus. Prog Med Virol 1992;39:116–138.

125. McLean JH, Shipley MT, Bernstein DI. Golgi-like transneuronal retrograde labeling with CNS injections of herpes simplex virus type 1. Brain Res Bull 1989;22:867–881.

126. Mendelsohn C, Wimmer E, Racaniello V. Cellular receptor for poliovirus: molecular cloning, nucleotide sequence, and expression of a new member of the immunoglobulin gene superfamily. Cell 1989;56:855–865.

127. Mims CA, Murphy FA, Taylor WP, et al. The pathogenesis of Rosss River virus infections in mice. I. Ependymal infection, cortical thinning and hydrocephalus. J Infect Dis 1973;127:121–128.

128. Mims CA, White DO. Viral pathogenesis and immunology. Oxford: Blackwell Scientific Publications, 1984.

129. Minor PD, Dunn G, Evans DMA, et al. The temperature sensitivity of the Sabin type 3 vaccine strain of poliovirus: molecular and structural effects of a mutation in the capsid protein VP3. J Gen Virol 1989;70:1117–1123.

130. Monath TP, Cropp C, Harrison A. Mode of entry of a neurotropic arbovirus into the central nervous system. Lab Invest 1983;48:399–410.

131. Morales JA, Herzog S, Kompter C, Frese K, Rott R. Axonal transport of Borna virus along olfactory pathways in spontaneously and experimentally infected rats. Med Microbiol Immunol 1988; 177: 51–68.

132. Morgensen S. Macrophages and age-dependent resistance to hepatitis induced by herpes simplex virus type 2. Infect Immunol 1978; 19:46–50.

133. Morgensen S. Role of macrophages in natural resistance to virus infection. Microbiol Rev 1979;43:1–26.

134. Morrison LA, Fields BN. Parallel mechanisms in neuropathogenesis of enteric virus infections. J Virol 1991;65:2767–2772.

135. Morrison LA, Sidman RL, Fields BN. Direct spread of reoviruses from the intestinal lumen to the central nervous system through vagal autonomic fibers. Proc Natl Acad Sci U S A 1991;88:3852–3856.

136. Moses AV, Bloom FE, Pauza CD, Nelson JA. Human immunodeficiency virus infection of human brain capillary endothelial cells occurs via a CD4/galactosylceramide-independent mechanism. Proc Natl Acad Sci U S A 1993;90:10474–10478.

137. Murphy FA. Rabies pathogenesis: brief review. Arch Virol 1977; 54:279–297.

138. Murphy FA, Bauer SP. Early street rabies virus infection in striated muscle and later progression to the central nervous system. Intervirology 1974;3:256–268.

139. Murphy FA, Harrison AK, Winn WCJR, Bauer SP. Comparative pathogenesis of rabies and rabies-like viruses: viral infection and transit from inoculation site to the central nervous system. Lab Invest 1973;29:1–16.

140. Murphy FA, Taylor W, Mims C, Marshall I. Pathogenesis of Ross River virus infection in mice. II. Muscle, heart, and brown fat lesions. J Infect Dis 1973;127:129–138.

141. Naniche D, Varior-Krishnan G, Cervoni F, et al. Human membrane cofactor protein (CD46) acts as a cellular receptor for measles virus. J Virol 1993;67:6025–6032.

142. Narayan O, Griffin D, Silverstein A. Slow virus infection: replication and mechanisms of persistence of visna virus in sheep. J Infect Dis 1977;135:800–806.

143. Nathanson N. Pathogenesis. In: Monath TP, ed. St. Louis encephalitis. Washington, DC: American Public Health Association, 1980: 201–236.

144. Nathanson N, Bodian D. Experimental poliomyelitis following intramuscular virus injection. I. The effect of neural block on a neurotropic and a pantropic strain. Bull Johns Hopkins Hosp 1961; 108:308–319.

145. Nomoto A, Omata T, Toyoda H, Kuge S, Horie H. Complete nucleotide sequence of the attenuated poliovirus Sabin 1 strain genome. Proc Natl Acad Sci U S A 1982;79:5793–5797.

146. Norrby E, Oxman MN. Measles virus. In: Fields BN, Knipe DM, eds. Virology. 2nd ed. New York: Raven Press, 1990:1013-1044.

147. Nuovo GJ, Gallery F, MacConnell P, Braun A. In situ detection of polymerase chain reaction–amplified HIV-1 nucleic acids and tumor necrosis factor α RNA in the central nervous system. Am J Pathol 1994;144:659–666.

148. Oakes J, Gray W, Lausch R. Herpes simplex virus type 1 DNA sequences which direct spread of virus from the cornea to central nervous system. Virology 1986;150:513–517.

149. Park BH, Lavi E, Blank KJ, Gaulton GN. Intracerebral hemorrhages and syncytium formation induced by endothelial cell infection with a murine leukemia virus. J Virol 1993;67:6015.

150. Park BH, Matuschke B, Lavi E, Gaulton G. A point mutation in the env gene of a murine leukemia virus induces syncytium formation and neurologic disease. J Virol 1994;68:7516–7524.

151. Pathak S, Webb HE. Possible mechanisms for the transport of Semiliki Forest virus into and within mouse brain: an electron microscopic study. J Neurol Sci 1974;23:175–184.

152. Peiris JS, Porterfield JS. Antibody-dependent enhancement of plaque formation on cell lines of macrophage origin: a sensitive assay for antiviral antibody. J Gen Virol 1981;57:119–125.

152a. Pekosz A, Griot C, Nathanson N, Gonzalez-Scarano F. Tropism of bunyaviruses: evidence for a GI glycoprotein-mediated entry pathway common to the California serogroup. Virology 1995;214:339–348.

153. Pekosz A, Griot C, Stillmock K, Nathanson N, Gonzalez-Scarano F. Protection from La Crosse virus encephalitis with recombinant glycoproteins: role of neutralizing anti-G1 antibodies. J Virol 1995;69: 3475–3481.

154. Peluso R, Haase AT, Stowring L, et al. A Trojan horse mechanism for the spread of visna in monocytes. Virology 1985;147:231–236.

155. Perlman S, Evans G, Afifi A. Effect of olfactory bulb ablation on spread of a neurotropic coronavirus into the mouse brain. J Exp Med 1990;172:1127–1132.

156. Perlman S, Jacobsen G, Afifi A. Spread of a neurotropic coronavirus into the CNS via the trigeminal and olfactory nerves. Virology 1989;170:556–560.

157. Peudenier S, Hery C, Montagnier J, Tardieu M. Human microglial cells: characterization in cerebral tissue and in primary culture, and study of their susceptibility to HIV-1 infection. Ann Neurology 1991;29:152–161.

158. Phillips PA, Alpers MP, Stanley NF. Hydrocephalus in mice inoculated neonatally by the oronasal route with reovirus type 1. Science 1970;168:858–859.

159. Pitts O, Powers M, Bilello J, Hoffman P. Ultrastructural changes associated with retroviral replication in central nervous system capillary endothelial cells. Lab Invest 1987;56:401–409.

160. Prather SL, Dagan R, Jenista JA, et al. The isolation of enteroviruses from the blood: a comparison of four processing methods. J Med Virol 1984;14:221–227.

161. Pulliam L, Herndier BG, Tang NM, McGrath MS. Human immunodeficiency virus-infected macrophages produce soluble factors that cause histological and neurochemical alterations in cultured brain cells. J Clin Invest 1991;87:503–512.

162. Pulliam L, West D, Haigwood N, Swanson RA. HIV-1 envelope gp120 alters astrocytes in human brain cultures. AIDS Res Hum Retroviruses 1993;9:439–444.

163. Rabin E, Jenson A, Melnick J. Herpes simplex virus in mice: electron microscopy of neural spread. Science 1968;162:126–129.

164. Racaniello VR, Baltimore D. Cloned poliovirus complementary DNA is infectious in mammalian cells. Science 1981;214:916–919.

165. Ratcliffe D, Migliorisi G, Cramer E. Translocation of influenza by migrating neutrophils. Cell Mol Biol 1992;38:63–70.

166. Reagan KJ, Wunner WH. Rabies virus interaction with various cell lines is independent of the acetylcholine receptor. Arch Virol 1985;84:277–282.

167. Reid H, Doherty P. Louping-ill encephalomyelitis in the sheep. I. The relationship of viremia and the antibody response to susceptibility. J Comp Pathol 1971;81:521–529.

168. Ren R, Costantini F, Gorgacz EJ, Lee JJ, Racaniello VR. Transgenic mice expressing a human poliovirus receptor: a new model for poliomyelitis. Cell 1990;63:353–362.

169. Ren R, Racaniello VR. Human poliovirus receptor gene expression and poliovirus tissue tropism in transgenic mice. J Virol 1992;66: 296-304.

170. Ren R, Racaniello VR. Poliovirus spreads from muscle to the central nervous system by neural pathways. J Infect Dis 1992;166:747–752.

171. Rossen DR, Smith CW, Laughter AH, et al. HIV-1 stimulated expression of CD11/CD18 integrins and ICAM-1: a possible mechanism for the extravascular dissemination of HIV-1 infected cells. Trans Assoc Am Phys 1989;102:117–130.

172. Sabatier JM, Vives E, Mabrouk K, et al. Evidence for neurotoxic activity of tat from HIV-1. J Virol 1991;65:961–967.

173. Sabin A. The nature and rate of centripetal progression of certain neurotropic viruses along peripheral nerves. Am J Pathol 1937;13: 615–617.

174. Sabin A, Olitsky P. Influence of host factors on neuroinvasiveness of vesicular stomatitis virus. J Exp Med 1937;66:15–34,35–57; 67:201–208,229–249.

175. Sabin A, Olitsky P. Pathological evidence of axonal and transsynaptic progression of vesicular stomatits and eastern equine encephalomyelitis viruses. Am J Pathol 1937;13:615.

176. Sellers M. Studies on the entry of viruses into the central nervous system of mice via the circulation: differential effects of vasoactive amines and CO on virus infectivity. J Exp Med 1969;129: 719–746.

177. Shankar V, Dietzschold B, Koprowski H. Direct entry of rabies virus into the central nervous system without prior local replication. J Virol 1991;65:2736–2738.

178. Sharma DP, Anderson M, Zink MC, et al. Derivation of neurotropic simian immunodeficiency virus from exclusively lymphocytotropic parental virus: pathogenesis of infection in macaques. J Virol 1992; 66:3550–3556.

179. Sharpless NE, O'Brien WA, Verdin E, Kufta CV, Chen ISY, Dubois-Dalcq M. Human immunodeficiency virus type 1 tropism for brain microglial cells is determined by a region of the env glycoprotein that also controls macrophage tropism. J Virol 1992;66: 2588–2593.

180. Shepley MP, Racaniello VR. A monoclonal antibody that blocks poliovirus attachment recognizes the lymphocyte homing receptor CD44. J Virol 1994;68:1301–1308.

181. Skinner MA, Racaniello VR, Dunn G, Cooper J, Minor PD, Almond JW. New model for the secondary structure of the 5' noncoding RNA of poliovirus is supported by biochemical and genetic data that also show that RNA secondary structure is important in neurovirulence. J Mol Biol 1989;207:379–392.

182. Spear PG. Entry of alphaherpesviruses into cells. Semin Virol 1993; 4:167-180.

183. Stanberry LR. Capsaicin interferes with the centrifugal spread of virus in primary and recurrent genital herpes simplex virus infections. J Infect Dis 1990;162:29–34.

184. Strack AM, Loewy AD. Pseudorabies virus: a highly specific transneuronal cell body marker in the sympathetic nervous system. J Neurosci 1990;10:2139–2147.

185. Sullivan JL, Barry DW, Lucas SJ, Albrecht P. Measles virus infection of human mononuclear cells: acute infection of peripheral blood lymphocytes and monocytes. J Exp Med 1975;142:773–784.

186. Summer BA, Griesen HA, Apper MG. Possible initiation of viral encephalomyelitis in dogs by migrating lymphocytes infected with distemper. Lancet 1978;1:187–189.

187. Superti F, Hauttercoeur B, Morelec MJ, et al. Involvement of gangliosides in rabies virus infection. J Gen Virol 1986;67:47–56.

188. Svitkin Y, Cammack N, Minor PD, Almond JW. Translation deficiency of the Sabin type 3 poliovirus genome: association with an attenuating mutation C474-U. Virology 1990;175:103–109.

189. Svitkin YV, Pestova TV, Maslova SV, Agol VI. Point mutations modify the response of poliovirus RNA to a translation initiation factor: a comparison of neurovirulent and attenuated strains. Virology 1988;166:394–404.

190. Tardieu ML, Weiner HL. Virus receptors on isolated murine and human ependymal cells. Science 1982;215:419–421.

191. Taylor-Wiedeman J, Sissons JGP, Borysiewicz LK, Sinclair JH. Monocytes are a major site of persistence of human cytomegalovirus in peripheral blood mononuclear cells. J Gen Virol 1991;72:2059–2064.

192. Thompson RL, Cook M, Devi-Rao G, Wagner E, Stevens J. Functional and molecular analysis of the avirulent wild-type herpes simplex virus type 1 strain KOS. J Virol 1986;58:203–211.

193. Tornatore CS, Chandra R, Berger J, Major EO. Infection of subcortical astrocytes in the pediatric central nervous system. Neurology 1994;44:481–487.

194. Tsiang H. Evidence for intraaxonal transport of fixed and street rabies virus. J Neuropathol Exp Neurol 1979;38:286–299.

195. Tsiang H. Pathophysiology of rabies virus infection of the nervous system. Adv Virus Res 1993;42:375–412.

196. Tsiang H, Ceccaldi PE, Lycke E. Rabies virus infection and transport in human sensory dorsal root ganglia neurons. J Gen Virol 1991;72:1191–1194.

197. Tsiang H, Lycke E, Ceccaldi PE, Ermine A, Hirardot X. The anterograde transport of rabies virus in rat sensory dorsal root ganglia neurons. J Gen Virol 1989;70:2075–2085.

198. Tyler KL. Host and viral factors that influence viral neurotropism. Trends Neurosci 1987;10:455–460,492–497.

199. Tyler KL, Fields BN. Pathogenesis of neurotropic viral infections. In: McKendall RR, Vinken PJ, Bruyn GW, eds. Viral disease. Handbook of clinical neurology, revised series. Vol 12. Amsterdam: Elsevier, 1989:25–49.

200. Tyler KL, McPhee DA. Molecular and genetic aspects of the pathogenesis of viral infections of the central nervous system. Crit Rev Neurobiol 1987;3:221–243.

201. Tyler K, McPhee D, Fields B. Distinct pathways of viral spread in the host determined by reovirus S1 gene segment. Science 1986; 233:770–774.

202. Ubol S, Tucker PC, Griffin DE, Hardwick JM. Neurovirulent strains of alphavirus induce apoptosis in bcl-2-expressing cells: role of a single amino acid change in the E2 glycoprotein. Proc Natl Acad Sci U S A 1994;91:5202–5206.

203. Ugolini G. Transneuronal transfer of herpes simplex virus type 1 (HSV 1) from mixed limb nerves to the CNS. I. Sequence of transfer from sensory, motor and sympathetic nerve fibres to the spinal cord. J Comp Neurol 1992;326:527–548.

204. Ugolini G, Kuypers HGJM, Simmons A. Retrograde transneuronal transfer of herpes simplex virus type 1 (HSV 1) from motoneurons. Brain Res 1987;422:242–256.

205. Ugolini G, Kuypers HGJM, Strick PL. Transneuronal transfer of herpes virus from peripheral nerves to cortex and brainstem. Science 1989;243:89–91.

206. Vahlne A, Nystrom B, Sandberg M, Hamberger A, Lycke E. Attachment of herpes simplex virus to neurons and glial cells. J Gen Virol 1978;40:359–371.

207. Vahlne A, Svennerholm B, Lycke E. Evidence of herpes simplex virus type-selective receptors on cellular plasma membranes. J Gen Virol 1979;44:217–225.

208. Verdin EM, King GL, Maratos-Flier E. Characterization of a common high-affinity receptor for reovirus serotypes 1 and 3 on endothelial cells. J Virol 1989;63:1318–1325.

209. Waldman WJ, Roberts WH, Davis DH, Williams MV, Sedmak DD, Stephens RE. Preservation of natural cytopathogenicity of cytomegalovirus by propagation in endothelial cells. Arch Virol 1991; 117:143–164.

210. Wang KS, Kuhn RJ, Strauss EG, Ou S, Strauss JH. High affinity laminin receptor is a receptor for Sindbis virus in mammalian cells. J Virol 1992;66:992–5001.

211. Watkins BA, Dorn HH, Kelly WB, et al. Specific tropism of HIV-1 for microglial cells in primary human brain cultures. Science 1990; 249:549–552.

212. Whealy ME, Card JP, Robbins AK, Dubin JR, Rziha H-J, Enquist LW. Specific pseudorabies virus infection of the rat visual system requires both gI and gp63 glycoproteins. J Virol 1993;67:3786–3797.

213. White DO, Fenner FJ. Medical virology. San Diego: Academic Press, 1994.

214. Wiley CA, Schrier RD, Nelson JA, Lampert PW, Oldstone MBA. Cellular localization of human immunodeficiency virus infection within the brains of acquired immune deficiency syndrome patients. Proc Natl Acad Sci U S A 1986;83:7089–7093.

215. Williams RK, Jiang G-S, Holmes KV. Receptor for mouse hepatitis virus is a member of the carcinoembryonic antigen family of glycoproteins. Proc Natl Acad Sci U S A 1991;88:5533–5536.

216. Wunner WH, Reagan KJ, Koprowski H. Characterization of saturable binding sites for rabies virus. J Virol 1984;50:691–697.

217. Yahi N, Baghdiguian S, Moreau H, Fantini J. Galactosyl ceramide (or a closely related molecule) is the receptor for human immunodeficiency virus type 1 on human colon epithelial HT29 cells. J Virol 1992;66:4848–4854.

218. Yuhasz SA, Stevens JG. Glycoprotein B is a specific determinant of herpes simplex virus type 1 neuroinvasiveness. J Virol 1993;67: 5948–5954.

219. Zack JA, Arrigo SJ, Weitsman SR, Go AS, Haislip A, Chen ISY. HIV-1 entry into quiescent primary lymphocytes: molecular analysis reveals a labile, latent viral structure. Cell 1990;61:213–222.

220. Ziegler R, Herman R. Peripheral infection in culture of rat sensory neurons by herpes simplex virus. Infect Immunol 1980;28:620–623.

221. Zisman B, Hirsch MS, Allison AC. Selective effects of anti-macrophage serum, silica and anti-lymphocyte serum on pathogenesis of herpes virus infection of young adult mice. J Immunol 1970;104:1155–1159.

222. Zurbriggen A, Fujinami R. Theiler's virus infection in nude mice: Viral RNA in vascular endothelial cells. J Virol 1988;62:3589–3596.

Viral Pathogenesis,
edited by Neal Nathanson, et al.
Lippincott–Raven Publishers, Philadelphia © 1997

CHAPTER 36

Viral Diseases of the Nervous System: Persistent Infections

Howard L. Lipton and Donald H. Gilden

INTRODUCTION

Many viral infections are characterized by persistence of the virus in the nervous system—that is, in the brain, spinal cord, and sensory ganglia—for months, years, or even the lifetime of the host. To establish a persistent infection, the virus must replicate over a long period without killing the host; it must be attenuated and restricted in its replicative capacity, and it must avoid elimination by the immune system. Because host survival is a prerequisite for persistence, there may be only minimal detectable tissue damage until late in the course of the infection. Tissues may be damaged directly, by virus-induced lysis of infected cells, or indirectly, by the immunopathology that results from prolonged exposure of the host immune system to the viral proteins synthesized. In general, persistence by RNA viruses tends to be associated with immunopathologic damage to neuronal and glial populations, whereas persistent DNA viruses are usually associated with cytolytic infection and neuronal or glial necrosis, although exceptions can be found. The molecular basis of persistence is complex and is still only partially understood.

The ability of a virus to persist in an immunocompetent host continues to intrigue investigators. Because of the importance of host defenses, in vitro studies cannot fully recapitulate viral persistence in an animal or human host. Several mechanisms by which viruses avoid immune surveillance have been demonstrated, and others have been proposed.[12,53,78,105] However, not all viruses can persist in an immunocompetent host. In contrast, immunodeficiency predictably leads to the persistence of most, if not all, viruses and often to the death of the host. Therefore, viral persistence in an immunodeficient host is a separate topic and is not covered in this chapter.

Three patterns of viral persistence in the nervous system are recognizable: latent, chronic defective, and chronic productive infection (Fig. 36-1). These patterns provide a framework to classify and compare the properties of the different viral infections. Table 36-1 lists the predominant persistent viral infections of the nervous system in the mammalian host. We discuss here examples of each of the three types of persistent infection, the molecular mechanisms involved, and the role of antiviral host immune defenses.

H. L. Lipton: Department of Neurology and Biochemistry, Molecular Biology and Cell Biology, Northwestern University, and Division of Neurology, Evanston Hospital, Evanston, Illinois 60201-1782.

D. H. Gilden: Departments of Neurology and Microbiology, University of Colorado Health Sciences Center, Denver, Colorado 80262.

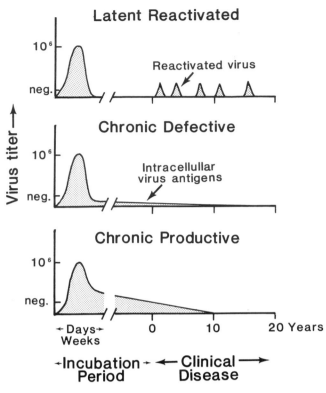

FIG. 36-1. Three patterns of persistent viral infection of the nervous system: latent, chronic defective, and chronic productive. The relative amount of virus is indicated on the ordinate and the time since infection on the abscissa.

HISTORY

Sigurdsson was the first to emphasize that viruses and other pathogens can persist in the central nervous system (CNS) and cause disease after a long latent period.[134] (Sigurdsson had actually studied three chronic diseases of sheep: maedi, a chronic interstitial pneumonitis caused by visna virus; Johne's disease, a chronic mycobacterial infection; and rida, the Icelandic term for scrapie.[75]) Sigurdsson applied the term "slow infection" to describe this delayed virus-host interaction and established several criteria: "(1) a very long initial period of latency lasting from several months to several years; (2) a rather regular protracted course after clinical signs have appeared, usually ending in serious disease or death; and (3) limitation of the infection to a single host species and anatomic lesions to only a single organ or tissue system."

Four decades later, these criteria still largely apply to the many extant persistent viral infections of the nervous system. However, it is now known that not all persistent infections lead to serious disease or death; some cause subclinical or asymptomatic infections and are eventually cleared. Although the consequences of the infection may be limited to a single organ or tissue system, many viruses persist both within and outside the nervous system (see Table 36-1). Some viruses also persist in more than a single host species, either naturally or after experimental infection. Although persistent viral infections fall within the rubric of slow infections, the latter term also denotes

chronic infections by unconventional spongiform agents (e.g., prions) and other microbes as well as conventional viruses. Here, we use the more accurate designation, persistent viral infection.

In the 1960s, the discovery of the viral origins of progressive multifocal leukoencephalopathy[109,158] and subacute sclerosing panencephalitis (SSPE)[110,143] focused attention on persistent viruses as a cause of chronic neurologic disease. At the same time, kuru and Creutzfeld-Jacob disease were successfully transmitted to primates, confirming their infectious nature. These events galvanized interest in viral persistence and in the emerging discipline of neurovirology. Subsequently, investigations have elucidated the virus-cell and virus-host interactions involved in the pathogenesis of many persistent viral infections (see Table 36-1). In addition, a number of new viruses have been shown to persist in the CNS and to cause neurologic disease, such as human immunodeficiency virus (HIV-1) and human T-lymphotropic virus. Persistent viral infection is also thought to underlie other chronic neurologic diseases, such as multiple sclerosis, Rasmussen's encephalitis, and Behçet's syndrome, although formal proof is still lacking.

SITES OF VIRAL PERSISTENCE

The preponderance of neurotropic viruses among those viruses causing persistent infections has led to the notion that the nervous system may offer a special milieu for virus-cell interactions. A heterogeneous, stable population of cells in which viruses can replicate, an extensive network of cellular processes (axons and dendrites) that sequester and promote the spread of the infection over long distances, and a blood-brain barrier that restricts access of antibodies and T cells from the blood have been noted as factors responsible for this special environment.[79] However, a substantial number of viruses persisting in the nervous system do not specifically target neurons or glia but persist in ordinary hematogenous cells, such as lymphocytes and macrophages, or in endogenous macrophages, known as microglia (Table 36-2). The immunologically privileged status of the nervous system also may not be absolute.[35] In addition, an increasing number of viruses have been discovered that persist extraneurally and produce chronic viremia. Therefore, it remains unclear whether the nervous system provides a special milieu for virus-cell interactions.

MACRODYNAMICS OF VIRUS-CELL INTERACTIONS

In any animal virus infection of an immunocompetent host, virus-specific neutralizing antibodies and cellular immune responses (as well as nonspecific inhibitors such as the interferons) that are induced early in the infection limit the growth and extracellular spread of virus. Except in latent virus infections, at least two additional aspects must be considered in persistent infections of an animal host.

The first is the reduced or restricted state of viral replication during persistence; by definition, a persistent RNA virus is restricted in replication. Obviously, an RNA virus cannot be highly lytic for the target cell population in which it persists. Either selection for genetic viral variants (quasispecies) that

TABLE 36-1. *Examples of persistent viral infections of the nervous system in mammalian hosts**

Absent or sporadic production of infectious virus				Regular production of infectious virus	
With episomal or integrated viral DNA (Viral Latency)		Without episomal or integrated viral DNA		Without episomal or integrated viral DNA	
Family	agent:host	Family	agent:host	Family	agent:host
Herpesviridae	**Herpes simplex virus:** human, mouse **Herpes viruses** (VZV, EBV, HHV6–8):human	*Paramyxoviridae*	(Measles virus:human, mouse) (**Canine distemper virus**:dog)	*Arenaviridae*	(LCMV:mouse) (Tamiami virus:rat) (Tacaribe virus:mouse)
Papovaviridae *Retroviridae*	JC virus:human† Murine leukemia virus:mouse Visna virus:sheep CAEV:goat HIV-1:human HTLV-I:human SIV:monkey	*Flaviviridae* *Coronaviridae*	(**Rubella virus**:human) (**JHMV/MHV-A59**:mouse, rat)	*Picornaviridae* *Flaviviridae* Unclassified	(**TMEV**:mouse) (Tickborne encephalitis virus:monkey) (Border disease virus:lamb)‡ (Borna disease virus:horse, rat)

*CAEV, caprine arthritis-encephalitis virus; EBV, Epstein-Barr virus; HIV, human immunodeficiency virus; HHV, human herpes viruses; HTLV, human T-lymphotropic virus; JHMV/MHV, mouse hepatitis virus; LCMV, lymphocytic choriomeningitis virus; SIV, simian immunodeficiency virus; TMEV, Theiler's murine encephalomyelitis virus; VZV, varicella-zoster virus.

Host is immunocompetent at the time of infection. Bold type indicates that the virus is found only in

TABLE 36-2. *Predominant sites of viral persistence in the nervous system*

Cell type	Virus	Investigators
Neuron	Herpes simplex virus	Cook et al, 1974[27]
	Varicella zoster virus	Gilden et al, 1987[51]; Hyman et al, 1983[69]; Sadzot-Delvaux et al, 1990[129]
	Measles virus	Herndon and Rubenstein, 1967[62]; Tellez-Nagel and Harter, 1966[143]
	Rubella virus	Townsend et al, 1976[145]
	LCMV*	Fazakerley et al, 1991[39]; Lehmann-Grube et al, 1983[82]
	Borna disease virus	Carbonne et al, 1989[14]
Oligodendrocyte	JC virus	Itoyama et al, 1982[70]; ZuRhein and Chow, 1965[158]
	Measles virus	Herndon and Rubenstein, 1967[62]; Tellez-Nagel and Harter, 1966[143]
	TMEV	Aubert et al, 1987[1]; Blakemore et al, 1988[8]; Rodriguez et al, 1983[123]
	Borna disease virus	Carbonne et al, 1989[14]
Astrocyte	HTLV-I	Lehky et al, 1995[81]
	MHV	Perlman and Ries, 1987[111]; Sun and Perlman, 1995[142]
Macrophage	Murine leukemia virus	Gravel et al, 1993[57]
	Visna virus	Gendelman et al, 1986[47]
	HIV-1	Eilbott et al, 1989[38]; Koenig et al, 1986[77]
	SIV	Simon et al, 1994[135]
	TMEV	Aubert et al, 1987[1]; Lipton et al, 1995[92]

LCMV, lymphocytic choriomeningitis virus; TMEV, Theiler's murine encephalomyelitis virus; HTLV-I, human T-cell lymphotrophic virus-I; MHV, mouse hepatitis virus; HIV-1, human immunodeficiency virus; SIV, simian immunodeficiency virus.

*LCMV persists to a much lesser extent in astrocytes, oligodendrocytes, ependyma, and endothelial cells.

are restricted in some replicative function occurs,[36] or host factors associated with the target cell restrict wild-type viral replication—that is, the cell itself is semipermissive for the virus. The molecular basis of restricted replication depends on the virus or the target host cell, or both. In either case, a stable equilibrium is reached between the virus and the infected cell population, usually involving infection of only a small fraction of the cells in a particular organ system in the host. Although such an equilibrium is easily envisioned for certain nonlytic viruses, such as lymphocytic choriomeningitis virus, Borna disease virus, and border disease virus, it may be more difficult to achieve and maintain for a lytic virus. The discovery that viruses kill cells by apoptosis has opened up a new area of research into the viral lytic process.[64,83,144] The inhibition of apoptosis by bcl-2 may promote viral persistence by enabling host cell survival—that is, by converting a lytic to a nonlytic, persistent infection. The molecular interactions of bcl-2 and other cell death pathways in virus infections is an area of intense investigation.

Persistent viruses commonly have a temperature-sensitive (ts) phenotype, largely because temperature sensitivity (which is associated with attenuation) results from mutation in almost any genome element or gene product, rather than from any fundamental role in persistence. Defective interfering variants,[67] which limit the growth of wild-type virus in high-density infections in cell culture, are not likely to play a significant role in a population dynamics involving infection of only a small fraction of the total cell population, such as persistence in animals and humans.

The second aspect of persistence relates to the mechanisms by which a persistent virus avoids elimination by the host immune system. The circumvention of immune clearance by viruses, including those that persist in the nervous system, is discussed in Chapter 9.

VIRUS-HOST PATTERNS OF VIRAL PERSISTENCE

Each of the three distinct patterns of persistent infection is postulated to follow an acute phase of logarithmic virus growth that is usually asymptomatic and may serve to amplify and disseminate the infection so that virus reaches the cellular site of persistence. In latent infections of the nervous system, as typified by herpes simplex virus (HSV) infection, the acute phase of replication occurs extraneurally; this may increase the number of axon endings exposed to virus and the number of neurons that become latently infected. Viral genetic information is maintained during latency in the cell nucleus in association with host DNA, in the absence of the production of infectious virus or viral gene products, and can be reactivated to produce infectious virus (see Fig. 36-1A). The virus persists in a form in which no identifiable proteins are present, a situation different from that seen with the other (chronic) forms of persistent viral infection. The identification of a latent virus therefore depends on detection of viral DNA by hybridization before or after polymerase chain reaction (PCR) amplification.

In many chronic defective and chronic productive infections, the acute phase of virus replication occurs in the nervous system, although the acute phase may be extraneural, as in lentiviral infections. The type of persistence of certain retroviruses, such as the lentiviruses (visna virus, caprine arthritis-encephalitis virus, HIV-1, and simian immunodeficiency virus), depends on their ability to integrate their genetic material into the host genome, but nonetheless they regularly produce infectious virus during persistence.

In chronic defective infections, viral proteins are readily detected in cells in the nervous system but are not assembled into infectious virions, although virus may be rescued by cocultivation techniques (see Fig. 36-1). By definition, therefore, a defective virus is highly cell-associated. This pattern of persistence is more common among enveloped RNA viruses that bud from internal or plasma membranes of host cells and spread by inducing fusion or syncytia. In this paradigm, the nervous system bears a relatively large viral antigenic load without actually yielding infectious virus. Viability of host cells may be jeopardized by a defective viral infection, or the cell may become a potential target of host humoral and cellular immune responses when virus antigens are present on the cell surface.

Chronic productive infections are characterized by the continued production of infectious virus (see Fig. 36-1B). In this form of persistence, low levels of infectious virus are released extracellularly within the nervous system, in contrast to the highly cell-associated nature of chronic defective infections. Both lytic and nonlytic viruses can cause chronic productive infections. They are characterized by a temporary stable equilibrium and a slow decline of virus levels, so that isolation or detection of infectious virus becomes increasingly difficult. However, even diminishingly small amounts of virus proteins may be a sufficient antigenic stimulus to drive and maintain immunopathologic tissue destruction. On the other hand, it is not completely clear whether antigen persistence is required for chronic immunopathology.

EXAMPLES OF PERSISTENT CENTRAL NERVOUS SYSTEM INFECTIONS

Latent Infections

Herpes Simplex Virus Infection in Humans

During latency, the virus genome is present, but infectious virus is not produced; virus may reactivate spontaneously (HSV, varicella-zoster virus [VZV]), or it can be rescued by explantation, cocultivation, or fusion of latently infected cells with indicator cells (HSV only). Virus particles cannot be seen ultrastructurally, and virus gene expression (both transcription and viral antigen production) is limited.

The notion that herpesvirus becomes latent in ganglia is almost 100 years old. In a series of 20 trigeminal ganglionectomies for trigeminal neuralgia, Cushing[29] in 1905 observed herpetic vesicles after surgery on the lip and nose of the unoperated side of one patient; in another patient, on whom supraorbital and infraorbital neurectomies had been performed, lesions were bilateral, on the unoperated side of the nose, lip, cheek, and angle of the jaw and on the operated side near the angle of the jaw. Because the skin rendered anesthetic by extirpation remained free of vesicles, Cushing cleverly concluded that the trigeminal ganglion was essential for the production of herpesvirus eruption. Goodpasture[54] later analyzed rabbits experimentally infected with HSV and confirmed the importance of pathways involving the trigeminal nerve and ganglion in the production of CNS disease. These observations led to a more complete analysis of activation of latent HSV in humans by trigeminal sensory root section: Carton and Kilbourne[15] found that 2 to 4 days after nerve section, HSV infection developed in 16 of 17 patients, and always in

the distribution of the ipsilateral maxillary or mandibular division, or both, of the trigeminal nerve; the ophthalmic division was spared. Less frequently, HSV-1 may be latent in other cranial nerve ganglia. Reactivation, triggered by factors such as stress or sunlight, produces lesions of the skin and mucous membranes on the face.

The physical state of HSV-1 DNA and RNA has been determined by analysis of latently infected ganglia removed from humans at autopsy and from animals (mice and rabbits) that survived experimental infection. Animals have also provided a model system to study pathogenesis and factors that cause virus to reactivate, such as skin irritation,[63] neurectomy,[148] and iontophoresis of epinephrine onto the cornea.[80] The intraaxonal spread of HSV from skin to ganglia was shown in mice,[28] and the first evidence that HSV is latent in ganglionic neurons came from studies of mice,[27] years before HSV latency in human ganglionic neurons was demonstrated.[140]

The initial isolation of HSV-1 from human trigeminal ganglia[6] was confirmed by two laboratories[5,150] and later extended to the isolation of HSV-1 from human superior cervical and vagus ganglia.[149] Although HSV-1 has not been isolated from ganglia below the neck, HSV-1 DNA has been amplified by PCR from normal human thoracic ganglia.[97] Although ganglia are the primary site of HSV latency and the only tissue from which HSV can be isolated, HSV DNA has also been detected in normal human brain by Southern blotting,[41] by in situ hybridization,[132] and most recently by PCR.[4,13,71,72,87] HSV has been successfully maintained in the latent state in neuronal cultures and reactivated after nerve growth factor deprivation[153]; such reactivation in vitro is enhanced on activation of second-messenger pathways.[136]

In an elegant study to determine the cell type that harbors HSV during latency, Cook and colleagues[27] used electron microscopy, immunofluorescence, and in situ hybridization analyses of latently infected mouse ganglia explanted and maintained in millipore chambers to show that HSV reactivated only from neurons, presumably the cell in which virus had established latency. In situ hybridization later showed that the HSV latency-associated transcript (LAT) is also present exclusively in neurons of latently infected ganglia.[55,141] The abundance of HSV DNA in latently infected human or mouse ganglia has been estimated to be one genome copy per 2.5 to 100 cells[37]; therefore, it is not surprising that HSV DNA has not yet been detected by in situ hybridization.

The physical state of HSV DNA in latently infected ganglia differs from that seen in acute infection or virions, because the HSV DNA termini are covalently linked,[121] indicating that virus DNA is circular or concatameric. Density gradient centrifugation further showed that latent HSV DNA is extrachromosomal[101] and, like eukaryotic chromatin, is associated with nucleosomes.[32]

HSV-1 transcription during latency is restricted to a 2-kb fragment of DNA within the repeat regions from which two mRNAs are transcribed, 2 and 1.5 kb in size.[141] These LATs are transcribed in the opposite direction to the immediate early gene ICP0. LATs are found exclusively in the nuclei of neurons.[55,139,141] LATs are less abundant during viral replication in cell culture than during latency.[137] LATs do not appear to play any essential role in establishing or maintaining latency,[74,131] although LAT deletion mutants of HSV-1 reactivate from the latent state with reduced frequency.[85] The potential functions and mechanisms of action of LATs were reviewed by Steiner and Kennedy[138] in 1995. Finally, a report of an immediate early 175-kD HSV-1 polypeptide in latently infected ganglia of rabbits[58] and the identification of an 80-kD HSV latency-associated antigen in latently infected neuronal cell cultures[34] remain to be confirmed.

Varicella-Zoster Virus Infection in Humans

VZV causes chickenpox (varicella). Virus then becomes latent in ganglia and reactivates decades later to produce shingles (zoster). Unlike HSV, VZV cannot be isolated from human ganglia,[114] although VZV DNA has been found in most human ganglia at all levels of the neuraxis.[52,96,97] Reactivation can produce lesions anywhere on the body, although the face and trunk are the most commonly involved sites, and vesicles (small blisters) are usually restricted to 1 to 3 dermatomes (localized zoster). Advancing age and immunosuppression predispose to VZV reactivation.

There is no animal model for VZV, but molecular virologic analysis of latently infected ganglia has revealed that multiple regions of the VZV genome are present during latency.[96] Transcription is limited to no less than four regions, corresponding to genes 21,[24,25] 29,[23,100] 62,[23,100] and 63.[23] The abundance of VZV DNA is 6 to 31 copies in every 100,000 ganglionic cells,[95] and most studies have found latent VZV exclusively in neurons.[51,69,94,129] The configuration of VZV DNA in latently infected ganglia is extrachromosomal and circular.[20] Finally, reports of expression of an immediate early protein encoded by VZV gene 63 during latency[31,94] remain to be confirmed. Table 36-3 compares clinical and virologic features of HSV and VZV latency and reactivation.

Chronic Defective Infection: Subacute Sclerosing Panencephalitis Infection in Humans

SSPE is a rare complication of measles that typically occurs late in the first decade of life. SSPE usually develops 5 to 10 years after acute measles infection; it begins with subtle impairment of psychological and intellectual functions, followed by sensory and motor signs. Ingravescent cerebral deterioration leads to death after months to years. The pattern of persistence is distinctly that of a chronic defective viral infection (see Fig. 36-1*B*), with an accumulation of measles virus (MV) nucleocapsids in the brain in the absence of complete infectious virus particles or formation of syncytia. The central issues in the pathogenesis of SSPE center on the molecular mechanism of persistence: How does a virus apparently defective in virion assembly and cell fusion spread and survive in the presence of extraordinarily high levels of MV neutralizing antibody?

Pathology

In SSPE, a panencephalitis preferentially involves the cerebrum and brain stem, producing gray matter destruction and demyelination accompanied by a striking inflammatory reaction. In the cortex and subcortical nuclei, nerve cells are lost or appear necrotic, and pleomorphic microglial cells are numerous. The inflammatory reaction in gray and white matter is characterized mainly by small lymphocytes and a few plasma cells, which infiltrate the leptomeninges and parenchyma and accumulate in perivascular sites. Astrocytic gliosis is variable, although at times it is diffuse and severe (i.e., sclerosing). Eosinophilic intranuclear inclusions (Cowdry type A) are seen in neurons and oligodendrocytes, which have been shown to contain typical paramyxovirus nucleocapsids by electron microscopy.[10,62,143] Nerve cell loss and demyelination appear to result from direct MV lysis of neurons and oligodendroglia rather than from immunopathology.

Cellular Sites of Persistence

Although MV is able to infect peripheral blood mononuclear cells (T cells, B cells, and monocytes) and has been isolated by cocultivation from lymph nodes of patients with SSPE,[66] neurons and oligodendrocytes appear to be the only targets of MV persistence in SSPE brain. The infection of both cell types was suggested by the discovery of inclusion bodies and confirmed by ultrastructural and immunohistochemical studies.[10,62,143] The lack of viral budding or evidence of mature measles virions within the extracellular spaces in brain by electron microscopy is consistent with the defective phenotype of this virus. Virus persistence may also depend on host cell factors and on the state of neuronal differentiation.[102] The fact that class I major histocompatibility (MHC) molecules required for cytotoxic T-lymphocyte recognition of viral antigens are not expressed on neurons may play a role in MV persistence in neurons.[76] Neurons may be able to provide a relatively safe haven for MV persistence, but oligodendrocytes that express class I MHC molecules would be subject to cytotoxic T-lymphocyte surveillance if infected.

TABLE 36-3. *Comparison of HSV–1 and VZV reactivation from latency*

Parameter	HSV-1	VZV
Site of latency	Cranial nerve ganglia	Ganglia at all levels of the neuraxis
Site of reactivation	Cranial nerve ganglia	Trunk > face > extremities
Frequency of reactivation (per lifetime)	Multiple times	Usually once
Factors affecting reactivation	Stress, sunlight	Age, immunodeficiency
Virus transcription during latency	A single latency-associated transcript	Multiple genes

HSV, herpes simplex virus; VZV, varicella-zoster virus.

Pathogenesis

MV probably enters the brain during acute infection, because almost one third of patients with uncomplicated measles have electroencephalographic abnormalities and cerebrospinal fluid pleocytosis.[61] Although an acute phase of CNS virus replication has not been documented, even in clinical cases of acute measles encephalitis,[104] early virus replication has been seen in rodents inoculated with the hamster neurotropic strain of MV, a model system that closely mimics SSPE.[11,118] An acute early phase of virus replication would also presumably favor the generation of mutants of MV, setting the stage for persistence. However, virtually nothing is known about the events leading to clinical disease. At least two possibilities exist. As suggested by Billeter and colleagues,[7] defective MV may spread by local cell fusion during the latent period, with clinical disease occurring after sufficient numbers of cells have been infected. Alternatively, widespread infection of neuronal and oligodendrocyte targets with infectious MV may occur on CNS invasion, defective MV may be selected, and MV proteins may slowly accumulate intracellularly, eventually leading to cell death and clinical disease.

Molecular Basis of Persistence

The molecular basis for defective MV gene expression in SSPE stems from the initial observation that MV could be rescued only by cocultivation of brain cells of SSPE patients with stable cell lines. Hall and colleagues[59,60] reported that SSPE patients mount high antibody titers against all MV proteins except the matrix (M) protein, and that the M protein was not detected in the brains of patients by antibodies against MV. The M protein is one of three MV envelope glycoproteins, the others being the fusion (F) and hemagglutinin (HA) proteins, transmembrane proteins responsible for membrane fusion and host-cell attachment, respectively. M protein is responsible for viral assembly, and it was postulated that loss of M protein expression may account for the lack of viral budding and favor persistence. The observation of reduced or absent antibody responses to the M protein was confirmed, and reports of defects in M gene transcription, translation, and M protein stability and function followed.[3,18,65] Subsequently, the sequencing of the M gene of MV strains that cause SSPE revealed mutations compared with wild-type MV.[2,3,19]

However, all five MV proteins, including M protein, have been demonstrated in frozen SSPE brain sections by immunofluorescence using labeled monoclonal antibodies,[106,107] and their mRNAs have been detected in SSPE brains by Northern blot analysis. Dhib-Jalbut and colleagues[33] quantitated antibodies specific for M and nucleocapsid (NC) proteins of SSPE patients by enzyme-linked immunosorbent assay and found substantial titers to M in the serum and cerebrospinal fluid, although the levels were lower than the titers to NC protein. Relatively normal T-cell proliferative responses to M, F, HA, and NC proteins were also observed by these investigators.[33] Thus, both the reduced expression of M protein in SSPE and its role in persistence were questioned.

Besides changes in the M gene, mutations have been demonstrated in other genes of MV strains that cause SSPE, including those encoding the F and HA proteins.[19,130] Abnormalities in F and HA gene expression have been reported[3,68]—for example, delayed cleavage activation of the F protein.[151] Presumably, a defect in the expression of any of the envelope proteins may result in MV persistence. It is unknown whether mutations in the envelope genes are the initial events after CNS invasion and are required for persistence and disease development, or whether the observed mutations are simply an epiphenomenon caused by the protracted host-cell interaction or by the high rates of mutation in RNA viruses that result from the lack of proofreading enzymes. A clear relation between specific mutations and MV persistence has not been established.

Role of the Host Immune Response

Markedly elevated levels of MV antibodies in serum and cerebrospinal fluid of patients provided the first clue to the cause of SSPE.[26] This raised the question of how MV evades neutralization to persist in the CNS. Fujinami and Oldstone[45,46] suggested that antibodies may actually aid persistence by reducing the expression of viral glycoproteins on the cell surface, thereby rendering the cell resistant to either antibody or T-cell–mediated lysis. Reduced or absent antibody responses to M protein were reported in SSPE and were thought to play a central role in disease pathogenesis; however, additional studies disputed this notion (see previous discussion). In fact, a neutralizing antibody response may be essential for MV persistence, because it has been shown that pretreatment of experimental animals with neutralizing antibodies to MV promotes persistence,[119,120,152] and monoclonal antibodies to HA decrease expression of M, F, and P proteins in MV-infected cells in culture.[44] Liebert and associates[86] reported that treatment of newborn rats with antibodies to HA but not to M, F, NC, or P proteins converts an acute encephalitis into a chronic defective infection. They also found transcriptional restriction of MV gene expression at the level of mRNA synthesis.[86] The potential ways in which antibodies reacting with the surface of infected cells may modulate intracellular replication of MV require further elucidation.

Chronic Productive Infection: Theiler's Murine Encephalomyelitis Virus Infection in Mice

The murine encephalomyelitis viruses are naturally occurring enteric pathogens of mice that belong to the cardiovirus genus in the family *Picornaviridae*. Discovered by Theiler in the early 1930s and originally termed murine polioviruses, these ubiquitous pathogens usually cause asymptomatic enteric infections in mice. Occasionally, the Theiler's murine encephalomyelitis viruses (TMEVs) spread beyond the intestinal tract and enter the CNS, presumably by means of a viremia, to induce a chronic productive CNS infection. The TMEVs have attracted additional attention because they provide one of the few available experimental animal models for multiple sclerosis.[89] TMEV-induced demyelinating disease is a highly relevant animal model for multiple sclerosis because (1) chronic pathologic involvement is limited to CNS white matter, (2) myelin breakdown accompanied by mononuclear inflammation is immune mediated, (3) demyelination results in clinical CNS disease, such as spastic paralysis, and (4) demyelinating disease is under multigenic control with a strong linkage to certain MHC genes.

Pathology

In the acute phase of infection, TMEV replicates in motor neurons in the spinal cord gray matter, leading to chromatolysis and neuronal death.[88] In the chronic phase, pathologic involvement shifts to the surrounding spinal cord white matter. During the persistence phase (2 to 6 months after infection), mononuclear inflammatory cells, consisting of lymphocytes, plasma cells, and macrophages, infiltrate the spinal cord leptomeninges and white matter.[8,30,123] The influx of macrophages in particular is closely related to the process of myelin breakdown. Macrophages have been observed to actively strip myelin loops or lamellae from normal-appearing axons and to contact myelin sheaths undergoing vesicular disruption. In the susceptible SJL strain, degenerating oligodendrocytes are rarely found, and oligodendroglial loops have been observed in close apposition to demyelinated axons, suggesting that myelin injury is not directly related to oligodendrocyte cytopathology.[30] In contrast, in susceptible CBA mice, degenerating oligodendrocytes have been detected.[8]

Cellular Sites of Persistence

TMEV persistence involves active virus replication, because infectious virus can readily be detected in the CNS by standard virologic assays for virtually the lifetime of the mouse. However, chronic TMEV replication has been shown to be restricted by a block at the level of minus-strand viral RNA synthesis.[17] Highly restricted virus production has also been demonstrated in macrophages isolated from the CNS of diseased mice,[22] but the finer details of the kinetics of replication remain to be elucidated. For example, it is not known whether an infected cell dies rapidly or remains viable and continues to produce infectious virus, nor whether the oligodendrocyte or the macrophage is the primary target of persisting virus. Some oligodendrocytes are infected early in the persistent phase,[30,123] and Blakemore and colleagues[8] observed by electron microscopy some oligodendrocytes that contained crystalline arrays of Theiler's virions in CBA mice. However, other evidence favors the macrophage as the predominant target cell for persistence, because as much as 90% of the viral load resides in these phagocytic cells.[22,84,92]

Pathogenesis of Demyelination

Appropriately timed immunosuppression can prevent the clinical signs and pathologic changes of TMEV-induced demyelinating disease, indicating that myelin breakdown is primarily immune mediated. If immunosuppression is induced too early, potentiation of the early neuronal infection is observed and may lead to encephalitis and high mortality.[42,90,91,126] Immunosuppression therefore is most effective if induced after the

first 1 to 2 weeks of infection. A number of different in vivo immunosuppressive modalities have been demonstrated to be effective, including cyclophosphamide, α-lymphocyte serum, tumor necrosis factor-alpha (TNF-α) antibodies, and monoclonal antibodies to Ia, CD4+, and CD8+ antigens.[103]

Several reports suggest that CD8+ T cells do not play a role in myelin breakdown. First, β-microglobulin–deficient mice, which do not express functional MHC class I proteins or produce significant numbers of CD8+ T cells when infected with the BeAn or DA strains of Theiler's virus, develop inflammatory demyelinating lesions, whereas control mice are resistant.[40,117,122] Second, mice rendered deficient in CD8+ cells by thymectomy and administration of CD8+ monoclonal antibodies before infection with BeAn virus were less efficient in clearing virus from the CNS, compared with intact mice, and also suffered from more severe demyelinating disease.[9] In addition, SJL mice infected with a dose of virus that normally produces a low incidence of disease were adoptively immunized with a TMEV VP2-specific CD4+ T-cell line, resulting in an increased incidence of demyelinating disease.[50] This observation provides further support for a role for CD4+ T cells in mediating TMEV-induced demyelinating disease.

The effector mechanism by which a nonbudding virus such as TMEV may lead to immune-mediated tissue injury is unknown. Because TMEV antigens have been found primarily in macrophages, it has been proposed that myelinated axons are damaged as a consequence of a virus-specific immune response through an innocent-bystander mechanism. In this instance, cytokines produced by MHC class II–restricted, TMEV-specific, delayed-type hypersensitivity (DTH) T cells (Th1 cells), primed by interaction with infected macrophages, are postulated to lead to the recruitment and activation of additional macrophages in the CNS, resulting in nonspecific macrophage-mediated demyelination (Fig. 36-2). Myelin damage could be initiated by the release from macrophages of enzymes (e.g., neutral proteases), cytokines (e.g., TNF), or free radicals. The specificity of the attack on myelin could also be imparted by preferential targeting of membrane-reactive terminal complement complexes to oligodendrocyte processes.[146] The innocent-bystander hypothesis is also consistent with the observation in several other model systems that antigen-specific T cells and T-cell lines cause bystander damage through macrophage activation.

Molecular Basis of Persistence

Recombinant TMEV, constructed by exchanging corresponding genomic regions between the highly virulent GDVII and less virulent BeAn or DA virus cDNAs, have been used to map a determinant or determinants for virus persistence (and demyelination) to the P1 sequences encoding the capsid proteins[12,43,99,125] (Fig. 36-3). However, conflicting results as to whether this determinant can include GDVII sequences have been reported.[43,125] Persistence of GDVII virus is difficult to assess directly because few or no infected animals survive long enough, even at relatively low inoculation doses.

Viral recombinants and mutants that contain largely GDVII sequences but do not persist indicate that GDVII lacks a per-

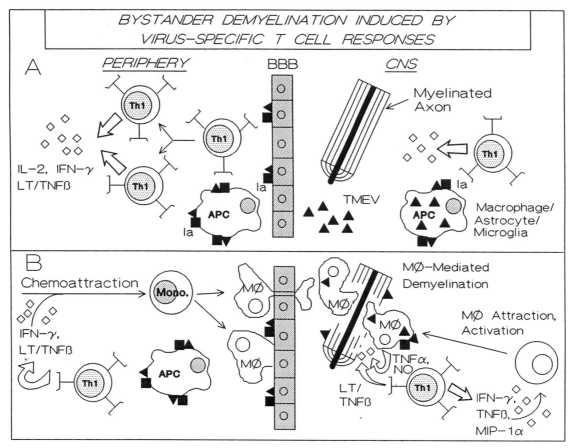

FIG. 36-2. Proposed model of demyelination induced by Theiler's murine encephalomyelitis virus (TMEV) through Th1 CD4+ T cell–mediated delayed-type hypersensitivity (DTH). **(A)** As a consequence of the infectious process, CD4+ Th1 TMEV-specific precursor T cells are triggered to clonally expand and differentiate into effector T cells in response to virus antigen presentation by antigen-presenting cells (APC). This process may occur systemically, as a result of the initial viremia, or inside the blood-brain barrier (BBB). The effector T cells may serve an important function in chronic stimulation of TMEV-specific DTH. **(B)** Release of cytokines—interleukin-2 (IL-2), interferon-γ (INF-γ), lymphotoxin (LT) or tumor necrosis factor-β (TNFβ) and chemokines (macrophage inhibitory factor-1α (MIP-1α)—by virus-specific Th1 CD4+ T cells leads to recruitment, activation, and accumulation of macrophages in the central nervous system (CNS). Macrophages (M0) cause demyelination, possibly by a nonspecific terminal response that results in stripping of myelin lamellae by processes of mononuclear cells and/or release of tumor necrosis factor-α (TNFα) or nitric oxide (NO). This hypothesis would account for the characteristic mononuclear cell infiltrates observed in areas of primary demyelination and provide a population of host cells in which TMEV persists.

sistence determinant[116] (see Fig. 36-3). The one exception is a GDVII-DA virus recombinant, designated GD1B-2C, which is partially neurovirulent and persists in the CNS.[43,125] GD1B-2C contains GDVII sequences in the carboxyl half of VP2 (amino acids 152 through 267) and in VP3 and VP1, and it was assembled using an *Nco1* restriction endonuclease site that lies between the sequences encoding VP2 puff A and puff B (Fig. 36-4). As a result, the recombinant virus has a hybrid VP2 puff structure. The GDVII *Nco1-AatII* or 1B-2C fragment was assembled into two parental DA cDNAs in different laboratories, so that the DA VP2 141 on the tip of puff A is either a lysine[108] or an asparagine[98] residue. The critical location of the *Nco1* site was revealed by Jarousse and associates,[73] who found that GD1B-2C persisted only in the former case.

The DA parental virus persisted with either amino acid in this position.

Pritchard and colleagues[115] constructed a series of TMEV recombinants in which BeAn sequences progressively replaced those of GDVII, starting at the 5' end of the capsid protein genes (see Fig. 36-3). The 3' ends of the inserted BeAn sequences end at various restriction sites, whose names were used for the viral nomenclature. As shown in Figure 36-3, the fact that χ1SM persists but χ1SA and χ1SS do not suggests that a conformation formed by the interaction of the VP2 puff A and B (nucleotides 1911 through 2048) with the VP1 CD loops (nucleotides 3219 through 3338) may be critical for CNS persistence. In χ1SA and χ1SS, the VP2 puff and VP1 CD loops consist of hybrid BeAn and GDVII sequences,

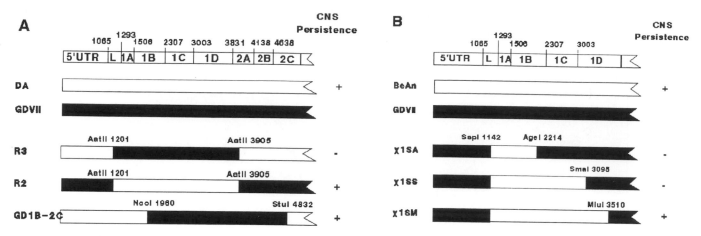

FIG. 36-3. Recombinant Theiler's murine encephalomyelitis viruses (TMEV) constructed by exchange of corresponding genomic regions between the highly virulent GDVII and the less virulent DA (**A**) or BeAn (**B**) cDNAs. These recombinants have been used to map a determinant for virus persistence to the P1 sequences encoding the capsid proteins. In **A**, the 5′ portion of the 8.1-kb TMEV RNA genome is represented at the top; the nucleotide positions are from the DA virus.[108] Representations of the DA and GDVII parental viruses are below. The GDVII-DA recombinant viruses R3 and R2[99] mapped the genetic elements for TMEV persistence to the less virulent (DA) virus capsid; similar GDVII-BeAn constructs have given the same results. GD1B-2C, a partially virulent GDVII-DA recombinant with virus persistence in surviving mice, is the only TMEV recombinant with a structure suggesting that capsid GDVII sequences may be involved in persistence.[73] The *Nco1* restriction endonuclease site in GD1B-2C lies between the sequences encoding VP2 puff A and puff B, forming a hybrid VP2 puff. In **B**, the format is the same, except that the nucleotides are numbered according to the BeAn sequence.[113] The fact that χ1SM persists but χ1SA and χ1SS do not suggests that the conformation formed by the interaction of the VP2 puff A and B (nucleotides 1911 to 2048) with the VP1 CD loops (nucleotides 3219 to 3338) is critical for persistence in the central nervous system (CNS).

which is not the case in χ1SM, and they probably have a different surface conformation.

Changes in the region of the VP2 puff may affect the conformation of its other parts or that of neighboring structures, such as VP1 CD loop II, which interacts with VP2 puff B.[56,93] VP1 CD loop II residue 101 has previously been shown to be important in persistence.[147,156,157] Therefore, TMEV persistence may involve a conformational determinant that includes the VP2 puff and VP1 CD loop II regions. Because residues involved in the virion receptor-binding or attachment site are located near these regions,[56,93] persistence may involve a receptor-mediated event that is affected by mutations in the adjacent loop structures. However, additional studies are required to confirm this hypothesis.

Role of the Host Immune Response

TMEV-infected mice mount a virus-specific humoral immune response (including neutralizing antibodies) during the first week, which peaks by 1 month after infection and is sustained thereafter.[112,127] Most antiviral immunoglobulin G (IgG) response in persistently infected susceptible mice is of the IgG2a subclass, whereas IgG1 antiviral antibodies appear to predominate in resistant and immunized mice.[16,112] Murine CD4+ T cells of the Th1 subset mediate DTH and regulate IgG2a production by production of interferon-gamma (IFN-γ), whereas CD4+ Th2 cells regulate IgG1 and IgE pro-

duction through interleukin-4 (IL-4). Therefore, the predominant IgG2a antiviral response in susceptible mice is an in vivo measure of preferential stimulation of a Th1-like pattern of cytokine synthesis.

Susceptible mouse strains also produce a robust virus-specific cellular immune response. T-cell proliferation and DTH appear by 2 weeks after infection and remain elevated for at least 6 months.[21] Both DTH and T-cell proliferation have been shown to be specific for TMEV and mediated by CD4+ MHC class II–restricted T cells.[21] A temporal correlation has also been found between the onset of demyelinating lesions and development of these virus-specific T-cell responses, as well as between high levels of virus-specific DTH and susceptibility of mice of different genetic backgrounds and crosses. DTH and T-cell proliferative responses in infected and immunized SJL mice are directed to the VP2 coat protein, and specifically to an epitope contained within the VP2 amino acids 70 through 85.[48,49] This immunodominant VP2 T-cell epitope, localized to amino acids 74 through 86, potentiates the development of demyelinating disease in infected mice immunized with the peptide before infection. Recently, two additional immunodominant T-cell epitopes have been mapped to the TMEV capsid, at VP1 residues 233 through 244 and VP3 residues 24 through 37.[154,155] VP1 233 through 244 has also been demonstrated to potentiate TMEV-induced demyelinating disease in SJL mice. Figure 36-4 shows the locations of these immunodominant T-cell epitopes within the polypeptide fold of the three capsid proteins.

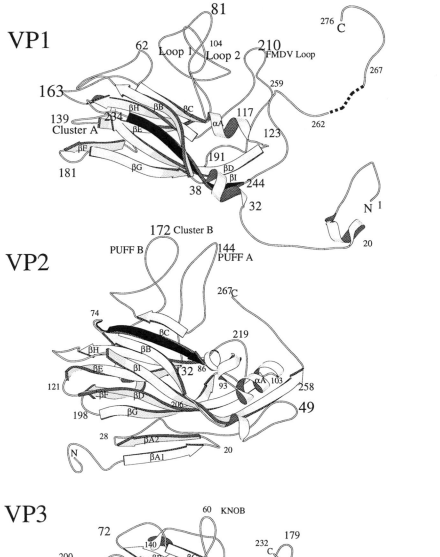

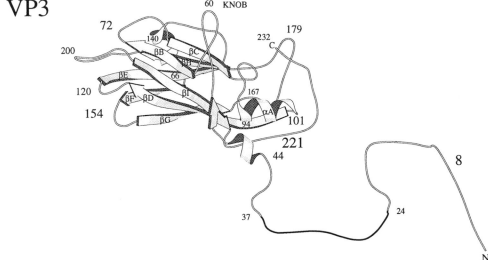

FIG. 36-4. Ribbon drawings showing the polypeptide fold of the three larger surface capsid proteins of Theiler's virus (TMEV). The locations of the three immunodominant TMEV T-cell epitopes that have been mapped to the capsid (VP1 βH strand, VP2 βC strand, and VP3 N-terminal) are indicated. The prominent VP1 loops I and II and VP2 puff A and B are shown.

Although virus-specific humoral and cellular immune responses mounted early after virus exposure cause peak virus titers to fall by 1000-fold to 10,000-fold, TMEVs somehow evade immune clearance to persist at low levels in the CNS, although not in extraneural sites. The precise mechanism by which TMEVs evade immune surveillance is not known, but it does not involve antigenic variation.[128] Although complement and virus-antibody deposition in the CNS parenchyma have not been detected,[124,133] extracellular transport of virus as infectious virus-antibody complexes could protect TMEVs from specific virus-immune responses and enable continued persistence.

In summary, after an acute phase of virus growth in neurons (e.g., anterior horn cells), TMEV persists as a chronic productive infection, largely in macrophages in the CNS white matter. TMEV replication in macrophages is highly restricted, probably as the result of host cell factors. Analysis of TMEV recombinant and mutant viruses suggests that persistence requires a specific capsid conformation involving the VP2 puff and VP1 loop II, which may influence persistence through virion receptor binding or attachment to host cells, such as macrophages. Virus persistence occurs despite the production of virus-specific humoral and cellular (CD4+ T-cell) immune responses. DTH and T-cell proliferative responses in infected SJL mice are directed to three immunodominant epitopes located in β-strands of VP1 (amino acids 233 through 244) and VP2 (amino acids 74 through 86), and in the N-terminus of VP3 (amino acids 24 through 37). It has been proposed that myelinated axons may be nonspecifically damaged as a consequence of a virus-specific CD4+ T-cell Th1 immune response through an innocent-bystander mechanism. In this instance, cytokines produced by CD4+, TMEV-specific Th1 cells primed by interaction with infected macrophages are postulated to lead to the recruitment and activation of additional macrophages in the CNS, resulting in nonspecific macrophage-mediated demyelination.

ABBREVIATIONS

CNS: central nervous system
DTH: delayed-type hypersensitivity
F: fusion protein (of MV envelope)
HA: hemagglutinin protein (of MV envelope)
HIV: human immunodeficiency virus
HSV: herpes simplex virus
IFN-γ: interferon-gamma
IgE, IgG, IgG1, IgG2a: immunoglobulins
IL-4: interleukin-4
LAT: latency-associated transcript (of HSV)
M: matrix protein (of MV envelope)
MHC: major histocompatibility complex
MV: measles virus
NC: nucleocapsid protein (of MV)
P: phosphoprotein (of MV)
PCR: polymerase chain reaction
SSPE: subacute sclerosing panencephalitis
TMEV: Theiler's murine encephalomyelitis virus
TNF: tumor necrosis factor
ts: temperature-sensitive (phenotype)
VSV: varicella-zoster virus

REFERENCES

1. Aubert C, Chamorro M, Brahic M. Identification of Theiler's virus infected cells in the central nervous system of the mouse during demyelinating disease. Microb Pathog 1987;3:319–326.
2. Ayata M, Hirano A, Wong TC. Structural defect linked to nonrandom mutations in the matrix gene of Biken strain of subacute sclerosing panencephalitis virus defined by cDNA cloning and expression of chimeric genes. J Virol 1989;63:1162–1173.
3. Baczko K, Liebert UG, Billeter M, Cattaneo R, Budka H, ter Meulen V. Expression of defective measles virus genes in brain tissues of patients with subacute sclerosing panencephalitis. J Virol 1986;59:472–478.
4. Baringer JR, Pisani P. Herpes simplex virus genomes in human nervous system tissue analyzed by polymerase chain reaction. Ann Neurol 1994;36:823–829.
5. Baringer JR, Swoveland P. Recovery of herpes-simplex virus from human trigeminal ganglions. N Engl J Med 1973;288:648–650.
6. Bastian FO, Rabson AS, Yee CL, Tralka TS. Herpesvirus hominis: isolation from human trigeminal ganglion. Science 1972;178:306–307.
7. Billeter MA, Cattaneo R, Spielhofer P, Kaelin K, Huber M, Schmid A, Baczko K, ter Meulen V. Generation and properties of measles virus mutations typically associated with subacute sclerosing panencephalitis. Ann N Y Acad Sci 1994;724:367–377.
8. Blakemore WF, Welsh CJ, Tonks P, Nash AA. Observations on demyelinating lesions induced by Theiler's virus in CBA mice. Acta Neuropathol (Berl) 1988;76:581–589.
9. Borrow P, Tonks P, Welsh CJ, Nash AA. The role of CD8+ T cells in the acute and chronic phases of Theiler's murine encephalomyelitis virus–induced disease in mice. J Gen Virol 1992;73:1861–1865.
10. Bouteille M, Fontaine C, Vedrenne C, Delarue J. Sur un cas d'encephalite subaigue a inclusions: etude anatomoclinique et ultrastructurale. Rev Neurol (Paris) 1965;113:454–458.
11. Burnstein T, Jensen JH, Waksman BH. The development of a neurotropic strain of measles virus in hamsters and mice. J Infect Dis 1995;114:265–272.
12. Calenoff MA, Faaberg KS, Lipton HL. Genomic regions of neurovirulence and attenuation in Theiler's murine encephalomyelitis. Proc Natl Acad Sci U S A 1990;87:978–982.
13. Cantin EM, Lange W, Openshaw H. Application of polymerase chain reaction assays to studies of herpes simplex virus latency. Intervirology 1991;32:93–100.
14. Carbone KM, Trapp BD, Griffin JW, Duchala CS, Narayan O. Astrocytes and Schwann cells are virus-host cells in the nervous system of rats with Borna disease. J Neuropath Exp Neurol 1989;48:631–644.
15. Carton CA, Kilbourne ED. Activation of latent herpes simplex by trigeminal sensory-root section. N Engl J Med 1952;246:172–176.
16. Cash E, Bandeira A, Chirinian S, Brahic M. Characterization of B lymphocytes present in the demyelinating lesions induced by Theiler's virus [published erratum appears in J Immunol 1989;143:2081]. J Immunol 1989;143:984–988.
17. Cash E, Chamorro M, Brahic M. Minus-strand RNA synthesis in the spinal cords of mice persistently infected with Theiler's virus. J Virol 1988;62:1824–1826.
18. Cattaneo R, Schmid A, Eschle D, Baczko K, ter Meulen V, Billeter M. Biased hypermutation and other genetic changes in defective measles viruses in human. Cell 1988;55:255–265.
19. Cattaneo R, Schmid A, Spielhofer P, et al. Mutated and hypermutated genes of persistent measles viruses which caused lethal human brain disease. Virology 1989;173:415–425.
20. Clarke P, Beer T, Cohrs R, Gilden DH. Configuration of latent varicella-zoster virus DNA. J Virol 1995;69:8151–8154.
21. Clatch RJ, Melvold RW, Miller SD, Lipton HL. Theiler's murine encephalomyelitis virus (TMEV)-induced demyelinating disease in mice is influenced by the H-2D region: correlation with TMEV-specific delayed-type hypersensitivity. J Immunol 1985;135:1408–1414.
22. Clatch RJ, Miller SD, Metzner R, Dal Canto MC, Lipton HL. Monocytes/macrophages isolated from the mouse central nervous system contain infectious Theiler's murine encephalomyelitis virus (TMEV). Virology 1990;176:244–254.
23. Cohrs RJ, Barbour M, Gilden DH. Varicella-zoster virus (VZV) transcription during latency in human ganglion: detection of transcripts mapping to genes 21, 29, 62 and 63 in a cDNA library enriched for VZV RNA. J Virol 1996;70:2789–2796.
24. Cohrs RJ, Barbour MB, Mahalingam R, Wellish M, Gilden DH. Varicella-zoster virus (VZV) transcription during latency in human ganglia: prevalence of VZV gene 21 transcripts in latently infected human ganglia. J Virol 1995;69:2674–2678.
25. Cohrs RJ, Shrock K, Barbour MB, et al. Varicella-zoster virus (VZV) transcription during latency in human ganglia: construction

of a cDNA library from latently infected human trigeminal ganglia and detection of a VZV transcript. J Virol 1994;68:7900–7908.

26. Connolly JH, Allen IV, Hurwitz LJ, Miller JHD. Measles virus antibody and antigen in subacute sclerosing panencephalitis. Lancet 1965;1:542–544.

27. Cook ML, Bastone VB, Stevens JB. Evidence that neurons harbor latent herpes simplex virus. Infect Immun 1974;9:946–951.

28. Cook ML, Stevens JG. Pathogenesis of herpetic neuritis and ganglionitis in mice: evidence for intra-axonal transport of infection. Infect Immun 1973;7:272–288.

29. Cushing H. The surgical aspects of major neuralgia of the trigeminal nerve. JAMA 1905;44:1002–1008.

30. Dal Canto MC, Lipton HL. Primary demyelination in Theiler's virus infection: an ultrastructural study. Lab Invest 1976;33:626–637.

31. Debrus S, Sadzot-Delvaux C, Nikkels AF, Piette J, Rentier B. Varicella-zoster virus gene 63 encodes an immediate-early protein that is abundantly expressed during latency. J Virol 1995;69:3240–3245.

32. Deshmane SL, Fraser NW. During latency, herpes simplex virus type 1 DNA is associated with nucleosomes in a chromatin structure. J Virol 1989;63:943–947.

33. Dhib-Jalbut S, McFarland HF, Mingioli ES, Sever JL, McFarlin DE. Humoral and cellular immune responses to matrix protein of measles virus in subacute sclerosing panencephalitis. J Virol 1988;62:2483–2489.

34. Doerig C, Pizer LI, Wilcox CL. An antigen encoded by the latency-associated transcript in neuronal cell cultures latently infected with herpes simplex virus type 1. J Virol 1991;65:2724–2727.

35. Doherty PC. Cell-mediated immunity in virus infections of the central nervous system. In: McKendall RR, Stroop WG, eds. Handbook of neurovirology. New York: Marcel Dekker, 1994:67–73.

36. Duarte EA, Novella IS, Weaver SC, et al. RNA virus quasispecies: significance for viral disease and epidemiology. Infect Agents Dis 1994;3:201–214. Review.

37. Efstathiou S, Minson AC, Field HJ, Anderson JR, Wildy P. Detection of herpes simplex virus-specific DNA sequences in latently infected mice and in humans. J Virol 1986;57:446–455.

38. Eilbott DJ, Peress N, Burger H, et al. Human immunodeficiency virus type 1 in spinal cords of acquired immunodeficiency syndrome patients with myelopathy: expression and replication in macrophages. Proc Natl Acad Sci U S A 1989;86:3337–3341.

39. Fazakerley JK, Southern P, Bloom F, Buchmeier MJ. High resolution in situ hybridization to determine the cellular distribution of lymphocytic choriomeningitis virus RNA in tissues of persistently infected mice: relevance to arenavirus disease and mechanism of viral persistence. J Gen Virol 1991;72:1611–1625.

40. Fiette L, Aubert C, Brahic M, Rossi CP. Theiler's virus infection of beta 2-microglobulin–deficient mice. J Virol 1993;67:589–592.

41. Fraser NW, Lawrence WC, Wroblewska Z, Gilden DH, Koprowski H. Herpes simplex type 1 DNA in human brain tissue. Proc Natl Acad Sci U S A 1981;78:6461–6465.

42. Friedmann A, Frankel G, Lorch Y, Steinman L. Monoclonal anti-I-A antibody reverses chronic paralysis and demyelination in Theiler's virus-infected mice: critical importance of timing of treatment. J Virol 1987;61:898–903.

43. Fu J, Stein S, Rosenstein L, et al. Neurovirulence determinants of genetically engineered Theiler's viruses. Proc Natl Acad Sci U S A 1990;87:4125–4129.

44. Fujinami RS, Norrby E, Oldstone MBA. Antigenic modulation induced by monoclonal antibodies: antibodies to measles virus hemagglutinin alters expression of other viral polypeptides in infected cells. J Immunol 1984;132:2618–2621.

45. Fujinami RS, Oldstone MBA. Alterations in expression of measles virus polypeptides by antibody: molecular events in antibody-induced antigenic modulation. J Immunol 1980;78–85.

46. Fujinami RS, Oldstone MBA. Antigenic modulation: a mechanism of viral persistence. Prog Brain Res 1983;59:105–111.

47. Gendelman HE, Narayan O, Kennedy-Stoskopf S, et al. Tropism of sheep lentiviruses for monocytes: susceptibility to infection and virus gene expression increase during maturation of monocytes to macrophages. J Virol 1986;58:67–74.

48. Gerety SJ, Clatch RJ, Lipton HL, Goswami RG, Rundell MK, Miller SD. Class II–restricted T cell responses in Theiler's murine encephalomyelitis virus–induced demyelinating disease. IV. Identification of an immunodominant T cell determinant on the N-termi-

49. Gerety SJ, Karpus WJ, Cubbon AR, et al. Class II–restricted T cell responses in Theiler's murine encephalomyelitis virus–induced demyelinating disease. V. Mapping of a dominant immunopathologic VP2 T cell epitope in susceptible SJL/J mice. J Immunol 1994;152:908–918.

50. Gerety SJ, Rundell KM, Dal Canto MC, Miller SD. Class II–restricted T cell responses in Theiler's murine encephalomyelitis virus–induced demyelinating disease. VI. Potentiation of demyelination with and characterization of an immunopathologic CD4⁺ T cell line specific for an immunodominant VP2 epitope. J Immunol 1994;152:919–929.

51. Gilden DH, Rozenman Y, Murray R, Devlin M. Detection of varicella-zoster virus nucleic acid in neurons of normal human thoracic ganglia. Ann Neurol 1987;22:377–380.

52. Gilden DH, Vafai A, Shtram Y, Becker Y, Devlin M, Wellish M. Varicella-zoster virus DNA in human sensory ganglia. Nature 1983;306:478–480.

53. Gooding LR. Virus proteins that counteract host defenses. Cell 1992;71:5–7. Minireview.

54. Goodpasture EW. Herpetic infection, with especial reference of involvement of nervous system. Medicine (Baltimore) 1929;8:223–243.

55. Gordon YJ, Johnson B, Romanowski E, Araullo-Cruz T. RNA complementary of herpes simplex virus type 1 ICPO gene demonstrated in neurons of human trigeminal ganglia. J Virol 1988;62:1832–1835.

56. Grant RA, Filman DJ, Fujinami RS, Icenogle JP, Hogle JM. Three-dimensional structure of Theiler's virus. Proc Natl Acad Sci U S A 1992;89:2061–2065.

57. Gravel C, Kay DG, Jolicoeur P. Identification of the infected target cell type in spongiform myeloencephalopathy induced by the neurotropic Cas-Br-E murine leukemia virus. J Virol 1993;67:6648–6658.

58. Green MT, Courtney RJ, Dunkel EC. Detection of an immediate early herpes simplex virus type 1 polypeptide in trigeminal ganglia from latently infected animals. Infect Immun 1981;34:987–992.

59. Hall WW, Choppin PW. Measles virus proteins in the brain tissue of patients with subacute sclerosing panencephalitis. N Engl J Med 1981;304:1152–1155.

60. Hall WW, Lamb RA, Choppin PW. Measles and subacute sclerosing panencephalitis virus proteins: lack of antibodies to the M protein in patients with subacute sclerosing panencephalitis. Proc Natl Acad Sci U S A 1979;76:2047–2051.

61. Hanninen P, Arstila P, Lang H, Salmi A, Panelius M. Involvement of the central nervous system in acute, uncomplicated measles virus infection. J Clin Microbiol 1980;11:610–613.

62. Herndon RM, Rubinstein LJ. Light and electron microscopy observations in the development of viral particles in the inclusions of Dawson's encephalitis (subacute sclerosing panencephalitis). Neurology 1967;18:8–20.

63. Hill TJ, Blyth WA, Harbour DA. Trauma to the skin causes recurrence of herpes simplex in the mouse. J Gen Virol 1978;39:21–28.

64. Hinshaw VS, Olsen CW, Dybdahl-Sissoko N, Evans D. Apoptosis: a mechanism of cell killing by influenza A and B viruses. J Virol 1994;68:3667–3673.

65. Hirano A, Ayata M, Wang AH, Wong TC. Functional analysis of matrix proteins expressed from cloned genes of measles virus variants that cause subacute sclerosing panencephalitis reveals a common defect in nucleocapsid binding. J Virol 1993;67:1848–1853.

66. Horta-Barbosa L, Hamilton R, Wittig B, Fuccillo DA, Sever JL, Vernon ML. Subacute sclerosing panencephalitis isolation of suppressed measles virus from lymph node biopsies. Science 1971;173:840–841.

67. Huang AS, Baltimore D. Defective interfering animal viruses. Compr Virol 1995;10:73–116.

68. Hummel KB, Vanchiere JA, Bellini WJ. Restriction of fusion protein mRNA as a mechanism of measles virus persistence. Virology 1994;202:665–672.

69. Hyman RW, Ecker JR, Tenser RB. Varicella-zoster virus RNA in human trigeminal ganglia. Lancet 1983;2:814–816.

70. Itoyama Y, Webster H deF, Sternberger NH, et al. Distribution of papovavirus, myelin-associated glycoprotein, and myelin basic protein

in progressive multifocal leukoencephalopathy lesions. Ann Neurol 1982;11:396–407.

71. Itzhaki RF, Maitland NJ, Wilcock GK, Yates CM, Jamieson GA. Detection by polymerase chain reaction of herpes simplex virus type 1 (HSV-1) DNA in brain of aged normals and Alzheimer's disease patients. In: Corain B, Iqbal K, Nicolini M, Winblad B, Wisniewski HM, Catta PF, eds. Alzheimer's disease: advances in clinical and basic research. New York: John Wiley, 1993:97–102.

72. Jamieson GA, Maitland NJ, Wilcock GK, Craske J, Itzhaki RF. Latent herpes simplex virus type 1 in normal and Alzheimer's disease brains. J Med Virol 1991;33:224–227.

73. Jarousse N, Grant RA, Hogle JM, et al. A single amino acid change determines persistence of a chimeric Theiler's virus. J Virol 1994; 68:3364–3368.

74. Javier RT, Stevens JG, Dissette VB, Wagner EK. A herpes simplex virus transcript abundant in latently infected neurons is dispensable for establishment of the latent state. Virology 1988;166:254–257.

75. Johnson RT. Slow infections: virus-host relationships. In: Zeiman W, Lennette EH, eds. Slow Virus Diseases. Baltimore: Williams and Wilkins, 1974:1–9.

76. Joly E, Mucre L, Oldstone MBA. Viral persistence in neurons explained by the lack of major histocompatibility class I expression. Science 1991;253:1283–1285.

77. Koenig S, Gendelman HE, Orenstein JM, et al. Detection of AIDS virus in macrophages in brain tissue from AIDS patients with encephalopathy. Science 1986;233:1089–1093.

78. Koup RA. Virus escape from CTL recognition. J Exp Med 1994; 180:779–782.

79. Kristensson K, Norrby E. Persistence of RNA viruses in the central nervous system. Ann Rev Microbiol 1995;40:159–184.

80. Kwon BS, Gangarosa LP, Green K, Hill JM. Kinetics of ocular herpes simplex virus shedding induced by epinephrine iontophoresis. Invest Ophthalmo Vis Sci 1982;22:818–821.

81. Lehky TJ, Fox CH, Koenig S, et al. Detection of human T-lymphotropic virus type I (HTLV-I) tax RNA in the central nervous system of HTLV-I–associated myelopathy/tropical spastic paraparesis patients by in situ hybridization. Ann Neurol 1995;37:167–175.

82. Lehmann-Grube L, Martinez-Peralta L, Bruns M, Lohler J. Lymphocytic choriomeningitis virus. In: Fraenkel-Conrat H, Wagner RR, eds. Comprehensive virology. New York: Plenum Press, 1983: 43–103.

83. Levine B, Huang Q, Issacs JT, Reed JC, Griffin DE, Hardwick JM. Conversion of lytic to persistent alphavirus infection by the bcl-2 cellular oncogene. Nature 1993;361:739–742.

84. Levy M, Aubert C, Brahic M. Theiler's virus replication in brain macrophages cultured in vitro. J Virol 1992;66:3188–3193.

85. Lieb DA, Bogard CL, Kosz-Vnenchak M, et al. A deletion mutant of the latency-associated transcript of herpes simplex virus type 1 reactivates from the latent state with reduced frequency. J Virol 1989; 63:2893–2900.

86. Liebert UG, Schneider-Schaulies S, Baczko K, ter Meulen V. Antibody-induced restriction of viral gene expression in measles encephalitis in rats. J Virol 1990;64:706–713.

87. Liedtke W, Opalka B, Zimmerman CS, Liquitz E. Age distribution of latent herpes simplex virus 1 and varicella-zoster virus genome in human nervous tissue. J Neurol Sci 1993;116:6–11.

88. Lipton HL. Theiler's virus infection in mice: an unusual biphasic disease process leading to demyelination. Infect Immun 1975;11: 1147–1155.

89. Lipton HL. Theiler's murine encephalomyelitis virus: animal models. In: McKendall RR, Stroop WG, eds. Handbook of neurovirology. New York: Marcel Dekker, 1994:521–528.

90. Lipton HL, Dal Canto MC. Theiler's virus-induced demyelination: prevention by immunosuppression. Science 1976;192:62–64.

91. Lipton HL, Dal Canto MC. Contrasting effects of immunosuppression on Theiler's virus infection in mice. Infect Immun 1977;15: 903–909.

92. Lipton HL, Twaddle G, Jelachich ML. The predominant virus antigen burden is present in macrophages in Theiler's murine encephalomyelitis virus (TMEV)–induced demyelinating disease. J Virol 1995;69:2525–2533.

93. Luo M, Cunheng H, Toth KS, Zhang CX, Lipton HL. Three-dimensional structure of Theiler's murine encephalomyelitis virus (BeAn strain). Proc Natl Acad Sci U S A 1992;89:2409–2413.

94. Mahalingam R, Wellish M, Cohrs R, et al. Expression of protein encoded by varicella-zoster virus open reading frame 63 in latently infected human ganglionic neurons. Proc Natl Acad Sci U S A 1996;93:2122–2124.

95. Mahalingam R, Wellish M, Lederer D, Forghani B, Cohrs R, Gilden D. Quantitation of latent varicella-zoster virus DNA in human trigeminal ganglia by polymerase chain reaction. J Virol 1993; 67:2381–2384.

96. Mahalingam R, Wellish M, Wolf W, et al. Latent varicella-zoster viral DNA in human trigeminal and thoracic ganglia. N Engl J Med 1990;323:627–631.

97. Mahalingam R, Wellish MC, Dueland AN, Cohrs R, Gilden DH. Localization of herpes simplex virus and varicella zoster virus DNA in human ganglia. Ann Neurol 1992;32:444–448.

98. McAllister A, Tangy F, Aubert C, Brahic M. Molecular cloning of the complete genome of Theiler's virus, strain DA, and production of infectious transcripts. Microb Pathog 1989;7:381–388.

99. McAllister A, Tangy F, Aubert C, Brahic M. Genetic mapping of the ability of Theiler's virus to persist and demyelinate [published erratum appears in J Virol 1993;67(4):2427]. J Virol 1990;64:4252–4257.

100. Meier JL, Holman RP, Croen KD, Smialek JE, Straus SE. Varicellazoster virus transcription in human trigeminal ganglia. Virology 1993;193:193–200.

101. Mellerick DM, Fraser NW. Physical state of the latent herpes simplex virus genome in a mouse model system: evidence suggesting an episomal state. Virology 1987;158:265–275.

102. Miller CA, Carrigan DR. Reversible repression and activation of measles virus infection in neural cells. Proc Natl Acad Sci U S A 1982;79:1629–1633.

103. Miller SD, Gerety SJ. Immunologic aspects of Theiler's murine encephalomyelitis virus (TMEV)–induced demyelinating disease. Semin Virol 1990;1:263–272.

104. Moench TR, Griffin DE, Obriecht CR, Vaisberg AJ. Acute measles in patients with and without neurological involvement: distribution of measles virus antigen and RNA. J Infect Dis 1988;158:433–442.

105. Moskophidis D, Zinkernagel RM. Immunobiology of cytotoxic T-cell escape mutants of lymphocytic choriomeningitis virus. J Virol 1995;69:2187–2193.

106. Norrby E, Kristensson K, Brzosko WJ, Kapsenberg JG. Measles virus matrix protein detected by immune fluorescence with monoclonal antibodies in the brain of patients with subacute sclerosing panencephalitis. J Virol 1985;56:337–340.

107. Norrby E, Kristensson K, Brzosko WJ, Kapsenberg JG. Identification of measles virus antigens in SSPE brain material by use of monoclonal antibodies. In: Bergamini F, Defanti CA, Ferrante P, eds. Subacute sclerosing panencephalitis. New York: Elsevier, 1986: 219–225.

108. Ohara Y, Stein S, Fu J, Stillman L, Klaman L, Roos RP. Molecular cloning and sequence determination of DA strain of Theiler's murine encephalomyelitis virus. Virology 1988;164:245–255.

109. Padgett BL, Walker DL, ZuRhein GM, Eckroade RJ. Cultivation of papova-like virus from human brain with progressive multifocal leukoencephalopathy. Lancet 1971;1:1257–1260.

110. Payne FE, Baublis JV, Itabashi HH. Isolation of measles virus from cell cultures of brain from a patient with subacute sclerosing panencephalitis. N Engl J Med 1969;281:585–589.

111. Perlman S, Ries D. The astrocyte is a target cell in mice persistently infected with mouse hepatitis virus, strain JHM. Microb Pathog 1987;3:309–314.

112. Peterson JD, Waltenbaugh C, Miller SD. IgG subclass responses to Theiler's murine encephalomyelitis virus infection and immunization suggest a dominant role for Th1 cells in susceptible mouse strains. Immunology 1992;75:652–658.

113. Pevear DC, Calenoff M, Rozhon E, Lipton HL. Analysis of the complete nucleotide sequence of the picornavirus Theiler's murine encephalomyelitis virus indicates that it is closely related to cardioviruses. J Virol 1987;61:1507–1516.

114. Plotkin SA, Stein S, Snyder M, Immesoete P. Attempts to recover varicella virus from ganglia. Ann Neurol 1977;2:249. Letter.

115. Pritchard A, Knauf T, Adami C, Lipton HL. Recombinant Theiler's viruses progressively replacing GDVII sequences in the capsid with those of BeAn indicate a role for a conformational determinant in central nervous system persistence (in preparation).

116. Pritchard AE, Bandyopadhyay PK, Calenoff MA, Lipton HL. Theiler's murine encephalomyelitis virus strain GDVII strain does not contain a determinant for central nervous system persistence. Virology 1995 (submitted).

117. Pullen M, Miller SD, Dal Canto MC, Kim BS. Class I deficient resistant mice intracerebrally inoculated with Theiler's virus show an increased T cell response to viral antigens and susceptibility to demyelination. Eur J Immunol 1993;23:2287–2293.

118. Rammohan K, McFarlin DE, McFarland HF. Chronic measles encephalitis in mice. J Infect Dis 1980;546–550.

119. Rammohan KW, McFarland HF, Bellini WJ, Gheuens J, McFarlin DE. Antibody-mediated modification of encephalitis induced by hamster neurotropic measles virus. J Infect Dis 1981;147:546–549.

120. Rammohan KW, McFarland HF, McFarlin DE. Induction of subacute murine measles encephalitis by monoclonal antibody to virus haemagglutinin. Nature 1981;290:588–589.

121. Rock DL, Fraser NW. Latent herpes simplex virus type 1 DNA contains two copies of the virion DNA joint region. J Virol 1985;55:849–852.

122. Rodriguez M, Dunkel AJ, Thiemann RL, Leibowitz J, Zijlstra M, Jaenisch R. Abrogation of resistance to Theiler's virus–induced demyelination in H-2b mice deficient in beta 2-microglobulin. J Immunol 1993;151:266–276.

123. Rodriguez M, Leibowitz JL, Lampert PW. Persistent infection of oligodendrocytes in Theiler's virus-induced encephalomyelitis. Ann Neurol 1983;13:426–433.

124. Rodriguez M, Lucchinetti CF, Clark RJ, Yakash TL, Markowitz H, Lennon VA. Immunoglobulins and complement in demyelination induced in mice by Theiler's virus. J Immunol 1988;140:800–806.

125. Rodriguez M, Roos RP. Pathogenesis of early and late disease in mice infected with Theiler's virus, using intratypic recombinant GDVII/DA viruses. J Virol 1992;66:217–225.

126. Rodriguez M, Sriram S. Successful therapy of Theiler's virus-induced demyelination (DA strain) with monoclonal anti-Lyt-2 antibody. J Immunol 1988;140:2950–2955.

127. Rossi CP, Cash E, Aubert C, Coutinho A. Role of the humoral immune response in resistance to Theiler's virus infection. J Virol 1991;65:3895–3899.

128. Rozhon EJ, Kratochvil JD, Lipton HL. Analysis of genetic variation in Theiler's virus during persistent infection in the mouse central nervous system. Virology 1983;128:16–32.

129. Sadzot-Delvaux C, Merville-Louis M, Delree P, et al. An in vivo model of varicella-zoster virus latent infection of dorsal root ganglia. J Neurosci Res 1990;26:83–89.

130. Schmid A, Spielhofer P, Cattaneo R, Baczko K, ter Meulen V, Billeter MA. Subacute sclerosing panencephalitis is typically characterized by alterations in the fusion protein cytoplasmic domain of the persisting measles virus. Virology 1992;188:910–915.

131. Sedarati F, Izumi KM, Wagner EK, Stevens JG. Herpes simplex virus type 1 latency-associated transcription plays no role in establishment or maintenance of a latent infection in murine sensory neurons. J Virol 1989;63:4455–4458.

132. Sequiera LW, Jennings LC, Carrasco LH, Lord MA, Curry A, Sutton RNP. Detection of herpes-simplex viral genome in brain tissue. Lancet 1979;2:609–612.

133. Sethi P, Lipton HL. Location and distribution of virus antigen in the central nervous system of mice persistently infected with Theiler's virus. Br J Exp Pathol 1983;64:57–65.

134. Sigurdsson B. Rida, a chronic encephalitis of sheep: with general remarks on infections which develop slowly and some of their special characteristics. Br Vet J 1954;110:341

135. Simon MA, Brodie SJ, Sasseville VG, Chalifoux LV, Desrosiers RC, Ringler DJ. Immunopathogenesis of SIV_mac. Virus Res 1994;32:227–251. Review.

136. Smith RL, Pizer LI, Johnson JEM, Wilcox CL. Activation of second-messenger pathways reactivates latent herpes simplex virus in neuronal cultures. Virology 1992;188:311–318.

137. Spivack JG, Fraser NW. Detection of herpes simplex virus type 1 transcripts during latent infection in mice. J Virol 1987;61: 3841–3847.

138. Steiner I, Kennedy PGE. Herpes simplex virus latent infection in the nervous system. J Neurovirol 1995;1:19–29.

139. Steiner I, Spivack JG, O'Boyle DR II, Lavi E, Fraser NW. Latent herpes simplex virus type 1 transcription in human trigeminal ganglia. J Virol 1988;62:3493–3496.

140. Stevens JG, Haarr L, Porter DD, Cook ML, Wagner EK. Prominence of the herpes simplex virus latency-associated transcript in trigeminal ganglia from seropositive humans. J Infect Dis 1988; 158:117–123.

141. Stevens JG, Wagner EK, Devi-Rao GB, Cook ML, Feldman LT. RNA complementary to a herpesvirus α gene mRNA is prominent in latently infected neurons. Science 1987;235:1056–1059.

142. Sun N, Perlman S. Spread of neurotropic coronaviruses to spinal cord white matter via neurons and astrocytes. J Virol 1995;69: 633– 641.

143. Tellez-Nagel I, Harter DH. Subacute sclerosing leukoencephalitis: ultrastructure of intranuclear and intracytoplasmic inclusions. Science 1966;154:899–901.

144. Tolskaya EA, Romanova LI, Kolesnickova MS, et al. Apoptosis-inducing and apoptosis-preventing functions of poliovirus. J Virol 1995;69:1181–1189.

145. Townsend JJ, Wolinsky JS, Baringer JR. The neuropathology of progressive rubella panencephalitis of late onset. Brain 1976;99:81–90.

146. Vanguri P, Shin ML. Hydrolysis of myelin basic protein in human myelin by terminal complement complexes. J Biol Chem 1988; 263:7228–7234.

147. Wada Y, Pierce ML, Fujinami RS. Importance of amino acid 101 within capsid protein VP1 for modulation of Theiler's virus–induced disease. J Virol 1994;68:1219–1223.

148. Walz MA, Price RW, Notkins AL. Latent ganglionic infection with herpes simplex virus types 1 and 2: viral reactivation in vivo after neurectomy. Science 1974;184:1185–1186.

149. Warren KG, Brown SM, Wroblewska Z, Gilden D, Koprowski H, Subak-Sharpe J. Isolation of latent herpes simplex virus from the superior cervical and vagus ganglions of human beings. N Engl J Med 1978;298:1068–1069.

150. Warren KG, Devlin M, Gilden DH, et al. Isolation of herpes simplex virus from human trigeminal ganglia, including ganglia from one patient with multiple sclerosis. Lancet 1977;2:637–639.

151. Watanabe M, Wang A, Gombart AF, et al. Delayed activation of altered fusion glycoprotein in a chronic measles virus variant that causes subacute sclerosing panencephalitis. J Neurovirol 1995;1: 177–188.

152. Wear DJ, Rapp F. Latent measles virus infection of the hamster central nervous system. J Immunol 1971;107:1593–1598.

153. Wilcox CL, Johnson JEM. Nerve growth factor deprivation results in the reactivation of latent herpes simplex virus in vitro. Virology 1987;61:2311–2315.

154. Yauch RL, Kerekes K, Saujani K, Kim BS. Identification of a major T-cell epitope within VP3 amino acid residues 24 to 37 of Theiler's virus in demyelination-susceptible SJL/J mice. J Virol 1995;69: 7315–7318.

155. Yauch RL, Kim BS. A predominant viral epitope recognized by T cells from the periphery and demyelinating lesions of SJL mice infected with Theiler's virus is located within VP1_{233-244}. J Immunol 1994;153:4508–4519.

156. Zurbriggen A, Fujinami RS. A neutralization-resistant Theiler's virus variant produces an altered disease pattern in the mouse central nervous system. J Virol 1989;63:1505–1513.

157. Zurbriggen A, Thomas C, Yamada M, Roos RP, Fujinami RS. Direct evidence of a role for amino acid 101 of VP-1 in central nervous system disease in Theiler's murine encephalomyelitis virus infection. J Virol 1991;65:1929–1937.

158. ZuRhein GM, Chow SM. Particles resembling papova viruses in human cerebral demyelinating disease. Science 1965;148:1477–1479.

Viral Pathogenesis,
edited by Neal Nathanson, et al.
Lippincott–Raven Publishers, Philadelphia © 1997

CHAPTER 37

Prion Diseases

Stanley B. Prusiner

S.B. Prusiner: Department of Neurology and Department of Biochemistry and Biophysics, University of California, San Francisco, California 94143.

INTRODUCTION

Prions cause a group of human and animal neurodegenerative diseases that are now classified together because their origin and pathogenesis involve modification of the prion protein (PrP).[393] Prion diseases are manifested as infectious, genetic, and sporadic disorders (Table 37-1). These diseases can be transmitted among mammals by the infectious particle designated "prion."[389] Despite intensive searches over the past three decades, no nucleic acid has been found within prions.[7,8,238,423] It has been established that a modified isoform of the host-encoded PrP, designated PrP^{Sc}, is essential for infectivity,[70,393,408,409,416] and considerable experimental data argue that prions are composed exclusively of PrP^{Sc}. Earlier terms used to describe the prion diseases included transmissible encephalopathies, spongiform encephalopathies, and slow virus diseases.[172,173,448]

The quartet of human (Hu) prion diseases are frequently referred to as kuru, Creutzfeldt-Jakob disease (CJD), Gerstmann-Sträussler-Scheinker disease (GSS), and fatal familial insomnia (FFI). Kuru was the first of the human prion diseases to be transmitted to experimental animals, and it has often been suggested that kuru spread among the Fore people of Papua New Guinea by ritualistic cannibalism.[172,175] The experimental and presumed human-to-human transmission of kuru led to the belief that prion diseases are infectious disorders caused by unusual viruses similar to those causing scrapie in sheep and goats. Yet, a paradox was presented by the occurrence of CJD in families, first reported almost 70 years ago,[268,325] which appeared to be a genetic disease. The significance of familial CJD remained unappreciated until mutations in the protein-coding region of the PrP gene were discovered.[228,397,455] The earlier finding that brain extracts from patients who had died of familial prion diseases, when inoculated into experimental animals, often transmitted disease posed a conundrum that was resolved with the genetic linkage of these diseases to mutations of the PrP gene.[310,392,467]

The most common form of prion disease in humans is sporadic CJD. Many attempts to show that the sporadic prion diseases are caused by infection have been unsuccessful.[53,104,218,297] The discovery that inherited prion diseases are caused by germ line mutation of the PrP gene raised the possibility that sporadic forms of these diseases may result from somatic mutation.[392] The discoveries that PrP^{Sc} is formed from the cellular isoform of the prion protein, PrP^{C}, by a posttranslational process[44] and that overexpression of wild-type (wt) PrP transgenes produces spongiform degeneration and infectivity de novo[483] raised the possibility that sporadic prion diseases result from spontaneous conversion of PrP^{C} into PrP^{Sc}.

CJD has a worldwide incidence of 1 case per 10^6 population per year.[313] Fewer than 1% of cases of CJD are infectious (and all of those appear to be iatrogenic), 10% to 15% are inherited, and the remaining cases are sporadic. Kuru was once the most common cause of death among New Guinea women in the Fore region of the Highlands,[175,177,178] but it has virtually disappeared with the cessation of ritualistic cannibalism.[12] Patients with CJD frequently present with dementia, but 10% of patients exhibit cerebellar dysfunction initially. Patients with kuru or GSS usually present with ataxia, whereas those with FFI manifest insomnia and autonomic dysfunction.[50,234,324]

PrP^{CJD} has been found in the brains of most patients studied who died of prion disease. In the brains of some patients with inherited prion diseases and in transgenic (Tg) mice expressing mouse (Mo) PrP with the human GSS point mutation (proline [Pro] → leucine [Leu]), detection of PrP^{Sc} has been problematic despite clinical and neuropathologic hallmarks of neurodegeneration.[232,235] Horizontal transmission of neurodegeneration from the brains of patients with inherited prion diseases to inoculated rodents has less frequently been achieved than with sporadic cases.[467] Whether a distinction between transmissible and nontransmissible inherited prion diseases will persist is unclear. Tg mice expressing a chimeric Hu/Mo PrP gene have been found to be highly susceptible to Hu prions from patients with sporadic or iatrogenic CJD[471] (see later discussion). These Tg(MHu2M) mice should make the use of apes and monkeys for the study of human prion diseases unnecessary and allow for tailoring of the PrP^{C} translated from the transgene to match the sequence of the PrP^{CJD} in the inoculum. The use of such Tg mice may enhance the ability to transmit human cases of inherited prion disease.

Scrapie is the most common natural prion disease of animals. An investigation into the cause of scrapie followed the vaccination of sheep for looping ill virus with formalin-treated extracts of ovine lymphoid tissue unknowingly contaminated with scrapie prions.[211] Two years later, scrapie had developed in more than 1500 sheep as a result of vaccination. Although the transmissibility of experimental scrapie became well established, the spread of natural scrapie within and among flocks of sheep remained puzzling. Parry argued that host genes were responsible for the development of scrapie in sheep. He was convinced that natural scrapie is a genetic disease that could be eradicated by proper breeding protocols.[370,372] He considered its transmission by inoculation of importance primarily for laboratory studies and communicable infection of little consequence in nature. Other investigators viewed natural scrapie as an infectious disease and argued that host genetics only modulates susceptibility to an endemic infectious agent.[135]

The offal of scrapied sheep in Great Britain is thought to be responsible for the current epidemic of bovine spongiform encephalopathy (BSE), or mad cow disease.[490] Prions in the offal from scrapie-infected sheep appear to have survived the rendering process which produced meat and bone meal that was fed to cattle as a nutritional supplement. After BSE was recognized, meat and bone meal produced from domestic animal offal was banned from further use. Since 1986, when BSE was first recognized, more than 160,000 cattle have died of BSE. Whether humans develop CJD after consuming beef from cattle with BSE prions is of considerable concern.

TABLE 37-1. *Human prion diseases*

Disease	Cause
Kuru	Infection
Creutzfeldt-Jakob disease	
Iatrogenic	Infection
Sporadic	Unknown
Familial	PrP mutation
Gerstmann-Sträussler-Scheinker disease	PrP mutation
Fatal familial insomnia	PrP mutation

Prions differ from all other known infectious pathogens in several respects. First, prions do not contain a nucleic acid genome that codes for their progeny. Viruses, viroids, bacteria, fungi, and parasites all have nucleic acid genomes that code for their progeny. Second, the only known component of the prion is a modified protein that is encoded by a cellular gene. Third, the major, and possibly only, component of the prion is PrP^{Sc}, which is a pathogenic conformer of PrP^{C}.

The fundamental event in prion diseases seems to be a conformational change in PrP. All attempts to identify a posttranslational chemical modification that distinguishes PrP^{Sc} from PrP^{C} have been unsuccessful to date.[458] PrP^{C} contains 45% α-helix and is virtually devoid of β-sheet.[369] Conversion to PrP^{Sc} creates a protein that contains 30% α-helix and 45% β-sheet. The mechanism by which PrP^{C} is converted into PrP^{Sc} remains unknown, but PrP^{C} appears to bind to PrP^{Sc} to form an intermediate complex during the formation of nascent PrP^{Sc}.

As our knowledge of the prion diseases increases and more is learned about the molecular and genetic characteristics of PrP, these disorders will undoubtedly undergo modification with respect to their classification. Indeed, the discovery of the PrP gene and the identification of pathogenic PrP gene mutations have already forced us to view these illnesses from perspectives not previously imagined.

DEVELOPMENT OF THE PRION CONCEPT

Hypotheses on the Nature of the Scrapie Agent

The published literature contains a fascinating record of the structural hypotheses for the scrapie agent proposed to explain the unusual features, first, of the disease and, later, of the infectious agent. Among the earliest hypotheses was the notion that scrapie was a disease of muscle caused by the parasite Sarcosporidia.[329,330] With the successful transmission of scrapie to animals, the hypothesis that scrapie is caused by a filterable virus became popular.[108,499] With the findings of Alper and her colleagues that scrapie infectivity resists inactivation by ultraviolet and ionizing radiation[7,8] a myriad of hypotheses on the chemical nature of the scrapie agent emerged. Among the structures proposed were a small DNA virus,[259] a replicating protein,[213,291,292,378] a replicating abnormal polysaccharide with membranes,[184,241] a DNA subvirus controlled by a transmissible linkage substance,[1,3] a provirus consisting of recessive genes generating RNA particles,[370,371] and a naked nucleic acid similar to those of plant viroids.[137]

The term unconventional virus was proposed, but no structural details were ever given with respect to how these unconventional virions differed from the conventional viral particles,[172] and some investigators have suggested that this term obscured the ignorance that continued to shroud the infectious scrapie agent.[376] Other suggestions included aggregated conventional virus with unusual properties,[433] replicating polysaccharide,[154] nucleoprotein complex,[289] nucleic acid surrounded by a polysaccharide coat,[2,342,447] spiroplasma-like organism,[23,237] multicomponent system with one component quite small,[240,454] membrane-bound DNA,[307] virino (viroid-like DNA complexed with host proteins), filamentous animal virus (SAF),[326] aluminum-silicate amyloid complex, and even a computer virus.[174]

Bioassays of Prion Infectivity

The experimental transmission of scrapie from sheep[211] to mice[87] gave investigators a more convenient laboratory model, one that yielded considerable information on the nature of the unusual infectious pathogen that causes scrapie.[7–9,184,331,378] Yet, progress was slow because quantitation of infectivity in a single sample required holding 60 mice for 1 year before accurate scoring could be accomplished.[87]

Attempts to develop a more economical bioassay by relating the titer to incubation times in mice were unsuccessful.[149,242] Some investigators used incubation times to characterize different "strains" of scrapie agent, and others determined the kinetics of prion replication in rodents.[128,131,261,262] However, these investigators refrained from trying to establish quantitative bioassays for prions based on incubation times, despite the successful application of such an approach for the measurement of picornaviruses and other viruses three decades earlier.[179] After scrapie incubation times were reported to be 50% shorter in Syrian golden hamsters (SHa) than in mice,[306] studies were undertaken to determine whether the incubation times in hamsters could be related to the titer of the inoculated sample. After it was found that there was an excellent correlation between the length of the incubation time and the dose of inoculated prions, a more rapid and economical bioassay for the scrapie agent was developed.[400,406] This improved bioassay accelerated purification of the infectious particles by a factor of almost 100.

Bioassays for human prions were initially performed in apes and monkeys.[188,190] Over the last 30 years, 300 cases of CJD, kuru, and GSS have been transmitted to a variety of apes and monkeys.[58] The scarcity of these primates, the expense of their long-term care, and the increasing ethical objections to such experiments have limited investigations. It has been stated that more than 90% of cases clinically and neuropathologically diagnosed as CJD transmit to nonhuman primates after prolonged incubation times.[58]

Because of the species barrier,[374] the initial passage of prions from humans to rodents requires prolonged incubation times, and illness develops in relatively few animals.[190,274,301,339,390,467] Subsequent passage in the same species occurs with high frequency and shortened incubation times. The molecular basis for the species barrier between Syrian hamster and mouse was found, with the use of Tg mice, to reside in the sequence of the PrP gene[442]: SHaPrP differs from MoPrP at 16 of 254 amino acid residues.[22,294]

Because mice expressing HuPrP transgenes have not shown abbreviated incubation times as Tg(SHaPrP) mice do when inoculated with homologous prions, a chimeric Hu/Mo transgene was constructed.[443] Human PrP differs from mouse PrP at 28 of 254 positions,[283] whereas chimeric Hu/Mo PrP, designated MHu2M, differs at 9 residues. The MHu2M transgenes are susceptible to Hu prions and exhibit abbreviated incubation times.[471]

Purification of Scrapie Infectivity

Many investigators attempted to purify the scrapie agent for several decades but with relatively little success. The slow, cumbersome, and tedious bioassays in sheep and later in mice greatly limited the number of samples that could be analyzed. Because the ease of purification of any biologically active macromolecule is directly related to the rapidity of the assay, it is not surprising that little progress was made with sheep and goats, where only very limited numbers of samples could be analyzed and incubation times exceeding 18 months were required.[238,376]

Experimental transmission of scrapie to mice allowed many more samples to be analyzed, but 1 year was required to complete the measurement of scrapie infectivity by end point titration using 60 animals to evaluate one sample.[87] Although some properties of the scrapie agent were determined by this rather cumbersome mouse bioassay, it was difficult to develop an effective purification protocol when the interval between execution of the experiment and the availability of the results was almost a year.[391,415,446] The resistance of scrapie infectivity to nondenaturing detergents, nucleases, proteases, and glycosidases[239,242,243,332] and the sedimentation properties of the agent were determined using end point titrations in mice.[410,411] Attempts to purify infectivity were complicated by the apparent size and charge heterogeneity of scrapie infectivity, which was interpreted to be a consequence of hydrophobic interactions.[412]

The Prion Concept

After an effective protocol was developed for preparation of partially purified fractions of scrapie agent from hamster brain, it became possible to demonstrate that those procedures that modify or hydrolyze proteins produce a diminution in scrapie infectivity.[389,417] At the same time, tests done in search of a scrapie-specific nucleic acid were unable to demonstrate any dependence of infectivity on a polynucleotide,[389] in agreement with earlier studies reporting the extreme resistance of infectivity to ultraviolet irradiation at 254 nm.[7]

Based on these findings, it seemed likely that the infectious pathogen capable of transmitting scrapie was neither a virus nor a viroid. For this reason the term prion was introduced to distinguish the **pro**teinaceous **in**fectious particles that cause scrapie, CJD, GSS, and kuru from both viroids and viruses.[389] Hypotheses for the structure of the infectious prion particle included proteins surrounding a nucleic acid encoding them (a virus), proteins associated with a small polynucleotide, and proteins devoid of nucleic acid.[389] Mechanisms postulated for the replication of infectious prion particles ranged from those used by viruses, to synthesis of polypeptides in the absence of a nucleic acid template, to posttranslational modifications of cellular proteins. Subsequent discoveries have narrowed hypotheses for both prion structure and the mechanism of replication.

Considerable evidence has accumulated over the past decade supporting the prion hypothesis.[393] Furthermore, the replication of prions and their mode of pathogenesis also appear to be without precedent. After a decade of severe criticism and serious doubt, the prion concept is now enjoying considerable acceptance.

Search for a Scrapie-Specific Nucleic Acid

The search for a scrapie-specific nucleic acid has been intense, thorough, and comprehensive, yet it has been unrewarding. The challenge to find a scrapie-specific polynucleotide was initiated by investigators who found that scrapie agent infectivity is highly resistant to ultraviolet and ionizing radiation.[7–9] Their results prompted speculation that the scrapie pathogen may be devoid of nucleic acid—a postulate initially dismissed by many scientists. Although some investigators have argued that the interpretation of these data was flawed,[429–432] they and others have failed to demonstrate the putative scrapie nucleic acid.

Based on the resistance of the scrapie agent to both ultraviolet and ionizing radiation, the possibility was raised that the scrapie agent may contain a small polynucleotide similar in size and properties to those of plant viroids.[137] Subsequently, evidence for a putative DNA-like viroid was published,[298,299,307] but the findings could not be confirmed,[404] and the properties of the scrapie agent were found to be incompatible with those of viroids.[138] Besides ultraviolet irradiation, reagents that specifically modify or damage nucleic acids, such as nucleases, psoralens, hydroxylamine, and zinc (Zn^{++}) ions, were found not to alter scrapie infectivity in homogenates,[389] microsomal fractions,[389] purified prion rod preparations, or detergent-lipid-protein complexes.[26,27,28,165,319,348]

Attempts to find a scrapie-specific polynucleotide using physical techniques such as polyacrylamide gel electrophoresis were as unsuccessful as molecular cloning approaches. Subtractive hybridization studies identified several cellular genes, the expression of which is increased in scrapie, but no unique sequence could be identified.[136,147,481] Extensively purified fractions were analyzed by a specially developed technique designated return refocusing gel electrophoresis, but no scrapie-specific nucleic acid was found.[327] These studies argue that, if such a molecule exists, its size is 80 nucleotides or less.[255,423] Attempts to use these highly enriched fractions to identify a scrapie-specific nucleic acid by molecular cloning were also unsuccessful.[354]

In spite of these studies, some investigators continue to champion the idea that scrapie is caused by a virus.[89,256] A few argue that the scrapie virus is similar to a retrovirus,[6,304,341,450,451,452,453] and others argue that the scrapie virus induces amyloid deposition in brain.[47,139,140] Some propose that scrapie is caused by a larger pathogen similar to *Spiroplasma bacterium*.[23,24] Still others contend that elongated protein polymers covered by DNA are the etiologic agents in scrapie.[343,344,345,346,347] DNA molecules similar to the D-loop DNA of mitochondria have also been suggested as the cause of scrapie.[4,5]

The search for a component within the prion particle other than PrP has focused largely on a nucleic acid, because some properties of prions are similar to those of viruses and a polynucleotide would most readily explain different isolates or strains of infectivity.[66,126,133,260] Specific scrapie isolates characterized by distinct incubation times retain this property when repeatedly passaged in mice or hamsters.[66,126,133,260] Although available data do not permit exclusion of a scrapie-specific polynucleotide, its existence seems increasingly unlikely. That prions may contain noncovalently bound cofactors such as peptides, oligosaccharides, fatty acids, sterols, or inorganic compounds deserves consideration.

DISCOVERY OF THE PRION PROTEIN

Copurification of Prion Infectivity and PrP^Sc

Data from several studies suggested that scrapie infectivity may depend on protein,[91,92,239,332] whereas other studies had demonstrated that infectivity was resistant to protease digestion.[307] Only after an effective protocol was developed for enriching fractions 100-fold for scrapie infectivity with respect to cellular protein[404,406] could the dependence of scrapie infectivity on protein be established.[417] Studies with partially purified fractions prepared from Syrian hamster brain showed loss of infectivity as a function of the concentration of protease and the time of digestion; these results demonstrated that a polypeptide is required for propagation of the infectious scrapie pathogen.[417]

Once the dependence of prion infectivity on protein was clear, the search for a scrapie-specific protein intensified. Although the insolubility of scrapie infectivity made purification problematic, my colleagues and I took advantage of this property along with its relative resistance to degradation by proteases to extend the degree of purification.[406,417] In subcellular fractions from hamster brain enriched for scrapie infectivity, a protease-resistant polypeptide of 27 to 30 kD, later designated PrP 27-30, was identified; it was absent from controls.[42,318,398] Radioiodination of partially purified fractions revealed a protein unique to preparations from scrapie-infected brains.[42,398] The existence of this protein was rapidly confirmed.[142]

Determination of the N-Terminal Sequence of PrP 27-30

Purification of PrP 27-30 to homogeneity allowed determination of its NH_2-terminal amino acid sequence.[405] These studies were particularly difficult because multiple signals were found in each cycle of the Edman degradation. Whether multiple proteins were present in these purified fractions or a single protein with a ragged NH_2-terminus was present was resolved only after data from five different preparations were compared. After the signals in each cycle were grouped according to their intensities (strong, intermediate, and weak), it became clear that a single protein with a ragged NH_2-terminal was being sequenced. Determination of a single, unique sequence for the NH_2-terminal of PrP 27-30 permitted the synthesis of an isocoding mixture of oligonucleotides that was subsequently used to identify incomplete PrP cDNA clones from hamster[356] and mouse.[90] cDNA clones encoding the entire open reading frames (ORFs) of SHa and Mo PrP were subsequently recovered.[22,294]

PrP is encoded by a chromosomal gene and not by a nucleic acid within the infectious scrapie prion particle.[22,356] Levels of PrP mRNA remain unchanged throughout the course of scrapie infection—an unpredicted observation which led to the identification of the normal PrP gene product, a protein of 33 to 35 kD designated PrP^C.[22,356] PrP^C is protease sensitive and soluble in nondenaturing detergents, whereas PrP 27-30 is the protease-resistant core of a 33- to 35-kD disease-specific protein, designated PrP^{Sc}, that is insoluble in detergents.[328] Progress in the study of prions was greatly accelerated by the discovery of PrP and determination of its N-terminal sequence.[42,398,405] Indeed, all of the elegant molecular genetic studies in humans and animals, as well as many highly informative transgenetic investigations, have their origin in the purification of PrP 27-30[416] and the determination of its N-terminal sequence.[405] PrP^C or a subset of PrP molecules are the substrate for PrP^{Sc} formation. Many lines of evidence argue that PrP^{Sc} is an essential component of the infectious prion particle (Table 37-2); all attempts to find a second component of the prion particle have been unsuccessful.

Prions Contain PrP^{Sc}

Much information on PrP^{Sc} in prion diseases indicates that prions are composed largely, if not entirely, of PrP^{Sc} molecules. Although some investigators contend that PrP^{Sc} is merely a pathologic product of scrapie infection and that PrP^{Sc} coincidentally purifies with the so-called scrapie virus, there are few data to support this view.[4,5,6,47,304,341,450,453] No infective fractions containing less than 1 PrP^{Sc} molecule per median infective dose unit (ID_{50}) have been found, arguing that PrP^{Sc} is required for infectivity. Some investigators report that PrP^{Sc} accumulation in hamsters occurs after the synthesis of many infective units,[110,111] but these results have been refuted.[248] In another study, the kinetics of PrP^{Sc} and infectivity production in mice inoculated with mouse-passaged CJD prions were similar in brain but were thought to be different in salivary gland.[438] The discrepancies between PrP^{Sc} and infectivity levels in these studies appear to result from comparisons of infectivity in crude homogenates with PrP^{Sc} concentrations in purified fractions. Other investigators claim to have dissociated scrapie infectivity from PrP 27-30 in brains of Syrian hamsters treated with amphotericin B and inoculated with the 263K isolate, but not if they were inoculated with the 139H isolate or with 139a prions.[501] No confirmation of these studies with amphotericin has been published.

The covalent structure of PrP^{Sc} remains uncertain because purified fractions contain 10^5 PrP 27-30 molecules per ID_{50} unit, the infectious dose at which 50% of the animals develop scrapie.[42,318,398] If fewer than 1% of the PrP^{Sc} molecules contained an amino acid substitution or posttranslational modification that conferred scrapie infectivity, our methods would not detect such a change.[458]

PrP Gene Structure and Organization

The entire ORF of all known mammalian and avian PrP genes is contained within a single exon[22,171,228,484] (Fig. 37-1). This feature of the PrP gene eliminates the possibility that PrP^{Sc} arises from alternative RNA splicing[22,484,485]; however, mechanisms such as RNA editing or protein splicing remain a possibility.[38,252] The two exons of the SHaPrP gene are separated by a 10-kb intron: exon 1 encodes a portion of the 5' untranslated leader sequence, and exon 2 encodes the ORF and 3' untranslated region.[22] The MoPrP and sheep PrP genes are comprised of three exons, with exon 3 analogous to exon 2 of the hamster.[482,485] The promoters of both the SHaPrP and MoPrP genes contain multiple copies of repeats rich in guanine-cytosine (G-C) and are devoid of TATA boxes. These G-C nonamers represent a motif that may function as a canonical binding site for the transcription factor Sp1.[322]

Mapping of PrP genes to the short arm of human chromosome 20 and the homologous region of Mo chromosome 2 argues for the existence of PrP genes before the speciation of mammals.[455] Hybridization studies demonstrated fewer than 0.002 PrP gene sequences per ID_{50} unit in purified prion fractions, indicating that a nucleic acid encoding PrP^{Sc} is not a component of the infectious prion particle.[356] This major fea-

TABLE 37-2. *Evidence that PrP^{Sc} is a major and essential component of the infectious prion*

Research result	Investigators
Copurification of PrP 27-30 and scrapie infectivity by biochemical methods concentration of PrP 27-30 is proportional to prion titer.	Bolton et al, 1982[42]; Hope et al, 1986[226]; Jendroska et al, 1991[248]; McKinley et al, 1983[318]; Prusiner et al, 1982[398]; Safar et al, 1990[437]; Turk et al, 1988[476]
Kinetics of proteolytic digestion of PrP 27-30 and infectivity are similar.	Bolton et al, 1982[42]; McKinley et al, 1983[318]; Prusiner et al, 1982[398]
Copurification of PrP^{Sc} and infectivity by immunoaffinity chromatography is shown; α-PrP antisera neutralize infectivity.	Gabizon et al, 1988[166]; Gabizon a Prusiner, 1990[169]
PrP^{Sc} is detected only in clones of cultured cells producing infectivity.	Butler et al, 1988[72]; McKinley et al, 1991[321]; Taraboulos et al, 1990[466]
PrP amyloid plaques are specific for prion diseases of animals and humans.	Bendheim et al, 1984[29]; DeArmond et al, 1985[117]; Kitamoto et al, 1986[275]; Roberts et al, 1988[425]
Deposition of PrP amyloid is controlled, at least in part, by the PrP sequence.	Prusiner et al, 1990[418]
PrP^{Sc} (or PrP^{CJD}) is specific for prion diseases of animals and humans.	Bockman et al, 1985[40]; Brown et al, 1986[56]; Serban et al, 1990[445]
Deposition of PrP^{Sc} precedes spongiform degeneration and reactive gliosis.	Carlson et al, 1994[75]; DeArmond et al, 1993[119]; Hecker et al, 1992[220]
Genetic linkage is shown between the PrP gene and scrapie incubation times in mice with short and long incubation times.	Carlson et al, 1988[76]; Carlson et al, 1986[77]; Hunter, 1987[245]; Race et al, 1990[420]
These genes encode PrP molecules differing at residues 108 and 189.	Westaway et al, 1987[484]
The length of the incubation time is determined by the level of PrP expression and the PrP sequence.	Carlson et al, 1994[75]
Expression of SHaPrP in Tg(SHaPrP) mice renders them susceptible to Sha prions.	Scott et al, 1989[442]
The primary structure of PrP^{Sc} in the inoculum governs the neuropathology and prion synthesis,	Prusiner et al, 1990[418]
Expression of a chimeric PrP in Tg(MHu2M) mice renders them susceptible to Hu prions.	Telling et al, 1994[471]
Genetic linkage between PrP gene point mutations at codons 102, 178, 198, or 200 and development of inherited prion diseases in humans is demonstrated.	Dlouhy et al, 1992[143]; Gabizon et al, 1993[170]; Hsiao et al, 1989[228]; Petersen et al, 1992[382]
Genetic linkage is established between the mutation insert of six additional octarepeats and familial CJD.	Poulter et al, 1992[387]
Mice expressing MoPrP transgenes with the P102L point mutation of GSS spontaneously develop neurologic dysfunction, spongiform brain degeneration, and astrocytic gliosis; serial transmission of neurodegeneration is initiated with brain extracts from these Tg mice.	Hsiao et al, 1990[235]
Ablation of the PrP gene in mice prevents scrapie and propagation of prions after intracerebral inoculation of prions.	Büeler et al, 1993[70]; Prusiner et al, 1993[409]
Mice expressing chimeric Mo/SHaPrP transgenes produce "artificial" prions with novel properties.	Scott et al, 1993[443]
Overexpression of MoPrP-B and SHaPrP produces spongiform degeneration, myopathy, and peripheral neuropathy in older transgenic mice; serial transmission of neurodegeneration is initiated with brain extracts.	Westaway et al, 1994[483]

ture distinguishes prions from viruses, including those retro-viruses that carry cellular oncogenes, and from plant satellite viruses that derive their coat proteins from other viruses.

Expression of the PrP Gene

Although PrP mRNA is constitutively expressed in the brains of adult animals,[90,356] it is highly regulated during de-velopment. In the septum, levels of PrP mRNA and choline acetyltransferase were found to increase in parallel during de-velopment.[334] In other brain regions, PrP gene expression oc-curred at an earlier age. In situ hybridization studies show that the highest levels of PrP mRNA are found in neurons.[282]

Because no antibodies are currently available to differenti-ate PrP^{C} from PrP^{Sc}, the former is usually measured in tissues from uninfected control animals, in which no PrP^{Sc} is found. PrP^{Sc} must be measured in tissues of infected animals, but af-

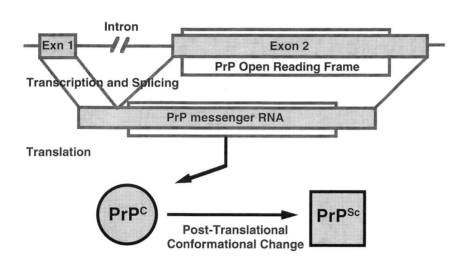

FIG. 37-1. Structure and organization of the chromosomal PrP gene. In all mammals examined, the entire open reading frame is contained within a single exon. The 5′ untranslated region of the PrP mRNA is derived from either one or two additional exons.[22,419,482,485] Only one PrP mRNA has been detected. PrPSc is thought to be derived from PrPC by a posttranslational process.[22,44,45,85,465] The amino acid sequence of PrPSc is identical to that predicted from the translated sequence of the DNA encoding the PrP gene,[22,458] and no unique posttranslational chemical modifications have been identified that differentiate PrPSc from PrPC. Therefore, it seems likely that PrPC undergoes a conformational change as it is converted to PrPSc. (From Prusiner SB. Prion diseases. In: Scriver CR, Beaudet AL, Sly WS, Valle D, eds. Metabolic basis of inherited disease. 7th ed. New York: McGraw-Hill, 1995.)

ter PrPC has been hydrolyzed by digestion with a proteolytic enzyme. PrPC expression in brain was defined by standard immunohistochemistry[118] and by histoblotting in the brains of uninfected controls[464] (Fig. 37-2). Immunostaining of PrPC in the SHa brain was most intense in the stratum radiatum and stratum oriens of the CA1 region of the hippocampus and was virtually absent from the granule cell layer of the dentate gyrus and the pyramidal cell layer throughout Ammon's horn. PrPSc staining was minimal in these regions, which were intensely stained for PrPC. A similar relation between PrPC and

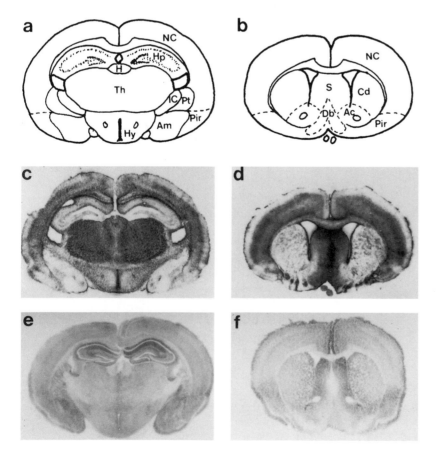

FIG. 37-2. Histoblots of Syrian hamster brain immunostained for PrPC or PrPSc. Coronal sections (**A**, **B**) were made through the hippocampus-thalamus (*left column*) and the septum-caudate (*right column*). Brain sections in **C** and **D** are from an animal that was clinically ill after inoculation with Sc237 prions and are immunostained for PrPSc; sections in **E** and **F** are from an uninfected control animal and are stained for PrPC. Ac, nucleus accumbens; Am, amygdala; Cd, caudate nucleus; Db, diagonal band of Broca; H, habenula; Hp, hippocampus; Hy, hypothalamus; IC, internal capsule; NC, neocortex; Pir, piriform cortex; Pt, putamen; S, septum; Th, thalamus. (From Taraboulos A, Jendroska K, Serban D, Yang S-L, DeArmond SJ, Prusiner SB. Regional mapping of prion proteins in brains. Proc Natl Acad Sci U S A 1992;89:7620–7624.)

PrP^{Sc} was found in the amygdala. In contrast, PrP^{Sc} accumulated in the medial habenular nucleus, the medial septal nuclei, and the diagonal band of Broca; these areas were virtually devoid of PrP^C. In the white matter, bundles of myelinated axons contained PrP^{Sc} but were devoid of PrP^C. These findings suggest that prions are transported along axons, in agreement with earlier findings in which scrapie infectivity was found to migrate in a pattern consistent with retrograde transport.[162,248,258] Although the rate of PrP^{Sc} synthesis appears to be a function of the level of PrP^C expression in Tg mice, the level to which PrP^{Sc} accumulates appears to be independent of PrP^C concentration.[418]

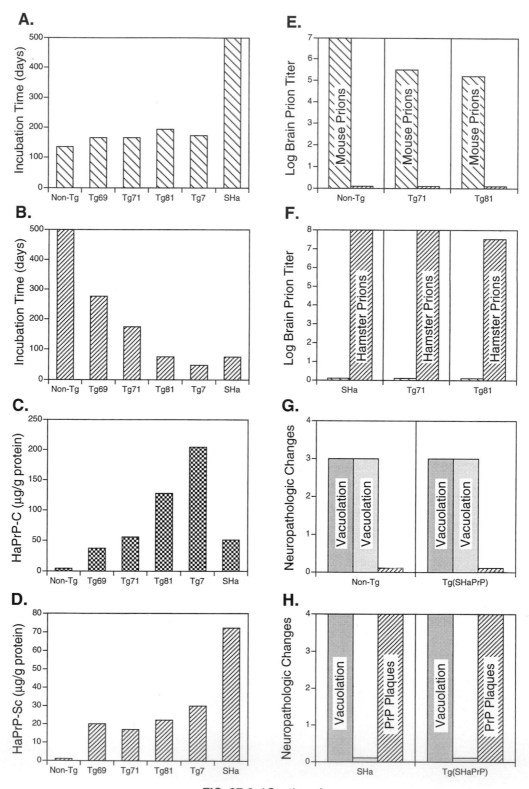

FIG. 37-3. (*Continued*)

PRP AMYLOID

The discovery of PrP 27-30 in fractions enriched for scrapie infectivity was accompanied by the identification of rod-shaped particles in the same fractions.[398,416] By both rotary shadowing and negative staining, the fine structure of these rod-shaped particles failed to reveal any regular substructure. The irregular ultrastructure of the prion rods differentiated them from viruses, which have regular, distinct structures,[496] and made them indistinguishable ultrastructurally from many purified amyloids.[95] This analogy was extended after the prion rods were found to display the tinctorial properties of amyloids.[416] These findings were followed by the demonstration that amyloid plaques in the brains of humans and other animals with prion diseases contain PrP, as determined by immunoreactivity and amino acid sequencing.[29,117,275,425,460]

The formation of prion rods requires limited proteolysis in the presence of detergent.[320] The prion rods in fractions enriched for scrapie infectivity are largely, if not entirely, artifacts of the purification protocol. Solubilization of PrP 27-30 into liposomes with retention of infectivity[167] demonstrated that large PrP polymers are not required for infectivity and permitted the immunoaffinity copurification of PrPSc and infectivity.[166,169] In scrapie-infected mouse neuroblastoma cells, immunocytochemical studies demonstrated PrPSc confined largely to secondary lysosomes; there was no ultrastructural evidence for polymers of PrP.[321] Numerous amyloid plaques were found in Tg(SHaPrP) mice inoculated with SHa prions, but none were observed if these mice were inoculated with Mo prions, indicating that amyloid formation is not an obligatory feature of prion diseases.[401,418] In accord with these Tg(SHaPrP) mouse studies, PrP plaques are consistently found in some inherited prion diseases[182] but are absent in others.[233]

TRANSGENETICS AND GENE TARGETING

Although transgenetic studies have yielded a wealth of new knowledge about infectious, genetic, and sporadic prion diseases, the laborious production of Tg mice limits the number of studies that can be performed. Transgenetic studies can yield an incomplete, and sometimes erroneous, interpretation of the data if the number of lines of mice examined expressing a particular construct is inadequate. Defining an adequate number of lines is difficult, but certainly comparisons of lines expressing high and low levels of a given PrP transgene have proved helpful.[232,418]

Species Barriers for Transmission of Prion Diseases

The passage of prions between species is a stochastic process characterized by prolonged incubation times.[374,375,378] Prions synthesized de novo reflect the sequence of the host PrP gene and not that of the PrPSc molecules in the inoculum.[41] On subsequent passage in a homologous host, the incubation time shortens to that recorded for all subsequent passages, and it becomes a nonstochastic process. The species barrier concept is of practical importance in assessing the risk to humans for development of CJD after consumption of scrapie-infected lamb or BSE-infected beef.[210,225,402,489,490]

To test the hypothesis that differences in PrP gene sequences may be responsible for the species barrier, Tg mice expressing SHaPrP were constructed.[418,442] The PrP genes of hamsters and mice encode proteins differing at 16 positions. Incubation times in four lines of Tg(SHaPrP) mice inoculated with Mo prions were prolonged compared to those observed in non-Tg control mice (Fig. 37-3A). Inoculation of Tg(SHaPrP) mice with SHa prions demonstrated abrogation of the species barrier, resulting in abbreviated incubation times as a result

FIG. 37-3. Transgenic (Tg) mice expressing Syrian hamster prion protein (SHaPrP) exhibit species-specific scrapie incubation times, infectious prion synthesis, and neuropathology.[418] (**A**) Scrapie incubation times in non-Tg and four lines of Tg mice expressing SHaPrP and Syrian hamsters (SHa) inoculated intracerebrally with ~10^6 median infective dose (ID_{50}) units of Chandler mouse prions serially passaged in Swiss mice. The four lines of Tg mice have different numbers of transgene copies: Tg69 and Tg71 mice have two to four copies of the SHaPrP transgene, whereas Tg81 have 30 to 50 and Tg7 mice have more than 60. The ordinate indicates the number of days from inoculation to onset of neurologic dysfunction. (**B**) Scrapie incubation times in mice and hamsters inoculated with ~10^7 ID_{50} units of Sc237 prions serially passaged in Syrian hamsters and as described in **A**. (**C**) Brain SHaPrPC levels in mice and hamsters, quantitated by an enzyme-linked immunoassay. (**D**) Brain SHaPrPSc levels as determined by immunoassay in mice and hamsters that were killed after exhibiting clinical signs of scrapie. (**E**) Prion titers in brains of clinically ill animals after inoculation with mouse prions. Brain extracts from non-Tg, Tg71, and Tg81 mice were bioassayed for prions in mice (*left bars*) and in hamsters (*right bars*). (**F**) Prion titers in brains of clinically ill animals after inoculation with hamster prions. Brain extracts from SHa and from Tg71 and Tg81 mice were bioassayed for prions in mice (*left bars*) and in hamsters (*right bars*). (**G**) Neuropathology in non-Tg mice and in Tg(SHaPrP) mice with clinical signs of scrapie after inoculation with mouse prions. Vacuolation was determined in gray matter (*left bars*) and white matter (*center bars*); presence of PrP amyloid plaques was also measured (*right bars*). Vacuolation score: 0, none; 1, rare; 2, modest; 3, moderate; 4, intense. (**H**) Neuropathology in hamsters and Tg mice inoculated with hamster prions. Degree of vacuolation and frequency of PrP amyloid plaques, as in **G**. (Adapted from Prusiner SB. Molecular biology of prion diseases. Science 1991;252: 1515–1522.)

of a nonstochastic process[418,442] (see Fig. 3*B*). The length of the incubation time after inoculation with SHa prions was inversely proportional to the level of SHaPrP^C in the brains of Tg(SHaPrP) mice[418] (Fig. 37-3*B* and *C*). SHaPrP^{Sc} levels in the brains of clinically ill mice were similar in all four Tg(SHaPrP) lines inoculated with SHa prions (see Fig. 37-3*D*). Bioassays of brain extracts from clinically ill Tg(SHaPrP) mice inoculated with Mo prions revealed that only Mo prions but no SHa prions were produced (see Fig. 37-3*E*). Conversely, inoculation of Tg(SHaPrP) mice with SHa prions led to the synthesis of only SHa prions (see Fig. 37-3*F*). Therefore, the de novo synthesis of prions is species specific and reflects the genetic origin of the inoculated prions. Similarly, the neuropathology of Tg(SHaPrP) mice is determined by the genetic origin of the prion inoculum. Mo prions injected into Tg(SHaPrP) mice produced a neuropathology characteristic of mice with scrapie. A moderate degree of vacuolation in both the gray and white matter was found, but amyloid plaques were rarely detected (see Fig. 37-3*G*; Table 37-3). Inoculation of Tg(SHaPrP) mice with SHa prions produced intense vacuolation of the gray matter, sparing of the white matter, and numerous SHaPrP amyloid plaques characteristic of scrapie in Syrian hamsters (Fig. 37-3*H*).

Overexpression of Wild-Type PrP Transgenes

During transgenetic studies, my colleagues and I discovered that uninoculated older mice harboring high copy numbers of wtPrP transgenes derived from Syrian hamsters, sheep, and PrP-B mice spontaneously developed truncal ataxia, hind-limb paralysis, and tremors.[482] These Tg mice exhibited a profound necrotizing myopathy involving skeletal muscle, a demyelinating polyneuropathy, and focal vacuolation of the CNS. Development of disease was dependent on transgene dosage. For example, Tg(SHaPrP$^{+/+}$)7 mice homozygous for the SHaPrP

transgene array regularly developed disease between 400 and 600 days of age, whereas hemizygous Tg(SHaPrP$^{+/0}$)7 mice also developed disease, but after more than 650 days.

Attempts to demonstrate PrP^{Sc} in either muscle or brain were unsuccessful, but transmission of disease with brain extracts from Tg(SHaPrP$^{+/+}$)7 mice inoculated into Syrian hamsters did occur. These Syrian hamsters had PrP^{Sc}, as detected by immunoblotting and spongiform degeneration (D Groth, SB Prusiner, unpublished data). Serial passage with brain extracts from these animals to recipients was observed. De novo synthesis of prions in Tg(SHaPrP$^{+/+}$)7 mice overexpressing wtSHaPrP^C provides support for the hypothesis that sporadic CJD does not result from infection but rather is a consequence of the spontaneous, although rare, conversion of PrP^C into PrP^{Sc}. Alternatively, a somatic mutation in which mutant SHaPrP^C is spontaneously converted into PrP^{Sc}, as in the inherited prion diseases, could also explain sporadic CJD. These findings as well as those described later for Tg(MoPrP-P101L) mice argue that prions are devoid of foreign nucleic acid, in accord with many earlier studies, already described, that used other experimental approaches.

Ablation of the PrP Gene

Ablation of the PrP gene in Tg (Prnp$^{0/0}$) mice has, unexpectedly, not affected the development of these animals.[71] In fact, they are healthy at almost 2 years of age. Prnp$^{0/0}$ mice are resistant to prions (Fig. 37-4) and do not propagate scrapie infectivity.[70,409] Prnp$^{0/0}$ mice were sacrificed 5, 60, 120, or 315 days after inoculation with RML prions passaged in CD-1 Swiss mice. Except for residual infectivity from the inoculum detected at 5 days after inoculation, no infectivity was detected in the brains of Prnp$^{0/0}$ mice (Table 37-4).

Prnp$^{0/0}$ mice crossed with Tg(SHaPrP) mice were rendered susceptible to SHa prions but remained resistant to Mo prions.[70,409] Because the absence of PrP^C expression does not pro-

TABLE 37-3. *Species-specific prion inocula determine the distribution of spongiform change and deposition of PrP amyloid plaques in transgenic mice**

| Animal | n | SHa prions | | | | n | Mo prions | | |
| | | Spongiform change | | PrP plaques | | | Spongiform change | | PrP plaques |
		Gray	White	Frequency	Diameter (mean±SE [no.])		Gray	White	Frequency
Non-Tg		N.D.		N.D.		10	+	+	−
Tg 69	6	+	−	Numerous	6.5±3.1 (389)	2	+	+	−
Tg 71	5	+	−	Numerous	8.1±3.6 (345)	2	+	+	−
Tg 81	7	+	−	Numerous	8.3±3.0 (439)	3	+	+	Few
Tg 7	3	+†	−	Numerous	14.0±8.3 (19)	4	+	+	−
SHa	3	+	−	Numerous	5.7±2.7 (247)		N.D.		N.D.

n, number of brains examined; N.D., not determined; +, present; −, not found; Tg, transgenic mouse; SHa, Syrian hamster.

*Spongiform change evaluated in hippocampus, thalamus, cerebral cortex, and brain stem for gray matter and the deep cerebellum for white matter. Plaques in the subcallosal region were stained with SHaPrP mAb 13A5, anti-PrP rabbit antisera R073, and trichrome stain.

†Focal: confirmed to the dorsal nucleus of the raphe.

From Prusiner SB. Molecular biology and genetics of neurodegenerative diseases caused by prions. Adv Virus Res 1992;41:241–280.

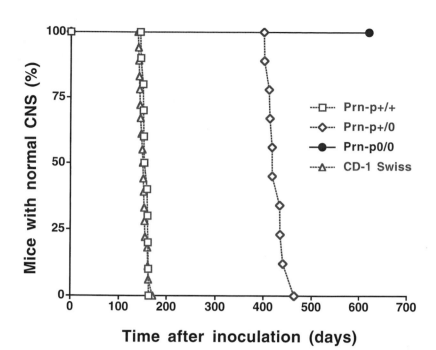

FIG. 37-4. Incubation times in PrP gene-ablated (Prnp[0/0]), hemizygous (Prnp[0/+]), wild-type (Prnp[+/+]), and CD-1 mice inoculated with RML mouse prions, which were heated and irradiated at 254 nm before intracerebral inoculation.

voke disease, it is likely that scrapie and other prion diseases are a consequence of PrP^Sc accumulation rather than an inhibition of PrP^C function.[71]

Mice heterozygous (Prnp[0/+]) for ablation of the PrP gene had prolonged incubation times when inoculated with Mo prions[409] (see Fig. 37-4). The Prnp[0/+] mice developed signs of neurologic dysfunction at 400 to 460 days after inoculation. These findings are in accord with studies on Tg(SHaPrP) mice, in which increased SHaPrP expression was accompanied by diminished incubation times[418] (see Fig. 37-3B).

Because Prnp[0/0] mice do not express PrP^C, they may more readily produce α-PrP antibodies. Prnp[0/0] mice immunized with Mo or SHa prion rods produced α-PrP antisera that bound Mo, SHa, and Hu PrP.[409] These findings contrast with earlier studies in which α-MoPrP antibodies could not be produced in mice, presumably because the mice had been rendered tolerant by the presence of MoPrP^C.[21,253,427] That Prnp[0/0] mice readily produce α-PrP antibodies is consistent with the hypothesis that the lack of an immune response in prion diseases is a result of the fact that PrP^C and PrP^Sc share many epitopes. Whether Prnp[0/0] mice produce α-PrP antibodies that specifically recognize conformation-dependent epitopes present on PrP^Sc but absent from PrP^C remains to be determined.

TABLE 37-4. *Prion titers in brains of Prnp[0/0] and Prnp[0/+] mice**

| Mouse | Time of sacrifice after inoculation with RML scrapie prions | | | | |
	5 days	60 days	120 days	315 days	500 days
Prnp[+/+]	<1	3.9±0.4	6.4±0.3		
	<1	4.8±0.3	7.1±0.1		
	<1	4.6±0.2	6.6±0.2		
Prnp[+/0]	<1	<1	5.1±0.2		
	0.6 ± 0.7	<1	5.2±0.6		
	1.2 ± 0.1†	3.4±0.2	2.8±0.1		
Prnp[0/0]	<1‡	<1	<1	<1	<1
	<1§	<1	<1	<1	<1
	<1				<1
					<1

*Log scrapie prion titers (median infective dose units/mL ± SE) are shown. Titers are for 10% (weight/volume) brain homogenates. Log titers of <1 reflect no signs of central nervous system dysfunction in CD-1 mice for >250 days after inoculation except as noted. Each entry represents a single mouse.

†3/9 mice developed scrapie between 208 and 210 days after inoculation.

‡2/9 mice developed scrapie between 208 and 225 days after inoculation.

§2/10 mice developed scrapie between 208 and 225 days after inoculation.

Modeling of GSS in Tg(MoPrP-P101L) Mice

The codon 102 point mutation found in GSS patients was introduced into the MoPrP gene and Tg(MoPrP-P101L)H mice were created; these animals express high (H) levels of the mutant transgene product. The two lines of Tg(MoPrP-P101L)H mice designated 174 and 87 spontaneously developed CNS degeneration, characterized by clinical signs indistinguishable from those of experimental murine scrapie and neuropathology consisting of widespread spongiform morphology, astrocytic gliosis,[235] and PrP amyloid plaques[232] (Fig. 37-5). By inference, these results contend that PrP gene mutations cause GSS, familial CJD, and FFI.

Brain extracts prepared from spontaneously ill Tg(MoPrP-P101L)H mice transmitted CNS degeneration to Tg196 mice. These mice express low levels of the mutant transgene product but do not develop spontaneous disease. In addition, some Syrian hamsters developed disease after inoculation with brain extracts from spontaneously ill Tg(MoPrP-P101L)H mice.[232] Many Tg196 mice and some Syrian hamsters developed CNS degeneration between 200 and 700 days after inoculation, whereas inoculated CD-1 Swiss mice remained well. Serial transmission of CNS degeneration in Tg196 mice required about 1 year, whereas serial transmission in Syrian hamsters occurred after 75 days.[232] Although brain extracts prepared from Tg(MoPrP-P101L)H mice transmitted CNS degeneration to some inoculated recipients, little or no PrP^{Sc} was detected by immunoassays after limited proteolysis. Undetectable or low levels of PrP^{Sc} in the brains of these Tg(MoPrP-P101L)H mice are consistent with the results of these transmission experiments, which suggest low titers of infectious prions. Although no PrP^{Sc} was detected in the brains of inoculated Tg196 mice exhibiting neurologic dysfunction by immunoassays after limited proteolysis, PrP

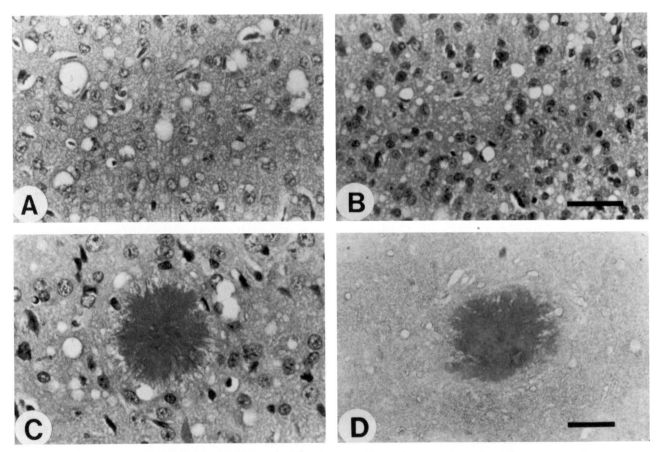

FIG. 37-5. Neuropathology of Tg(MoPrP-P101L) mice developing spontaneous neurodegeneration. The mice harbor transgenes carrying the PrP point mutation found in Gerstmann-Sträussler-Scheinker (GSS) disease of humans. (**A**) Vacuolation in cerebral cortex of a Swiss CD-1 mouse that exhibited signs of neurologic dysfunction at 138 days after intracerebral inoculation with ~10^6 median infective dose (ID$_{50}$) units of RML scrapie prions. (**B**) Vacuolation in cerebral cortex of a Tg(MoPrP-P101L) mouse that exhibited signs of neurologic dysfunction at 252 days of age. Bar in **B** = 50 μm and also applies to **A**. (**C**) Kuru-type PrP amyloid plaque stained with periodic acid-Schiff stain in the caudate nucleus of a Tg(MoPrP-P101L) mouse that exhibited signs of neurologic dysfunction. (**D**) PrP amyloid plaques stained with α-PrP antiserum (RO73) in the caudate nucleus of a Tg(MoPrP-P101L) mouse that exhibited signs of neurologic dysfunction. Bar in **D** = 25 μm and also applies to **C**. (From Prusiner SB. Transgenetics and cell biology of prion diseases: investigations of PrP^{Sc} synthesis and diversity. Br Med Bull 1993;49:873–912.)

amyloid plaques and spongiform degeneration were frequently found.

The neurodegeneration found in inoculated Tg196 mice probably results from a modification of mutant PrP^C that is initiated by mutant PrP^{Sc} present in the brain extracts prepared from ill Tg(MoPrP-P101L)H mice. In support of this explanation are the findings in some of the inherited human prion diseases that have been described, in which neither protease-resistant PrP[59,323] nor transmission to experimental rodents could be demonstrated.[467] Furthermore, transmission of disease from Tg(MoPrP-P101L)H mice to Tg196 mice but not to Swiss mice is consistent with earlier findings demonstrating that homotypic interactions between PrP^C and PrP^{Sc} markedly enhance the formation of PrP^{Sc}. Why Syrian hamsters are more permissive than Swiss mice for prion transmission from Tg(MoPrP-P101L)H mice is unknown. Presumably, transmission to hamsters reflects differences in tertiary structure between the two substrates SHaPrP^C and MoPrP^C.

In other studies, modification of the expression of mutant and wtPrP genes in Tg mice permitted experimental manipulation of the pathogenesis of both inherited and infectious prion diseases. Although overexpression of the wtPrP-A transgene 8-fold was not deleterious to the mice, it did shorten scrapie incubation times from 145 to 45 days after inoculation with Mo scrapie prions.[470a] In contrast, overexpression at the same level of a PrP-A transgene mutated at codon 101 produced spontaneous, fatal neurodegeneration between 150 and 300 days of age in two new lines of Tg(MoPrP-P101L) mice, designated 2866 and 2247. Genetic crosses of Tg(MoPrP-P101L)2866 mice with gene-targeted mice lacking both PrP alleles (Prnp$^{0/0}$) produced animals with a highly synchronous onset of spontaneous illness between 150 and 160 days of age. The Tg(MoPrP-P101L)2866/Prnp$^{0/0}$ mice had numerous PrP plaques and widespread spongiform degeneration, in contrast to the Tg2866 and Tg2247 mice, which exhibited spongiform degeneration but only a few PrP amyloid plaques. Another line of mice, designated Tg2862, overexpress the mutant transgene 32-fold and develop fatal neurodegeneration between 200 and 400 days of age. Tg2862 mice exhibited the most severe spongiform degeneration and had numerous, large PrP amyloid plaques.

Although mutant PrP^C(P101L) clearly produces neurodegeneration, wtPrP^C profoundly modifies both the age of onset of illness and the neuropathology for a given level of transgene expression. These findings and those from other studies[471] suggest that mutant and wtPrP interact, perhaps through a chaperone-like protein, to modify the pathogenesis of the dominantly inherited prion diseases.

SOME PROTEINS THAT ARE NOT ENCODED BY PrP GENES MAY MODIFY PRION DISEASES

As described previously, PrP transgenes can modulate virtually all aspects of scrapie, including prion propagation, incubation time length, synthesis of PrP^{Sc}, the species barrier, and neuropathologic lesions. Evidence for the role of proteins not encoded by PrP genes is now beginning to emerge. In particular, studies with Tg(MHu2M) and Tg(HuPrP) mice argue for the existence of a species-specific factor that has provisionally been designated protein X.[471] Investigations of prion strains in congenic mice suggest that a gene linked to but separate from PrP profoundly modifies the neuropathology of scrapie[75]; the product of this gene has provisionally been designated protein Y.

Protein X and the Transmission of Prions

Attempts to abrogate the prion species barrier between humans and mice by using an approach similar to that described for the abrogation of the species barrier between Syrian hamsters and mice were unsuccessful. Mice expressing HuPrP transgenes did not develop signs of CNS dysfunction more rapidly or frequently than non-Tg controls.[471]

The successful breaking of the species barrier between humans and mice had its origins in a set of studies with Tg mice expressing chimeric PrP genes derived from SHa and Mo PrP genes.[444] One SHa/MoPrP gene, designated MH2M PrP, contains five amino acid substitutions encoded by SHaPrP; another construct, designated MHM2 PrP, has two substitutions. Tg(MH2M PrP) mice were susceptible to both SHa or Mo prions, whereas three lines expressing MHM2 PrP were resistant to SHa prions.[443] The brains of Tg(MH2M PrP) mice dying of scrapie contained chimeric PrP^{Sc} and prions with an artificial host range favoring propagation in mice that express the corresponding chimeric PrP, and were also transmissible, at reduced efficiency, to non-Tg mice and hamsters. These findings provided additional genetic evidence for homophilic interactions between PrP^{Sc} in the inoculum and PrP^C synthesized by the host.

With the recognition that Tg(HuPrP) mice were not suitable recipients for the transmission of Hu prions, Tg(MHu2M) mice, analogous to the Tg(MH2M) mice just described, were constructed. Hu PrP differs from Mo PrP at 28 of 254 positions,[283] whereas chimeric MHu2MPrP differs at 9 residues. The mice expressing the MHu2M transgene are susceptible to human prions and exhibit abbreviated incubation times of 200 days.[471] In these initial studies, the chimeric MHu2M transgene encoded a methionine (Met) at codon 129, and all three of the patients were homozygous for Met at this residue. Two of the cases were sporadic CJD, and the third was an iatrogenic case that occurred after treatment with pituitary-derived human growth hormone (HGH). Whether it is necessary to match the PrP genotype of the Tg(MHu2M) mouse with that of the CJD patient from whom the inoculum is derived, or whether some variations in sequence can be tolerated, remains to be established.

From Tg(SHaPrP) mouse studies, prion propagation is thought to involve the formation of a complex between PrP^{Sc} and the homotypic substrate PrP^C.[418] Attempts to mix PrP^{Sc} with PrP^C have failed to produce nascent PrP^{Sc},[421] raising the possibility that proteins such as chaperones may be involved in catalyzing the conformational changes that feature in the formation of PrP^{Sc}.[369] One explanation for the difference in susceptibility of Tg(MHu2M) and Tg(HuPrP) mice to Hu prions in mice may be that mouse chaperones catalyzing the refolding of PrP^C into PrP^{Sc} can readily interact with the MHu2MPrP^C/HuPrP^{CJD} complex but not with HuPrP^C/HuPrP^{CJD}. The identification of protein X is an important avenue of research, because isolation of this protein or complex of proteins would presumably facilitate studies of PrP^{Sc} formation. To date, attempts to isolate specific proteins that bind to PrP have been disappointing.[355] Whether identification of protein X requires isolation of a ternary complex composed of PrP^C, PrP^Sc, and protein X remains to be determined.

The sensitivity of Tg(MHu2M) mice to Hu prions suggests that a similar approach to the construction of Tg mice susceptible to BSE and scrapie sheep prions may prove fruitful. The BSE epidemic has led to considerable concern about the safety for humans of consumption of beef and dairy products. Although epidemiologic studies over the past two decades argue that humans do not contract CJD from scrapie-infected sheep products,[53,104,218] it is unknown whether any of the seven amino acid substitutions that distinguish bovine from sheep PrP render bovine prions permissive in humans.[402] Whether Tg(MHu2M) mice are susceptible to bovine or sheep prions is unknown.

Protein Y and the Neuropathology of Prion Disease

Concurrent with many of the transgenic mouse studies already described, four lines of congenic mice were produced by crossing the PrP gene of the ILn/J mouse onto C57BL. The four lines of congenic mice were derived by backcrosses through 20 generations which are designated as follows: B6.I-4 for B6.I-*B2m^a*, B6.I-1 for B6.I-*Prnp^b*, B6.I-2 for B6.I-*Il-1a^d Prnp^b*, and B6.I-3 for B6.I-*B2m^a Prnp^b*.[74] Neuropathologic examination of B6.I-1, B6.I-2, ILn/J, and VM/Dk mice inoculated with 87V prions showed numerous PrP amyloid plaques, in accord with an earlier report on VM/Dk mice.[67] In B6.I-1 mice, intense spongiform degeneration, gliosis, and PrP immunostaining were found in the ventral posterior lateral nucleus of the thalamus, the habenula, and the raphe nuclei of the brain stem.[75] These same regions showed intense immunoreactivity for PrP^Sc on histoblots. Unexpectedly, B6.I-2 and ILn/J mice exhibited only mild vacuolation of the thalamus and brain stem. These findings suggest that a locus near *Prnp* influences the deposition of PrP^Sc, and thus vacuolation, in the thalamus, the habenula, and raphe nuclei. The product of this gene has provisionally been designated protein Y. The gene Y product appears to control, at least in part, neuronal vacuolation and presumably PrP^Sc deposition in mice inoculated with scrapie prions. Isolation of protein Y should be helpful in dissecting the molecular events in the pathogenesis of the prion diseases.

PRION DIVERSITY

Prion Strains and Variations in Patterns of Disease

For many years, studies of experimental scrapie were performed exclusively with sheep and goats. The disease was first transmitted by intraocular inoculation[108] and later by intracerebral, oral, subcutaneous, intramuscular, and intravenous injection of brain extracts from scrapied sheep. Incubation periods of 1 to 3 years were common, and many of the inoculated animals failed to develop disease.[134,214,215] Different breeds of sheep exhibited markedly different susceptibilities to scrapie

prions inoculated subcutaneously, suggesting that genetic background may influence host permissiveness.[212]

Length of incubation time has been used to distinguish prion strains inoculated into sheep, goats, mice, and hamsters. Dickinson and his colleagues developed a system for strain typing, by which mice with genetically determined short and long incubation times were used in combination with the F1 cross.[123,129,130] For example, C57BL mice exhibited short incubation times of 150 days if inoculated with either the Me7 or Chandler isolates; VM mice inoculated with these same isolates had prolonged incubation times of 300 days. The mouse gene controlling incubation times was labeled *Sinc*, and long incubation times were said to be a dominant trait because of prolonged incubation times in F1 mice. Prion strains were categorized into two groups: (1) those causing disease more rapidly in short-incubation C57BL mice and (2) those causing disease more rapidly in long-incubation VM mice. Noteworthy are the 22a and 87V prion strains, which can be passaged in VM mice while maintaining their distinct characteristics.

PrP Gene Dosage Controls the Length of the Scrapie Incubation Time

More than a decade of study was required to unravel the mechanism responsible for the dominance of long incubation times. As a result, long incubation times were found not to be dominant traits; instead, their apparent dominance is caused by a gene dosage effect.[75]

Studies by my group began with the identification of a widely available mouse strain with long incubation times. ILn/J mice inoculated with RML prions were found to have incubation times exceeding 200 days,[265] a finding that was confirmed by others.[80] After molecular clones of the PrP gene were available, we asked whether the PrP genes of short-incubation and long-incubation mice segregate with the incubation times. A restriction fragment length polymorphism of the PrP gene was used to follow the segregation of MoPrP genes (*Prnp*) from short-incubation NZW or C57BL mice with long-incubation ILn/J mice in F1 and F2 crosses. This approach permitted the demonstration of genetic linkage between *Prnp* and a gene modulating incubation times (*Prn-i*).[77] Other investigators have confirmed the genetic linkage, and one group has shown that the incubation time gene *Sinc* is also linked to PrP.[245,420] It now seems likely that the genes for PrP, *Prn-i*, and *Sinc* are all congruent; the term *Sinc* is no longer used.[353] The PrP sequences of NZW with short and long scrapie incubation times, respectively, differ at codons 108 (Leu → phenylalanine [Phe]) and 189 (threonine [Thr] → valine [Val]).[484]

Although the amino acid substitutions in PrP that distinguish *Prnp^a* from *Prnp^b* mice argued for the congruency of *Prnp* and *Prn-i*, experiments with *Prnp^a* mice expressing *Prnp^b* transgenes demonstrated shortening of incubation times.[485] It had been predicted that these Tg mice would exhibit a prolongation of the incubation time after inoculation with RML prions, based on (*Prnp^a* × *Prnp^b*) F1 mice, which do exhibit long incubation times. These findings were described as paradoxical shortening because my group and others had believed for many years that long incubation times were dominant traits.[77,130] From studies of congenic and transgenic mice expressing different numbers of the *a* and *b* alleles of *Prnp* (Table 37-5), it is now clear that these findings were not paradoxical; instead, they resulted from increased PrP gene dosage.[75] If the RML isolate was inoculated into congenic and Tg mice, an increase in the number of copies of the *a* allele was found to be the major determinant in reducing the incubation time; however, an increase in the number of copies of the *b* allele also reduced the incubation time, but not to the same extent as that seen with the *a* allele (see Table 37-5).

The discovery that incubation times are controlled by the relative dosage of *Prnp*[a] and *Prnp*[b] alleles was foreshadowed by studies of Tg(SHaPrP) mice in which the length of the incubation time after inoculation with SHa prions was inversely proportional to the level of the transgene product, SHaPrP[C].[418] Not only does the PrP gene dose determine the length of the incubation time, but so does the passage history of the inoculum, particularly in *Prnp*[b] mice (Table 37-6). The PrP[Sc] allotype in the inoculum produced the shortest incubation times when it was the same as that of PrP[C] in the host.[78] The term allotype is used to describe allelic variants of PrP. To address the issue of whether gene products other than PrP may be responsible for these findings, my colleagues and I inoculated B6 and B6.I-4 mice carrying *Prnp*[a/a], as well as I/Ln and B6.I-2 mice,[74,75] with RML prions passaged in mice homozygous for either the *a* or *b* allele of *Prnp* (see Table 37-6). CD-1 and NZW/LacJ mice produced prions containing PrP[Sc]-A encoded by *Prnp*[a], whereas ILn/J mice produced PrP[Sc]-B prions. The incubation times in the congenic mice reflected the PrP allotype rather than other factors acquired during prion passage.

The effect of the allotype barrier was small when measured in *Prnp*[a/a] mice but was clearly demonstrable in *Prnp*[b/b] mice. B6.I-2 congenic mice inoculated with prions from I/Ln mice had an incubation time of 237±18 days, compared with times of 360±116 days and 404±14 days for mice inoculated with prions passaged in CD-1 and NZW mice, respectively. Therefore, previous passage of prions in *Prnp*[b] mice shortened the incubation time by 40% when assayed in *Prnp*[b] mice, compared with passage in *Prnp*[a] mice.[78]

Overdominance

The phenomenon of overdominance, in which incubation times in F1 hybrids are longer than those of either parent,[128] contributed to the confusion surrounding control of scrapie incubation times. When the 22A scrapie isolate was inoculated into B6, B6.I-1, and (B6 × B6.I-1)F1 mice, overdominance was observed: the scrapie incubation time in B6 mice was 405±2 days, in B6.I mice 194±10 days, and in (B6 × B6.I-1)F1 mice 508±14 days (Table 37-7). Shorter incubation times were observed in Tg(MoPrP-B)15 mice that were either homozygous or hemizygous for the *Prnp*[b] transgene. Hemizygous Tg(MoPrP-B[+/0])15 mice exhibited a scrapie incubation time of 395±12 days, whereas the homozygous mice had an incubation time of 286±15 days.

As with the RML isolate (see Table 37-5), the findings with the 22A isolate can be explained on the basis of gene dosage; however, the relative effects of the *a* and *b* alleles differ in two

TABLE 37-5. *MoPrP-A expression is a major determinant of incubation times in mice inoculated with RML scrapie prions previously passaged in CD-1 (Prnp[a/a]) mice*

Mice	Prnp genotype (copies)	Prnp transgenes (copies)	Alleles		Incubation time* (days ± SEM)	Number of mice
			a	*b*		
Prnp[0/0]	0/0	—	0	0	>600	4
Prnp[+/0]	a/0	—	1	0	426±18	9*
B6.I-1	b/b	—	0	2	360±16	7†
B6.I-2	b/b	—	0	2	379±8	10†
B6.I-3	b/b	—	0	2	404±10	20
(B6 × B6.I-1)F1	a/b	—	1	1	268±4	7
B6.I-1 × Tg(MoPrP-B[0/0])15	a/b	—	1	1	255±7	11‡
B6.I-1 × Tg(MoPrP-B[0/0])15	a/b	—	1	1	274±3	9§
B6.I-1 × Tg(MoPrP-B[+/0])15	a/b	bbb/0	1	4	166±2	11‡
B6.I-1 × Tg(MoPrP-B[+/0])15	a/b	bbb/0	1	4	162±3	8§
C57BL/6J (B6)	a/a	—	2	0	143±4	8
B6.I-4	a/a	—	2	0	144±5	8
non-Tg(MoPrP-B[0/0])15	a/a	—	2	0	130±3	10
Tg(MoPrP-B[+/0])15	a/a	bbb/0	2	3	115±2	18
Tg(MoPrP-B[+/+])15	a/a	bbb/bbb	2	6	111±5	5
Tg(MoPrP-B[+/0])94	a/a	>30b	2	>30	75±2	15‖
Tg(MoPrP-A[+/0])B4053	a/a	>30a	>30	0	50±2	16

*Data from Prusiner et al, 1993.[409]

†Data from Carlson et al, 1993.[74]

‡The homozygous Tg(MoPrP-B[+/+])15 mice were maintained as a distinct subline selected for transgene homozygosity two generations removed from the (B6 × LT/Sv)F2 founder. Hemizygous Tg(MoPrP-B[+/0])15 mice were produed by crossing the Tg(MoPrP-B[+/+])15 line with B6 mice.

§Tg(MoPrP-B[+/0])15 mice were maintained by repeated backcrossing to B6 mice.

‖Data from Westaway et al, 1991.[485]

TABLE 37-6. *Mismatching of PrP allotypes between PrP^{Sc} in the inoculum and PrP^{C} in the inoculated host extends prion incubation times in congenic mice*

| Mice | Inoculum donor | | | Recipient host | |
	Genotype	Donor	Genotype	Incubation time	Number of mice
C57BL/6J (B6)	a/a	CD-1	a/a	143±4	8
B6.I-4	a/a	NZW	a/a	144±5	8
B6.I-4	a/a	I/Ln	b/b	150±6	6
B6.I-2	b/b	I/Ln	b/b	237±8	17
I/LnJ	b/b	I/Ln	b/b	193±6	16
B6.I-2	b/b	CD-1	a/a	360±16	8
B6.I-2	b/b	NZW	a/a	404±4	20
I/LnJ*	b/b	CD-1	a/a	314±13	11
I/LnJ	b/b	NZW	a/a	283±21	8

*I/LnJ results previously reported (Carlson et al, 1994[75]).

respects. First, the *b* allele is the major determinant of scrapie incubation time with the 22A isolate, not the *a* allele. Second, increasing the number of copies of the *a* allele does not diminish the incubation but prolongs it: the *a* allele is inhibitory with the 22A isolate (see Table 37-7). With the 87V prion isolate, the inhibitory effect of the *Prnp^a* allele is even more pronounced, because only a few *Prnp^a* and (*Prnp^a* × *Prnp^b*)F1 mice develop scrapie after more than 600 days since inoculation.[75]

The most interesting feature of the incubation time profile for 22A is the overdominance of the *a* allele of *Prnp* in prolonging incubation period. On the basis of overdominance, Dickinson and Outram put forth the replication site hypothesis, postulating that dimers of the *Sinc* gene product feature in the replication of the scrapie agent.[132] The results in Table 37-7 are compatible with the interpretation that the target for PrP^{Sc} may be a PrP^C dimer or multimer. The assumptions under this model are that PrP^C-B dimers are more readily converted to PrP^{Sc} than are PrP^C-A dimers and that PrP^C-A:PrP^C-B heterodimers are even more resistant to conversion to PrP^{Sc} than PrP^C-A dimers. Increasing the ratio of PrP-B to PrP-A would lead to shorter incubation times by favoring the formation of PrP^C-B homodimers (see Table 37-7). A similar mecha-

nism may account for the relative paucity of individuals heterozygous for the Met/Val polymorphism at codon 129 of the human PrP gene in spontaneous and iatrogenic CJD[366] (see later discussion). Alternatively, PrP^C-PrP^{Sc} interaction can be broken down to two distinct aspects: binding affinity and efficacy of conversion to PrP^{Sc}. If PrP-A has a higher affinity for 22A PrP^{Sc} than does PrP^C-B but is inefficiently converted to PrP^{Sc}, the exceptionally long incubation time of *Prnp$^{a/b}$* heterozygotes may reflect reduction in the supply of 22A prions available for interaction with the PrP^C-B product of the single *Prnp^b* allele. In addition, PrP^C-A may inhibit the interaction of 22A PrP^{Sc} with PrP^C-B, leading to prolongation of the incubation time. This interpretation is supported by prolonged incubation times in Tg(SHaPrP) mice inoculated with Mo prions, in which case SHaPrP^C is thought to inhibit the binding of MoPrP^{Sc} to the substrate MoPrP^C.[418]

Patterns of PrP^{Sc} Deposition

In addition to measurements of incubation time, profiles of spongiform degeneration have also been used to characterize different prion strains.[159,161] With the development of a new

Table 37-7. *MoPrP^C-A inhibits synthesis of 22A scrapie prions passaged in B6.I-1 mice before inoculation*

| Mice | Prnp genotype | Prnp transgenes (copies) | Alleles | | Incubation time (days ± SEM) | Number of mice |
| | | | *a* | *b* | | |
			(copies)			
B6.I-1	b/b	—	0	2	194±10	7
(B6 × B6.I-1)F1	a/b	—	1	1	508±14	7
C57BL/6J (B6)	a/a	—	2	0	405±2	8
non-Tg(MoPrP-B$^{0/0}$)15	a/a	—	2	0	378±8	3*
Tg(MoPrP-B$^{+/0}$)15	a/a	bbb/0	2	3	318±14	15*
Tg(MoPrP-B$^{+/0}$)15	a/a	bbb/0	2	3	395±12	6†
Tg(MoPrP-B$^{+/+}$)15	a/a	bbb/bbb	2	6	266±1	6*
Tg(MoPrP-B$^{+/+}$)15	a/a	bbb/bbb	2	6	286±15	5†

*The homozygous Tg(MoPrP-B$^{+/+}$)15 mice were maintained as a distinct subline selected for transgene homozygosity two generations removed from the (B6 × LT/Sv)F2 founder. Hemizygous Tg(MoPrP-B$^{+/0}$)15 mice were produced by crossing the Tg(MoPrP-B$^{+/+}$)15 line with B6 mice.

†Tg(MoPrP-B$^{+/0}$)15 mice were maintained by repeated backcrossing to B6 mice.

procedure for in situ detection of PrP[Sc], designated histoblotting,[464] it became possible to localize and quantify PrP[Sc] and to determine whether different strains produce different, reproducible patterns of PrP[Sc] accumulation (see Fig. 37-2).[119,220]

Histoblotting overcame two obstacles that plagued PrP[Sc] detection in brain by standard immunohistochemical techniques: the presence of PrP[C] and weak antigenicity of PrP[Sc].[118] The histoblot is made by pressing 10-μm thick cryostat sections of fresh frozen brain tissue to nitrocellulose paper. To localize protease-resistant PrP[Sc] in brain, the histoblot is digested with proteinase K to eliminate PrP[C], and then the undigested PrP[Sc] is denatured to enhance binding of PrP antibodies. Immunohistochemical staining yields a far more intense, specific, and reproducible PrP signal than can be achieved by immunohistochemistry on standard tissue sections. The intensity of immunostaining correlates well with neurochemical estimates of PrP[Sc] concentration in homogenates of dissected brain regions. PrP[C] can be localized in histoblots of uninfected, normal brains by eliminating the proteinase K digestion step.

Comparisons of PrP[Sc] accumulation on histoblots with histologic sections showed that PrP[Sc] deposition preceded vacuolation, and only those regions with PrP[Sc] underwent degeneration. Microdissection of individual brain regions confirmed the conclusions of the histoblot studies: those regions with high levels of PrP 27-30 had intense vacuolation.[82] It was therefore concluded that the deposition of PrP[Sc] is responsible for the neuropathologic changes found in the prion diseases.

Although studies with both mice and Syrian hamsters established that each isolate has a specific signature as defined by a specific pattern of PrP[Sc] accumulation in the brain,[75,119,220] comparisons must be done on an isogenic background.[232,443] When a single strain was inoculated in mice expressing different PrP genes, variations in the patterns of PrP[Sc] accumulation were found to be equally as great as those seen between two strains. Based on the initial studies, which were performed in animals of a single genotype, it was suggested that PrP[Sc] synthesis occurs in specific populations of cells for a given distinct prion isolate.

Prion Strain Specific Patterns of PrP[Sc] Accumulation

RML prions were inoculated into B6 or B6.I-1 congenic mice,[74,75] and the patterns of PrP[Sc] accumulation were compared (see Fig. 37-6A through F). First, the PrP[Sc] signal was more widely and more uniformly distributed in the neocortex and hippocampus in B6 mice (compare Figs. 6B and E). Second, the PrP[Sc] signal was more intense in the granule cell layer of the cerebellum in B6.I-1 mice (compare Figs. 37-6F and C). Third, PrP[Sc] accumulated preferentially in the cerebellar white matter in B6 mice but not in B6.I-1 mice (compare Figs. 6C and F). Other differences were also apparent, such as a weaker signal in the hypothalamus in B6.I-1 mice. These findings argue that the distribution of PrP[Sc] is influenced by both the infecting prion and the amino acid sequence of PrP[C].

Although the distributions of PrP[Sc] in the brains of B6.I-1 mice inoculated with RML or 22A were similar, clear differences were observed (see Figs. 6D through I). For example, there was a more intense PrP[Sc] signal in the molecular layer of the dentate gyrus with RML than with 22A, although the hy-

pothalamus contained more PrP[Sc] in the mice inoculated with 22A prions. The full thickness of the neocortex exhibited PrP[Sc] immunostaining with 22A prions, but only the inner layers stained with RML; this is reminiscent of the differences between Sc237 and 139H scrapie in Syrian hamsters.[220] The PrP[Sc] signal was more intense in the corpus callosum and in the white matter tracts coursing through the caudate nucleus with RML than with 22A (compare Figs. 37-6D and G). With both RML and 22A prions, there was intense PrP[Sc] staining in the granule cell layer of the cerebellum and a notable absence of PrP amyloid plaques.

PrP[Sc] deposition with 87V prions was markedly different from that with 22A or RML (see Figs. 37-6D through L) and was most intense in the thalamus, particularly in the ventral posterior lateral nucleus (see Fig. 37-6K), in the habenula (see Fig. 37-6K), and in the locus ceruleus and raphe nuclei of the brain stem (see Fig. 37-6L). Little or no PrP[Sc] accumulated in the neocortex, the hippocampus, or the hypothalamus. Relatively weak PrP[Sc] signals were distributed diffusely in the brain stem tegmentum, inferior colliculi, and amygdala. Multiple intense, punctate signals were located beneath the corpus callosum overlying the hippocampus (see Fig. 36-6K), in the caudate nucleus, and in the cerebellum. Histologic section staining with the periodic acid-Schiff method or α-PrP antibodies indicated that the punctate PrP[Sc] signals were kuru-type and primitive PrP amyloid plaques. Much of the intense PrP[Sc] signal in the raphe nuclei and locus ceruleus of the brain stem (see Fig. 37-6L) seems to be perivascular PrP plaques.

The development of Tg(MHu2M) mice that are highly susceptible to Hu prions offers a new approach to studying prion diversity. The patterns of PrP[Sc] in Tg(MHu2M) mice were remarkably similar for three inocula from humans who had died of CJD.[471] Two of the inocula were from patients who had died of sporadic CJD, and the third was from a patient previously treated with HGH who had died of iatrogenic CJD. Whether these three inocula all represented the same strain of prions or whether differences among them were obscured by passage in the Tg(MHu2M) mice remains to be established. PrP[CJD] accumulation was much greater in the cerebral cortex than in the cerebellum in the two patients with sporadic prion disease, whereas the distribution was reversed the patient with iatrogenic CJD.[121] Studies in rodents have shown that prion strains produce different patterns of PrP[Sc] accumulation,[119,220] which can be changed dramatically by the expression of different PrP sequences.[75,443] Transmission studies of Hu prions from patients dying of CJD or kuru to nonhuman primates suggest that each case may be caused by a different strain.[190]

Mice inoculated intracerebrally or intraperitoneally with Mo prions accumulated PrP[Sc] in follicular dendritic cells, but did not do so if inoculated with Hu prions.[270,317,338,340]

PrP Gene-Specific Patterns of PrP[Sc] Accumulation

Studies of a single isolate inoculated into mice expressing different PrP genes demonstrated that the PrP[Sc] accumulation could be profoundly altered by factors other than strain of prions. For example, the RML isolate inoculated into CD-1 mice and into Tg196 mice expressing the mutant MoPrP-P101L transgene produces much different patterns of PrP[Sc] accumu-

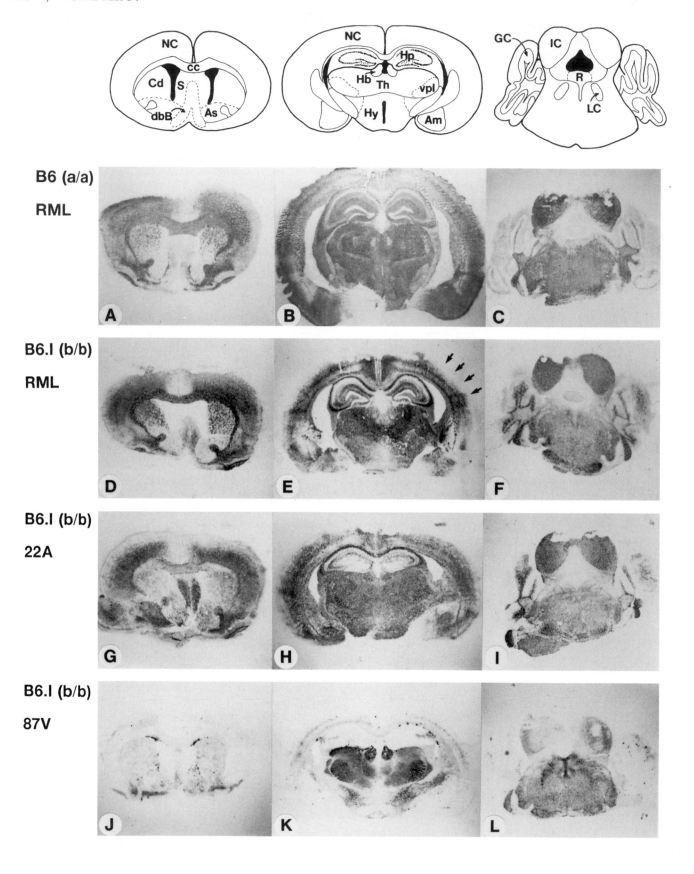

B6 (a/a)
RML

B6.I (b/b)
RML

B6.I (b/b)
22A

B6.I (b/b)
87V

lation. The deposition of PrPSc in the brains of CD-1 mice is widespread throughout the neocortex, hippocampus, thalamus, and caudate, whereas it is restricted to the thalamus and hypothalamus of Tg196 mice. In both CD-1 and Tg196 mice, RML prions seem to be propagated. The CD-1 mice have incubation times of 140 days, and extracts from their brains bioassayed in CD-1 mice have similar incubation times. The Tg196 mice have incubation times of 245 days after inoculation with RML prions, but extracts from their brains bioassayed in CD-1 mice have incubation times of only 140 days.[232] The prolonged incubation times in Tg196 mice indicate that the restricted pattern of PrPSc is not caused by an abbreviated illness in which the spread of PrPSc to other regions did not have sufficient time to occur. The mechanism by which PrPSc accumulation remains restricted to a few specific areas of the brain, as in the case of RML in Tg196 mice and 87V in B6.I-1 mice, is unknown. How the protein Y modulates the accumulation of PrPSc and thus neuronal vacuolation also remains to be established.

Mutations, Mixtures, and Cloning

The isolation of scrapie strains in mice usually has been performed with extracts prepared from the brains of scrapied sheep.[79,130] Cloning of new strains has been performed by limiting dilution in mice. Although many strains have been isolated, most of the studies were performed with only a few strains, and passaging was limited. For example, Me7 prions were passaged in C57BL mice,[124] which were later shown to have the *Prnp^a* allele, whereas 22a and 87V were passaged in VM mice, which have the *Prnp^b* allele. The *a* and *b* alleles of *Prnp* encode MoPrP molecules that differ at codons 108 and 189[484]; propagation of the Me7 strain was much more rapid in the *Prnp^a* mouse than in the *Prnp^b* mouse, but propagation of 22a and 87V was much faster in the *Prnp^b* mouse.[67,129] In other words, propagation of a particular strain was restricted by the PrP sequence in the host. It is noteworthy that a number of new strains have been isolated by passage of murine isolates into hamsters,[257,264] in which the PrP genes differ at 16 positions.[22,294]

Although mutation of scrapie isolates or strains has been reported, virtually nothing is known about the molecules that participate in this process. Low dilution of 87A was reported to give rise to 7D prions, but passage at high dilution pre-

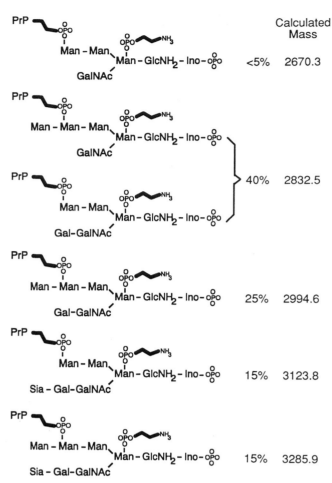

FIG. 37-7. Glycoinositol phospholipid (GPI) anchors of the prion protein (PrP). The proposed structures were determined for Syrian hamster PrPSc by mass spectrometry.[457] The percentages indicate an estimate of the approximate relative abundance of each glycoform. The calculated masses are based on the average molecular weight of each element in the GPI and include the mass of the C-terminal PrP (K12) peptide, which accounts for 1312.5 mass units of the total. (From Stahl N, Baldwin MA, Hecker R, Pan K-M, Burlingame AL, Prusiner SB. Glycosylinositol phospholipid anchors of the scrapie and cellular prion proteins contain sialic acid. Biochemistry 1992;31:5043–5053.)

FIG. 37-6. Histoblots showing PrPSc in coronal sections of mouse brain. Sections were cut at three levels: caudate and septal nuclei (*left column*), hippocampus and thalamus (*middle column*), and inferior colliculus (*right column*). B6 (**A–C**) and B6.1 (**D–L**) mice were inoculated with prions and sacrificed after showing clinical signs of scrapie. Mice in **A** through **F** were inoculated with RML, those in **G** through **I** with 22A, and those in **J** through **L** with 87V prions. Arrows in **E** indicate the outer surface of the cerebral cortex. Am, amygdala; As, accumbens septi; cc, corpus callosum; Cd, caudate nucleus; dbB, diagonal band of Broca; GC, granule cell layer of the cerebellar cortex; Hb, habenula; Hp, hippocampus; Hy, hypothalamus; IC, inferior colliculus; LC, locus ceruleus; NC, neocortex; R, raphe nuclei of the brain stem; S, septal nuclei; Th, thalamus; vpl, ventral posterior lateral nucleus of the thalamus. (From Carlson GA, Ebeling C, Yang S-L, et al. Prion isolate specified allotypic interactions between the cellular and scrapie prion proteins in congenic and transgenic mice. Proc Natl Acad Sci USA 1994;91:5690–5694.)

served the 87A properties.[65] Dickinson thought that it was important to prepare inocula from the smallest regions of individual brains in order to minimize contamination with other strains or mutants.

The construction of Tg(MH2MPrP) mice that are susceptible to both Mo and SHa prions has provided a new tool for the study of strains. The Tg(MH2MPrP) mice produce artificial prions, which infect Syrian hamsters as well as non-Tg and Tg(MH2MPrP) mice.[443]

Molecular Basis of Prion Strains

The mechanism by which isolate-specific information is carried by prions remains enigmatic; indeed, explaining the molecular basis of prion diversity seems to be a formidable challenge. Two hypotheses have been offered to explain distinct prion isolates: a second molecule may create prion diversity, or posttranslational modification of PrPSc may be responsible for the different properties of distinct prion isolates.[393]

Whether the PrPSc modification is chemical or only conformational remains to be established, but no candidate chemical modifications have been identified.[458] Structural studies of glycoinositol phospholipid (GPI) anchors of two SHa isolates have failed to reveal any differences. About 40% of the anchor glycans have sialic acid residues[457] (Fig. 37-7). A portion of the PrPC GPI anchors also have sialic acid residues; PrP is the first protein found to have sialic acid residues attached to GPI anchors.

The finding that the pattern of PrPSc accumulation in the CNS is characteristic for a particular strain offers a mechanism for the propagation of distinct prion isolates.[119,220] In this model, a different set of cells would propagate each isolate. Whether different asparagine (Asn)–linked carbohydrates (CHOs) function to target the PrPSc of a distinct isolate to a particular set of cells in which the same Asn-linked CHOs will be coupled to PrPC before its conversion to PrPSc remains to be established. The great diversity of Asn-linked CHOs makes them potential candidates for carrying isolate-specific information.[392] Even though this hypothesis is attractive, it must be

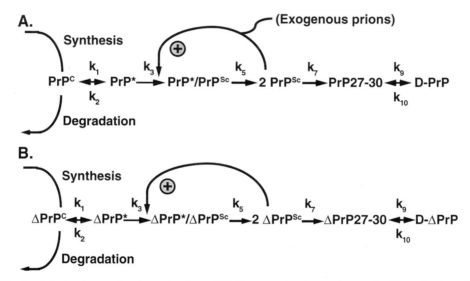

FIG. 37-8. Models for the replication of prions. (**A**) Proposed scheme for replication of prions in sporadic and infectious prion diseases. Wild-type PrPC is synthesized and degraded as part of the normal metabolism of many cells. Stochastic fluctuations in the structure of PrPC can create (k_1) a rare, partially unfolded, monomeric structure, PrP*, that is an intermediate in the formation of PrPSc but can revert (k_2) to PrPC or be degraded before conversion (k_3) into PrPSc. Normally, the concentration of PrP* is small and PrPSc formation is insignificant. In infectious prion diseases, exogenous prions enter the cell and stimulate conversion of PrP* into PrPSc. In the absence of exogenous prions, the concentration of PrPSc may eventually reach a threshold level in sporadic prion diseases, after which a positive feedback loop would stimulate the formation of PrPSc. Limited proteolysis of the N-terminal of PrPSc (k_7) produces PrP 27-30, which can also be generated in scrapie-infected cells from a recombinant vector encoding PrP truncated at the N-terminal.[428] Denaturation (k_9) of PrPSc or PrP 27-30 renders these molecules protease sensitive and abolishes scrapie infectivity; attempts to renature (k_{10}) these PrPSc or PrP 27-30 have been unsuccessful to date.[408,416] (**B**) Scheme for the replication of prions in genetic prion diseases. Mutant (Δ) PrPC is synthesized and degraded as part of the normal metabolism of many cells. Stochastic fluctuations in the structure of ΔPrPC are increased compared with wild-type PrPC, which creates (k_1) a partially unfolded, monomeric structure, ΔPrP*, that is an intermediate in the formation of ΔPrPSc but can revert (k_2) to DPrPC or be degraded before conversion (k_3) into ΔPrPSc. Limited proteolysis of the N-terminal of ΔPrPSc produces (k_7) ΔPrP 27-30, which in some cases may be less protease resistant than wild-type PrP 27-30.[335,413] (From Cohen FE, Pan K-M, Huang Z, Baldwin M, Fletterick RJ, Prusiner SB. Structural clues to prion replication. Science 1994;264:530–531.)

noted that PrP^{Sc} synthesis in scrapie-infected cells occurs in the presence of tunicamycin, which inhibits Asn-linked glycosylation, and with PrP molecules mutated at the Asn-linked glycosylation consensus sites.[466] Although the structures of Asn-linked CHOs have been analyzed for PrP^{Sc} of one isolate,[152] no data are available for PrP^{Sc} of other isolates or for PrP^C. The large number of Asn-linked CHOs found attached to the PrP 27-30 of Sc237 prions purified from Syrian hamster would seem to make it less likely that Asn-linked CHOs are responsible for strain variation, but experimental data addressing this point are still needed. Furthermore, as described previously, a single prion strain can produce markedly different patterns of PrP^{Sc} in mice expressing different prion protein allotypes.[443]

Are Prion Strains Different PrP^{Sc} Conformers?

Multiple prion strains may be explained by distinct PrP^{Sc} conformers that act as templates for the folding of de novo synthesized PrP^{Sc} molecules during prion replication (Fig. 37-8). Although it is clear that passage history can be responsible for the prolongation of incubation time if prions are passed between mice expressing different PrP allotypes[78] or between species,[418] many scrapie strains show distinct incubation times in the same inbred host.[68]

In recent studies, my colleagues and I inoculated three strains of prions into congenic and Tg mice harboring various numbers of the a and b alleles of $Prnp$.[75] The number of $Prnp^a$ genes was the major determinant of incubation times in mice inoculated with the RML prion isolate and was inversely related to the length of the incubation time (see Table 37-5). In contrast, the $Prnp^a$ allele prevented scrapie in mice inoculated with 87V prions. $Prnp^b$ genes were permissive for 87V prions and shortened incubation times in most mice inoculated with 22A prions (see Table 37-7). Experiments with the 87V isolate suggest that a genetic locus encoding protein Y, distinct from $Prnp$, controls the deposition of PrP^{Sc} and the attendant neuropathology. Although each prion isolate produced distinguishable patterns of PrP^{Sc} accumulation in brain, a comparison showed that RML and 22A prions in congenic $Prnp^b$ mice produced similar patterns, although RML prions caused very different patterns in $Prnp^a$ and $Prnp^b$ congenic mice. Therefore, both the PrP genotype and the specific prion isolate modify the distribution of PrP^{Sc} and the length of the incubation time. These findings suggest that prion strain-specific properties result from different affinities of PrP^{Sc} in the inocula for PrP^C-A and PrP^C-B allotypes encoded by the host.

Although the proposal for multiple PrP^{Sc} conformers is rather unorthodox, it is already known that PrP can assume at least two profoundly different conformations: PrP^C and PrP^{Sc}.[369] Of note, two different isolates from mink dying of transmissible mink encephalopathy exhibit different sensitivities of PrP^{Sc} to proteolytic digestion, supporting the suggestion that isolate-specific information may be carried by PrP^{Sc}.[35,36,305] How many conformations PrP^{Sc} can assume is unknown. The molecular weight of a PrP^{Sc} homodimer is consistent with the ionizing radiation target size of 55,000±9000 D as determined for infectious prion particles independent of their polymeric form.[28] If prions are oligomers of PrP^{Sc}, which

seems likely, then this offers another level of complexity, which in turn generates additional diversity.

SCRAPIE

Experimental Scrapie

For many years, studies of experimental scrapie were performed exclusively with sheep and goats. The disease was first transmitted by intraocular inoculation[108] and later by intracerebral, oral, subcutaneous, intramuscular, and intravenous injections of brain extracts from scrapied sheep. Incubation periods of 1 to 3 years were common, and many of the inoculated animals failed to develop disease.[134,214,215] Different breeds of sheep exhibited markedly different susceptibilities to scrapie prions inoculated subcutaneously, suggesting that the genetic background may influence host permissiveness.[212]

A crucial methodologic advance in experimental studies of scrapie was created by the demonstration that scrapie could be transmitted to mice,[87,88] which could be used for end point titrations of particular samples. In addition, pathogenesis experiments directed at elucidating factors governing incubation times and neuropathologic lesions were performed.[130,150,160]

Natural Scrapie in Sheep and Goats

Even though scrapie was recognized as a distinct disorder of sheep with respect to its clinical manifestations as early as 1738, the disease remained enigmatic for more than two centuries.[372] An investigation into the cause of scrapie followed the vaccination of sheep for looping ill virus with formalin-treated extracts of ovine lymphoid tissue unknowingly contaminated with scrapie prions.[211] Two years later, scrapie had developed in more than 1500 sheep as a result of this vaccine.

Communicability

Scrapie of sheep and goats appears to be unique among the prion diseases in that it is readily communicable within flocks. Although the transmissibility of scrapie seems to be well established, the mechanism of the natural spread of scrapie between sheep is so puzzling that it bears close scrutiny. The placenta has been implicated as one source of prions accounting for the horizontal spread of scrapie within flocks,[357,373,377,379] but the correctness of this view remains to be established. In Iceland, scrapied flocks of sheep were destroyed and the pastures left vacant for several years; however, reintroduction of sheep from flocks known to be free of scrapie for many years eventually resulted in scrapie.[368] The source of the scrapie prions that attacked the sheep from flocks without a history of scrapie is unknown.

Genetics of Sheep

Parry argued that host genes were responsible for the development of scrapie in sheep. He was convinced that natural scrapie is a genetic disease that can be eradicated by proper breeding protocols.[370,372] He considered its transmission by inoculation of importance primarily for laboratory studies and communicable infection of little consequence in nature. Other investigators viewed natural scrapie as an infectious disease and argued that host genetics only modulates susceptibility to an endemic infectious agent.[135] The incubation time gene for experimental scrapie in Cheviot sheep, called *Sip*, is said to be linked to a PrP gene restriction fragment length polymorphism,[244] a situation perhaps analogous to *Prn-i* and *Sinc* in mice; however, the null hypothesis of nonlinkage has yet to be tested, and this is important, especially in view of earlier studies indicating that susceptibility of sheep to scrapie is governed by a recessive gene.[370,372]

In Romanov and Ile-de-France breeds of sheep, a polymorphism in the PrP ORF was found at codon 136 (alanine [Ala] → Val) that seems to correlate with scrapie.[288] Sheep homozygous or heterozygous for Val at codon 136 were susceptible to scrapie but those that were homozygous for Ala were resistant. Only one of 74 scrapied autochthonous sheep had a Val at codon 136; these sheep were from three breeds, denoted Lacaune, Manech, and Presalpes.[286]

In Suffolk sheep, a polymorphism in the PrP ORF was found at codon 171 (glutamine [Gln] → arginine [Arg]).[208,209] Studies of natural scrapie in the United States have shown that 85% of the afflicted sheep are of the Suffolk breed. Only those Suffolk sheep homozygous for Gln at codon 171 were found with scrapie, although healthy control animals with QQ, QR, and RR genotypes were found.[486] These results argue that susceptibility in Suffolk sheep is governed by the PrP codon 171 polymorphism.

BOVINE SPONGIFORM ENCEPHALOPATHY

Epidemic of BSE

Beginning in 1986, an epidemic of a previously unknown disease appeared in cattle in the United Kingdom.[116,491,489,490,492] This disease, BSE (often called "mad cow disease" in the lay press), has been shown to be a prion disease. Based mainly on epidemiologic evidence, it has been proposed that BSE represents a gigantic common source epidemic, one which has caused more than 160,000 cases to date. In the United Kingdom, cattle, particularly dairy cows, are routinely fed meat and bone meal as a nutritional supplement. This supplement was prepared in the past by rendering of sheep and cattle offal, by a process that involved steam treatment and hydrocarbon extraction. In the late 1970s, many rendering plants in the United Kingdom altered their process by abandoning the use of hydrocarbon extraction, and it is postulated that sheep scrapie prions in the offal were no longer completely inactivated and were subsequently transmitted to cattle through consumption of contaminated meat and bone meal. Since 1988, the practice of feeding cattle dietary protein supplements derived from rendered sheep or cattle offal has been forbidden in the United Kingdom. Curiously, almost half of the BSE cases have occurred in herds in which only a single affected animal has been found; the occurrence of several cases of BSE in a single herd is infrequent.[116,491,492] Whether the distribution of BSE cases within herds will change as the epidemic progresses and whether BSE will disappear with the cessation of feeding rendered meat and bone meal are uncertain.

Crossing a Species Barrier

Assuming the above postulate is correct, then only sheep prions were present initially in the contaminated meat and bone meal. Because the species barrier depends, at least in part, on the amino acid sequences of PrP in the donor host and recipient, the similarity between bovine and sheep PrP was probably an important factor in initiation of the BSE epidemic. Bovine PrP differs from sheep PrP at only seven or eight residues, depending on the breed of sheep.[238,461] As the BSE epidemic expanded, infected bovine offal, which contained bovine prions, began to be rendered into meat and bone meal.

Transmission of BSE to Experimental Animals

Brain extracts from BSE cattle have transmitted disease to mice, cattle, sheep, and pigs after intracerebral inoculation.[64,114,115,163] Transmissions to mice and sheep suggest that cattle preferentially propagate a single strain of prions. Seven BSE brains all produced similar incubation times, as measured in each of three strains of inbred mice.[64]

Of particular importance to the BSE epidemic is the recent transmission of BSE to the marmoset, a nonhuman primate, after intracerebral inoculation followed by a prolonged incubation period.[20] The potential parallels with kuru of humans, confined to the Fore region of New Guinea,[172,175] are worthy of consideration. Once the most common cause of death among women and children in the Fore region, kuru has almost disappeared since the cessation of ritualistic cannibalism.[12] Although it seems likely that kuru was transmitted orally, as proposed for BSE among cattle, some investigators argue that nonoral routes were important because oral transmission of kuru prions to apes and monkeys has been difficult to demonstrate.[172,185]

There is no example of zoonotic transmission of prions from animals to humans, in spite of many epidemiologic studies that have attempted to implicate scrapie prions from sheep as a cause of CJD.[104,218,297] Whether BSE poses any risk to humans is unknown, but three teenagers and eight young adults in Britain and France have died of atypical CJD during the past year.[16,17,88a,439,492a]

Oral Transmission of BSE Prions

In addition to BSE, four other animal diseases appear to have arisen from the oral consumption of prions. It has been suggested that an outbreak of transmissible mink encephalopathy in 1985 arose from the use for feed of a cow with a sporadic case of BSE.[305] The source of prions in chronic wasting disease of captive mule deer and elk is unclear.[494,495] The prion-contaminated meat and bone meal thought to be the cause of BSE is also hypothesized to be the cause of feline spongiform encephalopathy (FSE) and exotic ungulate encephalopathy. FSE has been found in almost 30 domestic cats in Great Britain, as well as in a puma and a cheetah.[498] In three instances, FSE in domestic cats has been transmitted to laboratory mice and PrPSc has been identified in their brains by immunoblotting.[381] Prion disease has been found in the brains of the nyala, greater kudu, eland, gembok, and Arabian oryx in British zoos; all of these animals are exotic ungulates. Five of eight greater kudu born into a herd maintained in a London zoo since 1987 have developed prion disease. Except for the first case, none of the other kudu were exposed to feeds containing ruminant-derived meat and bone meal.[266] Brain extracts prepared from a nyala and a greater kudu have transmitted the disease to mice.[109,267] PrP of the greater kudu differs from the bovine protein at four residues; Arabian oryx PrP differs from the sheep PrP at only one residue.[386]

HUMAN PRION DISEASES

Clinical Manifestations of Human Prion Diseases

The human prion diseases are manifested as infectious, inherited diseases, and sporadic disorders and are often referred to as kuru, CJD, GSS, and FFI, depending on the clinical and neuropathologic findings (see Table 37-1).

Infectious forms of prion diseases result from the horizontal transmission of infectious prions, as occurs in iatrogenic CJD and kuru. Inherited forms, notably GSS, familial CJD, and FFI, comprise 10% to 15% of all cases of prion disease. A mutation in the ORF or protein-coding region of the PrP gene has been found in all reported kindreds with inherited human prion disease.* Sporadic forms of prion disease comprise most cases of CJD and possibly some cases of GSS.[313] How prions arise in patients with sporadic forms is unknown; hypotheses include horizontal transmission from humans or animals,[172] somatic mutation of the PrP gene ORF, and spontaneous conversion of PrPC into PrPSc.[233,392] Numerous attempts to establish an infectious link between sporadic CJD and a preexisting prion disease in animals or humans have been unrewarding.[39,53,104,218,297]

Diagnosis of Human Prion Diseases

Human prion disease should be considered in any patient who develops a progressive subacute or chronic decline in cognitive or motor function. Typically adults between 40 and 70 years of age, patients often exhibit clinical features that are helpful in providing a premorbid diagnosis of prion disease, particularly sporadic CJD.[52,434] There is as yet no specific diagnostic test for prion disease in the cerebrospinal fluid. A definitive diagnosis of human prion disease, which is invariably fatal, can often be made from examination of brain tissue. Over the past 4 years, knowledge of the molecular genetics of prion diseases has made it possible to diagnose inherited prion disease in living patients using peripheral tissues.

The broad spectrum of neuropathologic features in human prion diseases precludes a precise neuropathologic definition. The classic neuropathologic features of human prion disease

include spongiform degeneration, gliosis, and neuronal loss in the absence of an inflammatory reaction. If present, amyloid plaques that stain with α-PrP antibodies are diagnostic.

The presence of protease-resistant PrP (PrPSc or PrPCJD) in the infectious and sporadic forms and in most of the inherited forms of these diseases implicates prions in their pathogenesis. The absence of PrPCJD in a biopsy specimen may simply reflect regional variations in the concentration of the protein.[445] In some patients with inherited prion disease, PrPSc is barely detectable or undetectable[60,293,300,323]; this situation seems to be mimicked in transgenic mice, which express a mutant PrP gene and spontaneously develop neurologic illness indistinguishable from experimental murine scrapie.[232,235]

In humans and Tg mice that have no detectable protease-resistant PrP but express mutant PrP, neurodegeneration may be caused, at least in part, by abnormal metabolism of mutant PrP. Because molecular genetic analyses of PrP genes in patients with unusual dementing illnesses are readily performed, the diagnosis of inherited prion disease can often be established even in patients with little or no neuropathology,[99] atypical neurodegenerative disease,[323] or misdiagnosed neurodegenerative disease,[18,223] including Alzheimer's disease.

Although horizontal transmission of neurodegeneration to experimental hosts was for a time the gold standard of prion disease, it can no longer be used as such. Some investigators have reported that transmission of the inherited prion diseases from humans to rodents is frequently negative in spite of the presence of a pathogenic mutation in the PrP gene[467]; others state that this is not the case with apes and monkeys as hosts.[61] The discovery that Tg(MHu2M) mice are susceptible to Hu prions[471] promises to make feasible transmission studies that are not practical in apes and monkeys.[58]

The hallmark common to all of the prion diseases—whether sporadic, dominantly inherited, or acquired by infection—is that they involve aberrant metabolism of the prion protein.[393] A definitive diagnosis of human prion disease can rapidly be made if PrPSc can be detected immunologically. Frequently, PrPSc can be detected by either the dot blot method or Western immunoblot analysis of brain homogenates, in which samples are subjected to limited proteolysis to remove PrPC before immunostaining.[40,41,56,445] The dot blot method exploits enhancement of PrPSc immunoreactivity after denaturation in the chaotropic salt, guanidinium chloride. Because of regional variations in PrPSc concentration, methods using homogenates prepared from small brain regions can give false-negative results. Alternatively, PrPSc may be detected in situ in cryostat sections bound to nitrocellulose membranes followed by limited proteolysis to remove PrPC and guanidinium treatment to denature PrPSc and enhance its avidity for α-PrP antibodies[464] (see Figs. 37-2 and 37-6). Denaturation of PrPSc in situ before immunostaining has also been accomplished by autoclaving fixed tissue sections.[272]

In the familial forms of the prion diseases, molecular genetic analyses of PrP can be diagnostic and can be performed on DNA extracted from blood leucocytes antemortem. However, such testing is of little value in the diagnosis of the sporadic or infectious forms of prion disease. Although the first missense PrP mutation was discovered after the two PrP alleles of a patient with GSS were cloned from a genomic library and sequenced,[228] all subsequent novel missense and insertional mutations have been identified in PrP ORFs amplified

---

* References 34, 143, 145, 170, 203, 201, 202, 206, 228, 269, 271, 324, 382, 387

by polymerase chain reaction and sequenced. The 759 base pairs encoding the 253 amino acids of PrP reside in a single exon of the PrP gene, providing an ideal situation for the use of the polymerase chain reaction. Amplified PrP ORFs can be screened for known mutations by one of several methods, the most reliable of which is allele-specific oligonucleotide hybridization. If known mutations are absent, novel mutations may be found after the PrP ORF is sequenced.

If PrP amyloid plaques in brain are present, they are diagnostic for prion disease. However, they are thought to be present in only 10% of CJD cases, and by definition in all cases of GSS. The amyloid plaques in CJD are compact (kuru plaques). Those in GSS are either multicentric (diffuse) or compact. The amyloid plaques in prion diseases contain PrP.[275,425,426] The multicentric amyloid plaques that are pathognomonic for GSS may be difficult to distinguish from the neuritic plaques of Alzheimer's disease except by immunohistology.[182,246,352] In GSS kindreds, the diagnosis of Alzheimer's disease was excluded because the amyloid plaques failed to stain with β-amyloid antiserum but stained with α-PrP antiserum. In subsequent studies, missense mutations were found in the PrP genes of these kindreds.

In summary, the diagnosis of prion or prion protein disease may be made in patients on the basis of the presence of PrP^{Sc}, mutant PrP genotype, or appropriate immunohistology, and this diagnosis should not be excluded in patients with atypical neurodegenerative diseases until one or preferably two of these examinations have been performed.[97,99,285]

INFECTIOUS PRION DISEASES OF HUMANS

Kuru

For many decades, kuru devastated the lives of the Fore highlanders of Papua New Guinea.[172] The high incidence of the disease among women left a society of motherless children raised by their fathers (Table 37-8). It was unusual in the Fore region to see an older woman. With the cessation of traditional warfare, older men are now found, many of whom have had a succession of wives, each dying of kuru after leaving several children. Because contamination during ritualistic cannibalism appears to have been the mode of spread of kuru among the Fore people, and because cannibalism had ceased by 1960 in the Fore region, the patients now developing kuru presumably were exposed to the kuru agent more than three decades ago.[11,172] In many cases, histories from patients and their families of the episode in which they cannibalized the remains of a near relative who had died of kuru have been obtained, presumably accounting for the source of infection. That the kuru prions could remain apparently quiescent in these patients for two decades or more and then manifest in the form of a fatal neurologic disease is supported by incubation periods of more than 7.5 years in some monkeys inoculated with kuru agent.[185]

The uniform clinical presentation of kuru is remarkable.[10,177,178,226,227,449,502] In one study, the prodromal symptoms and the onset of disease were similar in all of the patients investigated.[403] Even the time interval between the prodromal symptoms of headache and joint pain and the onset of difficulty walking was always 6 to 12 weeks. In most cases, the disease progressed to death within 12 months, and all patients were dead within 2 years of onset. The average duration of ill-

Table 37-8. *Infectious prion diseases of humans*

Diseases	No. cases
KURU (1957–1982)	
Adult females	1739
Adult males	248
Children and adolescents	597
Total	2584
IATROGENIC CREUTZFELDT-JAKOB DISEASE	
Depth electrodes	2
Corneal transplants	1
Human pituitary growth hormone	79
Human pituitary gonadotropin	5
Dura mater grafts	23
Neurosurgical procedures	4
Total	114

ness for the 15 patients studied was 16 months.[403] Invariably, signs of cerebellar dysfunction dominated the clinical picture. All patients remained ambulatory with the aid of a stick for more than half of the clinical phase of their illness. These clinical characteristics were similar to those reported for adult patients at the peak of the kuru epidemic.[10,177,178,226,227,449]

Incubation Periods That Exceed Three Decades

No individual born in the South Fore after 1959 (i.e., since cannibalism ceased) has ever developed kuru.[12,11] Kuru has progressively disappeared, first among children and thereafter among adolescents. The number of deaths in adult females has decreased steadily, and adult male deaths have remained very infrequent. Each year, the youngest new patients are older than those of the previous year.

Of several hundred kuru orphans born since 1957 to mothers who later died of kuru, none has yet developed the disease. This indicates that the many children with kuru seen in the 1950s were not infected prenatally, perinatally, or neonatally by their mothers, in spite of evidence for prions in the placenta and colostrum of a pregnant woman who died of CJD.[462] Attempts to demonstrate consistent transmission of prion disease from mother to offspring in experimental animals have been unsuccessful.[14,303,336,377,461]

Although patients currently afflicted with kuru exhibit greatly prolonged incubation periods, children with kuru who were observed 30 years ago provide some information on the minimum incubation period. The youngest patient with kuru was 4 years old at the onset of the disease and died at age 5, but it is not known at what age young children were infected. CJD accidentally transmitted to humans has required only 18 months after intracerebral or intraoptic inoculation to manifest.[33,146] An incubation period of 18 months has also been found in chimpanzees inoculated intracerebrally with kuru prions.

Transmission by Cannibalism

Considerable evidence implicates ritualistic cannibalism as the mode of transmission for kuru among the Fore and neighboring tribes.[172] Oral transmission of kuru to monkeys has been documented.[185] Proposed transmission routes through laceration of the skin and rubbing of the eyes were suggested after early experiments on oral transmission to apes and monkeys failed, but documentation of nonoral transmission remains to be established.[172] The experimental results from oral transmission of scrapie to hamsters suggest that insufficient doses of kuru prions were used in those protocols.[399]

Origin of Kuru

It has been suggested that kuru began at the turn of the century as a spontaneous case of CJD that was propagated by ritualistic cannibalism.[11,172] It is not known whether the Fore peoples and their immediate neighbors provided an especially permissive genetic background on which kuru prions multiplied. Sequencing of the ORF of the PrP gene from three kuru patients failed to reveal any mutations.[195] Noteworthy is a case of CJD outside the kuru region in Papua New Guinea.

Transmission to Animals

Kuru has regularly been transmitted by intracerebral inoculation to apes and monkeys.[172,175,190] The prolonged incubation periods in experimental animals are similar to those observed with CJD and GSS (Table 37-9). Oral transmission of kuru to apes and monkeys has been difficult,[172] but recent studies have demonstrated transmission to monkeys.[185] Presumably, the difficulties in transmitting human kuru prions orally to apes and monkeys are caused by the inefficiency of this route and the necessity to cross a species barrier.[399] Although the number of differences in PrP amino acid sequences between humans and nonhuman primates is small, a few specific

amino acid changes could have a profound effect on susceptibility.[440]

Immunologic Studies

The kuru or amyloid plaques show intense immunostaining with α-PrP antiserum.[426] It has been estimated that 70% of patients dying of kuru have PrP amyloid plaques.[276] Protease-resistant immunoreactive proteins were reported in brain extracts from one of two patients who died of kuru.[55] Presumably, these two patients are included in a larger series, in which three out of four kuru patients were found to have the abnormal isoform of the prion protein.[56]

Iatrogenic Creutzfeldt-Jakob Disease

Accidental transmission of CJD to humans appears to have occurred as a result of corneal transplantation,[146] implantation of contaminated electroencephalography electrodes,[33] and surgical operations with contaminated instruments or apparatus[112,279,314,493] (see Table 37-8). A cornea removed from a donor who, unknowingly, had CJD was transplanted to an apparently healthy recipient, who developed CJD after a prolonged incubation period. Corneas of animals have significant levels of prions, making this scenario seem probable.[73] The same improperly decontaminated electrodes that caused CJD in two young patients with intractable epilepsy were found to cause CJD in a chimpanzee 18 months after their experimental implantation.[32,187] Surgical procedures may have resulted in accidental inoculation of patients with prions during their operations,[62,172,493] presumably because some instrument or apparatus in the operating theater became contaminated when a

Table 37-9. *Incubation periods and duration of illness in Creutzfeldt-Jakob disease (CJD) and Kuru*

Host	Incubation period*(months)		Duration of illness (months)	
	CJD	Kuru	CJD	Kuru
NATURAL				
Humans	18–360	60–360	1–55	3–12
EXPERIMENTAL				
Apes	11–71	10–82	1–6	1–15
Monkeys	4–73	8–92	1–27	1–23
Sheep	—			
Goats	36–48	39	2–6	—
Ferrets	—	18–71	—	—
Mink	—	45	—	—
Domestic cats	19–30	2–6	—	—
Guinea pigs	7–16	1	—	—
Hamsters	5–18	—	—	—
Mice	3–20	1–2	—	—

*Incubation period: from exposure to onset of illness.
From Prusiner SB, Hsiao KK, Bredesen DE, DeArmond SJ. Prion disease. In: Vinken PJ, Bruyn GW, Klawans HL, eds. Handbook of clinical neurology: viral disease. Vol 12 (56). Amsterdam: Elsevier, 1989: 543–580. (Data from references 11, 189, 190, 215, 301, 302, 314, and 469.)

CJD patient underwent surgery. Although the epidemiology of these studies is highly suggestive, no proof for such episodes exists.

Since 1988, 23 cases of CJD after implantation of dura mater grafts have been recorded.[†] Initially all of the grafts were thought to have been acquired from a single manufacturer, whose preparative procedures were inadequate to inactivate human prions.[62] One case of CJD occurred after repair of an eardrum perforation with a pericardium gray.[†463]

Thirty cases of CJD in physicians and health care workers have been reported[31]; however, no occupational link has been established.[422] Whether any of these cases represent infectious prion disease contracted during care of patients with CJD or processing of specimens from these patients remains uncertain.

Human Growth Hormone Therapy

The possibility of transmission of CJD from contaminated HGH preparations derived from human pituitaries has been raised by the occurrence of fatal cerebellar disorders with dementia in more than 79 patients, ranging in age from 10 to 41 years[48,62,69,158] (see Table 37-8). Although one case of spontaneous CJD in a 20-year-old woman has been reported,[48,192,365] CJD in patients younger than 40 years of age is very rare.[505] These patients received injections of HGH every 2 to 4 days for 4 to 12 years.[‡] Most of the patients presented with cerebellar syndromes that progressed over periods varying from 6 to 18 months. Some patients became demented during the terminal phases of their illnesses. This clinical course resembles kuru more than ataxic CJD in some respects.[403] Assuming these patients developed CJD from injections of prion-contaminated HGH preparations, the possible incubation periods range from 4 to 30 years.[62] The longest incubation periods are similar to those associated with cases of kuru in recent years.[176,277,403] Many patients received several common lots of HGH at various times during their prolonged therapies, but no single lot was administered to all the United States patients. An aliquot of one lot of HGH has been reported to transmit CNS disease to a squirrel monkey after a prolonged incubation period.[186] How many lots of the HGH may have been contaminated with prions is unknown.

CJD is a rare disease with an annual incidence of approximately 1 per 1,000,000 population.[314] If we assume that the average person lives 70 years, then the lifetime expectancy of developing CJD is about 1 per 10,000 (calculated as [70 years] $\times$ [1/10^6 person-years] = 1/10^4 persons). Because 10,000 human pituitaries were typically processed in a single HGH preparation, the possibility of hormone preparations contaminated with CJD prions is not remote.[49,54,57]

The concentration of CJD prions within infected human pituitaries is unknown; widespread degenerative changes have been observed in both the hypothalamus and pituitary of sheep with scrapie.[25] The forebrains from scrapie-infected mice have been added to human pituitary suspensions to determine whether prions and HGH copurify.[295] Bioassays in mice suggest that prions and HGH do not copurify with currently used protocols.[470] Although these results seem reassuring, especially for patients treated with HGH during much of the last decade, the relatively low titers of the murine scrapie prions used in these studies may not have provided an adequate test.[48] The extremely small size and charge heterogeneity exhibited by scrapie[8,43,407,412,416] and presumably by CJD prions[30,40] may complicate procedures designed to separate pituitary hormones from these slow infectious pathogens. Even though additional investigations argue for the efficacy of inactivating prions in HGH fractions prepared from human pituitaries using 6 M urea, it seems doubtful that such protocols will be used for purifying HGH, because recombinant HGH is available.[383]

Molecular genetic studies have shown that most patients in whom iatrogenic CJD develops after treatment with pituitary-derived HGH are homozygous for either Met or Val at codon 129 of the PrP gene.[54,101,122] Homozygosity at the codon 129 polymorphism has also been shown to predispose individuals to sporadic CJD.[366] Val homozygosity seems to be overrepresented in these HGH patients compared with the general population.

Five cases of CJD have occurred in women receiving human pituitary gonadotropin.[93,94,219]

INHERITED PRION DISEASES

Familial Prion Disease

The recognition that 10% of CJD cases are familial[§] posed a perplexing problem after it was established that CJD is transmissible.[188,191] Equally puzzling was the transmission of GSS to nonhuman primates[188,191,310] and mice,[469] because most cases of GSS are familial.[181] As with sheep scrapie, the relative contributions of genetic and infectious causes in the human prion diseases remained a conundrum until molecular clones of the PrP gene became available to probe the inherited aspects of these disorders.

PrP Mutations and Genetic Linkage

The discovery of the PrP gene raised the possibility that mutation may feature in the hereditary human prion diseases. A Pro → Leu mutation at codon 102 was shown to be linked genetically to development of GSS with a logarithm of odds (LOD) score exceeding 3[228] (Fig. 37-9). This mutation may be caused by the deamination of a methylated cytosine-phosphoguanine (CpG) in a germ line PrP gene resulting in the substitution of a thymine for cytosine. The P102L mutation has been found in ten different families in nine different countries, including the original GSS family.[145,206,207,280,281]

Patients with a dementing or telencephalic form of GSS have a mutation at codon 117. These patients as well as some in other families were once thought to have familial Alzheimer's disease but are now known to have prion disease on the basis of

---

[†] References 62, 308, 316, 333, 351, 358, 473, 497
[‡] References 15, 37, 107, 151, 192, 278, 296, 309, 350, 388, 474

[§]References 113, 164, 247, 268, 310, 311, 312, 325, 436, 459

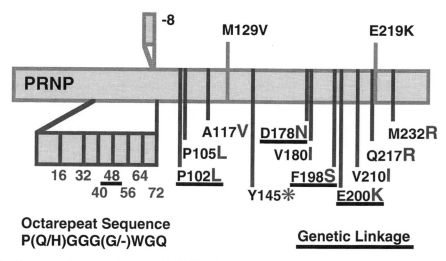

FIG. 37-9. Human prion protein gene (*PRNP*). The open reading frame is denoted by the large gray rectangle. Human *PRNP* wild-type coding polymorphisms are shown above the rectangle, and mutations that segregate with the inherited prion diseases are depicted below. The wild-type human PrP gene contains five octarepeat sequences, P(Q/H)GGG(G/−)WGQ, between codons 51 and 91.[283] Deletion of a single octarepeat at codon 81 or 82 is not associated with prion disease.[287,419,480] Whether this deletion alters the phenotypic characteristics of a prion disease is unknown. There are common polymorphisms at codons 117 (Ala→Ala) and 129 (Met→Val); homozygosity for Met or Val at codon 129 appears to increase susceptibility to sporadic Creutzfeldt-Jakob disease (CJD).[366] Octarepeat inserts of 16, 32, 40, 48, 56, 64, and 72 amino acids at codons 67, 75, or 83 are designated by the small rectangle below the open reading frame. These inserts segregate with familial CJD, and genetic linkage has been demonstrated when sufficient specimens from family members were available.[98,99,106,195,199,363,364,367] Point mutations are designated by the single-letter codes for the wild-type amino acid and the mutant residue, separated by the codon number (e.g., P102L). These point mutations segregate with the inherited prion diseases, and significant genetic linkage (underlined mutations) has been demonstrated when sufficient specimens from family members were available. Mutations at codons 102 (Pro→Leu), 117 (Ala→Val), 198 (Phe→Ser) and 217 (Gln→Arg) are found in patients with Gerstmann-Sträussler-Scheinker (GSS) disease.[145,195,196,204,206,228,229,231,234,468] Point mutations at codons 178 (Asp→Asn), 200 (Glu→Lys) and 210 (Val→Ile) are found in patients with familial CJD.[168,202,203,233,424] Point mutations at codons 198 (Phe→Ser) and 217 (Gln→Arg) are found in patients with GSS who have PrP amyloid plaques and neurofibrillary tangles.[143,230] Additional point mutations at codons 145 (Tyr→Stop), 105 (Pro→Leu), 180 (Val→Ile) and 232 (Met→Arg) have also been reported.[269,271] Single-letter code for amino acids is as follows: A, Ala; D, Asp; E, Glu; F, Phe; I, Ile; K, Lys; L, Leu; M, Met; N, Asn; P, Pro; Q, Gln; R, Arg; S, Ser; T, Thr; V, Val; Y, Tyr, *, Stop.

PrP immunostaining of amyloid plaques and PrP gene mutations.[153,182,183,352] Patients with GSS who have a Pro → Leu substitution at PrP codon 105 have been reported.[271]

An insert of 144 bp at codon 53, containing six octarepeats, has been described in patients with CJD from four families, all residing in southern England[97,98,99,106,361,363,364,387] (see Fig. 37-9). This mutation must have arisen through a complex series of events, because the human PrP gene contains only five octarepeats, indicating that a single recombination event could not have created the insert. Genealogic investigations have shown that all four families are related, arguing for a single founder born more than two centuries ago.[106] The LOD score for this extended pedigree exceeds 11. Studies from several laboratories have demonstrated that two, four, five, six, seven, eight, or nine octarepeats, in addition to the normal five, are found in individuals with inherited CJD,[51,98,99,199,362,363,364] whereas deletion of one octarepeat has been identified in an individual without the neurologic disease.[287,367,480]

For many years, the unusually high incidence of CJD among Israeli Jews of Libyan origin was thought to be caused by the consumption of lightly cooked sheep brain or eyeballs.[13,222,250,251,349,503] Recent studies have shown that some Libyan and Tunisian Jews in families with CJD have a PrP gene point mutation at codon 200 that results in a glutamate (Glu) → lysine (Lys) substitution.[168,204,233] One patient was homozygous for the E200K mutation, but her clinical presentation was similar to that of heterozygotes,[233] arguing that familial prion diseases are true autosomal dominant disorders, like Huntington's disease.[487] The E200K mutation has also been found in Slovaks originating from Orava in north central Czechoslovakia,[204] in a cluster of familial cases in Chile,[200] and in a large German family living in the United States.[34] Some investigators have argued that the E200K mutation originated in a Sephardic Jew whose descendants migrated from Spain and Portugal at the time of the Inquisition.[200] It is more likely that the E200K mutation has arisen independently multiple times by the deamidation of a methylated CpG, as described for the codon 102 mutation.[228,233] In support of this hypothesis are historical records of Libyan and Tunisian Jews indicating that they are descended from Jews living on the island of Jerba near the southern coast of Tunisia, where Jews first settled about 500 BC, and not from Sephardim.[477]

Many families with CJD have been found to have a point mutation at codon 178 that results in an aspartate (Asp) → Asn substitution.[59,156,198,202,216] In these patients and in those with the E200K mutation, PrP amyloid plaques are rare; the neuropathologic changes usually consist of widespread spongiform degeneration.

A new prion disease, FFI, has been described in three Italian families with the D178N mutation; the patients present with insomnia.[323] The neuropathology in these patients is restricted to selected nuclei of the thalamus. It is unclear whether all patients with the D178N mutation or only a subset present with sleep disturbances. It has been proposed that the allele with the D178N mutation encodes a Met at position 129 in FFI, whereas a Val is encoded at position 129 in familial CJD.[205] The discovery that FFI is an inherited prion disease widens the clinical spectrum of these disorders and raises the possibility that many other degenerative diseases of unknown origin may be caused by prions.[249,323] The D178N mutation has been linked to the development of prion disease, with a LOD score exceeding 5.[382] Studies of PrPSc in FFI and familial CJD caused by the D178N mutation show that after limited proteolysis the M_r of the FFI PrPSc is 1 kD smaller.[335] Whether this difference in protease resistance reflects distinct conformations of PrPSc that give rise to the different clinical and neuropathologic manifestations of these inherited prion diseases remains to be established.

Like the E200K and D178N(V129) mutations, a Val → isoleucine (Ile) mutation at PrP codon 210 produces CJD with classic symptoms and signs.[384,424] It appears that this V210I mutation is also incompletely penetrant.

Other point mutations at codons 105, 117, 145, 198, 217, and possibly 232 also segregate with inherited prion diseases.[51,145,230,229,269,271,273,475] Patients with the codon 198 mutation have numerous neurofibrillary tangles that stain with antibodies to the protein tau and amyloid plaques[153,182,183,352] that are composed largely of a PrP fragment extending from residues 58 to 150.[460] A genetic linkage study of one family produced an LOD score exceeding 6.[143] The neuropathology of two patients of Swedish ancestry with the codon 217 mutation[246] was similar to that of patients with the codon 198 mutation.

One patient with a prolonged neurologic illness spanning almost two decades who had PrP amyloid plaques was found to have an amber mutation of the PrP gene resulting in a stop codon at residue 145.[269,273] Staining of the plaques with α-PrP peptide antisera suggested that they may be composed exclusively of the truncated PrP molecules. That a PrP peptide ending at residue 145 polymerizes in amyloid filaments is to be expected, because an earlier study, noted previously in this chapter, showed that the major PrP peptide in plaques from patients with the F198S mutation was an 11-kD PrP peptide beginning at codon 58 and ending at 150.[460] Furthermore, synthetic PrP peptides adjacent to and including residues 109 to 122 readily polymerize into rod-shaped structures with the tinctorial properties of amyloid.[102,157,180,197]

PrP GENE POLYMORPHISMS IN HUMANS

Polymorphisms at Codons 129 and 219

At PrP codon 129, an amino acid polymorphism for the Met → Val has been identified.[360] This polymorphism appears able to influence prion disease expression, not only in inherited forms but also in iatrogenic and sporadic forms of prion disease. A second polymorphism, which results in an amino acid substitution at codon 219 (Glu → Lys), has been reported in the Japanese population, in which the K allele occurs with a frequency of 6%.[273]

Homozygosity at Codon 129 Predisposes to CJD in Whites But Not Asians

Studies of patients with sporadic CJD have shown that most are homozygous for Met or Val at codon 129.[366] This contrasts with the general population, in which frequencies for the codon 129 polymorphism in whites are 12% VV, 37% MM, and 51% MV.[101] The frequency of the Val allele in the Japanese population is much lower.[144]

Although no specific mutations have been identified in the PrP gene of patients with sporadic CJD,[195] homozygosity at codon 129 in sporadic CJD[217,366] is consistent with the results of Tg mouse studies. The finding that homozygosity at codon 129 predisposes to CJD supports a model of prion production that favors PrP interactions between homologous proteins, as appears to occur in Tg mice expressing SHaPrP inoculated with either SHa or Mo prions,[393,418,442] as well as in Tg mice expressing a chimeric mouse-hamster PrP transgene inoculated with artificial prions.[443]

Codon 129 May Influence Iatrogenic CJD

Susceptibility to infection may be partially determined by the PrP codon 129 genotype,[101] analogous in principle to the incubation-time alleles in mice.[77,101] In 16 patients (15 white, one Afro-American) from the United Kingdom, the United States, and France with iatrogenic CJD from contaminated HGH extracts, eight (50%) were VV, five (31%) were MM, and three (19%) were MV.[54,62,69,101,158,194] Therefore, a disproportionate number of patients with iatrogenic CJD were homozygous for valine at PrP codon 129, and heterozygosity at codon 129 may provide partial protection. Whether these associations are strongly significant awaits statistical analysis of larger samples. Thousands of children who received pituitary growth hormone extracts are still at risk for the development of CJD. The use of genetically engineered HGH eliminates this form of iatrogenic CJD.

Approximately 15% of patients with sporadic CJD develop ataxia as an early sign, accompanied by dementia.[63] Most, but not all, patients with ataxia have compact (kuru-like) plaques in the cerebellum.[380] Patients with ataxia and compact plaques exhibit a protracted clinical course which may last up to 3 years. The molecular basis for the differences between CJD of shorter and longer duration have not yet been fully elucidated; however, some preliminary analyses have suggested that patients with protracted, atypical clinical courses are more likely to be heterozygous at codon 129.[100,144]

Codon 129 and Inherited Prion Diseases

Homozygosity at codon 129 has been reported to be associated with an earlier age of onset in the inherited prion disease caused by the six-octarepeat insert, but not disease caused by the E200K mutation in Libyan Jews.[19,170] As noted previously, the FFI phenotype is found in patients with the D178N mutation who encode a Met at codon 129 on the mutant allele, whereas those with dementing illness (familial CJD) encode a Val at 129.[205] Homozygosity for either Met or Val at codon 129 is thought to be associated with an earlier age of onset in those with the D178N mutation.

THERAPEUTIC APPROACHES TO PRION DISEASES

There is no known effective therapy for treating or preventing CJD. There are no well documented cases of patients with CJD showing recovery, either spontaneously or after therapy, with one possible exception.[302] Because people at risk for inherited prion diseases can now be identified decades before neurologic dysfunction is evident, the development of an effective therapy is imperative.

Prenatal Screening for PrP Mutations

The inherited prion diseases can be prevented by genetic counseling coupled with prenatal DNA screening, but such testing presents ethical problems. For example, during the childbearing years, the parents are usually symptom free and may not want to know their own genotype. The apparent incomplete penetrance of some of the inherited prion diseases makes predicting the future for an asymptomatic individual uncertain.[170,233]

Gene Therapy and Antisense Oligonucleotides

Ablation of the PrP gene in Tg(Prnp[0/0]) mice has not affected the development of these animals, and they remain healthy at almost 2 years of age.[71] Because Prnp[0/0] mice are resistant to prions (see Fig. 37-4) and do not propagate scrapie infectivity (see Table 37-4),[70,409] gene therapy or antisense oligonucleotides may ultimately provide an effective therapeutic approach. Mice heterozygous (Prnp[0/+]) for ablation of the PrP gene had prolonged incubation times after inoculation with Mo prions.[409] This finding is in accord with studies on Tg(SHaPrP) mice, in which increased SHaPrP expression was accompanied by diminished incubation times.[418]

Inhibitors of β-Sheet Formation

Because the absence of PrP^C expression does not provoke disease, it seems reasonable to conclude that scrapie and other prion diseases are a consequence of PrP^{Sc} accumulation rather than an inhibition of PrP^C function.[71] The function of PrP^C remains unknown. These findings suggest that perhaps the most effective therapy may evolve from the development of drugs that block the conversion of PrP^C into PrP^{Sc}. Because the fundamental event in both the formation of PrP^{Sc} and the propagation of prions seems to be the unfolding of α-helices and their refolding into β-sheets,[369] drugs targeting this structural transformation may be efficacious.[96,236]

Whether dyes like Congo red which bind to PrP amyloid are effective in vivo in preventing the formation of PrP^{Sc} remains to be established. Congo red has been reported to inhibit the formation of PrP^{Sc} in cultured scrapie-infected mouse neuroblastoma cells,[84] but the mechanism by which this occurs is unknown.

Dextran sulfates have been used to delay the onset of scrapie in laboratory animals, but these compounds are effective only if given before or concurrently with the prion inoculum.[127,141,148] The inhibitory effect of dextrans on prion propagation has been most pronounced in animals inoculated intraperitoneally. The mechanism by which the sulphated sugar polymers inhibit PrP^{Sc} formation in cultured cells and animals is unknown.[86]

Injection of corticosteroids into mice at the time of intraperitoneal inoculation of prions results in prolongation of the incubation time.[359] These results suggested that the immune system plays a role in the initial phase of scrapie infection, as did studies with spleenless mice.[125] Studies with nude mice and, more recently, with SCID mice showed that incubation times were unaltered compared with controls after intracerebral inoculation; in contrast, SCID mice were not susceptible to prions inoculated intraperitoneally.[270] Studies of lymphoid tissues after intraperitoneal inoculation of prions showed that the follicular dendritic cells, which are thought to function in the presentation of antigens, selectively accumulate PrP^{Sc}. In SCID mice, no focal accumulations of PrP^{Sc} in lymphoid tissues have been found.[270]

Chronic treatment with the antifungal drug amphotericin, begun at the time of intracerebral inoculation, prolonged incubation periods in mice and hamsters.[81,385,501] Administration of amphotericin to humans with CJD had no therapeutic effect[315]; likewise, the antiviral drug amantidine was ineffective.[46,221,472] HPA-23 is an inhibitor of viral glycoprotein synthesis; if given to scrapie-infected animals at about the time of inoculation, but not later, it profoundly extends the length of the incubation period.[263] The effects in human CJD are uncertain.[83] Interferon has been used in experimental scrapie of rodents, but the incubation times were unaltered.[155,254,500]

Although antibodies have been raised against the scrapie PrP and these crossreact with PrPs in CJD human brains,[40] passive immunization or even vaccination would seem to be of little value. CJD and scrapie both progress in the absence of any immune response to the offending prions; however, neutralization of scrapie prion infectivity was accomplished when the infectious particles were dispersed into detergent-lipid-protein complexes.[165]

Resistant Breeds of Sheep

With the discovery that Suffolk sheep with QQ homozygosity at codon 171 are susceptible to scrapie but QR and RR sheep are resistant,[486] the notion of breeding scrapie-resistant sheep, as proposed by Parry, seems reasonable.[370] The screening procedures for identifying QQ sheep are simple and could be applied in an agricultural setting with ease.

CONCLUDING REMARKS

Prions Are Not Viruses

The study of prions has taken several unexpected directions over the past few years. The discovery that prion diseases in humans are uniquely both genetic and infectious has greatly strengthened and extended the prion concept. To date, 18 different mutations in the human PrP gene, all resulting in nonconservative substitutions, have been found either to be linked genetically to the inherited prion diseases or to segregate with them. Yet, the transmissible prion particle is composed largely, if not entirely, of an abnormal isoform of the prion protein designated PrP^{Sc}.[393] These findings argue that prion diseases should be considered pseudoinfections, because the particles transmitting disease appear to be devoid of a foreign nucleic acid and therefore differ from all known microorganisms, viruses, and viroids. Because much information, especially about scrapie of rodents, has been derived with the use of experimental protocols adapted from virology, we continue to use terms such as infection, incubation period, transmissibility, and end point titration in studies of prion diseases.

Do Prions Exist in Lower Organisms?

In *Saccharomyces cerevisiae*, ure2 and [URE3] mutants were described that can grow on ureidosuccinate under conditions of nitrogen repression such as the presence of glutamic acid and ammonia.[284] Mutants of uRE2 exhibit mendelian inheritance, whereas [URE3] is cytoplasmically inherited.[488] The [URE3] phenotype can be induced by ultraviolet radiation and by overexpression of ure2p, the gene product of ure2; deletion of ure2 abolishes [URE3]. The function of ure2p is unknown, but it has substantial homology with glutathione-S-transferase; attempts to demonstrate this enzymic activity with purified ure2p have not been successful.[103] Whether the [URE3] protein is a posttranslationally modified form of ure2p that acts on unmodified ure2p to produce more of itself remains to be established.

Another possible yeast prion is the [PSI] phenotype.[488] [PSI] is a nonmendelian inherited trait that can be induced by expression of the PNM2 gene.[105] Both [PSI] and [URE3] can be cured by exposure of the yeast to 3 mM GdnHCl. The mechanism responsible for abolishing [PSI] and [URE3] with a low concentration of GdnHCl is unknown. In the filamentous fungus, *Podospora anserina*, the het-s locus controls the vegetative incompatibility; conversion from the S^s to the s state seems to be a posttranslational, autocatalytic process.[120]

If any of these examples can be shown to function in a manner similar to prions in animals, then many new, more rapid, and economical approaches to prion diseases should be forthcoming.

Common Neurodegenerative Diseases

The knowledge accrued from the study of prion diseases may provide an effective strategy for defining the causes and dissecting the molecular pathogenesis of the more common neurodegenerative disorders such as Alzheimer's disease, Parkinson's disease, and amyotrophic lateral sclerosis. Advances in the molecular genetics of Alzheimer's disease and amyotrophic lateral sclerosis suggest that, as with the prion diseases, an important subset is caused by mutations that result in nonconservative amino acid substitutions in proteins expressed in the CNS.[193,290,337,435,441,456,478,479]

Future Studies

Tg mice expressing foreign or mutant PrP genes now permit virtually all facets of prion diseases to be studied and have created a framework for future investigations. Furthermore, the structure and organization of the PrP gene suggest that PrP^{Sc} is derived from PrP^C or a precursor by a posttranslational process. Studies with scrapie-infected cultured cells have provided much evidence that the conversion of PrP^C to PrP^{Sc} occurs within a subcellular compartment bounded by cholesterol-rich membranes. The molecular mechanism of PrP^{Sc} formation remains to be elucidated.

The study of prion biology and disease has emerged as a new area of biomedical investigation. Although prion biology has its roots in virology, neurology, and neuropathology, its relations to the disciplines of molecular and cell biology and protein chemistry are now evident. Learning how prions multiply and cause disease will open up new vistas in biochemistry and genetics.

ABBREVIATIONS

Ala: alanine (A)
Arg: arginine (R)
Asn: aspargine (N)
Asp: aspartate (D)
BSE: bovine spongiform encephalopathy
CHOs: carbohydrates
CJD: Creutzfeldt-Jakob disease
CpG: Cytosine-phosphoguanine
Cys: cysteine (C)
FFI: fatal familial insomnia
FSE: feline spongiform encephalopathy
Gln: glutamine (Q)
Glu: glutamate (E)
Gly: glycine (G)
GPI: glycoinositol phospholipid
GSS: Gerstmann-Sträussler-Scheinker disease
HGH: human growth hormone
Hu: human
ID$_{50}$: median infective dose unit
Ile: isoleucine (I)
Leu: leucine (L)
LOD: logarithm of odds (score)
Lys: lysine (K)

Met: methionine (M)
Mo: mouse
ORF: open reading frame
Phe: phenylalanine (F)
Pro: proline (P)
PrP 27-30: Protease-resistant polypeptide core of PrP^{Sc}
PrP: the prion (from **pro**teinaceous **in**fectious particle) protein
PrP^C: the normal cellular isoform of PrP
PrP^{CJD}: A pathogenic conformer found in brains of patients with prion disease
PrP^{Sc}: a pathogenic conformer of the host-encoded PrP^C
RML: Rocky Mountain Laboratory
Ser: serine (S)
SHa: Syrian golden hamster
Tg: transgenic
Thr: threonine (T)
Tyr: tyrosine (Y)
Val: valine (V)
wt: wild-type

ACKNOWLEDGMENTS

I thank M. Baldwin, D. Borchelt, G. Carlson, F. Cohen, C. Cooper, S. DeArmond, R. Fletterick, M. Gasset, R. Gabizon, D. Groth, R. Koehler, L. Hood, K. Hsiao, Z. Huang, V. Lingappa, K.-M. Pan, D. Riesner, M. Scott, A. Serban, N. Stahl, A. Taraboulos, M. Torchia, and D. Westaway for their help in these studies. Special thanks to L. Gallagher, who assembled this manuscript. Supported by grants from the National Institutes of Health (NS14069, AG08967, AG02132, NS22786, and AG10770) and the American Health Assistance Foundation, and by grants from Sherman Fairchild Foundation, Bernard Osher Foundation, and National Medical Enterprises.

REFERENCES

1. Adams DH. The nature of the scrapie agent: a review of recent progress. Pathol Biol 1970;18:559–577.
2. Adams DH, Caspary EA. Nature of the scrapie virus. Br Med J 1967;3:173.
3. Adams DH, Field EJ. The infective process in scrapie. Lancet 1968;2:714–716.
4. Aiken JM, Williamson JL, Borchardt LM, Marsh RF. Presence of mitochondrial D-loop DNA in scrapie-infected brain preparations enriched for the prion protein. J Virol 1990;64:3265–3268.
5. Aiken JM, Williamson JL, Marsh RF. Evidence of mitochondrial involvement in scrapie infection. J Virol 1989;63:1686–1694.
6. Akowitz A, Sklaviadis T, Manuelidis EE, Manuelidis L. Nuclease-resistant polyadenylated RNAs of significant size are detected by PCR in highly purified Creutzfeldt-Jakob disease preparations. Microb Pathog 1990;9:33–45.
7. Alper T, Cramp WA, Haig DA, Clarke MC. Does the agent of scrapie replicate without nucleic acid? Nature 1967;214:764–766.
8. Alper T, Haig DA, Clarke MC. The exceptionally small size of the scrapie agent. Biochem Biophys Res Commun 1966;22:278–284.
9. Alper T, Haig DA, Clarke MC. The scrapie agent: evidence against its dependence for replication on intrinsic nucleic acid. J Gen Virol 1978;41:503–516.
10. Alpers M. Kuru: a clinical study. In: Mimeographed Manuscript, Reissued. Bethesda: USDHEW, NIH, NINCDS, 1964;1–38.
11. Alpers MP. Epidemiology and ecology of kuru. In: Prusiner SB, Hadlow WJ, eds. Slow transmissible diseases of the nervous system. Vol 1. New York: Academic Press, 1979;67–90.
12. Alpers M. Epidemiology and clinical aspects of kuru. In: Prusiner SB, McKinley MP, eds. Prions: novel infectious pathogens causing scrapie and Creutzfeldt-Jakob disease. Orlando: Academic Press, 1987:451–465.
13. Alter M, Kahana E. Creutzfeldt-Jakob disease among Libyan Jews in Israel. Science 1976;192:428.
14. Amyx HL, Gibbs CJ Jr, Gajdusek DC, Greer WE. Absence of vertical transmission of subacute spongiform viral encephalopathies in experimental primates (41092). Proc Soc Exp Biol Med 1981;166:469–471.
15. Anderson JR, Allen CMC, Weller RO. Creutzfeldt-Jakob disease following human pituitary-derived growth hormone administration. Br Neuropathol Soc Proc 1990;16:543.
16. Anonymous. The first victim of mad cow disease? Daily Mail (London). 1993;Sept 13:1.
17. Anonymous. Second farmer's death raises fear of "mad cow" cover-up. London Times 1993;Aug 13:4.
18. Azzarelli B, Muller J, Ghetti B, Dyken M, Conneally PM. Cerebellar plaques in familial Alzheimer's disease (Gerstmann-Str(aua)ussler-Scheinker variant?). Acta Neuropathol (Berl) 1985;65:235–246.
19. Baker HF, Poulter M, Crow TJ, Frith CD, Lofthouse R, Ridley RM. Amino acid polymorphism in human prion protein and age at death in inherited prion disease. Lancet 1991;337:1286.
20. Baker HF, Ridley RM, Wells GAH. Experimental transmission of BSE and scrapie to the common marmoset. Vet Rec 1993; 132:403–406.
21. Barry RA, Prusiner SB. Monoclonal antibodies to the cellular and scrapie prion proteins. J Infect Dis 1986;154:518–521.
22. Basler K, Oesch B, Scott M, et al. Scrapie and cellular PrP isoforms are encoded by the same chromosomal gene. Cell 1986;46:417–428.
23. Bastian FO. Spiroplasma-like inclusions in Creutzfeldt-Jakob disease. Arch Pathol Lab Med 1979;103:665–669.
24. Bastian FO. Bovine spongiform encephalopathy: relationship to human disease and nature of the agent. ASM News 1993;59:235–240.
25. Beck E, Daniel PM, Parry HB. Degeneration of the cerebellar and hypothalamo-neurohypophysial systems in sheep with scrapie and its relationship to human system degenerations. Brain 1964;87:153–176.
26. Bellinger-Kawahara C, Cleaver JE, Diener TO, Prusiner SB. Purified scrapie prions resist inactivation by UV irradiation. J Virol 1987;61:159–166.
27. Bellinger-Kawahara C, Diener TO, McKinley MP, Groth DF, Smith DR, Prusiner SB. Purified scrapie prions resist inactivation by procedures that hydrolyze, modify, or shear nucleic acids. Virology 1987;160:271–274.
28. Bellinger-Kawahara CG, Kempner E, Groth DF, Gabizon R, Prusiner SB. Scrapie prion liposomes and rods exhibit target sizes of 55,000 Da. Virology 1988;164:537–541.
29. Bendheim PE, Barry RA, DeArmond SJ, Stites DP, Prusiner SB. Antibodies to a scrapie prion protein. Nature 1984;310:418–421.
30. Bendheim PE, Bockman JM, McKinley MP, Kingsbury DT, Prusiner SB. Scrapie and Creutzfeldt-Jakob disease prion proteins share physical properties and antigenic determinants. Proc Natl Acad Sci U S A 1985;82:997–1001.
31. Berger JR, David NJ. Creutzfeldt-Jakob disease in a physician: a review of the disorder in health care workers. Neurology 1993;43:205–206.
32. Bernouilli CC, Masters CL, Gajdusek DC, Gibbs CJ Jr, Harris JO. Early clinical features of Creutzfeldt-Jakob disease (subacute spongiform encephalopathy). In: Prusiner SB, Hadlow WJ, eds. Slow transmissible diseases of the nervous system. Vol 1. New York: Academic Press, 1979:229–251.
33. Bernouilli C, Siegfried J, Baumgartner G, et al. Danger of accidental person to person transmission of Creutzfeldt-Jakob disease by surgery. Lancet 1977;1:478–479.
34. Bertoni JM, Brown P, Goldfarb L, Gajdusek D, Omaha NE. Familial Creutzfeldt-Jakob disease with the PRNP codon 200^{Lys} mutation and supranuclear palsy but without myoclonus or periodic EEG complexes. Abstract. Neurology 1992;42(Suppl 3):350.
35. Bessen RA, Marsh RF. Biochemical and physical properties of the prion protein from two strains of the transmissible mink encephalopathy agent. J Virol 1992;66:2096–2101.

36. Bessen RA, Marsh RF. Identification of two biologically distinct strains of transmissible mink encephalopathy in hamsters. J Gen Virol 1992;73:329–334.

37. Billette de Villemeur T, Beauvais P, Gourmelon M, Richardet JM. Creutzfeldt-Jakob disease in children treated with growth hormone. Lancet 1991;337:864–865.

38. Blum B, Bakalara N, Simpson L. A model for RNA editing in kinetoplastid mitochondria: "guide" RNA molecules transcribed from maxicircle DNA provide edited information. Cell 1990;60:189–198.

39. Bobowick AR, Brody JA, Matthews MR, Roos R, Gajdusek DC. Creutzfeldt-Jakob disease: a case-control study. Am J Epidemiol 1973;98:381–394.

40. Bockman JM, Kingsbury DT, McKinley MP, Bendheim PE, Prusiner SB. Creutzfeldt-Jakob disease prion proteins in human brains. N Engl J Med 1985;312:73–78.

41. Bockman JM, Prusiner SB, Tateishi J, Kingsbury DT. Immunoblotting of Creutzfeldt-Jakob disease prion proteins: host species–specific epitopes. Ann Neurol 1987;21:589–595.

42. Bolton DC, McKinley MP, Prusiner SB. Identification of a protein that purifies with the scrapie prion. Science 1982;218:1309–1311.

43. Bolton DC, Meyer RK, Prusiner SB. Scrapie PrP 27-30 is a sialoglycoprotein. J Virol 1985;53:596–606.

44. Borchelt DR, Scott M, Taraboulos A, Stahl N, Prusiner SB. Scrapie and cellular prion proteins differ in their kinetics of synthesis and topology in cultured cells. J Cell Biol 1990;110:743–752.

45. Borchelt DR, Taraboulos A, Prusiner SB. Evidence for synthesis of scrapie prion proteins in the endocytic pathway. J Biol Chem 1992;267:16188–16199.

46. Braham J. Jakob-Creutzfeldt disease: treatment by amantadine. Br Med J 1971;4:212–213.

47. Braig H, Diringer H. Scrapie: concept of a virus-induced amyloidosis of the brain. EMBO J 1985;4:2309–2312.

48. Brown P. Virus sterility for human growth hormone. Lancet 1985;2:729–730.

49. Brown P. The decline and fall of Creutzfeldt-Jakob disease associated with human growth hormone therapy. Neurology 1988;38:1135–1137.

50. Brown P. The phenotypic expression of different mutations in transmissible human spongiform encephalopathy. Rev Neurol 1992;148:317–327.

51. Brown P. Infectious cerebral amyloidosis: clinical spectrum, risks and remedies. In: Brown F, ed. Developments in biological standardization. Basel, Switzerland: S Karger, 1993:91–101.

52. Brown P, Cathala F, Castaigne P, Gajdusek DC. Creutzfeldt-Jakob disease: clinical analysis of a consecutive series of 230 neuropathologically verified cases. Ann Neurol 1986;20:597–602.

53. Brown P, Cathala F, Raubertas RF, Gajdusek DC, Castaigne P. The epidemiology of Creutzfeldt-Jakob disease: conclusion of 15-year investigation in France and review of the world literature. Neurology 1987;37:895–904.

54. Brown P, Cerven(aaa)kov(aaa) L, Goldfarb LG, et al. Iatrogenic Creutzfeldt-Jakob disease: an example of the interplay between ancient genes and modern medicine. Neurology 1994;44:291–293.

55. Brown P, Coker-Vann M, Gajdusek DC. Immunological study of patients with Creutzfeldt-Jakob disease and other chronic neurological disorders: Western blot recognition of infection-specific proteins by scrapie virus antibody. In: Bignami A, Bolis CL, Gajdusek DC, eds. Molecular mechanisms of pathogenesis of central nervous system disorders. Geneva: Foundation for the Study of the Nervous System, 1986:107–109.

56. Brown P, Coker-Vann M, Pomeroy K, et al. Diagnosis of Creutzfeldt-Jakob disease by Western blot identification of marker protein in human brain tissue. N Engl J Med 1986;314:547–551.

57. Brown P, Gajdusek DC, Gibbs CJ Jr, Asher DM. Potential epidemic of Creutzfeldt-Jakob disease from human growth hormone therapy. N Engl J Med 1985;313:728–731.

58. Brown P, Gibbs CJ Jr, Rodgers-Johnson P, et al. Human spongiform encephalopathy: the National Institutes of Health series of 300 cases of experimentally transmitted disease. Ann Neurol 1994;35:513–529.

59. Brown P, Goldfarb LG, Kovanen J, et al. Phenotypic characteristics of familial Creutzfeldt-Jakob disease associated with the codon 178Asn PRNP mutation. Ann Neurol 1992;31:282–285.

60. Brown P, Goldfarb LG, McCombie WR, et al. Atypical Creutzfeldt-Jakob disease in an American family with an insert mutation in the PRNP amyloid precursor gene. Neurology 1992; 42:422–427.

61. Brown P, Kaur P, Sulima MP, Goldfarb LG, Gibbs CJJ, Gajdusek DC. Real and imagined clincopathological limits of "prion dementia." Lancet 1993;341:127–129.

62. Brown P, Preece MA, Will RG. "Friendly fire" in medicine: hormones, homografts, and Creutzfeldt-Jakob disease. Lancet 1992;340:24–27.

63. Brown P, Rodgers-Johnson P, Cathala F, Gibbs CJ Jr, Gajdusek DC. Creutzfeldt-Jakob disease of long duration: clinicopathological characteristics, transmissibility, and differential diagnosis. Ann Neurol 1984;16:295–304.

64. Bruce M, Chree A, McConnell I, Foster J, Fraser H. Transmissions of BSE, scrapie and related diseases to mice. In: IXth International Congress of Virology. Glasgow, Scotland, Aug. 8–13, 1993.1993: 93.

65. Bruce ME, Dickinson AG. Biological stability of different classes of scrapie agent. In: Prusiner SB, Hadlow WJ, eds. Slow transmissible diseases of the nervous system. Vol 2. New York: Academic Press, 1979:71–86.

66. Bruce ME, Dickinson AG. Biological evidence that the scrapie agent has an independent genome. J Gen Virol 1987;68:79–89.

67. Bruce ME, Dickinson AG, Fraser H. Cerebral amyloidosis in scrapie in the mouse: effect of agent strain and mouse genotype. Neuropathol Appl Neurobiol 1976;2:471–478.

68. Bruce ME, McConnell I, Fraser H, Dickinson AG. The disease characteristics of different strains of scrapie in Sinc congenic mouse lines: implications for the nature of the agent and host control of pathogenesis. J Gen Virol 1991;72:595–603.

69. Buchanan CR, Preece MA, Milner RDG. Mortality, neoplasia and Creutzfeldt-Jakob disease in patients treated with pituitary growth hormone in the United Kingdom. Br Med J 1991;302:824–828.

70. Büeler H, Aguzzi A, Sailer A, et al. Mice devoid of PrP are resistant to scrapie. Cell 1993;73:1339–1347.

71. Büeler H, Fischer M, Lang Y, et al. Normal development and behaviour of mice lacking the neuronal cell-surface PrP protein. Nature 1992;356:577–582.

72. Butler DA, Scott MRD, Bockman JM, et al. Scrapie-infected murine neuroblastoma cells produce protease-resistant prion proteins. J Virol 1988;62:1558–1564.

73. Buyukmihci N, Rorvik M, Marsh RF. Replication of the scrapie agent in ocular neural tissues. Proc Natl Acad Sci U S A 1980;77:1169–1171.

74. Carlson GA, Ebeling C, Torchia M, Westaway D, Prusiner SB. Delimiting the location of the scrapie prion incubation time gene on chromosome 2 of the mouse. Genetics 1993;133:979–988.

75. Carlson GA, Ebeling C, Yang S-L, et al. Prion isolate specified allotypic interactions between the cellular and scrapie prion proteins in congenic and transgenic mice. Proc Natl Acad Sci U S A 1994;91:5690–5694.

76. Carlson GA, Goodman PA, Lovett M, et al. Genetics and polymorphism of the mouse prion gene complex: the control of scrapie incubation time. Mol Cell Biol 1988;8:5528–5540.

77. Carlson GA, Kingsbury DT, Goodman PA, et al. Linkage of prion protein and scrapie incubation time genes. Cell 1986;46:503–511.

78. Carlson GA, Westaway D, DeArmond SJ, Peterson-Torchia M, Prusiner SB. Primary structure of prion protein may modify scrapie isolate properties. Proc Natl Acad Sci U S A 1989;86:7475–7479.

79. Carp RI, Callahan SM. Variation in the characteristics of 10 mouse-passaged scrapie lines derived from five scrapie-positive sheep. J Gen Virol 1991;72:293–298.

80. Carp RI, Moretz RC, Natelli M, Dickinson AG. Genetic control of scrapie: incubation period and plaque formation in mice. J Gen Virol 1987;68:401–407.

81. Casaccia P, Ladogana A, Xi YG, et al. Measurement of the concentration of amphotericin B in brain tissue of scrapie-infected hamsters with a simple and sensitive method. Antimicrob Agents Chemother 1991;35:1486–1488.

82. Casaccia-Bonnefil P, Kascsak RJ, Fersko R, Callahan S, Carp RI. Brain regional distribution of prion protein PrP27-30 in mice stereotaxically microinjected with different strains of scrapie. J Infect Dis 1993;167:7–12.

83. Cathala F, Baron H. Clinical aspects of Creutzfeldt-Jakob disease. In: Prusiner SB, McKinley MP, eds. Prions: novel infectious patho-

gens causing scrapie and Creutzfeldt-Jakob disease. Orlando: Academic Press, 1987:467–509.

84. Caughey B, Race RE. Potent inhibition of scrapie-associated PrP accumulation by Congo red. J Neurochem 1992;59:768–771.

85. Caughey B, Raymond GJ. The scrapie-associated form of PrP is made from a cell surface precursor that is both protease- and phospholipase-sensitive. J Biol Chem 1991;266:18217–18223.

86. Caughey B, Raymond GJ. Sulfated polyanion inhibition of scrapie-associated PrP accumulation in cultured cells. J Virol 1993;67: 643–650.

87. Chandler RL. Encephalopathy in mice produced by inoculation with scrapie brain material. Lancet 1961;1:1378–1379.

88. Chandler RL. Experimental scrapie in the mouse. Res Vet Sci 1963;4:276–285.

88a. Chazot G, Broussolle E, Lapras CI, Blättler T, Aguzzi A, Kopp N. New variant of Creutzfeldt-Jakob disease in a 26 year old French man. Lancet 1996;347:1181.

89. Chesebro B. PrP and the scrapie agent. Nature 1992;356:560.

90. Chesebro B, Race R, Wehrly K, et al. Identification of scrapie prion protein-specific mRNA in scrapie-infected and uninfected brain. Nature 1985;315:331–333.

91. Cho HJ. Requirement of a protein component for scrapie infectivity. Intervirology 1980;14:213–216.

92. Cho HJ. Inactivation of the scrapie agent by pronase. Can J Comp Med 1983;47:494–496.

93. Cochius JI, Hyman N, Esiri MM. Creutzfeldt-Jakob disease in a recipient of human pituitary-derived gonadotrophin: a second case. J Neurol Neurosurg Psychiatry 1992;55:1094–1095.

94. Cochius JI, Mack K, Burns RJ, Alderman CP, Blumbergs PC. Creutzfeldt-Jakob disease in a recipient of human pituitary-derived gonadotrophin. Aust N Z J Med 1990;20:592–593.

95. Cohen AS, Shirahama T, Skinner M. Electron microscopy of amyloid. In: Harris JR, ed. Electron microscopy of proteins. Vol 3. New York: Academic Press, 1982:165–206.

96. Cohen FE, Pan K-M, Huang Z, Baldwin M, Fletterick RJ, Prusiner SB. Structural clues to prion replication. Science 1994;264:530–531.

97. Collinge J, Brown J, Hardy J, et al. Inherited prion disease with 144 base pair gene insertion 2. Clinical and pathological features. Brain 1992;115:687–710.

98. Collinge J, Harding AE, Owen F, et al. Diagnosis of Gerstmann-Str(aua)ussler syndrome in familial dementia with prion protein gene analysis. Lancet 1989;2:15–17.

99. Collinge J, Owen F, Poulter H, et al. Prion dementia without characteristic pathology. Lancet 1990;336:7–9.

100. Collinge J, Palmer M. CJD discrepancy. Nature 1991;353:802.

101. Collinge J, Palmer MS, Dryden AJ. Genetic predisposition to iatrogenic Creutzfeldt-Jakob disease. Lancet 1991;337:1441–1442.

102. Come JH, Fraser PE, Lansbury PT Jr. A kinetic model for amyloid formation in the prion diseases: importance of seeding. Proc Natl Acad Sci U S A 1993;90:5959–5963.

103. Coschigano PW, Magasanik B. The URE2 gene product of Saccharomyces cerevisiae plays an important role in the cellular response to the nitrogen source and has homology to glutathione S-transferases. Mol Cell Biol 1991;11:822–832.

104. Cousens SN, Harries-Jones R, Knight R, Will RG, Smith PG, Matthews WB. Geographical distribution of cases of Creutzfeldt-Jakob disease in England and Wales 1970–84. J Neurol Neurosurg Psychiatry 1990;53:459–465.

105. Cox BS, Tuite MF, McLaughlin CS. The psi factor of yeast: a problem in inheritance. Yeast 1988;4:159–178.

106. Crow TJ, Collinge J, Ridley RM, et al. Mutations in the prion gene in human transmissible dementia. Seminar on Molecular Approaches to Research in Spongiform Encephalopathies in Man. Abstract. Medical Research Council, London, Dec 14, 1990.

107. Croxson M, Brown P, Synek B, et al. A new case of Creutzfeldt-Jakob disease associated with human growth hormone therapy in New Zealand. Neurology 1988;38:1128–1130.

108. Cuill´82 J, Chelle PL. Experimental transmission of trembling to the goat. CR Seances Acad Sci 1939;208:1058–1060.

109. Cunningham AA, Wells GAH, Scott AC, Kirkwood JK, Barnett JEF. Transmissible spongiform encephalopathy in greater kudu (Tragelaphus strepsiceros). Vet Rec 1993;132:68.

110. Czub M, Braig HR, Diringer H. Pathogenesis of scrapie: study of the temporal development of clinical symptoms of infectivity titres

and scrapie-associated fibrils in brains of hamsters infected intraperitoneally. J Gen Virol 1986;67:2005–2009.

111. Czub M, Braig HR, Diringer H. Replication of the scrapie agent in hamsters infected intracerebrally confirms the pathogenesis of an amyloid-inducing virosis. J Gen Virol 1988;69:1753–1756.

112. Davanipour Z, Goodman L, Alter M, Sobel E, Asher D, Gajdusek DC. Possible modes of transmission of Creutzfeldt-Jakob disease. N Engl J Med 1984;311:1582–1583.

113. Davison C, Rabiner AM. Spastic pseudosclerosis (disseminated encephalomyelopathy: corticopal-lidospinal degeneration): familial and nonfamilial incidence (a clinico-pathologic study). Arch Neurol Psychiatry 1940;44:578–598.

114. Dawson M, Wells GAH, Parker BNJ. Preliminary evidence of the experimental transmissibility of bovine spongiform encephalopathy to cattle. Vet Rec 1990;126:112–113.

115. Dawson M, Wells GAH, Parker BNJ, Scott AC. Primary parenteral transmission of bovine spongiform encephalopathy to the pig. Vet Rec 1990;Sept. 29:338.

116. Dealler SF, Lacey RW. Transmissible spongiform encephalopathies: the threat of BSE to man. Food Microbiol 1990;7:253–279.

117. DeArmond SJ, McKinley MP, Barry RA, Braunfeld MB, McColloch JR, Prusiner SB. Identification of prion amyloid filaments in scrapie-infected brain. Cell 1985;41:221–235.

118. DeArmond SJ, Mobley WC, DeMott DL, Barry RA, Beckstead JH, Prusiner SB. Changes in the localization of brain prion proteins during scrapie infection. Neurology 1987;37:1271–1280.

119. DeArmond SJ, Yang S-L, Lee A, et al. Three scrapie prion isolates exhibit different accumulation patterns of the prion protein scrapie isoform. Proc Natl Acad Sci U S A 1993;90:6449–6453.

120. Deleu C, Clav´82 C, B´82gueret J. A single amino acid difference is sufficient to elicit vegetative incompatibility in the fungus Podospora anserina. Genetics 1993;135:45–52.

121. Deslys J-P, Lasm´82zas C, Dormont D. Selection of specific strains in iatrogenic Creutzfeldt-Jakob disease. Lancet 1994;343:848–849.

122. Deslys J-P, Marc´82 D, Dormont D. Similar genetic susceptibility in iatrogenic and sporadic Creutzfeldt-Jakob disease. J Gen Virol 1994;75:23–27.

123. Dickinson AG, Bruce ME, Outram GW, Kimberlin RH. Scrapie strain differences: the implications of stability and mutation. In: Tateishi J, ed. Proceedings of Workshop on Slow Transmissible Diseases. Tokyo: Japanese Ministry of Health and Welfare, 1984; 105–118.

124. Dickinson AG, Fraser H. Genetical control of the concentration of ME7 scrapie agent in mouse spleen. J Comp Pathol 1969;79:363–366.

125. Dickinson AG, Fraser H. Scrapie: effect of Dh gene on the incubation period of extraneurally injected agent. Heredity 1972;29:91–93.

126. Dickinson AG, Fraser H. An assessment of the genetics of scrapie in sheep and mice. In: Prusiner SB, Hadlow WJ, eds. Slow transmissible diseases of the nervous system. Vol 1. New York: Academic Press, 1979:367–386.

127. Dickinson AG, Fraser H, Outram GW. Scrapie incubation time can exceed natural lifespan. Nature 1975;256:732–733.

128. Dickinson AG, Meikle VM. A comparison of some biological characteristics of the mouse-passaged scrapie agents, 22A and ME7. Genet Res 1969;13:213–225.

129. Dickinson AG, Meikle VMH. Host-genotype and agent effects in scrapie incubation: change in allelic interaction with different strains of agent. Mol Gen Genet 1971;112:73–79.

130. Dickinson AG, Meikle VMH, Fraser H. Identification of a gene which controls the incubation period of some strains of scrapie agent in mice. J Comp Pathol 1968;78:293–299.

131. Dickinson AG, Meikle VM, Fraser H. Genetical control of the concentration of ME7 scrapie agent in the brain of mice. J Comp Pathol 1969;79:15–22.

132. Dickinson AG, Outram GW. The scrapie replication-site hypothesis and its implications for pathogenesis. In: Prusiner SB, Hadlow WJ, eds. Slow transmissible diseases of the nervous system. Vol 2. New York: Academic Press, 1979:13–31.

133. Dickinson AG, Outram GW. Genetic aspects of unconventional virus infections: the basis of the virino hypothesis. In: Bock G, Marsh J, eds. Novel infectious agents and the central nervous system. Ciba Foundation Symposium 135. Chichester, UK: John Wiley & Sons, 1988;63–83.

134. Dickinson AG, Stamp JT. Experimental scrapie in Cheviot and Suffolk sheep. J Comp Pathol 1969;79:23–26.

135. Dickinson AG, Young GB, Stamp JT, Renwick CC. An analysis of natural scrapie in Suffolk sheep. Heredity 1965;20:485–503.

136. Diedrich J, Weitgrefe S, Zupancic M, et al. The molecular pathogenesis of astrogliosis in scrapie and Alzheimer's disease. Microb Pathog 1987;2:435–442.

137. Diener TO. Is the scrapie agent a viroid? Nature 1972;235:218–219.

138. Diener TO, McKinley MP, Prusiner SB. Viroids and prions. Proc Natl Acad Sci U S A 1982;79:5220–5224.

139. Diringer H. Transmissible spongiform encephalopathies (TSE) virus-induced amyloidoses of the central nervous system (CNS). Eur J Epidemiol 1991;7:562–566.

140. Diringer H. Hidden amyloidoses. Exp Clin Immunogenet 1992;9: 212–229.

141. Diringer H, Ehlers B. Chemoprophylaxis of scrapie in mice. J Gen Virol 1991;72:457–460.

142. Diringer H, Gelderblom H, Hilmert H, Ozel M, Edelbluth C, Kimberlin RH. Scrapie infectivity, fibrils and low molecular weight protein. Nature 1983;306:476–478.

143. Dlouhy SR, Hsiao K, Farlow MR, et al. Linkage of the Indiana kindred of Gerstmann-Str(aua)ussler-Scheinker disease to the prion protein gene. Nat Genet 1992;1:64–67.

144. Doh-ura K, Kitamoto T, Sakaki Y, Tateishi J. CJD discrepancy. Nature 1991;353:801–802.

145. Doh-ura K, Tateishi J, Sasaki H, Kitamoto T, Sakaki Y. Pro→Leu change at position 102 of prion protein is the most common but not the sole mutation related to Gerstmann-Str(aua)ussler syndrome. Biochem Biophys Res Commun 1989;163:974–979.

146. Duffy P, Wolf J, Collins G, Devoe A, Streeten B, Cowen D. Possible person to person transmission of Creutzfeldt-Jakob disease. N Engl J Med 1974;290:692–693.

147. Duguid JR, Rohwer RG, Seed B. Isolation of cDNAs of scrapie-modulated RNAs by subtractive hybridization of a cDNA library. Proc Natl Acad Sci U S A 1988;85:5738–5742.

148. Ehlers B, Diringer H. Dextran sulphate 500 delays and prevents mouse scrapie by impairment of agent replication in spleen. J Gen Virol 1984;65:1325–1330.

149. Eklund CM, Hadlow WJ, Kennedy RC. Some properties of the scrapie agent and its behavior in mice. Proc Soc Exp Biol Med 1963;112:974–979.

150. Eklund CM, Kennedy RC, Hadlow WJ. Pathogenesis of scrapie virus infection in the mouse. J Infect Dis 1967;117:15–22.

151. Ellis CJ, Katifi H, Weller RO. A further British case of growth hormone induced Creutzfeldt-Jakob disease. J Neurol Neurosurg Psychiatry 1992;55:1200–1202.

152. Endo T, Groth D, Prusiner SB, Kobata A. Diversity of oligosaccharide structures linked to asparagines of the scrapie prion protein. Biochemistry 1989;28:8380–8388.

153. Farlow MR, Yee RD, Dlouhy SR, Conneally PM, Azzarelli B, Ghetti B. Gerstmann-Str(aua)ussler-Scheinker disease. I. Extending the clinical spectrum. Neurology 1989;39:1446–1452.

154. Field EJ. The significance of astroglial hypertrophy in scrapie, kuru, multiple sclerosis and old age together with a note on the possible nature of the scrapie agent. Deutsch Z Nervenheilkd 1967;192: 265–274.

155. Field EJ, Joyce G, Keith A. Failure of interferon to modify scrapie in the mouse. J Gen Virol 1969;5:149–150.

156. Fink JK, Warren JT Jr., Drury I, Murman D, Peacock BA. Allele-specific sequencing confirms novel prion gene polymorphism in Creutzfeldt-Jakob disease. Neurology 1991;41:1647–1650.

157. Forloni G, Angeretti N, Chiesa R, et al. Neurotoxicity of a prion protein fragment. Nature 1993;362:543–546.

158. Fradkin JE, Schonberger LB, Mills JL, et al. Creutzfeldt-Jakob disease in pituitary growth hormone recipients in the United States. JAMA 1991;265:880–884.

159. Fraser H. Neuropathology of scrapie: the precision of the lesions and their diversity. In: Prusiner SB, Hadlow WJ, eds. Slow transmissible diseases of the nervous system. Vol 1. New York: Academic Press, 1979:387–406.

160. Fraser H, Dickinson AG. The sequential development of the brain lesions of scrapie in three strains of mice. J Comp Pathol 1968;78: 301–311.

161. Fraser H, Dickinson AG. Scrapie in mice. Agent-strain differences in the distribution and intensity of grey matter vacuolation. J Comp Pathol 1973;83:29–40.

162. Fraser H, Dickinson AG. Targeting of scrapie lesions and spread of agent via the retino-tectal projection. Brain Res 1985;346:32–41.

163. Fraser H, McConnell I, Wells GAH, Dawson M. Transmission of bovine spongiform encephalopathy to mice. Vet Rec 1988;123:472.

164. Friede RL, DeJong RN. Neuronal enzymatic failure in Creutzfeldt-Jakob disease:a familial study. Arch Neurol 1964;10:181–195.

165. Gabizon R, McKinley MP, Groth DF, Kenaga L, Prusiner SB. Properties of scrapie prion liposomes. J Biol Chem 1988;263:4950–4955.

166. Gabizon R, McKinley MP, Groth DF, Prusiner SB. Immunoaffinity purification and neutralization of scrapie prion infectivity. Proc Natl Acad Sci U S A 1988;85:6617–6621.

167. Gabizon R, McKinley MP, Prusiner SB. Purified prion proteins and scrapie infectivity copartition into liposomes. Proc Natl Acad Sci U S A 1987;84:4017–4021.

168. Gabizon R, Meiner Z, Cass C, et al. Prion protein gene mutation in Libyan Jews with Creutzfeldt-Jakob disease. Neurology 1991; 41:160.

169. Gabizon R, Prusiner SB. Prion liposomes. Biochem J 1990;266:1–14.

170. Gabizon R, Rosenmann H, Meiner Z, et al. Mutation and polymorphism of the prion protein gene in Libyan Jews with Creutzfeldt-Jakob disease. Am J Hum Genet 1993;33:828–835.

171. Gabriel J-M, Oesch B, Kretzschmar H, Scott M, Prusiner SB. Molecular cloning of a candidate chicken prion protein. Proc Natl Acad Sci U S A 1992;89:9097–9101.

172. Gajdusek DC. Unconventional viruses and the origin and disappearance of kuru. Science 1977;197:943–960.

173. Gajdusek DC. Subacute spongiform virus encephalopathies caused by unconventional viruses. In: Maramorosch K, McKelvey JJ Jr, eds. Subviral pathogens of plants and animals: viroids and prions. Orlando: Academic Press, 1985:483–544.

174. Gajdusek DC. Transmissible and non-transmissible amyloidoses: autocatalytic post-translational conversion of host precursor proteins to μl-pleated sheet configurations. J Neuroimmunol 1988; 20:95–110.

175. Gajdusek DC, Gibbs CJ Jr, Alpers M. Experimental transmission of a kuru-like syndrome to chimpanzees. Nature 1966;209:794–796.

176. Gajdusek DC, Gibbs CJ Jr, Asher DM, et al. Precautions in medical care of and in handling materials from patients with transmissible virus dementia (CJD). N Engl J Med 1977;297:1253–1258.

177. Gajdusek DC, Zigas V. Degenerative disease of the central nervous system in New Guinea: the endemic occurrence of "kuru" in the native population. N Engl J Med 1957;257:974–978.

178. Gajdusek DC, Zigas V. Clinical, pathological and epidemiological study of an acute progressive degenerative disease of the central nervous system among natives of the eastern highlands of New Guinea. Am J Med 1959;26:442–469.

179. Gard S. Encephalomyelitis of mice. II. A method for the measurement of virus activity. J Exp Med 1940;72:69–77.

180. Gasset M, Baldwin MA, Lloyd D, et al. Predicted α-helical regions of the prion protein when synthesized as peptides form amyloid. Proc Natl Acad Sci U S A 1992;89:10940–10944.

181. Gerstmann J, Str(aua)ussler E, Scheinker I. "9Aber eine eigenartige heredit(aua)r-famili(aua)re Erkrankung des Zentralnervensystems zugleich ein Beitrag zur frage des vorzeitigen lokalen Alterns. Z Neurol 1936;154:736–762.

182. Ghetti B, Tagliavini F, Masters CL, et al. Gerstmann-Str(aua)ussler-Scheinker disease. II. Neurofibrillary tangles and plaques with PrP-amyloid coexist in an affected family. Neurology 1989;39:1453–1461.

183. Giaccone G, Tagliavini F, Verga L, et al. Neurofibrillary tangles of the Indiana kindred of Gerstmann-Str(aua)ussler-Scheinker disease share antigenic determinants with those of Alzheimer disease. Brain Res 1990;530:325–329.

184. Gibbons RA, Hunter GD. Nature of the scrapie agent. Nature 1967; 215:1041–1043.

185. Gibbs CJ Jr, Amyx HL, Bacote A, Masters CL, Gajdusek DC. Oral transmission of kuru, Creutzfeldt-Jakob disease and scrapie to non-human primates. J Infect Dis 1980;142:205–208.

186. Gibbs CJ Jr, Asher DM, Brown PW, Fradkin JE, Gajdusek DC. Creutzfeldt-Jakob disease infectivity of growth hormone derived from human pituitary glands. N Engl J Med 1993;328: 358–359.

187. Gibbs CJ Jr, Asher DM, Kobrine A, Amyx HL, Sulima MP, Gajdusek DC. Transmission of Creutzfeldt-Jakob disease to a chimpanzee by electrodes contaminated during neurosurgery. J Neurol Neurosurg Psychiatry 1994;57:757–758.

188. Gibbs CJ Jr, Gajdusek DC. Infection as the etiology of spongiform encephalopathy. Science 1969;165:1023–1025.

189. Gibbs CJ Jr, Gajdusek DC. Experimental subacute spongiform virus encephalopathies in primates and other laboratory animals. Science 1973;182:67–68.

190. Gibbs CJ Jr, Gajdusek DC, Amyx H. Strain variation in the viruses of Creutzfeldt-Jakob disease and kuru. In: Prusiner SB, Hadlow WJ, eds. Slow transmissible diseases of the nervous system. Vol 2. New York: Academic Press, 1979:87–110.

191. Gibbs CJ Jr, Gajdusek DC, Asher DM, et al. Creutzfeldt-Jakob disease (spongiform encephalopathy): transmission to the chimpanzee. Science 1968;161:388–389.

192. Gibbs CJ Jr, Joy A, Heffner R, et al. Clinical and pathological features and laboratory confirmation of Creutzfeldt-Jakob disease in a recipient of pituitary-derived human growth hormone. N Engl J Med 1985;313:734–738.

193. Goate A, Chartier-Harlin M-C, Mullan M, et al. Segregation of a missense mutation in the amyloid precursor protein gene with familial Alzheimer's disease. Nature 1991;349:704–706.

194. Goldfarb LG, Brown P, Gajdusek DC. The molecular genetics of human transmissible spongiform encephalopathy. In: Prusiner SB, Collinge J, Powell J, Anderton B, eds. Prion diseases of humans and animals. London: Ellis Horwood, 1992:139–153.

195. Goldfarb LG, Brown P, Goldgaber D, et al. Creutzfeldt-Jakob disease and kuru patients lack a mutation consistently found in the Gerstmann-Str(aua)ussler-Scheinker syndrome. Exp Neurol 1990;108: 247–250.

196. Goldfarb L, Brown P, Goldgaber D, et al. Identical mutation in unrelated patients with Creutzfeldt-Jakob disease. Lancet 1990;336: 174–175.

197. Goldfarb LG, Brown P, Haltia M, Ghiso J, Frangione B, Gajdusek DC. Synthetic peptides corresponding to different mutated regions of the amyloid gene in familial Creutzfeldt-Jakob disease show enhanced in vitro formation of morphologically different amyloid fibrils. Proc Natl Acad Sci U S A 1993;90:4451–4454.

198. Goldfarb LG, Brown P, Haltia M, et al. Creutzfeldt-Jakob disease cosegregates with the codon 178Asn PRNP mutation in families of European origin. Ann Neurol 1992;31:274–281.

199. Goldfarb LG, Brown P, McCombie WR, et al. Transmissible familial Creutzfeldt-Jakob disease associated with five, seven, and eight extra octapeptide coding repeats in the PRNP gene. Proc Natl Acad Sci U S A 1991;88:10926–10930.

200. Goldfarb LG, Brown P, Mitrova E, et al. Creutzfeldt-Jacob disease associated with the PRNP codon 200Lys mutation: an analysis of 45 families. Eur J Epidemiol 1991;7:477–486.

201. Goldfarb LG, Brown P, Vrbovsk(aaa) A, et al. An insert mutation in the chromosome 20 amyloid precursor gene in a Gerstmann-Str(aua)ussler-Scheinker family. J Neurol Sci 1992;111:189–194.

202. Goldfarb LG, Haltia M, Brown P, et al. New mutation in scrapie amyloid precursor gene (at codon 178) in Finnish Creutzfeldt-Jakob kindred. Lancet 1991;337:425.

203. Goldfarb L, Korczyn A, Brown P, Chapman J, Gajdusek DC. Mutation in codon 200 of scrapie amyloid precursor gene linked to Creutzfeldt-Jakob disease in Sephardic Jews of Libyan and non-Libyan origin. Lancet 1990;336:637–638.

204. Goldfarb LG, Mitrova E, Brown P, Toh BH, Gajdusek DC. Mutation in codon 200 of scrapie amyloid protein gene in two clusters of Creutzfeldt-Jakob disease in Slovakia. Lancet 1990;336:514–515.

205. Goldfarb LG, Petersen RB, Tabaton M, et al. Fatal familial insomnia and familial Creutzfeldt-Jakob disease: disease phenotype determined by a DNA polymorphism. Science 1992;258:806–808.

206. Goldgaber D, Goldfarb LG, Brown P, et al. Mutations in familial Creutzfeldt-Jakob disease and Gerstmann-Str(aua)ussler-Scheinker's syndrome. Exp Neurol 1989;106:204–206.

207. Goldhammer Y, Gabizon R, Meiner Z, Sadeh M. An Israeli family with Gerstmann-Str(aua)ussler-Scheinker disease manifesting the codon 102 mutation in the prion protein gene. Neur 1993;43:2718–2719.

208. Goldmann W, Hunter N, Foster JD, Salbaum JM, Beyreuther K, Hope J. Two alleles of a neural protein gene linked to scrapie in sheep. Proc Natl Acad Sci U S A 1990;87:2476–2480.

209. Goldmann W, Hunter N, Manson J, Hope J. The PrP gene of the sheep, a natural host of scrapie. VIIIth International Congress of Virology, Berlin, Aug 26–31, 1990 [Abstr].

210. Goldmann W, Hunter N, Martin T, Dawson M, Hope J. Different forms of the bovine PrP gene have five or six copies of a short, G-C-rich element within the protein-coding exon. J Gen Virol 1991;72: 201–204.

211. Gordon WS. Advances in veterinary research. Vet Res 1946;58: 516–520.

212. Gordon WS. Variation in susceptibility of sheep to scrapie and genetic implications. In: Report of Scrapie Seminar, ARS 91-53. Washington, DC: US Department of Agriculture, 1966:53–67.

213. Griffith JS. Self-replication and scrapie. Nature 1967;215:1043–1044.

214. Hadlow WJ, Kennedy RC, Race RE. Natural infection of Suffolk sheep with scrapie virus. J Infect Dis 1982;146:657–664.

215. Hadlow WJ, Kennedy RC, Race RE, Eklund CM. Virologic and neurohistologic findings in dairy goats affected with natural scrapie. Vet Pathol 1980;17:187–199.

216. Haltia M, Kovanen J, Goldfarb LG, Brown P, Gajdusek DC. Familial Creutzfeldt-Jakob disease in Finland: Epidemiological, clinical, pathological and molecular genetic studies. Eur J Epidemiol 1991;7:494–500.

217. Hardy J. Prion dimers: a deadly duo. Trends Neurosci 1991;14:423–424.

218. Harries-Jones R, Knight R, Will RG, Cousens S, Smith PG, Matthews WB. Creutzfeldt-Jakob disease in England and Wales, 1980–1984: a case-control study of potential risk factors. J Neurol Neurosurg Psychiatry 1988;51:1113–1119.

219. Healy DL, Evans J. Creutzfeldt-Jakob disease after pituitary gonadotrophins. Br J Med 1993;307:517–518.

220. Hecker R, Taraboulos A, Scott M, et al. Replication of distinct prion isolates is region specific in brains of transgenic mice and hamsters. Genes Dev 1992;6:1213–1228.

221. Herishanu Y. Antiviral drugs in Jakob-Creutzfeldt disease. J Am Geriatr Soc 1973;21:229–231.

222. Herzberg L, Herzberg BN, Gibbs CJ Jr, Sullivan W, Amyx H, Gajdusek DC. Creutzfeldt-Jakob disease: hypothesis for high incidence in Libyan Jews in Israel. Science 1974;186:848.

223. Heston LL, Lowther DLW, Leventhal CM. Alzheimer's disease: a family study. Arch Neurol 1966;15:225–233.

224. Hope J, Morton LJD, Farquhar CF, Multhaup G, Beyreuther K, Kimberlin RH. The major polypeptide of scrapie-associated fibrils (SAF) has the same size, charge distribution and N-terminal protein sequence as predicted for the normal brain protein (PrP). EMBO J 1986;5:2591–2597.

225. Hope J, Reekie LJD, Hunter N, et al. Fibrils from brains of cows with new cattle disease contain scrapie-associated protein. Nature 1988;336:390–392.

226. Hornabrook RW. Kuru—a subacute cerebellar degeneration: the natural history and clinical features. Brain 1968;91:53–74.

227. Hornabrook RW. Kuru and clinical neurology. In: Prusiner SB, Hadlow WJ, eds. Slow transmissible diseases of the nervous system. Vol 1. New York: Academic Press, 1979:37–66.

228. Hsiao K, Baker HF, Crow TJ, et al. Linkage of a prion protein missense variant to Gerstmann-Str(aua)ussler syndrome. Nature 1989;338:342–345.

229. Hsiao KK, Cass C, Schellenberg GD, et al. A prion protein variant in a family with the telencephalic form of Gerstmann-Str(aua)ussler-Scheinker syndrome. Neurology 1991;41:681–684.

230. Hsiao K, Dlouhy S, Farlow MR, et al. Mutant prion proteins in Gerstmann-Str(aua)ussler-Scheinker disease with neurofibrillary tangles. Nat Genet 1992;1:68–71.

231. Hsiao KK, Doh-ura K, Kitamoto T, Tateishi J, Prusiner SB. A prion protein amino acid substitution in ataxic Gerstmann-Str(aua)ussler syndrome. Ann Neurol 1989;26:137.

232. Hsiao KK, Groth D, Scott M, et al. Serial transmission in rodents of neurodegeneration from transgenic mice expressing mutant prion protein. Proc Natl Acad Sci U S A 1994;91:9126–9130.

233. Hsiao K, Meiner Z, Kahana E, et al. Mutation of the prion protein in Libyan Jews with Creutzfeldt-Jakob disease. N Engl J Med 1991;324:1091–1097.

234. Hsiao K, Prusiner SB. Inherited human prion diseases. Neurology 1990;40:1820–1827.

235. Hsiao KK, Scott M, Foster D, Groth DF, DeArmond SJ, Prusiner SB. Spontaneous neurodegeneration in transgenic mice with mutant prion protein. Science 1990;250:1587–1590.

236. Huang Z, Gabriel J-M, Baldwin MA, Fletterick RJ, Prusiner SB, Cohen FE. Proposed three-dimensional structure for the cellular prion protein. Proc Natl Acad Sci U S A 1994;91:7139–7143.

237. Humphery-Smith I, Chastel C, Le Goff F. Spirosplasmas and spongiform encephalopathies. Med J Aust 1992;156:142.

238. Hunter GD. Scrapie: a prototype slow infection. J Infect Dis 1972;125:427–440.

239. Hunter GD, Gibbons RA, Kimberlin RH, Millson GC. Further studies of the infectivity and stability of extracts and homogenates derived from scrapie affected mouse brains. J Comp Pathol 1969;79:101–108.

240. Hunter GD, Kimberlin RH, Collis S, Millson GC. Viral and non-viral properties of the scrapie agent. Ann Clin Res 1973;5:262–267.

241. Hunter GD, Kimberlin RH, Gibbons RA. Scrapie: a modified membrane hypothesis. J Theor Biol 1968;20:355–357.

242. Hunter GD, Millson GC. Studies on the heat stability and chromatographic behavior of the scrapie agent. J Gen Microbiol 1964;37:251–258.

243. Hunter GD, Millson GC. Attempts to release the scrapie agent from tissue debris. J Comp Pathol 1967;77:301–307.

244. Hunter N, Foster JD, Dickinson AG, Hope J. Linkage of the gene for the scrapie-associated fibril protein (PrP) to the Sip gene in Cheviot sheep. Vet Rec 1989;124:364–366.

245. Hunter N, Hope J, McConnell I, Dickinson AG. Linkage of the scrapie-associated fibril protein (PrP) gene and Sinc using congenic mice and restriction fragment length polymorphism analysis. J Gen Virol 1987;68:2711–2716.

246. Ikeda S, Yanagisawa N, Allsop D, Glenner GG. A variant of Gerstmann-Str(aua)ussler-Scheinker disease with b-protein epitopes and dystrophic neurites in the peripheral regions of PrP: immunoreactive amyloid plaques. In: Natvig JB, Forre O, Husby G, et al, eds. Amyloid and amyloidosis 1990. Dordrecht: Kluwer Academic Publishers, 1991:737–740.

247. Jacob H, Pyrkosch W, Strube H. Die erbliche Form der Creutzfeldt-Jakobschen Krankheit. Arch Psychiatr Zeitsch Neurol 1950;184:653–674.

248. Jendroska K, Heinzel FP, Torchia M, et al. Proteinase-resistant prion protein accumulation in Syrian hamster brain correlates with regional pathology and scrapie infectivity. Neurology 1991;41:1482–1490.

249. Johnson RT. Prion disease. N Engl J Med 1992;326:486–487.

250. Kahana E, Milton A, Braham J, Sofer D. Creutzfeldt-Jakob disease: focus among Libyan Jews in Israel. Science 1974;183:90–91.

251. Kahana E, Zilber N, Abraham M. Do Creutzfeldt-Jakob disease patients of Jewish Libyan origin have unique clinical features? Neurology 1991;41:1390–1392.

252. Kane PM, Yamashiro CT, Wolczyk DF, Neff N, Goebl M, Stevens TH. Protein splicing converts the yeast TFP1 gene product to the 69-kD subunit of the vacuolar H+-adenosine triphosphatase. Science 1990;250:651–657.

253. Kascsak RJ, Rubenstein R, Merz PA, et al. Mouse polyclonal and monoclonal antibody to scrapie-associated fibril proteins. J Virol 1987;61:3688–3693.

254. Katz M, Koprowski H. Failure to demonstrate a relationship between scrapie and production of interferon in mice. Nature 1968;219:639–640.

255. Kellings K, Meyer N, Mirenda C, Prusiner SB, Riesner D. Further analysis of nucleic acids in purified scrapie prion preparations by improved return refocussing gel electrophoresis (RRGE). J Gen Virol 1992;73:1025–1029.

256. Kimberlin RH. Scrapie and possible relationships with viroids. Semin Virol 1990;1:153–162.

257. Kimberlin RH, Cole S, Walker CA. Temporary and permanent modifications to a single strain of mouse scrapie on transmission to rats and hamsters. J Gen Virol 1987;68:1875–1881.

258. Kimberlin RH, Field HJ, Walker CA. Pathogenesis of mouse scrapie: evidence for spread of infection from central to peripheral nervous system. J Gen Virol 1983;64:713–716.

259. Kimberlin RH, Hunter GD. DNA synthesis in scrapie-affected mouse brain. J Gen Virol 1967;1:115–124.

260. Kimberlin RH, Walker CA. Evidence that the transmission of one source of scrapie agent to hamsters involves separation of agent strains from a mixture. J Gen Virol 1978;39:487–496.

261. Kimberlin RH, Walker CA. Pathogenesis of mouse scrapie: effect of route of inoculation on infectivity titres and dose-response curves. J Comp Pathol 1978;88:39–47.

262. Kimberlin RH, Walker CA. Pathogenesis of mouse scrapie: dynamics of agent replication in spleen, spinal cord and brain after infection by different routes. J Comp Pathol 1979;89:551–562.

263. Kimberlin RH, Walker CA. The antiviral compound HPA-23 can prevent scrapie when administered at the time of infection. Arch Virol 1983;78:9–18.

264. Kimberlin RH, Walker CA, Fraser H. The genomic identity of different strains of mouse scrapie is expressed in hamsters and preserved on reisolation in mice. J Gen Virol 1989;70:2017–2025.

265. Kingsbury DT, Kasper KC, Stites DP, Watson JD, Hogan RN, Prusiner SB. Genetic control of scrapie and Creutzfeldt-Jakob disease in mice. J Immunol 1983;131:491–496.

266. Kirkwood JK, Cunningham AA, Wells GAH, Wilesmith JW, Barnett JEF. Spongiform encephalopathy in a herd of greater kudu (Tragelaphus strepsiceros): epidemiological observations. Vet Rec 1993;133:360–364.

267. Kirkwood JK, Wells GAH, Wilesmith JW, Cunningham AA, Jackson SI. Spongiform encephalopathy in an arabian oryx (Oryx leucoryx) and a greater kudu (Tragelaphus strepsiceros). Vet Rec 1990;127:418–420.

268. Kirschbaum WR. Zwei eigenartige Erkrankungen des Zentralnervensystems nach Art der spastischen Pseudosklerose (Jakob). Z Ges Neurol Psychiatr 1924;92:175–220.

269. Kitamoto T, Iizuka R, Tateishi J. An amber mutation of prion protein in Gerstmann-Str(aua)ussler syndrome with mutant PrP plaques. Biochem Biophys Res Commun 1993;192:525–531.

270. Kitamoto T, Muramoto T, Mohri S, Doh-ura K, Tateishi J. Abnormal isoform of prion protein accumulates in follicular dendritic cells in mice with Creutzfeldt-Jakob disease. J Virol 1991;65:6292–6295.

271. Kitamoto T, Ohta M, Doh-ura K, Hitoshi S, Terao Y, Tateishi J. Novel missense variants of prion protein in Creutzfeldt-Jakob disease or Gerstmann-Str(aua)ussler syndrome. Biochem Biophys Res Commun 1993;191:709–714.

272. Kitamoto T, Shin R-W, Doh-ura K, et al. Abnormal isoform of prion proteins accumulates in the synaptic structures of the central nervous system in patients with Creutzfeldt-Jakob disease. Am J Pathol 1992;140:1285–1294.

273. Kitamoto T, Tateishi J. Human prion diseases with variant prion protein. Phil Trans R Soc Lond B 1994;343:391–398.

274. Kitamoto T, Tateishi J, Sawa H, Doh-Ura K. Positive transmission of Creutzfeldt-Jakob disease verified by murine kuru plaques. Lab Invest 1989;60:507–512.

275. Kitamoto T, Tateishi J, Tashima I, et al. Amyloid plaques in Creutzfeldt-Jakob disease stain with prion protein antibodies. Ann Neurol 1986;20:204–208.

276. Klatzo I, Gajdusek DC, Zigas V. Pathology of kuru. Lab Invest 1959;8:799–847.

277. Klitzman RL, Alpers MP, Gajdusek DC. The natural incubation period of kuru and the episodes of transmission in three clusters of patients. Neuroepidemiology 1984;3:3–20.

278. Koch TK, Berg BO, DeArmond SJ, Gravina RF. Creutzfeldt-Jakob disease in a young adult with idiopathic hypopituitarism: possible relation to the administration of cadaveric human growth hormone. N Engl J Med 1985;313:731–733.

279. Kondo K, Kuroina Y. A case control study of Creutzfeldt-Jakob disease: association with physical injuries. Ann Neurol 1981;11:377–381.

280. Kretzschmar HA, Honold G, Seitelberger F, et al. Prion protein mutation in family first reported by Gerstmann, Straussler, and Scheinker. Lancet 1991;337:1160.

281. Kretzschmar HA, Kufer P, Riethm''81ller G, DeArmond SJ, Prusiner SB, Schiffer D. Prion protein mutation at codon 102 in an Italian family with Gerstmann-Str(aua)ussler-Scheinker syndrome. Neurology 1992;42:809–810.

282. Kretzschmar HA, Prusiner SB, Stowring LE, DeArmond SJ. Scrapie prion proteins are synthesized in neurons. Am J Pathol 1986; 122:1–5.

283. Kretzschmar HA, Stowring LE, Westaway D, Stubblebine WH, Prusiner SB, DeArmond SJ. Molecular cloning of a human prion protein cDNA. DNA 1986;5:315–324.

284. Lacroute F. Non-Mendelian mutation allowing ureidosuccinic acid uptake in yeast. J Bacteriol 1971;106:519–522.

285. Lantos PL, McGill IS, Janota I, et al. Prion protein immunocytochemistry helps to establish the true incidence of prion diseases. Neurosci Lett 1992;147:67–71.

286. Laplanche J, Chatelain J, Beaudry P, Dussaucy M, Bounneau C, Launay J. French autochthonous scrapied sheep without the 136Val PrP polymorphism. Mammalian Genome 1993;4:463–464.

287. Laplanche J-L, Chatelain J, Launay J-M, Gazengel C, Vidaud M. Deletion in prion protein gene in a Moroccan family. Nucleic Acids Res 1990;18:6745.

288. Laplanche JL, Chatelain J, Westaway D, et al. PrP polymorphisms associated with natural scrapie discovered by denaturing gradient gel electrophoresis. Genomics 1993;15:30–37.

289. Latarjet R, Muel B, Haig DA, Clarke MC, Alper T. Inactivation of the scrapie agent by near monochromatic ultraviolet light. Nature 1970;227:1341–1343.

290. Levy E, Carman MD, Fernandez-Madrid IJ, et al. Mutation of the Alzheimer's disease amyloid gene in hereditary cerebral hemorrhage, Dutch type. Science 1990;248:1124–1126.

291. Lewin P. Scrapie: an infective peptide? Lancet 1972;1:748.

292. Lewin P. Infectious peptides in slow virus infections: a hypothesis. Can Med Assoc J 1981;124:1436–1437.

293. Little BW, Brown PW, Rodgers-Johnson P, Perl DP, Gajdusek DC. Familial myoclonic dementia masquerading as Creutzfeldt-Jakob disease. Ann Neurol 1986;20:231–239.

294. Locht C, Chesebro B, Race R, Keith JM. Molecular cloning and complete sequence of prion protein cDNA from mouse brain infected with the scrapie agent. Proc Natl Acad Sci U S A 1986; 83:6372–6376.

295. Lumley Jones R, Benker G, Salacinski PR, Lloyd TJ, Lowry PJ. Large-scale preparation of highly purified pyrogen-free human growth hormone for clinical use. Br J Endocrinol 1979;82:77–86.

296. Macario ME, Vaisman M, Buescu A, Neto VM, Araujo HMM, Chagas C. Pituitary growth hormone and Creutzfeldt-Jakob disease. Br Med J 1991;302:1149.

297. Malmgren R, Kurland L, Mokri B, Kurtzke J. The epidemiology of Creutzfeldt-Jakob disease. In: Prusiner SB, Hadlow WJ, eds. Slow transmissible diseases of the nervous system. Vol 1. New York: Academic Press, 1979:93–112.

298. Malone TG, Marsh RF, Hanson RP, Semancik JS. Membrane-free scrapie activity. J Virol 1978;25:933–935.

299. Malone TG, Marsh RF, Hanson RP, Semancik JS. Evidence for the low molecular weight nature of the scrapie agent. Nature 1979;278: 575–576.

300. Manetto V, Medori R, Cortelli P, et al. Fatal familial insomnia: clinical and pathological study of five new cases. Neurology 1992; 42:312–319.

301. Manuelidis E, Gorgacz EJ, Manuelidis L. Interspecies transmission of Creutzfeldt-Jakob disease to Syrian hamsters with reference to clinical syndromes and strains of agent. Proc Natl Acad Sci U S A 1978;75:3422–3436.

302. Manuelidis E, Kim J, Angelo J, Manuelidis L. Serial propagation of Creutzfeldt-Jakob disease in guinea pigs. Proc Natl Acad Sci U S A 1976;73:223–227.

303. Manuelidis EE, Manuelidis L. Experiments on maternal transmission of Creutzfeldt-Jakob disease in guinea pigs. Proc Soc Biol Med 1979;160:233–236.

304. Manuelidis L, Manuelidis EE. Creutzfeldt-Jakob disease and dementias. Microb Pathog 1989;7:157–164.

305. Marsh RF, Bessen RA, Lehmann S, Hartsough GR. Epidemiological and experimental studies on a new incident of transmissible mink encephalopathy. J Gen Virol 1991;72:589–594.

306. Marsh RF, Kimberlin RH. Comparison of scrapie and transmissible mink encephalopathy in hamsters. II. Clinical signs, pathology and pathogenesis. J Infect Dis 1975;131:104–110.

307. Marsh RF, Malone TG, Semancik JS, Lancaster WD, Hanson RP. Evidence for an essential DNA component in the scrapie agent. Nature 1978;275:146–147.

308. Martinez-Lage JF, Sola J, Poza M, Esteban JA. Pediatric Creutzfeldt-Jakob disease: probable transmission by a dural graft. Child's Nerv Syst 1993;9:239–242.

309. Marzewski DJ, Towfighi J, Harrington MG, Merril CR, Brown P. Creutzfeldt-Jakob disease following pituitary-derived human growth hormone therapy: a new American case. Neurology 1988;38:1131–1133.

310. Masters CL, Gajdusek DC, Gibbs CJ Jr. Creutzfeldt-Jakob disease virus isolations from the Gerstmann-Str(aua)ussler syndrome. Brain 1981;104:559–588.

311. Masters CL, Gajdusek DC, Gibbs CJ Jr. The familial occurrence of Creutzfeldt-Jakob disease and Alzheimer's disease. Brain 1981; 104:535–558.

312. Masters CL, Gajdusek DC, Gibbs CJ Jr, Bernouilli C, Asher DM. Familial Creutzfeldt-Jakob disease and other familial dementias: an inquiry into possible models of virus-induced familial diseases. In: Prusiner SB, Hadlow WJ, eds. Slow transmissible diseases of the nervous system. Vol 1. New York: Academic Press, 1979:143–194.

313. Masters CL, Harris JO, Gajdusek DC, Gibbs CJ Jr, Bernouilli C, Asher DM. Creutzfeldt-Jakob disease: patterns of worldwide occurrence and the significance of familal and sporadic clustering. Ann Neurol 1978;5:177–188.

314. Masters CL, Richardson EP Jr. Subacute spongiform encephalopathy Creutzfeldt-Jakob disease: the nature and progression of spongiform change. Brain 1978;101:333–344.

315. Masullo C, Macchi G, Xi YG, Pocchiari M. Failure to ameliorate Creutzfeldt-Jakob disease with amphotericin B therapy. J Infect Dis 1992;165:784–785.

316. Masullo C, Pocchiari M, Macchi G, Alema G, Piazza G, Panzera MA. Transmission of Creutzfeldt-Jakob disease by dural cadaveric graft. J Neurosurg 1989;71:954.

317. McBride PA, Eikelenboom P, Kraal G, Fraser H, Bruce ME. PrP protein is associated with follicular dendritic cells of spleens and lymph nodes in uninfected and scrapie-infected mice. J Pathol 1992;168:413–418.

318. McKinley MP, Bolton DC, Prusiner SB. A protease-resistant protein is a structural component of the scrapie prion. Cell 1983;35:57–62.

319. McKinley MP, Masiarz FR, Isaacs ST, Hearst JE, Prusiner SB. Resistance of the scrapie agent to inactivation by psoralens. Photochem Photobiol 1983;37:539–545.

320. McKinley MP, Meyer R, Kenaga L, et al. Scrapie prion rod formation in vitro requires both detergent extraction and limited proteolysis. J Virol 1991;65:1440–1449.

321. McKinley MP, Taraboulos A, Kenaga L, et al. Ultrastructural localization of scrapie prion proteins in cytoplasmic vesicles of infected cultured cells. Lab Invest 1991;65:622–630.

322. McKnight S, Tjian R. Transcriptional selectivity of viral genes in mammalian cells. Cell 1986;46:795–805.

323. Medori R, Montagna P, Tritschler HJ, et al. Fatal familial insomnia: a second kindred with mutation of prion protein gene at codon 178. Neurology 1992;42:669–670.

324. Medori R, Tritschler H-J, LeBlanc A, et al. Fatal familial insomnia, a prion disease with a mutation at codon 178 of the prion protein gene. N Engl J Med 1992;326:444–449.

325. Meggendorfer F. Klinische und genealogische Beobachtungen bei einem Fall von spastischer Pseudosklerose Jakobs. Z Ges Neurol Psychiatr 1930;128:337–341.

326. Merz PA, Rohwer RG, Kascsak R, et al. Infection-specific particle from the unconventional slow virus diseases. Science 1984;225: 437–440.

327. Meyer N, Rosenbaum V, Schmidt B, et al. Search for a putative scrapie genome in purified prion fractions reveals a paucity of nucleic acids. J Gen Virol 1991;72:37–49.

328. Meyer RK, McKinley MP, Bowman KA, Braunfeld MB, Barry RA, Prusiner SB. Separation and properties of cellular and scrapie prion proteins. Proc Natl Acad Sci U S A 1986;83:2310–2314.

329. M'Fadyean J. Scrapie. J Comp Pathol 1918;31:102–131.

330. M'Gowan JP. Investigation into the disease of sheep called "scrapie." Edinburgh: William Blackwood & Sons, 1914:114.

331. Millson G, Hunter GD, Kimberlin RH. An experimental examination of the scrapie agent in cell membrane mixtures. II. The association of scrapie infectivity with membrane fractions. J Comp Pathol 1971;81:255–265.

332. Millson GC, Hunter GD, Kimberlin RH. The physico-chemical nature of the scrapie agent. In: Kimberlin RH, ed. Slow virus diseases of animals and man. New York: American Elsevier, 1976:243–266.

333. Miyashita K, Inuzuka T, Kondo H, et al. Creutzfeldt-Jakob disease in a patient with a cadaveric dural graft. Neurology 1991;41:940–941.

334. Mobley WC, Neve RL, Prusiner SB, McKinley MP. Nerve growth factor increases mRNA levels for the prion protein and the beta-amyloid protein precursor in developing hamster brain. Proc Natl Acad Sci U S A 1988;85:9811–9815.

335. Monari L, Chen SG, Brown P, et al. Fatal familial insomnia and familial Creutzfeldt-Jakob disease: different prion proteins determined by a DNA polymorphism. Proc Natl Acad Sci U S A 1994;91:2839–2842.

336. Morris JA, Gajdusek DC, Gibbs CJ Jr. Spread of scrapie from inoculated to uninoculated mice. Proc Soc Exp Biol Med 1965;120:108–110.

337. Mullan M, Houlden H, Windelspecht M, et al. A locus for familial early-onset Alzheimer's disease on the long arm of chromosome 14, proximal to the a1-antichymotrypsin gene. Nat Genet 1992;2:340–342.

338. Muramoto T, Kitamoto T, Hoque MZ, Tateishi J, Goto I. Species barrier prevents an abnormal isoform of prion protein from accumulating in follicular dendritic cells of mice with Creutzfeldt-Jakob disease. J Virol 1993;67:6808–6810.

339. Muramoto T, Kitamoto T, Tateishi J, Goto I. Successful transmission of Creutzfeldt-Jakob disease from human to mouse verified by prion protein accumulation in mouse brains. Brain Res 1992;599:309–316.

340. Muramoto T, Kitamoto T, Tateishi J, Goto I. Accumulation of abnormal prion protein in mice infected with Creutzfeldt-Jakob disease via intraperitoneal route: a sequential study. Am J Pathol 1993;143:1–10.

341. Murdoch GH, Sklaviadis T, Manuelidis EE, Manuelidis L. Potential retroviral RNAs in Creutzfeldt-Jakob disease. J Virol 1990;64:1477–1486.

342. Narang HK. Ruthenium red and lanthanum nitrate a possible tracer and negative stain for scrapie "particles?" Acta Neuropathol (Berl) 1974;29:37–43.

343. Narang HK. Relationship of protease-resistant protein, scrapie-associated fibrils and tubulofilamentous particles to the agent of spongiform encephalopathies. Res Virol 1992;143:381–386.

344. Narang HK. Scrapie-associated tubulofilamentous particles in human Creutzfeldt-Jakob disease. Res Virol 1992;143:387–395.

345. Narang HK, Asher DM, Gajdusek DC. Tubulofilaments in negatively stained scrapie-infected brains: relationship to scrapie-associated fibrils. Proc Natl Acad Sci U S A 1987;84:7730–7734.

346. Narang HK, Asher DM, Gajdusek DC. Evidence that DNA is present in abnormal tubulofilamentous structures found in scrapie. Proc Natl Acad Sci U S A 1988;85:3575–3579.

347. Narang HK, Asher DM, Pomeroy KL, Gajdusek DC. Abnormal tubulovesicular particles in brains of hamsters with scrapie. Proc Soc Exp Biol Med 1987;184:504–509.

348. Neary K, Caughey B, Ernst D, Race RE, Chesebro B. Protease sensitivity and nuclease resistance of the scrapie agent propagated in vitro in neuroblastoma-cells. J Virol 1991;65:1031–1034.

349. Neugut RH, Neugut AI, Kahana E, Stein Z, Alter M. Creutzfeldt-Jakob disease: familial clustering among Libyan-born Israelis. Neurology 1979;29:225–231.

350. New MI, Brown P, Temeck JW, Owens C, Hedley-Whyte ET, Richardson EP. Preclinical Creutzfeldt-Jakob disease discovered at autopsy in a human growth hormone recipient. Neurology 1988;38:1133–1134.

351. Nisbet TJ, MacDonaldson I, Bishara SN. Creutzfeldt-Jakob disease in a second patient who received a cadaveric dura mater graft. JAMA 1989;261:1118.

352. Nochlin D, Sumi SM, Bird TD, et al. Familial dementia with PrP-positive amyloid plaques: a variant of Gerstmann-Str(aua)ussler syndrome. Neurology 1989;39:910–918.

353. O'Brien SJ. In: Genetic maps: locus maps of complex genomes. 6th ed. Cold Spring Harbor, NY: Cold Spring Harbor Laboratory Press, 1993:4.42–4.45.

354. Oesch B, Groth DF, Prusiner SB, Weissmann C. Search for a scrapie-specific nucleic acid: a progress report. In: Bock G, Marsh J, eds. Novel infectious agents and the central nervous system. Ciba Foundation Symposium 135. Chichester, UK: John Wiley & Sons, 1988:209–223.

355. Oesch B, Teplow DB, Stahl N, Serban D, Hood LE, Prusiner SB. Identification of cellular proteins binding to the scrapie prion protein. Biochemistry 1990;29:5848–5855.

356. Oesch B, Westaway D, W(aua)lchli M, et al. A cellular gene encodes scrapie PrP 27-30 protein. Cell 1985;40:735–746.

357. Onodera T, Ikeda T, Muramatsu Y, Shinagawa M. Isolation of scrapie agent from the placenta of sheep with natural scrapie in Japan. Microbiol Immunol 1993;37:311–316.

358. Otto D. Jacob-Creutzfeldt disease associated with cadaveric dura. J Neurosurg 1987;67:149.

359. Outram G, Dickinson A, Fraser H. Reduced susceptibility of scrapie in mice after steroid administration. Nature 1974;249:855–856.

360. Owen F, Poulter M, Collinge J, Crow TJ. Codon 129 changes in the prion protein gene in Caucasians. Am J Hum Genet 1990;46:1215–1216.

361. Owen F, Poulter M, Collinge J, et al. Insertions in the prion protein gene in atypical dementias. Exp Neurol 1991;112:240–242.

362. Owen F, Poulter M, Collinge J, et al. A dementing illness associated with a novel insertion in the prion protein gene. Mol Brain Res 1992;13:155–157.

363. Owen F, Poulter M, Lofthouse R, et al. Insertion in prion protein gene in familial Creutzfeldt-Jakob disease. Lancet 1989;1:51–52.

364. Owen F, Poulter M, Shah T, et al. An in-frame insertion in the prion protein gene in familial Creutzfeldt-Jakob disease. Mol Brain Res 1990;7:273–276.

365. Packer RJ, Cornblath DR, Gonatas NK, Bruno LA, Asbury AK. Creutzfeldt-Jakob disease in a 20-year-old woman. Neurology 1980;30:492–496.

366. Palmer MS, Dryden AJ, Hughes JT, Collinge J. Homozygous prion protein genotype predisposes to sporadic Creutzfeldt-Jakob disease. Nature 1991;352:340–342.

367. Palmer MS, Mahal SP, Campbell TA, et al. Deletions in the prion protein gene are not associated with CJD. Hum Molec Genet 1993;2:541–544.

368. Palsson PA. Rida (scrapie) in Iceland and its epidemiology. In: Prusiner SB, Hadlow WJ, eds. Slow transmissible diseases of the nervous system. Vol 1. New York: Academic Press, 1979:357–366.

369. Pan K-M, Baldwin M, Nguyen J, et al. Conversion of α-helices into β-sheets features in the formation of the scrapie prion proteins. Proc Natl Acad Sci U S A 1993;90:10962–10966.

370. Parry HB. Scrapie: a transmissible and hereditary disease of sheep. Heredity 1962;17:75–105.

371. Parry HB. Scrapie: natural and experimental. In: Whitty CWM, Hughes JT, MacCallum FO, eds. Virus diseases and the nervous system. Oxford: Blackwell Publishing, 1969:99–105.

372. Parry HB. Scrapie disease in sheep. Oppenheimer DR, ed. New York: Academic Press, 1983.

373. Pattison IH. The spread of scrapie by contact between affected and healthy sheep, goats or mice. Vet Rec 1964;76:333–336.

374. Pattison IH. Experiments with scrapie with special reference to the nature of the agent and the pathology of the disease. In: Gajdusek DC, Gibbs CJ Jr, Alpers MP, eds. Slow, latent and temperate virus infections. NINDB Monograph 2. Washington, DC: US Government Printing, 1965:249–257.

375. Pattison IH. The relative susceptibility of sheep, goats and mice to two types of the goat scrapie agent. Res Vet Sci 1966;7:207–212.

376. Pattison IH. Fifty years with scrapie: a personal reminiscence. Vet Rec 1988;123:661–666.

377. Pattison IH, Hoare MN, Jebbett JN, Watson WA. Spread of scrapie to sheep and goats by oral dosing with foetal membranes from scrapie-affected sheep. Vet Rec 1972;90:465–468.

378. Pattison IH, Jones KM. The possible nature of the transmissible agent of scrapie. Vet Rec 1967;80:1–8.

379. Pattison IH, Millson GC. Experimental transmission of scrapie to goats and sheep by the oral route. J Comp Pathol 1961;71:171–176.

380. Pearlman RL, Towfighi J, Pezeshkpour GH, Tenser RB, Turel AP. Clinical significance of types of cerebellar amyloid plaques in human spongiform encephalopathies. Neurology 1988;38:1249–1254.

381. Pearson GR, Wyatt JM, Gruffydd-Jones TJ, et al. Feline spongiform encephalopathy: fibril and PrP studies. Vet Rec 1992;131:307–310.

382. Petersen RB, Tabaton M, Berg L, et al. Analysis of the prion protein gene in thalamic dementia. Neurology 1992;42:1859–1863.

383. Pocchiari M, Peano S, Conz A, et al. Combination ultrafiltration and 6 M urea treatment of human growth hormone effectively minimizes risk from potential Creutzfeldt-Jakob disease virus contamination. Horm Res 1991;35:161–166.

384. Pocchiari M, Salvatore M, Cutruzzola F, et al. A new point mutation of the prion protein gene in familial and sporadic cases of Creutzfeldt-Jakob disease. Ann Neurol 1993;34:802–807.

385. Pocchiari M, Salvatore M, Ladogana A, et al. Experimental drug treatment of scrapie: a pathogenetic basis for rationale therapeutics. Eur J Epidemiol 1991;7:556–561.

386. Poidinger M, Kirkwood J, Almond W. Sequence analysis of the PrP protein from two species of antelope susceptible to transmissible spongiform encephalopathy. Arch Virol 1993;131:193–199.

387. Poulter M, Baker HF, Frith CD, et al. Inherited prion disease with 144 base pair gene insertion. 1. Genealogical and molecular studies. Brain 1992;115:675–685.

388. Powell-Jackson J, Weller RO, Kennedy P, Preece MA, Whitcombe EM, Newsome-Davis J. Creutzfeldt-Jakob disease after administration of human growth hormone. Lancet 1985;2:244–246.

389. Prusiner SB. Novel proteinaceous infectious particles cause scrapie. Science 1982;216:136–144.

390. Prusiner SB. The biology of prion transmission and replication. In: Prusiner SB, McKinley MP, eds. Prions—novel infectious pathogens causing scrapie and Creutzfeldt-Jakob disease. Orlando: Academic Press, 1987:83–112.

391. Prusiner SB. Molecular structure, biology and genetics of prions. Adv Virus Res 1988;35:83–136.

392. Prusiner SB. Scrapie prions. Annu Rev Microbiol 1989;43:345–374.

393. Prusiner SB. Molecular biology of prion diseases. Science 1991;252:1515–1522.

394. Prusiner SB. Molecular biology and genetics of neurodegenerative diseases caused by prions. Adv Virus Res 1992;41:241–280.

395. Prusiner SB. Prion diseases. In: Scriver CR, Beaudet AL, Sly WS, Valle D, eds. Metabolic basis of inherited disease. 7th ed. New York: McGraw-Hill, 1993.

396. Prusiner SB. Transgenetics and cell biology of prion diseases: investigations of PrP^{Sc} synthesis and diversity. Br Med Bull 1993;49:873–912.

397. Prusiner SB. Inherited prion diseases. Proc Natl Acad Sci U S A 1994;91:4611–4614.

398. Prusiner SB, Bolton DC, Groth DF, Bowman KA, Cochran SP, McKinley MP. Further purification and characterization of scrapie prions. Biochemistry 1982;21:6942–6950.

399. Prusiner SB, Cochran SP, Alpers MP. Transmission of scrapie in hamsters. J Infect Dis 1985;152:971–978.

400. Prusiner SB, Cochran SP, Groth DF, Downey DE, Bowman KA, Martinez HM. Measurement of the scrapie agent using an incubation time interval assay. Ann Neurol 1982;11:353–358.

401. Prusiner SB, DeArmond SJ. Prion diseases and neurodegeneration. Annu Rev Neurosci 1994;17:311–339.

402. Prusiner SB, Fuzi M, Scott M, et al. Immunologic and molecular biological studies of prion proteins in bovine spongiform encephalopathy. J Infect Dis 1993;167:602–613.

403. Prusiner SB, Gajdusek DC, Alpers MP. Kuru with incubation periods exceeding two decades. Ann Neurol 1982;12:1–9.

404. Prusiner SB, Groth DF, Bildstein C, Masiarz FR, McKinley MP, Cochran SP. Electrophoretic properties of the scrapie agent in agarose gels. Proc Natl Acad Sci U S A 1980;77:2984–2988.

405. Prusiner SB, Groth DF, Bolton DC, Kent SB, Hood LE. Purification and structural studies of a major scrapie prion protein. Cell 1984;38:127–134.

406. Prusiner SB, Groth DF, Cochran SP, Masiarz FR, McKinley MP, Martinez HM. Molecular properties, partial purification, and assay by incubation period measurements of the hamster scrapie agent. Biochemistry 1980;19:4883–4891.

407. Prusiner SB, Groth DF, Cochran SP, McKinley MP, Masiarz FR. Gel electrophoresis and glass permeation chromatography of the hamster scrapie agent after enzymatic digestion and detergent extraction. Biochemistry 1980;19:4892–4898.

408. Prusiner SB, Groth D, Serban A, Stahl N, Gabizon R. Attempts to restore scrapie prion infectivity after exposure to protein denaturants. Proc Natl Acad Sci U S A 1993;90:2793–2797.

409. Prusiner SB, Groth D, Serban A, et al. Ablation of the prion protein (PrP) gene in mice prevents scrapie and facilitates production of anti-PrP antibodies. Proc Natl Acad Sci U S A 1993;90:10608–10612.

410. Prusiner SB, Hadlow WJ, Eklund CM, Race RE. Sedimentation properties of the scrapie agent. Proc Natl Acad Sci U S A 1977;74:4656–4660.

411. Prusiner SB, Hadlow WJ, Eklund CM, Race RE, Cochran SP. Sedimentation characteristics of the scrapie agent from murine spleen and brain. Biochemistry 1978;17:4987–4992.

412. Prusiner SB, Hadlow WJ, Garfin DE, et al. Partial purification and evidence for multiple molecular forms of the scrapie agent. Biochemistry 1978;17:4993–4997.

413. Prusiner SB, Hsiao KK. Human prion diseases. Ann Neurol 1994;35:385–395.

414. Prusiner SB, Hsiao KK, Bredesen DE, DeArmond SJ. Prion disease. In: Vinken PJ, Bruyn GW, Klawans HL, eds. Handbook of clinical neurology: viral disease. Vol 12(56). Amsterdam: Elsevier, 1989:543–580.

415. Prusiner SB, McKinley MP, Bolton DC, et al. Prions: methods for assay, purification and characterization. In: Maramorosch K, Koprowski H, eds. Methods in virology. New York: Academic Press, 1984:293–345.

416. Prusiner SB, McKinley MP, Bowman KA, et al. Scrapie prions aggregate to form amyloid-like birefringent rods. Cell 1983;35:349–358.

417. Prusiner SB, McKinley MP, Groth DF, et al. Scrapie agent contains a hydrophobic protein. Proc Natl Acad Sci U S A 1981;78:6675–6679.

418. Prusiner SB, Scott M, Foster D, et al. Transgenetic studies implicate interactions between homologous PrP isoforms in scrapie prion replication. Cell 1990;63:673–686.

419. Puckett C, Concannon P, Casey C, Hood L. Genomic structure of the human prion protein gene. Am J Hum Genet 1991;49:320–329.

420. Race RE, Graham K, Ernst D, Caughey B, Chesebro B. Analysis of linkage between scrapie incubation period and the prion protein gene in mice. J Gen Virol 1990;71:493–497.

421. Raeber AJ, Borchelt DR, Scott M, Prusiner SB. Attempts to convert the cellular prion protein into the scrapie isoform in cell-free systems. J Virol 1992;66:6155–6163.

422. Ridley RM, Baker HF. Occupational risk of Creutzfeldt-Jakob disease. Lancet 1993;341:641–642.

423. Riesner D, Kellings K, Meyer N, Mirenda C, Prusiner SB. Nucleic acids and scrapie prions. In: Prusiner SB, Collinge J, Powell J, Anderton B, eds. Prion diseases of humans and animals. London: Ellis Horwood, 1992:341–358.

424. Ripoll L, Laplanche J-L, Salzmann M, et al. A new point mutation in the prion protein gene at codon 210 in Creutzfeldt-Jakob disease. Neurology 1993;43:1934–1938.

425. Roberts GW, Lofthouse R, Allsop D, et al. CNS amyloid proteins in neurodegenerative diseases. Neurology 1988;38:1534–1540.

426. Roberts GW, Lofthouse R, Brown R, Crow TJ, Barry RA, Prusiner SB. Prion-protein immunoreactivity in human transmissible dementias. N Engl J Med 1986;315:1231–1233.

427. Rogers M, Serban D, Gyuris T, Scott M, Torchia T, Prusiner SB. Epitope mapping of the Syrian hamster prion protein utilizing chimeric and mutant genes in a vaccinia virus expression system. J Immunol 1991;147:3568–3574.

428. Rogers M, Yehiely F, Scott M, Prusiner SB. Conversion of truncated and elongated prion proteins into the scrapie isoform in cultured cells. Proc Natl Acad Sci U S A 1993;90:3182–3186.

429. Rohwer RG. Scrapie infectious agent is virus-like in size and susceptibility to inactivation. Nature 1984;308:658–662.

430. Rohwer RG. Virus-like sensitivity of the scrapie agent to heat inactivation. Science 1984;223:600–602.

431. Rohwer RG. Estimation of scrapie nucleic acid molecular weight from standard curves for virus sensitivity to ionizing radiation. Nature 1986;320:381.

432. Rohwer RG. The scrapie agent: "a virus by any other name." Curr Top Microbiol Immunol 1991;172:195–232.

433. Rohwer RG, Gajdusek DC. Scrapie: virus or viroid, the case for a virus. In: Boese A, ed. Search for the cause of multiple sclerosis and other chronic diseases of the central nervous system. Weinheim: Verlag Chemie, 1980;333–355.

434. Roos R, Gajdusek DC, Gibbs CJ Jr. The clinical characteristics of transmissible Creutzfeldt-Jakob disease. Brain 1973;96:1–20.

435. Rosen DR, Siddique T, Patterson D, et al. Mutations in Cu/Zn superoxide dismutase gene are associated with familial amyotrophic lateral slerosis. Nature 1993;362:59–62.

436. Rosenthal NP, Keesey J, Crandall B, Brown WJ. Familial neurological disease associated with spongiform encephalopathy. Arch Neurol 1976;33:252–259.

437. Safar J, Wang W, Padgett MP, et al. Molecular mass, biochemical composition, and physicochemical behavior of the infectious form of the scrapie precursor protein monomer. Proc Natl Acad Sci U S A 1990;87:6373–6377.

438. Sakaguchi S, Katamine S, Yamanouchi K, et al. Kinetics of infectivity are dissociated from PrP accumulation in salivary glands of Creutzfeldt-Jakob disease agent-inoculated mice. J Gen Virol 1993; 74:2117–2123.

439. Sawcer SJ, Yuill GM, Esmonde TFG, et al. Creutzfeldt-Jakob disease in an individual occupationally exposed to BSE. Lancet 1993;341:642.

440. Sch(aua)tzl HM, Da Costa M, Taylor L, Cohen FE, Prusiner SB. Prion protein gene variation among primates. J Mol Biol 1995; 245:362–374.

441. Schellenberg GD, Bird TD, Wijsman EM, et al. Genetic linkage evidence for a familial Alzheimer's disease locus on chromosome 14. Science 1992;258:668–671.

442. Scott M, Foster D, Mirenda C, et al. Transgenic mice expressing hamster prion protein produce species-specific scrapie infectivity and amyloid plaques. Cell 1989;59:847–857.

443. Scott M, Groth D, Foster D, et al. Propagation of prions with artificial properties in transgenic mice expressing chimeric PrP genes. Cell 1993;73:979–988.

444. Scott MR, K(auo)hler R, Foster D, Prusiner SB. Chimeric prion protein expression in cultured cells and transgenic mice. Protein Sci 1992;1:986–997.

445. Serban D, Taraboulos A, DeArmond SJ, Prusiner SB. Rapid detection of Creutzfeldt-Jakob disease and scrapie prion proteins. Neurology 1990;40:110–117.

446. Siakotos AN, Gajdusek DC, Gibbs CJ Jr, Traub RD, Bucana C. Partial purification of the scrapie agent from mouse brain by pressure disruption and zonal centrifugation in sucrose-sodium chloride gradients. Virology 1976;70:230–237.

447. Siakotos AN, Raveed D, Longa G. The discovery of a particle unique to brain and spleen subcellular fractions from scrapie-infected mice. J Gen Virol 1979;43:417–422.

448. Sigurdsson B. Rida, a chronic encephalitis of sheep with general remarks on infections which develop slowly and some of their special characteristics. Br Vet J 1954;110:341–354.

449. Simpson DA, Lander H, Robson HN. Observations on kuru. II. Clinical features. Aust Ann Med 1959;8:8–15.

450. Sklaviadis T, Akowitz A, Manuelidis EE, Manuelidis L. Nuclease treatment results in high specific purification of Creutzfeldt-Jakob disease infectivity with a density characteristic of nucleic acid-protein complexes. Arch Virol 1990;112:215–229.

451. Sklaviadis T, Akowitz A, Manuelidis EE, Manuelidis L. Nucleic acid binding proteins in highly purified Creutzfeldt-Jakob disease preparations. Proc Natl Acad Sci U S A 1993;90:5713–5717.

452. Sklaviadis T, Dreyer R, Manuelidis L. Analysis of Creutzfeldt-Jakob disease infectious fractions by gel permeation chromatography and sedimentation field flow fractionation. Virus Res 1992; 26:241–254.

453. Sklaviadis TK, Manuelidis L, Manuelidis EE. Physical properties of the Creutzfeldt-Jakob disease agent. J Virol 1989;63:1212–1222.

454. Somerville RA, Millson GC, Hunter GD. Changes in a protein-nucleic acid complex from synaptic plasma membrane of scrapie-infected mouse brain. Biochem Soc Trans 1976;4:1112–1114.

455. Sparkes RS, Simon M, Cohn VH, et al. Assignment of the human and mouse prion protein genes to homologous chromosomes. Proc Natl Acad Sci U S A 1986;83:7358–7362.

456. St George-Hyslop P, Haines J, Rogaev E, et al. Genetic evidence for a novel familial Alzheimer's disease locus on chromosome 14. Nat Genet 1992;2:330–334.

457. Stahl N, Baldwin MA, Hecker R, Pan K-M, Burlingame AL, Prusiner SB. Glycosylinositol phospholipid anchors of the scrapie and cellular prion proteins contain sialic acid. Biochemistry 1992;31:5043–5053.

458. Stahl N, Baldwin MA, Teplow DB, et al. Structural analysis of the scrapie prion protein using mass spectrometry and amino acid sequencing. Biochemistry 1993;32:1991–2002.

459. Stender A. Weitere Beitr(aua)ge zum Kapitel "Spastische Pseudosklerose Jakobs." Z Neurol Psychiat 1930;128:528–543.

460. Tagliavini F, Prelli F, Ghisto J, et al. Amyloid protein of Gerstmann-Str(aua)ussler-Scheinker disease (Indiana kindred) is an 11-kd fragment of prion protein with an N-terminal glycine at codon 58. EMBO J 1991;10:513–519.

461. Taguchi F, Tamai Y, Miura S. Experiments on maternal and paternal transmission of Creutzfeldt-Jakob disease in mice. Arch Virol 1993;130:219–224.

462. Tamai Y, Kojima H, Kitajima R, et al. Demonstration of the transmissible agent in tissue from a pregnant woman with Creutzfeldt-Jakob disease. N Engl J Med 1992;327:649.

463. Tange RA, Troost D, Limburg M. Progressive fatal dementia (Creutzfeldt-Jakob disease) in a patient who received homograft tissue for tympanic membrane closure. Eur Arch Otorhinolaryngol 1989;247:199–201.

464. Taraboulos A, Jendroska K, Serban D, Yang S-L, DeArmond SJ, Prusiner SB. Regional mapping of prion proteins in brains. Proc Natl Acad Sci U S A 1992;89:7620–7624.

465. Taraboulos A, Raeber AJ, Borchelt DR, Serban D, Prusiner SB. Synthesis and trafficking of prion proteins in cultured cells. Mol Biol Cell 1992;3:851–863.

466. Taraboulos A, Serban D, Prusiner SB. Scrapie prion proteins accumulate in the cytoplasm of persistently infected cultured cells. J Cell Biol 1990;110:2117–2132.

467. Tateishi J, Doh-ura K, Kitamoto T, et al. Prion protein gene analysis and transmission studies of Creutzfeldt-Jakob disease. In: Prusiner SB, Collinge J, Powell J, Anderton B, eds. Prion diseases of humans and animals. London: Ellis Horwood, 1992:129–134.

468. Tateishi J, Kitamoto T, Doh-ura K, et al. Immunochemical, molecular genetic, and transmission studies on a case of Gerstmann-Str(aua)ussler-Scheinker syndrome. Neurology 1990;40:1578–1581.

469. Tateishi J, Ohta M, Koga M, Sato Y, Kuroiwa Y. Transmission of chronic spongiform encephalopathy with kuru plaques from humans to small rodents. Ann Neurol 1979;5:581–584.

470. Taylor DM, Dickinson AG, Fraser H, Robertson PA, Salacinski PR, Lowry PJ. Preparation of growth hormone free from contamination with unconventional slow viruses. Lancet 1985;2:260–262.

470a. Telling GT, Haga T, Torchia M, Tremblay P, DeArmond SJ, Prusiner SB. Interactions between wild-type and mutant prion proteins modulate neurodegeneration in transgenic mice. Genes and Dev (in press).

471. Telling GC, Scott M, Hsiao KK, et al. Transmission of Creutzfeldt-Jakob disease from humans to transgenic mice expressing chimeric human-mouse prion protein. Proc Natl Acad Sci U S A 1994; 91:9936–9940.

472. Terzano MG, Montanari E, Calzetti S, Mancia D, Lechi A. The effect of amantadine on arousal and EEG patterns in Creutzfeldt-Jakob disease. Arch Neurol 1983;40:555–559.

473. Thadani V, Penar PL, Partington J, et al. Creutzfeldt-Jakob disease probably acquired from a cadaveric dura mater graft. Case report. J Neurosurg 1988;69:766–769.

474. Titner R, Brown P, Hedley-Whyte ET, Rappaport EB, Piccardo CP, Gajdusek DC. Neuropathologic verification of Creutzfeldt-Jakob disease in the exhumed American recipient of human pituitary growth hormone: epidemiologic and pathogenetic implications. Neurology 1986;36:932–936.

475. Tranchant C, Doh-ura K, Warter JM, et al. Gerstmann-Straussler-Scheinker disease in an Alsatian family: clinical and genetic studies. J Neurol Neurosurg Psychiatry 1992;55:185–187.

476. Turk E, Teplow DB, Hood LE, Prusiner SB. Purification and properties of the cellular and scrapie hamster prion proteins. Eur J Biochem 1988;176:21–30.

477. Udovitch AL, Valensi L. The Last Arab Jews: The Communities of Jerba, Tunisia. London: Harwood Academic Publishers, 1984: 178.

478. Van Broeckhoven C, Backhovens H, Cruts M, et al. Mapping of a gene predisposing to early-onset Alzheimer's disease to chromosome 14q24.3. Nat Genet 1992;2:335–339.

479. Van Broeckhoven C, Haan J, Bakker E, et al. Amyloid b protein precursor gene and hereditary cerebral hemorrhage with amyloidosis (Dutch). Science 1990;248:1120–1122.

480. Vnencak-Jones CL, Phillips JA. Identification of heterogeneous PrP gene deletions in controls by detection of allele-specific heteroduplexes (DASH). Am J Hum Genet 1992;50:871–872.

481. Weitgrefe S, Zupancic M, Haase A, et al. Cloning of a gene whose expression is increased in scrapie and in senile plaques. Science 1985;230:1177–1181.

482. Westaway D, Cooper C, Turner S, Da Costa M, Carlson GA, Prusiner SB. Structure and polymorphism of the mouse prion protein gene. Proc Natl Acad Sci U S A 1994;91:6418–6422.

483. Westaway D, DeArmond SJ, Cayetano-Canlas J, et al. Degeneration of skeletal muscle, peripheral nerves, and the central nervous system in transgenic mice overexpressing wild-type prion proteins. Cell 1994;76:117–129.

484. Westaway D, Goodman PA, Mirenda CA, McKinley MP, Carlson GA, Prusiner SB. Distinct prion proteins in short and long scrapie incubation period mice. Cell 1987;51:651662.

485. Westaway D, Mirenda CA, Foster D, et al. Paradoxical shortening of scrapie incubation times by expression of prion protein transgenes derived from long incubation period mice. Neuron 1991;7: 59–68.

486. Westaway D, Zuliani V, Cooper CM, et al. Homozygosity for prion protein alleles encoding glutamine-171 renders sheep susceptible to natural scrapie. Genes Dev 1994;8:959–969.

487. Wexler NS, Young AB, Tanzi RE, et al. Homozygotes for Huntington's disease. Nature 1987;326:194–197.

488. Wickner RB. Evidence for a prion analog in *S. cerevisiae*: the [URE3] non-Mendelian genetic element as an altered URE2 protein. Science 1994, in press.

489. Wilesmith JW, Hoinville LJ, Ryan JBM, Sayers AR. Bovine spongiform encephalopathy: aspects of the clinical picture and analyses of possible changes 1986–1990. Vet Rec 1992;130:197–201.

490. Wilesmith JW, Ryan JBM, Hueston WD, Hoinville LJ. Bovine spongiform encephalopathy: epidemiological features 1985 to 1990. Vet Rec 1992;130:90–94.

491. Wilesmith J, Wells GAH. Bovine spongiform encephalopathy. Curr Top Microbiol Immunol 1991;172:21–38.

492. Wilesmith JW, Wells GAH, Cranwell MP, Ryan JBM. Bovine spongiform encephalopathy: epidemiological studies. Vet Rec 1988; 123:638–644.

492a. Will RG, Ironside JW, Zeidler M, Cousens SN, Estibeiro K, Alperovitch A, Poser S, Pocchiari M, Hofman A, Smith PG. A new variant of Creutzfeldt-Jakob disease in the UK. Lancet 1996;347:921–925.

493. Will RG, Matthews WB. Evidence for case-to-case transmission of Creutzfeldt-Jakob disease. J Neurol Neurosurg Psychiatry 1982;45: 235–238.

494. Williams ES, Young S. Chronic wasting disease of captive mule deer: a spongiform encephalopathy. J Wildl Dis 1980;16:89–98.

495. Williams ES, Young S. Spongiform encephalopathy of Rocky Mountain Elk. J Wildl Dis 1982;18:465–471.

496. Williams RC. Electron microscopy of viruses. Adv Virus Res 1954; 2:183–239.

497. Willison HJ, Gale AN, McLaughlin JE. Creutzfeldt-Jakob disease following cadaveric dura mater graft. J Neurol Neurosurg Psychiatry 1991;54:940.

498. Willoughby K, Kelly DF, Lyon DG, Wells GAH. Spongiform encephalopathy in a captive puma (Felis concolor). Vet Rec 1992; 131:431–434.

499. Wilson DR, Anderson RD, Smith W. Studies in scrapie. J Comp Pathol 1950;60:267–282.

500. Worthington M. Interferon system in mice infected with the scrapie agent. Infect Immun 1972;6:643–645.

501. Xi YG, Ingrosso L, Ladogana A, Masullo C, Pocchiari M. Amphotericin B treatment dissociates in vivo replication of the scrapie agent from PrP accumulation. Nature 1992;356:598–601.

502. Zigas V, Gajdusek DC. Kuru: clinical study of a new syndrome resembling paralysis agitans in natives of the Eastern Highlands of Australian New Guinea. Med J Aust 1957;2:745–754.

503. Zilber N, Kahana E, Abraham MPH. The Libyan Creutzfeldt-Jakob disease focus in Israel: an epidemiologic evaluation. Neurology 1991;41:1385–1389.

Index